Radiology Review Manual

Fifth Edition

Radiology Review Manual

Fifth Edition

Wolfgang Dähnert, M.D.
Department of Radiology
Good Samaritan Regional Medical Center
Phoenix, Arizona

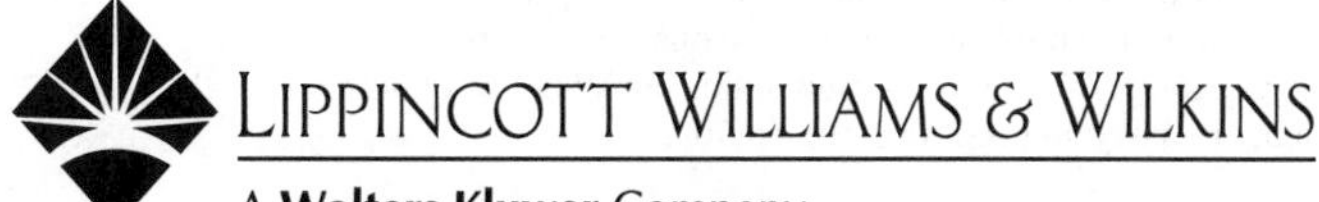
LIPPINCOTT WILLIAMS & WILKINS
A **Wolters Kluwer** Company
Philadelphia • Baltimore • New York • London
Buenos Aires • Hong Kong • Sydney • Tokyo

Acquisitions Editor: *Joyce-Rachel John*
Developmental Editor: *Anne Snyder*
Manufacturing Manager: *Tim Reynolds*

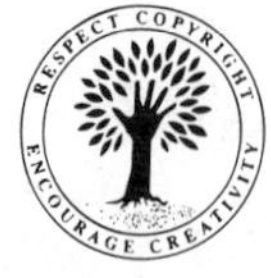

Printed in the United States of America
9 8 7 6 5 4 3 2 1

Library of Congress Cataloging-in-Publication Data

Dähnert, Wolfgang
Radiology review manual / Wolfgang Dähnert.—5th ed.
p. cm.
Includes index.
ISBN 0-7817-4822-4
1. Radiology, Medical—Outlines, syllabi, etc. 2. Diagnosis, Radioscopic—Outlines, syllabi, etc. I. Title.
RC78.17.D34 2002
616.07'57—dc21

2002034027

Care has been taken to confirm the accuracy of the information presented and to describe generally accepted practices. However, the authors, editors, and publisher are not responsible for errors or omissions or for any consequences from application of the information in this book and make no warranty, expressed or implied, with respect to the contents of this publication.

The authors, editors, and publisher have exerted every effort to ensure that drug selection and dosage set forth in this text are in accordance with current recommendations and practice at the time of publication. However, in view of ongoing research, changes in government regulations, and the constant flow of information relating to drug therapy and drug reactions, the reader is urged to check the package insert for each drug for any change in indications and dosage and for added warnings and precautions. This is particularly important when the recommended agent is a new or infrequently employed drug.

Some drugs and medical devices presented in this publication have Food and Drug Administration (FDA) clearance for limited use in restricted research settings. It is the responsibility of the health care provider to ascertain the FDA status of each drug or device planned for use in their clinical practice. →

"If a little knowledge is dangerous, where is the man who has so much to be out of danger!"

T.H. Huxley, 1825–1895
from Elementary Instruction in Physiology published in 1877

"It is the tragedy of the world that no one knows what he doesn't know — and the less a man knows, the more sure he is that he knows everything"

Jouce Cary, British author 1888–1957

*"Nothing in the world can take the place of persistence.
Talent will not; nothing is more common than unsuccessful men
with talent. Genius will not; unrewarded genius is almost a proverb.
Education will not; the world is full of educated derelicts.
Persistence and determination alone are omnipotent."*

Calvin Coolidge 1872–1933
Vice President 1921–1923
President 1923–1929

To my dear wife Sue,
to our children Mathias and Patrick
who mean so much to me

About the Author

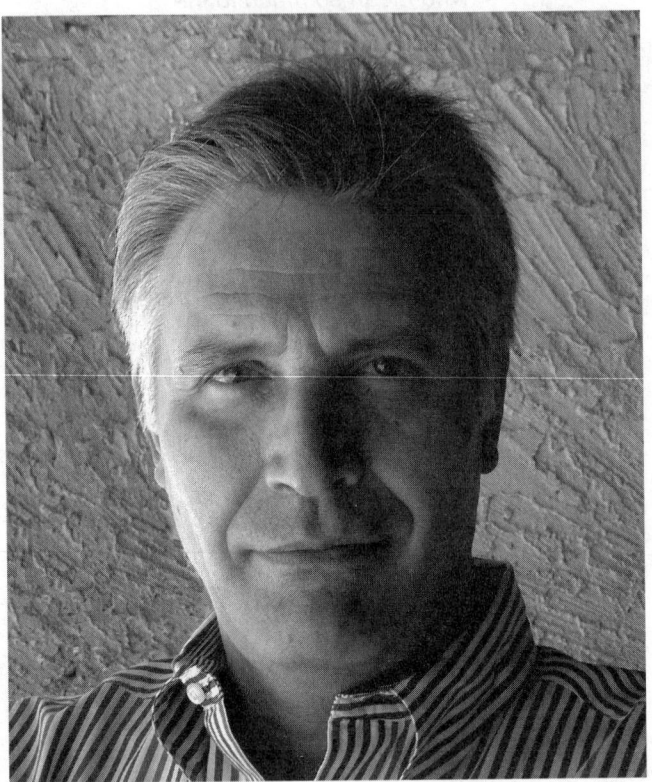

Wolfgang Dähnert, M.D.

Wolfgang Dähnert was born in Hamburg, Germany. He studied medicine at the universities of Düsseldorf and Mainz, where he graduated in 1975. After internship and a short surgical residency he enrolled in a 4-year radiology residency program at the Johannes-Gutenberg University in Mainz and received his German certification for radiology in 1982. In 1984 he started a 2-year fellowship in ultrasound and computed tomography at the Johns Hopkins Hospital in Baltimore and was appointed Clinical Instructor at the same institution in 1986. During his Hopkins years he sat for the FLEX exam, and the radiology specialty exam with the American Board of Radiology. During these three years the foundation of *Radiology Review Manual* was laid. Between 1987 and 1989 he worked as Assistant Professor of Radiology in ultrasound at Thomas Jefferson Hospital in Philadelphia. During these three years *Radiology Review Manual* was taken to fruition. Since December of 1989 he has been associated with Clinical Diagnostic Radiology & Nuclear Medicine, a large subspecialized radiology group practice in Phoenix, Arizona, providing radiology services to Good Samaritan Regional Medical Center, St. Joseph's Hospital and Medical Center, both tertiary care hospitals in Phoenix, Arizona Heart Hospital, and the Children's Hospital of Phoenix.

PREFACE

The depth of medical knowledge and scope of image interpretation expected from an average general radiologist has soared over the last two decades. The emergence of subspecialties within radiology is witness to this development. Books have become available on so many different imaging topics and in such a large number that it is impossible even for the avid reader to consume them all, catalogue them, and have instant access to them. While some radiologists have the luxury to practice exclusively in their area of special interest with impressive expertise, many practice a much broader scope of diagnostic radiology and find themselves occasionally in situations where recollections have become vague. I know that I regret my inability to recall many facts or – more frustrating – where to look them up. In a busy practice it is simply not possible to take time out and disappear in the library.

Radiology Review Manual has become my carry-on memory jogger, in an attempt to put into a single reference much of the information that is or could be relevant to my practice. I use it like a dictionary, always available at my workstation. It is published under the assumption that many colleagues practice like I do: trying to do a good job vis-à-vis significant time constraints. This concept has resonated well within the radiologic community. The popularity of the "green giant" or the "green bible", as it has been dubbed by residents, confirms the usefulness of this type of publication. At the time of this writing approximately 35,000 copies have been sold, one third outside the United States of America. *Radiology Review Manual* has received international attention. I was thrilled when I received a copy of the Portuguese translation published in Rio de Janeiro, Brazil.

The roots of this book can be traced to 1984, when I arrived at Johns Hopkins Hospital and started to collect radiologic tidbits on my first computer for my own personal use. Accordingly, none of the material in this book is of my own writing as is true for most textbooks of radiology. Our radiologic ancestors, mentors, teachers and scientists alike, throughout the world deserve our admiration and gratitude for the collective knowledge passed on to us for the benefit of our profession and our patients. The idea to publish these notes of a student of radiology originates with a former resident at the Johns Hopkins Hospital, now a well-known professor of radiology, who looked over my notes and liked the contents and its presentation. I have no doubt that the thought of compiling such a work has cropped up in the minds of many a resident, while preparing for the board exam. Yet, not until the first edition of Radiology Review Manual was released had anyone gathered the strength to go through with such a daunting project of labor. Not enough, it required the art of persuasion to find anyone who would want to publish the first timid steps of a review manual for the small eclectic readership of radiology residents. The success of review manuals in other medical specialties convinced one editor at Williams & Wilkins to give it a try.

Radiology Review Manual was created in preparation for the specialty exam as the "book under the pillow." Over the years, this material has been changed and expanded. Our voluminous field of diagnostic radiology makes it necessary to use an outline style for the sake of conserving space and thus provides only an extract of information. This may, at times, jeopardize the full meaning of statements when taken out of context or isolated from the fundamental knowledge of general radiology. It should be kept in mind that this book is not intended for the novice and that it requires familiarity with the subject of radiology and the background information of major textbooks.

How to use this book:
The organization of this book has caused a major headache as any topic can be looked at from various points of view. I have selected just one of many possibilities to avoid redundancy. The primary goal was to present the material anatomically from top to bottom but also in a manner that is in keeping with the topics of the current board exam. Unfortunately, this grouping is inconsistent, sectioning off by age (Pediatric Radiology) and image modality (Nuclear Medicine, Ultrasound). In order to avoid repetition, pediatric entities are subsumed within organ systems. Ultrasound and Nuclear Medicine are used from head to heel and consequently are mentioned in all body sections. However, Nuclear Medicine is treated in a separate section when emphasis is on technique and functional aspects not covered elsewhere. The book starts with disorders of the musculoskeletal system. The skull and spine, a crossing point of many subspecialties, are dealt with as the first part of the CNS section and closely follows the chapter on bone disease. While eye, ear, nose and throat imaging generally fall into the purview of neuroradiology readers, these body parts have deserved their own chapters to decrease the volume of the CNS chapter. Presented in sequence are then the topics of chest, breast, heart, liver, the gastrointestinal and genitourinary tract, and obstetrics and gynecology. Brief chapters on statistics and contrast media are added at the end. Labels printed along the page margins conveniently serve to locate the chapter of interest by simply thumbing along the free edge of the book.

The organization within the individual chapters follows the practical approach of reading films. The initial step of film interpretation is the description of radiologic patterns that serves to identify categories in which they belong. Therefore, radiologic patterns for differential diagnoses are found in the first portion of a chapter. Once the diagnostic possibilities have been reviewed in brief outline, one can look up detailed information about a disease entity in the last segment of a chapter. The disease entities are presented in alphabetical order. Both these segments are separated by a few pages of functional, anatomic, or embryologic aspects. Occasionally, important clinical signs and their differential diagnoses, relevant to the practice of radiology, are included in the first portion of a chapter. Mnemonics (which I personally abhor) have been liberally added by request. Accepted therapies for contrast reactions are printed on the inside of the back cover page for immediate access. A table of contents and abbreviations used throughout the book are found in front. A user-friendly index, which selectively refers to those pages with significant information concludes the manual. Notice that many systemic diseases will be mentioned in more than one chapter with some unavoidable redundancy. However, emphasized are those manifestations of the disease that occur within the organ under which it is listed. The index also includes so-called "buzz words" that are miraculously attached to diseases.

The backbone of the book are disease entities, radiologic symptoms, as well as lists of differential diagnosis. Disease entities are headed by their most commonly used name with other designations listed below. As a radiologic diagnosis should be entertained in context with its probability to be correct, percentages in regard to frequency of signs and symptoms are included liberally, often giving the lowest and the highest number found in the literature. The truth may be somewhere in between for a nonselected patient population, and occasionally a third number is provided between the high and low number as the most frequently cited. Arbitrary choices have been made in situations when different or contradictory results are found in the literature—unfortunately, an occurrence not at all infrequent.

Lists of differential diagnoses can be presented in many fashions. There is no right or wrong way, but there certainly is a chaotic versus an organized approach. An orderly thought process portrays familiarity with a problem. Examinees have always felt that "nailing" the diagnosis is secondary, but including it in one's consideration is paramount to a successful exam. Accordingly, an attempt is made to categorize differential diagnostic considerations or etiologies of certain diseases in a manner digestible for recapitulation. It is a common experience that this is not always possible, logically satisfactory, or complete.

Acknowledgement:
The information contained herein has been gathered over several years and stems from various sources. The most significant ones are the journals dedicated to imaging with brilliant review articles, in particular the practice-oriented publication of Radiographics, ACR syllabi, handouts from various CME courses, hand-written notes taken during lectures, as well as feed-back from candidates having taken the board exam. Anecdotal contributions can no longer be traced. I realize, in retrospect, that this may present a problem when certain statements appear unlikely and their verification has to be left to the user. For my defense, I can only say that I have tried to extract all data as diligently as possible.

The following textbooks have been particularly helpful and deserve mention: Barkovich AJ: Pediatric Neuroimaging; Burgener FA, Kormano M: Differential Diagnosis in Conventional Radiology; Chapman S, Nakielny R: Aids to Radiological Differential Diagnosis; Davidson AJ: Radiology of the Kidney; Eideken J: Roentgen Diagnosis of Diseases of Bone; Fraser RG, Pare JAP: Diagnosis of Diseases of the Chest; Gedgaudas E, Moller JH, Castaneda-Zuniga WR, Amplatz K: Cardiovascular Radiology; Harnsberger HR: Handbooks in Radiology, Head and Neck Imaging; Kadir S: Diagnostic Angiography; Kirks DR: Practical Pediatric Imaging; Margulis AR, Burhenne HJ: Computed Tomography of the Gastrointestinal Tract; Mittelstaedt CA: Abdominal Ultrasound; Newton TH, Hasso AN, Dillon WP: Computed Tomography of the Head and Neck in Modern Neuroradiology; Reed JC: Chest Radiology: Plain Film Patterns and Differential Diagnosis; Reeder MM, Felson B: Gamuts in Radiology; Romero R, Pilu G, Jeanty P, Ghidini A, Hobbins JC: Prenatal Diagnosis of Congenital Anomalies; Rumack CM, Wilson SR, Charboneau JW: Diagnostic Ultrasound; Resnick D, Niwayama G: Diagnosis of Bone and Joint Disorders; Sanders RC, James AE: Ultrasonography in Obstetrics and Gynecology; Swischuk LE: Plain Film Interpretation in Congenital Heart Disease; Tabár L, Dean PB: Teaching Atlas of Mammography; Taveras JM, Ferrucci JT: Radiology – Diagnosis – Imaging – Intervention.

I would like to acknowledge the input of numerous teachers, residents, and fellows at the Johns Hopkins Hospital in Baltimore, Thomas Jefferson University Hospital in Philadelphia as well as many colleagues that have helped subsequently. I am particularly indebted to the following individuals for reviewing the separate sections of this book: Christopher Canino, Thomas Chang, Adam E. Flanders, Keith Haidet, Charles Intenzo, David Karasick, Stephen Karasick, Alfred B. Kurtz, Esmond M. Mapp, Joel Raichlen, Paul Spirn, Robert M. Steiner, and C. Amy Wilson. My special thanks go to Flavius ("Buddy") Guglielmo, who supplied me with probably the largest collection of mnemonics in existence. While completing his training at Thomas Jefferson University Hospital, he compiled a long list of memory joggers together with Tom Helinek and Les Folio with contributions from Barbara McComb, Barry Tom, and Ron Wachsberg. Thomas S. Chang of Montefiori University Hospital in Pittsburgh has made valuable suggestions for improvement. My thanks also go to my former colleague Ross Levatter for his thorough review of the section on nuclear medicine.

Many of you have asked to have this book available in an electronic format as it allows your entry of personal comments and the use of swift search functions directly on your personal computer. The initial response was a CD-ROM version, first released in October of 1997. Plans are now under way to bring *Radiology Review Manual* into your Personal Digital Assistants.

I sincerely hope that *Radiology Review Manual* will serve you in your preparation for the board exam, teaching situations, and particularly in your daily work assignments.

Phoenix, September 2002

CONTENTS

ABBREVIATIONS

√	radiologic sign
•	clinical sign, symptom
=	equals, is
@	at anatomic location of
/	or, per
+	and, plus, with
±	with or without
<	less than
>	more than, over
◊	important comment
AAA	abdominal aortic aneurysm
ABC	aneurysmal bone cyst
AC	abdominal circumference
ACA	anterior cerebral artery
ACE	angiotensin I–converting enzyme
ACom	anterior communicating artery
ACTH	adrenocorticotropic hormone
ADEM	acute disseminated encephalo-myelitis
ADH	antidiuretic hormone
AFP	alpha-fetoprotein
AICA	anterior inferior cerebellar artery
AIDS	acquired immune deficiency syndrome
ALL	acute lymphoblastic leukemia
AMA	antimitochondrial antibody
AML	acute myeloblastic leukemia
AML	angiomyolipoma
aML	anterior mitral valve leaflet
ANA	antinuclear antibodies
Angio	angiography
ANT	anterior
Ao	aorta
AP	anteroposterior
APUD	amine precursor uptake and decarboxylation
APVR	anomalous pulmonary venous return
ARA-C	arabinoside C
ARDS	acute respiratory distress syndrome
AS	aortic stenosis
ASA	acetylsalicylic acid
ASD	atrial septal defect
ASH	asymmetric septal hypertrophy
aTL	anterior tricuspid valve leaflet
ATN	acute tubular necrosis
AV	arteriovenous; atrioventricular
AVF	arteriovenous fistula
AVM	arteriovenous malformation
AVN	avascular necrosis
AVNA	atrioventricular node artery

Ba	barium
BCDDP	breast cancer detection demonstration project
BCG	bacille Calmette-Guérin
BE	barium enema
BIDA	butyl iminodiacetic acid
BIH	benign intracranial hypertension
BKG	background
BOOP	Bronchiolitis obliterans organizing pneumonia
BP	blood pressure
BPD	biparietal diameter
BPH	benign prostatic hyperplasia
bpm	beats per minute
BPP	biophysical profile
BSA	body surface area
Bx	biopsy
Ca	calcium
CAD	coronary artery disease
CAM	cystic adenomatoid malformation
CBD	common bile duct
CC	craniocaudad
CCA	common carotid artery
CCAM	congenital cystic adenomatoid malformation
CCK	cholecystokinin
CDC	Center for Disease Control
CECT	contrast-enhanced computed tomography
CEMR	contrast-enhanced MR
CFI	color flow imaging
cGy	centigray = rad
CHD	common hepatic duct; congenital heart defect
CHF	congestive heart failure
CLL	chronic lymphatic leukemia
CMC	carpometacarpal
CML	chronic myelogenous leukemia
CMV	cytomegalovirus
CNS	central nervous system
CO	carbon monoxide
CoA	coarctation of aorta
COPD	chronic obstructive pulmonary disease
CPA	cerebellopontine angle
CPPD	calcium pyrophosphate dihydrate
CPR	cardiopulmonary resuscitation
CRF	chronic renal failure
CRT	cathode ray tube
CSF	cerebrospinal fluid
CST	contraction stress test
C/T	cardiothoracic ratio

CT	computed tomography
CVA	cerebrovascular accident
CWP	coal worker's pneumoconiosis
Cx	complication
CXR	chest x-ray
DCBE	double-contrast barium enema
DCIS	ductal carcinoma in situ
DDx	differential diagnosis
DES	diethylstilbestrol
DIC	disseminated intravascular coagulation
DIDA	diethyl iminodiacetic acid
DIL	drug-induced lupus erythematosus
DIP	desquamative interstitial pneumonia
DIP	distal interphalangeal
DISH	diffuse idiopathic skeletal hyperostosis
DISIDA	diisopropyl iminodiacetic acid
DIT	diiodotyrosine
DMSA	dimercaptosuccinic acid
DTPA	diethylenetriamine pentaacetic acid
DVT	deep vein thrombosis
Dx	diagnosis
EAC	external auditory canal
ECA	external carotid artery
ECD	endocardial cushion defect
ECF	extracellular fluid
ECG	electrocardiogram
ECHO	echocardiogram
ED	end-diastole
EDV	end-diastolic volume
EEG	electroencephalogram
EF	ejection fraction
EFW	estimated fetal weight
EG	eosinophilic granuloma
eg	exempli gratia
EHDP	ethylene hydroxydiphosphonate
ERC	endoscopic retrograde cholangiography
ERCP	endoscopic retrograde cholangiopancreatography
ES	end-systole
esp.	especially
ESR	erythrocyte sedimentation rate
ESV	end-systolic volume
F	female
FDA	Federal Drug Administration
FDG	fluorodeoxyglucose
FEV	forced expiratory volume

FIGO Fédération Internationale de Gynécologie et d'Obstétrique
FISP fast imaging with steady-state precession
FLASH fast low-angle shot
FN false negative
FNH follicular nodular hyperplasia
FP false positive
FRC functional residual capacity
FS fractional shortening
FSH follicle stimulating hormone
FUO fever of unknown origin
FWHM full-width at half-maximum

GA gestational age
GB gallbladder
GBM glioblastoma multiforme
GBS group B streptococcus
GCT giant cell tumor; granulosa cell tumor
Gd gadolinium
GE gastroesophageal
GER gastroesophageal reflux
GERD gastroesophageal reflux disease
GFR glomerular filtration rate
GI gastrointestinal
GIST gastrointestinal stromal tumor
GMRH germinal matrix–related hemorrhage
GN glomerulonephritis
GNRH gonadotropin releasing hormone
GRE gradient refocused echo
GU genitourinary

Hb hemoglobin
HC head circumference
hCG human chorionic gonadotropin
Hct hematocrit
HD Hodgkin disease
HIAA hydroxyindole acetic acid
HIDA hepatic 2,6-dimethyl iminodiacetic acid
HIP health insurance plan
Histo histology
HIV human immunodeficiency virus
HL Hodgkin lymphoma
HOCM hypertrophic obstructive cardiomyopathy; high-osmolarity contrast media
HPT hyperparathyroidism
HRCT high-resolution CT
HSA human serum albumin
HSE herpes simplex encephalitis
HSG hysterosalpingography
HSV herpes simplex virus
HTLV human T-cell lymphotropic virus
HU Hounsfield unit
HWP hepatic wedge pressure
Hx history

IAC internal auditory canal
ICA internal carotid artery
IDA iminodiacetic acid
IDDM insulin-dependent diabetes mellitus
IDM infant of diabetic mother
IDP iminodiphosphonate
ie id est
IHSS idiopathic hypertrophic subaortic stenosis
IM intramuscular
IMA inferior mesenteric artery
In indium
IPF idiopathic pulmonary fibrosis
IPH idiopathic pulmonary hemosiderosis
IR inversion recovery
IRP international reference preparation
IS ileosacral; international standard
IUD intrauterine device
IUGR intrauterine growth retardation
IV intravenous
IVC inferior vena cava
IVDA intravenous drug abuse
IVH intraventricular hemorrhage
IVP intravenous pyelogram
IVS intraventricular septum
IVU intravenous urogram

JAA juxtaposition of atrial appendages

KCC Kulchitzky cell carcinoma
KUB kidney + ureter + bladder on one film

L left
L-DOPA 3-(3,4-dihydroxyphenyl)-levo-alanin
LA left atrium
LAD left anterior descending
LAO left anterior oblique
LAT lateral
LATS long-acting thyroid stimulating
LAV lymphadenopathy-associated virus
LCA left coronary artery
LCH Langerhans cell histiocytosis
LCIS lobular carcinoma in situ
LCX left circumflex coronary artery
LDH lactate dehydrogenase
LE lupus erythematosus
LES lower esophageal sphincter
LGA large for gestational age
LH luteinizing hormone
LIP lymphocytic interstitial pneumonitis
LL lower lobes
LLL left lower lobe
LLQ left lower quadrant
Lnn lymph nodes
LOCM low-osmolarity contrast media
LPA left pulmonary artery
LPO left posterior oblique
LSD lysergic acid diethylamide
LUL left upper lobe
LUQ left upper quadrant
LV left ventricle
LVET left ventricular ejection time
$LVFT_2$ left ventricular slow filling time
LVOT left ventricular outflow tract
$LVFT_1$ left ventricular fast filling time

M male
MA menstrual age
MAA macroaggregated albumin
MAG mercaptoacetyltriglycine
MAI Mycobacterium avium intracellulare
MCA middle cerebral artery
MCDK multicystic dysplastic kidney
MCK multicystic kidney
MCP metacarpophalangeal
MDP methylene diphosphonate
MEA multiple endocrine adenomas
MEN multiple endocrine neoplasms
MFH malignant fibrous histiocytoma
MIBG metaiodobenzylguanidine
MID multi-infarct dementia
MIT monoiodotyrosine
ML middle lobe
MLCN multilocular cystic nephroma
MLO mediolateral oblique
MMAA mini-microaggregated albumin colloid
MMFR maximal midexpiratory flow rate
MoM multiple of mean
MPS mucopolysaccharidosis
MR magnetic resonance
MRCP Magnetic resonance cholangiopancreatography
MS-AFP maternal serum α-fetoprotein

MTP metatarsophalangeal
MUGA multiple gated acquisition
MV mitral valve
Myelo myelography

N.B. nota bene
NBS National Bureau of Standards
NEC necrotizing enterocolitis
NECT nonenhanced computed tomography
NF neurofibromatosis
NHL non-Hodgkin lymphoma
NIDDM non-insulin dependent diabetes mellitus
NPH normal pressure hydrocephalus
NPH nucleus pulposus herniation
npl neoplasm
NPO nulla per os
NSAID nonsteroidal anti-inflammatory drug
NST nonstress test
NTD neural tube defect
NUC nuclear medicine

OB-US obstetrical ultrasound
OCG oral cholecystogram
OCVM occult vascular malformation
OHP orthogonal-hole test pattern
OHSS ovarian hyperstimulation syndrome
OIH orthoiodohippurate

P phosphorus
PA posteroanterior; pulmonary artery
PAC premature atrial contraction
PAH para-aminohippurate; precapillary pulmonary arterial hypertension
PAP primary atypical pneumonia
PAP pulmonary alveolar proteinosis
PAPVR partial anomalous pulmonary venous return
PAS periodic acid Schiff
Path pathology
PAVM pulmonary arteriovenous malformation
PBF pulmonary blood flow
PCA posterior cerebral artery
PCAVC persistent complete atrioventricular canal
PCKD polycystic kidney disease
PCom posterior communicating artery
PCP Pneumocystis carinii pneumonia
PCWP pulmonary capillary wedge pressure
PD posterior descending artery
PDA patent ductus arteriosus
PE pulmonary embolism
PEEP positive end expiratory pressure
PEP preejection period
PET positron emission tomography
pHPT primary hyperparathyroidism
PICA posterior inferior cerebellar artery
PID pelvic inflammatory disease
PIE pulmonary infiltrate with eosinophilia; pulmonary interstitial emphysema
PIOPED prospective investigation of pulmonary embolus detection
PIP proximal interphalangeal
PIPIDA paraisopropyl iminodiacetic acid
PLES parallel-line–equal spacing
PM photomultiplier
PMF progressive massive fibrosis
PML progressive multifocal leukoencephalopathy
pML posterior mitral valve leaflet
PMN polymorphonuclear
PMT photomultiplier tube
PNET primitive neuroectodermal tumor
PO per oral
POST posterior
PPD purified protein derivative
PPG photoplethysmography
PPLO pleuropneumonia-like organism
ppm posterior papillary muscle
PS pulmonary stenosis
PSS progressive systemic sclerosis
PTC percutaneous transhepatic cholangiography
PTH parathyroid hormone
pTL posterior tricuspid valve leaflet
PTU propylthiouracil
PVC polyvinyl chloride
PVE periventricular echogenicity
PVH pulmonary venous hypertension
PVL periventricular leukomalacia
PVNS pigmented villonodular synovitis
PYP pyrophosphate
PVR pulse volume recording; postvoid residual

R right
RA rheumatoid arthritis
RA right atrium
RAO right anterior oblique
RBC red blood cell
RCA right coronary artery
RCC renal cell carcinoma
RDS respiratory distress syndrome
RES reticuloendothelial system
RI resistive index
RIND reversible ischemic neurologic deficit
RISA radioiodine serum albumin
RLL right lower lobe
RLQ right lower quadrant
RML right middle lobe
ROC receiver operating characteristic
ROI region of interest
RPA right pulmonary artery
RPF renal plasma flow
RPO right posterior oblique
RTA renal tubular acidosis
RUL right upper lobe
RV residual volume
RV right ventricle
RVOT right ventricular outflow tract
Rx therapy

S/P status post
SAE subcortical arteriosclerotic encephalopathy
SAG sagittal
SAH subarachnoid hemorrhage
SAM systolic anterior motion of mitral valve
SANA sinoatrial node artery
SBE subacute bacterial endocarditis
SBO salpingo-oophorectomy
SCBE single-contrast barium enema
SD standard deviation
SE spin echo
SGA small for gestational age
sHPT secondary hyperparathyroidism
SIJ sacroiliac joint
SFA superficial femoral artery
SLE systemic lupus erythematosus
SMA superior mesenteric artery
SMV superior mesenteric vein
Sn stannum

SNAT suspected nonaccidental trauma
SNHL sensorineural hearing loss
SOB small bowel obstruction
SONK spontaneous osteonecrosis of knee
S/P status post
SPECT single photon emission
SQ subcutaneous
STIR short tau inversion recovery
SV stroke volume
SVC superior vena cava

T1WI T1-weighted image
T2WI T2-weighted image
TAH total abdominal hysterectomy
TAPVR total anomalous pulmonary venous return
TB tuberculosis
TBG thyroxin-binding globulin
TBPA thyroxin-binding prealbumin
TCC transitional cell carcinoma
TDLU terminal ductal lobular unit
TE tracheoesophageal fistula
TGA transposition of great arteries
tHPT tertiary hyperparathyroidism
TIA transitory ischemic attack
TLC total lung capacity
TN true negative
TOA tubo-ovarian abscess
TOF tetralogy of Fallot
TORCH toxoplasmosis, rubella, cytomegalovirus, herpes virus
TP true positive
TR repetition time
TRH thyrotropin-releasing hormone
TRV transverse
TSH thyroid-stimulating hormone
TURP transurethral resection of prostate
TV tidal volume

UGI upper gastrointestinal series
UIP usual interstitial pneumonia
UL upper lobe
UPJ ureteropelvic junction
US ultrasound
USP XX United States Pharmacopoeia, 20th edition
UTI urinary tract infection
UVJ ureterovesical junction

VC vital capacity
VIP vasoactive intestinal peptides
VMA vanillylmandelic acid
V/Q ventilation perfusion
VS interventricular septum
VSD ventricular septal defect

WBC white blood cells
WDHA watery diarrhea, hypokalemia, achlorhydria
WDHH watery diarrhea, hypokalemia, hypochlorhydria
XGP xanthogranulomatous pyelonephritis

ACRONYMS AND MNEMONICS

MUSCULOSKELETAL SYSTEM

DIFFERENTIAL DIAGNOSIS OF MUSCULOSKELETAL DISORDERS

DIFFERENTIAL-DIAGNOSTIC GAMUT OF BONE DISORDERS

Conditions to be considered = "dissect bone disease with a DIATTOM"

Dysplasia + **D**ystrophy
Infection
Anomalies of development
Tumor + tumorlike conditions
Trauma
Osteochondritis + ischemic necrosis
Metabolic disease

DYSPLASIA = disturbance of bone growth
DYSTROPHY = disturbance of nutrition

LIMPING CHILD

1–4 Years

A. CONGENITAL
   1. Developmental dysplasia of hip
B. TRAUMATIC
   1. Toddler's fracture
   2. Nonaccidental trauma
   3. Other fractures
   4. Foreign body
C. INFLAMMATORY
   1. Diskitis
   2. Septic arthritis
   3. Osteomyelitis
   4. Transient synovitis of hip

4–10 Years

A. TRAUMATIC
B. INFLAMMATORY
   1. Septic arthritis
   2. Osteomyelitis
   3. Transient synovitis of hip
   4. Diskitis
   5. Juvenile rheumatoid arthritis
C. VASCULAR
   1. Legg-Perthes disease

10–15 Years

A. TRAUMATIC
   1. Stress fracture
   2. Osteochondritis dissecans
   3. Osgood-Schlatter disease
C. INFLAMMATORY
   1. Juvenile rheumatoid arthritis
   2. Ankylosing spondylitis
   3. Septic arthritis
   4. Osteomyelitis
D. HORMONAL
   1. Epiphyseolysis of femoral head

DELAYED BONE AGE

A. CONSTITUTIONAL
   1. Familial
   2. IUGR
B. METABOLIC
   1. Hypopituitarism
   2. Hypothyroidism
   3. Hypogonadism (Turner syndrome)
   4. Cushing disease, steroid therapy
   5. Diabetes mellitus
   6. Rickets
   7. Malnutrition
   8. Irradiation of brain (for cerebral tumor / ALL)
C. SYSTEMIC DISEASE
   1. Congenital heart disease
   2. Renal disease
   3. GI disease: celiac disease, Crohn disease, ulcerative colitis
   4. Anemia
   5. Bone marrow transplantation (<5 years of age)
D. SYNDROMES
   1. Trisomies
   2. Noonan disease
   3. Cornelia de Lange syndrome
   4. Cleidocranial dysplasia
   5. Lesch-Nyhan disease
   6. Metatrophic dwarfism

BONE SCLEROSIS

Diffuse Osteosclerosis

mnemonic: "5 M'S To PROoF"

Metastases
Myelofibrosis
Mastocytosis
Melorheostosis
Metabolic: hypervitaminosis D, fluorosis, hypothyroidism, phosphorus poisoning
Sickle cell disease
Tuberous sclerosis
Pyknodysostosis, **P**aget disease
Renal osteodystrophy
Osteopetrosis
Fluorosis

Constitutional Sclerosing Bone Disease

1. Engelmann-Camurati disease
2. Infantile cortical hyperostosis
3. Melorheostosis
4. Osteopathia striata
5. Osteopetrosis
6. Osteopoikilosis
7. Pachydermoperiostosis
8. Pyknodysostosis
9. Van Buchem disease
10. Williams syndrome

Sclerosing Bone Dysplasia

A. Dysplasias of ENDOCHONDRAL OSSIFICATION (PRIMARY SPONGIOSA)
   = failure in resorption + remodeling of primary immature spongiosa by osteoclasts
   √ accumulation of calcified cartilage matrix packing the medullary cavity
   Target sites: tubular + flat bones, vertebrae, skull base, ethmoids, ends of clavicle
   1. Osteopetrosis
   2. Pyknodysostosis
B. Dysplasias of ENDOCHONDRAL OSSIFICATION (SECONDARY SPONGIOSA)
   = errors in resorption + remodeling of secondary spongiosa
   √ focal densities / striations
   1. Enostosis
   2. Osteopoikilosis
   3. Osteopathia striata
C. Dysplasias of INTRAMEMBRANOUS OSSIFICATION
   = disequilibrium between periosteal bone formation + endosteal bone resorption
   Target sites: cortex of tubular + flat bones, calvaria, bones of upper face, tympanic parts of temporal bone, vomer, medial pterygoid
   1. Progressive diaphyseal dysplasia
   2. Hereditary multiple diaphyseal sclerosis (Ribbing disease)
   3. Hyperostosis corticalis generalisata
      – Van Buchem disease
      – Sclerosteosis (Truswell-Hansen disease)
      – Worth disease
      – Nakamura disease
   4. Diaphyseal dysplasia with anemia
   5. Oculodento-osseous dysplasia
   6. Trichodento-osseous dysplasia
   7. Kenny-Caffey syndrome
D. MIXED SCLEROSING DYSPLASIAS
   (a) predominantly endochondral disturbance
      1. Dysosteosclerosis
      2. Metaphyseal dysplasia (Pyle disease)
      3. Craniometaphyseal dysplasia
      4. Frontometaphyseal dysplasia
   (b) predominantly intramembranous defects
      1. Melorheostosis
      2. Craniodiaphyseal dysplasia
      3. Lenz-Majewski hyperostotic dwarfism
      4. Progressive diaphyseal dysplasia

Solitary Osteosclerotic Lesion

A. DEVELOPMENTAL
   1. Bone island
B. VASCULAR
   1. Old bone infarct
   2. Aseptic / ischemic / avascular necrosis
C. HEALING BONE LESION
   (a) trauma: callus formation in stress fracture
   (b) benign tumor: fibrous cortical defect / nonossifying fibroma, brown tumor; bone cyst
   (c) malignant tumor: lytic metastasis after radiation, chemo-, hormone therapy
D. INFECTION / INFLAMMATION
   (low-grade chronic infection / healing infection)
   1. Osteoid osteoma
   2. Chronic / healed osteomyelitis: bacterial, tuberculous, fungal
   3. Sclerosing osteomyelitis of Garré
   4. Granuloma
   5. Brodie abscess
E. BENIGN TUMOR
   1. Osteoma
   2. Osteoblastoma
   3. Ossifying fibroma
   4. Healed fibrous cortical defect
   5. Enchondroma / osteochondroma
F. MALIGNANT TUMOR
   1. Osteoblastic metastasis (prostate, breast)
   2. Lymphoma
   3. Sarcoma: osteo-, chondro-, Ewing sarcoma
G. OTHERS
   1. Sclerotic phase of Paget disease
   2. Fibrous dysplasia

Cortical Sclerotic Lesion in Child

1. Osteoid osteoma
2. Stress fracture
3. Chronic osteomyelitis
4. Healed fibrous cortical defect

Multiple Osteosclerotic Lesions

A. FAMILIAL
   1. Osteopoikilosis
   2. Enchondromatosis = Ollier disease
   3. Melorheostosis
   4. Multiple osteomas: associated with Gardner syndrome
   5. Osteopetrosis
   6. Pyknodysostosis
   7. Osteopathia striata
   8. Chondrodystrophia calcificans congenita = congenital stippled epiphyses
   9. Multiple epiphyseal dysplasia = Fairbank disease
B. SYSTEMIC DISEASE
   1. Mastocytosis = urticaria pigmentosa
   2. Tuberous sclerosis

Bone-within-bone Appearance

= endosteal new bone formation
1. Normal
   (a) thoracic + lumbar vertebrae (in infants)
   (b) growth recovery lines (after infancy)
2. Infantile cortical hyperostosis (Caffey)
3. Sickle cell disease / thalassemia
4. Congenital syphilis
5. Osteopetrosis / oxalosis
6. Radiation
7. Acromegaly
8. Paget disease

mnemonic: "BLT PLT RSD RSD"
Bismuth ingestion
Lead ingestion
Thorium ingestion
Petrosis (osteopetrosis)
Leukemia
Tuberculosis
Rickets
Scurvy
D toxicity (vitamin D)
RSD (reflex sympathetic dystrophy)

Dense Metaphyseal Bands

mnemonic: "DENSE LINES"
D-vitamin intoxication
Elemental arsenic and heavy metals (lead, bismuth, phosphorus)
Normal variant
Systemic illness
Estrogen to mother during pregnancy
Leukemia
Infection (TORCH), **I**diopathic hypercalcemia
Never forget healed rickets
Early hypothyroidism (cretinism)
Scurvy, congenital **S**yphilis, **S**ickle cell disease
also: methotrexate therapy

OSTEOPENIA

= decrease in bone quantity maintaining normal quality
√ increased radiolucency of bone:
- √ vertical striations in vertebral bodies
- √ accentuation of tensile + compressive trabeculae of proximal femur
- √ reinforcement lines (= bone bars) crossing marrow cavity about knee
- √ cortical resorption of 2nd metacarpal:
  - √ measuring outer cortical diameter (W) and width of medullary cavity (m) at midportion of bone and reporting combined cortical thickness (CCT)
- √ subperiosteal tunneling

Categories:
A. DIFFUSE OSTEOPENIA
1. Osteoporosis = decreased osteoid production
2. Osteomalacia = undermineralization of osteoid
3. Hyperparathyroidism
4. Multiple myeloma / diffuse metastases
5. Drugs
6. Mastocytosis
7. Osteogenesis imperfecta

B. REGIONAL OSTEOPENIA

Osteoporosis

= reduced bone mass of normal composition secondary to (a) osteoclastic resorption (85%) (trabecular, endosteal, intracortical, subperiosteal)
(b) osteocytic resorption (15%)

Incidence: 7% of all women aged 35–40 years; 1 in 3 women > age 65 years

Etiology:
A. CONGENITAL DISORDERS
1. Osteogenesis imperfecta
   ◊ The only osteoporosis with bending!
2. Homocystinuria

B. IDIOPATHIC (bone loss begins earlier + proceeds more rapidly in women)
1. Juvenile osteoporosis: <20 years
2. Adult osteoporosis: 20–40 years
3. Postmenopausal osteoporosis: >50 years (40–50% lower trabecular bone mineral density in elderly than in young women)
4. Senile osteoporosis: >60 years progressively decreasing bone density at a rate of 8% in females; 3% in males

C. NUTRITIONAL DISTURBANCES
scurvy; protein deficiency (malnutrition, nephrosis, chronic liver disease, alcoholism, anorexia nervosa, kwashiorkor, starvation), calcium deficiency

D. ENDOCRINOPATHY
Cushing disease, hypogonadism (Turner syndrome, eunuchoidism), hyperthyroidism, hyperparathyroidism, acromegaly, Addison disease, diabetes mellitus, pregnancy, paraneoplastic phenomenon in liver tumors

E. RENAL OSTEODYSTROPHY
decrease / same / increase in spinal trabecular bone; rapid loss in appendicular skeleton

F. IMMOBILIZATION = disuse osteoporosis

G. COLLAGEN DISEASE, RHEUMATOID ARTHRITIS

H. BONE MARROW REPLACEMENT
infiltration by lymphoma / leukemia (ALL), multiple myeloma, diffuse metastases, marrow hyperplasia secondary to hemolytic anemia

I. DRUG THERAPY
heparin (15,000–30,000 U for >6 months), methotrexate, corticosteroids, excessive alcohol consumption, smoking, Dilantin

J. RADIATION THERAPY

K. LOCALIZED OSTEOPOROSIS
Sudeck dystrophy, transient osteoporosis of hip, regional migratory osteoporosis of lower extremities

- serum calcium, phosphorus, alkaline phosphatase frequently normal
- hydroxyproline may be elevated during acute stage

Technique:
(1) SINGLE-PHOTON ABSORPTIOMETRY
measures primarily cortical bone of appendicular bones, single-energy I-125 radioisotope source
Site: distal radius (= wrist bone density), os calcis
Dose: 2–3 mrem
Precision: 1–3%

(2) DUAL-PHOTON ABSORPTIOMETRY
radioactive energy source with two photon peaks; should be reserved for patients <65 years of age because of interference from osteophytosis + vascular calcifications
Site: vertebrae, femoral neck
Dose: 5–10 mrem; Precision: 2–4%

(3) SINGLE X-RAY ABSORPTIOMETRY
= area projectional technique for quantitative bone density measurement
Site: distal radius, calcaneus
Dose: low
Precision: 0.5–2%

(4) DUAL ENERGY X-RAY ABSORPTIOMETRY (DEXA)
◊ Most widely used & most precise technique!
= quantitative digital radiography
= beams with two distinct energy levels allow identification of trabecular from cortical bone
• has replaced dual-photon absorptiometry and is produced by x-ray tube with higher radiation flux than radioisotope source
Site: lumbar spine, femoral neck, whole body, forearm
Dose: <3 mrem; Precision: 1–2%
Data collected:
BMD (bone marrow density) value (g/cm^2)
%BMD compared to young adults
%BMD compared to age-matched adults
T-score (SD of young-adult mean)
Z-score (SD of age-matched mean)

(5) QUANTITATIVE COMPUTED TOMOGRAPHY
= determines true volumetric density (mg/cm^3)
• high-turnover cancellous bone is important for vertebral strength and has high responsiveness
• trabecular bone + low-turnover compact bone can be measured separately
√ compared to external bone mineral reference phantom scanned simultaneously with patient to calibrate CT attenuation measurements
√ 10-mm–thick section with gantry angle correction through center of vertebral body
Site: vertebrae L1–L3, other sites
Use: assessment of vertebral fracture risk; measurement of age-related bone loss; follow-up of osteoporosis + metabolic bone disease
(a) single energy: 300–500 mrem; 6–25% precision
(b) dual energy: 750–800 mrem; 5–10% precision
◊ Most sensitive technique!

(6) PERIPHERAL QUANTITATIVE CT
= exact 3-dimensional localization of target volumes with multisection data acquisition capability covering a large volume of bone
Site: distal radius

DEXA Interpretation

Diagnosis	*T-score*	*Management*	*Follow-up*
Normal	>-1	prevention	3 years
Osteopenia	<-1 and >-2.5	prevention or therapy	2 years
Osteoporosis	<-2.5	therapy	1 year

Location: axial skeleton (lower dorsal + lumbar spine), proximal humerus, neck of femur, wrist, ribs
◊ Radiographs are insensitive prior to bone loss of 25–30%
◊ Bone scans do NOT show a diffuse increase in activity
√ decreased number + thickness of trabeculae
√ cortical thinning (endosteal + intracortical resorption)
√ juxtaarticular osteopenia with trabecular bone predominance
√ delayed fracture healing with poor callus formation (DDx: abundant callus formation in osteogenesis imperfecta + Cushing syndrome)
Cx: (1) Fractures at sites rich in labile trabecular bone (eg, vertebrae, wrist) in postmenopausal osteoporosis
(2) Fractures at sites containing cortical + trabecular bone (eg, hip) in senile osteoporosis
Rx: calcitonin, sodium fluoride, diphosphonates, parathyroid hormone supplements, estrogen replacement

Osteoporosis of Spine
√ diminished radiographic density
√ vertical striations (= marked thinning of transverse trabeculae with relative accentuation of vertical trabeculae along lines of stress)
√ accentuation of endplates
√ "picture framing" (= accentuation of cortical outline with preservation of external dimensions secondary to endosteal + intracortical resorption)
√ compression deformities with protrusion of intervertebral disks:
  √ biconcave vertebrae
  √ Schmorl nodes
  √ wedging
  √ decreased height of vertebrae
√ absence of osteophytes

Osteomalacia
= accumulation of excessive amounts of uncalcified osteoid with bone softening + insufficient mineralization of osteoid due to
(a) high remodeling rate: excessive osteoid formation + normal / little mineralization
(b) low remodeling rate: normal osteoid production + diminished mineralization

Etiology:
(1) dietary deficiency of vitamin D_3 + lack of solar irradiation
(2) deficiency of metabolism of vitamin D:
— chronic renal tubular disease
— chronic administration of phenobarbital (alternate liver pathway)
— diphenylhydantoin (interferes with vitamin D action on bowel)
(3) decreased absorption of vitamin D:
— malabsorption syndromes (most common)
— partial gastrectomy (self-restriction of fatty foods)

(4) decreased deposition of calcium in bone
— diphosphonates (for treatment of Paget disease)

Histo: excess of osteoid seams + decreased appositional rate

- bone pain / tenderness; muscular weakness
- serum calcium slightly low / normal
- decreased serum phosphorus
- elevated serum alkaline phosphatase

√ uniform osteopenia
√ fuzzy indistinct trabecular detail of endosteal surface
√ coarsened frayed trabeculae decreased in number + size
√ thin cortices of long bone
√ bone deformity from softening:
  √ hourglass thorax
  √ bowing of long bones
  √ acetabular protrusion
  √ buckled / compressed pelvis
  √ biconcave vertebral bodies
√ increased incidence of insufficiency fractures
√ pseudofractures = Looser zones
√ mottled skull

Localized / Regional Osteopenia

1. Disuse osteoporosis / atrophy
   Etiology: local immobilization secondary to
   (a) fracture (more pronounced distal to fracture site)
   (b) neural paralysis
   (c) muscular paralysis
2. Reflex sympathetic dystrophy = Sudeck dystrophy
3. Regional migratory osteoporosis, transient regional osteoporosis of hip
4. Rheumatologic disorders
5. Infection: osteomyelitis, tuberculosis
6. Osteolytic tumor
7. Lytic phase of Paget disease
8. Early phase of bone infarct and hemorrhage
9. Burns + frostbite

Bone Marrow Edema

= hypointensity on T1WI + hyperintensity on T2WI

1. Transient osteoporosis of hip
2. Osteonecrosis = early stage of AVN
3. Trauma
   (a) "bone bruise"
   (b) radiographically occult fracture in elderly women
4. Infection = osteomyelitis
5. Infiltrative neoplasm

Transverse Lucent Metaphyseal Lines

mnemonic: "LINING"

Leukemia
Illness, systemic (rickets, scurvy)
Normal variant
Infection, transplacental (congenital syphilis)
Neuroblastoma metastases
Growth lines

Frayed Metaphyses

mnemonic: "CHARMS"

Congenital infections (rubella, syphilis)
Hypophosphatasia
Achondroplasia
Rickets
Metaphyseal dysostosis
Scurvy

BONE TUMOR

Role of Radiologist

1. Is there a lesion?
2. Is it a bone tumor?
3. Is the tumor benign or malignant?
4. Is a biopsy necessary?
5. Is the histologic diagnosis consistent with the radiographic image?

Assessment of Aggressiveness

A. BENIGN
   1. Diagnosis certain: no further work-up necessary
   2. Asymptomatic lesion with highly probable benign diagnosis may be followed clinically
   3. Symptomatic lesion with highly probable benign diagnosis may be treated without further work-up
B. CONFUSING LESION
   not clearly categorized as benign or malignant; needs staging work-up
C. MALIGNANT: needs staging work-up

Staging work-up:

Bone scan: identifies polyostotic lesions (eg, multiple myeloma, metastatic disease, primary osteosarcoma with bone-forming metastases, histiocytosis, Paget disease)

Chest CT: identifies metastatic deposits + changes further work-up and therapy

Local staging with MR imaging:
(1) Margins: encapsulated / infiltrating
(2) Compartment: intra- / extracompartmental
(3) Intraosseous extent + skip lesions
(4) Soft-tissue extent (DDx: hematoma, edema)
(5) Joint involvement
(6) Neurovascular involvement

Local assessment with CT imaging:
√ matrix / rim calcifications

Tumorlike Conditions

1. Solitary bone cyst
2. Juxtaarticular ("synovial") cyst
3. Aneurysmal bone cyst
4. Nonossifying fibroma; cortical defect; cortical desmoid
5. Eosinophilic granuloma
6. Reparative giant cell granuloma
7. Fibrous dysplasia (monostotic; polyostotic)
8. Myositis ossificans
9. "Brown tumor" of hyperparathyroidism
10. Massive osteolysis

Pseudomalignant Appearance
1. Osteomyelitis
2. Aggressive osteoporosis

Pattern of Bone Destruction
A. GEOGRAPHIC BONE DESTRUCTION
Cause: (a) slow-growing usually benign tumor
(b) rarely malignant: plasma cell myeloma, metastasis
(c) infection: granulomatous osteomyelitis
√ well-defined smooth / irregular margin
√ short zone of transition

B. MOTH-EATEN BONE DESTRUCTION
Cause: (a) rapidly growing malignant bone tumor
(b) osteomyelitis
√ less well defined / demarcated lesional margin
√ longer zone of transition
mnemonic: "H LEMMON"
Histiocytosis X
Lymphoma
Ewing sarcoma
Metastasis
Multiple myeloma
Osteomyelitis
Neuroblastoma

C. PERMEATIVE BONE DESTRUCTION
Cause: aggressive bone tumor with rapid growth potential (eg, Ewing sarcoma)
√ poorly demarcated lesion imperceptibly merging with uninvolved bone
√ long zone of transition

Size, Shape, and Margin of Bone Lesion
◊ Primary malignant tumors are larger than benign tumors
√ elongated lesion (= greatest diameter of >1.5 times the least diameter): Ewing sarcoma, histiocytic lymphoma, chondrosarcoma, angiosarcoma
√ sclerotic margin (= reaction of host tissue to tumor)

Tumor Position in Transverse Plane
A. CENTRAL MEDULLARY LESION
1. Enchondroma
2. Solitary bone cyst

B. ECCENTRIC MEDULLARY LESION
1. Giant cell tumor
2. Osteogenic sarcoma, chondrosarcoma, fibrosarcoma
3. Chondromyxoid fibroma

C. CORTICAL LESION
1. Nonossifying fibroma
2. Osteoid osteoma

D. PERIOSTEAL / JUXTACORTICAL LESION
1. Juxtacortical chondroma / osteosarcoma
2. Osteochondroma
3. Parosteal osteogenic sarcoma

Tumor Position in Longitudinal Plane
A. EPIPHYSEAL LESION
1. Chondroblastoma (prior to closure of growth plate)
2. Intraosseous ganglion, subchondral cyst
3. Giant cell tumor (originating in metaphysis)
4. Clear cell chondrosarcoma
5. Fibrous dysplasia
6. Abscess

mnemonic: "CAGGIE"
Chondroblastoma
Aneurysmal bone cyst
Giant cell tumor
Geode
Infection
Eosinophilic granuloma
[after 40 years of age throw out "CEA" and insert metastases / myeloma]

B. METAPHYSEAL LESION
1. Nonossifying fibroma (close to growth plate)
2. Chondromyxoid fibroma (abutting growth plate)
3. Solitary bone cyst
4. Osteochondroma
5. Brodie abscess
6. Osteogenic sarcoma, chondrosarcoma

C. DIAPHYSEAL LESION
1. Round cell tumor (eg, Ewing sarcoma)
2. Nonossifying fibroma
3. Solitary bone cyst
4. Aneurysmal bone cyst
5. Enchondroma
6. Osteoblastoma
7. Fibrous dysplasia

mnemonic: "FEMALE"
Fibrous dysplasia
Eosinophilic granuloma
Metastasis
Adamantinoma
Leukemia, **L**ymphoma
Ewing sarcoma

Tumors Localizing to Hematopoietic Marrow
1. Metastases
2. Plasma cell myeloma
3. Ewing sarcoma
4. Histiocytic lymphoma

Diffuse Bone Marrow Abnormalities in Childhood
A. REPLACED BY TUMOR CELLS
(a) metastatic disease
1. Neuroblastoma (in young child)
2. Lymphoma (in older child)
3. Rhabdomyosarcoma (in older child)
(b) primary neoplasm
1. Leukemia

B. REPLACED BY RED CELLS
= **Red cell hyperplasia** = reconversion
(a) severe anemia: sickle cell disease, thalassemia, hereditary spherocytosis
(b) chronic severe blood loss

(c) marrow replacement by neoplasia
(d) treatment with granulocyte-macrophage colony stimulating factor

C. REPLACED BY FAT
1. Myeloid depletion = aplastic anemia

D. REPLACED BY FIBROUS TISSUE
1. Myelofibrosis

Age Incidence of Malignant Bone Tumors

◊ 80% of bone tumors are correctly determined on the basis of age alone!

Age [years]	*Tumor*
0.1	Neuroblastoma
0.1–10	Ewing tumor in tubular bones (diaphysis)
10 –30	Osteosarcoma (metaphysis); Ewing tumor in flat bones
30 –40	Reticulum cell sarcoma (similar histology to Ewing tumor); fibrosarcoma; malignant giant cell tumor (similar histology to fibrosarcoma); parosteal sarcoma; lymphoma
>40	Metastatic carcinoma; multiple myeloma; chondrosarcoma

SARCOMAS BY AGE:
mnemonic: "**E**very **O**ther **R**unner **F**eels **C**rampy **P**ain **O**n **M**oving"

Ewing sarcoma	0 –10 years
Osteogenic sarcoma	10–30 years
Reticulum cell sarcoma	20–40 years
Fibrosarcoma	20–40 years
Chondrosarcoma	40–50 years
Parosteal sarcoma	40–50 years
Osteosarcoma	60–70 years
Metastases	60–70 years

ROUND CELL TUMORS:
√ arise in midshaft
√ osteolytic lesion
√ reactive new bone formation
√ no tumor new bone
mnemonic: "LEMON"
Leukemia, **L**ymphoma
Ewing sarcoma, **E**osinophilic granuloma
Multiple myeloma
Osteomyelitis
Neuroblastoma

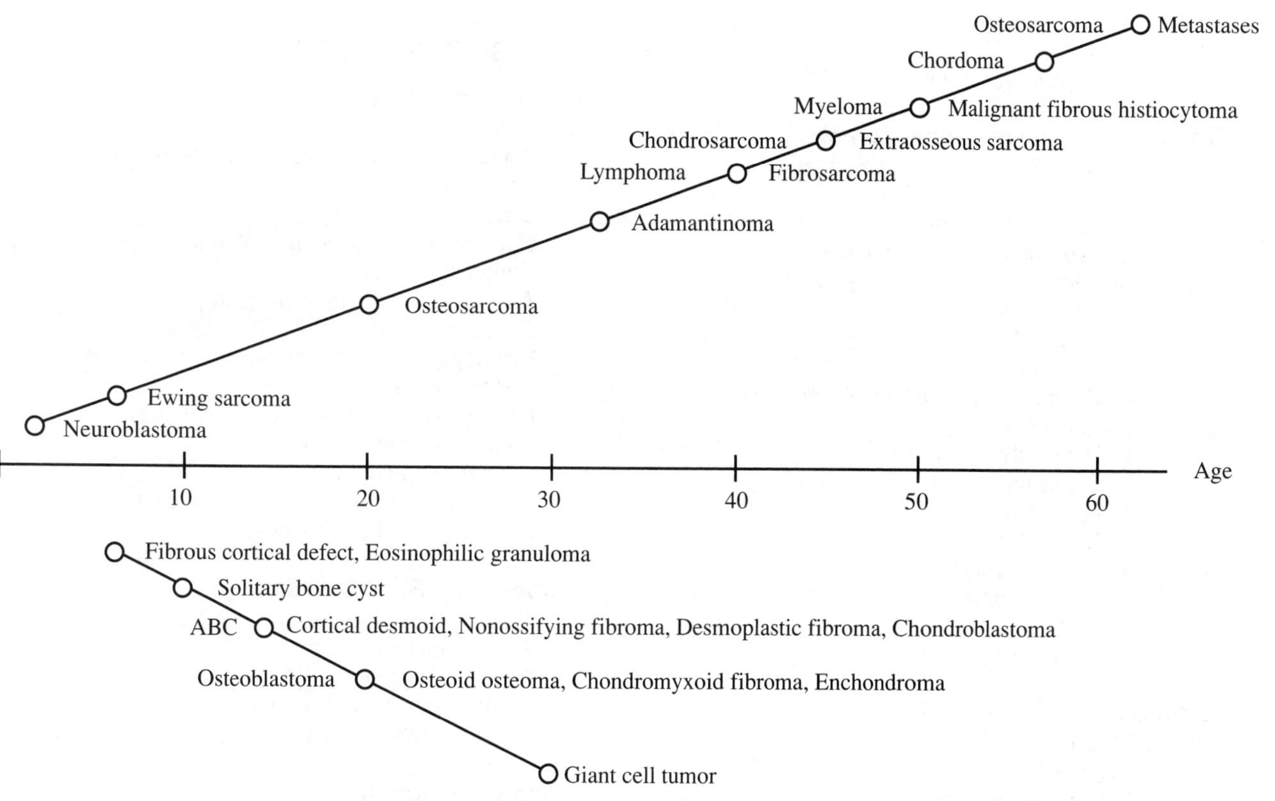

Average Age for Occurrence of Benign and Malignant Bone Tumors

MALIGNANCY WITH SOFT-TISSUE INVOLVEMENT

mnemonic: "**M**y **M**other **E**ats **Ch**ocolate **F**udge **O**ften"

Metastasis
Myeloma
Ewing sarcoma
Chondrosarcoma
Fibrosarcoma
Osteosarcoma

Tumor Matrix of Bone Tumors

Cartilage-forming Bone Tumors

√ centrally located ringlike / flocculent / flecklike radiodensities

A. BENIGN
1. Enchondroma
2. Parosteal chondroma
3. Chondroblastoma
4. Chondromyxoid fibroma
5. Osteochondroma

B. MALIGNANT
1. Chondrosarcoma
2. Chondroblastic osteosarcoma

Bone-forming Tumors

√ inhomogeneous / homogeneous radiodense collections of variable size + extent

A. BENIGN
1. Osteoma
2. Osteoid osteoma
3. Osteoblastoma
4. Ossifying fibroma

B. MALIGNANT
1. Osteogenic sarcoma

Fibrous Connective Tissue Tumors

A. BENIGN FIBROUS BONE LESIONS

(a) cortical
1. Benign cortical defect
2. Avulsion cortical irregularity

(b) medullary
1. Herniation pit
2. Nonossifying fibroma
3. Ossifying fibroma
4. Congenital generalized fibromatosis

(c) corticomedullary
1. Nonossifying fibroma
2. Ossifying fibroma
3. Fibrous dysplasia
4. Cherubism
5. Desmoplastic fibroma
6. Fibromyxoma

B. MALIGNANT
1. Fibrosarcoma

Tumors of Histiocytic Origin

A. LOCALLY AGGRESSIVE
1. Giant cell tumor
2. Benign fibrous histiocytoma

B. MALIGNANT
1. Malignant fibrous histiocytoma

Tumors of Fatty Tissue Origin

A. BENIGN
1. Intraosseous lipoma
2. Parosteal lipoma

B. MALIGNANT
1. Intraosseous liposarcoma

◊ Lipomas follow the signal intensity of subcutaneous fat in all sequences!

Tumors of Vascular Origin

<1% of all bone tumors

A. BENIGN
1. Hemangioma
2. Glomus tumor
3. Lymphangioma
4. Cystic angiomatosis
5. Hemangiopericytoma

B. MALIGNANT
1. Malignant hemangiopericytoma
2. Angiosarcoma = hemangioendothelioma
   Metastatic sites: lung, brain, lymph nodes, other bones

Tumors of Neural Origin

A. BENIGN
1. Solitary neurofibroma
2. Neurilemoma

B. MALIGNANT
1. Neurogenic sarcoma = malignant schwannoma

INTRAOSSEOUS LESION

Bubbly Bone Lesion

mnemonic: "FOG MACHINES"

Fibrous dysplasia, **F**ibrous cortical defect
Osteoblastoma
Giant cell tumor
Myeloma (plasmacytoma), **M**etastases from kidney, thyroid, breast
Aneurysmal bone cyst / **A**ngioma
Chondromyxoid fibroma, **C**hondroblastoma
Histiocytosis X, **H**yperparathyroid brown tumor, **H**emophilia
Infection (Brodie abscess, Echinococcus, coccidioidomycosis)
Nonossifying fibroma
Enchondroma, **E**pithelial inclusion cyst
Simple unilocular bone cyst

Infectious Bubbly Lesion

1. Brodie abscess (Staph. aureus)
2. Coccidioidomycosis
3. Echinococcus
4. Atypical mycobacterium
5. Cystic tuberculosis

Blowout Lesion

A. METASTASES
   Carcinoma of thyroid, kidney, breast

B. PRIMARY BONE TUMOR
   1. Fibrosarcoma
   2. Multiple myeloma (sometimes)
   3. Aneurysmal bone cyst
   4. Hemophilic pseudotumor

Nonexpansile Unilocular Well-demarcated Bone Defect

1. Fibrous cortical defect
2. Nonossifying fibroma
3. Simple unicameral bone cyst
4. Giant cell tumor
5. Brown tumor of HPT
6. Eosinophilic granuloma
7. Enchondroma
8. Epidermoid inclusion cyst
9. Posttraumatic / degenerative cyst
10. Pseudotumor of hemophilia
11. Intraosseous ganglion
12. Histiocytoma
13. Arthritic lesion
14. Endosteal pigmented villonodular synovitis
15. Fibrous dysplasia
16. Infectious lesion

Nonexpansile Multilocular Well-demarcated Bone Defect

1. Aneurysmal bone cyst
2. Giant cell tumor
3. Fibrous dysplasia
4. Simple bone cyst

Expansile Unilocular Well-demarcated Osteolysis

1. Simple unicameral bone cyst
2. Enchondroma
3. Aneurysmal bone cyst
4. Juxtacortical chondroma
5. Nonossifying fibroma
6. Eosinophilic granuloma
7. Brown tumor of HPT

Poorly Demarcated Osteolytic Lesion without Periosteal Reaction

A. NONEXPANSILE
   1. Metastases from any primary neoplasm
   2. Multiple myeloma
   3. Hemangioma

B. EXPANSILE
   1. Chondrosarcoma
   2. Giant cell tumor
   3. Metastasis from kidney / thyroid

Poorly Demarcated Osteolytic Lesion with Periosteal Reaction

1. Osteomyelitis
2. Ewing sarcoma
3. Osteosarcoma

Mixed Sclerotic and Lytic Lesion

A. WITH SEQUESTRUM: osteomyelitis

B. WITHOUT SEQUESTRUM:
   1. Osteomyelitis
   2. Tuberculosis
   3. Ewing sarcoma
   4. Metastasis
   5. Osteosarcoma

Trabeculated Bone Lesion

1. Giant cell tumor: delicate thin trabeculae
2. Chondromyxoid fibroma: coarse thick trabeculae
3. Nonossifying fibroma: lobulated
4. Aneurysmal bone cyst: delicate, horizontally oriented trabeculae
5. Hemangioma: striated radiating trabeculae

Lytic Bone Lesion Surrounded by Marked Sclerosis

mnemonic: "BOOST"

Brodie abscess
Osteoblastoma
Osteoid osteoma
Stress fracture
Tuberculosis

Multiple Lytic Lesions

mnemonic: "FEEMHI"

Fibrous dysplasia
Enchondromas
Eosinophilic granuloma
Metastases, **M**ultiple myeloma
Hyperparathyroidism (brown tumors), **H**emangiomas
Infection

Multiple Lytic Lesions in Child

1. Histiocytosis X
2. Metastatic neuroblastoma / leukemia
3. Fibrous dysplasia
4. Enchondromatosis
5. Rare: cystic angiomatosis, multifocal osteomyelitis

Lytic Bone Lesion in Patient <30 Years of Age

mnemonic: "CAINES"

Chondroblastoma
Aneurysmal bone cyst
Infection
Nonossifying fibroma
Eosinophilic granuloma
Solitary bone cyst

Lytic Bone Lesion on Both Sides of Joint

mnemonic: "SAC"

Synovioma
Angioma
Chondroid lesion

Multiple Bone Lesions & Soft-tissue Tumor
1. Neurofibromatosis & fibroxanthomas
2. Mafucci syndrome = enchondromatosis & hemangioma
3. Mazabraud syndrome = fibrous dysplasia & myxoma
4. Metastases
   (a) Multiple myeloma
   (b) Malignant melanoma
   (c) Lymphoma

Osteoblastic Bone Lesion
A. BENIGN
   1. Bone island
   2. Osteoma
   3. Osteoid osteoma
B. MALIGNANT
   1. Osteosarcoma
   2. Parosteal sarcoma

Widespread Osteosclerotic Lesions
1. Metastases: prostate, breast, lung, bladder, pancreas, stomach, colon, carcinoid, brain
2. Paget disease
3. Sarcoma
4. Myelofibrosis
5. Mastocytosis

DWARFISM
Classification:
(1) OSTEOCHONDRODYSPLASIA
   = abnormalities of cartilage / bone growth and development
   (a) identifiable at birth:
      — usually lethal: achondrogenesis, fibrochondrogenesis, thanatophoric dysplasia, short rib syndrome
      — usually nonlethal: chondrodysplasia punctata, camptomelic dysplasia, achondroplasia, diastrophic dysplasia, chondroectodermal dysplasia, Jeune syndrome, spondyloepiphyseal dysplasia congenita, mesomelic dysplasia, cleidocranial dysplasia, oto-palato-digital syndrome
   (b) identifiable in later life: hypochondroplasia, dyschondrosteosis, spondylometaphyseal dysplasia, acromicric dysplasia
   (c) abnormal bone density: osteopetrosis, pyknodysostosis, Melnick-Needles syndrome
(2) DYSOSTOSIS
   = malformation of individual bones singly / in combination
   (a) with cranial + facial involvement: craniosynostosis, craniofacial dysostosis (Crouzon), acrocephalosyndactyly, acrocephalopolysyndactyly, branchial arch syndromes (Treacher-Collins, Franceschetti, acrofacial dysostosis, oculo-auriculo-vertebral dysostosis, hemifacial microsomia, oculo-mandibulo-facial syndrome
   (b) with predominant axial involvement: vertebral segmentation defects (Klippel-Feil), Sprengel anomaly, spondylocostal dysostosis, oculovertebral syndrome
   (c) with predominant involvement of extremities: <u>acheiria</u> (= absence of hands), <u>apodia</u> (= absence of feet), polydactyly, syndactyly, camptodactyly, Rubinstein-Taybi syndrome, pancytopenia-dysmelia syndrome (Fanconi), Blackfan-Diamond anemia with thumb anomaly, thrombocytopenia-radial aplasia syndrome, cardiomelic syndromes (Holt-Oram), focal femoral deficiency, multiple synostoses
(3) IDIOPATHIC OSTEOLYSIS
   = disorders with multifocal resorption of bone
(4) CHROMOSOMAL ABERRATION
(5) PRIMARY METABOLIC DISORDER
   (a) calcium / phosphorus: hypophosphatasia
   (b) complex carbohydrates: mucopolysaccharidosis

Terminology:

Micromelia	= shortening involves entire limb (eg, humerus, radius + ulna, hand)
Rhizomelia	= shortening involves proximal segment (eg, humerus)
Mesomelia	= shortening involves intermediate segment (eg, radius + ulna)
Acromelia	= shortening involves distal segment (eg, hand)

Micromelic Dwarfism
= disproportionate shortening of entire leg
A. Mild micromelic dwarfism
   1. Jeune syndrome
   2. Ellis-van Creveld syndrome
      = chondroectodermal dysplasia
   3. Diastrophic dwarfism
B. Mild bowed micromelic dwarfism
   1. Camptomelic dysplasia
   2. Osteogenesis imperfecta, type III
C. Severe micromelic dwarfism
   1. Thanatophoric dysplasia
   2. Osteogenesis imperfecta, type II
   3. Homozygous achondroplasia
   4. Hypophosphatasia
   5. Short-rib polydactyly syndrome
   6. Fibrochondrogenesis

Acromelic Dwarfism
= distal shortening (hands, feet)
1. Asphyxiating thoracic dysplasia

Rhizomelic Dwarfism
= shortening of proximal segments (humerus, femur)
mnemonic: "MA CAT"
Metatrophic dwarfism
Achondrogenesis (most severe shortening)
Chondrodysplasia punctata (autosomal recessive)
Thanatophoric dysplasia
Achondroplasia, heterozygous

Osteochondrodysplasia
A. Failure of
- (a) articular cartilage: spondyloepiphyseal dysplasia
- (b) ossification center: multiple epiphyseal dysplasia
- (c) proliferating cartilage: achondroplasia
- (d) spongiosa formation: hypophosphatasia
- (e) spongiosa absorption: osteopetrosis
- (f) periosteal bone: osteogenesis imperfecta
- (g) endosteal bone: idiopathic osteoporosis

B. Excess of
- (a) articular cartilage: dysplasia epiphysealis hemimelica
- (b) hypertrophic cartilage: enchondromatosis
- (c) spongiosa: multiple exostosis
- (d) periosteal bone: progressive diaphyseal dysplasia
- (e) endosteal bone: hyperphosphatemia

Lethal Bone Dysplasia
in order of frequency
1. Thanatophoric dysplasia
2. Osteogenesis imperfecta type II
3. Achondrogenesis type I + II
4. Jeune syndrome (may be nonlethal)
5. Hypophosphatasia, congenital lethal form
6. Chondroectodermal dysplasia (usually nonlethal)
7. Chondrodysplasia punctata, rhizomelic type
8. Camptomelic dysplasia
9. Short-rib polydactyly syndrome
10. Homozygous achondroplasia

◊ Lethal short-limbed dysplasias typically are manifest on sonograms before 24 weeks MA!

Nonlethal Dwarfism
1. Achondroplasia (heterozygous)
2. Asphyxiating thoracic dysplasia
3. Chondroectodermal dysplasia
4. Chondrodysplasia punctata
5. Spondyloepiphyseal dysplasia (congenital)
6. Diastrophic dwarfism
7. Metatrophic dwarfism
8. Hypochondroplasia

Late-onset Dwarfism
1. Spondyloepiphyseal dysplasia tarda
2. Multiple epiphyseal dysplasia
3. Pseudoachondroplasia
4. Metaphyseal chondrodysplasia
5. Dyschondrosteosis
6. Cleidocranial dysostosis
7. Progressive diaphyseal dysplasia

Hypomineralization in Fetus
A. DIFFUSE
1. Osteogenesis imperfecta
2. Hypophosphatasia

B. SPINE
1. Achondrogenesis

Large Head in Fetus
1. Achondroplasia
2. Thanatophoric dysplasia

Narrow Chest in Fetus
1. Short-rib polydactyly syndrome
2. Asphyxiating thoracic dysplasia
3. Chondroectodermal dysplasia
4. Camptomelic dysplasia
5. Thanatophoric dwarfism
6. Homozygous achondroplasia
7. Achondrogenesis
8. Hypophosphatasia

Platyspondyly
1. Thanatophoric dysplasia
2. Osteogenesis imperfecta type II
3. Achondroplasia
4. Morquio syndrome

Bowed Long Bones in Fetus
1. Campomelic syndrome
2. Osteogenesis imperfecta
3. Thanatophoric dysplasia
4. Hypophosphatasia

Bone Fractures in Fetus
1. Osteogenesis imperfecta
2. Hypophosphatasia
3. Achondrogenesis

LIMB REDUCTION ANOMALIES
Amelia = absence of limb
Hemimelia = absence of distal parts
Phocomelia = proximal reduction with distal parts attached to trunk

Aplasia / Hypoplasia of Radius
mnemonic: "The **F**urry **C**at **H**it **M**y **D**og"
- **T**hrombocytopenia–absent radius syndrome
- **F**anconi anemia
- **C**ornelia de Lange syndrome
- **H**olt-Oram syndrome
- **M**yositis ossificans progressiva (thumb only)
- **D**iastrophic dwarfism ("hitchhiker's thumb")

Pubic Bone Maldevelopment
mnemonic: "CHIEF"
- **C**leidocranial dysostosis
- **H**ypospadia, epispadia
- **I**diopathic
- **E**xstrophy of bladder
- **F** for syringomyelia

BONE OVERGROWTH
Bone Overdevelopment
1. Marfan syndrome
2. Klippel-Trenaunay syndrome

3. Nerve territory-oriented macrodactyly
   (a) Macrodystrophia lipomatosa
   (b) Fibrolipomatous hamartoma with macrodactyly

Erlenmeyer Flask Deformity

= expansion of distal end of long bones, usually femur

1. Gaucher disease, Niemann-Pick disease
2. Anemia: thalassemia, sickle cell
3. Osteopetrosis
4. Heavy metal poisoning
5. Metaphyseal dysplasia = Pyle disease
6. Rickets
7. Fibrous dysplasia
8. Down syndrome
9. Achondroplasia
10. Rheumatoid arthritis
11. Hypophosphatasia

mnemonic: "TOP DOG"
Thalassemia
Osteopetrosis
Pyle disease
Diaphyseal aclasis
Ollier disease
Gaucher disease

PERIOSTEAL REACTION

1. Trauma, hemophilia
2. Infection
3. Inflammatory: arthritis
4. Neoplasm
5. Congenital: physiologic in newborn
6. Metabolic: hypertrophic osteoarthropathy, thyroid acropachy, hypervitaminosis A
7. Vascular: venous stasis

Solid Periosteal Reaction

= reaction to periosteal irritant
√ even + uniform thickness >1 mm
√ persistent + unchanged for weeks
Patterns:
(a) thin: eosinophilic granuloma, osteoid osteoma
(b) dense undulating: vascular disease
(c) thin undulating: pulmonary osteoarthropathy
(d) dense elliptical: osteoid osteoma; long-standing malignant disease (with destruction)
(e) cloaking: storage disease; chronic infection

Interrupted Periosteal Reaction

= pleomorphic, rapidly progressing process undergoing constant change
(a) buttressing = periosteal bone formation merges with underlying cortex: eosinophilic granuloma
(b) laminated = "onion skin": acute osteomyelitis; malignant tumor (osteosarcoma, Ewing sarcoma)
(c) radiating spicules = "sunburst": osteosarcoma; Ewing sarcoma; chondrosarcoma; fibrosarcoma; leukemia; metastasis; acute osteomyelitis
(d) perpendicular spicules = "hair-on-end": Ewing sarcoma
(e) amorphous: malignancy (deposits may represent extension of tumor / periosteal response); osteosarcoma
(f) Codman triangle: hemorrhage; malignancy (osteosarcoma, Ewing sarcoma); acute osteomyelitis; fracture

Symmetric Periosteal Reaction in Adulthood

1. Venous stasis (lower extremity)
2. Hypertrophic osteoarthropathy
3. Pachydermoperiostosis
4. Thyroid acropachy
5. Fluorosis
6. Rheumatoid arthritis
7. Psoriatic arthritis
8. Reiter syndrome
9. Idiopathic-degenerative

Periosteal Reaction in Childhood

(a) benign
1. Physiologic (up to 35%): symmetric involvement of diaphyses during first 1–6 months of life
2. Nonaccidental trauma = battered child syndrome
3. Infantile cortical hyperostosis: <6 months of age
4. Hypervitaminosis A
5. Scurvy
6. Osteogenesis imperfecta
7. Congenital syphilis

(b) malignant
1. Multicentric osteosarcoma
2. Metastases from neuroblastoma + retinoblastoma
3. Acute leukemia

mnemonic: "PERIOSTEAL SOCKS"
Physiologic, **P**rostaglandin
Eosinophilic granuloma
Rickets
Infantile cortical hyperostosis
Osteomyelitis
Scurvy
Trauma
Ewing sarcoma
A-hypervitaminosis
Leukemia + neuroblastoma
Syphilis
Osteosarcoma
Child abuse
Kinky hair syndrome
Sickle cell disease

Periosteal Reaction in Infant

– before 6 months of age
1. Infantile cortical hyperostosis
2. Physiologic
3. Extracorporeal membrane oxygenation

- after 6 months of age
  1. Hypervitaminosis A
  2. Scurvy
  3. Rickets
- anytime during infancy
  1. Nonaccidental trauma
  2. Syphilis
  3. Metastatic neuroblastoma / leukemia
  4. Prostaglandin therapy: within 40 days
  5. Sickle cell dactylitis

DDx: motion artifact

Enthesopathy

Enthesis = osseous attachment of tendon composed of 4 zones, ie, tendon itself + unmineralized fibrocartilage + mineralized fibrocartilage + bone

Cause:

1. Degenerative disorder
2. Seronegative arthropathies: ankylosing spondylitis, Reiter disease, psoriatic arthritis
3. Diffuse idiopathic skeletal hyperostosis
4. Acromegaly
5. Rheumatoid arthritis (occasionally)

Location: at site of tendon + ligament attachment

√ bone proliferation (enthesophyte)
√ calcification of tendon + ligament
√ erosion

BONE TRAUMA

Childhood Fractures

1. Greenstick fracture
2. Bowing fracture
3. Traumatic epiphyseolysis
4. Battered child syndrome
5. Epiphyseal plate injury

Pseudarthrosis in Long Bones

1. Nonunion of fracture
2. Fibrous dysplasia
3. Neurofibromatosis
4. Osteogenesis imperfecta
5. Congenital: clavicular pseudarthrosis

Exuberant Callus Formation

1. Steroid therapy / Cushing syndrome
2. Neuropathic arthropathy
3. Osteogenesis imperfecta
4. Congenital insensitivity to pain
5. Paralysis
6. Renal osteodystrophy
7. Multiple myeloma
8. Battered child syndrome

EPIPHYSIS

Premature Epiphyseal Ossification

@ Proximal femoral and humeral epiphyses

1. Jeune asphyxiating thoracic dysplasia
2. Ellis-van Creveld chondroectodermal dysplasia

Epiphyseal / Apophyseal Lesion

1. Chondroblastoma
2. Brodie abscess
3. Fungal / tuberculous infection
4. Langerhans cell histiocytosis
5. Osteoid osteoma
6. Chondromyxoid fibroma
7. Enchondroma
8. Bone cyst
9. Foreign-body granuloma

Subarticular Lesion

1. Giant cell tumor
2. Solitary subchondral cyst
3. Itraosseous ganglion
4. Brodie abscess
5. Clear cell chondrosarcoma

Stippled Epiphyses

1. Normal variant
2. Avascular necrosis
3. Hypothyroidism
4. Chondrodysplasia punctata
5. Multiple epiphyseal dysplasia
6. Spondyloepiphyseal dysplasia
7. Hypoparathyroidism
8. Down syndrome
9. Trisomy 18
10. Fetal warfarin syndrome
11. Homocystinuria (distal radial + ulnar epiphyses = pathognomonic)
12. Zellweger cerebrohepatorenal syndrome

Physeal / Metaphyseal Widening & Irregularity

1. Rickets
2. Hypophosphatasia
3. Metaphyseal chondroplasia

Epiphyseal Overgrowth

1. Juvenile rheumatoid arthritis
2. Hemophilia
3. Healed Legg-Perthes disease
4. Tuberculous arthritis
5. Pyogenic arthritis (chronic)
6. Fungal arthritis
7. Epiphyseal dysplasia hemimelica
8. Fibrous dysplasia of epiphysis
9. Winchester syndrome

Epiphyseolysis

= SLIPPED EPIPHYSIS (zone of maturing hypertrophic cartilage affected, not zone of proliferation)

1. Idiopathic / juvenile epiphyseolysis
   Age: 12–15 years (? puberty-related hormonal dysregulation)
   - adiposogenital type; tall stature
2. Renal osteodystrophy
3. Hyperparathyroidism in chronic renal disease
4. Hypothyroidism
5. Radiotherapy

JOINTS

Approach to Arthritis

mnemonic: "ABCDE'S"

Alignment
Bone mineralization
Cartilage loss
Distribution
Erosion
Soft tissues

Signs of Arthritis

Prevalence of arthritis: 15% of population in USA

Conventional x-ray:

- √ narrowing of radiologic joint space
  - (a) uniform = inflammatory arthritis
  - (b) nonuniform = degenerative arthritis
- √ evidence of disease on both sides of joint:
  - √ osteopenia
  - √ subchondral sclerosis
  - √ erosion
  - √ subchondral cyst formation
  - √ malalignment
- √ joint effusion
- √ joint bodies

NUC:

- √ increase in regional blood flow (active disease)
- √ distribution of disease

MR:

- √ irregularity + narrowing of articular cartilage
- √ Gd-DTPA enhancement of synovium (active disease)

Classification of Arthritides

A. SEPTIC ARTHRITIS
   1. Tuberculous
   2. Pyogenic
   3. Lyme arthritis
   4. Fungal arthritis: Candida, Coccidioides immitis, Blastomyces dermatitidis, Histoplasma capsulatum, Sporothrix schenckii, Cryptococcus neoformans, Aspergillus fumigatus

   N.B.: Tuberculous + fungal arthritis shows prominent osteoporosis + slower rate of destruction + less joint narrowing than a pyogenic infection (Phemister triad)

B. COLLAGEN / COLLAGEN-LIKE DISEASE
   1. Rheumatoid arthritis
   2. Ankylosing spondylitis
   3. Psoriatic arthritis
   4. Rheumatic fever
   5. Sarcoidosis

C. BIOCHEMICAL ARTHRITIS
   1. Gout
   2. Chondrocalcinosis
   3. Ochronosis
   4. Hemophilic arthritis

D. DEGENERATIVE JOINT DISEASE = Osteoarthritis

E. TRAUMATIC
   1. Secondary osteoarthritis
   2. Neurotrophic arthritis
   3. Pigmented villonodular synovitis

F. ENTEROPATHIC ARTHROPATHY
   (a) INFLAMMATORY BOWEL DISEASE
      1. Ulcerative colitis (in 10–20%)
      2. Crohn disease (in 5%): peripheral arthritis increases with colonic disease
      3. Whipple disease (in 60–90% transient intermittent polyarthritis: sacroiliitis, spondylitis)

      ◊ Resection of diseased bowel is associated with regression of arthritic symptomatology!

   (b) INFECTIOUS BOWEL DISEASE
      Infectious agents: Salmonella, Shigella, Yersinia

   (c) after intestinal bypass surgery

SPONDYLARTHRITIS + positive HLA-B 27 HISTOCOMPATIBILITY COMPLEX

1. Ankylosing spondylitis 95%
2. Reiter disease 80%
3. Arthropathy of inflammatory bowel disease 75%
4. Psoriatic spondylitis 70%
5. Normal population 10%

Monoarthritis

Destructive Monoarthritis

◊ Any destructive monoarthritis should be regarded as infection until proved otherwise!

A. Septic arthritis

B. Monoarticular presentation of a systemic arthritis
   1. Rheumatoid arthritis
   2. Gout
   3. Amyloidosis
   4. Seronegative arthritis

C. Joint tumor
   1. PVNS
   2. Synovial chondromatosis
   3. Articular hemangioma

Nonseptic Monoarthritis

1. Gout
2. Milwaukee shoulder
3. Rapidly destructive articular disease
4. Amyloid arthropathy
5. Hemophilic arthropathy
6. Primary synovial osteochondromatosis
7. Pigmented villonodular synovitis
8. Neuropathic arthropathy
9. Foreign-body synovitis

Arthritis without Demineralization

1. Gout
2. Neuropathic arthropathy
3. Psoriasis
4. Reiter disease
5. Pigmented villonodular synovitis

mnemonic: "PONGS"

Psoriatic arthritis
Osteoarthritis
Neuropathic joint
Gout
Sarcoidosis

Arthritis with Demineralization

mnemonic: "HORSE"

Hemophilia
Osteomyelitis
Rheumatoid arthritis, **R**eiter disease
Scleroderma
Erythematosus, systemic lupus

Deforming Nonerosive Arthropathy

1. Collagen-vascular disease, especially SLE
2. Rheumatoid arthritis (rare)
3. Rheumatic fever (Jaccoud arthritis) (rare)

Arthritis with Periostitis

1. Juvenile rheumatoid arthritis
2. Psoriatic arthritis
3. Reiter syndrome
4. Infectious arthritis

Premature Osteoarthritis

mnemonic: "COME CHAT"

Calcium pyrophosphate dihydrate arthropathy
Ochronosis
Marfan syndrome
Epiphyseal dysplasia
Charcot joint = neuroarthropathy
Hemophilic arthropathy
Acromegaly
Trauma

Synovial Disease with Decreased Signal Intensity

= hemosiderin deposition

1. Pigmented villonodular synovitis
2. Rheumatoid arthritis
3. Hemophilia

Chondrocalcinosis

mnemonic: "WHIP A DOG"

Wilson disease
Hemochromatosis, **H**emophilia, **H**ypothyroidism, 1° **H**yperparathyroidism (15%), **H**ypophosphatasia, Familial **H**ypomagnesemia
Idiopathic (aging)
Pseudogout (CPPD)
Arthritis (rheumatoid, postinfectious, traumatic, degenerative), **A**myloidosis, **A**cromegaly
Diabetes mellitus
Ochronosis
Gout

mnemonic: "3 C's"

Crystals	CPPD, sodium urate (gout)
Cations	calcium (any cause of hypercalcemia), copper, iron
Cartilage degeneration	osteoarthritis, acromegaly, ochronosis

Subchondral Cyst

= SYNOVIAL CYST = SUBARTICULAR PSEUDOCYST
= NECROTIC PSEUDOCYST = GEODES

Etiology: bone necrosis allows pressure-induced intrusion of synovial fluid into subchondral bone; in conditions with synovial inflammation

Cause:
1. Osteoarthritis
2. Rheumatoid arthritis
3. Osteonecrosis
4. CPPD

√ size of cyst usually 2–35 mm
√ may be large + expansile (especially in CPPD)

DDx:
(1) Giant cell tumor
(2) Pigmented villonodular synovitis
(3) Metastasis
(4) Intraosseous ganglion
(5) Hemophilia

Loose Intraarticular Bodies

1. Osteochondrosis dissecans
2. Synovial osteochondromatosis
3. Chip fracture from trauma
4. Severe degenerative joint disease
5. Neuropathic arthropathy

Intraarticular Process with Cortical Erosion

1. Pigmented villonodular synovitis
2. Synovial osteochondromatosis
3. Rheumatoid arthritis
4. Gout
5. Synovial hemangioma
6. Lipoma arborescens

Erosions of DIP Joints

1. Inflammatory osteoarthritis
2. Psoriatic arthritis
3. Gout
4. Multicentric reticulohistiocytosis
5. Hyperparathyroidism
6. Frostbite
7. Septic arthritis

Articular Disorders of Hand and Wrist

1. Osteoarthritis = degenerative joint disease
   = abnormal stress with minor + major traumatic episodes
   Target areas: DIP, PIP, 1st CMC, trapezioscaphoid; bilateral symmetric / asymmetric
   √ joint space narrowing
   √ subchondral eburnation
   √ marginal osteophytes + small ossicles
   √ radial subluxation of 1st metacarpal base
   ◊ Radiocarpal joint normal unless history of trauma
2. Erosive osteoarthritis = inflammatory osteoarthritis
   Age: predominantly middle-aged / postmenopausal women
   • acute inflammatory episodes
   Target areas: DIP, PIP, 1st CMC, trapezioscaphoid; bilateral symmetric / asymmetric

√ central erosions combined with osteophytes
= subchondral "gull wing" erosions
√ joint space narrowing + sclerosis
√ rare ankylosis

3. Psoriatic arthritis
= rheumatoid variant / seronegative spondyloarthropathy; peripheral manifestation in monarthritis / asymmetric oligoarthritis / symmetric polyarthritis

Target areas: all hand + wrist joints (commonly distal); bi- / unilateral asymmetric polyarticular changes
√ "mouse ears" marginal erosions
√ intraarticular osseous excrescences
√ new bone formation ± fusion
√ osteoporosis may be absent

4. Rheumatoid arthritis
= synovial proliferative granulation tissue = pannus

Target areas: PIP (early in 3rd), MCP (earliest changes in 2nd + 3rd), all wrist joints (early in RC, IRU), ulnar styloid; both hands in relative symmetric fashion
√ fusiform soft-tissue swelling
√ regional periarticular osteoporosis
√ diffuse loss of joint space
√ marginal + central poorly defined erosions
√ joint deformities

5. Gouty arthritis
• monosodium urate crystals in synovial fluid
• asymptomatic periods from months to years

Target areas: commonly CCMC + all hand joints
√ development of chronic tophaceous gout
= lobulated soft-tissue masses
√ well-defined eccentric erosions with overhanging edge (often periarticular) + sclerotic margins
√ preservation of joint spaces
√ absence of osteoporosis
√ most extensive changes in common carpometacarpal compartment:
√ scalloped erosions of bases of ulnar metacarpals

6. Calcium pyrophosphate dihydrate crystal deposition disease = CPPD

Target areas: MCP (2nd, 3rd), radiocarpal; bilateral symmetric / asymmetric changes
√ chondrocalcinosis + periarticular calcifications:
√ calcification of triangular fibrocartilage
√ "degenerative changes" in unusual locations:
√ narrowing ± obliteration of space between distal radius and scaphoid ± fragmentation of surfaces
√ scapholunate separation
√ destruction of trapezioscaphoid space
√ no erosions
√ + large osteophytes = hemochromatosis

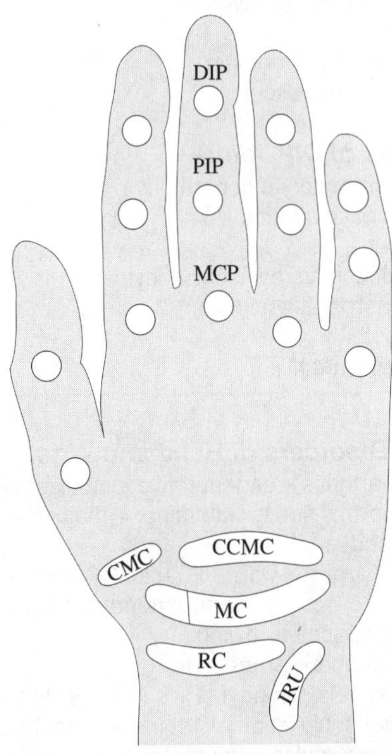

Articulations of Hand and Wrist

CCMC = common carpometacarpal
CMC = first carpometcarpal
DIP = distal interphalangeal
IRU = inferior radioulnar
MC = midcarpal (trapezioscaphoid region separated by vertical line)
MCP = metacarpophalangeal
PIP = proximal interphalangeal
RC = radiocarpal

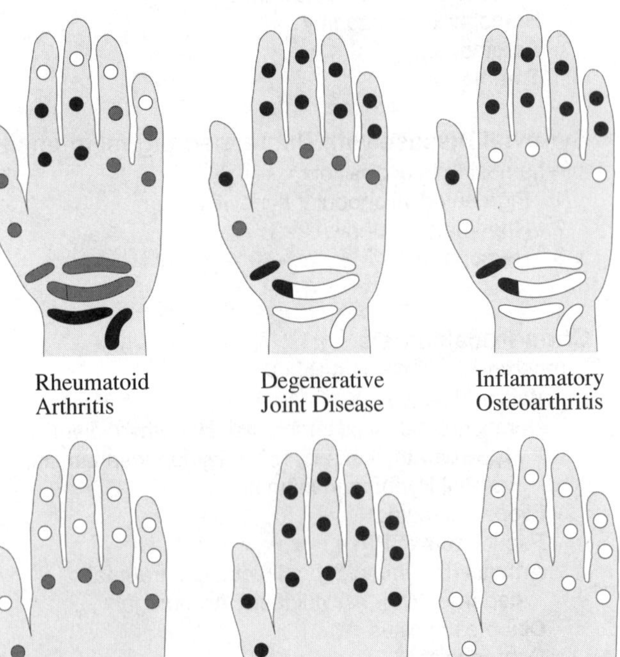

Distribution Pattern of Arthritic Lesions
(adapted from Donald Resnick, M.D.)

7. SLE
   = myositis, symmetric polyarthritis, deforming nonerosive arthropathy, osteonecrosis
   Target areas: PIP, MCP
   √ reversible deformities
8. Scleroderma = progressive systemic sclerosis (PSS)
   Target areas: DIP, PIP, 1st CMC
   √ tuft resorption
   √ soft-tissue calcifications

Arthritis Involving Distal Interphalangeal Joints

mnemonic: "POEM"

Psoriatic arthritis
Osteoarthritis
Erosive osteoarthritis
Multicentric reticulohistiocytosis

Ankylosis of Interphalangeal Joints

mnemonic: "S - Lesions"

1. P**s**oriatic arthritis
2. Ankylo**s**ing spondylitis
3. Ero**s**ive osteoarthritis
4. **S**till disease

Sacroiliitis

Joint anatomy:

- ligamentous portion (superior 2/3 to 1/2 of joint): formed by interosseous sacroiliac ligament
- synovial component (inferior 1/3 to 1/2 of joint): the sacral surface is lined by 3–5 mm-thick hyaline cartilage; the iliac surface of joint is lined by 1-mm-thick fibrocartilage
- 2–5 mm normal joint width

Positioning: oblique view + modified Ferguson view = AP projection with 23° cephalad angulation

√ findings predominate on the iliac side (thinner cartilage)

A. BILATERAL SYMMETRIC
   1. Ankylosing spondylitis
      √ small regular erosion = loss of definition of white cortical line on iliac side (initially)
      √ subchondral sclerosis + subsequent ankylosis
      √ ossification of interosseous ligaments
   2. Enteropathic arthropathy
      √ same signs as in ankylosing spondylitis
   3. Rheumatoid arthritis (in late stages)
      √ joint space narrowing without reparation
      √ osteoporosis
      √ ankylosis may occur
   4. Deposition arthropathy: gout, CPPD, ochronosis, acromegaly
      √ slow loss of cartilage
      √ subchondral reparative bone + osteophytes
   5. Osteitis condensans ilii
   DDx: Hyperparathyroidism (subchondral bone resorption on iliac side resembling erosion + widening of joint)

B. BILATERAL ASYMMETRIC
   1. Psoriatic arthritis
      √ large extensive erosion
      √ subchondral sclerosis + occasional ankylosis
   2. Reiter syndrome
   3. Juvenile rheumatoid arthritis

C. UNILATERAL
   1. Infection
   2. Osteoarthritis from abnormal mechanical stress
      √ no erosions
      √ irregular narrowing of joint space with subchondral sclerosis
      √ osteophytes at anterosuperior / -inferior aspect of joint (may resemble ankylosis)
   DDx: psoriatic arthritis, Reiter syndrome, trauma, gout, pigmented villonodular synovitis, osteitis condensans ilii

Sacroiliac Joint Widening

mnemonic: "CRAP TRAP"

Colitis
Rheumatoid arthritis
Abscess (infection)
Parathyroid disease
Trauma
Reiter syndrome
Ankylosing spondylitis
Psoriasis

Sacroiliac Joint Fusion

mnemonic: "CARPI"

Colitic spondylitis
Ankylosing spondylitis
Reiter syndrome
Psoriatic arthritis
Infection (TB)

Differential Diagnosis of Sacroiliac Joint Disease

	Osteoarthritis	*Ankylosing spondylitis*	*Osteitis condensans ilii*
Age	older	younger	younger
Sex	M, F	M > F	F > M
Distribution	bi- / unilateral symmetric	bilateral symmetric	bilateral
Sclerosis	iliac mild, focal	iliac ± extensive	iliac triangular
Erosions	absent	common	absent
Intraarticular ankylosis	rare	common	absent
Ligamentous ossification	less common	common	absent

Widened Symphysis Pubis

mnemonic: "EPOCH"

Exstrophy of the bladder
Prune belly syndrome
Osteogenesis imperfecta
Cleidocranial dysostosis
Hypothyroidism

Arthritis of Interphalangeal Joint of Great Toe

1. Psoriatic arthritis
2. Reiter disease
3. Gout
4. Degenerative joint disease

RIBS

Thoracic Deformity

Funnel Chest = Pectus Excavatum

= posterior depression of sternum compressing heart against spine

◊ Most frequently an isolated anomaly!

May be associated with:
prematurity, homocystinuria, Marfan syndrome, Noonan syndrome, fetal alcohol syndrome

√ depressed position of sternum (LATERAL)
√ indistinct right heart border mimicking right middle lobe process (FRONTAL)
√ decreased heart density (FRONTAL)
√ leftward displacement of heart mimicking cardiomegaly (FRONTAL)
√ horizontal course of posterior portion of ribs
√ accentuated downward course of anterior portions of ribs (FRONTAL)

Barrel Chest

= large sagittal diameter of thorax

Cause: COPD, emphysema

√ lateral segments of ribs elongated + straight pointing vertical (FRONTAL)
√ square shape on cross section (CT)

Congenital Rib Anomalies

Prevalence: 1.4%

1. Cervical rib (0.2–1–8%): M<F
   • usually asymptomatic
   • thoracic outlet syndrome (due to elevation of floor of scalene triangle with decrease of costoclavicular space):
     ◊ 10–20% of symptomatic patients have a responsible cervical rib
     ◊ 5–10% of complete cervical ribs cause symptoms

   May be associated with: Klippel-Feil anomaly
   √ uni- / bilateral
   √ may fuse with first ribs anteriorly
   √ adjacent transverse process angulated inferiorly
   Cx: aneurysmal dilatation of subclavian a.
   DDx: elongated transverse process of 7th cervical vertebra; hypoplastic 1st thoracic rib
2. Forked / bifid rib (0.6%) = duplication of anterior portion
   Location: 4th rib (most often)
   May be associated with: Gorlin basal cell nevus syndrome
   ◊ A single bifid rib is most commonly a normal incidental finding!
3. Rib fusion (0.3%)
   May be associated with: vertebral segmentation anomalies
   Location: 1st + 2nd rib / several adjacent ribs
   Site: posterior / anterior portion
4. Bone bridging = focal joining by bone outgrowth
   Cause: congenital / posttraumatic
   Location: anywhere along one pair of ribs / several adjacent ribs
   √ complete bridging / pseudarthrosis
5. Rudimentary / hypoplastic rib (0.2%)
   Location: 1st rib (usually)
   √ transverse process angulated superiorly
   DDx: cervical rib
6. Pseudarthrosis of 1st rib (0.1%)
   √ radiolucent line through midportion with dense sclerotic borders
7. Intrathoracic / pelvic rib (rare)
8. Abnormal number of ribs
   (a) supernumerary: trisomy 21, VATER syndrome
   (b) 11 pairs: normal individuals (5–8%); trisomy 21 (33%); cleidocranial dysplasia; campomelic dysplasia

Short Ribs

1. Thanatophoric dysplasia
2. Jeune asphyxiating thoracic dysplasia
3. Ellis-van Creveld chondroectodermal dysplasia
4. Short rib-polydactyly syndromes (Saldino-Noonan, Majewski, Verma-Naumoff)
5. Achondroplasia
6. Achondrogenesis
7. Mesomelic dwarfism
8. Spondyloepiphyseal dysplasia
9. Enchondromatosis

Rib Lesions

A. BENIGN RIB TUMOR
   1. Fibrous dysplasia (most common benign lesion)
      √ predominantly posterior location
   2. Osteochondroma / exostosis: at costochondral / costovertebral junction
      Associated with: spontaneous hemothorax
   3. Langerhans cell histiocytosis (eosinophilic granuloma)
   4. Benign cortical defect
   6. Hemangioma of bone
   7. Enchondroma: at costochondral / costovertebral junction
   8. Giant cell tumor
   9. Aneurysmal bone cyst
   10. Osteoblastoma
   11. Osteoid osteoma

12. Chondroblastoma
13. Enostosis = bone island (0.4%)
14. Paget disease
15. Brown tumor of HPT
16. Xanthogranuloma

B. PRIMARY MALIGNANT RIB TUMOR
1. Chondrosarcoma (calcified matrix): most common
2. Plasmacytoma
3. Lymphoma
4. Osteosarcoma (rare)
5. Fibrosarcoma
6. Primitive neuroectodermal tumor (= Askin tumor)

C. SECONDARY MALIGNANT RIB TUMOR
— in adult: 1. Metastasis (most common malignant lesion)
2. Multiple myeloma
3. Desmoid tumor
— in child: 1. Ewing sarcoma (most common malignant tumor affecting ribs of children + adolescents)
2. Metastatic neuroblastoma

D. TRAUMATIC RIB DISORDER
1. Healing fracture
2. Radiation osteitis
DDx: pulmonary nodule

E. AGGRESSIVE GRANULOMATOUS INFECTIONS = osteomyelitis

Expansile Rib Lesion

mnemonic: "O FEEL THE CLAMP"
Osteochondroma (25% of all benign rib tumors)
Fibrous dysplasia
Eosinophilic granuloma
Enchondroma (7% of all benign rib tumors)
Lymphoma / **L**eukemia
Tuberculosis
Hematopoiesis
Ewing sarcoma
Chondromyxoid fibroma
Lymphangiomatosis
Aneurysmal bone cyst
Metastases
Plasmacytoma

Abnormal Rib Shape

Rib Notching on Inferior Margin

= minimal concave scalloping / deep ridges along the neurovascular groove with reactive sclerosis
◊ Minor undulations in the inferior ribs are normal!
◊ The medial third of posterior ribs near transverse process of vertebrae may be notched normally!

A. ARTERIAL
Cause: intercostal aa. function as collaterals to descending aorta / lung
(a) Aorta: coarctation (usually affects ribs 4–8; rare before age 8 years), thrombosis
(b) Subclavian artery: Blalock-Taussig shunt
(c) Pulmonary artery: pulmonary stenosis, tetralogy of Fallot, absent pulmonary artery

B. VENOUS
Cause: enlargement of intercostal veins
(a) AV malformation of chest wall
(b) Superior vena cava obstruction

C. NEUROGENIC
1. Intercostal neuroma
2. Neurofibromatosis type 1
3. Poliomyelitis / quadriplegia / paraplegia

D. OSSEOUS
1. Hyperparathyroidism
2. Thalassemia
3. Melnick-Needles syndrome

UNILATERAL RIB NOTCHING ON INFERIOR MARGIN
1. Postoperative Blalock-Taussig shunt (subclavian to pulmonary artery)
2. Coarctation between origin of innominate a. + L subclavian a.
3. Coarctation proximal to aberrant subclavian a.

Rib Notching on Superior Margin
1. Rheumatoid arthritis
2. Scleroderma
3. Systemic lupus erythematosus
4. Hyperparathyroidism
5. Restrictive lung disease
6. Marfan syndrome

Dysplastic Twisted Ribbon Ribs
1. Osteogenesis imperfecta
2. Neurofibromatosis

Bulbous Enlargement of Costochondral Junction
1. Rachitic rosary
2. Scurvy
3. Achondroplasia
4. Hypophosphatasia
5. Metaphyseal chondrodysplasia
6. Acromegaly

Wide Ribs
1. Marrow hyperplasia (anemias)
2. Fibrous dysplasia
3. Paget disease
4. Achondroplasia
5. Mucopolysaccharidoses

Slender Ribs
1. Trisomy 18 syndrome
2. Neurofibromatosis

Dense Ribs
1. Tuberous sclerosis
2. Osteopetrosis
3. Mastocytosis
4. Fluorosis

5. Fibrous dysplasia
6. Chronic infection
7. Trauma
8. Subperiosteal rib resection

Hyperlucent Ribs

Congenitally Lucent Ribs

1. Osteogenesis imperfecta
2. Achondrogenesis
3. Hypophosphatasia
4. Campomelic dysplasia

Acquired Lucent Ribs

1. Cushing disease
2. Acromegaly
3. Scurvy

CLAVICLE

Absence of Outer End of Clavicle

1. Rheumatoid arthritis
2. Hyperparathyroidism
3. Posttraumatic osteolysis
4. Metastasis / multiple myeloma
5. Cleidocranial dysplasia
6. Gorlin basal cell nevus syndrome

Penciled Distal End of Clavicle

mnemonic: "SHIRT Pocket"

Scleroderma
Hyperparathyroidism
Infection
Rheumatoid arthritis
Trauma
Progeria

Destruction of Medial End of Clavicle

mnemonic: "MILERS"

Metastases
Infection
Lymphoma
Eosinophilic granuloma
Rheumatoid arthritis
Sarcoma

WRIST & HAND

Carpal Angle

= angle of 130° formed by tangents to proximal row of carpal bones

A. DECREASED CARPAL ANGLE (<124°)
   1. Turner syndrome
   2. Hurler syndrome
   3. Morquio syndrome
   4. Madelung deformity
B. INCREASED CARPAL ANGLE (>139°)
   1. Down syndrome
   2. Arthrogryposis
   3. Bone dysplasia with epiphyseal involvement

Metacarpal Sign

= relative shortening of 4th + 5th metacarpals
√ tangential line along heads of 5th + 4th metacarpals intersects 3rd metacarpal

1. Idiopathic
2. Pseudo- and pseudopseudohypoparathyroidism
3. Basal cell nevus syndrome
4. Multiple epiphyseal dysplasia
5. Beckwith-Wiedemann syndrome
6. Sickle cell anemia
7. Juvenile chronic arthritis
8. Gonadal dysgenesis: Turner syndrome, Klinefelter syndrome
9. Ectodermal dysplasia = Cornelia de Lange syndrome
10. Hereditary multiple exostoses
11. Peripheral dysostosis
12. Melorheostosis

mnemonic: "**P**ing **P**ong **I**s **T**ough **T**o **T**each"

Pseudohypoparathyroidism
Pseudopseudohypoparathyroidism
Idiopathic
Trauma
Turner syndrome
Trisomy 13–18

Lucent Lesion in Finger

A. BENIGN TUMOR
   1. Enchondroma
   2. Epidermoid inclusion cyst
   3. Giant cell tumor
   4. Reparative granuloma
   5. Sarcoidosis
   6 Glomus tumor (rare)

   others: aneurysmal bone cyst, brown tumor , hemophilic pseudotumor, solitary bone cyst, osteoblastoma
B. MALIGNANT TUMOR
   1. Osteosarcoma
   2. Fibrosarcoma
   3. Metastasis from lung, breast, malignant melanoma

mnemonic: "GAMES PAGES"

Glomus tumor
Arthritis (gout, rheumatoid)
Metastasis (lung, breast)
Enchondroma
Simple cyst (inclusion)
Pancreatitis
Aneurysmal bone cyst
Giant cell tumor
Epidermoid
Sarcoid

Dactylitis

= expansion of bone with cystic changes

1. Tuberculous dactylitis (= spina ventosa)
2. Pyogenic / fungal infection
3. Syphilitic dactylitis

4. Sarcoidosis
5. Hemoglobinopathies
6. Hyperparathyroidism
7. Leukemia

Resorption of Terminal Tufts

A. TRAUMA
   1. Amputation
   2. Burns, electric injury
   3. Frostbite
   4. Vinyl chloride poisoning

B. NEUROPATHIC
   1. Congenital indifference to pain
   2. Syringomyelia
   3. Myelomeningocele
   4. Diabetes mellitus
   5. Leprosy

C. COLLAGEN-VASCULAR DISEASE
   1. Scleroderma
   2. Dermatomyositis
   3. Raynaud disease

D. METABOLIC
   1. Hyperparathyroidism

E. INHERITED
   1. Familial acroosteolysis
   2. Pyknodysostosis
   3. Progeria = Werner syndrome
   4. Pachydermoperiostosis

F. OTHERS
   1. Sarcoidosis
   2. Psoriatic arthropathy
   3. Epidermolysis bullosa

Acroosteolysis

1. Acroosteolysis: (a) acquired, (b) familial
2. Massive osteolysis
3. Essential osteolysis
4. Ainhum disease

Acquired Acroosteolysis

mnemonic: "PETER's DIAPER SPLASH"

Psoriasis, **P**orphyria
Ehlers-Danlos syndrome
Thrombangitis obliterans
Ergot therapy
Raynaud disease
Diabetes, **D**ermatomyositis, **D**ilantin therapy
Injury (thermal + electrical burns, frostbite)
Arteriosclerosis obliterans
PVC (polyvinylchloride) worker
Epidermolysis bullosa
Rheumatoid arthritis, **R**eiter syndrome
Scleroderma, **S**arcoidosis
Progeria, **P**yknodysostosis
Leprosy, **L**esch-Nyhan syndrome
Absence of pain
Syringomyelia
Hyperparathyroidism

<u>also in</u>: yaws; Kaposi sarcoma; pachydermoperiostosis

√ lytic destructive process involving distal + middle phalanges
√ NO periosteal reaction
√ epiphyses resist osteolysis until late

Acroosteosclerosis

= focal opaque areas + endosteal thickening

1. Incidental in middle-aged women
2. Rheumatoid arthritis
3. Sarcoidosis
4. Scleroderma
5. Systemic lupus erythematosus
6. Hodgkin disease
7. Hematologic disorders

Fingertip Calcifications

1. Scleroderma / CREST syndrome
2. Raynaud disease
3. Systemic lupus erythematosus
4. Dermatomyositis
5. Calcinosis circumscripta universalis
6. Hyperparathyroidism

Brachydactyly

= shortening / broadening of metacarpals ± phalanges

1. Idiopathic
2. Trauma
3. Osteomyelitis
4. Arthritis
5. Turner syndrome
6. Osteochondrodysplasia
7. Pseudohypoparathyroidism, Pseudopseudohypoparathyroidism
8. Mucopolysaccharidoses
9. Cornelia de Lange syndrome
10. Basal cell nevus syndrome
11. Hereditary multiple exostoses

Clinodactyly

= curvature of finger in mediolateral plane

1. Normal variant
2. Down syndrome
3. Multiple dysplasia
4. Trauma, arthritis, contractures

Polydactyly

Frequently associated with:

1. Carpenter syndrome
2. Ellis-van Creveld syndrome
3. Meckel-Gruber syndrome
4. Polysyndactyly syndrome
5. Short rib-polydactyly syndrome
6. Trisomy 13

Syndactyly

= osseous ± cutaneous fusion of digits

1. Apert syndrome
2. Carpenter syndrome
3. Down syndrome

4. Neurofibromatosis
5. Poland syndrome
6. Others

HIP

Snapping Hip Syndrome

A. INTRAARTICULAR
 1. Osteocartilaginous bodies

B. EXTRAARTICULAR = tendon slippage
 1. fascia lata / gluteus maximus over greater trochanter
 2. iliopsoas tendon over iliopectineal eminence
 3. long head of biceps femoris over ischial tuberosity
 4. iliofemoral ligament over anterior portion of hip capsule

Increase in Teardrop Width

√ increase in distance between teardrop + femoral head
 Cause: hip joint effusion
√ increase in mediolateral size of teardrop
 Cause: hip dysplasia, chronic hip joint effusion during skeletal maturation

Protrusio Acetabuli

= acetabular floor bulging into pelvis
√ acetabular line projecting medially to ilioischial line by >3 mm (in males) / >6 mm (in females)
√ crossing of medial + lateral components of pelvic "teardrop" (U-shaped radiodense area medial to hip joint with (a) lateral aspect = acetabular articular surface (b) medial aspect = anteroinferior margin of quadrilateral surface of ilium)

A. UNILATERAL
 1. Tuberculous arthritis
 2. Trauma
 3. Fibrous dysplasia

B. BILATERAL
 1. Rheumatoid arthritis
 2. Paget disease
 3. Osteomalacia

mnemonic: "PROT"
 Paget disease
 Rheumatoid arthritis
 Osteomalacia (HPT)
 Trauma

Pain with Hip Prosthesis

Approximately 120,000 hip arthroplasties per year in USA

1. Heterotopic ossification
2. Trochanteric bursitis
3. Prosthetic fracture / periprosthetic fracture / cement fracture
4. Dislocation (due to capsular laxity / incorrect component placement)
5. Aseptic loosening
 Incidence: 50% of prostheses after 10 years
 Cause:
 (a) mechanical wear + tear
 (b) small-particle disease (= inflammatory-immune reaction to methylmethacrylate / metallic fragments activates phagocytes with secretion of cytokines + proteolytic enzymes leading to osteolysis)
 Rx: 30% require single-stage revision arthroplasty
6. Infection (= septic loosening)
 Incidence: 1–9%
 Organisms: Staphylococcus epidermidis (31%), Staphylococcus aureus (20%), Streptococcus viridans (11%), Escherichia coli (11%), Enterococcus faecalis (8%), group B streptococcus (5%)
 Time of onset: 33% within 3 months, 33% within 1 year, 33% >1 year after surgery
 Rx: excisional arthroplasty + protracted course of antimicrobial therapy + revision arthroplasty

Plain film:
 √ migration of prosthetic components compared to previous film:
  √ subsidence of prosthesis (up to 5 mm is normal for noncemented femoral component in first few months)
 √ cement / prosthesis fracture
 √ motion of components on stress views / fluoroscopy
 √ widening of prosthesis-cement interface
 √ lucency at cement-bone interface >2 mm
 √ progressive widening of cement-bone lucency after 12 postoperative months
 √ focal lytic area (due to particulate debris with foreign body granuloma / abscess)
 √ extensive periostitis (in infection, but rare)

NUC (83% sensitive, 88% specific):
 √ increased uptake of bone agent, gallium-67, indium-111–labeled leukocytes, complementary technetium-labeled sulfur colloid + combinations

Bone Scintigraphy:
 √ normal = strong evidence against a prosthetic abnormality (= high NPV)
 √ diffuse intense uptake around femoral component (= generalized osteolysis associated with aseptic loosening or infection)
 √ focal uptake at distal tip of femoral component in >1 year old prosthesis = aseptic loosening

Sequential bone-gallium scintigraphy:
 √ congruent spatial distribution of both tracers with gallium intensity less than bone tracer = no infection
 √ spatially incongruent / intensity of gallium exceeds that of bone agent = infection
 √ spatially congruent + similar intensity of both tracers = inconclusive

Combined labeled leukocyte–marrow scintigraphy:
Accuracy: >90%
Concept: Tc-99m sulfur colloid maps aberrantly located normal bone marrow as a point of reference for leukocyte tracer
√ spatially congruent distribution of both radiotracers = no infection
√ labeled leukocyte activity without corresponding sulfur colloid activity = infection

Arthrography:
√ irregularity of joint pseudocapsule
√ filling of nonbursal spaces / sinus tracts / abscess cavities

Aspiration of fluid under fluoroscopy (12–93% sensitive, 83–92% specific for infection):
√ injection of contrast material to confirm intraarticular location

Evaluation of Total Hip Arthroplasty

MEASUREMENTS

Reference line: transischial tuberosity line (R)

1. Leg length = vertical position of acetabular component
   = comparing level of greater / lesser tuberosity (T) with respect to line R
   High placement: shorter leg, less effective muscles crossing the hip joint
   Low placement: longer leg, muscles stretched to point of spasm with risk of dislocation
2. Vertical center of rotation
   = distance from center of femoral head (C) to line R
3. Horizontal center of rotation
   = distance from center of femoral head (C) to teardrop / other medial landmark
   Lateral position: iliopsoas tendon crosses medial to femoral head center of rotation increasing risk of dislocation
4. Lateral acetabular inclination = horizontal version
   = angle of cup in reference to line R (40° ± 10° desirable)
   Less angulation: stable hip, limited abduction
   Greater angulation: risk of hip dislocation
5. Varus / neutral / valgus stem position
   Varus position: tip of stem rests against lateral endosteum, increased risk for loosening
   Valgus position: tip of stem rests against medial endosteum, not a significant problem
6. Acetabular anteversion (15° ± 10° desirable)
   = lateral radiograph of groin
   Retroversion: risk of hip dislocation
7. Femoral neck anteversion
   works synergistically with acetabular anteversion, true angle assessed by CT

Radiographic findings

A. NORMAL
   √ irregular cement-bone interface
   = normal interdigitation of polymethylmethacrylate (PMMA) with adjacent bone remodeling providing a mechanical interlock
   ◊ PMMA is not a glue!
   √ thin lucent line along cement-bone interface
   = 0.1–1.5-mm thin connective tissue membrane (“demarcation”) along cement-bone interface accompanied by thin line of bone sclerosis
B. ABNORMAL
   √ wide lucent zone at cement-bone interface
   = ≥2-mm lucent line along bone-cement interface due to granulomatous membrane
   Cause: component loosening ± reaction to particulate debris (eg, PMMA, polyethylene)

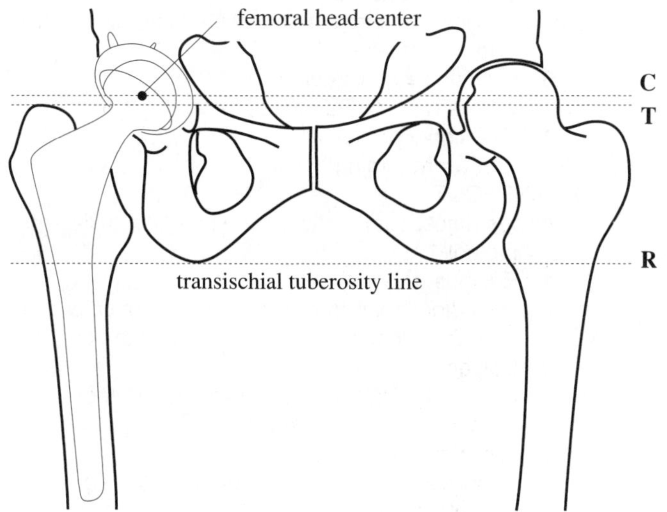

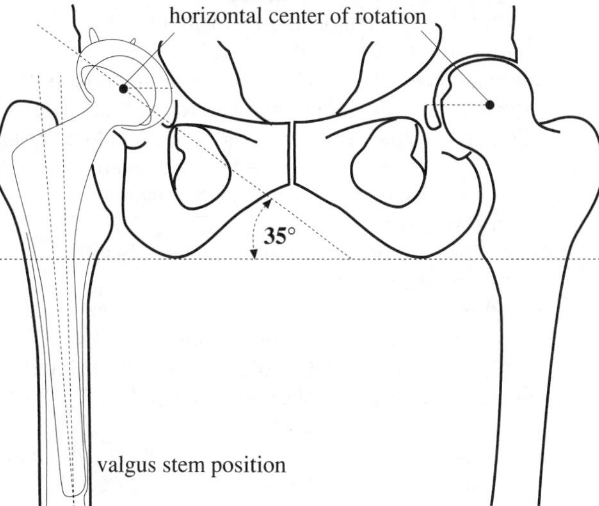

Initial Evaluation of Total Hip Arthroplasty

√ lucent zone at metal-cement interface along proximal lateral aspect of femoral stem
= suboptimal metal-cement contact at time of surgery / loosening

√ well-defined area of bone destruction (= histiocytic response, aggressive granulomatous disease)
Cause: granulomatous reaction as response to particulate debris / infection / tumor

√ asymmetric positioning of femoral head within acetabular component
Cause: acetabular wear / dislocation of femoral head / acetabular disruption / liner displacement / deformity

√ cement fracture
Cause: loosening

KNEE

Bone Contusion Pattern

√ edema of midportion of lateral femoral condyle
Cause: **pivot shift injury** = valgus load + external rotation of tibia / external rotation of femur applied to various states of flexion combined (noncontact injury)
Predisposed: skier, football player
Associated with injury of:
(1) anterior cruciate lig. (midsubstance > femoral attachment > tibial attachment site)
(2) posterior joint capsule + arcuate ligament
(3) posterior horn of lateral / medial meniscus
(4) medial collateral ligament

√ ± edema of posterior patellar surface
Cause: **dashboard injury** = force upon anterior proximal tibia with knee in flexed position
Associated with:
(1) rupture of posterior cruciate lig. (midsubstance > femoral attachment > tibial attachment site)
(2) tear of posterior joint capsule
(3) fracture / osteochondral injury of patella
(4) injury of hip

√ "kissing" bone contusion pattern = anterior aspect of tibial plateau + anterior aspect of femoral condyle
Cause: **hyperextension injury** = direct force upon anterior tibia while foot is planted / indirect force of forceful kicking motion
Associated with:
(1) injury to posterior / anterior cruciate lig.
(2) meniscal injury
(3) dislocation of knee
(4) popliteal neurovascular injury
(5) complete disruption of posterolateral complex

√ edema in lateral aspect of femoral condyle (secondary to direct blow)

√ small area of edema in medial femoral condyle (due to avulsive stress to medial collateral ligament)
Predisposed: football player
Cause: **clip injury** = pure valgus stress with knee in mild flexion
Associated with injury of:
(1) medial collateral ligament (at femoral attachment site
(2) anterior cruciate ligament
(3) medial meniscus
(4) combination of all three = **O'Donoghue triad**

√ anterolateral aspect of lateral femoral condyle

√ inferomedial aspect of patella
Predisposed: teenaged / young adult athletes with shallow trochlear groove
Cause: **lateral patellar dislocation** = twisting motion with knee in flexion + quadriceps contraction
Associated with injury of:
(1) medial retinaculum
(2) medial patellofemoral ligament (near femoral attachment site) most important stabilizing structure)
(3) medial patellotibial ligament

Unique Tibial Lesions

1. Fibrous dysplasia
2. Ossifying fibroma
3. Adamantinoma

Tibiotalar Slanting

= downward slanting of medial tibial plafond

1. Hemophilia
2. Still disease
3. Sickle cell disease
4. Epiphyseal dysplasia
5. Trauma

FOOT

Abnormal Foot Positions

A. FOREFOOT
1. Varus = adduction
   = axis of 1st metatarsal deviated medially relative to axis of talus
2. Valgus = abduction
   = axis of 1st metatarsal deviated laterally relative to axis of talus
3. Inversion = supination
   = inward turning of sole of foot
4. Eversion = pronation
   = outward turning of sole of foot

B. HINDFOOT
talipes (talus, pes) = any deformity of the ankle and hindfoot
1. Equinus
   = hindfoot abnormality with reversal of calcaneal pitch so that the heel cannot touch the ground
2. Calcaneal foot
   = very high calcaneal pitch so that forefoot cannot touch the ground
3. Pes planus = flatfoot
   = low calcaneal pitch + (usually) heel valgus + forefoot eversion
4. Pes cavus
   = high calcaneal pitch (fixed high arch)

Clubfoot = Talipes Equinovarus

Common severe congenital deformity characterized by

- equinus of heel (reversed calcaneal pitch)
- heel varus (talocalcaneal angle of almost zero on AP view with both bones parallel to each other)
- metatarsus adductus (axis of 1st metatarsal deviated medially relative to axis of talus)

1. Arthrogryposis multiplex congenita
2. Chondrodysplasia punctata
3. Neurofibromatosis
4. Spina bifida
5. Myelomeningocele

Rocker-bottom Foot = Vertical Talus

√ vertically oriented talus with increased talocalcaneal angle on lateral view
√ dorsal navicular dislocation at talonavicular joint
√ heel equinus
√ rigid deformity

Associated with: Arthrogryposis multiplex congenita; spina bifida; trisomy 13–18

Talar Beak = Hypertrophied Talar Ridge

1. Talocalcaneal type of tarsal coalition
2. Diffuse idiopathic skeletal hyperostosis (DISH)
3. Acromegaly
4. Rheumatoid arthritis

Heel Pad Thickening

= heel pad thickening >25 mm (normal <21 mm)

mnemonic: "MAD COP"

Myxedema
Acromegaly
Dilantin therapy
Callus
Obesity
Peripheral edema

Soft-tissue Masses of Foot + Ankle

A. NONTUMORAL
  (a) synovial proliferations
    1. Pigmented villonodular synovitis (PVNS)
    2. Giant cell tumor (GCT) of tendon sheath
  (b) posttraumatic
    1. Plantar fasciitis
  (c) inflammatory
  (d) uncertain origin
    1. Ganglion cyst
    2. Epidermoid cyst
    3. Morton neuroma
    4. Florid reactive periostitis
    6. Rheumatoid nodules
B. BENIGN TUMORS
  1. Plantar fibromatosis
  2. Deep fibromatosis
  3. Infantile digital fibromatosis
  4. Hemangioma
  5. Nerve sheath tumor
  6. Lipoma, angiolipoma

SOFT TISSUES

Histologic Classification of Soft-tissue Lesions

A. FATTY
  1. Lipoma
  2. Angiolipoma
  3. Liposarcoma
B. FIBROUS
  1. Fibroma
  2. Nodular fasciitis
  3. Aggressive fibromatosis / desmoid
  4. Fibrosarcoma
C. MUSCLE
  1. Rhabdomyoma
  2. Leiomyoma
  3. Rhabdomyosarcoma
  4. Leiomyosarcoma
D. VASCULAR
  1. Hemangioma
  2. Hemangiopericytoma
  3. Hemangiosarcoma
E. LYMPH
  1. Lymphangioma
  2. Lymphangiosarcoma
  3. Lymphadenopathy in lymphoma / metastasis
F. SYNOVIAL
  1. Nodular synovitis
  2. Pigmented villonodular synovitis
  3. Synovial sarcoma
G. NEURAL
  1. Neurofibroma
  2. Neurilemoma
  3. Ganglioneuroma
  4. Malignant neuroblastoma
  5. Neurofibrosarcoma
H. CARTILAGE AND BONE
  1. Myositis ossificans
  2. Extraskeletal osteoma
  3. Extraskeletal chondroma
  4. Extraskeletal chondrosarcoma
  5. Extraskeletal osteosarcoma

Fat-containing Soft-tissue Masses

A. BENIGN LIPOMATOUS TUMORS
  1. Lipoma
  2. Intra- / intermuscular lipoma
  3. Synovial lipoma
  4. Lipoma arborescens = diffuse synovial lipoma
  5. Neural fibrolipoma = fibrolipomatous tumor of nerve
  6. Macrodystrophia lipomatosa
B. LIPOMA VARIANTS
  1. Lipoblastoma (only in infancy + early childhood)
  2. **Lipomatosis** = diffuse overgrowth of mature adipose tissue infiltrating through the soft tissues of affected extremity / trunk
  3. **Hibernoma** = rare benign tumor of brown fat; often in peri- / interscapular region, axilla, thigh, chest wall
     √ marked hypervascularity

C. MALIGNANT LIPOMATOUS TUMOR
   1. Liposarcoma
D. OTHER FAT-CONTAINING TUMORS
   1. Hemangioma
   2. Elastofibroma
E. LESIONS MIMICKING FAT-CONTAINING TUMORS
   1. Myxoid tumors: intramuscular myxoma, extraskeletal myxoid chondrosarcoma, myxoid malignant fibrous histiocytoma
   2. Neural tumors: neurofibroma, neurilemoma, malignant schwannoma
      √ 73% have tissue attenuation less than muscle
   3. Hemorrhage

Extraskeletal Osseous + Cartilaginous Tumors

A. OSSEOUS SOFT-TISSUE TUMORS
   √ cloudlike "cumulus" type of calcification
   1. Myositis ossificans
   2. Fibrodysplasia ossificans progressiva
   3. Soft-tissue osteoma
   4. Extraskeletal osteosarcoma
   5. Myositis ossificans variants
      (a) Panniculitis ossificans
      (b) Fasciitis ossificans
      (c) Fibroosseous pseudotumor of digits
B. CARTILAGINOUS SOFT-TISSUE TUMORS
   √ arcs and rings, spicules and floccules of calcification
   1. Synovial osteochondromatosis
   2. Soft-tissue chondroma
   3. Extraskeletal chondrosarcoma

DDx:
(1) Synovial sarcoma
(2) Benign mesenchymoma
    = lipoma with chondroid / osseous metaplasia
(3) Malignant mesenchymoma
    = 2 or more unrelated sarcomatous components
(4) Calcified / ossified tophus of gout
(5) Ossified soft-tissue masses of melorheostosis
(6) **Pilomatricoma** = calcifying epithelioma of Malherbe
    • lesion arises from hair matrix cells with slow growth confined to the subcutaneous tissue of the face, neck, upper extremities
    √ central sandlike calcifications (84%)
    √ peripheral ossification (20%)
(7) Tumoral calcinosis

Soft-tissue Calcification

Metastatic Calcification

= deposit of calcium salts in previously normal tissue
(1) as a result of elevation of Ca x P product above 60–70
(2) with normal Ca x P product after renal transplant

Location: lung (alveolar septa, bronchial wall, vessel wall), kidney, gastric mucosa, heart, peripheral vessels

Cause:
(a) Skeletal deossification
   1. 1° HPT
   2. Ectopic HPT production (lung / kidney tumor)
   3. Renal osteodystrophy + 2° HPT
   4. Hypoparathyroidism
(b) Massive bone destruction
   1. Widespread bone metastases
   2. Plasma cell myeloma
   3. Leukemia
(c) Increased intestinal absorption
   1. Hypervitaminosis D
   2. Milk-alkali syndrome
   3. Excess ingestion / IV administration of calcium salts
   4. Prolonged immobilization
   5. Sarcoidosis
(d) Idiopathic hypercalcemia

Dystrophic Calcification

= in presence of normal serum Ca + P levels secondary to local electrolyte / enzyme alterations in areas of tissue injury

Cause:
(a) Metabolic disorder without hypercalcemia
   1. Renal osteodystrophy with 2° HPT
   2. Hypoparathyroidism
   3. Pseudohypoparathyroidism
   4. Pseudopseudohypoparathyroidism
   5. Gout
   6. Pseudogout = chondrocalcinosis
   7. Ochronosis = alkaptonuria
   8. Diabetes mellitus
(b) Connective tissue disorder
   1. Scleroderma
   2. Dermatomyositis
   3. Systemic lupus erythematosus
(c) Trauma
   1. Neuropathic calcifications
   2. Frostbite
   3. Myositis ossificans progressiva
   4. Calcific tendinitis / bursitis
(d) Infestation
   1. Cysticercosis
   2. Dracunculosis (guinea worm)
   3. Loiasis
   4. Bancroft filariasis
   5. Hydatid disease
   6. Leprosy
(e) Vascular disease
   1. Atherosclerosis
   2. Media sclerosis (Mönckeberg)
   3. Venous calcifications
   4. Tissue infarction (eg, myocardial infarction)
(f) Miscellaneous
   1. Ehlers-Danlos syndrome
   2. Pseudoxanthoma elasticum
   3. Werner syndrome = progeria

4. Calcinosis (circumscripta, universalis, tumoral calcinosis)
5. Necrotic tumor

Generalized Calcinosis

(a) Collagen vascular disorders
   1. Scleroderma
   2. Dermatomyositis
(b) Idiopathic tumoral calcinosis
(c) Idiopathic calcinosis universalis

Interstitial Calcinosis

Calcinosis Circumscripta

1. Acrosclerosis: granular deposits around joints of fingers + toes, fingertips
2. Scleroderma: acrosclerosis + absorption of ends of distal phalanges
3. Dermatomyositis: extensive subcutaneous deposits
4. Varicosities: particularly in calf
5. 1° Hyperparathyroidism: infrequently periarticular calcinosis
6. Renal osteodystrophy with 2° hyperparathyroidism: extensive vascular deposits even in young individuals
7. Hypoparathyroidism: occasionally around joints; symmetrical in basal ganglia
8. Vitamin D intoxication: periarticular in rheumatoid arthritis (puttylike); calcium deposit in tophi

Calcinosis Universalis

Progressive disease of unknown origin

Age: children + young adults

√ plaquelike calcium deposits in skin + subcutaneous tissues; sometimes in tendons + muscles

√ NO true bone formation

Soft-tissue Ossification

= formation of trabecular bone

1. Myositis ossificans progressiva / circumscripta
2. Paraosteoarthropathy
3. Soft-tissue osteosarcoma
4. Parosteal osteosarcoma
5. Posttraumatic periostitis = periosteoma
6. Surgical scar
7. Severely burned patient

Connective Tissue Disease

= CTD = [COLLAGEN VASCULAR DISEASE]

= group of disorders that share a number of clinical + laboratory features

- Features:
  (a) relatively specific: arthritis, myositis, Raynaud phenomenon with digital ulceration, tethered skin in extremities + trunk, malar rash sparing nasolabial folds, morning stiffness
  (b) relatively nonspecific: polyarthralgias (most common initial symptom), myalgias, mottling of extremities, muscle weakness + tenderness
- Laboratory findings:
  (a) relatively specific: ANA in peripheral rim / nucleolar pattern, anti-DNA, elevated muscle enzyme
  (b) relatively nonspecific: ANA in homogeneous pattern, anti-single-stranded DNA, positive rheumatoid factor

Types and most distinctive features:

1. Rheumatoid arthritis
   positive rheumatoid factor, prominent morning stiffness, symmetric erosive arthritis
2. Systemic lupus erythematosus
   malar rash, photosensitivity, serositis, renal disorders with hemolytic anemia, leukopenia, lymphopenia, thrombocytopenia, positive ANA
3. Sjögren syndrome
   dry eyes + mouth, abnormal Schirmer test
4. Scleroderma
   Raynaud phenomenon, skin thickening of distal extremities proceeding to include proximal extremities + chest + abdomen, positive ANA in a nucleolar pattern
5. Polymyositis, dermatomyositis
   heliotrope rash over eyes, proximal muscle weakness, elevated muscle enzymes, inflammation at muscle biopsy

Mixed Connective Tissue Disease

= disorder that shares distinctive features of ≥2 different connective tissue diseases in same patient (eg, overlapping features of SLE, PSS, polymyositis)

- pulmonary hypertension (due to interstitial pulmonary fibrosis / intimal proliferation of pulmonary arterioles)

Muscle

MR signal intensity of normal muscle:

√ higher than water + lower than fat on T1WI

√ much lower than water + fat on T2WI

Intramuscular Mass

A. NEOPLASM
B. INFECTION / INFLAMMATION
   1. Intramuscular abscess
   2. Focal myositis = benign inflammatory pseudotumor
   3. Necrotizing fasciitis
   4. Sarcoidosis
      √ nodules with central star-shaped area of fibrosis surrounded by granuloma
C. MYONECROSIS
   1. Sickle cell crisis
   2. Poorly controlled diabetes
   3. Compartment syndrome
   4. Crush injury
   5. Severe ischemia
   6. Intraarterial chemotherapy

7. **Rhabdomyolysis** = severe muscle injury with loss of integrity of muscle cell membranes
Cause: trauma, severe exercise, ischemia, burn, toxin, IV heparin therapy, autoimmune inflammation
Cx: renal damage from myoglobulinemia, tetany, compartment syndrome

D. TRAUMA
1. Intramuscular hematoma (eg, severe muscle strain, laceration, contusion, spontaneous)
2. Myositis ossificans traumatica

Muscle Edema

√ muscle hyperintensity on STIR images

A. INFLAMMATION
1. Dermatomyositis
2. Polymyositis
4. Radiation therapy: straight sharp margins, involves muscle + subcutaneous fat
5. Early stage of myositis ossificans

B. CELLULAR INFILTRATE
1. Lymphoma

C. INFECTION
1. Bacterial / infectious myositis
(a) direct extension from adjacent infection (eg, osteomyelitis, subcutaneous abscess)
(b) hematogenous
2. Inclusion body myositis (probably due to paramyxovirus infection) resembling polymyositis

D. RHABDOMYOLYSIS
1. Sport / electric injury
2. Diabetic muscular infarction
3. Focal nodular myositis
4. Metabolic myopathy: eg, phosphofructokinase deficiency, hypokalemia, alcohol overdose
5. Viral myositis

E. TRAUMA
1. **Subacute muscle denervation**
Time of onset: 2–4 weeks after denervation
Mechanism: spinal cord injury, poliomyelitis, peripheral nerve injury / compression (ganglion cyst, bone spur), Graves disease, neuritis
2. Muscle contusion (from direct blow)
3. Muscle strain (= injury at musculotendinous junction from overly forceful muscle contraction)
Predilection for: hamstring, gastrocnemius m., biceps brachii m.)
4. Delayed-onset muscle soreness
= overuse injury becoming symptomatic hours / days after overuse episode)
5. **Compartment syndrome**
= increased pressure within indistensible space of confining fascia leading to venous occlusion, muscle + nerve ischemia, arterial occlusion, tissue necrosis
Cause: trauma, burns, heavy exercise, extrinsic pressure, intramuscular hemorrhage
• severe pain
• dysfunction of sensory + motor nerves passing through affected compartment
6. Sickle cell crisis

Fatty Infiltration of Muscle

1. Chronic stage of muscle denervation (eg, poliomyelitis, stroke, peripheral nerve injury)
2. Chronic disuse (eg, chronic tendon tear, severe osteoarthritis)
3. Late stage of severe muscle injury
4. Long-term high-dose corticosteroid medication affecting truncal muscles

FIXATION DEVICES

Internal Fixation Devices

A. Screws
1. Cortical screw = shallow finely threaded over entire length, blunt tip
Use: fixation of plates
2. Cancellous screw = wide thread diameter with varying length of smooth shank between head + threads
Use: compression across fracture site
3. Malleolar screw = partially threaded
4. Interference screw = short, fully threaded, cancellous thread pattern, self-tapping tip, recessed head
Use: within tunnel holding bone graft of ACL and PCL reconstruction
5. Cannulated screw = hollow screw inserted over guide pin
Use: fracture of femoral neck
6. Herbert screw = cannulated screw threaded on both ends with different pitches, no screw head
Use: scaphoid fracture

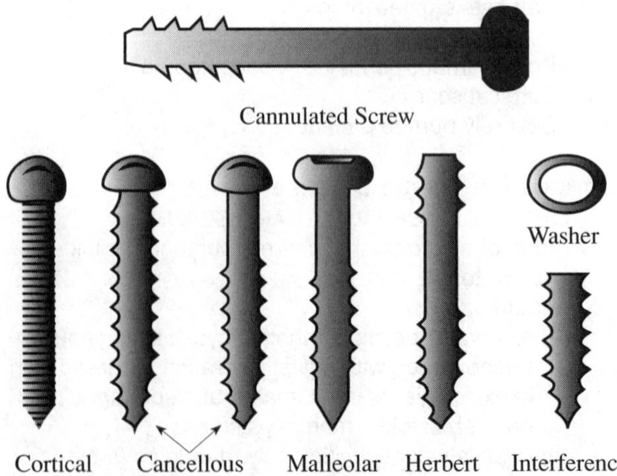

Screws

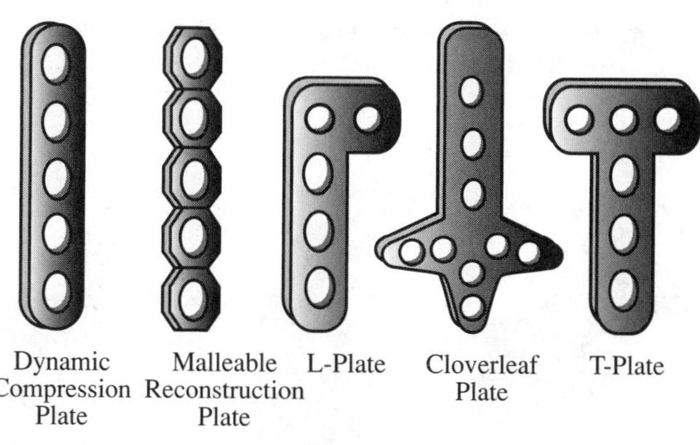

Plates

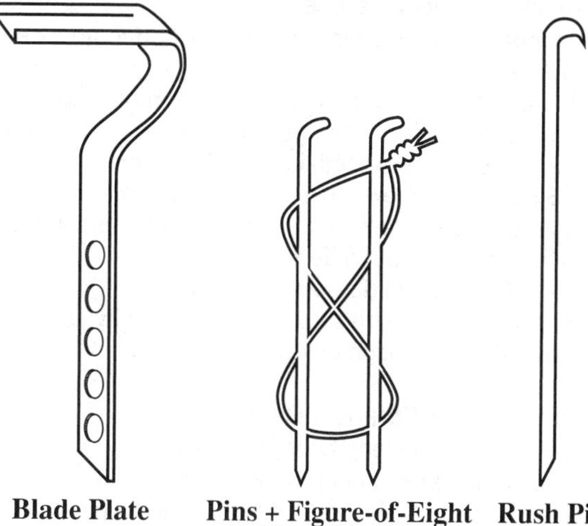

7. Dynamic hip screw = screw free to slide within barrel of side plate allowing impaction of fracture during healing without perforation of subarticular cortex
   Use: subcapital, intertrochanteric, subtrochanteric fracture

B. Washer
1. Flat washer = increase surface area over which force is distributed
2. Serrated washer = spiked edges used for affixing avulsed ligaments

C. Plates
— compression plate
  Use: compression of stable fractures
— neutralization plate = protects fracture from bending, rotation + axial-loading forces
— buttress plate = support of unstable fractures in compression / axial loading
1. Straight plate
   (a) straight plate with round holes
   (b) dynamic compression plate = oval holes
   (c) tubular plate = thin pliable plate with concave inner surface
   (d) reconstruction plate = thin pliable plate to allow bending, twisting, contouring
2. Special plates
   T-shaped, L-shaped, Y-shaped, cloverleaf, spoon, cobra, condylar blade plate, dynamic compression screw system

D. Staples
Fixation = bone = epiphyseal = fracture staples with smooth / barbed surface
— Coventry = stepped osteotomy staple
— stone = table staple

E. Wires
1. K wire = unthreaded segments of extruded wire of variable thickness
   Use: temporary fixation
2. Cerclage wiring = wire placed around bone
   Use: fixation of comminuted patellar fracture, holding bone grafts in position
3. Tension band wiring = figure-of-eight wire placed on tension side of bone
   Use: olecranon / patellar fractures

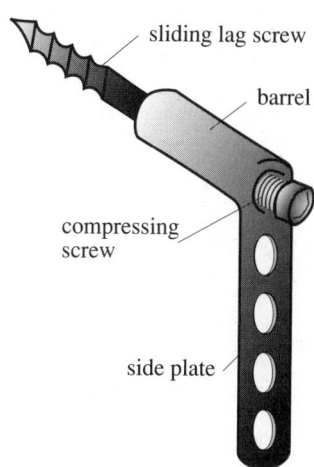

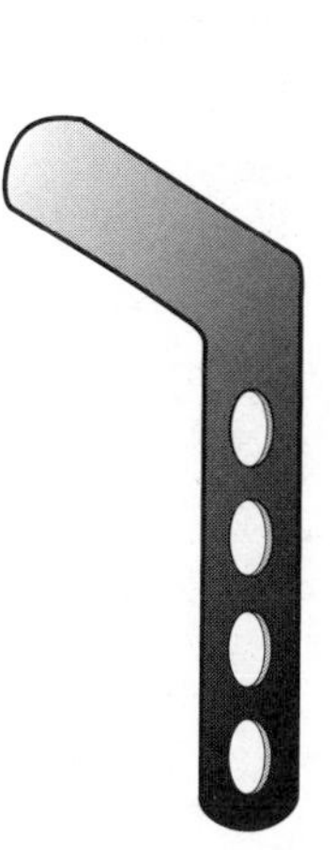

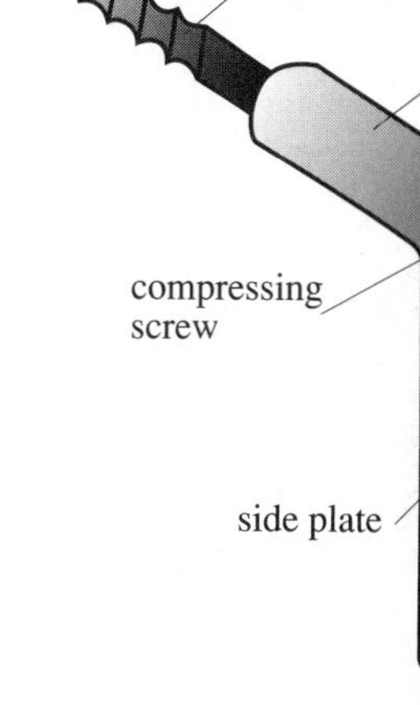

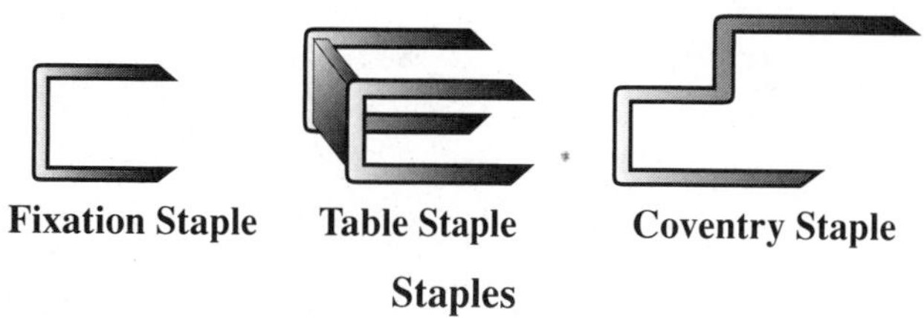

Staples

External Fixation Devices

= smooth / threaded pins / wires attached to an external frame

(a) unilateral pin = enters bone only from one side
   1. Steinmann pin = large-caliber wire with pointed tip
   2. Rush pin = smooth intramedullary pin
   3. Schanz screw = pin threaded at one end to engage cortex, smooth at other end to connect to external fixation device
   4. Knowles pin (for femoral neck fracture)

(b) transfixing pin = passes through extremity supported by external fixation device on both ends

Intramedullary Fixation Devices

Use: diaphyseal long bone fractures

(a) nail = driven into bone without reaming

(b) rod = solid / hollow device with blunted tip driven into reamed channel (reaming disrupts blood supply and may decrease the rate of fracture healing)

(c) interlocking nail = accessory pins / screws / deployable fins placed to prevent rotation

1. Rush pin = beveled end + hooked end
2. Ender nail = oval in cross section
3. Sampson rod = slightly curved rigid rod with fluted surface
4. Küntscher nail = cloverleaf in cross section with rounded tip

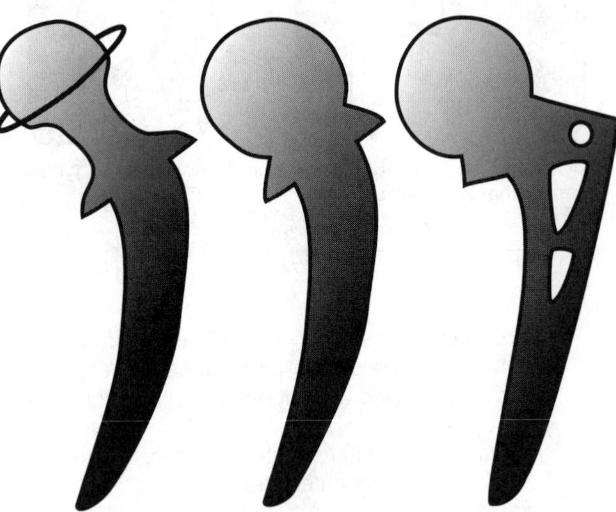

Hip Prostheses

ANATOMY AND METABOLISM OF BONE

BONE MINERALS

Calcium

A. 99% in bone
B. serum calcium
  (a) protein-bound fraction (albumin)
  (b) ionic (pH-dependent) 3% as calcium citrate / phosphate in serum

Absorption: facilitated by vitamin D
Excretion: related to dietary intake; >500 mg/24 hours = hypercalciuria

Phosphorus

Absorption: requires sodium; decreased by aluminum hydroxide gel in gut
Excretion: increased by estrogen, parathormone decreased by vitamin D, growth hormone, glucocorticoids

HORMONES

Parathormone

Major stimulus: low levels of serum calcium ions (action requires vitamin D presence)
Target organs:
(a) BONE: increase in osteocytic + osteoclastic activity mobilizes calcium + phosphate = bone resorption
(b) KIDNEY: (1) increase in tubular reabsorption of calcium
  (2) decrease in tubular reabsorption of phosphate (+ amino acids) = phosphate diuresis
(c) GUT: increased absorption of calcium + phosphorus

Major function:
- increase of serum calcium levels
- increase in serum alkaline phosphatase (50%)

Vitamin D Metabolism

required for
(1) adequate calcium absorption from gut
(2) synthesis of calcium-binding protein in intestinal mucosa
(3) parathormone effects (stimulation of osteoclastic + osteocytic resorption of bone)

Biochemistry:
inactive form of vitamin D_3 present through diet / exposure to sunlight; vitamin D_3 is converted into 25-OH-vitamin D_3 by liver and then converted into 1,25-OH vitamin D_3 (= hormone) by kidney
Stimulus for conversion: (1) hypophosphatemia
  (2) PTH elevation

Action:
(a) INTESTINE: (1) increased absorption of calcium from bowel
  (2) increased absorption of phosphate from distal small bowel
(b) BONE: (1) proper mineralization of osteoid
  (2) mobilization of calcium + phosphate (potentiates parathormone action)
(c) KIDNEY: (1) increased absorption of calcium from renal tubule
  (2) increased absorption of phosphate from renal tubule

Calcitonin

secreted by parafollicular cells of thyroid
Major stimulus: increase in serum calcium
Target organs:
(a) BONE: (1) inhibits parathormone-induced osteoclasis by reducing number of osteoclasts
  (2) enhances deposition of calcium phosphate; responsible for sclerosis in renal osteodystrophy
(b) KIDNEY: inhibits phosphate reabsorption in renal tubule
(c) GUT: increases excretion of sodium + water into gut

Major function: decreases serum calcium + phosphate

PHYSIS

Four distinct zones of cartilage in longitudinal layers
(1) Germinal zone = small cells adjacent to epiphyseal ossification center
(2) Proliferating zone = flattened cells arranged in columns
(3) Hypertrophic zone = swollen vacuolated cells
(4) Zone of provisional calcification

Parathormone Function

	PTH Action	*Net Effect*	
Principal:	(1) phosphate diuresis (2) resorption of Ca + P from bone	(1) Serum:	increase in Ca decrease in P
Secondary:	(3) resorption of Ca from gut (4) reabsorption of Ca from renal tubule	(2) Urine:	increase in Ca increase in P

NORMAL SHOULDER JOINT ANATOMY

Glenoid Labrum

= 4-mm–wide fibrocartilaginous ring with considerable variation in shape attached to glenoid rim
√ triangular / rounded shape on cross-sectional image
√ blends superiorly with biceps tendon

Biceps Tendon

= long head of biceps muscle
√ attached to anterosuperior aspect of glenoid rim with fibers to
(a) anterosuperior labrum (labral-bicipital complex)
(b) posterosuperior labrum (labral-bicipital complex)
(c) supraglenoid tubercle
(d) base of coracoid process
√ exits joint through intertubercular groove
√ secured to intertubercular groove by transverse lig.

Glenohumeral Ligaments

= thickened bands of joint capsule functioning as shoulder stabilizers

Superior Glenohumeral Ligament

= most consistently identified
√ arises from anterosuperior labrum / tendon attachment of long head of biceps / middle glenohumeral ligament
√ courses in plane perpendicular to middle glenohumeral ligament + parallel to coracoid process
√ best visualized on transverse CT / MR

Middle Glenohumeral Ligament

= varies most in size + attachment; may be absent
√ courses obliquely from superomedial to inferolateral
√ attaches medially on glenoid neck / superior portion of anterior glenoid rim
√ ligament stretched through external arm rotated
√ may be thick + cordlike
√ best visualized on sagittal / transverse CT / MR

Inferior Glenohumeral Ligament

= important stabilizer of anterior shoulder joint
1. Anterior band
   √ inserts along inferior 2/3 of anterior glenoid labrum
   √ usually quite prominent, in 25% very thin
2. Posterior band (usually thinner)

Normal Anatomic Variants of Shoulder

Superior Sublabral Recess

= variations in depth of sulcus between glenoid rim + labrum
Location: 12 o'clock position at the site of biceps tendon attachment
type I = no sulcus
type II = small sulcus
type III = deep probe-patent sulcus
√ may be continuous with sublabral foramen
√ best visualized on coronal CT / MR
DDx: type II SLAP lesion

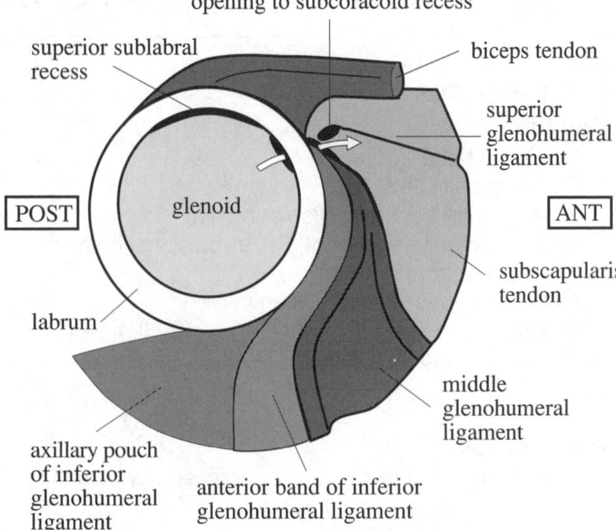

Normal Anatomy of Right Shoulder En Face
(arrow in sublabral foramen)

Sublabral Foramen

= sublabral hole between labrum + glenoid
Incidence: 11% of individuals
Location: 2 o'clock position anterior to biceps tendon attachment
√ may coexist with sublabral recess
DDx: labral tear

Buford Complex

= cordlike thickening of middle glenohumeral ligament directly attaching to anterosuperior glenoid + absence of anterosuperior labrum
Incidence: 1.5% of individuals
Location: 2 o'clock position anterior to biceps tendon attachment
√ may coexist with sublabral recess
DDx: displaced labral fragment

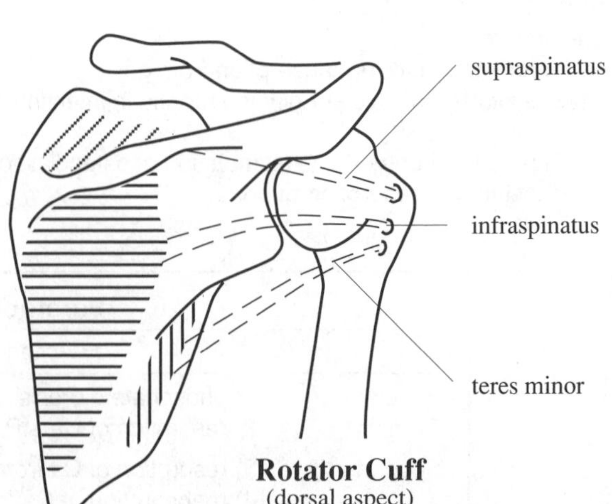

Rotator Cuff
(dorsal aspect)

ROTATOR CUFF MUSCLES

mnemonic: "SITS"

Supraspinatus
Infraspinatus
Teres minor
Subscapularis

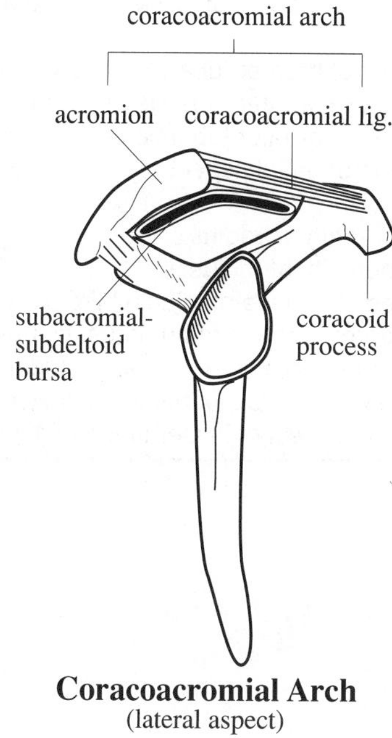

Coracoacromial Arch
(lateral aspect)

OCCURRENCE OF BONE CENTERS AT ELBOW

mnemonic: "CRITOE"

Capitellum	1 year	(3–6 months)
Radial head	4 years	(3–6 years)
Internal humeral epicondyle	7 years	(5–7 years, last to fuse)
Trochlea	10 years	(9–10 years)
Olecranon	10 years	(6–10 years)
External humeral epicondyle	11 years	(9–13 years)

mnemonic: "Nelson's X: 1, 7, 10, 11 years"

LAT MED 11 7 1 10

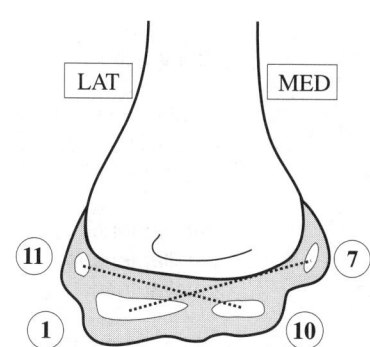

Occurrence of Bone Centers
(numbers in years)

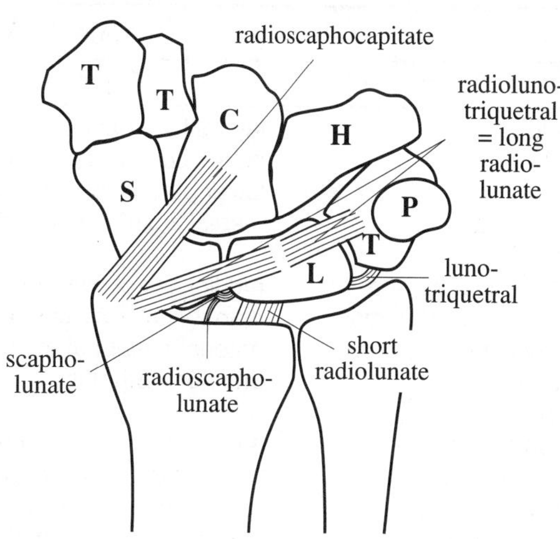

Carpal Bones and Ligaments
(volar aspect)

CARPAL BONES

mnemonic: "**S**ome **L**overs **T**ry **P**ositions **T**hat **T**hey **C**an't **H**andle"

proximal row	distal row
Scaphoid	**T**rapezium
Lunate	**T**rapezoid
Triquetrum	**C**apitate
Pisiform	**H**amate

◊ Remember that trapezium comes before trapezoid in the dictionary as well!

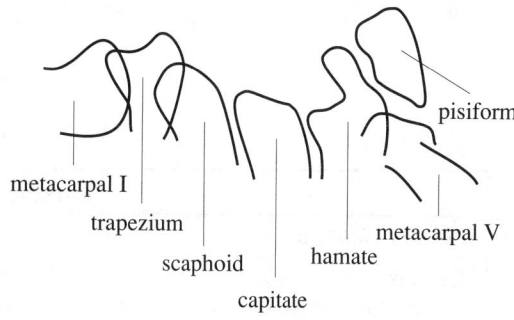

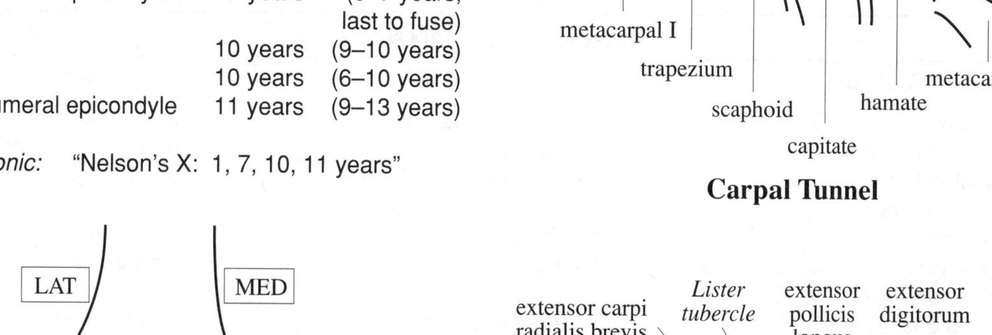

Carpal Tunnel

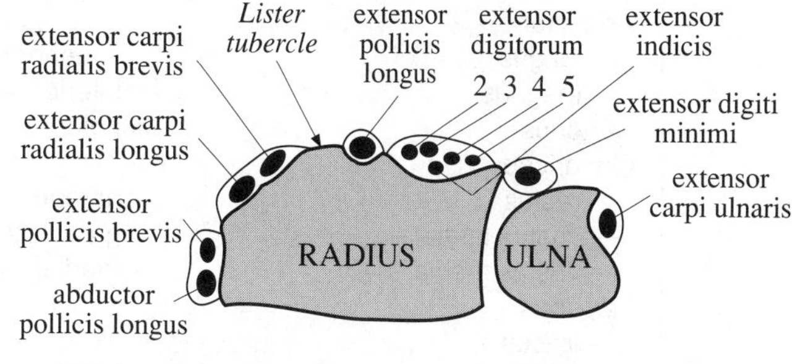

Wrist Cross Section of Distal Radioulnar Joint with the 6 Extensor Compartments

Muscle Attachments of Shoulder		
Name of Muscle	*Origin*	*Insertion*
Deltoid	lateral third of clavicle	deltoid tuberosity of humerus
	lateral border of acromion	deltoid tuberosity of humerus
	lower part of spinous process of scapula	deltoid tuberosity of humerus
Subscapularis	medial 2/3 of costal surface of scapula	superior aspect of lesser tubercle of humerus
Pectoralis major		
– clavicular portion	medial half of clavicle	crest of greater tubercle of humerus
– sternocostal portion	manubrium + corpus of sternum	crest of greater tubercle of humerus
– abdominal portion	anterior sheath of rectus abdominis	crest of greater tubercle of humerus
Pectoralis minor	2nd / 3rd–5th ribs	superomedial aspect of coracoid process
Biceps brachii		
– long head	supraglenoid tubercle of scapula	tuberosity of radius
– short head	tip of coracoid process	tuberosity of radius
Coracobrachialis	tip of coracoid process	medial surface of middle third of humerus
Supraspinatus	supraspinatus fossa of scapula	greater tubercle of humerus, highest facet
Infraspinatus	infraspinatus fossa of scapula	greater tubercle of humerus, middle facet
Teres minor	upper 2/3 of lateral border of scapula	greater tubercle of humerus, lower facet
Teres major	dorsum of inferior angle of scapula	inferior crest of lesser tubercle of humerus

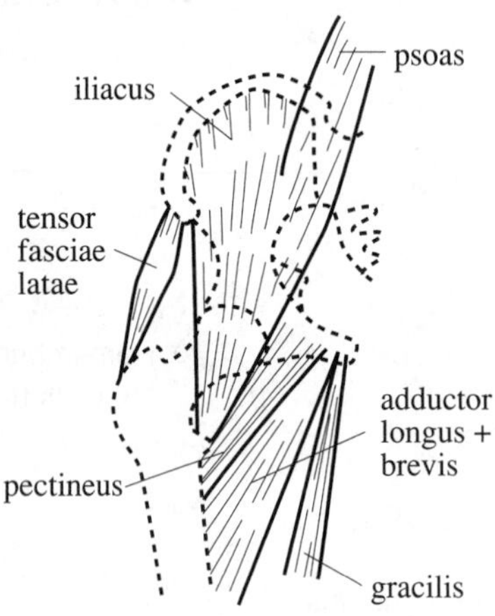

Hip Flexors

Muscle Attachments of Thigh		
Name of Muscle	*Origin*	*Insertion*
Gracilis	inferior pubic ramus	pes anserinus
Semimembranosus	ischial tuberosity	medial tibial condyle
Semitendinosus	ischial tuberosity	pes anserinus
Biceps femoris		
– long head	ischial tuberosity	fibular head
– short head	lateral linea aspera	fibular head
Adductor		
– longus	superior pubic ramus	medial linea aspera
– magnus	inferior pubic ramus	medial linea aspera
Sartorius	anterior superior iliac spine	pes anserinus
Quadriceps		
– rectus	anterior inferior iliac spine	patellar tendon
– vastus lateralis	greater trochanter	patellar tendon
– vastus medialis	medial intertrochanteric line	patellar tendon
Iliopsoas		
– iliacus	ilium	lesser trochanter
– psoas	lumbar spine	lesser trochanter
Tensor fasciae latae	anterior superior iliac spine	anterolateral tibia

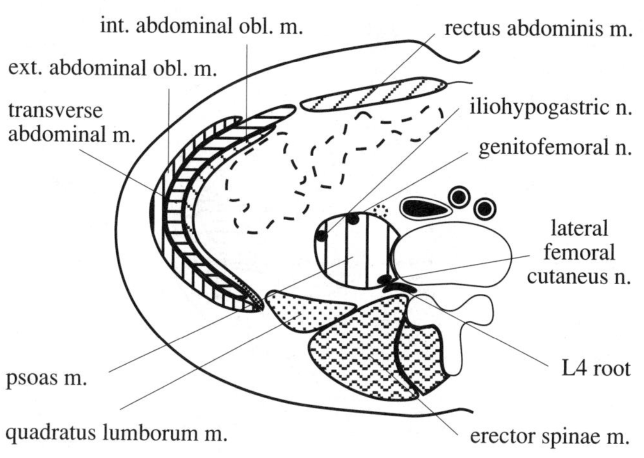

Cross Section through L4-5

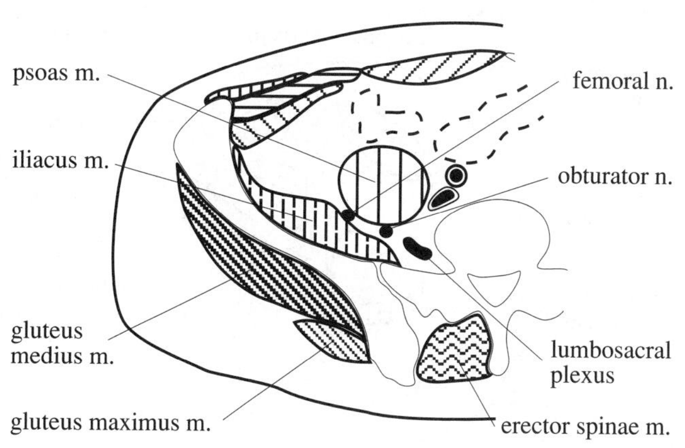

Cross Section through L5-S1

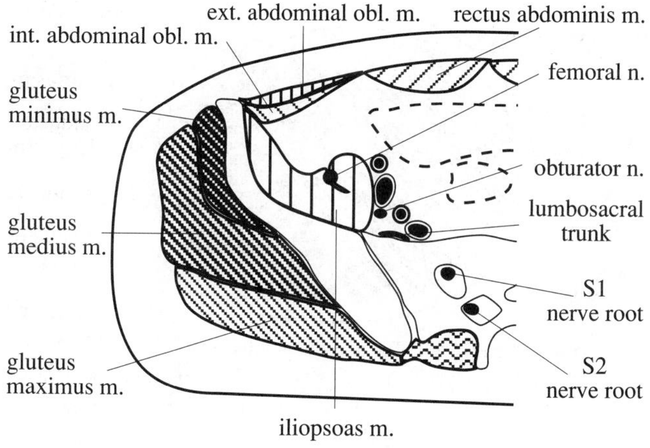

Cross Section through S1-2

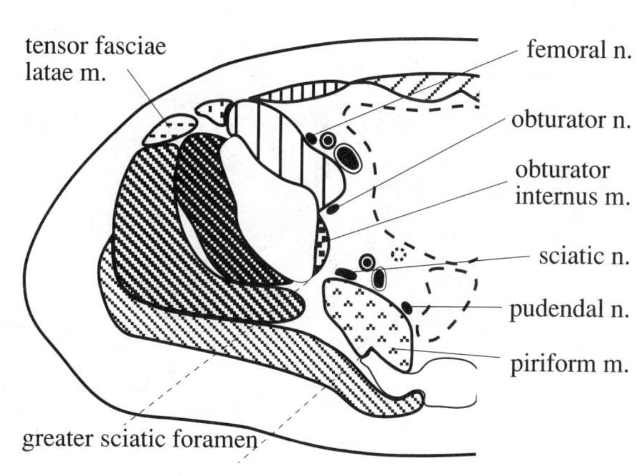

Cross Section through S4

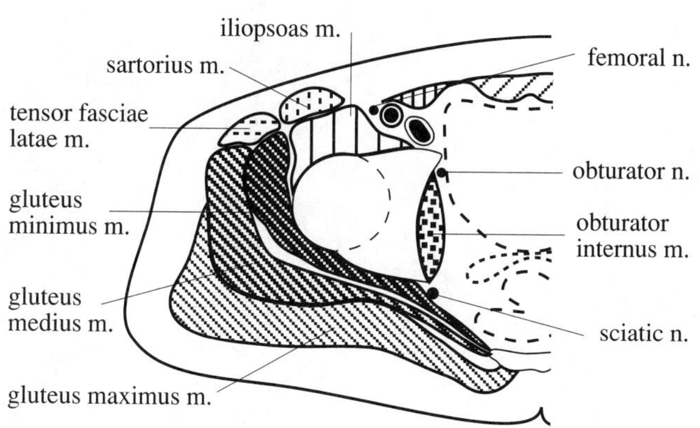

Cross Section through Actabular Roof

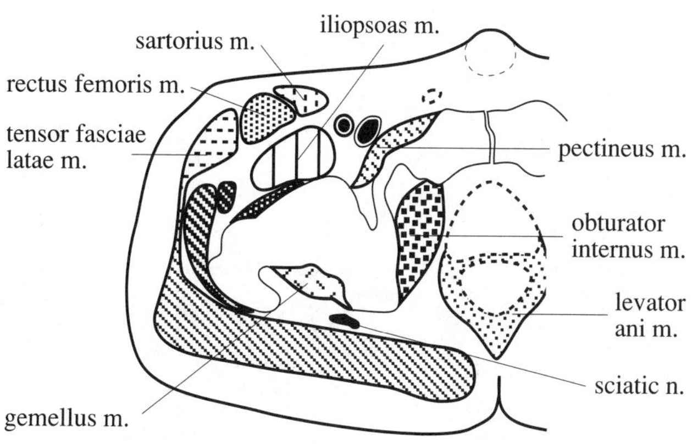

Cross Section through Greater Trochanter

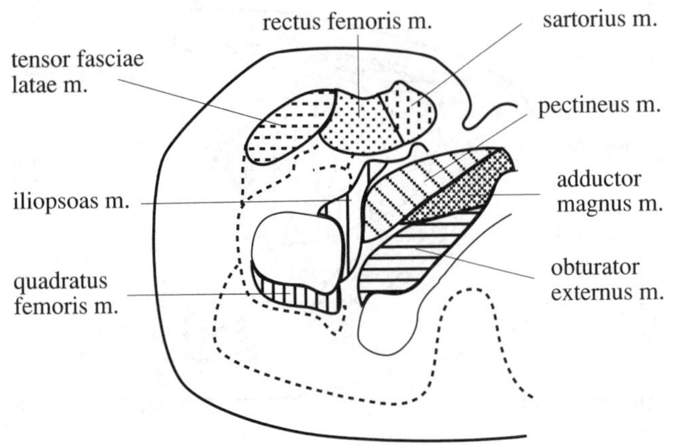

Cross Section through Level of Obturator Foramen

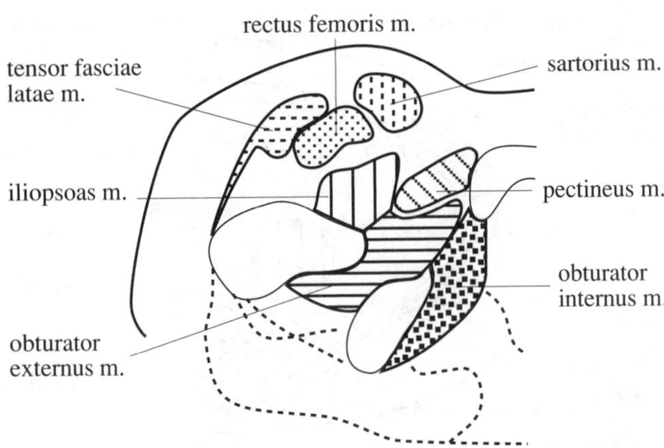

Cross Section through Level of Minor Trochanter

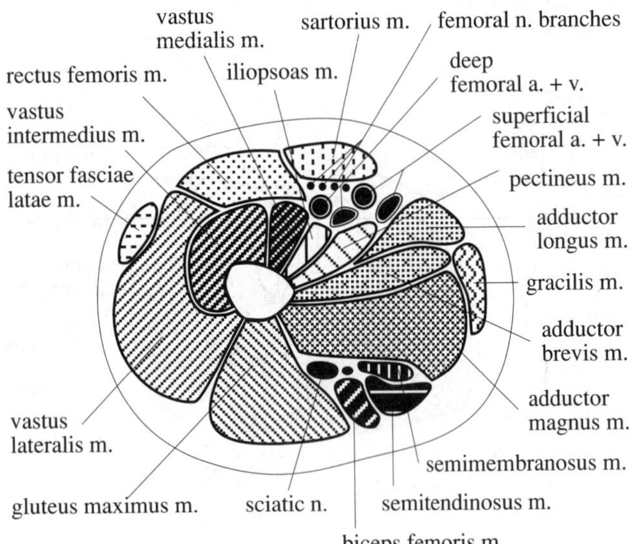

Cross Section through Level of Proximal Thigh

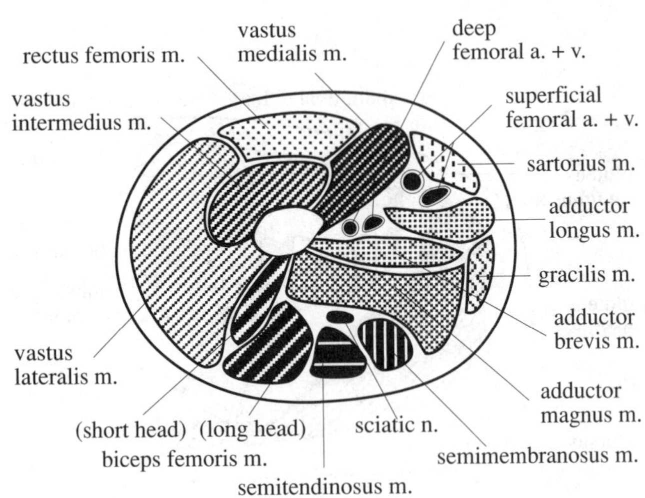

Cross Section through Level of Mid Thigh

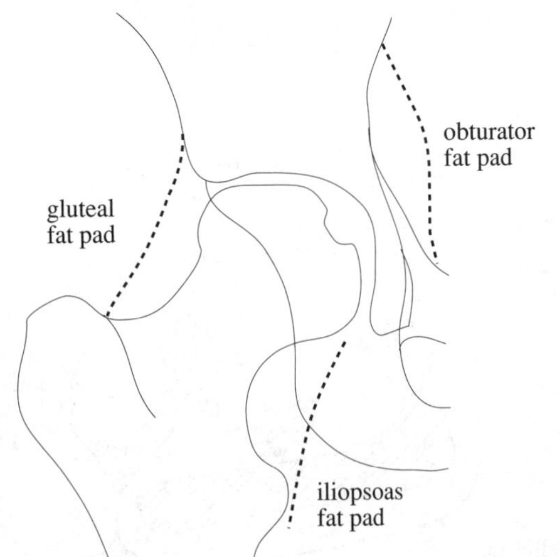

Fat Pads of the Rigth Hip in Perfect AP Position

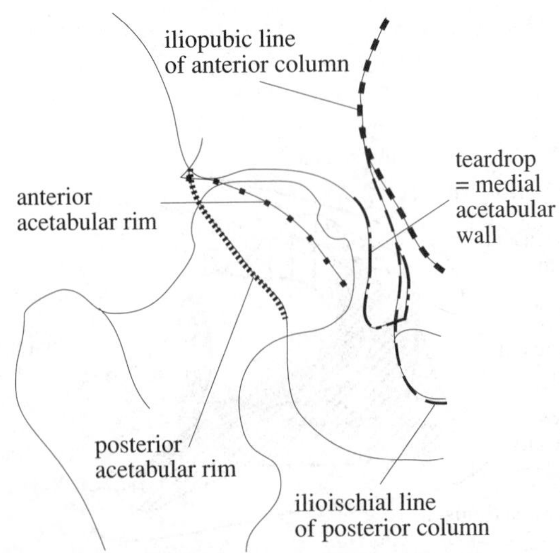

Bony Landmarks of the Rigth Hip in Perfect AP Position

LOWER EXTREMITY

Pes Anserinus

= [*pes*, Latin = foot; *anser*, Latin = goose]
= tendinous configuration of 3 flexors + medial rotators of knee joint attaching inferomedially to tibial tuberosity

mnemonic: "**Sa**y **Gra**c**Se** before eating goose"

1. Sartorius tendon (anterior)
2. Gracilis tendon (middle)
3. Semitendinosus tendon (posterior)

Iliotibial Tract

= strong stabilizing band of deep fascia composed of the fusion of aponeurotic coverings of:

1. Tensor fascia lata
2. Gluteus maximus m.
3. Gluteus medius m.

Insertion:
(a) supracondylar tubercle of lateral femoral condyle
(b) lateral tubercle of tibia = Gerdy tubercle (main site)
(c) patella + patellar ligament

Hamstrings

(a) medial hamstring
1. Semimembranosus m.
2. Semitendinosus m.
Function: flexion + medial rotation of knee joint

(b) lateral hamstring
= long + short head of biceps femoris m.
Function: flexion + lateral rotation of knee joint

Cruciate Ligaments

◊ Both cruciate ligaments are intracapsular but extrasynovial!

Anterior Cruciate Ligament (ACL)

Function: limits anterior tibial translation
Origin: inner face of lateral femoral condyle
Insertion: noncartilaginous region of anterior aspect of intercondylar eminence of tibia
Anatomy: several distinct bundles of fibers
(1) posterior bulk = spiraling together at femoral origin
(2) anteromedial bundle diverging at tibial insertion

√ thin solid taut dark band (sagittal MR with knee in extension) almost parallel to intercondylar roof (= Blumensaat line)
√ thin hypointense band parallel to inner aspect of lateral femoral condyle + fanlike configuration toward tibial spine (coronal MR)
√ thin ovoid hypointense band proximally, elliptical configuration distally with higher intensity (axial MR)
√ greater signal intensity than posterior cruciate ligament (due to anatomy)

Posterior Cruciate Ligament (PCL)

Function: limits posterior tibial translation
Origin: in a depression posterior to intercondylar region of tibia below joint surface
Insertion: most distal + anterior aspect of inner face of medial femoral condyle

√ thick dark band slightly posteriorly convex (arclike course on sagittal MR with knee in extension)
√ medial to ACL (coronal MR)

Collateral Ligaments of Knee Joint

Medial (Tibial) Collateral Ligament

Origin: just distal to adductor tubercle of femur
Insertion: anteromedial face of tibia distal to level of tibial tubercle about 5 cm below joint line

(a) deep portion:
– meniscofemoral ligament
– meniscotibial ligaments

(b) superficial portion
– vertical band from femoral epicondyle to pes anserinus
– posterior oblique ligament = posterior oblique band from femoral epicondyle to semimembranosus tendon

√ deep and superficial dark bands separated by a thin bursa + fatty tissue (on coronal MR)

Lateral (Fibular) Collateral Ligament

Origin: lateral aspect of lateral femoral condyle
Insertion: styloid process of fibular head

√ bicipital tendon + iliotibial band join lateral collateral ligament

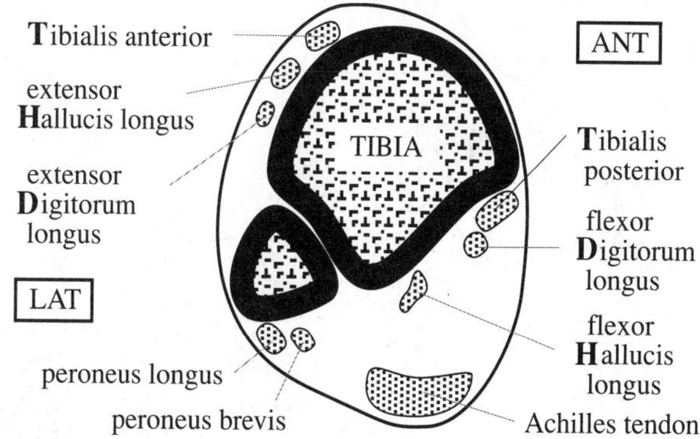

Cross Section through Distal Right Leg

mnemonic for posterior tendons: "**T**om, **D**ick and **H**arry"
Tibialis posterior
Digitorum longus (flexor)
Hallucis longus (flexor)

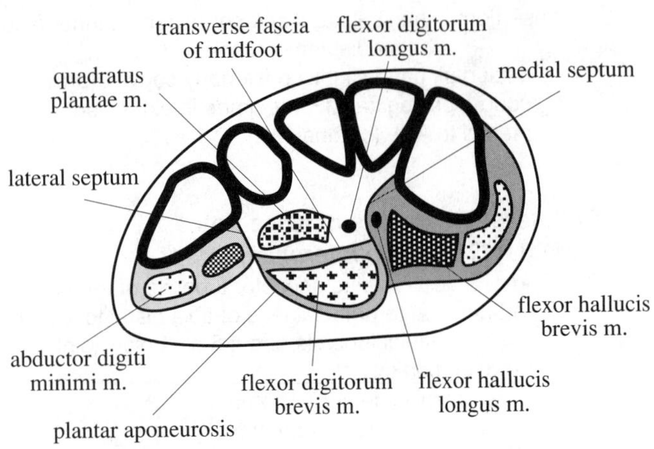

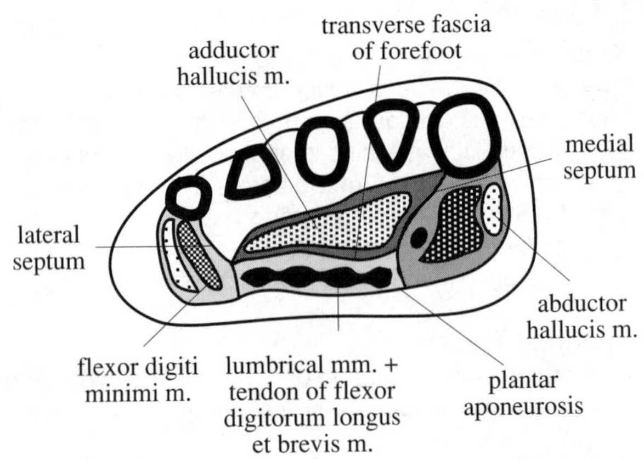

Plantar Compartments of the Midfoot **Plantar Compartments of the Forefoot**

Medial compartment = bordered by medial septum (extending from plantar aponeurosis to navicular bone, medial cuneiform bone, and lateral border of plantar surface of 1st metatarsal bone);
contains abductor hallucis m. + flexor hallucis brevis m. + flexor hallucis longus tendon

Lateral compartment = bordered by lateral septum (extending from plantar aponeurosis to medial surface of 5th metatarsal bone);
contains abductor m. + short flexor m. + opponens m. of 5th toe

Central compartment = bordered by medial + lateral septa; communicates directly with posterior compartment of calf;
subdivided by horizontal septa: adductor hallucis m. separated from quadratus plantae m.
contains flexor digitorum brevis m. + flexor digitorum longus tendon + quadratus plantae m. + lumbricales mm.. + adductor hallucis m.

Deep subcompartment = bordered by transverse fascia of forefoot; separated from quadratus plantae m.; contains adductor hallucis m.

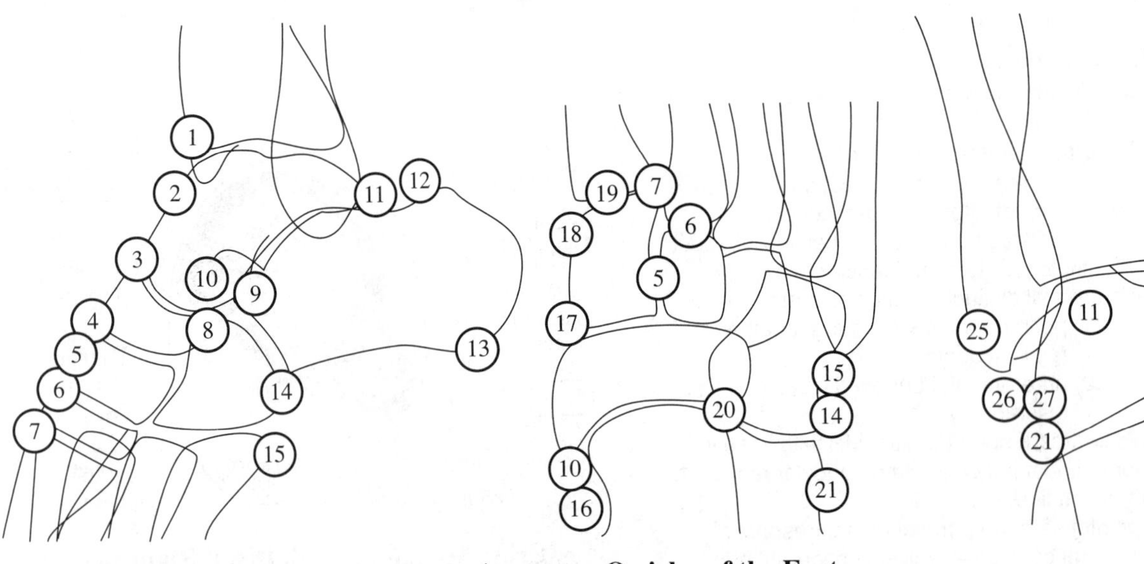

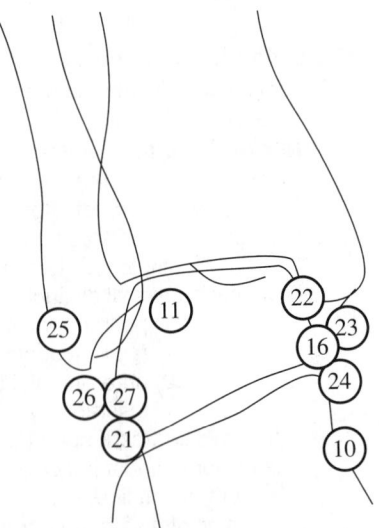

Accessory Ossicles of the Foot

1 Os talotibiale
2 Os supratalare
3 Os supranaviculare
4 Os infranaviculare
5 Os intercuneiforme
6 Os cuneometatarsale II dorsale
7 Os intermetatarsale
8 Secondary cuboid
9 Calcaneus secundarius
10 Os tibiale externum
11 Trigonum
12 Os accessorium supracalcaneum
13 Os subcalcis
14 Os peroneum
15 Os vesalianum
16 Talus accessorius
17 Os cuneonaviculare mediale
18 Sesamum tibiale anterius
19 Os cuneometatarsale I plantare
20 Cuboides secundarium
21 Os trochleare calcanei
22 Sesamoid talus - int. malleolus
23 Os subtibiale
24 Os sustentaculi
25 Os retinaculi
26 Os subfibulare
27 Talus secundarius

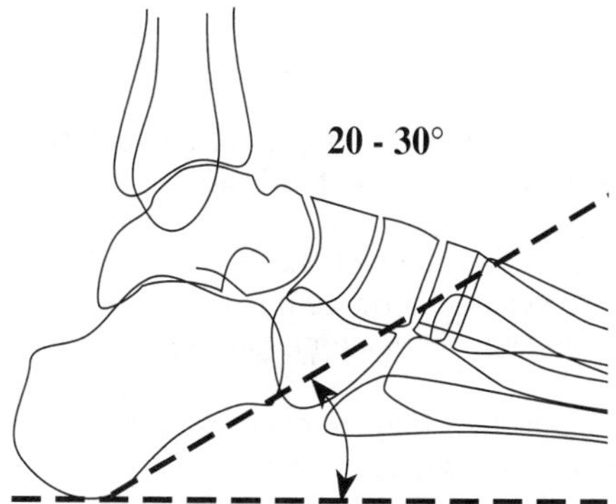

Calcaneal Pitch
= Calcaneal Inclination Angle
= determines longitudinal arch of foot; angle between line drawn along the inferior border of calcaneus connecting the anterior and posterior prominences + line representing the horizontal surface

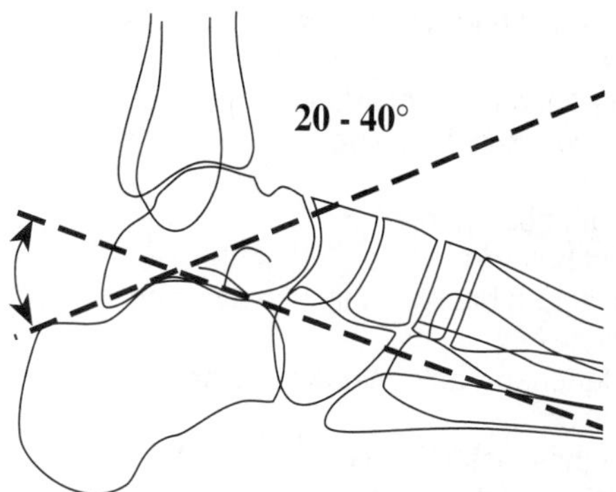

Boehler Angle
= angle between first line drawn from posterosuperior prominence of calcaneus anteriorly to sustentaculum tali + second line drawn from anterosuperior prominence posteriorly to sustentaculum tali; measures integrity of calcaneus

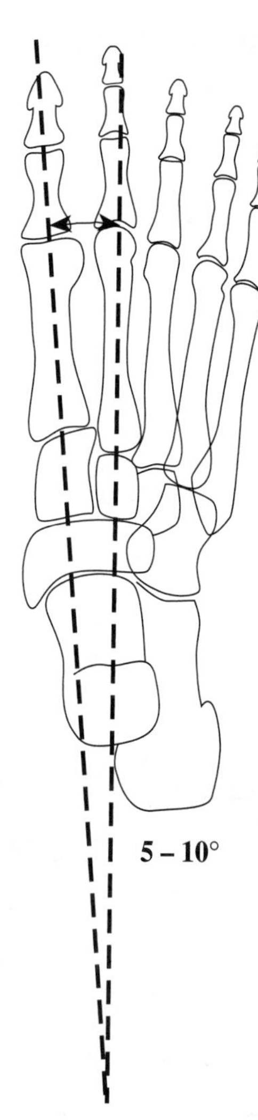

Intermetatarsal Angle
= amount that 1st + 2nd metatarsals diverge from each other

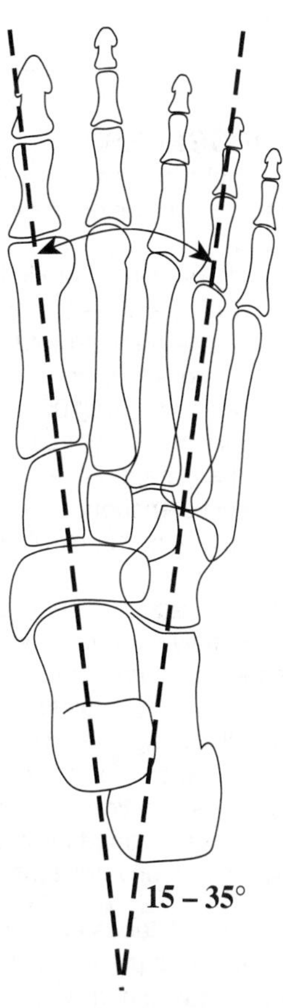

Talocalcaneal Angle on AP View
= KITE ANGLE = the midtalar and midcalcaneal lines parallel the 1st + 4th metatarsals; angle is greater in infants

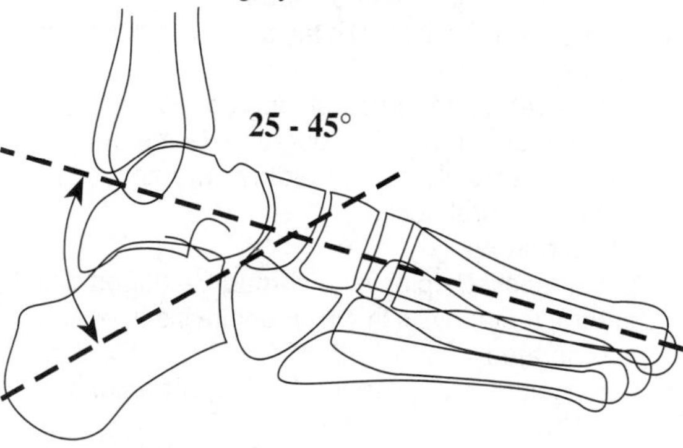

Talocalcaneal Angle on LAT View
= angle between lines drawn through mid-transverse planes of talus + calcaneus; the midtalar line parallels the longitudinal axis of the first metatarsal

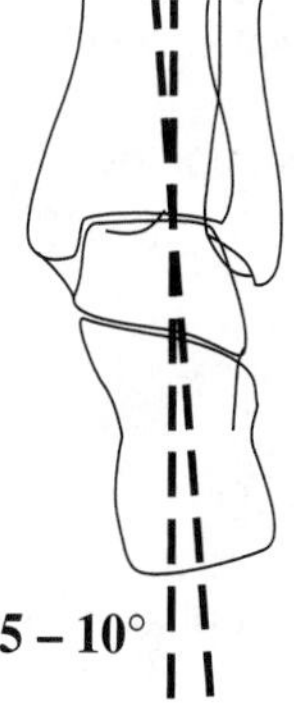

Heel Valgus
cannot be measured directly on radiographs but inferred from the talocalcaneal angle and estimated on coronal CT sections

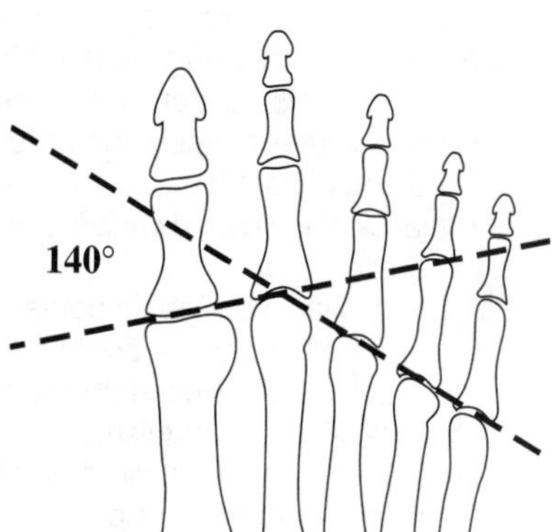

Angle of Metatarsal Heads
= obtuse angle formed by lines tangential to metatarsal heads

BONE AND SOFT-TISSUE DISORDERS

ACHONDROGENESIS

= autosomal recessive lethal chondrodystrophy characterized by extreme micromelia, short trunk, large cranium

TRIAD: (1) severe short-limb dwarfism
(2) lack of vertebral calcification
(3) large head with normal / decreased calvarial ossification

Birth prevalence: 2.3:100,000

Path: disorganization of cartilage

A. TYPE I = Parenti-Fraccaro disease
= defective enchondral + membranous ossification
√ complete lack of ossification of calvarium + spine + pelvis
√ absent sacrum + pubic bone
√ extremely short long bones without bowing, especially femur, radius, ulna
√ thin ribs with multiple fractures (frequent)

B. TYPE II = Langer-Saldino disease
= defective enchondral ossification only
√ good ossification of skull vault
√ nonossification of lower lumbar vertebrae + sacrum
√ short + stubby horizontal ribs without fractures

• often subcutaneous edema
√ irregular flared metaphyses (esp. humerus)
√ short trunk with narrow chest + protruding abdomen
√ redundant soft tissues
√ polyhydramnios (common)
√ increase in HC:AC ratio

Prognosis: lethal often in utero / within few hours or days after birth (respiratory failure)

DDx: often confused with thanatophoric dwarfism

ACHONDROPLASIA

Heterozygous Achondroplasia

◊ Prototype of rhizomelic dwarfism!

= autosomal dominant / sporadic (80%) disease with quantitatively defective endochondral bone formation; related to advanced paternal age; epiphyseal maturation + ossification unaffected

Incidence: 1:26,000–66,000 births, most common of lethal bone dysplasias; M < F

• normal intelligence + motor function
• neurologic defects
• classically circus dwarfs

@ Skull
• flat nasal bridge (hypoplastic base of skull)
• macrocephaly + brachycephaly with enlarged bulging forehead (nonprogressive hydrocephalus)
• relative prognathism
√ large calvarium with frontal bossing
√ depression of nasion
√ broad mandible
√ constricted basicranium + small foramen magnum:
√ communicating hydrocephalus caused by obstruction of basal cisterns + aqueduct

Cx: apnea + sudden death (due to compression of spinal cord + lower brain stem)

@ Chest
√ anteroposterior narrowing of chest
√ short anteriorly flared concave ribs
√ squaring of inferior scapular margin

@ Spine
√ hypoplastic bullet- / wedge-shaped vertebra:
√ rounded anterior beaking of vertebra in upper lumbar spine (DDx: Hurler disease)
√ decreased vertebral height
√ scalloped posteriorly concave vertebral margin
√ scoliosis:
√ thoracolumbar angular kyphosis (gibbus)
√ exaggerated sacral lordosis
√ stenosis of lumbar spine:
√ narrowing of interpedicular space due to laminar thickening
√ ventrodorsal narrowing of spine due to short pedicles
√ bulging / herniation of intervertebral disks
√ wide intervertebral foramina

@ Pelvis
• protuberant abdomen
• prominent buttocks
• rolling gait from backward tilt of pelvis and hip joints
√ square flattened iliac bones = tombstone configuration
√ "champagne glass"-shaped pelvic inlet
√ lack of flaring of iliac wings
√ horizontal acetabula (= flat acetabular angle)
√ small sacrosciatic notch

@ Extremities
• short stubby limbs + fingers
• trident hand = separation of 2nd + 3rd digit and inability to approximate 3rd + 4th finger
• limited range of motion of elbow
√ predominantly rhizomelic micromelia of long bones (femur, humerus):
√ "trumpet" appearance of long bones = shortening with disproportionate metaphyseal flaring (actually normal width of metaphysis)
√ short femoral necks
√ limb bowing
√ "ball-in-socket" epiphysis = broad V-shaped distal femoral metaphysis in which epiphysis is incorporated
√ high position of fibular head (= disproportionately long fibula)
√ short ulna with thick proximal + slender distal end
√ brachydactyly (short tubular bones of hand + feet), especially short proximal + middle phalanges

OB-US (diagnosable >21–27th week GA):
√ shortening of proximal long bones: femur length <99th percentile between 21 and 27 weeks MA

√ increased BPD, HC, HC:AC ratio
√ decreased FL:BPD ratio
√ normal mineralization, no fractures
√ normal thorax + normal cardiothoracic ratio
√ three-pronged (= trident) hand = 2nd + 3rd + 4th finger of similarly short length without completely approximating each other (= PATHOGNOMONIC)

Cx:
(1) Hydrocephalus + syringomyelia (small foramen magnum)
(2) Recurrent ear infection (poorly developed facial bones)
(3) Neurologic complications (compression of spinal cord, lower brainstem, cauda equina, nerve roots): apnea and sudden death
(4) Crowded dentition + malocclusion

Prognosis: long life
DDx: various mucopolysaccharidoses

Homozygous Achondroplasia

= hereditary autosomal dominant disease with severe features of achondroplasia (disproportionate limb shortening, more marked proximally than distally)
Risk: marriage of two achondroplasts to each other

√ large cranium with short base + small face
√ flattened nose bridge
√ short ribs with flared ends
√ hypoplastic vertebral bodies
√ decreased interpedicular distance
√ short squared innominate bones
√ flattened acetabular roof
√ small sciatic notch
√ short limb bones with flared metaphyses
√ short, broad, widely spaced tubular bones of hand

Prognosis: often stillborn; lethal in neonatal period (from respiratory failure)
DDx: thanatophoric dysplasia

ACROCEPHALOSYNDACTYLY

= syndrome characterized by
(1) increased height of skull vault due to generalized craniosynostosis (= acrocephaly, oxycephaly)
(2) syndactyly of fingers / toes

Type I : Apert syndrome = acrocephalosyndactyly
Type II : Vogt cephalosyndactyly
Type III : Acrocephalosyndactyly with asymmetry of skull + mild syndactyly
Type IV : Wardenburg type
Type V : Pfeiffer type

ACROOSTEOLYSIS, FAMILIAL

dominant inheritance
Age: onset in 2nd decade; M:F = 3:1
• sensory changes in hands + feet
• destruction of nails
• joint hypermobility
• swelling of plantar of foot with deep wide ulcer + ejection of bone fragments

@ Skull
√ wormian bones
√ craniosynostosis
√ basilar impression
√ protuberant occiput
√ resorption of alveolar processes + loss of teeth

@ Spine
√ spinal osteoporosis ± fracture
√ kyphoscoliosis + progressive decrease in height

ACROMEGALY

Etiology: excess growth hormone due to eosinophilic adenoma / hyperplasia in anterior pituitary
• gigantism in children: advanced bone age + excessive height (DDx: **Soto syndrome** of cerebral gigantism = large skull, mental retardation, cerebral atrophy, advanced bone age)
√ osseous enlargement (phalangeal tufts, vertebrae)
√ flared ends of long bone
√ cystic changes in carpals, femoral trochanters
√ osteoporosis

@ Hand
• spadelike hand
√ widening of terminal tufts

@ Skull
√ prognathism (= elongation of mandible) in few cases
√ sellar enlargement + erosion
√ enlargement of paranasal sinuses: large frontal sinuses (75%)
√ calvarial hyperostosis (especially inner table)
√ enlarged occipital protuberance

@ Vertebrae
√ posterior scalloping in 30% (secondary to pressure of enlarged soft tissue)
√ anterior new bone
√ loss of disk space (weakening of cartilage)

@ Soft tissue
√ heel pad >25 mm

@ Joints
√ premature osteoarthritis (commonly knees)

ACTINOMYCOSIS

= chronic suppurative infection characterized by formation of multiple abscesses, draining sinuses, abundant granulation tissue
Organism: Actinomyces israelii, Gram-positive anaerobic pleomorphic small bacterium with proteolytic activity, superficially resembling the morphology of a hyphal fungus (Gomori methenamine silver stain-positive filaments); closely related to mycobacteria
Histo: mycelial form in tissue; rod-shaped bacterial form normally inhabiting oropharynx (dental caries, gingival margins, tonsillar crypts) + GI tract
Predisposed: individuals with very poor dental hygiene, immunosuppressed patients
Location: mandibulofacial > intestinal > lung
Types:
(1) Mandibulo- / cervicofacial actinomycosis (55%)
Cause: poor oral hygiene

- draining cutaneous sinuses
- "sulfur granules" in sputum / exudate = colonies of organisms arranged in circular fashion = mycelial clumps with thin hyphae 1–2 mm in diameter

√ osteomyelitis of mandible (most frequent bone involved) with destruction of mandible around tooth socket
√ no new-bone formation
√ spread to soft tissues at angle of jaw + into neck

(2) Abdominopelvic / ileocecal actinomycosis (20%)
Cause: rupture / surgery of appendix; IUD use
Location: initially localized to cecum / appendix
- fever, leukocytosis, mild anemia
- weight loss, nausea, vomiting, pain
- chronic sinus in groin

√ fold thickening + ulcerations (resembling Crohn disease)
√ rupture of abdominal viscus (usually appendix)
√ fistula formation
√ abscess in liver (15%), retroperitoneum, psoas muscle (containing yellow "sulfur granules" = 1–2-mm colony of gram-positive bacilli)

(3) Pleuropulmonary actinomycosis (15%)
Cause: aspiration of infected material from oropharynx / hematogenous spread
Predisposed: alcoholics
Histo: masses of PMN leukocytes containing round actinomycotic / sulfur granules surrounded by a rim of granulation tissue

@ Lung
- draining chest wall sinuses (spread through fascial planes)

√ enhancing extensive transfissural chronic segmental consolidation (acute airspace pneumonia rare); usually unilateral + upper lobe predominance
√ cavitary lesion (abscess) with ringlike enhancement
√ fibrotic pleuritis
√ chronic pleural effusion / empyema
CT:
√ central areas of low attenuation within consolidation
√ adjacent pleural thickening
DDx: carcinoma, tuberculosis, bacterial / fungal pneumonia

@ Vertebra + ribs
√ destruction of vertebra with preservation of disk + small paravertebral abscess without calcification (DDx to tuberculosis: disk destroyed, large abscess with calcium)
√ thickening of cervical vertebrae around margins
√ destruction / thickening of ribs

(4) Mixed organs (10%)
@ Tubular bones of hands
√ destructive lesion of mottled permeating type
√ cartilage destruction + subarticular erosive defects in joints (simulating TB)
@ Skin, brain, pericardium

Rx: surgical débridement + penicillin

ADAMANTINOMA

= (MALIGNANT) ANGIOBLASTOMA
= locally aggressive / malignant lesion
Histo: pseudoepithelial cell masses with peripheral columnar cells in a palisade pattern with varying amounts of fibrous stroma; areas of squamous / tubular / alveolar / vessel transformation; prominent vascularity; resembles ameloblastoma of the jaw
Age: 25–50 years, commonest in 3rd–4th decade
- frequently history of trauma
- local swelling ± pain

Location: middle 1/3 of tibia (90%), fibula, ulna, carpals, metacarpals, humerus, shaft of femur
√ eccentric round osteolytic lesion with sclerotic margin, may have additional foci in continuity with major lesion (CHARACTERISTIC)
√ may show mottled density
√ bone expansion frequent
√ often multiple
Prognosis: tendency to recur after local excision; after several recurrences pulmonary metastases may develop
DDx: fibrous dysplasia (possibly related)

AINHUM DISEASE

= DACTYLOLYSIS SPONTANEA
[ainhum = fissure, saw, sword]
Etiology: unknown
Histo: hyperkeratotic epidermis with fibrotic thickening of collagen bundles below; chronic lymphocytic inflammatory reaction may be present; arterial walls may be thickened with narrowed vessel lumina
Incidence: up to 2%
Age: usually in males in 4th + 5th decades; Blacks (West Africa) + their American descendants; M > F
- deep soft-tissue groove forming on medial aspect of plantar surface of proximal phalanx with edema distally
- painful ulceration may develop

Location: mostly 5th / 4th toe (rarely finger); near interphalangeal joint; mostly bilateral
√ sharply demarcated progressive bone resorption of distal / middle phalanx with tapering of proximal phalanx to complete autoamputation (after an average of 5 years)
√ osteoporosis
Rx: early surgical resection of groove with Z-plasty
DDx: (1) Neuropathic disorders (diabetes, leprosy, syphilis)
(2) Trauma (burns, frostbite)
(3) Acroosteolysis from inflammatory arthritis, infection, polyvinyl chloride exposure
(4) Congenitally constricting bands in amniotic band syndrome

AMYLOIDOSIS

= extracellular deposition of a chemically diverse group of protein polysaccharides in body tissues (β_2-microglobulin); tends to form around capillaries + endothelial cells of larger blood vessels causing ultimately vascular obliteration with infarction

β_2-microglobulin = low-molecular-weight serum protein not filtered by standard dialysis membranes

Path: stains with Congo red

At risk: patients on long-term hemodialysis

- bone pain (eg, shoulder pain)
- periarticular rubbery soft-tissue swelling + stiffness (shoulders, hips, fingers)
  - carpal-tunnel syndrome (commonly bilateral)
- Bence Jones protein (without myeloma)

1. Synovial-articular pattern = **amyloid arthropathy**
   Location: cervical spine, hip, shoulder, elbow
   √ juxtaarticular soft-tissue swelling (amyloid deposited in synovium, joint capsule, tendons, ligaments) ± extrinsic osseous erosion
   √ mild periarticular osteoporosis
   √ subchondral cysts + well-defined sclerotic margin
   √ joint space preserved until late in course of disease
   √ subluxation of proximal humerus + femoral neck
   MR:
   √ extensive deposition of abnormal soft tissue of low to intermediate signal intensity on T1WI + T2WI covering synovial membrane, filling subchondral defects, extending into periarticular tissue
   √ joint effusion
   DDx: inflammatory arthritis

2. Diffuse marrow deposition
   √ generalized osteoporosis
   √ coarse trabecular pattern (DDx: sarcoidosis)
   √ pathologic collapse of vertebral body may occur

3. Localized destructive lesion (rarest form)
   Location: appendicular > axial skeleton
   √ focal medullary lytic lesion with endosteal scalloping (± secondary invasion + erosion of articular bone) = **amyloidoma**
   Cx: pathologic fracture

ANEURYSMAL BONE CYST

= expansile lesion of bone containing thin-walled blood-filled cystic cavities; name derived from roentgen appearance

Etiology:
(a) primary ABC (65–99%)
local circulatory disturbance as a result of trauma
(b) secondary ABC (1–35%)
arising in preexisting bone tumor causing venous obstruction / arteriovenous fistula: giant cell tumor (39%), osteoblastoma, chondroblastoma, angioma, telangiectatic osteosarcoma, solitary bone cyst, fibrous dysplasia, xanthoma, chondromyxoid fibroma, nonossifying fibroma, metastatic carcinoma

Histo: "intraosseous arteriovenous malformation" with honeycombed spaces filled with blood + lined by granulation tissue / osteoid; areas of free hemorrhage; sometimes multinucleated giant cells; solid component predominates in 5–7%

Types:
1. INTRAOSSEOUS ABC
   = primary cystic / telangiectatic tumor of giant cell family, originating in bone marrow cavity, slow expansion of cortex; rarely related to history of trauma
2. EXTRAOSSEOUS ABC
   = posttraumatic hemorrhagic cyst; originating on surface of bones, erosion through cortex into marrow

Age: peak age 16 years (range 10–30 years); in 75% <20 years; F > M

- pain of relatively acute onset with rapid increase of severity over 6–12 weeks
- ± history of trauma
- neurologic signs (radiculopathy to quadriplegia) if in spine

Location: (a) spine (12–30%) with slight predilection for posterior elements; thoracic > lumbar > cervical spine (22%); involvement of vertebral body (40–90%); may involve two contiguous vertebrae (25%)
(b) long bones: eccentric in metaphysis of femur, tibia, humerus, fibula; pelvis

√ purely lytic eccentric radiolucency
√ aggressive expansile ballooning lesion of "soap-bubble" pattern + thin internal trabeculations
√ rapid progression within 6 weeks to 3 months
√ sclerotic inner portion
√ almost invisible thin cortex (CT shows integrity)
√ tumor respects epiphyseal plate
√ no periosteal reaction (except when fractured)

CT:
√ "blood-filled sponge" = fluid-fluid / hematocrit levels due to blood sedimentation (in 10–35%)

MR:
√ multiple cysts of different signal intensity representing different stages of blood by-products
√ low-signal intensity rim = intact thickened periosteal membrane

NUC:
√ "doughnut sign" = peripheral increased uptake (64%)

Angio:
√ hypervascularity in lesion periphery (in 75%)

Prognosis: 20–30% recurrence rate

Rx: preoperative embolotherapy; complete resection; radiation therapy (subsequent sarcoma possible)

Cx: (1) pathologic fracture (frequent)
(2) extradural block with paraplegia

DDx: (1) Giant cell tumor (particularly in spine)
(2) Hemorrhagic cyst (end of bone / epiphysis, not expansile)
(3) Enchondroma
(4) Metastasis (renal cell + thyroid carcinoma)
(5) Plasmacytoma
(6) Chondro- and fibrosarcoma
(7) Fibrous dysplasia
(8) Hemophilic pseudotumor
(9) Hydatid cyst

ANGIOMATOSIS

= diffuse infiltration of bone / soft tissue by hemangiomatous / lymphangiomatous lesions

Age: first 3 decades of life

May be associated with:
chylothorax, chyloperitoneum, lymphedema, hepatosplenomegaly, cystic hygroma

A. OSSEOUS ANGIOMATOSIS (30–40%)
- indolent course

Location: femur > ribs > spine > pelvis > humerus > scapula > other long bones > clavicle

√ osteolysis with honeycomb / latticework ("hole-within-hole") appearance
√ may occur on both sides of joint

DDx: solitary osseous hemangioma

B. CYSTIC ANGIOMATOSIS
= extensive involvement of bone

Histo: endothelium-lined cysts in bone

Age: peak 10–15 years; range of 3 months to 55 years

Location: long bones, skull, flat bones

√ multiple osteolytic metaphyseal lesions of 1–2 mm to several cm with fine sclerotic margins + relative sparing of medullary cavity
√ may show overgrowth of long bone
√ endosteal thickening
√ sometimes associated with soft-tissue mass ± phleboliths
√ chylous pleural effusion suggests fatal prognosis

DDx: (other polyostotic diseases such as) histiocytosis X, fibrous dysplasia, metastases, Gaucher disease, congenital fibromatosis, Maffuci syndrome, neurofibromatosis, enchondromatosis

C. SOFT-TISSUE ANGIOMATOSIS (60–70%)
= VISCERAL ANGIOMATOSIS
- poor prognosis

D. ANGIOMATOUS SYNDROMES
1. Maffuci syndrome
2. Osler-Weber-Rendu syndrome
3. Klippel-Trenaunay-Weber disease
4. Kasabach-Merritt syndrome
5. Gorham disease

ANGIOSARCOMA

= aggressive vascular malignancy with frequent local recurrence + distant metastasis

Histo: vascular channels surrounded by hemangiomatous / lymphomatous cellular elements with high degree of anaplasia

Age: M:F = 2:1

Associated with: **Stewart-Treves syndrome**
= angiosarcoma with chronic lymphedema developing in postmastectomy patients

Location: skin (33%); soft tissue (24%); bone (6%): tibia (23%), femur (18%), humerus (13%), pelvis (7%)

DDx: hemangioendothelioma, hemangiopericytoma

ANKYLOSING SPONDYLITIS

= autoimmune disease of unknown etiology primarily affecting axial skeleton

Age: 15–35 years; M:F = 3:1–10:1; Caucasians:Blacks = 3:1

Associated with: (1) ulcerative colitis, regional enteritis
(2) iritis in 25%
(3) aortic insufficiency + atrioventricular conduction defect

- HLA-B 27 positive in 96%
- insidious onset of low back pain + stiffness

Path: involves synovial + cartilaginous joints and sites of ligamentous attachment

Location:
(a) axial skeleton: sacroiliac joints, thoracolumbar + lumbosacral junctions
◊ HALLMARK is sacroiliac joint involvement!
(b) peripheral skeleton (10–20%): sternal joint, symphysis pubis, hip, glenohumeral joint
(c) tendinous insertions in pelvis + proximal femur

Temporal course: initial abnormalities of sacroiliac joints + thoracolumbar junction with gradual involvement of remainder of spine

@ Skull
√ temporomandibular joint space narrowing, erosions, osteophytosis

@ Hand (30%)
Target area: MCP, PIP, DIP
√ exuberant osseous proliferation
√ osteoporosis, joint space narrowing, osseous erosions (deformities less striking than in rheumatoid arthritis)

@ Sacroiliac joint / symphysis pubis
√ initially sclerosis of joint margins primarily on iliac side (<u>bilateral + symmetric</u> late in disease, may be unilateral + asymmetric early in disease)
√ later irregularities + widening of joint (cartilage destruction)
√ bony fusion

@ Pelvis
√ periostitic "whiskering": ischial tuberosity, iliac crest, ischiopubic rami, greater femoral trochanter, external occipital protuberance, calcaneus

@ Spine
√ squaring = straightened / convex anterior vertebral margins = erosive osteitis of anterior corners
√ "shiny corner" = reactive sclerosis of corners of vertebral bodies
√ diskitis = erosive abnormalities of diskovertebral junction
√ "diskal ballooning" = biconvex shape of intervertebral disk related to osteoporotic deformity ± diskal calcification
√ marginal <u>syndesmophyte</u> formation = thin vertical radiodense spicules bridging the vertebral bodies = ossification of outer fibers of annulus fibrosus (NOT anterior longitudinal ligament)
√ "bamboo spine" on AP view = undulating contour due to syndesmophytosis

Cx: prone to fracture resulting in <u>pseudarthrosis</u>

√ asymmetric erosions of laminar + spinous processes of lumbar spine
√ ossification of supraspinous + interspinous ligaments:
  √ "dagger sign" = single radiodense line on AP view
  √ "trolley-track" sign on AP view = central line of ossification with two lateral lines of ossification (apophyseal joint capsules)
√ apophyseal + costovertebral joint ankylosis (on oblique views)
√ dorsal arachnoid diverticula in lumbar spine with erosion of posterior elements (Cx: cauda equina syndrome)
√ atlantoaxial subluxation

@ Chest
Incidence: 1% of patients with ankylosing spondylitis
Histo: interstitial + pleural fibrosis with foci of dense collagen deposition, NO granulomas
• bone manifestations obvious + severe
Location: apices / upper lung fields
√ sternomanubrial joint irregularities + sclerosis
√ uni- / bilateral coarse upper lobe pulmonary fibrosis with upward retraction of hila (DDx: tuberculosis)
√ reticulonodular progressively confluent opacities in lung apices
√ apical bullae + cavitation (mimicking TB)
HRCT:
  √ peripheral interstitial lung disease
  √ bronchiectasis
  √ paraseptal emphysema
  √ apical fibrosis
Cx: superinfection, especially with aspergillosis (mycetoma formation) / atypical mycobacteria
DDx: other causes of pulmonary apical fibrosis (primary infection by fungi / mycobacteria; cancer)

@ Cardiovascular
1. Aortitis (5%) of ascending aorta ± aortic valve insufficiency

Prognosis: 20% progress to significant disability; occasionally death from cervical spine fracture / aortitis
DDx: (1) Reiter syndrome (unilateral asymmetric SI joint involvement, paravertebral ossifications)
(2) Psoriatic arthritis (unilateral asymmetric SI joint involvement, paravertebral ossifications)
(3) Inflammatory bowel disease
(4) Sternocostoclavicular hyperostosis (pustulosis palmaris et plantaris)

ANTERIOR TIBIAL BOWING

= WEISMANN-NETTER SYNDROME
= congenital painless nonprogressive bilateral anterior leg bowing
Age: beginning in early childhood
• may be accompanied by mental retardation, goiter, anemia
√ anterior bowing of tibia + fibula, bilaterally, symmetrically at middiaphysis
√ thickening of posterior tibial + fibular cortices
√ minor radioulnar bowing
√ kyphoscoliosis
√ extensive dural calcification
DDx: Luetic saber shin (bowing at lower end of tibia + anterior cortical thickening)

APERT SYNDROME

= ACROCEPHALOSYNDACTYLY type I
Frequency: 5.5:1,000,000 neonates
Etiology: autosomal dominant with incomplete penetrance; sporadic (in majority)
Associated with CNS anomalies:
megalocephaly, gyral abnormalities, hypoplastic white matter, heterotopic gray matter, frontal encephalocele, corpus callosal agenesis, Kleeblattschädel, cleft palate, ventriculomegaly (? related to skull base hypoplasia, rarely progressive)
• IQ varies depending on CNS anomalies (in 50% normal)
• otitis media (high prevalence)
• bifid uvula
• conductive hearing loss (common due to external + middle ear malformations)

@ Skull
• downturned mouth
√ brachycephalic skull (due to coronal craniosynostosis) + flat occiput
√ widened metopic + sagittal sutures extending from glabella to posterior fontanel (closing between 2 to 4 years)
√ hypoplastic / retruded midface:
  √ hypertelorism
  √ shallow orbits with proptosis
  √ underdeveloped paranasal sinuses
  √ underdeveloped maxilla with prognathism
√ high pointed arch of palate
√ prominent vertical crest in middle of forehead (increased intracranial pressure)
√ V-shaped anterior fossa due to elevation of lateral margins of lesser sphenoid
√ sella may be enlarged
√ stylohyoid ligament calcification (38–88%)
√ cervical spine fusion (in up to 71%), commonly of 5th and 6th vertebrae
√ choanal stenosis

@ Hand & feet
√ severe symmetric syndactyly = fusion of distal portions of phalanges, metacarpals / carpals (most often of 2nd, 3rd + 4th digit)
√ absence of middle phalanges
√ missing / supernumerary carpal / tarsal bones
√ pseudarthroses

@ GU (10%)
• cryptorchidism
√ hydronephrosis
√ polycystic kidneys (rare)
√ bicornuate uterus (rare)

ARTERIOVENOUS FISTULA OF BONE

Etiology: (a) acquired (usually gunshot wound)
(b) congenital

Location: lower extremity most frequent

√ soft-tissue mass
√ presence of large vessels
√ phleboliths (DDx: long-standing varicosity)
√ accelerated bone growth
√ cortical osteolytic defect (= pathway for large vessels into medulla)
√ increased bone density

ARTHROGRYPOSIS

= ARTHROGRYPOSIS MULTIPLEX CONGENITA
= nonprogressive congenital syndrome complex characterized by poorly developed + contracted muscles, deformed joints with thickened periarticular capsule and intact sensory system

Pathophysiology:
congenital / acquired defect of motor unit (anterior horn cells, nerve roots, peripheral nerves, motor end plates, muscle) early in fetal life with immobilization of joints at various stages in their development

Cause: ? neurotropic agents, toxic chemicals, hard drugs, hyperthermia, neuromuscular blocking agents, mytotic abnormalities, mechanical immobilization

Incidence: 0.03% of newborn infants; 5% risk of recurrence in sibling

Path: diminution in size of muscle fibers + fat deposits in fibrous tissue

Associated with:
(1) neurogenic disorders (90%)
(2) myopathic disorders
(3) skeletal dysplasias
(4) intrauterine limitation of movement (myomata, amniotic band, twin, oligohydramnios)
(5) connective tissue disorders

Distribution: all extremities (46%), lower extremities only (43%), upper extremities only (11%); peripheral joints >> proximal joints; symmetrical

• clubfoot
• congenital dislocation of hip
• claw hand
• diminished muscle mass
• skin webs

√ flexion + extension contractures
√ osteopenia ± pathologic fractures
√ congenital dislocation of hip
√ carpal coalition
√ vertical talus
√ calcaneal valgus deformity

ASPHYXIATING THORACIC DYSPLASIA

= JEUNE DISEASE
= autosomal recessive dysplasia

Incidence: 100 cases

Associated with: renal anomalies (hydroureter), PDA

• respiratory distress due to reduced thoracic mobility (abdominal breathing) + frequent pulmonary infections
• progressive renal failure + hypertension

@ Chest
√ markedly narrow + elongated bell-shaped chest:
√ chest diameter significantly decreased compared with that of the abdomen
√ normal size of heart leaving little room for lungs
√ horizontal clavicles at level of 6th cervical vertebra
√ short horizontal ribs + irregular bulbous costochondral junction

@ Pelvis
√ trident pelvis (retardation of ossification of triradiate cartilage)
√ small iliac wings flared + shortened in cephalocaudal diameter ("wineglass" pelvis)
√ short ischial + pubic bones
√ reduced acetabular angle + acetabular spurs
√ premature ossification of capital femoral epiphysis

@ Extremities
√ rhizomelic brachymelia (humerus, femur) = long bones shorter + wider than normal
√ metaphyseal irregularity
√ postaxial hexadactyly (occasionally)
√ shortening of distal phalanges + cone-shaped epiphyses in hands + feet
√ proximal humeral + femoral epiphyses ossified at birth (frequently)

@ Kidneys
√ medullary cystic renal disease = enlarged kidneys with linear streaking on nephrogram (in adulthood)

OB-US:
√ proportionate shortening of long bones
√ small thorax with decreased circumference
√ increased cardiothoracic ratio
√ occasionally polydactyly
√ polyhydramnios

Prognosis: neonatal death in 80% (respiratory failure + infections)

DDx: Ellis-van Creveld syndrome

AVASCULAR NECROSIS

= AVN = OSTEONECROSIS = ASEPTIC NECROSIS
= consequence of interrupted blood supply to bone with death of cellular elements

Histo:
(a) cellular ischemia leading to death of hematopoietic cells (in 6–12 hours), osteocytes (in 12–48 hours) and lipocytes (in 2–5 days)
(b) necrotic debris in intertrabecular spaces + proliferation and infiltration by mesenchymal cells + capillaries
(c) mesenchymal cells differentiate to osteoblasts on the surface of dead trabeculae synthesizing new bone layers + resulting in trabecular thickening

Pathogenesis:
(1) obstruction of extra- and intraosseous vessels by arterial embolism, venous thrombosis, traumatic disruption, external compression (increased marrow space pressure)
(2) cumulative stress from cytotoxic factors

Cause:
A. Traumatic interruption of arteries
  @ femoral head:
    1. Femoral neck fracture (60–75%)
    2. Dislocation of hip joint (25%)
    3. Slipped capital femoral epiphysis (15–40%)
  @ carpal scaphoid:
    4–6 months after fracture (in 10–15%), in 30–40% of nonunion of scaphoid fracture
    Site: proximal fragment (most common)
  @ humeral head (infrequent)
B. Embolization of arteries
  1. Hemoglobinopathy: sickle-cell disease
  2. Nitrogen bubbles: Caisson disease
C. Vasculitis
  1. Collagen-vascular disease: SLE
  2. Radiation exposure
D. Abnormal accumulation of cells
  1. Lipid-containing histiocytes: Gaucher disease
  2. Fat cells: steroid therapy
E. Idiopathic
  1. Spontaneous osteonecrosis of knee
  2. Legg-Calvé-Perthes disease
  3. Freiberg disease

mnemonic: "PLASTIC RAGS"
Pancreatitis, **P**regnancy
Legg-Perthes disease, **L**upus erythematosus
Alcoholism, **A**therosclerosis
Steroids
Trauma (femoral neck fracture, hip dislocation)
Idiopathic (Legg-Perthes disease), **I**nfection
Caisson disease, **C**ollagen disease (SLE)
Rheumatoid arthritis, **R**adiation treatment
Amyloid
Gaucher disease
Sickle cell disease

mnemonic: "GIVE INFARCTS"
Gaucher disease
Idiopathic (Legg-Calvé-Perthes, Köhler, Chandler)
Vasculitis (SLE, polyarteritis nodosa, rheumatoid arthritis)
Environmental (frostbite, thermal injury)
Irradiation
Neoplasia (-associated coagulopathy)
Fat (prolonged corticosteroid use increases marrow)
Alcoholism
Renal failure + dialysis
Caisson disease
Trauma (femoral neck fracture, hip dislocation)
Sickle cell disease

NO predisposing factors in 25%!

Location: femoral head (most common), humeral head, femoral condyles

Avascular Necrosis of Hip

◊ Involvement of one hip increases risk to contralateral hip to 70%!

Age: 20–50 years

• hip / groin / thigh / knee pain
• limited range of motion

Plain film (positive only several months after symptoms):
√ subtle relative sclerosis of femoral head secondary to resorption of surrounding vascularized bone (earliest sign)
√ radiolucent crescent parallel to articular surface in weight-bearing portion secondary to subchondral structural collapse of necrotic segment
  Site: anterosuperior portion of femoral head (best seen on frogleg view)
√ preservation of joint space (DDx: arthritis)
√ flattening of articular surface
√ increased density of femoral head (compression of bony trabeculae following microfracture of nonviable bone, calcification of dendritic marrow, creeping substitution = deposition of new bone)

Classification (Steinberg):

Stage 0	=	normal
Stage I	=	normal / barely detectable trabecular mottling; abnormal bone scan / MRI
Stage IIA	=	focal sclerosis + osteopenia
Stage IIB	=	distinct sclerosis + osteoporosis + early crescent sign
Stage IIIA	=	subchondral undermining ("crescent sign") + cyst formation
Stage IIIB	=	mild alteration in femoral head contour / subchondral fracture + normal joint space
Stage IV	=	marked collapse of femoral head + significant acetabular involvement
Stage V	=	joint space narrowing + acetabular degenerative changes

NUC (80–85% sensitivity):
◊ Bone marrow imaging (with radiocolloid) more sensitive than bone imaging (with diphosphonates)
◊ More sensitive than plain films in early AVN (evidence of ischemia seen as much as 1 year earlier)
◊ Less sensitive than MR

Technique: imaging improved with double counts, pinhole collimation

√ early: cold = photopenic defect (interrupted blood supply)
√ late: "doughnut sign" = cold spot surrounded by increased uptake secondary to
  (a) capillary revascularization + new-bone synthesis
  (b) degenerative osteoarthritis

CT (utilized for staging of known disease):
√ staging upgrades in 30% compared with plain films

MR (90–100% sensitive, 85% specific for symptomatic disease):

Prevalence of clinically occult disease: 6%

◊ MR imaging changes reflect the death of marrow fat cells (not death of osteocytes with empty lacunae)!

◊ Sagittal images particularly useful!

Classification (Mitchell):

Stage	*T1*	*T2*	*Analogous to*
A	high	intermediate	fat
B	high	high	subacute blood
C	low	high	fluid / edema
D	low	low	fibrosis

EARLY AVN:
- √ decreased Gd-enhancement on short-inversion-recovery (STIR) images (very early)
- √ low-signal intensity band with sharp inner interface + blurred outer margin on T1WI within 12–48 hours (= mesenchymal + fibrous repair tissue, amorphous cellular debris, thickened trabecular bone) seen as
  (a) band extending to subchondral bone plate
  (b) complete ring (less frequent)
- √ "double-line sign" on T2WI (in 80%) [MORE SPECIFIC] = juxtaposition of inner hyperintense band (granulation tissue) + outer hypointense band (chemical shift artifact / fibrosis + sclerosis)

ADVANCED AVN:
- √ "pseudohomogeneous edema pattern" = inhomogeneous large areas of mostly decreased signal intensity on T1WI
- √ hypo- to hyperintense lesion on T2WI
- √ contrast-enhancement of interface + surrounding marrow + within lesion

SUBCHONDRAL FRACTURE:
- √ predilection for anterosuperior portion of femoral head (sagittal images!)
- √ cleft of low-signal intensity running parallel to the subchondral bone plate within areas of fatlike signal intensity on T1WI
- √ hyperintense band (= fracture cleft filled with articular fluid / edema) within the intermediate- or low-signal-intensity necrotic marrow on T2WI
- √ lack of enhancement within + around fracture cleft

EPIPHYSEAL COLLAPSE:
- √ focal depression of subchondral bone

Cx: early osteoarthritis through collapse of femoral head + joint incongruity in 3–5 years if left untreated

Rx:
(1) core decompression (for grade 0–II): most successful with <25% involvement of femoral head
(2) osteotomy (for grade 0–II)
(3) arthroplasty / arthrodesis / total hip replacement (for grade >III)

DDx: bone marrow edema (ill-delimited marrow changes, no reactive interface); epiphyseal fracture (speckled / linear hypointense areas, focal depression of epiphyseal contour); spondyloarthropathy

Blount Disease

= TIBIA VARA
= avascular necrosis of medial tibial condyle
Age: >6 years
- • limping, lateral bowing of leg
- √ medial tibial condyle enlarged + deformed (DDx: Turner syndrome)
- √ irregularity of metaphysis (medially + posteriorly prolonged with beak)

Calvé-Kümmel-Verneuil Disease

= VERTEBRAL OSTEOCHONDROSIS = VERTEBRA PLANA
= avascular necrosis of vertebral body
Age: 2–15 years
- √ uniform collapse of vertebral body into flat thin disk
- √ increased density of vertebra
- √ neural arches NOT affected
- √ disks are normal with normal intervertebral disk space
- √ intravertebral vacuum cleft sign (PATHOGNOMONIC)

DDx: eosinophilic granuloma, metastatic disease

Freiberg Disease

[Albert Henry Freiberg (1868–1940), orthopedic surgeon in Cincinnati, Ohio]
= osteochondrosis of head of 2nd (3rd / 4th) metatarsal
Age: 10–18 years; M:F = 1:3
- • metatarsalgia, swelling, tenderness

Early:
- √ flattening, increased density, cystic lesions of metatarsal head
- √ widening of metatarsophalangeal joint

Late:
- √ osteochondral fragment
- √ sclerosis + flattening of metatarsal head
- √ increased cortical thickening

Kienböck Disease

= LUNATOMALACIA
[Robert Kienböck (1871–1953), radiologist in Vienna, Austria]
= avascular necrosis of lunate bone
Predisposed: individuals engaged in manual labor with repeated / single episode of trauma
Age: 20–40 years
Associated with: ulna minus variant (short ulna) in 75%
- • progressive pain + soft-tissue swelling of wrist

Location: uni- > bilateral (usually right hand)
- √ initially normal radiograph
- √ osteonecrotic fracture of carpal lunate
- √ increased density + altered shape + collapse of lunate

Cx: scapholunate separation, ulnar deviation of triquetrum, degenerative joint disease in radiocarpal / midcarpal compartments
Rx: ulnar lengthening / radial shortening, lunate replacement

Köhler Disease

= avascular necrosis of tarsal scaphoid
Age: 3–10 years; boys
√ irregular outline
√ fragmentation
√ disklike compression in AP direction
√ increased density
√ joint space maintained
√ decreased / increased uptake on radionuclide study

Legg-Calvé-Perthes Disease

= COXA PLANA
= idiopathic avascular necrosis of femoral head in children; one of the most common sites of AVN; in 5–10% bilateral
Age: (a) 2–12 (peak, 4–8) years: M:F = 5:1
(b) adulthood: **Chandler disease**
Cause: trauma in 30% (subcapital fracture, epiphyseolysis, esp. posterior dislocation), closed reduction of congenital hip dislocation, prolonged interval between injury and reduction
Pathophysiology:
insufficient femoral head blood supply (epiphyseal plate acts as a barrier in ages 4–10; ligamentum teres vessels become nonfunctional; blood supply is from medial circumflex artery + lateral epiphyseal artery only)
Stages:
I = histologic + clinical diagnosis without radiographic findings
II = sclerosis ± cystic changes with preservation of contour + surface of femoral head
III = loss of structural integrity of femoral head
IV = in addition loss of structural integrity of acetabulum

• 1 week–6 months (mean 2.7 months) duration of symptoms prior to initial presentation: limp, pain
NUC (may assist in early diagnosis):
√ decreased uptake (early) in femoral head = interruption of blood supply
√ increased uptake (late) in femoral head =
(a) revascularization + bone repair
(b) degenerative osteoarthritis
√ increased acetabular activity with associated degenerative joint disease

X-RAY:
Early signs:
√ femoral epiphysis smaller than on contralateral side (96%)
√ sclerosis of femoral head epiphysis (sequestration + compression) (82%)
√ slight widening of joint space due to thickening of cartilage, failure of epiphyseal growth, presence of joint fluid, joint laxity (60%)
√ ipsilateral bone demineralization (46%)
√ alteration of pericapsular soft-tissue outline due to atrophy of ipsilateral periarticular soft tissues (73%)
√ rarefaction of lateral + medial metaphyseal areas of neck
√ NEVER destruction of articular cortex as in bacterial arthritis
Late signs:
√ delayed osseous maturation of a mild degree
√ "radiolucent crescent line" of subchondral fracture = small archlike subcortical lucency (32%)
√ subcortical fracture on anterior articular surface (best seen on frogleg view)
√ femoral head fragmentation
√ femoral neck cysts (from intramedullary hemorrhage in response to stress fractures)
√ loose bodies (only found in males)
Regenerative signs:
√ coxa plana = flattened collection of sclerotic fragments (over 18 months)
√ coxa magna = remodeling of femoral head to become wider + flatter in mushroom configuration to match widened metaphysis + epiphyseal plate
CT:
√ loss of "asterisk" sign (= starlike pattern of crossing trabeculae in center of femoral head) with distortion of asterisk and extension to surface of femoral head
MR:
√ normal signal intensity in marrow of femoral epiphysis replaced by low signal intensity on T1WI + high signal intensity on T2WI = "asterisk" sign
√ "double-line" sign (80%) = sclerotic nonsignal rim producing line between necrotic + viable bone edged by a hyperintense rim of granulation tissue
√ fluid within fracture plane
√ hip joint incongruity: lateral femoral head uncovering, labral inversion, femoral head deformity
Cx: severe degenerative joint disease in early adulthood
Rx: bed rest, abduction bracing (to reduce stress on infarcted head)

Panner Disease

= osteonecrosis of capitellum

Preiser Disease

= nontraumatic osteonecrosis of scaphoid

Spontaneous Osteonecrosis of Knee

= SONK
Cause: ? meniscal tear (78%), trauma with resultant microfractures, vascular insufficiency, degenerative joint disease, severe chondromalacia, gout, rheumatoid arthritis, joint bodies, intraarticular steroid injection (45–85%)

Age: 7th decade (range 13–83 years)
- acute onset of pain

Location: weight-bearing medial condyle more toward epicondylus (95%), lateral condyle (5%), may involve tibial plateau

√ radiographs usually normal (within 3 months after onset)
√ positive bone scan within 5 weeks (most sensitive)
√ flattening of weight-bearing segment of medial femoral epicondyle
√ radiolucent focus in subchondral bone + peripheral zone of osteosclerosis
√ horizontal subchondral fracture (within 6–9 months) + osteochondral fragment
√ periosteal reaction along medial side of femoral shaft (30–50%)

Cx: osteoarthritis

BASAL CELL NEVUS SYNDROME

= NEVOID BASAL CELL CARCINOMA SYNDROME = GORLIN SYNDROME
= syndrome of autosomal dominant inheritance characterized by
(1) multiple cutaneous basal cell carcinomas during childhood
(2) odontogenic keratocysts of mandible
(3) ectopic calcifications
(4) skeletal anomalies

- multiple nevoid basal cell carcinomas (nose, mouth, chest, back) at mean age of 19 years; after puberty aggressive, may metastasize
- pitlike defects in palms + soles
- mental retardation

Association: high incidence of medulloblastoma in children; ovarian fibroma (in 17%); cardiac fibroma (in 14%)

√ mandibular hypoplasia:
  √ multiple mandibular + maxillary cysts (dentigerous cysts + ectopic dentition)
√ anomalies of upper 5 ribs:
  √ forked = bifid rib (most commonly 4th rib)
  √ agenesis / supernumerary ribs
  √ fusion of adjacent ribs
  √ dysplastic distorted ribs
√ bifid spinous processes, spina bifida
√ scoliosis (cervical + upper thoracic)
√ hemivertebrae + block vertebrae
√ Sprengel deformity (scapula elevated, hypoplastic, bowed)
√ deficiency of lateral clavicle
√ brachydactyly
√ extensive calcification of falx + tentorium
√ ectopic calcifications of subcutaneous tissue, ovaries, sacrotuberous ligaments, mesentery
√ bony bridging of sella turcica
√ macrocephaly

BATTERED CHILD SYNDROME

= CAFFEY-KEMPE SYNDROME = CHILD ABUSE = PARENT - INFANT TRAUMATIC STRESS SYNDROME = NON-ACCIDENTAL TRAUMA

◊ Most common cause of serious intracranial injuries in children <1 year of age; 3rd most common cause of death in children after sudden infant death syndrome + true accidents

Prevalence: 1.7 million cases reported + 833,000 substantiated in United States in 1990 (45% neglected children, 25% physically abused, 16% sexually abused children); resulting in 2,500–5,000 deaths/year; 5–10% of children seen in emergency rooms

Age: usually <2 years

- skin burns, bruising, lacerations, hematomas (SNAT = suspected nonaccidental trauma)

@ Skeletal trauma (50–80%)
Site: multiple ribs, costochondral / costovertebral separation, acromion, skull, anterior-superior wedging of vertebra, tibia, metacarpus
Unusual sites: transverse fracture of sternum, lateral end of clavicles, scapula, vertebral compression, vertebral fracture dislocation, disk space narrowing, spinous processes
Other clues: bilateral acute fractures, fractures of lower extremities in children not yet walking

√ multiple asymmetric fractures in different stages of healing (repeated injury = HALLMARK)
√ exuberant callus formation at fracture sites
√ avulsion fracture of ligamentous insertion; frequently seen without periosteal reaction

@ Epiphysis
  √ separation of distal epiphysis

@ Metaphysis
  √ marked irregularity + fragmentation of metaphyses (DDx: osteochondritis stage of congenital syphilis; infractions of scurvy)
  √ "corner" fracture (11%) = "bucket-handle" fracture = avulsion of an arcuate metaphyseal fragment overlying the lucent epiphyseal cartilage
  Cause: sudden twisting motion of extremity (periosteum easily pulled away from diaphysis but tightly attached to metaphysis)
  Location: knee, elbow, distal tibia, fibula, radius, ulna

@ Diaphysis
  √ isolated spiral fracture (15%) of diaphysis secondary to external rotatory force applied to femur / humerus
  √ extensive periosteal reaction from large subperiosteal hematoma apparent after 7–14 days following injury (DDx: scurvy, copper deficiency)

√ cortical hyperostosis extending to epiphyseal plate (DDx: not in infantile cortical hyperostosis)

@ Head trauma (13–25%)
Most common cause of death + physical disability
(1) Impact injury with translational force: skull fracture (flexible calvaria + meninges decrease likelihood of skull fractures), subdural hematoma, brain contusion, cerebral hemorrhage, infarction, generalized edema
(2) Whiplash injury with rotational force: shearing injuries + associated subarachnoid hemorrhage
• bulging fontanels, convulsions
• ocular lesions, retinal detachment
Skull film (associated fracture in 1%):
√ linear fracture > comminuted fracture > diastases (conspicuously absent)
CT:
√ subdural hemorrhage (most common): interhemispheric location most common
√ subarachnoid hemorrhage
√ epidural hemorrhage (uncommon)
√ cerebral edema (focal, multifocal, diffuse)
√ acute cerebral contusion as ovoid collection of intraparenchymal blood with surrounding edema
MR: more sensitive in identifying hematomas of differing ages
√ white matter shearing injuries as areas of prolonged T1 + T2 at corticomedullary junction, centrum semiovale, corpus callosum

@ Viscera (3%)
◊ Second leading cause of death in child abuse
Cause: crushing blow to abdomen (punch, kick)
Age: often >2 years
√ small bowel / gastric rupture
√ hematoma of duodenum / jejunum
√ contusion / laceration of lung, pancreas, liver, spleen, kidneys
√ traumatic pancreatic pseudocyst

Cx: (1) Brain atrophy (up to 100%)
(2) Infarction (50%)
(3) Subdural hygroma
(4) Encephalomalacia
(5) Porencephaly

DDx: normal periostitis of infancy, long-term ventilator therapy in prematurity, osteogenesis imperfecta, congenital insensitivity to pain, infantile cortical hyperostosis, Menkes kinky hair syndrome, Schmid-type chondrometaphyseal dysplasia, scurvy, congenital syphilitic metaphysitis

BENIGN CORTICAL DEFECT

= developmental intracortical bone defect
Age: usually 1st–2nd decade; uncommon in boys <2 years of age; uncommon in girls <4 years of age
• asymptomatic
Site: metaphysis of long bone
√ well-defined intracortical round / oval lucency
√ usually <2 cm long
√ sclerotic margins

Cx: pathologic / avulsion fracture following minor trauma (infrequent)

Prognosis: (1) Spontaneous healing resulting in sclerosis / disappearance
(2) Ballooning of endosteal surface of cortex = fibrous cortical defect
(3) Medullary extension resulting in nonossifying fibroma

BONE INFARCT

Etiology:
A. Occlusion of vessel:
(a) thrombus: thromboembolic disease, sickle cell anemia (SS + SC hemoglobin), polycythemia rubra vera
(b) fat: pancreatitis (intramedullary fat necrosis from circulating lipase), alcoholism
(c) gas: Caisson disease, astronauts
B. Vessel wall disease:
1. Arteritis: SLE, rheumatoid arthritis, polyarteritis nodosa, sarcoidosis
2. Arteriosclerosis
C. Vascular compression by deposition of:
(a) fat: corticosteroid therapy (eg, renal transplant, Cushing disease)
(b) blood: trauma (fractures + dislocations)
(c) inflammatory cells: osteomyelitis, infection, histiocytosis X
(d) edema: radiation therapy, hypothyroidism, frostbite
(e) substances: Gaucher disease (vascular compression by lipid-filled histiocytes), gout
D. Others: idiopathic, hypopituitarism, pheochromocytoma (microscopic thrombotic disease), osteochondroses

Medullary Infarction

◊ Nutrient artery is the sole blood supply for diaphysis!
Location: distal femur, proximal tibia, iliac wings, ribs, humeri
(a) Acute phase:
√ NO radiographic changes without cortical involvement
√ area of rarefaction
√ bone marrow scan: diminished uptake in medullary RES for long period of time
√ bone scan: photon-deficient lesion within 24–48 hours; increased uptake after collateral circulation established
(b) Healing phase (complete healing / fibrosis / calcification):
√ demarcation by zone of serpiginous / linear calcification + ossification parallel to cortex
√ dense bone indicating revascularization

Cortical Infarction

◊ Requires compromise of
(a) nutrient artery and (b) periosteal vessels!
Age: particularly in childhood where periosteum is easily elevated by edema

√ avascular necrosis = osteonecrosis
√ osteochondrosis dissecans
Cx: (1) Growth disturbances
√ cupped / triangular / coned epiphyses
√ "H-shaped" vertebral bodies
(2) Fibrosarcoma (most common), malignant fibrous histiocytoma, benign cysts
(3) Osteoarthritis

BONE ISLAND

= ENOSTOSIS = ENDOSTEOMA = COMPACT ISLAND = FOCAL SCLEROSIS = SCLEROTIC BONE ISLAND = CALCIFIED MEDULLARY DEFECT
= focal lesion of densely sclerotic (compact) bone nesting within spongiosa
Age: any age (mostly 20–80 years of age); grows more rapidly in children
Histo: nest of lamellar compacted bone with haversian system embedded within medullary canal
Pathogenesis:
? misplaced cortical hamartoma, ? developmental error of endochondral ossification as a coalescence of mature bone trabeculae with failure to undergo remodeling; not inherited
• asymptomatic
Location: ilium + proximal femur (88–92%), ribs, spine (1–14%), humerus, phalanges (not in skull)
√ round / oval / oblong solitary osteoblastic lesion with abrupt transition to surrounding normal trabecular bone
√ long axis of bone island parallels long axis of bone
√ usually 2–10 mm in size; lesion >2 cm in longest axis = **giant bone island**
√ "brush border" = "thorny radiations" = sharply demarcated margins with feathery peripheral radiations (HALLMARK) blending with trabeculae of surrounding spongiosa
√ may show activity on bone scan, esp. if large (33%)
√ may demonstrate slow growth / decrease in size (32%)
√ NO involvement of cortex / radiolucencies / periosteal reaction
Prognosis: may increase to 8–12 cm over years (40%); may decrease / disappear
DDx: (1) Osteoblastic metastasis (aggressive, break through cortex, periosteal reaction)
(2) Low-grade osteosarcoma (cortical thickening, extension beyond medullary cavity)
(3) Osteoid osteoma (pain relieved by aspirin, nidus)
(4) Benign osteoblastoma
(5) Involuted nonossifying fibroma replaced by dense bone scar
(6) Eccentric focus of monostotic fibrous dysplasia
(7) Osteoma (surface lesion)

BRUCELLOSIS

= multisystemic zoonosis of worldwide distribution; endemic in Saudi Arabia, Arabian Peninsula, South America, Spain, Italy (secondary to ingestion of raw milk / milk products)
Organism: small Gram-negative nonmotile, nonsporing, aflagellate, nonencapsulated coccobacilli: Brucella abortus, B. suis, B. canis, B. melitensis
Histo: small intracellular pathogens shed in excreta of infected animals (urine, stool, milk, products of conception) cause small noncaseating granuloma within RES
Location: commonest site of involvement is reticuloendothelial system; musculoskeletal system
• 1–3 weeks between initial infection + symptoms
◊ Radiologic evidence of disease in 69% of symptomatic sites!
@ Brucellar spondylitis (53%)
Age: 40 years is average age at onset
• pain, localized tenderness, radiculopathy, myelopathy
Location: lumbar (71%) > thoracolumbar (10%) > lumbosacral (8%) > cervical (7%) > thoracic (4%)
(a) focal form
√ bone destruction at diskovertebral junction (anterior aspect of superior endplate)
√ associated with bone sclerosis + anterior osteophyte formation + small amount of gas
(b) diffuse form: entire vertebral endplate / whole vertebral body affected with spread to adjacent disks + vertebral bodies
√ bone destruction associated with sclerosis
√ small amount of disk gas (25–30%)
√ obliteration of paraspinal muscle-fat planes
√ no / minimal epidural extension
DDx: TB (paraspinal abscess, gibbus)
@ Extraspinal disease
(a) Brucellar synovitis (81%)
Location: knee > sacroiliac joint > shoulder > hip > sternoclavicular joint > ankle > elbow
Site: organism localized in synovial membrane
• serosanguinous sterile joint effusion
(b) Brucellar destructive arthritis (9%)
√ indistinguishable from tuberculous / pyogenic arthritis
(c) Brucellar osteomyelitis (2%)
• pain, tenderness, swelling
(d) Brucellar myositis (2%)
Dx: serologic tests (enzyme-linked immunosorbent assay, counterimmunoelectrophoresis, rose bengal plate test
Rx: combination of aminoglycosides + tetracyclines
DDx: fibrous dysplasia, benign tumor, osteoid osteoma

CAISSON DISEASE

= DECOMPRESSION SICKNESS = THE BENDS
Etiology: during too rapid decompression = reduction of surrounding pressure (ascent from dive, exit from caisson / hyperbaric chamber, ascent to altitude) nitrogen bubbles form (nitrogen more soluble in fat of panniculus adiposus, spinal cord, brain, bones containing fatty marrow)
• "the bends" = local pain in knee, elbow, shoulder, hip
• neurologic symptoms (paresthesia, major cerebral / spinal involvement)
• "chokes" = substernal discomfort + coughing (embolization of pulmonary vessels)

Location: mostly in long tubular bones of lower extremity (distal end of shaft + epiphyseal portion); symmetrical lesions
√ early: area of rarefaction
√ healing phase: irregular new-bone formation with greater density
√ peripheral zone of calcification / ossification
√ ischemic necrosis of articular surface with secondary osteoarthritis

CALCIUM PYROPHOSPHATE DIHYDRATE CRYSTAL DEPOSITION DISEASE

= CPPD = PSEUDOGOUT = FAMILIAL CHONDROCALCINOSIS
◊ Most common crystalline arthropathy
Types: 1. Osteoarthritic form (35–60%)
2. Pseudogout = acute synovitis (10–20%)
3. Rheumatoid form (2–6%)
4. Pseudoneuropathic arthropathy (2%)
5. Asymptomatic with tophaceous pseudogout (common)

Associated with: **h**yperparathyroidism, **h**ypothyroidism, **h**emochromatosis, **h**ypomagnesemia
Prevalence: widespread in older population; M:F = 3:2
• calcium pyrophosphate crystals in synovial fluid + within leukocytes (characteristic weakly positive birefringent diffraction pattern)
• acute / subacute / chronic joint inflammation
Location: (a) knee (especially meniscus + cartilage of patellofemoral joint)
(b) wrist (triangular fibrocartilage in distal radioulnar joint bilaterally)
(c) pelvis (sacroiliac joint, symphysis)
(d) spine (annulus fibrosis of lumbar intervertebral disk; NEVER in nucleus pulposus as in ochronosis)
(e) shoulder (glenoid), hip (labrum), elbow, ankle, acromioclavicular joint
√ polyarticular chondrocalcinosis (in fibro- and hyaline cartilage)
√ large subchondral cyst (HALLMARK)
√ numerous intraarticular bodies (fragmentation of subchondral bone)
√ involvement of tendons, bursae, pinnae of the ear
N.B.: pyrophosphate arthropathy resembles osteoarthritis: joint space narrowing + extensive subchondral sclerosis

@ Hand
Site: radiocarpal compartment; trapezioscaphoid joint + 1 CMC; 2,3 MCP joints; bilateral symmetric
√ resembling degenerative joint disease (without DIP and PIP involvement)
√ extensive narrowing / obliteration of joint space between distal radius + scaphoid:
√ incorporation of scaphoid into articular surface of radius
√ prominent cysts
√ calcification of triangular fibrocartilage
√ scapholunate separation
√ destruction of trapezioscaphoid space

@ Knee
√ medial femorotibial + patellofemoral compartments commonly involved simultaneously (as in osteoarthritis) but with greater osseous destruction + fragmentation
√ disproportionate narrowing of patellofemoral joint
@ Spine
√ chondrocalcinosis / calcifications of outer fibers of annulus fibrosus resembling syndesmophytes
√ vertical radiodense line in symphysis pubis

CAMPOMELIC DYSPLASIA

= sporadic / autosomal recessive dwarfism
Incidence: 0.05:10,000 births
Associated with:
1. Hydrocephalus (23%)
2. Congenital heart disease (30%): VSD, ASD, tetralogy, AS
3. Hydronephrosis (30%)

• pretibial dimple
√ macrocephaly, cleft palate, micrognathia (90–99%)
@ Chest & spine
√ hypoplastic scapulae (92%)
√ narrow bell-shaped chest
√ hypoplastic vertebral bodies + nonmineralized pedicles (especially lower cervical spine)
@ Pelvis
√ vertically narrowed iliac bones
√ vertical inclination of ischii
√ wide symphysis
√ narrow iliac bones with small wings
√ shallow acetabulum
@ Extremities (lower extremity more severely affected)
√ dislocation of hips + knees
√ anterior bowing (= campo) of long bones: marked in tibia + moderate in femur
√ hypoplastic fibula
√ small secondary ossification center of knee
√ small primary ossification center of talus
√ clubfoot
OB-US:
√ bowing of tibia + femur
√ decreased thoracic circumference
√ hypoplastic scapulae
√ ± cleft palate
Prognosis: death usually <5 months of age (within first year in 97%) due to respiratory insufficiency

CARPAL TUNNEL SYNDROME

= entrapment syndrome caused by chronic pressure on the median nerve within the carpal tunnel
Cause: repetitive wrist / finger flexion; carpal tunnel crowding by cyst / mass / flexor tendon tendinitis or tenosynovitis / anomalous origin of lumbrical muscles
Pathogenesis: probably ischemia with venous congestion (stage 1), nerve edema from anoxic damage to capillary endothelium (stage 2), impairment of venous + arterial blood supply (stage 3)

- nocturnal hand discomfort
- weakness, clumsiness, finger paresthesias

MR:
- √ "pseudoneuroma" of median nerve = swelling of median nerve proximal to carpal tunnel
- √ swelling of nerve within carpal tunnel
- √ increased signal intensity of nerve on T2WI
- √ volar bowing of flexor retinaculum
- √ swelling of tendon sheath (due to tenosynovitis)
- √ mass(es) within carpal tunnel
- √ marked enhancement (nerve edema = breakdown of blood-nerve barrier)
- √ no enhancement (ischemia) provoked by wrist held in an extended / flexed position

CARPENTER SYNDROME

= ACROCEPHALOPOLYSYNDACTYLY type 2

autosomal recessive
- retardation
- hypogonadism
- √ patent ductus arteriosus
- √ acro(oxy)cephaly
- √ preaxial polysyndactyly + soft-tissue syndactyly

CEREBROCOSTOMANDIBULAR SYNDROME

= rare bone disorder of uncertain transmission
- respiratory distress (due to flail chest + airway abnormalities)
- √ 11 pairs of ribs:
  - √ abnormal costovertebral articulations
  - √ posterior ossification gaps resembling fractures
- √ microcephaly
- √ micrognathia
- √ congenital heart disease

DDx: multiple fractures

CHONDROBLASTOMA

= CODMAN TUMOR = BENIGN CHONDROBLASTOMA
= CARTILAGE-CONTAINING GIANT CELL TUMOR

Incidence: 1% of primary bone neoplasms (700 cases in world literature)

Age: peak in 2nd decade (range of 8–59 years); 10–26 years (90%); M:F = 2:1; occurs before cessation of enchondral bone growth

Path: derived from primitive cartilage cells

Histo: polyhedral chondroblasts + multinucleated giant cells + nodules of pink amorphous material (= chondroid) = epiphyseal chondromatous giant cell tumor (resembles chondromyxoid fibroma); "chicken wire" calcification = pericellular deposition of calcification is virtually PATHOGNOMONIC

- symptomatic for months to years prior to treatment
- mild joint pain, tenderness, swelling (joint effusion)
- limitation of motion

Location:
- (a) long bones (80%): proximal femur + greater trochanter (23%), distal femur (20%), proximal tibia (17%), proximal humerus (17%)
  - ◊ 2/3 in lower extremity, 50% about knee
  - ◊ may occur in apophyses (minor + greater trochanter, patella, greater tuberosity of humerus)
- (b) flat bones: near triradiate cartilage of innominate bone, rib (3%)
- (c) short tubular bones of hand + feet

Site: eccentric medullary, subarticular location with open growth plate (98% begin within epiphysis); tumor growth may continue to involve metaphysis (50%) + rarely diaphysis

- √ oval / round eccentrically placed lytic lesion of epiphysis
- √ 1–4 cm in diameter occupying < one-half of epiphysis
- √ well-defined sclerotic margin, lobulated in 50%
- √ stippled / irregular calcifications in 25–30–50% (cartilaginous clumps better visualized by CT)
- √ intact scalloped cortical border
- √ thick periosteal reaction in metaphysis (50%) / joint involvement
- √ periostitis of adjacent metaphysis / diaphysis (30–50%)
- √ open growth plate in majority of patients

MR:
- ◊ MR tends to overestimate extent + aggressiveness due to large area of reactive edema!
- √ intermediate to low signal intensity on T2WI relative to fat
- √ extensive intramedullary signal abnormalities consistent with bone marrow edema
- √ peripheral rim of very low signal intensity
- √ hypointense changes on T1WI + hyperintense on T2WI in adjacent soft tissues (muscle edema) in 50%
- √ ± joint effusion

Prognosis: almost always benign; may become locally aggressive; rarely metastasizes

Dx: surgical biopsy

Rx: curettage + bone chip grafting (recurrence in 25%)

DDx:
(1) Ischemic necrosis of femoral head (may be indistinguishable, more irregular configuration)
(2) Giant cell tumor (usually larger + less well demarcated, not calcified, older age group with closed growth plate)
(3) Chondromyxoid fibroma
(4) Enchondroma
(5) Osteomyelitis (less well-defined, variable margins)
(6) Aneurysmal bone cyst
(7) Intraosseous ganglion
(8) Langerhans cell histiocytosis (less well-defined, variable margins)
(9) Primary bone sarcoma

CHONDRODYSPLASIA PUNCTATA

= CONGENITAL STIPPLED EPIPHYSES = DYSPLASIA EPIPHYSEALIS PUNCTATA = CHONDRODYSTROPHIA CALCIFICANS CONGENITA

= proportional / mesomelic dwarfism

Etiology: peroxisomal disorder characterized by fibroblast plasmalogen deficiency

Incidence: 1:110,000 births

A. AUTOSOMAL RECESSIVE CHONDRODYSPLASIA PUNCTATA = RHIZOMELIC TYPE
Associated with: CHD (common)
- flat face
- congenital cataracts
- ichthyotic skin thickening
- mental retardation
- cleft palate

√ multiple small punctate calcifications of varying size in epiphyses (knee, hip, shoulder, wrist), in base of skull, in posterior elements of vertebrae, in respiratory cartilage and soft tissues (neck, rib ends) before appearance of ossification centers
√ prominent symmetrical shortening of femur + humerus (rarely all limbs symmetrically affected)
√ congenital dislocation of hip
√ flexion contractures of extremities
√ clubfeet
√ metaphyseal splaying of proximal tubular bones (in particular about knee)
√ thickening of diaphyses
√ prominent vertebral + paravertebral calcifications
√ coronal clefts in vertebral bodies
Prognosis: death usually <1 year of age
DDx: Zellweger syndrome

B. CONRADI-HÜNERMANN DISEASE = NONRHIZOMELIC TYPE
more common milder nonlethal variety;
autosomal dominant
- normal intelligence

√ more widespread but milder involvement as above
Prognosis: survival often into adulthood

Cx: respiratory failure (severe underdevelopment of ribs), tracheal stenosis, spinal cord compression
DDx: (1) Cretinism (may show epiphyseal fragmentation, much larger calcifications within epiphysis)
(2) Warfarin embryopathy
(3) Zellweger syndrome

CHONDROECTODERMAL DYSPLASIA

= ELLIS-VAN CREVELD SYNDROME = MESODERMAL DYSPLASIA
= autosomal recessive acromesomelic dwarfism
Incidence: 120 cases; in inbred Amish communities
Associated with: congenital heart disease in 50% (single atrium, ASD, VSD)
- ectodermal dysplasia:
  - absent / hypoplastic brittle spoon-shaped nails
  - irregular + pointed dysplastic teeth, partial anodontia, teeth may be present at birth
  - scant / fine hair
- obliteration of maxillary mucobuccal space (thick frenula between alveolar mucosa + upper lip)
- strabismus
- genital malformations: epispadia, hypospadia, hypoplastic external genitalia, undescended testicles

√ hepatosplenomegaly
√ accelerated skeletal maturation
√ normal spine

@ Skull
√ wormian bones
√ cleft lip
@ Chest
√ elongated narrow thorax in AP + transverse dimensions exaggerating the heart size
√ cardiomegaly (frequently ASD / single atrium)
√ short horizontal ribs + anterior osseous expansion
√ elevated clavicles
@ Pelvis
√ small flattened ilium
√ trident shape of acetabulum with indentation in roof + bony spur (almost pathognomonic)
√ acetabular + tibial exostoses
@ Extremities
√ variety of micromelia (= thickening + shortening of all long bones):
√ acromelia = hypoplasia / absence of terminal phalanges
√ mesomelia = shortening of forearms + lower legs (radius + tibia > humerus + femur)
√ cone-shaped epiphyses
√ premature ossification of proximal humeral + femoral epiphyses
@ Upper extremity
√ "drumstick" forearm = swelling of proximal end of ulna + distal end of radius
√ anterior dislocation of radial head (due to shortening of ulna)
√ carpal / tarsal fusion = frequent fusion of two / more carpal (hamate + capitate) + tarsal bones (after complete ossification)
√ supernumerary carpal bones
√ postaxial polydactyly common (usually finger, rarely toe) ± syndactyly of hands + feet
@ Lower extremity
√ genu valgum:
√ slanting of proximal tibial metahysis (= delayed development of tibial plateau)
√ excessive shortening of fibula
√ widening of proximal tibial shaft
√ medial tibial diaphyseal exostosis

OB-US:
√ proportional shortening of long bones
√ small thorax with decreased circumference
√ increased cardiothoracic ratio
√ ASD
√ polydactyly
Prognosis: death within first month of life in 33–50% (due to respiratory / cardiac complications)
DDx: asphyxiating thoracic dysplasia (difficult distinction); rhizomelic achondroplasia

CHONDROMALACIA PATELLAE

= pathologic softening of patellar cartilage
Cause: trauma, tracking abnormality of patella
- anterior knee pain
- asymptomatic (incidental arthroscopic diagnosis)

Classification of Chondromalacia Patellae

Grade	*Arthroscopic pathology*	*T1WI of MRI*
1	softening + swelling of articular cartilage	focal hypointense areas not extending to cartilage surface / subcondral bone
2	blistering of articular cartilage producing deformity of surface	focal hypointense areas extending to cartilage surface with preservation of sharp cartilage margins
3	surface irregularity + cartilage fibrillation with minimal extension to subchondral bone ("brush-border sign")	focal hypointense areas extending to articular surface but not to osseous surface; loss of sharp dark margin between articular cartilage of patella + trochlea
4	ulceration with exposure of subchondral bone	focal hypointense areas extending from subchondral bone to cartilage surface; cartilage thinned to subchondral bone

CHONDROMYXOID FIBROMA

Rare benign cartilaginous tumor; initially arising in cortex

Incidence: <1% of all bone tumors

Histo: chondroid + fibrous + myxoid tissue (related to chondroblastoma); may be mistaken for chondrosarcoma

Age: peak 2nd–3rd decade (range of 5–79 years); M:F = 1:1

- slowly progressive local pain, swelling, restriction of motion

Location: (a) long bones (60%): about knee (50%), proximal tibia (82% of tibial lesions), distal femur (71% of femoral lesions), fibula
(b) short tubular bones of hand + feet (20%)
(c) flat bones: pelvis, ribs (classic but uncommon)

Site: eccentric, metaphyseal (47–53%), metadiaphyseal (20–43%), metaepiphyseal (26%), diaphyseal (1–10%), epiphyseal (3%)

√ expansile ovoid lesion with radiolucent center + oval shape at each end of lesion
√ long axis parallel to long axis of host bone (1–10 cm in length and 4–7 cm in width)
√ geographic bone destruction (100%)
√ well-defined sclerotic margin (86%)
√ expanded shell = bulged + thinned overlying cortex (68%)
√ partial cortical erosion (68%)
√ scalloped margin (58%)
√ septations (57%) may mimic trabeculations
√ stippled calcifications within tumor in advanced lesions (7%)
√ NO periosteal reaction (unless fractured)

Prognosis: 25% recurrence rate following curettage

Cx: malignant degeneration distinctly unusual

DDx: (1) Aneurysmal bone cyst
(2) Simple bone cyst
(3) Nonossifying fibroma
(4) Fibrous dysplasia
(5) Enchondroma
(6) Chondroblastoma
(7) Eosinophilic granuloma
(8) Fibrous cortical defect
(9) Giant cell tumor

CHONDROSARCOMA

A. PRIMARY CHONDROSARCOMA
no preexisting bone lesion

B. SECONDARY CHONDROSARCOMA
as a complication of a preexisting skeletal abnormality such as
1. Osteochondroma
2. Enchondroma
3. Parosteal chondroma

Spread: via marrow cavity / periosteum

Metastases (uncommon) to: lung, epidural space

CT:
√ chondroid matrix mineralization of "rings and arcs" (CHARACTERISTIC) in 70%
√ nonmineralized portion of tumor hypodense to muscle (high water content of hyaline cartilage)
√ extension into soft-tissues

MR:
√ low to intermediate signal intensity on T1WI
√ high signal intensity on T2WI + hypointense areas (due to mineralization / fibrous septa)
√ enhancement of fibrous septations

Central Chondrosarcoma

= INTRAMEDULLARY CHONDROSARCOMA = ENDOSTEAL CHONDROSARCOMA

Incidence: 3rd most common primary bone tumor (1st multiple myeloma, 2nd osteosarcoma); 8–17% of biopsied primary bone tumors

Path: lobular morphology with variable amounts of calcium; presence of fibrous bands at tumor-marrow interface suggests malignancy (DDx from atypical enchondroma)

Histo: arises from chondroblasts (tumor osteoid is never formed)

Age: median 45 years; 50% >40 years; 10% in children (rapidly fatal); M:F = 2:1

- hyperglycemia as paraneoplastic syndrome (85%)

Location: neck of femur, pubic rami, proximal humerus, ribs (19%), skull (sphenoid bone, cerebellopontine angle, mandible), sternum, spine (3–12%)

Site: central within medullary canal + meta- / diaphysis
√ expansile osteolytic lesion 1 to several cm in size
√ short transition zone ± sclerotic margin (well defined from host bone)
√ ± small irregular punctate / snowflake type of calcification; single / multiple
√ late: loss of definition + break through cortex
√ endosteal cortical thickening, sometimes at a distance from the tumor (due to invasion of haversian system)
√ presence of large soft-tissue mass
DDx: benign enchondroma, osteochondroma, osteosarcoma, fibrosarcoma

Peripheral Chondrosarcoma

= EXOSTOTIC CHONDROSARCOMA
= malignant degeneration of hereditary multiple osteochondromatosis and rarely of a solitary exostosis (beginning in cartilaginous cap of exostosis)
Frequency: 8% of all chondrosarcomas
Average age: 50–55 years for solitary exostosis; 25–30 years for hereditary multiple osteochondromatosis; M:F = 1.5:1
Histo: low histologic grade in 67–85%
• growth after skeletal maturity
• gradually increasing pain, often worse at night
• local swelling / palpable mass (45%)
Location: pelvis, hip, scapula, sternum, ribs, ends of humerus / femur, skull, facial bones
√ growth of a previously unchanged osteochondroma in a skeletally mature patient
√ unusually large soft-tissue mass (= hyaline cartilage cap) containing flocculent / streaky chondroid calcifications (CHARACTERISTIC):
  √ cartilage cap 1.5–12 cm (average, 5.5–6 cm) thick
    ◊ >1.5 cm is suspect of malignant transformation
√ irregular / indistinct lesion surface:
  √ dense radiopaque center with streaks radiating to periphery with loss of smooth margin
√ focal regions of radiolucency in interior of lesion
√ erosion / destruction of adjacent bone
Metastases: in 3–7%, most commonly to lung
Rx: wide resection
Prognosis: 70–90% long-term survival
DDx: (1) Osteochondroma (densely calcified with multiple punctate calcifications)
(2) Parosteal osteosarcoma (more homogeneous density of calcified osteoid)

Clear Cell Chondrosarcoma

◊ Usually mistaken for chondroblastoma because of low grade malignancy (may be related)!
Histo: small lobules of tissue composed of cells with centrally filled vesicular nuclei surrounded by large clear cytoplasm
Age: 19–68 years, predominantly after epiphyseal fusion
Location: proximal femur, proximal humerus, proximal ulna, lamina vertebrae (5%); pubic ramus
Site: epiphysis
√ single lobulated oval / round sharply marginated lesion of 1–2 cm in size
√ surrounding increased bone density
√ aggressive rapid growth over 3 cm
√ may contain calcifications
√ bone often enlarged
√ indistinguishable from conventional chondrosarcoma / chondroblastoma (slow growth over years)

Extraskeletal Chondrosarcoma

Incidence: 2% of all soft-tissue sarcomas

Myxoid Extraskeletal Chondrosarcoma

(most common)
Mean age: 50 years (range 4–92 years); M > F

Enchondroma versus Chondrosarcoma in Appendicular Skeleton

	Enchondroma	*Intramedullary Chondrosarcoma*
Mean age and sex	40 years; M:F = 2:3	50 years; M:F = 11:9
Palpable mass	28%	82%
Pain	40% (fracture associated)	95% (longer duration + increasing severity)
Lesion location	hands, feet	axial skeleton (spine, pelvis)
Site	diaphysis	metaphysis, epiphysis
Lesion size	<5 cm	>5–6 cm
Endosteal scalloping		
relative to cortical thickness	90% <2/3 of cortical thickness	90% >2/3 of cortical thickness,
relative to lesion length	66% along <2/3 of lesion	79% along >2/3 of lesion
Cortical remodeling (radiography)	15%	47%
Cortical thickening (radiography)	17%	47%
Perisoteal reaction (radiography)	3%	47%
Pathologic fracture (radiography)	5%	27%
Matrix mineralization (CT)	100% (more extensive)	94% (less extensive)
Cortical destruction (CT)	8%	88%
Soft-tissue extension (MR)	3%	76%
Small hyperintense foci (T1WI)	65%	35%

Histo: surrounded by fibrous capsule + divided into multiple lobules by fibrous septa; delicate strands of small elongated chondroblasts are suspended in an abundant myxoid matrix; foci of mature hyaline cartilage are rare

- slowly growing soft-tissue mass
- pain + tenderness (33%)

◊ Metastatic in 40–45% at time of presentation!

Location: extremities (thigh most common)

Site: deep soft tissues; subcutis (25%)

√ lobulated soft-tissue mass WITHOUT calcification / ossification

√ usually between 4 and 7 cm in diameter

MR:

√ approximately equal to muscle on T1WI + equal to fat on T2WI

√ may mimic a cyst / myxoma

Prognosis: 45% 10-year survival rate; 5–15 years survival after development of metastases

Extraskeletal Mesenchymal Chondrosarcoma

◊ 50% of all mesenchymal chondrosarcomas arise in soft tissues

Histo: proliferation of small primitive mesenchymal cells with scattered islands of cartilage; hemangiopericytoma-like vascular pattern

Bimodal age distribution: M = F

(a) tumors of head + neck in 3rd decade (common): meninges, periorbital region

(b) tumors of thigh + trunk in 5th decade

- frequently metastasized to lungs + lymph nodes

√ matrix mineralization (50–100%) characterized as rings + arcs / flocculent + stippled calcification / dense mineralization

MR:

√ approximately equal to muscle on T1WI + equal to fat on T2WI

√ signal voids from calcifications

√ homogeneous enhancement

Prognosis: 25% 10-year survival rate

CLEIDOCRANIAL DYSOSTOSIS

= CLEIDOCRANIAL DYSPLASIA = MUTATIONAL DYSOSTOSIS

= delayed ossification of midline structures (particularly of membranous bone)

Autosomal dominant disease

@ Skull

- large head

√ diminished / absent ossification of skull (in early infancy)

√ wormian bones

√ widened fontanels + sutures with delayed closure

√ persistent metopic suture

√ brachycephaly + prominent bossing

√ large mandible

√ high narrow palate (± cleft)

√ hypoplastic paranasal sinuses

√ delayed / defective dentition

@ Chest

√ hypoplasia / absence (10%) of clavicles (defective development usually of lateral portion, R > L (DDx: congenital pseudarthrosis of clavicle)

√ thorax may be narrowed + bell-shaped

√ supernumerary ribs

√ incompletely ossified sternum

√ hemivertebrae, spondylosis (frequent)

@ Pelvis

√ delayed ossification of bones forming symphysis pubis (DDx: bladder exstrophy)

√ hypoplastic iliac bones

@ Extremities

√ radius short / absent

√ elongated second metacarpals

√ pseudoepiphyses of metacarpal bases

√ short hypoplastic distal phalanges of hand

√ pointed terminal tufts

√ coned epiphyses

√ coxa vara = deformed / absent femoral necks

√ accessory epiphyses in hands + feet (common)

OB-US:

√ cephalopelvic disproportion (large fetal head + narrow birth canal of affected maternal pelvis) necessitates cesarean section

COCCIDIOIDOMYCOSIS

Histo: chronic granulomatous process in bones, joints, periarticular structures

Location: (a) bones: most frequently in metaphyses of long bones + medial end of clavicle, spine, ribs, pelvis / bony prominences of patella, tibial tuberosity, calcaneus, olecranon, acromion

(b) weight-bearing joints (33%): ankle, knee, wrist, elbow

- "desert rheumatism" = immune-complex–mediated arthritis

(c) tenosynovitis of hand, bursitis

√ focal areas of destruction, formation of cavities (early) = bubbly bone lesion

√ bone sclerosis surrounding osteolysis (later, rare)

√ proliferation of overlying periosteum

√ destruction of vertebra with preservation of disk space

√ psoas abscess indistinguishable from tuberculosis, may calcify

√ joints rarely infected (usually monoarticular from direct extension of osteomyelitic focus): synovial effusion, osteopenia, joint space narrowing, bone destruction, ankylosis

√ soft-tissue abscesses common

DDx: tuberculosis

CONGENITAL INSENSITIVITY TO PAIN WITH ANHYDROSIS

= rare autosomal recessive disorder presumably on the basis of abnormal neural crest development

Age: presenting at birth

Incidence: 15 reported cases

Path: absence of dorsal + sympathetic ganglia, deficiency of neural fibers <6 μm in diameter + disproportionate number of fibers of 6–10 μm in diameter

• history of painless injuries + burns (DDx: familial dysautonomia, congenital sensory neuropathy, hereditary sensory radicular neuropathy, acquired sensory neuropathy, syringomyelia)
• abnormal pain + temperature perception
• burns, bruises, infections are common
• biting injuries of fingers, lips, tongue
• absence of sweating
• mental retardation

CRITERIA: (1) defect must be present at birth
(2) general insensitivity to pain
(3) general mental / physical retardation

√ epiphyseal separation in infancy (epiphyseal injuries result in growth problems)
√ metaphyseal fractures in early childhood
√ diaphyseal fractures in late childhood
√ Charcot joints = neurotrophic joints (usually weight-bearing joints) with effusions + synovial thickening
√ ligamentous laxity
√ bizarre deformities + gross displacement + considerable hemorrhage (unnoticed fractures + dislocations)
√ osteomyelitis + septic arthritis may occur + progress extensively

DDx: (1) sensory neuropathies (eg, diabetes mellitus)
(2) hysteria
(3) syphilis
(4) mental deficiency,
(5) syringomyelia
(6) organic brain disease

CORNELIA DE LANGE SYNDROME

= AMSTERDAM DWARFISM

• mental retardation (IQ <50)
• hirsutism; hypoplastic genitalia
• feeble growling cry
• high forehead; short neck
• arched palate
• bushy eyebrows meeting in midline + long curved eyelashes
• small nose with depressed bridge; upward tilted nostrils; excessive distance between nose + upper lip

√ small + brachycephalic skull
√ hypoplasia of long bones (upper extremity more involved)
√ forearm bones may be absent
√ short radius + elbow dislocation
√ thumbs placed proximally (hypoplastic 1st metacarpal)
√ short phalanges + clinodactyly of 5th finger

CORTICAL DESMOID

= AVULSIVE CORTICAL IRREGULARITY = PERIOSTEAL / SUBPERIOSTEAL DESMOID = SUBPERIOSTEAL / CORTICAL ABRASION = SUBPERIOSTEAL CORTICAL DEFECT

= rare fibrous lesion of the periosteum

Age: peak 14–16 years (range of 3–17 years); M:F = 3:1

Histo: shallow defect filled with proliferating fibroblasts, multiple small fragments of resorbing bone (microavulsions) at tendinous insertions

• no localizing signs / symptoms

Location: posteromedial aspect of medial femoral epicondyle along medial ridge of linea aspera at attachment of adductor magnus aponeurosis; 1/3 bilateral

√ area of cortical thickening
√ 1–2 cm irregular, shallow, concave saucerlike crater with sharp margin
√ lamellated periosteal reaction
√ localized cortical hyperostosis proximally (healing phase)

◊ May be confused with a malignant tumor (eg, osteosarcoma) / osteomyelitis!

CRI-DU-CHAT SYNDROME

= deletion of short arm of 5th chromosome (5 p)

• generalized dwarfism due to marked growth retardation
• failure to thrive
• peculiar high-pitched cat cry (hypoplastic larynx)
• antimongoloid palpebral fissures
• strabismus
• profound mental retardation
• round facies
• low-set ears

Associated with: congenital heart disease (obtain CXR!)

√ agenesis of corpus callosum
√ microcephaly
√ hypertelorism
√ small mandible
√ faulty long-bone development
√ short 3rd, 4th, 5th metacarpals
√ long 2nd, 3rd, 4th, 5th proximal phalanges
√ horseshoe kidney

Dx: made clinically

CROUZON SYNDROME

= CRANIOFACIAL SYNOSTOSIS / DYSOSTOSIS

= Apert syndrome without syndactyly

= skull + cranial base deformities characterized by craniosynostosis, maxillary hypoplasia, shallow orbits, ocular proptosis, bifid uvula, cleft palate

Prevalence: 1:25,000

Etiology: autosomal dominant inheritance (in 67%)

Associated intracranial anomalies:
anomalous venous drainage, hydrocephalus (often progressive), Chiari I malformation (71%)

• parrot-beak nose
• strabismus
• deafness
• mental retardation
• dental abnormalities
• bifid uvula
• acanthosis nigrans (= hyperpigmented hyperkeratotic lesions on neck + near joint flexures)

√ premature craniosynostosis: acro(oxy)cephaly / brachycephaly / scaphocephaly / trigonocephaly / "cloverleaf" skull

√ hypertelorism + exophthalmos (due to shallow orbits)
√ hypoplastic maxilla (relative prominence of mandible)
√ cleft palate
√ calcification of stylohyoid ligament (in 50% of patients >4 years of age)
√ C2 to C5 spine abnormalities (in up to 40%)
√ elbow malformation (18%)
√ minor hand deformities (10%)
√ visceral anomalies (7%)
√ musculoskeletal deformities (7%)

OB-US:
- √ cloverleaf appearance (coronal view) + bilateral frontal indentations (axial view) of skull
- √ increased interorbital distance + ocular proptosis
- √ mild ventriculomegaly

CRUCIATE LIGAMENT INJURY

A. COMPLETE TEAR
- √ failure to identify ligament
- √ amorphous areas of high signal intensity on T1WI + T2WI with inability to define ligamentous fibers
- √ focal discrete complete disruption of all visible fibers

B. PARTIAL / INTRASUBSTANCE TEAR
- √ abnormal signal intensity within substance of ligament with some intact + some discontinuous fibers

Anterior Cruciate Ligament Injury (ACL)

◊ If the ACL appears intact in one of the sagittal oblique sequences discordant findings in other sequences can be disregarded!

Site: intrasubstance tear near insertion of femoral condyle (frequently); bone avulsion (rarely)

√ hyperintense signal (= focal fluid collection / soft-tissue edema) replacing the tendon substance in acute tear
√ mass (hematoma + torn fibers) in intercondylar notch near femoral attachment
√ concavity of anterior margin of ligament

Indirect findings:
- ◊ The indirect signs of ACL injury have a low sensitivity but high specificity!
- √ bone bruise in lateral compartment (posterolateral tibia + mid lateral femur) in >50%
- √ deepening of lateral femoral sulcus >1.5 mm
- √ posterior displacement of posterior horn of lateral meniscus >3.5 mm behind tibial plateau
- √ anterior translation of tibia (= anterior drawer sign)
- √ PCL bowing = angle between proximal + distal limbs of PCL <105°

False-positive Dx:
(1) slice thickness / interslice gap too great
(2) adjacent fluid / synovial proliferation
(3) cruciate ganglion / synovial cyst

Associated injuries:
meniscal tear (lateral > medial) in 65%

Chronic ACL Tear

√ often complete absence of ligament
√ bridging fibrous scar within intercondylar notch (simulating an intact ligament)

Partial ACL Tear *(15%)*

◊ Extremely difficult to diagnose! 40–50% of partial tears are missed on MR!
• positive Lachman test (in 12–30%)
√ MR primary signs positive for injury (in 33–43%)

Posterior Cruciate Ligament Injury (PCL)

Prevalence: 2–23% of all knee injuries
√ midsubstance of PCL most frequently involved (best seen on sagittal images)
√ bone avulsion from posterior tibial insertion (<10%), best seen on lateral plain film

Mechanism:
(1) Direct blow to proximal anterior tibia with knee flexed (dashboard accident)
- √ midsubstance PCL tear
- √ injury to posterior joint capsule
- √ bone contusion at anterior tibial plateau + femoral condyles farther posteriorly

(2) Hyperextension of knee
- √ avulsion of tibial attachment of PCL (with preservation of PCL substance)
- √ ± ACL rupture
- √ bone contusion in anterior tibial plateau + anterior aspect of femoral condyles

(3) Severe ab- / adduction + rotational forces
- √ + injury to collateral ligaments

Associated with: coexistent ligamentous injury in 70%

anterior cruciate ligament	27–38%
medial collateral ligament	20–23%
lateral collateral ligament	6–7%
medial meniscal tear	32–35%
lateral meniscal tear	28–30%
bone marrow injury	35–36%
effusion	64–65%

◊ In 30% of cases injury of PCL is isolated!
• posterior tibial laxity
• difficult to evaluate arthroscopically unless ACL torn

DEEP FIBROMATOSES

Aggressive Infantile Fibromatosis

= childhood equivalent of deep fibromatosis

Age: first 2 years of life; rarely >5 years of age; M > F
Histo: may mimic infantile fibrosarcoma
• firm nodular soft-tissue mass within skeletal muscle / fascia / periosteum

Location: head, neck (tongue, mandible, mastoid), shoulder, thigh, foot

Extraabdominal Desmoid Tumor

= AGGRESSIVE FIBROMATOSIS = DEEP FIBROMATOSIS = MUSCULOAPONEUROTIC FIBROMATOSIS
= common benign aggressively growing soft-tissue tumor arising from connective tissue of muscle, fascia, aponeurosis outside abdominal cavity

Peak age: 25–35 years

Histo: parallel halo arrays of uniform-appearing fibroblasts surrounded by highly variable amounts of collagen fibers with infiltrative growth pattern

• painless soft-tissue mass

Location: extremities (70%); shoulder (20%), chest wall + back (15%), thigh (12%), mesentery (10%), neck (10%), knee (7%); solitary (majority) / synchronous multicentricity in same extremity (10–15%)

◊ Most common benign soft-tissue tumor of the foot

Site: fascia in / around muscle

√ mostly <10 cm in diameter

@ Bone

√ Erlenmeyer flask deformity in multicentric fibromatosis (infrequent)

@ Abdominal wall

Prevalence: in 87% in females of childbearing age

Predilection: for female patients taking birth control pills / during or after pregnancy

Location: aponeurosis of rectus abdominis, internal oblique muscle

MR:

√ poorly defined (with invasion of fat / muscle) / lobulated well-defined lesion

√ hypo- / isointense to muscle on T1WI

√ hyperintense (hypercellular) / hyperintense with areas of low intensity (intermixed with fibrous components) / hypointense (hypocellular) on T2WI

Cx: compresses / engulfs adjacent structures

Prognosis: 75% recurrence within 2 years after surgical excision (up to 87% local recurrence in <30 years of age; 20% recurrence rate in >20 years of age)

Abdominal Desmoid Tumor

= DESMOID TUMOR

= uncommon benign tumor of the subgroup of fibromatoses consisting of fibrous tissue with insidious growth [*desmos* , Greek = band / tendon]

Location: mesentery (most common mesenteric primary), musculoaponeurosis of rectus, internal oblique muscle; occasionally external oblique muscle

Age: peak age in 3rd decade, 70% between 20 and 40 years of age; M:F = 1:3

Path: poorly circumscribed coarsely trabeculated tumor resembling scar tissue, confined to musculature + overlying aponeurosis

Histo: elongated spindle-shaped cells of uniform appearance, septated by dense bands of collagen, infiltration of adjacent tissue (DDx: low-grade fibrosarcoma, reactive fibrosis)

Associated with: Gardner syndrome, multiple pregnancies, prior trauma

• firm slowly growing deep-seated mass

Size: 5–20 cm in diameter

MR:

√ hypointense to muscle on T1WI + variable intensity on T2WI

CT:

√ ill-defined / well-circumscribed mass

√ usually higher attenuation than muscle

√ ± enhancement

√ retraction, angulation, distortion of small / large bowel with mesenteric infiltration

US:

√ sharply defined + smoothly marginated mass of low / medium / high echogenicity

Cx: compression / displacement of bowel / ureter, intestinal perforation

Prognosis: locally aggressive growth; 25–65% recurrence rate

Rx: local resection + radiotherapy, antiestrogen therapy

DDx: (1) Malignant tumor: metastasis, fibrosarcoma, rhabdomyosarcoma, synoviosarcoma, liposarcoma, fibrous histiocytoma, lymphoma,
(2) Benign tumor: neurofibroma, neuroma, leiomyoma
(3) Acute hematoma

Infantile Myofibromatosis

= GENERALIZED HAMARTOMATOSIS = CONGENITAL MULTIPLE FIBROMATOSIS = MULTIPLE VASCULAR LEIOMYOMAS = DESMOFIBROMATOSIS

= rare disorder characterized by proliferation of fibroblasts

Cause: unknown

Frequency: most common fibromatosis in childhood

Age: at birth (in 60%), <2 years (in 89%); M:F = 1.7:1

Path: well-marginated soft-tissue lesion 0.5–3 cm in diameter with scarlike consistency ± infiltration of surrounding tissues

Histo: spindle-shaped cells in short bundles and fascicles in periphery of lesion with features of both smooth muscle + fibroblasts; hemangiopericytoma-like pattern in center with necrosis, hyalinization, calcification

(1) Solitary lesion (50–75%)

Location: dermis, subcutis, muscle (86%); head, neck, trunk, bone (9%), GI tract (4%)

Prognosis: spontaneous regression in 100%; recurrence after surgical excision in 7–10%

(2) Multicentric disease (25–50%)

Location: skin (98%), subcutis (98%), muscle (98%), bone (57%), viscera (25–37%): lung (28%), heart (16%), GI tract (14%), pancreas (9%), liver (8%)

Prognosis: related to extent + location of visceral lesions with cardiopulmonary + GI involvement as harbingers of poor prognosis (death in 75–80%); spontaneous regression (33%)

• firm nodules in skin, subcutis, muscle

• ± overlying scarring of skin with ulceration

@ Skeleton
Location: any bone may be involved; commonly in femur, tibia, rib, pelvis, vertebral bodies, calvarium; often symmetric
Site: metaphysis of long bones
√ eccentric lobulated lytic foci with smooth margins 0.5 –1.0 cm in size
√ well-defined with narrow zone of transition
√ initially no sclerosis; sclerotic margin with healing
√ osseous foci may increase in size and number
√ healing leaves little residual abnormality
√ unusual osseous findings:
√ periosteal reaction, pathologic fracture
√ vertebra plana, kyphoscoliosis with posterior scalloping of vertebral bodies
NUC (bone scan):
√ increased / little radiotracer uptake
DDx: (1) Langerhans cell histiocytosis (skin lesions)
(2) Neurofibromatosis (multiple masses)
(3) Osseous hemangiomas / lymphangiomatosis / lipomatosis
(4) Metastatic neuroblastoma
(5) Multiple nonossifying fibromas
(6) Enchondromatosis
(7) Hematogenous osteomyelitis (unusual organism)
(8) Fibrous dysplasia
@ Soft tissue
√ solid mass with central necrosis
√ central / peripheral solitary / multiple calcifications
√ prominent vascularity of skin lesions resembles hemangiomas
CT:
√ attenuation increased compared to muscle, before + after contrast enhancement
MR:
√ hypo- to hyperintense mass on T1WI + T2WI
DDx: (1) Neurofibromatosis
(2) Infantile fibrosarcoma, leiomyosarcoma
(3) Angiomatosis
@ Lung
√ interstitial fibrosis, reticulonodular infiltrates
√ discrete mass
√ generalized bronchopneumonia
@ GI tract
√ diffuse narrowing / multiple small filling defects

DERMATOMYOSITIS

= autoimmune inflammatory myopathy with diffuse nonsuppurative inflammation of striated muscle + skin
Cause: cell-mediated (type IV) autoimmune attack on striated muscle
Pathophysiology: damaged chondroitin sulfate no longer inhibits calcification
Path: atrophy of muscle bundles followed by edema and coagulation necrosis, fibrosis, calcification
Histo: mucoid degeneration with round cell infiltrates concentrated around blood vessels
Age: bimodal: 5–15 and 50–60 years; M:F = 1:2

• gradual onset of muscle weakness
• elevated muscle enzymes (creatinine kinase, aldolase)
• myositis-specific autoantibodies: anti-Jo-1
(a) anti-aminoacyl-tRNA synthetase
• arthritis, Raynaud phenomenon, fever, fatigue
• interstitial lung disease
Prognosis: requires prolonged treatment
(b) anti-Mi-2 antibodies:
• V-shaped chest rash (= shawl rash)
• cuticular overgrowth
Prognosis: good response to medication
(c) anti-signal recognition particle antibodies
• abrupt onset myositis ± heart involvement
@ Skeletal musculature
Location: thigh (vastus lateralis + intermedius m. with relative sparing of rectus + biceps femoris m.) > pelvic girdle > upper extremity > neck flexors > pharyngeal muscles
√ bilateral symmetric edema in pelvic + thigh muscles
√ fatty infiltration + muscle atrophy (over months to years)
√ sheetlike confluent calcifications in soft tissues of extremities (quadriceps, deltoid, calf muscles), elbows, knees, hands, abdominal wall, chest wall, axilla, inguinal region) in 75%
@ Skeleton
√ pointing + resorption of terminal tufts
√ rheumatoid-like arthritis (rare)
√ "floppy-thumb" sign
Cx: flexion contractures; soft-tissue ulceration
@ Chest
• respiratory muscle weakness
√ disseminated pulmonary infiltrates (reminiscent of scleroderma)
√ diaphragmatic elevation with reduced lung volumes + basilar atelectasis
√ interstitial fibrosis (5–30%), most severely at lung bases:
√ fine reticular pattern progressing to coarse reticulonodular pattern + honeycombing
√ bronchiolitis obliterans organizing pneumonia
√ diffuse alveolar damage
HRCT:
√ predominantly linear abnormalities + ground-glass attenuation
√ air-space consolidation in middle + lower lung zones with peribronchial + subpleural distribution
Cx: aspiration pneumonia (most common finding due to pharyngeal muscle weakness)
@ Myocardium
√ changes similar to skeletal muscle
@ GI tract
• progressive weakness of proximal striated muscle:
• dysphagia
√ atony + dilatation of esophagus
√ atony of small intestines + colon

ACUTE FORM = childhood-onset form
• fever, joint pain, lymphadenopathy, splenomegaly, subcutaneous edema

√ more severe dermatomyositis
Prognosis: death within a few months

CHRONIC FORM = adult-onset form
= insidious onset with periods of spontaneous remission and relapse
• low-grade fever, muscular aches + pains, edema
• muscle weakness (due to active inflammation, necrosis, muscle atrophy with fatty replacement, steroid-induced myopathy)
◊ first symptom in 50%
• skin erythema: heliotrope rash (= dusky erythema of eyelids) with periorbital edema, Gottron sign (= scaly erythematous papules of knuckles, major joints and upper body)
◊ first symptom in 25%
Cx: increased prevalence of malignant neoplasms of breast, prostate, lung, ovary, GI tract, kidney
Dx: muscle biopsy (normal in up to 15%)

Polymyositis

= involves skeletal muscle only
Age: 4th decade

DESMOPLASTIC FIBROMA

= INTRAOSSEOUS DESMOID TUMOR
= rare locally aggressive benign neoplasm of bone with borderline malignancy resembling soft-tissue desmoids / musculoaponeurotic fibromatosis
Incidence: 107 cases in world literature
Histo: intracellular collagenous material in fibroblasts with small nuclei
Age: mean of 21 years (range 15 months to 75 years); in 90% <30 years; M:F = 1:1
• slowly progressive pain + local tenderness
• palpable mass
Location: mandible (26%), ilium (14%), >50% in long bones (femur [14%], humerus [11%], radius [9%], tibia [7%], clavicle), scapula, vertebra, calcaneus
Site: central meta- / diaphyseal (if growth plate open); may extend into epiphysis with subarticular location (if growth plate closed)
√ geographic (96%) / moth-eaten (4%) bone destruction without matrix mineralization
√ narrow (96%) / poorly defined (4%) zone of transition
√ no marginal sclerosis (94%)
√ residual columns of bone with "pseudotrabeculae" are CLASSIC (91%)
√ bone expansion (89%); may grow to massive size (simulating aneurysmal bone cyst / metastatic renal cell carcinoma)
√ breach of cortex + soft-tissue mass (29%)
Cx: pathologic fracture (9%)

Prognosis: 52% rate of local recurrence
Rx: wide excision
DDx: (1) Giant cell tumor (round rather than oval, may extend into epiphysis + subchondral bone plate)
(2) Fibrous dysplasia (occupies longer bone, contains mineralized matrix, often with sclerotic rim)
(3) Aneurysmal bone cyst (eccentric blowout appearance rather than fusiform)
(4) Chondromyxoid fibroma (eccentric with delicate marginal sclerosis + scalloped border)

DEVELOPMENTAL DYSPLASIA OF HIP (DDH)

= CONGENITAL DYSPLASIA OF HIP
= deformity of acetabulum due to disrupted relationship between femoral head and acetabulum
◊ Acetabular dysplasia (without femoral subluxation / dislocation) can be determined only by imaging!
Etiology:
A. Late intrauterine event (98%)
(a) mechanical:
— oligohydramnios (restricted space in utero)
— firstborn (tight maternal musculature)
◊ in 60% of patients with DDH
— breech position (hip hyperflexion results in shortening of iliopsoas muscle; L:R = 4:1)
◊ in 30–50% of patients with DDH
◊ only 2–4% of deliveries are breech
(b) physiologic (females are more sensitive to):
— maternal estrogen (not inactivated by immature fetal liver) blocks cross-linkage of collagen fibrils
– pregnancy hormone relaxin
B. Teratologic (2%) due to a neuromuscular disorder (myelodysplasia, arthrogryposis) occurring during 12th–18th week GA
C. Postnatal onset (<1%)
Incidence: 0.15% of neonates (Australia 1%, Netherlands 3.7%, Poland 3.9%, Israel 5.9%, Austria 6.6%, Norway 16.9%)
Age: most dislocations probably occur after birth; M:F = 1:4–1:8; Caucasians > Blacks
Increased risk:
(1) infants born in frank breech position (25%; risk of breech:vertex = 6–8:1)
(2) congenital torticollis (10–20%)
(3) skull-molding deformities; scoliosis; generalized joint laxity (Larsen syndrome, Ehlers-Danlos syndrome, Down syndrome [5%]); neuromuscular disorders (eg, myelodysplasia, spina bifida, sacral agenesis, arthrogryposis multiplex)
(4) family history of DDH (6–20%): 6% risk for subsequent sibling of normal parents, 36% risk for subsequent sibling of one affected parent; 12% risk for patient's own children
(5) foot deformities [metatarsus adductus, clubfoot](2%)
(6) neonatal hyperextension of hips: swaddling of infants in hip extension / strapping to cradle board
Anatomy: acetabulum has a small bony component + a large cartilaginous component at birth; acetabulum highly susceptible for modeling within first 6 weeks of age + minimally susceptible >16 weeks of age

Classification:
1. Normal hip
2. Lax = subluxable hip
   ◊ subluxability up to 6 mm is normal in newborns (still under influence of maternal hormones); decreasing to 3 mm by 2nd day of life
3. Concentric DISLOCATABLE UNSTABLE HIP
   = joint laxity allowing nondisplaced femoral head to become subluxed / dislocated under stress
   Incidence: 0.25–0.85% of all newborn infants (2/3 are firstborns)
   • Barlow positive
   √ slight increase in femoral anteversion
   √ mild marginal abnormalities in acetabular cartilage
   √ early labral eversion
   Prognosis: 60% will become stable after 1 week; 88% will become stable by age of 2 months
4. Decentered SUBLUXED HIP
   = femoral head shallow in location
   √ loss of femoral head sphericity
   √ increased femoral anteversion
   √ early labral inversion
   √ shallow acetabulum
5. Eccentric DISLOCATED HIP
   = femoral head frankly displaced out of acetabulum
   (a) reducible = Ortolani positive
   (b) irreducible = Ortolani negative
   √ accentuated flattening of femoral head
   √ shallow acetabulum
   √ limbus formation (= inward growth + hypertrophy of labrum)

• "hip click" = usually result of joint capsule and tendon stretching + snapping (often confused with "hip clunk")
• positive examination result (up to 3 months of age):
  • positive **Ortolani reduction test** = reduction of proximal femur into the acetabulum by progressive abduction of flexed hips and knees ± associated with audible "clunk"
  • positive **Barlow dislocation test** = displacement of proximal femur by progressive adduction with downward pressure (piston maneuver) on flexed hips and knees associated with audible "clunk"
• warning signs on physical examination:
  • limited hip abduction on affected side
  • shortening of thigh on affected side:
    • asymmetric thigh / buttock creases
    • Allis sign = Galeazzi sign = affected knee is lower with knees bent in supine position
    • Trendelenburg test = visible drooping + shortening on dislocated side with child standing on both feet, then one foot

Location: left:right:bilateral = 11:1:4

Radiologic lines:
1. Line of Hilgenreiner
   = line connecting superolateral margins of triradiate cartilage

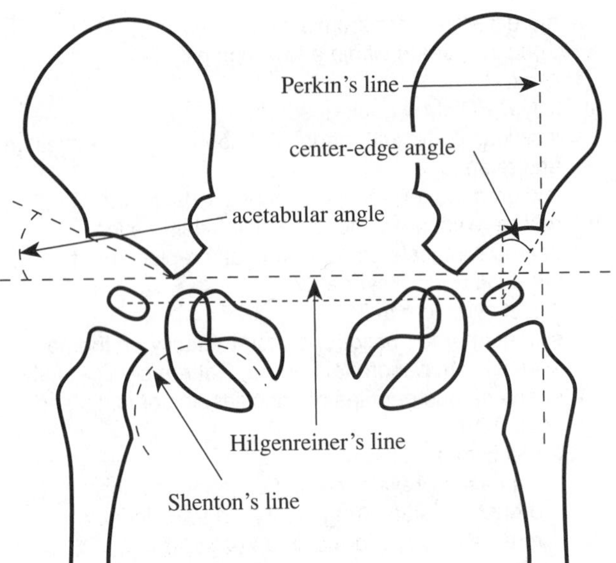

Radiographic Lines of Hip Joint Position

2. Acetabular angle / index
   = slope of acetabular roof = angle that lies between Hilgenreiner's line and a line drawn from most superolateral ossified edge of acetabulum to superolateral margin of triradiate cartilage
3. Perkin's line
   = vertical line to Hilgenreiner's line through the lateral rim of acetabulum
4. Shenton's curved line
   = arc formed by inferior surface of superior pubic ramus (= top of obturator foramen) + medial surface of proximal femoral metaphysis to level of lesser trochanter
   √ disruption of line (DDx: coxa valga)
5. Center-edge angle
   = angle subtended by one line drawn from the acetabular edge to center of femoral head + second line perpendicular to line connecting centers of femoral heads
   √ <25° suggests femoral head instability

AP pelvic radiograph: >6–8 weeks of age (von Rosen view = legs abducted 45° + thighs internally rotated)
◊ Not reliable first 3 months of life!
√ proximal + lateral migration of femoral neck:
  √ eccentric position of proximal femoral epiphysis (position estimated by a circle drawn with a diameter equivalent to width of femoral neck)
  √ interrupted discontinuous arc of Shenton's line
  √ line drawn along axis of femoral shaft will not pass through upper edge of acetabulum but intersect the anterior-superior iliac spine (during Barlow maneuver)
  √ apex of metaphysis lateral to edge of acetabulum
  √ femoral shaft above horizontal line drawn through the Y-synchondroses

√ unilateral shortening of vertical distance from femoral ossific nucleus / femoral metaphysis to Hilgenreiner's line
√ femoral ossific nucleus / medial beak of femoral metaphysis outside inner lower quadrant of coordinates established by Hilgenreiner's + Perkin's lines

√ acetabular dysplasia = shallow incompletely developed acetabulum:
√ acetabular angle >30° strongly suggests dysplasia
√ development of false acetabulum
√ delayed ossification of femoral epiphysis (usually evident between 2nd and 8th month of life)

US (practical only up to 4–6 months of age):
◊ Too sensitive during first 2 weeks of life!
(1) static evaluation (popularized in Europe by Graf)
(2) dynamic evaluation (popularized in USA by Harcke)
@ Relationship of femoral head & acetabulum
√ femoral head position at rest in neutral position:
√ hip instability under motion + stress maneuvers:
√ dislocated (= eccentric) hip can be reduced (Ortolani positive):
√ hypoechoic femoral head not centered over triradiate cartilage between pubis + ischium (on transverse view)
√ increased amount of soft-tissue echoes ("pulvinar") between femoral head and acetabulum
√ cartilaginous acetabular labrum interposed between head and acetabulum (inverted labrum)
√ posterior + superior dislocation of head against ilium
√ equator sign = <50% of femoral head lies medial to line drawn along iliac bone (on coronal view): >58% coverage is normal; 58% to 33% coverage is indeterminate; <33% coverage is abnormal
@ Femoral head
√ disparity in size of directly visualized unossified femoral head
√ disparity in presence + size of ossific nucleus
@ Acetabulum
√ delayed ossification of acetabular corner
√ wavy contour of bony acetabulum with only slight curvature
√ abnormally acute alpha angle (= angle between straight lateral edge of ilium + bony acetabular margin)
√ α >60° in an infant is normal
√ α 55–60° can be normal <4 weeks of age
√ α <55° occurs in an immature acetabulum
◊ 4°–6° interobserver variation!

Prognosis: alpha-angle <50° at birth / 50°–59° after 3 months indicates significant risk for dislocation without treatment; follow-up at 4-week intervals are recommended

CT:
sector angle = angle between line drawn from center of femoral head to acetabular rim + horizontal axis of pelvis (= reflection of acetabular support)
√ anterior acetabular sector angle <50°
√ posterior acetabular sector angle <90°

Sonographic Hip Types

Type	*Description*	*α Angle*	*β Angle*
1	mature hip	>60°	
1A	narrow cartilaginous roof		<55°
1B	wide cartilaginous roof		>55°
2	deficient bony acetabulum		
2A	physiologic <3 months	50 – 59°	
2B	delayed ossification >3 months		
2C	concentric but unstable; *critical range*	43 – 49°	70 – 77°
2D	decentered = subluxed		>77°
3	eccentric = dislocated	<43°	
4	severe dysplasia with inverted labrum		

(1) α **angle** = angle between straight lateral edge of ilium + bony acetabular margin (on coronal view); determines sonographic hip type
(2) β **angle** = angle between straight lateral edge of ilium + fibrocartilaginous acetabulum; determines nuances of sonographic hip type

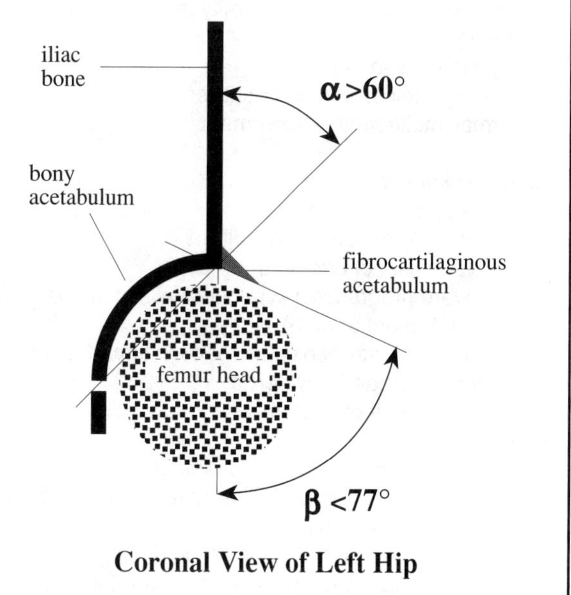

Coronal View of Left Hip

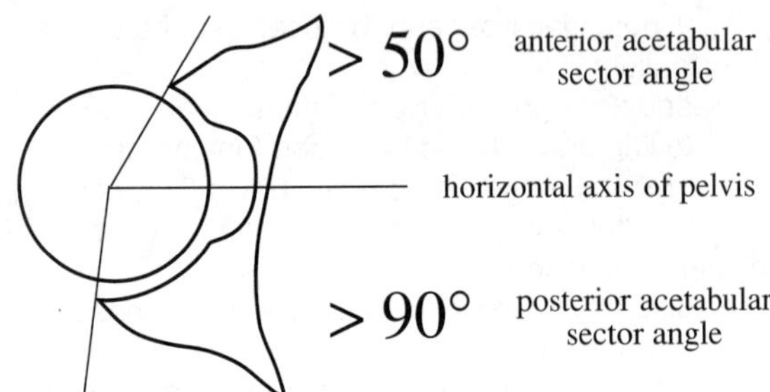

Acetabular Sector Angles (in normal right hip)

Cx: (1) Avascular necrosis of femoral head
(2) Intraarticular obstacle to reduction
(a) pulvinar = fibrofatty tissue at apex of acetabulum
(b) hypertrophy of ligamentum teres
(c) labral hypertrophy / inversion
(3) Extraarticular obstacle to reduction
iliopsoas tendon impingement on anterior joint capsule with infolding of joint capsule

Prognosis: 78% of hips become spontaneously normal by 4th week + 90% by 9th week

Rx: (1) Flexion-abduction-external rotation brace (Pavlik harness) / splint / spica cast
(2) Femoral varus osteotomy
(3) Pelvic (Salter) / acetabular rotation
(4) Increase in acetabular depth (Pemberton)
(5) Medialization of femoral head (Chiari)

DIASTROPHIC DYSPLASIA

= DIASTROPHIC DWARFISM = EPIPHYSEAL DYSOSTOSIS
= autosomal recessive severe rhizomelic dwarfism secondary to generalized disorder of cartilage followed by fibrous scars + ossifications

- diastrophic = "twisted" habitus
- "cauliflower ear" = ear deformity from inflammation of pinna
- laryngomalacia
- lax + rigid joints with contractures
- normal intellectual development

@ Axial skeleton
√ cleft palate (25%)
√ cervical spina bifida occulta
√ hypoplasia of odontoid
√ severe progressive kyphoscoliosis of lumbar spine (not present at birth)
√ narrowed interpedicular space in lumbar spine
√ short + broad bony pelvis
√ posterior tilt of sacrum

@ Extremities
√ severe micromelia (predominantly rhizomelic = humerus + femur shorter than distal long bones
√ widened metaphysis
√ flattened epiphysis (retardation of epiphyseal ossification) with invagination of ossification centers into distal ends of femora
√ multiple joint flexion contractures (notably of major joints)
√ dislocation of one / more large joints (hip, elbow), lateral dislocation of patella
√ coxa vara (common)
√ medially bowed metatarsals
√ clubfoot = severe talipes equinovarus
√ ulnar deviation of hands
√ oval + hypoplastic 1st metacarpal bone + abducted proximally positioned thumb = "hitchhiker's thumb" (CHARACTERISTIC)
√ bizarre carpal bones with supernumerary centers
√ widely spaced fingers

OB-US:
√ proportionately shortened long bones
√ hitchhiker thumb
√ clubfeet
√ joint contractures
√ abnormal spinal curvature

Prognosis: death in infancy (due to abnormal softening of tracheal cartilage)

DIFFUSE IDIOPATHIC SKELETAL HYPEROSTOSIS

= DISH = FORESTIER DISEASE = ANKYLOSING HYPEROSTOSIS
= common ossifying diathesis characterized by bone proliferation at sites of tendinous + ligamentous attachment (enthesis)

Etiology:
(1) may be caused by altered vitamin A metabolism (elevated plasma levels of unbound retinol)
(2) long-term ingestion of retinoid derivatives for treatment of acne (eg, Accutane®);
? hypertrophic variant of spondylosis deformans

Age: >50 years; M:F = 3:1

- pain, tenderness in extraspinal locations
- restricted motion of vertebral column
- hyperglycemia
- positive HLA-B27 in 34%

√ increased incidence of hyperostosis frontalis interna

@ Spine
Location: middle + lower thoracic > lower cervical > entire lumbar spine
√ <u>flowing</u> ossification of <u>at least 4</u> contiguous vertebral bodies:
√ osteophytes located anteriorly + laterally on right side (not on left because of aorta)
√ osteophytes largest at level of intervertebral disk
√ radiolucency beneath deposited bone
√ disk spaces well preserved, no apophyseal ankylosis, no sacroiliitis

@ Pelvis
√ bridge across superior aspect of symphysis pubis
√ ossification of iliolumbar + sacrotuberous + sacroiliac ligaments (high probability for presence of spinal DISH, DDx: fluorosis)
√ "whiskering" at iliac crest, ischial tuberosity, trochanters
√ broad osteophytes at lateral acetabular edge, inferior portions of sacroiliac joints

@ Extremities
- √ big heel spurs (on plantar + posterior surface of calcaneus)
- √ spur of olecranon process of ulna
- √ spur on anterior surface of patella
- √ ossification of coracoclavicular ligament, patellar ligament, tibial tuberosity, interosseous membranes

Cx: postoperative heterotopic bone formation (hip)

DDx:
(1) Fluorosis (increased skeletal density)
(2) Acromegaly (posterior scalloping, skull features)
(3) Hypoparathyroidism
(4) X-linked hypophosphatemic vitamin D–resistant rickets
(5) Ankylosing spondylitis (squaring of vertebral bodies, coarser syndesmophytes, sacroiliitis, apophyseal alteration)
(6) Intervertebral osteochondrosis (vacuum phenomenon, vertebral body marginal sclerosis, decreased intervertebral disk height)

DISLOCATION

Hip Dislocation

Incidence: 5% of all dislocations

A. POSTERIOR HIP DISLOCATION (80–85%)
Mechanism: classical dashboard injury (= flexed knee strikes dashboard)
Associated with: fractures of posterior rim of acetabulum, femoral head

B. ANTERIOR HIP DISLOCATION (5–10%)
1. anterior obturator dislocation
2. superoanterior / pubic hip dislocation

Associated with: fractures of acetabular rim, greater trochanter, femoral neck, femoral head (characteristic depression on posterosuperior and lateral portion)

C. CENTRAL ACETABULAR FRACTURE - DISLOCATION
Mechanism: force applied to lateral side of trochanter

Patellar Dislocation

= TRANSIENT LATERAL PATELLAR DISLOCATION

Incidence: 2–3% of all knee injuries

Mechanism: during attempt to slow forward motion while pivoting medially on a planted foot; internal rotation of femur on fixed tibia while knee is flexed + quadriceps contraction produces a net lateral force

At risk: shallow trochlear groove

Associated with: medial meniscal tear / major ligamentous injury in 31%

Age: young physically active people

- hemarthrosis (most common cause of hemarthrosis in young conscripts)
- swelling + tenderness of medial retinaculum

◊ >50% not clinically diagnosed initially!

- √ increased signal intensity / thickening / disruption of medial patellar retinaculum
- √ lateral patellar tilt
- √ contusion / microfracture / osteochondral injury of nonarticular surface of lateral femoral condyle + medial articular surface of patella
- √ hemarthrosis

MR:
- √ bone contusion of anterolateral aspect of lateral femoral condyle + inferomedial aspect of patella
- √ sprain / disruption / avulsion of medial retinaculum + medial patellofemoral ligament + medial patellotibial ligament
- √ elevation of vastus medialis obliquus muscle

Rx:
(1) Temporary immobilization + rehabilitation: successful in 75%
(2) Surgery: fixation of osteochondral fragments, medial capsule repair, lateral retinacular release, vastus medialis et lateralis rearrangement, medial retinaculum reefing

Shoulder Dislocation

Sternoclavicular Dislocation (3%)

Acromioclavicular Dislocation (12%)

grade 1 = soft-tissue swelling + no joint widening
grade 2 = subluxation with elevation of clavicle of <5 mm (weight-bearing!)
grade 3 = dislocation with wide AC joint + increased coracoclavicular distance

Glenohumeral Dislocation (85%)

◊ Glenohumeral joint dislocations make up >50% of all dislocations!

ANTERIOR / SUBCORACOID SHOULDER DISLOCATION (96%)

Types: subcoracoid, subglenoid, subclavicular, intrathoracic

Mechanism: external rotation + abduction; 40% recurrent

Age: in younger individuals

May be associated with:
- √ fracture of greater tuberosity (15%)
- √ Bankart lesion = anterior tear of glenoid labrum (originally only referring to injury of anterior band of glenohumeral ligament)
[Arthur Sydney Blundell Bankart (1879–1951), British orthopedic surgeon]

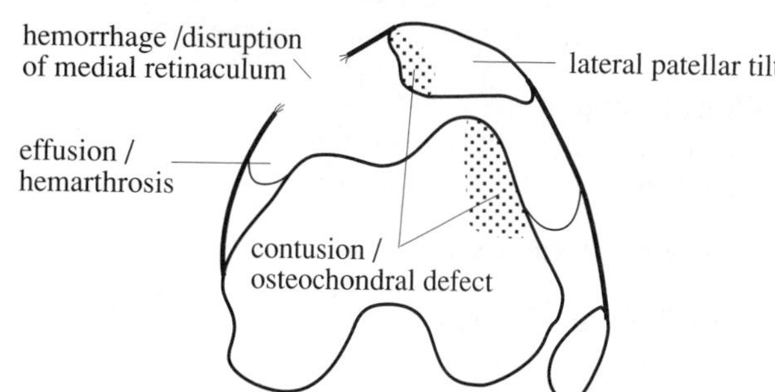

MR Imaging Signs of Patellar Dislocation

√ fracture of anterior rim of glenoid
√ Hill-Sachs defect (50%) = depression / impacted fracture of posterolateral surface of humeral head at / above level of coracoid process (due to impaction against anterior edge of glenoid rim in subglenoid type)
[Harold Arthur Hill (1901–1973) and Maurice David Sachs (1909–1987), radiologists in San Francisco, California]
Cx: recurrent dislocations

Posterior Shoulder Dislocation (2–4%)
Cause: (a) traumatic: convulsive disorders / electric shock therapy
(b) nontraumatic: voluntary, involuntary, congenital, developmental
Types: subacromial, subglenoid, subspinous
◊ In >50% unrecognized initially + subsequently misdiagnosed as frozen shoulder!
◊ Average interval between injury and diagnosis is 1 year!
√ rim sign (66%) = distance between medial border of humeral head + anterior glenoid rim <6 mm
May be associated with:
√ trough sign (75%) = "reverse Hill-Sachs" = compression fracture of anteromedial humeral head (tangential Grashey view of glenoid!)
√ fracture of posterior glenoid rim
√ avulsion fracture of lesser tuberosity

Inferior Shoulder Dislocation (1–2%)
= LUXATIO ERECTA
= extremity held over head in fixed position with elbow flexed
Mechanism: severe hyperabduction of arm resulting in impingement of humeral head against acromion
√ humeral articular surface faces inferiorly
Cx: rotator cuff tear; fracture of acromion ± inferior glenoid fossa ± greater tuberosity; neurovascular injury

Superior Shoulder Dislocation (<1%)
= humeral head driven upward through rotator cuff
May be associated with: fracture of humerus, clavicle, acromion
DDx: drooping shoulder (transient phenomenon after fracture of surgical neck of humerus due to hemarthrosis / muscle imbalance)

Wrist Dislocation
Mechanism: fall on outstretched hand
Incidence: 10% of all carpal injuries

Lunate Dislocation

Perilunate Dislocation
2–3 times more common than lunate dislocation accompanied by fracture in 75% (= transscaphoid perilunate dislocation)
√ most commonly dorsal dislocation

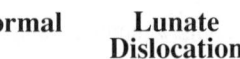

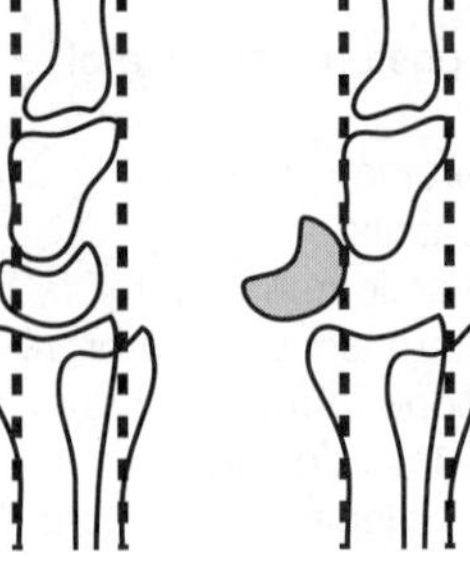
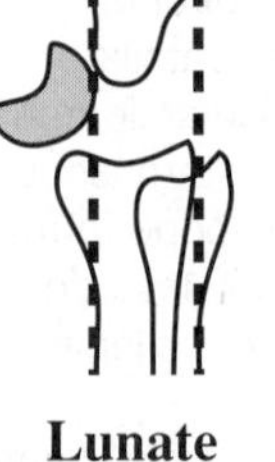
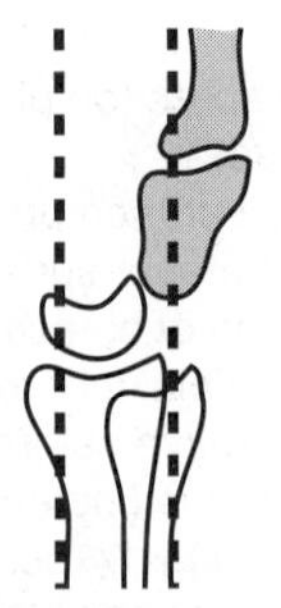
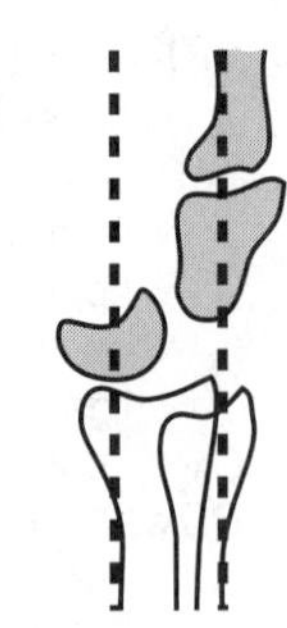

Rotary Subluxation of Scaphoid
= tearing of interosseous ligaments of lunate, scaphoid, capitate
Mechanism: acute dorsiflexion of wrist; may be associated with rheumatoid arthritis
√ gap >4 mm between scaphoid + lunate (PA view)
√ foreshortening of scaphoid
√ ring sign of distal pole of scaphoid

Midcarpal Dislocation

DOWN SYNDROME
= MONGOLISM = TRISOMY 21
Chromosomes: 95% nondisjunction, 5% translocation
Incidence: 1:870 liveborn infants, most common karyotype / chromosomal abnormality in USA
• mental retardation
• hypotonia in infancy
• characteristic facies
• Simian crease
@ Skull
√ hypotelorism
√ persistent metopic suture (40–79%) after age 10
√ hypoplasia of sinuses + facial bones
√ microcrania (brachycephaly)
√ delayed closure of sutures + fontanels
√ dental abnormalities (underdeveloped tooth No. 2)
√ flat-bridged nose
@ Axial skeleton
√ atlantoaxial subluxation (25%)
√ anterior scalloping of vertebral bodies
√ "squared vertebral bodies" = centra high and narrow = positive lateral lumbar index (ratio of horizontal to vertical diameters of L2)
@ Chest
√ congenital heart disease (40%): endocardial cushion defect, VSD, tetralogy of Fallot
√ hypersegmentation of manubrium = 2–3 ossification centers (90%)
√ gracile ribs; 11 pairs of ribs (25%)
@ Pelvis (frontal view)
√ flaring of iliac wings (= rotation of iliac wings toward coronal plane at sacroiliac joints) = "Mickey Mouse ears" / "elephant ears":
√ decreased iliac angle + index (in 70–80%)
√ flattening of acetabular roof (small acetabular angle)

√ elongated + tapered ischia

@ Extremities
- √ metaphyseal flaring
- √ clinodactyly (50%); widened space between first two digits of hands + feet
- √ hypoplastic and triangular middle + distal phalanges of 5th finger = acromicria (DDx: normal individuals, cretins, achondroplastic dwarfs)
- √ pseudoepiphyses of 1st + 2nd metacarpals

@ Gastrointestinal
- √ umbilical hernia
- √ "double bubble" sign (8–10%) = duodenal atresia / stenosis / annular pancreas
- √ tracheoesophageal fistula
- √ anorectal anomalies
- √ Hirschsprung disease

OB-US:
- • **triple-marker screening test**:
  - • low (0.7 MoM) maternal alpha-fetoprotein (20–30%)
  - • increased (2.04 MoM) hCG (DDx: decreased in trisomy 18)
  - • decreased (0.79 MoM) unconjugated estriol (ue3)
  - • dimeric inhibin A (= new additional analyte)
  - ◊ Detects 60% + 75% of all Down syndrome pregnancies in women <35 years + >35 years
  - ◊ Most accurate between 16 and 18 weeks!
- • advanced maternal age
  - ◊ In 1:385 live births for women >35 years of age
  - ◊ HOWEVER: 80% of fetuses with Down syndrome are born to mothers <35 years of age
- √ major structural malformations:
  - √ VSD / complete AV canal (50%)
  - √ cystic hygroma, resolved by 20th week MA
  - √ omphalocele
  - √ double bubble of duodenal atresia (8–10%), not apparent before 22 weeks GA
  - √ hydrothorax
  - √ mild cerebral ventricular dilatation
  - √ agenesis of corpus callosum
  - √ imperforate anus
- √ occipital-nuchal skin thickening ≥5 mm during 14–18 weeks / ≥6 mm during 19–24 weeks
- √ mild fetal pyelectasis (17–25%)
- √ hyperechoic bowel at <20 weeks GA (15%, in 0.6% of normals)
- √ intracardiac echogenic focus, usually in left ventricle = thickening of papillary muscle (18%, in 5% of normals)
- √ ratio of measured-to-expected femur length ≤0.91 [expected femur length: –9.3105 + 0.9028 x BPD] (sensitivity 40%, specificity 95%, false-positive rate of 2–7%, 0.3% PPV for low-risk population [1:700], 1% PPV for high-risk population [1:250])
- √ elevated BPD / femur ratio (secondary to short femur)
- √ ratio of measured-to-expected humerus length ≤0.90 [expected humerus length: –7.9404 + 0.8492 x BPD] (1–2% PPV for low-risk population; 3% PPV for high-risk population)
- √ sandal-gap deformity = separation of great toe (45%)
- √ hypoplasia of middle phalanx of 5th digit resulting in clinodactyly (= inward curve) in 60%
- √ flared ilium = iliac wings rotated toward coronal plane:
  - √ mean iliac angle at superiormost level of 95.6 ± 11.7° (compared to 76.4 ± 16.8° for euploid fetuses)
- √ brachycephaly
- √ small cerebellum
- √ IUGR (in 30%)
- √ polyhydramnios

Cx: leukemia (increased frequency 3–20 x)

DYSCHONDROSTEOSIS

= LÉRI-LAYANI-WEILL SYNDROME

= mesomelic long-bone shortening (forearm + leg); autosomal dominant

M:F = 1:4

- • limited motion of elbow + wrist
- √ bilateral Madelung deformity:
  - √ radial shortening in relation to ulna
  - √ bowing of radius laterally + dorsally
  - √ dorsal subluxation of distal end of ulna
  - √ carpal wedging between radius + ulna (due to triangular shape of distal radial epiphysis + underdevelopment of ulna)

DDx: pseudo-Madelung deformity (from trauma / infection)

DYSPLASIA EPIPHYSEALIS HEMIMELICA

= TREVOR DISEASE = TARSOEPIPHYSEAL ACLASIS

= uncommon skeletal developmental disorder representing an epiphyseal osteochondroma

Incidence: 1:1,000,000

Age: 2–4 years; M:F = 3:1

Cause: failure of normal progression of cellular cartilage breakdown (= aclasis); spontaneous occurrence

Path: lobulated mass protruding from epiphysis with a cartilaginous cap

Histo: normal bone + hyaline cartilage with abundant enchondral ossification (= abnormal cellular activity at cartilaginous ossification center)

Forms:

(1) Localized form = monostotic involvement: usually hindfoot and ankle

(2) Classic form (>66%) = more than one area of involvement in a single extremity with characteristic hemimelic distribution: talus, distal femur, distal tibia

(3) Generalized / severe form = disease involving the whole lower extremity
- √ pelvic involvement: femoral head, symphysis pubis, triradiate cartilage
- √ hypertrophy of ipsilateral iliac bone

- • antalgic (= pain-avoiding) gait; palpable mass
- • varus / valgus deformity; limb length discrepancy
- • limited joint mobility and function

Location: lower extremity (tarsus, knee, ankle); rare in upper extremity (humerus, ulna, scapula)

Site: restricted to medial OR lateral side of limb (= hemimelic), ie, medial:lateral = 2:1

@ Infant & toddler
  √ premature appearance of an eccentric, lobulated, overgrown, asymmetric ossification center
  √ stippled calcification of anomalous cartilage
@ Childhood
  √ disorganized epiphyseal calcification accompanied by irregular ossification
  √ osteochondroma-like growth from one side of epiphysis
  √ premature closure of physis results in limb deformity and limb length discrepancy
  √ irregular articular surface combined with angular deformity
  √ undertubulation of bone as a consequence of secondary involvement of metaphysis

Cx: premature secondary osteoarthritis
DDx: osteochondroma

ECHINOCOCCUS OF BONE

Occurs occasionally in the USA; usually in foreign-born individuals; bone involvement in 1%

Histo: no connective tissue barrier; daughter cysts extend directly into bone

@ Pelvis, sacrum, rarely long tubular bones
  √ round / irregular regions of rarefaction
  √ multiloculated lesion (bunch of grapes)
  √ no sharp demarcation (DDx: chondroma, giant cell tumor) with secondary infection:
    √ thickening of trabeculae with generalized perifocal condensation
    √ cortical breakthrough with soft-tissue mass
@ Vertebra
  √ sclerosis without pathologic fracture
  √ intervertebral disks not affected
  √ vertebral lamina often involved
  √ frequently involvement of adjacent ribs

EHLERS-DANLOS SYNDROME

= group of autosomal dominant diseases of connective tissue characterized by abnormal collagen synthesis

Types: 10 types have been described that differ clinically, biochemically, and genetically
Age: present at birth; predominantly in males

• hyperelasticity of skin
• fragile brittle skin with gaping wounds and poor healing
• molluscoid pseudotumors over pressure points
• hyperextensibility of joints
• joint contractures with advanced age
• bleeding tendency (fragility of blood vessels)
• blue sclera, microcornea, myopia, keratoconus, ectopia lentis

@ Soft tissues
  √ multiple ovoid calcifications (2–10 mm) in subcutis / in fatty cysts ("spheroids"), most frequently in periarticular areas of legs
  √ ectopic bone formation
@ Skeleton
  √ hemarthrosis (particularly in knee)
  √ malalignment / subluxation / dislocation of joints on stress radiographs
  √ recurrent dislocations (hip, patella, shoulder, radius, clavicle)
  √ precocious osteoarthrosis (predominantly in knees)
  √ ulnar synostosis
  √ kyphoscoliosis
  √ spondylolisthesis
  √ spina bifida occulta
@ Chest
  √ diaphragmatic hernia
  √ panacinar emphysema + bulla formation
  √ tracheobronchomegaly + bronchiectasis
@ Arteries
  √ aneurysm of great vessels, aortic dissection, tortuosity of arch, ectasia of pulmonary arteries
  ◊ AORTOGRAPHY CONTRAINDICATED! (Cx following arteriography: aortic rupture, hematomas)
@ GI tract
  √ ectasia of gastrointestinal tract

ELASTOFIBROMA

= benign tumorlike lesion forming as a reaction to mechanical friction

Incidence: in 24% of women + 11% of men >55 years (autopsy study)
Age: elderly; M:F = 1:2
Histo: enlarged irregular serrated elastic hypereosinophilic fibers, collagen, scattered fibroblasts, occasional lobules of adipose tissue

• asymptomatic
• may remain clinically inapparent

Location: between inferior margin of scapula + posterior chest wall; bilateral in 25%

√ inhomogeneous poorly defined lesion of soft-tissue attenuation similar to muscle
√ well-defined intermediate-signal intensity lesion with interlaced areas of fat-intensity signal on T1WI + T2WI

ENCHONDROMA

= benign cartilaginous growth in medullary cavity; bones preformed in cartilage are affected (NOT skull)

Incidence: 3–17% of biopsied primary bone tumors
  ◊ Second most common cartilage-containing tumor!
Etiology: continued growth of residual benign rests of cartilage displaced from the growth plate
Age: 10–30 years; M:F = 1:1
Histo: lobules of pure hyaline cartilage

• usually asymptomatic, painless swelling

Location: (usually solitary; multiple = enchondromatosis)
  (a) in 40% small tubular bones of wrists + hand (most frequent tumor here), distal + mid aspects of metacarpals, proximal / middle phalanges
  (b) proximal femur, proximal humerus, tibia, radius, ulna, foot, rib (3%)

Site: central within medullary canal + metaphyseal; epiphysis only affected after closure of growth plate

√ oval / round area of geographic destruction with lobulated contour + fine marginal line

√ cortical endosteal scalloping
√ ground-glass appearance
√ dystrophic calcifications within small cartilage nodules / fragments of lamellar bone: pinhead, stippled, flocculent, "rings and arcs" pattern
√ bulbous expansion of bone with thinning of cortex in small tubular bones of phalanx, rib, fibula
√ Madelung deformity = bowing deformities of limb, discrepant length
√ NO cortical breakthrough / periosteal reaction

MR:
- √ low- to intermediate-signal intensity on T1WI + high-signal intensity on T2WI
- √ low-signal intensity matrix calcifications
- √ normal fat marrow interspersed between cartilage nodules
- √ peripheral enhancement pattern

Cx: (1) Pathologic fracture
(2) Malignant degeneration in long-bone enchondromas in 15–20% (gradually increasing pain in an adult patient)

DDx: (1) Epidermoid inclusion cyst (phalangeal tuft, history of trauma, more lucent)
(2) Unicameral bone cyst (rare in hands, more radiolucent)
(3) Giant cell tumor of tendon sheath (commonly erodes bone, soft-tissue mass outside bone)
(4) Fibrous dysplasia (rare in hand, mostly polyostotic)
(5) Bone infarct
(6) Chondrosarcoma (exceedingly rare in phalanges, metacarpals, metatarsals)

ENCHONDROMATOSIS

= OLLIER DISEASE = DYSCHONDROPLASIA = MULTIPLE ENCHONDROMATOSIS
= nonhereditary failure of cartilage ossification

Cause: derangement of cartilaginous growth resulting in migration of cartilaginous rests from epiphyseal plate into metaphysis where they proliferate

Age: early childhood presentation

Association: juvenile granulosa cell tumor of ovary

- growth disparity with leg / arm shortening
- hand + feet deformity

Location: predominantly unilateral monomelic distribution (a) localized (b) regional (c) generalized

√ well-demarcated rounded radiolucencies / columnar streaks of decreased density from epiphyseal plate into diaphysis of long bones = cartilaginous rests
√ expansile remodeling of affected bone:
- √ clublike deformity / expansion of metaphyseal region
- √ predominant thinning of cortex + endosteal scalloping
- √ bony spurs pointing toward the joint (DDx: exostosis points away from it)

√ cartilaginous areas show punctate calcifications with age:
- √ matrix mineralization with TYPICAL arc-and-ring appearance of chondroid lesions

√ associated with dwarfing of the involved bone due to impairment of epiphyseal fusion
√ bowing deformities of limb bones
√ discrepancy in length = Madelung deformity (radius, ulna)
√ small bones of feet + hands: aggressive deforming tumors that may break through cortex secondary to tendency to continue to proliferate
√ fanlike radiation of cartilage from center to crest of ilium

Cx: sarcomatous transformation (in 25–30%): osteosarcoma (young adults); chondro- / fibrosarcoma (in older patients)

Maffuci Syndrome

= nonhereditary mesodermal dysplasia characterized by enchondromatosis + multiple soft-tissue cavernous hemangiomas + less commonly lymphangiomas

Age: 25% during 1st year of life; 45% prior to 6 years; 78% before puberty; M > F

Association: juvenile granulosa cell tumor of ovary

- multiple blue subcutaneous nodules particularly on digits + extremities (cavernous hemangiomas)
- normal intelligence

Location: unilateral involvement (50%) / marked asymmetry; distinct predilection for tubular bones of hands + feet

√ phleboliths may be present
√ striking tendency for enchondromata to be very large projecting into soft tissues
√ growth disturbance of long bones (common)

Cx: (a) malignant transformation of
(1) Enchondroma to chondrosarcoma / fibrosarcoma (15–20%)
(2) Cavernous hemangioma to hemangiosarcoma / hemangioendothelioma / lymphangiosarcoma (in 3–5%)
(b) increased prevalence of ovarian carcinoma, pancreatic carcinoma, CNS glioma, gastrointestinal adenocarcinoma

Prevalence of malignancy: 23–100%

DDx: Ollier disease (without hemangiomas)

ENGELMANN-CAMURATI DISEASE

= PROGRESSIVE DIAPHYSEAL DYSPLASIA = CAMURATI-ENGELMANN DISEASE

Cause: autosomal dominant; disturbance in intramembranous bone formation + modeling (as occurs in cortex of long bones, calvaria, mandible, facial bones, midsegment of clavicle)

Age: 5–25 years (primarily in childhood); M > F

- neuromuscular dystrophy = delayed walking (18–24 months) with wide-based waddling gait; often misdiagnosed as muscular dystrophy / poliomyelitis
- weakness + easy fatigability in legs
- bone pain + tenderness usually in midshaft of long bones
- underdevelopment of muscles secondary to malnutrition
- NORMAL laboratory values

Location: usually symmetrical; NO involvement of hands, feet, ribs, scapulae

@ Skull (initially affected)
- √ amorphous increase in density at base of skull
- √ encroachment of frontal + sphenoid sinus; sparing of maxillary sinus

@ Long bones (bilateral symmetrical distribution)
Site: tibia > femur > fibula > humerus > ulna > radius
- √ fusiform enlargement of diaphyses with cortical thickening (endosteal + periosteal accretion of mottled new bone) and progressive obliteration of medullary cavity
- √ progression of lesions along long axis of bone toward either end
- √ abrupt demarcation of lesions (metaphyses + epiphyses spared)
- √ relative elongation of extremities

DDx: (1) Chronic osteomyelitis (single bone)
(2) Hyperphosphatasemia (high alkaline phosphatase levels)
(3) Paget disease (age, new-bone formation, increased alkaline phosphatase)
(4) Infantile cortical hyperostosis (fever; mandible, rib, clavicles; regresses, <1 year of age)
(5) Fibrous dysplasia (predominantly unilateral, subperiosteal new bone)
(6) Osteopetrosis (very little bony enlargement)
(7) Vitamin A poisoning

EPIDERMOID CYST

= INFUNDIBULAR CYST
= proliferation of surface epidermal cells within the dermis
Histo: production of keratin within closed space lined by surface epidermis
Associated with: nevoid basal cell syndrome (Gorlin syndrome) patients have a high prevalence of epidermoid / dermoid cysts
- √ isointense / slightly hyperintense relative to muscle on T1WI
- √ hyperintense with focal areas of decreased signal on T2WI

Epidermoid Inclusion Cyst

= INTRAOSSEOUS KERATIN CYST = IMPLANTATION CYST
Age: 2nd–4th decade; M > F
Histo: stratified squamous epithelium, keratin, cholesterol crystals (soft white cheesy contents)
- • history of trauma (implantation of epithelium under skin with secondary bone erosion)
- • asymptomatic

Location: superficially situated bones such as calvarium (typically in frontal / parietal bone), phalanx (usually terminal tuft of middle finger), L > R hand, occasionally in foot
- √ well-defined round osteolysis with sclerotic margin
- √ cortex frequently expanded + thinned
- √ NO calcifications / periosteal reaction / soft-tissue swelling
- √ pathologic fracture often without periosteal reaction

DDx: (a) in finger: glomus tumor, enchondroma (rare in terminal phalanx)
(b) in skull: infection, metastasis (poorly defined), eosinophilic granuloma (beveled margin)

EPIPHYSEOLYSIS OF FEMORAL HEAD

= SLIPPED CAPITAL FEMORAL EPIPHYSIS
= atraumatic fracture through hypertrophic zone of physeal plate
Frequency: 2:100,000 people
Etiology: growth spurt, renal osteodystrophy, rickets, childhood irradiation, growth hormone therapy, trauma (Salter-Harris type I epiphyseal injury)
Pathogenesis: widening of physeal plate during growth spurt + change in orientation of physis from horizontal to oblique increases shear forces
Age: overweight 8–17 year old boys (mean age for boys 13, for girls 11 years); M:F = 3:1; black > white
Associated with:
(a) malnutrition, endocrine abnormality, developmental dysplasia of hip (during adolescence)
(b) delayed skeletal maturation (after adolescence)
- • hip pain (50%) / knee pain (25%) for 2–3 weeks

Location: usually unilateral; bilateral in 20–37% (at initial presentation in 9–18%)
- √ widening of epiphyseal growth plate (preslip phase):
  - √ irregularity + blurring of physeal physis
  - √ demineralization of neck metaphysis
- √ posteromedial displacement of head (acute slip):
  - √ decrease in neck-shaft angle with alignment change in the growth plate to a more vertical orientation
  - √ line of Klein (= line drawn along superior edge of femoral neck) fails to intersect the femoral head
  - √ epiphysis appears smaller due to posterior slippage: early slips are best seen on cross-table LAT view
    CAVE: positioning into a frogleg view may cause further displacement
- √ sclerosis + irregularity of widened physis (chronic slip):
  - √ metaphyseal blanch sign = area of increased opacity in proximal part of metaphysis (healing response)

Grading (based on femoral head position):
mild = displaced by <1/3 of metaphyseal diameter
moderate = displaced by 1/3–2/3 of diameter
severe = displaced by >2/3 of metaphyseal diameter

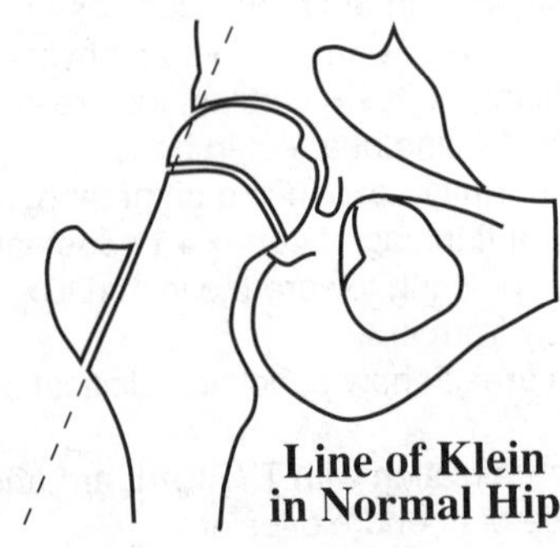
Line of Klein in Normal Hip

Cx: (1) Chondrolysis = acute cartilage necrosis (7–10%)
= rapid loss of >50% of thickness of cartilage
√ joint space <3 mm
(2) Avascular necrosis of femoral head (10–15%): risk increases with advanced degree of slip, delayed surgery for acute slip, anterior pin placement, large number of fixation pins, subcapital osteotomy
(3) Pistol-grip deformity = broadening + shortening of femoral neck in varus deformity
(4) Degenerative osteoarthritis (90%)
(5) Limb-length discrepancy due to premature physeal closure

Rx: (1) limitation of activity, (2) prophylactic pinning
(3) osteotomy
Attempted reductions increase risk of AVN!

ESSENTIAL OSTEOLYSIS

= progressive slow bone-resorptive disease

Histo: proliferation + hyperplasia of smooth muscle cells of synovial arterioles

√ progressive osteolysis of carpal + tarsal bones
√ thinned pointed proximal ends of metacarpals + metatarsals
√ elbows show same type of destruction
√ bathyrocephalic depression of base of skull

DDx: (1) Massive osteolysis = Gorham disease (local destruction of contiguous bones, usually not affecting hands / feet)
(9) Mutilating forms of rheumatoid arthritis
(2) Tabes dorsalis
(3) Leprosy
(4) Syringomyelia
(5) Scleroderma
(6) Raynaud disease
(7) Regional posttraumatic osteolysis
(8) Ulcero-mutilating acropathy
(9) Mutilating forms of rheumatoid arthritis
(10) Acrodynia mutilante (nonhereditary)

EWING SARCOMA

= EWING TUMOR

Incidence: 4–10% of all bone tumors (less common than osteo- / chondrosarcoma); most common malignant bone tumor in children; 4th most common bone tumor overall

◊ Clinically, radiologically, and histologically very similar to PNET!

Histo:
small round cells, uniformly sized + solidly packed (DDx: lymphoma, osteosarcoma, myeloma, neuroblastoma, carcinoma, eosinophilic granuloma) invading medullary cavity and entering subperiosteum via Haversian canals producing periostitis, soft-tissue mass, osteolysis; glycogen granules present (DDx to reticulum cell sarcoma); absence of alkaline phosphatase (DDx to osteosarcoma); MIC2 cell surface immunoreactivity (in 100%)

Age: peak 15 years (range 5 months to 54 years); in 95% 4–25 years; in 30% <10 years; in 39% 11–15 years; in 31% >15 years; in 50% <20 years; M:F = 1:2; Caucasians in 96%

• severe localized pain
• soft-tissue mass
• fever, leukocytosis, anemia (in early metastases) simulating infection

Location:
femur (25%), pelvis-ilium (14%), tibia (11%), humerus (10%), fibula (8%), ribs (6–10%)
(a) long bones in 60%:
metadiaphysis (44%), middiaphysis (33%), metaphysis (15%), metaepiphyseal (6%), epiphyseal (2%); usually no involvement of epiphysis as tumor originates in medullary cavity with invasion of Haversian system
(b) flat bones in 40%: pelvis, scapula, skull, vertebrae (in 3–10%; sacrum > lumbar > thoracic > cervical spine); ribs (in 7% > age 10; in 30% < age 10)
◊ >20 years of age predominantly in flat bones
◊ <20 years of age predominantly in cylindrical bones (tumor derived from red marrow)

√ 8–10 cm long lytic lesion in shaft of long bone (62% lytic, 23% mixed density, 15% dense)
√ mottled "moth-eaten" destructive permeative lesion (72%) (late finding)
√ penetration into soft tissue (55%) with preservation of tissue planes (DDx: osteomyelitis with diffuse soft-tissue swelling)
√ early fusiform lamellated "onionskin" periosteal reaction (53%) / spiculated = "sunburst" / "hair-on-end" (23%), Codman triangle
√ cortical thickening (16%)
√ cortical destruction (18%)
√ ± cortical sequestration
√ reactive sclerotic new bone (30%)
√ bone expansion (12%)

@ Ewing sarcoma of rib:
√ primarily lytic / sclerotic / mixture of lysis + sclerosis
√ disproportionately large inhomogeneous soft-tissue mass
√ large intrathoracic + minimal extrathoracic component
√ may spread into spinal canal via intervertebral foramen

Metastases to: lung, bones, regional lymph nodes in 11–30% at time of diagnosis, in 40–45% within 2 years of diagnosis

Cx: pathologic fracture (5–14%)

Prognosis: 60–75% 5-year survival

DDx: (1) Multiple myeloma (older age group)
(2) Osteomyelitis (duration of pain <2 weeks)
(3) Eosinophilic granuloma (solid periosteal reaction)
(4) Osteosarcoma (ossification in soft tissue, near age 20, no lamellar periosteal reaction)
(5) Reticulum cell sarcoma (clinically healthy, between 30 and 50 years, no glycogen)
(6) Neuroblastoma (< age 5)
(7) Anaplastic metastatic carcinoma (>30 years of age)

(8) Osteosarcoma
(9) Hodgkin disease

EXTRAMEDULLARY HEMATOPOIESIS

= compensatory response to deficient bone marrow blood cell production

Etiology: prolonged erythrocyte deficiency due to
(1) destruction of RBC:
congenital hemolytic anemia (thalassemia, hereditary spherocytosis, sickle cell anemia), acquired hemolytic anemia, idiopathic severe anemia, erythroblastosis fetalis
(2) inability of normal blood-forming organs to produce erythrocytes:
iron deficiency anemia, pernicious anemia, myelofibrosis, myelosclerosis, polycythemia vera, carcinomatous / lymphomatous replacement of bone marrow (chronic myelogenous leukemia, Hodgkin disease)
◊ NO hematologic disease in 25%

• absence of pain, bone erosion, calcification
• chronic anemia

Sites: in areas of fetal erythropoiesis
@ spleen
√ splenomegaly
√ focal isodense masses on enhanced CT
@ liver, lymph nodes
@ thorax: mediastinum, heart, thymus, lung
√ uni- / bilateral smooth lobulated paraspinal masses between T8 and T12
√ anterior rib ends expanded by masses
@ Spine
◊ Most commonly afflicted in thalassemia
• back pain, symptoms of spinal cord compression
√ coarsened trabeculation
√ extramedullary hematopoiesis in epidural space
@ adrenal glands
@ renal pelvis
@ gastrointestinal lymphatics
@ dura mater (falx cerebri and over brain convexity)
@ cartilage, broad ligaments
@ thrombi, adipose tissue
√ lack of calcification / bone erosion

FAMILIAL IDIOPATHIC ACROOSTEOLYSIS

= HAJDU-CHENEY SYNDROME
= rare bizarre entity of unknown etiology

Location: may be unilateral

• fingernails remain intact
• sensory changes + plantar ulcers rare

√ pseudoclubbing of fingers + toes with osteolysis of terminal + more proximal phalanges
√ genu varum / valgum
√ hypoplasia of proximal end of radius
√ subluxation of radial head
√ scaphocephaly, basilar impression
√ wide sutures, persistent metopic suture, Wormian bones, poorly developed sinuses
√ kyphoscoliosis
√ severe osteoporosis + fractures at multiple sites (esp. of spine)
√ protrusio acetabuli

FANCONI ANEMIA

= autosomal recessive disease with severe hypoplastic anemia + skin pigmentation + skeletal and urogenital anomalies

• skin pigmentation (melanin deposits) in 74% (trunk, axilla, groin, neck)
• anemia onset between 17 months and 22 years of age
• bleeding tendency (pancytopenia)
• hypogonadism (40%)
• microphthalmia (20%)

√ anomalies of radial component of upper extremity (strongly suggestive):
√ absent / hypoplastic / supernumerary thumb
√ hypoplastic / absent radius
√ absent / hypoplastic navicular / greater multangular bone
√ slight / moderate dwarfism
√ minimal microcephaly
√ renal anomalies (30%): renal aplasia, ectopia, horseshoe kidney

Prognosis: fatal within 5 years after onset of anemia; patient's family shows high incidence of leukemia

FARBER DISEASE

= DISSEMINATED LIPOGRANULOMATOSIS

Histo: foam cell granulomas; lipid storage of neuronal tissue (accumulation of ceramide + gangliosides)

• hoarse weak cry
• swelling of extremities; generalized joint swelling
• subcutaneous + periarticular granulomas
• intermittent fever, dyspnea
• lymphadenopathy

√ capsular distension of multiple joints (hand, elbow, knee)
√ juxtaarticular bone erosions from soft-tissue granulomas
√ subluxation / dislocation
√ disuse / steroid deossification

Prognosis: death from respiratory failure within 2 years

FIBROCHONDROGENESIS

= autosomal recessive lethal short-limb skeletal dysplasia

Incidence: 5 cases

√ severe micromelia + broad dumbbell-shaped metaphyses
√ flat + clefted pear-shaped vertebral bodies
√ short + cupped ribs
√ frontal bossing
√ low-set abnormally formed ears

Prognosis: stillbirth / death shortly after birth

DDx: (1) Thanatophoric dysplasia
(2) Metatropic dysplasia
(3) Spondyloepiphyseal dysplasia

FIBRODYSPLASIA OSSIFICANS PROGRESSIVA

= MYOSITIS OSSIFICANS PROGRESSIVA (misnomer since primarily connective tissues are affected)
= rare slowly progressive sporadic / autosomal dominant disease with variable penetrance characterized by remissions + exacerbations of fibroblastic proliferation, subsequent calcification + ossification of subcutaneous fat, skeletal muscle, tendons, aponeuroses, ligaments

Histo: edema with proliferating fibroblasts in a loose myxoid matrix; subsequent collagen deposition plus calcification + ossification of collagenized fibrous tissue in the center of nodules

Age: presenting by age 2 years (50%)

• initially subcutaneous painful masses on neck, shoulders, upper extremities
• progressive involvement of remaining musculature of back, chest, abdomen, lower extremities
• lesions may ulcerate and bleed
• muscles of back + proximal extremities become rigid followed by thoracic kyphosis
• inanition secondary to jaw trismus (masseter, temporal muscle)
• "wry neck" = torticollis (due to restriction of sternocleidomastoid muscle)
• respiratory failure (thoracic muscles affected)
• conductive hearing loss (fusion of middle ear ossicles)

A. ECTOPIC OSSIFICATION
√ rounded / linear calcification in neck / shoulders, paravertebral region, hips, proximal extremity, trunk, palmar + plantar fascia forming ossified bars + bony bridges
√ ossification of voluntary muscles, complete by 20–25 years (sparing of sphincters + head)

B. SKELETAL ANOMALIES
may appear before ectopic ossification
• clinodactyly
√ microdactyly of big toes (90%) and thumbs (50%) = usually only one large phalanx present / synostosis of metacarpal + proximal phalanx (first sign)
√ phalangeal shortening of hand + foot (middle phalanx of 5th digit)
√ shortened 1st metatarsal + hallux valgus (75%)
√ shortened metacarpals + metatarsals
√ shallow acetabulum
√ short widened femoral neck
√ thickening of medial cortex of tibia
√ progressive fusion of posterior arches of cervical spine
√ narrowed AP diameter of cervical + lumbar vertebral bodies
√ ± bony ankylosis

CAVE: surgery is hazardous causing accelerated ossification at the surgical site

FIBROMA OF SOFT TISSUE

Histo: hypocellular highly collagenic tumor

Age: 3rd and 4th decades; M > F

Location: tendon sheath of distal upper extremity

√ slowly growing lesion 1–5 cm in size

MR:
√ small hypointense nodule on all pulse sequences

FIBROSARCOMA

Incidence: 4% of all primary bone neoplasm

Etiology:
A. PRIMARY FIBROSARCOMA (70%)
B. SECONDARY FIBROSARCOMA (30%)
1. following radiotherapy of giant cell tumor / lymphoma / breast cancer
2. underlying benign lesion: Paget disease (common); giant cell tumor, bone infarct, osteomyelitis, desmoplastic fibroma, enchondroma, fibrous dysplasia (rare)
3. dedifferentiation of low-grade chondrosarcoma

Histo: spectrum of well to poorly differentiated fibrous tissue proliferation; will not produce osteoid / chondroid / osseous matrix

Age: predominantly in 3rd–5th decade (range of 8–88 years); M:F = 1:1

Metastases to: lung, lymph nodes

• localized painful mass

Location: tubular bones in young, flat bones in older patients; femur (40%), tibia (16%) (about knee in 30–50%), jaw, pelvis (9%); rare in small bones of hand + feet or spinal column

Site: eccentric at diaphyseal-metaphyseal junction into metaphysis; intramedullary / periosteal

A. CENTRAL FIBROSARCOMA
= intramedullary
√ well-defined lucent bone lesion
√ thin expanded cortex
√ aggressive osteolysis with geographic / ragged / permeative bone destruction + wide zone of transition
√ occasionally large osteolytic lesion with cortical destruction, periosteal reaction + soft-tissue invasion
√ sequestration of bone may be present (DDx: eosinophilic granuloma, bacterial granuloma)
√ sparse periosteal proliferation (uncommon)
√ intramedullary discontinuous spread
√ no calcification

DDx: malignant fibrous histiocytoma, myeloma, telangiectatic osteosarcoma, lymphoma, desmoplastic fibroma, osteolytic metastasis

B. PERIOSTEAL FIBROSARCOMA
= rare tumor arising from periosteal connective tissue

Location: long bones of lower extremity, jaw
√ contour irregularity of cortical border
√ periosteal reaction with perpendicular bone formation may be present
√ rarely extension into medullary cavity

Cx: pathologic fracture (uncommon)

Prognosis: 20% 10-year survival

DDx:
(1) Osteolytic osteosarcoma (2nd–3rd decade)
(2) Chondrosarcoma (usually contains characteristic calcifications)
(3) Aneurysmal bone cyst (eccentric blown-out appearance with rapid progression)
(4) Malignant giant cell tumor (begins in metaphysis extending toward joint)

FIBROUS CORTICAL DEFECT

Incidence: 30% of children; M:F = 2:1
Age: peak age of 7–8 years (range of 2–10 years); mostly before epiphyseal closure
Histo: fibrous tissue from periosteum invading underlying cortex
• asymptomatic

Location: metaphyseal cortex of long bone; posterior medial aspect of distal femur, proximal tibia, proximal femur, proximal humerus, ribs, ilium, fibula
√ round when small, average diameter of 1–2 cm
√ oval, extending parallel to long axis of host bone
√ cortical thinning + expansion may occur
√ smooth, well-defined / scalloped margins
√ larger lesions are multilocular
√ involution over 2–4 years
Prognosis:
(a) potential to grow and encroach on the medullary cavity leading to nonossifying fibroma
(b) bone islands in the adult may be residue of incompletely involuted cortical defect

FIBROUS DYSPLASIA

= LICHTENSTEIN-JAFFÉ DISEASE
= benign fibroosseous developmental anomaly of the mesenchymal precursor of bone, manifested as a defect in osteoblastic differentiation and maturation
Cause: probable gene mutation during embryogenesis
Age: 1st–2nd decade (highest incidence between 3 and 15 years), 75% before age 30; progresses until growth ceases; M:F = 1:1
Histo: medullary cavity replaced by immature matrix of collagen with small irregularly shaped trabeculae of immature "woven" bone + inadequate mineralization; never replaced by mature lamellar bone
Types:
A. MONOSTOTIC FORM (70–80%)
• usually asymptomatic until 2nd–3rd decade
Location: ribs (28%), proximal femur (23%), craniofacial bones (10–25%)
B. POLYOSTOTIC FORM (20–30%)
Age: mean age of 8 years
• 2/3 symptomatic by age 10
• leg pain, limp, pathologic fracture (75%)
• abnormal vaginal bleeding (25%)
Location: unilateral + asymmetric; femur (91%), tibia (81%), pelvis (78%), foot (73%), ribs, skull + facial bones (50%), upper extremities, lumbar spine (14%), clavicle (10%), cervical spine (7%)
Site: metadiaphysis
√ leg length discrepancy (70%)
√ "shepherd's crook" deformity (35%)
√ facial asymmetry
√ tibial bowing
√ rib deformity
C. CRANIOFACIAL FORM = LEONTIASIS OSSEA
Incidence: in 10–25% of monostotic form / in 50% of polyostotic form / isolated
• cranial asymmetry
• facial deformity
• exophthalmos
• visual impairment
Location: sphenoid, frontal, maxillary, ethmoid bones > occipital, temporal bones
√ unilateral overgrowth of facial bones + calvarium (NO extracranial lesions)
√ outward expansion of outer table maintaining convexity (DDx: Paget disease with destruction of inner + outer table)
√ prominence of external occipital protuberance
Cx: neurologic deficit secondary to narrowed cranial foramina (eg, blindness)
D. CHERUBISM (special variant)
= FAMILIAL FIBROUS DYSPLASIA
= autosomal dominant disorder of variable penetrance
Age: childhood; more severe in males
• bilateral jaw fullness + slight upward turning of eyes
√ bilateral expansile multiloculated cystic masses with symmetric involvement of mandible + maxilla
Cx: problems with dentition after perforation of cortex
Prognosis: regression after adolescence

May be associated with:
(a) endocrine disorders:
— precocious puberty in girls
— hyperthyroidism
— hyperparathyroidism: renal stones, calcinosis
— acromegaly
— diabetes mellitus
— Cushing syndrome: osteoporosis, acne
— growth retardation
(b) soft-tissue myxoma (rare) = **Mazabraud syndrome**: typically multiple intramuscular lesions in vicinity of most severely affected bone

VARIANT: **McCune-Albright syndrome** (10%)
(1) polyostotic unilateral fibrous dysplasia
(2) "coast of Maine" café-au-lait spots (35%)
(3) endocrine dysfunction: peripheral sexual precocity (menarche in infancy [20%]), hyperthyroidism

• swelling + tenderness
• limp, pain (± pathologic fracture)
• increased alkaline phosphatase
• advanced skeletal + somatic maturation (early)
• coast of Maine café-au-lait spots = yellowish to brownish patches of cutaneous pigmentation with irregular / serrated border, predominantly on back of trunk (30–50%), buttocks, neck, shoulders; often ipsilateral to bone lesions (DDx: "coast of California" spots of neurofibromatosis)
Common location:
rib cage (30%), craniofacial bones [calvarium, mandible] (25%), femoral neck + tibia (25%), pelvis

Site: metaphysis is primary site with extension into diaphysis (rarely entire length)
√ normal bone architecture altered + remodeled
√ lesions in medullary cavity: radiolucent / "ground-glass" appearance / increased density
√ trabeculated appearance due to reinforced subperiosteal bone ridges in wall of lesion
√ expansion of bones (ribs, skull, long bones)
√ well-defined sclerotic margin of reactive bone = rind
√ endosteal scalloping with thinned / lost cortex (ribs, long bones) and intervening normal cortex is HALLMARK
√ lesion may undergo calcification + enchondral bone formation = fibrocartilaginous dysplasia
√ increased activity on bone scan during early perfusion + on delayed images

MR:
- √ homogeneous / mildly heterogeneous marrow lesions hyperintense to fat (60%) / of intermediate / of low signal intensity on T2WI
- √ marrow lesions hypointense to muscle on T1WI

@ Skull
- • skull deformity with cranial nerve compromise
- • proptosis

Location: frontal bone > sphenoid bone; hemicranial involvement (DDx: Paget disease is bilateral)
- √ sclerotic skull base, may narrow neural foramina (visual + hearing loss)
- √ widened diploic space with displacement of outer table, inner table spared (DDx: Paget disease, inner table involved)
- √ obliteration of sphenoid + frontal sinuses due to encroachment by fibrous dysplastic bone
- √ inferolateral displacement of orbit
- √ sclerosis of orbital plate + small orbit + hypoplasia of frontal sinuses (DDx: Paget disease, meningioma en plaque)
- √ occipital thickening
- √ cystic calvarial lesions, commonly crossing sutures
- √ mandibular cystic lesion (very common) = osteocementoma, ossifying fibroma

@ Pelvis + ribs
- √ cystic lesions (extremely common)
- √ fusiform enlargement of ribs + loss of normal trabecular pattern + thin preserved cortex (in up to 30%)
  - ◊ Fibrous dysplasia is the most common cause of a benign expansile lesion of a rib!
  - ◊ A rib is the most common site of monostotic fibrous dysplasia!
- √ protrusio acetabuli

@ Extremities
- • short stature as adult / dwarfism
- √ premature fusion of ossification centers
- √ epiphysis rarely affected before closure of growth plate
- √ bowing deformities + discrepant limb length (tibia, femur) due to stress of normal weight bearing
- √ "shepherd's crook" deformity of femoral neck = coxa vara
- √ pseudarthrosis in infancy = osteofibrous dysplasia (DDx: neurofibromatosis)
- √ premature onset of arthritis

Cx:
(1) Transformation into osteo- / chondro- / fibrosarcoma or malignant fibrous histiocytoma (0.5–1%, more often in polyostotic form)
- • increasing pain
- √ enlarging soft-tissue mass
- √ previously mineralized lesion turns lytic

(2) Pathologic fractures: transformation of woven into lamellar bone may be seen, subperiosteal healing without endosteal healing

DDx:
(1) HPT (chemical changes, generalized deossification, subperiosteal resorption)
(2) Neurofibromatosis (rarely osseous lesions, cystic intraosseous neurofibroma rare, café-au-lait spots smooth, familial disease)
(3) Paget disease (mosaic pattern histologically, radiographically identical to monostotic cranial lesion)
(4) Osteofibrous dysplasia (almost exclusively in tibia of infants, monostotic, lesion begins in cortex)
(5) Nonossifying fibroma
(6) Simple bone cyst
(7) Giant cell tumor (no sclerotic margin)
(8) Enchondromatosis
(9) Eosinophilic granuloma
(10) Osteoblastoma
(11) Hemangioma
(12) Meningioma

FIBROUS HISTIOCYTOMA

Benign fibrous histiocytoma

Incidence: 0.1% of all bone tumors
Histo: interlacing bundles of fibrous tissue in storiform pattern (whorled / woven) interspersed with mono- / multinucleated cells resembling histiocytes, benign giant cells, and lipid-laden macrophages; resembles nonossifying fibroma / fibroxanthoma
Age: 23–60 years
• localized intermittently painful soft-tissue swelling
Location: long bone, pelvis, vertebra (rare)
Site: typically in epiphysis / epiphyseal equivalent
√ well-defined radiolucent lesion with septa / soap-bubble appearance / no definable matrix
√ may have reactive sclerotic rim
√ narrow transition zone (= nonaggressive lesion)
√ no periosteal reaction
Rx: curettage
DDx: nonossifying fibroma (childhood / adolescence, asymptomatic, eccentric metaphyseal location)

Atypical Benign Fibrous Histiocytoma

Histo: "atypical aggressive" features = mitotic figures present
√ lytic defect with irregular edges
Prognosis: may metastasize

Malignant Fibrous Histiocytoma

= MFH = MALIGNANT FIBROUS XANTHOMA = XANTHOSARCOMA = MALIGNANT HISTIOCYTOMA = FIBROSARCOMA VARIANT

Histo: spindle-cell neoplasm of a mixture of fibroblasts + giant cells resembling histiocytes with nuclear atypia and pleomorphism in pinwheel arrangement; closely resembles high-grade fibrosarcoma (= fibroblastic cells arranged in uniform pattern separated by collagen fibers)
(a) pleomorphic-storiform subtype (50–60%)
(b) myxoid subtype (25%)
(c) giant cell subtype (5–10%)
(d) inflammatory subtype (5–10%)
(e) angiomatoid subtype (<5%)

Age: 10–90 (average 50) years; peak prevalence in 5th decade; more frequent in Caucasians; M:F = 3:2

Location: potential to arise in any organ (ubiquitous mesenchymal tissue); soft tissues >> bone

Soft-tissue MFH

Incidence: 20–30% of all soft-tissue sarcomas; most common primary malignant soft-tissue tumor of late adult life

◊ Any deep-seated invasive intramuscular mass in a patient >50 years of age is most likely MFH!

Location: extremities (75%), [lower extremity (50%), upper extremity (25%)], retroperitoneum (15%), head + neck (5%)

Site: within large muscle groups

• large painless soft-tissue mass with progressive enlargement over several months

√ mass usually 5–10 cm in size with increase over months / years

√ poorly defined curvilinear / punctate peripheral calcifications / ossifications (in 5–20%)

√ cortical erosion of adjacent bone (HIGHLY SUGGESTIVE FEATURE)

CT:

√ well-defined soft-tissue mass with central hypodense area = myxoid MFH (DDx: hemorrhage, necrosis, leiomyosarcoma with necrosis, myxoid lipo- / chondrosarcoma)

√ enhancement of solid components

MR:

√ inhomogeneous poorly defined lesion iso- / hyperintense to muscle on T1WI + hyperintense on T2WI

Prognosis:
larger + more deeply located tumors have a worse prognosis; 2-year survival rate of 60%; 5-year survival rate of 50%; local recurrence rate of 44%; metastatic rate of 42% (lung, lymph nodes, liver, bone)

DDx: (1) Liposarcoma (younger patient, presence of fat in >40%, calcifications rare)
(2) Rhabdomyosarcoma
(3) Synovial sarcoma (cortical erosion)

Osseous MFH

Prevalence: 5% of all primary malignant bone tumors

• painful, tender, rapidly enlarging mass

• pathologic fracture (20%)

Associated with:
prior radiation therapy, bone infarcts, Paget disease, fibrous dysplasia, osteonecrosis, fibroxanthoma (= nonossifying fibroma), enchondroma, chronic osteomyelitis

◊ 20% of all osseous MFH arise in areas of abnormal bone!

Location: femur (45%), tibia (20%), 50% about knee; humerus (10%); ilium (10%); spine; sternum; clavicle; rarely small bones of hand + feet

Site: central metaphysis of long bones (90%); eccentric in diaphysis of long bones (10%)

√ radiolucent defect with ill-defined margins (2.5–10 cm in diameter)

√ extensive mineralization / small areas of focal metaplastic calcification

√ permeation + cortical destruction

√ expansion in smaller bones (ribs, sternum, fibula, clavicle)

√ occasionally lamellated periosteal reaction (especially in presence of pathologic fracture)

√ soft-tissue extension

Cx: pathologic fracture (30–50%)

DDx: (1) Metastasis
(2) Fibrosarcoma (often with sequestrum)
(3) Reticulum cell sarcoma
(4) Osteosarcoma
(5) Giant cell tumor
(6) Plasmacytoma

Pulmonary MFH *(extremely rare)*

√ solitary pulmonary nodule without calcification

√ diffuse infiltrate

NUC:

√ increased uptake of Tc-99m MDP (mechanism not understood)

√ increased uptake of Ga-67 citrate

US:

√ well-defined mass with hyperechoic + hypoechoic (necrotic) areas

CT:

√ mass of muscle density with hypodense areas (necrosis)

√ invasion of abdominal musculature, but not IVC / renal veins (DDx to renal cell carcinoma)

Angio:

√ hypervascularity + early venous return

FOCAL FIBROCARTILAGINOUS DYSPLASIA OF TIBIA

Associated with: tibia vara

Age: 9–28 months

Histo: dense hypocellular fibrous tissue resembling tendon with lacuna formation

• slight shortening of affected leg

Location: insertion of pes anserinus (= tendinous insertion of gracilis, sartorius, semitendinosus muscles) distal to proximal tibial physis; unilateral involvement

√ unilateral tibia vara
√ well-defined elliptic obliquely oriented lucent defect in medial tibial metadiaphyseal cortex
√ sclerosis along lateral border of lesion
√ absence of bone margin superomedially

Prognosis: resolution in 1–4 years

DDx: (1) Unilateral Blount disease (typically bilateral in infants, varus angulation of upper tibia, decreased height of medial tibial metaphysis, irregular physis)
(2) Chondromyxoid fibroma, eosinophilic granuloma, osteoid osteoma, osteoma, fibroma, chondroma (not associated with tibia vara, soft-tissue mass)

FRACTURE

= soft-tissue injury in which there is a break in the continuity of bone or cartilage

General description:

(1) OPEN / [CLOSED]
open Fx = communication between fractured bone + skin

(2) [COMPLETE] / INCOMPLETE
complete Fx = all cortical surfaces disrupted
incomplete Fx = partial separation of bone
greenstick Fx = break of one cortical margin only with intact periosteum due to tension on soft growing bone
buckle / torus Fx = buckling of cortex due to compression
bowing Fx = plastic deformity of thin long bone (clavicle, ulna, fibula)
lead-pipe Fx = combination of greenstick + torus Fx

(3) SIMPLE / COMMINUTED
simple Fx = noncomminuted
comminuted Fx = >2 fragments
segmental Fx = isolated segment of shaft
butterfly fragment = V-shaped fragment not completely circumscribed by cortex

(4) DIRECTION OF FRACTURE LINE in relation to long axis of bone:
transverse, oblique, oblique-transverse, spiral

Special terminology:

avulsion Fx = fragment pulled off by tendon / ligament from parent bone
transchondral Fx = cartilaginous surface involved
chondral Fx = cartilage alone involved
osteochondral Fx = cartilage + subjacent bone involved

Description of anatomic positional changes:

= change in position of distal fracture fragment in relation to proximal fracture fragment

LENGTH
= longitudinal change of fragments
distraction = increase from original anatomic length
shortening = decrease from original anatomic length
— impacted = fragments driven into each other
— overriding = also includes latitudinal changes
— overlapping = bayonet apposition

DISPLACEMENT
= latitudinal change of anatomic axis:
— undisplaced
— anterior, posterior, medial / ulnar, lateral / radial

ANGULATION / TILT
= long axes of fragments intersect at the fracture apex:
— medial / lateral, ventral / dorsal
— varus = angular deviation of distal fragment toward midline on frontal projection
— valgus = angular deviation of distal fragment away from midline on frontal projection
eg, "ventral angulation of fracture apex"
eg, "in anatomic / near anatomic alignment"

ROTATION
◊ Difficult to detect radiographically!
√ differences in diameters of apposing fragments
√ mismatch of fracture line geometry
— internal / external rotation

NUC:

Typical time course:

1. Acute phase (3–4 weeks)
abnormal in 80% <24 hours, in 95% <72 hours
◊ Elderly patients show delayed appearance of positive scan
√ broad area of increased tracer uptake (wider than fracture line)
2. Subacute phase (2–3 months) = time of most intense tracer accumulation
√ more focal increased tracer uptake corresponding to fracture line
3. Chronic phase (1–2 years)
√ slow decline in tracer accumulation
√ in 65% normal after 1 year; >95% normal after 3 years

Return to normal:

◊ Non–weight-bearing bone returns to normal more quickly than weight-bearing bone
◊ Rib fractures return to normal most rapidly
◊ Complicated fractures with orthopedic fixation devices take longest to return to normal

1. Simple fractures: 90% normal by 2 years
2. Open reduction / fixation: <50% normal by 3 years
3. Delayed union: slower than normal for type of fracture
4. Nonunion: persistent intense uptake in 80%
5. Complicated union (true pseudarthrosis, soft-tissue interposition, impaired blood supply, presence of infection)
√ intense uptake at fracture ends
√ decreased uptake at fracture site
6. Vertebral compression fractures: 60% normal by 1 year; 90% by 2 years; 97% by 3 years

Types of Fractures

Type	Bone Quality	Load
Traumatic	normal	single large
Fatigue (stress)	normal	repetitive
Insufficiency (stress)	abnormal (metabolic)	minimal
Pathologic	abnormal (tumor)	minimal

Pathologic Fracture

= fracture at site of preexisting osseous abnormality

Cause: tumor, osteoporosis, infection, metabolic disorder

Stress Fracture

= fractures produced as a result of repetitive prolonged muscular action on bone that has not accommodated itself to such action

Insufficiency Stress Fracture

= normal physiologic stress applied to bone with abnormal elastic resistance / deficient mineralization

Cause:
1. Osteoporosis
2. Rheumatoid arthritis
3. Paget disease
4. Fibrous dysplasia
5. Osteogenesis imperfecta
6. Osteopetrosis
7. Osteomalacia / rickets
8. Hyperparathyroidism
9. Renal osteodystrophy
10. Radiation therapy
11. Prolonged corticosteroid treatment
12. Tumor treatment with ifosfamide, methotrexate

Location: lower extremity (calcaneus, tibia, fibula), thoracic vertebra, sacrum, ilium, pubic bone

Plain film / CT (1–2 weeks after onset of fracture):
- √ cortical lucency (due to disruption)
- √ periosteal new bone formation
- √ medullary sclerosis (endosteal callus formation)

MR:
- √ marrow edema (hypointense on T1WI)
- √ cortical fracture line

NUC (bone scan):
- √ increased abnormal uptake

Pelvic Insufficiency Stress Fracture

- severe pain in lower back + sacroiliac joints; radiates to buttocks, hips, groin, legs; worsens with weight bearing
- walking ability impaired

Incidence: 1.8–5% of women >55 years

Predisposed: postmenopausal women

Location: sacral ala, parasymphyseal region of os pubis, pubic rami, supraacetabular region, iliac blades, superomedial portion of ilium

Types:

(a) occult fracture:
- Site: sacrum > supraacetabulum, ilium
- √ sclerotic band, cortical disruption, fracture line
- ◊ Often obscured by overlying bowel gas + osteopenia!

(b) aggressive fracture:
- Site: parasymphysis, pubic rami
- √ exuberant callus formation, osteolysis + fragments (with prolonged or delayed healing / chronic nonunion)
- CAVE: fracture may be misdiagnosed as neoplasm; interpretation also histologically difficult

NUC:
- √ butterfly / H-shaped ("Honda sign") / asymmetric incomplete H-shaped pattern of sacral uptake
- √ pelvic outlet view for parasymphyseal fx

CT and MR (most accurate modalities):
- √ sclerotic band, linear fracture line, cortical disruption, fragmentation, displacement
- √ bone marrow edema
- ◊ Excludes bone destruction + soft-tissue masses!

Prognosis: healing in 12–30 months

Femoral Insufficiency Fracture

Site: subcapital
- √ subtle femoral neck angulation
- √ trabecular angulation
- √ subcapital impaction line

Fatigue Stress Fracture

= normal bone subjected to repetitive stresses (none of which is singularly capable of producing a fracture) leading to mechanical failure over time

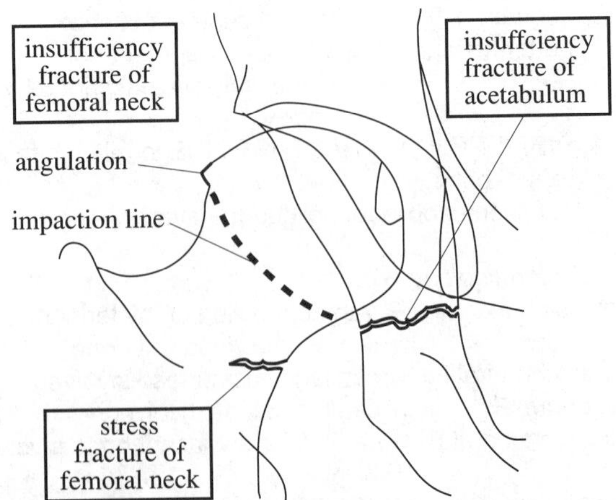

Fatigue (Stress) and Insufficiency Fracture of Hip

Risk factors: new / different / rigorous repetitive activity; female sex; increased age; Caucasian race; low bone mineral density; low calcium intake; fluoride treatment for osteoporosis; condition resulting in altered gait

- activity-related pain abating with rest
- constant pain with continued activity

1. **Clay shoveler's fracture**: spinous process of lower cervical / upper thoracic spine
2. **Clavicle**: postoperative (radical neck dissection)
3. **Coracoid process of scapula**: trap shooting
4. **Ribs**: carrying heavy pack, golf, coughing
5. **Distal shaft of humerus**: throwing ball
6. **Coronoid process of ulna**: pitching ball, throwing javelin, pitchfork work, propelling wheelchairs
7. **Hook of hamate**: swinging golf club / tennis racquet / baseball bat
8. **Spondylolysis** = pars interarticularis of lumbar vertebrae: ballet, lifting heavy objects, scrubbing floors
9. **Femoral neck**: ballet, long-distance running
   Site: medial femoral neck
   √ subtle lucency / sclerosis (= acute fracture)
   √ lucent line surrounded by sclerosis (= subacute fracture)
10. **Femoral shaft**: ballet, marching, long-distance running, gymnastics
11. **Obturator ring of pelvis**: stooping, bowling, gymnastics
    Site: superior / inferior pubic ramus
12. **Sacrum** (<2%): long-distance runner, military recruits
    Site: unilateral (? due to leg length discrepancy)
13. **Patella**: hurdling
14. **Tibial shaft**: ballet, jogging
15. **Fibula**: long-distance running, jumping, parachuting
16. **Calcaneus**: jumping, parachuting, prolonged standing, recent immobilization
17. **Navicular**: stomping on ground, marching, prolonged standing, ballet
18. **Metatarsal** (commonly 2nd MT): marching, stomping on ground, prolonged standing, ballet, postoperative bunionectomy
19. **Sesamoids of metatarsal**: prolonged standing

X-RAY (15% sensitive in early fractures, increasing to 50% on follow-up):
- cancellous (trabecular) bone (notoriously difficult to detect)
  √ subtle blurring of trabecular margins
  √ faint sclerotic radiopaque area of peritrabecular callus (50% change in bone density needed)
  √ sclerotic band (due to trabecular compression + callus formation) usually perpendicular to cortex
- compact (cortical) bone
  √ "gray cortex sign" = subtle ill definition of cortex
  √ intracortical radiolucent striations (early)
  √ solid thick lamellar periosteal new bone formation
  √ endosteal thickening (later)

√ follow-up radiography after 2–3 weeks of conservative therapy

NUC ("gold standard" = almost 100% sensitive):
√ abnormal uptake within 6–72 hours of injury (prior to radiographic abnormality)
√ "stress reaction" = focus of subtly increased uptake
√ focal fusiform area of intense cortical uptake
√ abnormal uptake persists for months

MR (very sensitive modality; fat saturation technique most sensitive to detect increase in water content of medullary edema / hemorrhage):
√ diminished marrow signal intensity on T1WI of fracture line
√ increased marrow signal intensity on T2WI (edema may obscure the fracture line), resolves within 6 months in 90%
√ low-intensity band contiguous with cortex on T2WI = fracture line of more advanced lesion

CT (least sensitive modality):
helpful in: longitudinal stress fracture of tibia; in confusing pediatric stress fracture (to detect endosteal bone formation)

DDx:
(1) Shin splints (activity not increased in angiographic / blood-pool phase)
   √ long linear uptake on posteromedial (soleus muscle) / anterolateral (tibialis anterior muscle) tibial cortex on delayed images (from stress to periosteum at muscle insertion site)
(2) Osteoid osteoma (eccentric, nidus, solid periosteal reaction, night pain)
(3) Chronic sclerosing osteomyelitis (dense, sclerotic, involving entire circumference, little change on serial radiographs)
(4) Osteomalacia (bowed long bones, looser zones, gross fractures, demineralization)
(5) Osteogenic sarcoma (metaphyseal, aggressive periosteal reaction)
(6) Ewing tumor (lytic destructive appearance with soft-tissue component, little change on serial radiographs)

Epiphyseal Plate Injury

Prevalence: 6–18–30% of bone injuries in children <16 years of age
Peak age: 12 years
Location: distal radius (28%), phalanges of hand (26%), distal tibia (10%), distal phalanges of foot (7%), distal humerus (7%), distal ulna (4%), proximal radius (4%), metacarpals (4%), distal fibula (3%)

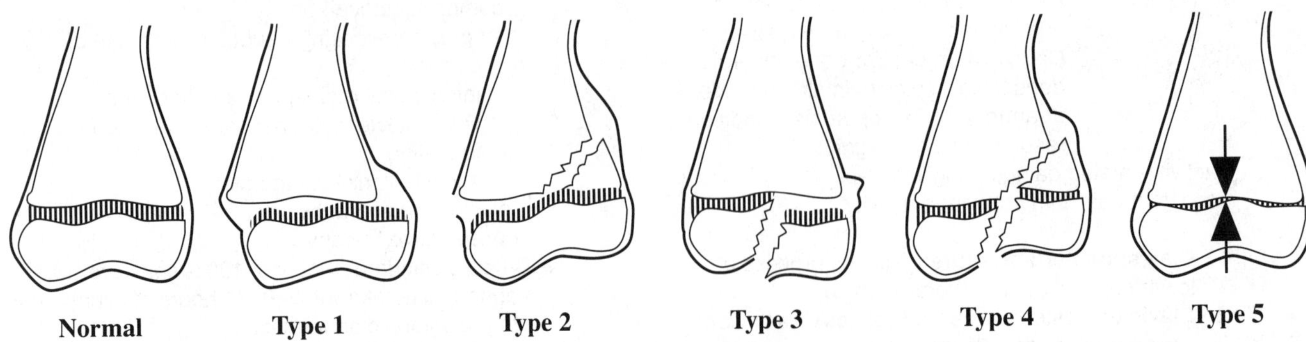

Salter-Harris Classification of Epiphyseal Plate Injuries

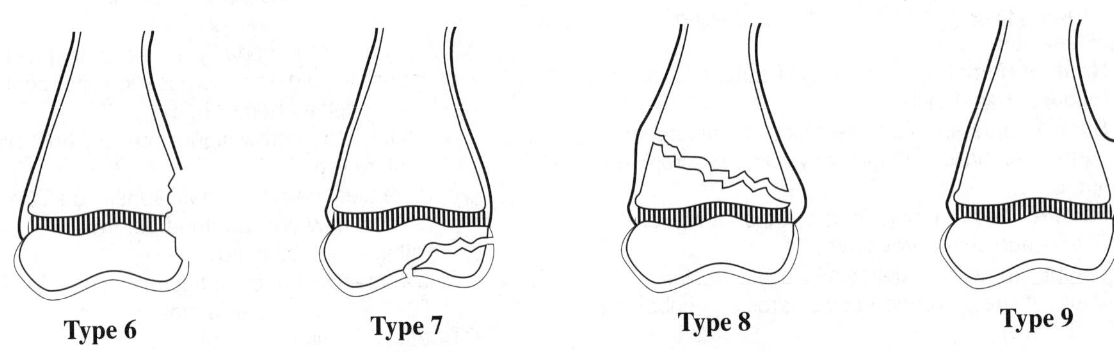

Rang and Ogden's Additions to Salter-Harris

Mechanism: 80% shearing force; 20% compression
Resistance to trauma: ligament > bone > physis (hypertrophic zone most vulnerable)

Salter-Harris classification (considering probability of growth disturbance)

[Robert Bruce Salter (1924–) and W. Robert Harris (1922–), orthopedic surgeons in Toronto, Canada]

◊ Prognosis is worse in lower extremities (ankle + knee) irrespective of Salter-Harris type!

mnemonic: "SALTR"
Slip of physis = type 1
Above physis = type 2
Lower than physis = type 3
Through physis = type 4
Rammed physis = type 5

Salter Type 1 *(6–8.5%)*

= slip of epiphysis due to shearing force separating epiphysis from physis

Line of cleavage: confined to physis

Location: most commonly in phalanges, distal radius (includes: apophyseal avulsion, slipped capital femoral epiphysis)

√ displacement of epiphyseal ossification center

Prognosis: favorable irrespective of location

Salter Type 2 *(73–75%)*

= shearing force splits growth plate

Line of fracture: through physis + extending through margin of metaphysis separating a triangular metaphyseal fragment (= "corner sign")

Location: distal radius (33–50%), distal tibia + fibula, phalanges

Prognosis: good, may result in minimal shortening

Salter Type 3 *(6.5–8%)*

= intraarticular fracture, often occurring after partial closure of physis

Line of fracture: vertically / obliquely through epiphysis + extending horizontally to periphery of physis

Location: distal tibia, distal phalanx, rarely distal femur

√ epiphysis split vertically

Prognosis: fair (imprecise reduction leads to alteration in linearity of articular plane)

Salter Type 4 *(10–12%)*

Location: lateral condyle of humerus, distal tibia

√ fracture involves metaphysis + physis + epiphysis

Prognosis: guarded (may result in deformity + angulation)

Salter Type 5 (<1%)

= crush injury with injury to vascular supply
Location: distal femur, proximal tibia, distal tibia
Often associated with: fracture of adjacent shaft
√ no immediate radiographic finding
√ shortening of bone + cone epiphysis / angular deformity on follow-up
Prognosis: poor (impairment of growth in 100%)

Triplane Fracture (6%)

Location: distal tibia, lateral condyle of distal humerus
√ vertical fracture of epiphysis + horizontal cleavage plane within physis + oblique fracture of adjacent metaphysis

MR:
√ focal dark linear area (= line of cleavage) within bright physis on gradient echo images (GRE)

Cx:
(1) progressive angular deformity from segmental arrest of germinal zone growth with formation of a bone bridge across physis = "bone bar"
(2) limb length discrepancy from total cessation of growth
(3) articular incongruity from disruption of articular surface
(4) Bone infarction in metaphysis / epiphysis

Apophyseal Injury

Mechanism: avulsive force
◊ Physis under secondary ossification center is weakest part!
At risk: hurdlers, sprinters, cheerleaders (repetitive to and fro adduction / abduction + flexion / extension)
• pain, point tenderness, swelling

Location	Muscle Origin / Insertion
Anterior superior iliac spine	sartorius muscle + tensor fasciae femoris m.
Anterior inferior iliac spine	rectus femoris muscle
Lesser trochanter	psoas muscle
Ischial tuberosity	hamstring muscle
Greater trochanter	gluteal muscle
Iliac crest	abdominal muscle
Symphysis pubis	adductor muscle

√ irregularity at site of avulsion
√ displaced pieces of bone of variable size:
  √ crescentic ossific opacity if viewed on tangent
  √ very subtle disk-shaped opacity if seen en face
√ abnormal foci of heterotopic ossification (later)

Hand Fracture

Bennett Fracture

[Edward Hallaran Bennett (1837–1907), surgeon in Dublin, Ireland]
Mechanism: forced abduction of thumb
√ intraarticular fracture-dislocation of base of 1st metacarpal
√ small fragment of 1st metacarpal continues to articulate with trapezium
√ lateral retraction of 1st metacarpal shaft by abductor pollicis longus
Rx: anatomic reduction important, difficult to keep in anatomic alignment
Cx: pseudarthrosis

Boxer's Fracture

Mechanism: direct blow with clenched fist
√ transverse fracture of distal metacarpal (usually 5th)

Gamekeeper's Thumb

= SKIER'S THUMB
originally described as chronic lesion in hunters strangling rabbits
Incidence: 6% of all skiing injuries; 50% of skiing injuries to the hand
Mechanism: violent abduction of thumb with injury to ulnar collateral ligament (UCL) in 1st MCP (faulty handling of ski pole)
√ disruption of ulnar collateral ligament of 1st MCP joint, usually occurring distally near insertion on proximal phalanx
√ radial stress examination necessary to document ligamentous disruption
√ displacement of UCL superficial to aponeurosis of adductor pollicis (= Stener lesion) [torn end of UCL may be marked by avulsed bone fragment]

Navicular Fracture

= SCAPHOID FRACTURE
◊ Most frequent (90%) of all carpal bones fractures!
Mechanism: fall on dorsiflexed outstretched hand
• pain + tenderness at anatomic snuff box
Radiographic misses: 25–33–65%
N.B.: If initial radiograph negative, reexamine in 2 + 6 weeks after treatment with short-arm spica cast!
MR: high sensitivity
Bone scan: up to 100% sensitive, 93% PPV after 2–3 days
Prognosis: dependent on following factors
√ fracture displacement = >1 mm offset / angulation / rotation of fragments (less favorable)
√ location (blood supply derived from distal part):
  – distal 1/3 (10%) = usually fragments reunite
  – middle 1/3 (70%) = failure to reunite in 30%
  – proximal 1/3 (20%) = failure to reunite in 90%
√ orientation of fracture
  – transverse / horizontal oblique = relatively stable
  – vertical oblique (less common) = unstable
◊ Good prognosis with distal fracture + no displacement + no ligamentous injury!
◊ Less favorable prognosis with displaced / comminuted fracture + proximal pole fracture!
Cx: avascular necrosis of proximal fragment

Rolando Fracture
[Silvio Rolando (?–1931?), surgeon in Genoa, Italy]
√ comminuted Y- / T-shaped intraarticular fracture-dislocation through base of thumb metacarpal
Prognosis: worse than Bennett's fracture (difficult to reduce)

Forearm Fracture
Barton Fracture
[John Rhea Barton (1794–1871), orthopedic surgeon at Pennsylvania Hospital, Philadelphia]
Mechanism: fall on outstretched hand
√ intraarticular oblique fracture of ventral / dorsal lip of distal radius
√ carpus dislocates with distal fragment up and back on radius

Chauffeur Fracture
= HUTCHINSON FRACTURE = BACKFIRE FRACTURE = LORRY DRIVER FRACTURE
[Jonathan Hutchinson (1828–1913), British surgeon]
= name derived from direct trauma to radial side of wrist sustained from recoil of crank used in era of hand cranking to start automobiles
Mechanism: acute dorsiflexion + abduction of hand
√ triangular fracture of radial styloid process

Colles Fracture
[Abraham Colles (1773–1843), surgeon in Dublin, Ireland]
= POUTEAU FRACTURE (term used in France)
[Claude Pouteau (1725–1775), surgeon in Lyon, France]
◊ Most common fracture of forearm!
Mechanism: fall on outstretched hand
√ nonarticular radial fracture in distal 2 cm
√ dorsal displacement of distal fragment + volar angulation of fracture apex
√ ± ulnar styloid fracture
√ "silver-fork" deformity
Cx: posttraumatic arthritis
Rx: anatomic reduction important

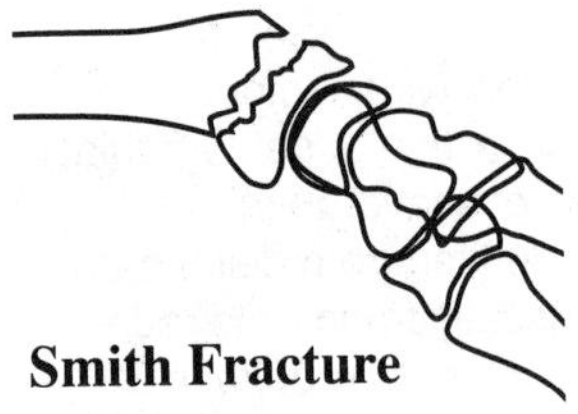
Smith Fracture

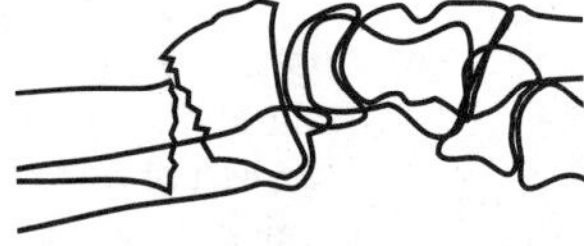
Colles Fracture

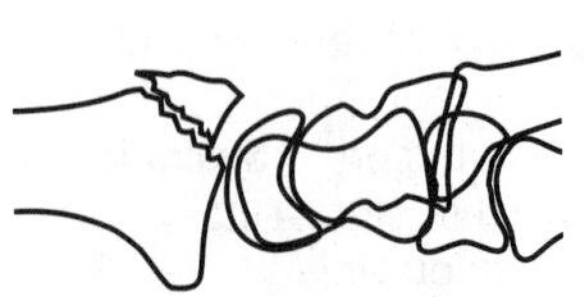
Barton Fracture

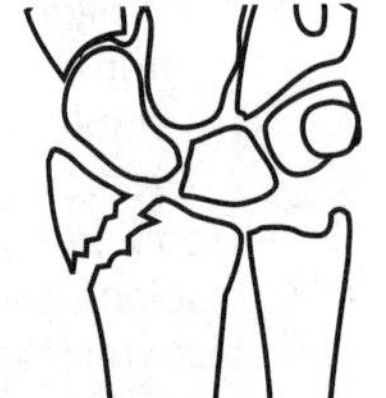
Chauffeur Fracture

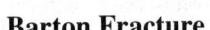

Significant postreduction deformity:
1. Residual positive ulnar variance >5 mm indicates unsatisfactory outcome in 40%
2. Dorsal angulation of palmar tilt >15° decreases grip strength + endurance in >50%

Essex-Lopresti Fracture
[Peter Gordon Essex-Lopresti (1918–1951), surgeon at Birmingham Accident Center, England]
√ comminuted displaced radial head fracture
√ dislocation of distal radioulnar joint

Galeazzi Fracture
[Ricardo Galeazzi (1866–1952), orthopedic surgeon in Italy]
= PIEDMONT FRACTURE
Mechanism: fall on outstretched hand with elbow flexed
√ radial shaft fracture (most commonly) at junction of distal to middle third with dorsal angulation
√ subluxation / dislocation of distal radioulnar joint
√ ulnar plus variance (= radial shortening) of >10 mm implies complete disruption of interosseous membrane = complete instability of radioulnar joint
Cx: (1) High incidence of nonunion, delayed union, malunion (unstable fracture)
(2) Limitation of pronation / supination

Monteggia-type Fracture
= fracture of ulnar shaft + dislocation of radial head
Bado Classification:
[Jose Luis Bado (1903–1977), orthopedic surgeon from Uruguay]

Type I = **classic Monteggia fracture**
[Giovanni Battista Monteggia (1762–1815), Italian surgeon]
Mechanism: direct blow to the forearm
√ anteriorly angulated proximal ulnar fracture
√ anterior dislocation of radial head
√ may have associated wrist injury
Cx: nonunion, limitation of motion at elbow, nerve abnormalities

Type II = reverse Monteggia fracture
√ radial head displaced posteriorly / posterolaterally
√ dorsally angulated proximal ulnar fracture

Type III
√ anterior / anterolateral dislocation of radial head
√ ulnar metaphyseal fracture

Type IV
√ anterior displacement of radial head
√ fracture of proximal third of radius + ulna at the same level

Smith Fracture
= REVERSE COLLES FRACTURE = REVERSE BARTON FRACTURE = GOYRAND FRACTURE (term used in France)
[Robert William Smith (1807–1873), succeeding Colles as professor of surgery at Trinity College in Dublin, Ireland]

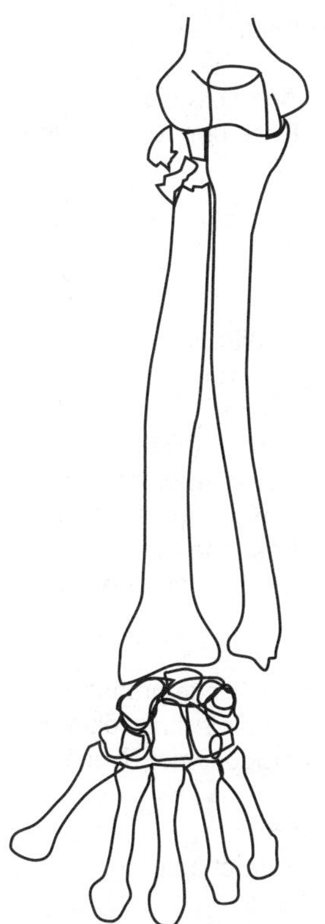

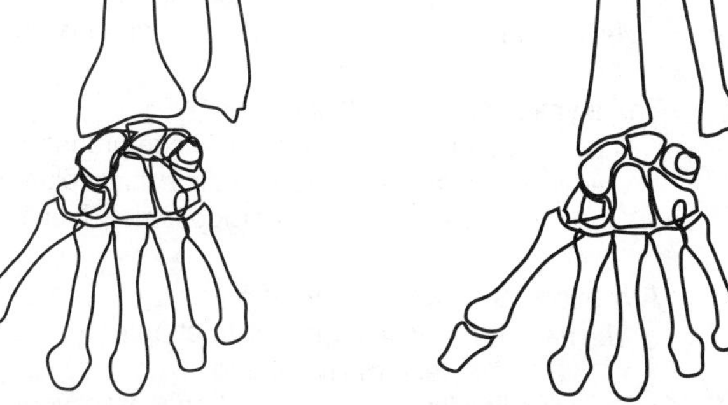

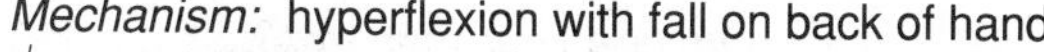

Essex-Lopresti Fracture **Galeazzi Fracture**

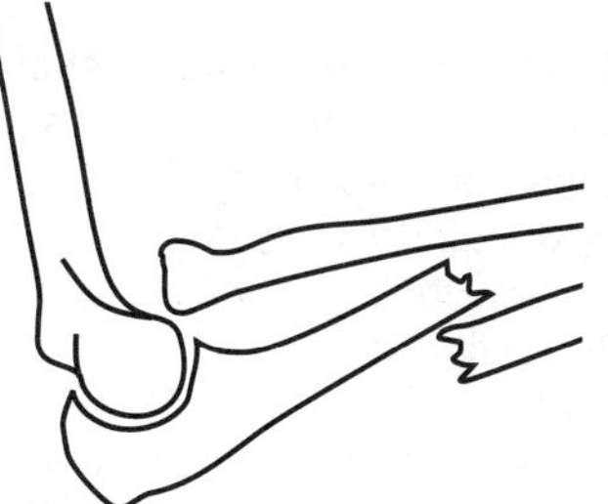

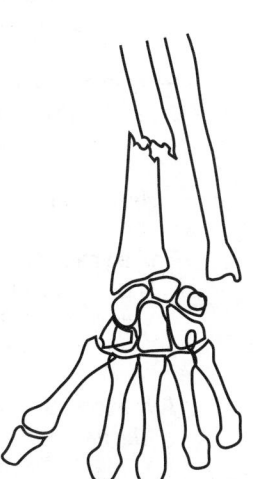

Bado Type I

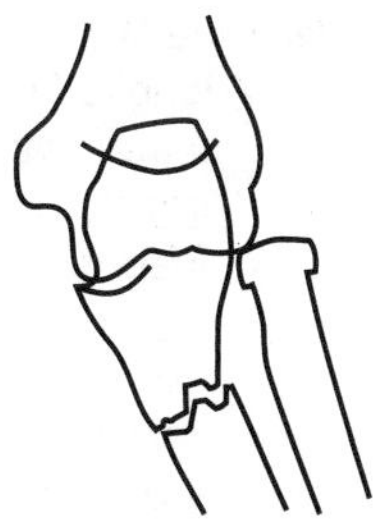

Bado Type III

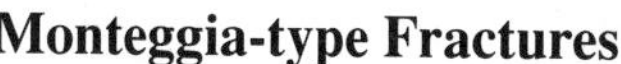

Monteggia-type Fractures

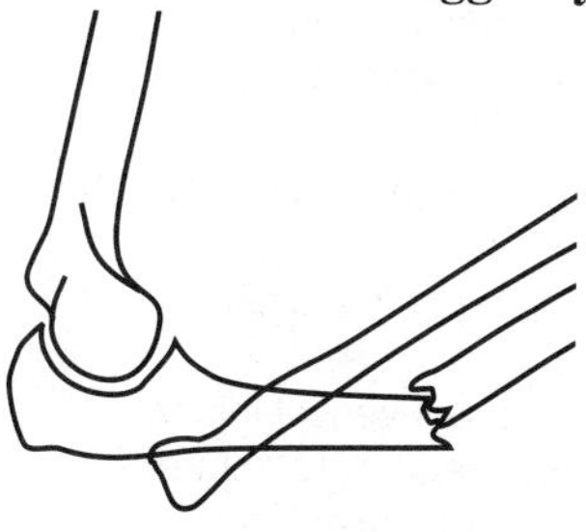

Bado Type II

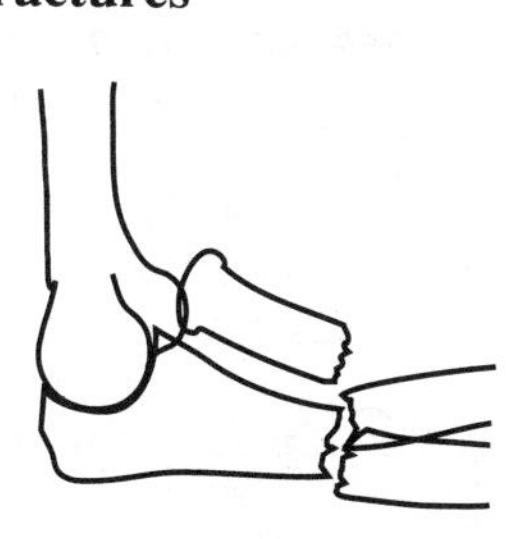

Bado Type IV

Mechanism: hyperflexion with fall on back of hand
√ nonarticular distal radial fracture
√ ventral displacement of fragment
√ radial deviation of hand
√ "garden spade" deformity
Cx: altered function of carpus

Elbow Fracture

common among children 2–14 years of age

@ Soft-tissue
- √ displacement of anterior + posterior fat pads (= elbow joint effusion with supracondylar / lateral condylar / proximal ulnar fractures)
- √ supinator fat pad (= fracture of proximal radius)
- √ focal edema medially (= medial epicondyle fx) / laterally (= lateral condyle fx)

@ Humerus (80%)

Supracondylar fracture (55%)
Mechanism: hyperextension with vertical stress
- √ transverse fracture line
- √ distal fragment posteriorly displaced / tilted
- √ anterior humeral line intersecting anterior to posterior third of capitellum (on lateral x-ray)

Lateral condylar fracture (20%)
Mechanism: hyperextension with varus stress
- √ fracture line between lateral condyle + trochlea / through capitellum

Medial epicondylar fracture (5%)
Mechanism: hyperextension with valgus stress
- √ avulsion of medial epicondyle (by flexor muscles of forearm)
- √ may become trapped in joint space (after reduction of concomitant elbow dislocation)

@ Radius (10%)
Mechanism: hyperextension with valgus stress
- √ Salter-Harris type II / IV fracture
- √ transverse metaphyseal / radial neck fracture

Mechanism: hyperextension with varus stress
- √ dislocation as part of Monteggia fracture (from rupture of annular ligament)

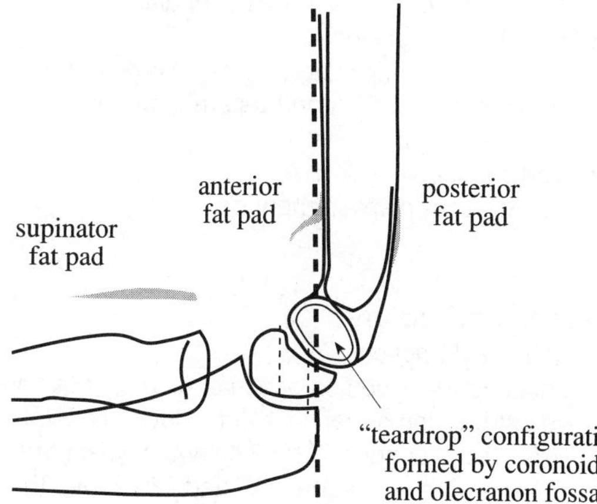

Anterior Humeral Line and Elbow Fat Pads

@ Ulna (10%)
√ longitudinal linear fracture through proximal shaft
Mechanism: hyperextension with vertical stress
√ transverse fracture through olecranon
Mechanism: hyperextension with valgus / varus stress; blow to posterior elbow in flexed position
√ coronoid process avulsion
Mechanism: hyperextension-rotation associated with forceful contraction of brachial m.

Rib Fracture

Associated with: pneumothorax, hemothorax, lung contusion / laceration

@ 1st rib
◊ Indicates substantial trauma (due to protected location)
Cause: acute trauma / fatigue fracture (from carrying a heavy back pack)
Associated with: aortic / great vessel injury; thoracic vertebral fracture; scapular fracture

@ Lower ribs
Associated with: injury to upper abdominal organs / diaphragm

Flail Chest

= fracture of >4 contiguous ribs
• paradoxic motion of chest wall with respiration
• respiratory failure

Cough Fracture

Location: 4–9th rib in anterior axillary line

Pelvic Fracture

Unstable pelvic fractures
(a) anterior compression
1. Bilateral vertical pubic rami fractures
2. Symphysis + sacroiliac joint diastasis
(b) lateral compression
1. Malgaigne (ipsilateral anterior + posterior fx)
2. Bucket-handle (contralateral anterior + posterior fx)
(c) vertical shear
1. Superior displacement of pelvis

Acetabular Fracture

Anatomy & Function:
most important portion of acetabulum is roof / dome; weight-bearing surface for entire lower limb is derived + supported by 2 columns which are oriented in an inverted "Y" and join above the acetabular roof at an angle of 60°:
(a) anterior iliopubic column of acetabulum
(b) posterior ilioischial column of acetabulum

Classification (Judet and Letournel):
A. Elementary fractures

Posterior wall	27%	Anterior column	5%
Transverse	9%	Posterior column	4%
Anterior wall	2%		

B. Associated fractures

Transverse + posterior wall	27%
Both columns	19%
T-shaped	6%
Anterior wall + posterior hemitransverse	5%
Posterior column + posterior wall	3%

POSTERIOR WALL (LIP / RIM) FRACTURE (27%)
Mechanism: indirect force transmitted through length of femur with flexed hip joint (knee strikes dashboard)
Associated with: posterior dislocation of femur

TRANSVERSE FRACTURE (9%)
N.B.: most difficult to diagnose + comprehend
√ transects both the iliopubic + ilioischial columns with fracture line in an anteroposterior direction

ANTERIOR COLUMN FRACTURE (5%)
Mechanism: blow to greater trochanter with hip externally rotated
Associated with: posterior column / transverse fracture
√ fracture begins between anterior iliac spines + traverses the acetabular fossa + ends in the ischiopubic ramus

POSTERIOR COLUMN FRACTURE (4%)
Mechanism: indirect force transmitted through length of femur with hip abducted
Associated with: posterior dislocation of femur + sciatic nerve injury
√ fracture begins at greater sciatic notch + traverses the posterior aspect of acetabular fossa + ends in the ischiopubic ramus

ANTERIOR WALL FRACTURE (2%)
Mechanism: force transmitted through greater trochanter
Associated with: posterior dislocation of femur + sciatic nerve injury
√ fracture begins on anterior rim of acetabulum + emerges on lateral aspect of superior pubic ramus

Malgaigne Fracture

[Joseph Francois Malgaigne (1806–1865), French surgical historian, published first comprehensive book on fractures]
= fracture-dislocation of one side of the pelvis with anterior + posterior disruption of pelvic ring
Mechanism: direct trauma
• shortening of involved extremity
√ vertical fractures through one side of pelvic ring
(1) superior to acetabulum (ilium)

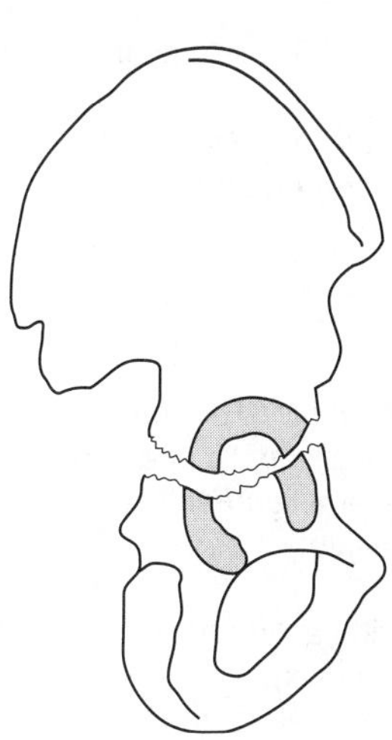

Transverse Fracture 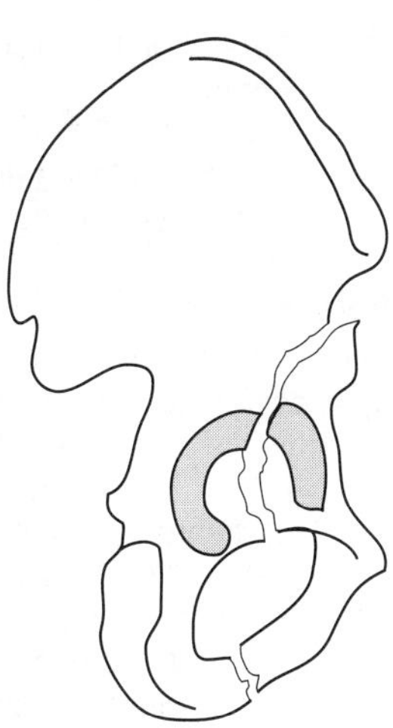 **Anterior Column Fracture** 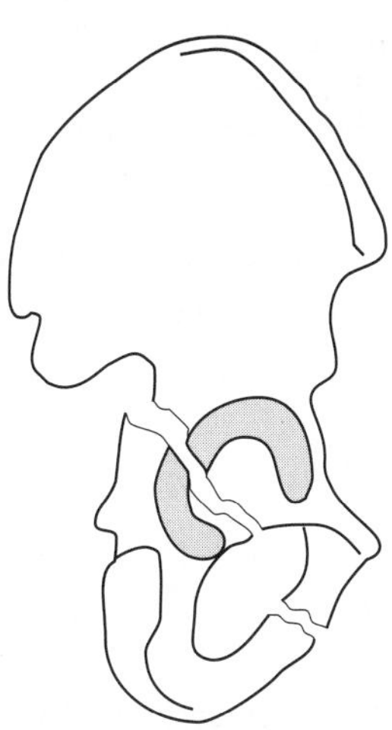 **Posterior Column Fracture** 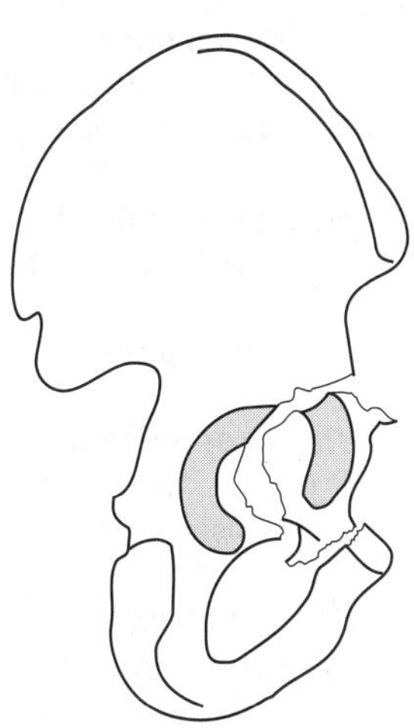 **Anterior Wall Fracture**

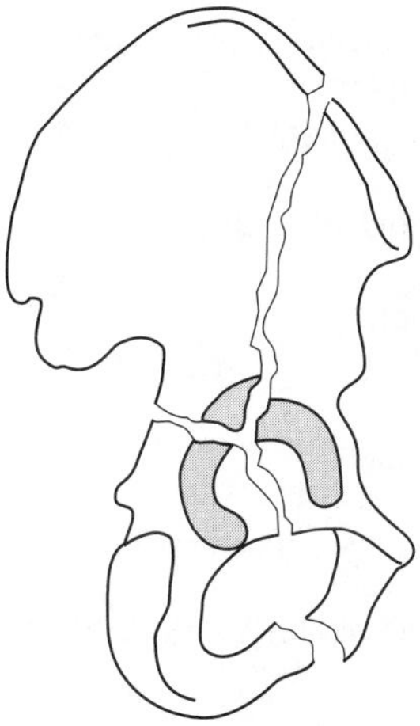

Fracture of Both Columns 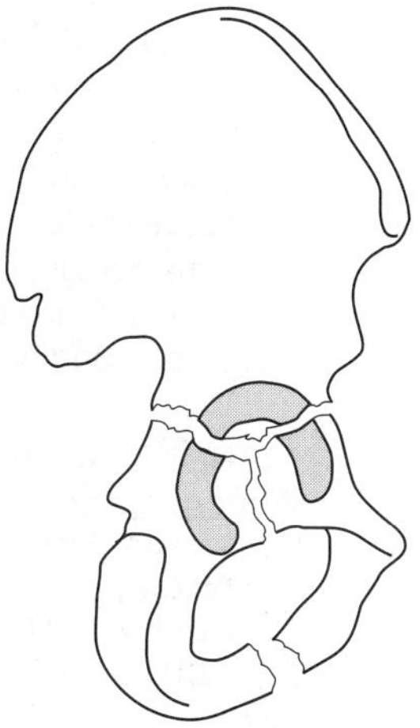 **T-shaped Fracture** 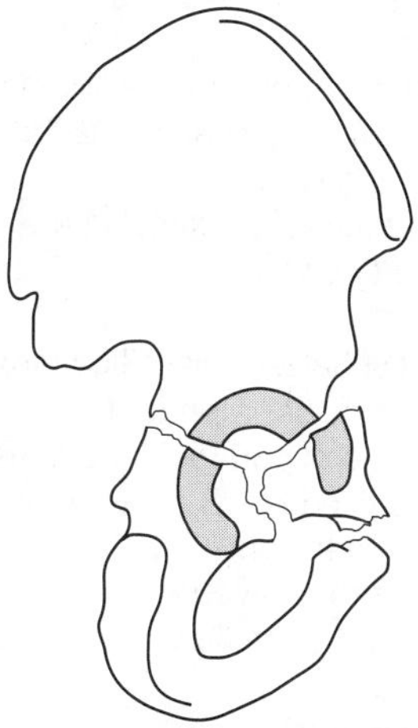 **Anterior Wall + Posterior Hemitransverse Fracture** 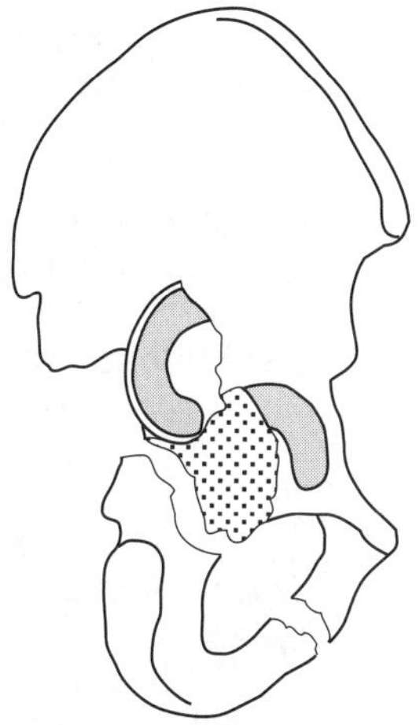 **Posterior Wall + Posterior Column Fracture**

Fractures of the Acetabulum

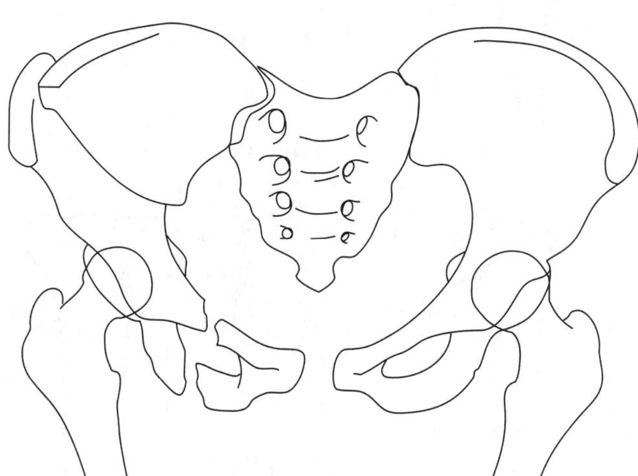

Malgaigne Fracture

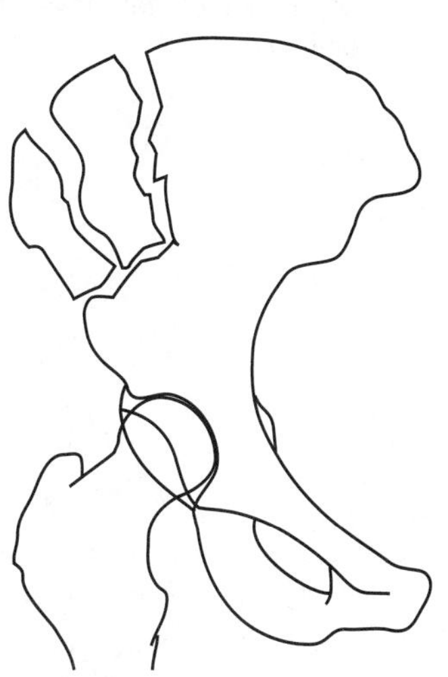

Duverney Fracture

(2) inferior to acetabulum (pubic rami)
(3) ± sacroiliac dislocation / fracture
√ lateral unstable fragment contains acetabulum

Bucket Handle Fracture

√ double vertical fracture through superior and inferior pubic rami + sacroiliac joint dislocation on contralateral side

Duverney Fracture

[Joseph Guichard Duverney (1648–1730), French surgeon]
√ isolated fracture of iliac wing

Knee Fracture

Segond Fracture

[Paul Ferdinand Segond (1851–1912), surgeon in chief at Salpêtrière in Paris, France]

Mechanism: external rotation + varus stress causing excessive tension on the lateral capsular ligament

Associated with: lesion of anterior cruciate ligament (75–100%), meniscal tear (67%)

- anterolateral instability of the knee

√ small cortical avulsion fracture of proximal lateral tibial rim just distal to lateral plateau

Tibial Plateau Fracture (Schatzker classification)

Mechanism: valgus force ("bumper / fender fracture" from lateral force of automobile against a pedestrian's fixed knee) / compression force often in extension

Type I	= wedge-shaped pure cleavage fracture	6%
Type II	= combined cleavage + median compression fracture	25%
Type III	= pure compression fracture	36%
Type IV	= medial plateau fracture with a split / depressed comminution	10%
Type V	= bicondylar fracture, often with inverted Y appearance	3%
Type VI	= transverse / oblique fracture with separation of metaphysis from diaphysis	20%

◊ Lateral plateau fractures (type I–III) are most common!
◊ Fractures of medial plateau are associated with greater violence and higher percentage of associated injuries!

Foot Fracture

Ankle Fracture

Incidence: ankle injuries account for 10% of all emergency room visits; 85% of all ankle sprains involve lateral ligaments

Ligamentous connections at ankle:
(a) binding tibia + fibula
1. anterior inferior tibiofibular ligament (= tibiofibular syndesmosis)
2. posterior inferior tibiofibular ligament
3. transverse tibiofibular ligament
4. interosseous membrane

(b) lateral malleolus
85% of all ankle sprains involve these ligaments:
1. anterior talofibular ligament
2. posterior talofibular ligament
3. calcaneofibular ligament

(c) medial malleolus = deltoid ligament with
1. navicular portion
2. sustentaculum portion
3. talar portion

Lateral Malleolar Fractures

Weber Type A

[Bernhard Georg Weber (1929–), orthopedic surgeon in St. Gall, Switzerland]
= SUPINATION-ADDUCTION INJURY = INVERSION-ADDUCTION INJURY

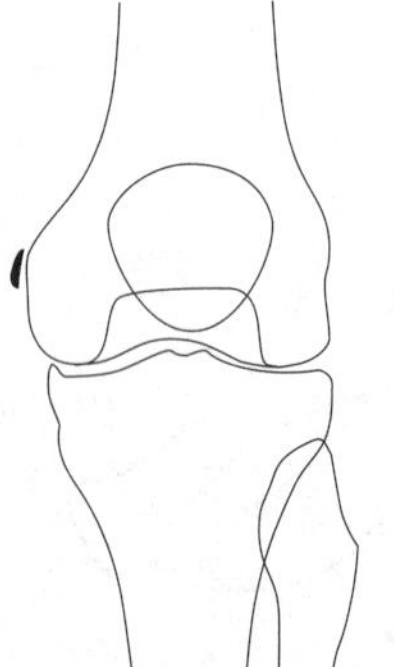

Pellegrini-Stieda Disease

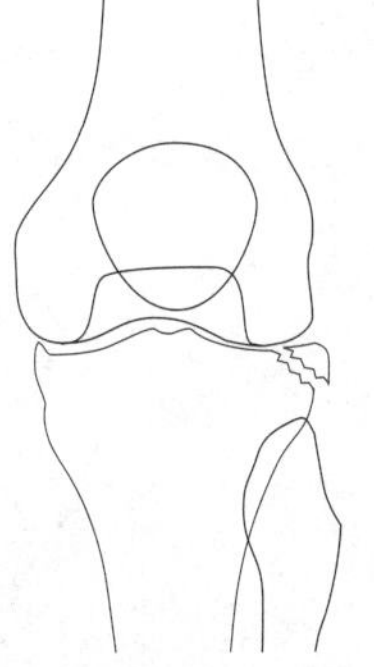

Segond Fracture

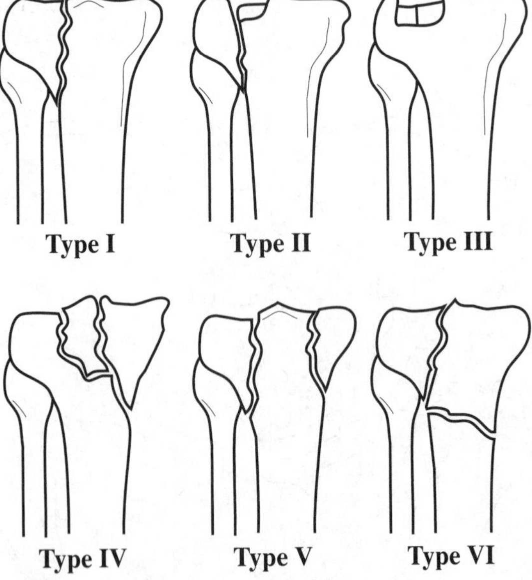

Tibial Plateau Fractures

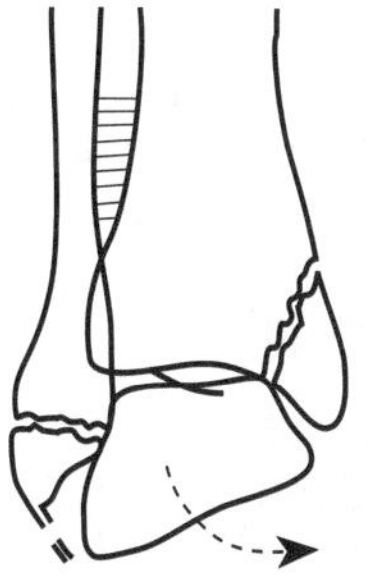
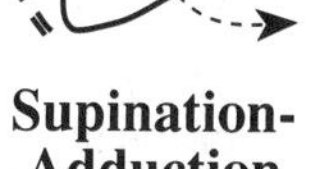
Supination-Adduction

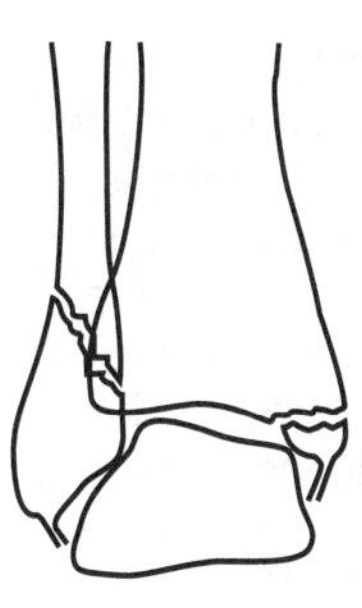
Supination-Abduction

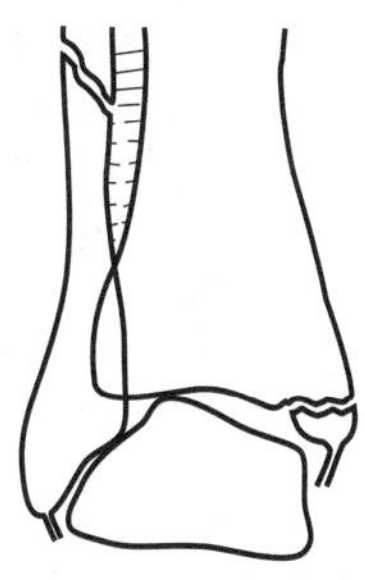
Pronation-External Rotation

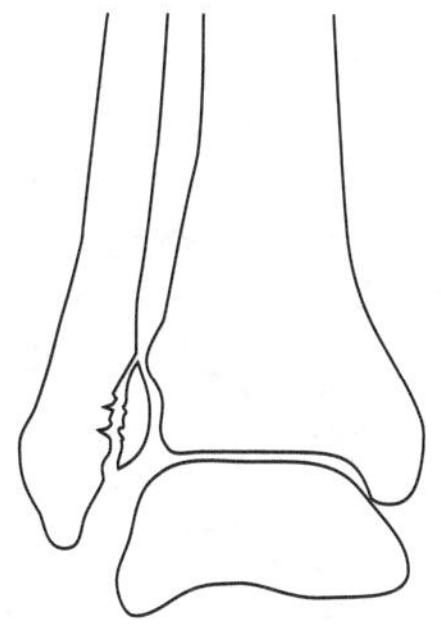
LeFort Ankle Fracture

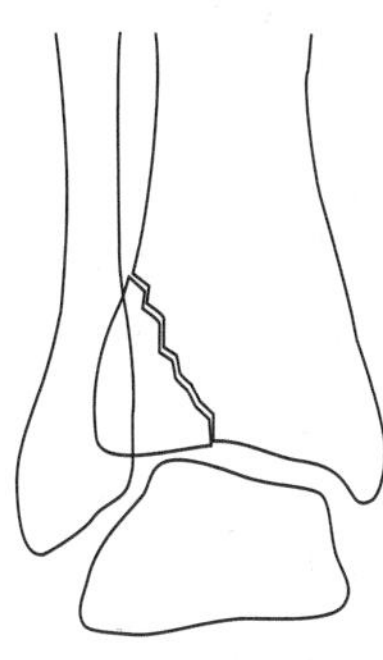
Tillaux Fracture

Mechanism:
(1) avulsive forces affect lateral ankle structures
(2) impactive forces secondary to talar shift stress medial structures

√ sprain / rupture of lateral collateral ligament
◊ Anterior tibiofibular ligament ruptures alone in 66%
◊ Injury of all 3 lateral ligaments in 20%
Prognosis: chronic lateral ankle instability in 10–20%

√ transverse avulsion of malleolus sparing tibiofibular ligaments
√ ± oblique fracture of medial malleolus
√ ± posterior tibial lip fracture

Weber Type B

= SUPINATION-ABDUCTION INJURY = EVERSION-EXTERNAL ROTATION

Mechanism:
(1) avulsive forces on medial structures
(2) impacting forces on lateral structures (talar impact)

√ oblique / spiral fracture of lateral malleolus starting at level of joint space extending proximally
√ lateral subluxation of talus
√ partial disruption of tibiofibular ligament
√ ± sprain / rupture / avulsion of deltoid ligament
√ ± transverse fracture of medial malleolus

(a) **Dupuytren Fracture**
[Guillaume Dupuytren (1777–1835), French surgeon]
√ fracture of distal fibula above a disrupted tibiofibular ligament + disruption of deltoid ligament

(b) **Le Fort Fracture of Ankle**
[Léon Clement Le Fort (1829–1893), French surgeon]
√ vertical fracture of anterior medial portion of distal fibula
√ avulsion of anterior tibiofibular ligament

Weber Type C

= PRONATION-EXTERNAL ROTATION = EVERSION + EXTERNAL ROTATION

√ fibular fracture higher than ankle joint (Maisonneuve fracture if around knee)
√ ± deltoid ligament tear
√ ± medial malleolar fracture
√ tear of tibiofibular ligament / avulsion of anterior tubercle (Tillaux-Chaput) / avulsion of posterior tubercle (Volkmann)
√ tear of interosseous membrane = lateral instability

(a) **Tillaux Fracture**
[Paul Jules Tillaux (1834–1904), French surgeon and anatomist]
√ avulsion injury of anterior tibial tubercle at attachment of distal anterior tibiofibular ligament

(b) **Maisonneuve Fracture**
[Jacques Gilles Maisonneuve (1809–1897), student of Dupuytren]
√ tear of distal tibiofibular syndesmosis + interosseous membrane
√ spiral fracture of upper third of fibula
√ associated fracture of medial malleolus / rupture of deep deltoid ligament

Chopart Fracture

[Francois Chopart (1743–1795), surgeon in Paris, France]

√ fracture-dislocation through midtarsal / Chopart (calcaneocuboid + talonavicular) joint
√ commonly associated with fractures of the bones abutting the joint

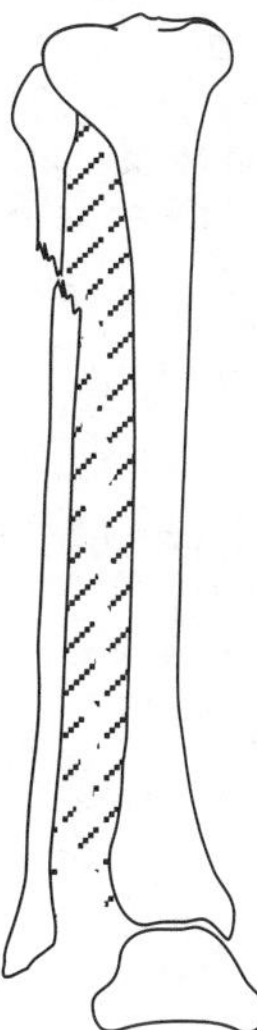
Maisonneuve Fracture

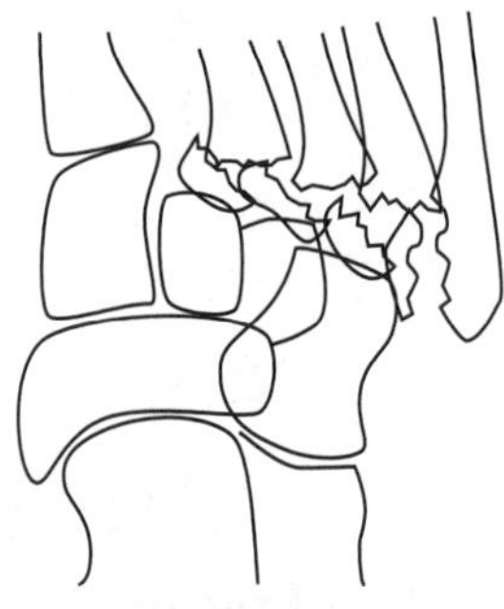

Lisfranc Fracture-Dislocation

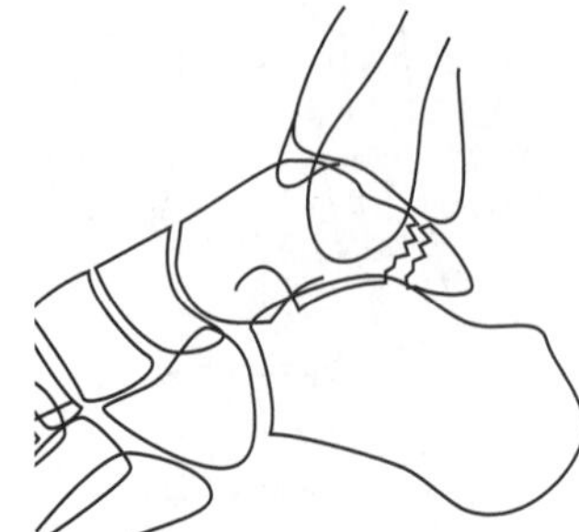

Shepherd Fracture

Jones Fracture

[Robert Jones (1857–1933), British orthopedic surgeon and pioneer in radiology]

√ transverse fracture at base of 5th metatarsal distal to metatarsal tuberosity >1.5 cm from proximal tip

Peroneus Brevis Avulsion Fracture

= METATARSAL 5 TUBEROSITY FRACTURE

Mechanism: plantar flexion + inversion (stepping off a curb)

√ transverse avulsion fracture of base of 5th metatarsal proximal to metatarsal tuberosity (insertion of peroneus brevis tendon)

DDx: Jones fracture (slightly different location)

Lisfranc Fracture

[Jacques Lisfranc De Saint Martin (1790–1847), surgeon in Napoleon's army]

Mechanism: metatarsal heads fixed and hindfoot forced plantarward and into rotation

√ fracture-dislocation / fracture-subluxation of tarsometatarsal joints (typically 2 through 5)

√ lateral displacement of metatarsals

Shepherd Fracture

[Francis J. Shepherd (1851–1929), demonstrator in anatomy at McGill University in Montreal, Canada]

√ fracture of lateral tubercle of posterior process of talus

DDx: os trigonum

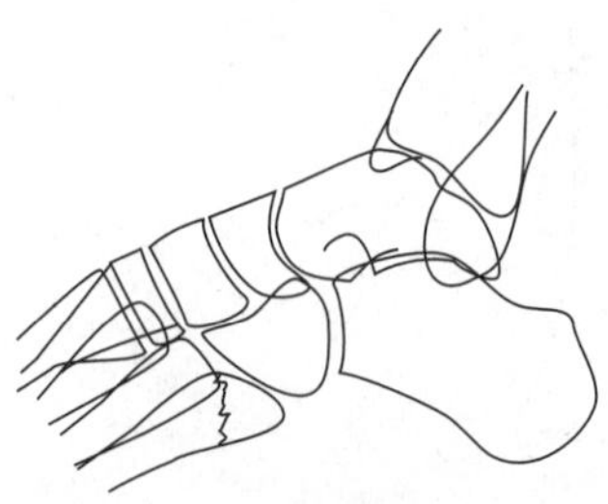

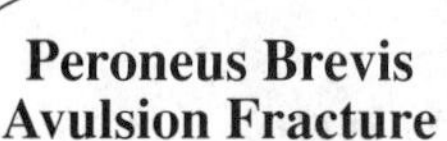

Peroneus Brevis Avulsion Fracture

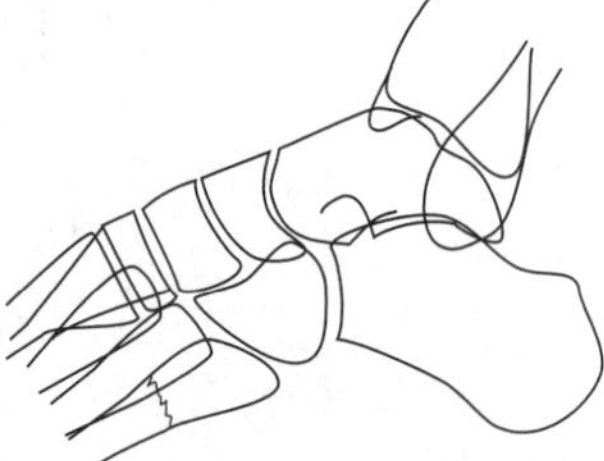

Jones Fracture

Calcaneal Fracture

Incidence: most commonly fractured tarsal bone; 60% of all tarsal fractures; 2% of all fractures in the body; commonly bilateral

Mechanism: fall from heights

May be associated with: lumbar vertebral fracture

Age: 95% in adults, 5% in children

— adulthood: intraarticular (75%), extraarticular (25%)

— childhood: extraarticular (63–92%)

Classification:

(a) extraarticular fracture of calcaneal tuberosity: beak type, vertical, horizontal, medial avulsion

(b) intraarticular fracture

— subtalar joint involvement: undisplaced, displaced, comminuted

— calcaneocuboid joint involvement

√ apex of lateral talar process does not point to "crucial angle" of Gissane

√ Boehler angle decreased below 28°–40°

FROSTBITE

Cause: (1) cellular injury + necrosis from freezing process

(2) cessation of circulation secondary to cellular aggregates + thrombi forming as a result of exposure to low temperatures below –13° C (usually cold air)

• firm white numb areas in cutis (separation of epidermal-dermal interface)

Location: feet, hands (thumb commonly spared due to protection by clenched fist)

Early changes:

√ soft-tissue swelling + loss of tissue at tips of digits

CHILD

√ fragmentation / premature fusion / destruction of distal phalangeal epiphyses

√ secondary infection, articular cartilage injury, joint space narrowing, sclerosis, osteophytosis of DIP

√ shortening + deviation / deformity of fingers

ADULT

√ osteoporosis (4–10 weeks after injury)

√ periostitis

√ acromutilation (secondary to osteomyelitis + surgical removal) + tuftal resorption (result of soft-tissue loss)

√ small round punched-out areas near edge of joint

√ interphalangeal joint abnormalities (simulating osteoarthritis)

√ calcification / ossification of pinna

Angio:

√ vasospasm, stenosis, occlusion

√ proliferation of arterial + venous collaterals (in recovery phase)

Bone scintigraphy:

√ persistent absence of uptake (= lack of vascular perfusion) indicates nonviable tissue

Rx: selective angiography with intraarterial reserpine

GANGLION

Ganglion cyst = mucin-containing cyst arising from tendon sheath / joint capsule / bursa / subchondral bone lined by flat spindle-shaped cells

Synovial cyst = cyst continuous with joint capsule lined by synovial cells (term is used by some synonymously with ganglion)

Soft-tissue Ganglion

= cystic tumorlike lesion usually attached to a tendon sheath

Origin: synovial herniation / coalescence of smaller cysts formed by myxomatous degeneration of periarticular connective tissue

- asymptomatic / pain
- uni- / multilocular swelling

Location: hand, wrist, foot (over dorsum)

Site: arise from tendon, muscle, semilunar cartilage

√ soft-tissue mass with surface bone resorption
√ periosteal new-bone formation
√ arthrography may demonstrate communication with joint / tendon sheath
√ internal septations, lobulated configuration
√ low to intermediate signal intensity on T1WI
√ high signal intensity on T2WI

Prognosis: may resolve spontaneously

Rx: steroid injection may improve symptomatology

Intraosseous Ganglion

= benign subchondral radiolucent lesion WITHOUT degenerative arthritis

- mild localized pain (4% of patients with unexplained wrist pain)

Age: middle age

Origin: (1) mucoid degeneration of intraosseous connective tissue perhaps due to trauma / ischemia
(2) penetration of juxtaosseous soft-tissue ganglion (= synovial herniation) into underlying bone (occasionally)

Path: uni- / multilocular cyst surrounded by fibrous lining, containing gelatinous material

Location: epiphysis of long bone (medial malleolus, femoral head, proximal tibia, carpal bones) / subarticular flat bone (acetabulum)

√ well-demarcated solitary 0.6–6 cm lytic lesion
√ sclerotic margin
√ NO communication with joint
√ increased radiotracer uptake on bone scintigraphy (in 10%)

DDx: posttraumatic / degenerative cyst

Periosteal Ganglion

= cystic structure with viscid / mucinous contents

Incidence: 11 cases in literature

Age: 39–50 years; M > F

- swelling, mild tenderness

Location: long tubular bones of lower extremity

√ cortical erosion / scalloping / reactive bone formation
√ NO intraosseous component (endosteal surface intact)

CT:
√ well-defined soft-tissue mass adjacent to bone cortex with fluid contents

MR:
√ homogeneous isointense signal to muscle on T1WI
√ homogeneous hyperintense signal to fat on T2WI
√ NO internal septations (DDx to soft-tissue ganglion)

DDx: periosteal chondroma without matrix calcification, cortical desmoid, subperiosteal aneurysmal bone cyst, acute subperiosteal hematoma (history of trauma / blood dyscrasia), subperiosteal abscess (involvement of adjacent bone marrow)

Rx: surgical excision (local recurrence possible)

GARDNER SYNDROME

= autosomal dominant syndrome characterized by (1) osteomas (2) soft-tissue tumors (3) colonic polyps

Location of osteomas: paranasal sinuses; outer table of skull (frequent); mandible (at angle)

√ endosteal cortical thickening / osteomas in any bone
√ may have solid periosteal cortical thickening
√ osteomas / exostoses may protrude from periosteal surface
√ wavy cortical thickening of superior aspect of ribs
√ polyps: colon, stomach, duodenum, ampulla of Vater, small intestine

Cx: high incidence of carcinoma of duodenum / ampulla of Vater

GAUCHER DISEASE

= rare autosomal recessive / dominant (in a few) lipid storage disorder; common among Ashkenazi Jews; M = F

Etiology: deficiency of lysosomal hydrolase acid ß-glycosidase (= glucocerebrosidase) leads to accumulation of glucosylceramide (glucocerebroside) within macrophages of RES (liver, spleen, bone marrow, lung, lymph nodes)

Histo: bone-marrow aspirate shows Gaucher cells (kerasin-laden histiocytes) of 20–100 μm in diameter with a foamy appearance

Types:

(1) Adult / chronic nonneuropathic form = type 1 (most common form in USA)
Age of onset: 3rd–4th decade
Prognosis: longest time of survival; pulmonary involvement / hepatic failure may lead to early death

(2) Rapidly fatal infantile / acute neuropathic form = type 2
Age of onset: 1–12 months
- early onset of significant hepatosplenomegaly
- severe progressive neurologic symptoms: seizures, mental retardation, strabismus, spasticity

√ skeletal manifestations are rare
Prognosis: fatal during first 2 years of life

(3) Juvenile / subacute neuropathic form = type 3 (rarest type)
Age of onset: 2–6 years

• hepatosplenomegaly
• mild neurologic involvement
√ delayed onset of skeletal manifestations
Prognosis: survival into adolescence

• hepatosplenomegaly, impairment of liver function, ascites
• elevated serum acid phosphatase
• pancytopenia, anemia, leukopenia, thrombocytopenia (hypersplenism)
• hemochromatosis (yellowish brown pigmentation of conjunctiva + skin)
• dull bone pain; bone involvement in 75%

Location: predominantly long tubular bones (distal femur), axial skeleton, hip, shoulder, pelvis; bilateral

√ generalized osteopenia (decrease in trabecular bone density):
  √ striking cortical thinning + bone widening
  √ endosteal scalloping (due to marrow packing)
√ numerous sharply circumscribed lytic lesions resembling metastases / multiple myeloma (marrow replacement)
√ periosteal reaction = cloaking
√ Erlenmeyer flask deformity of distal femur + proximal tibia (2° to marrow infiltration) MOST CHARACTERISTIC
√ weakening of subchondral bone:
  √ osteonecrosis (common), frequently of femoral head
  √ degenerative arthritis
√ bone infarction in long-bone metaphyses (common):
  √ focal / serpentine areas of sclerosis
  √ bone-within-bone appearance
√ H-shaped / "step-off" / biconcave "fish-mouth" vertebrae (DDx: sickle cell disease)

@ Liver
  √ hepatomegaly
  √ nonspecific fatty + cirrhotic changes

@ Spleen
  √ splenomegaly + lymphadenopathy
  √ multiple nodular lesions (= clusters of RES cells laden with glucosylceramide):
    √ hypodense without enhancement on CT
    √ hypoechoic / hyperechoic on US
    √ isointense on T1WI + hyperintense on T2WI
  √ splenic infarction leading to fibrosis

@ Lung
  √ diffuse reticulonodular infiltrates at lung bases (= infiltration with Gaucher cells)

Cx: ◊ >90% have orthopedic complications at some time
  (1) pathologic fractures + compression fractures of vertebrae
  (2) avascular necrosis of femoral head, humeral head, wrist, ankle (common)
  (3) osteomyelitis (increased incidence)
  (4) myelosclerosis in long-standing disease
  (5) repeated pulmonary infections

Prognosis: highly variable clinical course; strong relationship between splenic volume and disease severity

DDx: metastatic disease, multiple myeloma, leukemia, sickle-cell disease, fibrous dysplasia

GIANT CELL REPARATIVE GRANULOMA

= GIANT CELL REACTION = GIANT CELL GRANULOMA

Cause: ? reactive inflammatory process to trauma / infection (not a true neoplasm)

Histo: numerous giant cells in exuberant fibrous matrix arranged in clusters around foci of hemorrhage + commonly exhibiting osteoid formation (unusual in giant cell tumor); indistinguishable from brown tumor of HPT; cystic degeneration + ABC components distinctly uncommon

Peak age: 2nd + 3rd decade (ranging from childhood to 76 years); 74% <30 years of age; M:F = 1:1

May be associated with: enchondromatosis, Goltz syndrome, fibrous dysplasia, Paget disease

Location:

@ Gnathic (1–7% of all benign oral tumors): gingiva + alveolar mucosa of mandible, maxilla
  (a) central type = in bone
  (b) peripheral type = in gingival soft tissue
  M:F = 1:2
  • nonspecific pain + swelling (increasing during pregnancy)
  √ expansile remodeling of bone with multilocular appearance
  √ thinned usually intact cortex
  DDx: indistinguishable from odontogenic cyst, ABC, ameloblastoma, odontogenic myxoma, odontogenic fibroma

@ Small bones of hand + feet (less common): phalanges of hand > metcarpals > metatarsals > carpal bones > tarsal bones > phalanges of foot
  M:F = 1:1
  • nonspecific pain + swelling for months to years
  Site: metaphysis ± extension into diaphysis; extension into epiphysis is UNCOMMON
  √ expansile lytic defect of 2–2.5 cm in diameter with internal trabeculations
  √ thinning of overlying cortex
  √ matrix mineralization may be seen (DDx to GCT)
  √ periosteal reaction is unusual (as in GCT)
  √ extension beyond cortex is unusual

@ Other locations (rare):
  ethmoid sinus, sphenoid sinus, temporal bone, skull, spine, clavicle, tibia, humerus, ribs, femur

Cx: pathologic fracture

Prognosis: may recur; no malignant transformation

Rx: curettage (22–50% recurrence rate) / local excision

DDx:
  (1) Enchondroma (same location, matrix calcification)
  (2) Aneurysmal bone cyst (rare in small bones of hand + feet, typically prior to epiphyseal closure)
  (3) Giant cell tumor (more aggressive appearance)
  (4) Infection (clinical)
  (5) Brown tumor of HPT (periosteal bone resorption, abnormal Ca + P levels)

GIANT CELL TUMOR

= OSTEOCLASTOMA = OSTEOBLASTOCLASTOMA = TUMOR OF MYELOPLAXUS = MYELOID SARCOMA

= nonmineralized lytic eccentric metaepiphyseal lesion involving a long bone with extension to subarticular bone in the skeletally mature patient

Origin: probably arise from zone of intense osteoclastic activity (of endochondral ossification) in skeletally immature patients

Incidence: 4–9.5% of all primary bone tumors; 18–23% of benign skeletal tumors; unusually high prevalence in China + southern India

Path: friable vascular stroma of numerous thin-walled capillaries with necrosis + hemorrhage + cyst formation (DDx: aneurysmal bone cyst without solid areas)

Histo: large number of multinucleated osteoclastic giant cells in a diffuse distribution in a background of mononuclear cells intermixed throughout a spindle cell stroma (DDx: giant cells characteristic of all reactive bone disease as in pigmented villonodular synovitis, benign chondroblastoma, nonosteogenic fibroma, chondromyxoid fibroma, fibrous dysplasia)

Age: peaks in 3rd decade; 1–3% < age 14; 80% between 20 and 50 years; 9–13% > age 50; M:F = 1:1.1 to 1:1.5 (in spine 1:2.5)

May be associated with: Paget disease (in 50–60% located in skull + facial bones)

Staging:
- Stage 1 indolent radiographic + histologic appearance (10–15%)
- Stage 2 more aggressive radiographic appearance with expansile remodeling (70–80%)
- Stage 3 extension into adjacent soft tissues with histologically benign appearance (10–15%)

• pain at affected site (most common – in 10% pathologic fracture)
• local swelling + tenderness
• weakness + sensory deficits (if in spine)

Location:
@ long bones (75–85–90%)
— lower extremity (50–65% about knee):
distal end of femur (23–30%) > proximal end of tibia (20–25%) > proximal femur (4%) > distal tibia (2–5%) > proximal fibula (3–4%) > foot (1–2%)
- RARE in patella (the largest sesamoid bone) + greater trochanter (epiphyseal equivalent)
— upper extremity (away from elbow):
distal end of radius (10–12%) > proximal end of humerus (4–8%) > hand and wrist (1–5%)
@ flat bones (15%)
- pelvis: sacrum near SIJ (4%), iliac bone (3%)
- spine (3–6%): thoracic > cervical > lumbar spine (tumor frequency 2nd only to chordoma)
- rib (anterior / posterior end)
- skull (sphenoid bone)

Site: eccentric (42–93%) in <u>metaphysis</u> of long bones adjacent to ossified epiphyseal line; extension to within 1 cm of subarticular bone (84–99%) after fusion of epiphyseal plate (MOST TYPICAL) with possible transarticular spread

◊ The open epiphyseal plate acts as a barrier to tumor growth!

√ well-circumscribed expansile solitary lytic bone lesion with a narrow zone of transition:
  √ wide zone of transition (10–20%)
  √ large lesions are more centrally located
√ "soap bubble" appearance (47–60%) = expansile remodeling with multiloculated appearance:
  √ NO internal mineralization of tumor matrix
  √ prominent trabeculation (33–57%):
    (a) reactive with appositional bone growth
    (b) pseudotrabeculation of osseous ridges in endosteal scalloping
√ no sclerosis (80–85%) / periosteal reaction (10–30%) due to aggressive rapid growth in absence of fracture
√ cortical penetration (33–50%):
  √ cortical thinning
  √ soft-tissue invasion (25%)
  √ complete / incomplete pathologic fracture (11–37%)
√ destruction of vertebral body with secondary invasion of posterior elements (DDx: ABC, osteoblastoma)
√ frequently vertebral collapse
√ involves adjacent vertebral disks + vertebrae, crosses sacroiliac joint
√ may cross joint space in long bones (exceedingly rare)

NUC:
  √ diffusely increased uptake ± "doughnut" sign (57%) of central photopenia on delayed bone scintigraphy
  √ increased uptake across an articulation + in adjacent joints (62%) due to increased blood flow + disuse osteoporosis and NOT tumor extension

Angio:
  √ hypervascular (60–65%) / hypovascular (20%) / avascular (10%) lesion

CT:
  √ tumor of soft-tissue attenuation similar to muscle with foci of low attenuation (hemorrhage / necrosis):
    √ NO matrix mineralization
  √ well-defined margins ± thin rim of sclerosis (in up to 20%)
  √ soft-tissue extension (33–44%) usually at metaphyseal end of tumor
  √ aneurysmal bone cyst components (in 14%) of low density with fluid levels
  √ joint involvement is unusual except for sacroiliac joint (38%) with sacral lesion
  √ significant enhancement

MR:
  √ relatively well-defined lesion of heterogeneous signal intensity with <u>low to intermediate intensity</u> on T1WI + T2WI (63–96%) due to increased cellularity + high collagen content + hemosiderin
    ◊ HELPFUL feature to distinguish from other subarticular lesions (solitary subchondral cyst, intraosseous ganglion, Brodie abscess, clear cell chondrosarcoma with hyperintense matrix on T2WI)
  √ focal aneurysmal bone cyst components (in 14%) in tumor center with marked hyperintensity on T2WI
    ◊ Direct biopsy to peripheral solid-tissue component to prevent misdiagnosis!

√ low-signal-intensity margin (= osseous sclerosis / pseudocapsule
√ significant enhancement of solid-tissue component

Cx: in 5–10% malignant transformation within first 5 years (M:F = 3:1); metastases to lung

Prognosis: locally aggressive; 80–90% recurrence rate within first 3 years after initial treatment

Rx: currettage + bone grafting (40–60% recurrence); currettage with filling of void with high-speed burr + polymethylmeth-acrylate (2–25% recurrence); wide resection (7% recurrence) and reconstruction with allografts / metal prosthesis; radiation therapy for inoperable GCT (39–63% recurrence)

DDx: (1) Aneurysmal bone cyst (contains only cystic regions; in posterior elements of spine)
(2) Brown tumor of HPT (lab values)
(3) Osteoblastoma
(4) Cartilage tumor: chondroblastoma, enchondroma (not epiphyseal), chondromyxoid fibroma, chondrosarcoma
(5) Nonossifying fibroma
(6) Bone abscess
(7) Hemangioma
(8) Fibrous dysplasia
(9) Giant cell reparative granuloma

Multifocal Giant Cell Tumor

= additional GCTs (up to a maximum of 20) developing synchronously / metachronously for up to 20 years without increased risk of pulmonary metastases

Incidence: <1% of all GCT cases

Age: 25 years (range, 11–62 years); M<F

May be associated with:
Paget disease, usually polyostotic (GCT develops at a mean age of 61 years + after an average time lapse of 12 years) with involvement of skull + facial bones

Location: increased prevalence of hands + feet

Malignant Giant Cell Tumor

= group of giant cell–containing lesions capable of malignant behavior + pulmonary metastases

Prevalence: 5–10% of all GCTs

Age: older than patients with benign GCTs

Types:

(1) Benign metastasizing GCT
Prevalence: 1–5%
√ pulmonary metastases may remain stable / regress spontaneously
√ pulmonary nodules may show peripheral ossification
Prognosis: death in 13%

(2) Primary malignant transformation of GCT
= malignant tumor of bone composed of a sarcomatous growth juxtaposed to zones of typical benign GCT without a history of radiation therapy / repeated currettage / resection
Prognosis: median survival time of 4 years

(3) Secondary malignant GCT (86%)
= sarcomatous growth that occurs at a site of previously documented GCT usually after radiation therapy (80%) / repeated resections
Prognosis: median survival time of 1 year

(4) Osteoclastic (giant cell) sarcoma
= highly malignant tumor composed of anaplastic osteoclast-like giant cells without tumor osteoid / bone / cartilage

GLOMUS TUMOR

= hamartoma composed of cells derived from neuromyoarterial apparatus (regulating blood flow in skin)

Glomus body = encapsulated oval organ of 300 µm length; located in reticular dermis (= deepest layer of skin); concentrated in tips of digits (93–501/cm^2); composed of an afferent arteriole, an anastomotic vessel (= Sucquet-Hoyer canal lined by endothelium + surrounded by smooth muscle fibers), a primary collecting vein, the intraglomerular reticulum + capsule

Histo: (a) vascular (b) myxoid (c) solid form

Prevalence: 1–5% of soft-tissue tumors of hand

Age: mostly in 4–5th decade

- joint tenderness + pain (on average of 4–7 years duration prior to diagnosis)
- Love test = eliciting pain by applying precise pressure with a pencil tip
- Hildreth sign = disappearance of pain after application of a tourniquet proximally on arm (PATHOGNOMONIC)

@ SUBUNGUAL GLOMUS TUMOR
√ increased distance between dorsum of phalanx + underside of nail (25%)
√ extrinsic bone erosion (14–25–65%), often with sclerotic border
√ small hypoechoic tumor by US (>3 mm detectable)
√ homogeneously high-signal–intensity lesion on T2WI (detectable if >2 mm in diameter)

@ GLOMUS TUMOR OF BONE occasionally within bone
√ resembles enchondroma

DDx: (1) Mucoid cyst (painless, in proximal nail fold, communicating with DIP joint, associated with osteoarthritis)
(2) Angioma (more superficially located)

GOUT

= characterized by derangement of purine metabolism manifested by:
(1) hyperuricemia
(2) deposition of positively birefringent monosodium urate monohydrate crystals in synovial fluid leukocytes
(3) gross deposits of sodium urate in periarticular soft tissues (synovial membranes, articular cartilage, ligaments, bursae)
(4) recurrent episodes of arthritis

Age: >40 years; males (in women gout may occur after menopause)

Cause:

A. Primary Gout (90%)

Incidence: 0.3%; M:F = 20:1;
5% in postmenopausal women

Disturbance:

- overproduction of uric acid due to inborn error of metabolism
- inherited defect in renal urate excretion

(a) Idiopathic (99%)
- normal urinary excretion (80–90%)
- increased urinary excretion (10–20%)

(b) Specific enzyme / metabolic defect (1%)
(1) increased activity of PP-ribose-P synthetase
(2) partial deficiency of hypoxanthine-guanine phosphoribosyltransferase

B. Secondary Gout (10%)

◊ Rarely cause for radiographically apparent disease

(a) increased turnover of nucleic acids:
(1) Myeloproliferative disorders + sequelae of their treatment: polycythemia vera, leukemia, lymphoma, multiple myeloma
(2) Blood dyscrasias: chronic hemolysis

(b) increase in purine synthesis de novo due to enzyme defects:
(1) Glycogen storage disease Type I (von Gierke = glucose-6-phosphatase deficiency)
(2) Lesch-Nyhan syndrome (choreoathetosis, spasticity, mental retardation, self-mutilation of lips + fingertips) due to absence of hypoxanthine-guanine phosphoribosyltransferase

(c) acquired defect in renal excretion of urates (due to reduction in renal function):
(1) Chronic renal failure
(2) Drugs, toxins: lead poisoning
(3) Endocrinologic: myxedema, hypo- / hyperparathyroidism
(4) Vascular: myocardial infarction, hypertension

Histo: tophus (PATHOGNOMONIC LESION) composed of crystalline / amorphous urates surrounded by highly vascularized inflammatory tissue rich in histiocytes, lymphocytes, fibroblasts, foreign-body giant cells (similar to a foreign-body granuloma)

Clinical stages in chronologic order:

(1) **Asymptomatic hyperuricemia**

(2) **Acute gouty arthritis**

◊ Gout accounts for 5% of all cases of arthritis

Precipitated by: trauma, surgery, alcohol, dietary indiscretion, systemic infection

- monoarticular (90%)
- polyarticular (10%): any joint may be affected

Prognosis: usually self-limited (pain resolving within a few hours / days) without treatment

(3) **Chronic tophaceous gout**

= multiple large urate deposits in intraarticular, extraarticular, intraosseous location

Prevalence: <50% of patients experiencing acute attacks; M:F = 20:1

Histo: cartilage degeneration + destruction, synovial proliferation + pannus, destruction of subarticular bone + proliferation of marginal bone

Distribution: symmetric polyarticular disease (resembling rheumatoid arthritis), asymmetric polyarticular disease, monoarticular disease

- more severe prolonged attacks
- may ulcerate expressing whitish chalky material

Cx: tendon rupture, nerve compression / paralysis

(4) **Gouty nephropathy / nephrolithiasis**

(a) Acute urate nephropathy
(b) Uric acid urolithiasis

◊ May precede arthritis in up to 20% of cases!

- renal hypertension
- isosthenuria (inability to concentrate urine)
- proteinuria
- pyelonephritis

Cx: increased incidence of calcium oxalate stones (urate crystals serve as a nidus)

Location:

(a) joints: hands + feet (1st MTP joint most commonly affected = podagra) > ankles > heels > wrists (carpometacarpal compartment especially common and severe) > fingers > elbows; knees; shoulder; sacroiliac joint (15%, unilateral);
◊ involvement of hip + spine is rare
(b) bones, tendon, bursa, bones
(c) external ear; pressure points over elbow, forearms, knees, feet

◊ Radiologic features usually not seen until 6–12 years after initial attack

◊ Radiologic features present in 45% of inflicted patients

@ Soft tissues

√ eccentric juxtaarticular lobulated soft-tissue masses (hand, foot, ankle, elbow, knee)
Site: tendency for extensor tendons, eg, quadriceps, triceps, Achilles tendon

√ calcific deposits in periphery of gouty tophi in 50% (sodium urate crystals are not radiopaque, tophi radiographically visible only after calcium deposition of an underlying abnormality of calcium metabolism)

√ bilateral effusion of bursae olecrani (PATHOGNOMONIC), prepatellar bursa

√ aural calcification

@ Joint

√ joint effusion (earliest sign)

√ periarticular swelling (in acute monoarticular gout)

√ preservation of joint space until late in disease (IMPORTANT CLUE):
√ cartilage destruction (late in course of disease)

√ absence of periarticular demineralization (due to short duration of attacks; important DDx for rheumatoid arthritis)

√ eccentric erosions with thin sclerotic margins:
√ scalloped erosion of bases of ulnar metacarpals

√ chondrocalcinosis (5%):
Location: menisci (fibrocartilage only)
◊ Patients with gout have a predisposition for calcium pyrophosphate dihydrate deposition disease (CPPD)
Cx: secondary osteoarthritis
√ round / oval well-marginated subarticular cysts (pseudotumor) up to 3 cm (containing tophus / urate crystal-rich fluid)
DDx: rheumatoid arthritis (marginal erosions without sclerotic rim, periarticular demineralization)

@ Bone
√ "punched-out" lytic bone lesion ± sclerosis of margin = "mouse / rat bite" from erosion of long-standing soft-tissue tophus
√ "overhanging margin" (40%) = elevated osseous spicule separating tophaceous nodule from adjacent erosion (in intra- and extraarticular locations) (HALLMARK)
√ proliferative bone changes:
√ club-shaped metatarsals, metacarpals, phalanges
√ enlargement of ulnar styloid process
√ diaphyseal thickening
√ ischemic necrosis of femoral / humeral heads
√ intraosseous calcification:
√ punctate / circular calcifications of subchondral / subligamentous regions (DDx: enchondroma)
√ bone infarction due to deposits at vascular basement membrane (DDx: bone island)

@ Kidney
√ renal stones (in up to 20%):
– pure uric acid stones (84%): radiolucent on radiographs, hyperdense on CT
– uric acid + calcium oxalate (4%)
– pure calcium oxalate / calcium phosphate (12%)

MR:
√ tophus (most frequently) isointense to muscle on T1WI
√ low or intermediate signal intensity on T2WI
√ homogeneous intense enhancement

Rx: colchicine, allopurinol (effective treatment usually does not improve roentgenograms)

DDx:
(1) CPPD (pseudogout symptomatology, polyarticular chondrocalcinosis involving hyaline and fibrocartilage + degenerative arthropathy with joint space narrowing)
(2) Psoriasis (progressive joint space destruction, paravertebral ossification, sacroiliac joint involvement)
(3) Rheumatoid arthritis (nonproliferative marginal bone erosions, fusiform soft-tissue swelling, symmetric distribution, early joint-space narrowing, osteopenia)
(4) Joint infection (rapid destruction of joint space, loss of articular cortex over a continuous segment)
(5) Amyloidosis (bilateral symmetric involvement, periarticular osteopenia)
(6) Xanthomatosis (laboratory work-up)
(7) Osteoarthritis (symmetric distribution, elderly women)

GRANULOCYTIC SARCOMA

= CHLOROMA = MYELOBLASTOMA
= extramedullary solid tumor consisting of primitive precursors of the granulocytic series of WBCs (myeloblasts, promyelocytes, myelocytes)

Clinical setting:
(1) patient with acute myelogenous leukemia (in 3–8%)
(2) harbinger of AML in nonleukemic patient (usually developing within 1 year)
(3) indicator of impending blast crisis in CML (in 1%) / leukemic transformation in myelodysplastic syndromes (polycythemia rubra vera, myelofibrosis with myeloid metaplasia, hypereosinophilic syndrome)
(4) isolated event

• 60% are of green color (chloroma) due to high levels of myeloperoxidase (30% are white / gray / brown depending on preponderance of cell type + oxidative state of myeloperoxidase)

Location: orbit, soft tissue, skin, paranasal sinus, lymph node, periosteum, organs, bowel; often multiple
Site: propensity for bone marrow (arises from bone marrow traversing haversian canal + reaching the periosteum), perineural + epidural tissue
√ osteolysis with ill-defined margins
√ homogeneous enhancement on CT / MR (DDx to hematoma / abscess)

MR:
√ isointense to brain / bone marrow / muscle on T1WI + T2WI

Prognosis: resolution under chemotherapy ± radiation therapy; recurrence rate of 23%
DDx: osteomyelitis, histiocytosis X, neuroblastoma, lymphoma, multiple myeloma

GUNSHOT INJURY

Firearms: handgun, rifle (great energy), shotgun
Projectiles:
(a) bullet:
– jacketed bullet with mantle of copper
– semijacketed bullet = exposed lead at tip
– nonjacketed bullet
(b) pellets of steel / lead:
– birdshot = small pellets
– buckshot =large pellets

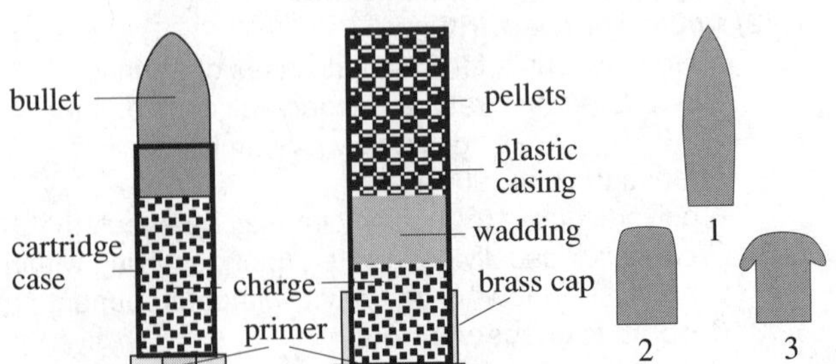

Projectiles
1 = fully jacketed rifle bullet, 2 = soft-point bullet, 3 = hollow-point bullet

Assessment:
(1) Type of projectile
√ fully jacketed bullets show no trail of lead fragments
√ semi- / nonjacketed bullets distribute lead fragments along bullet track
√ hollow-point bullets transform into mushroom shape
√ "lead snowstorm" of high-velocity soft-point rifle bullets:
√ conical distribution with apex pointing toward entry site
√ steel pellets remain round, lead pellets become deformed + fragmented
(2) Path of projectile
√ bullet tips points to entry wound (after tumbling through 180°):
√ impact deformation of bullet modifies tumbling
√ bullet + bone fragments deposited along track
√ bone fracture beveled toward the direction of travel
(3) Extent of injury
Cx: pellet embolization, magnetization in MRI

HEMANGIOENDOTHELIAL SARCOMA

= HEMANGIOENDOTHELIOMA = HEMANGIOEPITHELIOMA
= neoplasm of vascular endothelial cells of intermediate aggressiveness with either benign or malignant behavior
Histo: irregular anastomosing vascular channels lined by one / several layers of atypical anaplastic endothelial cells
Age: 4th–5th decade; M:F = 2:1
• history of trauma / irradiation

Soft-tissue Hemangioendothelioma (common)

Location: deep tissues of extremities
Site: in 50% closely related to a vessel (often a vein)

Osseous Hemangioendothelioma (rare)

Age: 2nd–3rd decade of life; M > F
Location: calvarium, spine, femur, tibia, humerus, pelvis; multicentric lesions in 30% often with regional distribution (less aggressive)
√ eccentric lesion in metaphysis of long bones
√ osteolytic aggressively destructive area with indistinct margins (high grade)
√ well-demarcated margins with scattered bony trabeculae (low grade)
√ osteoblastic area in vertebrae, contiguous through several vertebrae
Metastases to: lung (early)
Prognosis: 26% 5-year survival rate
DDx: aneurysmal bone cyst, poorly differentiated fibrosarcoma, highly vascular metastasis, alveolar rhabdomyosarcoma

HEMANGIOMA

◊ Most common benign soft-tissue tumor of vascular origin!
Histo: frequently containing variable amounts of nonvascular elements: fat, smooth muscle, fibrous tissue, bone, hemosiderin, thrombus
◊ Fat overgrowth may be so extensive that some lesion may be misdiagnosed as a lipoma!

A. CAPILLARY HEMANGIOMA (most common)
= small-caliber vessels lined by flattened epithelium
Site: skin, subcutaneous tissue; vertebral body
Age: first few years of life
(a) Juvenile capillary hemangioma = strawberry nevus
Prevalence: 1:200 births; in 20% multiple
Prognosis: involutes in 75–90% by age 7 years
(b) Verrucous capillary hemangioma
(c) Senile capillary hemangioma
√ enlarged arteries + arteriovenous shunting
√ pooling of contrast material

B. CAVERNOUS HEMANGIOMA
= dilated blood-filled spaces lined by flattened endothelium
Site: deeper soft tissues, frequently intramuscular; calvarium
Age: childhood
√ phleboliths = dystrophic calcification in organizing thrombus (in nearly 50%)
√ large cystic spaces
√ enlarged arteries + arteriovenous shunting
√ pooling of contrast material
Prognosis: NO involution

C. ARTERIOVENOUS HEMANGIOMA
= persistence of fetal capillary bed with abnormal communications of an increased number of normal / abnormal arteries and veins
Etiology: (?) congenital arteriovenous malformation
Age: young patients
Site: soft tissues
(a) superficial lesion without arteriovenous shunting
(b) deep lesion with arteriovenous shunting
• limb enlargement, bruit
• distended veins, overlying skin warmth
• Branham sign = reflex bradycardia after compression
√ large tortuous serpentine feeding vessels
√ fast blood flow + dense staining
√ early draining veins

D. VENOUS HEMANGIOMA
= thick-walled vessels containing muscle
Site: deep soft tissues of retroperitoneum, mesentery, muscles of lower extremities
Age: adulthood
√ ± phleboliths
√ serpentine vessels with slow blood flow
√ vessels oriented along long axis of extremity (in 78%) + neurovascular bundle (in 64%)
√ multifocal involvement (in 37%)
√ muscle atrophy with increased subcutaneous fat
√ may be normal on arterial angiography

Osseous Hemangioma

Incidence: 10%
Histo: mostly cavernous; capillary type is rare
Age: 4th–5th decade; M:F = 2:1
• usually asymptomatic
@ Vertebra (28% of all skeletal hemangiomas)
Incidence: in 5–11% of all autopsies; multiple in 1/3
Histo: capillary hemangioma interspersed in fatty matrix
◊ The larger the degree of fat overgrowth, the less likely the lesion will be symptomatic!
Age: >40 years; female
Location: in lower thoracic / upper lumbar spine
√ "accordion" / "corduroy" / "honeycomb" vertebra = coarse vertical trabeculae with osseous reinforcement adjacent to bone resorption caused by vascular channels (also in multiple myeloma, lymphoma, metastasis)
√ bulge of posterior cortex
√ extraosseous extension beyond bony lesion into spinal canal (with cord compression) / neural foramina
√ paravertebral soft-tissue extension
√ lesion enhancement (due to hypervascularity)
CT:
√ polka-dot appearance = small punctate areas of sclerosis (= thickened vertical trabeculae)
MR:
√ mottled pattern of low-to-high intensity on T1WI + very-high intensity on T2WI depending on degree of adipose tissue (CHARACTERISTIC)
Cx: vertebral collapse (unusual), spinal cord compression
@ Calvarium (20% of all hemangiomas)
Location: frontal / parietal region
Site: diploe
√ <4 cm round osteolytic lesion with sunburst / weblike / spoke-wheel appearance of trabecular thickening
√ expansion of outer table to a greater extent than inner table producing palpable lump
@ Flat bones & long bones (rare)
– ribs, clavicle, mandible, zygoma, nasal bones, metaphyseal ends of long bones (tibia, femur, humerus)
√ radiating trabecular thickening
√ bubbly bone lysis creating honeycomb / latticelike / "hole-within-hole" appearance
MR:
√ serpentine vascular channels with low signal intensity on T1WI + high signal intensity on T2WI (= slow blood flow) / low signal intensity on all sequences (= high blood flow)
NUC (bone / RBC-labeled scintigraphy):
√ photopenia / moderate increased activity

Soft-tissue Hemangioma

Incidence: 7% of all benign tumors; most frequent tumor of infancy + childhood
Age: primarily in children; M < F
May be associated with:
Maffuci syndrome (= multiple cavernous hemangiomas + enchondromas)
• intermittent change in size
• painful
• bluish discoloration of overlying skin (rare)
• may dramatically increase in size during pregnancy
Location: usually intramuscular; synovia (<1% of all hemangiomas); common in head and neck
√ nonspecific soft-tissue mass
√ may extend into bone creating subtle rounded / linear areas of hyperlucency (rare)
√ ± longitudinal / axial bone overgrowth (secondary to chronic hyperemia)
√ may contain phleboliths (30% of lesions, SPECIFIC)
√ nonspecific curvilinear / amorphous calcifications
√ may contain such large amounts of fat as to be indistinguishable from lipoma
CT:
√ poorly defined mass with attenuation similar to muscle
√ areas of decreased attenuation approximating subcutaneous fat (= fat overgrowth) most prominent in periphery of lesion
MR:
√ poorly marginated mass hypo- / isointense to muscle on T1WI
√ areas with increased signal intensity on T1WI in periphery of lesion extending into septations (= fat)
√ well-marginated markedly hyperintense mass on T2WI (increased free water content in stagnant blood) with striated / septated configuration
√ tubular structures with blood flow characteristics (flow void / inflow enhancement; marked contrast enhancement)
√ phleboliths as low-intensity areas inside lesion
√ high-signal-intensity areas on T1WI + T2WI (= hemorrhage)
US:
√ complex mass
√ low-resistance arterial signal (occasionally)

Synovial Hemangioma

• repetitive bleeding into joint
Location: knee (60%), elbow (30%)
DDx: hemophilic arthropathy (polyarticular)

HEMANGIOPERICYTOMA

= borderline tumor with benign / locally aggressive / malignant behavior (counterpart of glomus tumor)
Age: 4th–5th decade; M:F = 1:1
Path: large vessels predominantly in tumor periphery
Histo: cells packed around vascular channels containing cystic + necrotic areas; arising from cells of Zimmerman that are located around vessels
@ Soft tissue
= deep-seated well-circumscribed lesion arising in muscle
Location: lower extremity in 35% (thigh), pelvic cavity, retroperitoneum

- painless slowly growing mass up to 20 cm

@ Bone (rare)
Location: lower extremity, vertebrae, pelvis, skull (dura similar to meningioma)
√ osteolytic lesions in metaphysis of long / flat bone
√ subperiosteal large blowout lesion (similar to aneurysmal bone cyst)

Angio:
√ displacement of main artery
√ pedicle of tumor feeder arteries
√ spider-shaped arrangement of vessels encircling tumor
√ small corkscrew arteries
√ dense tumor stain

DDx: hemangioendothelioma, angiosarcoma

HEMOCHROMATOSIS

1. PRIMARY HEMOCHROMATOSIS
   = autosomal recessive / indeterminate inheritance (abnormal iron-loading gene) in thalassemia, sideroblastic anemia
2. SECONDARY HEMOCHROMATOSIS
   = excessive iron absorption in anemias, myelofibrosis, portacaval shunt, exogenous administration of iron, porphyria cutanea tarda, beer brewed in iron vessels + deposition of excessive iron in liver, pancreas, spleen, GI tract, kidney, gonads, heart, endocrine glands (pituitary, hypothalamus)

Age: >40 years; M:F = 10:1 (females protected by menstruation)

- cirrhosis
- "bronzed diabetes"
- congestive heart failure
- skin pigmentation
- hypogonadism
- arthritic symptoms (30%)
- increase in serum iron

@ Skeleton
Site: most commonly in hands (metacarpal heads, particularly 2nd + 3rd MCP joints), carpal + proximal interphalangeal joints, knees, hips
√ generalized osteoporosis
√ small subchondral cystlike rarefactions with fine rim of sclerosis (metacarpal heads)
√ arthropathy in 50% with iron deposition in synovium
√ uniform joint space narrowing
√ enlargement of metacarpal heads
√ eventually osteophyte formation
√ chondrocalcinosis in >60%, knees most commonly affected
(a) calcium pyrophosphate deposition (inhibition of pyrophosphatase enzyme within cartilage which hydrolyzes pyrophosphate to soluble orthophosphate)
(b) calcification of triangular cartilage of wrist, menisci, annulus fibrosus, ligamentum flavum, symphysis pubis, Achilles tendon, plantar fascia

@ Brain MRI:
√ marked loss in signal intensity of anterior lobe of pituitary gland (iron deposition)

Cx: hepatoma (in 30%)

Prognosis: death from CHF (30%), death from hepatic failure (25%)

DDx:
(1) Pseudogout (no arthropathy)
(2) Psoriatic arthritis (skin + nail changes)
(3) Osteoarthritis (predominantly distal joints in hands)
(4) Rheumatoid arthritis
(5) Gout (may also have chondrocalcinosis)

HEMOPHILIA

= X-linked deficiency / functional abnormality of coagulation factor VIII (= hemophilia A) in >80% / factor IX (= hemophilia B = Christmas disease)

Incidence: 1:10,000 males

Hemophilic Arthropathy (most common)

Cause: repeated bleeding into synovial joint

Path: pannus formation erodes cartilage with loss of subchondral bone plate and formation of subarticular cysts

Histo: synovial hyperplasia, chronic inflammatory changes, fibrosis, siderosis of synovial membrane

Age: 1st and 2nd decade

- tense red warm joint with decreased range of motion (muscle spasm)
- fever, elevated WBC (DDx: septic arthritis)

Location: knee > ankle > elbow > shoulder; commonly bilateral although bleeding episodes tend to recur within same joint
√ joint effusion (= hemarthrosis)
√ enlargement of epiphysis (secondary to synovial inflammation + hyperemia)
√ juxtaarticular osteoporosis (secondary to synovial inflammation + hyperemia)
√ joint space narrowing (particularly patella) secondary to cartilaginous denudation
√ erosion of articular surface with multiple subchondral cysts

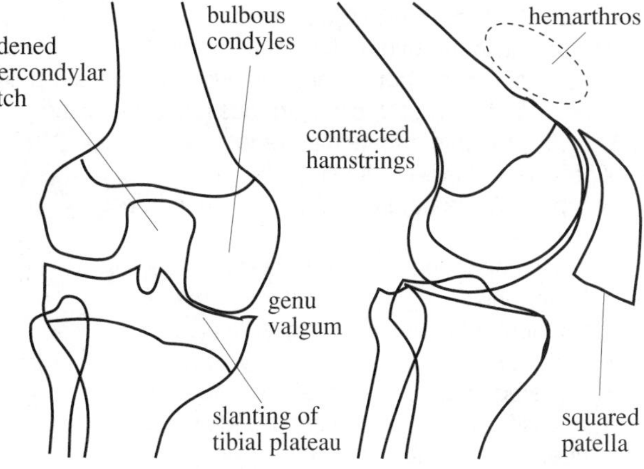

Hemophiliac Arthritis

√ sclerosis + osteophytosis (secondary to superimposed degenerative joint disease)

@ Knee

√ "squared" patella
√ widening of intercondylar notch
√ flattening of condylar surface
√ medial "slanting" of tibiotalar joint

MR:

√ low signal intensity of hypertrophied synovial membrane on all pulse sequences (due to magnetic susceptibility effect of hemosiderin)
√ varying intensity of subarticular defects (depending on substrate: fluid / soft tissue / hemosiderin)

Hemophilic Pseudotumor (1–2%)

= posthemorrhagic cystic swelling within muscle + bone characterized by pressure necrosis + destruction

(a) juvenile form = usually multiple intramedullary expansile lesions without soft-tissue mass in small bones of hand / feet (before epiphyseal closure)
(b) adult form = usually single intramedullary expansile lesion with large soft-tissue mass in ilium / femur
(c) soft-tissue involvement of retroperitoneum (psoas muscle), bowel wall, renal collecting system

√ mixed cystic expansile lesion
√ bone erosion + pathologic fracture

CT:

√ sometimes encapsulated mass containing areas of low attenuation + calcifications

MR:

√ hemorrhage of varying age

Cx: joint contracture (after repeated bleeding into muscle)

N.B.: Needle aspiration / biopsy / excision may cause fistulae / infection / uncontrolled bleeding!

Rx: palliative radiation therapy (destroys vessels prone to bleed) + transfusion of procoagulation factor concentrate

HEREDITARY HYPERPHOSPHATASIA

= "JUVENILE PAGET DISEASE"

= rare autosomal recessive disease with sustained elevation of serum alkaline phosphatase, especially in individuals of Puerto Rican descent

Histo: rapid turnover of lamellar bone without formation of cortical bone; immature woven bone is rapidly laid down, but simultaneous rapid destruction prevents normal maturation

Age: 1st–3rd year; usually stillborn

- rapid enlargement of calvarium + long bones
- dwarfism
- cranial nerve deficit (blind, deaf)
- hypertension
- frequent respiratory infections
- pseudoxanthoma elasticum
- elevated alkaline phosphatase

√ deossification = decreased density of long bones with coarse trabecular pattern
√ metaphyseal growth deficiency
√ wide irregular epiphyseal lines (resembling rickets in childhood), persistent metaphyseal defects (40% of adults)
√ bowing of long bones + fractures with irregular callus
√ widened medullary canal with cortical thinning (cortex modeled from trabecular bone)
√ skull greatly thickened with wide tables, cotton wool appearance
√ vertebra plana

OB-US:

√ diagnosis suspected in utero in 20%

Cx: pathologic fractures; vertebra plana universalis

DDx:
(1) Osteogenesis imperfecta
(2) Polyostotic fibrous dysplasia
(3) Paget disease (> age 20, not generalized)
(4) Pyle disease (spares midshaft)
(5) van Buchem syndrome (only diaphyses > age 20, no long-bone bowing)
(6) Engelmann syndrome (lower limbs)

HEREDITARY MULTIPLE DIAPHYSEAL SCLEROSIS

= RIBBING DISEASE

= autosomal recessive disorder similar to Engelmann-Camurati disease

Age: after puberty

- mild neuromuscular symptoms

Location: long bones only

√ unilateral asymmetric / asynchronous bilateral sclerosis

DDx: Engelmann-Camurati disease (begins in childhood, severe neuromuscular symptoms, symmetric bilateral sclerosis of long bones, skull involved)

HEREDITARY SPHEROCYTOSIS

= autosomal dominant congenital hemolytic anemia

Age: anemia begins in early infancy to late adulthood

- rarely severe anemia
- jaundice
- spherocytes in peripheral smear

√ bone changes rare (due to mild anemia); long bones rarely affected
√ widening of diploe with displacement + thinning of outer table
√ hair-on-end appearance

Rx: splenectomy corrects anemia even though spherocytemia persists

√ improvement in skeletal alterations following splenectomy

HERNIATION PIT

= SYNOVIAL HERNIATION PIT = CONVERSION DEFECT

= ingrowth of fibrous + cartilaginous elements from adjacent joint through perforation in cortex

Histo: fibroalveolar tissue

Age: usually in older individuals

- may be symptomatic
- no clinical significance

Location: anterior superolateral aspect of proximal femoral neck; uni- or bilateral

Site: subcortical

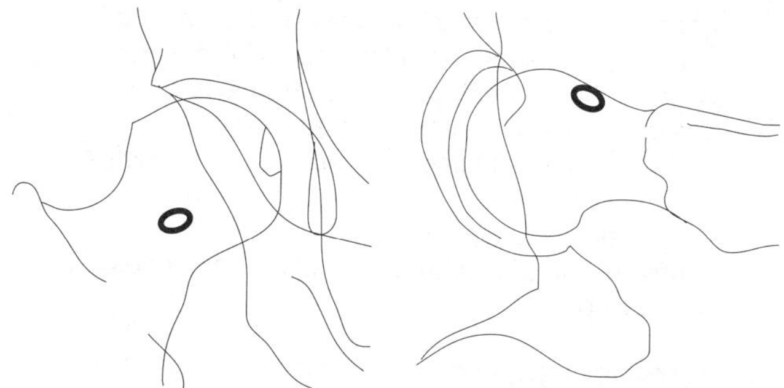

Herniation Pit on AP and LAT radiographs

- √ well-circumscribed round lucency
- √ usually <1 cm in diameter; may enlarge over time
- √ reactive thin sclerotic border
- √ hyperintense area on T2WI (= fluid signal intensity)
- √ bone scan may be positive

HOLT-ORAM SYNDROME

Autosomal dominant; M < F

Associated with CHD: secundum type ASD (most common), VSD, persistent left SVC, tetralogy, coarctation

- • intermittent cardiac arrhythmia
- • bradycardia (50–60/min)

Location: upper extremity only involved; symmetry of lesions is the rule; left side may be more severely affected

- √ aplasia / hypoplasia of radial structures: thumb, 1st metacarpal, carpal bones, radius
- √ "fingerized" hypoplastic thumb / triphalangeal thumb
- √ slender elongated hypoplastic carpals + metacarpals
- √ hypoplastic radius; absent radial styloid
- √ shallow glenoid fossa (voluntary dislocation of shoulder common)
- √ hypoplastic clavicula
- √ high arched palate
- √ cervical scoliosis
- √ pectus excavatum

HOMOCYSTINURIA

Autosomal recessive disorder

Etiology: cystathionine B synthetase deficiency results in defective methionine metabolism with accumulation of homocystine + homocysteine in blood and urine; causes defect in collagen / elastin structure

- • thromboembolic phenomena due to stickiness of platelets
- • ligamentous laxity
- • downward + inward dislocation of lens (DDx: upward + outward dislocation in Marfan syndrome)
- • mild / moderate mental retardation
- • crowding of maxillary teeth and protrusion of incisors
- • malar flush
- √ arachnodactyly in 1/3 (DDx: Marfan syndrome)
- √ microcephaly

	Marfan Syndrome	*Homocystinuria*
Inheritance	autosomal dominant	autosomal recessive
Biochemical defect	not known	cystathionine synthetase
Osteoporosis	no	yes
Spine	scoliosis	biconcave vertebrae
Lens dislocation	upward	downward
Arachnodactyly	100%	33%

- √ enlarged paranasal sinuses
- √ osteoporosis of vertebrae (biconcave / flattened / widened vertebrae)
- √ scoliosis
- √ pectus excavatum / carinatum (75%)
- √ osteoporosis of long bones (75%) with bowing + fracture
- √ children: metaphyseal cupping (50%); enlargement of ossification centers in 50% (knee, carpal bones); epiphyseal calcifications (esp. in wrist, resembling phenylketonuria); delayed ossification
- √ Harris lines = multiple growth lines
- √ genu valgum, coxa valga, coxa magna, pes cavus
- √ premature vascular calcifications

Prognosis: death from occlusive vascular disease / minor vascular trauma

HYPERPARATHYROIDISM

= uncontrolled production of parathyroid hormone

Age: 3rd–5th decade; M:F = 1:3

Histo: decreased bone mass secondary to increased number of osteoclasts, increased osteoid volume (defect in mineralization), slightly increased number of osteoblasts

- • increase in parathyroid hormone (100%)
- • increase in serum alkaline phosphatase (50%)
- • elevation of serum calcium (due to accelerated bone turnover and increased calcium absorption) + decrease in serum phosphate (30%)
- • hypotonicity of muscles, weakness, constipation, difficulty in swallowing, duodenal / gastric peptic ulcer disease (secondary to hypercalcemia)
- • polyuria, polydipsia (hypercalciuria + hyperphosphaturia)
- • renal colic + renal insufficiency (nephrocalculosis + nephrocalcinosis)
- • rheumatic bone pain + tenderness (particularly at site of brown tumor), pathologic fracture secondary to brown tumor

A. BONE RESORPTION

(a) subperiosteal (most constant + specific finding; virtually PATHOGNOMONIC of hyperparathyroidism):

- √ lacelike irregularity of cortical margin; may progress to scalloping / spiculation (pseudoperiostitis)

Site: phalangeal tufts (earliest involvement), radial aspect of middle phalanx of 2nd + 3rd finger beginning in proximal metaphyseal region (early involvement), bandlike zone of resorption in middle / base of terminal tuft, distal end of clavicles, medial tibia plateau, medial humerus neck, medial femoral neck, distal ulna, superior + inferior margins of ribs in midclavicular line, lamina dura of skull and teeth

(b) subchondral:
- √ pseudowidening of joint space
- √ collapse of cortical bone + overlying cartilage with development of erosion, cyst, joint narrowing (similar to rheumatoid arthritis)

Site: DIP joint (most commonly 4th + 5th digit), MCP joint, PIP joint, distal clavicle, acromioclavicular joint (clavicular side), "pseudowidening" of sacroiliac joint (iliac side), sternoclavicular joint, symphysis pubis, "scalloping" of posterior surface of patella, Schmorl nodes; typically polyarticular

(c) cortical (due to osteoclastic activity within haversian canal):
- √ intracortical tunneling
- √ scalloping along inner cortical surface (endosteal resorption)

(d) trabecular:
- √ spotty deossification with indistinct + coarse trabecular pattern
- √ granular salt and pepper skull
- √ loss of distinction between inner and outer table
- √ ground-glass appearance

(e) subligamentous:
- √ bone resorption with smooth scalloped / irregular ill-defined margins

Site: inferior surface of calcaneus (long plantar tendons + aponeurosis), inferior aspect of distal clavicle (coracoclavicular ligament), greater trochanter (hip abductors), lesser trochanter (iliopsoas), anterior inferior iliac spine (rectus femoris), humeral tuberosity (rotator cuff), ischial tuberosity (hamstrings), proximal extensor surface of ulna (anconeus), posterior olecranon (triceps)

B. BONE SOFTENING
- √ basilar impression of skull
- √ wedged vertebrae, kyphoscoliosis, biconcave vertebral deformities
- √ bowing of long bones
- √ slipped capital femoral epiphysis

C. BROWN TUMOR
= OSTEOCLASTOMA

Cause: PTH-stimulated osteoclastic activity (more frequent in 1° HPT; in 1.5% of 2° HPT)

Path: localized replacement of bone by vascularized fibrous tissue (osteitis fibrosa cystica) containing giant cells; lesions may become cystic following necrosis + liquefaction

Location: jaw, pelvis, rib, metaphyses of long bones (femur), facial bones, axial skeleton

Site: often eccentric / cortical; frequently solitary
- √ expansile lytic well-marginated cystlike lesion (DDx: giant cell tumor) without adjacent reactive bone formation
- √ endosteal scalloping
- √ destruction of midportions of distal phalanges with telescoping

D. OSTEOSCLEROSIS
More frequent in 2° HPT

Cause: ? PTH-stimulated osteoblastic activity, ? role of calcitonin (poorly understood)

Site: strong predilection for axial skeleton, pelvis, ribs, clavicles, metaphysis + epiphysis of appendicular skeleton
- √ "rugger jersey spine"

E. SOFT-TISSUE CALCIFICATION
More frequent in 2° HPT; metastatic calcification when Ca x P product >70 mg/dL

(a) cornea, viscera (lung, stomach, kidney)
(b) periarticular in hip, knee, shoulder, wrist
(c) arterial tunica media (resembling diabetes mellitus)
(d) chondrocalcinosis (15–18%) = calcification of hyaline / fibrous cartilage in menisci, wrist, shoulder, hip, elbow

F. EROSIVE ARTHROPATHY
- • asymptomatic
- √ simulates rheumatoid arthritis with preserved joint spaces

G. PERIOSTEAL NEW-BONE FORMATION

Cause: PTH-stimulation of osteoblasts

Site: pubic ramus along iliopectineal line (most frequent), humerus, femur, tibia, radius, ulna, metacarpals, metatarsals, phalanges
- √ linear new bone paralleling cortical surface; may be laminated; often separated from cortex by radiolucent zone
- √ increase in cortical thickness (if periosteal reaction becomes incorporated into adjacent bone)

Sequelae:
1. Renal stones / nephrocalcinosis (70%)
2. Increased osteoblastic activity (25%)
   - • increased alkaline phosphatase
   - (a) osteitis fibrosa cystica
     - √ subperiosteal bone resorption + cortical tunneling
     - √ brown tumors (primary HPT)
   - (b) bone softening
     - √ fractures
3. Peptic ulcer disease (increased gastric secretion from gastrinoma)
4. Calcific pancreatitis
5. Soft-tissue calcifications (2° HPT)
6. Marginal joint erosions + subarticular collapse (DIP, PIP, MCP)

Primary Hyperparathyroidism

= pHPT = 1° HPT = hypercalcemia due to uncontrolled secretion of parathormone by one / more hyperfunctioning parathyroid glands featuring
(1) brown tumor
(2) chondrocalcinosis (20–30%)

◊ requires surgical Rx

Incidence: 25:100,000 per year; incidence of bone lesions in HPT is 25–40%

Etiology:
(1) Parathyroid adenoma (87%): single (80%); multiple (7%)
(2) Parathyroid hyperplasia (10%): chief cell (5%); clear cell (5%)
(3) Parathyroid carcinoma (3%)

Histo: increased number of osteoclasts, increased osteoid volume (defect in mineralization), slightly increased osteoblasts = decreased bone mass

Age: 3rd–5th decade; M:F = 1:3

Associated with:
(a) Wermer syndrome = MEA I (+ pituitary adenoma + pancreatic islet cell tumor)
(b) Sipple syndrome = MEA II (+ medullary thyroid carcinoma + pheochromocytoma)

X-RAY (skeletal involvement in 10–20%):
√ thin cortices with lacy cortical pattern (subperiosteal bone resorption)
√ brown tumor (particularly in jaw + long bones)
√ osteitis cystica fibrosa (= intertrabecular fibrous connective tissue)

NUC:
√ normal bone scan in 80%
√ foci of abnormal uptake: calvarium (especially periphery), mandible, sternum, acromioclavicular joint, lateral humeral epicondyles, hands
√ increased uptake in brown tumors
√ extraskeletal uptake: cornea, cartilage, joint capsules, tendons, periarticular areas, lungs, stomach
√ normal renal excretion [except in stone disease / calcium nephropathy (10%)]

Rx: pathologic glands identified by experienced surgeons in 90–95% on initial neck exploration (ectopic + supernumerary glands often overlooked at operation; recurrent hypercalcemia in 3–10%)

<u>Surgical risk for repeat surgery</u>

6.6%	recurrent laryngeal nerve injury
20.0%	permanent hypoparathyroidism
<1.0%	perioperative mortality

Secondary Hyperparathyroidism

= sHPT = 2° HPT = diffuse / adenomatous hyperplasia of all four parathyroid glands as a compensatory mechanism in any state of hypocalcemia featuring (1) soft-tissue calcifications (2) osteosclerosis

◊ requires medical Rx

Etiology:
(a) renal osteodystrophy (renal insufficiency + osteomalacia / rickets)

Skeletal Findings	*1° HPT*	*2° HPT*
Osteopenia, diffuse	present	present
Osteosclerosis, regional / diffuse	rare	common
Bone resorption	common	common
Brown tumor	common	less common
Soft-tissue calcification	not infrequent	common
Chondrocalcinosis	not infrequent	rare

(b) calcium deprivation, maternal hypoparathyroidism, pregnancy, hypovitaminosis D
(c) rise in serum phosphate leading to decrease in calcium by feedback mechanism

• low to normal calcium levels
• Ca^{2+} PO_4^{2-} solubility product often exceeded

NUC:
√ "superscan" in 2° HPT:
  √ absent kidney sign
  √ increased bone-to-soft tissue uptake ratio
  √ increased uptake in calvarium, mandible, acromioclavicular region, sternum, vertebrae, distal third of long bones, ribs
√ diffuse Tc-99m MDP uptake in lungs (60%)

Tertiary Hyperparathyroidism

= tHPT = 3° HPT = development of autonomous PTH adenoma in patients with chronically overstimulated hyperplastic parathyroid glands (renal insufficiency + prolonged renal dialysis)

◊ requires surgical Rx

Clue: (a) intractable hypercalcemia
(b) inability to control osteomalacia by vitamin D administration

Ectopic Parathormone Production

= pseudohyperparathyroidism as paraneoplastic syndrome in bronchogenic carcinoma + renal cell carcinoma

HYPERTROPHIC OSTEOARTHROPATHY

= HYPERTROPHIC PULMONARY OSTEOARTHROPATHY

Etiology:
(1) Release of vasodilators which are not metabolized by lung
(2) Increased flow through AV shunts
(3) Reflex peripheral vasodilation (vagal impulses)
(4) Hormones: estrogen, growth hormone, prostaglandin

A. THORACIC CAUSES
(a) malignant tumor (0.7–12%): bronchogenic carcinoma (88%), mesothelioma, lymphoma, pulmonary metastasis from osteogenic sarcoma, melanoma, renal cell carcinoma, breast cancer
(b) benign tumor: benign pleural fibroma, tumor of ribs, thymoma, esophageal leiomyoma, pulmonary hemangioma, pulmonary congenital cyst

(c) chronic infection / inflammation: pulmonary abscess, bronchiectasis, blastomycosis, TB (very rare); cystic fibrosis, interstitial fibrosis
(d) congenital heart disease with R-to-L shunt

B. EXTRATHORACIC CAUSES
(a) GI tract: ulcerative colitis, amebic + bacillary dysentery, intestinal TB, Whipple disease, Crohn disease, gastric ulcer, bowel lymphoma, gastric carcinoma
(b) liver disease: biliary + alcoholic cirrhosis, posthepatic cirrhosis, chronic active hepatitis, bile duct carcinoma, benign bile duct stricture, amyloidosis, liver abscess
(c) undifferentiated nasopharyngeal carcinoma, pancreatic carcinoma, chronic myelogenous leukemia

- burning pain, painful swelling of limbs, and stiffness of joints: ankles (88%), wrists (83%), knees (75%), elbows (17%), shoulders (10%), fingers (7%)
- peripheral neurovascular disorders: local cyanosis, areas of increased sweating, paresthesia, chronic erythema, flushing + blanching of skin
- hippocratic fingers + toes (clubbing)
- hypertrophy of extremities (soft-tissue swelling)

Location: tibia + fibula (75%), radius + ulna (80%), proximal phalanges (60%), femur (50%), metacarpus + metatarsus (40%), humerus + distal phalanges (25%), pelvis (5%); unilateral (rare)
Site: in diametaphyseal regions
√ cortical thickening
√ lamellar periosteal proliferation of new bone, at first smooth then undulating + rough
  Site: most conspicuous on concavity of long bones (dorsal + medial aspects)
√ soft-tissue swelling ("clubbing") of distal phalanges
√ regression of periosteal reaction after thoracotomy

Bone scan (reveals changes early with greater sensitivity + clarity):
  √ symmetric diffusely increased uptake along cortical margins of diaphysis + metaphysis of tubular bones of the extremities with irregularities
  √ increased periarticular uptake (= synovitis)
  √ scapular involvement in 2/3
  √ mandible ± maxilla abnormal in 40%

HYPERVITAMINOSIS A

Age: usually infants + children
Cause: overdosing vitamin A, 13-cis-retinoic acid (treatment for neuroblastoma)
- anorexia, irritability
- loss of hair, dry skin, pruritus, fissures of lips
- jaundice, enlargement of liver

√ separation of cranial sutures secondary to hydrocephalus (coronal > lambdoid) in children <10 years of age, may appear within a few days
√ symmetrical solid periosteal new-bone formation along shafts of long + short bones (ulna, clavicle)
√ premature epiphyseal closure + thinning of epiphyseal plates
√ accelerated growth
√ tendinous, ligamentous, pericapsular calcifications
√ changes usually disappear after cessation of vitamin A ingestion
DDx: infantile cortical hyperostosis (mandible involved)

HYPERVITAMINOSIS D

= excessive ingestion of vitamin D (large doses act like parathormone)
- loss of appetite, diarrhea, drowsiness, headaches
- polyuria, polydipsia, renal damage
- convulsions
- excessive phosphaturia (parathormone decreases tubular absorption)
- hypercalcemia + hypercalciuria; anemia

√ deossification
√ widening of provisional zone of calcification
√ cortical + trabecular thickening
√ alternating bands of increased + decreased density near / in epiphysis (zone of provisional calcification)
√ vertebra outlined by dense band of bone + adjacent radiolucent line within
√ dense calvarium
√ metastatic calcinosis in
  (a) arterial walls (between age 20 and 30)
  (b) kidneys = nephrocalcinosis
  (c) periarticular tissue (puttylike)
  (d) premature calcification of falx cerebri (most consistent sign!)

HYPOPARATHYROIDISM

- tetany = hypocalcemic neuromuscular excitability (numbness, cramps, carpopedal spasm, laryngeal stridor, generalized convulsions)
- hypocalcemia + hyperphosphatemia
- normal / low serum alkaline phosphatase

√ premature closure of epiphyses
√ hypoplasia of tooth enamel + dentine; blunting of roots
√ generalized increase in bone density in 9%:
  √ localized thickening of skull

	HypoPT	*Pseudo HypoPT*	*Pseudopseudo HypoPT*
Serum Ca	↓	↓	↔
Serum P	↑	↑	↔
AlkaPhos	↓ or ↔	↓ or ↔	↔

Response to PTH-Injection	*Norm / HypoPT*	*PseudoHypoPT*
Urine AMP	↑	↔
Urine P	↑	↔
Plasma AMP	↑	↔

√ sacroiliac sclerosis
√ bandlike density in metaphysis of long bones (25%), iliac crest, vertebral bodies
√ thickened lamina dura (inner table) + widened diploe
√ deformed hips with thickening + sclerosis of femoral head + acetabulum

@ Soft tissue
√ intracranial calcifications in basal ganglia, choroid plexus, occasionally in cerebellum
√ calcification of spinal and other ligaments
√ subcutaneous calcifications
√ ossification of muscle insertions
√ ectopic bone formation

Idiopathic Hypoparathyroidism

= rare condition of unknown cause
• round face, short dwarflike, obese
• mental retardation
• cataracts
• dry scaly skin, atrophy of nails
• dental hypoplasia (delayed tooth eruption, impaction of teeth, supernumerary teeth)

Secondary Hypoparathyroidism

= accidental removal / damage to parathyroid glands in thyroid surgery / radical neck dissection (5%); I-131 therapy (rare); external beam radiation; hemorrhage; infection; thyroid carcinoma; hemochromatosis (iron deposition)

HYPOPHOSPHATASIA

= autosomal recessive congenital disease with low activity of serum-, bone-, liver-alkaline phosphatase resulting in poor mineralization (deficient generation of bone crystals)

Incidence: 1:100,000
Histo: indistinguishable from rickets
• phosphoethanolamine in urine as precursor of alkaline phosphatase
• normal serum calcium + phosphorus

A. GROUP I = neonatal = congenital lethal form
√ marked demineralization of calvarium ("caput membranaceum" = soft skull)
√ lack of calcification of metaphyseal end of long bones
√ streaky irregular spotty margins of calcification
√ cupping of metaphysis
√ angulated shaft fractures with abundant callus formation
√ short poorly ossified ribs
√ poorly ossified vertebrae (especially neural arches)
√ small pelvic bones
OB-US:
√ high incidence of intrauterine fetal demise
√ increased echogenicity of falx (enhanced sound transmission secondary to poorly mineralized calvarium)
√ poorly mineralized short bowed tubular bones + multiple fractures
√ poorly mineralized spine
√ short poorly ossified ribs
√ polyhydramnios
Prognosis: death within 6 months

B. GROUP II = juvenile severe form
onset of symptoms within weeks to months
• moderate / severe dwarfism
• delayed weight bearing
√ resembles rickets
√ separated cranial sutures; craniostenosis in 2nd year
Prognosis: 50% mortality

C. GROUP III = adult mild form
recognized later in childhood / adolescence / adulthood
• dwarfism
√ clubfoot, genu valgum
√ demineralization of ossification centers (at birth / 3–4 months of age):
√ widened metaphyses
√ wormian bones
Prognosis: excellent; after 1 year no further progression

D. GROUP IV = latent form
heterozygous state
• normal / borderline levels of alkaline phosphatase
• patients are small for age
• disturbance of primary dentition
√ bone fragility + healed fractures
√ enlarged chondral ends of ribs
√ metaphyseal notching of long bones
√ Erlenmeyer flask deformity of femur

HYPOTHYROIDISM

A. Childhood = CRETINISM
Frequency: 1:4,000 live births have congenital hypothyroidism
Cause: sporadic hypoplasia / ectopia of thyroid
√ delayed skeletal maturation (appearance + growth of ossification centers, epiphyseal closure)
√ fragmented stippled epiphyses
√ wide sutures / fontanels with delayed closure
√ delayed dentition
√ delayed / decreased pneumatization of sinuses + mastoids
√ hypertelorism
√ dense vertebral margins
√ demineralization
√ hypoplastic phalanges of 5th finger
MR:
√ reduced myelination of brain (usually beginning during midgestation)
OB-US:
√ fetal goiter (especially in hyperthyroid mothers treated with methimazole / propylthiouracil / I-131)

B. Adulthood
√ calvarial thickening / sclerosis
√ wedging of dorsolumbar vertebral bodies
√ coxa vara with flattened femoral head
√ premature atherosclerosis
◊ No skeletal changes with adult onset!

INFANTILE CORTICAL HYPEROSTOSIS

= CAFFEY DISEASE
= uncommon self-limiting proliferative bone disease of infancy; remission + exacerbations are common

Cause: ? infectious; ? autosomal dominant with variable expression + incomplete penetrance / sporadic occurrence (rare)

Age: <6 months, reported in utero; M:F = 1:1

Histo: inflammation of periosteal membrane, proliferation of osteoblasts + connective tissue cells, deposition of immature bony trabeculae

• sudden, hard, extremely tender soft-tissue swellings over bone
• irritability, fever
• ± elevated ESR, increased alkaline phosphatase
• leukocytosis, anemia

Location: mandible (80%) > clavicle > ulna + others (except phalanges + vertebrae + round bones of wrists and ankles)

Site: hyperostosis affects diaphysis of tubular bones asymmetrically, epiphyses spared

√ massive periosteal new-bone formation + perifocal soft-tissue swelling
√ "double-exposed" ribs
√ narrowing of medullary space (= proliferation of endosteum)
√ bone expansion with remodeling of old cortex

Prognosis: usually complete recovery by 30 months

Rx: mild analgesics, steroids

Chronic Infantile Hyperostosis

• disease may persist or recur intermittently for years
• delayed muscular development, crippling deformities
√ bowing deformities, osseous bridging, diaphyseal expansion

DDx: (1) Hypervitaminosis A (rarely <1 year of age)
(2) Periostitis of prematurity
(3) Healing rickets
(4) Scurvy (uncommon <4 months of age)
(5) Syphilis (focal destruction)
(6) Child abuse
(7) Prostaglandin administration (usually following 4–6 weeks of therapy)
(8) Osteomyelitis
(9) Leukemia
(10) Neuroblastoma
(11) Kinky hair syndrome
(12) Hereditary hyperphosphatasia

IRON DEFICIENCY ANEMIA

Age: infants affected

Cause:
(1) inadequate iron stores at birth
(2) deficient iron in diet
(3) impaired gastrointestinal absorption of iron
(4) excessive iron demands from blood loss
(5) polycythemia vera (6) cyanotic CHD

√ widening of diploe + thinning of tables with sparing of occiput (no red marrow)
√ hair-on-end appearance of skull
√ osteoporosis in long bones (most prominent in hands)
√ absence of facial bone involvement

JACCOUD ARTHROPATHY

After subsidence of frequent severe attacks of rheumatic fever

Path: periarticular fascial + tendon fibrosis without synovitis

• rheumatic valve disease

Location: primarily involvement of hands; occasionally in great toe

√ muscular atrophy
√ periarticular swelling of small joints of hands + feet
√ ulnar deviation + flexion of MCP joints most marked in 4th + 5th finger
√ NO joint narrowing / erosion

KLINEFELTER SYNDROME

47,XXY (rarely XXYY) chromosomal abnormality

Incidence: 1:750 live births (probably commonest chromosomal aberration)

• testicular atrophy (hyalinization of seminiferous tubules) = small / absent testes, sterility (azoospermia)
• eunuchoid constitution: gynecomastia; paucity of hair on face + chest; female pubic escutcheon
• mild mental retardation
• high level of urinary gonadotropins + low level of 17-ketosteroids after puberty

◊ NO distinctive radiological findings!

√ may have delayed bone maturation
√ failure of frontal sinus to develop
√ small bridged sella turcica
√ ± scoliosis, kyphosis
√ ± coxa valga
√ ± metacarpal sign (short 4th metacarpal)
√ accessory epiphyses of 2nd metacarpal bilaterally

47,XXX = Superfemale Syndrome

• usually over 6 feet tall; subnormal intelligence; frequently antisocial behavior

KLIPPEL-TRENAUNAY SYNDROME

= sporadic (nonhereditary) rare mesodermal abnormality that usually affects a single lower limb characterized by a triad of:
(1) port-wine nevus = unilateral large flat infiltrative cutaneous capillary hemangioma often in dermatomal distribution on affected limb; may fade in 2nd–3rd decade
(2) gigantism = overgrowth of distal digits / entire extremity (especially during adolescent growth spurt) involving soft-tissue + bone
(3) varicose veins on lateral aspect of affected limb; usually ipsilateral to hemangioma

Pathogenesis:
superficial lateral venous channel of large caliber thought to represent the fetal lateral limb bud vein that has failed to regress; tissue overgrowth is secondary to impaired venous return

Age: usually in children; M:F = 1:1
Associated with:
— polydactyly, syndactyly, clinodactyly, oligodactyly, ectrodactyly, congenital dislocation of hip
— hemangiomas of colon / bladder (3–10%)
— spinal hemangiomas + AVMs
— hemangiomas in liver / spleen
— lymphangiomas of limb

Location: lower extremity (10–15 x more common than upper extremity); bilateral in <5%; extension into trunk may occur
• extremity pain
• spontaneous cutaneous hemorrhage
• chronic venous insufficiency
• cutaneous lymphatic vesicles, lymphorrhea

√ elongation of bones:
 √ leg length discrepancy
 √ increased metatarsal / metacarpal + phalangeal size
√ cortical thickening
√ soft-tissue hypertrophy (at birth / later in life)
√ punctate calcifications (phleboliths) in pelvis (bowel wall, urinary bladder)
√ pulmonary vein varicosities
√ cystic lung lesions
Venogram:
 √ extensive dilation of superficial veins
 √ enlarged perforating veins
 √ aplasia / hypoplasia of lower extremity veins (18–40%): ? selective flow of contrast material up the lateral venous channel may fail to opacify the deep venous system
 √ incompetent valveless collateral venous channels (? persistent lateral limb bud vein = Klippel-Trenaunay vein) arises near the ankle + extends a variable distance up the extremity + drains into deep femoral vein / iliac veins (in >66%)
Color Doppler US:
 √ normal deep veins
Lymphangiography:
 √ hypoplasia of lymphatic system
Cx: thrombophlebitis, deep venous thrombosis, pulmonary embolism, lymphangitis
Rx: (1) conservative: application of graded compressive stockings, pneumatic compression devices, percutaneous sclerosis of localized venous malformations / superficial varicosities
 (2) surgical: epiphysiodesis, excision of soft-tissue hypertrophy, vein stripping
DDx: (1) **Parke-Weber syndrome**
 = congenital persistence of multiple microscopic AV fistulas + spectrum of Klippel-Trenaunay-Weber syndrome (pulsatility, thrill, bruit)
 (2) Neurofibromatosis (café-au-lait spots, axillary freckling, cutaneous neurofibromas, macrodactyly secondary to plexiform neurofibromas, wavy cortical reaction, early fusion of growth plate, limb hypertrophy not as extensive / bilateral)
 (3) Beckwith-Wiedemann syndrome (aniridia, macroglossia, cryptorchidism, Wilms tumor, broad metaphyses, thickened long-bone cortex, advanced bone age, periosteal new-bone formation, hemihypertrophy)
 (4) Macrodystrophia lipomatosis (hyperlucency of fat, distal phalanges most commonly affected, overgrowth ceases with puberty, usually limited to digits)
 (5) Maffuci syndrome (cavernous hemangiomas, soft tissue hypertrophy, phleboliths, multiple enchondromas)

LABRAL TEARS OF SHOULDER

Anterior Labral Tear

Location: anteroinferior labrum > entire anterior labrum > isolated tear of anterosuperior labrum
Subtypes of anteroinferior labral tears:
 (1) Bankart lesion
 (2) Anterior labroligamentous periosteal sleeve avulsion
 (3) Perthes lesion
√ absence / detachment of labrum
√ frayed labrum with irregular margin
DDx: (1) Middle + inferior glenohumeral ligaments closely apposed to anterior labrum
 (2) Recess between anterior labrum + glenoid rim
 (3) Recess between middle + inferior ligaments

SLAP Lesion

= anterior-to-posterior lesion of the superior labrum centered at biceps tendon attachment
Mechanism: sports activity with overhead arm motion, fall on an outstretched hand
• pain, clicking sensation
Type I = small tear / irregularity confined to superior labrum; common in elderly as a degenerative tear
Type II = detachment of superior labral-bicipital complex from glenoid rim
 DDx: superior sublabral recess (less distance between labrum + glenoid, no irregular appearance, no lateral extension of defect)
Type III = detachment of superior portion of labrum from glenoid + biceps tendon (similar to bucket-handle tear of knee meniscus)
Type IV = type III + tear extending into biceps tendon

LANGERHANS CELL HISTIOCYTOSIS

= LCH = HISTIOCYTOSIS X (former name)
= poorly understood group of disorders characterized by proliferation of Langerhans cells (normally responsible for first-line immunologic defense in the skin)
Cause: uncertain (? primary proliferative disorder possibly due to defect in immunoregulation; neoplasm)

Path: influx of eosinophilic leukocytes simulating inflammation; reticulum cells accumulate cholesterol + lipids (= foam cells); sheets or nodules of histiocytes may fuse to form giant cells, cytoplasm contains (? viral) Langerhans bodies

Histo: Langerhans cells are similar to mononuclear macrophages + dendritic cells as the two major types of nonlymphoid mononuclear cells involved in immune + nonimmune inflammatory response; derived from promonocytes (= bone marrow stem cell)

Age: any age, mostly presenting at 1–4 years; M:F = 1:1

Location: bone + bone marrow, lymph nodes, thymus, ear, liver and spleen, gallbladder, GI tract, endocrine system

DDx: osteomyelitis, Ewing sarcoma, leukemia, lymphoma, metastatic neuroblastoma

Clinical manifestations:

A. Localized LCH (70%)
   = eosinophilic granuloma
B. Disseminated LCH (30%)
   1. Chronic disseminated LCH (20%)
      = Hand-Schüller-Christian disease
   2. Fulminant disseminated LCH (10%)
      = Letterer-Siwe disease

Eosinophilic Granuloma (70%)

= most benign variety of LCH localized to bone

Age: 5–10 years (highest frequency); range 2–30 years; <20 years (in 75%); M:F = 3:2

Path: bone lesions arise within medullary canal (RES)

Histo: considerable number of eosinophils in addition to the dominant Langerhans cell constituent

• eosinophilia in blood + CSF

Location: bone (in children) or lung (in adults)

Sites: monostotic involvement in 50–75%;
- (a) flat bones: calvarium > mandible > ribs > pelvis > vertebrae (rarely posterior elements)
- (b) long bones: diaphyseal (58%) + metaphyseal (28%) + metadiaphyseal (12%) + epiphyseal (2%) in humerus, femur, tibia

√ bone lesions 1–15 cm in diameter:
- • often accompanied by tender soft-tissue mass
- √ geographic / permeative / moth-eaten configuration
- √ well- / poorly defined borders

  DDx: neuroblastoma metastases , leukemia, lymphoma

@ Skull (50%)

Site: diploic space of parietal bone (most commonly involved) + temporal bone (petrous ridge, mastoid)

√ round / ovoid punched-out lesion:

DDx: venous lake, arachnoid granulation, parietal foramen, epidermoid cyst, hemangioma

- √ beveled edge / "hole-within-hole" appearance (due to asymmetric destruction of inner + outer tables)
- √ sharply marginated without sclerotic rim (DDx: epidermoid with bone sclerosis)
- √ sclerotic margin during healing phase (50%)
- √ "button sequestrum" = remnants of bone as a central bone density within a lytic lesion
- √ soft-tissue mass overlying the lytic process in calvarium (often palpable)
- √ isodense homogeneously enhancing mass in hypothalamus / pituitary gland

@ Orbit
- √ benign focal mass ± infiltration of orbital bones

@ Mastoid process
- • intractable otitis media with chronically draining ear (in temporal bone involvement)
- √ destructive lesion near mastoid antrum

DDx: mastoiditis, cholesteatoma, metastasis

Cx: extension to middle ear may destroy ossicles leading to deafness

@ Jaw
- • gingival + contiguous soft-tissue swelling
- √ "floating" teeth = destruction of alveolar bone
- √ mandibular fracture

@ Axial skeleton (25%)
- √ "vertebra plana" = "coin on edge" = Calvé disease (6%) = collapse of vertebra (most commonly thoracic):
  - ◊ Most common cause of vertebra plana in children
  - √ preserved disk space
  - √ rare involvement of posterior elements
  - √ no kyphosis
- √ lytic lesion in supraacetabular region

@ Proximal long bones (15%)
- • painful bone lesion + swelling

Site: mostly diaphyseal; epiphyseal lesions are uncommon

- √ expansile lytic lesion with ill-defined / sclerotic edges
- √ endosteal scalloping, widening of medullary cavity
- √ cortical thinning, intracortical tunneling
- √ erosion of cortex + soft-tissue mass
- √ laminated periosteal reaction (frequent), may show interruptions
- √ may appear rapidly within 3 weeks
- √ lesions respect joint space + growth plate

@ Lung involvement (20%)

Incidence: 0.05–0.5:100,000 annually

Age: peak between 20 and 40 years

- ◊ Strong association between smoking + primary pulmonary Langerhans cell histiocytosis!
- √ 3–10 mm nodules
- √ reticulonodular pattern with predilection for apices
- √ may develop into honeycomb lung
- √ recurrent pneumothoraces (25%)
- √ rib lesions with fractures (common)
- √ pleural effusion, hilar adenopathy (unusual)

NUC:
- √ negative bone scans in 35% (radiographs more sensitive)
- √ bone lesions generally not Ga-67 avid
- √ Ga-67 may be helpful for detecting nonosseous lesions

Prognosis: excellent with spontaneous resolution of bone lesions in 6–18 months

Hand-Schüller-Christian Disease (20%)

= chronic disseminated form of LCH characterized by CLASSIC TRIAD (in 10–15%) of
(1) exophthalmos (mass effect on orbital bone)
(2) diabetes insipidus (basilar skull disease / direct infiltration of posterior pituitary gland)
(3) destructive bone lesions (often of calvaria)

Path: proliferation of histiocytes, may simulate Ewing sarcoma

Age at onset: <5 years (range from birth to 40 years); M:F = 1:1

- diabetes insipidus (30–50%) often with large lytic lesion in sphenoid bone / panhypopituitarism
- otitis media with mastoid + inner ear invasion
- exophthalmos (33%), sometimes with orbital wall destruction
- generalized eczematoid skin lesions (30%)
- ulcers of mucous membranes (gingiva, palate)

Sites: bone, liver, spleen, lymph nodes, skin

@ Bone
√ osteolytic skull lesions with overlying soft-tissue nodules
√ "geographic skull" = ovoid / serpiginous destruction of large area
√ "floating teeth" with mandibular involvement
√ destruction of petrous ridge + mastoids + sella turcica

@ Orbit
√ diffuse orbital disease with multiple osteolytic bone lesions

@ Liver
√ hepatosplenomegaly (rare)
√ scattered echogenic / hypoattenuating liver granuloma
√ lymphadenopathy (may be massive)
√ gallbladder wall thickening (from infiltration)

@ Lung
√ cyst + bleb formation with spontaneous pneumothorax (25%)
√ ill-defined diffuse nodular infiltration often progressing to fibrosis + honeycomb lung

@ Thymus
√ enlarged thymus + punctate calcifications

Prognosis: spontaneous remissions + exacerbations; fatal in 15%

Letterer-Siwe Disease (10%)

= acute disseminated, fulminant form of LCH characterized by wasting, pancytopenia (from bone marrow dysfunction), generalized lymphadenopathy, hepatosplenomegaly

Incidence: 1: 2,000,000

Age: several weeks after birth to 2 years

Path: generalized involvement of reticulum cells; may be confused with leukemia

- hemorrhage, purpura (secondary to coagulopathy)
- severe progressive anemia / pancytopenia
- intermittent fever
- failure to grow / malabsorption + hypoalbuminemia
- skin rash: scaly erythematous seborrhea-like brown to red papules
  Location: especially pronounced behind ears, in axillary, inguinal, and perineal areas

Sites: liver, spleen, bone marrow, lymph nodes, skin

√ hepatosplenomegaly + lymphadenopathy (most often cervical)
√ obstructive jaundice

@ Bone involvement (50%):
√ widespread multiple lytic lesions; "raindrop" pattern in calvarium

Prognosis: rapidly progressive with 70% mortality rate

LAURENCE-MOON-BIEDL SYNDROME

- retardation
- obesity
- hypogonadism

√ craniosynostosis
√ polysyndactyly

LEAD POISONING

= PLUMBISM

Path: lead concentrates in metaphyses of growing bones (distal femur > both ends of tibia > distal radius) leading to failure of removal of calcified cartilaginous trabeculae in provisional zone

- loss of appetite, vomiting, constipation, abdominal cramps
- peripheral neuritis (adults), meningoencephalitis (children)
- anemia
- lead line at gums (adults)

√ bands of increased density at metaphyses of tubular bones (only in growing bone)
√ lead lines may persist
√ clubbing if poisoning severe (anemia)
√ bone-in-bone appearance

DDx: (1) Healed rickets
(2) Normal increased density in infants <3 years of age

LEPROSY

= HANSEN DISEASE

Organism: Mycobacterium leprae

Types:
(1) lepromatous: in cutis, mucous membranes, viscera
(2) neural: enlarged indurated nodular nerve trunks; anesthesia, muscular atrophy, neurotrophic changes
(3) mixed form

@ Osseous changes (in 15–54% of patients)
√ specific signs:
Location: center of distal end of phalanges / eccentric
√ ill-defined areas of decalcification, reticulated trabecular pattern, small rounded osteolytic lesions, cortical erosions

√ joint spaces preserved
√ healing phase: complete resolution / bone defect with sclerotic rim + endosteal thickening
√ nasal spine absorption + destruction of maxilla, nasal bone, alveolar ridge
√ enlarged nutrient foramina in clawlike hand
√ erosive changes of ungual tufts
√ nonspecific signs:
√ soft-tissue swelling; calcification of nerves
√ contractures / deep ulcerations
√ neurotrophic joints (distal phalanges in hands, MTP in feet, Charcot joints in tarsus)

LEUKEMIA OF BONE

A. CHILDHOOD
most common malignancy of childhood:
1/3 of all pediatric malignancies
Histo: acute lymphocytic leukemia (in 75%)
Peak age: 4 years
- migratory paraarticular arthralgias (25–50%) due to adjacent metaphyseal lesions (may be confused with acute rheumatic fever / rheumatoid arthritis)
- low-grade fever, bruising, fatigue, bone pain
- elevated erythrocyte sedimentation rate, anemia
- hepatosplenomegaly, occasionally lymphadenopathy

◊ Peripheral blood smears may be negative in aleukemic form!
Skeletal manifestations in 50–90%:
Location: proximal + distal metaphyses of long bones, flat bones, spine
(a) Diffuse osteopenia (most common pattern)
√ diffuse demineralization of spine + long bones (= leukemic infiltration of bone marrow + catabolic protein / mineral metabolism)
√ coarse trabeculation of spongiosa (due to destruction of finer trabeculae)
√ multiple biconcave / partially collapsed vertebrae (14%)
(b) "Leukemic lines" (40–53% in acute lymphoblastic leukemia):
√ transverse radiolucent metaphyseal bands, uniform + regular across the width of metaphysis (= leukemic infiltration of bone marrow / osteoporosis at sites of rapid growth)
Location: large joints (proximal tibia, distal femur, proximal humerus, distal radius + ulna)
√ horizontal / curvilinear bands in vertebral bodies + edges of iliac crest
√ dense metaphyseal lines after treatment
(c) Focal destruction of flat / tubular bones:
√ multiple small clearly defined ovoid / spheroid osteolytic lesions (destruction of spongiosa, later cortex) in 30–60%
√ moth-eaten appearance, sutural widening, prominent convolutional markings of skull
◊ Lytic lesions distal to knee / elbow in children are suggestive of leukemia (rather than metastases)!
(d) Isolated periostitis of long bones (infrequent):
√ smooth / lamellated / sunburst pattern of periosteal reaction (cortical penetration by sheets of leukemic cells into subperiosteum) in 12–25%
(e) Metaphyseal osteosclerosis + focal osteoblastic lesion (very rare)
√ osteosclerotic lesions (late in disease due to reactive osteoblastic proliferation)
√ mixed lesions (lytic + bone-forming) in 18%
Dx: sternal marrow / peripheral blood smear
Cx: proliferation of leukemic cells in marrow leads to extraskeletal hematopoiesis
DDx: metastatic neuroblastoma, Langerhans cell histiocytosis

B. ADULTHOOD
◊ Death usually occurs before skeletal abnormalities manifest
√ osteoporosis
√ solitary radiolucent foci (vertebral collapse)
√ permeating radiolucent mottling (proximal humerus)

LIPOBLASTOMA

= postnatal proliferation of mesenchymal cells with a spectrum of differentiation ranging from prelipoblasts (spindle cells) to mature adipocytes
Path: immature adipose tissue separated by septa into multiple lobules
Histo: uni- and multivacuolated lipoblasts interspersed between spindle / stellate mesenchymal cells; suspended in myxoid stroma
Age: <3 years of age; M:F = 2:1
Location: subcutaneous tissue of extremities, neck, trunk, perineum, retroperitoneum
√ fatty tumor with enhancing soft-tissue component
DDx: liposarcoma (extremely rare in children)

LIPOMA OF BONE

= INTRAOSSEOUS LIPOMA
Incidence: <1:1,000 primary bone tumors
Age: any (4th–6th decade); M:F = 1:1
May be associated with: hyperlipoproteinemia
- asymptomatic / localized bone pain

Location: calcaneus, extremities (proximal femur > tibia, fibula, humerus), ilium, skull, mandible, maxilla, ribs, vertebrae, sacrum, coccyx, radius
Site: metaphysis
√ expansile nonaggressive radiolucent lesion
√ loculated / septated appearance (trabeculae)
√ thin well-defined sclerotic border
√ ± thinned cortex (NO cortical destruction)
√ NO periosteal reaction
√ may contain clump of calcification centrally (= dystrophic calcification from fat necrosis)
◊ VIRTUALLY DIAGNOSTIC:
@ Calcaneus
√ in triangular region between major trabecular groups (LAT projection)
√ calcified / ossified nidus

@ Proximal femur
√ on / above intertrochanteric line
√ marked ossification of margins of lesion

◊ Radiographic appearance similar to unicameral bone cyst (infarcted lipoma = unicameral bone cyst ?)

DDx: fibrous dysplasia, simple bone cyst, posttraumatic cyst, giant cell tumor, desmoplastic fibroma, chondromyxoid fibroma, osteoblastoma

LIPOMA OF SOFT TISSUE

Most common mesenchymal tumor composed of mature adipose tissue

Histo: mature fat cells (adipocytes) that are uniform in size + shape, occasionally have fibrous connective tissue as septations; fat unavailable for systemic metabolism

• stable size after initial period of discernible growth

Age: 5th–6th decade; M > F

Location:
(a) superficial = subcutaneous lipoma (more common) in posterior trunk, neck, proximal extremities
(b) deep lipoma in retroperitoneum, chest wall, deep soft tissue of hands + feet; multiple in 5–7% (up to several hundred tumors)

√ mass of fat opacity / density / intensity identical to subcutaneous fat
√ cortical thickening (with adjacent parosteal lipoma)

CT:
√ well-defined + homogeneous tumor with low attenuation coefficient (–65 to –120 HU)
√ no enhancement following IV contrast material

MR:
√ well-defined + homogeneous, often with septations
√ signal intensity characteristics similar to subcutaneous fat: hyperintense on T1WI + moderately intense on T2WI
√ differentiation from other lesions by fat suppression technique

Angiolipoma

= lesion composed of fat separated by small branching vessels

Age: 2nd + 3rd decade; 5% familial incidence

• tender

Location: upper extremity, trunk

√ signal characteristics of fat + mixed with varying numbers of large / small vessels
√ mostly encapsulated lesion, may infiltrate

Benign Mesenchymoma

= long-standing lipoma with chondroid + osseous metaplasia

Infiltrating Lipoma

= INTRAMUSCULAR LIPOMA
= relatively common benign lipomatous tumor extending between muscle fibers that become variably atrophic

Peak age: 5th–6th decade; M > F

Location: thigh (50%), shoulder, upper arm

Lipoma Arborescens

= DIFFUSE SYNOVIAL LIPOMA
= lipoma-like lesion composed of hypertrophic synovial villi distended with fat, probably reactive process to chronic synovitis

Location: knee; monoarticular

Frequently associated with:
degenerative joint disease, chronic rheumatoid arthritis, prior trauma

Neural Fibrolipoma

= FIBROLIPOMATOUS HAMARTOMA OF NERVE
= rare tumorlike condition characterized by sausage-shaped / fusiform enlargement of a nerve by fibrofatty tissue

Age: early adulthood before age 30 years / at birth

Histo: infiltration of epineurium + perineurium by fibrofatty tissue with separation of nerve bundles

• soft slowly enlarging mass
• pain, tenderness, decreased sensation, paresthesia

Location: volar aspect of hand, wrist, forearm

Site: median n. (most frequently), ulnar n., radial n., brachial plexus;

May be associated with:
macrodactyly (in 2/3) = **macrodystrophia lipomatosa**

√ may not be visible radiographically

MR:
√ longitudinally oriented, cylindrical, linear / serpiginous structures of signal void about 3 mm in diameter (= nerve fascicles with epi- and perineural fibrosis) separated by areas of fat signal intensity (= mature fat infiltrating the interfascicular connective tissue)

US:
√ "cablelike appearance" = alternating hyper- and hypoechoic bands on US

DDx: cyst, ganglion, lipoma, traumatic neuroma, plexiform neurofibroma, vascular malformation

LIPOSARCOMA

Malignant tumor of mesenchymal origin with bulk of tumor tissue differentiating into adipose tissue

Incidence: 12–18% of all malignant soft-tissue tumors; 2nd most common soft-tissue sarcoma in adults (after malignant fibrous histiocytoma)

Age: 5th–6th decade

Histo:
rarely arising from lipoma
(a) myxoid type (most common, in 40–50%): varying degrees of mucin + fibrous tissue + relatively little lipid (<10%) = intermediate differentiation
√ radiodensity between water + muscle
(b) lipogenic type: malignant lipoblasts with large amounts of lipid + scanty myxoid matrix
= well-differentiated
√ radiodensity of fat with thick + poorly defined streaks of high attenuation
(c) pleomorphic type (least common): marked cellular pleomorphism, paucity of lipid + mucin
= highly undifferentiated

√ radiodensity of muscle (no distinguishing imaging features from other soft-tissue sarcomas)

• usually painless mass (may be painful in 10–15%)

Location: lower extremity (45%), abdominal cavity + retroperitoneum (14%), trunk (14%), upper extremity (7.6%), head & neck (6.5%), miscellaneous (13.5 %)

Spread: hematogenous to lung, visceral organs; myxoid liposarcoma shows tendency for serosal + pleural surfaces, subcutaneous tissue, bone

√ nonspecific soft-tissue mass (frequently fat is radiologically not detectable)

√ inhomogeneous mass with soft-tissue + fatty components

√ enhancement after IV contrast material (contradistinction to lipoma)

√ concomitant mass in retroperitoneum / thigh (in up to 10% of myxoid liposarcomas) as multicentric lesion / metastasis

√ mass of near water density / hypoechoic / hypointense on T1WI + hyperintense on T2WI in myxoid liposarcoma (high content of myxoid cells)

LYME ARTHRITIS

Agent: spirochete Borrelia burgdorferi; transmitted by tick Ixodes dammini

Histo: inflammatory synovial fluid, hypertrophic synovia with vascular proliferation + cellular infiltration

• history of erythema chronicum migrans

• endemic areas: Lyme, Connecticut, first recognized location; now also throughout United States, Europe, Australia

• recurrent attacks of arthralgias within days to 2 years after tick bite (80%)

Location: mono- / oligoarthritis of large joints (especially knee)

√ erosion of cartilage / bone (4%)

Rx: antibiotics

DDx: (1) Rheumatic fever (2) Rheumatoid arthritis (3) Gonococcal arthritis (4) Reiter syndrome

LYMPHANGIOMA

= sequestered noncommunicating lymphoid tissue lined by lymphatic endothelium

Cause: congenital obstruction of lymphatic drainage

Subtypes:

(1) Capillary lymphangioma (rare)
  Location: subcutaneous tissue

(2) Cavernous lymphangioma
  Location: about the mouth + tongue

(3) Cystic lymphangioma (most common)
  = cystic hygroma
  Associated with: hydrops fetalis, Turner syndrome
  Location: head, neck (75%), axilla (20%), extension into mediastinum (3–10%)
  • soft fluctuant mass
  ◊ Lymphangiomas are frequently a mixture of subtypes!

Age: found at birth (50–65%); within first 2 years of life (90%)

Location: soft tissue; bone (rare)

√ multilocular cystic lesion with fibrous septations

√ occasionally serpentine vascular channels

√ opacification during lymphangiography / direct puncture

√ clear / milky fluid on aspiration

DDx: hemangioma (blood on aspiration)

LYMPHOMA OF BONE

= RETICULUM CELL SARCOMA = HISTIOCYTIC LYMPHOMA = PRIMARY LYMPHOMA OF BONE

◊ the generalized form of reticulum cell sarcoma is lymphoma

Prevalence: 2–6% of all primary malignant bone tumors in children

Incidence of bone marrow involvement:

5–15% in Hodgkin disease;
25–40% in non-Hodgkin lymphoma

◊ Bone marrow involvement indicates progression of disease

◊ Bone marrow imaging-guidance for biopsy!

NUC: 40% sensitivity; 88% specificity
MR: 65% sensitivity; 90% specificity

Histo: sheets of reticulum cells, larger than those in Ewing sarcoma (DDx: myeloma, inflammation, osteosarcoma, eosinophilic granuloma)

Age: any age; peak age in 3rd–5th decade; 50% <40 years; 35% <30 years; M:F = 2:1

• striking contrast between size of lesion + patient's well-being

Location: lower femur, upper tibia (40% about knee), humerus, pelvis, scapula, ribs, vertebra

Site: dia- / metaphysis

√ cancellous bone erosion (earliest sign)

√ mottled permeative pattern of separate coalescent areas

√ late cortical destruction

√ lamellated / sunburst periosteal response (less than in Ewing sarcoma)

√ lytic / reactive new-bone formation

√ associated soft-tissue mass without calcification

√ synovitis of knee joint common

Cx: pathologic fracture (most common among malignant bone tumors)

Prognosis: 50% 5-year survival

DDx: (1) Osteosarcoma (less medullary extension, younger patients)
(2) Ewing tumor (systemic symptoms, debility, younger patients)
(3) Metastatic malignancy (multiple bones involved, more destructive)

MACRODYSTROPHIA LIPOMATOSA

= rare nonhereditary congenital form of localized gigantism = neural fibrolipoma with macrodactyly

Path: striking increase in adipose tissue in a fine fibrous network involving periosteum, bone marrow, nerve sheath, muscle, subcutaneous tissue

May be associated with: syn-, clino-, polydactyly
- painless

Location: 2nd or 3rd digit of hand / foot; unilateral; one / few adjacent digits may be involved in the distribution of the median / plantar nerves

√ long + broad splayed phalanges with endosteal + periosteal bone deposition
√ overgrowth of soft tissue, greatest at volar + distal aspects
√ slanting of articular surfaces
√ lucent areas of fat (DIAGNOSTIC)

Prognosis: accelerated maturation possible; growth stops at puberty

DDx: fibrolipomatous hamartoma associated with macrodystrophia lipomatosa (indistinguishable), Klippel-Trenaunay-Weber syndrome, lymphangiomatosis, hemangiomatosis, neurofibromatosis, chronic vascular stimulation, Proteus syndrome

MARFAN SYNDROME

= ARACHNODACTYLY
= autosomal dominant familial disorder of connective tissue with high penetrance but extremely variable expression, new mutations in 15%

Etiology: fibrillin gene defect on chromosome 15 resulting in abnormal cross-linking of collagen fibers

Prevalence: 5:100,000; M:F = 1:1

A. MUSCULOSKELETAL MANIFESTATIONS
- tall thin stature with long limbs, arm span greater than height
- muscular hypoplasia + hypotonicity
- scarcity of subcutaneous fat (emaciated look)

√ generalized osteopenia

@ Skull
- elongated face

√ dolichocephaly
√ prominent jaw
√ high arched palate

@ Hand
- Steinberg sign = protrusion of thumb beyond the confines of the clenched fist (found in 1.1% of normal population)
- metacarpal index (averaging the 4 ratios of length of 2nd through 5th metacarpals divided by their respective middiaphyseal width) >8.8 (male) or 9.4 (female)

√ arachnodactyly = elongation of phalanges + metacarpals
√ flexion deformity of 5th finger

@ Foot
√ pes planus
√ clubfoot
√ hallux valgus
√ hammer toes
√ disproportionate elongation of 1st digit of foot

@ Spine
- ratio of measurement between symphysis and floor + crown and floor >0.45

√ pectus carinatum / excavatum (common)
√ scoliosis / kyphoscoliosis (45–60%)
√ increased incidence of Scheuermann disease and spondylosis
√ dural ectasia
√ increased interpedicular distance
√ posterior scalloping
√ presacral + lateral sacral meningoceles
√ expansion of sacral spinal canal
√ enlargement of sacral foramina
√ winged scapulae

@ Joints
- ligamentous laxity + hypermobility + instability

√ premature osteoarthritis
√ patella alta
√ genu recurvatum
√ recurrent dislocations of patella, hip, clavicle, mandible
√ slipped capital femoral epiphysis
√ progressive protrusio acetabuli (50%), bilateral > unilateral, F > M

B. OCULAR MANIFESTATIONS
- bilateral ectopia lentis, usually upward + outward (secondary to poor zonular attachments)
- glaucoma, macrophthalmia
- hypoplasia of iris + ciliary body
- contracted pupils (absence of dilator muscle)
- myopia, retinal detachment
- strabismus, ptosis
- blue sclera
- megalocornea = flat enlarged thickened cornea

C. CARDIOVASCULAR MANIFESTATIONS (60–98%) affecting mitral valve, ascending aorta, pulmonary artery, splenic + mesenteric arteries (occasionally)

◊ Cause of death in 93%!
- chest pain, palpitations, shortness of breath, fatigue
- mid-to-late systolic murmur + one / more clicks

Associated with congenital heart defect (33%): incomplete coarctation, ASD

@ Aorta (cause of death in 55%)

Histo: myxomatous degeneration of aortic annulus

√ "tulip bulb aorta" = symmetrical dilatation of aortic sinuses of Valsalva slightly extending into ascending aorta (58%)
√ annuloaortic ectasia = combination of aortic root dilatation + aortic regurgitation
√ fusiform aneurysm of ascending aorta, rarely beyond innominate artery (due to cystic medial necrosis)
√ aortic wall calcification rare

Cx: (1) Aortic regurgitation (in 81% if root diameter >5 cm; in 100% if root diameter >6 cm (2) Aortic dissection (3) Aortic rupture (secondary to progressive aortic root dilatation)

@ Mitral valve
Histo: myxomatous degeneration of valve leads to redundancy + laxness
• mid-to-late systolic murmur + one / more clicks
√ "floppy valve syndrome" (95%) = redundant chordae tendineae with mitral valve prolapse + regurgitation
Cx: (1) Mitral regurgitation
(2) Rupture of chordae tendineae (rare)
@ Coarctation (mostly not severe)
@ Pulmonary artery aneurysm + dilatation of pulmonary arterial root (43%)
@ Cor pulmonale (secondary to chest deformity)

D. PULMONARY MANIFESTATIONS
√ cystic lung disease
√ recurrent spontaneous pneumothoraces

E. ABDOMINAL MANIFESTATION
√ recurrent biliary obstruction

DDx: (1) Homocystinuria (osteoporosis)
(2) Ehlers-Danlos syndrome
(3) Congenital contractural arachnodactyly (ear deformities, NO ocular / cardiac abnormalities)
(4) Type III MEN (medullary thyroid carcinoma, mucosal neuromas, pheochromocytoma, marfanoid habitus)

MASSIVE OSTEOLYSIS

= GORHAM DISEASE = "VANISHING BONE" SYNDROME = PHANTOM BONE = HEMANGIOMA OF BONE = LYMPHANGIOMATOSIS OF BONE
= infrequent disorder of unknown etiology with unpredictable course + progression
Incidence: >100 cases described
Histo: massive proliferation of hemangiomatous / lymphangiomatous tissue with large sinusoid spaces + fibrosis
Age: children + adults <40 years
Associated with: soft-tissue hemangiomas without calcifications
• frequently history of severe trauma (50%)
• little / no pain

Location: any bone; most commonly major long bones (humerus, shoulder, mandible), innominate bone, spine, thorax, short tubular bones of hand + feet (unusual)

√ progressive relentless destruction of bone
√ lack of reaction (no periosteal reaction, no repair)
√ advancing edge of destruction not sharply delineated
√ tapering margins of bone ends at sites of osteolysis with conelike spicule of bone (early changes)
√ no respect for joints
√ may destroy all bones in a particular area
DDx: Langerhans cell histiocytosis, fibrous dysplasia, brown tumor of hyperparathyroidism

MELORHEOSTOSIS

Nonhereditary disease of unknown etiology; often incidental finding
Age: slow chronic course in adults; rapid progression in children
Associated with: osteopoikilosis, osteopathia striata, tumors / malformations of blood vessels (hemangioma, vascular nevi, glomus tumor, AVM, aneurysm, lymphedema, lymphangiectasia)
• severe pain + limited joint motion (bone may encroach on nerves, blood vessels, or joints)
• thickening + fibrosis of overlying skin (resembling scleroderma)
• muscle atrophy (frequent)

Location: diaphysis, usually monomelic with at least two bones involved in dermatomal distribution (follows spinal sensory nerve sclerotomes); entire cortex / limited to one side of cortex; more common in lower limb; skull, spine, ribs rarely involved
√ "candle wax dripping" = continuous / interrupted streaks / blotches of sclerosis along tubular bone beginning at proximal end extending distally with slow progression
√ may cross joint with joint fusion
√ small opacities in scapula + hemipelvis (similar to osteopoikilosis)
√ discrepant limb length
√ flexion contractures of hip + knee
√ genu valgum / varus
√ dislocated patella
√ ossified soft-tissue masses (27%)

DDx: (1) Osteopoikilosis (generalized)
(2) Fibrous dysplasia (normal bone structure not lost, not as dense)
(3) Engelmann disease
(4) Hyperostosis of neurofibromatosis, tuberous sclerosis, hemangiomas
(5) Osteoarthropathy

MENISCAL TEAR

Type of tear:
A. LONGITUDINAL TEAR
1. Horizontal cleavage tear
Cause: usually degenerative
Associated with: meniscal cyst
Site: primarily involving the central horizontal plane of meniscus beginning at inner margin
2. Bucket handle tear
Cause: traumatic
Site: usually in medial rarely in lateral meniscus
√ longitudinal vertical tear with unstable displaced inner fragment
3. Peripheral tear
Cause: traumatic
√ vertical tear in peripheral third of meniscus

B. OBLIQUE TEAR
Site: common in midportion of medial meniscus
√ both horizontal and vertical components
√ commonly extending to inferior surface of meniscus
1. Parrot beak tear
Cause: usually degenerative
Site: in body of lateral meniscus near the junction of body + posterior horn
√ fraying of free edge
2. Flap tear = oblique + incomplete tear
Cause: traumatic, at times degenerative

C. TRANSVERSE TEAR = RADIAL TEAR
Site: posterior + midportion of lateral meniscus
√ peripheral displacement of meniscus
√ "absent" / gray meniscus posteriorly
Cx: lack of resistance to hoop stresses

D. MENISCOCAPSULAR SEPARATION
= tearing of peripheral attachments of meniscus
√ linear regions of fluid separating meniscus from capsule
√ uncovering of a portion of tibial plateau owing to inward movement of separated meniscus

MR Classification

Grade	*Type*	*MR Finding*	*PPV for Tear*
0	0	normal meniscus	1%
1	I	globular / punctate intrameniscal signal	2%
2	II	linear signal not extending to surface	5%
	III	short tapered apex of meniscus	23%
	IV	truncated / blunted apex of meniscus	71%
3	V	signal extending to only one surface	85%
3	VI	signal extending to both surfaces	95%
3	VII	comminuted reticulated signal pattern	82%

◊ Diagnosis of tear hinges on surface involvement!
◊ Intrameniscal signal may be a sign of persistent vascularity in children + young adults (type VII)!
◊ Truncation artifact + magic angle artifact may cause increased intrameniscal signal!
◊ Grade 3 signal identified only on a single image is unlikely to be confirmed as a tear at surgery!

Site of injury:
(a) medial meniscus in 45%: no isolated tears of body / anterior horn
(b) lateral meniscus in 22%: posterior horn involved in 80% of all lateral meniscal tears
(c) both menisci involved in 33%

Associated with: ligamentous injury
• asymptomatic in up to 20% of older individuals
√ signal extending to articular surface (type V + VI)
√ notch sign = linear signal intensity becoming wider as it extends toward meniscal surface indicates type V finding (tapering toward surface = type II finding)
√ meniscal cyst = implies presence of meniscal tear
DDx: synovial cyst, tendon sheath fluid, fluid within normal synovial recess, fluid collection remote from meniscus

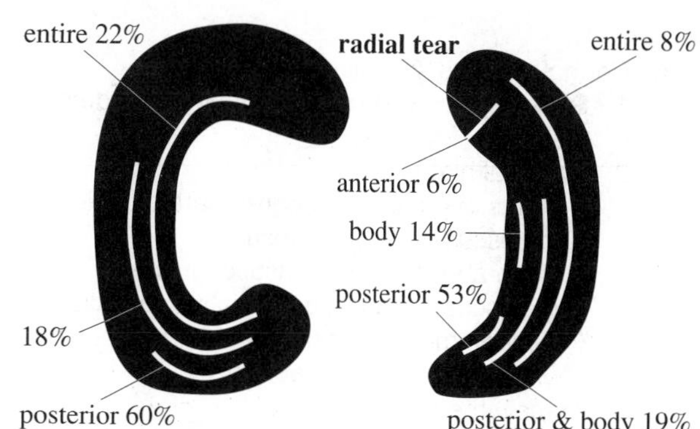

Medial Meniscus Tears **Lateral Meniscus Tears**

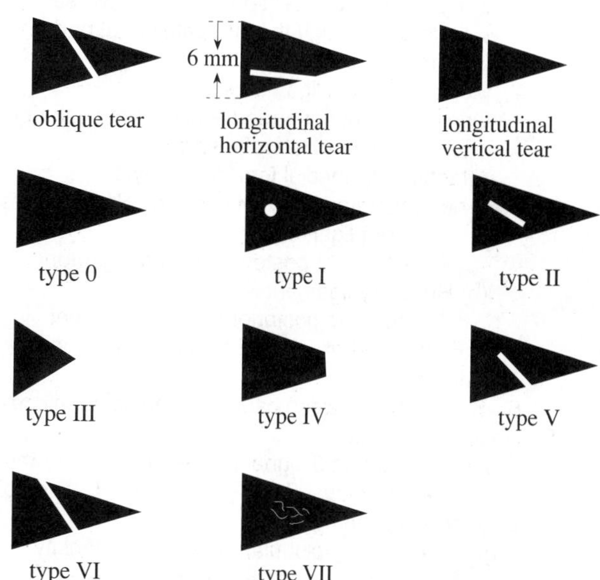

Types of Meniscal Injury

MR sensitivity, specificity, and accuracy:

Tear of	*Sensitivity*	*Specificity*	*Accuracy*
Medial meniscus	95%	88%	59–92%
Lateral meniscus	81%	96%	87–92%
Anterior cruciate lig.			91–96%
Posterior cruciate lig.			up to 99%

◊ MR has a high negative predictive value!
◊ 60–97% accuracy for arthrography
◊ 84–99% accuracy for arthroscopy (poor at posterior horn of medial meniscus)

Interpretative errors (12% for experienced radiologist):
Lateral meniscus: 5.0% FN (middle + posterior horn)
1.5% FP (posterior horn)
Medial meniscus: 2.5% FN (posterior horn)
2.5% FP (posterior horn)

PITFALLS:

A. Normal variants simulating tears:
   1. Superior recess on posterior horn of medial meniscus
   2. Popliteal hiatus
      √ hiatus of popliteal tendon separates lateral meniscus from joint capsule
      ◊ Seen above posterior aspect of lateral meniscus on most superficial sagittal slice!
      ◊ Tendon moves behind + inferior to meniscus on adjacent deeper sections!
   3. Transverse ligament
      Course: connects anterior horns of both menisci
      √ overrides superior aspect of menisci before completely fusing to menisci
      ◊ Trace the cross section of the transverse ligament through the infrapatellar fat pad on more central images!
   4. Meniscofemoral ligaments
      Origin: superior + medial aspect of posterior horn of lateral meniscus
      Attachment: medial femoral condyle
      √ demonstrated in 1/3 of cases on SAG images
      (a) Wrisberg ligament
         √ posterior to posterior cruciate ligament
      (b) Humphry ligament
         √ anterior to posterior cruciate ligament
      ◊ Finding usually limited to single most medial image!
   5. Soft tissue between capsule + medial meniscus

B. Healed meniscus
   √ persistent grade 3 signal at least up to 6 months
   √ S/P meniscectomy (false-positive type IV finding)

C. Degenerative changes
   √ grade 1 signal = globular increase in intensity
   √ grade 2 signal = linear signal not extending to articular surface

D. Diskoid meniscus
   = abnormally shaped enlarged diskus-like meniscus
   Prevalence: in 1.5–15.5%
   Age: children, adolescents
   Side: lateral >> medial meniscus
   √ centrally displaced fragment with meniscus apparently of normal size (coronal images)

MESOMELIC DWARFISM

= heritable bone dysplasia with shortening of intermediate segments (radius + ulna or tibia + fibula)

A. **Langer type** — autosomal recessive
   • mental impairment
   √ mesomelic shortening of limbs
   √ hypoplasia of ulna + fibula
   √ hypoplasia of mandible with short condyles

B. **Nievergelt type** — autosomal dominant
   √ severe mesomelic shortening of lower limbs
   √ marked thickening of tibia + fibula in central portion
   √ clubfoot (frequent)

C. Reinhardt type: — autosomal dominant

D. Robinow type: — autosomal dominant

E. Werner type: — autosomal dominant

F. **Lamy-Bienenfeld type** — autosomal dominant
   • ligamentous laxity
   √ shortening of radius + ulna + tibia
   √ absent fibula
   √ normal femur + humerus

√ shortening of all long bones at birth, most marked in tibia + radius
√ modeling deformity with widening of diaphysis
√ mild to moderate bowing
√ hypoplasia of fibula with absent lateral malleolus
√ short + thick ulna with hypoplastic distal end
√ Madelung deformity of wrist
√ hypoplasia of a vertebral body may be present

METAPHYSEAL CHONDRODYSPLASIA

= severe short-limbed dwarfism
√ metaphyseal flaring (Erlenmeyer flask deformity) extending into diaphysis

A. **Schmid type** (most common)
   autosomal dominant
   • waddling gate
   Distribution: more marked in lower limbs; mild involvement of hands + wrists
   √ shortened bowed long bones
   √ widened epiphyseal growth plates
   √ irregular widened cupped metaphyses
   √ coxa vara
   √ genu varum
   DDx: vitamin D–refractory rickets

B. **McKusick type**
   autosomal recessive (eg, in Amish)
   • sparse brittle hair, deficient pigmentation
   • normal intelligence
   √ shortening of long bones with normal width
   √ cupped + widened metaphyses with lucent defects
   √ short middle phalanges + narrow distal phalanges becoming triangular and bullet-shaped (more frequent in hands than feet)
   √ widened costochondral junctions + cystic lucencies

C. **Jansen type** (less common)
   sporadic occurrence with wide spectrum
   • intelligence normal / retarded
   • serum calcium levels often elevated
   Distribution: symmetrical involvement of all long + short tubular bones
   √ widened epiphyseal plates
   √ expanded irregular + fragmented metaphyses (unossified cartilage extending into diaphyses)
   DDx: rickets

D. **Pyle disease** = Metaphyseal dysplasia
   • often tall
   • often asymptomatic
   Distribution: major long bones, tubular bones of hands, medial end of clavicle, sternal end of ribs, innominate bone
   √ splaying of proximal + distal ends of long bones with thinned cortex

√ relative constriction of central portion of shafts
√ craniofacial hyperostosis
√ genu valgum

METASTASES TO BONE

◊ 15–100 times more common than primary skeletal neoplasms!

Frequency:

If primary known		*If primary unknown*	
Breast	35%	Prostate	25%
Prostate	30%	Lymphoma	15%
Lung	10%	Breast	10%
Kidney	5%	Lung	10%
Uterus	2%	Thyroid	2%
Stomach	2%	Colon	1%
Others	13%		

METASTASES OF PRIMARY BONE TUMORS

1. Osteosarcoma: 2% with distant metastases, adjuvant therapy has changed the natural history of the disease in that bone metastases occur in 10% of osteosarcomas without metastases to the lung
2. Ewing sarcoma: 13% with distant metastases

SOLITARY BONE LESION

◊ Of all causes only 7% are due to metastasis
◊ In patients with known malignancy solitary bone lesions are due to metastasis (55%), due to trauma (25%), due to infection (10%)

Location: axial skeleton (64–68%), ribs (45%), extremities (24%), skull (12%)

mnemonic: "**S**everal **K**inds **O**f **H**orribly **N**asty **T**umors **L**eap **P**romptly **T**o **B**one"

Sarcoma, **S**quamous cell carcinoma
Kidney tumor
Ovarian cancer
Hodgkin disease
Neuroblastoma
Testicular cancer
Lung cancer
Prostate cancer
Thyroid cancer
Breast cancer

Breast cancer: extensive osteolytic lesions; involvement of entire skeleton; pathologic fractures common

Thyroid / kidney: often solitary; rapid progression with bone expansion (bubbly); frequently associated with soft-tissue mass (distinctive)

Rectum / colon: may resemble osteosarcoma with sunburst pattern + osteoblastic reaction

Hodgkin tumor: upper lumbar + lower thoracic spine, pelvis, ribs; osteolytic / occasionally osteoblastic lesions

Ewing tumor: extensive osteolytic / osteoblastic reaction

Neuroblastoma: extensive destruction, resembles leukemia (metaphyseal band of rarefaction), mottled skull destruction + increased intracranial pressure, perpendicular spicules of bone

Mode of spread: through bloodstream / lymphatics / direct extension

Location: predilection for marrow-containing skeleton (skull, spine, ribs, pelvis, humeri, femora)

√ single / multiple lesions of variable size
√ usually nonexpansile
√ joint spaces + intervertebral spaces preserved (cartilage resistant to invasion)

Osteolytic Bone Metastases

Most common cause: neuroblastoma (in childhood); lung cancer (in adult male); breast cancer (in adult female), thyroid cancer; kidney; colon

√ may begin in spongy bone (associated with soft tissue mass in ribs)
√ vertebral pedicles often involved (not in multiple myeloma)

Osteoblastic Bone Metastases

= evidence of slow-growing neoplasm

Primary: prostate, breast, lymphoma, malignant carcinoid, medulloblastoma, mucinous adenocarcinoma of GI tract, TCC of bladder, pancreas, neuroblastoma

Most common cause: prostate cancer (in adult male); breast cancer (in adult female)

mnemonic: "5 **B**ees **L**ick **P**ollen"

Brain (medulloblastoma)
Bronchus
Breast
Bowel (especially carcinoid)
Bladder
Lymphoma
Prostate

√ frequent in vertebrae + pelvis
√ may be indistinguishable from Paget disease

Mixed Bone Metastases

breast, prostate, lymphoma

Expansile / Bubbly Bone Metastases

kidney, thyroid

Permeative Bone Metastases

Burkitt lymphoma, mycosis fungoides

Bone Metastases with "Sunburst" Periosteal Reaction (infrequent)

prostatic carcinoma, retinoblastoma, neuroblastoma (skull), GI tract

Bone Metastases with Soft-tissue Mass

thyroid, kidney

Calcifying Bone Metastases

mnemonic: "BOTTOM"

Breast
Osteosarcoma
Testicular
Thyroid
Ovary
Mucinous adenocarcinoma of GI tract

Skeletal Metastases in Children

1. Neuroblastoma (most often)
2. Retinoblastoma
3. Embryonal rhabdomyosarcoma
4. Hepatoma
5. Ewing tumor

Skeletal Metastases in Adult

mnemonic: "**C**ommon **B**one **L**esions **C**an **K**ill **T**he **P**atient"

Colon
Breast
Lung
Carcinoid
Kidney
Thyroid
Prostate

Role of Bone Scintigraphy in Bone Metastases

Pathophysiology: accumulation of tracer at sites of reactive bone formation

False-negative scan: very aggressive metastases

False-positive scan: degeneration, healing fractures, metabolic disorders

Baseline bone scan:

(a) high sensitivity for many metastatic tumors to bone (particularly carcinoma of breast, lung, prostate); 5% of metastases have normal scan; 5–40% occur in appendicular skeleton
(b) substantially less sensitive than radiographs in infiltrative marrow lesions (multiple myeloma, neuroblastoma, histiocytosis)
(c) screening of asymptomatic patients
— useful in: prostate cancer, breast cancer
— not useful in: non–small-cell bronchogenic carcinoma, gynecologic malignancy, head and neck cancer

√ multiple asymmetric areas of increased uptake
√ axial > appendicular skeleton (dependent on distribution of bone marrow); vertebrae, ribs, pelvis involved in 80%
√ superscan in diffuse bony metastases

Follow-up bone scan:

√ stable scan = suggestive of relatively good prognosis
√ increased activity in:
(a) enlargement of bone lesions / appearance of new lesions indicate progression of the disease
(b) "healing flare" phenomenon (in 20–61%) = transient increase in lesion activity secondary to healing under antineoplastic treatment concomitant with increased sclerosis, detected at 3.2 ± 1.4 months after initiation of hormonal / chemotherapy, of no additional favorable prognostic value
(c) avascular necrosis particularly in hips, knees, shoulders caused by steroid therapy
(d) osteoradionecrosis / radiation-induced osteosarcoma

√ decreased activity in:
(a) predominately osteolytic destruction
(b) metastases under radiotherapy; as early as 2–4 months with minimum of 2000 rads

ROLE OF BONE SCAN IN BREAST CANCER

Routine preoperative bone scan not justified:

Stage I : unsuspected metastases in 2%, mostly single lesion
Stage II : unsuspected metastases in 6%
Stage III : unsuspected metastases in 14%

Follow-up bone scan:

At 12 months no new cases; at 28 months in 5% new metastases; at 30 months in 29% new metastases

Conversion from normal: Stage I : in 7%
Stage II : in 25%
Stage III : in 58%

◊ With axillary lymph node involvement conversion rate 2.5 x that of those without!
◊ Serial follow-up examinations are important to assess therapeutic efficacy + prognosis!

ROLE OF BONE SCAN IN PROSTATE CANCER

Stage B : 5% with skeletal metastases
Stage C : 10% with skeletal metastases
Stage D : 20% with skeletal metastases

Test sensitivities for detection of osseous metastases:
(a) scintigraphy 1.0
(b) radiographic survey 0.68
(c) alkaline phosphatase 0.5
(d) acid phosphatase 0.5

DDx: pulmonary metastasis (SPECT helpful in distinguishing nonosseous lung from overlying rib uptake)

Role of Magnetic Resonance Imaging in Bone Metastases

ideal for bone marrow imaging due to high contrast between bone marrow fat + water-containing metastatic deposits

(1) Focal lytic lesion:
√ hypointense on T1WI + hyperintense on T2WI
(2) Focal sclerotic lesion:
√ hypointense on T1WI + T2WI

(3) Diffuse inhomogeneous lesions:
√ inhomogeneously hypointense on T1WI + hyperintense on T2WI
(4) Diffuse homogeneous lesions:
√ homogeneously hypointense on T1WI + hyperintense on T2WI

METATROPHIC DYSPLASIA

= HYPERPLASTIC ACHONDROPLASIA = METATROPHIC DWARFISM
metatrophic = "changeable" (change in proportions of trunk to limbs over time secondary to developing kyphoscoliosis in childhood)
• longitudinal double skin fold overlying coccyx
√ long bones short with dumbbell-like / trumpet-shaped configuration (exaggerated metaphyseal flaring)
√ "hourglass" phalanges (short with widened ends)
√ wide separation of major joint spaces (thick articular cartilage)
√ delayed ossification of flat irregular epiphyses
@ Chest
√ cylindrical narrowed elongated thorax
√ short + wide ribs
√ pectus carinatum
@ Vertebrae
√ odontoid hypoplasia with atlantoaxial instability
√ progressive kyphoscoliosis
√ platyspondyly + very wide intervertebral spaces
√ wedge- / keel-shaped vertebral bodies
@ Pelvis
√ coccygeal appendage similar to a tail (rare but CHARACTERISTIC)
√ short squared iliac bones + irregular acetabula
√ narrowed greater sciatic notch
Prognosis: compatible with life, increased disability from kyphoscoliosis
DDx: achondroplasia, mucopolysaccharidoses

METHOTREXATE OSTEOPATHY

= syndrome that consists of
(1) bone pain
(2) osteopenia
(3) pathologic fractures
Methotrexate
= dihydrofolate reductase inhibitor most often used in children for treatment of ALL / osteosarcoma / brain tumor
◊ Radiographic findings similar to scurvy:
√ osteopenia
√ dense provisional zones of calcification
√ pathologic fractures (most often metaphyseal)
√ sharply outlined epiphyses
√ NO massive subperiosteal hemorrhage
√ impaired healing of fractures

MORTON NEUROMA

= INTERDIGITAL NEUROMA
M:F = 1:4
Path: perineural fibrosis involving + entrapping a plantar digital nerve
Histo: dense collagenous + fibrous tissue
• burning / electric forefoot pain during walking
Location: typically 3rd intermetatarsal space
MR:
√ small lesion of intermediate signal intensity on T1WI + low signal intensity on T2WI
√ ± fluid in intermetatarsal bursa
Rx: conservative treatment; surgical excision

MUCOPOLYSACCHARIDOSES

= lysosomal storage disorder from deficiency of specific lysosomal enzymes involved in degradation of mucopolysaccharides

Type I = Hurler	Type V = Scheie
Type II = Hunter	Type VI = Maroteaux-Lamy
Type III = Sanfilippo	Type VII = Sly
Type IV = Morquio	

◊ All autosomal recessive except for Hunter (X-linked)!
Associated with: valvular heart disease
• corneal clouding
• retardation (prominent in types I, II, III, VII)
• skeletal involvement dominates in types IV and VI
√ scaphocephaly, macrocephaly; thick calvarium; hypertelorism
√ platyspondyly with kyphosis + dwarfism
√ irregularity at anterior aspect of vertebral bodies
√ atlantoaxial subluxation + instability (laxity of transverse ligament / hypoplasia or absence of odontoid)
√ limb contractures
√ broad hands + brachydactyly
√ hepatosplenomegaly
@ Brain
√ brain atrophy
√ varying degree of hydrocephalus
√ multiple white matter changes within cerebral hemispheres (diffuse hypodense areas, prolongation of T1 + T2)
Cx: cord compression at atlantoaxial joint (types IV + VI)
Dx: combination of clinical features, radiographic abnormalities correlated with genetic + biochemical studies
Prenatal Dx: occasionally successful analysis of fibroblasts cultured from amniotic fluid
DDx: Gaucher disease, Niemann-Pick disease

Hurler Syndrome

= GARGOYLISM = PFAUNDLER-HURLER DISEASE = MPS I-H
= autosomal recessive disease
Cause: homozygous for MPS III gene with excess chondroitin sulfate B due to deficient X-L iduronidase (= Hurler corrective factor)
Incidence: 1:10,000 births
Age: usually appears >1st year
• dwarfism
• progressive mental deterioration after 1–3 years
• large head; sunken bridge of nose; hypertelorism
• early corneal clouding progressing to blindness

Mucopolysaccharidoses

Type	Eponym	Inheritance	Enzyme Deficiency	Urinary Glycosaminoglycan	Neurologic Signs
I-H	Hurler	autosomal recessive	alpha-L-iduronidase	dermatan sulfate	marked
II	Hunter	X-linked recessive	iduronate sulfatase	dermatan / heparan sulfate	mild to moderate
III	Sanfilippo	autosomal recessive		heparan sulfate	mental deterioration
	A		heparan sulfate sulfatase		
	B		N-acetyl-alpha-D-glucosaminidase		
	C		alpha-glucosamine-N-acetyl-transferase		
	D		N-acetylglucosamine-6-sulfate sulfatase		
IV	Morquio A–D	autosomal recessive	N-acetylgalactosamine-6-sulfate sulfatase beta-galactosidase	keratan sulfate	none
I-S(V)	Scheie	autosomal recessive	alpha-L-iduronidase	heparan sulfate	none
VI	Maroteaux-Lamy	autosomal recessive	arylsulfatase B	dermatan sulfate	none
VII	Sly	autosomal recessive	beta-glucuronidase	dermatan sulfate heparan sulfate	variable

- "gargoyle" features = everted lips + protruding tongue
- teeth widely separated + poorly formed
- progressive narrowing of nasopharyngeal airway
- protuberant abdomen (secondary to dorsolumbar kyphosis + hepatosplenomegaly)
- urinary excretion of chondroitin sulfate B (dermatan sulfate) + heparan sulfate
- Reilly bodies (metachromic granules) in white blood cells or bone marrow cells

@ Skull (earliest changes >6 months of age)
- √ frontal bossing
- √ calvarial thickening
- √ premature fusion of sagittal + lambdoid sutures
- √ deepening of optic chiasm
- √ enlarged J-shaped sella (undermining of anterior clinoid process)
- √ small facial bones
- √ wide mandibular angle + underdevelopment of condyles
- √ communicating hydrocephalus

@ Extremities
- √ thick periosteal cloaking of long-bone diaphyses (early changes)
- √ swelling / enlargement of diaphyses + cortical thinning (due to dilatation of medullary canal) + tapering of either end: distal humerus, radius, ulna, proximal ends of metacarpals
- √ deossification with heterogenous bone density + course trabeculation (due to deposition of accumulated precursor metabolites in bone marrow)
- √ flexion deformities of knees + hips
- √ trident hands; clawing (occasionally)
- √ delayed maturation of irregular carpal bones

@ Spine
- √ thoracolumbar kyphosis with lumbar gibbus
- √ oval centra with normal / increased height + anterior beak at T12/L1/L2
- √ long slender pedicles
- √ proximally long slender ribs at level of neck + wide distally = spatulate rib configuration

@ Pelvis
- √ widely flared iliac wings with inferior tapering
- √ constriction of iliac bones
- √ coxa valga

Prognosis: death by age 10–15 years

Morquio Syndrome

= KERATOSULFATURIA = MPS IV
= autosomal recessive; excess keratosulfate

Incidence: 1:40,000 births

Etiology: N-acetylgalactosamine-6-sulfatase deficiency resulting in defective degradation of keratin sulfate (mainly in cartilage, nucleus pulposus, cornea)

Age: normal at birth; skeletal changes manifest within first 18 months

- excessive urinary excretion of keratan sulfate
- normal intelligence
- weakness + hypotonia
- dwarfism with short trunk (<4 feet tall)
- head thrust forward + sunken between high shoulders
- normal intelligence
- corneal opacities evident around age 10
- progressive deafness
- short nose, wide mouth, spacing between teeth

- semicrouching stance + knock knees from flexion deformities of knees + hips

@ Skull
- √ mild dolichocephaly
- √ hypertelorism
- √ poor mastoid air cell development
- √ short nose + depression of bridge of nose
- √ prominent maxilla

@ Chest
- √ increased AP diameter + marked pectus carinatum
- √ slight lordosis with wide short ribs
- √ bulbous costochondral junctions
- √ failure of fusion of sternal segments

@ Spine
- √ hypoplasia / absence of odontoid process of C2
- √ C1-C2 instability with anterior subluxation
- √ thick C2-body with narrowing of vertebral canal
- √ atlas close to occiput / posterior arch of C1 within foramen magnum
- √ platyspondyly = universal vertebra plana esp. affecting lumbar spine (DDx: normal height in Hurler syndrome)
- √ ovoid vertebral bodies with central anterior beak / tongue at lower thoracic / upper lumbar vertebrae
- √ mild gibbus at thoracolumbar transition = low dorsal kyphosis
- √ exaggerated lumbar lordosis
- √ widened intervertebral disk spaces

@ Pelvis
- √ "goblet-shaped" / "wineglass" pelvis = constricted iliac bodies + elongated pelvic inlet + flared iliac wings
- √ oblique hypoplastic acetabular roofs

@ Femur
- √ initially well-formed femoral head epiphysis, then involution + fragmentation by age 3–6 years
- √ lateral subluxation of femoral heads; later hip dislocation
- √ wide femoral neck + coxa valga deformity

@ Tibia
- √ delayed ossification of lateral proximal tibial epiphysis
- √ sloping of superior margin of tibia plateau laterally + severe genu valgum

@ Hand & foot
- √ short bones of forearm with widening of proximal ends
- √ delayed appearance + irregularity of carpal centers
- √ small irregular carpal bones
- √ proximally pointed short metacarpals 2–5
- √ enlarged joints; hand + foot deformities (flat feet)
- √ ulnar deviation of hand

Cx: cervical myelopathy (traumatic quadriplegia / leg pains / subtle neurologic abnormality) most common cause of death secondary to C2 abnormality; frequent respiratory infections (from respiratory paralysis)

Rx: early fusion of C1–C2

Prognosis: may live to adulthood

DDx:
(1) Hurler syndrome (normal / increased vertebral height; vertebral beak inferior)
(2) Spondyloepiphyseal dysplasia (autosomal dominant, present at birth, absent flared ilia / deficient acetabular ossification, small acetabular angle, deficient ossification of pubic bones, varus deformity of femoral neck, minimal involvement of hand + foot, myopia)

MULTIPLE EPIPHYSEAL DYSPLASIA

= FAIRBANK DISEASE

= ? tarda form of chondrodystrophia calcificans congenita

- √ mild limb shortening
- √ irregular mottled calcifications of epiphyses (in childhood + adolescence)
- √ epiphyseal irregularities + premature degenerative joint disease, especially of hips (in adulthood)
- √ short phalanges

DDx: Legg-Perthes disease, hypothyroidism

MULTIPLE MYELOMA

◊ Most common primary malignant neoplasm in adults!

Histo: normal / pleomorphic plasma cells (not pathognomonic), may be mistaken for lymphocytes (lymphosarcoma, reticulum cell sarcoma, Ewing tumor, neuroblastoma)
(a) diffuse infiltration: myeloma cells intimately admixed with hematopoietic cells
(b) tumor nodules: displacement of hematopoietic cells by masses entirely composed of myeloma cells

Age: usually 5th–8th decade; 98% >40 years; rare <30 years of age; M:F = 2:1
(a) DISSEMINATED FORM: >40 years of age (98%); M:F = 3:2
(b) SOLITARY FORM: mean age 50 years

- bone pain (68%)
- normochromic normocytic anemia (62%)
- RBC rouleau formation
- renal insufficiency (55%)
- hypercalcemia (30–50%)
- proteinuria (88%)
- Bence Jones proteinuria (50%)
- increased globulin production (monoclonal gammopathy)

Location:

A. DISSEMINATED FORM:
scattered; axial skeleton predominant site; vertebrae (50%) > ribs > skull > pelvis > long bones (distribution correlates with normal sites of red marrow)

B. SOLITARY PLASMACYTOMA OF BONE:
vertebrae > pelvis > skull > sternum > ribs

C. SPINAL PLASMA CELL MYELOMA
- √ sparing of posterior elements (no red marrow) (DDx: metastatic disease)
- √ paraspinal soft-tissue mass with extradural extension
- √ scalloping of anterior margin of vertebral bodies (osseous pressure from adjacent enlarged lymph nodes)

√ generalized osteopenia only (15%) with accentuation of trabecular pattern, especially in spine (early)
√ punched out appearance of widespread osteolytic lesions (skull, long bones) with endosteal scalloping and of uniform size
√ diffuse osteolysis (pelvis, sacrum)
√ expansile osteolytic lesions (ballooning) in ribs, pelvis, long bones
√ soft-tissue mass adjacent to bone destruction (= extrapleural + paraspinal mass adjacent to ribs / vertebral column)
√ periosteal new-bone formation exceedingly rare
√ involvement of mandible (rarely affected by metastatic disease)
√ sclerosis may occur after chemotherapy, radiotherapy, fluoride administration
√ sclerotic form of multiple myeloma (1–3%)
(a) solitary sclerotic lesion: frequently in spine
(b) diffuse sclerosis
Associated with **POEMS syndrome**:
Polyneuropathy
Organomegaly
Endocrine abnormalities
Myeloma, sclerotic
Skin changes

MR (recognition dependent on knowledge of normal range of bone marrow appearance for age):
√ hypointense focal areas on T1WI (25%)
√ hyperintense focal areas on T2WI (53%)
√ absence of fatty infiltration (nonspecific)

SENSITIVITY OF BONE SCANS VS. RADIOGRAPHS
Radiographs : in 90% of patients and 80% of sites
Bone scan : in 75% of patients and 24–54% of sites
Gallium scan : in 55% of patients and 40% of sites
◊ 30% of lesions only detected on radiographs
◊ 10% of lesions only detected on bone scans

Cx: (1) Renal involvement frequent
(2) Predilection for recurrent pneumonias (leukopenia)
(3) Secondary amyloidosis in 6–15%
(4) Pathologic fractures occur often

Prognosis: 20% 5-year survival; death from renal insufficiency, bacterial infection, thromboembolism

DDx:
— with osteopenia: (1) Postmenopausal osteoporosis
(2) Hyperparathyroidism
— with lytic lesion: (1) Metastatic disease
(2) Amyloidosis
(3) Myeloid metaplasia
— with sclerotic lesion: (1) Osteopoikilosis
(2) Lymphoma
(3) Osteoblastic metastasis
(4) Mastocytosis
(5) Myelosclerosis
(6) Fluorosis
(7) Lymphoma
(8) Renal osteodystrophy

Myelomatosis
√ generalized deossification without discrete tumors
√ vertebral flattening

MUSCULOTENDINOUS INJURY

Muscle Contusion
Cause: direct trauma, usually by blunt object
Site: deep within muscle belly
• injury at point of impact
√ NO architectural changes
√ feathery appearance of diffuse muscle edema
√ increased muscle girth
√ deep intramuscular hematoma (with severe trauma resulting in disruption of muscle fibers)

Myotendinous Strain
Cause: single traumatic event from excessive stretching
Susceptibility factors:
(1) muscle composed of (fast contracting) type II fibers
(2) fusiform shape of muscle
(3) extension across two joints
(4) superficial location of muscle
(5) eccentric muscle action

Site: myotendinous junction (= weakest point of musculotendinous unit)
Classification:
1° degree = stretch injury (some fiber disruptions)
• no loss of muscle function
Path: interstitial edema + hemorrhage at myotendinous junction with extension into adjacent muscle fibers
√ feathery appearance of muscle
2° degree = partial tear without retraction
• mild loss of muscle function
√ hematoma at myotendinous junction
√ perifascial fluid collection
3° degree = complete rupture
• complete loss of muscle function
√ retracted muscle tendon
√ hematoma at myotendinous junction

Acute Avulsion Injury
Cause: forceful unbalanced often eccentric muscle contraction
Path: periosteal stripping with hematoma at tendon attachment site
Site: at tendon insertion
• loss of function, severe tenderness
√ waviness + retraction of the torn end of tendon with fragment of bone / cartilage

MYELOFIBROSIS
= MYELOSCLEROSIS = AGNOGENIC MYELOID METAPLASIA
= MYELO-PROLIFERATIVE SYNDROME
= PSEUDOLEUKEMIA
= hematologic disorder of unknown etiology with gradual replacement of bone marrow elements by fibrotic tissue

Characterized by
(1) extramedullary hematopoiesis
(2) progressive splenomegaly
(3) anemia
(4) variable changes in number of granulocytes + platelets; often predated by polycythemia vera

Cause:
(a) primary: rare in children
(b) secondary: radiation therapy, chemotherapy

Age: usually >50 years
Path: fibrous / bony replacement of bone marrow; extramedullary hematopoiesis
Associated with: metastatic carcinoma, chemical poisoning, chronic infection (TB), acute myelogenous leukemia, polycythemia vera, McCune-Albright syndrome, histiocytosis

• dyspnea, weakness, fatigue, weight loss, hemorrhage
• normochromic normocytic anemia; polycythemia may precede myelosclerosis in 59%
• dry marrow aspirate

Location: red marrow–containing bones in 40% (thoracic cage, pelvis, femora, humeral shafts, lumbar spine, skull, peripheral bones)

√ splenomegaly
√ widespread diffuse increase in density (ground glass)
√ "jail-bar" ribs
√ sandwich / rugger jersey spine
√ generalized increase in bone density in skull + obliteration of diploic space; scattered small rounded radiolucent lesions; or combination of both

MR:
√ hypointense marrow on T1WI + fat-suppression

NUC:
√ diffuse increased uptake of bone tracer in affected skeleton, possibly "superscan"
√ increased uptake at ends of long bones

DDx: (1) With splenomegaly: chronic leukemia, lymphoma, mastocytosis
(2) Without splenomegaly: osteoblastic metastases, fluorine poisoning, osteopetrosis, chronic renal disease

MYELOID DEPLETION

= APLASTIC ANEMIA

Cause: idiopathic; ? sequelae of viral infection, medication, toxin, chemo- / radiation therapy
Path: normal marrow replaced by fat cells

MR:
√ high signal intensity on T1WI
√ low signal intensity on fat-suppressed T2WI
◊ Best seen in areas with high percentage of hematopoietic marrow: proximal femoral metaphyses, spine

MYELOPROLIFERATIVE DISORDERS

= autonomous clonal disorder initiated by an acquired pluripotential hematopoietic stem cell

Types:
1. Polycythemia vera
2. Chronic granulomatous leukemia = chronic myelogenous leukemia
3. Essential idiopathic thrombocytopenia
4. Agnogenic myeloid metaplasia (= primary myelofibrosis + extramedullary hematopoiesis in liver + spleen)

Pathophysiology:
— self-perpetuating intra- and extramedullary hematopoietic cell proliferation without stimulus
— trilinear panmyelosis (RBCs, WBCs, platelets)
— myelofibrosis with progression to myelosclerosis
— myeloid metaplasia = extramedullary hematopoiesis (normocytic anemia, leukoerythroblastic anemia, reticulocytosis, low platelet count, normal / reduced WBC count)

MYOSITIS OSSIFICANS

= PSEUDOMALIGNANT OSSEOUS TUMOR OF SOFT TISSUE = EXTRAOSSEOUS LOCALIZED NONNEOPLASTIC BONE AND CARTILAGE FORMATION = MYOSITIS OSSIFICANS CIRCUMSCRIPTA = HETEROTOPIC OSSIFICATION
= benign solitary self-limiting ossifying soft-tissue mass typically occurring within skeletal muscle
◊ Myositis is a misnomer for lack of inflammation!

Cause: direct trauma (75%), paralysis, burn, tetanus, intramuscular hematoma, spontaneous
Age: adolescents, young athletic adults; M > F
Path: lesion rimmed by compressed fibrous connective tissue + surrounded by atrophic skeletal muscle (myositis = misnomer since no primary inflammation of muscle present)

Histo:
(a) early: focal hemorrhage + degeneration + necrosis of damaged muscle; histiocytic invasion; central nonossified core of proliferating benign fibroblasts + myofibroblasts; mesenchymal cells enclosed in ground substance assume characteristics of osteoblasts with subsequent mineralization + peripheral bone formation
(b) intermediate age (3–6 weeks): "zone phenomenon" with central area of cellular variation and atypical mitotic figures (impossible to differentiate from soft-tissue sarcoma); middle zone of immature osteoid; outer zone of well-formed mature trabeculated dense bone

• pain, tenderness, soft-tissue mass

Location: large muscles of extremities (80%)
(a) within muscle: anterolateral aspect of thigh + arm; temporal muscle; small muscles of hands; gluteal muscle; **"rider's bone"** (adductor longus); **"fencer's bone"** (brachialis); **"dancer's bone"** (soleus); breast, elbow, knee
(b) periosteal at tendon insertion: **Pellegrini-Stieda disease** (in / near medial (tibial) collateral ligament of knee) as a result of Stieda fracture (= avulsion injury from medial femoral condyle at origin of tibial collateral ligament)
[Augusto Pellegrini (1877–1958), surgeon in Florence, Italy]
[Alfred Stieda (1869–1945), surgeon in Königsberg, Germany]

√ faint calcifications develop in 2–6 weeks after onset of symptoms
√ well-defined partially ossified soft-tissue mass apparent by 6–8 weeks, becoming smaller + mature by 5–6 months
√ radiolucent zone separating lesion from bone (DDx: periosteal sarcoma on stalk)
√ ± periosteal reaction

MR:
- √ initially heterogenous muscle edema
- √ progression to masslike region of high-signal intensity on T2WI (during first days to weeks after injury)

CT:
- √ well-defined mineralization at periphery of lesion after 4–6 weeks + less distinct lucent center (DDx: sarcoma with ill-defined periphery + calcified ossific center)
- √ diffuse ossification in mature lesion

MR:
- Early phase:
  - √ mass with poorly defined margins
  - √ inhomogeneously hyperintense to fat on T2WI
  - √ isointense to muscle on T1WI
  - √ contrast enhancement
- Intermediate phase:
  - √ isointense / slightly hyperintense core on T1WI, increasing in intensity on T2WI
  - √ rim of curvilinear areas of decreased signal intensity surrounding the lesion (= peripheral mineralization / ossification)
  - √ increased peritumoral signal intensity on T2WI (= edema of diffuse myositis)
  - √ focal signal abnormality within bone marrow (= marrow edema)
- Mature phase:
  - √ well-defined inhomogeneous mass with signal intensity approximating fat
  - √ decreased signal intensity surrounding lesion + within (dense ossification + fibrosis, hemosiderin from previous hemorrhage)

NUC:
- √ intense tracer accumulation on bone scan (directly related to deposition of calcium in damaged muscle)
- √ in phase of mature ossification activity becomes reduced + surgery may be performed with little risk of recurrence

Angio:
- √ diffuse tumor blush + fine neovascularity in early active phase
- √ avascular mass in mature healing phase

Prognosis: ? resorption in 1 year

DDx:
◊ In early stages difficult to differentiate histologically + radiologically from soft-tissue sarcomas!
(1) Osteosarcoma
(2) Synovial sarcoma
(3) Fibrosarcoma
(4) Chondrosarcoma
(5) Rhabdomyosarcoma
(6) Parosteal sarcoma (usually metaphyseal with thick densely mineralized attachment to bone)
(7) Posttraumatic periostitis (ossification of subperiosteal hematoma with broad-based attachment to bone)
(8) Acute osteomyelitis (substantial soft-tissue edema + early periosteal reaction)
(9) Tumoral calcinosis (periarticular calcific masses of lobular pattern with interspersed lucent soft-tissue septa)
(10) Osteochondroma (stalk contiguous with normal adjacent cortex + medullary space)

Myositis Ossificans Variants

Panniculitis Ossificans

Location: subcutis of mostly upper extremities
√ less prominent zoning phenomenon

Fasciitis Ossificans

Location: fascia

Fibroosseous Pseudotumor of Digits

= FLORID REACTIVE PERIOSTITIS
= nonneoplastic solitary self-limiting process of unknown pathogenesis, probably related to trauma

Age: mean age of 32 years (range 4 –64 years); M:F = 1:2

• fusiform soft-tissue swelling / mass

Location: predominantly tubular bones of hand + foot: fingers (2nd > 3rd > 5th)

Site: proximal > distal > middle phalanx

√ radiopaque soft-tissue mass with radiolucent band between mass + cortex
√ visible calcifications (50%)
√ focal periosteal thickening (50%)
√ cortical erosion (occasionally)

Rx: local excision

DDx: parosteal / periosteal osteogenic sarcoma, peripheral chondrosarcoma, periosteal chondroma, soft-tissue chondroma

NAIL-PATELLA SYNDROME

= FONG DISEASE = ILIAC HORNS = FAMILIAL / HEREDITARY OSTEO-ONYCHODYSPLASIA = OSTEO-ONYCHODYS-OSTOSIS = HOOD SYNDROME = ELBOW-PATELLA SYNDROME
= rare autosomal dominant disorder characterized by symmetrical meso- and ectodermal anomalies

Etiology: ? enzymatic defect in collagen metabolism

Age: evident in 2nd + 3rd decades

• aplasia / hypoplasia of thumb + index fingernails
• bilateral spooning / splitting / ridging of fingernails
• abnormal gait
• abnormal pigmentation of iris
• renal dysfunction (secondary to abnormal glomerular basement membrane): proteinuria, hematuria, failure later in life

√ bilateral posterior iliac horns in 80% (occasionally capped by an epiphysis) DIAGNOSTIC

√ flared iliac crest with protuberant anterior iliac spines
√ genu valgum due to asymmetrical development of femoral condyles
√ prominent tibial tubercles
√ fragmentation / hypoplasia / absence of patella; frequently with recurrent lateral dislocations
√ radial head / capitellum hypoplasia with subluxation / dislocation of radial head dorsally and increased carrying angle of elbow (DDx: congenital dislocation of radial head)
√ clinodactyly of 5th finger
√ short 5th metacarpal
√ flexion contractures of hip, knee, elbow, fingers, foot
√ deltoid, triceps, quadriceps hypoplasia
√ mandibular cysts (occasionally)
√ scoliosis
√ renal osteodystrophy

DDx: (1) Seckel syndrome = bird-headed dwarfism
(2) Popliteal pterygium syndrome (absence of patella, toenail dysplasia)

NECROTIZING FASCIITIS

Incidence: 500 cases in literature
Age: 58 ± 14 years; M>F
Cause: deep internal infection / malignancy (perforated duodenal ulcer / retroperitoneal appendix, retroperitoneal / perirectal infection, infiltrating rectal / sigmoid carcinoma
Predisposed: patients with diabetes, cancer, alcohol / drug abuse, poor nutrition
Organism: Staphylococcus, E. coli, Bacteroides, Streptococcus, Peptostreptococcus, Klebsiella, Proteus, C. perfringens (5–15%) (multiple organisms in 75%)
Histo: necrotic superficial fascia, leukocytic infiltration of deep fascial layers; fibrinoid thrombosis of arterioles + venules with vessel wall necrosis; microbial infiltration of destroyed fascia

• indolent (1–21 days delay before diagnosis)
• nonspecific symptoms: severe pain, fever, leukocytosis, shock, altered mental status
• crepitus (50%), overlying skin may be completely intact

Location: lower extremity, arm, neck, back, male perineum / scrotum (= Fournier gangrene)
√ asymmetric fascial thickening with fat stranding (80%) from fluid
√ gas in soft-tissues dissecting along fascial planes from gas-forming organisms (in 55%)
√ associated deep abscess (35%)
√ ± secondary muscle involvement

Prognosis: poor with delay in diagnosis
Rx: extensive surgical débridement
DDx: (1) Myonecrosis (infection originating in muscle)
(2) Fasciitis-panniculitis syndromes (chronic swelling of skin + underlying soft tissues + fascial planes in arm + calf)
(3) Soft-tissue edema of CHF / cirrhosis (symmetrical diffuse fat stranding)

NEUROPATHIC OSTEOARTHROPATHY

= NEUROTROPHIC JOINT = CHARCOT JOINT
= traumatic arthritis due associated with loss of sensation + proprioception of affected limb

Pathogenesis: (1) decreased pain sensation produces repetitive trauma
(2) sympathetic dysfunction results in local hyperemia + bone resorption

Cause:
A. Congenital
1. Myelomeningocele
2. Congenital indifference to pain = asymbolia
3. Familial dysautonomia (Riley-Day syndrome)
4. Hereditary sensory and motor neuropathy (Charcot-Marie-Tooth disease)

B. Acquired
(a) central neuropathy
1. Injury to brain / spinal cord
2. Syringomyelia (in 1/3 of patients): shoulder, elbow
3. Neurosyphilis = tabes dorsalis (in 15–20% of patients): hip, knee, ankle, tarsals
4. Spinal cord tumors / infection
5. Extrinsic compression of spinal cord
6. Multiple sclerosis
7. Alcoholism

(b) peripheral neuropathy
1. Diabetes mellitus (most common cause, although incidence low): ankle, foot, hand
2. Peripheral nerve injury
3. Peripheral nerve tumor
4. Leprosy (Hansen disease)
5. Poliomyelitis

(c) others
1. Scleroderma, Raynaud disease, Ehlers-Danlos syndrome
2. Rheumatoid arthritis, psoriasis
3. Amyloid infiltration of nerves, adrenal hypercorticism
4. Uremia
5. Pernicious anemia

C. Iatrogenic
1. Prolonged use of pain-relieving drugs
2. Intraarticular / systemic steroid injections

mnemonic: "DS6"
Diabetes
Syphilis
Steroids
Spinal cord injury
Spina bifida
Syringomyelia
Scleroderma

Pathophysiology:
Loss of proprioception with sensory deficits arising in the spinal cord / peripheral nerves
(1) Neurotraumatic theory
= repetitive trauma with absence of normal protective sensory feedback

(2) Neurovascular theory
= absence of neural stimuli leads to a loss of sympathetic tone resulting in vasodilatation and hyperemia, which promotes bone resorption + weakening of subchondral bone

Pathology:
(a) atrophic pattern (most common):
osseous resorption in which osteoclasts + macrophages remove bone + cartilage debris making bone susceptible to fractures
Associated with: syringomyelia, peripheral nerve lesion
Location: non-weight-bearing joints of upper extremity
DDx: surgical amputation, septic arthritis
(b) hypertrophic pattern:
joint destruction + fragmentation, osseous sclerosis, osteophyte formation (early attaining enormous size)
DDx: severe osteoarthritis
(c) mixed pattern
(d) common to both:
joint disorganization, large persistent bloody joint effusion

- no history of trauma
- swollen + warm joint with normal WBC count + ESR (infection may coexist)
- usually painless joint; pain at presentation (in 1/3) with decreased response to deep pain + proprioception
- joint changes frequently precede neurologic deficit
- synovial fluid: frequently xanthochromic / bloody, lipid crystals (from bone marrow)

√ persistent joint effusion (first sign)
√ narrowing of joint space
√ speckled calcification in soft tissue (= calcification of synovial membrane)
√ fragmentation of eburnated subchondral bone
√ NO juxtaarticular osteoporosis (unless infected)
√ "bag-of-bones" appearance in late stage (= marked deformities around joint)
mnemonic: "6 Ds"
√ **D**ense subchondral bone (= sclerosis)
√ **D**egeneration (= attempted repair by osteophytes)
√ **D**estruction of articular cortex (with sharp margins resembling those of surgical amputation)
√ **D**eformity ("pencil point" deformity of metatarsal heads)
√ **D**ebris (loose bodies)
√ **D**islocation (nontraumatic)
√ subluxation of joints (laxity of periarticular soft tissues)
√ progressive rapid bone resorption
√ joint distension (by fluid, hypertrophic synovitis, osteophytes, subluxation)
√ fracture: healing with exuberant bizarre callus formation

MR:
√ decreased signal intensity in bone marrow on T1WI + T2WI (due to osteosclerotic changes)

@ Shoulder
Cause: syringomyelia, cord trauma with paraplegia
- shoulder mass (due to fluid distension)

√ amputated appearance of proximal humerus
√ dislocation
√ large joint effusion
√ fragmented osseous debris in joint capsule + subacromial-subdeltoid bursa
DDx: chondrosarcoma

@ Hands + feet
Cause: leprosy (due to trauma + secondary bacterial infection)
√ claw hand / claw toes
√ licked candy stick phalanx = tapered phalanx (due to concentric bone atrophy with decrease in bone length + width)
DDx: diabetes mellitus, frostbite, pernicious anemia, scleroderma, syringomyelia, tabes dorsalis, familial sensory neuropathy

@ Spine (involved in 6–21%):
Cause: traumatic spinal cord injury, inadequately treated syphilis, amyloidosis, congenital insensitivity to pain, diabetes mellitus
Site: thoracolumbar junction, lumbar spine
√ disk space narrowing
√ osteolysis / sclerosis of vertebrae + facet joints
√ subluxation
√ abrupt curvature
√ scoliosis
√ paraspinous soft-tissue calcification
√ large hypertrophic beaking endplate osteophytes
√ extensive osseous fragmentation with extension beyond confines of vertebral body margin into paraspinous musculature + into spinal canal
DDx: vertebral osteomyelitis, metastasis, granulomatous infection

@ Foot + ankle
Cause: long-term poorly controlled diabetes mellitus, syphilis
- soft-tissue swelling, warmth, erythema

Site: often begins in midfoot
√ vascular calcifications
√ subluxation (starting at 2nd tarsometatarsal joint)
√ avulasion fracture of posterior tubercle of calcaneus
√ subchondral fracture of head of 2nd metatarsal
√ talonavicular displacement with midfoot arthropathy

NODULAR TENOSYNOVITIS

= GIANT CELL TUMOR OF TENDON SHEATH
= benign proliferative lesion of synovial origin viewed as an extraarticular form of PVNS

Age: young adult
Path: very cellular tumor with a capsule that separates the tumor into lobules
Histo: multinucleated giant cells, macrophages, fibroblasts, xanthoma cells, varying amounts of hemosiderin

Location: hand, occasionally ankle / foot
◊ One of the most common tumors of the hand!
Site: tendon sheath, joint capsule, bursa, ligament

√ lobulated lesion with well-defined nodules up to 4 cm in size
√ located along tendon sheath (CHARACTERISTIC)
√ bone erosion (15%)
MR:
√ low signal intensity on T1WI + T2WI (hemosiderin deposition)
√ homogeneous contrast enhancement
DDx: (1) Florid proliferative synovitis (diffuse infiltrative form of GCT = extraarticular subtype of PVNS)
(2) Pigmented villonodular synovitis
(3) Desmoid tumor
(4) Malignant fibrous histiocytoma

NONOSSIFYING FIBROMA

= FIBROXANTHOMA = NONOSTEOGENIC FIBROMA
= XANTHOMA = XANTHOGRANULOMA OF BONE
= FIBROUS METAPHYSEAL-DIAPHYSEAL DEFECT
= FIBROUS MEDULLARY DEFECT
Incidence: up to 40% of all children >2 years of age
Etiology: lesion resulting from proliferative activity of a fibrous cortical defect that has expanded into medullary cavity
Histo: interlacing whorled bundles of spindle-shaped fibroblasts + scattered multinucleated giant cells + foamy xanthomatous cells, variable degree of hemosiderin; usually cellular with only small amounts of collagen
Age: 8–20 years; 75% in 2nd decade of life
• usually asymptomatic; pain if large
Location: shaft of long bone; mostly in bones of lower extremity, especially about knee (distal femur + proximal tibia); distal tibia; fibula
Site: eccentric metaphyseal, several cm shaftward from epiphysis, mostly intramedullary, rarely purely diaphyseal
Multiple fibroxanthomas (in 8–10%):
Associated with: neurofibromatosis, fibrous dysplasia, Jaffé-Campanacci syndrome

√ multilocular ovoid bubbly osteolytic area
√ alignment along long axis of bone, about 2 cm in length
√ dense sclerotic border toward medulla; V- or U-shaped at one end
√ endosteal scalloping + thinning ± overlying bulge
√ migrates toward center of diaphysis
√ resolves with age
NUC: √ minimal / mild uptake on bone scan
MR:
√ 80% hypointense on T1WI + T2WI (extensive hypocellular fibrous tissue, hemosiderin pigment)
√ 20% hypointense on T1WI + hyperintense on T2WI (massive aggregation of foamy histiocytes)
√ peripheral hypointense rim + internal septation (marginal reactive sclerosis + trabeculation)
√ intense contrast enhancement (in 80%) / marginal septal enhancement (in 20%) on T1WI
CAVE: lesions >33 mm long involving >50% of the transverse bone diameter need observation

Prognosis: spontaneous healing in most cases
Cx: (1) Pathologic fracture (not uncommon)
(2) Hypophosphatemic vitamin D–resistant rickets + osteomalacia (tumor may secrete substance that increases renal tubular resorption of phosphorus)
DDx: (1) Adamantinoma (midshaft of tibia)
(2) Chondromyxoid fibroma (bulging of cortex more striking, hyperintense on T2WI)
(3) Fibrous dysplasia (internal septations rare)
(4) Aneurysmal bone cyst (heterogeneously hyperintense with fluid-fluid levels)
(5) Intraosseous ganglion (hyperintense on T2WI)

Jaffé-Campanacci Syndrome

= nonossifying fibroma with extraskeletal manifestations in children
• mental retardation
• hypogonadism
• ocular defect
• cardiovascular congenital defect
• café-au-lait spots

NOONAN SYNDROME

= PSEUDO–TURNER = MALE TURNER SYNDROME
= phenotype similar to Turner syndrome but with normal karyotype (occurs in both males + females)
Striking familial incidence
• short / may have normal height
• webbed neck
• agonadism / normal gonads
• delayed puberty
• mental retardation
√ osteoporosis
√ retarded bone age
√ cubitus valgus
@ Skull
√ mandibular hypoplasia with dental malocclusion
√ hypertelorism
√ biparietal foramina
√ dolichocephaly, microcephaly / cranial enlargement
√ webbed neck
@ Chest
√ sternal deformity: pectus excavatum / carinatum
√ right-sided congenital heart disease (valvar pulmonic stenosis, ASD, eccentric hypertrophy of left ventricle, PDA, VSD)
√ coronal clefts of spine
√ may have pulmonary lymphangiectasis
@ Gastrointestinal tract
√ intestinal lymphangiectasia
√ eventration of diaphragm
√ renal malrotation, renal duplication, hydronephrosis, large redundant extrarenal pelvis
DDx: Turner syndrome (mental retardation rare, renal anomalies frequent)

OCHRONOSIS

= ALKAPTONURIA

= inherited absence of homogentisic acid oxidase with excessive homogentisic acid production + deposition in connective tissue including cartilage, synovium, and bone

Histo: black-pigmented cartilage subject to deterioration resulting in calcification + denudation of cartilaginous tissue

M:F = 2:1

- black pigment in soft tissues (in 2nd decade): yellowish skin; gray pigmentation of sclera; bluish tinge of ears + nose cartilage
- alkaptonuria with black staining of diapers
- heart failure, renal failure (pigment deposition)

@ Spine
  Age: middle age
  Site: lumbar region with progressive ascension
  √ laminated calcification of multiple intervertebral disks
  √ severe narrowing of intervertebral disk space
  √ multiple "vacuum" phenomena (common)
  √ osteoporosis of adjoining vertebrae
  √ massive osteophytosis + ankylosis of spine (in older patient)
  √ spotty calcifications in tissue anterior to vertebral bodies

@ Joints
  √ hypertrophic changes in humeral head
  √ severe premature progressive osteoarthritic changes in shoulder, knee, hip, spine of young patients
  √ intraarticular osseous bodies
  √ small calcifications in paraarticular soft tissues + tendon insertions

ORODIGITOFACIAL SYNDROME

= OROFACIODIGITAL SYNDROME
= group of heterogeneous defects, probably representing varying expressivity, involving face, oral cavity, and limbs

Etiology: autosomal trisomy of chromosome No. 1 with 47 chromosomes; X-linked dominant
Sex: nuclear chromatin pattern female (lethal in male)
Associated with: renal polycystic disease

- mental retardation
- hypertelorism
- cleft lip + tongue, lingual hamartoma
- bifid nasal tip

√ cleft in palate + jaw bone
√ hypoplasia of mandible (micrognathia) + occiput of skull
√ hypodontia
√ clinodactyly, syndactyly, brachydactyly (metacarpals may be elongated), polysyndactyly, duplication of hallux

OSGOOD-SCHLATTER DISEASE

[Robert B. Osgood (1873–1956), Boston orthopedic surgeon]
[Carl Schlatter (1864–1934), surgeon in Zurich, Switzerland]

= traumatically induced disruption of the attachment of the patellar ligament to the tibial tuberosity (chronic fatigue injury, NOT osteonecrosis); bilateral in 25%

Age: 10–15 years; M > F
Cause: trauma (common in sports that involve jumping, kicking, squatting) = ? cartilaginous avulsion fracture, ? tendinitis

- local pain + tenderness on pressure
- swelling of overlying soft tissue

√ soft-tissue swelling in front of tuberosity (= edema of skin + subcutaneous tissue)
√ thickening of distal portion of patellar tendon
√ indistinct margin of patellar tendon
√ increased radiodensity of infrapatellar fat pad
√ avulsion with separation of small ossicles from the developing ossification center of tibial tuberosity
√ single / multiple ossifications in avulsed fragment
√ comparison with other side (irregular development normal)

MR:
  √ increased signal intensity at tibial insertion site of patellar tendon on T1WI + T2WI
  √ distension of deep infrapatellar bursa
  √ bone marrow signal changes in tibial tuberosity + tibial apophysis (rare)

Cx: nonunion of bone fragment, patellar subluxation, chondromalacia, avulsion of patellar tendon, genu recurvatum
Rx: immobilization / steroid injection
DDx: (1) Normal ossification pattern of tibial tuberosity between ages 8–14 (no symptoms)
(2) Osteitis: tuberculous / syphilitic
(3) Soft-tissue sarcoma with calcifications

OSSIFYING FIBROMA

Closely related to fibrous dysplasia + adamantinoma

Age: 2nd–4th decade; M < F
Histo: maturing cellular fibrous spindle cells with osteoblastic activity producing many calcific cartilaginous + bone densities

Location: frequently in face

@ Mandible, maxilla
  - painless expansion of tooth-bearing portion of jaw
  √ 1–5 cm well-circumscribed round / oval tumor
  √ moderate expansion of intact cortex
  √ homogeneous tumor matrix
  √ dislodgment of teeth

@ Tibia
  √ eccentric ground-glass lesion (resembling fibrous dysplasia)

Cx: frequent recurrences

OSTEITIS CONDENSANS ILII

Incidence: 2% of population
Cause: chronic stress secondary to instability of pubic symphysis
Age: young multiparous women

- associated with low back pain when instability of pubic symphysis present

√ triangular area of sclerosis along inferior anterior aspect of ileum adjacent to SI joint (joint space uninvolved)
√ similar triangle of reparative bone on sacral side
√ usually bilateral + symmetric; occasionally unilateral
√ sclerosis dissolves in 3–20 years following stabilization of pubic symphysis

DDx: (1) Ankylosing spondylitis (affects ilium + sacrum, joint space narrowing, involvement of other bones)
(2) Rheumatoid arthritis (asymmetric, joint destruction)
(3) Paget disease (thickened trabecular pattern)

OSTEOARTHRITIS

= DEGENERATIVE JOINT DISEASE
= predominantly noninflammatory degeneration of cartilage in synovial joints

Cause: (1) abnormal forces acting on a normal joint (eg, slipped capital femoral epiphysis)
(2) normal forces acting on abnormal joint due to
(a) cartilage abnormality
(b) subchondral bone abnormality

Path: decreased chondroitin sulfate with age creates unsupported collagen fibrils followed by irreversible hyaline cartilage degeneration (= inability for regeneration)

Stages:
I cartilage swelling + softening from damage to collagen matrix resulting in decreased proteoglycan content and aggregate size + increase in water content
II increased cartilage thickness from proliferation of chondrocytes with increase in anabolic + catabolic activity
III cartilage loss with continued damage due to decrease in cellular proliferation of chondrocytes resulting in fibrillation + erosion + cracking of articular cartilage

√ joint space narrowing (stage III) = inaccurate indicator of cartilage integrity
√ subchondral sclerosis / eburnation in areas of stress
√ subchondral cyst formation (geodes)
√ increased joint fluid
√ synovial inflammation (in severe osteoarthritis)
√ osteophytosis at articular margin / nonstressed area

MR:
√ increased signal intensity of abnormal cartilage on T2WI (= increased amount of free water)
√ morphologic defects on surface of cartilage (best seen on fat-suppressed spoiled gradient-echo MR)

@ Hand + foot
Target area: 1st MCP; trapezioscaphoid; DIP > PIP; 1st MTP
√ loss of joint space, subchondral eburnation, marginal osteophytes, small ossicles in DIP + PIP:
√ Bouchard nodes = osteophytosis at PIP joint
√ Heberden nodes = osteophytosis at DIP joint: M:F = 1:10
√ radial subluxation of 1st metacarpal base
√ joint space narrowing + eburnation of trapezioscaphoid area

@ Shoulder
√ elevation of humeral head + lack of significant glenohumeral joint involvement (DDx to rheumatoid arthritis)

@ Hip
√ femoral + acetabular osteophytes, sclerosis, subchondral cyst formation
√ thickening / buttressing of medial femoral cortex / calcar
√ migration of femoral head
√ superolateral subluxation of femoral head
√ medial / axial subluxation ± protrusio acetabuli (in 20%)
√ primary hereditary protrusio = Otto pelvis (M < F)

@ Knee
Location: medial > lateral femorotibial > patellofemoral compartment
√ varus deformity (M>>F)

@ Spine
√ sclerosis + narrowing of intervertebral apophyseal joints
√ osteophytosis usually associated with diskogenic disease

@ Sacroiliac joint
◊ Most common disorder of sacroiliac joints
Location: bi- / unilateral (<u>contralateral</u> SIJ with bad hip)
√ diffuse joint space loss
√ vacuum phenomenon
√ well-defined line of sclerosis, especially on iliac side of articulation
√ prominent bridging osteophyte at superior + inferior limits of joint
DDx: osteoblastic metastasis

Erosive Osteoarthritis

= inflammatory form of osteoarthrosis
Predisposed: postmenopausal females
Site: distribution identical to noninflammatory osteoarthritis: DIP > PIP > MCP joints of hands; radial aspect of wrist; bilateral + symmetric
√ "bird-wing" / "sea-gull" joint configuration = central erosions + osteophytosis
√ may lead to bony ankylosis
DDx: Rheumatoid arthritis, Wilson disease, chronic liver disease, hemochromatosis

Early Osteoarthritis

mnemonic: "**E**arly **O**steo**A**rthritis"
Epiphyseal dysplasia, multiple
Ochronosis
Acromegaly

Milwaukee Shoulder

= association of
(1) complete rotator cuff tear
(2) osteoarthritic changes
(3) noninflammatory joint effusion containing calcium hydroxyapatite and calcium pyrophosphate dihydrate (CPPD) crystals
(4) hyperplasia of synovium
(5) destruction of cartilage + subchondral bone
(6) multiple osteochondral loose bodies

Age: older women
• frequent history of trauma

- rapidly progressive arthritis of shoulder

Radiograph:
- √ joint space narrowing
- √ subchondral sclerosis + cyst formation
- √ destruction of subchondral bone
- √ soft-tissue swelling
- √ capsular calcifications
- √ intraarticular loose bodies

MR:
- √ large effusion
- √ complete rotator cuff tear
- √ narrowing of glenohumeral joint

Rapidly Destructive Articular Disease

= unusual form of osteoarthritis typically involving the hip (almost always unilateral)

Age: elderly women

Associated with: conventional osteoarthritis in hands, wrists, knees, opposite hip

- hip pain
- √ progressive loss of joint space
- √ loss of subchondral bone in femoral head + acetabulum resulting in "hatchet" deformity of femoral head
- √ superolateral subluxation of femoral head / intrusion deformity within ilium
- √ no / small osteophytes

Prognosis: rapid destruction of hip within 14 months after onset of symptoms

Rx: total joint replacement

DDx: osteonecrosis, septic arthritis, neuroarthropathy, crystal-induced arthropathy

OSTEOBLASTOMA

= GIANT OSTEOID OSTEOMA = OSTEOGENIC FIBROMA OF BONE = OSSIFYING FIBROMA

= rare benign tumor with unlimited growth potential + capability of malignant transformation

Incidence: <1% of all primary bone tumors; 3% of all benign bone tumors

Age: mean age of 16–19 years; 6–30 years (90%); 2nd decade (55%); 3rd decade (20%); M:F = 2:1

Path: lesion >1.5 cm; smaller lesions are classified as osteoid osteoma

Histo: numerous multinucleated giant cells (osteoclasts), irregularly arranged osteoid + bone; very vascular connective tissue stroma with interconnecting trabecular bone; trabeculae broader + longer than in osteoid osteoma

- asymptomatic in <2%
- dull localized pain of insidious onset (84%), worse at night in 7–13%
- response to salicylates in 7%
- localized swelling, tenderness, decreased range of motion (29%)
- painful scoliosis in 50% (with spinal / rib location) secondary to muscle spasm, may be convex toward side of tumor
- paresthesias, mild muscle weakness, paraparesis, paraplegia (due to cord compression)
- occasional systemic toxicity (high WBC, fever)

Location: (rarely multifocal)
- (a) spine (33–37%): 62–94% in posterior elements, secondary extension into vertebral body (28–42%); cervical spine (31%), thoracic spine (34%), lumbar spine (31%), sacrum (3%)
- (b) long bones (26–32%): femur (50%), tibia (19%), humerus (19%), radius (8%), fibula (4%); unusual in neck of femur
- (c) small bones of hand + feet (15–26%): dorsal talus neck (62%), calcaneus (4%), scaphoid (8%), metacarpals (8%), metatarsals (8%)
- (d) calvarium + mandible (= cementoblastoma)

Site: diaphyseal (58%), metaphyseal (42%); eccentric (46%), intracortical (42%), centric (12%), may be periosteal

- √ similar to osteoid osteoma:
  - √ radiolucent nidus >2 cm (range of 2–12 cm) in size
  - √ well demarcated (83%)
  - √ ± stippled / ringlike small flecks of matrix calcification
  - √ reactive sclerosis (22–91%) / no sclerosis (9–56%)
- √ progressive expansile lesion that may rapidly increase in size (25%):
  - √ cortical expansion (75–94%) / destruction (20–22%)
  - √ tumor matrix radiolucent (25–64%) / ossified (36–72%)
  - √ sharply defined soft-tissue component
  - √ thin shell of periosteal new bone (58–77%) / no periosteal reaction
- √ scoliosis (35%)
- √ osteoporosis due to disuse + hyperemia in talar location
- √ rapid calcification after radiotherapy

CT:
- √ multifocal matrix mineralization, sclerosis
- √ expansile bone remodeling, thin osseous shell

NUC:
- √ intense focal accumulation of bone agent (100%)

Angio:
- √ tumor blush in capillary phase (50%)

MR:
- √ low to intermediate signal intensity on T1WI
- √ mixed intermediate to high intensity on T2WI
- √ surrounding edema

Prognosis: 10% recurrence after excision; incomplete curettage can effect cure due to cartilage production + trapping of host lamellar bone

DDx:
1. (1) Osteo- / chondrosarcoma (periosteal new bone)
2. (2) Osteoid osteoma (dense calcification + halo of bone sclerosis, stable lesion size <2 cm due to limited growth potential)
3. (3) Cartilaginous tumors (lumpy matrix calcification
4. (4) Giant cell tumor (no calcification, epiphyseal involvement)
5. (5) Aneurysmal bone cyst
6. (6) Osteomyelitis
7. (7) Hemangioma
8. (8) Lipoma
9. (9) Epidermoid
10. (10) Fibrous dysplasia

(11) Metastasis
(12) Ewing sarcoma

OSTEOCHONDROMA

= OSTEOCARTILAGINOUS EXOSTOSIS
= developmental hyperplastic / dysplastic bone disturbance; growth ends when nearest epiphyseal plate fuses
◊ Most common benign growth of the skeleton!
◊ Most common benign cartilage-containing tumor!

Etiology: separation of a fragment of physeal cartilage herniating through periosteal bone cuff that surrounds the growth plate (encoche of Ranvier); the fragment continues to grow and undergoes enchondral ossification
(a) microtrauma / Salter-Harris injury with in vivo transplantation of physeal tissue
(b) radiation therapy (in 6–24%) with latency period of 3–17 years in patients between 8 months and 11 years of age receiving 1,500–5,500 cGy (frequently for treatment of neuroblastoma / Wilms tumor)
◊ Most common benign radiation-induced tumor

Path: continuity of lesion with marrow + cortex of host bone (HALLMARK)
Histo: hyaline cartilage cap containing a basal surface with enchondral ossification (thin cortex + trabecular bone + marrow space)

√ continuity of bone cortex with host bone cortex
√ continuity of medullary marrow space with host bone
√ hyaline cartilaginous cap:
  √ arcs / rings / flocculent calcifications on radiographs
√ growth pointing away from nearest joint + toward center of shaft:
  √ at right angle on diaphyseal side of stalk
  √ slope on epiphyseal side

CT:
  √ optimal depiction of cortical + marrow continuity with host bone (PATHOGNOMONIC)
  √ nonmineralized cartilage cap hypodense to muscle (in 75–80%):
    √ 6–8 mm thick in skeletally mature patients
    √ up to 30 mm thick in skeletally immature patients

MR:
  √ cortical + medullary continuity (MR best modality)
  √ hyaline cartilage cap very hyperintense on T2WI + of intermediate intensity on T1WI:
    √ hypointense mineralized areas of cartilage
    √ hypointense periphery = perichondrium
    √ slight septal + peripheral enhancement

US:
  √ hypoechoic nonmineralized cartilaginous cap easily distinguished from muscle and fat
  √ posterior acoustic shadowing for mineralized portion

NUC:
  √ active lesion (predominantly in young patient)
  √ quiescent lesion in older patient

Prognosis: exostosis begins in childhood; stops growing when nearest epiphyseal center fuses

Rx: surgical excision (2% recurrence rate, 13% complication rate [neuropraxia, arterial laceration, compartment syndrome, fracture])

Cx:
(1) Osseous and cosmetic deformity (most frequent)
  • mechanical limitation of joint movement
  • snapping tendon / ligament
  • hematuria (irritating pubic osteochondroma)
  √ saucerization / scalloping of cortex of adjacent bone due to extrinsic pressure erosion (of paired tubular bones)
  √ premature osteoarthritis
  √ pleural effusion / spontaneous hemothorax (due to irritating rib lesion)
(2) Fracture through stalk of osteochondroma
(3) Vascular compromise
  – venous / arterial stenosis
  – arterial occlusion / venous thrombosis
  – pseudoaneurysm formation:
    Cause: repetitive trauma to vessel wall
    Age: near end of normal skeletal growth
    Location: popliteal a., brachial a., superficial femoral a., posterior tibial a.
(4) Neurologic compromise
  – peripheral nerve compression with entrapment neuropathy: foot drop with peroneal nerve involvement (most frequent)
  – central nerve compression: cranial nerve deficit, radiculopathy, cauda equina syndrome, cord compression with myelomalacia
    √ often very narrow stalk of attachment
    √ difficult imaging diagnosis owing to complex anatomy of skull base (21% TP)
    √ spinal canal osteochondroma (15% FN)
(5) Reactive bursa formation (in 1.5%)
  • enlarging mass overlying an osteochondroma simulating malignant transformation
  Location: scapula (>50%), lesser trochanter, shoulder
  √ fluid-filled mass ± chondral filling defects:
    √ mineralization of intrabursal chondral bodies may mimic a thick cartilage cap with growth
  Cx: inflammation, infection, hemorrhage into bursa, secondary synovial chondromatosis
(6) Malignant transformation into secondary / peripheral chondrosarcoma / osteosarcoma
  Frequency: 1% in solitary osteochondroma; <5% in hereditary multiple osteochondromatosis
  Location: iliac bone commonest site
  ◊ Any cartilage cap >1.5 cm thick is suspect of malignant transformation!
  mnemonic: "GLAD PAST"
  Growth after physeal closure
  Lucency (new radiolucency)
  Additional scintigraphic activity
  Destruction (cortical)
  Pain after puberty
  And
  Soft-tissue mass
  Thickened cartilaginous cap >1.5 cm

OSTEOCHONDROMA VARIANTS
1. Dysplasia epiphysealis hemimelica
2. Subungual exostosis
3. Turret exostosis
4. Traction exostosis (at tendinous attachments)
5. Bizarre parosteal osteochondromatous proliferation = Nora lesion
6. Florid reactive periostitis

Solitary Osteochondroma

Frequency: 1–2%; M:F = 1.6:1–3.4:1
20–50% of benign bone tumors;
10–15% of all bone tumors

Age: 1st–3rd decade; M:F = 1.5:1

- incidental nontender painless mass near joints
- symptomatic (in 75% before the age of 20 years)

Site: metaphysis of long bones; rarely diaphysis

Location: in any bone that develops by enchondromal calcification; femur (30%), tibia (15–20%), about knee (40%), humerus (10–20%), hands and feet (10%), pelvis (5%), scapula (4%), rib (3%), spine (2%, cervical [esp. C2] > thoracic [T8 > T4] > lumbar)

Type: (a) pedunculated osteochondroma = narrow stalk
(b) sessile osteochondroma = broad base

Hereditary Multiple Exostoses

= DIAPHYSEAL ACLASIS (ACLASIA) = MULTIPLE OSTEOCHONDROMAS = FAMILIAL OSTEOCHONDROMATOSIS
= most common of osteochondrodysplasias characterized by formation of multiple exostoses

Prevalence: 1:50,000–1:100,000;
1:1,000 on Guam / Mariana Islands

Genetics: autosomal dominant (incomplete penetrance in females); 3 distinct loci on chromosomes 8, 11, 19
◊ 2/3 of affected individuals have a positive family history

Age: forms shortly after birth; virtually all patients discovered by 12 years of age; M:F = 1.5:1.0

- short stature (40%) due to development of exostoses at the expense of longitudinal bone growth

Location: multiple + usually bilateral; knee (70–98%), humerus (50–98%), scapula + rib (40%), elbow (35–40%), hip (30–90%), wrist (30–60%), ankle (25–54%), hand (20–30%), foot (10–25%), pelvis (5–15%), vertebra (7%)

Site: metaphyses of long bones near epiphyseal plate (distance to epiphyseal line increases with growth)

√ disproportionate shortening of an extremity (50%)

@ Upper extremity
- √ pseudo-Madelung deformity:
  - √ ulnar shortening + longer bowed radius
  - √ ulnar tilt of distal radial articular surface
  - √ ulnar deviation of hand
- √ dislocation of radial head
- √ radioulnar synostosis
- √ shortening of 4th + 5th metacarpals
- √ supernumerary fingers / toes

@ Lower extremity
- √ coxa valga (25%)
- √ genu valgus (20–40%)
- √ valgus deformity of ankle = tibiotalar tilt (45–54%)
- √ undertubulation with widened metadiaphyseal junction:
  - √ Erlenmeyer flask deformity of distal femur

CT:
- √ wavy pelvis sign = small sessile lesion create undulating cortical contour

OSTEOCHONDROSIS DISSECANS

= OSTEOCHONDRITIS DISSECANS
= OSTEOCHONDRAL FRACTURE
= fragmentation + possible separation of a portion of the articular surface

Etiology:
(1) subchondral fatigue fracture as a result of shearing, rotatory / tangentially aligned impaction forces
(2) ? autosomal dominant trait associated with short stature, endocrine dysfunction, Scheuermann disease, Osgood-Schlatter disease, tibia vara, carpal tunnel syndrome

Age: adolescence; M > F

- asymptomatic / vague complaints
- clicking, locking, limitation of motion
- swelling, pain aggravated by movement

Location: (a) knee: medial (in 10% lateral) femoral condyle close to fossa intercondylaris; bilateral in 20–30%
(b) humeral head
(c) capitellum of elbow
(d) talus

√ purely cartilaginous fragment unrecognized on plain film
√ fracture line parallels joint surface
√ mouse = osteochondrotic fragment
Location: posterior region of knee joint, olecranon fossa, axillary / subscapular recess of glenohumeral joint
√ mouse bed = sclerosed pit in articular surface
√ soft-tissue swelling, joint effusion

DDx: spontaneous osteonecrosis, neuroarthropathy, degenerative joint disease, synovial osteochondromatosis

OSTEOFIBROUS DYSPLASIA

= entity previously mistaken for fibrous dysplasia

Age: newborn up to 5 years

Histo: fibrous tissue surrounding trabeculae in a whorled storiform pattern

Location: normally confined to tibia (middiaphysis in 50%), lesion begins in anterior cortex; ipsilateral fibula affected in 20%

√ enlargement of tibia with anterior bowing
√ cortex thin / invisible
√ periosteal expansion
√ sclerotic margin (DDx: nonosteogenic fibroma, chondromyxoid fibroma)
√ spontaneous regression in 1/3

Cx: pathologic fracture in 25%, fractures will heal with immobilization; infrequently complicated by pseudarthrosis

DDx: fibrous dysplasia, Paget disease

OSTEOGENESIS IMPERFECTA

= PSATHYROSIS = FRAGILITAS OSSIUM = LOBSTEIN DISEASE

= heterogeneous group of a generalized connective tissue disorder leading to micromelic dwarfism characterized by bone fragility, blue sclerae, and dentinogenesis imperfecta

Incidence: overall in 1:28,500 (1:20,000–1:60,000) live births; M:F = 1:1

Histo: immature collagen matrix

Clinical types:

1. OSTEOGENESIS IMPERFECTA CONGENITA
   = disease manifest at birth (occurring in utero); autosomal dominant; corresponds to type II; lethal variety
2. OSTEOGENESIS IMPERFECTA TARDA
   = usually not manifest at birth; recessive / sporadic corresponds to type I + IV; nonlethal variety

- soft skull (caput membranaceum)
- hyperlaxity of joints
- blue sclerae
- poor dentition
- otosclerosis
- thin loose skin

√ diffuse demineralization, deficient trabecular structure, cortical thinning
√ defective cortical bone: increase in diameter of proximal ends of humeri + femora; slender fragile bone; multiple cystlike areas
√ multiple fractures + pseudarthrosis with bowing (vertebral bodies, long bones)
√ normal / exuberant callus formation
√ rib thinning / notching
√ thin calvarium
√ sinus + mastoid cell enlargement
√ thickened undermineralized otic capsule (= otosclerosis)
√ wormian bones persisting into adulthood
√ basilar impression (= platybasia)
√ biconcave vertebral bodies + Schmorl nodes, increased height of intervertebral disk space
√ bowing deformities after child begins to walk

Cx: (1) Impaired hearing / deafness from otosclerosis (20–60%)
(2) Death from intracranial hemorrhage (abnormal platelet function)

Dx: chorionic villous sampling

Osteogenesis Imperfecta Type I

Transmission: autosomal dominant; compatible with life

Age at presentation: 2–6 years

- blue sclerae
- presenile deafness
- normal / abnormal dentinogenesis

√ infants of normal weight + length
√ osteoporosis
√ fractures in neonate (occurring during delivery)

OB-US:
√ marked bowing of long bones
√ NO IUGR

Osteogenesis Imperfecta Type II

= CONGENITAL LETHAL OI

= perinatal lethal form

Transmission: sporadic new dominant mutations / autosomal recessive

Incidence: 1:54,000 births; most frequent variety

- blue sclerae
- ligamentous laxity + loose skin

√ shortened broad crumpled long bones
√ bone angulations, bowing, demineralization
√ localized bone thickening from callus formation
√ thin beaded ribs ± fractures resulting in bell-shaped / narrow chest
√ thin poorly ossified skull
√ wormian bones (present in most cases)
√ spinal osteopenia
√ platyspondyly

OB-US:
◊ A normal sonogram after 17 weeks MA excludes the diagnosis!
√ increased through-transmission of skull (extremely poor mineralization):
  √ unusually good visualization of brain surface
  √ unusually good visualization of orbits
  √ increased visualization of intracranial arterial pulsations
√ abnormal compressibility of skull vault with transducer
√ decreased visualization of skeleton
√ multiple fetal fractures + deformities of long bones + ribs:
  √ wrinkled appearance of bone (= more than one fracture in single bone)
  √ beaded ribs (callus formation around fractures)
√ abnormally short limbs
√ small thorax (collapse of thoracic cage)
√ decreased fetal movement
√ infants small for gestational age (frequent)
√ polyhydramnios + nonimmune hydrops

Prognosis: stillborn / death shortly after birth due to pulmonary hypoplasia

DDx: congenital hypophosphatasia; achondrogenesis type I; campomelic dysplasia

Osteogenesis Imperfecta Type III

= SEVERE PROGRESSIVELY DEFORMING OI

Transmission: autosomal recessive; progressively deforming disorder compatible with life

- bluish sclerae during infancy that turn pale with time
- joint hyperlaxity (50%)

√ decreased ossification of skull
√ normal vertebrae + pelvis
√ shortened + bowed long bones

√ progressive deformities of limbs + spine into adulthood
√ ± rib fractures
√ multiple fractures present at birth in 2/3 of cases
√ fractures heal well

OB-US:
- √ short + bowed long bones
- √ fractures
- √ humerus almost normal in shape
- √ normal thoracic circumference

Prognosis: progressive limb + spine deformities during childhood / adolescence

Osteogenesis Imperfecta Type IV

Transmission: autosomal dominant; mildest form with best prognosis

- normal scleral color
- little tendency to develop hearing loss

√ tubular bones of normal length; mild femoral bowing may occur
√ osteoporosis

OB-US:
- √ bowing of long bones

OSTEOID OSTEOMA

= benign skeletal neoplasm composed of osteoid + woven bone less than 1.5 cm in diameter per definition

Incidence: 12% of benign skeletal neoplasms
Etiology: ? inflammatory response
Histo: small nidus of osteoid-laden interconnected trabeculae with a background of highly vascularized fibrous connective tissue surrounded by zone of reactive bone sclerosis; osteoblastic rimming; indistinguishable from osteoblastoma
Age: 10–20 years (51%); 2nd + 3rd decade (73%); 5–25 years (90%); range of 19 months–56 years; uncommon <5 and >40 years of age; M:F = 2:1; uncommon in Blacks

- tender to touch + pressure
- local pain (95–98%), weeks to years in duration, worse at night, decreased by activity
- salicylates give relief in 20–30 minutes in 75–90%
- prostaglandin E2 elevated 100–1000 x normal within nidus (probable cause of pain and vasodilatation)

Location:
- (a) meta- / diaphysis of long bones (73%): upper end of femur (43%), hands (8%), feet (4%); frequent in proximal tibia + femoral neck, fibula, humerus; no bone exempt
- (b) spine (10–14%): predominantly in posterior elements (50% in pedicle + lamina + spinous process; 20% in articular process) of lumbar (59%), cervical (27%), thoracic (12%), sacral (2%) segments
  - painful scoliosis, focal / radicular pain
  - gait disturbance, muscle atrophy
- (c) skull, rib, ischium, mandible, patella

Classification:

Cortical osteoid osteoma (most common)
= nidus within cortex
√ solid / laminated periosteal reaction
√ fusiform sclerotic cortical thickening in shaft of long bone
√ radiolucent area within center of osteosclerosis

Cancellous Osteoid Osteoma (intermediate frequency)
= intramedullary
◊ Intraarticular lesion difficult to identify with delay in diagnosis of 4 months–5 years!
Site: juxta- / intraarticular at femoral neck, vertebral posterior elements, small bones of hands + feet
√ little osteosclerosis / sclerotic cortex distant to nidus (functional difference of intraarticular periosteum)
√ joint space widened (effusion, synovitis)

Subperiosteal Osteoid Osteoma (rare)
= round soft-tissue mass adjacent to bone
Site: juxta- / intraarticular at medial aspect of femoral neck, hands, feet (neck of talus)
√ juxtacortical mass excavating the cortex (bony pressure atrophy) with almost no reactive sclerosis

√ round / oval radiolucent nidus (75%) of <1.5 cm in size
√ variable surrounding sclerosis ± central calcification
√ painful scoliosis concave toward lesion / kyphoscoliosis / hyperlordosis / torticollis with spinal location (due to spasm)
√ may show extensive synovitis + effusion + premature loss of cartilage with intraarticular site (lymphofollicular synovitis)
√ osteoarthritis (50%) with intraarticular site 1.5–22 years after onset of symptomatology
√ regional osteoporosis (probably due to disuse)
◊ Radiographically difficult areas: vertebral column, femoral neck, small bones of hand + feet

NUC:
- √ intensely increased radiotracer uptake (increased blood flow + new-bone formation)
- √ double density sign = small area of focal activity (nidus) superimposed on larger area of increased tracer uptake

CT (for detection + precise localization of nidus):
- √ small well-defined round / oval nidus surrounded by variable amount of sclerosis
- √ nidus enhances on dynamic scan
- √ nidus with variable amount of mineralization (50%): punctate / amorphous / ringlike / dense

MR (diminished conspicuity of lesion compared with CT):
- √ nidus isointense to muscle on T1WI
- √ signal intensity increases to between that of muscle + fat / remains low on T2WI
- √ perinidal inflammation of bone marrow (63%)
- √ perinidal soft-tissue inflammation / edema (47%)
- √ synovitis + joint effusion with intraarticular site

Angio:
- √ highly vascularized nidus with intense circumscribed blush appearing in early arterial phase + persisting late into venous phase

Prognosis: no growth progression, infrequent regression

Rx: (1) complete surgical excision of nidus (reactive bone regresses subsequently)
(2) percutaneous CT-guided removal
(3) percutaneous ablation with radio-frequency electrode / laser / alcohol

DDx:
(1) Cortical osteoid osteoma: Brodie abscess, sclerosing osteomyelitis, syphilis, bone island, stress fracture, osteosarcoma, Ewing sarcoma, osteoblastic metastasis, lymphoma, subperiosteal aneurysmal bone cyst, osteoblastoma (progressive growth)
(2) Intraarticular osteoid osteoma: inflammatory / septic / tuberculous / rheumatoid arthritis, nonspecific synovitis / Legg-Calvé-Perthes disease

OSTEOMA

= benign tumor of membranous bone (hamartoma)
Age: adult life
Associated with: Gardner syndrome (multiple osteomas + colonic polyposis)
Location: inner / outer table of calvarium (usually from external table), paranasal sinuses (frontal / ethmoid sinuses), mandible, nasal bones
√ well-circumscribed round extremely dense structureless lesion usually <2 cm in size

Fibrous Osteoma

Probably a form of fibrous dysplasia
Age: childhood
√ less dense than osteoma / radiolucent
√ expanding external table without affecting internal table
DDx: endostoma, bone island, bone infarct (located in medulla)

OSTEOMYELITIS

Acute Osteomyelitis

Age: most commonly affects children
Organisms:
(a) newborns: S. aureus, group B streptococcus, Escherichia coli
(b) children: S. aureus (blood cultures in 50% positive)
(c) adults: S. aureus (60%), enteric species (29%), Streptococcus (8%)
(d) drug addicts: Pseudomonas (86%), Klebsiella, Enterobacteriae; (57 days average delay in diagnosis)
(e) sickle cell disease: S. aureus, Salmonella

Cause:
(1) genitourinary tract infection (72%)
(2) lung infection (14%)
(3) dermal infection (14%): direct contamination from a soft-tissue lesion in diabetic patient

Pathogenesis:
(a) hematogenous spread
(b) direct implantation from a traumatic / iatrogenic source
(c) extension from adjacent soft-tissue infection

Location:
@ Lower extremity (75%)
over pressure points in diabetic foot
@ Vertebrae (53%)
lumbar (75%) > thoracic > cervical (= infectious spondylitis)
@ Radial styloid (24%)
@ Sacroiliac joint (18%)

• leukocytosis + fever (66%)

A. ACUTE NEONATAL OSTEOMYELITIS
Age: onset <30 days of age
• little / no systemic disturbance
√ multicentric involvement more common; often joint involvement
√ bone scan falsely negative / equivocal in 70%

B. ACUTE OSTEOMYELITIS IN INFANCY
Age: <18 months of age
Pathomechanism: spread to epiphysis because transphyseal vessels cross growth plate into <u>epiphysis</u>
√ striking soft-tissue component
√ subperiosteal abscess with extensive periosteal new bone
Cx: frequent joint involvement
Prognosis: rapid healing

C. ACUTE OSTEOMYELITIS IN CHILDHOOD
Age: 2–16 years of age
Pathomechanism:
transphyseal vessels closed; metaphyseal vessels adjacent to growth plate loop back toward metaphysis locating the primary focus of infection into <u>metaphysis</u>; abscess formation in medulla with cortical spread
Location: femur, tibia
√ sequestration frequent
√ periosteal elevation (with disruption of periosteal blood supply)
√ small single / multiple osteolytic areas in metaphysis
√ extensive periosteal reaction parallel to shaft (after 3–6 weeks); may be "lamellar nodular" (DDx: osteoblastoma, eosinophilic granuloma)
√ shortening of bone with destruction of epiphyseal cartilage
√ growth stimulation by hyperemia + premature maturation of adjacent epiphysis
√ midshaft osteomyelitis less frequent site
√ serpiginous tract with small sclerotic rim (PATHOGNOMONIC)

D. ACUTE OSTEOMYELITIS IN ADULTHOOD
Associated with: soft-tissue abscess, pathological fracture
Risk factors: IV drug use, previous trauma, immunosuppressed state, diabetes
√ delicate periosteal new bone
√ joint involvement common

Conventional radiographs (insensitive):
- √ initial radiographs often normal (notoriously poor in early phase of infection for as long as 10–14 days)
- √ localized soft-tissue swelling adjacent to metaphysis with obliteration of usual fat planes (after 3–10 days)
- √ permeative metaphyseal osteolysis (lags 7–14 days behind pathologic changes)
- √ endosteal erosion
- √ intracortical fissuring
- √ involucrum = cloak of laminated / spiculated periosteal reaction (develops after 20 days)
- √ sequestrum = detached necrotic cortical bone (develops after 30 days)
- √ cloaca formation = space in which dead bone resides

CT:
- √ marrow density of >+20 HU difference to healthy side indicates marrow infection

MR:
- √ bone marrow hypointense on T1WI + hyperintense on T2WI (= water-rich inflammatory tissue)
  DDx: neuropathic osteoarthropathy, aseptic arthritis, acute fracture, recent surgery
- √ focal / linear cortical involvement hyperintense on T2WI
- √ hyperintense halo surrounding cortex on T2WI = subperiosteal infection
- √ hyperintense line on T2WI extending from bone to skin surface + enhancement of borders (= sinus tract)

Abscess characteristics:
- √ hyperintense enhancing rim (= hyperemic zone) around a central focus of low intensity (= necrotic / devitalized tissue) on contrast-enhanced T1WI
- √ hyperintense fluid collection surrounded by hypointense pseudocapsule on T2WI + contrast enhancement of granulation tissue
- √ hyperintense adjacent soft tissues on T2WI
- √ fat-suppressed contrast-enhanced imaging (88% sensitive + 93% specific compared with 79% + 53% for nonenhanced MR imaging)

NUC (accuracy approx. 90%):
(1) Ga-67 scans: 100% sensitivity; increased uptake 1 day earlier than for Tc-99m MDP
  ◊ Gallium helpful for chronic osteomyelitis!
(2) Static Tc-99m diphosphonate: 83% sensitivity 5–60% false-negative rate in neonates + children because of (a) masking effect of epiphyseal plates, (b) early diminished blood flow with infection, (c) spectrum of uptake pattern from hot to cold
(3) Three-phase skeletal scintigraphy: 92% sensitivity, 87% specificity
  Phase 1: Radionuclide angiography = perfusion phase of regional blood flow
  Phase 2: "blood pool" images
  Phase 3: "bone uptake"
  Limitations: diagnostic difficulties in children, in posttraumatic / postoperative state, diabetic neuropathy (poor blood supply), neoplasia, septic arthritis, Paget disease, healed osteomyelitis, noninfectious inflammatory process
  DDx: cellulitis (decrease in activity over time)
(4) WBC-scan:
  (a) In-111–labeled leukocytes: best agent for acute infections
  (b) Tc-99m labeled leukocytes: preferred over In-111–leukocyte imaging especially in extremities
  ◊ WBC scans have largely replaced gallium imaging for acute osteomyelitis due to improved photon flux + improved dosimetry (higher dose allowed relative to In-111) allowing faster imaging + greater resolution

- √ "cold" area in early osteomyelitis subsequently becoming "hot" if localized to long bones / pelvis (not seen in vertebral bodies)
- √ local increase in radiopharmaceutical uptake (positive within 24–72 hours)

Cx:
(1) Soft-tissue abscess
(2) Fistula formation
(3) Pathologic fracture
(4) Extension into joint
(5) Growth disturbance due to epiphyseal involvement
(6) Neoplasm
(7) Amyloidosis
(8) Severe deformity with delayed treatment

Chronic Osteomyelitis
- √ thick irregular sclerotic bone with radiolucencies, elevated periosteum, chronic draining sinus

Sclerosing Osteomyelitis of Garré
= STERILE OSTEOMYELITIS
= low-grade nonnecrotic nonpurulent infection
Location: mandible (most commonly)
- √ focal bulge of thickened cortex (sclerosing periosteal reaction)

DDx: osteoid osteoma, stress fracture

Chronic Recurrent Multifocal Osteomyelitis
= benign self-limited disease of unknown etiology
Age: children + adolescents; M:F = 1:2
Histo: nonspecific subacute / chronic osteomyelitis
- • pain, soft-tissue swelling, limited motion

Location: tibia > femur > clavicle > fibula
Site: metaphyses of long bones; often symmetric
- √ small areas of bone lysis, often confluent

Brodie Abscess
= subacute pyogenic osteomyelitis (smoldering indolent infection)
Organism: S. aureus (most common)
Histo: granulation tissue + eburnation

Age: more common in children; M > F
Location: predilection for ends of tubular bones (proximal / distal tibial metaphysis most common); carpal + tarsal bones
Site: metaphysis, rarely traversing the open growth plate; epiphysis (children + infants)
√ central area of lucency surrounded by dense rim of reactive sclerosis
√ lucent tortuous channel extending toward growth plate (PATHOGNOMONIC)
√ periosteal new-bone formation
√ ± adjacent soft-tissue swelling
√ may persist for many months
MR:
√ "double line" effect = high signal intensity of granulation tissue surrounded by low signal intensity of bone sclerosis on T2WI
√ well-defined low- to intermediate-signal lesion outlined by low-signal rim on T1WI
DDx: Osteoid osteoma

Epidermoid Carcinoma

Etiology: complication of chronic osteomyelitis (0.2–1.7%)
Histo: squamous cell carcinoma (90%); occasionally: basal cell carcinoma, adenocarcinoma, fibrosarcoma, angiosarcoma, reticulum cell sarcoma, spindle cell sarcoma, rhabdomyosarcoma, parosteal osteosarcoma, plasmacytoma
Age: 30–80 (mean 55) years; M >> F
Latent period: 20–30 (range of 1.5–72) years
• history of childhood osteomyelitis
• exacerbation of symptoms with increasing pain, enlarging mass
• change in character / amount of sinus drainage
Location: at site of chronically / intermittently draining sinus; tibia (50%), femur (21%)
√ lytic lesion superimposed on changes of chronic osteomyelitis
√ soft-tissue mass
√ pathologic fracture
Prognosis:
(1) Early metastases in 14–20–40% (within 18 months)
(2) No recurrence in 80%

OSTEOPATHIA STRIATA

= VOORHOEVE DISEASE
= autosomal dominant / sporadic inherited disorder
• usually asymptomatic (similar to osteopoikilosis)
Location: all long bones affected; the only bone sclerosis primarily involving metaphysis (with extension into epi- and diaphysis)
√ longitudinal striations of dense bone in metaphysis
√ radiating densities of "sunburst" appearance from acetabulum into ileum

OSTEOPETROSIS

= ALBERS-SCHÖNBERG DISEASE = MARBLE BONE DISEASE = rare hereditary disorder

Path: defective osteoclast function with failure of proper reabsorption + remodeling of primary spongiosa; bone sclerotic + thick but structurally weak + brittle

A. INFANTILE AUTOSOMAL RECESSIVE TYPE
= congenital more severe form
Cause: defect on chromosome 11q13
• failure to thrive
• premature senile appearance of facies
• severe dental caries
• pancytopenia (= anemia, leukocytopenia, thrombocytopenia) due to severe marrow depression
• cranial nerve compression (optic atrophy, deafness)
• hepatosplenomegaly (extramedullary hematopoiesis)
• lymphadenopathy
• subarachnoid hemorrhage (due to thrombocytopenia)
May be associated with:
renal tubular acidosis + cerebral calcification
√ dense skeleton
√ splayed metaphyses + costochondral junctions
√ fractures from minor trauma (due to brittle bones)
Prognosis: stillbirth, survival beyond middle life uncommon (death due to recurrent infection, massive hemorrhage, terminal leukemia)
DDx: chronic renal failure, oxalosis, pyknodysostosis, physiologic sclerosis

B. BENIGN ADULT AUTOSOMAL DOMINANT TYPE
Cause: defect on chromosome 1p21
• 50% asymptomatic
• recurrent fractures, mild anemia
• occasionally cranial nerve palsy
√ Erlenmeyer flask deformity = clublike long bones due to lack of tubulization + flaring of ends
Phenotype I:
√ diffuse osteosclerosis = generalized dense amorphous structureless bones with obliteration of normal trabecular pattern; mandible least commonly involved
√ cortical thickening with medullary encroachment
Phenotype II:
√ bone-within-bone appearance (= endobones)
√ "sandwich" vertebrae / rugger-jersey spine
√ alternating sclerotic + radiolucent transverse metaphyseal lines (phalanges, ilium) as indicators of fluctuating course of disease
√ longitudinal metaphyseal striations
√ obliteration of mastoid cells, paranasal sinuses, basal foramina by osteosclerosis
√ sclerosis predominantly involving base of skull; calvaria often spared
Prognosis: normal life expectancy

Cx: (1) Usually transverse fractures (common because of brittle bones) with abundant callus + normal healing
(2) Crowding of marrow (myelophthisic anemia + extramedullary hematopoiesis)
(3) Frequently terminates in acute leukemia

Rx: bone marrow transplant
DDx: (1) Heavy metal poisoning
(2) Melorheostosis (limited to one extremity)
(3) Hypervitaminosis D
(4) Pyknodysostosis
(5) Fibrous dysplasia of skull / face

OSTEOPOIKILOSIS

= OSTEOPATHIA CONDENSANS DISSEMINATA
= autosomal-dominant disorder; M > F
Associated with: dermatofibrosis lenticularis disseminata
• asymptomatic
Histo: compact bone islands
Location: in most metaphyses + epiphyses (rarely extending into midshaft); concentrated at glenoid + acetabulum, wrist, ankle, pelvis; rare in skull, ribs, vertebral centra, mandible
√ multiple ovoid / lenticular bone islands (2–10 mm) in cancellous bone
√ long axis of lesions parallel to long axis of bone
√ scintigraphic activity rare
Prognosis: not progressive, no change after cessation of growth
DDx: (1) Epiphyseal dysplasia (metaphyses normal)
(2) Melorheostosis (diaphyseal involvement)

OSTEOSARCOMA

Most common malignant primary bone tumor in young adults + children; 2nd most common primary malignant bone tumor after multiple myeloma
Prevalence: 4–5:1,000,000; 15% of all primary bone tumors confirmed at biopsy
Types & Frequency:

A. Conventional osteosarcoma:		
– high-grade intramedullary		75%
– telangiectatic		4.5–11%
– low-grade intraosseous		4–5%
– small cell		1–4%
– osteosarcomatosis		3–4%
– gnathic		6–9%
B. Surface / juxtacortical osteosarcoma:		4–10%
– intracortical	rare	
– parosteal	65%	
– periosteal	25%	
– high-grade surface	10%	
C. Extraskeletal		4%
D. Secondary osteosarcoma		5–7%

Prognosis: dependent on age, sex, tumor size, site, classification; best predictor is degree of tissue necrosis in postresection specimen following chemotherapy (91% survival with tumor necrosis >90%, 14% survival with <90% tumor necrosis)

Extraskeletal Osteosarcoma

= located within soft tissue without attachment to bone / periosteum
Incidence: 1% of soft-tissue sarcomas
Histo: variable amounts of neoplastic osteoid + bone + cartilage; frequently associated with fibrosarcoma, malignant fibrous histiocytoma, malignant peripheral nerve sheath tumor
Mean age: 50 years; 94% >30 years of age; M > F
Location: lower extremity (thigh in 42–47%), upper extremity (12–23%), retroperitoneum (8–17%), buttock, back, orbit, submental, axilla, abdomen, neck, kidney, breast
• slowly growing soft-tissue mass
• painful + tender (25–50%)
• history of trauma (12–31%): in preexisting myositis ossificans / site of intramuscular injection
√ often deep-seated + fixed soft-tissue tumor (average diameter of 9 cm)
√ focal / massive area of mineralization (>50%)
√ increased radionuclide uptake on bone scan
Prognosis:
(1) multiple local recurrences (in 80–90%) after interval of 2 months to 10 years
(2) metastases after interval of 1 month to 4 years: lungs (81–100%), lymph nodes (25%), bone, subcutis, liver
(3) death within 2–3 years (>50%) with tumor size as major predictor

High-grade Intramedullary Osteosarcoma

= CENTRAL OSTEOSARCOMA = CONVENTIONAL OSTEOSARCOMA
Histo: arising from undifferentiated mesenchymal tissue; forming fibrous / cartilaginous / osseous matrix (mostly mixed) that produces osteoid / immature bone
(a) osteoblastic (50–80%)
(b) chondroblastic (5–25%)
(c) fibroblastic-fibrohistiocytic (7–25%)
Age: bimodal distribution 10– 25 years and >60 years; 21% <10 years; 68% <15 years; 70% between 10 and 30 years; M:F = 3:2 to 2:1; >35 years: related to preexisting condition
• painful swelling (1–2 months' duration)
• fever (frequent)
• slight elevation of alkaline phosphatase
• diabetes mellitus (paraneoplastic syndrome) in 25%
Location: long bones (70–80%), femur (40–45%), tibia (16–20%); 50–55% about knee; proximal humerus (10–15%); facial bones (8%); cylindrical bone <30 years; flat bone (ilium) >50 years
Site: origin in metaphysis (90–95%) / diaphysis (2–11%) /epiphysis (<1%); growth through open physis with extension into epiphysis (75–88%)
Doubling time: 20–30 day
√ usually large bone lesion of >5–6 cm when first detected
√ cloudlike density (90%) / almost normal density / osteolytic (fibroblastic type)
√ aggressive periosteal reaction: sunburst / hair-on-end / onion-peel = laminated / Codman triangle
√ moth-eaten bone destruction + cortical disruption

√ soft-tissue mass with tumor new bone (osseous / cartilaginous type)
√ transphyseal spread before plate closure (75–88%); physis does NOT act as a barrier to tumor spread
√ spontaneous pneumothorax (due to subpleural metastases)

NUC (bone scintigraphy):
√ intensely increased activity on blood flow, blood pool, delayed images (hypervascularity, new-bone formation)
√ soft-tissue extension demonstrated, especially with SPECT
√ bone scan establishes local extent (extent of involvement easily overestimated due to intensity of uptake), skip lesions, metastases to bone + soft tissues

CT:
√ soft-tissue attenuation (nonmineralized portion) replacing fatty bone marrow
√ low attenuation (higher water content of chondroblastic component / hemorrhage / necrosis)
√ very high attenuation (mineralized matrix)

MR (preferred modality):
√ tumor of intermediate signal intensity on T1WI + high signal intensity on T2WI
√ clearly defines marrow extent (best on T1WI), vascular involvement, soft-tissue component (best on T2WI)

Evaluate for:
(1) extent of marrow + soft-tissue involvement
(2) invasion of epiphysis
(3) joint (19–24%) + neurovascular involvement
(4) viable tumor + mineralized matrix for biopsy

Metastases (in 2% at presentation):
(a) hematogenous lung metastases (15%): calcifying; spontaneous pneumothorax secondary to subpleural cavitating nodules rupturing into pleural space
(b) lymph nodes, liver, brain (may be calcified)
(c) skeletal metastases uncommon (unlike Ewing sarcoma); skip lesions = discontinuous tumor foci in marrow cavity in 1–25%

Cx: (1) pathologic fracture (15–20%)
(2) radiation-induced osteosarcoma (30 years delay)

Rx: chemotherapy followed by wide surgical resection

Prognosis: 60–80% 5-year survival
(1) amputation: 20% 5-year survival; 15% develop skeletal metastases; 75% dead within <2 years
(2) multidrug chemotherapy: 55% 4-year survival more proximal lesions carry higher mortality (0% 2-year survival for axial primary)

Predictors of poor outcome:
metastasis at presentation, soft-tissue mass >20 cm, pathologic fracture, skip lesions in marrow

Predictors of poor response to chemotherapy:
no change / increase in size of soft-tissue mass, increase in bone destruction

DDx: Osteoid osteoma, sclerosing osteomyelitis, Charcot joint

High-grade Surface Osteosarcoma

Location: femur, humerus, fibula
Site: diaphysis
√ similar to periosteal osteosarcoma
√ often involve entire circumference of bone
√ frequent invasion of medullary canal

Prognosis: identical to conventional intramedullary osteosarcoma

Intracortical Osteosarcoma

Rarest form of osteosarcoma

Histo: sclerosing variant of osteosarcoma which may contain small foci of chondro- or fibrosarcoma

Location: femur, tibia
√ tumor <4 cm in diameter
√ intracortical geographic bone lysis
√ tumor margin may be well defined with thickening of surrounding cortex
√ metastases in 29%

Low-grade Intraosseous Osteosarcoma

= WELL-DIFFERENTIATED / SCLEROSING OSTEOSARCOMA

Path: penetration among bony trabeculae; fibrous stroma sometimes lacking nuclear atypia + pleomorphism; highly variable amount of tumor osteoid production; may be misinterpreted as fibrous dysplasia

Age: most frequently 3rd decade; M:F = 1:1

• protracted clinical course with nonspecific symptoms

Location: about the knee; femur involved in 50%
Site: metaphysis; often with extension into epiphysis
√ may have well-defined margins + sclerotic rim
√ diffuse sclerosis
√ expansile remodeling of bone
√ subtle signs of aggressiveness: bone lysis, focally indistinct margin, cortical destruction, soft-tissue mass, periosteal reaction

N.B.: the relatively benign appearance has resulted in misdiagnosis as a benign entity!

Cx: transformation into high-grade osteosarcoma

Prognosis: similar to parosteal osteosarcoma; 80–90% 5-year survival rate; local recurrence in 10% (due to inadequate resection)

DDx: fibrous dysplasia, nonossifying fibroma, chondrosarcoma, chondromyxoid fibroma

Osteosarcoma of Jaw

= GNATHIC OSTEOSARCOMA

Average age: 34 years (10–15 years older than in conventional osteosarcoma)

Histo: chondroblastic predominance (~50%), osteoblastic predominance (~25%); better differentiated (grade 2 or 3) than conventional osteosarcoma (grade 3 or 4)

• simulating periodontal disease: rapidly enlarging mass, lump, swelling

- paresthesia (if inferior alveolar nerve involved)
- painful / loose teeth, bleeding gum

Location: body of mandible (lytic), alveolar ridge of maxilla (sclerotic), maxillary antrum

√ osteolytic / osteoblastic / mixed pattern
√ osteoid matrix (60–80%)
√ aggressive periosteal reaction for mandibular lesion
√ soft-tissue mass (100%)
√ opacification of maxillary sinus (frequent in maxillary lesions)

Prognosis: 40% 5-year survival rate (lower probability of metastases, lower grade)

DDx: metastatic disease (lung, breast, kidney), multiple myeloma, direct invasion by contiguous tumor from oral cavity, Ewing sarcoma, primary lymphoma of bone, chondrosarcoma, fibrosarcoma, acute osteomyelitis, ameloblastoma, Langerhans cell histiocytosis, giant cell reparative granuloma, "brown tumor" of HPT

Osteosarcomatosis

= MULTIFOCAL OSTEOSARCOMA = MULTIPLE SCLEROTIC OSTEOSARCOMA

Frequency: 2.7–4.2% of osteosarcomas

Etiology: (a) multicentric type of osteosarcoma
(b) multiple metastatic bone lesions

Classification (Amstutz):

Type I multiple synchronous bone lesions occurring within 5 months of diagnosis + patient ≤18 years of age

Type II multiple synchronous bone lesions occurring within 5 months of presentation + patient >18 years of age

Type IIIa early metachronous metastatic osteosarcoma occurring 5 to 24 months after diagnosis

Type IIIb late metachronous metastatic osteosarcoma occurring >24 months after diagnosis

Age: Amstutz type I = 4–18 (mean 11) years
Amstutz type II = 19–63 (mean 30) years

Site: metaphysis of long bones; may extend into epiphyseal plate / begin in epiphysis

√ multicentric simultaneously appearing lesions with a radiologically dominant tumor (97%)
√ smaller lesions are densely opaque (osteoblastic)
√ lesions bilateral + symmetrical
√ early: bone islands
√ late: entire metaphysis fills with sclerotic lesions breaking through cortex
√ lesions are of same size
√ lung metastases (62%)

Prognosis: uniformly poor with mean survival of 12 (range, 6–37) months

DDx: heavy metal poisoning, sclerosing osteitis, progressive diaphyseal dysplasia, melorheostosis, osteopoikilosis, bone infarction, osteopetrosis

Parosteal Osteosarcoma

Frequency: 4% of all osteosarcomas; 65% of all juxtacortical osteosarcomas

Origin: outer layer of periosteum; slowly growing lesion with fulminating course if tumor reaches medullary canal

Histo: low-grade lesion with higher-grade regions (22–64%), invasion of medullary canal (8–59%); fibrous stroma + extensive osteoid with small foci of cartilage

Age: peak age 38 years (range of 12–58 years); 50% > age 30 (for central osteosarcoma 75% < age 30); M:F = 2:3

Location: posterior aspect of distal femur (50–65%), either end of tibia, proximal humerus, fibula, rare in other long bones

Site: metaphysis (80–90%)

- palpable mass

√ large lobulated "cauliflower-like" homogeneous ossific mass extending away from cortex
√ "string sign" = initially fine radiolucent line separating tumor mass from cortex (30–40%)
√ tumor stalk (= attachment to cortex) grows with tumor obliterating the radiolucent cleavage plane
√ cortical thickening without aggressive periosteal reaction
√ tumor periphery less dense than center (DDx: myositis ossificans with periphery more dense than center + without attachment to cortex)
√ large soft-tissue component with osseous + cartilaginous elements

Prognosis: 80–90% 5- and 10-year survival rates (best prognosis of all osteosarcomas)

DDx: osteochondroma, myositis ossificans, juxtacortical hematoma, extraosseous osteosarcoma

Periosteal Osteosarcoma

Origin: deep layer of periosteum

Histo: intermediate-grade lesion; highly chondroblastic lesion with smaller areas of osteoid formation

Age: peak 10–20 years (range of 13–70 years)

Location: femur and tibia (85–95%), ulna and humerus (5–10%)

Site: diaphysis / metadiaphysis of long bone; limited to periphery of cortex with normal endosteal margin + medullary canal (resembles parosteal sarcoma)

√ tumor 7–12 cm in length, 2–4 cm in width, involving 50% of osseous circumference
√ tumor base closely attached to cortex over entire extent of tumor
√ tumor lies in apparent depression on bone surface causing scalloped surface of thickened diaphyseal cortex
√ short spicules of new bone perpendicular to shaft extending into broad-based elliptical soft-tissue mass
√ solid (cortical thickening) / aggressive periosteal reaction (Codman triangle) at upper and lower margins of lesion
√ NO cortical destruction / medullary cavity invasion

√ chondroblastic areas of low attenuation on CT, hypointense on T1WI, very hyperintense on T2WI

Prognosis: 80–90% cure rate (better prognosis than central osteosarcoma with 50% 5-year survival but worse than parosteal osteosarcoma)

DDx: juxtacortical chondrosarcoma

Secondary Osteosarcoma

Cause: malignant transformation within benign process

(1) Paget disease (67–90%)

◊ 0.2–7.5% of patients with Paget disease develop osteosarcoma dependent on extent of disease

(2) Sequelae of irradiation (6–22%) 2–40 years ago (malignant fibrous histiocytoma most common; fibrosarcoma 3rd most common)

◊ 0.02–4% of patients with radiation therapy develop osteosarcoma related to exposure dose (usually >1,000 cGy)

(3) Osteonecrosis, fibrous dysplasia, metallic implants, osteogenesis imperfecta, chronic osteomyelitis, retinoblastoma (familial bilateral type)

Path: high-grade anaplastic tissue with little / no mineralization

Age: middle-aged / late adulthood

√ aggressive bone destruction in area of preexisting condition associated with large soft-tissue mass

Prognosis: <5% 5-year survival rate

Small-cell Osteosarcoma

Age: similar to conventional osteosarcoma; M:F = 1:1

Histo: small round blue cells (similar to Ewing sarcoma) lacking cellular uniformity and consistently producing fine reticular osteoid

Location: distal femur

Site: metaphysis with frequent extension into epiphysis; diaphysis (in 15%)

√ predominantly permeative lytic medullary lesion
√ cortical breakthrough
√ aggressive periosteal reaction
√ associated soft-tissue mass

Prognosis: extremely poor

Telangiectatic Osteosarcoma

= MALIGNANT BONE ANEURYSM

Frequency: 4–11% of all osteosarcomas

Age: 3–67 (mean 20) years; M:F = 3:2

Path: malignant osteoid-forming sarcoma of bone with large blood-filled vascular channels

Histo: hemorrhagic + cystic + necrotic spaces occupying >90% of the lesion before therapy; blood-filled cavernous vessels lined with osteoclastic giant cells

Location: about knee (62%); distal femur (48%), proximal tibia (14%), proximal humerus (16%)

Site: metaphysis (90%); extension into epiphysis (87%)

√ geographic bone destruction with a wide zone of transition
√ marked aneurysmal expansion of bone (19%)
√ fluid-fluid levels (90%)
√ nodular calcific foci of osteoid (61–81%)
√ "doughnut sign" = peripherally increased uptake with central photopenia on bone scan

DDx: aneurysmal bone cyst (no enhancing rim of viable tumor along lesion periphery)

OXALOSIS

Rare inborn error of metabolism

Etiology: excessive amounts of oxalic acid combine with calcium and deposit throughout body (kidneys, soft tissue, bone)

• hyperoxaluria = urinary excretion of oxalic acid >50 mg/ day
• progressive renal failure

√ osteoporosis = cystic rarefaction + sclerotic margins in tubular bones on metaphyseal side, may extend throughout diaphysis
√ erosions on concave side of metaphysis near epiphysis (DDx: hyperparathyroidism)
√ bone-within-bone appearance of spine
√ nephrocalcinosis (2° HPT: subperiosteal resorption, rugger jersey spine, sclerotic metaphyseal bands)

Cx: pathologic fractures

PACHYDERMOPERIOSTOSIS

= OSTEODERMOPATHIA HYPERTROPHICANS (TOURAINE-SOLENTE-GOLE) = PRIMARY HYPERTROPHIC OSTEOARTHROPATHY

Autosomal dominant

Age: 3–38 years with progression into late 20s / 30s; M >> F

• large skin folds of face + scalp

Location: epiphyses + diametaphyseal region of tubular bones; distal third of bones of legs + forearms (early); distal phalanges rarely involved

√ enlargement of paranasal sinuses
√ irregular periosteal proliferation of phalanges + distal long bones (hand + feet) beginning in epiphyseal region at tendon / ligament insertions
√ thick cortex, BUT NO narrowing of medulla
√ clubbing
√ may have acroosteolysis

Prognosis: progression ceases after several years

DDx: pulmonary osteoarthropathy, thyroid acropachy

PAGET DISEASE

= OSTEITIS DEFORMANS

= multifocal chronic skeletal disease characterized by disordered and exaggerated bone remodeling

Etiology: ? chronic paramyxoviral infection

Prevalence: 3% of individuals >40 years; 10% of persons >80 years; higher prevalence in northern latitudes; 2nd most common disease (after osteoporosis) affecting older individuals

Age: Caucasian >55 years (in 3%); >85 years (in 10%); unusual <40 years; M:F = 2:1

Histo: increased resorption + increased bone formation; newly formed bone is abnormally soft with disorganized trabecular pattern ("mosaic pattern") causing deformity

(a) ACTIVE PHASE = OSTEOLYTIC PHASE
= intense osteoclastic activity = aggressive bone resorption with lytic lesions
Path: replacement of hematopoietic bone marrow by fibrous connective tissue with numerous large vascular channels
√ osteoporosis circumscripta of skull
√ flame-shaped radiolucency

(b) MIDDLE / MIXED PHASE (common)
= decreased osteoclastic activity + increased osteoblastic activity
√ coexistence of lytic + sclerotic phases

(c) INACTIVE / LATE PHASE = QUIESCENT PHASE
= diminished osteoblastic activity with decreased bone turnover
Path: loss of excessive vascularity
√ osteosclerosis + cortical accretion (eg, ivory vertebral body)

- asymptomatic (1/5 – 3/4)
- fatigue
- enlarged hat size
- peripheral nerve compression
- neurologic disorders from compression of brainstem (basilar invagination)
- hearing loss, blindness, facial palsy (narrowing of neural foramina) — rare
- pain from (a) primary disease process — rare
  (b) pathologic fracture
  (c) malignant transformation
  (d) degenerative joint disease / rheumatic disorder aggravated by skeletal deformity
- local hyperthermia of overlying skin
- high-output congestive heart failure from markedly increased perfusion (rare)
- increased alkaline phosphatase (increased bone formation)
- hydroxyproline increased (increased bone resorption)
- normal serum calcium + phosphorus

Sites: usually polyostotic + asymmetric; pelvis (75%) > lumbar spine > thoracic spine > proximal femur > calvarium > scapula > distal femur > proximal tibia > proximal humerus

Sensitivity: scintigraphy + radiography (60%)
scintigraphy only (27–94%)
radiography only (13–74%)

√ osseous expansion
√ trabecular coarsening
√ cortical thickening
√ cystlike areas (fat-filled marrow cavity / blood-filled sinusoids / liquefactive degeneration + necrosis of proliferating fibrous tissue)

@ Skull (involvement in 29–65%)
√ inner + outer table involved
√ diploic widening
√ osteoporosis circumscripta = well-defined lysis, most commonly in calvarium anteriorly, occasionally in long bones (destructive active stage)
√ "cotton wool" appearance = mixed lytic + blastic pattern of thickened calvarium (late stage)
√ basilar impression with encroachment on foramen magnum
√ deossification + sclerosis in maxilla
√ sclerosis of base of skull

@ Long bones (almost invariable at end of bone; rarely in diaphysis)
√ "candle flame" / "blade of grass" lysis = advancing tip of V-shaped lytic defect in diaphysis of long bone originating in subarticular site (CHARACTERISTIC)
√ lateral curvature of femur, anterior curvature of tibia (commonly resulting in fracture)

@ Ribs (1–4%)

@ Small / flat bones
√ bubbly destruction + periosteal successive layering

@ Pelvis
√ thickened trabeculae in sacrum, ilium; rarefaction in central portion of ilium
√ thickening of iliopectineal line
√ acetabular protrusion (DDx: metastatic disease not deforming) + secondary degenerative joint disease

@ Spine (upper cervical, low dorsal, midlumbar)
√ lytic / coarse trabeculations at periphery of bone
√ "picture-frame vertebra" = bone-within-bone appearance = enlarged square vertebral body with reinforced peripheral trabeculae + radiolucent inner aspect, typically in lumbar spine
√ "ivory vertebra" = blastic vertebra with increased density
√ ossification of spinal ligaments, paravertebral soft tissue, disk spaces

Bone scan (94% sensitive):
√ usually markedly increased uptake (symptomatic lesions strikingly positive due to increased blood flow + osteoblastic activity)
√ normal scan in some sclerotic burned-out lesions
√ marginal uptake in lytic lesions
√ enlargement + deformity of bones

Bone marrow scan:
√ sulfur colloid bone marrow uptake is decreased (marrow replacement by cellular fibrovascular tissue)

MR:
Indications: imaging of complications (spinal stenosis, basilar impression, tumor staging)
√ areas of decreased signal intensity within marrow on T1WI + increased intensity on T2WI (= fibrovascular tissue resembling granulation tissue)
√ hypointense area / area of signal void on T1WI + T2WI (cortical thickening, coarse trabeculation)
√ reduction in size + signal intensity of medullary cavity (replacement of high-signal-intensity fatty marrow by increased medullary bone formation)

√ focal areas of higher signal intensity than fatty marrow (= cystlike fat-filled marrow spaces)
√ widening of bone

Cx: (1) Associated neoplasia (0.7–1–20%)
(a) sarcomatous transformation into osteosarcoma (22–90%), fibrosarcoma / malignant fibrous histiocytoma (29–51%), chondrosarcoma (1–15%)
√ osteolysis in pelvis, femur, humerus
Prognosis: <10% 5-year survival
(b) multicentric giant cell tumor (3–10%)
√ lytic expansile lesion in skull, facial bones
(c) lymphoma, plasma cell myeloma
(2) Insufficiency fracture
(a) "banana fracture" = tiny horizontal cortical infractions on convex surfaces of lower extremity long bones (lateral bowing of femur, anterior bowing of tibia);
(b) compression fractures of vertebrae (soft bone despite increased density)
(3) Neurologic entrapment
(a) basilar impression with obstructive hydrocephalus + brainstem compression + syringomyelia
(b) spinal stenosis with extradural spinal block (osseous expansion / osteosarcoma / vertebral retropulsion owing to compression fracture)
(4) Early-onset osteoarthritis
Pathogenesis: altered biomechanics across affected articulations

Rx: calcitonin, biphosphonates, mithramycin
Detection of recurrence:
(a) in 1/3 detected by bone scan
(b) in 1/3 detected by biomarkers (alkaline phosphatase, urine hydroxyproline)
(c) in 1/3 by scan + biomarkers simultaneously
√ diffuse (most common) / focal increase in tracer uptake
√ extension of uptake beyond boundaries of initial lesion
DDx: osteosclerotic metastasis, osteolytic metastasis, Hodgkin disease, vertebral hemangioma

PARAOSTEOARTHROPATHY

= HETEROTOPIC BONE FORMATION = ECTOPIC OSSIFICATION = MYOSITIS OSSIFICANS

Common complication following surgical manipulation, total hip replacement (62%) and chronic immobilization (spinal cord injury / neuromuscular disorders)

Mechanism: pluripotent mesenchymal cell lays down matrix for formation of heterotopic bone similar to endosteal bone

Causes: para- / quadriplegia (40–50%), myelomeningocele, poliomyelitis, severe head injury, cerebrovascular disease, CNS infections (tetanus, rabies), surgery (commonly following total hip replacement)

Evolution: calcifications seen 4–10 weeks following insult; progression for 6–14 months; trabeculations by 2–3 months; stable lamellar bone ankylosis in 5% by 12–18 months

√ largest quantity of calcifications around joints, especially hip, along fascial planes
√ disuse osteoporosis of lower extremities
√ renal calculi (elevation of serum calcium levels)

Radiographic grading system (Brooker):
0 no soft-tissue ossification
I separate small foci of ossification
II >1 cm gap between opposing bone surfaces of heterotopic ossifications
III <1 cm gap between opposing bone surfaces
IV bridging ossification

Bone scan:
√ tracer accumulation in ectopic bone
√ assessment of maturity for optimal time of surgical resection (indicated by same amount of uptake as normal bone)

Cx: ankylosis in 5%
Rx: 1000–2000 rad within 4 days following surgical removal

PHENYLKETONURIA

High incidence of x-ray changes in phenylalanine-restricted infants:
√ metaphyseal cupping of long bones (30–50%), especially wrist
√ calcific spicules extending vertically from metaphysis into epiphyseal cartilage (DDx to rickets)
√ sclerotic metaphyseal margins
√ osteoporosis
√ delayed skeletal maturation
DDx: homocystinuria

PHOSPHORUS POISONING

Etiology: (1) ingestion of metallic phosphorus (yellow phosphorus)
(2) treatment of rachitis or TB with phosphorized cod liver oil

Location: long tubular bones, ilium
√ multiple transverse lines (intermittent treatment with phosphorus)
√ lines disappear after some years

PIERRE ROBIN SYNDROME

May be associated with: CHD, defects of eye and ear, hydrocephalus, microcephaly
• glossoptosis
√ micrognathia = hypoplastic receding mandible
√ arched ± cleft palate
√ rib pseudarthrosis
Cx: airway obstruction (relatively large tongue), aspiration

PIGMENTED VILLONODULAR SYNOVITIS

= PVNS = benign tumor of histiocytic origin / inflammatory process with extensive intraarticular highly vascular synovial proliferation

Cause: frequently history of antecedent trauma

Path: many villous / frondlike synovial proliferations

Histo: (1) hyperplasia of undifferentiated connective tissue with multinucleated large cells ingesting hemosiderin / lipoid (foam / giant cells)
(2) villonodular appearance of synovial membrane ± fibrosis
(3) pressure erosion / invasion of adjoining bone

Age: mainly 3rd–4th decade (range 12–68 years); 50% <40 years; M:F=1:1

- hemorrhagic "chocolate" / serosanguinous / xanthochromic joint effusion without trauma
- insidious onset of swelling, pain of long duration
- joint stiffness with decreased range of motion, joint locking

Location: knee (80%) > hip > ankle > shoulder > elbow > tarsal + carpal joints; predominantly monoarticular (DDx: degenerative arthritis)

√ soft-tissue swelling around joint (effusion + synovial proliferation):
  √ joint effusion in knee, but not relevant in other joints
√ dense soft tissues (hemosiderin deposits)
√ subchondral pressure erosion (56%) at margins of joint on both sides of joint
√ multiple sites of irregular cystlike radiolucent defects due to invasion of bone
√ NO calcifications, osteoporosis, joint space narrowing (until late)

CT:
  √ small radiographically invisible erosions
  √ juxtaarticular soft-tissue mass with high attenuation

MR:
  √ masses of synovial tissue in a joint with effusion
  √ scalloping / truncation of prefemoral fat pad
  √ predominantly low signal intensity on all sequences (due to presence of iron) is CHARACTERISTIC
  √ often heterogeneous low + high signal intensity on T2WI:
    √ low-signal intensity on T2WI in periphery of lesions (magnetic susceptibility effect of hemosiderin)
    DDx: hemosiderin deposits in other diseases (eg, rheumatoid arthritis)
    √ high-signal intensity areas (due to fat, effusion, edema, inflammation)

Rx: synovectomy (50% recurrence rate), arthrodesis, arthroplasty, radiation

DDx: (1) Degenerative / traumatic arthritis
(2) Synovial sarcoma (solitary calcified mass outside joint)
(3) Sclerosing hemangioma
(4) Benign xanthoma
(5) Xanthogranuloma

Intraarticular Localized Nodular Synovitis

= synovial lining without hemosiderin

Tenosynovial Giant Cell Tumor

= localized form of PVNS only involving the tendon sheath

POLAND SYNDROME

May be associated with: aplasia of mamilla / breast

Autosomal recessive

√ unilateral absence of the sternocostal head of the pectoralis major muscle
√ ipsilateral syndactyly + brachydactyly
√ rib anomalies

POLIOMYELITIS

√ osteoporosis
√ soft-tissue calcification / ossification
√ intervertebral disk calcification
√ rib erosion commonly on superior margin of 3rd + 4th rib (secondary to pressure from scapula)
√ "bamboo" spine (resembling ankylosing spondylitis)
√ sacroiliac joint narrowing

POPLITEAL CYST

= BAKER CYST
= synovial cyst in the posterior aspect of knee joint communicating with posterior joint capsule

Prevalence: 19% in general orthopedic patients, 61% in patients with rheumatoid arthritis

Pathophysiology:
formed by escape of synovial effusion into one of the bursae; fluid trapped by one-way valvular mechanism
(a) Bunsen-type valve = expanding cyst compresses the communicating channel
(b) ball-type valve = ball composed of fibrin + cellular debris plugs the communication channel

Etiology: (1) Arthritis (rheumatoid arthritis most common)
(2) Internal derangement (meniscal / anterior cruciate ligament tears)
(3) Pigmented villonodular synovitis

- pseudothrombophlebitis syndrome (= pain + swelling in calf)
- cellulitis (after leakage / rupture)

Location: (a) gastrocnemio-semimembranous bursa = posterior to gastrocnemius muscle at level of medial condyle
(b) supralateral bursa = between lateral head of gastrocnemius muscle + distal end of biceps muscle superior to lateral condyle (uncommon)
(c) popliteal bursa = beneath lateral meniscus + anterior to popliteal muscle (uncommon)

√ communication with bursa (documented on arthrogram)
√ hypointense collection on T1WI + hyperintense on T2WI

Types:
1. Intact cyst
   √ smooth contour
2. Dissected cyst
   √ smooth contour extending along fascial planes (usually between gastrocnemius + soleus)
3. Ruptured cyst
   √ leakage into calf tissues

DDx of other synovial cysts about the knee:
(1) Meniscal cyst (at lateral / medial side of joint line; associated with horizontal cleavage tears)
(2) Tibiofibular cyst (at proximal tibiofibular joint, which communicates with knee joint in 10%)
(3) Cruciate cyst (surrounding anterior / posterior cruciate ligaments following ligamentous injury)

PROGERIA

= HUTCHINSON-GILFORD SYNDROME
= autosomal recessive inheritance; most commonly in populations with consanguineous marriages (Japanese, Jewish)
Age: shortly after adolescence; M:F = 1:1

Characteristic habitus + stature:
- symmetric retardation of growth
- absent adolescent growth spurt
- dwarf with short stature + light body weight
- spindly extremities with stocky trunk
- beak-shaped nose + shallow orbits

Premature senescence:
- birdlike appearance
- graying of hair + premature baldness
- hyperpigmentation
- voice alteration
- diffuse arteriosclerosis
- bilateral cataracts
- osteoporosis

Scleroderma-like skin changes:
- atrophic skin + muscles
- circumscribed hyperkeratosis
- telangiectasia
- tight skin
- cutaneous ulcerations
- localized soft-tissue calcifications

Endocrine abnormalities:
- diabetes
- hypogonadism

√ generalized osteoporosis
@ Skull
√ thin cranial vault
√ delayed sutural closure + wormian bones
√ hypoplastic facial bones (maxilla + mandible)
@ Chest
√ narrow thorax + slender ribs
√ progressive resorption with fibrous replacement of outer portions of thinned clavicles (HALLMARK)
√ coronary artery + heart valve calcifications with cardiac enlargement
@ Extremities & joints
√ short + slender long bones
√ coxa valga
√ valgus of humeral head
√ acroosteolysis of terminal phalanges (occasionally)
√ flexion + extension deformities of toes (hallux valgus, pes planus)
√ excessive degenerative joint disease of major + peripheral joints
√ neurotrophic joint lesions (feet)
√ widespread osteomyelitis + septic arthritis (hands, feet, limbs)
@ Soft tissue
√ soft-tissue atrophy of extremities
√ soft-tissue calcifications around bony prominences (ankle, wrist, elbow, knee)
√ peripheral vascular calcifications = premature atherosclerosis

Prognosis: most patients die in their 30s / 40s from complications of arteriosclerosis (myocardial infarction, stroke) or neoplasm (sarcoma, meningioma, thyroid carcinoma)
DDx: Cockayne syndrome (mental retardation, retinal atrophy, deafness, family history)

PSEUDOACHONDROPLASIA

- normal face + head

√ limb shortening
√ irregular epiphyses
√ scoliosis
√ coxa vara
√ marked shortening of bones in hands + feet

PSEUDOFRACTURES

= LOOSER LINES = LOOSER ZONES = OSTEOID SEAMS = MILKMAN SYNDROME
= insufficiency stress fractures + nonunion (incomplete healing due to mineral deficiency)
Path: area of unmineralized woven bone occurring at sites of mechanical stress / nutrient vessel entry
Associated with:
(1) Osteomalacia / rickets
(2) Paget disease ("banana fracture")
(3) Osteogenesis imperfecta tarda
(4) Fibrous dysplasia
(5) Organic renal disease in 1%
(6) Renal tubular dysfunction
(7) Congenital hypophosphatasia
(8) Congenital hyperphosphatasia ("juvenile Paget disease")
(9) Vitamin D malabsorption / deficiency
(10) Neurofibromatosis

mnemonic: "POOF"
Paget disease
Osteomalacia
Osteogenesis imperfecta
Fibrous dysplasia

Common locations:
scapulae (axillary margin, lateral + superior margin), medial femoral neck + shaft, pubic + ischial rami, ribs, lesser trochanter, ischial tuberosity, proximal 1/3 of ulna, distal 1/3 of radius, phalanges, metatarsals, metacarpals, clavicle
√ typically bilateral + symmetric at right angles to bone margin
√ paralleled by marginal sclerosis in later stages
√ healing fracture with little or no callus response

	PHypoPT	PPHypoPT
√ calcification of basal ganglia	44%	8%
√ soft-tissue calcifications	55%	40%
√ metacarpal shortening (4 + 5 always involved)	75%	90%
√ metatarsal shortening (3 + 4 involved)	70%	99%

√ 2–3-mm stripe of lucency at right angle to cortex (= osteoid seams formed within stress-induced infractions (PATHOGNOMONIC) + nonunion (= incomplete healing due to mineral deficiency)

PSEUDOHYPOPARATHYROIDISM

= PHypoPT = congenital X-linked dominant abnormality with renal + skeletal resistance to PTH due to (1) end-organ resistance, (2) presence of antienzymes, (3) defective hormone

May be associated with: hyperparathyroidism due to hypocalcemia; F > M

- short obese stature, round face
- mental retardation
- corneal + lenticular opacity
- abnormal dentition (hypoplasia, delayed eruption, excessive caries)
- hypocalcemia + hyperphosphatemia (resistant to PTH injection)
- normal levels of PTH

√ brachydactyly in bones in which epiphysis appears latest (metacarpal, metatarsal bones I, IV, V) (75%)
√ accelerated epiphyseal maturation resulting in dwarfism + coxa vara / valga
√ multiple diaphyseal exostoses (occasionally)
√ calcification of basal ganglia + dentate nucleus
√ calcification / ossification of skin + subcutaneous tissue

PSEUDOPSEUDOHYPOPARATHYROIDISM

= PPHypoPT = different expression of same familial disturbance with identical clinical + radiographic features as pseudohypoparathyroidism but normocalcemic

Cause: end-organ resistance to PTH

- short stature, round facies
- NO blood chemical changes (normal calcium + phosphorus)
- normal response to injection of PTH

√ brachydactyly

PSEUDOXANTHOMA ELASTICUM

= recessive hereditary systemic disorder characterized by degeneration of elastic tissue

@ Skin
- redundant skin folds, particularly in flexor regions
- yellowish xanthomatous papules

√ large amorphous calcific deposits in soft tissue about the joints

@ Eyes
- diminished visual acuity due to alteration of chorioretinal structure
- angioid streaks = reddish brown serrated lines extending from optic disk in a spoke-wheel fashion

@ Arteries
- claudication + decreased pulses

Histo: tissue degeneration of internal elastic lamina + medial thickening

√ lobulated appearance of arteries (similar to fibromuscular hyperplasia)
√ aneurysm formation
√ vessel calcification at early age

Cx: GI tract hemorrhage

PSORIATIC ARTHRITIS

Uncommon disease involving synovium + ligamentous attachments with propensity for sacroiliitis / spondylitis classified as seronegative spondyloarthropathy 6/c

Incidence: 20% of patients with psoriasis (peripheral arthritis in 5%, sacroiliitis in 29%, peripheral arthritis + sacroiliitis in 10%)

Path: synovial inflammation (less prominent than in rheumatoid arthritis) with early fibrosis of proliferative synovium; bony proliferation at joint margins / tendon insertions / subperiosteum

Types:
(1) true psoriatic arthritis (31%)
(2) psoriatic arthritis resembling rheumatoid arthritis (38%)
(3) concomitant rheumatoid + psoriatic arthritis (31%)

- skin rash precedes / develops simultaneously with onset of arthritis in 85%
  ◊ Arthritis antedates dermatological changes by an interval of up to 20 years!
- pitting, discoloration, hyperkeratosis, subungual separation, ridging of nails (in 80%)
- positive HLA-B27 in 80%
- negative rheumatoid factor

Location: widely variable distribution + asymmetry with involvement of lower + upper extremities; distinctive pattern: terminal interphalangeal joints, ray distribution, unilateral polyarticular asymmetrical distribution

√ NO / minimal juxtaarticular osteoporosis (early stage); frequent osteoporosis (later stages)
√ marginal erosions
√ periosteal reaction frequent
√ intraarticular osseous excrescences

@ Hand + foot

Target area: DIP, PIP, MCP

√ "sausage digit" = soft-tissue swelling of entire digit
√ destruction of distal interphalangeal joints (erosive polyarthritis) + osseous resorption
√ bony ankylosis (10%)
√ "pencil-in-cup" deformity = erosions with ill-defined margins + adjacent proliferation of periosteal new bone (CHARACTERISTIC)

√ ivory phalanx = sclerosis of terminal phalanx (28%)
√ destruction of interphalangeal joint of 1st toe with exuberant periosteal reaction + bony proliferation at distal phalangeal base (PATHOGNOMONIC)
√ poorly defined diffuse new bone formation at attachment of Achilles tendon + plantar aponeurosis
√ erosions at superior / posterior margin of calcaneus (20%)
√ acroosteolysis (occasionally)

@ Axial skeleton
√ "floating" osteophyte = large bulky vertically oriented paravertebral soft-tissue ossification (AP view):
√ ill-defined excrescence sweeping across the diskovertebral junction from midportion of one vertebra to the next
Location: lower cervical, thoracic, upper lumbar spine; asymmetric / unilateral
√ squaring of vertebrae in lumbar region
√ sacroiliitis (40%) = (most commonly) bilateral + symmetric sacroiliac joint widening, increased density, fusion
√ apophyseal joint narrowing + sclerosis
√ atlantoaxial subluxation + odontoid abnormalities

DDx: (1) Reiter syndrome (affects only lower extremity)
(2) Ankylosing spondylitis
(3) Rheumatoid arthritis (bilaterally symmetric well-defined erosions, juxtaarticular osteoporosis)

PYKNODYSOSTOSIS

= MAROTEAUX-LAMY DISEASE
= autosomal recessive inherited disease; probably variant of cleidocranial dysostosis

Cause: mutation in cathepsin-K gene
Age: children; M:F = 2:1

• dwarfism
• mental retardation (10%)
• widened hands + feet
• dystrophic nails
• yellowish discoloration of teeth
• characteristic facies (beaked nose, receding jaw)

√ brachycephaly + platybasia
√ wide cranial sutures, wormian bones
√ thick skull base
√ hypoplasia of mandible + obtuse mandibular angle
√ hypoplasia + nonpneumatization of paranasal sinuses
√ nonsegmentation of C1/2 and L5/S1
√ generalized increased density of long bones with thickened cortices (resembling osteopetrosis but with preservation of medullary canal)
√ clavicular dysplasia
√ hypoplastic tapered terminal tufts (=acroosteolysis)
√ multiple spontaneous fractures

DDx: (1) Osteopetrosis (no dwarfism, no mandibular / skull abnormality, no phalangeal hypoplasia, no transverse metaphyseal bands, anemia, Erlenmeyer flask deformity; "bone-within-bone" appearance)
(2) Cleidocranial dysostosis (no dense bones / terminal phalangeal hypoplasia, short stature)

RADIATION INJURY TO BONE

Pathogenesis: vascular compromise with obliterative endarteritis + periarteritis followed by damage to osteoblasts + osteoclasts with decreased matrix production (growing bone + periosteal new bone most sensitive)

Dose effects:
depend on age of patient, absorbed dose, size of radiation field, beam energy, fractionation

>300 rad:	microscopic changes
>400 rad:	growth retardation
<600–1200 rad:	histological recovery retained
>1200 rad:	pronounced cellular damage to chondrocytes; bone marrow atrophy + cartilage degeneration after >6 months; vascular fibrosis

A. BONE GROWTH DISTURBANCE
@ Appendicular skeleton
√ joint space widening (due to cartilage hypertrophy) after 8–10 months
√ growth plate widening in 1–2 months, often returning to normal by 6 months
√ permanent alteration in bone length / size (due to premature fusion of physis)
√ metaphyseal bowing
√ sclerotic metaphyseal bands
√ metaphyseal irregularity + fraying resembling rickets
√ longitudinal striations
√ overtubulation (= abnormal narrowing of the diaphyseal shaft)
Cx: slippage of femoral / humeral epiphysis ± ischemic necrosis (after doses of >25 Gy)
@ Axial skeleton (dose of <15 Gy)
√ "bone-within-bone" appearance after 9–12 months
√ irreversible scalloping + irregularity of vertebral endplate with decreased height of vertebra (= failure of vertical growth)
√ scoliosis concave to the side of irradiation (due to asymmetric vertebral growth + muscular fibrosis)
√ hypoplasia of ilium + ribs
√ acetabular dysplasia, coxa vara / valga

B. RADIATION OSTEITIS = OSTEORADIONECROSIS
= RADIATION NECROSIS
= bone mottling due to osteopenia + coarse trabeculation + focally increased bone density (due to attempts of osseous repair with deposition of new bone on ischemic trabeculae)
Dose: >6,000 cGy in adults; >2,000 cGy in children
Time of onset: 1–3 years following radiation therapy
Location: mandible, ribs, clavicle, humerus, spine, pelvis, femur
√ focal lytic area with abnormal bone matrix:
√ radiolucency confined to radiation field with narrow zone of transition
√ periostitis
√ increased fragility with sclerosis (= pathologic insufficiency fx)
√ ± cortical thinning from chronic infection

MR:
√ increased intensity of spinal bone marrow on T1WI + T2WI corresponding to radiation port (fatty infiltration)

NUC:
√ bone scan with decreased uptake in radiation field

Cx: increased susceptibility of irradiated bone to infection

DDx: recurrent malignancy, radiation-induced sarcoma (soft-tissue mass), infection

C. BENIGN NEOPLASM
Most likely in patients <2 years of age at treatment; with doses of 1600–6425 rads
Latent period: 1.5–5–14 years
1. Osteochondroma = exostosis (exclusively in children under 2 years of age during treatment)
2. Osteoblastoma

D. MALIGNANT NEOPLASM
= RADIATION-INDUCED SARCOMA
Latency period: 3–55 (average of 11–14) years
Minimum dose: 1,660–3,000 rad
Criteria: (a) malignancy occurring within irradiated field
(b) latency period of >5 years
(c) histologic proof of sarcoma
(d) microscopic evidence of altered histology of the original lesion
Histo: 1. Osteosarcoma (90%) = 4–11% of all osteogenic sarcomas
2. Fibrosarcoma > chondrosarcoma > malignant fibrous histiocytoma
- pain, soft-tissue mass, rapid progression of lesion

REFLEX SYMPATHETIC DYSTROPHY

= CAUSALGIA = SHOULDER-HAND SYNDROME = POSTTRAUMATIC OSTEOPOROSIS = SUDECK DYSTROPHY
= serious + potentially disabling condition with poorly understood origin + cause

Etiology:
(1) Trauma in >50% (fracture, frostbite; may be trivial)
◊ Affects 0.01% of all trauma patients
(2) Idiopathic in 27% (immobilization, infection)
(3) Myocardial ischemia in 6%
(4) CNS disorders in 6%
◊ Affects 12–21% of patients with hemiplegia
(5) Diskogenic disease in 5%

- burning pain, tenderness, allodynia, hyperpathia
- soft-tissue swelling ± pitting edema out of proportion to degree of injury
- dystrophic skin + nail changes
- sudomotor changes: hyperhidrosis + hypertrichosis
- vasomotor instability (Raynaud phenomenon, local vasoconstriction / -dilatation)
- end-stage (after 6–12 months): contractures, atrophy of skin + soft tissues

Location: hands and feet distal to injury
√ periarticular soft-tissue swelling
√ patchy osteopenia (50%) as early as 2–3 weeks after onset of symptoms (DDx: disuse osteopenia)
√ generalized osteopenia = ground-glass appearance with endosteal + intracortical excavation:
√ subperiosteal bone resorption
√ lysis of juxtaarticular + subchondral bone
√ preservation of joint space (DDx: rheumatoid / septic arthritis)

NUC (3-phase bone scan):
√ increased flow + increased blood pool + increase in periarticular uptake on delayed images in affected part (60%)
√ diminished flow / delayed uptake (15–20%)

Rx: sympathetic block, α- / β-adrenergic blocking agents, nonsteroidal antiinflammatory drugs, radiation therapy, hypnosis, acupuncture, acupressure, transcutaneous nerve stimulation, physiotherapy, calcitonin, corticosteroids, early mobilization

REITER SYNDROME

= triad of (1) arthritis (2) uveitis (3) urethritis; 98% male

Types:
(1) endemic (venereal)
(2) epidemic (postdysenteric)

- history of sexual exposure / diarrhea 3–11 days before onset of urethritis
- mucocutaneous lesions (keratosis blennorrhagia, balanitis circinata sicca)
- uveitis, conjunctivitis
- positive HLA-B27 in 76%

Location: asymmetric mono- / pauciarticular
√ polyarthritis
√ articular soft-tissue swelling + joint space narrowing in 50% (particularly knees, ankles, feet)
√ widening + inflammation of Achilles + patella tendons
√ "fluffy" periosteal reaction (DISTINCTIVE) at metatarsal necks, proximal phalanges, calcaneal spur, tibia + fibula at ankle and knee
√ juxtaarticular osteoporosis (rare in acute stage)

CHRONIC CHANGES
- recurrent joint attacks in a few cases

√ calcaneal spur at insertion of plantar fascia + Achilles tendon
√ periarticular deossification
√ marginal erosions, loss of joint space
√ bilateral sacroiliac changes indistinguishable from ankylosing / psoriatic spondylitis (in 10–40%)
√ paravertebral ossification = isolated "floating osteophyte" usually in thoracolumbar area

Cx: gastric ulcer + hemorrhage; aortic incompetence; heart block; amyloidosis

RELAPSING POLYCHONDRITIS

= rare disorder characterized by generalized recurring inflammation + destruction of cartilage in joints, ears, nose, larynx, airways

Etiology: acquired metabolic disorder (? abnormal acid mucopolysaccharide metabolism) / hypersensitivity / autoimmune process (antibodies directed against type II collagen)

Histo: loss of cytoplasm in chondrocytes; plasma cell + lymphocyte infiltration
Age: 40–60 years (no age predilection)
- nasal chondritis = saddle-nose deformity
- bilateral auricular chondritis = swollen + tender ears, cauliflower ears
- hearing loss (obstruction of external auditory meatus / audiovestibular damage)
- ocular inflammation
- cough, hoarseness, dyspnea (collapse of trachea)
- nonerosive seronegative inflammatory polyarthritis = arthralgia

@ Head
√ calcification of pinna of ear
@ Chest
√ manubriosternal / costochondral arthropathy (30%)
@ Respiratory tract (in up to 70%)
√ ectasia + collapsibility (cartilaginous destruction) of trachea and mainstem bronchi with focal thickening (mucosal edema) + luminal narrowing (fibrosis)
√ bronchiectasis
√ generalized + localized emphysema
@ Cardiovascular (in 15–46%)
√ aortic aneurysm (4–10%), mostly in ascending aorta, may be multiple / dissecting
√ aortic / mitral valve insufficiency (8%)
√ systemic vasculitis (13%)
@ Bone
√ periarticular osteoporosis
√ erosive changes in carpal bones resembling rheumatoid arthritis
√ soft-tissue swelling around joints + styloid process of ulna
√ erosive irregularities in sacroiliac joints
√ disk space erosion + increased density of articular plates

Rx: corticosteroids, immunosuppression
Prognosis: 74% 5-year survival rate; 55% 10-year survival rate; median survival time of 11 years; airway complications account for >50% of deaths

RENAL OSTEODYSTROPHY

= constellation of musculoskeletal abnormalities that occur with chronic renal failure as a combination of
(a) osteomalacia (adults) / rickets (children)
(b) 2° HPT with osteitis cystica fibrosa + soft-tissue calcifications
(c) osteosclerosis
(d) soft-tissue + vascular calcifications

Classification:
(1) Glomerular form = acquired renal disease: chronic glomerulonephritis (common)
(2) Tubular form = congenital renal osteodystrophy:
1. Vitamin D–resistant rickets = hypophosphatemic rickets
2. Fanconi syndrome = impaired resorption of glucose, phosphate, amino acids, bicarbonate, uric acid, sodium, water
3. Renal tubular acidosis

Pathogenesis:
(1) Renal insufficiency causes a decrease in vitamin D conversion into the active 1,25$(OH)_2D_3$ (done by 25-OH-D-1-a hydroxylase, which is exclusive to renal tissue mitochondria); vitamin D deficiency slows intestinal calcium absorption; *vitamin D resistance predominates* and calcium levels stay low (Ca x P product remains almost normal secondary to hyperphosphatemia); low calcium levels lead to OSTEOMALACIA; additional factors responsible for osteomalacia are inhibitors to calcification produced in the uremic state, aluminum toxicity, dysfunction of hepatic enzyme system
(2) Renal insufficiency with diminished filtration results in phosphate retention; maintenance of Ca x P product lowers serum calcium directly, which in turn increases PTH production (2° HPT); *2° HPT predominates* associated with mild vitamin D resistance and leads to an increase in Ca x P product with SOFT-TISSUE CALCIFICATION in kidney, lung, joints, bursae, blood vessels, heart as well as OSTEITIS FIBROSA
(3) Mixture of (a) and (b): increased serum phosphate inhibits vitamin D activation via feedback regulation

- phosphate retention
- hypocalcemia

A. OSTEOPENIA (in 0–25–83%)
= diminution in number of trabeculae + thickening of stressed trabeculae = increased trabecular pattern
Cause: combined effect of
(1) Osteomalacia (reduced bone mineralization due to acquired insensitivity to vitamin D / antivitamin D factor)
(2) Osteitis fibrosa cystica (bone resorption)
(3) Osteoporosis (decrease in bone quantity)
Contributing factors:
chronic metabolic acidosis, poor nutritional status, pre- and posttransplantation azotemia, use of steroids, hyperparathyroidism, low vitamin D levels
Cx: fracture predisposition (lessened structural strength) with minor trauma / spontaneously; fracture prevalence increases with duration of hemodialysis + remains unchanged after renal transplantation
Site: vertebral body (3–25%), pubic ramus, rib (5–25%)
√ Milkman fracture / Looser zones (in 1%)
√ metaphyseal fractures
Prognosis: osteopenia may remain unchanged / worsen after renal transplantation + during hemodialysis

B. RICKETS (children)
Cause: in CRF normal vessels fail to develop in an orderly way along cartilage columns in zone of provisional calcification; this results in disorganized proliferation of the zone of maturing + hypertrophying cartilage and disturbed endochondral calcification

Location: most apparent in areas of rapid growth such as knee joints
√ diffuse bone demineralization
√ widening of growth plate
√ irregular zone of provisional calcification
√ metaphyseal cupping + fraying
√ bowing of long bones, scoliosis
√ diffuse concave impression at multiple vertebral end plates, basilar invagination
√ slipped epiphysis (10%): capital femoral, proximal humerus, distal femur, distal radius, heads of metacarpals + metatarsals
√ general delay in bone age

C. SECONDARY HPT (in 6–66%)
Cause: inability of kidneys to adequately excrete phosphate leads to hyperplasia of parathyroid chief cells (2° HPT); excess PTH affects the development of osteoclasts, osteoblasts, osteocytes
• hyperphosphatemia
• hypocalcemia
• increased PTH levels
√ subperiosteal, cortical, subchondral, trabecular, endosteal, subligamentous bone resorption
√ osteoclastoma = brown tumor = osteitis fibrosa cystica in 1.5–1.7% (due to PTH-stimulated osteoclastic activity; more common in 1° HPT)
√ periosteal new-bone formation (8–25%)
√ chondrocalcinosis (more common in 1° HPT)

D. OSTEOSCLEROSIS (9–34%)
◊ One of the most common radiologic manifestations; most commonly with chronic glomerulonephritis; may be the sole manifestation of renal osteodystrophy
√ diffuse chalky density: thoracolumbar spine in 60% (rugger jersey spine); also in pelvis, ribs, long bones, facial bones, base of skull (children)
Prognosis: may increase / regress after renal transplantation

E. SOFT-TISSUE CALCIFICATIONS
(a) metastatic
secondary to hyperphosphatemia (solubility product for calcium + phosphate [Ca^{2+} x PO_4^{-2}] exceeds 60–75 mg/dL in extracellular fluid), hypercalcemia, alkalosis with precipitation of calcium salts
(b) dystrophic
secondary to local tissue injury
Location:
— arterial (27–83%):
in medial + intimal elastic tissue
Location: dorsal pedis a., forearm, hand, wrist, leg
√ pipestem appearance without prominent luminal involvement
— periarticular (0–52%):
multifocal, frequently symmetric, may extend into adjacent joint
• chalky fluid / pastelike material
• inflammatory response in surrounding tenosynovial tissue
√ discrete cloudlike dense areas
√ fluid-fluid level in tumoral calcinosis
Prognosis: often regresses with treatment
— visceral (79%): heart, lung, stomach, kidney
√ fluffy amorphous "tumoral" calcification

Rx:
1. Decrease of phosphorus absorption in bowel (in hyperphosphatemia)
2. Vitamin D_3 administration (if vitamin D resistance predominates)
3. Parathyroidectomy for 3° HPT (= autonomous HPT)

Dialysis-related Disorders
1. Osteomyelitis
2. Osteonecrosis
3. Crystal deposition
4. Destructive spondyloarthropathy
5. Amyloidosis
6. Dialysis cysts

Congenital Renal Osteodystrophy
Vitamin D–Resistant Rickets
= PHOSPHATE DIABETES = PRIMARY HYPOPHOSPHATEMIA = FAMILIAL HYPOPHOSPHATEMIC RICKETS
= rare X-linked dominant disorder of renal tubular reabsorption characterized by
(a) impaired resorption of phosphate in proximal renal tubule (due to defect in renal brush-border membrane)
(b) inappropriately low synthesis of 1,25-dihydroxyvitamin D_3 [$1,25(OH)_2D_3$] in renal tubules resulting in decreased intestinal resorption of calcium + phosphate
Age: <1 year
• hypophosphatemia + hyperphosphaturia
• elevated serum alkaline phosphatase
• normal plasma + urine calcium
• normal / low serum $1,25(OH)_2D_3$
√ classic rachitic changes
√ skeletal deformity, particularly bowed legs
√ retarded bone age; dwarfism if untreated
√ osteosclerosis / bone thickening (from overabundance of incompletely calcified matrix)
Rx: phosphate infusion + large doses of vitamin D
DDx: vitamin-D–deficient and –dependent rickets (absence of muscle weakness + seizures + tetany)

Fanconi Syndrome
Triad of
(1) Hyperphosphaturia
(2) Amino aciduria
(3) Renal glucosuria (normal blood glucose)
Etiology: renal tubular defect
√ rickets, osteomalacia, osteitis fibrosa, osteosclerosis

Prognosis: functional renal impairment likely when bone changes occur
Rx: large doses of vitamin D + alkalinization

Renal Tubular Acidosis

• systemic acidosis, bone lesions
√ rickets, osteomalacia, pseudofractures, nephrocalcinosis, osteitis fibrosa (rare)
(a) Lightwood syndrome = salt-losing nephritis (transient self-limited form)
  • NO nephrocalcinosis
(b) Butler-Albright syndrome (severe form)
  • nephrocalcinosis

RHEUMATOID ARTHRITIS

= generalized connective tissue disease
= type III hypersensitivity = delayed hypersensitivity
= immune complex disease (= formation of antigen-antibody complexes with complement fixation)

Prevalence: 1% of population
Cause: genetic predisposition; ? reaction to antigen from Epstein-Barr virus / certain strains of E. coli
Age: highest incidence 40–50 years; M:F = 1:3 if <40 years; M:F = 1:1 if >40 years
Pathogenesis: injury to synovial endothelial cells; synovitis with synovial hypertrophy leads to impaired nutrition with chondronecrosis, joint narrowing, subluxation, and ankylosis
Diagnostic criteria of American Rheumatism Association (at least 4 criteria should be present):
(1) morning stiffness for ≥1 hour
(2) swelling of ≥3 joints, particularly of wrist, metatarsophalangeal or proximal interphalangeal joints for >6 weeks
(3) symmetric swelling
(4) typical radiographic changes
(5) rheumatoid nodules
(6) positive rheumatoid factor

• morning stiffness
• fatigue, weight loss, anemia
• carpal tunnel syndrome
• rheumatoid factor (positive in 85–94%) = IgM-antibody = agglutination of sensitized sheep RBCs closely correlating with disease severity;
  false positive: normal (5%), asbestos workers with fibrosing alveolitis (25%), viral / bacterial / parasitic infection, other inflammatory diseases
• antinuclear antibodies (positive in many)
• LE cells (positive in some)
• positive latex flocculation test
• hormonal influence:
  (a) decrease in activity during pregnancy
  (b) men with RA have low testosterone levels

Location: symmetric involvement of diarthrodial joints

EARLY SIGNS:
√ fusiform periarticular soft-tissue swelling (result of effusion)
√ regional osteoporosis (disuse + local hyperthermia)
√ widened joint space
√ giant synovial cyst

LATE SIGNS:
√ diffuse loss of interosseous space
√ marked destruction + fractures of joint space
√ extensive destruction of bone ends
√ bony fusion

@ Hand & wrist
  Target areas:
  all five MCP, PIP, interphalangeal joint of thumb, all wrist compartments (especially radiocarpal, inferior radioulnar, pisiform-triquetral joints); earliest changes seen in 2 + 3 MCP, 3 PIP
  √ marginal + central bone erosions (less common in large joints); site of first erosion is classically base of proximal phalanx of 4th finger
  √ changes in the ulnar styloid + distal radioulnar joint (early sign)
  √ flexion + extension contractures with ulnar subluxation + dislocation

@ Cervical spine
  √ erosions of odontoid process (1) between anterior arch of atlas + dens, (2) between transverse ligament of atlas + dens, (3) at tip of odontoid process
  √ anterior atlantoaxial subluxation (in >6%): >2.5 mm in adults, >4.5 mm in children during neck flexion
  √ "cranial settling" = odontoid process projects into skull base due to significant disease of atlanto-occipital and atlantoaxial joints
  √ lateral head tilt = lateral subluxation = asymmetry between odontoid process + lateral masses of atlas
  √ "stepladder appearance" of cervical spine due to subaxial subluxations + absence of osteophytosis:
    √ destruction + narrowing of disk spaces
    √ irregular vertebral body outlines
    √ erosion + destruction of zygapophyseal joints
    √ resorption of spinous processes
  √ osteoporosis

@ Ribs
  √ erosion of superior margins of posterior portions of ribs 3–5

@ Shoulder
  √ symmetric loss of glenohumeral joint space:
    √ marginal erosions at superolateral aspect of humeral head
    √ osteoporosis
    √ elevation of humeral heads = narrowing of acromiohumeral distance (2° to tear / atrophy of rotator cuff)
  √ widened acromioclavicular joint:
    √ erosions at acromial + clavicular end
    √ tapered margins of distal clavicle
  √ scalloped erosion on undersurface of distal clavicle opposite the coracoid process (attachment of coracoclavicular ligament)

@ Hip
  √ often appears normal during early disease process
  √ pannus formation (MR imaging)

√ symmetric loss of joint space with axial migration of femoral head
√ marginal + central erosions, cysts, localized sclerosis
√ decompression of joint effusion into iliopsoas bursa through weak anterior capsule displacing muscle + vasculature
√ rupture of gluteal tendon
√ protrusio acetabuli (from osteoporosis)

@ Knee
Location: medial + lateral femorotibial compartments; bilateral symmetric
√ diffuse loss of joint space
√ osteoporosis
√ superficial + deep marginal + central erosions
√ subchondral sclerosis (especially in tibia)
√ synovial herniation + cysts (eg, popliteal cyst)
√ varus / valgus angulation (due to crumbling of osteoporotic bone of tibia + ligamentous abnormalities)

@ Foot
Target areas:
medial aspect of MT heads (2,3,4), medial + lateral aspect of MT5 (earliest sign); interphalangeal joints of foot (esp. great toe); bilateral + symmetric
√ calcaneal plantar spur

DDx: SLE, psoriatic arthritis, seronegative spondylarthropathies

EXTRA-ARTICULAR MANIFESTATIONS (76%)

(a) **Felty syndrome** (<1%)
= rheumatoid arthritis (present for >10 years) + splenomegaly + neutropenia
Age: 40–70 years; F > M; rare in Blacks
• rapid weight loss
• therapy refractory leg ulcers
• brown pigmentation over exposed surfaces of extremities

(b) Sjögren syndrome (15%)
= keratoconjunctivitis + xerostomia + rheumatoid arthritis

(c) Pulmonary manifestations
√ pleural effusion, mostly unilateral, without change for months, usually not associated with parenchymal disease
√ interstitial fibrosis with lower lobe predominance
Prevalence: 2–9% of rheumatoid patients
√ rheumatoid nodules (30%): well-circumscribed, peripheral, with frequent cavitation
√ Caplan syndrome (= hyperimmune reactivity to silica inhalation with rapidly developing multiple pulmonary nodules)
√ pulmonary hypertension secondary to arteritis

(d) Subcutaneous nodules
(in 5–35% with active arthritis) over extensor surfaces of forearm + other pressure points (eg, olecranon) without calcifications (DDx to gout)

(e) Cardiovascular involvement
1. Pericarditis (20–50%)
2. Myocarditis (arrhythmia, heart block)
3. Aortitis (5%) of ascending aorta ± aortic valve insufficiency

(f) Rheumatoid vasculitis
= leukocytoclastic lesion of small venules mimicking periarteritis nodosa
• polyneuropathy, cutaneous ulceration, gangrene, polymyopathy, myocardial / visceral infarction

(g) Neurologic sequelae
1. Distal neuropathy (related to vasculitis)
2. Nerve entrapment (atlantoaxial subluxation, carpal tunnel syndrome, Baker cyst)

(h) Lymphadenopathy (up to 25%)
√ splenomegaly (1–5%)

Cystic Rheumatoid Arthritis

= intraosseous cystic lesions as dominant feature
Pathogenesis: increased pressure in synovial space from joint effusion decompresses through microfractures of weakened marginal cortex into subarticular bone
◊ Increase in size + extent of cysts correlates with increased level of activity + absence of synovial cysts
Age: as above; M:F = 1:1
• seronegative in 50%
√ juxtaarticular subcortical lytic lesions with well-defined sclerotic margins
√ relative lack of cartilage loss, osteoporosis, joint disruption
DDx: gout (presence of urate crystals), pigmented villonodular synovitis (monoarticular)

Juvenile Rheumatoid Arthritis

= rheumatoid arthritis in patients <16 years of age; M < F
Classification:
(1) <u>Juvenile-onset adult type</u> (10%)
• IgM RA factor positive; age 8–9; poor prognosis
√ erosive changes; perfuse periosteal reaction; hip disease with protrusio
(2) <u>Polyarthritis of the ankylosing spondylitic type</u>
• iridocyclitis; boys age 9–11 years
√ peripheral arthritis; fusion of greater trochanter; complete fusion of both hips; heel spur
(3) **Still disease**
(a) systemic
(b) polyarticular
(c) pauciarticular + iridocyclitis (30%)
• fever, rash, lymphadenopathy, hepatosplenomegaly; pericarditis, dwarfism
• fatal kidney disease in 20%
Age: 2–4 and 8–11 years of age; M < F
Location: involvement of carpometacarpal joints ("squashed carpi" in adulthood), hind foot, hip (40–50%)
√ periosteal reaction of phalanges; broadening of bones; accelerated bone maturation + early fusion (stunting of growth)

• morning stiffness, arthralgia
• subcutaneous nodules (10%)

- skin rash (50%)
- fever, lymphadenopathy

Location: early involvement of large joints (hips, knees, ankles, wrists, elbows); later of hands + feet

√ radiologic signs similar to rheumatoid arthritis (except for involvement of large joints first, late onset of bony changes, more ankylosis, wide metaphyses)
√ periarticular soft-tissue swelling
√ thinning of joint cartilage
√ large cystlike lesions removed from articular surface (invasion of bone by inflammatory pannus); rare in children
√ articular erosions at ligamentous + tendinous insertion sites
√ joint destruction may resemble neuropathic joints
√ juxtaarticular osteoporosis
√ "balloon epiphyses" + "gracile bones" (epiphyseal overgrowth + early fusion with bone shortening secondary to hyperemia)

@ Hand / foot
√ "rectangular" phalanges (periostitis + cortical thickening)
√ ankylosis in carpal joints

@ Axial skeleton
Location: predominantly upper cervical spine
√ ankylosis of cervical spine (apophyseal joints), sacroiliac joints
√ decreased size of vertebral bodies + atrophic intervertebral disks
√ subluxation of atlantoaxial joint (66%)
√ thoracic spinal compression fractures

@ Chest
√ ribbon ribs
√ pleural + pericardial effusions
√ interstitial pulmonary lesions (simulating scleroderma, dermatomyositis)
√ solitary pulmonary nodules, may cavitate

Prognosis: complete recovery (30%); secondary amyloidosis

RICKETS

= osteomalacia during enchondral bone growth

Age: 4–18 months

Histo: zone of preparatory calcification does not form, heap up of maturing cartilage cells; failure of osteoid mineralization also in shafts so that osteoid production elevates periosteum

- irritability, bone pain, tenderness
- craniotabes
- rachitic rosary
- bowed legs
- delayed dentition
- swelling of wrists + ankles

Location: metaphyses of long bones subjected to stress are particularly involved (wrists, ankles, knees)

√ poorly mineralized epiphyseal centers with delayed appearance
√ irregular widened epiphyseal plates (increased osteoid)
√ increase in distance between end of shaft and epiphyseal center
√ cupping + fraying of metaphysis with threadlike shadows into epiphyseal cartilage (weight-bearing bones)
√ cortical spurs projecting at right angles to metaphysis
√ coarse trabeculation (NO ground-glass pattern as in scurvy)
√ periosteal reaction may be present
√ deformities common (bowing of soft diaphysis, molding of epiphysis, fractures)
√ bowing of long bones
√ frontal bossing

mnemonic: "RICKETS"
Reaction of periosteum may occur
Indistinct cortex
Coarse trabeculation
Knees + wrists + ankles mainly affected
Epiphyseal plates widened + irregular
Tremendous metaphysis (fraying, splaying, cupping)
Spur (metaphyseal)

Causes of Rickets

I. *ABNORMALITY IN VITAMIN D METABOLISM*
Associated with reactive hyperparathyroidism
  A. VITAMIN D DEFICIENCY
    1. Dietary lack of vitamin D
       = famine osteomalacia
    2. Lack of sunshine exposure
    3. Malabsorption of vitamin D
       = gastroenterogenous rickets due to
       (1) Pancreatitis + biliary tract disease
       (2) Steatorrhea, celiac disease, postgastrectomy
       (3) Inflammatory bowel disease
  B. DEFECTIVE CONVERSION OF VITAMIN D TO 25-OH-CHOLECALCIFEROL IN LIVER
    1. Liver disease
    2. Anticonvulsant drug therapy (= induction of hepatic enzymes that accelerate degradation of biologically active vitamin D metabolites)
  C. DEFECTIVE CONVERSION OF 25-OH-D3 TO 1,25-OH-D3 IN KIDNEY
    1. Chronic renal failure = renal osteodystrophy
    2. Vitamin D–dependent rickets = autosomal recessive enzyme defect of 1-OHase

II. *ABNORMALITY IN PHOSPHATE METABOLISM*
not associated with hyperparathyroidism secondary to normal serum calcium
  A. PHOSPHATE DEFICIENCY
    1. Intestinal malabsorption of phosphates
    2. Ingestion of aluminum salts [$Al(OH)_2$] forming insoluble complexes with phosphate
    3. Low phosphate feeding in prematurely born infants
    4. Severe malabsorption state
    5. Parenteral hyperalimentation
  B. DISORDERS OF RENAL TUBULAR REABSORPTION OF PHOSPHATE
    1. Renal tubular acidosis (renal loss of alkali)

2. deToni-Debré-Fanconi syndrome = hypophosphatemia, glucosuria, aminoaciduria
3. Vitamin D–resistant rickets
4. Cystinosis
5. Tyrosinosis
6. Lowe syndrome
7. Ifosfamide nephrotoxicity (for the treatment of rhabdomyosarcoma, Wilms tumor)

C. HYPOPHOSPHATEMIA WITH NONENDOCRINE TUMORS
= Oncogenic rickets = elaboration of humeral substance which inhibits tubular reabsorption of phosphates (paraneoplastic phenomenon)
1. Nonossifying fibroma
2. Sclerosing hemangioma
3. Hemangiopericytoma
4. Ossifying mesenchymal tumor

D. HYPOPHOSPHATASIA

III. *CALCIUM DEFICIENCY*
1. Dietary rickets = milk-free diet (extremely rare)
2. Malabsorption
3. Consumption of substances forming chelates with calcium

Classification of Rickets

I. Primary vitamin D–deficiency rickets
II. Gastrointestinal malabsorption
   A. Partial gastrectomy
   B. Small intestinal disease: gluten-sensitive enteropathy / regional enteritis
   C. Hepatobiliary disease: chronic biliary obstruction / biliary cirrhosis
   D. Pancreatic disease: chronic pancreatitis
III. Primary hypophosphatemia; vitamin D–deficiency rickets
IV. Renal disease
   A. Chronic renal failure
   B. Renal tubular disorders: renal tubular acidosis
   C. Multiple renal defects
V. Hypophosphatasia + pseudohypophosphatasia
VI. Fibrogenesis imperfecta osseum
VII. Axial osteomalacia
VIII. Miscellaneous
   Hypoparathyroidism, hyperparathyroidism, thyrotoxicosis, osteoporosis, Paget disease, fluoride ingestion, ureterosigmoidostomy, neurofibromatosis, osteopetrosis, macroglobulinemia, malignancy

ROTATOR CUFF LESIONS

Subacromial Pain Syndrome

(1) Impingement syndrome
(2) Rotator cuff tendinitis
(3) Degeneration without impingement
(4) Shoulder instability with secondary impingement
(5) Instability without impingement

Impingement Syndrome

= lateral shoulder pain with abduction; common cause of rotator cuff tears; NOT radiographic diagnosis

Age: lifelong process; 1st stage <25 years; 2nd stage 25–40 years; complete rotator cuff tear >40 years

Pathophysiology:
movement of humerus impinges rotator cuff tendons against coracoacromial arch resulting in microtrauma, which causes inflammation of subacromial bursa (= fibrous thickening of subacromial bursa) / rotator cuff (critical zone of rotator cuff = supraspinatus tendon 2 cm from its attachment to humerus)
◊ Impingement pathophysiology may be secondary to primary instability!

Impingement anatomy:
narrowing of subacromial space secondary to
(1) acquired degenerative subacromial osteophyte / enthesophyte from
   (a) bony outgrowth along coracoacromial ligament
   (b) acromioclavicular joint osteoarthritis
(2) congenital subacromial hook of anterior acromion (= subacromial spur)
◊ Impingement syndrome may exist without impingement anatomy!

• painful arc of motion
√ subacromial enthesophyte
√ alteration in acromial shape + orientation
√ thickening of coracoacromial ligament

Cx: (1) partial / complete tear (may be precipitated by acute traumatic event on preexisting degenerative changes)
(2) cuff tendinitis / degenerative tendinosis

Dx: Lidocaine impingement test (= subacromial lidocaine injection relieves pain)

Rx: acromioplasty (= removal of a portion of the acromion), removal of subacromial osteophytes, removal / lysis / débridement of coracoacromial ligament, resection of distal clavicle, removal of acromioclavicular joint osteophytes

Glenohumeral Instability

Glenohumeral stability is dependent on a functional anatomic unit (= anterior capsular mechanism) formed by: glenoid labrum, joint capsule, superior + middle + anteroinferior + posteroinferior glenohumeral ligaments, coracohumeral ligament, subscapularis tendon, rotator cuff

Age: <35 years
Frequency: acute, recurrent, fixed
Cause: traumatic, microtraumatic, atraumatic
Direction: anterior > multidirectional > inferior > posterior

Type of lesions:
labral abnormalities (compression, avulsion, shearing), capsular / ligamentous tear / avulsion

Associated lesions:
Hill-Sachs fracture, trough line fracture, glenoid fracture, labral cyst
◊ Normal clefts may exist within labrum!

False positive for labral separation:
(1) Articular cartilage deep to labrum
(2) Glenohumeral ligaments passing adjacent to labrum

Rotator Cuff Tear

Etiology: (1) Attritional change + tendon degeneration due to aging, repeated microtrauma as a result of impingement between humeral head + coracoacromial arch, overuse of shoulder from professional / athletic activities
(2) Acute trauma (rare)
Age: most commonly >50 years
Location: "critical zone" of supraspinatus tendon 1 cm medial to tendon attachment (area of relative hypovascularity)

Classification:
EXTENT OF TEAR
(a) incomplete rupture = **partial tear** involves either bursal or synovial surface or remains intratendinous
(b) complete rupture = **full-thickness tear** bridging subacromial bursa and glenohumeral joint
— pure transverse tear
— pure vertical / longitudinal tear
— tear with retraction of tendon edges
— global tear = **massive tear** / avulsion of cuff involving more than one of the tendons
TOPOGRAPHY OF TEAR
(a) extent in frontal plane: nondisplaced, minimally displaced, dramatically displaced
(b) extent in anterior direction: supraspinatus tendon + coracohumeral ligament + subscapularis tendon
(c) extent in posterior direction: supraspinatus tendon + infraspinatus + teres minor tendon

Arthrography (71–100% sensitive, 71–100% specific for combined full + partial thickness tears):
√ opacification of subacromial-subdeltoid bursa
MR (41–100% sensitive and 79–100% specific for combined full + partial thickness tears):
√ discontinuity of cuff with retraction of musculotendinous junction
√ focal / generalized intense / markedly increased signal intensity on T2WI (= fluid within cuff defect) in <50%
√ fluid within subacromial-subdeltoid bursa (MOST SENSITIVE)
√ low / moderate signal intensity on T2WI (= severely degenerated tendon, intact bursal / synovial surface, granulation / scar tissue filling the region of torn tendinous fibers)
√ cuff defect with contour irregularity
√ abrupt change in the signal character at boundary of the lesion
√ supraspinatus muscle atrophy (MOST SPECIFIC)
Pitfalls:
√ hyperintense focus in distal supraspinatus tendon
√ gray signal isointense to muscle on all pulse sequences
(a) partial volume averaging with superior + lateral infraspinatus tendon
(b) vascular "watershed" area
(c) magic angle effect = orientation of collagen fibers at 55° relative to main magnetic field
√ hyperintense focus within rotator cuff on T2WI
(a) partial volume averaging with fluid in biceps tendon sheath / subscapularis bursa
(b) partial volume averaging with fat of peribursal fat
(c) motion artifacts: respiration, vascular pulsation, patient movement
√ fatty atrophy of muscle
(a) impingement of axillary / suprascapular nn. = quadrilateral space syndrome
US (scans in hyperextended position, 75–100% sensitive, 43–97% specific, 65–95% negative predictive value, 55–75% positive predictive value):
√ nonvisualization of rotator cuff (large tear), most reliable sign:
√ deltoid muscle directly on top of humeral head
√ defect filled with hypoechoic thickened bursa + fat (with hypervascularity on color Doppler) between deltoid and humeral head
√ focal nonvisualization of rotator cuff, reliable sign:
√ "naked tuberosity sign" = retracted tendon leaves a bare area of bone
√ folding of bursal + peribursal fat tissue into focal defect
√ discontinuity of rotator cuff filled with joint fluid / hypoechoic reactive tissue
√ abrupt + sharply demarcated focal thinning
√ small comma-shaped area of hyperechogenicity (small tear filled with granulation tissue / hypertrophied synovium)
False negative: longitudinal tear, partial tear
False positive: intraarticular biceps tendon, soft-tissue calcification, small scar / fibrous tissue

Subacromial-Subdeltoid Bursitis

common finding in rotator cuff tears
√ peribursal fat totally / partially obliterated + replaced by low-signal-intensity tissue on all pulse sequences
√ fluid accumulation within bursa

Supraspinatus Tendinopathy / Tendinosis

Cause: impingement, acute / chronic stress
Histo: mucinous + myxoid degeneration
√ increase in signal intensity in tendon on proton-density images without disruption of tendon
√ tendinous enlargement + inhomogeneous signal pattern

RUBELLA

= GERMAN MEASLES
Incidence: endemic rate of 0.1%
Age: infants (in utero transmission)
• neonatal dwarfism (intrauterine growth retardation)
• failure to thrive
• retinopathy, cataracts, deafness
• mental deficiency with encephalitis + microcephaly

- thrombocytopenic purpura, petechiae, anemia
√ "celery-stalk" sign (50%) = metaphyseal irregular margins + coarsened trabeculae extending longitudinally from epiphysis; distal end of femur > proximal end of tibia, humerus
√ no periosteal reaction
√ hepatosplenomegaly + adenopathy
√ pneumonitis
@ Cardiovascular:
 √ congenital heart disease (PDA)
 √ peripheral pulmonary artery stenosis
 √ necrosis of myocardium
@ CNS
 √ punctate / nodular calcifications
 √ porencephalic cysts
 √ occasionally microcephaly
Prognosis: osseous manifestations disappear in 1–3 months
DDx: (1) CMV
 (2) Congenital syphilis (diaphysitis + epiphysitis)
 (3) Toxoplasmosis

RUBINSTEIN-TAYBI SYNDROME

= BROAD THUMB SYNDROME
= rare sporadic syndrome without known chromosomal / biochemical markers; M:F = 1:1
- small stature
- mental, motor, language retardation
@ Characteristic facies
 - beaked / straight nose ± low nasal septum
 - antimongoloid slant of palpebral fissures
 - epicanthic folds
 - broad fleshy nasal bridge
 - high-arched palate
 - dental abnormalities
@ Ophthalmologic findings
 - strabismus, ptosis, refractive errors
@ Cutaneous findings
 - keloids, hirsutism, simian crease
 - flat capillary hemangioma on forehead / neck
@ Musculoskeletal findings
 √ short broad "spatulate" terminal phalanges of thumb and great toe ± angulation deformity (MOST CONSISTENT + CHARACTERISTIC FINDING)
 √ radial angulation of distal phalanx (50%) caused by trapezoid / delta shape of proximal phalanx
 √ tufted "mushroom-shaped" fingers + webbing
 √ thin tubular bones of hand + feet
 √ club feet
 √ skeletal maturation retardation
 √ dysplastic ribs
 √ spina bifida occulta
 √ scoliosis
 √ flat acetabular angle + flaring of ilia
@ Genitourinary tract anomalies
 √ bilateral renal duplication
 √ renal agenesis
 √ bifid ureter
 √ incomplete / delayed descent of testes
@ Cardiovascular abnormalities
 √ atrial septal defect
 √ patent ductus arteriosus
 √ coarctation of aorta
 √ valvular aortic stenosis
 √ pulmonic stenosis
OB-US:
 √ decreased head circumference
 √ small for gestational age
Cx in infancy: obstipation, feeding problems, recurrent upper respiratory infection

SAPHO SYNDROME

= **S**ynovitis, **A**cne, **P**almoplantar pustulosis, **H**yperostosis, **O**steitis
= PUSTULOTIC ARTHROSTEITIS
= STERNOCLAVICULAR HYPEROSTOSIS
= association between rheumatologic and cutaneous lesions (= seronegative spondyloarthropathy)
◊ Delay of several years can separate osseous from cutaneous lesions!
Etiology: ? variant of psoriasis
Age: young to middle-aged adults; M:F = 1:1
- palmoplantar pustulosis (52%) = chronic eruption of yellowish intradermal sterile pustules on palms + soles
- severe acne (15%) = acne fulminans, acne conglobata
- pain, soft-tissue swelling, limitation of motion at skeletal site of involvement
@ Sternoclavicular joint (70–90%)
 Site: insertion of costoclavicular ligament, clavicles, manubrium sterni
 √ osteolysis at beginning of disease
 √ hyperostosis + osteosclerosis
 √ arthritis + ankylosis of sternoclavicular joint
@ Axial skeleton (33%)
 √ osteosclerosis of one / more vertebral bodies
 √ disk space narrowing + endplate erosion
 √ paravertebral ossifications (mimicking marginal / nonmarginal syndesmophytes / massive bridging)
 √ unilateral sacroiliitis + associated osteosclerosis of adjacent iliac bone
@ Appendicular skeleton (30%)
 Location: distal femur, proximal tibia, fibula, humerus, radius, ulna
 Site: metaphysis
 √ osteosclerosis / osteolysis + periosteal new bone formation with aggressive appearance
@ Joints
 Location: knee, hip, ankle, DIP of hand
 √ synovial inflammation with juxtaarticular osteoporosis (early)
 √ joint narrowing, marginal erosion, hyperostosis, enthesopathy (later)
Prognosis: chronic course with unpredictable exacerbations + remissions
Rx: nonsteroidal antiinflammatory drugs, corticosteroids, analgesics, cyclosporine
DDx: infectious osteomyelitis / spondylitis, osteosarcoma, Ewing sarcoma, metastasis, Paget disease, aseptic necrosis of clavicle

SARCOIDOSIS

Osseous involvement in 6–15–20%
• unimpaired joint function, joints are rarely involved
Location: small bones of hands + feet (middle + distal phalanges)
√ reticulated "lacelike" trabecular pattern in metaphyseal ends of middle + distal phalanges, metacarpals, metatarsals
√ well-defined cystlike lesions of varying size
√ neuropathy-like destruction of terminal phalanges (DDx: scleroderma)
√ phalangeal endosteal sclerosis + periosteal new bone (infrequent)
√ vertebral involvement unusual: destructive lesions with sclerotic margin
√ diffuse sclerosis of multiple vertebral bodies
√ paravertebral soft-tissue mass (DDx: indistinguishable from tuberculosis)
√ osteolytic changes in skull

SCURVY

= BARLOW DISEASE = HYPOVITAMNOSIS C
= vitamin C (= ascorbic acid) deficiency with defective osteogenesis from abnormal osteoblast function

Infantile Scurvy

Age: 6–9 months (maternal vitamin C protects for first 6 months)
Predisposed: feeding with pasteurized / boiled milk
Pathogenesis: abnormal collagen formation
• irritability
• tenderness + weakness of lower limbs
• scorbutic rosary of ribs
• bleeding of gums (teething)
• legs drawn up + widely spread = pseudoparalysis
Location: distal femur (esp. medial side), proximal and distal tibia + fibula, distal radius + ulna, proximal humerus, sternal end of ribs
√ "ground-glass" osteoporosis (CHARACTERISTIC)
√ cortical thinning
√ soft-tissue edema (rare)
@ Metaphysis
√ white line of Fränkel = metaphyseal zone of preparatory calcification (DDx: lead / phosphorus poisoning, bismuth treatment, healing rickets)
√ Trümmerfeld zone = radiolucent zone on shaft side of Fränkel's white line (site of subepiphyseal infraction)
√ Pelkan spurs = metaphyseal spurs projecting at right angles to shaft axis
√ Parke corner sign = subepiphyseal infraction / comminution resulting in mushrooming / cupping of epiphysis (DDx: syphilis, rickets)
@ Epiphysis
√ Wimberger ring = sclerotic ring around low-density epiphysis (due to osteopenia of epiphysis)
@ Diaphysis
√ subperiosteal hematoma with calcification of elevated periosteum (sure sign of healing)
@ Teeth
√ cyst formation + hemorrhage in enamel
DDx: TORCH infections, leukemia, neuroblastoma

Adult Scurvy

Incidence: rare
√ hemarthroses + bleeding at synchondroses

SEPTIC ARTHRITIS

N.B.: MEDICAL EMERGENCY = immediate treatment necessary to prevent permanent joint damage!
Organism:
most often due to Staphylococcus aureus; gonorrhea (multifocal septic arthritis in young adults; indistinguishable from tuberculous arthritis, but more rapid); brucellar arthritis (indistinguishable from tuberculosis, slow infection); Salmonella (commonly associated with sickle cell disease / Gaucher disease)
(a) neonates, infants: group D streptococcus
(b) <4 years of age: Hemophilus influenzae, Streptococcus pyogenes, S. aureus,
(c) >4 years of age: S. aureus
(d) >10 years of age: S. aureus, Neisseria gonorrheae
(e) adults: S. aureus
Pathophysiology:
(a) lytic enzymes in purulent articular fluid destroy articular + epiphyseal cartilages
(b) pus increases intraarticular pressure and compromises blood flow to epiphysis resulting in osteonecrosis
Mode of infection:
(1) hematogenous spread (most common; IV drug abuser, immunocompromised patient):
(a) hip, knee in children
(b) the five "S" joints in adults:
Shoulder (AC joint)
Sternoclavicular joint
Spine
SI joint
Symphysis pubis
(2) contiguous spread from focus of osteomyelitis
(a) metaphyseal focus: hip, elbow, shoulder, ankle have intraarticular metaphyses (children)
(b) epiphyseal focus: growth plate perforated by vascular channels in children <1 year of age
(3) direct inoculation of joint from penetrating wound: small joints of hand + feet; unusual organisms like Pseudomonas + Klebsiella
Age: most prevalent in the young
Location: lower extremity (75%) with hip + knee in 90%
• pain, limp, pseudoparalysis
• warmth, swelling
• septic clinical picture
• bacteremia, leukocytosis

ACUTE SIGNS:
√ initial radiographs frequently normal
√ soft-tissue swelling (first sign secondary to local hyperemia + edema)

√ joint distension (effusion) ± subluxation of hip and humerus in children (early)
√ joint space narrowing = rapid development of destruction of articular cartilage (not in tuberculous arthritis)
√ rapid periarticular osteoporosis
US:
√ detection + follow-up of hip effusion
NUC:
√ increased activity in joint + adjacent osteomyelitis
√ occasionally decreased activity simulating avascular necrosis (2° to joint effusion, vascular spasm, vascular compression)
MR:
√ hypointense signal in bone marrow on T1WI
√ enhancement of abnormal bone marrow on fat-suppressed T1WI
√ hyperintense signal in bone marrow on fat-suppressed T2WI

SUBACUTE SIGNS after 8–10 days:
√ small marginal + central erosions in articular cortex / loss of entire cortical outline (marginal erosions in tuberculosis)
√ reactive bone sclerosis in underlying bone
√ subchondral bone destruction (by synovial proliferation)
√ defective reparation / ankylosis (if entire cartilage is destroyed)
√ local bone atrophy (immobility)
√ metaphyseal bone destruction (if osteomyelitis is source of septic joint)

Dx: (1) prompt arthrocentesis:
- turbid / frankly purulent synovial fluid
- fluid WBC >20,000/mm^3 with predominance of PMNs
- positive result of Gram stain

(2) blood culture
Cx: (1) bone growth disturbance (lengthening, shortening, angulation)
(2) chronic degenerative arthritis
(3) ankylosis
(4) osteonecrosis = avascular necrosis

SHIN SPLINTS
= SHIN SORENESS = MEDIAL TIBIAL STRESS SYNDROME = SOLEUS SYNDROME
= nonspecific term describing exertional lower leg pain
Incidence: 75% of exertional leg pain
Cause: ? atypical stress fracture, traction periostitis, compartment syndrome
- diffuse tenderness along posteromedial tibia in its middle to distal aspect

Location: posterior / posteromedial tibial cortex
Plain radiographs:
√ normal / longitudinal periosteal new bone
Bone scintigraphy:
√ normal radionuclide angiogram + blood-pool phase (DDx to stress fracture)
√ linear longitudinal uptake on delayed images
MR:
√ marrow edema / hemorrhage
√ periosteal fluid

SHORT–RIB POLYDACTYLY SYNDROME
= group of autosomal recessive disorders characterized by short limb dysplasia, constricted thorax, postaxial polydactyly (on ulnar / fibular side)
TYPE I = SALDINO-NOONAN SYNDROME
TYPE II = MAJEWSKI TYPE
TYPE III = NAUMOFF TYPE
TYPE BEEMER

√ severe micromelia
√ pointed femurs at both ends (type I); widened metaphyses (type III)
√ narrow thorax
√ extremely short horizontally oriented ribs
√ distorted underossified vertebral bodies + incomplete coronal clefts
√ polydactyly
√ cleft lip / palate
Prognosis: uniformly lethal

SICKLE CELL DISEASE
Abnormal hemoglobins:
HbS = DNA mutation substituting glutamic acid in position 6 on β-chain with valine
HbC = DNA mutation substituting glutamic acid in position 6 on β-chain with lysine
(a) homozygous = HbSS = sickle cell anemia
(b) heterozygous = HbSA = sickling trait but no anemia
(c) heterozygous variants:
— HbSC (less severe form)
— HbS β-thalassemia anemia (seen occasionally)
Incidence: 8–13% of American Blacks carry sickling factor (HbS); 1:40 with sickle cell trait will manifest sickle cell anemia (HbSS); 1:120 with sickle cell trait will manifest HbSC disease
Pathogenesis:
altered shape + plasticity of RBCs under lowered oxygen tension lead to increased blood viscosity, stasis, "log jam" occlusion of small blood vessels, infarction, necrosis, superinfection; damage of intima occurs most frequently in vessels with high flow rates (terminal ICA); sickling occurs in areas of
(a) slow flow (spleen, liver, renal medulla)
(b) rapid metabolism (brain, muscle, fetal placenta)
- chronic hemolytic anemia (increased sequestration of sickled RBCs in spleen), jaundice
- chronic leg ulcers, priapism
- abdominal crisis
- rheumatism-like joint pain
- skeletal pain (osteomyelitis, cellulitis, bone marrow infarction)
- splenomegaly (in children + infants), later organ atrophy

Cx: high incidence of infections (lung, bone, brain)
Prognosis: death <40 years

(1) DEOSSIFICATION DUE TO MARROW HYPERPLASIA
√ porous decrease in bone density of skull (25%)
√ widening of diploe with decrease in width of outer table (22%)
√ vertical hair-on-end striations (5%)
√ osteoporosis with thinning of trabeculae
√ biconcave "fish" vertebrae (bone softening) in 70%
√ widening of medullary space + thinning of cortices
√ coarsening of trabecular pattern in long + flat bones
√ rib notching
√ pathologic fractures

(2) THROMBOSIS AND INFARCTION
Location: in diaphysis of small tubular bones (children); in metaphysis + subchondrium of long bones (adults)
√ osteolysis (in ACUTE infarction)
√ dystrophic medullary calcification
√ periosteal reaction (bone-within-bone appearance)
√ juxtacortical sclerosis
√ Lincoln log = Reynold sign = H-vertebrae = steplike endplate depression
√ articular disintegration
√ collapse of femoral head (DDx: Perthes with involvement of metaphysis)
MR:
√ diffusely decreased signal of marrow on short + long TR/TE images (= hematopoietic marrow replacing fatty marrow)
√ focal areas of decreased signal intensity on short TR/TE + increased intensity on long TR/TE (= acute marrow infarction)
√ focal areas of decreased signal intensity on short TR/TE + long TR/TE images (= old infarction / fibrosis)

(3) SECONDARY OSTEOMYELITIS
Organism: Salmonella in unusual frequency, also Staphylococcus
√ periostitis (DDx: indistinguishable from bone infarction)
√ dactylitis = hand-foot syndrome

(4) GROWTH EFFECTS (secondary to diminished blood supply)
Location: particularly in metacarpal / phalanx
√ bone shortening = premature epiphyseal fusion
√ epiphyseal deformity with cupped metaphysis
√ cup / peg-in-hole defect of distal femur
√ diminution in vertebral height (shortening of stature + kyphoscoliosis)

@ Brain
Pathophysiology:
chronic anemia produces cerebral hyperemia, hypervolemia, impaired autoregulation
(a) cerebral blood flow cannot be increased leading to infarction in time of crisis
(b) increased cerebral blood flow produces epithelial hyperplasia of large intracranial vessels (terminal ICA / proximal MCA) resulting in thrombus formation
• stroke (5–17%): ischemic infarction (70%), ischemia of deep white matter (25%), hemorrhage (20%), embolic infarction
Angio (in 87% abnormal):
√ arterial stenosis / occlusion of supraclinoid portion of ICA + proximal segments of ACA and MCA
√ moyamoya syndrome (35%)
√ distal branch occlusion (secondary to thrombosis / embolism)
√ aneurysm (rare)
CT:
√ cerebral infarction (mean age of 7.7 years)
√ subarachnoid hemorrhage (mean age of 27 years)

@ Chest
√ cardiomegaly + CHF

@ Gallbladder
√ cholelithiasis

@ Kidney
• hematuria
• hyposthenuria
• nephrotic syndrome
• renal tubular acidosis (distal)
• hyperuricemia
• progressive renal insufficiency
√ normal urogram (70%)
√ papillary necrosis (20%)
√ focal renal scarring (20%)
√ smooth large kidney (4%)
MR:
√ decreased cortical signal on T2-weighted images (renal cortical iron deposition)

@ Spleen
√ splenomegaly < age 10 (in patients with heterozygous sickle cell disease)
Cx: splenic rupture
√ splenic infarction
√ hemosiderosis

Functional Asplenia
= anatomically present nonfunctional spleen
• Howell-Jolly bodies, siderocytes, anisocytosis, irreversibly sickled cells
√ normal-sized / enlarged spleen on CT
√ absence of tracer uptake on sulfur colloid scan

Autosplenectomy
= autoinfarction of spleen in homozygous sickle cell disease (function lost by age 5)
Histo: extensive perivascular fibrosis with deposition of hemosiderin + calcium
√ small (as small as 5–10 mm) densely calcified spleen

Acute Splenic Sequestration Crisis
= sudden trapping of large amount of blood in spleen

Cause: obstruction of small intrasplenic veins / sinusoids; unknown trigger event

Age: (a) homozygous: infancy / childhood
(b) heterozygous: any age

- LUQ pain
- sudden massive splenic enlargement
- rapid drop in hemoglobin, hematocrit, platelets (spleen traps large volumes of blood)
- rise in reticulocytes

√ enlarged spleen
√ multiple lesions at periphery of spleen: hypoechoic by US, of low attenuation by CT
√ hyperdense areas (due to acute hemorrhage)
√ hyperintense areas on T1WI + T2WI (due to subacute hemorrhage)
√ main splenic vessels patent by Doppler US

Prognosis: in 50% death <2 years of age (due to hypovolemic shock)

Bone marrow scintigraphy:

√ usually symmetric marked expansion of hematopoietic marrow beyond age 20 involving entire femur, calvarium, small bones of hand + feet (normally only in axial skeleton + proximal femur and humerus)
√ bone marrow defects indicative of acute / old infarction

Tc-99m diphosphonate scan:

√ increased overall skeletal uptake (high bone-to-soft tissue ratio)
√ prominent activities at knees, ankles, proximal humerus (delayed epiphyseal closure / increased blood flow to bone marrow)
√ bone marrow expansion (calvarial thickening with relative decrease in activity along falx insertion)
√ decreased / normal uptake on bone scan within 24 hours in acute infarction / posthealing phase following infarction (cyst formation)
√ increased uptake on bone scan after 2–10 days persistent for several weeks in healing infarction
√ increased uptake on bone scan within 24–48 hours in osteomyelitis
√ increased blood-pool activity + normal delayed image on bone scan in cellulitis
√ renal enlargement with marked retention of tracer in renal parenchyma (medullary ischemia + failure of countercurrent system) in 50%
√ persistent splenic uptake (secondary to degeneration, atrophy, fibrosis, calcifications)

Sickle Cell Trait

Hb SA carrier; mild disease with few episodes of crisis + infection; sickling provoked only under extreme stress (unpressurized aircraft, anoxia with CHD, prolonged anesthesia, marathon running)

Incidence: in 8–10% of American Blacks

- may have normal blood count
- recurrent gross hematuria

√ splenic infarction

SC Disease

Hb SC carrier

Incidence: 3% of American Blacks

- retinal hemorrhages
- hematuria due to multiple infarctions

√ aseptic necrosis of hip

Sickle-Thal Disease

Resembling clinically Hb SS patients

- anemia (no normal adult hemoglobin)

√ persistent splenomegaly

SINDING-LARSEN-JOHANSSON DISEASE

= osteochondrosis of inferior pole of patella, often bilateral (NOT osteonecrosis / epiphysitis / osteochondritis)

Cause: traction with contusion + subsequent tendinitis / traumatic avulsion of bone; repeated subluxation ± dislocation of patella

Age: adolescents (often 10–14 years)

Predisposed: cerebrospastic children

- tenderness + soft-tissue swelling over lower pole of patella

√ peripatellar soft-tissue swelling
√ calcification / ossification of patellar tendon
√ small bone fragments at lower pole of patella (LAT view)

MR:

√ hypointense area on T1WI + hyperintense on T2WI in inferior pole of patella + surrounding soft tissues

SMALLPOX

5% of infants

Location: elbow bilateral; metaphysis of long bones

√ rapid bone destruction spreading along shaft
√ periosteal reaction
√ endosteal + cortical sclerosis frequent
√ premature epiphyseal fusion with severe deformity
√ ankylosis is frequent

SOFT-TISSUE CHONDROMA

= EXTRASKELETAL CHONDROMA = CHONDROMA OF SOFT PARTS

Incidence: 1.5% of all benign soft-tissue tumors

Age: 30–60 years (range 1–85 years); M:F = 1.2:1

Histo: adult-type hyaline cartilage with areas of calcification + ossification; myxoid change; regions of increased cellularity + cytologic atypia

- slow-growing soft-tissue mass
- occasionally pain + tenderness

Location: hand (54–64%) + foot (20–28%)

√ lobulated well-defined extraskeletal mass <2 cm in size
√ may contain calcifications (33–70%) with ringlike appearance / ossifications
√ scalloping of adjacent bone with sclerotic reaction

MR:

√ high signal intensity on T2WI
√ intermediate signal intensity on T1WI

Rx: local excision

Prognosis: 15–25% recurrence rate

DDx: (1) Extraskeletal myxoid chondrosarcoma (deep-seated in large muscles of upper + lower extremities, pelvic + shoulder girdles)
(2) Periosteal chondroma

SOFT-TISSUE OSTEOMA

= OSTEOMA OF SOFT PARTS (extremely rare)

Histo: mature lamellar bone with well-defined haversian system; bone marrow, myxoid, vascular, fibrous connective tissue between bone trabeculae; collagenous capsule blending into benign hyaline cartilage

Location: head (usually posterior part of tongue), thigh

√ ossified mass

NUC:
- √ intense tracer accumulation, greater than adjacent bone

SOLITARY BONE CYST

= UNICAMERAL / SIMPLE BONE CYST

Incidence: up to 5% of primary bone lesions

Etiology: ? trauma (synovial entrapment at capsular reflection), ? vascular anomaly (blockage of interstitial drainage)

Histo: cyst filled with clear yellowish fluid often under pressure, wall lined with fibrous tissue + hemosiderin, giant cells may be present

Age: 3–19 years (80%); occurs during active phase of bone growth; M:F = 3:1

• asymptomatic, unless fractured

Location: proximal femur + proximal humerus (60–75%), fibula, at base of calcaneal neck (4%, >12 years of age), talus; rare in ribs, ilium, small bones of hand + feet (rare), NOT in spine / calvarium; solitary lesion

Site: intramedullary centric metaphyseal, adjacent to epiphyseal cartilage (during active phase) / migrating into diaphysis with growth (during latent phase), does not cross epiphyseal plate

√ 2–3 cm oval radiolucency with long axis parallel to long axis of host bone

√ fine sclerotic boundary

√ scalloping + erosion of internal aspect of underlying cortex

√ photopenic area on bone scan (if not fractured)

√ "fallen fragment" sign if fractured (20%) = centrally dislodged fragment falls into a dependent position

Prognosis: mostly spontaneous regression

Cx: pathologic fracture (65%)

DDx: (1) Enchondroma (calcific stipplings)
(2) Fibrous dysplasia (more irregular lucency)
(3) Eosinophilic granuloma
(4) Chondroblastoma (epiphyseal)
(5) Chondromyxoid fibroma (more eccentric + expansile)
(6) Giant cell tumor
(7) Aneurysmal bone cyst (eccentric)
(8) Hemorrhagic cyst
(9) Brown tumor

SOLITARY PLASMACYTOMA OF BONE

= represents early stage of multiple myeloma, precedes multiple myeloma by 1–20 years

Age: 5th–7th decade

• negative marrow aspiration; no IgG spike in serum / urine

A. SOLITARY MYELOMA OF BONE

Site: thoracic / lumbar spine (most common) > pelvis > ribs > sternum, skull, femora, humeri

√ solitary "bubbly" osteolytic grossly expansile lesion

√ poorly defined margins, Swiss-cheese pattern

√ frequently pathologic fracture (collapse of vertebra)

DDx: giant cell tumor, aneurysmal bone cyst, osteoblastoma, solitary metastasis from renal cell / thyroid carcinoma

B. EXTRAMEDULLARY PLASMACYTOMA

Location: majority in head + neck; 80% in nasal cavity, paranasal sinuses, upper airways of trachea, lung parenchyma

SPONDYLOEPIPHYSEAL DYSPLASIA

Spondyloepiphyseal Dysplasia Congenita

Autosomal dominant / sporadic (most)

• disproportionate dwarfism with spine + hips more involved than extremities
• waddling gait + muscular weakness
• flat facies
• short neck
• deafness

√ cleft palate

@ Axial skeleton
- √ ovoid vertebral bodies + severe platyspondyly (incomplete fusion of ossification centers + flattening of vertebral bodies)
- √ hypoplasia of odontoid process (Cx: cervical myelopathy)
- √ progressive kyphoscoliosis (short trunk) involving thoracic + lumbar spine
- √ narrowing of disk spaces (resulting in short trunk)
- √ broad iliac bases + deficient ossification of pubis
- √ flat acetabular roof

@ Chest
- √ bell-shaped thorax
- √ pectus carinatum

@ Extremities
- √ normal / slightly shortened limbs
- √ severe coxa vara + genu valgum
- √ multiple accessory epiphyses in hands + feet
- √ talipes equinovarus

Cx: (1) Retinal detachment, myopia (50%)
(2) Secondary arthritis in weight-bearing joints

Spondyloepiphyseal Dysplasia Tarda

= sex-linked recessive form with milder manifestation + later clinical onset

Age: apparent by 10 years; exclusive to males

√ hyperostotic new bone along posterior 2/3 of vertebral end plate (PATHOGNOMONIC)

√ platyspondyly with depression of anterior 1/3 of vertebral body

√ narrowing with calcification of disk spaces + spondylitic bridging
√ short trunk
√ dysplastic joints (eg, flattened femoral heads)
√ premature osteoarthritis
DDx: Ochronosis

SPRENGEL DEFORMITY

= failure of descent of scapula secondary to fibrous / osseous omovertebral connection
Associated with: Klippel-Feil syndrome, renal anomalies
• webbed neck
• shoulder immobility
√ elevation + medial rotation of scapula

SUBUNGUAL EXOSTOSIS

= DUPUYTREN EXOSTOSIS
Cause: repetitive trauma (14–25%)
Age: 2nd – 3rd decade (range, 7–58 years)
Histo: proliferating fibroblasts developing into fibrocartilage + bone
Location: toes (86–90%, great toe in 77–80%), thumb + index finger (10–14%, dominant hand in 75%)
Site: dorsal / dorsomedial aspect of distal phalanx
• mass under / adjacent to nail bed ± rapid growth
• may be painful with overlying skin ulceration
√ ossific mass distal to physeal scar:
  √ NO continuity to cortex / medulla of host bone
  √ broad / narrow base
√ indistinct / well-demarcated cartilage cap larger than base
Rx: complete surgical excision
Prognosis: 11–53% recurrence rate
DDx: osteochondroma (exostosis continuous with cortex and medulla of host bone)

SUPERFICIAL FIBROMATOSES

Infantile Digital Fibromatosis

= REYE TUMOR = INFANTILE DIGITAL FIBROMA
= INFANTILE DIGITAL MYOFIBROBLASTOMA
= single / multiple nodular dermal protrusion of fibrous tissue on extensor surface of digits
Age: 1st year of life (>80%); 30% congenital
Histo: intracytoplasmic perinuclear inclusion bodies
Location: fingers (60%) , toes (40%)
Site: lateral aspect of distal / middle phalanx
√ nonspecific soft-tissue mass involving a digit
√ infrequently bone involvement
Prognosis: spontaneous regression (in 8%); 60% recurrence rate after excision

Juvenile Aponeurotic Fibroma

= CALCIFIED APONEUROTIC FIBROMA
= rare locally aggressive benign fibrous tumor
Histo: cellular dense fibrous tissue with focal chondral elements infiltrating adjacent structures (= cartilaginous tumor)
Age: children + adolescents (within first 2 decades of life); M:F = 2:1
• slow-growing asymptomatic soft-tissue mass
Location: deep palmar fascia of hand + wrist (67%); soles of feet
√ nonspecific soft-tissue mass overlying inflamed bursa (often mistaken for calcified bursitis)
√ stippled calcifications (frequent)
√ interosseous soft-tissue mass of forearm + wrist
√ erosion / scalloping of bone may occur
Prognosis: recurrence rate of >50% after resection
Dx: biopsy (to differentiate from synovial sarcoma)
DDx: synovial sarcoma (commonly calcifies, bone erosion), chondroma, fibrosarcoma, osteosarcoma, myositis ossificans

Palmar Fibromatosis

= DUPUYTREN DISEASE
Prevalence: 1–2%
Age: in 24% of people >65 years; M:F = 4:1
• subcutaneous nodules on palmar surface of distal crease of hand progressing to cords and bands
• flexion contractures of digits (2° to fibrous attachment to flexor tendons)
Location: 4th + 5th (most commonly) > 2nd + 3rd digit; bilateral in 42–60%
√ predominantly hypointense on T2WI + low to intermediate intensity on T1WI (in hypocellular lesions)
√ intermediate signal intensity on T2WI (proliferative hypercellular lesions)

Plantar Fibromatosis

= PLANTAR FASCIITIS = LEDDERHOSE DISEASE
= common form of superficial fibromatosis
Cause: trauma
Age: 30–50 years
Path: abnormal fibrous tissue replacing the plantar aponeurosis and infiltrating subcutaneous tissue + skin
Histo: nonencapsulated proliferation of fibroblasts separated by variable amounts of collagen
At risk: runners, obese patients
Associated with (in 50%): Dupuytren contracture (10–65%), Peyronie disease
• heel pain (one of the most common causes)
• one / multiple firm fixed subcutaneous nodules
Location: proximal / central portion of plantar aponeurosis; bilateral in 20–50%
Site: medial aspect of aponeurosis
√ calcaneal spur
MR:
  √ single or multiple nodules / poorly defined infiltrative mass iso- / hypointense compared to plantar muscles on T1WI + T2WI
  √ marked contrast enhancement in 50%
  √ ± subcutaneous edema

SYNOVIAL OSTEOCHONDROMATOSIS

= SYNOVIAL CHONDROMATOSIS = JOINT CHONDROMA

Primary Synovial Osteochondromatosis

= benign self-limiting monoarticular disorder characterized by proliferation + metaplastic transformation of the synovium with formation of multiple intrasynovial cartilaginous / osteocartilaginous nodules

Cause: hyperplastic synovium with cartilage metaplasia (foci <2–3 cm); loose body may remain free floating / conglomerate with other loose bodies into large mass / reattach to synovium with either reabsorption or continued growth

Histo: foci of hyaline cartilage with mineralized chondroid matrix beneath synovial surface + within subsynovial connective tissue; hypercellularity + nuclear atypia may be confused with malignancy

Composition of cartilaginous bodies:
cartilage alone / cartilage + bone / mature bone + fatty marrow

Age: presents in 3rd–5th decade; M:F = 2–4:1

• slow-growing soft-tissue mass in joint
• progressive joint pain for several years with limitation of motion / locking
• ± hemorrhagic joint effusion

Location: knee (most common with >50%, in 10% bilateral) elbow > hip > shoulder > ankle > wrist; usually monoarticular, occasionally bilateral

Sites: joint / tendon sheath / ganglion / bursa

√ multiple calcified / ossified loose bodies in a single joint
(bony shell of remodeled lamellar bone is rare)
√ size of nodules varies between a few mm to several cm
√ varying degrees of bone mineralization (25–30% of chondromas show no radiopacity)
√ pressure erosion of adjacent bone in joints with tight capsule (eg, hip)
√ widening of joint space (from accumulation of loose bodies)
√ joint effusion uncommon
√ NO osteoporosis

CT:
√ multiple calcified / ossified intraarticular bodies
√ intraarticular soft-tissue mass of near-water attenuation containing multiple small calcifications

MR:
√ lobulated intraarticular mass isointense to muscle on T1WI + hyperintense to muscle on T2WI containing multiple foci of low signal intensity
DDx: large effusion, soft-tissue tumor
√ peripheral contrast enhancement of chondral lesions
√ central area of high-signal intensity on T1WI for intraarticular bodies with fatty marrow

Cx: (1) Long-standing disease may lead to degenerative arthritis (from chronic mechanical irritation + destruction of articular cartilage by loose bodies)
(2) Malignant dedifferentiation to chondrosarcoma

Rx: removal of loose bodies (recurrence is common)

DDx: (1) Synovial sarcoma, chondrosarcoma
(2) Osteochondral fracture (history of trauma), osteochondritis dissecans, osteonecrosis
(3) Secondary osteochondromatosis
(4) Pigmented villonodular synovitis, synovial hemangioma, lipoma arborescens

Secondary Synovial Osteochondromatosis

= joint surface disintegration

Cause: trauma, osteonecrosis, rheumatoid arthritis, neuropathic arthropathy, tuberculous arthritis, degenerative joint disease

√ intraarticular bodies tend to be larger, less numerous, more varied in size compared to primary synovial osteochondromatosis
√ prominent osteoarthritis

SYNOVIOMA

= SYNOVIAL SARCOMA
= slow-growing expansile malignant tumor originating in the synovial lining / bursa / tendon sheath; uncommonly intraarticular

Incidence: 10% of soft-tissue sarcomas

Histo: fibrosarcomatous + synovial component

Age: 3rd–5th decade; M:F = 2:3

• painful soft-tissue mass

Location: knee (most common), hip, ankle, elbow, wrist, hands, feet; usually solitary

√ large spheroid well-defined soft-tissue mass
√ lesion about 1 cm removed from joint cartilage
√ amorphous calcifications (1/3), often at periphery
√ involvement of adjacent bone (11–20%):
 √ periosteal reaction
 √ bone remodeling (pressure from tumor)
 √ invasion of cortex with wide zone of transition
√ juxtaarticular osteoporosis

MR:
√ low signal intensity on T1WI
√ inhomogeneously increased signal intensity on T2WI
√ multilocular appearance with internal septation
√ fluid-fluid levels (previous hemorrhage)

Rx: local excision / amputation + radiation / chemotherapy

SYPHILIS OF BONE

Congenital Syphilis

◊ Transplacental transmission cannot occur <16 weeks gestational age

• positive rapid plasma reagin (measures quantity of antibodies to assess new infection / efficacy of Rx)
• positive microhemagglutination test for Treponema pallidum (remains reactive for life)

√ pneumonia alba
√ hepatomegaly

Location: symmetrical bilateral osteomyelitis involving multiple bones (HALLMARK)

A. Early phase
◊ Skeletal radiography abnormal in 19% of infected newborns without overt disease!
1. Metaphysitis
√ lucent metaphyseal band adjacent to thin / widened zone of provisional calcification (disturbance in enchondral bone growth)
√ frayed edge of metaphyseal-physeal junction (osteochondritis) = erosions + lytic defects
2. Diaphyseal periostitis = "luetic diaphysitis"
√ solid / lamellated periosteal new-bone growth = bone-within-bone appearance
3. Spontaneous epiphyseal fractures causing Parrot pseudopalsy (DDx: battered child syndrome)
4. Bone destruction
√ marginal destruction of spongiosa + cortex along side of shaft with widening of medullary canal (in short tubular bones)
√ patchy rarefaction in diaphysis
5. Wimberger sign
√ symmetrical focal bone destruction of medial portion of proximal tibial metaphysis (ALMOST PATHOGNOMONIC)

B. Late phase
• Hutchinson triad = dental abnormality, interstitial keratitis, 8th nerve deafness
√ frontal bossing of Parrot = diffuse thickening of outer table
√ saddle nose + high palate (syphilitic chondritis + rhinitis)
√ short maxilla (maxillary osteitis)
√ thickening at sternal end of clavicle
√ "saber-shin" deformity = anteriorly convex bowing in upper 2/3 of tibia with bone thickening

Acquired Syphilis

= TERTIARY SYPHILIS resembles chronic osteomyelitis
√ dense bone sclerosis of long bones
√ irregular periosteal proliferation + endosteal thickening with narrow medulla
√ extensive calvarial bone proliferation with mottled pattern (anterior half + lateral skull) in outer table (DDx: fibrous dysplasia, Paget disease)
√ ill-defined lytic destruction in skull, spine, long bones (gumma formation)
√ enlargement of clavicle (cortical + endosteal new bone)
√ Charcot arthropathy of lower extremities + spine

TARSAL COALITION

= abnormal fibrous / cartilaginous / osseous fusion of two or more tarsal ossification bones
◊ Clinically most important congenital problem of calcaneus
Prevalence: 1–2% of population
Cause: abnormal segmentation of primitive mesenchyme with lack of joint formation
Age: fibrous coalition at birth, ossification during 2nd decade of life with onset of symptoms; M:F = 1:1
• asymptomatic; often first noted after antecedent trauma / weight gain / increase in athletic activity
• peroneal spastic / rigid pes planus (=flatfoot) in adjustment for calcaneus valgus (= heel valgus)
• hindfoot / tarsal pain or stiffness
√ both feet affected in 20–50%
√ osseous bars between bones of hindfoot / bones in close proximity with irregular surfaces

MR (of joint space):
√ bone marrow contiguity (osseous coalition)
√ fluid- / cartilage-intensity (cartilaginous coalition)
√ intermediate- to low-signal intensity (fibrous coalition)
√ reactive periarticular bone changes
√ bone marrow edema along fused joint (STIR images)

Types:
(1) Calcaneonavicular coalition (45%)
Age: 8–12 years (due to earlier ossification)
• rigid flat foot ± pain in 2nd decade of life
Radiographs:
√ narrowed calcaneonavicular joint with indistinct articular margins (bones that usually do not articulate)
√ widening / flattening of anteromedial calcaneus
√ "anteater's nose" = elongation of anterior dorsal calcaneus on lateral radiograph
√ hypoplastic talar head
CT (axial scan):
√ broadening of medial aspect of anterodorsal calcaneus in apposition to navicular
√ narrowing of space between the 2 bones + minimal marginal reactive sclerosis
Dx: mostly diagnosed on 45° internal oblique films

(2) Talocalcaneal coalition (45%)
Age: 12–16 years
• painful peroneal spastic flat foot, relieved by rest
Site: middle facet at level of sustentaculum tali (most frequently)
Secondary radiographic signs (due to alteration in hindfoot biomechanics):
√ prominent talar beak (66%) arising from dorsal aspect of head / neck of talus (due to impaired subtalar joint motion)
√ rounding of the lateral talar process
√ narrowing of posterior subtalar joint
√ lack of depiction of middle facets
√ asymmetric anterior talocalcaneal joint
√ "ball-in-socket" ankle mortise in severe cases
√ "C sign" = C-shaped outline of the medial talar dome + posteroinferior sustentaculum on lateral radiograph (from bone bridge between talar dome + sustentaculum)
CT (coronal scan):
√ bony bar bridging the middle facet of subtalar joint
√ narrowed middle facet with reactive cystic + hypertrophic changes
√ downward or horizontal slope of sustentaculum, instead of upward
Dx: requires cross-sectional imaging for diagnosis

(3) Talonavicular coalition
(4) Calcaneocuboid coalition
(5) Cubonavicular coalition

Rx: orthotics, casting, NSAID, steroid injections, physical therapy, resection, arthrodesis

DDx: acquired intertarsal ankylosis (infection, trauma, arthritis, surgery)

THALASSEMIA SYNDROMES

= inherited disorders of hemoglobin synthesis typically seen in individuals of Mediterranean descent

Physiologic hemoglobins:

(a) in adulthood:
  Hb A (98% = 2 α- and 2 β-chains);
  Hb A_2 (2% = 2 α- and 2 δ-chains)

(b) in fetal life, rapidly decreasing up to 3 months of newborn period:
  Hb F (= 2 α- and 2 γ-chains)

A. ALPHA-THALASSEMIA
  = decreased synthesis of a-chains leading to excess of β-chains + γ-chains (Hb H = 4 β-chains; Hb Bart = 4 γ-chains)
  • disease begins in intrauterine life as no fetal hemoglobin is produced
  • homozygosity is lethal (lack of oxygen transport)

B. BETA-THALASSEMIA
  = decreased synthesis of β-chains leading to excess of α-chains + γ-chains (= fetal hemoglobin)
  • disease manifest in early infancy
  (a) homozygous defect = thalassemia major = Cooley anemia
  (b) heterozygous defect = thalassemia minor

Thalassemia Major

= COOLEY ANEMIA = MEDITERRANEAN ANEMIA
= HEREDITARY LEPTOCYTOSIS = β-THALASSEMIA
= most severe form with trait inherited from both parents (= homozygous form)

Incidence: 1% for American Blacks; 7.4% for Greek population; 10% for certain Italian populations

Age: develops after newborn period within first 2 years of life

• retarded growth
• elevated serum bilirubin
• hyperpigmentation of skin
• hyperuricemia
• secondary sexual characteristics retarded, normal menstruation rare (primary gonadotropin insufficiency from iron overload in pituitary gland)
• hypochromic microcytic anemia (Hb 2–3 g/dL), nucleated RBC, target cells, reticulocytosis, decrease in RBC survival, leukocytosis
• susceptible to infection (leukopenia secondary to splenomegaly)
• bleeding diathesis (secondary to thrombocytopenia)

@ Skull:
  • mongoloid facies
  √ marrow expansion of diploe:
    √ widening of diploic space with coarsened trabeculations and displacement (from marrow hyperplasia = extramedullary hematopoiesis)
    √ thinning of outer table
    √ frontal bossing
    √ severe hair-on-end appearance (frontal bone, NOT inferior to internal occipital protuberance)
  √ marrow expansion in paranasal sinuses:
    √ impaired pneumatization of maxillary antra + mastoid sinuses
    √ narrowing of nasal cavity
    √ rodent facies = ventral displacement of incisors (marrow overgrowth in maxillary bone) with dental malocclusion
  √ lateral displacement of orbits

@ Peripheral skeleton:
  • earliest changes in small bones of hands + feet (>6 months of age)
  √ diffuse osteopenia:
    √ atrophy + coarsening of trabeculae (from marrow hyperplasia)
    √ prominence of nutrient foramina
  √ widened medullary spaces with thinning of cortices:
    √ Erlenmeyer flask deformity = bulging of normally concave outline of metaphyses
  √ premature fusion of epiphyses (10%), usually at proximal humerus + distal femur
  √ arthropathy (secondary to hemochromatosis + CPPD + acute gouty arthritis)
  √ regression of peripheral skeletal changes (as red marrow becomes yellow)

@ Chest:
  √ cardiac enlargement + congestive heart failure (secondary to anemia)
  √ paravertebral masses (= extramedullary hematopoiesis)

@ Ribs
  √ costal osteomas = bulbous widening of posterior aspect of ribs with thinned cortices
  √ undertubulated broad ribs
  √ heterogenous rib ossification:
    √ localized lucencies
    √ cortical erosion
    √ rib-within-rib appearance

@ Abdomen:
  √ hepatosplenomegaly
  √ gallstones

Cx: (1) Pathologic fractures
(2) Iron overload + hemosiderosis from frequent blood transfusion therapy (absent puberty, diabetes mellitus, adrenal insufficiency, myocardial insufficiency)

Prognosis: usually death within 1st decade

Rx: systematic transfusion has lessened the severity of skeletal abnormalities

DDx: chronic anemia, storage diseases, fibrous dysplasia

Thalassemia Intermedia

= subgroup of homozygous form
• milder clinical presentation

- not requiring hypertransfusion to maintain an adequate hematocrit

Prognosis: longer life expectancy

Thalassemia Minor

= beta-thalassemia trait inherited from one parent (= heterozygous)

- usually asymptomatic except for periods of stress (pregnancy, infection)
- microcytic hypochromic anemia (Hb 9–11 g/dL)
- occasionally jaundice + splenomegaly

THANATOPHORIC DYSPLASIA

= sporadic lethal skeletal dysplasia characterized by severe rhizomelia (micromelic dwarfism) transmitted by a dominant gene mutation

Incidence: 6.9:100,000 births; 1:6,400–16,700 births;
◊ Most common lethal bone dysplasia after osteogenesis imperfecta type II

- severe respiratory distress (early in life)
- hypotonic infants
- protuberant abdomen
- extended arms + abducted externally rotated thighs

@ Head
- √ large head with short base of skull + prominent frontal bone
- √ occasionally trilobed cloverleaf skull = "Kleeblattschädel"

@ Chest radiograph (PATHOGNOMONIC)
- √ narrow chest
- √ short horizontal ribs:
  - √ not extending beyond anterior axillary line
  - √ cupped anterior ends
- √ short curved "telephone handle" humeri
- √ H- / U-shaped vertebra plana
- √ small scapula + normal clavicles

@ Spine
- √ normal length of trunk
- √ reduction of interpediculate space of last few lumbar vertebrae
- √ extreme generalized platyspondyly = severe H- / U-shaped vertebra plana
- √ excessive intervertebral space height

@ Pelvis (hypoplastic iliac bones)
- √ iliac wings small + square (vertical shortening but wide horizontally)
- √ flat acetabulum
- √ narrow sacrosciatic notch
- √ short pubic bones

@ Extremities
- √ severe micromelia + bowing of extremities
- √ metaphyseal flaring = "telephone handle" appearance of long bones
- √ thornlike projections in metaphyseal area
- √ polydactyly

OB-US (findings may be seen very early in pregnancy):
- √ polyhydramnios (71%)
- √ short-limbed dwarfism with extremely short + bowed "telephone receiver"-like femurs
- √ extremely small hypoplastic thorax with short ribs + narrowed in anteroposterior dimension
- √ protuberant abdomen
- √ macrocrania with frontal bossing ± hydrocephalus (increased HC:AC ratio)
- √ "cloverleaf skull" (in 14%) (DDx: encephalocele)
- √ diffuse platyspondyly
- √ redundant soft tissues

Prognosis: often stillborn; uniformly fatal within a few hours / days after birth (respiratory failure)

DDx:
(1) Ellis-van Creveld syndrome (extra digit, acromesomelic short limbs)
(2) Asphyxiating thoracic dysplasia (less marked bone shortening, vertebrae spared)
(3) Short-rib polydactyly syndrome
(4) Homozygous achondroplasia
(5) Achondrogenesis

THROMBOCYTOPENIA-ABSENT RADIUS SYNDROME

= TAR SYNDROME
= rare autosomal recessive disorder

Age: presentation at birth

May be associated with: CHD (33%): ASD, tetralogy

- platelet count <100,000/mm^3 (decreased production by bone marrow)
- √ usually bilateral radial aplasia / hypoplasia
- √ uni- / bilaterally hypoplastic / absent ulna / humerus
- √ defects of hands, feet, legs

Prognosis: death in 50% in early infancy (hemorrhage)

THYROID ACROPACHY

Onset: after 18 months following thyroidectomy for hyperthyroidism (does not occur with antithyroid medication)

Incidence: 0.5–1% of patients with thyrotoxicosis

- clubbing, soft-tissue swelling
- eu- / hypo- / hyperthyroid state

Location: diaphyses of phalanges + metacarpals of hand; less commonly feet, lower legs, forearms

- √ thick spiculated lacy "feathery" periosteal reaction

DDx:
(1) Pulmonary osteoarthropathy (painful)
(2) Pachydermoperiostosis
(3) Fluorosis (ligamentous calcifications)

TRANSIENT REGIONAL OSTEOPOROSIS

= TRANSIENT BONE MARROW EDEMA

Cause: unknown; ? overactivity of sympathetic nervous system + local hyperemia similar to reflex sympathetic dystrophy syndrome, trauma, synovitis, transient ischemia

Regional Migratory Osteoporosis

= rapid onset of self-limiting episodes of severe localized osteoporosis and pain but repetitive occurrence of same symptoms in other regions of the same or opposite lower extremity

- rapid onset of local pain
- diffuse erythema, swelling, increased heat
- significant disability due to severe pain on weight bearing

Age: middle-aged males
Location: usually lower extremity (ie, ankle, knee, hip, foot)
√ rapid localized osteoporosis within 4–8 weeks after onset migrating from one joint to another; may affect trabecular / cortical bone
√ linear / wavy periosteal reaction
√ preservation of subchondral cortical bone
√ no joint space narrowing, bone erosion
MR:
√ affected area has low signal intensity on T1WI, high signal intensity on T2WI (= bone marrow edema)
NUC:
√ increased activity
Prognosis: persists for 6–9 months in one area; cycle of symptoms may last for several years
Rx: variable response to analgesics / corticosteroids

Partial Transient Osteoporosis

= variant of regional migratory osteoporosis with more focal pattern of osteoporosis, which may eventually become more generalized
(a) Zonal form = portion of bone involved, ie, one femoral condyle / one quadrant of femoral head
(b) Radial form = only one / two rays of hand / foot involved

Transient Osteoporosis of Hip

= self-limiting disease of unknown etiology
Age: typically in middle-aged males / in 3rd trimester of pregnancy in females involving left hip; M > F

- spontaneous onset of hip and groin pain, usually progressive over several weeks
- painful swelling of joint followed by progressive demineralization
- rapid development of disability, limp, decreased range of motion

Site: hip most commonly affected; generally only one joint at a time
√ progressive marked osteoporosis of femoral head, neck, acetabulum (3–8 weeks after onset of illness)
√ virtually PATHOGNOMONIC striking loss of subchondral cortex of femoral head + neck region
√ NO joint space narrowing / subchondral bone collapse
NUC:
√ markedly increased uptake on bone scan without cold spots / inhomogeneities (positive before radiograph)
MR:
√ diffuse bone marrow edema involving femoral head + neck + sometimes intertrochanteric region
√ small joint effusion
Cx: pathologic fracture common
Prognosis: spontaneous recovery within 2–6 months; recurrence in another joint within 2 years possible

DDx: (1) AVN (cystic + sclerotic changes, early subchondral undermining)
(2) Septic / tuberculous arthritis (joint aspiration!)
(3) Monoarticular rheumatoid arthritis
(4) Metastasis
(5) Reflex sympathetic dystrophy
(6) Disuse atrophy
(7) Synovial chondromatosis
(8) Villonodular synovitis

TRANSIENT SYNOVITIS OF HIP

= OBSERVATION HIP = TRANSITORY SYNOVITIS = TOXIC SYNOVITIS = COXITIS FUGAX
= nonspecific inflammatory reaction
◊ Most common nontraumatic cause of acute limp in a child
Etiology: unknown; no organism on joint aspiration
Age: 5–10 (average 6) years; M:F = 2:1

- history of recent viral illness (65%)
- developing limp over 1–2 days
- pain in hip, thigh, knee
- mild fever (25%), mildly elevated ESR (50%)

√ radiographs usually normal
√ joint effusion:
√ displacement of femur from acetabulum
√ displacement of psoas line
√ lateral displacement of gluteal line (least sensitive + least reliable)
√ regional osteoporosis (? hyperemia, disuse)
NUC:
√ normal / slight increase in activity (excluding osteomyelitis + avascular necrosis)
Prognosis: complete recovery within a few weeks
Dx: per exclusion
Rx: non–weight-bearing treatment
DDx: trauma, Legg-Perthes disease, acute rheumatoid arthritis, acute rheumatic fever, septic arthritis, tuberculosis, malignancy

TREACHER-COLLINS SYNDROME

= MANDIBULOFACIAL DYSOSTOSIS
= autosomal dominant disease (with new mutations in 60%) characterized by bilateral malformations of eyes, malar bones, mandible, and ears resulting in birdlike face
Incidence: 1:50,000 births
Cause: defect in growth of 1st + 3rd branchial arches before the 7th to 8th week of gestation
◊ NO limb anomalies (important DDx!)

- extension of scalp hair growth onto cheek
- microstomia

√ craniosynostosis
√ narrowing of retropharyngeal space (apnea, speech difficulties)
@ Eyes
- antimongoloid eye slant (drooping lateral lower eyelids due to hypoplasia of lateral canthal tendon of orbicular muscle)
- sparse / absent eye lashes / coloboma in lower lids

√ egg-shaped orbits = drooping of outer inferior orbital rim
√ hypoplasia of lateral wall of orbits + shallow / incomplete orbital floor

@ Nose
- broad / protruded nose

√ choanal shortening

@ Malar bone
√ sunken cheek due to marked hypoplasia / agenesis of zygomatic arches (= malar hypoplasia)

@ Maxilla
√ hypoplasia of maxilla + maxillary sinus
√ narrow / overprojected maxilla
√ high-arched / narrow palate

@ Mandible
- retruded chin, retrognathism
- dental malocclusion

√ pronounced micrognathia = mandibular hypoplasia with broad concave curve on lower border of body

@ Ear
- dysplastic low-set auricles
- preauricular skin tags / fistulas
- conductive hearing loss (common)

√ microtia with small middle ear cavity
√ deformed / fused / absent auditory ossicles
√ atresia / stenosis of external auditory canal

OB-US:
√ polyhydramnios (from swallowing difficulty)

Prognosis: early respiratory problems (tongue relatively too large for hypoplastic mandible)

Rx: surgical correction

DDx: (1) Goldenhar-Gorlin syndrome (unilateral microtia + midface anomalies, hemivertebrae, block vertebrae, vertebral hypoplasia, microphthalmia, coloboma of upper lid)
(2) Acrofacial dysplasia (limb malformations)
(3) Crouzon disease (maxillary hypoplasia with protrusion of mandible, hypertelorism, exophthalmos, craniosynostosis)

TRISOMY D SYNDROME

= Trisomy 13–15 group syndrome

Etiology: additional chromosome in D group; high maternal age

- severe mental retardation
- hypertonic infant
- cleft lip + palate

Associated with: capillary hemangioma of face + upper trunk

- hypotelorism
- coloboma, cataract, microphthalmia
- malformed ear with hypoplastic external auditory canal
- hyperconvex nails

√ postaxial polydactyly

@ Skull
√ deficient ossification of skull
√ cleft / absent midline structures of facial bones
√ poorly formed orbits
√ slanting of frontal bones
√ microcephaly
√ arrhinencephaly
√ holoprosencephaly

@ Chest
√ thin malformed ribs
√ diaphragmatic hernia (frequent)
√ congenital heart disease

Prognosis: death within 6 months of age

TRISOMY E SYNDROME

= Trisomy 16–18 group syndrome

Etiology: additional chromosome at 18 or E group location

Sex: usually female

◊ Marked phenotypic variability!

- hypertonic spastic infants
- mental + psychomotor retardation
- typical facies: micrognathia, high narrow palate with small buccal cavity, low-set deformed ears
- flexed ulnar-deviated fingers + short adducted thumb
- 2nd finger overlapping of 3rd (CHARACTERISTIC)

Associated with: congenital heart disease in 100% (PDA, VSD); hernias; renal anomalies; eventration of diaphragm

√ stippled epiphyses

@ Skull
√ thin calvarium
√ persistent metopic suture
√ dolichocephaly with prominent occiput
√ micrognathia due to hypoplastic mandible (most constant feature) + maxilla

@ Chest
√ increase in AP diameter of thorax
√ "shield deformity" due to hypoplastic short sternum
√ hypoplastic clavicles (DDx: cleidocranial dysostosis)
√ 11 rib pairs with slender hypoplastic + tapered ribs
√ diaphragmatic eventration (common)

@ Pelvis
√ small pelvis with forward rotation of iliac wings
√ increased obliquity of acetabulum
√ acute iliac angle (DIAGNOSTIC)

@ Hand & foot
√ adducted thumb = short 1st metacarpal + phalanges (DIAGNOSTIC)
√ overlap of 2nd on 3rd finger (DIAGNOSTIC)
√ flexed ulnar-deviated fingers
√ short 1st toe
√ varus deformities of forefoot + dorsiflexion of toes
√ rocker bottom foot / extreme pes planus (frequent)

OB-US:
√ hydrocephalus
√ cystic hygroma
√ diaphragmatic hernia
√ clubfoot
√ overlapping index finger
√ choroid plexus cyst (30%)

Prognosis: child rarely survives beyond 6 months of age

DDx: osteogenesis imperfecta, trisomy 13 syndrome, Cockayne syndrome, Werdnig-Hoffmann disease

TUBERCULOSIS OF BONE

Incidence: 1–3–5% of tuberculous patients, 30% in patients with extrapulmonary tuberculosis

Age: any, rare in 1st year of life, M:F = 1:1

- negative skin test excludes diagnosis
- history of active pulmonary disease (in 50%)

Location: vertebral column, hip, knee, wrist, elbow

Associated with: concurrent active intrathoracic tuberculosis in <50%

Pathogenesis:

1. Hematogenous spread from
   (a) primary infection of lung (particularly in children)
   (b) quiescent primary pulmonary site / extraosseous focus
2. Reactivation: especially in hip

Tuberculous Arthritis

= joint involvement usually secondary to adjacent osteomyelitis / hematogenous dissemination

Incidence: 84% of skeletal tuberculosis

Pathophysiology: synovitis with pannus formation leads to chondronecrosis

Age: middle-aged / elderly

- chronic pain, weakness, muscle wasting
- soft-tissue swelling, draining sinus
- joint fluid: high WBC count, low glucose level, poor mucin clot formation (similar to rheumatoid arthritis)

Location: hip, knee (large weight-bearing joints) >> elbow, wrist, sacroiliac joint, glenohumeral, articulation of hand + foot

◊ Monoarticular involvement is typical!

√ **Phemister triad**:

1. Gradual narrowing of joint space due to slow cartilage destruction (DDx: cartilage destruction in pyogenic arthritis is much quicker)
2. Peripherally located (= marginal) bone erosions
3. Juxtaarticular osteoporosis

(DDx: fungal disease, rheumatoid arthritis)

Early radiographs:

√ joint effusion (hip in 0%, knee in 60%, ankle in 80%)

√ extensive periarticular osteopenia (deossification) adjacent to primarily weight-bearing joints

√ soft tissues normal

Late radiographs:

√ small cystlike erosions along joint margins in non–weight-bearing line opposing one another (DDx: pyogenic arthritis erodes articular cartilage)

√ no joint space narrowing for months (CLASSIC!)

√ articular cortical bone destruction earlier in joints with little unopposed surfaces (hip, shoulder)

√ "kissing sequestra" = wedge-shaped areas of necrosis on both sides of the joint due to infection of subchondral bone

√ increased density with extensive soft-tissue calcifications in healing phase

Cx: fibrous ankylosis, leg shortening

Dx: synovial biopsy (in 90% positive), culture of synovial fluid (in 80% positive)

DDx: pyogenic arthritis (central erosion of articular cartilage, early joint space narrowing, bony ankylosis)

Tuberculous Osteomyelitis

Incidence: 16% of skeletal tuberculosis

Age: children <5 years (0.5–14%), rare in adults

- painless swelling of hand / foot

Location: femur, tibia, small bones of hand + foot (most common); any bone may be involved

Site: (a) metaphysis (TYPICALLY) with transphyseal spread (in child) (DDx: pyogenic infections usually do not extend across physis)
(b) epiphysis with spread to joint / spread from adjacent affected joint
(c) diaphysis (<1%)

√ initially round / oval poorly defined lytic lesion with minimal / no surrounding sclerosis

√ varying amounts of eburnation + periostitis

√ advanced epiphyseal maturity / overgrowth (due to hyperemia) ± limb shortening from premature physeal fusion

√ **cystic tuberculosis** = well-marginated round / oval radiolucent lesions with variable amount of sclerosis
(a) in children (frequent): in peripheral skeleton, ± symmetric distribution, no sclerosis
(b) in adults (rare): in skull / shoulder / pelvis / spine, with sclerosis
(DDx: eosinophilic granuloma, sarcoidosis, cystic angiomatosis, plasma cell myeloma, chordoma, fungal infections, metastases)

√ tuberculous dactylitis = digit with exuberant lamellated / solid periosteal new-bone formation and fusiform soft-tissue swelling (children >> adults):

√ **spina ventosa** ("wind-filled sail") = ballooning dactylitis forming an enlarging cystlike cavity with erosion of endosteal cortex (end-stage disease)

DDx: (1) pyogenic osteomyelitis (no transphyseal spread)
(2) syphilitic dactylitis (bilateral symmetric involvement, less soft-tissue swelling and sequestration)
(3) Sarcoidosis, hemoglobinopathies, hyperparathyroidism, leukemia

Tuberculous Spondylitis

= POTT DISEASE

[Percival Pott (1714–1788), surgeon in London, England associated cancer of the scrotum with coal tar in chimney sweeps]

= destruction of vertebral body + intervertebral disk by tuberculous mycobacterium

Incidence: <1% of patients with tuberculosis; 25–50–60% of all skeletal tuberculosis

Age: children / adults; M > F

- insidious onset of back pain, stiffness
- local tenderness
- NO pulmonary lesions in 50%

Location: upper lumbar + lower thoracic spine (L1 most common); TYPICALLY more than one vertebra affected
Site: vertebral body (82%) with predilection for anterior part adjacent to superior / inferior endplate >> posterior elements (18%)

Spread:
(a) hematogenous spread via paravertebral venous plexus of Batson: separate foci in 1–4%
(b) contiguous into disk by penetrating subchondral endplate + cartilaginous endplate
(c) subligamentous spread beneath anterior / posterior longitudinal ligaments to adjacent vertebral bodies

√ collapse of intervertebral disk space
  N.B.: vertebral disk space maintained longer than in pyogenic arthritis (disk itself preserved but fragmented)
√ demineralization (= resorption of dense margin) of vertebral endplates:
  √ "gouge defect" = mild contour irregularity of anterior and lateral aspect of vertebral body (= erosion from subligamentous extension of tuberculous abscess)
  √ reactive sclerosis / periosteal reaction TYPICALLY absent
√ collapse of vertebral body:
  √ vertebra plana in children
  √ angular kyphotic deformity (= gibbus) due to preferential anterior involvement in adults
√ vertebra within a vertebra (= growth recovery lines)
√ ivory vertebra (= reossification as healing response to osteonecrosis)
√ paraspinal infection:
  √ large cold fusiform abscess in paravertebral gutters / psoas, commonly bilateral ± anterolateral scalloping of vertebral bodies
  √ amorphous / teardrop-shaped calcification in paraspinal area between L1 + L5
  (DDx: nontuberculous abscess rarely calcifies)
  √ abscess may extend into groin / thigh

Cx: angular kyphosis (= gibbus deformity), scoliosis, ankylosis, osteonecrosis, paralysis (spinal cord compression from abscess, granulation tissue, bone fragments, arachnoiditis)

Prognosis: 26–30% mortality rate

DDx: (1) Pyogenic spondylitis (rapid destruction, multiple abscess cavities, no thickening / calcification of abscess rim, little new-bone formation, posterior elements not involved)
(2) Brucellosis (gas within disk, minimal paraspinal mass, no kyphosis, predilection for lower lumbar spine)
(3) Sarcoidosis
(4) Neoplasia (multiple noncontiguous lesions, no disk destruction, little soft-tissue involvement)

TUMORAL CALCINOSIS

= LIPOCALCINOGRANULOMATOSIS
= rare disease with progressive large nodular juxtaarticular calcified soft-tissue masses in patients with normal serum calcium + phosphorus and no evidence of renal, metabolic, or collagen-vascular disease

Etiology: autosomal dominant (1/3) with variable clinical expressivity; unknown biochemical defect of phosphorus metabolism responsible for abnormal phosphate reabsorption + 1,25-dihydroxy-vitamin D formation
Path: multilocular cystic lesions with creamy white fluid (hydroxyapatite) + many giant cells (granulomatous foreign body reaction) surrounded by fibrous capsule
Age: onset mostly within 1st / 2nd decade (range of 1–79 years); M:F = 1:1; predominantly in Blacks

- progressive painful / painless soft-tissue mass with overlying skin ulceration + sinus tract draining chalky milklike fluid
- swelling
- limitation of motion
- hyperphosphatemia + hypervitaminosis D
- normal serum calcium, alkaline phosphatase, renal function, parathyroid hormone

@ Soft tissue
  Location: paraarticular in hips > elbows > shoulders > feet, ribs, ischial spines; single / multiple joints; ALMOST NEVER knees; usually along extensor surface of joints (? initially a calcific bursitis)
  √ dense loculated multiglobular homogeneously calcified soft-tissue mass of 1–20 cm in size
  √ radiolucent septa (= connective tissue)
  √ ± fluid-fluid levels with milk-of-calcium consistency
  √ underlying bones NORMAL
  √ increased tracer uptake of soft-tissue masses on bone scan
@ Bone
  √ diaphyseal periosteal reaction (diaphysitis)
  √ patchy areas of calcification in medullary cavity (calcific myelitis)
@ Teeth
  √ bulbous root enlargement
  √ pulp stones = intrapulp calcifications
@ Pseudoxanthoma elasticum-like features
  √ calcinosis cutis = skin calcifications
  √ vascular calcifications
  √ angioid streaks of retina

Prognosis: tendency for recurrence after incomplete excision
Rx: phosphate depletion
DDx: Chronic renal failure on hemodialysis, CPPD, paraosteoarthropathy, hyperparathyroidism

TURNER SYNDROME

= due to nondisjunction of sex chromosomes as
(1) complete monosomy (45,XO)

(2) partial monosomy (structurally altered second X chromosome)
(3) mosaicism (XO + another sex karyotype)

Incidence: 1:3,000–5,000 livebirths

Associated with: coarctation, aortic stenosis, horseshoe kidney (most common)

- sexual infantilism (spontaneous puberty in 5–15%):
  - primary amenorrhea
  - absent secondary sex characteristics
- short stature; absence of prepubertal growth spurt
- webbed neck; low irregular nuchal hair line
- shield-shaped chest + widely spaced nipples
- mental deficiency (occasionally)
- high palate; thyromegaly
- multiple pigmented nevi; keloid formation
- idiopathic hypertension; elevated urinary gonadotropins

@ General
- √ normal skeletal maturation with growth arrest at skeletal age of 15 years
- √ delayed fusion of epiphyses > age 20 years
- √ osteoporosis during / after 2nd decade (gonadal hormone deficiency)
- √ coarctation of aorta (10%); aortic stenosis
- √ renal ectopia / horseshoe kidney
- √ lymphedema

@ Skull
- √ basilar impression; basal angle >140°
- √ parietal thinning
- √ small bridged sella
- √ hypertelorism

@ Axial skeleton
- √ hypoplasia of odontoid process + C1
- √ osteochondrosis of vertebral plates
- √ squared lumbar vertebrae; kyphoscoliosis
- √ deossification of vertebrae
- √ small iliac wings; late fusion of iliac crests
- √ android pelvic inlet with narrowed pubic arch + small sacrosciatic notches

@ Chest
- √ thinning of lateral aspects of clavicles
- √ thinned + narrowed ribs with pseudonotching

@ Hand + arm
- √ positive metacarpal sign = relative shortening of 3rd + 4th metacarpal
- √ positive carpal sign = narrowing of scaphoid-lunate-triquetrum angle <117°
- √ phalangeal preponderance = length of proximal + distal phalanx exceeds length of 4th metacarpal by >3 mm
- √ shortening of 2nd + 5th middle phalanx (also in Down syndrome)
- √ "drumstick" distal phalanges = slender shaft + large distal head
- √ "insetting" of epiphyses into bases of adjacent metaphyses (phalanges + metacarpals)
- √ Madelung deformity = shortening of ulna / absence of ulnar styloid process
- √ cubitus valgus = bilateral radial tilt of articular surface of trochlea
- √ deossification of carpal bones

@ Knee
- √ tibia vara = enlarged medial femoral condyle + depression of medial tibial plateau (DDx: Blount disease)
- √ small exostosis-like projection from medial border of proximal tibial metaphysis

@ Foot
- √ deossification of tarsal bones
- √ shortening of 1st, 4th, and 5th metatarsals
- √ pes cavus

US:
- √ prepubertal uterus
- √ nonvisualized / streaky ovaries (in complete monosomy); normal ovaries (in mosaic karyotype)

OB-US:
- √ large nuchal cystic hygroma
- √ lymphangiectasia with generalized hydrops
- √ symmetrical edema of dorsum of feet
- √ CHD (20%): coarctation of aorta (70%), left heart lesions
- √ horseshoe kidney

Bonnevie-Ullrich Syndrome

= infantile form of Turner syndrome
(1) congenital webbed neck
(2) widely separated nipples
(3) lymphedema of hands + feet

TURRET EXOSTOSIS

Cause: trauma with formation of subperiosteal hematoma

- immobile, occasionally painful lump on dorsum of finger
- reduced ability to flex finger (= ossified hematoma diminishes excursion of extensor tendon)

Location: dorsum of proximal / middle phalanx of hand

√ smooth dome-shaped extracortical mass

VAN BUCHEM DISEASE

= GENERALIZED CORTICAL HYPEROSTOSIS
= autosomal recessive disease; may be related to hyperphosphatasemia

Cause: defect on chromosome 17

- paralysis of facial nerve
- auditory + ocular disturbances (in late teens secondary to foraminal encroachment)
- increased alkaline phosphatase

Location: skull, mandible, clavicles, ribs, long-bone diaphyses

- √ symmetrical generalized sclerosis + thickening of endosteal cortex
- √ obliteration of diploe
- √ spinous processes thickened + sclerotic

DDx: (1) Osteopetrosis (sclerosis of all bones, not confined to diaphyses)
(2) Generalized hyperostosis with pachydermia (involves entire long bones, considerable pain, skin changes)

(3) Hyperphosphatasia (infancy, widened bones but decreased cortical density)
(4) Engelmann disease (rarely generalized, involves lower limbs)
(5) Pyle disease (does not involve middiaphyses)
(6) Polyostotic fibrous dysplasia (rarely symmetrically generalized, paranasal sinuses abnormal, skull involvement)
(7) Sclerosteosis = Truswell-Hansen disease (syndactyly of 2nd + 3rd fingers, nail dysplasia)

WILLIAMS SYNDROME

= IDIOPATHIC HYPERCALCEMIA OF INFANCY

- peculiar elfinlike facies, dysplastic dentition
- neonatal hypercalcemia (not in all patients)
- mental + physical retardation

@ Skeletal manifestations
- √ osteosclerosis (secondary to trabecular thickening)
- √ dense broad zone of provisional calcification
- √ radiolucent metaphyseal bands
- √ dense vertebral end plates + acetabular roofs
- √ bone islands in spongiosa
- √ metastatic calcification
- √ craniostenosis

@ Cardiovascular manifestations
- √ supravalvular aortic stenosis (33%), aortic hypoplasia
- √ valvular + peripheral pulmonary artery stenosis
- √ ASD, VSD
- √ stenoses of major vessels (innominate, carotids, renal arteries)

@ GI and GU tract:
- √ colonic diverticula
- √ bladder diverticula

Prognosis: spontaneous resolution after 1 year in most
Rx: withhold vitamin D + calcium
DDx: Hypervitaminosis D

WILSON DISEASE

= HEPATOLENTICULAR DEGENERATION
= autosomal recessive disease with excessive copper retention (= copper toxicosis)

Prevalence: 1:33,000–200,000; 1:90 persons is a heterozygous carrier

Cause: alteration of chromosome 13 resulting in inability of liver to excrete copper into bile; hypothetically due to either
(a) lysosomal defect in hepatocytes, or
(b) deficiency of biliary copper-binding proteins, or
(c) persistence of fetal mode of copper metabolism, or
(d) hepatic synthesis of high-affinity copper-binding proteins)

Age of onset: 7–50 years; hepatic manifestations predominate in children; neuropsychiatric manifestations predominate in adolescents + adults

Histo: macrovesicular fat deposition in hepatocytes, glycogen degeneration of hepatocyte nuclei, Kupffer cell hypertrophy

Stage 1 asymptomatic copper accumulation in hepatocytic cytosol
Stage 2 redistribution of copper into hepatic lysosomes + circulation from saturated hepatocytic cytosol
(a) gradual redistribution is asymptomatic
(b) rapid redistribution causes fulminant hepatic failure / acute intravascular hemolysis
Stage 3 cirrhosis, neurologic, ophthalmologic, renal dysfunction may be reversible with therapy

- tremor, rigidity, dysarthria, dysphagia (excessive copper deposition in lenticular region of brain)
- intellectual impairment, emotional disturbance
- Kayser-Fleischer ring (= green pigmentation surrounding limbus corneae) is DIAGNOSTIC
- jaundice / portal hypertension (liver cirrhosis)
- elevated copper concentration in serum ceruloplasmin (BEST SCREENING TEST)
- decreased incorporation of orally administered radiolabeled copper into newly synthesized ceruloplasmin

Skeletal manifestations (in 2/3):
- √ generalized deossification may produce pathologic fractures

@ Joints: shoulder (frequent), knee, hip, wrist, 2nd–4th MCP joints
- • articular symptoms in 75%: pain, stiffness, gelling of joints
- √ subarticular cysts
- √ premature osteoarthritis (narrowing of joint space + osteophyte formation)
- √ osteochondritis dissecans
- √ chondrocalcinosis
- √ premature osteoarthrosis of spine, prominent Schmorl nodes, wedging of vertebrae, irregularities of vertebral plates

@ Liver (in children)
- √ normal hepatic attenuation (fatty infiltration + copper deposition cancel each other out)
- √ normal T1 relaxation time (in spite of paramagnetic effects of copper)

@ Brain (adolescents + adults)
Location: basal ganglia, rarely thalamus
- √ cerebral white matter atrophy
- √ hypodensities, prolongation of T1 + T2

Cx: rickets + osteomalacia (secondary to renal tubular dysfunction) in minority of patients
Rx: life-long pharmacologic therapy with chelation agents (penicillamine / trientine / zinc); liver transplantation

DIFFERENTIAL DIAGNOSIS OF SKULL AND SPINE DISORDERS

LOW BACK PAIN

Low Back Pain in Childhood

1. Spondylosis, spondylolisthesis
2. Osteomyelitis, diskitis
3. Leukemia
4. Histiocytosis X
5. Osteoid osteoma

Lumbosacral Postsurgical Syndrome

= FAILED BACK SURGERY SYNDROME
= signs of dysfunction and disability + pain and paresthesia following surgery
◊ Interpretation in immediate postoperative period difficult, stabilization of findings occurs in 2–6 months
Frequency: failure of improvement in 5–15%

A. OSSEOUS CAUSES
  1. Spondylolisthesis
  2. Central stenosis
  3. Foraminal stenosis
  4. Pseudarthrosis
B. SOFT-TISSUE CAUSES
  1. Perioperative intraspinal hemorrhage (onset <1 week)
  2. Residual disk herniation (onset <1 week)
  3. Recurrent disk herniation (onset 1 week – 1 month)
     √ no enhancement on early T1WI (appears enhanced ≥30 minutes post injection)
  4. Spinal / meningeal / neural inflammation / infection (onset 1 week – 1 month)
  5. Intraspinal scar formation (onset >1 month)
     (a) Epidural fibrosis (scarring)
        √ enhancing epidural plaque / mass
        √ heterogeneous enhancement on early T1WI (maximum at about 5 minutes post injection)
     (b) Fibrosing arachnoiditis = adhesive arachnoiditis
        √ thickened irregular clumped nerve roots
        √ adhesion of roots to wall of thecal sac
        √ abnormal enhancement of thickened meninges + matted nerve roots
C. SURGICAL ERRORS
  1. Wrong level / side of surgery
  2. Direct nerve injury
D. Remote phenomena unrelated to spine

mnemonic: "ABCDEF"
Arachnoiditis
Bleeding
Contamination (infection)
Disk (residual / recurrent / new level)
Error (wrong disk excised)
Fibrosis (scar)

Cauda Equina Syndrome

= constellation of signs + symptoms resulting from compressive lesion in lower lumbar spinal canal
Cause:
  (1) displaced disk fragment
  (2) intra- / extramedullary tumor
  (3) osseous: Paget disease, osteomyelitis, osteoarthrosis of facet joints, complication of ankylosing spondylitis

• diminished sensation in lower lumbar + sacral dermatomes
• wasting + weakness of muscles
• decreased ankle reflexes
• impotence
• disturbed sphincter function + overflow incontinence
• decreased sphincter tone

SKULL

Sutural Abnormalities

Wide Sutures

= >10 mm at birth, >3 mm at 2 years, >2 mm at 3 years of age; (sutures are splittable up to age 12–15; complete closure by age 30)

A. NORMAL VARIANT
   in neonate + prematurity; growth spurt occurs at 2–3 years and 5–7 years
B. CONGENITAL UNDEROSSIFICATION
   osteogenesis imperfecta, hypophosphatasia, rickets, hypothyroidism, pyknodysostosis, cleidocranial dysplasia
C. METABOLIC DISEASE
   hypoparathyroidism; lead intoxication; hypo- / hypervitaminosis A
D. RAISED INTRACRANIAL PRESSURE
   Cause: (1) intracerebral tumor (2) subdural hematoma (3) hydrocephalus
   Age: seen only if <10 years of age
   Location: coronal > sagittal > lambdoid > squamosal suture
E. INFILTRATION OF SUTURES
   Cause: metastases to meninges from
   (1) neuroblastoma
   (2) leukemia
   (3) lymphoma
   √ poorly defined margins
F. RECOVERY
   from (1) deprivational dwarfism
   (2) chronic illness
   (3) prematurity
   (4) hypothyroidism

Craniosynostosis

= CRANIOSTENOSIS = premature closure of sutures (normally at about 30 years of age)
Age: often present at birth; M:F = 4:1

Etiology:
- A. Primary craniosynostosis
- B. Secondary craniosynostosis
  - (a) hematologic: sickle cell anemia, thalassemia
  - (b) metabolic: rickets, hypercalcemia, hyperthyroidism, hypervitaminosis D
  - (c) bone dysplasia: hypophosphatasia, achondroplasia, metaphyseal dysplasia, mongolism, Hurler disease, skull hyperostosis, Rubinstein-Taybi syndrome
  - (d) syndromes: Crouzon, Apert, Carpenter, Treacher-Collins, cloverleaf skull, craniotelencephalic dysplasia, arrhinencephaly
  - (e) microcephaly: brain atrophy / dysgenesis
  - (f) after shunting procedures

Types:
Sagittal suture most commonly affected followed by coronal suture
1. **Scaphocephaly** = **Dolichocephaly** (55%) premature closure of sagittal suture (long skull)
2. **Brachycephaly** = **Turricephaly** (10%) premature closure of coronal / lambdoid sutures (short tall skull)
3. **Plagiocephaly** (7%) unilateral early fusion of coronal + lambdoidal suture (lopsided skull)
4. **Trigonocephaly**: premature closure of metopic suture (forward pointing skull)
5. **Oxycephaly**: premature closure of coronal, sagittal, lambdoid sutures
6. **Cloverleaf skull** = Kleeblattschädel: intrauterine premature closure of sagittal, coronal, lambdoid sutures;
   May be associated with: thanatophoric dysplasia

√ sharply defined thickened sclerotic suture margins
√ delayed growth of BPD in early pregnancy

Wormian Bones

= intrasutural ossicles in lambdoid, posterior sagittal, temporosquamosal sutures; normal up to 6 months of age (most frequently)

mnemonic: "PORK CHOPS I"
- **P**yknodysostosis
- **O**steogenesis imperfecta
- **R**ickets in healing phase
- **K**inky hair syndrome
- **C**leidocranial dysostosis
- **H**ypothyroidism / **H**ypophosphatasia
- **O**topalatodigital syndrome
- **P**rimary acroosteolysis (Hajdu-Cheney) / **P**achydermoperiostosis / **P**rogeria
- **S**yndrome of Down
- **I**diopathic

Increased Skull Thickness

A. GENERALIZED
1. Chronic severe anemia (eg, thalassemia, sickle cell disease)
2. Cerebral atrophy following shunting of hydrocephalus
3. Engelmann disease: mainly skull base
4. Hyperparathyroidism
5. Acromegaly
6. Osteopetrosis

B. FOCAL
1. Meningioma
2. Fibrous dysplasia
3. Paget disease
4. Dyke-Davidoff-Mason syndrome
5. Hyperostosis frontalis interna
   = dense hyperostosis of inner table of frontal bone; M < F

mnemonic: "HIPFAM"
- **H**yperostosis frontalis interna
- **I**diopathic
- **P**aget disease
- **F**ibrous dysplasia
- **A**nemia (sickle cell, iron deficiency, thalassemia, spherocytosis)
- **M**etastases

Hair-on-end Skull

mnemonic: "HI NEST"
- **H**ereditary spherocytosis
- **I**ron deficiency anemia
- **N**euroblastoma
- **E**nzyme deficiency (glucose-6-phosphate dehydrogenase deficiency causes hemolytic anemia)
- **S**ickle cell disease
- **T**halassemia major

Leontiasis Ossea

= overgrowth of facial bones causing leonine (lionlike) facies
1. Fibrous dysplasia
2. Paget disease
3. Craniometaphyseal dysplasia
4. Hyperphosphatasia

Abnormally Thin Skull

A. GENERALIZED
1. Obstructive hydrocephalus
2. Cleidocranial dysostosis
3. Progeria
4. Rickets
5. Osteogenesis imperfecta
6. Craniolacunia

B. FOCAL
1. Neurofibromatosis
2. Chronic subdural hematoma
3. Arachnoid cyst

Inadequate Calvarial Calcification

1. Achondroplasia
2. Osteogenesis imperfecta
3. Hypophosphatasia

Osteolytic Lesion of Skull

A. NORMAL VARIANT
   1. Emissary vein
      connecting venous systems inside + outside skull
      √ bony channel <2 mm in width
   2. Venous lake
      = outpouching of diploic vein
      √ extremely variable in size, shape, and number
      √ irregular well-demarcated contour
   3. Pacchionian granulations
      √ usually multiple lesions with irregular contour in parasagittal location (within 3 cm of superior sagittal sinus) primarily involving the inner table
      Associated with: impressions by arachnoid granulations
   4. Parietal foramina
      nonossification of embryonal rests in parietal fissure; bilateral at superior posterior angles of parietal bone; hereditary transmission

B. TRAUMA
   1. Surgical burr hole
   2. Leptomeningeal cyst

C. INFECTION
   1. Osteomyelitis
   2. Hydatid disease
   3. Syphilis
   4. Tuberculosis

D. CONGENITAL
   1. Epidermoid / dermoid
   2. Neurofibromatosis (asterion defect)
   3. Meningoencephalocele
   4. Fibrous dysplasia
   5. Osteoporosis circumscripta of Paget disease

E. BENIGN TUMOR
   1. Hemangioma
   2. Brown tumor
   3. Eosinophilic granuloma

F. MALIGNANT TUMOR
   1. Solitary / multiple metastases
   2. Multiple myeloma
   3. Leukemia
   4. Neuroblastoma

Solitary Lytic Lesion in Skull

mnemonic: "HELP MFT HOLE"
Hemangioma
Epidermoid / dermoid
Leptomeningeal cyst
Postop, **P**aget disease
Metastasis, **M**yeloma
Fibrous dysplasia
Tuberculosis
Hyperparathyroidism
Osteomyelitis
Lambdoid defect (neurofibromatosis)
Eosinophilic granuloma

Multiple Lytic Lesions in Skull

mnemonic: "BAMMAH"
Brown tumor
AVM
Myeloma
Metastases
Amyloidosis
Histiocytosis

Lytic Area in Bone Flap

mnemonic: "RATI"
Radiation necrosis
Avascular necrosis
Tumor
Infection

Button Sequestrum

mnemonic: "TORE ME"
Tuberculosis
Osteomyelitis
Radiation
Eosinophilic granuloma
Metastasis
Epidermoid

Absent Greater Sphenoid Wing

mnemonic: "M FOR MARINE"
Meningioma
Fibrous dysplasia
Optic glioma
Relapsing hematoma
Metastasis
Aneurysm
Retinoblastoma
Idiopathic
Neurofibromatosis
Eosinophilic granuloma

Absence of Innominate Line

= OBLIQUE CAROTID LINE
= vertical line projecting into orbit (on PA skull film) produced by orbital process of sphenoid

A. CONGENITAL
   1. Fibrous dysplasia
   2. Neurofibromatosis
B. INFECTION
C. TUMOR

Widened Superior Orbital Fissure

mnemonic: "A FAN"
Aneurysm (internal carotid artery)
Fistula (cavernous sinus)
Adenoma (pituitary)
Neurofibroma

Tumors of Central Skull Base

A. DEVELOPMENTAL
   1. Encephalocele

B. INFECTION / INFLAMMATION
1. Extension from paranasal sinus / mastoid infection
2. Complication of trauma
3. Fungal disease: mucormycosis in diabetics, aspergillosis in immunosuppressed patients
4. Sinus + nasopharyngeal sarcoidosis
5. Radiation necrosis

C. BENIGN
1. Juvenile angiofibroma
2. Meningioma
3. Chordoma
4. Pituitary tumor
5. Paget disease
6. Fibrous dysplasia

D. MALIGNANT
1. Metastasis: prostate, lung, breast
2. Chondrosarcoma
3. Nasopharyngeal carcinoma
4. Rhabdomyosarcoma
5. Perineural tumor spread: head + neck neoplasm

Craniofacial Syndromes

= developmental malformations of the face + skull associated with CNS malformations
1. Midfacial clefts
2. Goldenhaar syndrome
3. Apert syndrome
4. Crouzon syndrome
5. Treacher Collins syndrome

MAXILLA AND MANDIBLE

Maxillary Hypoplasia

1. Down syndrome
2. Drugs (alcohol, dilantin, valproate)
3. Apert / Crouzon syndrome
4. Achondroplasia
5. Cleft lip/palate

Mandibular Hypoplasia = Micrognathia

A. WITH ABNORMAL EARS
1. Treacher-Collins syndrome
2. Goldenhar syndrome (hemifacial microsomia) = facio-auriculo-vertebral spectrum (x-rays of vertebrae!)
3. Langer-Giedion syndrome (IUGR, protruding ears)

B. ABNORMALITIES OF EARS + OTHER ORGANS
1. Miller syndrome (severe postaxial hand anomalies)
2. Velo-cardio-facial syndrome (hand + cardiac lesions)
3. Otopalatodigital syndrome - type II (hand abnormalities)
4. Stickler syndrome (ear anomalies not severe)
5. Pierre-Robin syndrome (large fleshy ears)

C. NO EAR ANOMALIES
1. Pyknodysostosis

D. OTHERS
1. Seckel syndrome (bird-headed dwarfism)
2. Multiple pterygium syndrome
3. Pena-Shokeir syndrome
4. Beckwith-Wiedemann syndrome
5. Arthrogryposis
6. Skeletal dysplasias
7. Trisomy 13, 18, 9 (abnormal karyotype in 25%)

Destruction of Temporomandibular Joint

mnemonic: "HIRT"
Hyperparathyroidism
Infection
Rheumatoid arthritis
Trauma

Radiolucent Lesion of Mandible

A. SHARPLY MARGINATED LESION
(a) around apex of tooth
1. Radicular cyst
2. Cementoma

(b) around unerupted tooth
1. Dentigerous cyst
2. Ameloblastoma

(c) unrelated to tooth
1. Simple bone cyst
2. Fong disease
3. Basal cell nevus syndrome

B. POORLY MARGINATED LESIONS
√ "floating teeth": suggestive of primary / secondary malignancy
√ resorption of tooth root: hallmark of benign process
(a) infection
1. Osteomyelitis: actinomycosis

(b) radiotherapy
1. Osteoradionecrosis

(c) malignant neoplasm
1. Osteosarcoma (1/3 lytic, 1/3 sclerotic, 1/3 mixed)
2. Local invasion from gingival / buccal neoplasms (more common)
3. Metastasis from breast, lung, kidney in 1% (in 70% adenocarcinoma)

(d) other
1. Eosinophilic granuloma: "floating tooth"
2. Fibrous dysplasia
3. Osteocementoma
4. Ossifying fibroma (very common)

Cystic Lesion of Jaw

A. ODONTOGENIC WITHOUT MINERALIZATION
= mostly benign lesion developing during / after formation of teeth
• asymptomatic / pain ± swelling
• paresthesia, tooth displacement / mobility
√ radiolucent

1. **Ameloblastoma = adamantinoma of jaw**
 = benign locally aggressive epithelial neoplasm
 Prevalence: 10% of odontogenic tumors
 Origin: enamel-type epithelial tissue elements around tooth; 30–50% arise from epithelium of dentigerous cyst (= mural ameloblastoma)
 Age: 3rd–5th decade; M:F = 1:1
 • slow-growing painless mass
 Location: ramus + posterior body of mandible (75%), maxilla (25%)
 Site: in region of bicuspids + molars (angle of mandible commonly affected)
 √ well-defined well-corticated unilocular lucent lesion (DDx: odontogenic keratocyst, dentigerous cyst)
 √ multilocular lesion with internal septations (honeycomb / soap bubble appearance)
 √ typically expansile with scalloped margin
 √ may perforate the lingual cortex + infiltrate adjacent soft tissues
 √ often associated with the crown of an impacted / unerupted tooth
 √ resorption of the root of a tooth
 Prognosis: frequently local recurrence even more aggressive after excision
2. **Odontogenic keratocyst**
 Origin: dental lamina + other sources of odontogenic epithelium
 Prevalence: 5–15% of all jaw cysts
 Age: 2nd–4th decade
 Path: daughter cysts + nests of cystic epithelia in vicinity (high rate of recurrence)
 Histo: parakeratinized lining epithelium + "cheesy" material in lumen of lesion
 Location: body + ramus of mandible (most often); may be anywhere in mandible / maxilla
 √ unilocular lucent lesion with smooth corticated border
 √ often associated with impacted tooth
 √ ± undulating borders / multilocular appearance
 √ ± cortical thinning, tooth displacement, root resorption
 DDx: indistinguishable from dentigerous cyst / ameloblastoma
3. **Dentigerous cyst = follicular cyst**
 Prevalence: most common type of noninflammatory odontogenic cyst
 Path: epithelial-lined cyst from odontogenic epithelium developing around unerupted tooth
 Histo: forms within lining of dental follicle
 Age: adolescent / young adult
 • typically painfree
 Location: mandible, maxilla (may expand into maxillary sinus)
 Site: around the crown of an unerupted tooth (usually 3rd molar)
 √ cystic expansile pericoronal lesion containing impacted tooth
 √ root of tooth often outside lesion
 √ well-defined round / ovoid corticated lucent lesion ± mandibular expansion
 Cx: may degenerate into mural ameloblastoma (rare)
 DDx: unilocular odontogenic keratocyst
4. **Radicular cyst = periapical cyst**
 Prevalence: most common cyst of the jaw
 Cause: periapical inflammatory lesion secondary to pulpal necrosis in deep carious lesion / deep filling / trauma
 Age: 30–50 years
 Site: intimately associated with apex of nonvital tooth
 √ round / pear-shaped unilocular periapical lucent lesion, usually <1 cm in diameter
 √ bordered by thin rim of cortical bone
 √ ± displacement of adjacent teeth
 √ ± mild root resorption
 DDx: periapical granuloma

B. ODONTOGENIC WITH MINERALIZATION
 = elaborate enamel, dentin, cementum
 √ varying degrees of opacity
 1. **Odontoma**
  = odontogenic hamartomatous malformation
  Prevalence: most common odontogenic mass (67%)
  Age: 2nd decade
  √ 1–3 cm in diameter
  √ may be surrounded by lucent follicle
  Types:
  (a) compound odontoma (more common)
   √ multiple teeth / tooth-like structures
  (b) complex odontoma
   = multiple masses of dental tissue
   √ well-defined lesion with amorphous calcifications
  Cx: impaction, malpositioning, resorption of adjacent teeth
  DDx: focal cemento-osseous dysplasia, ameloblastic fibro-odontoma, adenomatoid odontogenic tumor
 2. **Odontogenic myxoma**
  Prevalence: 3–6% of odontogenic tumors
  Origin: mesenchymal odontogenic tissue
  Age: 10–30 years; M < F
  • usually painless
  Location: maxilla > mandible
  √ well-demarcated / ill-defined lytic lesion of varying size
  √ often multilocular with honeycomblike internal structure
  √ foci of irregular calcifications (frequent)
  Cx: can be locally aggressive causing considerable destruction of adjacent bone + soft-tissue infiltration
  DDx: malignancy, traumatic bone cyst, central giant cell granuloma, calcifying epithelial odontogenic tumor

C. NONODONTOGENIC

1. **Ossifying fibroma** (conventional slow-growing ossifying fibroma, juvenile active aggressive ossifying fibroma)
   = encapsulated circumscribed benign neoplasm
   Histo: highly cellular fibrous connective tissue containing varying amounts of osteoid, bone, cementum, cementumlike calcified tissue
   • asymptomatic
   • facial asymmetry due to bone expansion
   • tooth displacement
   √ initially lucent + later often opaque lesion (depending on degree of calcification)
   √ surrounded by thin line of lucency (= fibrous capsule) + in turn surrounded by thin sclerotic rim of reactive bone
   √ intense focal uptake on bone scan
   DDx: odontoma, sequestrum, fibrous dysplasia, vascular lesion
2. **Focal cemento-osseous dysplasia**
   = nonneoplastic benign fibro-osseous lesion
   Age: adult life
   • asymptomatic
   Location: mandible >> maxilla
   √ one / more, closely apposed / confluent, round / ovoid lucent lesion with varying amounts of opacity
   √ initially cystic lucency + later progressively more opaque internally
   √ no extension into adjacent bone
   √ no cortical expansion
   DDx: periapical periodontitis, ossifying fibroma
3. **Periapical cemento-osseous dysplasia** (= **cementoma**) = fibro-osteoma
   Age: 30–40 years of age; most common in women
   • asymptomatic
   Location: in anterior portion of mandible
   Site: at apex of vital tooth
   √ often multicentric
   √ mixed lucent + sclerotic lesion with little expansion, calcifies with time
   DDx: ossifying fibroma, fibrous dysplasia, Paget disease
4. **Florid osseous dysplasia**
   Age: adult life
   • asymptomatic
   √ diffuse multiquadrant distribution of mixed lucent-opaque osseous changes
5. **Traumatic bone cyst**
   = not a true cyst for lack of epithelial lining
   Cause: ? response to trauma
   Age: 2nd decade
   • asymptomatic
   Location: mandible
   √ unilocular sharply marginated lucent defect
   √ scalloped superior margin with fingerlike projections extending between roots of teeth
   √ ± thinning of mandibular cortex ± osseous expansion
   DDx: vascular lesion, central giant cell granuloma, ossifying fibroma
6. **Lingual salivary gland inclusion defect**
   = well-defined depression in lingual surface of mandible (= Stafne cyst)
   Path: aberrant lobe of submandibular gland / fat
   • asymptomatic
   Location: usually near mandibular angle
   Site: just above inferior border of mandible, anterior to angle of jaw, inferior to mandibular canal, posterior to 3rd molar
   √ oval / rectangular well-defined area of lucency
   √ border surrounded by an opaque line
   √ may extend to buccal cortex
   DDx: arteriovenous malformation
7. **Central giant cell granuloma** (common)
   Age: <30 years (75%)
   • painless swelling, tenderness on palpation
   Location: mandible:maxilla = 2:1
   Site: anterior to 1st molar (= deciduous teeth); propensity for crossing midline (especially in maxilla)
   √ unilocular area of lucency (early)
   √ multilocular with wispy internal septa (later)
   √ expansion of bone + displacement of teeth
   √ usually well-defined border
   DDx: brown tumor of HPT (histologically similar)
8. **Brown tumor of hyperparathyroidism**
   = osteoclastoma = central giant cell lesion in patients with long-standing HPT
   • hypercalcemia, hypophosphatemia
   • elevated levels of parathyroid hormone
   √ variably defined margin ± cortical expansion
   √ generalized demineralization of medullary bones of jaw
   √ loss of lamina dura around roots of teeth
9. **Arteriovenous malformation**
   ◊ Tooth extraction can result in lethal exsanguination!
   • occasionally pulsatile soft-tissue swelling
   Location: ramus + posterior body of mandible
   √ cystlike due to bone resorption ± calcifications
   √ ± multilocular ± bone expansion
   √ ± erosive margins
   √ angiogram confirms diagnosis
   DDx: traumatic bone cyst, central giant cell granuloma, ossifying fibroma
10. Mucoepidermoid carcinoma

Tooth Mass

A. CYSTIC LESION
1. Radicular cyst = periapical cyst
2. Ameloblastoma = adamantinoma of jaw
3. Giant cell reparative granuloma
4. Primordial cyst
   arising from follicle of tooth that never developed
5. Traumatic bone cyst

6. Dentigerous cyst = follicular cyst
7. Odontogenic keratocyst

B. SCLEROTIC LESION
1. Cementoma
2. True cementoma = benign cementoblastoma
3. Gigantiform cementoma
4. **Hypercementosis**
   = bulbous enlargement of a root
   (a) idiopathic
   (b) associated with Paget disease
5. Benign fibro-osseous lesions
   (a) ossifying fibroma: young adults; mandible > maxilla
   (b) monostotic fibrous dysplasia: M < F, younger patients
   (c) condensing osteitis = focal chronic sclerosing osteitis
   √ near apex of nonvital tooth
6. Paget disease
   involvement of jaw in 20%; maxilla > mandible
   Location: bilateral, symmetric involvement
   √ widened alveolar ridges
   √ flat palate
   √ loosening of teeth
   √ hypercementosis
   √ may cause destruction of lamina dura
7. **Torus mandibularis** = exostosis
   Site: midline of hard palate; lingual surface of mandible in region of bicuspids

CRANIOVERTEBRAL JUNCTION

Craniovertebral Junction Anomaly

Basilar Invagination

= primary developmental anomaly with abnormally high position of vertebral column prolapsing into skull base

Associated with: Chiari malformation, syringohydromyelia in 25–35%

Cause:
1. Condylus tertius = ossicle at distal end of clivus
   √ pseudojoint with odontoid process / anterior arch of C1
2. Condylar hypoplasia
   √ lateral masses of atlas may be fused to condyles
   √ violation of Chamberlain line
   √ widening of atlantooccipital joint axis angle
   √ tip of odontoid >10 mm above bimastoid line
3. Basiocciput hypoplasia
   √ shortening of clivus
   √ violation of Chamberlain line
   √ clivus-canal angle typically decreased
4. Atlantooccipital assimilation
   = complete / partial failure of segmentation between skull + 1st cervical vertebra
   √ violation of Chamberlain line
   √ clivus-canal angle decreased
   May be associated with: fusion of C2 + C3
   Cx: atlantoaxial subluxation (50%); sudden death

• limitation in range of motion of CVJ
√ abnormal craniometry
√ C-spine + foramen magnum bulge into cranial cavity
√ elevation of posterior arch of C1

Basilar Impression

= acquired form of basilar invagination with bulging of C-spine and foramen magnum into cranial cavity
√ tip of odontoid process projects >5 mm above Chamberlain line (= line between hard palate + opisthion)

Cause: Paget disease, osteomalacia, rickets, fibrous dysplasia, hyperparathyroidism, Hurler syndrome, osteogenesis imperfecta, skull base infection

mnemonic: "PF ROACH"
- **P**aget disease
- **F**ibrous dysplasia
- **R**ickets
- **O**steogenesis imperfecta, **O**steomalacia
- **A**chondroplasia
- **C**leidocranial dysplasia
- **H**yperparathyroidism, **H**urler syndrome

Platybasia

= anthropometric term referring to flattening of skull base

May be associated with: basilar invagination

• cord symptoms
√ craniovertebral = clivus-canal angle becomes acute (<150°)
√ Welcher basal angle = sphenoid angle >140°
√ bowstring deformity of cervicomedullary junction

ATLAS AND AXIS

Atlas Anomalies

A. POSTERIOR ARCH ANOMALIES
1. Posterior atlas arch rachischisis (4%)
   Location: midline (97%), lateral through sulcus of vertebral artery (3%)
   √ absence of arch-canal line (LAT view)
   √ superimposed on odontoid process / axis body simulating a fracture (open-mouth odontoid view)
2. Total aplasia of posterior atlas arch
3. Keller-type aplasia with persistence of posterior tubercle
4. Aplasia with uni- / bilateral remnant + midline rachischisis
5. Partial / total hemiaplasia of posterior arch

B. ANTERIOR ARCH ANOMALIES
1. Isolated anterior arch rachischisis (0.1%)
2. Split atlas = anterior + posterior arch rachischisis
   √ plump rounded anterior arch overlapping the odontoid process making identification of predental space impossible (LAT view)
   √ duplicated anterior margins (LAT view)

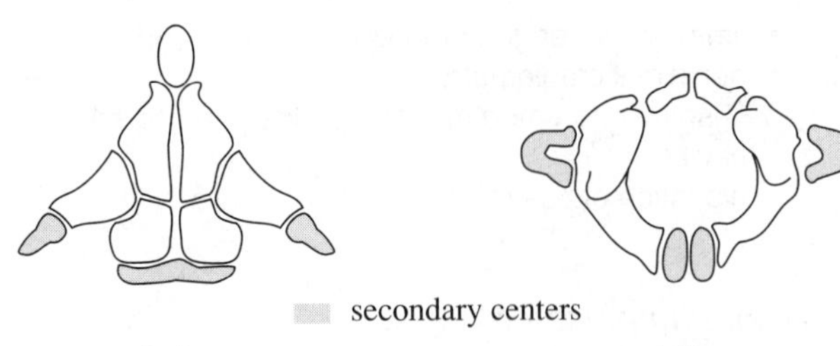

Primary and Secondary Ossification Centers

Axis Anomalies

1. Persistent ossiculum terminale = Bergman ossicle
   √ unfused odontoid process >12 years of age
   DDx: type 1 odontoid fracture
2. Odontoid aplasia (extremely rare)
3. Os odontoideum
   = independent os cephalad to axis body in location of odontoid process
   √ absence of odontoid process
   √ anterior arch of atlas hypertrophic + situated too far posterior in relation to axis body
   Cx: atlantoaxial instability
   DDx: type 2 odontoid fracture (uncorticated margin)

Odontoid Erosion

mnemonic: "P LARD"
Psoriasis
Lupus erythematosus
Ankylosing spondylitis
Rheumatoid arthritis
Down syndrome

Atlantoaxial Subluxation

= displacement of atlas with respect to axis
(1) Posterior atlantoaxial subluxation (rare)
(2) Anterior atlantoaxial subluxation (common)
= distance between dens + anterior arch of C1 (measurement along midplane of atlas on lateral view):
(a) predental space: >2.5 mm; >4.5 mm (in children)
(b) retrodental space: <18 mm

Causes of subluxation:
(a) Congenital
1. Occipitalization of atlas
   0.75% of population; fusion of basion + anterior arch of atlas
2. Congenital insufficiency of transverse ligament
3. Os odontoideum / aplasia of dens
4. Down syndrome (20%)
5. Morquio syndrome
6. Bone dysplasia

(b) Arthritis
due to laxity of transverse ligament or erosion of dens
1. Rheumatoid arthritis
2. Psoriatic arthritis
3. Reiter syndrome
4. Ankylosing spondylitis
5. SLE

rare: in gout + CPPD

(c) Inflammatory process
Pharyngeal infection in childhood, retropharyngeal abscess, coryza, otitis media, mastoiditis, cervical adenitis, parotitis, alveolar abscess
√ dislocation 8–10 days after onset of symptoms
(d) Trauma (very rare without odontoid fracture)
(e) Marfan disease

mnemonic: "JAP LARD"
Juvenile rheumatoid arthritis
Ankylosing spondylitis
Psoriatic arthritis
Lupus erythematosus
Accident (trauma)
Retropharyngeal abscess, **R**heumatoid arthritis
Down syndrome

PSEUDOSUBLUXATION
= ligamentous laxity in infants allows for movement of the vertebral bodies on each other, esp. C2 on C3

SPINAL DYSRAPHISM

= abnormal / incomplete fusion of midline embryologic mesenchymal, neurologic, bony structures
External signs (in 50%):
- subcutaneous lipoma
- hypertrichosis
- pigmented nevi
- skin dimple
- bladder + bowel dysfunction
- pathologic plantar response
- spastic gait disturbance
- foot deformities
- absent tendon reflexes
- sinus tract

Spina Bifida

= incomplete closure of bony elements of the spine (lamina + spinous processes) posteriorly

Spina Bifida Occulta

= OCCULT SPINAL DYSRAPHISM
= cleft / tethered cord WITH skin cover
Frequency: 15% of spinal dysraphism
- rarely leads to neurologic deficit in itself

Associated with:
(a) vertebral defect (85 – 90%)
(b) lumbosacral dermal lesion (80%): hairy tuft (= hypertrichosis), dimple, sinus tract, nevus, hyperpigmentation, hemangioma, subcutaneous mass
1. Diastematomyelia
2. Lipomeningocele
3. Tethered cord syndrome
4. Filum terminale lipoma

5. Intraspinal dermoid
6. Epidermoid cyst
7. Myelocystocele
8. Split notochord syndrome
9. Meningocele
10. Dorsal dermal sinus
11. Tight filum terminale syndrome

Spina Bifida Aperta

= SPINA BIFIDA CYSTICA
= posterior protrusion of all / parts of the contents of the spinal canal through a bony spinal defect
Frequency: 85% of spinal dysraphism
◊ Most severe form of midline fusion defect
• neural placode WITHOUT skin cover
• associated with neurologic deficit in >90%

1. Simple meningocele
   = herniation of CSF-filled sac without neural elements
2. Myelocele
   = midline plaque of neural tissue lying exposed at the skin surface
3. Myelomeningocele
   = a myelocele elevated above skin surface by expansion of subarachnoid space ventral to neural plaque
4. Myeloschisis
   = surface presentation of neural elements completely uncovered by meninges

Caudal Spinal Anomalies

= malformation of distal spine and cord in associated with hindgut, renal, and genitourinary anomalies

1. Terminal myelocystocele
2. Lateral meningocele
3. Caudal regression

Segmentation Anomalies of Vertebral Bodies

during 9 – 12th week of gestation two ossification centers form for the ventral + dorsal half of vertebral body

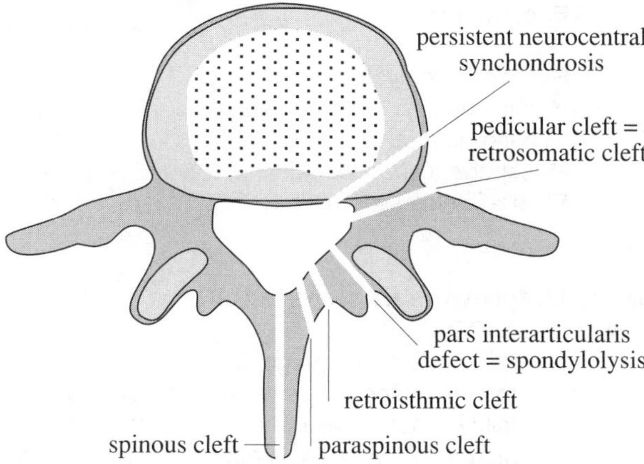

Clefts in Neural Arch

1. **Asomia** = agenesis of vertebral body
   √ complete absence of vertebral body
   √ hypoplastic posterior elements may be present
2. **Hemivertebra**
   (a) Unilateral wedge vertebra
      √ right / left hemivertebra
      √ scoliosis at birth
   (b) Dorsal hemivertebra
      √ rapidly progressive kyphoscoliosis
   (c) Ventral hemivertebra (extremely rare)
3. **Coronal cleft**
   = failure of fusion of anterior + posterior ossification centers
   May be associated with: premature male infant, Chondrodystrophia calcificans congenita
   Location: usually in lower thoracic + lumbar spine
   √ vertical radiolucent band just behind midportion of vertebral body; disappears mostly by 6 months of life
4. **Butterfly vertebra**
   = failure of fusion of lateral halves secondary to persistence of notochordal tissue
   May be associated with: anterior spina bifida ± anterior meningocele
   √ widened vertebral body with butterfly configuration (AP view)
   √ adaptation of vertebral endplates of adjacent vertebral bodies
5. **Block vertebra**
   = congenital vertebral fusion
   Location: lumbar / cervical
   √ height of fused vertebral bodies equals the sum of heights of involved bodies + intervertebral disk
   √ "waist" at level of intervertebral disk space
6. Hypoplastic vertebra
7. Klippel-Feil syndrome

VERTEBRAL BODY

Destruction of Vertebral Body

A. NEOPLASM
   1. Metastasis
   2. Primary neoplasm: lymphoma, multiple myeloma, chordoma
B. INFECTION
   1. Pyogenic vertebral osteomyelitis
   2. Tuberculous spondylitis
   3. Brucellosis
   4. Fungal disease
   5. Echinococcosis
   6. Sarcoidosis

Small Vertebral Body

1. Radiation therapy
   during early childhood in excess of 1,000 rads
2. Juvenile rheumatoid arthritis
   Location: cervical spine
   √ atlantoaxial subluxation may be present
   √ vertebral fusion may occur

3. Eosinophilic granuloma
   Location: lumbar / lower thoracic spine
   √ compression deformity / vertebra plana
4. Gaucher disease
   = deposits of glucocerebrosides within RES
   √ compression deformity
5. Platyspondyly generalisata
   = flattened vertebral bodies associated with many hereditary systemic disorders (achondroplasia, spondyloepiphyseal dysplasia tarda, mucopolysaccharidosis, osteopetrosis, neurofibromatosis, osteogenesis imperfecta, thanatophoric dwarfism)
   √ disk spaces of normal height

Vertebra Plana

mnemonic: " FETISH"

Fracture (trauma, osteogenesis imperfecta)
Eosinophilic granuloma
Tumor (metastasis, myeloma, leukemia)
Infection
Steroids (avascular necrosis)
Hemangioma

Signs of Acute Vertebral Collapse on MRI

1. OSTEOPOROSIS
   √ retropulsion of posterior bone fragment
2. MALIGNANCY
   √ epidural soft-tissue mass
   √ no residual normal marrow signal intensity
   √ abnormal enhancement

Enlarged Vertebral Body

1. Paget disease
   √ "picture framing"; bone sclerosis
2. Gigantism
   √ increase in height of body + disk
3. Myositis ossificans progressiva
   √ bodies greater in height than width
   √ osteoporosis
   √ ossification of ligamentum nuchae

Enlarged Vertebral Foramen

1. Neurofibroma
2. Congenital absence / hypoplasia of pedicle
3. Dural ectasia (Marfan syndrome, Ehlers-Danlos syndrome)
4. Intraspinal neoplasm
5. Metastatic destruction of pedicle

Cervical Spine Fusion

mnemonic: "SPAR BIT"

Senile hypertrophic ankylosis (DISH)
Psoriasis, **P**rogressive myositis ossificans
Ankylosing spondylitis
Reiter disease, **R**heumatoid arthritis (juvenile)
Block vertebra (Klippel-Feil)
Infection (TB)
Trauma

Vertebral Border Abnormality

Straightening of Anterior Border

1. Ankylosing spondylitis
2. Paget disease
3. Psoriatic arthritis
4. Reiter disease
5. Rheumatoid arthritis
6. Normal variant

Anterior Scalloping of Vertebrae

1. Aortic aneurysm
2. Lymphadenopathy
3. Tuberculosis
4. Multiple myeloma (paravertebral soft-tissue mass)

Posterior Scalloping of Vertebrae

in conditions associated with dural ectasia

A. INCREASED INTRASPINAL PRESSURE
   1. Communicating hydrocephalus
   2. Ependymoma
B. MESENCHYMAL TISSUE LAXITY (dural ectasia)
   1. Neurofibromatosis
   2. Marfan syndrome
   3. Ehlers-Danlos syndrome
   4. Posterior meningocele
C. BONE SOFTENING
   1. Mucopolysaccharidoses: Hurler, Morquio, Sanfilippo
   2. Achondroplasia
   3. Acromegaly (lumbar vertebrae)
   4. Ankylosing spondylitis (lax dura acting on osteoporotic vertebrae)

mnemonic: "DAMN MALE SHAME"

Dermoid
Ankylosing spondylitis
Meningioma
Neurofibromatosis

Marfan syndrome
Acromegaly
Lipoma
Ependymoma

Syringohydromyelia
Hydrocephalus
Achondroplasia
Mucopolysaccharidoses
Ehlers-Danlos syndrome

Bony Outgrowths from Vertebra

A. CHILDHOOD
   1. Hurler syndrome = gargoylism
      √ rounded appearance of vertebral bodies
      √ mild kyphotic curve with smaller vertebral body at apex of kyphosis displaying tonguelike beak at anterior half (usually at T12 / L1)
      √ "step-off" deformities along anterior margins

2. Hunter syndrome
   less severe changes than in Hurler syndrome
3. Morquio disease
   √ flattened + widened vertebral bodies
   √ anterior "tonguelike" elongation of central portion of vertebral bodies
4. Hypothyroidism = cretinism
   √ small flat vertebral bodies
   √ anterior "tonguelike" deformity (in children only)
   √ widened disk spaces + irregular endplates

B. ADULTS
1. Spondylosis deformans
   √ osteophytosis along anterior + lateral aspects of endplates with horizontal + vertical course as a result of shearing of the outer annular fibers (Sharpey fibers connecting the annulus fibrosus to adjacent vertebral body)
2. Diffuse idiopathic skeletal hyperostosis (DISH)
   √ flowing calcifications + ossifications along anterolateral aspect of >4 contiguous thoracic vertebral bodies ± osteophytosis
3. Ankylosing spondylitis
   √ bilateral symmetric syndesmophytes (ossification of annulus fibrosus)
   √ "bamboo spine"
   √ "diskal ballooning" = biconvex intervertebral disks secondary to osteoporotic deformity of endplates
   √ straightening of anterior margins of vertebral bodies (erosion)
   √ ossification of paraspinal ligaments
4. Fluorosis
   √ vertebral osteophytosis + hyperostosis
   √ sclerotic vertebral bodies + kyphoscoliosis
   √ calcification of paraspinal ligaments
5. Acromegaly
   √ increase in anteroposterior diameter of vertebrae + concavity on posterior portion
   √ enlargement of intervertebral disk
6. Hypoparathyroidism
7. Neuropathic arthropathy
8. Sternoclavicular hyperostosis

Spine Ossification

1. Syndesmophyte = ossification of annulus fibrosus
   √ thin slender vertical outgrowth extending from margin of one vertebral body to next
   Associated with: ankylosing spondylitis, ochronosis

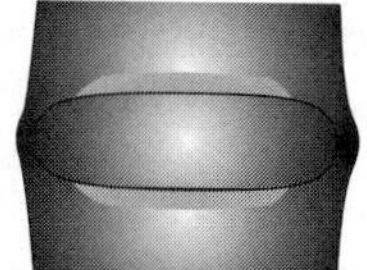

Ankylosing Spondylitis

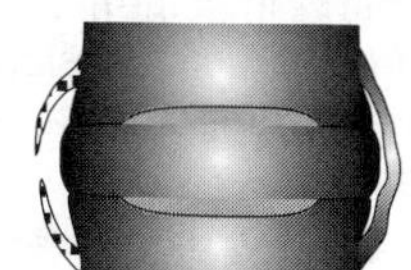

Psoriasis Reiter Syndrome

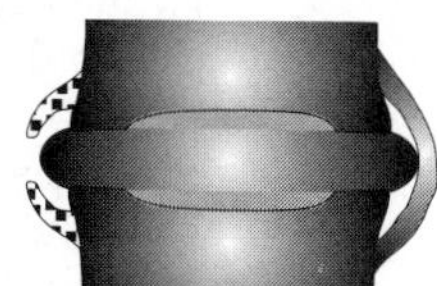

Spondylosis Deformans

Syndesmophytes

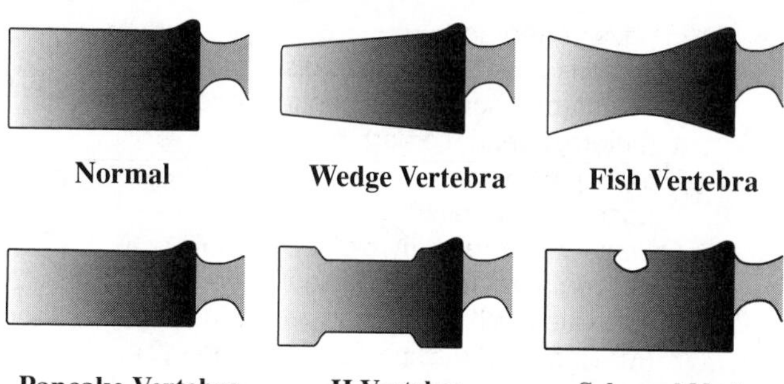

Vertebral Endplate Abnormalities

2. Osteophyte
   = ossification of anterior longitudinal ligament
   √ initially triangular outgrowth several millimeters from edge of vertebral body
   Associated with: osteoarthritis
3. Flowing anterior ossification
   = ossification of disk, anterior longitudinal ligament, paravertebral soft tissues
   Associated with: diffuse idiopathic skeletal hyperostosis
4. Paravertebral ossification
   √ initially irregular / poorly defined paravertebral ossification eventually merging with vertebral body
   Associated with: psoriatic arthritis, Reiter syndrome

Vertebral Endplate Abnormality

1. Cupid's bow vertebra
   Cause: ? (normal variant)
   Location: 3–5th lumbar vertebra
   √ two parasagittal posterior concavities on inferior aspect of vertebral body (viewed on AP)
2. Osteoporosis (senile / steroid-induced)
   (a) "fish / fish-mouth vertebrae"
   Cause: osteomalacia, Paget disease, hyperparathyroidism, Gaucher disease
   √ biconcave vertebrae
   √ bone sclerosis along endplates
   (b) wedge-shaped vertebrae
   √ anterior border height reduced by >4 mm compared to posterior border height
   (c) "pancake" vertebrae
   √ overall flattening of vertebra
3. "H-vertebrae"
   Cause: sickle cell + other anemias, Gaucher disease
   = compression of central portions from subchondral infarcts
4. Schmorl / cartilaginous node
   = intraosseous herniation of nucleus pulposus at center of weakened endplate
   Cause: Scheuermann disease, trauma, hyperparathyroidism, osteochondrosis
5. Butterfly vertebra
   Cause: congenital defect

6. Limbus vertebrae
   = intraosseous herniation of disk material at junction of vertebral bony rim of centra + endplate (anterosuperior corner)
7. "Ring" epiphysis
8. "Rugger-jersey spine"
   Cause: hyperparathyroidism, myelofibrosis
   √ horizontal sclerosis subjacent to vertebral endplates with intervening normal osseous density (resembling the stripes on rugby jerseys)
9. "Sandwich" / "hamburger" vertebrae
   Cause: osteopetrosis, myelofibrosis
   √ sclerotic endplates alternate with radiolucent midportions of vertebral bodies

Ring Epiphysis

= normal aspect of developing vertebra (between 6 and 12 years of age)

√ small steplike recess at corner of anterior edge of vertebral body

1. Severe osteoporosis
2. Healing rickets
3. Scurvy

Bullet-shaped Vertebral Body

mnemonic: "HAM"

Hypothyroidism
Achondroplasia
Morquio syndrome

Bone-within-bone Vertebra

= "ghost vertebra" following stressful event during vertebral growth phase in childhood

1. Stress line of unknown cause
2. Leukemia
3. Heavy metal poisoning
4. Thorotrast injection, TB
5. Rickets
6. Scurvy
7. Hypothyroidism
8. Hypoparathyroidism

Ivory Vertebra

mnemonic: "LOST FROM CHOMP"

Lymphoma
Osteopetrosis
Sickle cell disease
Trauma, **T**uberculous spondylitis
Fluorosis
Renal osteodystrophy
Osteoblastic metastasis
Myelosclerosis
Chronic sclerosing osteomyelitis, **C**hordoma
Hemangioma
Osteosarcoma
Myeloma
Paget disease

Sclerotic Pedicle

1. Osteoid osteoma
2. Unilateral spondylolysis
3. Contralateral congenitally absent pedicle

TUMORS OF VERTEBRA

Expansile Lesion of Vertebrae

A. INVOLVEMENT OF MULTIPLE VERTEBRAE
   Metastases, multiple myeloma / plasmacytoma, lymphoma, hemangioma, Paget disease, angiosarcoma, eosinophilic granuloma

B. INVOLVEMENT OF TWO / MORE CONTIGUOUS VERTEBRAE
   Osteochondroma, chordoma, aneurysmal bone cyst, myeloma

C. BENIGN LESION
   1. Osteochondroma (1–5% with solitary osteochondromas, 7–9% with hereditary multiple exostoses) commonly cervical, esp. C2; commonly rising from posterior elements
   2. Osteoblastoma (30–40% in spine)
      M:F = 2:1; equal distribution in spine; posterior elements (lamina, pedicle), may involve body if large; expansile lesion with sclerotic / shell-like rim, foci of calcified tumor matrix in 50%
   3. Giant cell tumor (5–7% in spine)
      commonly sacrum, expansile lytic lesion of vertebral body with well-defined borders; secondary invasion of posterior elements; malignant degeneration in 5–20% after radiation therapy
   4. Osteoid osteoma (10–25% in spine)
      commonly lower thoracic / upper lumbar spine, posterior elements (pedicle, lamina, spinous process), painful scoliosis with concavity toward lesion
   5. Aneurysmal bone cyst (12–30% in spine)
      thoracic > lumbar > cervical spine, posterior elements with frequent extension into vertebral bodies, well-defined margins, may arise from primary bone lesion (giant cell tumor, fibrous dysplasia) in 50%, may involve two contiguous vertebrae
   6. Hemangioma (30% in spine)
      10% incidence in general population; commonly lower thoracic / upper lumbar spine, vertebral body, "accordion" / "corduroy" appearance
   7. Hydatid cyst (1% in spine)
      slow-growing destructive lesion, well-defined sclerotic borders, endemic areas
   8. Paget disease
      vertebral body ± posterior elements, enlargement of bone, "picture framing"; bone sclerosis
   9. Eosinophilic granuloma (6% in spine)
      most often cervical / lumbar spine, vertebral body, "vertebra plana"; multiple involvement common

10. Fibrous dysplasia (1% in spine)
    vertebral body, nonhomogeneous trabecular "ground-glass" appearance
11. Enostosis (1–14% in spine)
    Location: T1–T7 > L2–L3

D. MALIGNANT
1. Chordoma (15% in spine)
   most common nonlymphoproliferative primary malignant tumor of the spine in adults; particularly C2, within vertebral body; violates disk space
2. Metastases (especially from lung, breast)
   Age: >50 years of age;
   Clue: pedicles often destroyed
3. Multiple myeloma / plasmacytoma
   Clue: vertebral pedicles usually spared
4. Angiosarcoma
   10% involve spine, most commonly lumbar
5. Chondrosarcoma (3–12% in spine)
   2nd most common nonlymphoproliferative primary malignant tumor of the spine in adults
   Site: vertebral body (15%), posterior elements (40%), both (45%)
   √ involvement of adjacent vertebra by extension through disk (35%)
6. Ewing sarcoma and PNET
   most common nonlymphoproliferative primary malignant tumor of the spine in children; metastases more common than primary
   Site: vertebral body with extension to posterior elements
   √ diffuse sclerosis + osteonecrosis (69%)
7. Osteosarcoma (0.6–3.2% in spine)
   Average age: 4th decade
   Location: lumbosacral segments
   Site: vertebral body, posterior elements (10–17%)
   √ may present as "ivory vertebra"
8. Lymphoma

Blowout Lesion of Posterior Elements

mnemonic: "GO APE"

Giant cell tumor
Osteoblastoma
Aneurysmal bone cyst
Plasmacytoma
Eosinophilic granuloma

Bone Tumors Favoring Vertebral Bodies

mnemonic: "CALL HOME"

Chordoma
Aneurysmal bone cyst
Leukemia
Lymphoma
Hemangioma
Osteoid osteoma, **O**steoblastoma
Myeloma, **M**etastasis
Eosinophilic granuloma

Primary Vertebral Tumors in Children

in order of frequency:
1. Osteoid osteoma
2. Benign osteoblastoma
3. Aneurysmal bone cyst
4. Ewing sarcoma

Primary Tumor of Posterior Elements

mnemonic: "A HOG"

Aneurysmal bone cyst
Hydatid cyst, **H**emangioma
Osteoblastoma, **O**steoid osteoma
Giant cell tumor

SACRUM

Destructive Sacral Lesion

mnemonic: "SPACEMON"

Sarcoma
Plasmacytoma
Aneurysmal bone cyst
Chordoma
Ependymoma
Metastasis
Osteomyelitis
Neuroblastoma

Sacral Tumor

Sacral Bone Tumor

A. BENIGN
1. Giant cell tumor (2nd most common primary)
2. Aneurysmal bone cyst (rare)
3. Cavernous hemangioma (very rare)
4. Osteoid osteoma / osteoblastoma (very rare)

B. MALIGNANT
1. Metastases (most common sacral neoplasm):
   - hematogenous: lung, breast, kidney, prostate
   - contiguous: rectum, uterus, bladder
2. Plasmacytoma, multiple myeloma
3. Lymphoma, leukemia
4. Chordoma (most common primary)
   ◊ 2–4% of malignant osseous neoplasms!
5. Sacrococcygeal teratoma
6. Ewing sarcoma (rare)

Sacral Canal Tumor (less common)

A. BENIGN
1. Neurofibroma: multiple suggestive of NF
2. Schwannoma (rare)
3. Meningioma (very rare)

B. MALIGNANT
1. Ependymoma
2. Drop metastases
3. Carcinoid tumor

INTERVERTEBRAL DISK

Loss of Disk Space

1. Degenerative disk disease
2. Neuropathic osteoarthropathy
3. Dialysis spondyloarthropathy with amyloidosis
4. Ochronosis
5. Ankylosing spondylitis with pseudarthrosis
6. Sarcoidosis

Spinal Vacuum Phenomena

(a) nucleus pulposus	Osteochondrosis
(b) annulus fibrosus	Spondylosis deformans
(c) disk within vertebral body	Cartilaginous node
(d) disk within spinal canal	Intraspinal disk herniation
(e) apophyseal joint	Osteoarthritis
(f) vertebral body	Ischemic necrosis

Vacuum Phenomenon in Intervertebral Disk Space

= liberation of nitrogen gas from surrounding tissues into clefts with an abnormal nucleus or annulus attachment

Prevalence: in up to 20% of plain radiographs / in up to 50% of spinal CT in patients > age 40

Cause:

1. Primary / secondary degeneration of nucleus pulposus
2. Intraosseous herniation of disk (= Schmorl node)
3. Spondylosis deformans (gas in annulus fibrosus)
4. Adjacent vertebral metastatic disease with vertebral collapse
5. Infection (extremely rare)

Intervertebral Disk Calcification

mnemonic: " A DISK SO WHITE"

Amyloidosis, **A**cromegaly
Degenerative
Infection
Spinal fusion
CPPD
Spondylitis ankylosing
Ochronosis
Wilson disease
Hemochromatosis, **H**omocystinuria, **H**yperparathyroidism
Idiopathic skeletal hyperostosis
Traumatic
Etceteras: Gout and other causes of chondrocalcinosis

Intervertebral Disk Ossification

Associated with: fusion of vertebral bodies

1. Ankylosing spondylitis
2. Ochronosis
3. Sequelae of trauma
4. Sequelae of disk-space infection
5. Degenerative disease

Schmorl = Cartilaginous Node

= superior / inferior intravertebral herniation of disk material through weakened area of vertebral endplate

Pathogenesis: disruption of cartilaginous plate of vertebral body left during regression of chorda dorsalis, ossification gaps, previous vascular channels

Cause:

(a) osseous: osteoporosis, osteomalacia, Paget disease, hyperparathyroidism, infection, neoplasm
(b) cartilaginous: intervertebral osteochondrosis, disk infection, juvenile kyphosis

√ concave defects at upper and lower vertebral endplates with sharp margins

MR:

√ node of similar signal intensity as disk
√ low signal intensity of rim
√ associated with narrowed disk space

DDx: *mnemonic:* "SHOOT"

Scheuermann disease
Hyperparathyroidism
Osteoporosis
Osteomalacia
Trauma

SPINAL CORD

◊ Most spinal cord neoplasms are malignant!
◊ 90–95% are classified as gliomas

Intramedullary Lesion

Prevalence: 4–10% of all CNS tumors; 20% of all intraspinal tumors in adults (35% in children)

A. TUMOR

√ expansion of cord
√ heterogenous signal on T2WI
√ cysts + necrosis
√ variable enhancement (vast majority with some enhancement)

(a) primary:

1. Ependymoma (60% of all spinal cord tumors)
   ◊ The most common glial tumor in adults
2. Astrocytoma (25%)
   ◊ The most common intramedullary tumor in children
3. Hemangioblastoma (5%)
4. Oligodendroglioma (3%)
5. Epidermoid, dermoid, teratoma (1–2%)
6. Ganglioglioma (1%)
7. Lipoma (1%)

Location:
— cervical region: astrocytoma
— thoracic region: teratoma-dermoid, astrocytoma
— lumbar region: ependymoma, dermoid

(b) metastatic: eg, malignant melanoma, breast, lung

B. CYSTIC LESION
√ fluid isointense to CSF
√ smooth well-defined internal margins
√ thinned adjacent parenchyma
√ cord atrophy
√ no contrast enhancement
(a) peritumoral cyst = syringomyelia
√ polar / satellite cysts = rostral / caudal cysts representing reactive dilatation of central canal
◊ A higher location within spinal canal raises the likelihood of syrinx development
Prevalence: in 60% of all intramedullary tumors
1. Syringomyelia
2. Hydromyelia
3. Reactive cyst
(b) tumoral cyst
√ shows peripheral enhancement
1. Ganglioglioma (in 46%)
2. Astrocytoma (in 20%)
3. Ependymoma (in 3%)
4. Hemangioblastoma (2–4%)

C. VASCULAR
1. Cord concussion = reversible local edema
2. Hemorrhagic contusion
3. Cord transection
4. AVM

D. CHRONIC INFECTION
1. Sarcoid
2. Transverse myelitis
3. Multiple sclerosis

mnemonic: "I'M ASHAMED"
Inflammation (multiple sclerosis, sarcoidosis, myelitis)
Medulloblastoma
Astrocytoma
Syringomyelia / hydromyelia
Hematoma, **H**emangioblastoma
Arteriovenous malformation
Metastasis
Ependymoma
Dermoid

Intramedullary Neoplastic Lesion

A. GLIAL NEOPLASM
1. Ependymoma (60%)
2. Astrocytoma (33%)
3. Ganglioglioma (1%)

B. NONGLIAL NEOPLASM
(a) highly vascular lesions:
1. Hemangioblastoma
2. Paraganglioma
(b) rare lesions:
3. Metastasis
4. Lymphoma
5. Primitive neuroectodermal tumor

C. EXTRAMEDULLARY NEOPLASM
1. Intramedullary meningioma
2. Intramedullary schwannoma

Intramedullary Nonneoplastic Mass

1. Epidermoid
2. Congenital lipoma
3. Posttraumatic pseudocyst
4. Wegener granuloma
5. Cavernous malformation
6. Abscess

Intramedullary Nonneoplastic Lesion

Prevalence: 4%
√ no cord expansion
1. Demyelinating disease
2. Sarcoidosis
3. Amyloid angiopathy
4. Pseudotumor
5. Dural arteriovenous fistula
6. Cord infarction
7. Chronic arachnoiditis
8. Cystic myelomalacia

Intradural Extramedullary Mass

1. Nerve sheath tumor (35%)
2. Meningioma (25%)
3. Lipoma
4. Dermoid
commonly conus / cauda equina; associated with spinal dysraphism (1/3)
5. Ependymoma
commonly filum terminale; NO spinal dysraphism
6. "Drop metastases" from CNS tumors
7. Metastases from outside CNS
8. Arachnoid cyst
9. Neurenteric cyst
10. Hemangioblastoma
11. Paraganglioma

mnemonic: "MAMA N"
Metastasis
Arachnoiditis
Meningioma
AVM, **A**rachnoid cyst
Neurofibroma

Epidural Extramedullary Lesion

Prevalence: 30% of all spinal tumors
A. TUMOR
(a) benign
1. Dermoid, epidermoid
2. Lipoma: over several segments
3. Fibroma
4. Neurinoma (with intradural component)
5. Meningioma (with intradural component)
6. Ganglioneuroblastoma, ganglioneuroma
(b) malignant
1. Hodgkin disease
2. Lymphoma: most commonly in dorsal space
3. Metastasis: breast, lung — most commonly from involved vertebrae without extension through dura
4. Paravertebral neuroblastoma

B. DISK DISEASE
  1. Bulging disk
  2. Herniated nucleus pulposus
  3. Sequestered nucleus pulposus
C. BONE: spinal stenosis, spondylosis
D. INFECTION: epidural abscess
E. BLOOD: hematoma
F. OTHERS: synovial cyst, arachnoid cyst, extradural lipomatosis, extramedullary hematopoiesis

mnemonic: "MANDELIN"
Metastasis (drop mets from CNS tumor), **M**eningioma
Arachnoiditis, **A**rachnoid cyst
Neurofibroma
Dermoid / epidermoid
Ependymoma
Lipoma
Infection (TB, cysticercosis)
Normal but tortuous roots

Cord Lesions

A. INFLAMMATION
  1. Multiple sclerosis
  2. Acute disseminated encephalomyelitis
  3. Acute transverse myelitis
     √ involves half the cross-sectional area of cord
  4. Lyme disease
  5. Devic syndrome
B. INFECTION
  1. Cytomegalovirus
  2. Progressive multifocal leukoencephalopathy
  3. HIV
C. VASCULAR
  1. Anterior spinal artery infarct
     √ affects central gray matter first
     √ extends to anterior two-thirds of cord
  2. Venous infarct / ischemia
     √ starts centrally progressing centripetally
D. NEOPLASM

Cord Atrophy

1. Multiple sclerosis
2. Amyotrophic lateral sclerosis
3. Cervical spondylosis
4. Sequelae of trauma
5. Ischemia
6. Radiation therapy
7. AVM of cord

Delayed Uptake of Water-Soluble Contrast in Cord Lesion

1. Syringohydromyelia
2. Cystic tumor of cord
3. Osteomalacia

exceedingly rare:
4. Demyelinating disease
5. Infection
6. Infarction

Extraarachnoid Myelography

A. SUBDURAL INJECTION
  √ spinal cord, nerve roots, blood vessels not outlined
  √ irregular filling defects
  √ slow flow of contrast material
  √ CSF pulsations diminished
  √ contrast material pools at injection site within anterior / posterior compartments
B. EPIDURAL INJECTION
  √ contrast extravasation along nerve roots
  √ contrast material lies near periphery of spinal canal
  √ intraspinal structures are not well outlined

MUSCULOSKELETAL NEUROGENIC TUMORS

A. BENIGN NEUROGENIC TUMOR
  1. Traumatic neuroma
  2. Morton neuroma
  3. Neural fibrolipoma
  4. Nerve sheath ganglion
  5. Benign peripheral nerve sheath tumors (PNST)
B. MALIGNANT NEUROGENIC NEOPLASM
  = malignant peripheral nerve sheath tumor (PNST)

Benign Tumor of Nerve Sheath

= BENIGN PERIPHERAL NERVE SHEATH TUMOR (PNST)
= NEURINOMA

contains cellular elements closely related to Schwann cell
Schwann cell = cell that surrounds cranial, spinal, and peripheral nerves producing myelin sheath around axons thus providing mechanical protection, serving as a tract for nerve regeneration

◊ NOTE that myelin sheaths within brain substance are made by oligodendrocytes!

Plain film:
  √ fusiform mass delineated by surrounding fat
  √ soft-tissue and osseous overgrowth
  √ bone involvement + mineralization (osteoid / chondroid / amorphous) only in larger lesions

Angio:
  √ displacement of major vascular structures
  √ corkscrew-type vessels at upper / lower pole of tumor (= hypertrophy of nutrient nerve vasculature)

MR, CT:
  √ fusiform mass in a typical nerve distribution (94%):
    √ entering + exiting nerve (intradural / extradural)
    √ dumbbell shape with extension into enlarged neural foramen (intra- and extradural)
    √ low attenuation (as low as 5–25 HU) due to
      (a) high lipid content of myelin from Schwann cells
      (b) entrapped fat
      (c) endoneural myxoid tissue with high water content (Antoni B areas)
    √ isointense to muscle on T1WI + hyperintense to fat on T2WI
    √ well-defined hyperdense / hypointense margins
    √ hypointense on T2WI in diffuse neurofibromas:

√ "target sign":
√ hypo- to isointense center + hyperintense periphery on T2WI (almost PATHOGNOMONIC)
√ hyperdense center + hypodense periphery
√ "fascicular sign" = multiple small ringlike structures with peripheral higher signal intensity on T2WI
√ "split-fat sign" = rim of fat surrounding mass suggests a tumor origin in the intermuscular space
√ marked uniform enhancement (most helpful for intradural lesions)
√ muscle atrophy with striated increased fat content (in 23%)

Ga-67 scintigraphy:
√ significant uptake in malignant PNST

Schwannoma = Neurilemmoma

= usually solitary well-encapsulated benign slowly growing neoplasm arising from Schwann cells displacing nerve fibers eccentrically

◊ Nerve root NOT incorporated

Prevalence: 5–10% of all benign soft-tissue tumors
Age: 20–30 years
Path: fusiform mass with entering + exiting nerve surrounded by a true capsule of epineurium; in large nerves mass is eccentric to involved nerve with nerve fibers splayed about the neoplasm
Histo: S-100 protein positive

(a) cellular component (**Antoni type A** tissue): more organized area composed of densely packed cellular spindle cells arranged in short bundles / interlacing fascicles
Location: posterior mediastinum, retroperitoneum, 25% of extremity lesions
√ hypointense on T2WI

(b) myxoid component (**Antoni type B** tissue): less organized loosely arranged area of hypocellular myxoid tissue with high water content
√ hyperintense on T2WI

(c) ancient schwannoma: degenerative changes of cyst formation, calcification, hemorrhage, fibrosis

Location: spinal + sympathetic nerve roots

(a) extracranial: neck, flexor surfaces of upper + lower extremities, posterior mediastinum, retroperitoneum
Site: spinal and sympathetic nerve roots, ulnar n., peroneal n.
◊ Usually solitary, but in 5% associated with neurofibromatosis type 1 (= >2 schwannomas / one plexiform neurofibroma)

(b) intracranial: mostly from sensory nerves, vestibulocochlear (VIII) cranial nerve (most common) > trigeminal (V) cranial nerve (2nd most common) > VII
◊ Usually sporadic tumor, but 5–20% of patients with solitary intracranial schwannomas have neurofibromatosis type 2!

• painless, fairly mobile mass
• ± neurologic symptoms

√ solitary fusiform well-encapsulated <5 cm lesion
√ slow growth

MR:
√ well-delineated mass of intermediate signal intensity on T1WI
√ heterogeneous mass of high signal intensity on T2WI
√ frequently low-signal-intensity rim (= capsule)
√ heterogenous enhancement in 33%
√ peritumoral edema in 33%

DDx: may appear similar to meningioma

Rx: excision (affected nerve usually separable from neoplasm after incision of epineurium)

Neurofibroma

= usually multiple often infiltrative tumors of nerve sheath separating nerve fibers resulting in fusiform enlargement of nerve

Prevalence: 5% of all benign soft-tissue tumors
Histo: swirls of neuronal elements containing Schwann cells, nerve fibers, fibroblasts, collagen
Associated with: neurofibromatosis type 1
Age: 20–30 years; M:F = 1:1

◊ Malignant transformation exceedingly rare!
◊ The spinal neurofibroma is rarely sporadic and usually a sign of type 1 neurofibromatosis!
◊ Only 10% of patients with neurofibromas have von Recklinghausen disease!

Location: any level, but particularly cervical

(a) peripheral nerves
√ nonencapsulated well-circumscribed fusiform mass of peripheral nerves

(b) intradural extramedullary mass
√ well-defined mass with dumbbell configuration (= extradural component extends through neural foramen)
√ widening of intervertebral foramen + erosion of pedicles
√ scalloping of vertebral bodies
√ hypodense (CHARACTERISTIC) approaching characteristics of water / isodense to skeletal muscle
√ usually NO contrast enhancement

MR:
√ homogeneous mass isointense to cord / muscle on T1WI
√ hyperintense tumor on T2WI compared with surrounding fat
√ "target sign" = low signal-intensity center on T2WI (due to collagen + condensed Schwann cells) in 70% of extracranial neurofibromas
√ ± muscular atrophy

DDx: conjoined nerve root sleeve
Rx: surgical resection with sacrifice of nerve (tumor not separable from normal nerve)

Localized Neurofibroma

Prevalence: 90% of all neurofibromas
Path: fusiform tumor, often remaining within epineurium as a true capsule
Histo: interlacing fascicles of wavy elongated cells containing abundant amounts of collagen
Location: affecting primarily superficial cutaneous nerves, occasionally deep-seated larger nerves
√ mostly solitary slow-growing lesion <5 cm in size

Diffuse Neurofibroma

Age: children + young adults
Path: poorly defined lesion within subcutaneous fat, infiltrating along connective tissue septa, inseparable from normal nerve tissue
Histo: very uniform prominent fibrillary collagen
Location: most frequently in subcutaneous tissues of head + neck
• plaquelike elevation of skin with thickening of entire subcutis
√ isolated lesion in 90% unassociated with NF1
√ always indistinct infiltrative margins due to subcutaneous spread along connective tissue septa

Plexiform Neurofibroma

= involvement of long segment of nerve + branches extending into adjacent muscle, fat, subcutaneous tissue
= PATHOGNOMONIC of neurofibromatosis type 1
√ serpentine "bag of worms" appearance = tortuous tangles / fusiform enlargement of peripheral nerves
√ reticulated linear branching pattern within subcutaneous tissue

Malignant Tumor of Nerve Sheath

= PERIPHERAL MALIGNANT NERVE SHEATH TUMOR (PNST) = NEUROGENIC SPINDLE CELL SARCOMA
Prevalence: 5–10% of all soft-tissue sarcomas
Age: 20–50 years; M:F = 8:1
Associated with: neurofibromatosis type 1 (in 25–70%), radiation therapy (in 11% of all malignant PNSTs after a latent period of 10–20 years)
Histo: tumor cells arranged in fascicles resembling fibrosarcoma; additional heterotopic foci with mature cartilage and bone, rhabdomyosarcoma elements, glandular and epithelial components (in 10–15%)
• pain, motor weakness, sensory deficits
Location: major nerve trunks (sciatic n., brachial plexus, sacral plexus)
Metastases: lung, bone, pleura, retroperitoneum (60%); regional lymph nodes (9%)
√ fusiform mass with entering + exiting nerve
√ frequently indistinct margins
√ sudden increase in size of a previously stable neurofibroma
√ frequently areas of hemorrhage + necrosis
Rx: resection + adjuvant chemo- and radiation therapy with local recurrence in 40%
Prognosis: 44% 5-year survival rate

SPINAL FIXATION DEVICES

Function: (1) to restore anatomic alignment in fractures (fracture reduction)
(2) to stabilize degenerative disease
(3) to correct congenital deformities (scoliosis)
(4) to replace diseased / abnormal vertebrae (infection, tumor)

Posterior Fixation Devices

using paired / unpaired rods attached with

1. Sublaminar wiring
   = passing a wire around lamina + rod
2. Interspinous wiring
   = passing a wire through a hole in the spinous process; a Drummond button prevents the wire from pulling through the bone
3. Subpars wiring
   = passing a wire around the pars interarticularis
4. Laminar / sublaminar hooks
   used on rods for compression / distraction forces to be applied to pedicles / laminae
   (a) upgoing hook curves under lamina
   (b) downgoing hook curves over lamina
5. Pedicle / transpedical screws
6. Rods
   (a) Luque rod = straight / L-shaped smooth rod 6–8 mm in diameter
   (b) O-ring fixator, rhomboid-shaped bar, Luque rectangle, segmental rectangle = preshaped loop to form a flat rectangle
   (c) Harrington distraction rod
   (d) Harrington compression rod
   (e) Knodt rod = threaded distraction rod with a central fixed nut (turnbuckle) and opposing thread pattern
   (f) Cotrel-Dubousset rods = a pair of rods with a serrated surface connected by a cross-link with ≥4 laminar hooks / pedicle screws
7. Plates
   (a) Roy-Camille plates
   = simple straight plates with round holes
   (b) Luque plates
   = long oval holes with clips encircling the plate
   (c) Steffee plates = straight plates with long slots

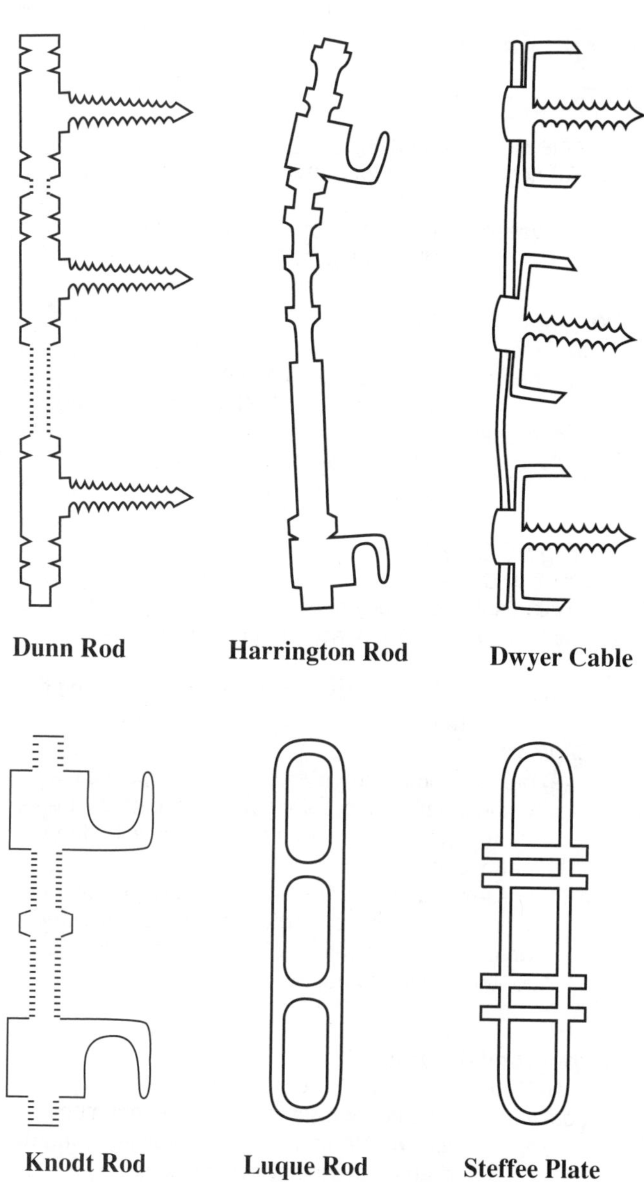

Spinal Fixation Devices

Cotrel-Dubousset Rods and Pedicle Screws

8. Translaminar screw
   = cancellous screws for single level fusion
9. Percutaneous pinning
   = (hollow) interference screws placed across disk level

Anterior Fixation Devices

1. Dwyer device
   = screws threaded into vertebral body over staples embedded into vertebral body connected by braided titanium wire; placed on convex side of spine
2. Zielke device
   = modified Dwyer system replacing cable with solid rod
3. Kaneda device
   = 2 curved vertebral plates with staples attached to vertebral bodies with screws, plates connected by 2 threaded rods attached to screw heads
4. Dunn device
   (similar to Kaneda device, discontinued)

ANATOMY OF SKULL AND SPINE

FORAMINA OF BASE OF SKULL

on inner aspect of middle cranial fossa 3 foramina are oriented along an oblique line in the greater sphenoidal wing from anteromedial behind the superior orbital fissure to posterolateral

mnemonic: "rotos"
- foramen **rot**undum
- foramen **o**vale
- foramen **s**pinosum

Foramen Rotundum

= canal within greater sphenoid wing connecting middle cranial fossa + pterygopalatine fossa

Location: inferior and lateral to superior orbital fissure

Course: extends obliquely forward + slightly inferiorly in a sagittal direction parallel to superior orbital fissure

Contents:
- (a) nerves: V_2 (maxillary nerve)
- (b) vessels: (1) artery of foramen rotundum
  (2) emissary vv.

√ best visualized by coronal CT

Foramen Ovale

= canal connecting middle cranial fossa + infratemporal fossa

Location: medial aspect of sphenoid body, situated posterolateral to foramen rotundum (endocranial aspect) + at base of lateral pterygoid plate (exocranial aspect)

Contents:
- (a) nerves: (1) V_3 (mandibular nerve)
  (2) lesser petrosal nerve (occasionally)
- (b) vessels: (1) accessory meningeal artery
  (2) emissary vv.

Foramen Spinosum

Location: on greater sphenoid wing posterolateral to foramen ovale (endocranial aspect) + lateral to eustachian tube (exocranial aspect)

Contents:
- (a) nerves: (1) recurrent meningeal branch of mandibular nerve
  (2) lesser superficial petrosal nerve
- (b) vessels: (1) middle meningeal a.
  (2) middle meningeal v.

Foramen Lacerum

Fibrocartilage cover (occasionally), carotid artery rests on endocranial aspect of fibrocartilage

Location: at base of medial pterygoid plate

Contents: (inconstant)
- (a) nerve: nerve of pterygoid canal (actually pierces cartilage)
- (b) vessel: meningeal branch of ascending pharyngeal a.

Foramen Magnum

Contents:
- (a) nerves: (1) medulla oblongata
  (2) cranial nerve XI (spinal accessory n.)
- (b) vessels: (1) vertebral a.
  (2) anterior spinal a.
  (3) posterior spinal a.

Pterygoid Canal

= VIDIAN CANAL

= within sphenoid body connecting pterygopalatine fossa anteriorly to foramen lacerum posteriorly

Location: at base of pterygoid plate below foramen rotundum

Contents:
- (a) nerves: vidian nerve = nerve of pterygoid canal
  = continuation of greater superficial petrosal nerve (from cranial nerve VII) after its union with deep petrosal nerve
- (b) vessel: vidian artery = artery of pterygoid canal
  = branch of terminal portion of internal maxillary a.
  arises in pterygopalatine fossa + passes through foramen lacerum posterior to Vidian n.

Hypoglossal Canal

= ANTERIOR CONDYLAR CANAL

Location: in posterior cranial fossa anteriorly above condyle starting above anterolateral part of foramen magnum, continuing in an anterolateral direction + exiting medial to jugular foramen

Contents:
- (a) nerves: cranial nerve XII (hypoglossal nerve)
- (b) vessels: (1) pharyngeal artery
  (2) branches of meningeal artery

Jugular Foramen

Location: at the posterior end of petro-occipital suture directly posterior to carotid orifice

- (a) anterior part:
  (1) inferior petrosal sinus
  (2) meningeal branches of pharyngeal artery + occipital artery
- (b) intermediate part:
  (1) cranial nerve IX (glossopharyngeal nerve)
  (2) cranial nerve X (vagus nerve)
  (3) cranial nerve XI (spinal accessory nerve)
- (c) posterior part: internal jugular vein

CRANIOVERTEBRAL JUNCTION

Craniometry:

— LATERAL VIEW

1. **Chamberlain line** = line between posterior pole of hard palate + opisthion (= posterior margin of foramen magnum)
   √ tip of odontoid process usually lies below / tangent to Chamberlain line
   √ tip of odontoid process may lie up to 1 ± 6.6 mm above the Chamberlain line
2. **McGregor line** = line between posterior pole of hard palate + most caudal portion of occipital squamosal surface
   ◊ Substitute to Chamberlain line if opisthion not visible
   √ tip of odontoid <5 mm above this line

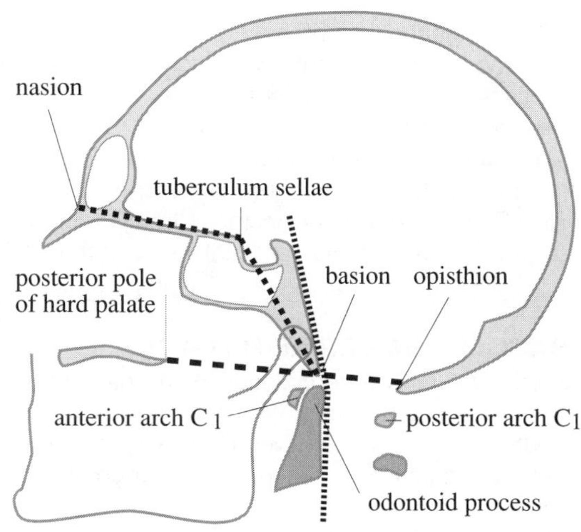

Skull Base Lines on Lateral View

3. **Wackenheim clivus baseline**
   = BASILAR LINE = line along clivus
   √ usually falls tangent to posterior aspect of tip of odontoid process
4. **Craniovertebral angle** = clivus-canal angle
   = angle formed by line along posterior surface of axis body and odontoid process + basilar line
   √ ranges from 150° in flexion to 180° in extension
   √ ventral spinal cord compression may occur at <150°
5. **Welcher basal angle**
   = formed by nasion-tuberculum line and tuberculum-basion line
   √ angle averages 132° (should be <140°)
6. **McRae line** = line between anterior lip (= basion) to posterior lip (= opisthion) of foramen magnum
   √ tip of odontoid below this line

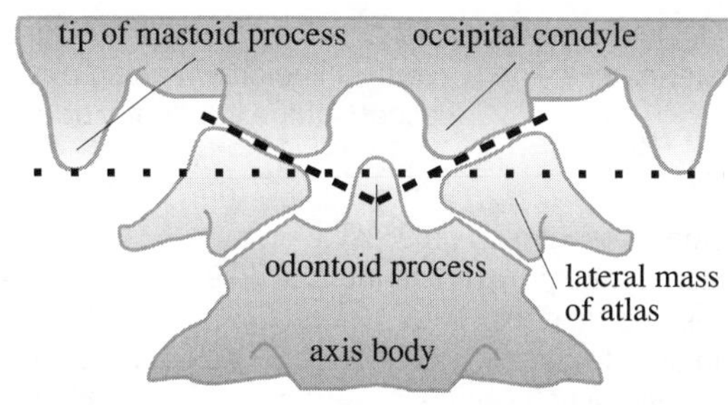

Open-Mouth Odontoid View

— ANTEROPOSTERIOR VIEW (= "open-mouth" / odontoid view)

7. **Atlantooccipital joint axis angle**
   = formed by lines drawn parallel to both atlanto-occipital joints
   √ lines intersect at center of odontoid process
   √ average angle of 125° (range of 124° to 127°)
8. **Digastric line** = line between incisurae mastoideae (origin of digastric muscles)
   √ tip of odontoid below this line
9. **Bimastoid line** = line connecting the tips of both mastoid processes
   √ tip of odontoid <10 mm above this line

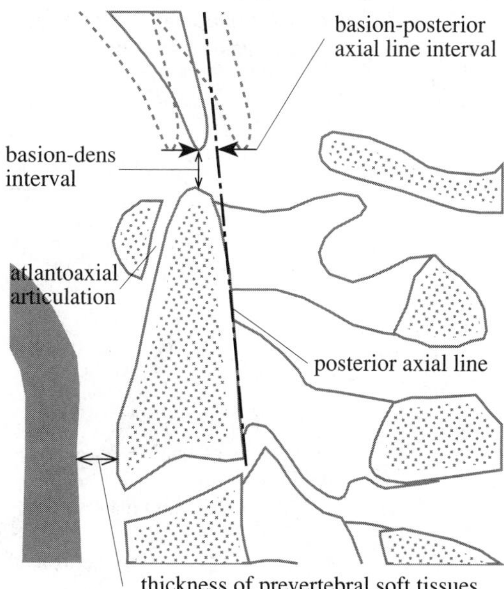

Normal Relationship of Craniocervical Junction
(range of the two extreme normal positions of the basion is drawn in dashes)

Normal dimensions for adults:

[posterior axial line = vertical line drawn along posterior aspect of the subdental body of C2]

Basion-dens interval (in 95%) .... <12 mm
Basion-posterior axial line interval (in 98%)
  posterior to dens .... <12 mm
  anterior to dens .... <4 mm
Prevertebral soft tissues at C2 .... <6 mm
Anterior atlanto-dens interval .... <2 mm
Lateral atlanto-dens interval (side-to-side) ... <3 mm
Atlanto-occipital articulation .... <2 mm
Atlantoaxial articulation .... <3 mm

MENINGES OF SPINAL CORD

A. PERIOSTEUM
   = continuation of outer layer of cerebral dura mater
B. EPIDURAL SPACE
   = space between dura mater + bone containing rich plexus of epidural veins, lymphatic channels, connective tissue, fat
   (a) cervical + thoracic spine: spacious posteriorly, potential space anteriorly
      √ normal thickness of epidural fat 3–6 mm at T7
   (b) lower lumbar + sacral spine: may occupy more than half of cross-sectional area
C. DURA
   = continuation of meningeal / inner layer of cerebral dura mater; ends at 2nd sacral vertebra + forms coccygeal ligament around filum terminale; sends tubular extensions around spinal nerves; is continuous with epineurium of peripheral nerves
   Attachment: at circumference of foramen magnum, bodies of 2nd + 3rd cervical vertebrae, posterior longitudinal ligament (by connective tissue strands)
D. SUBARACHNOID SPACE
   = space between arachnoid and pia mater containing CSF, reaching as far lateral as spinal ganglia
   dentate ligament partially divides CSF space into an anterior + posterior compartment extending from foramen magnum to 1st lumbar vertebra, is continuous with pia mater of cord medially + dura mater laterally (between exiting nerves)
   dorsal subarachnoid septum connects the arachnoid to the pia mater (cribriform septum)
E. PIA MATER
   = firm vascular membrane intimately adherent to spinal cord, blends with dura mater in intervertebral foramina around spinal ganglia, forms filum terminale, fuses with periosteum of 1st coccygeal segment

THORACIC SPINE

- 12 load-bearing vertebrae
- posterior arch (= pedicles, laminae, facets, transverse processes) handles tensional forces
- vertebral bodies:
  (a) height of vertebrae anteriorly 2–3 mm less than posteriorly = mild kyphotic curvature
  (b) AP diameter: gradual increase from T1 to T12
  (c) transverse diameter: gradual increase from T3 to T12

THORACOLUMBAR SPINE (T11–L2)

- anterior column = anterior longitudinal ligament, anterior annulus fibrosus, anterior vertebral body
- middle column = posterior longitudinal ligament, posterior annulus fibrosus, posterior vertebral body margin
  ◊ Integrity of the middle column is synonymous with stability!
- posterior column = posterior elements + ligaments

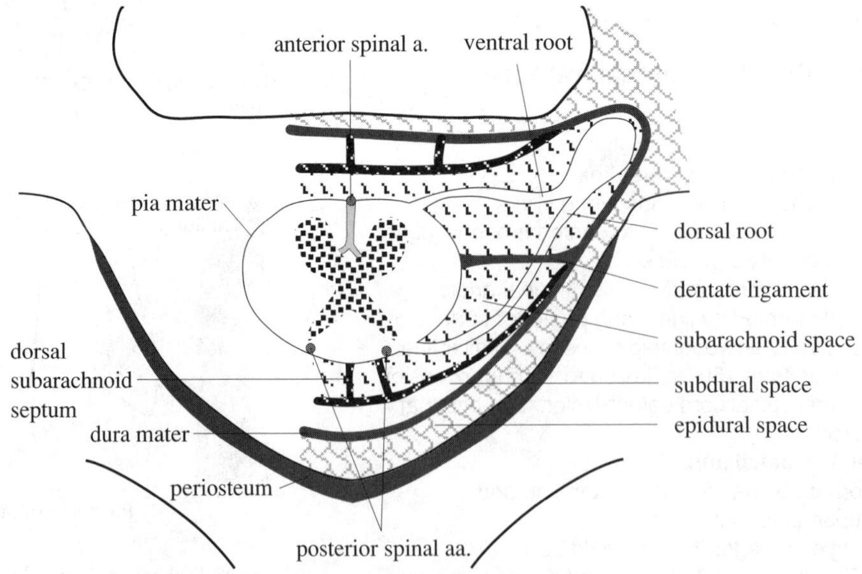

Meninges of Spinal Cord

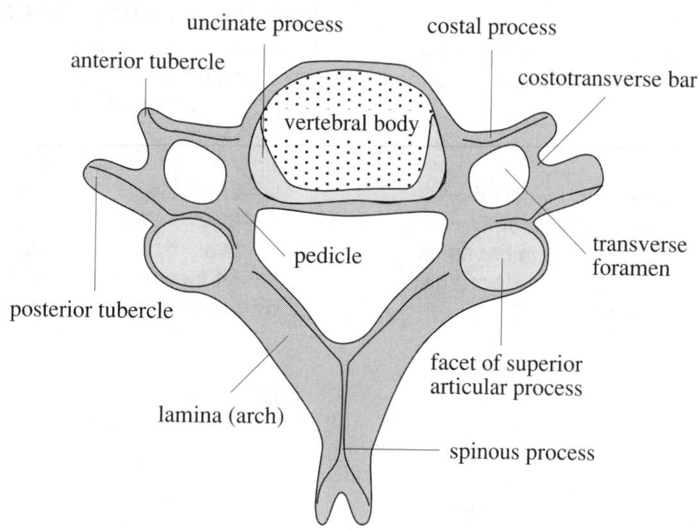

Typical Cervical Vertebra
(cranial aspect)

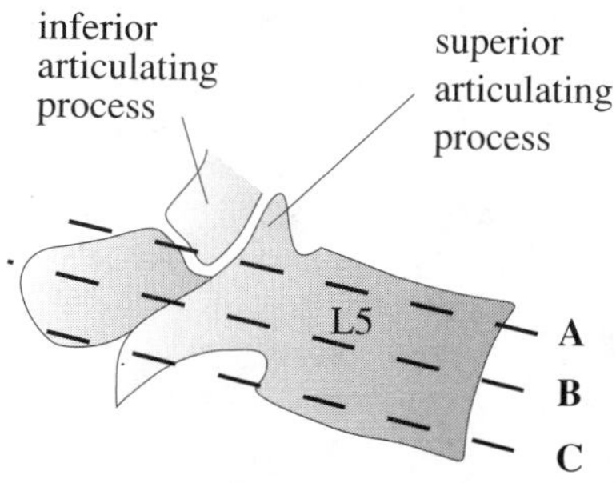

Lateral Scout View of L5

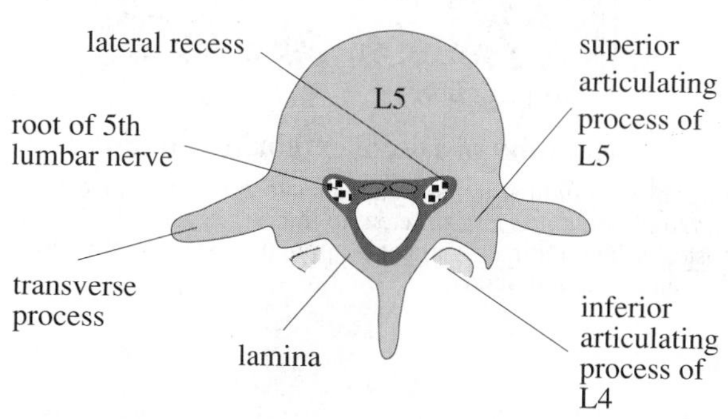

Cross Section through (A)

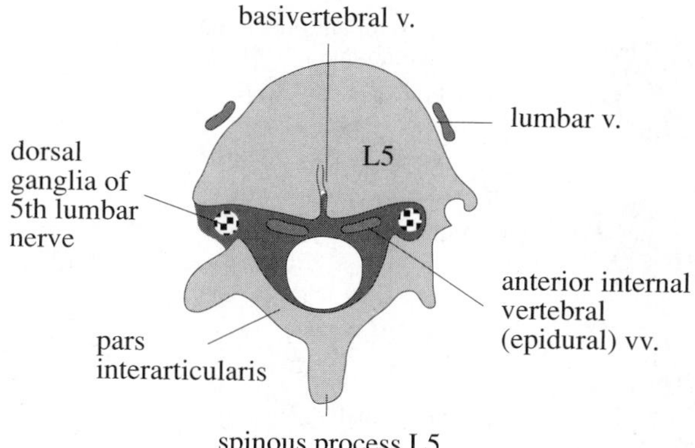

Cross Section through (B)

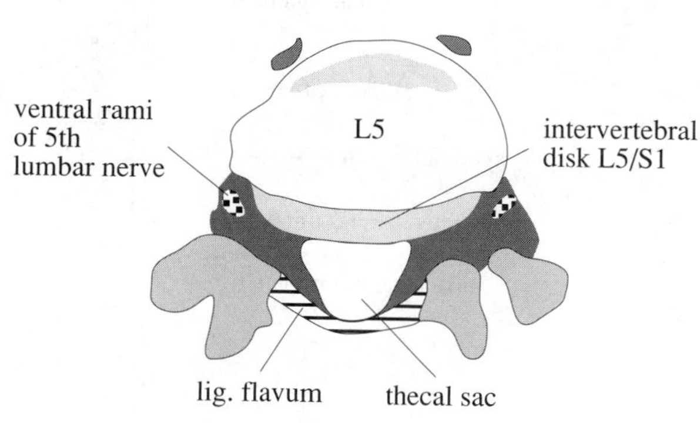

Cross Section through (C)

Cross Sections through 5th Lumbar Vertebra

TRANSITIONAL VERTEBRA

= vertebra retaining partial features of segments below and above; total number of vertebrae usually unchanged

Prevalence: 20%

• incidental finding

Location:

often at sacrococcygeal + lumbosacral junction

√ "sacralized L5" = L5 incorporated into sacrum

√ "lumbarized S1" = S1 incorporated into lumbar spine

Cx: confusion over labeling / assignment of vertebral levels during treatment planning

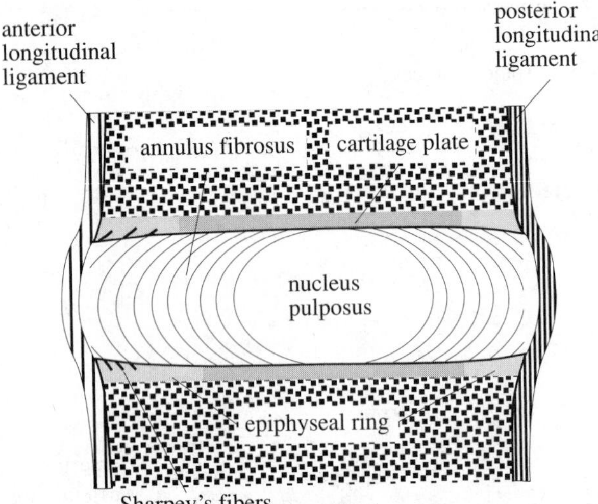

Anatomy of Discovertebral Junction

anterior longitudinal ligament attaches to anterior surface of vertebral body; it is less adherent to intervertebral disk; posterior longitudinal ligament is applied to back of intervertebral disk and vertebral bodies

NORMAL POSITION OF CONUS MEDULLARIS

◊ Vertebral bodies grow more quickly than spinal cord during fetal period of <19 weeks MA!

◊ No significant difference regardless of age!

Inferior-most aspect of conus:

L1–L2 level:	normal (range T12 to L3)
L2–L3 or higher:	in 97.8%
L3 level:	indeterminate (in 1.8%)
L3–L4 / lower:	abnormal
by 3 month:	above inferior endplate of L2 (in 98%)

N.B.: If conus is at / below L3 level, a search should be made for tethering mass, bony spur, thick filum!

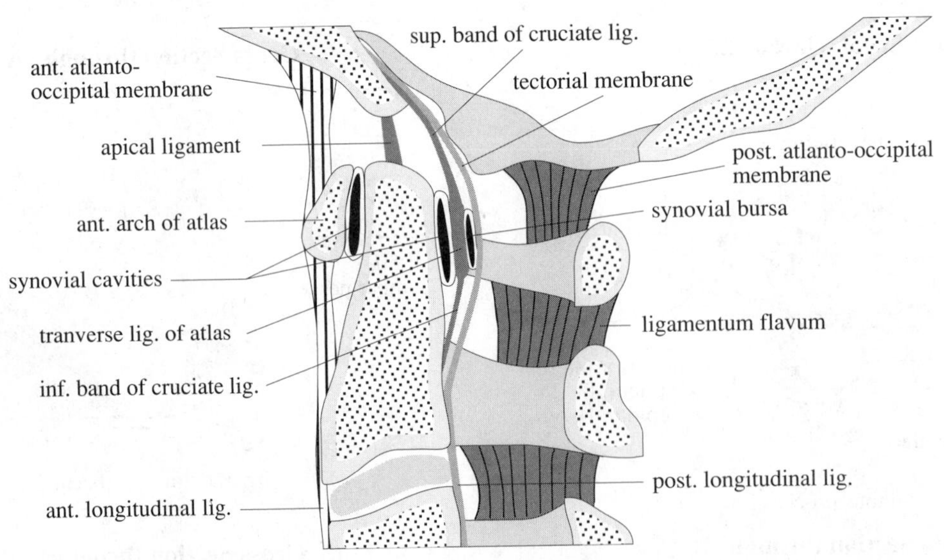

Joints and Ligaments of Occipito-Atlanto-Axial Region

SKULL AND SPINE DISORDERS

ARACHNOIDITIS

Etiology: trauma, back surgery, meningitis, subarachnoid hemorrhage, pantopaque myelography (inflammatory effect potentiated by blood), idiopathic

Associated with: syrinx

Myelo:

√ blunting of nerve root sleeves
√ blocked nerve roots without cord displacement (2/3)
√ streaking + clumping of contrast

CT:

√ fusion / clumping of nerve roots
√ intradural pseudomass
√ intradural cysts
√ "empty thecal sac" = featureless empty-looking sac with individual nerve roots adherent to wall (final stage)

ARACHNOID CYST OF SPINE

Location: dorsal to cord in thoracic region

Site:

(a) extradural cyst secondary to congenital / acquired dural defect
(b) intradural secondary to congenital deficiency within arachnoid (= true arachnoid cyst) / adhesion from prior infection or trauma (= arachnoid loculation)

√ oval sharply demarcated extramedullary mass
√ immediate / delayed contrast filling depending upon size of opening between cyst + subarachnoid space
√ local displacement + compression of spinal cord
√ higher signal intensity than CSF (from relative lack of CSF pulsations)

ARACHNOID DIVERTICULUM

= widening of root sheath with arachnoid space occupying >50% of total transverse diameter of root + sheath together

Cause: ? congenital / traumatic, arachnoiditis, infection

Pathogenesis: hydrostatic pressure of CSF

√ scalloping of posterior margins of vertebral bodies
√ myelographic contrast material fills diverticula

ARTERIOVENOUS MALFORMATION OF SPINAL CORD

Classification:

1. True intramedullary AVM
   = nidus of abnormal intermediary arteriovenous structure with multiple shunts
   Age: 2nd–3rd decade
   Cx: subarachnoid hemorrhage, paraplegia
   Prognosis: poor (especially in midthoracic location)
2. Intradural arteriovenous fistula
   = single shunt between one / several medullary arteries + single perimedullary vein
3. Dural arteriovenous fistula
   = single shunt between meningeal arteries + intradural vein
4. Metameric angiomatosis

ATLANTOAXIAL ROTARY FIXATION

• history of insignificant cervical spine trauma / upper respiratory tract infection
• limited painful neck motion
• head held in "cock-robin" position + inability to turn head

√ atlanto-odontoid asymmetry (open mouth odontoid view):
  √ decrease in atlanto-odontoid space + widening of lateral mass on side ipsilateral to rotation
  √ increase in atlanto-odontoid space + narrowing of lateral mass on side contralateral to rotation
√ atlantoaxial asymmetry remains constant with head turned into neutral position

Types:

I <3 mm anterior displacement of atlas on axis
II 3–5 mm anterior displacement
III >5 mm anterior displacement
IV posterior displacement of atlas on axis

DDx: torticollis (atlantoaxial symmetry reverts to normal with head turned into neutral position)

BRACHIAL PLEXUS INJURY

1. Erb-Duchenne: adduction injury affecting C5/6 (downward displacement of shoulder)
2. Klumpke: abduction injury at C7, C8, T1 (arm stretched over head)

√ pouchlike root sleeve at site of avulsion
√ asymmetrical nerve roots
√ contrast extravasation collecting in axilla
√ metrizamide in neural foramina (CT myelography)

CAUDAL REGRESSION SYNDROME

= SACRAL AGENESIS
= midline closure defect of neural tube with a spectrum of anomalies

Etiology: disturbance of caudal mesoderm <4th week of gestation from toxic / infectious / ischemic insult

Prevalence: 1:7,500 births; 0.005–0.01% of population; 0.1–0.2% in children of diabetic mothers

Predisposed: infants of diabetic mothers (16–22% of children with sacral agenesis have mothers with diabetes mellitus!)

◊ NOT associated with VATER syndrome!

A. Musculoskeletal anomalies
   @ Lower extremity
   • symptoms from minor muscle weakness to complete sensorimotor paralysis of both lower extremities
   √ hip dislocation
   √ foot deformities
   √ hypoplasia of extremities

@ Lumbosacral spine = SACRAL AGENESIS
Spectrum:
Type 1 = unilateral partial agenesis localized to sacrum / coccyx
Type 2 = bilateral partial symmetric defects of sacrum + iliosacral articulation
Type 3 = total sacral agenesis + iliolumbar articulation
Type 4 = total sacral agenesis + ilioilial fusion posteriorly
√ fusion of caudal-most 2 or 3 vertebrae
√ spina bifida (lipomyelomeningocele often not in combination with hydrocephalus)
√ narrowing of spinal canal rostral to last intact vertebra

B. Spinal cord anomalies
√ characteristic club- / wedge-shaped configuration of conus medullaris (hypoplasia of distal spinal cord)
√ ± tethered spinal cord
√ ± dural sac stenosis with high termination
√ ± spinal cord lipoma, teratoma, cauda equina cyst
√ ± syrinx

C. Genitourinary anomalies
• neurogenic bladder (if >2 segments are missing)
• malformed external genitalia
• lack of bowel control
√ ± bilateral renal aplasia with pulmonary hypoplasia + Potter facies
√ anal atresia

OB-US:
• normal / imperforate anus
√ normal / mildly dilated urinary system
√ normal / increased amniotic fluid
√ 2 umbilical arteries
√ 2 hypoplastic nonfused lower extremities
√ sacral agenesis, absent vertebrae from lower thoracic / upper lumbar spine caudally

Sirenomelia

= recently considered a distinct separate entity from caudal regression syndrome
◊ NOT associated with maternal diabetes mellitus!
• Potter facies
• absence of anus
• absent genitalia
√ bilateral renal agenesis / dysgenesis (lethal)
√ marked oligohydramnios
√ single aberrant umbilical artery
√ single / fused lower extremity
√ sacral agenesis, absent pelvis, lumbosacral "tail", lumbar rachischisis
Prognosis: incompatible with life

CHORDOMA

◊ Chordoma is the most common primary malignant tumor of the spine in adults excluding lymphoproliferative neoplasms!

Prevalence: 1:2,000,000; 1–2–4% of all primary malignant neoplasms of bone; 1% of all intracranial tumors
Etiology: originates from embryonic remnants of notochord / ectopic cordal foci (notochord appears between 4th and 7th week of embryonic development, extends from Rathke pouch to coccyx and forms nucleus pulposus)
Age: 30–70 years (peak age in 6th decade); M:F = 2:1; highly malignant in children
Path: lobulated tumor contained within pseudocapsule
Histo:
(1) typical chordoma: cords + clusters of large bubblelike vacuolated (physaliferous) cells containing intracytoplasmic mucous droplets; abundant extracellular mucus deposition + areas of hemorrhage
(2) chondroid chordoma: cartilage instead of mucinous extracellular matrix

Location: (a) 50% in sacrum (b) 35% in clivus (c) 15% in vertebrae (d) other sites (5%) in mandible, maxilla, scapula
√ enhancement after contrast administration
CT:
√ low-attenuation within soft-tissue mass (due to myxoid-type tissue)
√ higher attenuation fibrous pseudocapsule
MR (modality of choice):
√ low to intermediate intensity on T1WI, occasionally hyperintense (due to high protein content):
√ heterogeneous internal texture due to calcification, necrosis, gelatinous mucoid collections
√ very high signal intensity on T2WI (similar to nucleus pulposus with high water content)
Angio:
√ prominent vascular stain
NUC:
√ cold lesion on bone scan
√ no uptake on gallium scan
Metastases (in 5–43%) to: liver, lung, regional lymph nodes, peritoneum, skin (late), heart
Prognosis: almost 100% recurrence rate despite radical surgery

Sacrococcygeal Chordoma (50–70%)

◊ Most common primary malignant sacral tumor; 2–4% of all malignant osseous neoplasms!
Peak age: 40–60 years; M:F = 2:1
• low back pain (70%)
• constipation / fecal incontinence
• rectal bleeding (42%)
• sciatica
• frequency, urgency, straining on micturition
• sacral mass (17%)
Location: esp. in 4th + 5th sacral segment
√ presacral mass with average size of 10 cm extending superiorly + inferiorly; rarely posterior location
√ displacement of rectum + bladder
√ solid tumor with cystic areas (in 50%)

√ osteolytic midline mass in sacrum + coccyx
√ amorphous peripheral calcifications (15–89%)
√ secondary bone sclerosis in tumor periphery (50%)
√ honeycomb pattern with trabeculations (10–15%)
√ may cross sacroiliac joint

Prognosis: 8–10 years average survival; 66% 5-year survival rate (adulthood)

DDx: Giant cell tumor, plasmacytoma, lymphoma, metastatic adenocarcinoma, aneurysmal bone cyst, atypical hemangioma, chondrosarcoma, osteomyelitis, ependymoma

Spheno-occipital Chordoma (15–35%)

Age: younger patient (peak age of 20–40 years); M:F - 1:1

• orbitofrontal headache
• visual disturbances, ptosis
• 6th nerve palsy / paraplegia

Location: clivus, spheno-occipital synchondrosis

√ bone destruction (in 90%): clivus > sella > petrous bone > orbit > floor of middle cranial fossa > jugular fossa > atlas > foramen magnum
√ reactive bone sclerosis (rare)
√ calcifications / bone fragments (20–70%)
√ soft-tissue extension into nasopharynx (common), into sphenoid + ethmoid sinuses (occasionally), may reach nasal cavity + maxillary antrum
√ variable degree of enhancement

MR:
- √ large intraosseous mass extending into prepontine cistern, sphenoid sinus, middle cranial fossa, nasopharynx
- √ posterior displacement of brainstem
- √ usually isointense to brain / occasionally inhomogeneously hyperintense on T1WI
- √ hyperintense on T2WI

Prognosis: 4–5 years average survival

DDx: meningioma, metastasis, plasmacytoma, giant cell tumor, sphenoid sinus cyst, nasopharyngeal carcinoma, chondrosarcoma

Vertebral / Spinal Chordoma (15–20%)

more aggressive than sacral / cranial chordomas

Age: younger patient; M:F = 2:1

• low back pain + radiculopathy

Location: cervical (8% – particularly C2), thoracic spine (4%), lumbar spine (3%)

√ solitary midline spinal mass
√ tumor calcification in 30%
√ sclerosis / "ivory vertebra" in 43–62%
√ total destruction of vertebra, initially unaccompanied by collapse
√ variable extension into spinal canal
√ violates disk space to involve adjacent bodies (10–14%) simulating infection
√ anterior soft-tissue mass

Cx: complete spinal block

Prognosis: 4–5 years average survival

DDx: metastasis, primary bone tumor, primary soft-tissue tumor, neuroma, meningioma

CSF FISTULA

Cause:
(1) Trauma to skull base (most commonly)
◊ 2% of all head injuries develop CSF fistula
(2) Tumor: especially those arising from pituitary gland
(3) Congenital anomalies: encephalocele

• traumatic leak: usually unilateral; onset within 48 hours after trauma, usually scanty; resolve in 1 week
• nontraumatic leak: profuse flow; may persist for years
• anosmia (in 78% of trauma cases)

Location: fractures through frontoethmoidal complex + middle cranial fossa (most commonly)

√ high-resolution thin-section CT in coronal plane followed by rescanning after low-dose intrathecal contrast material instilled into lumbar subarachnoid space

Cx: infection (in 25–50% of untreated cases)

DEGENERATIVE DISK DISEASE

◊ Therapeutic decision-making should be based on clinical assessment alone!
◊ There are no prognostic indicators on images in patients with acute lumbar radiculopathy!
35% of individuals without back trouble have abnormal findings (HNP, disk bulging, facet degeneration, spinal stenosis)
◊ Imaging is only justified in patients for whom surgery is considered!

Pathophysiology:
loss of disk height leads to stress on facet joints + uncovertebral joints (= uncinate process), exaggerated joint motion with misalignment (= rostrocaudal subluxation) of facet joints, spine instability with arthritis, capsular hypertrophy, hypertrophy of posterior ligaments, facet fracture

Plain film:
- √ **intervertebral osteochondrosis** = disease of nucleus pulposus (desiccation = loss of disk water):
  - √ narrowing of disk space
  - √ vacuum disk phenomenon = radiolucent interspace accumulation of nitrogen gas at sites of negative pressure
  - √ disk calcification
  - √ bone sclerosis of adjacent vertebral bodies
- √ **spondylosis deformans** = degeneration of the outer fibers of the annulus fibrosus:
  - √ endplate osteophytosis growing initially horizontally + then vertically several millimeters from disko-vertebral junction (2° to displacement of nucleus pulposus in anterior + anterolateral direction producing traction on osseous attachment of annulus fibrosus [= fibers of Sharpey])
  - √ enlargement of uncinate processes
- √ **osteoarthritis** = degenerative disease of synovium-lined apophyseal / costovertebral joints:
  - √ degenerative spondylolisthesis
- √ cartilaginous node = intraosseous disk herniation

Myelography:
- √ delineation of thecal sac, spinal cord, exiting nerve roots

CT (accuracy >90%):
- √ facet joint disease (marginal sclerosis, joint narrowing, cyst formation, bony overgrowth)
- √ uncovertebral joint disease of cervical spine (osteophytes project into lateral spinal canal + neuroforamen)

MR:
- √ scalloping of cord (T2W FSE / GRE images):
  - √ anterior encroachment by disk / spondylosis
  - √ posterior encroachment by ligamentum flavum hypertrophy
- √ loss of disk signal (due to desiccation)
- √ disk collapse
- √ **endplate + marrow changes** (Modic & DeRoos):
  - (a) Type I (4%) hypointense on T1WI + hyperintense on T2WI (= bone marrow edema + vascular congestion), contrast-enhancement of marrow
  - (b) Type II (16%) hyperintense on T1WI + iso- to hypointense on T2WI (= local fatty replacement of marrow)
  - (c) Type III hypointense signal on T1WI + T2WI (= advanced sclerosis after a few years)
- √ juxtaarticular **synovial cyst** in posterolateral spinal canal (most frequently at L4-5):
  - √ smooth well-defined extradural mass adjacent to facet joint
  - √ variable signal pattern (due to serous, mucinous, gelatinous fluid components, air, hemorrhage)
  - √ hypointense perimeter (= fibrous capsule with calcium + hemosiderin) with contrast enhancement

NUC:
SPECT imaging of vertebrae can aid in localizing increased uptake to vertebral bodies, posterior elements, etc.
- √ eccentrically placed increased uptake on either side of an intervertebral space (osteophytes, diskogenic sclerosis)

Sequelae: (1) disk bulging
(2) disk herniation
(3) spinal stenosis
(4) facet joint disease

DDx: **Idiopathic segmental sclerosis of vertebral body** (middle-aged / young patient, hemispherical sclerosis in anteroinferior aspect of lower lumbar vertebrae with small osteolytic focus, only slight narrowing of intervertebral disk; unknown cause)

TERMINOLOGY:
1. Disk bulge
   = concentric smooth circumferential expansion of softened disk material beyond the confines of endplates after lengthening of annular fibers
2. Disk protrusion
   = focal eccentric protrusion of disk material maintaining broad base with parent disk due to focally weakened / ruptured annulus but intact posterior longitudinal ligament; <3 mm beyond vertebral margin
3. Disk herniation
   = disk protrusion that exceeds >3 mm beyond vertebral body margin
4. Disk extrusion
   = prominent focal extension of disk material through the annulus with only an isthmus of connection to parent disk + intact / ruptured posterior longitudinal ligament
5. Free fragment
   = frank separation of disk material from parent disk
6. Free fragment migration
   = separated disk material travels above / below intervertebral disk space

Bulging Disk

= broad-based disk extension outward in all directions with weakened but intact annulus fibrosus + posterior longitudinal ligament

Age: common finding in individuals >40 years of age
Location: lumbar, cervical spine
- √ rounded symmetric defect localized to disk space level
- √ concave anterior margin of thecal sac
- √ encroachment on inferior portion of neuroforamen

MR:
- √ nucleus pulposus hypointense on T1WI + hyperintense on T2WI (water loss through degeneration)

Herniation of Nucleus Pulposus

= HNP = focal protrusion of disk material >3 mm beyond margins of adjacent vertebral endplates secondary to rupture of annulus fibrosus confined within posterior longitudinal ligament

◊ 21% of asymptomatic population has disk herniation!
- local somatic spinal pain = sharp / aching, deep, localized
- centrifugal radiating pain = sharp, well-circumscribed, superficial, "electric," confined to dermatome
- centrifugal referred pain = dull, ill-defined, deep or superficial, aching or boring, confined to somatome (= dermatome + myotome + sclerotome)

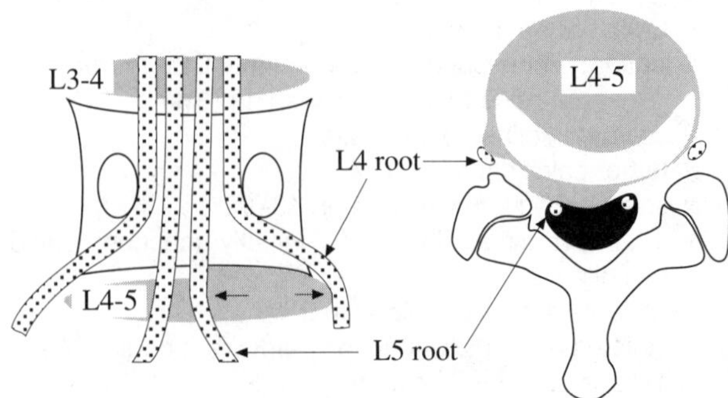

Lateral Disk Herniation
Nerve compression usually occurs posterolaterally (here at L4-5); therefore an atypical lateral compression (here of L4 root) directs surgery to the wrong more cephalad level (L3-4 disk)

Site:
(a) posterolateral (49%) = weakest point along posterolateral margin of disk at lateral recess of spinal canal (posterior longitudinal ligament tightly adherent to posterior margins of disk)
(b) posterocentral (8%)
(c) bilateral (on both sides of posterior ligament)
(d) lateral / foraminal (<10%)
(e) intraosseous / vertical = Schmorl node (14%)
(f) extraforaminal = anterior (commonly overlooked) (29%)

Myelography:
√ sharply angular indentation on lateral aspect of thecal sac with extension above or below level of disk space (ipsilateral oblique projection best view)
√ asymmetry of posterior disk margin
√ double contour secondary to superimposed normal + abnormal side (horizontal beam lateral view)
√ narrowing of intervertebral disk space (most commonly a sign of disk degeneration)
√ deviation of nerve root / root sleeve
√ enlargement of nerve root secondary to edema ("trumpet sign")
√ amputated / truncated nerve root (nonfilling of root sleeve)

MR:
√ herniated disk material of low signal intensity displaces the posterior longitudinal ligament and epidural fat of relative high signal intensity on T1WI
√ "squeezed toothpaste" effect = hourglass appearance of herniated disk at posterior disk margin on sagittal image
√ asymmetry of posterior disk margin on axial image

Cx: spinal stenosis
Prognosis:
conservative therapy reduces size of herniation by
0–50% in 11% of patients,
50–75% in 36% of patients,
75–100% in 46% of patients
(secondary to growth of granulation tissue)

Free Fragment Herniation

= DISK SEQUESTRATION
= complete separation of disk material with rupture through posterior longitudinal ligament into epidural space
◊ Missed free fragments are a common cause of failed back surgery!
√ migration superiorly / inferiorly away from disk space with compression of nerve root above / below level of disk herniation
√ disk material noted >9 mm away from intervertebral disk space
√ soft-tissue density with higher value than thecal sac

DDx: (1) Postoperative scarring (retraction of thecal sac to side of surgery)
(2) Epidural abscess
(3) Epidural tumor
(4) Conjoined nerve root (2 nerve roots arising from thecal sac simultaneously representing mass in ventrolateral aspect of spinal canal; normal variant in 1–3% of population)
(5) Tarlov cyst (dilated nerve root sleeve)

Cervical Disk Herniation

Peak age: 3rd–4th decade
• neck stiffness, muscle splinting
• dermatomic sensory loss
• weakness + muscle atrophy
• reflex loss

Sites: C6-7 (69%); C5-6 (19%); C7-T1 (10%); C4-5 (2%)
Sequelae: (1) compression of exiting nerve roots with pain radiating to shoulder, arm, hand
(2) cord compression (spinal stenosis + massive disk rupture)

Thoracic Disk Herniation

Prevalence: 1% of all disk herniations
Sites: T11/12
√ calcification of disk fragments + parent disk (frequent)

Lumbar Disk Herniation

• sciatica =
(1) stiffness in back
(2) pain radiating down to thigh / calf / foot
(3) paresthesia / weakness / reflex changes
• pain exaggerated by coughing, sneezing, physical activity + worse while sitting / straightening of leg

Sites: L4/5 (35%) > L5/S1 (27%) > L3/4 (19%) > L2/3 (14%) > L1/2 (5%)

DERMOID OF SPINE

= uni- / multilocular cystic tumor lined by squamous epithelium containing skin appendages (hair follicles, sweat glands, sebaceous glands)

Cause:
(a) congenital dermal rest / focal expansion of dermal sinus
(b) acquired from implantation of viable dermal tissue (by spinal needle without trocar)

Prevalence: 1% of spinal cord tumors
Age at presentation: <20 years; M:F = 1:1
May be associated with: dermal sinus (in 20%)
• slowly progressive myelopathy
• acute onset of chemical meningitis (secondary to rupture of inflammatory cholesterol crystals from cyst into CSF)

Location: lumbosacral (60%), cauda equina (20%)
Site: extramedullary (60%), intramedullary (40%)
√ almost always complete spinal block on myelography
√ intensity of fat
√ occasionally hypointense on T1WI + hypodense on CT (secretions from sweat glands within tumor)
√ NO contrast enhancement
√ CT myelography facilitates detection

DIASTEMATOMYELIA

= SPLIT CORD = MYELOSCHISIS
= sagittal division of spinal cord into two hemicords, each of which contains a central canal, one dorsal horn + one ventral horn

Etiology: congenital malformation as a result of adhesions between ectoderm and endoderm; M:F = 1:3

Path:
(a) 2 hemicords each covered by layer of pia within single subarachnoid space + dural sac (60%); not accompanied by bony spur / fibrous band
(b) 2 hemicords each with its own pial, subarachnoidal + dural sheath (40%); accompanied by fibrous band (in 25%), cartilaginous / bony spurs (in 75%)

Associated with: myelomeningocele

- hypertrichosis, nevus, lipoma, dimple, hemangioma overlying the spine (26–81%)
- clubfoot (50%)
- muscle wasting, ankle weakness in one leg

Location: lower thoracic / upper lumbar > upper thoracic > cervical spine

√ sagittal cleft in spinal cord resulting in 2 asymmetric hemicords
√ the 2 hemicords usually reunite caudal to cleft
√ occasionally 2 coni medullaris
√ eccentric central canal within both hemicords
√ bony spur through center of spinal canal arising from posterior aspect of centra (<50%)
√ thickened filum terminale >2 mm (>50%)
√ tethered cord (>50%)
√ low conus medullaris below L2 level (>75%)
√ defect in thecal sac on myelogram

@ Vertebrae
√ congenital scoliosis (50–75%)
◊ 5% of patients with congenital scoliosis have diastematomyelia
√ spina bifida over multiple levels
√ anteroposterior narrowing of vertebral bodies
√ widening of interpediculate distance
√ narrowed disk space with hemivertebra, butterfly vertebra, block vertebra
√ fusion + thickening of adjacent laminae (90%)
(a) fusion to ipsilateral lamina at adjacent levels
(b) diagonal fusion to contralateral adjacent lamina = intersegmental laminar fusion

Cx: progressive spinal cord dysfunction

DISKITIS

◊ Most common pediatric spine problem!

Etiology:
(1) Bloodborne bacterial invasion of vertebrae infecting disk via communicating vessels through endplate
◊ Vertebral osteomyelitis + diskitis may be the same entity!
(2) Invasive procedure: surgery, diskography, myelography, chemonucleolysis

Agents:
(a) pyogenic: Staphylococcus aureus (by far most common), Gram-negative rods (in IV drug abusers / immunocompromised patients)
(b) nonpyogenic: tuberculosis, coccidioidomycosis
◊ TB has a propensity to extend beneath longitudinal ligaments with involvement of multiple vertebral levels

Pathogenesis: infection starts in disk (still vascularized in children) / in anterior inferior corner of vertebral body (in adults) with spread across disk to adjacent vertebral endplate

Age peak: 6 months to 4 years and 10–14 years; average age of 6 years at presentation

- over 2–4 weeks gradually progressing irritability, malaise, low-grade fever
- back / referred hip pain, limp
- refusal to bear weight
- elevated sedimentation rate, WBC count often normal

Location: L3/4, L4/5, unusual above T9; usually one disk space (occasionally 2) involved

Plain film (positive 2–4 weeks after onset of symptoms):
√ decrease in disk space height (earliest sign)
= intraosseous herniation of nucleus pulposus into vertebral body through weakened endplate
√ indistinctness of adjacent endplates with destruction
√ endplate sclerosis (during healing phase beginning anywhere from 8 weeks to 8 months after onset)
√ bone fusion (after 6 months to 2 years)

CT:
√ paravertebral inflammatory mass
√ epidural soft-tissue extension with deformity of thecal sac

MR (preferred modality; 93% sensitive, 97% specific, 95% accurate):
◊ Very sensitive modality early on in disease process (especially enhanced T1WI + fat suppression)
√ decreased marrow intensity on T1WI in two contiguous vertebrae
√ in early stage preserved disk height with variable intensity on T2WI (often increased)
√ in later stages loss of disk height with increased intensity on T2WI

NUC (41% sensitive, 93% specific, 68% accurate on Tc-99m MDP + Tc-99m WBC scans):
√ positive before radiographs
√ increased uptake in vertebral endplate adjacent to disk
√ bone scan usually positive in adjacent vertebrae (until age 20) secondary to vascular supply via endplates; may be negative after age 20

Cx: epidural / paravertebral abscess, kyphosis

Rx: immobilization in body cast for ~4 weeks

DDx: neoplastic disease (no breach of endplate, disk space often intact)

Postoperative Diskitis

Frequency: 0.75–2.8%

Organism: Staphylococcus aureus; many times no organism recovered

- severe recurrent back pain 7–28 days after surgery accompanied by decreased back motion, muscle spasm, positive straight leg raising test
- fever (33%)
- wound infection (8%)
- persistently elevated / increasing ESR

MR:
√ decreased signal intensity within disk + adjacent vertebral body marrow on T1WI
√ increased signal intensity in disk + adjacent marrow on T2WI often with obliteration of intranuclear cleft
√ contrast-enhancement of vertebral bone marrow ± disk space

DDx: degenerative disk disease type I (no gadolinium-enhancement of disk)

DISLOCATION OF SPINE

Atlanto-occipital Dislocation

= ATLANTO-OCCIPITAL DISTRACTION INJURY
= disruption of tectorial membrane + paired alar ligaments resulting in grossly unstable injury

Cause: rapid deceleration with either hyperextension or hyperflexion

Age: childhood (due to larger size of head relative to body, increased laxity of ligaments, horizontally oriented occipito-atlanto-axial joint, hypoplastic occipital condyles)

May be associated with: occipital condyle fracture

- neurologic symptoms: range from respiratory arrest with quadriplegia to normal neurologic exam
- discomfort, stiffness

Lateral radiograph:
√ >10 mm soft-tissue swelling anterior to C2 + pathologic convexity of soft tissues (80%)
√ basion-dens interval (BD) >12 mm without traction placed on head / neck
√ basion-posterior axial line interval >12 mm anterior / >4 mm posterior to axial line
√ BC/OA ratio >1 = ratio of distance between basion + posterior arch of C1 divided by distance between opisthion + anterior arch of C1

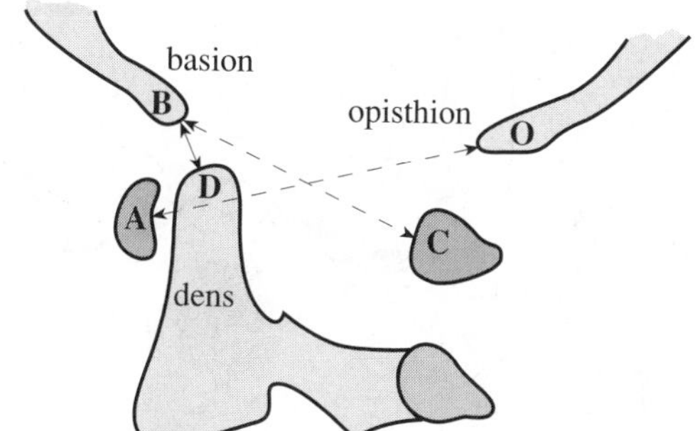

Atlanto-occipital Landmarks on Lateral Radiograph

CT:
√ blood in region of tectorial membrane + alar ligaments
√ condylar fracture ± fracture extension through hypoglossal canal (for cranial nerve XII)
√ widening / incongruity of articulation between occipital condyles + lateral masses of C1

MR:
√ fluid in articular capsules, nuchal ligament, interspinous ligament

Cx:
(1) Injury to caudal cranial nerves + upper 3 cervical nerves
(2) Epidural hematoma with brainstem compression + upper spinal cord injury
(3) Vasospasm / dissection of internal carotid and vertebral arteries

Atlantoaxial Distraction

= injury to transverse atlantal ligament, alar ligament, tectorial membrane between C1 and C2, disruption of articular capsules

May be associated with: type 1 dens fracture
√ prevertebral soft-tissue swelling
√ subluxation with enlargement of predental space to >5 mm in children <9 years of age >3 mm in adults
√ widening of C1-C2 facets

MR:
√ prevertebral, interspinous, nuchal ligament edema
√ facet widening / fluid
√ increased signal intensity of spinal cord
√ ± epidural hematoma

DORSAL DERMAL SINUS

= epithelium-lined dural tube extending from skin surface to intracanalicular space + frequently communicating with CNS / its coverings

Cause: focal point of incomplete separation of cutaneous ectoderm from neural ectoderm during neurulation

Age: encountered in early childhood–3rd decade; M:F = 1:1

- small midline dimple / pinpoint ostium
- hyperpigmented patch / hairy nevus / capillary angioma

Location: lumbosacral (60%), occipital (25%), thoracic (10%), cervical (2%), sacrococcygeal (1%), ventral (8%)

Course: in a craniad direction from skin level toward cord (due to ascension of cord relative to spinal canal during embryogenesis)

◊ 50% of dorsal dermal sinuses end in dermoid / epidermoid cysts!
◊ 20–30% of dermoid cysts / dermoid tumors are associated with dermal sinus tracts!

CT myelography (best modality to define intraspinal anatomy):
√ groove in upper surface of spinous process + lamina of vertebra
√ hypoplastic spinous process
√ single bifid spinous process
√ focal multilevel spina bifida
√ laminar defect
√ dorsal tenting of dura + arachnoid

CNS

√ sinus may terminate in conus medullaris / filum terminale / nerve root / fibrous nodule on dorsal aspect of cord / dermoid / epidermoid
√ nerve roots bound down to capsule of dermoid / epidermoid cyst
√ displacement / compression of cord by extramedullary dermoids / epidermoids
√ expansion of cord by intramedullary dermoids / epidermoids
√ clumping of nerve roots from adhesive arachnoiditis

Cx: (1) Meningitis (bacterial / chemical)
(2) Subcutaneous / epidural / subdural / subarachnoid / subpial abscess (bacterial ascent)
◊ Dermal sinus accounts for up to 3% of spinal cord abscesses!
(3) Compression of neural structures

DDx: pilonidal sinus / simple sacral dimple (no extension to neural structures)

EPIDERMOID OF SPINE

= cystic tumor lined by a membrane composed of epidermal elements of skin

Cause:
(a) congenital dermal rest / focal expansion of dermal sinus
(b) acquired from implantation of viable epidermal tissue (by spinal needle without trocar)

Prevalence: 1% of spinal cord tumors
Age at presentation: 3rd–5th decade; M > F
May be associated with: dermal sinus

- slowly progressive myelopathy
- acute onset of chemical meningitis (secondary to rupture of inflammatory cholesterol crystals from cyst into CSF)

Location: upper thoracic (17%), lower thoracic (26%), lumbosacral (22%), cauda equina (35%)
Site: extramedullary (60%), intramedullary (40%)
√ almost always complete spinal block on myelography
√ displacement of spinal cord / nerve roots
√ small tumors isointense to CSF
√ NO contrast enhancement
√ CT myelography facilitates detection

EPIDURAL ABSCESS OF SPINE

Cause: diskitis, osteomyelitis, idiopathic
- back pain, radicular pain
- fever, leukocytosis

MR:
√ thickening of epidural tissues (early stage):
 √ isointense on T1WI
 √ moderately hyperintense on T2WI
√ liquefied abscess cavity oval-shaped on axial images:
 √ hypointense on T1WI + hyperintense on T2WI
√ cellulitis surrounding abscess:
 √ best seen on with contrast enhancement (inflamed hypervascular tissue) + fat suppression

EPIDURAL HEMATOMA OF SPINE

Etiology: (1) vertebral fracture / dislocation (2) traumatic lumbar puncture (3) hypertension (4) AVM (5) vertebral hemangioma (6) bleeding diathesis / anticoagulation / hemophilia (7) idiopathic (45%)
Peak age: 40–50 years
- acute radicular pain
- paraplegia

Location: thoracic spine (most common)
√ compression of posterior aspect of cord
√ high attenuation lesion on CT

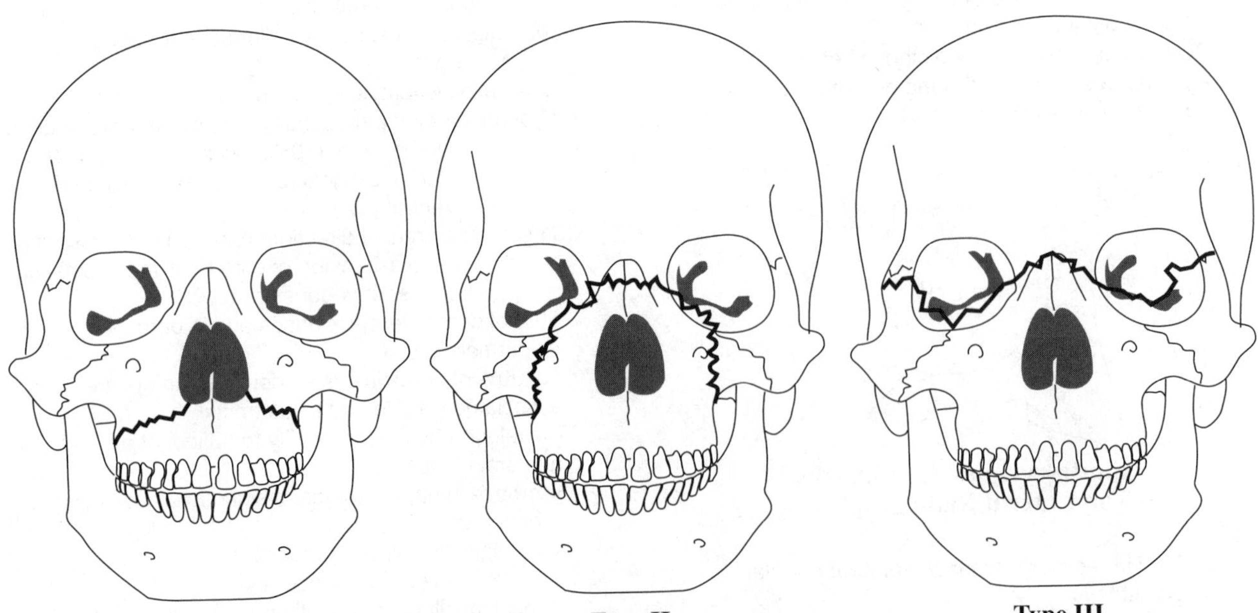

Le Fort Fractures

√ iso- / slightly hypointense lesion on T1WI with marked increase in intensity on T2WI

FRACTURES OF SKULL

1. Linear fracture (most common type)
   √ deeply black sharply defined line
   DDx: (1) vascular groove, esp. temporal artery (gray line, slightly sclerotic margin, branching like a tree, typical location (temporal artery projects behind dorsum sellae)
   (2) suture
2. Depressed fracture
   • often palpable
   √ bone-on-bone density
   Rx: surgery indicated if depression >3–5 mm (due to arachnoid tear / brain injury)
   N.B.: CT / MR mandatory to assess extent of underlying brain injury
3. Skull-base fracture = **basilar skull fracture**
   • rhinorrhea (CSF)
   • otorrhea (CSF / hemotympanum)
   • raccoon eyes = periorbital ecchymosis
   √ pneumocephalus
     √ air in sulci
     √ air-fluid level in sinuses
   Cx: infection, acute / delayed cranial nerve deficit, vascular laceration / dissection / occlusion / infarction
4. **Healing skull fracture**
   @ infants: in 3–6 months without a trace
   @ children (5–12 years): in 12 months
   @ adults: in 2–3 years
     √ persistent lucency mimicking vascular groove
   Cx: leptomeningeal cyst (= growing fracture)

LeFort Fracture

[Rene Le Fort (1869–1951), French surgeon]

◊ All LeFort fractures involve the pterygoid process!

A. LeFort I = transverse (horizontal) maxillary fracture caused by blow to premaxilla
   Fracture line: (a) alveolar ridge
   (b) lateral aperture of nose
   (c) inferior wall of maxillary sinus
   √ detachment of alveolar process of maxilla
   √ teeth contained in detached fragment
B. LeFort II = "pyramidal fracture"
   ◊ May be unilateral
   Fracture line: arch through
   (a) posterior alveolar ridge
   (b) medial orbital rim
   (c) across nasal bones
   √ separation of midportion of face
   √ floor of orbit + hard palate + nasal cavity involved
C. LeFort III = "craniofacial disjunction"
   Fracture line: horizontal course through
   (a) nasofrontal suture
   (b) maxillo-frontal suture
   (c) orbital wall
   (d) zygomatic arch
   √ separation of entire face from base of skull

Sphenoid Bone Fracture

Prevalence: involved in 15% of skull-base fractures

• CSF rhinorrhea / otorrhea
• hemotympanum
• battle sign = mastoid region ecchymosis
• raccoon eyes = periorbital ecchymosis
• 7th / 8th nerve palsy
• muscular dysfunction: problems with ocular motility, mastication, speech, swallowing, eustachian tube function

√ air-fluid level in sinuses + mastoid
√ axial thin-slice high-resolution CT for best delineation of fractures
√ water-soluble intrathecal contrast material for CSF fistula

Temporal Bone Fracture

Longitudinal Fracture of Temporal Bone (75%)

= fracture parallel to the axis of petrous pyramid arising in squamosa of temporal bone through tegmen tympani, EAC (external auditory canal), middle ear, terminating in foramen lacerum

• bleeding from EAC (disruption of tympanic membrane)
• otorrhea (CSF leak with ruptured tympanic membrane; rare)
• conductive hearing loss (dislocation of auditory ossicles — most commonly incus as the least anchored ossicle)
  • NO neurosensory hearing loss
• facial nerve palsy (10–20%) due to edema / fracture of facial canal near geniculate ganglion; frequent spontaneous recovery

√ pneumocephalus
√ herniation of temporal lobe
√ incudostapedial joint dislocation (weakest joint):
  √ "ice cream" (malleus) has fallen off the "cone" (incus) on direct coronal CT scan
  √ fracture of "molar tooth" on direct sagittal CT scan
√ mastoid air cells opaque / with air-fluid level

Plain film views: Stenvers / Owens projection

Transverse Fracture of Temporal Bone (25%)

= fracture perpendicular to axis of petrous pyramid originating in occipital bone extending anteriorly across the base of skull + across the petrous pyramid

• irreversible neurosensory hearing loss (fracture line across apex of IAC / labyrinthine capsule with injury to both parts of cranial nerve VIII)
• persistent vertigo
• facial (cranial nerve VII) nerve palsy in 50% (injury in IAC); less frequent spontaneous recovery because of disruption of nerve fibers
• rhinorrhea (CSF leak with intact tympanic membrane)
• bleeding into middle ear

Plain film views: posteroanterior (transorbital) + Towne projection

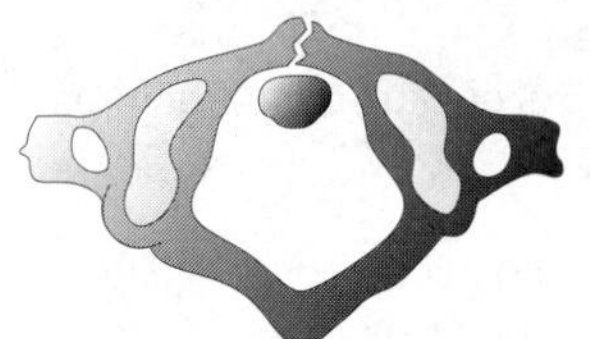
Anterior Arch Fracture

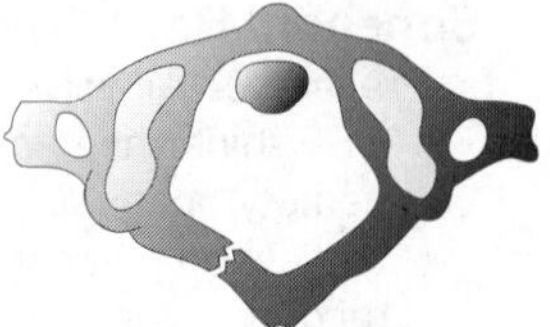
Posterior Arch Fracture

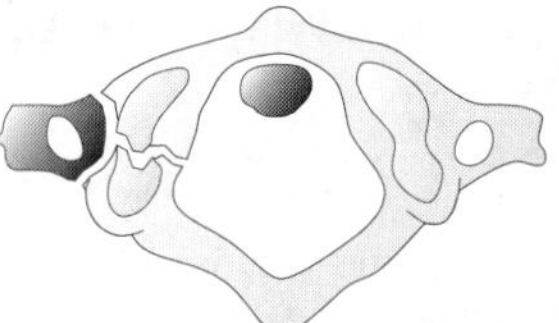
Lateral Mass Fracture

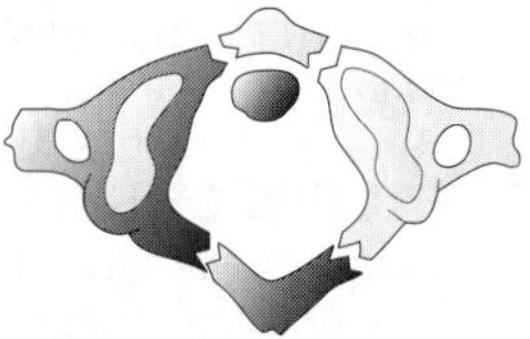
Jefferson Fracture

Atlas Fractures

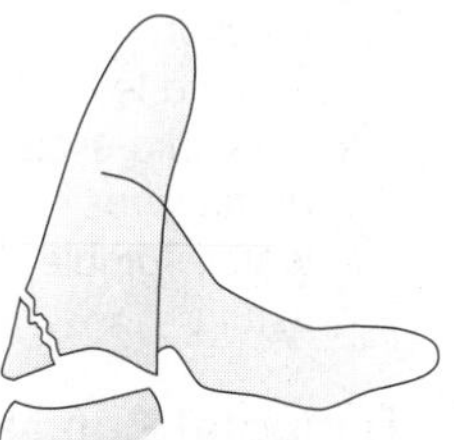
Teardrop Fracture

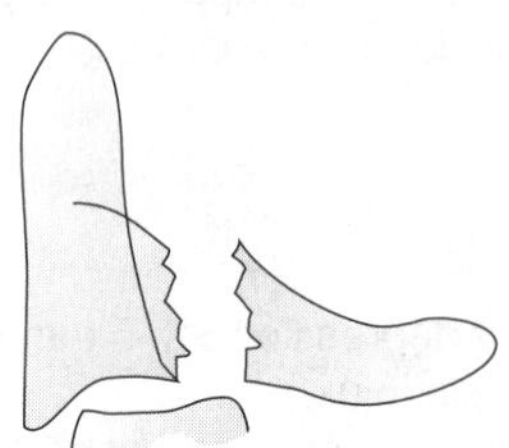
Hangman's Fracture

Axis Fractures

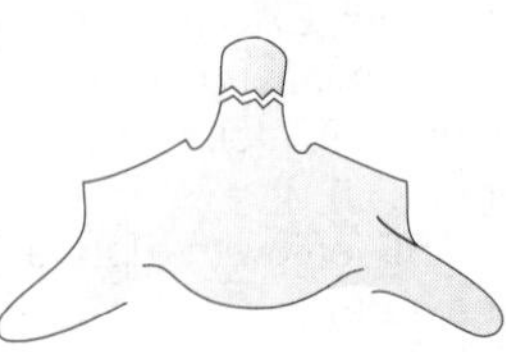
Type I

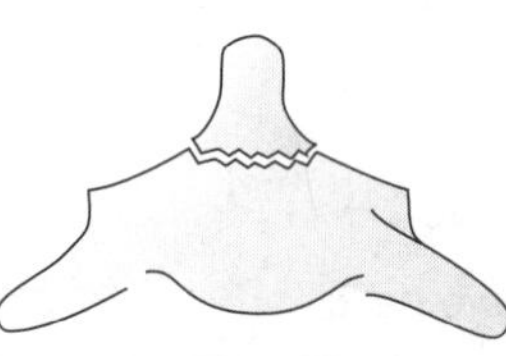
Type II

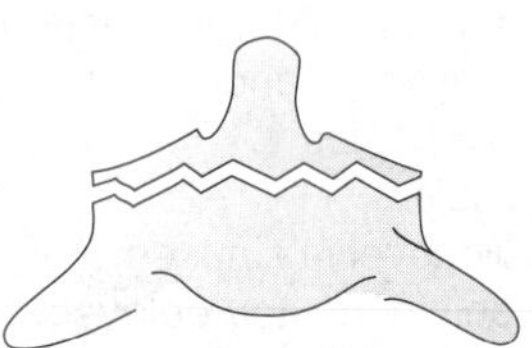
Type III

Dens Fractures

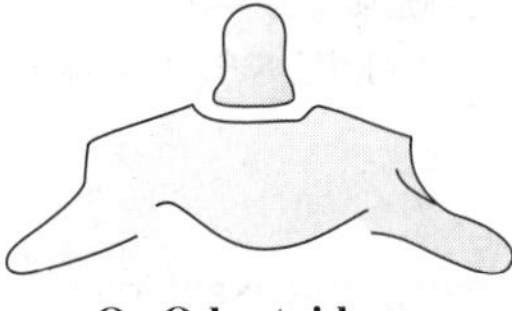
Os Odontoideum

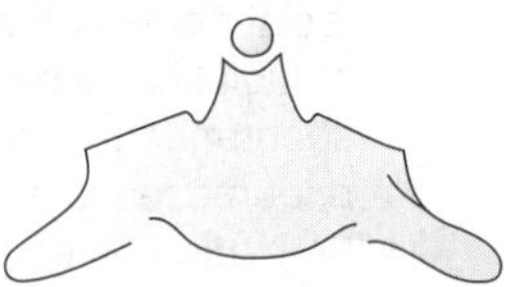
Ossiculum Terminale

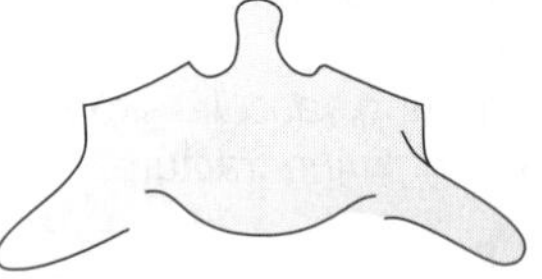
Hypoplasia of Dens

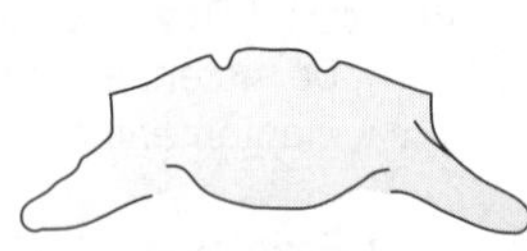
Aplasia of Dens

Dens Variants

Zygomaticomaxillary Fracture

= "TRIPOD" FRACTURE = MALAR / ZYGOMATIC COMPLEX FRACTURE

Cause: direct blow to malar eminence

- loss of sensibility of face below orbit
- deficient mastication
- double vision / ophthalmoplegia
- facial deformity

Fracture line:
(a) lateral wall of maxillary sinus
(b) orbital rim close to infraorbital foramen
(c) floor of orbit (d) zygomatico-frontal suture / zygomatic arch

Blowout Fracture

= isolated fracture of orbital floor

Cause: sudden direct blow to globe (ball or fist) with increase in intraorbital pressure transmitted to the weak orbital floor

- diplopia on upward gaze (entrapment of inferior rectus + inferior oblique muscles)
- enophthalmos
- facial anesthesia

Associated with: fracture of the thin lamina papyracea (= medial orbital wall) in 20–50%

√ soft-tissue mass extending into maxillary sinus (= herniation of orbital fat)
√ complete opacification of maxillary sinus (edema + hemorrhage)
√ depression of orbital floor (= orbital process of maxilla)
√ posttraumatic atrophy of orbital fat leads to enophthalmos
√ opacification of adjacent ethmoid air cells
√ disruption of lacrimal duct

FRACTURES OF CERVICAL SPINE

Factors associated with higher risk of fracture:
(1) Glasgow Coma Score <14

(2) Neck tenderness
(3) Loss of consciousness
(4) Neurologic deficit
(5) Drug ingestion
(6) Specific mechanism of injury: motor vehicle accident, fall from a height >3 m

Indications for screening CT of cervical spine:
high-risk adult patients (= >5% pretest probability of injury) defined by:
(1) High-speed (>35 mph) motor vehicle accident
(2) Crash resulting in death at scene of accident
(3) Fall from height >3 m (10 feet)
(4) Significant closed head injury (intracranial hemorrhage seen on CT)
(5) Neurologic signs / symptoms referred to C-spine
(6) Pelvic / multiple extremity fractures

Frequency: 1–3% of all trauma cases;
C2, C6 > C5, C7 > C3, C4 > C1
◊ Cervical spine trauma accounts for 2/3 of all spinal cord injuries!

• neurologic / spinal cord damage (39–50%)

Location:
(a) upper cervical spine = C1/2 (19–25%): atlas (4%), odontoid (6%)
(b) lower cervical spine = C3–7 (75–81%)
(c) cervicothoracic junction (9–18%)
(d) multiple noncontiguous spine fractures (15–20%)

Site: vertebral arch (50%), vertebral body (30%), intervertebral disk (25%), posterior ligaments (16%), dens (14%), locked facets (12%), anterior ligament (2%)

Associated with injury to:
head (70%), thoracic spine (15%), lumbar spine (10%), thorax (35%), pelvis (15%), upper extremity (10%), lower extremity (30%)

N.B.: 5–8% of patients with fractures may have normal radiographs!
◊ Most missed fractures involve C1 (8%), C2 (34%), C4 (12%), C6-7 (14%), occipital condyles !
◊ C7–T1 space not visualized in at least 26% of all trauma patients

Cx: neurologic deterioration with delay in diagnosis

A. HYPERFLEXION INJURY (46–79%)
1. Odontoid fracture
2. Simple wedge fracture (stable)
3. **Flexion teardrop fracture** = avulsion of anteroinferior corner by anterior ligament (unstable)
   ◊ Most severe + unstable injury of C-spine
   Location: C5, C6, C7
   √ triangular fragment in soft tissues anterior to vertebral body
   √ retrolisthesis
   √ widening of facets
   √ narrowing of spinal canal
   √ mild kyphosis
   Associated with: ligamentous tears, spinal cord compression
4. Anterior subluxation
5. **Bilateral facet lock** = interlocking of articular surfaces (unstable)
   √ anterolisthesis of affected vertebra by 1/2 vertebral body width
   √ mild focal kyphosis
   √ soft-tissue swelling
   √ no rotation
6. Anterior disk space narrowing
7. Spinous process fracture = clay shoveler's fracture = sudden load on flexed spine with avulsion fracture of C6 / C7 / T1 (stable)
8. Flexion instability = isolated rupture of posterior ligaments
   ◊ Dx may be missed without delayed flexion views
   √ no fracture
   √ interspinous widening
   √ loss of facet parallelism
   √ widening of posterior portion of disk
   √ anterolisthesis >3 mm
   √ focal kyphosis

B. HYPEREXTENSION INJURY (20–38%)
◊ High risk for neurologic deficit!
◊ Radiographs may be completely normal!
1. Anteriorly widened disk space
2. Prevertebral swelling
3. **Extension teardrop fracture**
   Location: C2, C3
4. Neural arch fracture of C1 (stable = anterior ring + transverse ligament intact)
5. Subluxation (anterior / posterior)
6. **Hangman's fracture** (unstable)
   = TRAUMATIC SPONDYLOLISTHESIS
   √ bilateral pars fracture of C2

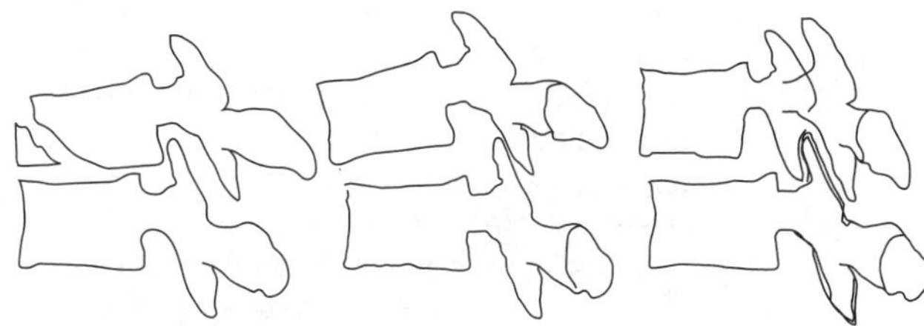

Teardrop Fracture **Flexion Instability** **Unilateral Facet Lock**

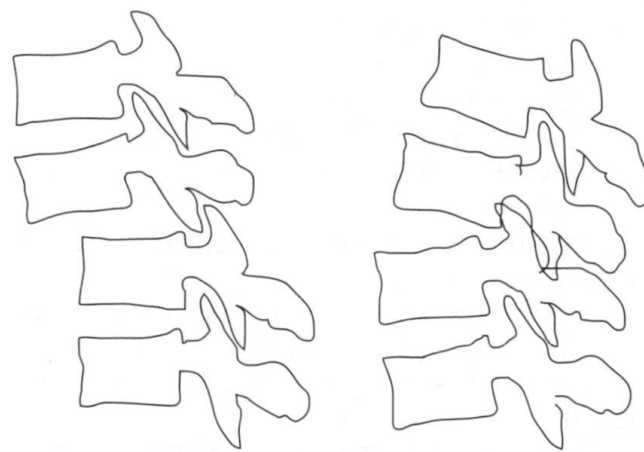

Bilateral Facet Lock **Hyperextension Dislocation**

Spine Injury

√ prevertebral soft-tissue swelling >5 mm at anterior-inferior margin of C2
√ anterior subluxation of C2 on C3:
√ disruption of C1–C2 spinolaminar line
√ disruption of C2–C3 posterior vertebral body line
√ avulsion of anteroinferior corner of C2 (rupture of anterior longitudinal ligament)

C. FLEXION-ROTATION INJURY (12%)
1. **Unilateral facet lock** (oblique views!, stable)
√ anterolisthesis <1/4 vertebral body width
√ "bow-tie" sign = the 4 rotated facets on LAT view
√ decrease in spinolaminar space
√ rotation of spinous process (on AP view)
√ "naked facet" (on CT)

D. VERTICAL COMPRESSION (4%)
1. **Jefferson fracture**
[Sir Geofrey Jefferson (1886–1961), neurosurgeon in Manchester, England]
√ comminuted burst fracture of ring of C1 (unstable) with uni- / bilateral ipsilateral anterior + posterior fractures
√ lateral displacement of lateral masses (self-decompressing) on AP view
(*DDx:* Pseudo-Jefferson fracture = lateral offset of lateral masses of atlas without fracture in fusion anomalies of anterior / posterior arches of C1, in children as lateral masses of atlas ossify earlier than C2)
2. **Burst fracture** = intervertebral disk driven into vertebral body below (stable)
√ loss of posterior vertebral body height with several fragments:
√ sagittal fracture component extending to inferior endplate
√ retropulsed fragment from posterior superior margin in spinal canal
√ interpedicular widening
√ posterior element fracture
Associated with: widening of apophyseal joints, fracture of posterior vertebral arches

E. LATERAL FLEXION / SHEARING (4–6%)
1. Uncinate fracture
2. Isolated pillar fracture
3. Transverse process fracture
4. Lateral vertebral compression

Significant Signs of Cervical Vertebral Trauma
(a) most reliable + specific:
√ widening of interspinous space (43%)
√ widening of facet joint (39%)
√ displacement of prevertebral fat stripe (18%)
(b) reliable but nonspecific:
√ wide retropharyngeal space >7 mm (31%)
(DDx: mediastinal hemorrhage of other cause, crying in children, S/P difficult intubation)
(c) nonspecific:
√ loss of lordosis (63%)
√ anterolisthesis / retrolisthesis (36%)
√ kyphotic angulation (21%)
√ tracheal deviation (13%)
√ disk space: narrow (24%), wide (8%)

Atlas Fracture
Prevalence: 4% of cervical spine injuries
Site: posterior arch, anterior arch, massa lateralis, Jefferson fracture
Associated with: fractures of C7 (25%), C2 pedicle (15%), extraspinal fractures (58%)

Axis Fracture
Prevalence: 6% of cervical spine injuries
Associated with: fractures of C1 in 8%
Type I = avulsion of tip of odontoid (5–8%)
√ difficult to detect
Type II = fracture through base of dens (54–67%)
Cx: nonunion
◊ Axial CT alone misses >50%!
Type III = subdental fracture (30–33%)
Prognosis: good
DDx: os odontoideum, ossiculum terminale, hypoplasia of dens, aplasia of dens

FRACTURES OF THORACOLUMBAR SPINE
◊ 40% of all vertebral fractures that cause neurologic deficit; mostly complex (body + posterior elements involved)
Location: 2/3 at thoracolumbar junction
√ diastasis of apophyseal joints
√ disruption of interspinal ligament
√ retropulsion of body fragments into spinal canal
√ "burst" fragments at superior surface of body

Fracture of Upper Thoracic Spine (T1 to T10)
Frequency: in 3% of all blunt chest trauma
Types:
1. compression / axial loading fracture (most common)
√ wedging of vertebral body
√ retropulsion of bone fragments
√ posttraumatic disk herniation
2. burst fracture
√ associated fracture of posterior neural arch
√ comminuted retropulsed bone fragments
3. sagittal slice fracture
√ vertebra above telescopes into vertebra below, displacing it laterally
4. anterior / posterior dislocation
√ torn anterior / posterior longitudinal ligament
√ facet dislocation

◊ Relatively stable fractures due to rib cage + strong costovertebral ligaments + more horizontal orientation of facet joints!
◊ Only 51% detected on initial CXR!
Often associated with: fracture of sternum
√ widening of paraspinal lines

√ mediastinal widening
√ loss of height of vertebral body
√ obscuration of pedicle
√ left apical cap
√ deviation of nasogastric tube

Signs of spinal instability:
= inability to maintain normal associations between vertebral segments while under physiologic load
√ displaced vertebra
√ widening of interspinous / interlaminar distance
√ facet dislocation
√ disruption of posterior vertebral body line

Fracture of Thoracolumbar Junction (T11 to L2)

= area of transition between a stiff + mobile segment of the spine
• neurologic deficit (in up to 40%)
Classification based on injury to the middle column:
(1) Hyperflexion injury (most common)
= compression of anterior column + distraction of posterior spinal elements
(a) hyperflexion-compression fracture
√ loss of height of vertebral body anteriorly + laterally
√ focal kyphosis / scoliosis
√ fracture of anterosuperior endplate
(b) flexion-rotation injury (unusual)
◊ Very unstable!
• catastrophic neurologic sequelae: paraplegia
√ subluxation / dislocation
√ widening of interspinous distance
√ fractures of lamina, transverse process, facets, adjacent ribs
(c) shearing fracture-dislocation
= damage of all 3 columns secondary to horizontally impacting force
(d) flexion-distraction injury: Chance fracture
2. Hyperextension injury (extremely uncommon)
√ widened disk space anteriorly
√ posterior subluxation
√ vertebral anterior superior corner avulsion
√ posterior arch fracture
3. Axial compression fracture
◊ Unstable!
√ burst fracture with herniation of intervertebral disk through endplates + comminution of vertebral body
√ marked anterior vertebral body wedging
√ retropulsed bone fragment
√ increase in interpediculate distance
√ ± vertical fracture through vertebral body, pedicle, lamina

Chance Fracture

= SEATBELT FRACTURE
[George Quentin Chance, British radiologist in Manchester, England]
Mechanism: shearing flexion-distraction injury (lap-type seatbelt injury in back-seat passengers)
• neurologic deficit infrequent (20%)
Location: L2 or L3
√ horizontal splitting of spinous process, pedicles, laminae + superior portion of vertebral body
√ disruption of ligaments
√ distraction of intervertebral disk + facet joints
◊ Fracture often unstable!
Often associated with:
(1) other bone injury
rib fractures along the course of diagonal strap; sternal fractures; clavicular fractures
(2) soft-tissue injury
transverse tear of rectus abdominis muscle; anterior peritoneal tear; diaphragmatic rupture
(3) vascular injury
mesenteric vascular tear; transection of common carotid artery; injury to internal carotid artery, subclavian artery, superior vena cava; thoracic aortic tear; abdominal aortic transection
(4) visceral injury
perforation of jejunum + ileum > large intestine > duodenum (free intraperitoneal fluid in 100%, mesenteric infiltration in 88%, thickened bowel wall in 75%, extraluminal air in 56%); laceration / rupture of liver, spleen, kidneys, pancreas, distended urinary bladder; uterine injury

Chance Equivalent

= purely ligamentous disruption leading to lumbar subluxation / dislocation
√ mild widening of posterior aspect of affected disk space
√ widened facet joints
√ splaying of spinous processes = "empty hole sign" on AP view

Holdsworth Fracture

[Sir Frank Wild Holdsworth (1904–1969), British pioneering orthopedist in rehabilitation of spinal injuries]
Location: thoracolumbar junction
√ unstable spinal column fracture-dislocation with fracture through vertebral body + articular processes
√ rupture of posterior spinal ligaments

Seatbelt Injury

= injury caused by three-point restraint type (combined lap and shoulder belt device)
• bruise in subcutaneous tissue + fat of anterior chest wall
• skin abrasions are associated with significant internal injuries (in 30%)
@ Skeleton
sternum, ribs (along diagonal course of shoulder harness), clavicle, transverse processes of C7 or T1
@ Cardiovascular
aortic transection, cardiac contusion, ventricular rupture, subclavian artery, SVC

@ Airways
tracheal / laryngeal tear, diaphragmatic rupture

Transverse Process Fracture of Lumbar Spine

Cause: direct trauma, violent lateral flexion-extension forces, avulsion of psoas muscle, Malgaigne fracture
Frequency: 7%
In 21–51% associated injury:
genitourinary injury, hepatic + splenic laceration
Location: L3 > L2 > L1 > L4 > L5; L:R = 2:1; multiple:single = 2:1; unilateral:bilateral = 20:1
√ vertical:horizontal (94%:6%) fractures
√ associated lumbar burst / compression fracture
◊ Detection by conventional radiography in 40% only!
Prognosis: minor and stable injury; 10% mortality

Sacral Fracture

Zone 1 = fracture lateral to sacral foramina
• significant neurologic deficit (uncommon)
Zone 2 = fracture through ≥1 foramina
• unilateral lumbar / sacral radiculopathy (rare)
Zone 3 = fracture through central canal
• significant bilateral neurologic damage (frequent): bowel / bladder incontinence
Cx: chronic disability (in up to 50%)

GLIOMA OF SPINAL CORD

Astrocytoma of Spinal Cord

◊ Most common intramedullary spinal neoplasm in children!
Frequency: 30% of spinal cord tumors; 2nd in prevalence to ependymoma in adults
Mean age: 29 years; M:F = 58:42
Path: ill-defined fusiform cord enlargement without cleavage plane / capsule
Histo: hypercellularity with infiltrative growth along the scaffold of normal astrocytes, oligodendrocytes and axons;
Grade I pilocytic astrocytoma (75%), usually most common in cerebellum
Grade II fibrillary type
Grade III anaplastic astrocytoma with necrosis (up to 25%)
Grade IV glioblastoma multiforme with endothelial proliferation (0.2–1.5%)
Location: thoracic cord (67%), cervical cord (49%), conus medullaris (3%); on average over 7 vertebral segments involved; holocord presentation (in up to 60% in children); often extending into lower brainstem
• pain + sensory deficit (54%)
• motor dysfunction (41%)
• gait abnormalities (27%)
• torticollis (27%)
Radiographs:
√ scoliosis (24%)
√ widened interpedicular distance
√ bone erosion
MR:
√ usually homogeneous extensive ill-defined cord tumor with widening of spinal cord:
√ iso- / hypointense to cord on T1WI
√ hyperintense on T2WI
√ poorly defined margins
√ eccentric location within spinal cord (57%)
√ dilated veins on surface of cord
√ patchy irregular Gd enhancement on MR
√ eccentric irregular tumor cysts + polar cysts + syrinx (common):
√ water-soluble myelographic contrast enters cystic space on delayed CT images
√ leptomeningeal spread (in 60% of glioblastoma multiforme)
Rx: tumor debulking + radiation therapy
Prognosis: 95% 5-year survival in low-grade tumors; higher mortality rate than for ependymoma
DDx: ependymoma (cap sign, central location, well defined, hemorrhage common, focal intense enhancement, predilection for conus)

Ependymoma of Spinal Cord

◊ Most common intramedullary spinal neoplasm in adults!
Frequency: 40–60% of primary spinal cord tumors; 90% of primary tumors in the filum terminale
Mean age: 39 years; M:F = 57:43
Origin: ependymal cells lining the central canal (62–76%)
Path: symmetric cord expansion with displacement of neural tissue
Histo: perivascular pseudorosettes; cystic degeneration (50%); hemorrhage at superior + inferior tumor margins
Subtypes: cellular (most common), papillary, clear cell, tanycytic, myxopapillary (along filum terminale), melanotic
Location: cervical cord alone (44%) / with extension into thoracic cord (23%); thoracic cord alone (26%); conus medullaris (7%); extends over several vertebral segments (on average 3.6 segments involved)
ectopic: sacrococcygeal region, broad ligament of ovary (associated with spina bifida occulta [33%])
• long antecedent history (mean duration of 37 months):
• back / neck pain (67%) = compression / interruption of central spinothalamic tracts first
• sensory deficits (52%), motor weakness (46%)
• bowel / bladder dysfunction (15%)
Metastases to: lung, retroperitoneum, lymph nodes

√ well-demarcated / diffusely infiltrating cord tumor
√ associated with at least one cyst (in 78–84%):
√ polar cysts (62%)
√ tumoral cysts (4–50%)
√ syringohydromyelia (9–50%)
Radiographs:
√ scoliosis (16%)

√ widening of spinal canal (11%):
  √ scalloping of vertebral body
  √ pedicle erosion, laminar thinning

Myelography:
√ enlarged cord with complete / partial block to flow of contrast material

CT:
√ iso- / slightly hyperattenuating cord mass
√ intense enhancement

MR:
√ iso- / hypointense (rarely hyperintense from hemorrhage) mass relative to spinal cord on T1WI
√ hyper- / isointense on T2WI
√ "cap sign" = extremely hypointense rim at the tumor poles on T2WI (in 20–33%) due to hemorrhage
√ cord edema (60%)
√ mostly intense homogeneous enhancement on Gd-enhanced MR (84%)
√ well-defined margins on contrast-enhanced images (89%)

Prognosis: 82% 5-year survival rate
DDx: astrocytoma (pediatric tumor, eccentric location, ill defined, hemorrhage uncommon, patchy irregular enhancement)

Ganglioglioma of Spinal Cord

= GANGLIOGLIONEUROMA = GANGLIONIC NEUROMA = NEUROASTROCYTOMA = NEUROGANGLIOMA = GANGLIONIC GLIOMA = = NEUROGLIOMA = NEUROMA GANGLIOCELLULARE

Prevalence: 0.4–6.2% of all CNS tumors; 1.1% of all spinal neoplasms
Mean age: 19 years; children > adults; M:F = 1:1
Histo: mixture of irregularly oriented neoplastic mature neuronal elements (neurons / ganglion cells) + glial elements (neoplastic astrocytes), arranged in clusters = grade I or II lesions
Location: cervical cord (48%), thoracic cord (22%), conus, holocord; usually supratentorial (temporal lobe)

• duration of symptoms between 1 month and 5 years

√ scoliosis (44%), spinal remodeling (93%)
√ eccentric
√ small tumoral cysts (in 46%)
√ calcifications (rare compared with intracranial tumor)

MR:
√ mixed tumor signal intensities on T1WI (in 84%)
√ tumor homogeneously hyperintense on T2WI
√ surrounding edema (less common)
√ patchy tumor enhancement (65%), no enhancement (15%)
√ enhancement of pial surface (58%)

Cx: malignant transformation (10%)
Prognosis: slow growth; 89% 5-year and 83% 10-year survival rate ; 27% recurrence rate

Myxopapillary Ependymoma of Spinal Cord

= special variant of ependymoma of lower spinal cord

Prevalence: 13% of all spinal ependymomas; most common neoplasm of conus medullaris (83%)
Mean age: 35 years; M>F
Origin: ependymal glia of filum terminale
Path: heterogenous tumor with generous mucin production

• lower back / leg / sacral pain
• weakness / sphincter dysfunction

Location: conus medullaris, filum terminale; occasionally multiple (14–43%)

√ isointense on T1Wi + hyperintense on T2WI
√ occasionally hyperintense on T1WI + T2WI due to mucin content / hemorrhage
√ almost always contrast enhancing
√ occasionally large lytic area of bone destruction

Subependymoma of Spinal Cord

= variant of CNS ependymoma

Origin: tanycytes [*tanyos* , Greek = stretch] that bridge pial + ependymal layers
Mean age: 42 years; M:F = 74:26
Histo: sparsely dispersed ependymal cells among predominant fibrillar astrocytes

• 52 months mean duration of symptoms:
  • pain, sensory + motor dysfunction
  • atrophy of one / both distal upper extremities (83%)

Location: ventricular system of brain, some in cervical cord

√ fusiform dilatation of spinal cord:
  √ enhancing lesion with well-defined borders (50%)
  √ nonenhancing lesion with diffuse symmetric cord enlargement
√ eccentrically located mass
√ ± edema

HEMANGIOBLASTOMA OF SPINE

= ANGIOBLASTOMA = ANGIORETICULOMA

Prevalence: 1–7.2% of all spinal cord tumors; mostly sporadic
Associated with: von Hippel-Lindau disease (in 1/3)
Recommendation: screening MR imaging of brain + spine in patients with von Hippel-Lindau syndrome
Age: middle age; M:F = 1:1
Path: highly vascular discrete nodular masses abutting leptomeninges with prominent dilated + tortuous vessels on posterior cord surface
Histo: large pale stromal cells packed between blood vessels of varying sizes
Location: intramedullary (75%), radicular (20%), intradural extramedullary (5%); thoracic cord (50%), cervical cord (40%); solitary in >80%, multiple lesions indicate von Hippel-Lindau syndrome

• mean duration of symptoms is 38 months:
  • sensory changes (39%): impaired proprioception
  • motor dysfunction (31%), pain (31%)

√ increased interpediculate distance (mass effect)

Angio:
- √ highly vascular mass with dense prolonged blush
- √ large draining veins form sinuous mass along posterior aspect of cord

MR:
- √ iso- (50%) / hyperintense (25%) diffuse cord expansion on T1WI
- √ hyperintense lesion with intermixed focal flow voids on T2WI:
  - √ curvilinear area of signal void
- √ cyst formation / syringohydromyelia (in up to 100%):
  - √ intratumoral cystic component (50–60%)
  - √ occasionally cystic mass with enhancing mural nodule (CLASSIC for cerebellar hemangioblastoma)
  - √ densely staining tumor nodule
- √ ± surrounding edema and cap sign
- √ well-demarcated Gd-enhancing mass

Cx: intramedullary hemorrhage, hematomyelia, subarachnoid hemorrhage (rare)

DDx: arteriovenous fistula (not well circumscribed, heterogenous signal intensity)

KLIPPEL-FEIL SYNDROME

= BREVICOLLIS

= synostosis of two / more cervical segments

May be associated with:
platybasia, syringomyelia, encephalocele, facial + cranial asymmetry, Sprengel deformity (25–40%), syndactyly, clubbed foot, hypoplastic lumbar vertebrae; renal anomalies in 50% (agenesis, dysgenesis, malrotation, duplication, renal ectopia); congenital heart disease in 5% (atrial septal defect, coarctation)

- • clinical triad of
  - (1) short neck
  - (2) restriction of cervical motion
  - (3) low posterior hairline
- • deafness (30%)
- • webbed neck

Location: cervical spine

- √ fusion of vertebral bodies and posterior elements
- √ ± hemivertebrae
- √ may have cervicothoracic / cervical / atlanto-occipital fusion
- √ torticollis
- √ scoliosis
- √ rib fusion
- √ Sprengel deformity (25–40%)
- √ ear anomalies: absent auditory canal, microtia, deformed ossicles, underdevelopment of bony labyrinth

KÜMMELL DISEASE

= intravertebral vacuum phenomenon

Cause:
1. Osteonecrosis
2. Weeks to months following acute fracture

Pathophysiology: likely to represent gaseous release into bony clefts within a nonhealed fracture underneath endplate

Age: >50 years

Location: most commonly at thoracolumbar junction

- √ gas collection increasing with extension + traction, decreasing with flexion

LEPTOMENINGEAL CYST

= "Growing" fracture = loculation of CSF into / through skull

Prevalence: 1% of all pediatric skull fractures

Pathogenesis: skull fracture with dural tear leads to arachnoid herniation into dural defect; CSF pulsations produce fracture diastasis + erosion of bone margins (apparent 2–3 months after injury)

- √ skull defect with indistinct scalloped margins
- √ CSF-density cyst adjacent to / in skull, may contain cerebral tissue

MR:
- √ cyst isointense with CSF + communicating with subarachnoid space
- √ area of encephalomalacia underlying fracture (frequent)
- √ intracranial tissue extending between edges of bone

LIPOMA OF SPINE

= partially encapsulated mass of fat + connective tissue in continuity with leptomeninges / spinal cord

- • skin-coated subcutaneous back mass, occasionally associated with hemangiomatous / hairy lesion
- • sensory deficiency, paresis, neurogenic bladder

Types:
- (a) lipomyelomeningocele (84%)
- (b) fibrolipoma of filum terminale (12%)
- (c) intradural lipoma (4%)

Location: lumbosacral region

◊ Intradural lipomas + lipomyelomeningoceles represent 35% of skin-covered lumbosacral masses + 20–50% of occult spinal dysraphism!

Intradural Lipoma

= subpial juxtamedullary mass totally enclosed in intact dural sac

Prevalence: <1% of primary intraspinal tumors

Age peaks: first 5 years of life (24%), 2nd + 3rd decade (55%), 5th decade (16%)

- • slow ascending mono- / paraparesis, spasticity, cutaneous sensory loss, defective deep sensation (with cervical + thoracic intradural lipoma)
- • flaccid paralysis of legs, sphincter dysfunction (with lumbosacral intradural lipoma)
- • overlying skin most often normal
- • elevation of protein in CSF (30%)

Location: cervical (12%) / cervicothoracic (24%) / thoracic (30%); dorsal aspect of cord (75%), lateral / anterolateral (25%)

- √ spinal cord open in midline dorsally
- √ lipoma in opening between lips of placode
- √ exophytic component at upper / lower pole of lipoma
- √ syringohydromyelia (2%)
- √ focal enlargement of spinal canal ± adjacent neural foramina
- √ narrow localized spina bifida

Lipomyelomeningocele

= lipoma tightly attached to exposed dorsal surface of neural placode blending with subcutaneous fat

Prevalence: 20% of skin-covered lumbosacral masses; up to 50% of occult spinal dysraphism

Age: typically <6 months of age; M < F

- semifluctuant lumbosacral mass with overlying skin intact
- sensory loss in sacral dermatomes, motor loss, bladder dysfunction
- foot deformities, leg pain

Location: lumbosacral; longitudinal extension over entire length of spinal canal (in 7%)

√ lipoma dorsally continuous with subcutaneous fat
√ lipoma may enter central canal and extend rostrally (= "intradural intramedullary lipoma")
√ lipoma may extend upward within spinal canal external to dura (= "epidural lipoma")
√ deformed undulating spinal cord with dorsal cleft
√ tethered cord
√ ventral + dorsal nerve roots leave neural placode ventrally
√ dilated subarachnoid space

US:
√ echogenic intraspinal mass adjacent to deformed spinal cord + continuous with slightly hypoechoic subcutaneous fat

@ Vertebral changes
√ large spinal canal
√ erosion of vertebral body + pedicles
√ posterior scalloping of vertebral bodies (50%)
√ focal spina bifida
√ segmental anomalies / butterfly vertebra (up to 43%)
√ confluent sacral foramina / partial sacral agenesis (up to 50%)

Fibrolipoma of Filum Terminale

Prevalence: 6% of autopsies

- asymptomatic

Location: intradural filum, extradural filum, involvement of both portions

Prognosis: potential for development of symptoms of tethered cord

LÜCKENSCHÄDEL

= CRANIOLACUNIA = LACUNAR SKULL
= mesenchymal dysplasia of calvarial ossification (developmental disturbance)

Age: present at birth

Associated with: (1) meningocele / myelomeningocele (2) encephalocele (3) spina bifida (4) cleft palate (5) Arnold-Chiari II malformation

- normal intracranial pressure

Location: particularly upper parietal area

√ honeycombed appearance about 2 cm in diameter (thinning of diploic space)
√ premature closure of sutures (turricephaly / scaphocephaly)

Prognosis: spontaneous regression within first 6 months of life

DDx: (1) Convolutional impressions = "digital" markings (visible at 2 years, maximally apparent at 4 years, disappear by 8 years of age)
(2) "Hammered silver" appearance of increased intracranial pressure

LYMPHOMA OF SPINAL CORD

Prevalence: 3.3% of CNS lymphoma, 1% of all lymphomas

Mean age: 47 years; M<F

Histo: monotonous collection of lymphocytes packed tightly into perivascular space; predominantly B-cell lymphocyte population

- weakness, numbness, progressive difficulty in ambulation

Location: cervical > thoracic > lumbar cord

√ mostly solitary, rarely multicentric
√ isointense relative to cord on T1WI
√ high signal intensity on T2WI (in contrast to characteristic low signal intensity of intracranial lesions)
√ extensive cord edema
√ hetero- / homogeneous enhancement

MENINGEAL CYST

= abnormal dilatation of meninges within sacral canal / foramina

Prevalence: 5%

√ remodeling erosion of sacral canal / foramen (due to CSF pulsations)
√ thinned cortical margins

Perineural Sacral Cyst / Tarlov Cyst

= dilated nerve-root sleeve as normal variant

Location: posterior rootlets (S2 + S3 most common)

- neurologic symptoms if large

√ cyst communicates freely with subarachnoid space

Sacral Meningeal / Arachnoid Cyst (less common)

= OCCULT INTRASACRAL MENINGOCELE

- usually asymptomatic

√ cyst does not communicate with subarachnoid space

MENINGIOMA OF SPINE

Prevalence: 25–45% of all spine tumors; 2–3% of pediatric spinal tumors; 12% of all meningiomas

Age: >40 years + female (80%)

Location: thoracic region (82%); cervical spine on anterior cord surface near foramen magnum (2nd most common location); 90% on lateral aspect

Site: intradural extramedullary (50%); entirely epidural; intradural + epidural

- spinal cord / nerve root compression

√ bone erosion in <10%
√ scalloping of posterior aspect of vertebral body
√ widening of interpedicular distance

√ enlargement of intervertebral foramen
√ may calcify (not as readily as intracranial meningioma)
CT:
√ solid smoothly marginated mass isodense to skeletal muscle
√ marked enhancement
MR:
√ isointense to gray matter on T1WI + T2WI
√ rapid + dense enhancement after Gd-DTPA
DDx: nerve sheath tumor

METASTASES TO VERTEBRA

Source:
(a) Metastatic tumors: lung, breast, prostate, kidney, lymphoma, malignant melanoma
(b) Primary tumor: multiple myeloma
Pathogenesis: hematogenous spread to vertebral bodies (bones with greatest vascularity)
MR:
√ patchy multifocal relatively well-defined lesions
√ diminished signal on T1WI on background of high-signal appearance of marrow fat
√ increased signal on T2WI (except for blastic metastases with diminished T1 + T2 signals)
√ contrast enhancement on T1WI (majority)
√ pathologic compression fracture:
√ fracture only after all vertebral body fat replaced
√ hyperintense on diffusion-weighted images (DDx: hypointense benign fracture)
DDx: (1) Infection (centered around disk space)
(2) Primary vertebral tumor (rare in older patients, almost always benign in patients <21 years of age)

METASTASES TO SPINAL CORD

Intramedullary Metastasis

Prevalence: 0.9–2.1% (autoptic)
Origin: lung (40–85%), breast (11%), melanoma (5%), renal cell (4%), colorectal (3%), lymphoma (3%), cerebellar medulloblastoma; 5% of unknown origin
Spread:
(a) common: hematogenous (via arterial supply) / direct extension from leptomeninges
(b) rare: dissemination along central canal / extension along Batson venous plexus from retroperitoneal primary tumor / extension along perineural lymphatic ducts
• symptomatic for <1 month (in 75%):
• motor weakness, bowel / bladder dysfunction (60%)
• pain (70%), paresthesia (50%)
Location: cervical (45%), thoracic (35%), lumbar cord (8%)
Myelography (up to 40% undetected)
MR:
√ mild cord expansion over several segments (average length of 2–3 vertebral segments)
√ central area of low signal intensity (mimicking syrinx) on T1WI
√ high signal intensity on T2WI (reflecting edema / tumor infiltration)
√ intense homogeneous enhancement
√ disproportionately large amount of surrounding edema
Prognosis: 66% die within 6 months
Rx: radiation therapy, corticosteroids

Intradural Tumor Seeding

√ focal nodular masses varying substantially in size from a few mm to >10 mm
√ enlarged cord (from diffuse coating of outer wall of spinal cord) simulating an intramedullary lesion
√ thickening of meninges
√ thickened + nodular matted nerve roots
√ nodular + irregularly narrowed thecal sac
√ Gd-DTPA enhancement

Metastases from Outside CNS

(a) with subarachnoid hemorrhage: malignant melanoma, choriocarcinoma, hypernephroma, bronchogenic carcinoma
(b) others: breast, lymphoma
√ predominantly dorsal location

Drop Metastases

= CSF SEEDING OF INTRACRANIAL NEOPLASMS
Age: occurs more frequently in pediatric age group than in adults
Location: lumbosacral + dorsal thoracic spine (due to CSF flow / gravitation)
Site: on spinal arachnoid / pia mater
CNS tumors causing drop metastases:
1. Primitive neuroectodermal tumor
2. Medulloblastoma: up to 33%
3. Anaplastic glioma
4. Ependymoma: after local recurrence, more common in infra- than supratentorial ependymomas
5. Germinoma
6. Pineoblastoma, pineocytoma

Less common: choroid plexus carcinoma, teratoma, angioblastic meningioma
mnemonic: "MEGO TP"
Medulloblastoma
Ependymoma
Glioblastoma multiforme
Oligodendroglioma
Teratoma
Pineoblastoma, **P**NET

MYELOCYSTOCELE

= SYRINGOCELE
= hydromyelic spinal cord + arachnoid herniated through posterior spina bifida; least common form of spinal dysraphism
May be associated with: GI tract anomalies, GU tract anomalies

- cystic skin-covered mass over spine
- cloacal exstrophy (frequent)

Location: lower spine > cervical > thoracic spine

√ direct continuity of meningocele with subarachnoid space

√ cyst communicating with widened central canal of spinal cord typically posteriorly + inferiorly to meningocele

√ lordosis, scoliosis, partial sacral agenesis (common)

MYELOMENINGOCELE

= sac covered by leptomeninges containing CSF + variable amount of neural tissue; herniated through a defect in the posterior / anterior elements of spine

Prevalence: 1:1,000–2,000 births (in Great Britain 1:200 births); twice as common in infants of mothers >35 years of age; Caucasians > Blacks > Orientals; most common congenital anomaly of CNS

Etiology: localized defect of closure of caudal neuropore (usually closed by 28 days); persistence of neural placode causes derangement in the development of mesenchymal + ectodermal structures

- positive family history in 10%
- neural placode = reddish neural tissue in the middle of back made up of open spinal cord
- normal skin / cutaneous abnormality: pigmented nevus, abnormal distribution of hair, skin dimple, angioma, lipoma
- MS-AFP (≥ 2.5 S.D. over mean) permits detection in 80% (positive predictive value of 2–5%) if defect not covered by full skin thickness

Recurrence rate: 3–7% chance of NTD with previously affected sibling / in fetus of affected parent

Associated with:

(1) Hydrocephalus (70–90%): requiring ventriculoperitoneal shunt in 90%
  ◊ 25% of patients with hydrocephalus have spina bifida!

(2) Chiari II malformation (99%)

(3) Congenital / acquired kyphoscoliosis (90%)

(4) Vertebral anomalies (vertebral body fusion, hemivertebrae, cleft vertebrae, butterfly vertebrae)

(5) Diastematomyelia (20–46%): spinal cord split above (31%), below (25%), at the same level (22%) as the myelomeningocele

(6) Duplication of central canal (5%) cephalic to + at level of placode

(7) **Hemimyelocele** (10%) = two hemicords in separate dural tubes separated by fibrous / bony spur: one hemicord with myelomeningocele on one side of midline, one hemicord normal / with smaller myelomeningocele at a lower level
  - impaired neurological function on side of hemimyelocele

(8) Hydromyelia (29–77%) cranial to placode as a result of disturbed CSF circulation

(9) Chromosomal anomalies (10–17%): trisomy 18, trisomy 13, triploidy, unbalanced translocation
  ◊ In 20% no detectable associated anomalies!

(10) Tethering of spinal cord (70–90%)

(11) Arachnoid cyst (2%) due to developmental deficiency during formation of arachnoid / dura mater with a subdural location

Distribution: thoracic (2%), thoracolumbar (32%), lumbar (22%), lumbosacral (44%)

Location:

(a) **dorsal / posterior meningocele**:
  - lumbosacral (70% below L2): may be associated with tethered cord, partial sacral agenesis
  - suboccipital

(b) **anterior sacral meningocele** = prolapse through anterior sacral bony defect; occasionally associated with neurofibromatosis type 1, Marfan syndrome, partial sacral agenesis, imperforate anus, anal stenosis, tethered spinal cord, GU tract / colonic anomalies; M:F = 1:4

(c) **lateral thoracic meningocele** through enlarged intervertebral foramen into extrapleural aspect of thorax; right > left side, in 10% bilateral; often associated with neurofibromatosis (85%) + sharply angled scoliosis convex to meningocele
  √ expanded spinal canal
  √ erosion of posterior surface of vertebral body
  √ thinning of neural arch
  √ enlarged neural foramen

(d) **lateral lumbar meningocele** through enlarged neural foramina into subcutaneous tissue / retroperitoneum; often associated with Marfan / Ehlers-Danlos syndrome / neurofibromatosis
  √ expanded spinal canal
  √ erosion of posterior surface of vertebral body
  √ thinning of neural arch
  √ enlarged neural foramen

(e) **traumatic meningocele** = avulsion of spinal nerve roots secondary to tear in meningeal root sheath; in C-spine after brachial plexus injury (most commonly)
  √ small irregular arachnoid diverticulum with extension outside the spinal canal

(f) cranial meningocele = encephalocele

OB-US:

detection rate of 85–90%; sensitivity dependent on GA (fetal spine may be adequately visualized after 16–20 weeks GA); false-negative rate of 24%

√ spinal level estimated by counting up from last sacral ossification center = S4 in 2nd trimester + S5 in 3rd trimester (79% accuracy for ± spinal level)

√ may have clubfoot / rocker-bottom foot

√ polyhydramnios

@ Spine:
  √ loss of dorsal epidermal integrity
  √ soft-tissue mass protruding posteriorly + visualization of sac

√ widening of lumbar spine with fusiform enlargement of spinal canal:
  √ splaying (= divergent position) of ossification centers of laminae with cup- / wedge-shaped pattern (in transverse plane = most important section for diagnosis)
  √ absence of posterior line = posterior vertebral elements (in sagittal plane)
  √ gross irregularity in parallelism of lines representing laminae of vertebrae (in coronal plane)
√ anomalies of segmentation / hemivertebrae (33%) with short-radius kyphoscoliosis
√ tethered cord (with lumbar / lumbosacral myelomeningocele)

@ Head:
√ "lemon sign" = concave / linear frontal contour abnormality located at coronal suture associated with nonskin-covered myelomeningocele (PPV of 81–84%, in 0.7–1.3% of normal fetuses)
Prevalence: in 98% of fetuses ≤24 weeks; in 13% of fetuses >24 weeks; disappears in 3rd trimester
√ "banana sign"
Prevalence: in 96% of fetuses ≤24 weeks; in 91% of fetuses >24 weeks

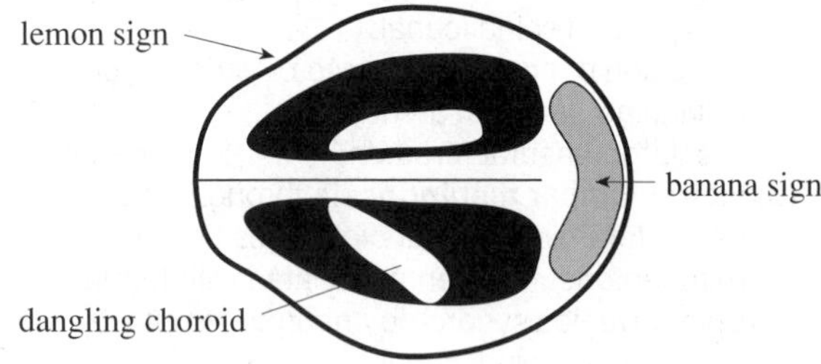

√ "nonvisualization" of cerebellum
√ effaced cisterna magna (100% sensitivity)
  ◊ A normal cisterna magna is 3–10 mm deep and usually visualized in 97% at 15–25 weeks GA
√ BPD <5th percentile during 2nd trimester (65–79% sensitivity)
√ HC <5th percentile (35% sensitivity)
√ ventriculomegaly (40–90%) with choroid plexus incompletely filling the ventricles (54–63% sensitivity) = "dangling" choroid on dependent side
Prevalence: in 44% of myelomeningoceles <24 weeks GA; in 94% of myelomeningoceles during 3rd trimester

Plain films:
√ bony defect in neural arch
√ deformity + failure of fusion of lamina
√ absent spinous process
√ widened interpedicular distance
√ widened spinal canal

Rx: (1) Possibly elective cesarean section at 36–38 weeks GA (may decrease risk of contaminating / rupturing the meningomyelocele sac)
(2) Repair within 48 hours

Postoperative complications:
(1) Postoperative tethering of spinal cord by placode / scar
(2) Constricting dural ring
(3) Cord compression by lipoma / dermoid / epidermoid cyst
(4) Ischemia from vascular compromise
(5) Syringohydromyelia

Prognosis:
(1) Mortality 15% by age 10 years
(2) Intelligence: IQ <80 (27%); IQ >100 (27%); learning disability (50%)
(3) Urinary incontinence: 85% achieve social continence (scheduled intermittent catheterization)
(4) Motor function: some deficit (100%); improvement after repair (37%)
(5) Hindbrain dysfunction associated with Chiari II malformation (32%)
(6) Ventriculitis: 7% in initial repair within 48 hours, more common in delayed repair >48 hours

NEURENTERIC CYST

= incomplete separation of foregut and notochord with persistence of canal of Kovalevski between yolk sac + notochord; cyst connected to meninges through midline defect

Incidence: rarest of bronchopulmonary foregut malformations (pulmonary sequestration, bronchogenic cyst, enteric cyst)

Associated with: neurofibromatosis; meningocele; spinal malformation (stalk connects cyst and neural canal; usually no stalk between cyst and esophagus)

Location: anterior to spinal canal on mesenteric side of gut

√ posterior mediastinal mass
√ air-fluid level (if communicating with GI tract through diaphragmatic defect)
√ spinal dysraphism at the same level:
  √ midline cleft in centra (accommodates stalk)
  √ anterior / posterior spina bifida
  √ vertebral body anomalies: absent vertebra, butterfly vertebra, hemivertebra, scoliosis
  √ diastematomyelia
  √ thoracic myelomeningocele

OSSIFYING FIBROMA

Peak incidence: first 2 decades of life

Histo: areas of osseous tissue intermixed with a highly cellular fibrous tissue

Sites: maxilla > frontal > ethmoid bone > mandible (rarely seen elsewhere)

√ areas of increased + decreased attenuation
√ intact inner + outer table
√ slow-growing expansile lesion
√ usually unilateral + monostotic

DDx: may be impossible to differentiate from fibrous dysplasia

OSTEOMYELITIS OF VERTEBRA

Prevalence: 2–10% of all cases of osteomyelitis

Causes:

(1) direct penetrating trauma (most common); following surgical removal of nucleus pulposus

(2) hematogenous: associated with urinary tract infections / following GU surgery / instrumentation; diabetes mellitus; drug abuse

Pathophysiology: infection begins in low-flow end-vascular arcades adjacent to subchondral plate

Organism: Staphylococcus aureus, Salmonella

Peak age: 5th–7th decade

- pain in back, neck, chest, abdomen, flank, hip
- neurologic deficit
- fever (most common presenting symptom), leukocytosis
- increased erythrocyte sedimentation rate
- positive blood / urine culture

√ disk space narrowing (earliest radiographic sign)
√ demineralization of adjacent vertebral endplates
√ bulging of paraspinal lines
√ tracer uptake in adjacent portions of two vertebral bodies
√ decreased marrow signal on T1WI
√ iso- / hyperintense marrow signal on T2WI

Cx: secondary infection of intervertebral disk is frequent

Rx: >4 weeks course of IV antibiotics

DDx: diskitis

PARAGANGLIOMA

Mean age: 46 years; M > F

Path: soft encapsulated (75%) slightly hemorrhagic mass supplied by numerous feeding arteries

Histo: chief cells + sustentacular cells surrounded by fibrovascular stroma; nests of chief cells in classic "Zellballen" configuration

- mean duration of symptoms for 4 years:
  - lower back pain, sciatica

Location: cauda equina , filum terminale

Site: intradural extramedullary compartment

CT:

√ bone erosion of spine

MR:

√ 3.3 (range, 1.5–10.0) cm average tumor size
√ well-circumscribed mass isointense to cord on T1WI
√ iso- to hyperintense on T2WI:
  √ cap sign = low-signal–intensity rim on T2WI from hemorrhage
  √ ± "salt-and-pepper" appearance
√ intense enhancement
√ serpentine flow voids along surface + within tumor nodule
√ ± syringohydromyelia

Angio:

√ intense early blush persisting well into late arterial + early venous phase

PRIMITIVE NEUROECTODERMAL TUMOR OF SPINAL CORD

Prevalence: 20 cases reported in literature

Location: spinal cord, intradural-extramedullary compartment, extradural compartment

Age: more common in adults than children; M:F = 6:4

Histo: small round blue cells with hyperchromatic nuclei + scanty cytoplasm, frequent mitoses

- weakness, paresthesia, gait disturbance, pain

Spread: throughout CSF space into cranium, lung, bone, lymph node

√ T1 and T2 prolongation

Prognosis: in >50% death within 2 years

SACROCOCCYGEAL TERATOMA

Prevalence: 1:40,000 livebirths; type I + II (80%); most common congenital solid tumor in the newborn; M:F = 1:4

Pathogenesis:

(1) growth of residual primitive pluripotential cells derived from the primitive streak + knot (Hensen node) of very early embryonic development

(2) attempt at twinning
- increased prevalence of twins in family

Histo:

(1) Mature teratoma (55–75%) with elements from glia, bowel, pancreas, bronchial mucosa, skin appendages, striated + smooth muscle, bowel loops, bone components (metacarpal bones + digits), well-formed teeth, choroid plexus structures (production of CSF)
  ◊ MATURE TERATOMA = benign tumor composed of tissues foreign to the anatomic site in which they arise, usually containing tissues from at least 2 germ cell layers

(2) Immature teratoma (11–28%): admixed with primitive neuroepithelial / renal tissue
  ◊ IMMATURE TERATOMA = benign teratoma with embryonic elements

(3) Malignant germ cell tumor
  (a) mixed malignant teratoma (7–17%): elements of endodermal sinus tumor (= yolk sac tumor) + either form of teratoma
  (b) pure endodermal sinus tumor (rare)
  (c) seminoma (dysgerminoma), embryonal carcinoma, choriocarcinoma (extremely rare)
  Metastases to: lung, bone, lymph nodes (inguinal, retroperitoneal), liver, brain

Age: 50–70% during first few days of life; 80% by 6 months of age; <10% >2 years of age; rare in adulthood; M:F = 1:4

Classification (Altman):

Type I predominantly external lesion covered by skin with only minimal presacral component (47%)

Type II predominantly external tumor with significant presacral component (35%)

Type III predominantly sacral component + external extension (8%)

Type IV presacral tumor with no external component (10%)

Associated with: other congenital anomalies (in 18%):
(1) musculoskeletal (5–16%): spinal dysraphism, sacral agenesis, dislocation of hip
(2) renal anomalies: hydronephrosis, renal cystic dysplasia, Potter syndrome
(3) GI tract: imperforate anus, gastroschisis, constipation
(4) fetal hydrops (due to high-output cardiac failure)
(5) placentomegaly (due to fetal hydrops)
(6) curvilinear sacrococcygeal defect (rare autosomal dominant inheritance with equal sex incidence, low malignant potential, absence of calcifications) + anorectal stenosis / atresia, vesicoureteral reflux

- AFP elevated with mixed malignant teratoma + endodermal sinus tumor (CAVE: fetal + newborn serum contains AFP, which does not reach adult levels until about 8 months of age)
- premature labor (due to polyhydramnios + large mass)
- uterus large for dates
- radicular pain, constipation, urinary frequency / incontinence

Plain film:
√ amorphous, punctate, spiculated calcifications, possibly resembling bone (36–50%); suggestive of benign tumor
√ soft-tissue mass in pelvis protruding anteriorly + inferiorly

BE:
√ anterosuperior displacement of rectum
√ luminal constriction

IVP:
√ displacement of bladder anterosuperiorly
√ development of bladder neck obstruction

Myelography:
√ intraspinal component may be present

Angio:
√ neovascularity (arterial supply by middle + lateral sacral + gluteal branches of internal iliac artery, branches of profunda femoris artery)
√ enlargement of feeding vessels
√ arterial encasement
√ arteriovenous shunting
√ early venous filling with serpiginous dilated tumor veins

US / CT:
√ solid (25%) / mixed (60%) / cystic (15%) sacral mass
√ 1–30 cm (average size of 8 cm) in diameter
√ polyhydramnios (2/3)
√ oligohydramnios, fetal hydronephrosis, fetal hydrops with ascites, pleural effusions, skin edema, placentomegaly are poor prognostic factors

MR:
√ lobulated + sharply demarcated tumor extremely heterogeneous on T1WI as a result of high signal from fat, intermediate signal from soft tissue, low signal from calcium
√ best modality to detect spinal canal invasion

Prognosis: prevalence of malignant germ cell tumors increases with patient's age
◊ predominantly fatty tissue tumors are usually benign
◊ hemorrhage / necrosis is suggestive of malignancy
◊ cystic lesions are less likely malignant
◊ sacral destruction indicates malignancy
◊ patients >2 months of age have a malignant tumor with a 50–90% probability

Cx: (1) dystocia in 6–13%
(2) massive intratumoral hemorrhage
(3) fetal death in utero / stillbirth

Rx: 1. Complete tumor resection + coccygectomy + reconstruction of pelvic floor: up to 37% recurrence rate, esp. without coccygectomy
2. Multiagent chemotherapy (in malignancy) with long-term survival rate of 50%

DDx: (1) Myelomeningocele (superior to sacrococcygeal region, not septated, axial bone changes)
(2) Rectal duplication, anterior meningocele (purely cystic)
(3) Hemangioma, lymphangioma, lipomeningocele, lipoma, epidermal cyst, chordoma, sarcoma, ependymoma, neuroblastoma

SCHEUERMANN DISEASE

= SPINAL OSTEOCHONDROSIS = KYPHOSIS DORSALIS JUVENILIS = VERTEBRAL EPIPHYSITIS
= disorder consisting of vertebral wedging + endplate irregularity + narrowing of intervertebral disk space

Prevalence: in 31% of male + 21% of female patients with back pain
Age: onset at puberty
Location: lower thoracic / upper lumbar vertebrae; in mild cases limited to 3–4 vertebral bodies
√ anterior wedging of vertebral body of >5°
√ increased anteroposterior diameter of vertebral body
√ slight narrowing of disk space
√ kyphosis of >40°/ loss of lordosis; scoliosis
√ Schmorl nodes (intravertebral herniation of nucleus pulposus into vertebral body) = depression in contour of endplate in posterior half of vertebral body; found in up to 30% of adolescents + young adults
√ flattened area in superior surface of epiphyseal ring anteriorly = avulsion fracture of ring apophysis due to migration of nucleus pulposus through weak point between ring apophysis + vertebral endplate (fusion of ring apophysis usually occurs at about 18 years of age)
√ detached epiphyseal ring anteriorly

DDx: (1) Developmental notching of anterior vertebrae (NO wedging or Schmorl nodes)
(2) Osteochondrodystrophy (earlier in life, extremities show same changes)

SPINAL STENOSIS

= encroachment on central spinal canal, lateral recess, or neuroforamen by bone / soft tissue

Cause:
A. Congenitally short pedicles
(a) idiopathic

(b) developmental: Down syndrome, achondroplasia, hypochondroplasia, Morquio disease

B. Acquired:

1. Hypertrophy of ligamentum flavum = buckling of ligament secondary to joint slippage in facet joint osteoarthritis (most common)
2. Facet joint hypertrophy
3. Degenerated bulging / herniated disk
4. Spondylosis, spondylolisthesis
5. Surgical fusion
6. Fracture
7. Ossification of posterior longitudinal ligament
8. Paget disease
9. Epidural lipomatosis

Age: middle-aged for congenital cause / elderly during 6th–8th decade for acquired cause; M > F

Location: generally involves lumbar spinal canal; cervical spinal canal may be similarly affected

√ obliteration of epidural fat
√ interpedicular distance <25 mm
◊ Measurements are not a valid indicator of disease!

Cervical Spinal Stenosis

Location: multiple levels in mid- and lower cervical spine

√ sagittal diameter of cervical spinal canal <13 mm
√ hourglass narrowing of thecal sac with scalloping of the dorsal + ventral margins of the cord
√ greater degree of stenosis in hyperextended position (due to buckling of ligamenta flava):
√ may appear as spinal block in hyperextended neck on AP views

Lumbar Spinal Stenosis

Cause:

1. Achondroplasia:
   √ narrowed interpediculate distance progressive toward lumbar spine
2. Paget disease: bony overgrowth
3. Spondylolisthesis
4. Operative posterior spinal fusion
5. Herniated disk
6. Metastasis to vertebrae
7. Developmental / congenital

Age: presentation between 30 and 50 years of age

- often asymptomatic until middle age (until development of secondary degenerative changes)
- low back pain
- "neurogenic / spinal claudication" = bilateral lower extremity pain, numbness, weakness worse during walking / standing + relieved in supine position and flexion
- cauda equina syndrome: paraparesis, incontinence, sensory findings in saddlelike pattern, areflexia

√ sagittal diameter of spinal canal <16 mm (normal range in adults: 15–23 mm)
√ dural sac area <100 mm^2
√ diminished amount of CSF + crowding of nerve roots
√ unusual small quantity of contrast material to fill thecal sac
√ anteroposterior + interpediculate diameter spinal canal constricted
√ hourglass configuration of thecal sac (SAG view)
√ triangular / trefoil shape of thecal sac (AXIAL view)
√ redundant serpiginous nerve roots above + below stenosis
√ thickened articular process, pedicles, laminae, ligaments
√ bulging disks

SPLIT NOTOCHORD SYNDROME

= spectrum of anomalies with persistent connection between gut + dorsal ectoderm

Etiology: failure of complete separation of ectoderm from endoderm with subsequent splitting of notochord and mesoderm around the adhesion about 3rd week of gestation

√ fistula / isolated diverticula / duplication / cyst / fibrous cord / sinus along the tract

Types:

1. **Dorsal enteric fistula**
   = fistula between intestinal cavity + dorsal midline skin traversing prevertebral soft tissue, vertebral body, spinal canal, posterior elements of spine
   - bowel ostium / exposed pad of mucous membrane in dorsal midline in newborn
   - opening passes meconium + feces

   √ dorsal bowel hernia into a skin- / membrane-covered dorsal sac after passing through a combined anterior + posterior spina bifida
2. **Dorsal enteric sinus**
   = blind remnant of posterior part of tract with midline opening to dorsal external skin surface
3. **Dorsal enteric enterogenous cyst**
   = prevertebral / postvertebral / intraspinal enteric-lined cyst derived from intermediate part of tract

   Intraspinal enteric cyst

   Age at presentation: 20–40 years
   - intermittent local / radicular pain worsened by elevation of intraspinal pressure

   Location: intraspinal in lower cervical / upper thoracic region

   √ enlarged spinal canal at site of cyst
   √ hemivertebrae, segmentation defect, partial fusion, scoliosis in region of cyst
4. **Dorsal enteric diverticulum**
   = tubular / spherical diverticulum arising from dorsal mesenteric border of bowel as a persistent portion of tract between gut + vertebral column
5. **Dorsal enteric cyst**
   = involution of portion of diverticulum near gut
   - mass in abdomen / mediastinum (due to bowel rotation)

SPONDYLOLISTHESIS

= forward displacement of one vertebra over another

Prevalence: 4% of general population

Location: L5/S1 or L4/L5

Grades I–IV (Meyerding method): each grade equals 1/4 anterior subluxation of superior on inferior vertebral body

Isthmic Spondylolisthesis = open-arch type

Cause: usually bilateral spondylolysis

= separation of anterior part (vertebral body, pedicles, transverse processes, superior articular facet) slipping forward from posterior part (inferior facet, laminae, dorsal spinous process)

Age: often <45 years

• symptomatic if intervertebral disk + posterosuperior aspect of vertebral body encroaches on superior portion of neuroforamen

√ elongation of spinal canal in anteroposterior diameter

√ bilobed configuration of neuroforamen

√ ratio of maximum anteroposterior diameter of spinal canal at any level divided by diameter at L1 >1.25

Degenerative Spondylolisthesis = closed-arch type

= PSEUDOSPONDYLOLISTHESIS

Cause: degenerative / inflammatory joint disease (eg, rheumatoid arthritis)

Pathophysiology: excess motion of facet joints allowing forward / posterior movement

Age: usually >60 years; M < F (at L4-5)

• commonly symptomatic due to spinal stenosis + narrowing of neuroforamen

√ narrowing of spinal canal

√ hypertrophy of facet joints

√ ratio of maximum anteroposterior diameter of spinal canal at any level divided by diameter at L1 <1.25

SPONDYLOLYSIS

= pars interarticularis defect between superior + inferior articulating processes as the weakest portion of spinal unit

Prevalence: 3–7% of population; in 30–70% other family members afflicted

Age: early childhood; M:F = 3:1; Whites:Blacks = 3:1

Cause:

(a) pseudarthrosis following stress (fatigue) fracture of pars (in most) from repetitive minor trauma; common in gymnastics (30%), diving, contact sports (football, soccer, hockey, lacrosse)

(b) hereditary hypoplasia of pars leads to insufficiency fracture; eg, pars defect in 34% of Eskimos

(c) secondary spondylolysis: neoplasm, osteomyelitis, Paget disease, osteomalacia, osteogenesis imperfecta

(d) congenital malformation: frequently associated with spina bifida occulta of S1, dorsally wedge-shaped body of L5, hypoplasia of L5; HOWEVER: no pars defects have been identified in fetal cadavers

• symptomatic in 50% (if associated with degenerative disk disease / spondylolisthesis)

Location: L5 (67–95%); L4 (15–30%); L3 (1–2%); in 75% bilateral

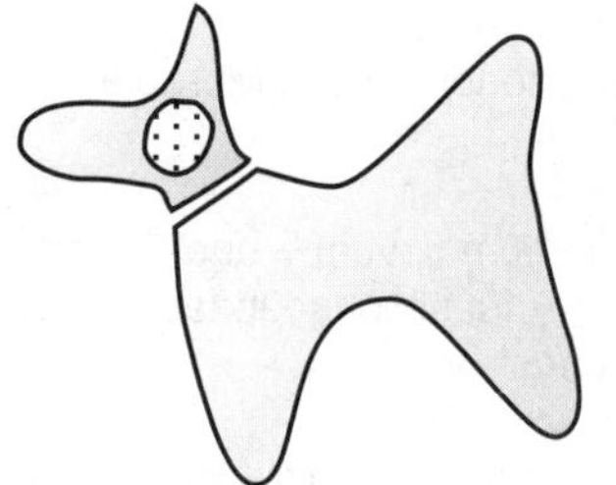

Oblique Radiograph of L5

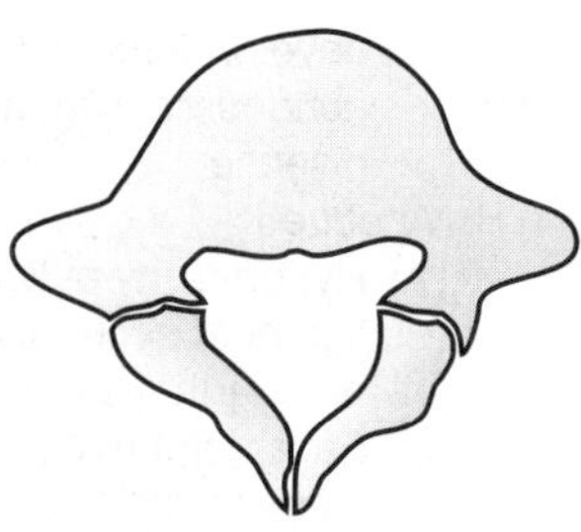

CT Scan through Mid-Vertebral Body

Spondylolysis

Plain film:

√ radiolucent band ± sclerotic margin resembling the collar of the "Scottie dog" (on oblique view)

√ may be associated with spondylolisthesis

√ subluxation of involved vertebra (if pars defect bilateral)

√ Wilkinson syndrome = reactive sclerosis + bony hypertrophy of contralateral pedicle + lamina (produced by stress changes related to weakening of neural arch in unilateral pars defect)

◊ Planar / SPECT bone scintigraphy may be useful!

CT:

√ pars defect located 10–15 mm above disk space

√ inner contour of spinal canal interrupted

Spondylolysis of Cervical Spine

= progressive degeneration of intervertebral disks leading to proliferative changes of bone + meninges; more common than disk herniation as a cause for cervical radiculopathy

Prevalence: 5–10% at age 20–30; >50% at age 45; >90% by age 60

• spastic gait disorder

• neck pain

Location: C4-5, C5-6, C6-7 (greater normal cervical motion at these levels)

Sequelae:
(a) direct compression of spinal cord
(b) neural foraminal stenosis
(c) ischemia due to vascular compromise
(d) repeated trauma from normal flexion / extension

DDx of myelopathy:

rheumatoid arthritis, congenital anomalies of craniocervical junction, intradural extramedullary tumor, spine metastases, cervical spinal cord tumor, arteriovenous malformation, amyotrophic lateral sclerosis, multiple sclerosis, neurosyphilis

SYRINGOHYDROMYELIA

= SYRINGOMYELIA = SYRINX (used in a general manner reflecting difficulty in classification)

= longitudinally oriented CSF-filled cavities + gliosis within spinal cord frequently involving both parenchyma + central canal

Age: primarily childhood / early adult life

Cause: Chiari I malformation (41%), trauma (28%), neoplasm (15%), idiopathic (15%)

• loss of sensation to pain + temperature (interruption of spinothalamic tracts)
• trophic changes [skin lesions; Charcot joints in 25% (shoulder, elbow, wrist)]
• muscle weakness (anterior horn cell involvement)
• spasticity, hyperreflexia (upper motor neuron involvement)
• abnormal plantar reflexes (pyramidal tract involvement)

Location: predominantly lower end of cervical cord; extension into brainstem (= syringobulbia)

CT:
√ distinct area of decreased attenuation within spinal cord (100%)
√ swollen / normal-sized / atrophic cord
√ no contrast enhancement
√ flattened vertebral border (rare) with increased transverse diameter of cord
√ change in shape + size of cord with change in position (rare)
√ filling of syringohydromyelia with intrathecal contrast
  (a) early filling via direct communication with subarachnoid space
  (b) late filling after 4–8 hours (80–90%) secondary to permeation of contrast material

Myelography:
√ enlarged cord (DDx: intramedullary tumor)
√ "collapsing cord sign" = collapsing of cord with gas myelography as fluid content moves caudad in the erect position (rare)

MR:
√ cystic area of low signal intensity on T1WI, increased intensity on T2WI
√ presence of CSF flow-void (= low signal on T2WI) within cavity from pulsations
√ beaded cavity from multiple incomplete septations
√ cord enlargement

Hydromyelia
= PRIMARY / CONGENITAL SYRINGOHYDROMYELIA
= dilatation of persistent central canal of spinal cord (in 70–80% obliterated), which communicates with 4th ventricle (= communicating syringomyelia)

Histo: lined by ependymal tissue

Associated with:
(1) Chiari malformation in 20–70%
  √ metameric haustrations within syrinx on sagittal T1WI
(2) Spinal dysraphism
(3) Myelocele
(4) Dandy-Walker syndrome
(5) Diastematomyelia
(6) Scoliosis in 48–87%
(7) Klippel-Feil syndrome
(8) Spinal segmentation defects
(9) Tethered cord (in up to 25%)

DDx: transient dilatation of the central canal (transient finding in newborns during the first weeks in life)

Syringomyelia
= ACQUIRED / SECONDARY SYRINGOHYDROMYELIA
= any cavity within substance of spinal cord that may communicate with the central canal, usually extending over several vertebral segments

Histo: not lined by ependymal tissue

Pathophysiology: interrupted flow of CSF through the perivascular spaces of cord between subarachnoid space + central canal

Cause:
1. <u>Posttraumatic syringomyelia</u>
   Prevalence: in 3.2% after spinal cord injury
   Location: 68% in thoracic cord
   √ 0.5–40 cm (average 6 cm) in length
   √ syrinx may be septated (parallel areas of cavitation) on transverse T1WI
   √ loss of sharp cord-CSF interface (obliteration of arachnoid space by adhesions)
   √ in 44% associated with arachnoid loculations (extramedullary arachnoid cysts) at upper aspect of syrinx
2. <u>Postinflammatory syringomyelia</u>
   subarachnoid hemorrhage, arachnoid adhesions, S/P surgery, infection (tuberculosis, syphilis)
3. <u>Tumor-associated syringomyelia</u>
   spinal cord tumors, herniated disk; secondary to circulatory disturbance + thoracic spinal cord atrophy
4. <u>Vascular insufficiency</u>

Reactive Cyst
= POSTTRAUMATIC SPINAL CORD CYST
= CSF-filled cyst adjacent to level of trauma; usually single (75%)

• late deterioration in patients with spinal cord injury (not related to severity of original injury)

Rx: shunting leads to clinical improvement

TERATOMA OF SPINE
= neoplasm containing tissue belonging to all 3 germinal layers at sites where these tissues do not normally occur

Prevalence: 0.15% (excluding sacrococcygeal teratoma)
Age: all ages; M:F = 1:1
Path: solid, thin- / thick-walled partially / wholly cystic with clear / milky / dark cyst fluid, uni- / multilocular, presence of bone / cartilage

Location: intra- / extramedullary
√ complete block at myelography
√ syringomyelia above level of tumor
√ spinal canal may be focally widened

TERMINAL MYELOCYSTOCELE
= combination of posterior spina bifida + meningocele + tethered cord + hydromyelia + cystic dilatation of the distal central canal

Cause: disturbed CSF circulation resulting in dilatation of ventriculus terminalis + disruption of dorsal mesenchyme

Associated with: anorectal + genitourinary + vertebral anomalies (anal atresia, cloacal exstrophy, scoliosis, sacral agenesis)
• skin-covered mass in lumbosacral region
√ spinal cord surrounded dorsally + ventrally by dilated subarachnoid space of the meningocele
√ nerve root exit ventrally
√ bifid spinal cord
√ hydromyelia

TETHERED CORD

= TIGHT FILUM TERMINALE SYNDROME = LOW CONUS MEDULLARIS
= abnormally short + thickened filum terminale with position of conus medullaris below L2/3 (normal location of tip of conus medullaris: L 4/5 at 16 weeks of gestation, L 2/3 at birth, L1/2 >3 months of age)
◊ RULE OF THREES: above L3 by age 3 months!

Etiology: incomplete involution of distal spinal cord with failure of ascent of conus
Pathophysiology: stretching of cord leads to vascular insufficiency at level of conus
Age at presentation: 5–15 years (in years of growth spurt); M:F = 2:3
Associated with: filar lipoma in 29–78%, filar cyst, diastematomyelia, imperforate anus
• dorsal nevus, dermal sinus tract, hair patch (50%)
• bowel + bladder dysfunction in childhood
• spastic gait with muscle stiffness
• lower extremity weakness + muscle atrophy
• asymmetric hyporeflexia + fasciculations
• orthopedic anomalies: scoliosis, pes cavus, tight Achilles tendon
• hypalgesia, dysesthesia
• paraplegia, paraparesis
• radiculopathy (adults)
• hyperactive deep tendon reflexes
• extensor plantar responses
• anal / perineal pain (in adults)
• back pain (particularly with exertion)

@ Tight filum
√ diameter of filum terminale >2 mm (normal range of 0.5 to 2 mm) at L5–S1 level (55%)
√ small fibrolipoma within thickened filum (23%)
√ small filar cyst (3%)
√ spinal cord ending in a small lipoma (13%)
@ Tethered cord (100%)
√ conus medullaris below level of L3 at birth and below L2 by age 12 (86%)
√ abnormal dorsal fixation of cord adjacent to vertebral arches (in prone position)
√ reduced / absent pulsatile movement of the cord + nerve roots (on M-mode scanning)
√ widened triangular thecal sac tented posteriorly (thecal sac pulled posteriorly by filum)
√ abnormal lateral course of nerve roots (>15° angle relative to spinal cord)
@ Vertebrae
√ lumbar spina bifida occulta with interpedicular widening
√ scoliosis (20%)
MR:
√ prolonged T1 relaxation in center of spinal cord on T1WI in 25% (? myelomalacia / mild hydromyelia)
Rx: decompressive laminectomy / partial removal of lipoma ± freeing of cord
Dx: tip of conus medullaris below L2-3

TRAUMATIC NEUROMA

= nonneoplastic proliferation of the proximal end of a severed / partially transected injured nerve
Histo: nonencapsulated tangled multidirectional regenerating axonal masses + Schwann cells + endo- and perineural cells in dense collagenous matrix with surrounding fibroblasts
Types:
(a) spindle neuroma = internal focal fusiform swelling
Cause: chronic friction / irritation of nondisrupted injured but intact nerve trunk
(b) lateral / terminal neuroma
Cause: severe trauma with partial avulsion / disruption / total transection of nerve
Time of onset: 1–12 months after injury
• pain
• Tinel sign = palpation / tapping on lesion reproduces pain
Location: lower extremity (after amputation), head and neck (after tooth extraction), radial nerve, brachial plexus
√ fusiform mass / focal enlargement with entering and exiting nerve (spindle type)
√ bulbous mass in continuity with normal nerve proximally (lateral / terminal type)
MR:
√ isointense to muscle on T1WI
√ heterogeneous intermediate to high signal intensity on T2WI
√ "fascicular sign" = heterogeneous ringlike pattern on T2WI
Rx: acupuncture, cortisone injection, transcutaneous / direct nerve stimulation, physical therapy, surgical resection

VENTRICULUS TERMINALIS

= small ependyma-lined oval cyst at the transition from the tip of the conus medullaris to the origin of the filum terminale
Origin: result of canalization and regressive differentiation of the caudal end of the developing spinal cord during embryogenesis
Size: 8–10 mm long, 2–4 mm in diameter
◊ Regresses during the first weeks after birth

DIFFERENTIAL DIAGNOSIS OF BRAIN DISORDERS

BIRTH TRAUMA

1. **Caput succedaneum**
   = localized edema in presenting portion of scalp, frequently associated with microscopic hemorrhage + subcutaneous hyperemia
   Cause: common after vaginal delivery
   • soft superficial pitting edema
   √ crosses suture lines
2. **Subgaleal hemorrhage**
   = hemorrhage between galea aponeurotica (= central fascia formed by occipitofrontal + temporoparietal muscles) and periosteum of outer table
   • may become symptomatic secondary to significant blood loss in children
   • firm fluctuant mass increasing in size after birth
   • may dissect into subcutaneous tissue of neck
   • usually resolves over 2–3 weeks
   ◊ Occasionally due to spontaneous decompression of intracranial (epidural) hematoma
3. **Cephalohematoma**
   = hematoma beneath outer layer of periosteum
   Cause: incorrect application of obstetric forceps / skull fracture during birth
   Incidence: 1–2% of all deliveries
   Location: most commonly parietal
   • firm tense mass
   • usually increase in size after birth
   • resolution in few weeks to months
   √ crescent-shaped lesion adjacent to outer table of skull
   √ will not cross cranial suture line
   √ may calcify / ossify causing thickening of diploe
4. Skull fracture
   Incidence: 1% of all deliveries
   √ CT shows associated intracranial hemorrhage
5. Subdural hemorrhage
   (a) convexity hematoma (b) interhemispheric hematoma (c) posterior fossa hematoma
6. **Benign subdural effusion**
   = benign condition that resolves spontaneously
   • clear / xanthochromic fluid with elevated protein level
   √ extracerebral fluid collection accompanied by ventricular dilatation (= communicating hydrocephalus caused by impaired CSF absorption of these subdural fluid collections)

Glasgow Coma Scale

• eye opening: (1–5)
• motor response: (1–5)
• verbal response: (1–5)
Total: 3–15

INCREASED INTRACRANIAL PRESSURE

1. Intracranial mass
2. Hydrocephalus
3. Malignant hypertension
4. Diffuse cerebral edema
5. Increased venous pressure
6. Elevated CSF protein
7. Pseudotumor cerebri

• papilledema
√ enlargement of perioptic nerve subarachnoid space

PROLACTIN ELEVATION

Normal level: up to 25 ng/mL
Cause:
1. Interference with hypothalamic-pituitary axis:
   (a) hypothalamic tumor
   (b) parasellar tumor
   (c) pituitary adenoma
   (d) sarcoidosis
   (e) histiocytosis
   (f) traumatic infundibular transection
2. Pharmacologic agents
   alpha-methyldopa, reserpine, phenothiazine, butyrophenone, tricyclic antidepressants, oral contraceptives
3. Hypothyroidism (TRH also stimulates prolactin)
4. Renal failure
5. Cirrhosis
6. Stress / recent surgery
7. Breast examination
8. Pregnancy
9. Lactation

STROKE

= generic term designating a heterogeneous group of cerebrovascular disorders
Incidence:
3rd leading cause of death in United States (after heart disease + cancer); 2nd leading cause of death due to cardiovascular disease in U.S.; 2nd leading cause of death in patients >75 years of age; 450,000 new cases per year; 160 new strokes per 100,000 population per year; leading cause of death in Orient
Age: >55 years (12% occur in young adults); M:F = 2:1
Risk factors: heredity, hypertension (50%), smoking, diabetes (15%), obesity, familial hypercholesterolemia, myocardial infarction, atrial fibrillation, congestive heart failure, alcoholic excess, substance abuse, oral contraceptives, pregnancy, high anxiety + stress
Etiology:
A. NONVASCULAR (5%): eg, tumor, hypoxia
B. VASCULAR (95%)
   1. Brain infarction = ischemic stroke (80%)
      (a) Occlusive atheromatous disease of extracranial (35%) / intracranial (10%) arteries
          = large vessel disease between aorta + penetrating arterioles
          — critical stenosis, thrombosis,
          — plaque hemorrhage / ulceration / embolism

(b) Small vessel disease of penetrating arteries (25%) = lacunar infarct
(c) Cardiogenic emboli (6–15–23%)
— Ischemic heart disease with mural thrombus
- acute myocardial infarction (3% risk/ year)
- cardiac arrhythmia
— Valvular heart disease
- postinflammatory (rheumatic) valvulitis
- infective endocarditis (20% risk/year)
- nonbacterial thrombotic endocarditis (30% risk/year)
- mitral valve prolapse (low risk)
- mitral stenosis (20% risk/year)
- prosthetic valves (1–4% risk/year)
— Nonvalvular atrial fibrillation (6% risk/year)
— Left atrial myxoma (27–55% risk/year)
(d) Nonatheromatous disease (5%)
— elongation, coil, kinks (up to 20%)
— fibromuscular dysplasia (typically spares origin + proximal segment of ICA)
— aneurysm (rare) may occur in cervical / petrous portion / intracranially
— dissection: traumatic / spontaneous (2%); up to 15% of strokes in young adults
— cerebral arteritis (Takayasu, collagen disease, lymphoid granulomatosis, temporal arteritis, Behçet disease, chronic meningitis, syphilis)
— postendarterectomy thrombosis / embolism / restenosis
(e) Overactive coagulation (5%)
2. Hemorrhagic stroke (20%)
(a) Primary intracerebral hemorrhage (15%)
— Hypertensive hemorrhage (40–60%)
— Amyloid angiopathy (15–25%)
— Vascular malformation (10–15%)
— Drugs: eg, anticoagulants (1–2%)
— Bleeding diathesis (<1%): eg, hemophilia
(b) Vasospasm due to nontraumatic SAH (4%)
— Ruptured aneurysm (75–80%)
— Vascular malformation (10–15%)
— "Nonaneurysmal" SAH (5–15%)
(c) Veno-occlusive disease (1%): sinus thrombosis

May be preceded by TIA
◊ 10–14% of all strokes are preceded by TIA!
◊ 60% of all strokes ascribed to carotid disease are preceded by TIA!

Prognosis:
(1) death during hospitalization (25%): alteration in consciousness, gaze preference, dense hemiplegia have a 40% mortality rate
(2) survival with varying degrees of neurologic deficit (75%)
(3) good functional recovery (40%)
◊ Hypodensity involving >50% of MCA territory has a fatal outcome in 85%!

◊ Clinical diagnosis inaccurate in 13%!

Role of imaging:
1. Confirm clinical diagnosis
2. Identify primary intracerebral hemorrhage
3. Detect structural lesions mimicking stroke: tumor, vascular malformation, subdural hematoma
4. Detect early complications of stroke: cerebral herniation, hemorrhagic transformation

Indications for cerebrovascular testing:
1. TIA = transient ischemic attack
2. Progression of carotid disease to 95–98% stenosis
3. Cardiogenic cerebral emboli

Temporal classification:
1. **TIA** = transient ischemic attack
2. **RIND** = reversible ischemic neurologic deficit
= fully reversible prolonged ischemic event resulting in minor neurologic dysfunction for >24 hours and <8 weeks
Incidence: 16 per 100,000 population per year
3. **Progressing stroke** = stepwise / gradually progressing accumulative neurologic deficit evolving over hours / days
4. **Slow stroke** = rare clinical syndrome presenting as developing neuronal fatigue with weakness in lower / proximal upper extremity after exercise; occurs in patients with occluded internal carotid artery
5. **Completed stroke** = severe + persistent stable neurologic deficit = cerebral infarction (death of neuronal tissue) as end stage of prolonged ischemia >21 days
• level of consciousness correlates well with size of infarction
Prognosis: 6–11% recurrent stroke rate

TRANSIENT ISCHEMIC ATTACK

= brief episode of transient focal neurological deficit owing to ischemia of <24 hours duration with return to pre-attack status

Incidence: 31 per 100,000 population per year; increasing with age up to 300; 105,000 new cases per year in United States; M > F

Cause:
(1) embolic: usually from ulcerative plaque at carotid bifurcation
(2) hemodynamic: fall in perfusion pressure distal to a high-grade stenosis / occlusion

Risk factors:
(1) Hypertension (linear increase in probability of stroke with increase in diastolic blood pressure)
(2) Cardiac disorders (prior myocardial infarction, angina pectoris, valvular heart disease, dysrhythmia, congestive heart failure)
(3) Diabetes mellitus
(4) Cigarette smoking (weak)

Prognosis: 5.3% stroke rate per year for 5 years after first TIA; per year 12% increase of stroke / myocardial infarction / death; complete stroke in 33% within 5 years; complete stroke in 5% in 1 month

A. CAROTID TIA (2/3)
- carotid attacks <6 hours in 90%
- transient weakness / sensory dysfunction CLASSICALLY in
  (a) hand / face with embolic event
  (b) proximal arm + lower extremity with hemodynamic event (watershed area)
- — motor dysfunction = weakness, paralysis, clumsiness of one / both limbs on same side
- — sensory alteration = numbness, loss of sensation, paresthesia of one / both limbs on same side
- — speech / language disturbance = difficulty in speaking (dys- / aphasia) / writing, in comprehension of language / reading / performing calculations
- — visual disturbance = loss of vision in one eye, homonymous hemianopia, amaurosis fugax
  - paresis (mono-, hemiparesis) in 61%
  - paresthesia (mono-, hemiparesthesia) in 57%
  - amaurosis fugax (= transient premonitory attack of impaired vision due to retinal ischemia) in 12% caused by transient hypotension or emboli of platelets / cholesterol crystals, which may be revealed by funduscopy
  - facial paresthesia in 30%

B. VERTEBROBASILAR TIA (1/3)
- vertebrobasilar events <2 hours in 90%
- — motor dysfunction = as with carotid TIA but sometimes changing from side to side including quadriplegia, diplopia, dysarthria, dysphagia
- — sensory alteration = as with carotid TIA usually involving one / both sides of face / mouth / tongue
- — visual loss = as with carotid TIA including uni- / bilateral homonymous hemianopia
- — disequilibrium of gait / postural disturbance, ataxia, imbalance / unsteadiness
- — drop attack = sudden fall to the ground without loss of consciousness
- binocular visual disturbance in 57%
- vertigo in 50%
- paresthesia in 40%
- diplopia in 38%
- ataxia in 33%
- paresis in 33%
- headaches in 25%
- seizures in 1.5%

Accelerating / crescendo TIA

= repeated periodic events of neurologic dysfunction with complete recovery to normal in interphase

Rx:
1. Carotid endarterectomy (1% mortality, 5% stroke)
2. Anticoagulation
3. Antiplatelet agent: aspirin, ticlopidine (Ticlid®)
   — in patients with recently symptomatic TIA / minor stroke + >70% carotid artery stenosis: prophylactic carotid endarterectomy + chronic low-dose aspirin therapy

DEMENTIA
1. Alzheimer disease
2. Pick disease
3. Normal pressure hydrocephalus
4. Subdural hematoma
5. Brain mass

TRIGEMINAL NEUROPATHY
- facial pain, numbness, weakness of masticatory muscles, trismus
- diminished / absent corneal reflex
- abnormal jaw reflex
- decreased pain / touch / temperature sensation
- atrophy of masticatory muscles
- **tic douloureux** = paroxysmal facial pain (usually confined to V_2 and V_3) mainly caused by neurovascular compression (tortuous elongated superior cerebellar artery / anterior inferior cerebellar artery / vertebrobasilar dolichoectasia / venous compression)

A. BRAINSTEM LESION
1. Vascular: infarct, AVM
2. Neoplastic: glioma, metastasis
3. Inflammatory: multiple sclerosis (1–8%), herpes rhombencephalitis
4. Other: syringobulbia

B. CISTERNAL CAUSES
1. Vascular: aneurysm, AVM, vascular compression
2. Neoplastic: acoustic schwannoma, meningioma, trigeminal schwannoma, epidermoid cyst, lipoma, metastasis
3. Inflammatory: neuritis

C. MECKEL CAVE + CAVERNOUS SINUS
1. Vascular: carotid aneurysm
2. Neoplastic: meningioma, trigeminal schwannoma, epidermoid cyst, lipoma, pituitary adenoma, base of skull neoplasm, metastasis, perineural tumor spread
3. Inflammatory: Tolosa-Hunt syndrome

D. EXTRACRANIAL
1. Neoplastic: neurogenic tumor, squamous cell carcinoma, adenocarcinoma, lymphoma, adenoid cystic carcinoma, mucoepidermoid carcinoma, melanoma, metastasis, perineural tumor spread
2. Inflammatory: sinusitis
3. Other: masticator space abscess, trauma

CLASSIFICATION OF CNS ANOMALIES

A. DORSAL INDUCTION ANOMALY
= defects of neural tube closure
1. Anencephaly
2. Cephalocele: at 4 weeks
3. Chiari malformation: at 4 weeks
4. Spinal dysraphism
5. Hydromyelia

B. VENTRAL INDUCTION ANOMALY
= defects in formation of brain vesicles + face
1. Holoprosencephaly: 5 – 6 weeks
2. Septo-optic dysplasia: 6 – 7 weeks
3. Dandy-Walker malformation: 7 – 10 weeks
4. Agenesis of septum pellucidum

C. NEURONAL PROLIFERATION & HISTOGENESIS
1. Neurofibromatosis: 5 weeks – 6 months
2. Tuberous sclerosis: 5 weeks – 6 months
3. Primary hydranencephaly: >3 months
4. Neoplasia
5. Vascular malformation (vein of Galen, AVM, hemangioma)

D. NEURONAL MIGRATION ANOMALY
due to infection, ischemia, metabolic disorders
1. Schizencephaly: 2 months
2. Agyria + pachygyria: 3 months
3. Gray matter heterotopia: 5 months
4. Dysgenesis of corpus callosum: 2 – 5 months
5. Lissencephaly
6. Polymicrogyria
7. Unilateral megalencephaly

E. DESTRUCTIVE LESIONS
1. Hydranencephaly
2. Porencephaly
3. Hypoxia: periventricular leukomalacia, germinal matrix hemorrhage
4. Toxicosis
5. Infections (TORCH)
   (a) **T**oxoplasmosis
   (b) **O**ther: syphilis, hepatitis, zoster
   (c) **R**ubella
      √ punctate / nodular calcifications
      √ porencephalic cysts
      √ occasionally microcephaly
   (d) **C**ytomegalovirus inclusion disease
      √ typically punctate / stippled / curvilinear periventricular calcifications
      √ often hydrocephalus
   (e) **H**erpes simplex

Absence of Septum Pellucidum
1. Holoprosencephaly
2. Callosal agenesis
3. Septo-optic dysplasia
4. Schizencephaly
5. Severe chronic hydrocephalus
6. Destructive porencephaly

Phakomatoses
phako (Greek) = lens / lentil-shaped object
= NEUROCUTANEOUS SYNDROMES
= NEUROECTODERMAL DYSPLASIAS
= development of benign tumors / malformations especially in organs of ectodermal origin
1. Neurofibromatosis
2. Tuberous sclerosis
3. von Hippel-Lindau disease
4. Sturge-Weber-Dimitri syndrome
5. Ataxia-telangiectasia

DEGENERATIVE DISEASES OF CEREBRAL HEMISPHERES
= progressive fatal disease characterized by destruction / alteration of gray and white matter

Etiology: genetic; viral infection; nutritional disorders (eg, anorexia nervosa, Cushing syndrome); immune system disorders (eg, AIDS); exposure to toxins (eg, CO); exposure to drugs (eg, alcohol, methotrexate + radiation)

Leukodystrophy
= degenerative diffuse sclerosis with symmetrical bilateral white matter lesions

Leukoencephalopathy
= disease of white matter

A. MYELINOCLASTIC / DEMYELINATING DISEASE
= disease that destroys normally formed myelin
◊ Usually affects older children / adults
(a) infectious
   1. Progressive multifocal leukoencephalopathy
   2. Subacute sclerosing panencephalitis (SSPE)
   3. Acute disseminated encephalomyelitis (ADE)
(b) noninfectious
   1. Radiation
   2. Anoxia
   3. Hypertensive encephalopathy
   4. Disseminated necrotizing leukoencephalopathy (from methotrexate therapy)
(c) others
   1. Multiple sclerosis (most frequent primary demyelinating disease)
   2. Alzheimer disease (most common of diffuse gray matter degenerative diseases)
   3. Parkinson disease (most common subcortical degenerative disease)
   4. Creutzfeldt-Jakob disease
   5. Menkes disease (sex-linked recessive disorder of copper metabolism)
   6. Globoid cell leukodystrophy
   7. Spongiform degeneration
   8. Cockayne syndrome
   9. Spongiform leukoencephalopathy
   10. Myelinoclastic diffuse sclerosis (Schilder disease)

B. DYSMYELINATING DISEASE
= metabolic disorder (= enzyme deficiency) resulting in deficient / absent myelin sheaths
◊ Usually presents in first 2 years / 1st decade of life!
◊ Associated with white matter atrophy
(a) macrencephalic:
   1. Alexander disease (frontal areas affected first)
   2. Canavan disease (white matter diffusely affected)
(b) hyperdense thalami, caudate nuclei, corona radiata
   1. Krabbe disease
(c) family history (X-linked recessive)
   1. X-linked adrenoleukodystrophy
   2. Pelizaeus-Merzbacher disease
(d) others
   1. Metachromatic leukodystrophy (most common hereditary leukodystrophy)

2. Binswanger disease (SAE)
3. Multi-infarct dementia (MID)
4. Pick disease
5. Huntington disease
6. Wilson disease
7. Reye syndrome
8. Mineralizing microangiopathy
9. Diffuse sclerosis

BRAIN ATROPHY

Cerebral Atrophy

= irreversible loss of brain substance + subsequent enlargement of intra- and extracerebral CSF-containing spaces (hydrocephalus ex vacuo = ventriculomegaly)

A. DIFFUSE BRAIN ATROPHY
Cause:
(a) Trauma, radiation therapy
(b) Drugs (dilantin, steroids, methotrexate, marijuana, hard drugs, chemotherapy), alcoholism, hypoxia
(c) Demyelinating disease (multiple sclerosis, encephalitis)
(d) Degenerative disease
eg, Alzheimer disease, Pick disease, Jakob-Creutzfeldt disease
(e) Cerebrovascular disease + multiple infarcts
(f) Advancing age, anorexia, renal failure
√ enlarged ventricles + sulci

B. FOCAL BRAIN ATROPHY
Cause: vascular / chemical / metabolic / traumatic / idiopathic (Dyke-Davidoff-Mason syndrome)

C. REVERSIBLE PROCESS SIMULATING ATROPHY (in younger people)
Cause: anorexia nervosa, alcoholism, catabolic steroid treatment, pediatric malignancy

√ prominent sulci
√ ipsilateral dilatation of basal cisterns + ventricles
√ ex vacuo dilatation of ventricles
√ thinning of gyri

Cerebellar Atrophy

A. WITH CEREBRAL ATROPHY
= generalized senile brain atrophy

B. WITHOUT CEREBRAL ATROPHY
1. Olivopontocerebellar degeneration / Marie ataxia / Friedreich ataxia
 • onset of ataxia in young adulthood
2. Ataxia-telangiectasia
3. Ethanol toxicity: predominantly affecting midline (vermis)
4. Phenytoin toxicity: predominantly affecting cerebellar hemispheres
5. Idiopathic degeneration secondary to carcinoma (= paraneoplastic), usually oat cell carcinoma of lung
6. Radiotherapy
7. Focal cerebellar atrophy:
(a) infarction (b) traumatic injury

Intra- versus Extraaxial Mass

	Intraaxial	*Extraaxial*
Relationship to dura	no attachment until advanced	contiguous
Local bony changes	uncommon	common
Cortex displaced	toward bone	away from bone, buckling of gray + white matter, displacement of vessels
Subarachnoid cistern	effaced	widened, CSF cleft
Feeding arteries	pial	dural

Hippocampal Atrophy

1. Alzheimer Disease
2. Mesial temporal sclerosis
 • complex partial seizures
3. Normal in octogenarians

EXTRAAXIAL LESIONS

Extraaxial Tumor

mnemonic: "MABEL"
Meningioma
Arachnoid cyst
Bony lesion
Epidermoid
Leukemic / lymphomatous infiltration

Leptomeningeal Disease

A. INFLAMMATION
1. Langerhans cell histiocytosis
2. Sarcoidosis
3. Wegener granulomatosis
4. Chemical meningitis: rupture of epidermoid

B. INFECTION
1. Bacterial meningitis
2. Tuberculous meningitis
3. Fungal meningitis
4. Neurosyphilis

C. TUMOR
(a) Primary meningeal tumor
1. Meningioma
2. Glioma: primary leptomeningeal glioblastomatosis / gliosarcomatosis
3. Melanoma / melanocytoma
4. Sarcoma
5. Lymphoma
(b) CSF-spread from primary CNS tumor
1. Medulloblastoma
2. Germinoma
3. Pineoblastoma

(c) Metastasis
1. Breast carcinoma
2. Lymphoma / leukemia
3. Lung carcinoma
4. Malignant melanoma
5. Gastrointestinal carcinoma
6. Genitourinary carcinoma

D. TRAUMA
1. Old subarachnoid hemorrhage
2. Surgical scarring from craniotomy
3. Lumbar puncture

Pericerebral Fluid Collection in Childhood

A. ENLARGED SUBARACHNOID SPACE
(a) due to macrocephaly
(b) due to brain atrophy
√ superficial cortical veins cross subarachnoid space to reach superior sagittal sinus
√ wide sulci, normal configuration of gyri
√ normal / prominent size of ventricles

B. SUBDURAL FLUID COLLECTION
(1) Subdural hygroma
(2) Subdural empyema / abscess (due to meningitis)
(3) Subdural hematoma
√ superficial cortical veins are prevented from crossing tge subarachnoid space by the presence of arachnoid / neomembrane
√ wide interhemispheric fissure

Subdural Fluid Collection

A. Hyperdense = acute subdural hematoma
B. Isodense = subacute subdural hematoma
C. Hypodense
1. Chronic subdural hematoma
2. Subdural hygroma
3. Effusion from meningo-encephalitis

HYPODENSE BRAIN LESIONS

Diffusely Swollen Hemispheres

A. METABOLIC
1. Metabolic encephalopathy: eg, uremia, Reye syndrome, ketoacidosis
2. Anoxia: cardiopulmonary arrest, near-drowning, smoke inhalation, ARDS

B. NEUROVASCULAR
1. Hypertensive encephalopathy
2. Superior sagittal sinus thrombosis
3. Head trauma
4. Pseudotumor cerebri

C. INFLAMMATION
eg, herpes encephalitis, CMV, toxoplasmosis

Brain Edema

= increase in brain volume due to increased tissue-water content (80% for gray matter + 68% for white matter is normal)

Etiology:

(a) Cytotoxic edema
reversible increase in intracellular water content secondary to ischemia / anoxia (axonal pallor)

(b) Vasogenic edema (most common form)
increase in pinocytotic activity with passage of protein across vessel wall into intercellular space (lack of contrast enhancement means breakdown of blood-brain barrier is not the cause); associated with primary brain neoplasm, metastases, hemorrhage, infarction, inflammation

Types:

1. Hydrostatic edema
rapid increase / decrease in intracranial pressure
2. Interstitial edema
increase in periventricular interstitial spaces secondary to transependymal flow of CSF with elevated intraventricular pressure
3. Hypoosmotic edema
produced by overhydration from IV fluid / inappropriate secretion of antidiuretic hormone
4. Congestive brain swelling
rapid accumulation of extravascular water as a result of head trauma; may become irreversible (brain death) if intracranial pressure equals systolic blood pressure

√ decreased distinction between gray + white matter
√ compressed slitlike lateral ventricles
√ compression of cerebral sulci + perimesencephalic cisterns

CT:
√ areas of hypodensity
◊ Edema is always greatest in white matter!
√ mass effect: flattening of gyri, displacement + deformation of ventricles, midline shift
√ return to normal from nonhemorrhagic edema / brain atrophy from white matter shearing injury

MR:
√ decreased intensity on T1WI, increased intensity on T2WI
√ enhancement with gadolinium

US:
√ generalized / focal increase of parenchymal echogenicity with featureless appearance
√ decreased resistive indices

Brain Herniation

1. Subfalcine
contralateral shift of midline structures under falx cerebri
2. Transtentorial
(a) upward (superior vermian): displacement of cerebellum through tentorial incisura
(b) downward
– anterior: uncal herniation (most common) caused by lesions in anterior half of brain
– posterior: herniation of parahippocampal gyrus
– total: herniation of entire hippocampus
3. Retroalar
herniation of frontal lobe posteriorly across edge of sphenoid ridge

4. Transforaminal
   herniation of inferior mesial portions of cerebellum downward through foramen magnum (= inferior tonsillar)

Cholesterol-containing CNS Lesions

1. Epidermoid inclusion cyst
2. Cholesterol granuloma
3. Acquired epidermoid of middle ear
4. Congenital cholesteatoma of middle ear
5. Craniopharyngioma

Cyst with Mural Nodule

1. Pilocytic astrocytoma (childhood)
2. Ganglioglioma
3. Pleomorphic xanthoastrocytoma
4. Glioblastoma multiforme
5. Hemangioblastoma (posterior fossa, spinal cord)

Midline Cyst

1. **Cavum septi pellucidi** = "5th ventricle"
   = thin triangular membrane consisting of two glial layers covered laterally with ependyma separating the frontal horns of lateral ventricles
   Incidence: in 80% of term infants; in 15% of adults
   Location: posterior to genu of corpus callosum, inferior to body of corpus callosum, anterosuperior to anterior pillar of fornix
   √ extends to foramen of Monro
   √ may dilate + cause obstructive hydrocephalus (rare)
2. **Cavum vergae** = "6th ventricle"
   = cavity posterior to columns of fornix; contracts after about 6th gestational month
   Incidence: in 30% of term infants; in 15% of adults
   Location: posterior to fornix, anterior to splenium of corpus callosum, inferior to body of corpus callosum, superior to transverse fornix
   √ posterior midline continuation of cavum septi pellucidi beyond foramen of Monro
3. **Cavum veli interpositi**
   = extension of quadrigeminal plate cistern above 3rd ventricle to foramen of Monro, laterally bounded by columns of fornix + thalamus
4. Colloid cyst: anterior + superior to cavum septi pellucidi
5. Arachnoid cyst: in region of quadrigeminal plate cistern
   √ curvilinear margins

Posterior Fossa Cystic Malformation

1. Dandy-Walker malformation
2. Dandy-Walker variant
3. Megacisterna magna
4. Arachnoid pouch

Suprasellar Low-density Lesion with Hydrocephalus

A. CYST
   1. Arachnoid cyst
   2. Ependymal cyst of 3rd ventricle
   3. Parasitic cyst of 3rd ventricle (cysticercosis)
   4. Dilated 3rd ventricle (in aqueductal stenosis)

B. CYSTIC MASS
   1. Epidermoid
   2. Hypothalamic pilocytic astrocytoma
   3. Cystic craniopharyngioma

N.B.: Cystic lesion may be inapparent within surrounding CSF; metrizamide cisternography is helpful in detection + to exclude aqueduct stenosis

Multiple Tiny CNS Cysts

A. DIFFUSE DEGENERATIVE DISEASE
B. DIFFUSE INFLAMMATORY PROCESS
C. LOW-GRADE CYSTIC NEOPLASM
   1. Ganglioglioma
   2. Pyelocytic astrocytoma
   3. Pleomorphic xanthoastrocytoma

Mesencephalic Low-density Lesion

1. Normal: decussation of superior cerebellar peduncles at level of inferior colliculi
2. Syringobulbia
   found in conjunction with syringomyelia, Arnold-Chiari malformation, trauma
   √ CSF density centrally
   √ intrathecal contrast enters central cavity
3. Brainstem infarction
   √ abnormal contrast enhancement after 1 week
   √ well-defined low-attenuation region without enhancement after 2–4 weeks
4. Central pontine myelinolysis
5. Brainstem glioma
   √ mass with indistinct margins + vague enhancement
6. Metastasis
   √ well-defined contrast enhancement
7. Granuloma in TB / sarcoidosis (rare)

Intracranial Pneumocephalus

Cause:

A. TRAUMA (74%):
   (a) blunt trauma
      in 3% of all skull fractures; in 8% of fractures involving paranasal sinuses (frontal > ethmoid > sphenoid > mastoid) or base of skull
   (b) penetrating injury

B. NEOPLASM INVADING SINUS (13%):
   1. Osteoma of frontal / ethmoid sinus
   2. Pituitary adenoma
   3. Mucocele, epidermoid
   4. Malignancy of paranasal sinuses

C. INFECTION WITH GAS-FORMING ORGANISM (9%):
   in mastoiditis, sinusitis

D. SURGERY (4%):
   hypophysectomy, paranasal sinus surgery

Mechanism (dural laceration):
(1) ball-valve mechanism during straining, coughing, sneezing
(2) vacuum phenomenon secondary to loss of CSF

Time of onset: on initial presentation (25%), usually seen within 4–5 days, delay up to 6 months (33%)
Mortality: 15%
Cx: (1) CSF rhinorrhea (50%)
(2) Meningitis / epidural / brain abscess (25%)
(3) Extracranial pneumocephalus = air collection in subaponeurotic space

HYPERDENSE INTRACRANIAL LESIONS

Intracranial Calcifications

mnemonic: "PINEEAL"
Physiologic
Infection
Neoplasm
Endocrine
Embryologic
Arteriovenous
Leftover Ls

A. PHYSIOLOGIC INTRACRANIAL CALCIFICATIONS
B. INFECTION
TORCH (toxoplasmosis, others [syphilis, hepatitis, zoster], CMV, rubella, herpes), healed abscess, hydatid cyst, granuloma (tuberculoma, actinomycosis, coccidioidomycosis, cryptococcosis, mucormycosis), cysticercosis, trichinosis, paragonimiasis
mnemonic:
CM**V** calcifications are **c**ircum**v**entricular
Toxoplasma calcifications are in**t**raparenchymal
C. NEOPLASM
Craniopharyngioma (40–80%), oligodendroglioma (50–70%), chordoma (25–40%), choroid plexus papilloma (10%), meningioma (20%), pituitary adenoma (3–5%), pinealoma (10–20%), dermoid (20%), lipoma of corpus callosum, ependymoma (50%), astrocytoma (15%), after radiotherapy, metastases (1–2%, lung > breast > GI tract)
N.B.: astrocytomas calcify less frequently but are the most common tumor
mnemonic: "Ca^{2+} COME"
Craniopharyngioma
Astrocytoma, **A**neurysm,
Choroid plexus papilloma
Oligodendroglioma
Meningioma, **M**edulloblastoma
Ependymoma
D. ENDOCRINE
Hyperparathyroidism, hypervitaminosis D, hypoparathyroidism, pseudohypoparathyroidism, CO poisoning, lead poisoning
E. EMBRYOLOGIC
Neurocutaneous syndromes (tuberous sclerosis, Sturge-Weber, neurofibromatosis), Fahr disease, Cockayne syndrome, basal cell nevus syndrome
F. ARTERIOVENOUS
Atherosclerosis, aneurysm, AVM, occult vascular malformation, hemangioma, subdural + epidural hematomas, intracerebral hemorrhage
G. LEFTOVER Ls
Lipoma, lipoid proteinosis, lissencephaly

Physiologic Intracranial Calcification

1. Pineal calcification
Age: no calcification <5 years of age, in 8–10% at 8–14 years of age, in 40% by 20 years of age, 2/3 of adult population
√ amorphous / ringlike calcification <3 mm from midline usually <10 mm in diameter
√ approximately 30 mm above highest posterior elevation of pyramids
CAVE: pineal calcification >14 mm suggests pineal neoplasm (teratoma / pinealoma)
2. Habenula
Incidence: approximately in 1/3 of population
Age: >10 years of age
√ posteriorly open C-shaped calcification 4–6 mm anterior to pineal gland
3. Choroid plexus
may calcify in all ventricles: most commonly in glomus within atrium of lateral ventricles, near foramen of Monro, tela choroidea of 3rd ventricle, roof of 4th ventricle, along foramina of Luschka
Age: >3 years of age
√ 20–30 mm behind + slightly below pineal on lateral projection, symmetrical on AP projection
DDx: neurofibromatosis
4. Dura, falx cerebri, falx cerebelli, tentorium
Incidence: 10% of population
Age: >3 years of age
DDx: basal cell nevus syndrome (Gorlin syndrome), pseudoxanthoma elasticum, congenital myotonic dystrophy
5. Petroclinoid ligament (= reflection of tentorium) between tip of dorsum sellae and apex of petrous bone
Age: >5 years of age
6. Interclinoid ligament
= interclinoid bridging
7. Arteriosclerosis: particularly intracavernous segment of ICA, basilar a., vertebral a.
8. Basal ganglia

Increased Density of Falx

1. Subarachnoid hemorrhage
2. Interhemispheric subdural hematoma
3. Diffuse cerebral edema (= increased density relative to low-density brain)
4. Dural calcifications (hypercalcemia from chronic renal failure, basal cell nevus syndrome, hyperparathyroidism)
5. Normal falx (can be normal in pediatric population)

Intraparenchymal Hemorrhage

mnemonic: "ITHACANS"

Infarction (hemorrhagic)
Trauma
Hypertensive hemorrhage
Arteriovenous malformation
Coagulopathy
Aneurysm, **A**myloid angiopathy
Neoplasm: metastasis / primary neoplasm
Sinus thrombosis

Dense Cerebral Mass

Substrate: calcification / hemorrhage / dense protein

A. VESSEL
   1. Aneurysm
   2. Arteriovenous malformation
   3. Hematoma (acute / subacute)

B. TUMOR
   1. Lymphoma
   2. Medulloblastoma
   3. Meningioma
   4. Metastasis
      (a) from mucinous-producing adenocarcinoma
      (b) hemorrhagic metastases: melanoma, choriocarcinoma, hypernephroma, bronchogenic carcinoma, breast carcinoma (rarely)

Dense Lesion near Foramen of Monro

A. INTRAVENTRICULAR LESION
   1. Colloid cyst
   2. Meningioma
   3. Choroid plexus tumor / granuloma
   4. AVM of septal, thalamostriate, internal cerebral veins

B. PERIVENTRICULAR MASS
   1. Primary CNS lymphoma
   2. Tuberous sclerosis
      (a) subependymal tuber
      (b) giant cell astrocytoma
   3. Metastasis from mucin-producing adenocarcinoma / hemorrhagic metastasis (melanoma, choriocarcinoma, hypernephroma, bronchogenic carcinoma, breast carcinoma)
   4. Glioblastoma of septum pellucidum

C. MASSES PROJECTING SUPERIORLY FROM SKULL BASE
   1. Pituitary adenoma
   2. Craniopharyngioma
   3. Aneurysm
   4. Dolichoectatic basilar artery

BRAIN MASSES

Classification of Primary CNS Tumors

A. TUMORS OF BRAIN AND MENINGES
   (a) Gliomas
      ASTROCYTOMA (50%)
         1. Astrocytoma (astrocytoma grades I–II)
         2. Glioblastoma (astrocytoma grades III–IV)
      OLIGODENDROGLIOMA
      PARAGLIOMA
         1. Ependymoma
         2. Choroid plexus papilloma
      GANGLIOGLIOMA
      MEDULLOBLASTOMA
   (b) Pineal tumor
      1. Germinoma
      2. Teratoma
      3. Pineocytoma
      4. Pineoblastoma
   (c) Pituitary tumor
      1. Pituitary adenoma
      2. Pituitary carcinoma
   (d) Meningioma
   (e) Nerve sheath tumor
      1. Schwannoma
      2. Neurofibroma
   (f) Miscellaneous
      1. Sarcoma
      2. Lipoma
      3. Hemangioblastoma

B. TUMORS OF EMBRYONAL REMNANTS
   (a) Craniopharyngioma
   (b) Colloid cyst
   (c) Teratoid tumor
      1. Epidermoid
      2. Dermoid
      3. Teratoma

Incidence of Brain Tumors

= 9% of all primary neoplasms (5th most common primary neoplasm); 5–10 cases per 100,000 population per year; account for 1.2% of autopsied deaths

Incidence of Brain Tumors

All Age Groups		*Pediatric Age Group*	
Glioma	34%	Astrocytoma	50%
Meningioma	17%	Medulloblastoma	15%
Metastasis	12%	Ependymoma	10%
Pituitary adenoma	6%	Craniopharyngioma	6%
Neurinoma	4%	Choroid plexus papilloma	2%
Sarcoma	3%		
Granuloma	3%		
Craniopharyngioma	2%		
Hemangioblastoma	2%		

CNS Tumors Presenting at Birth

1. Hypothalamic astrocytoma
2. Choroid plexus papilloma / carcinoma
3. Teratoma
4. Primitive neuroectodermal tumor
5. Medulloblastoma
6. Ependymoma
7. Craniopharyngioma

CNS Tumors in Pediatric Age Group

Incidence:
2.4:100,000 (<15 years of age); 2nd most common pediatric tumor (after leukemia); 15% of all pediatric neoplasms; 15–20% of all primary brain tumors; M > F

- increased intracranial pressure
- increasing head size

A. SUPRATENTORIAL (50%)
Age: first 2–3 years of life

Covering of brain	dural sarcoma, schwannoma, meningioma (3%)
Cerebral hemisphere	astrocytoma (37%), oligodendroglioma
Corpus callosum	astrocytoma
3rd ventricle	colloid cyst, ependymoma
Lateral ventricle	ependymoma (5%), choroid plexus papilloma (12%)
Optic chiasm	craniopharyngioma (12%), optic nerve glioma (13%), teratoma, pituitary adenoma
Hypothalamus	glioma (8%), hamartoma
Pineal region	germinoma, pinealoma, teratoma (8%)

B. INFRATENTORIAL (50%)
Age: 4–11 years

Cerebellum	astrocytoma (31–33%), PNET / medulloblastoma (26–31%)
Brainstem	glioma (16–21%)
4th ventricle	ependymoma (6–14%), choroid plexus papilloma

mnemonic: "BE MACHO"
Brainstem glioma
Ependymoma
Medulloblastoma
AVM
Cystic astrocytoma
Hemangioblastoma
Other

	PNET	*Ependymoma*	*Astrocytoma*
CT	hyper	iso	hypo
T2WI	intermed.	intermed.	increased
Enhancement	moderate	minimal	nodule
Calcification	10–15%	40–50%	<10%
Cyst formation	rare	common	typical
CSF seeding	15–40%	rare	rare
Foraminal spread	no	yes	no

Supratentorial Midline Tumors

1. Optic + hypothalamic glioma (39%)
2. Craniopharyngioma (20%)
3. Astrocytoma (9%)
4. Pineoblastoma (9%)
5. Germinoma (6%)
6. Lipoma (6%)
7. Teratoma (3.5%)
8. Pituitary adenoma (3.5%)
9. Meningioma (2%)
10. Choroid plexus papilloma (2%)

Supratentorial Intraventricular Tumors

(a) Lateral ventricle (3/4)
1. Choroid plexus tumor (44%)
2. Giant cell astrocytoma in tuberous sclerosis (19%)
3. Hemangioma in Sturge-Weber syndrome (12%)

(b) Third ventricle (1/4)
1. Astrocytoma (13%)
2. Choroid plexus tumor (6%)
3. Meningioma (6%)

CLASSIFICATION BY HISTOLOGY
1. Astrocytic tumors (33.5%)
2. "Primitive" neuroectodermal tumor = PNET (21%)
highly malignant neoplasms originating from germinal matrix + containing glial + neural elements
   — Medulloblastoma (16%)
   — Ependymoblastoma (2.5%)
   — PNET of cerebral hemisphere (2.5%)
3. Mixed gliomas (16%)
4. Malformative tumors (11.5%)
   — Craniopharyngioma (5.5%)
   — Lipoma (4.5%)
   — Dermoid cyst (1%)
   — Epidermal cyst (0.5%)
5. Choroid plexus tumors (4%)
6. Ependymal tumors (4%)
7. Tumors of meningeal tissues (3.5%)
   — Meningioma (3%)
   — Meningeal sarcoma (0.5%)
8. Germ cell tumors (2.5%)
   — Germinoma (1.5%)
   — Teratomatous tumor (1%)
9. Neuronal tumors
   — Gangliocytoma (1.5%)
10. Tumors of neuroendocrine origin
   — Pituitary adenoma (1%)
11. Oligodendroglial tumors (0.5%)
12. Tumors of blood vessel
   — Hemangioma (1%)

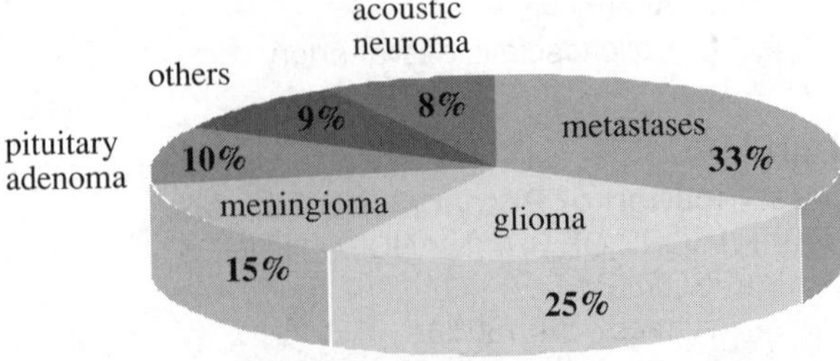

Intracranial Tumors in Adult Population

Superficial Gliomas

= peripherally located cortical neoplasms serving as a seizure focus

1. Ganglioglioma
2. Desmoplastic infantile ganglioglioma
3. Gangliocytoma
4. Dysplastic cerebellar gangliocytoma
5. Pleomorphic xanthoastrocytoma
6. Dysembryoplastic neuroepithelial tumor

Multifocal CNS Tumors

A. METASTASES FROM PRIMARY CNS TUMOR
   (a) via commissural pathways: corpus callosum, internal capsule, massa intermedia
   (b) via CSF: ventricles / subarachnoid cisterns
   (c) satellite metastases
B. MULTICENTRIC CNS TUMOR
   (a) true multicentric gliomas (4%)
   (b) concurrent tumors of different histology (coincidental)
C. MULTICENTRIC MENINGIOMAS (3%) without neurofibromatosis
D. MULTICENTRIC PRIMARY CNS LYMPHOMA
E. PHAKOMATOSES
   1. Generalized neurofibromatosis:
      meningiomatosis, bilateral acoustic neuromas, bilateral optic nerve gliomas, cerebral gliomas, choroid plexus papillomas, multiple spine tumors, AVMs
   2. Tuberous sclerosis:
      subependymal tubers, intraventricular gliomas (giant cell astrocytoma), ependymomas
   3. von Hippel-Lindau disease:
      retinal angiomatosis, hemangioblastomas, congenital cysts of pancreas + liver, benign renal tumors, cardiac rhabdomyomas

CNS Tumors Metastasizing Outside CNS

mnemonic: "MEGO"

Medulloblastoma
Ependymoma
Glioblastoma multiforme
Oligodendroglioma

Calcified Intracranial Mass

mnemonic: "Ca^{2+} COME"

Craniopharyngioma
Astrocytoma, **A**neurysm
Choroid plexus papilloma
Oligodendroglioma
Meningioma
Ependymoma

Avascular Mass of Brain

mnemonic: "TEACH"

Tumor: astrocytoma, metastasis, oligodendroglioma
Edema
Abscess
Cyst, **C**ontusion
Hematoma, **H**erpes

Jugular Foramen Mass

A. NONNEOPLASTIC ENTITIES
   1. Asymmetrically enlarged jugular foramen
   2. High-riding jugular bulb
   3. **Dehiscent jugular bulb**
      • pulsatile tinnitus
      • vascular tympanic membrane
      √ middle ear soft-tissue mass contiguous with jugular foramen (= jugular bulb bulging into middle ear cavity)
      √ absence of bony plate separating jugular bulb from posteroinferior middle ear cavity
      DDx: Jugular megabulb (rises above floor of EAC but with preservation of bony plate)
   4. Jugular vein thrombosis
B. NEOPLASM
   1. Paraganglioma = glomus tumor
   2. Nerve sheath tumor = neuroma
   3. Meningioma
   4. Vascular metastasis (renal / thyroid cancer)
C. PRIMARY BONE LESION
   1. Multiple myeloma
   2. Lymphoma
   3. Langerhans cell histiocytosis

Dumbbell Mass Spanning Petrous Apex

1. Large trigeminal schwannoma
2. Meningioma
3. Epidermoid cyst

Posterior Fossa Tumor In Adult

Extraaxial	*Intraaxial*
1. Acoustic neuroma	1. Metastasis (lung, breast)
2. Meningioma	2. Hemangioblastoma
3. Chordoma	3. Lymphoma
4. Choroid plexus papilloma	4. Lipoma
5. Epidermoid	5. Glioma

Cerebellopontine Angle Tumor

= extraaxial tumor arising in CSF-filled space bound by pons + cerebellar hemisphere + petrous bone

Incidence: 5–10% of all intracranial tumors

• cranial neuropathy: high frequency hearing loss (n. VIII), tinnitus + facial motor dysfunction (n. V II), facial sensory dysfunction (n. V), taste disturbance (chorda tympani)
• signs of posterior fossa mass effect: headache, nausea, vomiting, disequilibrium, ataxia
• hemifacial spasm, trigeminal neuralgia (tic douloureux)
√ may widen CSF space (cistern) in 25%
√ bone erosion / hyperostosis
√ sharp margination with brain

Types:

1. Acoustic neuroma = schwannoma (80–90%): from intracanalicular portion of 8th cranial nerve

2. Meningioma (10–18%)
   2nd most common extraaxial mass in posterior fossa; <5% of all intracranial meningiomas; larger + more hemispheric in shape + more homogeneously enhancing than acoustic neuroma
3. Epidermoid inclusion cyst (5–9%)
4. Arachnoid cyst (<1%)
5. Aneurysm of basilar / vertebral / posterior inferior cerebellar artery:
   congenital berry aneurysm / saccular aneurysm / atherosclerotic dolichoectasia
6. Choroid plexus papilloma
7. Ependymoma
8. Trigeminal neuroma
   from gasserian ganglion within Meckel cave in the most anteromedial portion of petrous pyramid / trigeminal nerve root
9. Glomus jugulare tumor
   within adventitia of bulb of jugular vein at base of petrous bone with invasion of posterior fossa
10. Chordoma
11. Exophytic brainstem glioma
    Histo: usually diffuse fibrillary astrocytoma
12. Metastasis (0.2–2%)
13. Lipoma (<1%)

mnemonic: "**E**ver **G**rave **C**erebello**P**ontine **A**ngle **M**asses"

Epidermoid
Glomus jugulare tumor
Chondroma, **C**hordoma, **C**holesteatoma
Pituitary tumor, **P**ontine glioma (exophytic)
Acoustic + trigeminal neuroma, **A**neurysm of basilar / vertebral artery, **A**rachnoid cyst
Meningioma, **M**etastasis

	Meningioma	*Schwannoma*
Angle with dura	obtuse	acute
Dural tail	frequent	rare
Calcification	20%	rare
Cystic/necrotic	rare	10%
IAC involvement	rare	80%
NECT	hyperdense	isodense
Enhancement	uniform	32% nonuniform

Low-attenuation Extraaxial Lesion

1. Acoustic schwannoma (occasionally low-density mass)
2. Epidermoid tumor
3. Arachnoid cyst

	Epidermoid	*Arachnoid Cyst*
CT density	± hyperdense to CSF	CSF-like
Margins	scalloped	smooth
Vessels	encased	displaced
Proton density	deviates from CSF	CSF-like
Diffusion	restricted	CSF-like

Cystic Mass in Cerebellar Hemisphere

1. Hemangioblastoma
2. Cerebellar astrocytoma
3. Metastasis
4. Lateral medulloblastoma (= "cerebellar sarcoma")
5. Choroid plexus papilloma with lateral extension

Lesion Expanding Cavernous Sinus

A. TUMOR
   1. Trigeminal schwannoma
   2. Pituitary adenoma
   3. Parasellar meningioma
   4. Parasellar metastasis
   5. Invasion by tumor of skull base
B. VESSEL
   1. Internal carotid artery aneurysm
   2. Carotid-cavernous fistula
   3. Cavernous sinus thrombosis
C. TOLOSA-HUNT SYNDROME
   = granulomatous invasion of cavernous sinus

Corpus Callosum Lesion

A. TUMOR
   1. GBM
   2. Lymphoma
   3. Metastasis
B. TRAUMA
   1. Shearing injury
C. WHITE MATTER DISEASE
   1. Multiple sclerosis
   2. Progressive multifocal leukoencephalopathy
   3. Adrenoleukodystrophy
   4. Marchiafava-Bignami disease
C. INFECTION
   1. Toxoplasmosis

Ring-enhancing Lesion Crossing Corpus Callosum

mnemonic: "GAL"

Glioblastoma multiforme (butterfly glioma)
Astrocytoma
Lymphoma

ENHANCING BRAIN LESIONS

Gyral Enhancement

A. MENINGEAL TUMOR
   (a) Meningeal carcinomatosis from systemic tumor: eg, breast carcinoma, small cell carcinoma of lung, malignant melanoma, lymphoma / leukemia
   (b) Seeding primary CNS tumor:
      1. Medulloblastoma
      2. Pineoblastoma
      3. Ependymoma
B. MENINGITIS
   pyogenic, tuberculous, fungal, cysticercosis, sarcoidosis

C. SEQUELAE OF SUBARACHNOID HEMORRHAGE (from fibroblastic proliferation)
D. SUBACUTE BRAIN INFARCT

mnemonic: "CAL MICE"
Cerebritis
Arteriovenous malformation
Lymphoma
Meningitis
Infarct
Carcinomatosis
Encephalitis

Solitary Ring-enhancing Lesion of Brain

Cause:

A. NEOPLASM
1. Primary neoplasm: high-grade glioma, meningioma, lymphoma, leukemia, pituitary macroadenoma, acoustic neuroma, craniopharyngioma
2. Metastatic carcinoma + sarcoma

B. ABSCESS
1. Abscess: bacterial, fungal, parasitic
2. Empyema of epidural / subdural / intraventricular spaces

C. HEMORRHAGIC-ISCHEMIC LESION
1. Resolving infarction
2. Aging hematoma
3. Operative bed following resection
4. Thrombosed aneurysm

D. DEMYELINATING DISORDER
1. Radiation necrosis
2. Tumefactive demyelinating lesion ("singular sclerosis")
3. Necrotizing leukoencephalopathy after methotrexate

Pathogenesis:
(1) hypervascular margin of lesion = granulation tissue / peripheral vascular channels / hypervascular tumor capsule
(2) breakdown of blood-brain barrier = leakage of contrast out of abnormally permeable vessels into extracellular fluid space
(3) hypodense center = avascular / hypovascular (requires time to fill) / cystic degeneration

Incidence of ring blush:
abscess (in 73%); glioblastoma (in 48%); metastasis (in 33%); grade II astrocytoma (in 26%) [NOT in grade I astrocytoma]

mnemonic: "MAGICAL DR"
Metastasis
Abscess / cerebritis
Glioblastoma multiforme, **G**lioma
Infarct (resolving), **I**mpact
Contusion
AIDS toxoplasmosis
Lymphoma (often AIDS-related)
Demyelinating disease
Radiation necrosis, **R**esolving hematoma

Small Spherical Ring-enhancing Lesion at Corticomedullary Margin + Substantial Amount of Vasogenic Edema

1. Metastasis
2. Abscess of brain
   (a) bacterial, fungal, granulomatous
   (b) parasitic: cysticercosis, paragonimiasis, echinococcus
3. Subacute infarction
4. Resolving hematoma

Dense & Enhancing Lesions

1. Aneurysm
2. Meningioma
3. CNS lymphoma
4. Medulloblastoma
5. Metastasis

Multifocal Enhancing Lesions

1. Multiple infarctions
2. Arteriovenous malformations
3. Multifocal primary / secondary neoplasms
4. Multifocal infectious processes
5. Demyelinating diseases: eg, multiple sclerosis

Innumerable Small Enhancing Cerebral Nodules

A. METASTASES
B. PRIMARY CNS LYMPHOMA
C. DISSEMINATED INFECTION
1. Cysticercosis
2. Histoplasmosis
3. Tuberculosis

D. INFLAMMATION
1. Sarcoidosis
2. Multiple sclerosis

E. SUBACUTE MULTIFOCAL INFARCTION
from hypoperfusion, multiple emboli, cerebral vasculitis (SLE), meningitis, cortical vein thrombosis

Enhancing Lesion in Internal Auditory Canal

A. NEOPLASTIC
1. Acoustic schwannoma
2. Ossifying hemangioma

B. NONNEOPLASTIC
1. Sarcoidosis
2. Meningitis
3. Postmeningitic / postcraniotomy fibrosis
4. Vascular loop of anterior inferior cerebellar a.

VASCULAR DISEASE OF BRAIN

Classification of Vascular CNS Anomalies

A. VASCULAR MALFORMATION
(a) arterial = arteriovenous malformation (AVM)
   1. Facial / brain arteriovenous malformation
   2. Vein of Galen malformation

(b) capillary = telangiectasia
   1. Facial port wine stain
   • commonly asymptomatic

(c) venous = venous malformation
= tangle of abnormal varices of a "caput-medusae" / "spoked-wheel" configuration draining into a dilated cortical vein
- soft + compressible without thrills / pulsations
- distension with Valsalva maneuver
- commonly asymptomatic

Location: white matter with normal intervening brain parenchyma

Cx (uncommon): hemorrhage, ischemia
1. Venous angioma
2. Sinus pericranii

(d) lymphatic
1. Cystic hygroma

(e) combinations
1. Sturge-Weber disease
2. Rendu-Osler-Weber disease

B. VASCULAR TUMOR
1. Hemangioma
   (a) capillary hemangioma: seen in children, involution by 7 years of age in 95%
   (b) cavernous hemangioma: seen in adults, no involution
   √ thrombosed blood + hemosiderin
   √ normal angiogram
2. Hemangiopericytoma
3. Hemangioendothelioma
4. Angiosarcoma

<u>Occult / cryptic vascular malformation</u>
1. Cavernous hemangioma
2. Capillary telangiectasia

Occlusive Vascular Disease

(a) Embolic state:
√ single vascular territory

(b) Hypoperfusive state:
√ multiple vascular territories

Cause:
1. Vasospasm from subarachnoid hemorrhage
2. Embolic infarction (50%)
   (a) thrombus (atrial fibrillation, valvular disease, Atheromatous plaques of extracerebral arteries, fibromuscular dysplasia, intracranial aneurysm, surgery, paradoxic emboli, sickle cell disease, atherosclerosis, thrombotic thrombocytopenic purpura)
   - fluctuating blood pressures
   - hypercoagulability
   √ cerebral petechial hemorrhage within cortical / basal gray matter during 2nd week (from fragments of embolus) in up to 40%; initial ischemia is followed by reperfusion (= HALLMARK of embolic infarction)
   √ "supernormal artery" on NECT = high-density material lodged in cerebral vessel near major bifurcations
   √ atheromatous narrowing of vessels
   (b) fat
   (c) nitrogen
3. Watershed infarct
   involving deep white matter between two adjacent vascular beds in global hypoperfusion secondary to poor cardiac output / cervical carotid artery occlusion
   ◊ 6% of cerebral infarcts have hemorrhage (red infarct)
   - stroke (3rd most common cause of death in USA, 5% of stroke syndromes are caused by underlying tumor)
   - TIA = transitory ischemic attack: clears within 24 hours
   - RIND = reversible ischemic neurologic deficit: still evident >24 hours with eventual total recovery
   - amaurosis fugax = transient monocular blindness
   - weakness / numbness in an extremity
   - aphasia
   - dizziness, diplopia, dysarthria (vertebrobasilar ischemia)
4. Hypertension
   (a) Hypertensive encephalopathy
   √ diffuse white matter hypodensity (edema secondary to arterial spasm)
   (b) Hypertensive hemorrhage
   Location: basal ganglia (putamen, external capsule), thalamus, pons, cerebellum
   (c) Lacunar infarction
   (d) Subcortical arteriosclerotic encephalopathy
5. Amyloidosis
   involvement of small- + medium-sized arteries of meninges + cortex
   - normotensive patient >65 years of age
   √ multiple simultaneous / recurrent cortical hemorrhages
6. Vasculitis
   (a) Bacterial meningitis, TB, syphilis, fungus, virus, rickettsia
   (b) Collagen-vascular disease: Wegener granulomatosis, polyarteritis nodosa, SLE, scleroderma, dermatomyositis
   (c) Granulomatous angitis: giant cell arteritis, sarcoidosis, Takayasu disease, temporal arteritis
   (d) Inflammatory arteritis: rheumatoid arteritis, hypersensitivity arteritis, Behçet disease, lymphomatoid granulomatosis
   (e) Drug-induced: IV amphetamine, ergot preparations, oral contraceptives
   (f) Radiation arteritis = mineralizing microangiopathy
   (g) Moyamoya disease
7. Anoxic encephalopathy
   cardiorespiratory arrest, near-drowning, drug overdose, CO poisoning
8. Venous thrombosis

Multiple Infarctions

◊ Typical in extracranial occlusive disease, cardiac output problems, small vessel disease; in 6% from a shower of emboli

Location: usually bilateral + supratentorial (3/4); supra- and infratentorial (1/4)

Displacement of Vessels

A. ARTERIAL SHIFT
   (a) Pericallosal arteries
      1. Round shift = frontal lesion anterior to coronal suture
      2. Square shift = lesion behind foramen of Monro in lower half of hemisphere
      3. Distal shift = posterior to coronal suture in upper half of hemisphere
      4. Proximal shift = basifrontal lesion / anterior middle cranial fossa including anterior temporal lobe
   (b) Sylvian triangle
      = branches of MCA within sylvian fissure on outer surface of insula form a loop upon reaching the upper margin of the insula; serves as angiographic landmark for localizing supratentorial masses

      Location of lesion:

– anterior sylvian	frontal region
– suprasylvian	posterior frontal + parietal
– retrosylvian	occipital, parieto-occipital
– infrasylvian	temporal lobe + extracerebral region
– intrasylvian	usually due to meningioma
– lateral sylvian	frontal, frontotemporal, parietotemporal
– central sylvian	deep posterior frontal, basal ganglia

B. CEREBRAL VEINS
   = indicate the midline of the posterior part of the forebrain showing the exact location of the roof of the 3rd ventricle

BRAIN VENTRICLES

Ventriculomegaly

A. MACROCEPHALY
   • increased intraventricular pressure
   (a) Obstruction to CSF flow
      1. Communicating hydrocephalus
      2. Noncommunicating hydrocephalus
   (b) Overproduction of CSF = nonobstructive hydrocephalus
   (c) Neoplasm

B. MICROCEPHALY
   • normal intraventricular pressure
   (a) Primary failure of brain growth
      — dysgenesis
         1. Holoprosencephaly
         2. Aneuploidy syndromes (trisomies)
         3. Migrational (<6 layers)
      — environment: alcohol, drugs, toxins
      — infection: TORCH

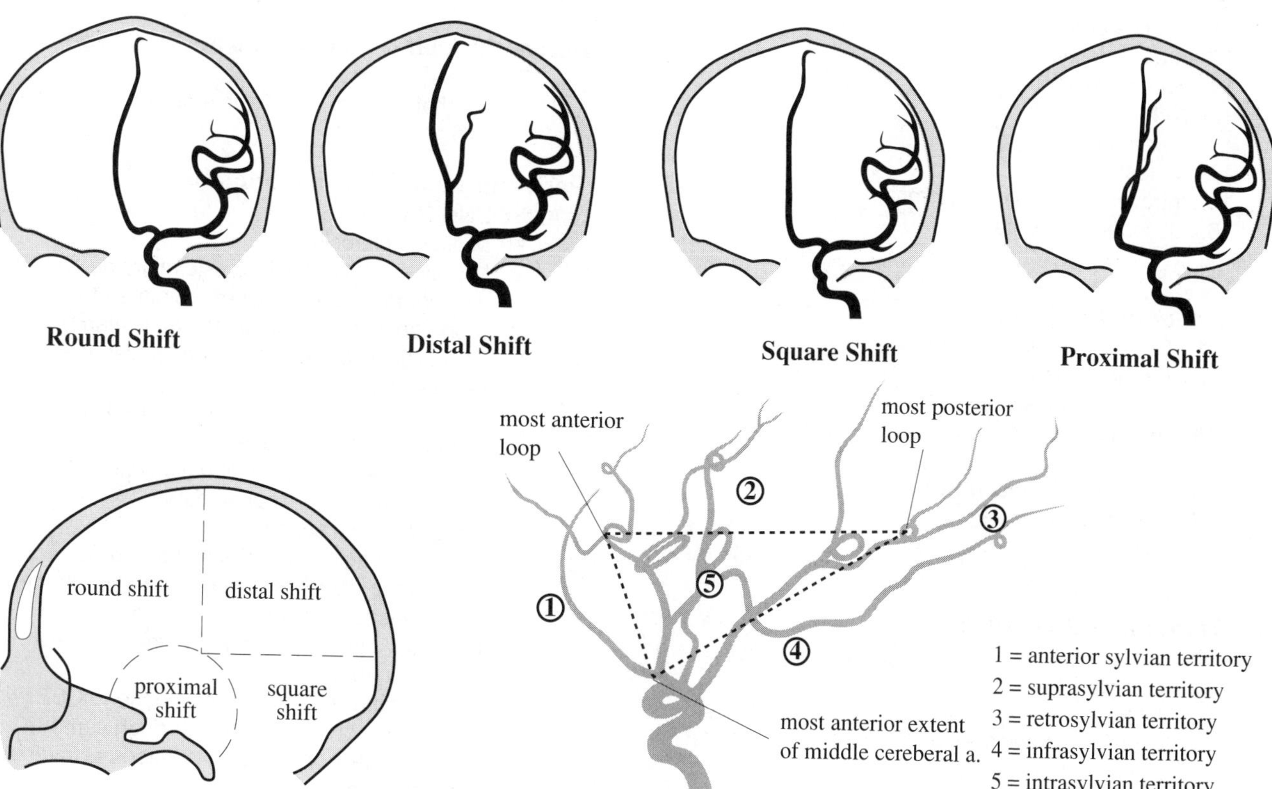

Sylvian Triangle and Intracranial Shifts

(b) Loss of brain mantle
— Infection: TORCH
— Vascular accident:
1. Hydranencephaly
2. Schizencephaly
3. Porencephaly
— Hemorrhage:
1. Porencephaly
2. Leukomalacia

C. NORMOCEPHALY

Colpocephaly

= dilatation of trigones + occipital horns + posterior temporal horns of lateral ventricles

1. Agenesis of corpus callosum
2. Arnold-Chiari malformation
3. Holoprosencephaly

Intraventricular Tumor

Prevalence: 10% of all intracranial neoplasms

1. Ependymoma	20%
2. Astrocytoma	18%
3. Colloid cyst	12%
4. Meningioma	11%
5. Choroid plexus papilloma	7%
6. Epidermoid / dermoid	6%
7. Craniopharyngioma	6%
8. Medulloblastoma	5%
9. Cysticercosis	5%
10. Arachnoid cyst	4%
11. Subependymoma	2%
12. AVM	2%
13. Teratoma	1%
14. Metastasis	
15. Intraventricular neurocytoma	
16. Oligodendroglioma	

Tumor in 4th Ventricle

1. Choroid plexus papilloma
2. Ependymoma / glioma
3. Hemangioblastoma
4. Vermian metastasis
5. AVM
6. Epidermoid tumor (rare)
7. Inflammatory mass
8. Cyst

Tumor in 3rd Ventricle

1. Colloid cyst
2. Glioma
3. Aneurysm
4. Craniopharyngioma
5. Ependymoma
6. Meningioma
7. Choroid plexus papilloma
8. Intraventricular neurocytoma

PERIVENTRICULAR REGION

Periventricular Hypodensity

1. Encephalomalacia
√ slightly denser than CSF
2. Porencephaly
= cavity communicating with ventricle / cistern from intracerebral hemorrhage
Associated with: dilated ventricle, sulci, and fissures
√ CSF density
3. Resolving hematoma
• history of previously demonstrated hematoma
√ may show ring enhancement + compression of adjacent structures
4. Cystic tumor
√ mass effect + contrast enhancement

Enhancing Ventricular Margins

(a) Subependymal spread of metastatic tumor
1. Bronchogenic carcinoma (especially small cell carcinoma)
2. Melanoma
3. Breast carcinoma

(b) Subependymal seeding of CNS primary
1. Glioma
2. Ependymoma

(c) Ependymal seeding of CNS primary
1. Medulloblastoma
2. Germinoma

(d) Primary CNS lymphoma / systemic lymphoma

(e) Inflammatory ventriculitis

Periventricular Calcifications in Childhood

1. Tuberous sclerosis
2. Congenital infection: CMV, toxoplasmosis

Periventricular T2WI-hyperintense Lesions

A. YOUNG PATIENTS
1. Multiple sclerosis
2. Migraine: in 41% with classic migraine, in 57% with complicated migraine; presumed to represent vasculitis-induced small infarcts
3. Vasculitic disorder: SLE, Behçet disease, sickle cell disease
√ triad of deep white matter lesions + cortical infarcts + hemorrhage
4. Acute disseminated encephalomyelitis (ADE)
= postviral leukoencephalopathy
5. Virchow-Robin space
= small invaginations of subarachnoid space following pia mater along perforating nutrient end vessels into brain substance
Location: inferior third of putamen; usually bilateral
√ 1–2-mm round lesions isointense to CSF (well seen on coronal sections through centrum semiovale + on low-axial sections at level of anterior commissure)
6. Leukodystrophy: in children
√ symmetric diffuse confluent involvement

7. Ependymitis granularis
   = symmetrically focal areas of hyperintensity on T2WI anterior + lateral to frontal horns in normal individuals
   Histo: patchy loss of ependyma with paucity of hydrophobic myelin, which allows migration of fluid out of the ventricle into interstitium

B. ELDERLY
1. **État criblé** (sievelike) / gliosis
   = deep white matter ischemia
   = extensive number of perivascular fluid spaces predominantly at arteriolar level as part of subacute arteriosclerotic encephalopathy
   Cause: chronic ischemia due to arteriosclerosis of long penetrating arteries arising from circle of Willis (lenticulostriate + thalamo-perforators) = small vessel disease
   Predisposed: cigarette smoker, hypertensive patient
   Histo: lipohyalin deposits within vessel walls followed by partial demyelination, gliosis, interstitial edema
   Incidence: in 10% without risk factors, in 84% with risk factors and symptoms
   Age: >60 years (in 30–60%)
   Location: periventricular white matter > optic radiation > basal ganglia > centrum semiovale > brainstem (usually spares corpus callosum + subcortical U-fibers)
   √ multiple focal lesions <2 mm
2. Lacunar infarction

C. PATIENTS WITH AIDS
1. HIV encephalitis:
   √ well-defined "patchy" / ill-defined "dirty white matter"
   √ central atrophy
2. Toxoplasmosis
3. Lymphoma
4. Progressive multifocal leukoencephalopathy (PML)

D. PATIENTS WITH TRAUMA
1. Diffuse axonal / shearing injury
2. Diffuse white matter injury
   = radiation-induced demyelination of periventricular white matter
   Cause: whole-brain irradiation
   • subclinical
3. Diffuse necrotizing leukoencephalopathy
   Cause: intrathecal methotrexate ± whole brain irradiation
   • rapidly deteriorating clinical course
   √ confluent pattern with scalloped margins within periventricular white matter extending out to subcortical U-fibers

E. PATIENTS WITH HYDROCEPHALUS
1. Transependymal CSF flow
   √ smooth halo of even thickness

BASAL GANGLIA

Bilateral Basal Ganglia Lesions in Childhood

◊ Basal ganglia are susceptible to damage during childhood because of high energy requirements (ATP) mandating a rich blood supply + high concentration of trace metals (iron, copper, manganese)
• increased irritability, lethargy, dystonia
• seizure, behavioral changes
√ bilateral necrosis of basal ganglia

ACUTE CAUSES
A. Compromise of vascular supply
   1. Hemolytic-uremic syndrome causing microthrombosis of basal ganglia, thalami, hippocampi, cortex
   2. Encephalitis (usually viral agents)
B. Compromise of nutrient supply
   1. Hypoxia: respiratory arrest, near drowning, strangling, barbiturate intoxication
   2. Hypoglycemia
      √ hemorrhage rarely seen
   3. Osmotic myelinolysis
      √ associated central pontine location common
C. Acute poisoning
   1. Carbon monoxide
      √ preferentially affects globus pallidus

   rare in children:
   2. Hydrogen sulfide
   3. Cyanide poisoning
   4. Methanol poisoning

CHRONIC CAUSES
A. Inborn errors of metabolism
   1. Leigh disease
      = subacute necrotizing encephalomyelopathy
      = autosomal recessive disorder characterized by deficiencies in pyruvate carboxylase, pyruvate dehydrogenase complex, cytochrome *c* oxidase resulting in anaerobic ATP production
      • lactic acidosis (elevated ratio of lactate to pyruvate in CSF + serum)
      √ propensity to involve putamen
   2. Wilson disease
      = hepatolenticular degeneration
      = increased deposition of copper in brain + liver
      • decreased levels of serum copper + ceruloplasmin
      • increased urinary copper excretion
      √ cell damage of lenticular nucleus (= lenslike configuration of putamen + globus pallidus)
   3. Mitochondrial encephalomyelopathies
      = subset of lactic acidemias with structurally abnormal mitochondria
      • "ragged red" fibers in muscle biopsy
   4. Maple syrup urine disease
      = inability to catabolize branched-chain amino acids (leucine, isoleucine, valine)
      • urine smells of maple syrup

5. Methylmalonic acidemia
   = group of genetically distinct autosomal recessive disorders of organic acid metabolism affecting conversion of methylmalonyl-CoA to succinyl-CoA
   • accumulation of methylmalonic acid in blood + urine

B. Degenerative disease
   1. Huntington disease
   2. Dystrophic calcifications

C. Dysmyelinating disease
   basal ganglia are a mixture of gray + white matter
   1. Canavan disease
   2. Metachromatic leukodystrophy

D. Others
   1. Neurofibromatosis type 1

Low-attenuation Lesion in Basal Ganglia

1. Poisoning: carbon monoxide, barbiturate intoxication, hydrogen sulfide poisoning, cyanide poisoning, methanol intoxication
2. Hypoxia
3. Hypoglycemia
4. Hypotension (lacunar infarcts)
5. Wilson disease

Basal Ganglia Calcification

Prevalence in children: 1.1–1.6%

A. PHYSIOLOGIC WITH AGING

B. ENDOCRINE
   1. Hypoparathyroidism, pseudo~, pseudopseudo~ (60%)
   2. Hyperparathyroidism
   3. Hypothyroidism

C. METABOLIC
   1. Leigh disease
   2. Mitochondrial cytopathy
      (a) Kearns-Sayre syndrome = ophthalmoplegia, retinal pigmentary degeneration, complete heart block, short stature, mental deterioration
      (b) MELAS = **M**itochondrial myopathy, **E**ncephalopathy, **L**actic acidosis, **A**nd **S**troke
      (c) MERRF = **M**yoclonic **E**pilepsy with **R**agged **R**ed **F**ibers
   3. Fahr disease = familial cerebrovascular ferrocalcinosis

D. CONGENITAL / DEVELOPMENTAL
   1. Familial idiopathic symmetric basal ganglia calcification
   2. Hastings-James syndrome
   3. Cockayne syndrome
   4. Lipoid proteinosis = hyalinosis cutis
   5. Neurofibromatosis
   6. Tuberous sclerosis
   7. Oculocraniosomatic disease
   8. Methemoglobinopathy
   9. Down syndrome

E. INFLAMMATION / INFECTION
   1. Toxoplasmosis, congenital rubella, CMV
   2. Measles, chicken pox
   3. Pertussis, Coxsackie B virus
   4. Cysticercosis
   5. Systemic lupus erythematosus
   6. AIDS

F. TRAUMA
   1. Childhood leukemia following methotrexate therapy
   2. S/P radiation therapy
   3. Birth anoxia, hypoxia
   4. Cardiovascular event

G. TOXIC
   1. Carbon monoxide poisoning
   2. Lead intoxication
   3. Nephrotic syndrome

mnemonic: "BIRTH"
Birth anoxia
Idiopathic (most common), **I**nfarct
Radiation therapy
Toxoplasmosis / CMV
Hypoparathyroidism / pseudoHPT

Linear Echogenic Foci in Thalamus + Basal Ganglia

A. IN UTERO INFECTION
   = **mineralizing vasculopathy** = destruction of wall of lenticulostriate arteries + replacement by deposits of amorphous granular basophilic material
   1. TORCH agents: Toxoplasma, others (syphilis, hepatitis, zoster), rubella virus, cytomegalovirus, herpes virus
   2. Syphilis
   3. Human immunodeficiency virus

B. CHROMOSOMAL ABNORMALITY
   1. Down syndrome
   2. Trisomy 13

C. OTHERS (anoxic injury?)
   1. Perinatal asphyxia, respiratory distress syndrome, cyanotic congenital heart disease, necrotizing enterocolitis
   2. Fetal alcohol syndrome
   3. Nonimmune hydrops

Eye-of-the-Tiger Sign

= markedly hypointense globus pallidus on T2WI surrounding a higher-intensity center

Cause: excess iron accumulation + central gliosis

Associated with: Hallervorden-Spatz syndrome (Hallervorden-Spatz disease, dementia, tetraparesis, neurofibrillary tangles, retinitis pigmentosa, acanthocytosis, pallidal degeneration, X-linked disorders with mental retardation + Dandy-Walker malformation, disorders with Lewy bodies); extrapyramidal parkinsonian disorders

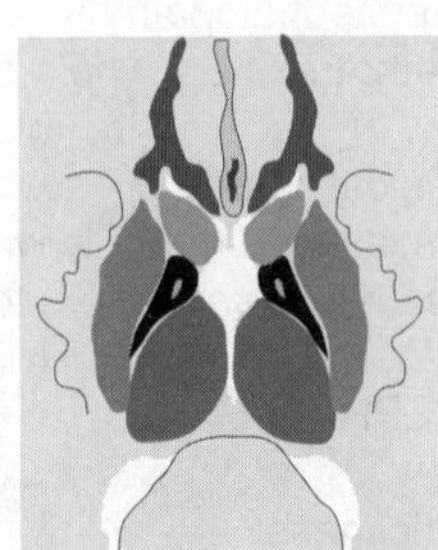

SELLA

Destruction of Sella

1. Pituitary adenoma
2. Suprasellar tumor
3. Carcinoma of sphenoid + posterior ethmoid sinus
   √ opacification of sinus + destruction of walls
   √ associated with nasopharyngeal mass (common)
4. Nasopharyngeal carcinoma
   (a) squamous cell carcinoma
   (b) lymphoepithelioma = Schmincke tumor = non-keratinizing form of squamous cell carcinoma
   √ sclerosis of adjacent bone
5. Metastasis to sphenoid
   from breast, kidney, thyroid, colon, prostate, lung, esophagus
6. Primary tumor of sphenoid bone (rare)
   osteogenic sarcoma, giant cell tumor, plasmacytoma
7. Chordoma
8. Mucocele of sphenoid sinus (uncommon)
9. Enlarged 3rd ventricle
   aqueductal stenosis from infratentorial mass, maldevelopment

J-shaped Sella

mnemonic: "CONMAN"

Chronic hydrocephalus
Optic glioma, **O**steogenesis imperfecta
Neurofibromatosis
Mucopolysaccharidosis
Achondroplasia
Normal variant

Enlarged Sella

A. PRIMARY TUMOR
   1. Pituitary adenoma
   2. Craniopharyngioma
   3. Meningioma: hyperostosis
   4. Optic glioma: J-shaped sella
B. PITUITARY HYPERPLASIA
   1. Hypothyroidism
   2. Hypogonadism
   3. Nelson syndrome (occurring in 7% of patients subsequent to adrenalectomy)
C. CSF SPACE
   1. Enlarged 3rd ventricle
   2. Hydrocephalus
   3. Empty sella
D. VESSEL
   1. Arterial aneurysm
   2. Ectatic internal carotid artery

mnemonic: "CHAMPS"

Craniopharyngioma
Hydrocephalus (empty sella)
AVM, **A**neurysm
Meningioma
Pituitary adenoma
Sarcoidosis, TB

Pituitary Gland Enlargement

1. Neoplasm: eg, pituitary gland adenoma
2. Hypertrophy: primary precocious puberty, primary hypothyroidism
3. Lymphocytic hypophysitis
4. Infection
5. Severe dural AV fistula

Intrasellar Mass

1. Pituitary adenoma / carcinoma (most common cause)
2. Craniopharyngioma (2nd most common cause)
3. Meningioma: from surface of diaphragm / tuberculum sellae
4. Chordoma
5. Metastasis: lung, breast, prostate, kidney, GI tract, spread from nasopharynx
6. Intracavernous ICA aneurysm: bilateral in 25%
7. Pituitary abscess: rapidly expanding mass associated with meningitis
8. Empty sella
9. Rathke cleft cyst: commonly at junction of anterior + posterior pituitary gland
10. Granular cell tumor = myeloblastoma: benign neoplasm of posterior pituitary gland
11. Granuloma: sarcoidosis, giant cell granuloma, TB, syphilis, eosinophilic granuloma
12. Lymphoid adenohypophysitis
13. Pituitary hyperplasia, eg, in Nelson syndrome

Hypointense Lesion of Sella

1. Empty sella
2. Pituitary stone (= pituilith)
   = sequelae of autonecrosis of pituitary adenoma
3. Intrasellar aneurysm
4. Persistent trigeminal artery
5. Calcified meningioma
6. Pituitary hemochromatosis (anterior pituitary lobe only)

Parasellar Mass

1. Meningioma: tentorium cerebelli
2. Neurinoma (III, IV, V_1, V_2, VI)
3. Metastasis: lung, breast, kidney, GI tract, spread from nasopharynx
4. Epidermoid
5. Aneurysm
6. Carotid-cavernous fistula

mnemonic: "SATCHMO"

Sella neoplasm with superior extension, **S**arcoidosis
Aneurysm, ectatic carotid, carotid-cavernous sinus fistula, **A**rachnoid cyst
Teratoma: dysgerminoma (usually), dermoid, epidermoid
Craniopharyngioma, **C**hordoma
Hypothalamic glioma, **H**istiocytoma, **H**amartoma
Metastatic disease, **M**eningioma, **M**ucocele
Optic nerve glioma, neuroma

Suprasellar Mass

1. Meningioma
2. Craniopharyngioma: in 80% suprasellar
3. Chiasmal + optic nerve glioma
   in 38% of neurofibromatosis; adolescent girls;
   DDx: chiasmal neuritis
4. Hypothalamic glioma
5. Hamartoma of tuber cinereum
6. Infundibular tumor
   metastasis (esp. breast); glioma; lymphoma / leukemia; histiocytosis X; sarcoidosis, tuberculosis
   √ diameter of infundibulum >4.5 mm immediately above level of dorsum; cone-shaped (on coronal scan)
7. Germinoma
   = malignant tumor similar to seminoma (= "ectopic pinealoma")
   √ frequently calcified (teratoma)
   √ CSF spread (germinoma + teratocarcinoma)
   √ enhancement on CECT (common)
8. Epidermoid / dermoid
   √ cystic lesion containing calcifications + fat
   √ minimal / no contrast enhancement
9. Arachnoid cyst
   • hydrocephalus (common), visual impairment
   • endocrine dysfunction
   Age: most common in infancy
10. Enlarged 3rd ventricle extending into pituitary fossa
11. Suprasellar aneurysm
    √ rim calcification + eccentric position

Suprasellar Mass with Low Attenuation

1. Craniopharyngioma
2. Dermoid / epidermoid
3. Arachnoid cyst
4. Lipoma
5. Simple pituitary cyst
6. Glioma of hypothalamus

Suprasellar Mass with Mixed Attenuation

A. IN CHILDREN
   1. Hypothalamic-chiasmatic glioma
   2. Craniopharyngioma
   3. Hamartoma of tuber cinereum
   4. Histiocytosis

B. IN ADULTS
   1. Suprasellar extension of pituitary adenoma
   2. Craniopharyngioma
   3. Epidermoid cyst
   4. Thrombosed aneurysm
   5. Low-grade hypothalamic / optic glioma
   6. Inflammatory lesion: sarcoidosis, TB, sphenoid mucocele

Suprasellar Mass with Calcification

A. CURVILINEAR
   1. Giant carotid aneurysm
   2. Craniopharyngioma

B. GRANULAR
   1. Craniopharyngioma
   2. Meningioma
   3. Granuloma
   4. Dermoid cyst / teratoma
   5. Optic / hypothalamic glioma (rare)

Enhancing Supra- and Intrasellar Mass

1. Pituitary adenoma
2. Meningioma
3. Germinoma
4. Hypothalamic glioma
5. Craniopharyngioma

Perisellar Vascular Lesion

1. ICA aneurysm
   Giant aneurysms are >2.5 cm in diameter
   √ destruction of bony sella / superior orbital fissure
   √ calcified wall / thrombus
   √ CECT enhancement, nonuniform with thrombosis
2. Ectatic carotid artery
   √ curvilinear calcifications
   √ encroachment upon sella turcica
3. Carotid-cavernous sinus fistula

PINEAL GLAND

Classification of Pineal Gland Tumors

Incidence of pineal mass:
<1% of all intracranial tumors, 4% of all childhood intracranial masses, 9% of all intracranial masses in Asia

A. PRIMARY TUMOR
   (a) Germ cell origin (2/3)
   — forming embryonic tissue
      1. Germinoma (40–50%)
      2. Embryonal cell carcinoma
      3. Teratoma (15%): benign mature teratoma, benign immature teratoma, malignant teratoma
   — forming extraembryonic tissue
      4. Choriocarcinoma (<5%)
      5. Endodermal sinus tumor = yolk sac tumor
   (b) Pineal parenchymal cell origin (<15%)
      1. Pineocytoma
      2. Pineoblastoma
   (c) Other cell origin
      1. Retinoblastoma (trilateral retinoblastoma = left eye + right eye + pineal gland
      2. Astrocytoma
      3. Ependymoma
      4. Meningioma
      5. Hemangiopericytoma
      6. Pineal + tectal glioma
      7. Cavernous hemangioma
      8. Meningioma
   (d) Cysts
      1. Pineal cyst
      2. Malignant teratoma

3. AVM, vein of Galen aneurysm
4. Arachnoid cyst
5. Inclusion cyst (dermoid / epidermoid)

B. SECONDARY TUMOR
Metastasis: eg, lung carcinoma

DDx considerations:

— female:	likely NOT germ cell tumor
— hypodense matrix:	likely NOT pineal cell tumor
— distinct tumor margins:	probably pineocytoma / teratoma / germinoma
— calcification:	likely NOT teratocarcinoma, metastasis, germinoma
— CSF seeding:	NOT teratoma
— intense enhancement:	likely NOT teratoma

Serum markers:

choriocarcinoma	– β-HCG
embryonal cell carcinoma	– α-FP and β-HCG
endodermal sinus tumor	– α-FP
teratoma	– β-HCG and α-FP
germinoma	– placental alkaline phosphatase

Intensely Enhancing Mass in Pineal Region

1. Germinoma
2. Pineocytoma / -blastoma
3. Pineal teratocarcinoma
4. Glioma of brainstem / thalamus
5. Subsplenial meningioma
6. Vein of Galen aneurysm

ANATOMY OF BRAIN

EMBRYOLOGY

Neurulation

neural plate = CNS originates as a plate of thickened ectoderm on the dorsal aspect of the embryo
neural crest = elevation of the lateral margins of the neural plate; forms the peripheral nervous system
neural tube = invagination between the two neural crests; its wall forms the brain + spinal cord; its lumen forms the ventricles + spinal canal
4.6 weeks MA: formation of neural tube
5.6 weeks MA: rostral neuropore closes
5.9 weeks MA: caudal neuropore closes
6.0 weeks MA: 3 primary brain vesicles develop (prosencephalon, mesencephalon, rhombencephalon) development of cervical flexure
7.0 weeks MA: 2 additional primary brain vesicles form out of rhombencephalon (pontine flexure divides into myelencephalon, metencephalon)
15 weeks MA: dorsal portion of alar plates bulging into 4th ventricle have fused in midline to form cerebellar vermis

Brain Growth

= increase in thickness of brain mantle with relative constant ventricular width
◊ Most rapid brain growth from 12 to 24 weeks MA!

Neuronal Migration

7th week subependymal neuronal proliferation = germinal matrix
8th week radial migration to cortex along radial glial fibers

Myelination

Progression: caudal to cranial; posterior to anterior
MR: T1WI if <7 months of age;
T2WI if >7 months of age
Milestones:
term birth: brainstem, cerebellum, posterior limb of internal capsule
2 months: anterior limb of internal capsule
3 months: splenium of corpus callosum
6 months: genu of corpus callosum
Occipital white matter:
√ central at 5 months (T1WI), 14 months (T2WI)
√ peripheral at 7 months (T1WI), 15 months (T2WI)
Frontal white matter:
√ central at 6 months (T1WI), 16 months (T2WI)
√ peripheral at 11 months (T1WI), 18 months (T2WI)

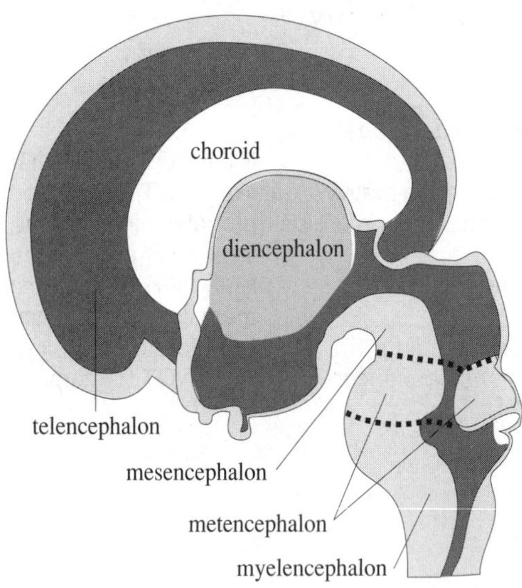

Sagittal Section through Brain at 10–11 Weeks GA

CLASSIFICATION OF BRAIN ANATOMY

A. PROSENCEPHALON = forebrain
√ cerebrum, lateral ventricles, choroid, thalami, cerebellum sonographically visible at 12 weeks MA
1. **Telencephalon** = cerebrum
= cerebral hemispheres, putamen, caudate nucleus
2. **Diencephalon**
= thalamus, hypothalamus, epithalamus (= pineal gland + habenula), globus pallidus

B. MESENCEPHALON = midbrain
= short segment of brainstem above pons; traverses the hiatus in tentorium cerebelli; contains cerebral peduncles, tectum, colliculi (corpora quadrigemina)

C. RHOMBENCEPHALON = hindbrain
√ posterior cystic space of 4th ventricle sonographically detectable between 8 and 10 weeks MA
1. **Metencephalon** = cerebellar hemispheres, vermis
2. **Myelencephalon** = medulla oblongata, pons

D. BRAINSTEM = mesencephalon + myelencephalon contains
(a) cranial nerve nuclei
(b) sensory and motor tracts between thalamus, cerebral cortex, and spinal cord
(c) reticular formation controlling respiration, blood pressure, gastrointestinal function, centers for arousal and wakefulness

SCALP

◊ The outer 3 layers are often torn off as a unit in accidents; wounds do not gape if epicranius not involved

A. SKIN

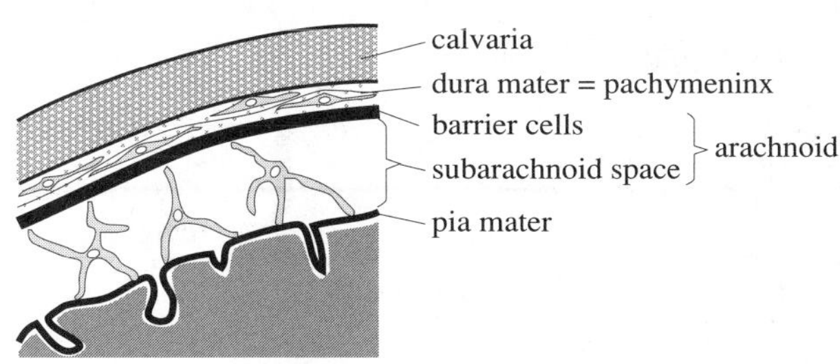

Meninges of Brain

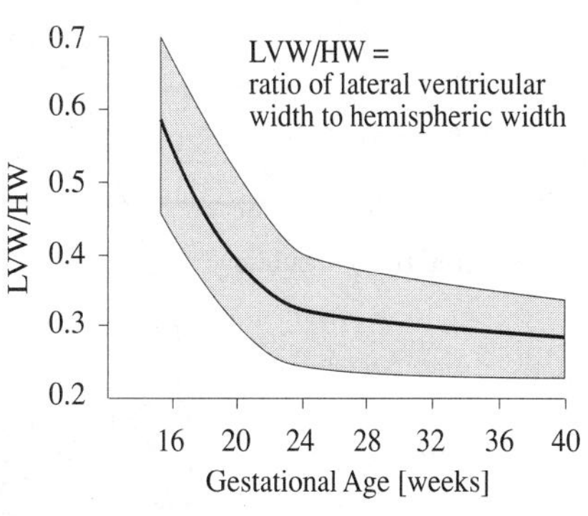

Lateral Ventricular Width to Hemispheric Width during Gestation

B. SUBCUTIS
 = fibro-adipose tissue closely adherent to skin and underlying epicranius
C. EPICRANIUS + GALEA APONEUROTICA
 = occipitofrontal + temporoparietal muscles forming centrally the epicranial aponeurosis
D. SUBGALEAL SPACE
 = subaponeurotic areolar tissue between periosteum of outer table and galea
E. PERICRANIUM = periosteum of outer table
F. SUBPERIOSTEAL SPACE
 = created when periosteum of outer table becomes detached from calvaria (= **cephalohematoma**)

MENINGES OF BRAIN

A. CALVARIA = upper part of cranium enclosing the brain
 (a) outer table of resilient compact bone
 (b) diploë = trabecular bone containing red bone marrow
 (c) inner table of thin and brittle compact bone
B. EPIDURAL SPACE
 = created when outer layer of dura (periosteum of inner table) becomes detached from calvaria
C. PACHYMENINGES = DURA MATER
 (a) outer dural layer
  = highly vascularized periosteum of inner table
 (b) space for venous sinuses
 (c) inner dural layer
  = meningeal layer derived from meninx
D. SUBDURAL SPACE
 = cleft formed in pathologic states within inner layer of dura
E. LEPTOMENINGES
 1. Arachnoid
  = closely applied to inner surface of dura
 2. Subarachnoid space
  Histo: fine connective tissue + cellular septa link pia and arachnoid
  – contains CSF that drains through the valves of arachnoid granulations into venous sinuses
  – forms basal cisterns
 3. Pia mater
F. SUBPIAL SPACE
 = perivascular (Virchow-Robin) space
G. EPENDYMA

CEREBROSPINAL FLUID

Total volume:
 50 mL in newborn, 150 mL in adult
Composition:
 inorganic salts like those in plasma, traces of protein + glucose
Production:
 0.3 – 0.4 mL/min resulting in 500 mL/day; secreted into ventricles by choroid plexuses (80–90%), 10–20% formed by parenchyma of the cerebrum + spinal cord
Circulation:
 from ventricles through foramina of Magendie + Luschka of 4th ventricle into cisterna magna + basilar cisterns; 80% of CSF flows initially into suprasellar cistern + cistern of lamina terminalis, the ambient / superior cerebellar cisterns, eventually ascending over superolateral aspects of each hemisphere; 20% initially enters spinal subarachnoid space + eventually recirculates into cerebral subarachnoid space
Absorption:
 into venous system by
 (a) arachnoid villi of superior sagittal sinus (villi behave as one-way valves with an opening pressure between 20–50 mm of CSF)
 (b) cranial + spinal nerves with eventual absorption by lymphatics (50%)
 (c) prelymphatic channels of capillaries within brain parenchyma
 (d) vertebral venous plexuses, intervertebral veins, posterior intercostal + upper lumbar veins into azygos + hemiazygos veins

Cerebral Aqueduct

pulsatile flow (due to brain motion during cardiac cycle) + net outflow into 4th ventricle; diameter of 2.6–4.2 mm; peak outflow velocity of 6–51 mm/sec; inflow velocity of 3–28 mm/sec

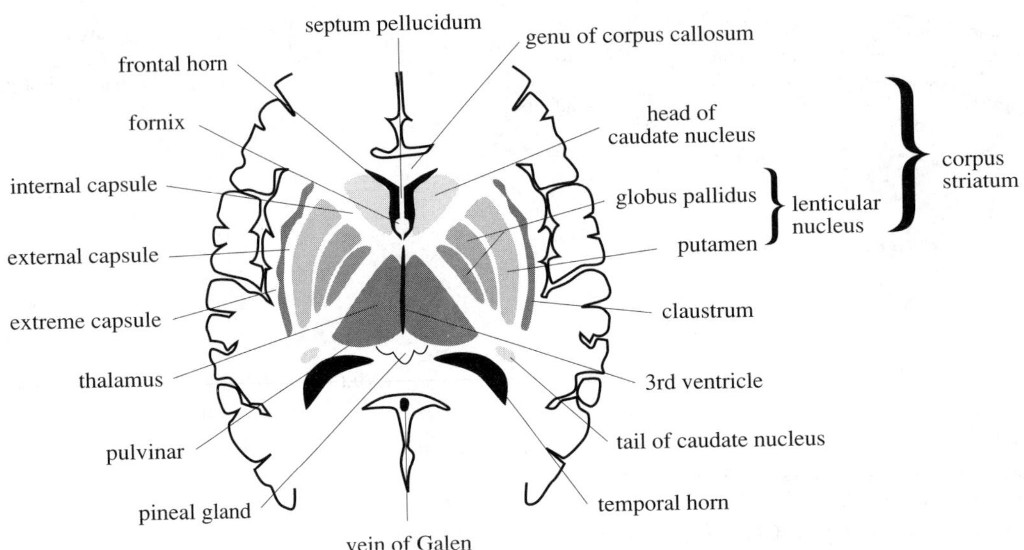

Axial Section through Level of Third Ventricle

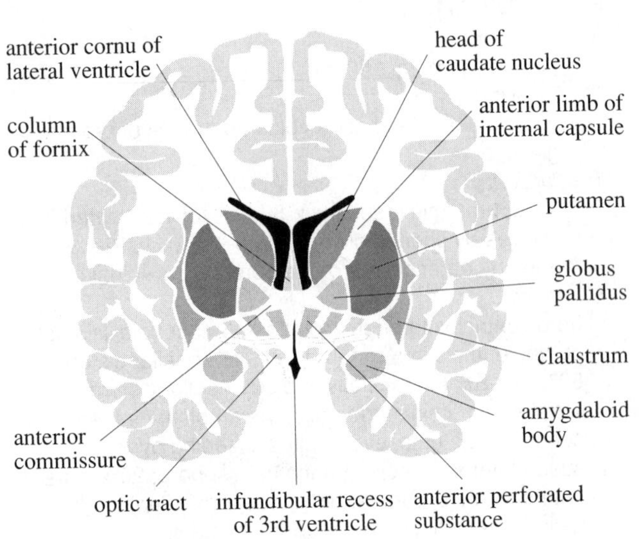

Coronal Section through Anterior Commisssure

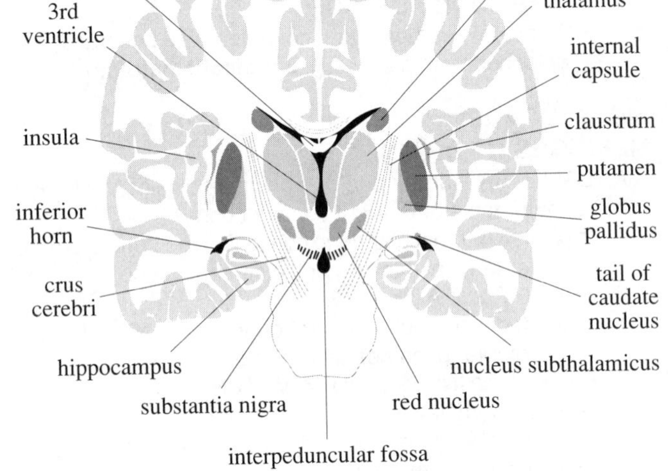

Coronal Section through Ventral Part of Pons

BASAL NUCLEI

= BASAL GANGLIA (earlier incorrect designation)

A. Amygdaloid body
B. Claustrum
C. Corpus striatum
   (1) Caudate
   (2) Lentiform nucleus
      (a) pallidum = globus pallidus
      (b) putamen

PITUITARY GLAND

= HYPOPHYSIS CEREBRI within hypophyseal fossa of sphenoid, covered superiorly by sellar diaphragm (= dura mater) which has an aperture for the infundibulum centrally

Size:
adult size is achieved at puberty
Height in adult females = 7 (range 4–10) mm
Height in adult males = 5 (range 3– 7) mm

Shape:
√ flat / downwardly convex superior border
√ upwardly convex during puberty, pregnancy, in hypothyroidism (due to hyperplasia)

A. ANTERIOR LOBE
= larger anterior portion of adenohypophysis comprising 80% of pituitary gland volume
Origin: ectodermal derivative of stomadeum

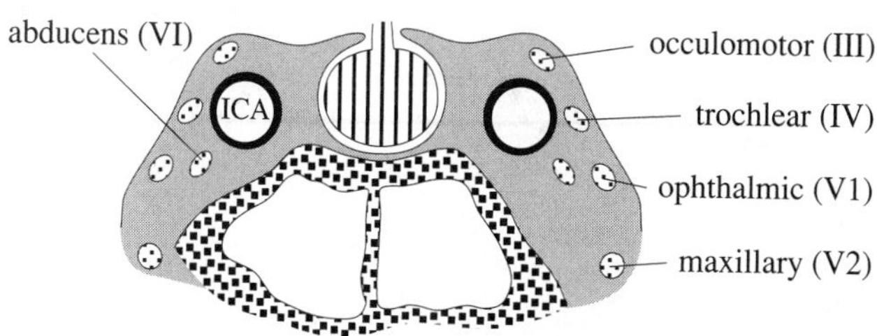

Cavernous Sinus
(coronal view)

Function:
(a) chromophil cells
1. acidophil cells = α cells
growth hormone = somatotropin (STH), prolactin = lactogenic hormone (LTH)
2. basophil cells = β cells
adrenocorticotropin = adrenocorticotropic hormone (ACTH), thyrotropin = thyroid-stimulating hormone (TSH), follicle-stimulating hormone (FSH), interstitial-cell-stimulating hormone (ICSH), luteinizing hormone (LH), melanocyte-stimulating hormone (MSH)

(b) chromophobe cells = 50% of epithelial cell population, of unknown significance

MRI:
- √ larger homogeneous component isointense to white matter on T1WI + T2WI
- √ prominent contrast enhancement (during first 3 minutes) due to lack of blood-brain barrier
- √ hyperintense in the newborn fading to normal adult signal by 2nd month of life

B. PARS INTERMEDIA
= posterior portion of adenohypophysis; separated from anterior lobe by hypophyseal cleft in fetal life
Origin: Rathke cleft / pouch within intermediate lobe of pituitary gland
Function: termination point of short hypothalamic axons elaborating tropic hormones (= releasing factors + prolactin inhibiting factor), which are carried to anterior lobe via the portal system
√ not visible with imaging techniques

C. POSTERIOR LOBE
= major portion of neurohypophysis
Origin: diencephalic outgrowth (termination point of axons from supraoptic + paraventricular nuclei of hypothalamus)
Function: storage site for vasopressin (= antidiuretic hormone [ADH]) + oxytocin transported from paraventricular + supraoptic nuclei of hypothalamus along neurosecretory hypothalamohypophyseal tract

MRI:
- √ hyperintense on T1WI + isointense on T2WI in comparison with anterior lobe (? due to relaxing agent of phospholipid / neurosecretory granules / vasopressin)
- √ isointense in 10% of normal individuals

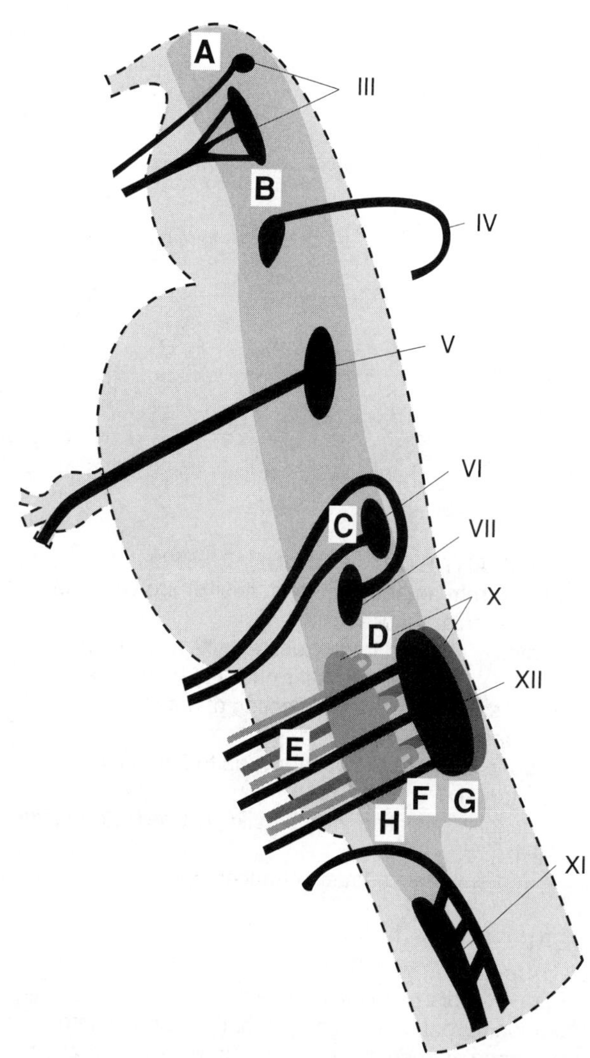

Cranial Nuclei of Brainstem and Reticular Formation
A = sleep, wakefulness, consciousness
B = visual spatial orientation, higher autonomic coordination of food intake
C = pneumotaxic center, coordination of breathing and circulation
D = swallowing
E = blood pressure, cardiac activity, vascular tone
F = expiration
G = area postrema = trigger zone for vomiting
H = inspiration

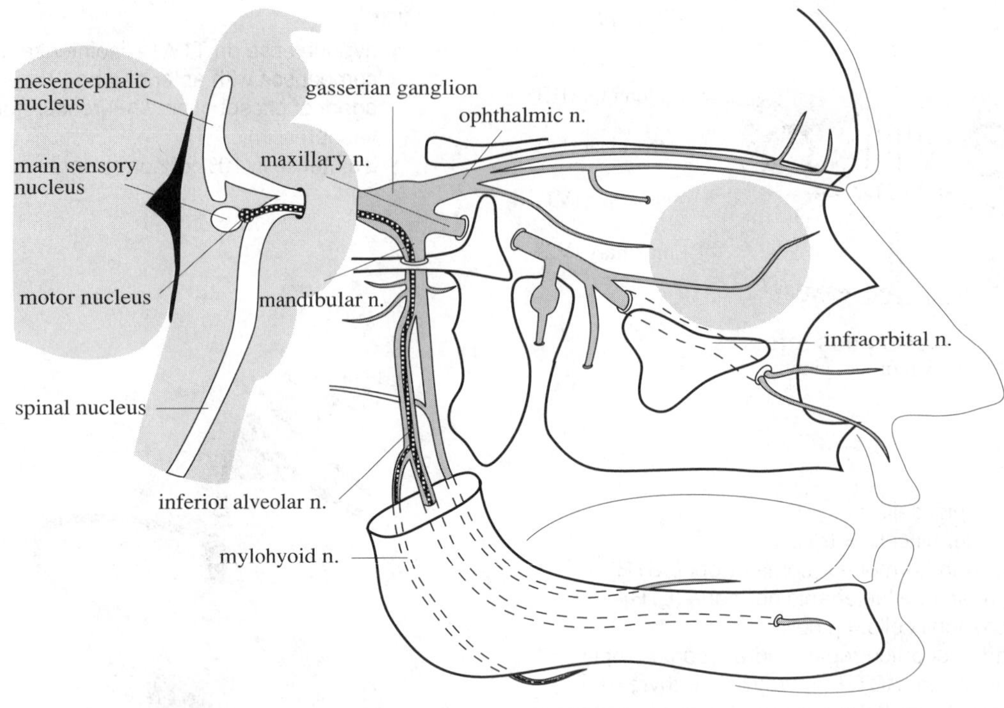

Trigeminal Nerve

D. PITUITARY STALK = INFUNDIBULUM
arises from anterior aspect of floor of 3rd ventricle (infundibular recess)
Histo: formed from axons of cells lying in supraoptic + paraventricular nuclei of hypothalamus
√ joins posterior lobe at junction of anterior + posterior lobes
√ up to 3 mm thick superiorly, up to 2 mm thick inferiorly
√ usually in midline, may be slightly tilted to one side
MRI:
√ prominent contrast enhancement

PINEAL GLAND

Development:
from area of ependymal thickening at the most caudal portion of roof of 3rd ventricle that evaginates into a pinecone-shaped mass during 7th week of gestation; initially contains ependyma lining in central cavity that connects with 3rd ventricle

Function:
1. Regulation of long-term biologic rhythm (eg, onset of puberty)
2. Regulation of short-term biologic rhythm (eg, diurnal / circadian) due to photoperiodic clues via accessory optic pathway

Histo:
(a) pinealocytes with dendritic processes (= neuronal cells) make up 95% of population
(b) neuroglial supporting cells make up 5% of population

Location: attached to upper aspect of posterior border of 3rd ventricle, lies within CSF of quadrigeminal cistern, anterior to pineal gland is cistern of velum interpositum (= cistern of transverse fissure)
Size: 8 mm long, 4 mm wide

TRIGEMINAL NERVE (V)

Nuclei:
(1) mesencephalic nucleus: proprioception extends to level of inferior colliculus
(2) main sensory nucleus: tactile sensation
(3) motor nucleus: motor innervation
(4) spinal nucleus: pain + temperature sensation extends to level of 2nd cervical vertebra
Location: in tegmentum of lateral pons, along anterolateral aspect of 4th ventricle

Course:
— through prepontine cistern
— exits through porus trigeminus (= opening in dura)
— enters Meckel cave with dura mater + leptomeninges forming trigeminal cistern (= CSF-filled subarachnoid space) at the most anteromedial portion of the petrous pyramid
— forms gasserian ganglion (= trigeminal ganglion), which contains cell bodies of sensory fibers except those for proprioception

Trifurcation into 3 principal branches:

(1) **ophthalmic nerve** (V_1)
 Course: in lateral wall of cavernous sinus
 Exit: superior orbital fissure
 Supply: sensory innervation of scalp, forehead, nose, globe
 • mediates afferent aspect of corneal reflex

(2) **maxillary nerve** (V_2)
 Course: between lateral dural wall of cavernous sinus + skull base
 Exit: through foramen rotundum into pterygopalatine fossa
 Supply: sensory innervation of middle third of face, upper teeth
 Main trunk: infraorbital nerve

(3) **mandibular nerve** (V_3)
 Course: NOT through cavernous sinus
 Exit: through foramen ovale into masticator space
 Supply: (a) sensory innervation of lower third of face, tongue, floor of mouth, jaw
 (b) motor innervation of muscles of mastication (masseter, temporalis, medial + lateral pterygoid), mylohyoid m., anterior belly of digastric m., tensor tympani m., tensor veli palatini m.

FACIAL NERVE (VII)

Function:

1. Lacrimation (via greater superficial petrosal nerve)
2. Stapedius reflex: sound damping
3. Taste of anterior 2/3 of tongue (via chorda tympani nerve to lingual nerve)
4. Facial expression (platysma)
5. Secretion of lacrimal + submandibular + sublingual glands (via nervus intermedius)

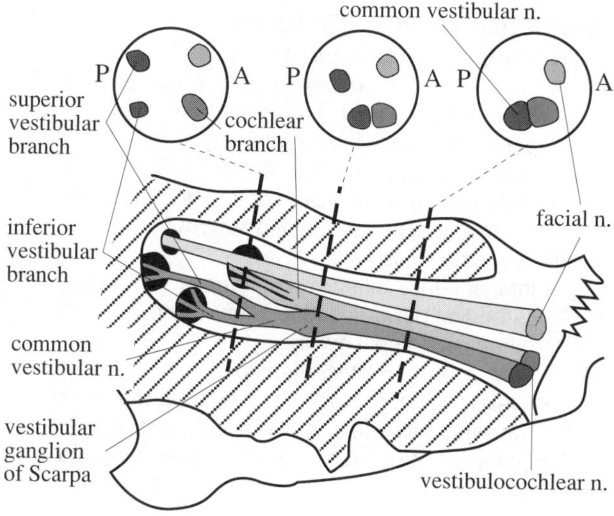

Internal Auditory Canal

Posterior wall of IAC is removed; cross sections through IAC are displayed above; A = anterior, P = posterior

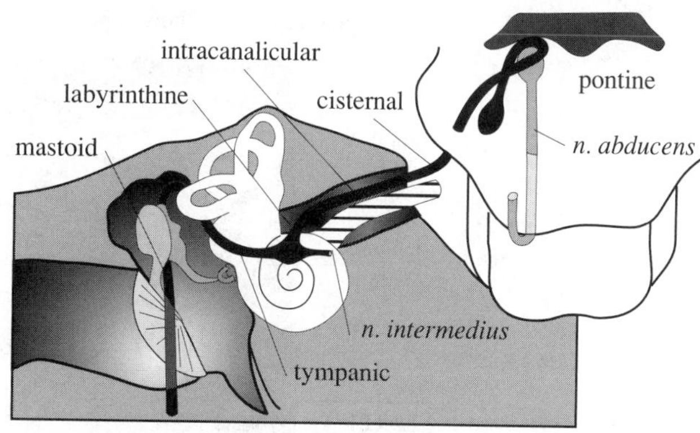

Segmental Anatomy of Facial Nerve Intracranially
(viewed from anteriorly)

Nuclei:

(1) Motor nucleus: ventrolateral deep in reticular formation of the caudal part of the pons
 Intrapontine course:
 — dorsomedially towards 4th ventricle
 — curving anterolaterally around upper pole of abducens nucleus (= **geniculum**)
 — descending anterolaterally through reticular formation
 Innervation to: stapedius m., stylohyoid m., posterior belly of digastric m., occipitalis m., buccinator, muscles of facial expression, platysma

(2) Nucleus solitarius (sensory nucleus):
 — **nervus intermedius**: sensation from anterior 2/3 of tongue, skin on + adjacent to ear

(3) Superior salivatory nucleus (parasympathetic secretomotor innervation)
 – greater petrosal n.: secretion of lacrimal glands, nasal cavity, paranasal sinuses
 — chorda tympani: submandibular gland, sublingual glands

Course & Segments:

(a) intracranial segment
 from brainstem to porus acusticus internus:
 — pontine segment: motor root fibers of facial n. hook around the abducens nucleus forming the facial colliculus (= elevation in the floor of the 4th ventricle); the nerve continues laterally from the corticospinal tract
 — cisternal segment: facial n. emerges from lateral aspect of pontomedullary junction + courses anterolaterally in cerebellopontine angle cistern to internal auditory canal (IAC)

(b) intracanalicular segment
 = motor root of facial n. within internal auditory canal in anterosuperior groove of vestibulocochlear n. with nervus intermedius between them
 mnemonic: "seven up"

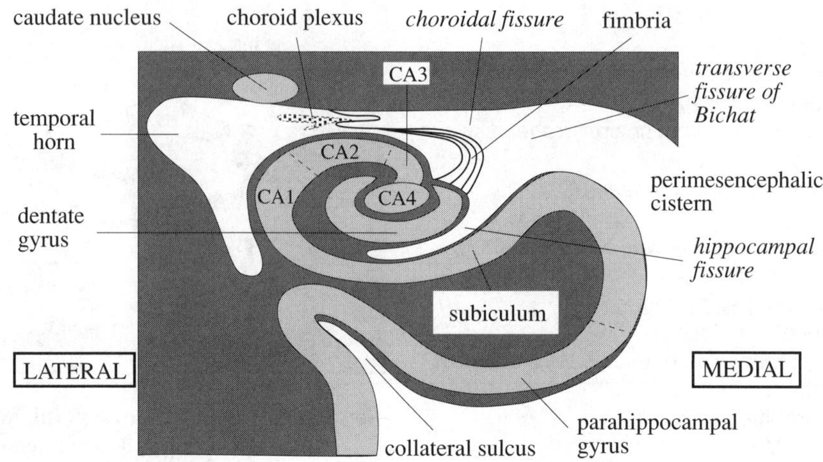

Coronal Section through the Right Mesial Temporal Lobe
(CA1 through CA4 = hippocampus)

(c) labyrinthine segment
short segment of facial n. travels within its own bony canal (= **fallopian canal**) curving anteriorly over top of cochlea; terminates in anteromedial genu (**geniculate ganglion)**

(d) tympanic segment
= segment from anterior to posterior genu just underneath lateral semicircular canal
— horizontal segment: facial n. makes a 130° turn posteriorly and horizontally along medial wall of mesotympanum lateral to vestibule between lateral semicircular canal (above) and oval window (below)
— pyramidal segment: facial n. turns inferiorly at **second genu** in pyramidal eminence; gives off the nerve for the stapedius muscle

(e) mastoid segment
facial n. descends from posterior genu through anterior mastoid (= medial wall of aditus ad antrum) and gives off chorda tympani just prior to exit from skull base through stylomastoid foramen

(f) parotid / extracranial segment
facial n. travels forward between superficial + deep lobes of parotid gland lateral to styloid process + external carotid a. + retromandibular v.

Branches:

(1) **Greater superficial petrosal nerve**
(parasympathetic + motor fibers) arises from geniculate ganglion, runs anteromedially, and exits at the facial hiatus on the anterior surface of the temporal bone + passes under Meckel cave near foramen lacerum
— forms **vidian nerve** after receiving sympathetic fibers from deep petrosal nerve, which surrounds the internal carotid artery

(2) **Stapedial nerve** (motor fibers) arises from proximal descending facial n.

(3) **Chorda tympani** (sensory + parasympathetic fibers) leaves facial n. about 6 mm above stylomastoid foramen
— ascends forward in a bony canal (= posterior canaliculus)
— perforates posterior wall of tympanic cavity
— crosses medial to handle of the malleolus underneath mucosa of tympanic cavity
— reenters bone at medial end of petrotympanic fissure (= posterior canaliculus)
— joins the lingual nerve (= branch of V_3) containing sensory fibers from anterior 2/3 of tongue + secretomotor fibers for submandibular and sublingual glands

PERIHIPPOCAMPAL FISSURES

1. Transverse fissure of Bichat
= lateral extension of perimesencephalic cistern separating thalamus superiorly from parahippocampal gyrus inferiorly
2. Choroidal fissure
= superior lateral extension of transverse fissure extending superior to hippocampus
3. Hippocampal fissure
= inferior lateral extension of transverse fissure extending between hippocampus and parahippocampal gyrus
4. Temporal horn of lateral ventricle
= lateral margin of hippocampus; separated from transverse fissure by fimbria + choroid plexus
◊ Does not communicate with transverse fissure

CEREBRAL VESSELS

Common Carotid Artery

- 70% of blood flow is delivered to ICA

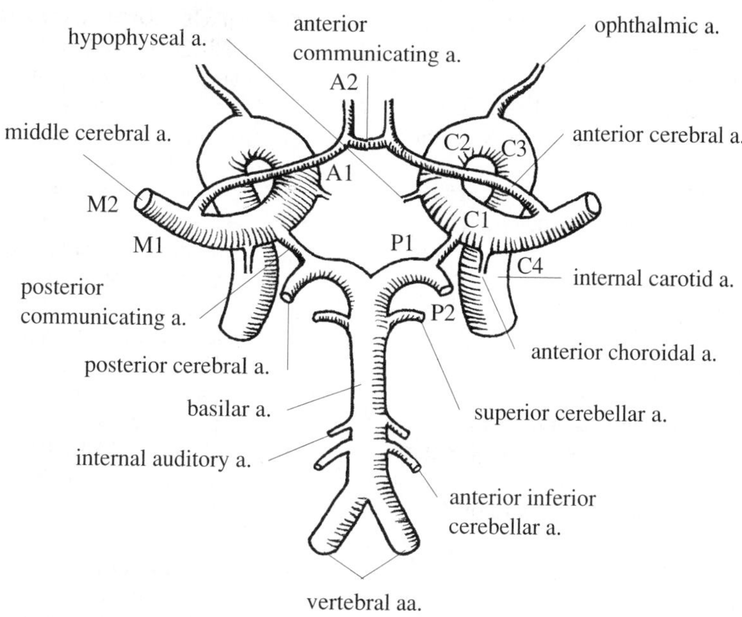

Circle of Willis

√ shares waveform characteristics of both internal + external carotid arteries
√ velocity increases toward the aorta (9 cm/sec for each cm of distance from the carotid bifurcation)

Carotid Bifurcation

= physiologic stenosis due to inertial forces of blood flow diverting main-flow stream from midvessel to a path along vessel margin at flow divider

Location: lateral to upper border of thyroid cartilage; at level of C3-4 intervertebral disk

Branches: ECA arises anterior + medial to ICA (95%)

External Carotid Artery Branches

mnemonic: "**A**ll **S**ummer **L**ong **E**mily **O**gled **P**eter's **S**porty **I**suzu"

Ascending pharyngeal artery
Superior thyroid artery
Lingual artery
External maxillary = facial artery
Occipital artery
Posterior auricular artery
Superficial temporal artery
Internal maxillary artery

Internal Carotid Artery

A. CERVICAL SEGMENT
ascends posterior and medial to ECA; enters carotid canal of petrous bone; NO branches

Carotid bulb = carotid sinus:
= dilated proximal part of ICA with thinner media + thicker adventitia containing many receptor endings of glossopharyngeal nerve

Function: baroreceptor responsive to changes in arterial blood pressure

• hypersensitive carotid sinus
= slight touch / head movement initiates
(a) vasodilatation with drop in blood pressure
(b) vagal stimulation with sinoatrial / atrioventricular cardiac block

√ stagnant eddy that rotates at outer vessel margin

Cervical Segment

ascends posterior and medial to ECA; enters carotid canal of petrous bone; NO branches

B. PETROUS SEGMENT
ascends briefly, in carotid canal bends anteromedially in a horizontal course (anterior to tympanic cavity + cochlea); exits near petrous apex through posterior portion of foramen lacerum; ascends to juxtasellar location where it pierces dural layer of cavernous sinus

Branches:
1. **Caroticotympanic a.**: to tympanic cavity, anastomoses with anterior tympanic branch of maxillary a. + stylomastoid a.
2. **Pterygoid (vidian) a.**: through pterygoid canal; anastomoses with recurrent branch of greater palatine a.

C. CAVERNOUS SEGMENT
ascends to posterior clinoid process, then turns anteriorly + superomedially through cavernous sinus; exits medial to anterior clinoid process piercing dura

Branches:
1. **Meningohypophyseal trunk**
(a) tentorial branch
(b) dorsal meningeal branch
(c) inferior hypophyseal branch

2. **Anterior meningeal a.**: supplies dura of anterior fossa; anastomoses with meningeal branch of posterior ethmoidal a.
3. Cavernous rami supply trigeminal ganglion, walls of cavernous + inferior petrosal sinuses

D. SUPRACLINOID SEGMENT
ascends posterior + lateral between oculomotor + optic nerve
Branches:
mnemonic: "OPA"
Ophthalmic a.
Posterior communicating a.
Anterior choroidal a.

1. **Ophthalmic a.** exits from ICA medial to anterior clinoid process, travels through optic canal inferolateral to optic nerve
   - (a) recurrent meningeal branch: dura of anterior middle cranial fossa
   - (b) posterior ethmoidal a.: supplies dura of planum sphenoidale
   - (c) anterior ethmoidal a.
2. **Superior hypophyseal a.**: optic chiasm, anterior lobe of pituitary
3. **Posterior communicating a.** (pCom)
4. **Anterior choroidal a.**
5. **Middle + anterior cerebral arteries** (MCA, ACA)

Carotid Siphon

flow direction: C4–C1
(a) C4 segment = before origin of ophthalmic a.
(b) C3 segment = genu of ICA
(c) C2 segment = supraclinoid segment after origin of ophthalmic a.
(d) C1 segment = terminal segment of ICA between pCom + ACA

Anterior Cerebral Artery (ACA)

A. HORIZONTAL PORTION = A 1 SEGMENT
= segment between origin and anterior communicating a. (aCom)
(a) Inferior branches
supply superior surface of optic nerve + chiasm
(b) superior branches
penetrate brain to supply anterior hypothalamus, septum pellucidum, anterior commissure, fornix columns, anterior inferior portion of corpus striatum (largest striatal artery = medial lenticulostriate artery = recurrent **artery of Heubner** for anteroinferior portion of head of caudate, putamen, anterior limb of internal capsule)

B. INTERHEMISPHERIC PORTION = A 2 SEGMENT
= segment after origin of anterior communicating a. (aCom); ascends in cistern of lamina terminalis
Branches:

1. **Medial orbitofrontal a.**: along gyrus rectus
2. **Frontopolar a.**
3. **Callosomarginal a.**: within cingulus gyrus
4. **Pericallosal a.**: over corpus callosum within callosal cistern
   - (a) Superior internal parietal a.: anterior portion of precuneus + convexity of superior parietal lobule
   - (b) Inferior internal parietal a.
   - (c) Posterior pericallosal a.

   from callosomarginal / pericallosal artery:
   - — Anterior + middle + posterior internal frontal aa.
   - — Paracentral a.: supplies precentral + postcentral gyri

Supply: anterior 2/3 of medial cerebral surface + 1 cm of superomedial brain over convexity

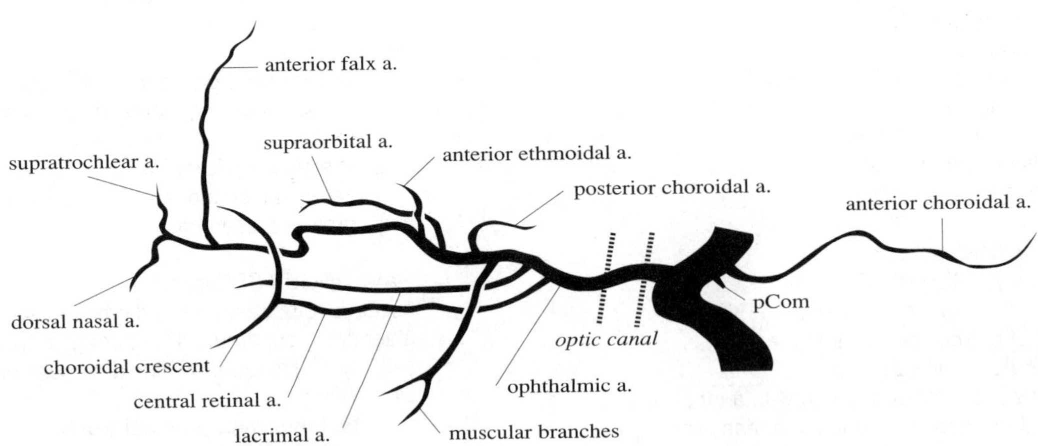

Ophthalmic Artery

Middle Cerebral Artery

= largest branch of ICA arising lateral to optic chiasm; passes horizontal in lateral direction just ventral to anterior perforated substance to enter sylvian fissure where it divides into 2 / 3 / 4 branches

Branches:
1. **Anterior temporal a.**
2. **Ascending frontal a.** (candelabra) / prefrontal a.
3. **Precentral a.** = pre-Rolandic a.
4. **Central a.** = Rolandic a.
5. **Anterior parietal a.** = post-Rolandic a.
6. **Posterior parietal a.**
7. **Angular a.**
8. **Middle temporal a.**
9. **Posterior temporal a.**
10. **Temporo-occipital a.**

Supply: lateral cerebrum, insula, anterior + lateral temporal lobe

Posterior Cerebral Artery

originates from bifurcation of basilar artery within interpeduncular cistern (in 15% as a direct continuation of posterior communicating artery); lies above oculomotor nerve and circles midbrain above the tentorium cerebelli

Branches:
1. Mesencephalic perforating branches: tectum + cerebral peduncles
2. Posterior thalamoperforating aa.: midline of thalamus + hypothalamus
3. Thalamogeniculate aa.: geniculate bodies + pulvinar
4. Posterior medial choroidal a.: circles midbrain parallel to PCA; enters lateral aspect of quadrigeminal cistern;
   passes laterally and above pineal gland and enters roof of 3rd ventricle; supplies quadrigeminal plate + pineal gland
5. Posterior lateral choroidal a.: courses laterally and enters choroidal fissure; anterior branch to temporal horn + posterior branch to choroid plexus of trigone and lateral ventricle + lateral geniculate body
6. Cortical branches: (a) Anterior inferior temporal a.
   (b) Posterior inferior temporal a.
   (c) Parieto-occipital a.
   (d) Calcarine a.
   (e) Posterior pericallosal a.

Supply: medial + posterior temporal lobe, medial parietal lobe, occipital lobe

Arterial Anastomoses of the Brain

ANASTOMOSES VIA THE ARTERIES AT THE BASE OF THE BRAIN

A. Circle of Willis
   1. Right ICA ↔ right ACA ↔ aCom ↔ left ACA ↔ left ICA
   2. ICA ↔ pCom ↔ basilar a.
   3. ICA ↔ anterior choroidal a. ↔ posterior choroidal a. ↔ PCA ↔ basilar a.

B. Developmental anomaly
   three transient embryonal carotid-basilar anastomoses appearing consecutively in fetal life:

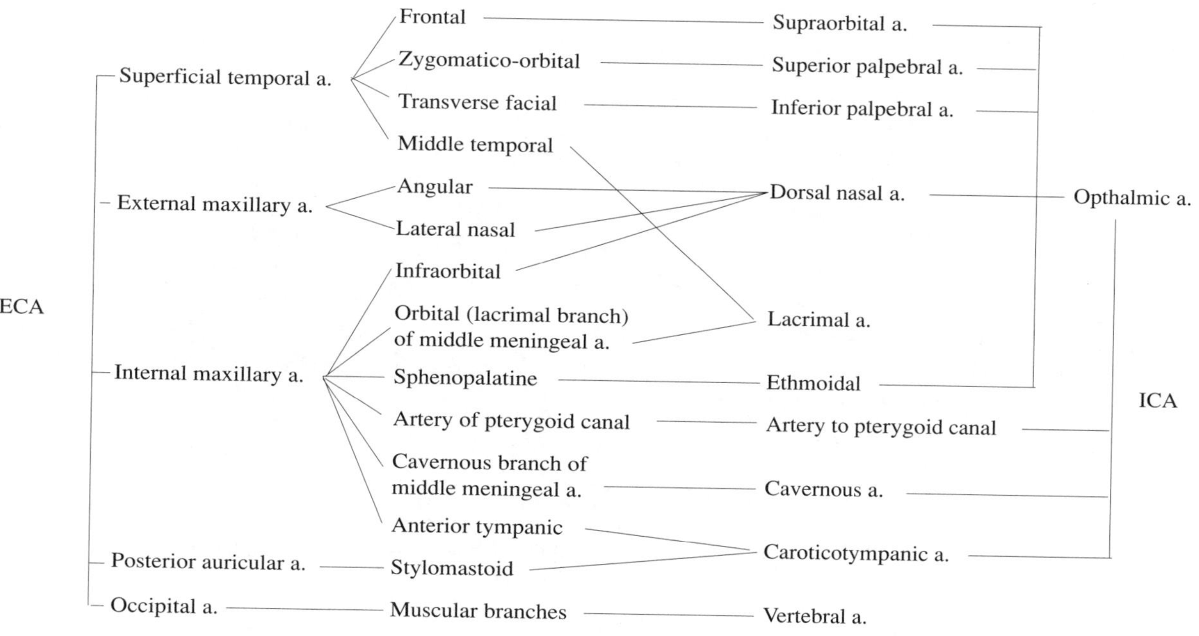

Anastomoses between ICA and ECA and Vertebral Artery

CNS

1. **Primitive hypoglossal artery**
   = arterial connection between the intrapetrosal portion of ICA and proximal portion of basilar artery
2. **Primitive acoustic (otic) artery**
   = arterial connection between cervical portion of ICA + vertebral artery in region of 12th nerve
3. **Persistent primitive trigeminal artery**
   Incidence: 1–2 / 1,000 angiograms
   √ short wide connection between the cavernous portion of ICA and upper third of basilar artery (beneath posterior communicating artery)
   √ enlargement of ipsilateral ICA
   √ ectopic vessel crossing the pontine cistern to anastomose with basilar artery

ANASTOMOSES VIA SURFACE VESSELS
A. Leptomeningeal anastomoses of the cerebrum: ACA ↔ MCA ↔ PCA
B. Leptomeningeal anastomoses of the cerebellum: Superior cerebellar a. ↔ AICA ↔ PICA

RETE MIRABILE
ECA ↔ middle meningeal a. / superficial temporal a. ↔ leptomeningeal aa. ↔ ACA / MCA

Cerebral Veins

Important vascular markers:
1. Pontomesencephalic v. = anterior border of brainstem
2. Precentral cerebellar v. = position of tectum
   ◊ Colliculocentral point = midpoint of Twining's line at knee of precentral cerebellar vein
3. Venous angle = acute angle at junction of thalamostriate with internal cerebral v. = posterior aspect of foramen of Monro
4. Internal cerebral vv. = demarcate caudad border of splenium of corpus callosum superiorly + pineal gland inferiorly
5. Copular point = junction of inferior + superior retrotonsillar tributaries draining cerebellar tonsils in region of copular pyramids of vermis

CEREBELLAR VESSELS

Vertebral Artery

originates from subclavian a. proximal to thyrocervical trunk; left vertebral a. usually greater than right cerebral a.; left vertebral a. may originate directly from aorta (5%)

A. PREVERTEBRAL SEGMENT
   ascends posterosuperiorly between longus colli + anterior scalene muscle; enters transverse foramina at C6
   Branches: muscular branches
B. CERVICAL SEGMENT
   ascends through transverse foramina in close proximity to uncinate processes
   Branches: 1. **Anterior meningeal a.**
C. ATLANTIC SEGMENT
   exits transverse foramen of atlas; passes posteriorly in a groove on superior surface of posterior arch of atlas; pierces atlanto-occipital membrane + dura mater to enter cranial cavity
   Branches: 1. **Posterior meningeal branch** to posterior falx + tentorium

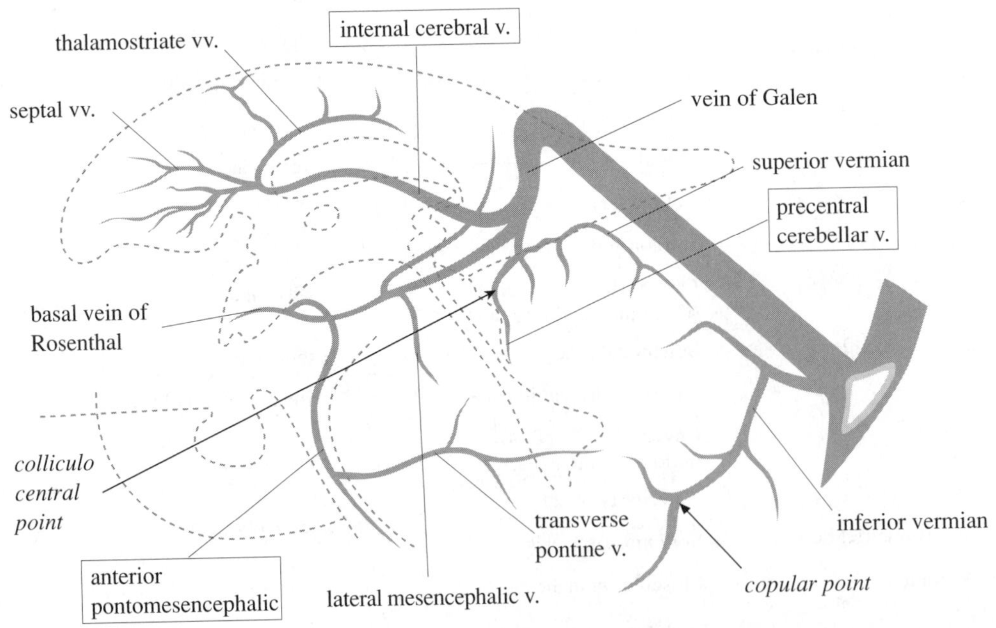

Cerebral Veins

D. INTRACRANIAL SEGMENT
ascends anteriorly + laterally around medulla to reach midline at pontomedullary junction; anastomoses with contralateral side to form basilar artery at clivus
Branches:
1. **Anterior + posterior spinal a.**
2. **Posterior inferior cerebellar a.** (PICA)
3. **Anterior inferior cerebellar a.** (AICA)
4. **Internal auditory a.**
5. **Superior cerebellar a.**
6. **Posterior cerebral a.** (PCA)
7. Medullary + pontine perforating branches

◊ May terminate in common AICA-PICA trunk

Anterior Inferior Cerebellar Artery

= AICA = first branch of basilar artery
Supply:
lateroinferior part of pons, middle cerebellar peduncle, floccular region, anterior petrosal surface of cerebellar hemisphere

◊ Quite variable course + vascular supply with reciprocal relation between vascular territories of AICA + PICA!

Posterior Inferior Cerebellar Artery

= PICA = last and largest branch of vertebral artery
Supply:
inferoposterior surface of cerebellar hemisphere adjacent to occipital bone, ipsilateral part of inferior vermis, inferior portion of deep white matter only

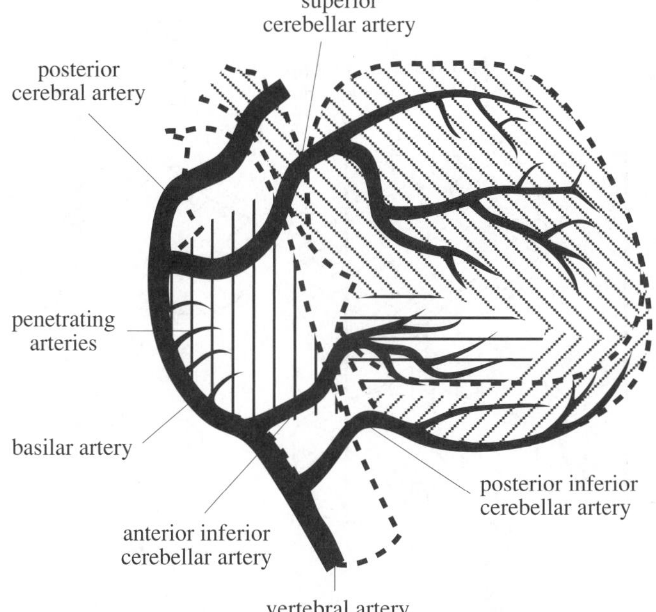

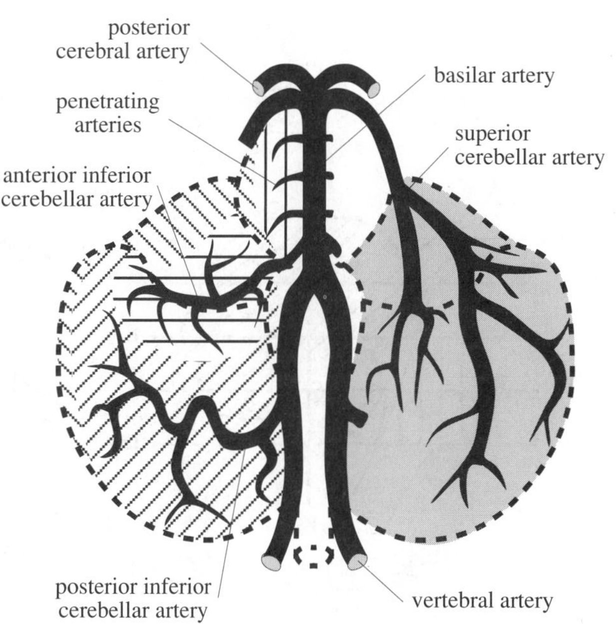

Blood Supply of the Cerebellum

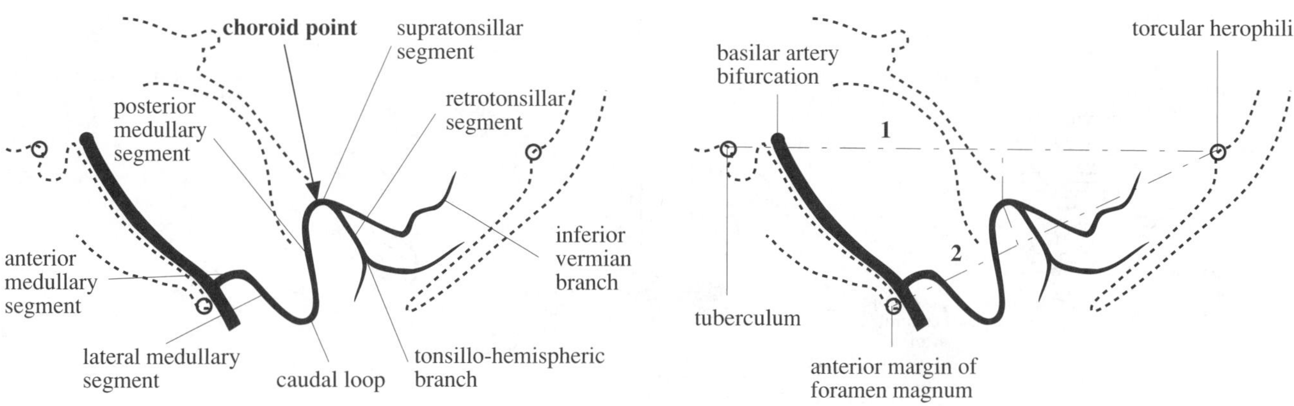

Posterior Inferior Cerebellar Artery
1, 2 = lines to establish orthotopic choroid point (see text)

Parts:

1. Premedullar segment = caudal loop around medulla, may descend below level of foramen magnum
2. Retromedullar segment = ascending portion up to the level of 4th ventricle and tonsils
3. Supratonsillar segment = the most cranial point is the choroidal point

P1 segment = horizontal segment between origin of PICA + pCom

P2 segment = segment downstream from pCom take-off

Variations: commonly asymmetric; hypoplastic / absent in 20% [vascular supply then provided by anterior inferior cerebellar artery (AICA)]

Orthotopic **choroid point** established by:

1. perpendicular line from choroid point onto Twining's line = TTT-line (Twining's Tuberculum-Torcular line) bisects TTT-line (length of anterior portion 52–60%)
2. perpendicular line from choroid point cuts CT-line (Clivus-Torcular line) <1 mm anterior / <3 mm posterior to junction of anterior and middle thirds of CT-line

Superior Cerebellar Artery

= SCA = last but one branch of basilar artery

Supply:

superior aspect of cerebellar hemisphere (tentorial surface), ipsilateral superior vermis, largest part of deep white matter including dentate nucleus, pons

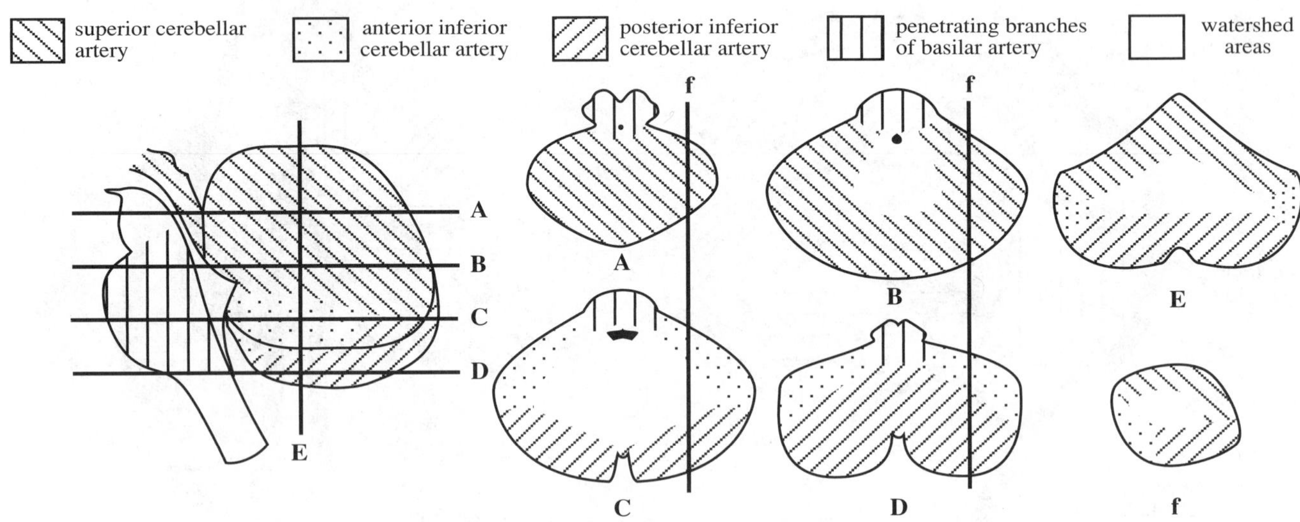

Vascular Territories of Cerebellum

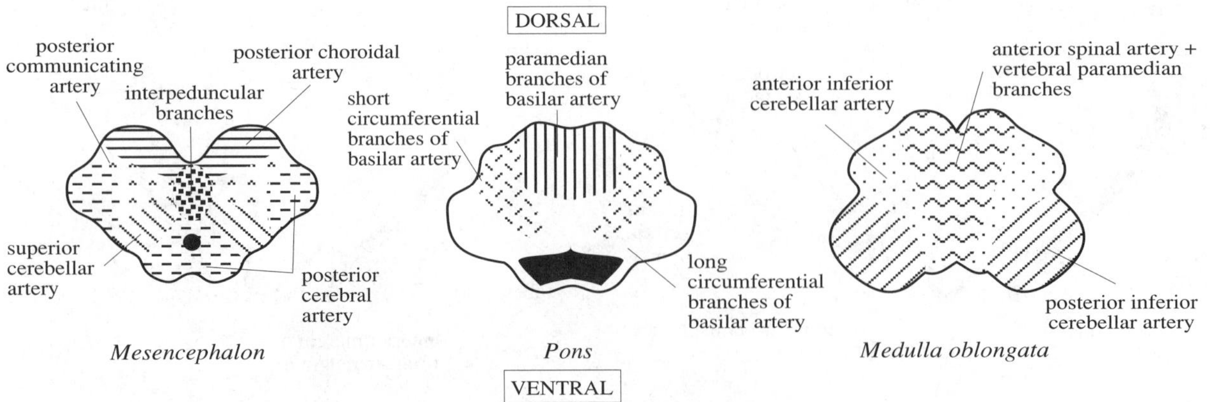

Vascular Territories of Brainstem

BRAIN DISORDERS

ABSCESS OF BRAIN

Pyogenic Abscess

= focal area of necrosis beginning in area of cerebritis with formation of surrounding membrane

Cause:
1. Extension from paranasal sinus infection (41%) / mastoiditis / otitis media (5%) / facial soft-tissue infection / dental abscess
2. Generalized septicemia (32%):
   (a) lung (most common): bronchiectasis, empyema, lung abscess, bronchopleural fistula, pneumonia
   (b) heart (less common): CHD with R-L shunt (in children >60%), AVM, bacterial endocarditis
   (c) osteomyelitis
3. Penetrating trauma or surgery
4. Cryptogenic (25%)

Predisposed: diabetes mellitus, patients on steroids / immunosuppressive drugs, congenital / acquired immunologic deficiency

Organism: anaerobic streptococcus (most common), bacteroides, staphylococcus; in 20% multiple organisms; in 25% sterile contents

Pathophysiology:
- Stage I: vascular congestion, petechial hemorrhage, edema
- Stage II: cerebral softening + necrosis
- Stage III: (after 2–3 weeks) liquefaction, cavitation + capsule consisting of inner layer of granulation tissue, a middle collagenous layer and an outer astroglial layer; edema outside abscess capsule

• headache, drowsiness, confusion, seizure
• focal neurologic deficit
• fever, leukocytosis (resolves with encapsulation)

Location: typically at corticomedullary junction; frontal + temporal lobes; supratentorial : infratentorial = 2:1

NCCT:
- √ zone of low density with mass effect (92%)
- √ slightly increased rim density (4%), development of collagen layer takes 10–14 days
- √ gas within lesion (4%) is diagnostic of gas-forming organism

CECT:
- √ ring enhancement (90%) with peripheral zone of edema
- √ homogeneous enhancement in lesions <0.5 cm
- √ edema + contrast enhancement suppressed by steroids
- √ smooth regular 1–3-mm thick wall with relative thinning of medial wall (secondary to poorer blood supply of white matter)
- √ multiloculation + subjacent daughter abscess in white matter

MR: (most sensitive modality)
- √ centrally increased / variable intensity with hypointense rim on T2WI
- √ outside border of increased signal intensity on T2WI (edema)

Cx:
(1) Development of daughter abscesses toward white matter
(2) Rupture into ventricular system / subarachnoid space (thinner abscess capsule formation on medial wall of abscess related to fewer blood vessels) producing ventriculitis ± meningitis

Dx helpful features:
- multiple lesions at gray-white matter border
- clinical history of altered immune status
- R-to-L shunt: eg, pulmonary AV fistula
- foreign travel
- high-risk behavior: eg, IV drug abuse

DDx: primary / metastatic neoplasm, subacute infarction, resolving hematoma

Granulomatous Abscess

1. Tuberculoma
2. Sarcoid abscess
3. Fungal abscess: coccidioidomycosis, mucormycosis (in diabetics), aspergillosis, cryptococcus

Predisposed: immunocompromised host
- √ enhancement of leptomeningeal surface
- √ nodular / ring-enhancing parenchymal lesion

Cx: Communicating hydrocephalus (secondary to thick exudate blocking basal cisterns)

ACRANIA

= EXENCEPHALY
= developmental anomaly characterized by partial / complete absence of membranous neurocranium + complete but abnormal development of brain tissue

Incidence: 25 cases reported

Cause: impaired migration of mesenchyme to its normal location under the calvarial ectoderm resulting in failure for development of dura mater + skull + musculature

Time: develops after closure of anterior neuropore during 4th week

May be associated with:
cleft lip, bilateral absence of orbital floors, metatarsus varus, talipes, cervicothoracic spina bifida

• ± elevation of maternal serum AFP
- √ absence of calvarium
- √ normal ossification of chondrocranium (face, skull base)
- √ hemispheres surrounded by thin membrane

Prognosis: uniformly lethal; progression to anencephaly (brain destruction secondary to exposure to amniotic fluid + mechanical trauma)

DDx: encephalocele, anencephaly, osteogenesis imperfecta, hypophosphatasia

ADRENOLEUKODYSTROPHY

= BRONZED SCLEROSING ENCEPHALOMYELITIS
= inherited metabolic disorder characterized by progressive demyelination of cerebral white matter + adrenal insufficiency

Etiology: defective peroxisomal fatty acid oxidation due to impaired function of lignoceryl-coenzyme A ligase with accumulation of saturated very long chain fatty acids (cholesterol esters) in white matter + adrenal cortex + testes

Dx: assay of plasma, red cells, cultured skin fibroblasts for the presence of increased amounts of very long chain fatty acids

Mode of inheritance:
(a) X-linked recessive in boys (common)
(b) autosomal recessive in neonates (uncommon)

Histo: PAS cytoplasmic inclusions in brain, adrenals, other tissues

Age: 3–10 years (X-linked recessive)

- deteriorating vision (27%), loss of hearing (50%)
- ataxia
- optic disk pallor
- adrenal gland insufficiency (abnormal increased pigmentation, elevated ACTH levels)
- altered behavior, attention disorder, mental deterioration, death

Location: disease process usually starts in central occipital white matter, advances anteriorly through internal + external capsules + centrum semiovale, centripetal progression to involve subcortical white matter, interhemispheric spread via corpus callosum particularly splenium, involvement of optic radiation ± auditory system ± pyramidal tract

CT:
√ large symmetric low-density lesions in occipitoparietotemporal white matter (80%) advancing toward frontal lobes + cerebellum
√ thin curvilinear / serrated enhancing rims near edges of lesion
√ initial frontal lobe involvement (12%)
√ calcifications within hypodense areas (7%)
√ cerebral atrophy in late stage (progressive loss of cortical neurons)

MR:
√ hypointensity on T1WI in affected areas (hypointense atrophic splenium of corpus callosum)
√ hyperintense bilateral confluent areas on T2WI

Prognosis: usually fatal within several years after onset of symptoms

Adrenomyeloneuropathy

= clinically milder form with later age of onset
- symptoms of spinal cord demyelination + peripheral neuropathy

AGENESIS OF CORPUS CALLOSUM

= COMPLETE DYSGENESIS OF CORPUS CALLOSUM
= failure of formation of corpus callosum originating from the lamina terminalis at 7–13 weeks from where a phalanx of callosal tissue extends backward arching over the diencephalon; usually developed by 20 weeks

Incidence: 0.7–5.3%

Cause: congenital, acquired (infarction of ACA)

Histo: axons from cerebral hemispheres that would normally cross continue along medial walls of lateral ventricles as longitudinal callosal bundles of Probst that terminate randomly in occipital + temporal lobes

Associated with:
(a) CNS anomalies (85%):
1. Dandy-Walker cyst (11%)
2. Interhemispheric arachnoid cyst may be continuous with 3rd and lateral ventricles
3. Hydrocephalus (30%)
4. Midline intracerebral lipoma of corpus callosum often surrounded with ring of calcium (10%)
5. Arnold-Chiari II malformation (7%)
6. Midline encephalocele
7. Porencephaly
8. Holoprosencephaly
9. Hypertelorism median cleft syndrome
10. Polymicrogyria, gray-matter heterotopia

(b) Cardiovascular, gastrointestinal, genitourinary anomalies (62%)
(c) Abnormal karyotype (trisomy 13, 15, 18)

- normal brain function in isolated agenesis
- intellectual impairment; seizures

√ absence of septum pellucidum + corpus callosum + cavum septi pellucidi
√ longitudinal bundles of Probst create crescentic lateral ventricles:
  √ colpocephaly (= dilatation of trigones + occipital horns + posterior temporal horns in the absence of splenium
  √ "bat-wing" appearance of lateral ventricles (= wide separation of lateral ventricles with straight parallel parasagittal orientation with absent callosal body)
  √ laterally convex frontal horns in case of absent genu of corpus callosum
√ "high-riding third ventricle" = upward displacement of widened 3rd ventricle often to level of bodies of lateral ventricle
√ anterior interhemispheric fissure adjoins elevated 3rd ventricle ± communication (PATHOGNOMONIC)
√ "interhemispheric cyst" = interhemispheric CSF collection as an upward extension of 3rd ventricle
√ enlarged foramina of Monro
√ "sunburst gyral pattern" = dysgenesis of cingulate gyrus with characteristic radial orientation of cerebral sulci from the roof of the 3rd ventricle (on sagittal images)
√ failure of normal convergence of calcarine + parieto-occipital sulci
√ persistent eversion of cingulate gyrus (rotated inferiorly + laterally) with absence on midsagittal images
√ incomplete formation of Ammon's horn in the hippocampus

OB-US (>22 weeks GA):
√ absence of septum pellucidum
√ "teardrop" ventriculomegaly = disproportionate enlargement of occipital horns = colpocephaly
√ dilated + elevated 3rd ventricle
√ radial array pattern of medial cerebral sulci

Angio:
√ wandering straight posterior course of pericallosal arteries (lateral view)
√ wide separation of pericallosal arteries secondary to intervening 3rd ventricle (anterior view)
√ separation of internal cerebral veins
√ loss of U-shape in vein of Galen

DDx: (1) Prominent cavum septi pellucidi + cavum vergae (should not be mistaken for 3rd ventricle)
(2) Arachnoid cyst in midline (suprasellar, collicular plate) raising and deforming the 3rd ventricle and causing hydrocephalus

Partial Agenesis of Corpus Callosum

= milder form of callosal dysgenesis (best seen on MR) depending on time of arrested growth (anteroposterior development of genu + body + splenium, however, rostrum forming last)
(a) genu only
(b) genu + part of the body
(c) genu + entire body
(d) genu + body + splenium (without rostrum)

AIDS

= DNA retrovirus infection attacking monocytes + macrophages, which leads to deficient cell-mediated immunity

Incidence: 1% of population in United States is HIV-seropositive; 187,000 new cases in 1991

Histo: formation of microglial nodules instead of granulomas in 75–80% of autopsied brains

• neurologic symptoms as initial complaint in 10%, ultimately afflict up to 40–60%: headache, memory loss, confusion, dementia, focal deficit from mass lesion

◊ Any male with neurologic symptoms between age 20 and 50 has AIDS until proven otherwise

◊ Unusual presentations are clues to HIV infection: pan-sinusitis, mastoiditis, parotid cysts, cervical adenopathy, hypointense spine

DIFFUSE CHANGES:
(1) HIV / CMV encephalopathy (most common complication)
both viruses occur always in combination
• dementia in up to 60% during course of disease
• cognitive dysfunction in up to 90%
√ patchy white matter lesions (= subacute leukoencephalitis) in 31%

FOCAL CHANGES:
(1) Toxoplasmosis (50–70%)
(2) Primary CNS lymphoma (20–30%)
Prevalence: in 75% at autopsy
◊ Initial manifestation in 0.6% of AIDS patients
◊ 2% of AIDS patients develop primary CNS lymphoma at some point during their illness
(3) Progressive multifocal leukoencephalopathy (10–20%)
(4) Fungal, granulomatous, viral, bacterial infection
(a) Cryptococcosis
Location: extension along Virchow-Robin spaces
√ hydrocephalus + cortical / central atrophy (with inadequate immune response)
√ enhancing granulomatous meningitis (with sufficient immune response)
√ bilateral nonenhancing hyperintense abnormalities in lenticulostriate region (= gelatinous pseudocyst) on T2WI
(b) Other opportunistic CNS infections: tuberculosis, neurosyphilis

◊ With multiple CNS lesions toxoplasmic encephalitis is the more likely diagnosis!

◊ With a single CNS lesion the probability of lymphoma is at least equal to toxoplasmosis!

Rx: azidothymidine (AZT)

ALEXANDER DISEASE

= FIBRINOID LEUKODYSTROPHY

Age: as early as first few weeks of life
• macrocephaly
• failure to attain developmental milestones
• progressive spastic quadriparesis
• intellectual failure

Location: frontal white matter gradually extending posteriorly into parietal region + internal capsule

CT:
√ low-density white matter lesion
√ contrast enhancement near tip of frontal horn

MR:
√ prolonged T1 + T2 relaxation times

Prognosis: death in infancy / early childhood

ALZHEIMER DISEASE

= diffuse gray matter disease with large loss of cells from cerebral cortex + other areas

◊ Most common of dementing disorders in elderly!

Incidence: 10% of people >65 years of age; 50% of people >85 years of age

• slowly progressing memory loss, dementia (large overlap with other dementias of elderly)

√ "cracked walnut" appearance = symmetrically enlarged sulci in high-convexity area
√ focal atrophic change in medial temporal lobe (82% sensitive, 75% specific, 80% accurate):
√ volume loss of hippocampus + parahippocampal gyrus
√ enlargement of perihippocampal fissures
√ smooth periventricular halo of hyperintensity (50%)

AMYOTROPHIC LATERAL SCLEROSIS

= most common form of motor neuron disease (without autonomic / sensory / cognitive involvement)

Cause: free radical damage to neurons / autoimmune process / heavy metal toxicity

Age: middle – late adulthood; M > F

Path: atrophy of precentral gyrus

Histo: loss of pyramidal + Betz cells in motor cortex; loss of anterior horn cells in spinal cord; swelling of proximal axons of neuronal cells

- progressive neurodegenerative disorder
  - upper neuronal symptoms: hyperreflexia, spasticity
  - lower neuronal symptoms: fasciculation, atrophy

MR:

√ hyperintense corticospinal tracts (corona radiata, corpus callosum, posterior limb of internal capsule, ventral aspect of brain stem, anterolateral column of spinal cord) on T2WI

√ low signal intensity in motor cortex on T2WI (due to iron deposition)

DDx: Friedreich ataxia, vitamin B_{12} deficiency (abnormal signal limited to internal capsule)

ANENCEPHALY

= lethal anomaly with failure of closure of the rostral end of the neural tube by 5.6 weeks MA

◊ Associated with highest AF-AFP and MS-AFP values; >90% will be detected with MS-AFP ≥2.5 MoM

Incidence: 1:1,000 births (3.5:1,000 in South Wales); M:F = 1:4; most common congenital defect of CNS; 50% of all neural tube defects

Recurrence rate: 3–4%

Etiology: multifactorial (genetic + environmental)

Path: absence of cerebral hemispheres + cranial vault; partial / complete absence of diencephalic + mesencephalic structures; hypophysis + rhombencephalic structures usually preserved

Risk factors: family history of neural tube defect; twin pregnancy

Associated anomalies:

spinal dysraphism (17–50%), cleft lip / palate (2%), clubfoot (2%), umbilical hernia, amniotic band syndrome

√ absence of bony calvarium cephalad to orbits

√ ± cranial soft-tissue mass (= angiomatous stroma)

√ bulging froglike eyes

√ short neck

√ polyhydramnios (40–50%) after 26 weeks GA (due to failure of normal fetal swallowing) / oligohydramnios

Dx: in 100% >14 weeks GA

Prognosis: uniformly fatal within hours to days of life; in 53% premature birth; in 68% stillbirth

DDx: acrania, encephalocele, amniotic band syndrome

ANEURYSM OF CNS

Etiology:

(a) congenital (97%) = "berry aneurysm" in 2% of population (in 20% multiple); associated with aortic coarctation + adult polycystic kidney disease
(b) infectious (3%) = mycotic aneurysm
(c) arteriosclerotic: fusiform shape
(d) traumatic
(e) neoplastic
(f) fibromuscular disease
(g) collagen vascular disease

Risk factors:

(1) family history for aneurysms in 1st- / 2nd-degree relatives
(2) female gender
(3) age >50 years
(4) cigarette smoking
(5) oral contraceptives / pregnancy
(6) Marfan syndrome, pseudoxanthoma elasticum, Ehlers-Danlos syndrome, neurofibromatosis type 1
(7) polycystic kidney disease
(8) asymmetry of circle of Willis
(9) cerebral arteriovenous malformation

Pathogenesis: arterial wall deficient in tunica media + external elastic lamina (natural occurrence with advancing age)

Location of aneurysm:

A. by autopsy:
  (a) circle of Willis (85%):
  aCom (25%), pCom (18%), MCA bifurcation (25%), distal ACA (5%), ICA at bifurcation (4%), ophthalmic a. (4%), anterior choroidal a. (4%)
  (b) posterior fossa (15%)
  basilar bifurcation (7%), basilar trunk (3%), vertebral-PICA (3%), PCA (2%)

B. by angiography (= symptomatic aneurysms):
  pCom (38%) > aCom (36%) > MCA bifurcation (21%) > ICA bifurcation > tip of basilar artery (2.8%)

C. by risk of bleeding: 1–2% per year
  aCom (70% bleed), pCom (2nd highest risk)
  ◊ Aneurysms at bifurcations / branching points are at greatest risk for rupture!

MULTIPLE ANEURYSMS

Cause: congenital in 20–30%, mycotic in 22%

mnemonic: "FECAL P"

Fibromuscular dysplasia
Ehlers-Danlos syndrome
Coarctation
Arteriovenous malformation
Lupus erythematosus
Polycystic kidney disease (adult)

◊ 35% of patients with one MCA aneurysm have one on the contralateral side (= mirror image aneurysms)!

◊ Simultaneous aneurysm + AVM in 4–15%

CECT: detection rate of aneurysms at pCom (40%), aCom / MCA, basilar artery (80%)

Angio (all 4 cerebral vessels):

√ contrast outpouching

√ <2 mm infundibuli typically occur at pCom / anterior choroidal a. origin

√ mass effect in thrombosed aneurysm

◊ 2nd arteriogram within 1–2 weeks detects aneurysm in 10–20% following negative 1st angiogram!

Prognosis:
(1) Death in 10% within 24 hours from concomitant intracerebral hemorrhage, extensive brain herniation, massive infarcts + hemorrhage within brainstem; 45% mortality within 30 days (25% prior to admission)
(2) Complete recovery in 58% of survivors
(3) Cerebral ischemia + infarction
(4) Rebleeding rate: 12–20% within 2 weeks, 11–22% within 30 days, up to 50% within 6 months (increased mortality); thereafter 1–2–4% risk/year

Surgical mortality rate: 50% for ruptured, 1–3% for unruptured aneurysms

Cx: subdural hematoma

Ruptured Berry Aneurysm

Incidence: 28,000 cases/year = 10 cases/10,000 people/year
Age: 50–60 years of age; M:F = 1:2
Rupture size: 5–15 mm

- "worst headache of one's life"
- neck stiffness, nausea, vomiting
- sudden loss of consciousness (in up to 45%)
- history of warning leak / sentinel hemorrhage hours to days earlier

Clues for which aneurysm is bleeding:
(a) the largest aneurysm (87%)
(b) anterior communicating artery (70%)
(c) contralateral side of all visualized aneurysms (60%), nonvisualization due to spasm

mnemonic: "BISH"
Biggest
Irregular contour
Spasm (adjacent)
Hematoma location

Location of blood suggesting accurately in 70% the site of the ruptured aneurysm:
(a) according to location of subarachnoid hemorrhage:
1. Anterior chiasmatic cistern : aCom
2. Septum pellucidum : aCom
3. Interhemispheric fissure : aCom
4. Intraventricular : aCom, ICA, MCA
5. Sylvian fissure : MCA, ICA, pCom
6. Anterior pericallosal cistern : ACA, aCom
7. Prepontine cistern : basilar a.
8. Foramen magnum : PICA
9. Symmetric distribution in subarachnoid space : ACA + basilar a.

(b) according to location of cerebral hematoma:
1. Inferomedial frontal lobe : aCom
2. Temporal lobe : MCA
3. Corpus callosum : pericallosal artery

(c) intraventricular hemorrhage
from aneurysms at aCom, MCA, pericallosal artery (CAVE: blood may have entered in retrograde manner from subarachnoid location)

Giant Aneurysm

= aneurysm larger than 2.5 cm in diameter, usually presenting with intracranial mass effect
Incidence: 25% of all aneurysms
Age: no age predilection; M:F = 2:1
Location: (arise from arteries at the base of the brain)
(a) middle fossa: cavernous segment of ICA (43%), supraclinoid segment of ICA, terminal bifurcation of ICA, middle cerebral artery
(b) posterior fossa: at tip of basilar artery, AICA, vertebral artery

Skull film:
√ predominantly peripheral curvilinear calcification (22%)
√ bone erosion (44%)
√ pressure changes on sella turcica (18%)

CECT:
√ "target sign" = centrally opacified vessel lumen + ring of thrombus + enhanced fibrous outer wall
√ simple ring-blush (75%) of fibrous outer wall with total thrombosis
√ little / no surrounding edema

MR:
√ mixed signal intensity (combination of subacute + chronic hemorrhage, calcification)

Cx: subarachnoid hemorrhage in <30%

Mycotic Aneurysm

= 3% of all intracranial aneurysms, multiple in 20%
Source: subacute bacterial endocarditis (65%), acute bacterial endocarditis (9%), meningitis (9%), septic thrombophlebitis (9%), myxoma
Location: peripheral to first bifurcation of major vessel (64%); often located near surface of brain especially over convexities
(a) suprasellar cistern = circle of Willis
(b) inferolateral sylvian fissure = middle cerebral artery trifurcation
(c) genu of corpus callosum = origin of callosomarginal artery
(d) bottom of 3rd ventricle = pericallosal a.

NCCT:
√ aneurysm rarely visualized; indirect evidence from focal hematoma secondary to rupture
√ zone of increased density / calcification
√ increased density in subarachnoid, intraventricular, intracerebral spaces (extravasated blood)
√ focal / diffuse lucency of brain (edema / infarction / vasospasm)

CECT:
√ intense homogeneous enhancement within round / oval mass contiguous to vessels
√ incomplete opacification with mural thrombus

Cx: develop recurrent bleeding more frequently than congenital aneurysms

Supraclinoid Carotid Aneurysm

= 38% of intracranial aneurysms

Site: (a) at origin of pCom (65%)
(b) at bifurcation of internal carotid artery (23%)
(c) at origin of ophthalmic artery (12%) medial to anterior clinoid process; most likely to become giant aneurysm

Presentation: bitemporal hemianopia (extrinsic compression on chiasm)

√ calcification is rare (frequent in atherosclerotic cavernous sinus aneurysm)

Cavernous Sinus Aneurysm

Age: 20–70 years, peak 5th–6th decade; F >> M
Cause: sinus thrombophlebitis

- progressive visual impairment
- cavernous sinus syndrome: trigeminal nerve pain, oculomotor nerve paralysis

Site: extradural portion of cavernous sinus ICA

√ undercutting of anterior clinoid process
√ erosion of lateral half of sella
√ erosion of posterior clinoid process
√ invasion of middle cranial fossa
√ enlargement of superior orbital fissure
√ erosion of tip of petrous pyramid
√ rimlike calcification (33%)
√ displacement of thin bony margins without sclerosis

Rx: often inoperable; balloon embolization ± parent artery occlusion

AQUEDUCTAL STENOSIS

= focal reduction in size of aqueduct at level of superior colliculi / intercollicular sulcus (normal range of 0.2–1.8 mm^2)

Embryology:
aqueduct develops about the 6th week of gestation + decreases in size until birth due to growth pressure from adjacent mesencephalic structures

Incidence: 0.5–1:1,000 births; most frequent cause of congenital hydrocephalus (20–43%); recurrence rate in siblings of 1–4.5%; M:F = 2:1

Etiology:
(a) postinflammatory (50%): secondary to perinatal infection (toxoplasmosis, CMV, syphilis, mumps, influenza virus) or intracranial hemorrhage
= destruction of ependymal lining of aqueduct with adjacent marked fibrillary gliosis
(b) developmental: aqueductal forking (= marked branching of aqueduct into channels) / narrowing / transverse septum (X-linked recessive inheritance in 25% of males)
(c) neoplastic (extremely rare): pinealoma, meningioma, tectal astrocytoma (may be missed on routine CT scans, easily differentiated by MR)

May be associated with: other congenital anomalies (16%): thumb deformities

√ enlargement of lateral + 3rd ventricles with normal-sized 4th ventricle (4th ventricle may be normal with communicating hydrocephalus)

Prognosis: 11–30% mortality

ARACHNOID CYST

= CSF-containing intraarachnoid cyst without ventricular communication / brain maldevelopment

Incidence: 1% of all intracranial masses

Origin:
(1) congenital: arising from clefts / duplication / "splitting" of arachnoid membrane with expansion by CSF due to secretory activity of arachnoid cells
= **true arachnoid cyst**
(2) acquired: following surgery / trauma / subarachnoid hemorrhage / infection in neonatal period / associated with extraaxial neoplasm = loculation of CSF surrounded by arachnoidal scarring with expansion by osmotic filtration / ball-valve mechanism = **leptomeningeal cyst** = **secondary arachnoid cyst** = **acquired arachnoid cyst**

Histo: cyst filled with clear fluid, thin wall composed of cleaved arachnoid membrane lined by ependymal / meningothelial cells

Age: presentation at any time during life

- often asymptomatic
- symptomatic due to mass effect, hydrocephalus, seizures, headaches, hemiparesis, intracranial hypertension, craniomegaly, developmental delay, visual loss, precocious puberty, bobble-head doll syndrome

Location: (arise in CSF cisterns between brain + dura)
(a) floor of middle fossa near tip of temporal lobe (sylvian fissure) in 50%
(b) suprasellar / chiasmatic cistern (may produce endocrinopathy) in 10%
(c) posterior fossa (1/3): cerebellopontine angle (11%), quadrigeminal plate cistern (10%), in relationship to vermis (9%), prepontine / interpeduncular cistern (3%)
(d) interhemispheric fissure, cerebral convexity, anterior infratentorial midline

√ forward bowing of anterior wall of cranial fossa + elevation of sphenoid ridge
√ extraaxial unilocular thin-walled CSF-density cyst with well-defined smooth angular margins
√ compression of subarachnoid space + subjacent brain (minimal mass effect)
√ may erode inner table of calvarium
√ NO enhancement (intrathecal contrast penetrates into cyst on delayed scans)
√ NO calcifications

MR (best modality):
√ well-circumscribed lesion with same uniform signal intensity as CSF ± mass effect

Cx: (1) hydrocephalus (30–60%)
(2) concurrent subdural / intracystic hemorrhage

Prognosis: favorable if removed before onset of irreversible brain damage

Rx: fenestration / cyst-peritoneal shunting

CT-DDx:
epidermoid cyst, dermoid, subdural hygroma, infarction, porencephaly

US-DDx:
choroid plexus cyst, porencephalic cyst (communicates with ventricle), cystic tumor (solid components), midline cyst associated with agenesis of corpus callosum, dorsal cyst associated with holoprosencephaly, Dandy-Walker cyst (extension of 4th ventricle, developmental delay), vein of Galen aneurysm

ARTERIOVENOUS FISTULA

= abnormal communication between artery + vein resulting in tremendous amount of flow due to high pressure gradient; leading to enlargement + elongation of draining veins

Cause:
(1) Vessel laceration (delay between trauma + clinical manifestation due to delayed lysis of hematoma surrounding arterial laceration)
(2) Angiodysplasia: fibromuscular disease, neurofibromatosis, Ehlers-Danlos syndrome
(3) Congenital fistula

- pulsatile mass + thrill / bruit
- ± neurologic symptoms / deficit (due to arterial steal)

Location:
(a) carotid-cavernous sinus fistula (most common)
(b) vertebral artery fistula
(c) external carotid fistula (rare)

ARTERIOVENOUS MALFORMATION

= congenital abnormality consisting of a nidus of abnormal dilated tortuous arteries + veins with racemose tangle of closely packed pathologic vessels resulting in shunting of blood from arterial to venous side without intermediary capillary bed

Prevalence: most common vascular lesion

Histo: affected arteries have thin walls (no elastica, small amount of muscularis); intervening gliotic brain parenchyma between vessels

Age: 80% by end of 4th decade; 20% <20 years of age

- headaches, seizures (nonfocal in 40%), mental deterioration
- progressive hemispheric neurologic deficit (50%)
- ictus from acute intracranial hemorrhage (50%)

Location:
(a) supratentorial (90%): parietal > frontal > temporal lobe > paraventricular > intraventricular region > occipital lobe
(b) infratentorial (10%)

Vascular supply:
(a) pial branches of ICA in 73% of supratentorial location, in 50% of posterior fossa location
(b) dural branches of ECA in 27% with infratentorial lesions

√ NO mass effect

Skull film:
√ speckled / ringlike calcifications (15–30%)
√ thinning / thickening of skull at contact area with AVM
√ prominent vascular grooves on inner table of skull (dilated feeding arteries + draining veins) in 27%

NCCT:
√ irregular lesion with large feeding arteries + draining veins
√ mixed density (60%): dense large vessels + hemorrhage + calcifications
√ isodense lesion (15%): may be recognizable by mass effect
√ low density (15%): brain atrophy due to ischemia
√ not visualized (10%)

CECT:
√ serpiginous dense enhancement in 80% (tortuous dilated vessels)
√ No enhancement in thrombosed AVM
√ No avascular spaces within AVM
√ lack of mass effect / edema (unless thrombosed / bleeding)
√ rapid shunting
√ thickened arachnoid covering
√ adjacent atrophic brain

MR:
√ flow void (imaging with GRASS gradient echo + long TR sequences)

Angio:
√ grossly dilated efferent + afferent vessels with a racemose tangle ("bag of worms")
√ arteriovenous shunting into at least one early draining vein
√ negative angiogram (compression by hematoma / thrombosis)

Cx: (1) Hemorrhage (common): bleeding on venous side due to increased pressure / ruptured aneurysm (5%)
(2) Infarction

Prognosis: 10% mortality; 30% morbidity; 2–3% yearly chance of bleeding increasing to 6% in year following 1st bleed + 25% in year following 2nd bleed

Wyburn-Mason Syndrome

= telangiectasias of skin + retinal cirsoid aneurysm + AVM involving entire optic tract (optic nerve, thalamus, geniculate bodies, calcarine cortex);

May be associated with: AVMs of posterior fossa, neck, mandible / maxilla presenting in childhood

ASTROCYTOMA

Incidence: 70–75% of all primary intracranial tumors; most common brain tumor in children (40–50% of all primary pediatric intracranial neoplasms)

Location:
cerebral hemisphere (lobar), thalamus, pons, midbrain, may spread across corpus callosum (incidence of occurrence proportional to amount of white matter); no particular lobar distribution;
(a) in adults: central white matter of cerebrum (15–30% of all gliomas)

(b) in children: cerebellum (40%) + brainstem (20%), supratentorial (30%)

Well-differentiated = Low-grade Astrocytoma

Incidence: 9% of all primary intracranial tumors; 10–15% of gliomas
Age: 20– 40 years; M > F
Path: benign nonmetastasizing; poorly defined borders with infiltration of white matter + basal ganglia + cortex; NO significant tumor vascularity / necrosis / hemorrhage; blood-brain barrier may remain intact
Histo: homogeneous relatively uniform appearance with proliferation of well-differentiated multipolar fibrillary / protoplasmic astrocytes; mild nuclear pleomorphism + mild hypercellularity; mitoses rare
Location: posterior fossa in children, supratentorial in adults (typically lobar); distribution proportional to amount of white matter
√ may develop a cyst with high-protein content (rare)
CT:
- √ usually hypodense lesion with minimal mass effect + minimal / NO peritumoral edema
- √ well-defined tumor margins
- √ central calcifications (15–20%)
- √ minimal / no contrast enhancement (normal capillary endothelial cells)

MR:
- √ well-defined hypointense lesion with little mass effect / vasogenic edema / heterogeneity on T1WI
- √ hyperintense on T2WI
- √ little / no enhancement on Gd-DTPA
- √ cyst with content hyperintense to CSF (protein content)
- √ hyperintense area within tumor mass (paramagnetic effect of methemoglobin)
- √ inhomogeneous gadolinium-DTPA enhancement of tumor nodule

Angio:
- √ majority avascular

Prognosis: 3–10 years postoperative survival; occasionally converting into more malignant form several years after presentation

Anaplastic Astrocytoma

Incidence: 11% of all primary intracranial neoplasms; 25% of gliomas
Path: frequently vasogenic edema; NO necrosis / hemorrhage
Histo: less well differentiated with greater degree of hypercellularity + pleomorphism, multipolar fibrillary / protoplasmic astrocytes; mitoses + vascular endothelial proliferation common
Location: typically frontal + temporal lobes
Distribution: proportional to amount of white matter
MR:
- √ moderate mass effect
- √ well-defined slightly heterogeneous hypointense lesion on T1WI with prevalent vasogenic edema
- √ hyperintense on T2WI
- √ ± enhancement on Gd-DTPA

Prognosis: 2 years postoperative survival

Pilocytic Astrocytoma

= JUVENILE PILOCYTIC ASTROCYTOMA
= most benign histologic subtype of astrocytoma without progression to high-grade glioma
◊ Most common infratentorial neoplasm in pediatric age group
Histo: alternating pattern of compact bipolar pilocytic (hairlike) astrocytes arranged mostly around vessels + loosely aggregated protoplasmic astrocytes undergoing microcystic degeneration
Age: predominantly in children + young adults; peak age between birth and 9 years of age; M:F = 1:1
Associated with: neurofibromatosis type 1
Location: cerebellum, hypothalamus (around 3rd ventricle), optic nerve / chiasm
√ micro- / macrocysts in cerebellar location (in 60–80%)
√ mural tumor nodule located in wall of cerebellar cyst

WHO Classification of Astrocytomas

Grade	Type	Features
Grade I	Circumscribed astrocytoma	generally benign well-circumscribed tumor, specific unique histologic features for each tumor, **pilocytic astrocytoma** (most common), subependymal **giant cell astrocytoma**; no tendency to progress to higher grade; low rate of recurrence
Grade II	Astrocytoma	diffusely infiltrating; well-differentiated; minimal pleomorphism or nuclear atypia; no vascular proliferation / necrosis
Grade III	Anaplastic astrocytoma	pleomorphism and nuclear atypia; increased cellularity; mitotic activity; vascular proliferation + necrosis absent
Grade IV	Glioblastoma multiforme	marked vascular proliferation and necrosis; increased cellularity; anaplasia + pleomorphism; variable mitotic activity; cell type may be poorly differentiated, fusiform, round or multinucleated

√ multilobulated / dumbbell appearance along optic pathway
√ rarely calcifies
√ increased heterogeneous signal intensity on early Gd-DTPA-enhanced T1WI; homogeneous enhancement on delayed images

Prognosis: relatively benign clinical course, almost never recurs after surgical excision; >90% postsurgical 5-year survival; NO malignant transformation to anaplastic form

DDx: metastasis, hemangioblastoma, atypical medulloblastoma

Pleomorphic Xanthoastrocytoma

= superficially located supratentorial tumor that involves leptomeninges

Prevalence: 1% of all brain neoplasms

Age: average age of 26 years (range, 5–82 years)

Path: circumscribed tumor attached to meninges with infiltration into surrounding brain

Histo: pleomorphic spindled tumor cells (reactive to glial fibrillary acidic protein) with intracytoplasmic lipid (xanthomatous) deposits in a dense intercellular reticulin network; giant cells; eosinophilic granular bodies; WHO grade II tumor

• long history of seizures (71%)

Location: supratentorial (98%): temporal (49%) / parietal (17%) / frontal (10%) / occipital (7%) lobe; thalamus; cerebellum; spinal cord
◊ Its peripheral location is the single most consistent imaging feature

√ cystic (48%) supratentorial mass with mural nodule
√ intense enhancement of solid portions
√ CHARACTERISTIC involvement of leptomeninges (71%)
√ peritumoral vasogenic edema / calcification / skull erosion are uncommon

CT:
√ hypo- / isoattenuating mass

MR:
√ hypo- to isointense relative to gray matter on T1WI
√ hyper- to isointense on T2WI

Rx: surgical resection (unresponsive to chemotherapy + radiation therapy)

Prognosis: 81% 5-year survival rate; 70% 10-year survival rate; high rate of recurrence; malignant transformation in 20%

DDx: meningioma, glioblastoma multiforme, oligodendroglioma, metastatic disease, infection

ATAXIA-TELANGIECTASIA

= autosomal recessive disorder characterized by telangiectasias of skin + eye, cerebellar ataxia, sinus + pulmonary infections, immunodeficiencies, propensity to develop malignancies

Incidence: 1:40,000 livebirths

Path: neuronal degradation + atrophy of cerebellar cortex (? from vascular anomalies)

• cerebellar ataxia at beginning of walking age
• progressive neurologic deterioration
• oculomotor abnormalities, dysarthric speech, choreoathetosis, myoclonic jerks
• mucocutaneous telangiectasias: bulbar conjunctiva, ears, face, neck, palate, dorsum of hands, antecubital + popliteal fossa
• recurrent bacterial + viral sinopulmonary infections

√ cerebellar cortical atrophy: diminished cerebellar size, dilatation of 4th ventricle, increased cerebellar sulcal prominence
√ cerebral hemorrhage (rupture of telangiectatic vessels)
√ cerebral infarct (emboli shunted through vascular malformations in lung)

Cx:
(1) Bronchiectasis + pulmonary failure (most common cause of death)
(2) Malignancies (10–15%): lymphoma, leukemia, epithelial malignancies

BINSWANGER DISEASE

= ENCEPHALOPATHIA SUBCORTICALIS PROGRESSIVA
= LEUKOARIAOSIS = SUBCORTICAL ARTERIOSCLEROTIC ENCEPHALOPATHY (SAE)

Cause: arteriosclerosis affecting the poorly collateralized distal penetrating arteries (perforating medullary arteries, thalamoperforators, lenticulostriates, pontine perforators); positive correlation with hypertension + aging

Path: ischemic demyelination / infarction

Age: >60 years

• psychiatric changes, intellectual impairment, slowly progressive dementia, transient neurologic deficits, seizures, spasticity, syncope

Location: periventricular white matter, centrum semiovale, basal ganglia; subcortical white matter "U" fibers + corpus callosum are spared

√ multifocal hypodense lesions (periventricular, centrum semiovale) with sparing of U fibers
√ lacunar infarcts in basal ganglia
√ sulcal enlargement + dilated lateral ventricles (brain atrophy)

MR:
√ focal areas of increased signal intensity on T2WI (= "unidentified bright objects")

DDx: leukodystrophy, progressive multifocal leukoencephalopathy, multiple sclerosis

CANAVAN DISEASE

= SPONGIFORM LEUKODYSTROPHY
= rare form of leukodystrophy as an autosomal recessive disorder, most common in Ashkenazi Jews

Incidence: <100 reported cases

Cause: deficiency of aspartoacyclase leading to accumulation of *N*-acetylaspartic acid in brain, plasma, urine, CSF

Histo: spongy degeneration of white matter with astrocytic swelling + mitochondrial elongation

Age: 3–6 months

• marked hypotonia

- progressive megalencephaly
- seizures
- failure to attain motor milestones
- spasticity
- intellectual failure
- optic atrophy with blindness
- swallowing impairment

√ diffuse symmetric white matter abnormality
√ may involve basal ganglia
√ cortical atrophy

CT:
√ low-density white matter

MR:
√ white matter hypointense on T1WI + hyperintense on T2WI

Prognosis: death in 2nd–5th year of life

Dx: (1) elevation of *N*-acetylaspartic acid in urine
(2) deficiency of aspartoacyclase in cultured skin fibroblasts

CAPILLARY TELANGIECTASIA

= CAPILLARY ANGIOMA
= abnormal dilated capillaries separated by normal neural tissue; commonly "cryptic"

May be associated with:
hereditary Rendu-Osler-Weber syndrome, ataxia-telangiectasia syndrome, irradiation (latency period of 5 months to 22 years)

Age: typically in elderly

- usually asymptomatic (incidental finding at necropsy)

Location: mostly in pons / midbrain; usually multiple / may be solitary

√ poorly defined area of dilated vessels (resembling petechiae)
√ best delineated with MR (due to hemorrhage)

Cx: punctate hemorrhage (uncommon), gliosis + calcifications (rare)

Prognosis: bleeding in pons usually fatal

DDx: cavernous angioma (identical on images)

CAVERNOUS HEMANGIOMA OF BRAIN

= CAVERNOUS ANGIOMA = CAVERNOMA

Path: well-circumscribed nodule of honeycomblike large sinusoidal vascular spaces separated by fibrous collagenous bands <u>without</u> intervening neural tissue; slow blood flow in vascular channels

Age: 3rd–6th decade; M > F

- seizures (commonly presenting symptom)

Location: cerebrum (mainly subcortical) > pons > cerebellum; solitary > multiple

√ NO obvious mass effect / edema

NCCT:
√ extensive calcifications = hemangioma calcificans (20%)
√ small round hyperdense region (CLUE)
√ minimal surrounding edema

CECT:
√ minimal / intense enhancement
√ low-attenuation areas due to thrombosed portions

MR:
√ well-defined area of mixed signal intensity centrally (= "mulberry"-shaped lesion) with a mixture of
√ increased signal intensity (= extracellular methemoglobin / slow blood flow / thrombosis)
√ decreased intensity (= deoxyhemoglobin / intracellular methemoglobin / hemosiderin / calcification)
√ surrounded by hypointense rim (= hemosiderin) on T2WI

Angio:
√ negative = "cryptic / occult vascular malformation"

Cx: hemorrhage of varying ages

DDx: (1) Hemorrhagic neoplasm (edema, mass effect)
(2) Small AVM (thrombosed / small feeding vessels, associated hemorrhage)
(3) Capillary angioma (no difference)

CENTRAL PONTINE MYELINOLYSIS

= OSMOTIC MYELINOLYSIS = OSMOTIC DEMYELINATION SYNDROME

Etiology:
unknown; osmotic insult + metabolic compromise: comatose patient receiving rapid correction / overcorrection of severe hyponatremia >12 mmol/L/day (following prolonged IV fluid administration; 60–70% in chronic alcoholics)

Pathophysiology:
rapid correction of sodium releases myelinotoxic compounds by gray matter components resulting in destruction of myelin sheaths (osmotic myelinolysis) with preservation of neurons + axons

- spastic quadriparesis + pseudobulbar palsy
- acute mental status change
- progression to pseudocoma (locked-in syndrome) in 3–5 days

Location: (a) isolated pons lesion (most commonly)
(b) combined type: central + extrapontine areas: basal ganglia, cerebellar white matter, thalamus, caudate nucleus, subcortical cerebral white matter, corona radiata, lateral geniculate body

CT:
√ diminished attenuation in central region of pons

MR (positive 1–2 weeks post-onset of symptoms):
√ single central symmetric midline pons lesion:
√ trident-shaped / round (coronal scan) + bat-wing configuration (sagittal scan)
√ hypointense on T1WI + hyperintense on T2WI
√ bilateral symmetric well-demarcated lesions in basal ganglia ± other extrapontine sites

Prognosis: 5–10% survival rate beyond 6 months

DDx: hypoxia, Leigh disease, Wilson disease

CEPHALOCELE

= mesodermal defect in skull + dura with extracranial extension of intracranial structures with persistent connection to subarachnoid space

CRANIAL MENINGOCELE = herniation of meninges + CSF only

ENCEPHALOCELE = herniation of meninges + CSF + neural tissue

Prevalence:
1–4 per 10,000 livebirths; 5–6–20% of all craniospinal malformations; predominant neural axis anomaly in fetuses spontaneously aborted <20 weeks GA;
3% of fetal anomalies detected with MS-AFP screening;
6% of all detected neural tube defects in fetuses

Cause:
failure of surface ectoderm to separate from neuroectoderm early in embryonic development
@ Skull base
(1) faulty closure of neural tube (without mesenchyme membranous cranial bone cannot develop)
(2) failure of basilar ossification centers to unite
@ Calvarium
(1) defective induction of bone
(2) pressure erosion of bone by intracranial mass / cyst

In 60% associated with:
1. Spina bifida (7–30%)
2. Corpus callosum dys- / agenesis
3. Chiari malformation
4. Dandy-Walker malformation
5. Cerebellar hypoplasia
6. Amniotic band syndrome: multiple irregular asymmetric off-midline encephaloceles
7. Migrational abnormalities
8. Chromosomal anomalies in 44% (trisomy 18)

• MS-AFP elevated in 3% (skin-covered in 60%)
• CSF rhinorrhea
• meningitis

Prognosis: dependent on associated malformations + size and content of lesion; 21% liveborn; 50% survival in liveborns, 74% retarded
◊ Outcome poorer the larger the brain volume

Risk of recurrence: 3% (25% with Meckel syndrome)

DDx: teratoma, cystic hygroma, iniencephaly, scalp edema, hemangioma, branchial cleft cyst, cloverleaf skull

Nomenclature:
based on origin of their roof + floor, eg
frontonasal: frontal bone = roof, nasal bone = floor

Occipital Encephalocele (75%)

Most common encephalocele in Western Hemisphere

Associated with:
(1) Meckel-Gruber syndrome
= occipital encephalocele + microcephaly + cystic dysplastic kidneys + polydactyly
(2) Dandy-Walker malformation
(3) Chiari malformation

• external occipital mass

Location: supra- and infratentorial structures involved with equal frequency

√ skull defect (visualized in 80%)
√ flattening of basiocciput
√ ventriculomegaly
√ lemon sign = inward depression of frontal bones (33%)
√ cyst-within-a-cyst (ventriculocele = herniation of 4th ventricle into cephalocele)
√ acute angle between mass + skin line of neck and occiput

DDx: cystic hygroma

Sincipital Encephalocele (13–15%)

Most common variety in Southeast Asia!

Location: midface about dorsum of nose, orbits, and forehead

Cause: failure of anterior neuropore located near optic recess to close normally at 4th week GA

Types:
1. Frontonasal (40–60%)
= herniation of dura mater through foramen cecum + fonticulus frontalis
2. Nasoethmoidal (30%)
= persistent herniation of dural diverticulum through foramen cecum into prenasal space
3. Combination of both (10%)

Associated with: midline craniofacial dysraphism (dysgenesis of corpus callosum, interhemispheric lipoma, anomalies of neural migration, facial cleft, schizencephaly)

• obvious mass, broad nasal root, hypertelorism
• nasal stuffiness, rhinorrhea
• change in size during crying / Valsalva maneuver
• positive Fürstenberg test = change in size during jugular compression

√ soft-tissue mass extending to glabella / nasal cavity
√ pedunculated intranasal mass extending from superomedial nasal cavity downward
√ enlarged foramen cecum

OB:
√ widened interorbital distance

CT:
√ bifid / absent crista galli
√ absent cribriform plate / frontal bone

MR:
√ isointense relative to gray matter
√ may be hyperintense on T2WI (due to gliosis)

N.B.: biopsy is CONTRAINDICATED (due to potential for CSF leaks, seizures, meningitis)

Risk of recurrence: 6% of congenital CNS abnormalities for younger siblings

Rx: complete surgical resection with repair of dura mater (NO neurologic deficit due to abnormal function of herniated brain)

DDx:
(1) Dacryocystocele / nasolacrimal mucocele
(2) Nasal glioma (no subarachnoid connection on cisternography)

Sphenoidal Encephalocele (10%)

= BASAL ENCEPHALOCELE

Age: present at end of first decade of life

• clinically occult

- mass in nasal cavity, nasopharynx, mouth, posterior portion of orbit
- mouth breathing due to nasopharyngeal obstruction
- nasopharyngeal mass increasing with Valsalva
- diminished visual acuity with hypoplasia of optic discs
- hypothalamic-pituitary dysfunction

Associated with: agenesis of corpus callosum (80%)

Types:
(a) sphenopharyngeal = through sphenoid body
(b) spheno-orbital = through superior orbital fissure
(c) sphenoethmoidal = through sphenoid + ethmoid
(d) transethmoidal = through cribriform plate
(e) sphenomaxillary = through maxillary sinus

Parietal Encephalocele (10–12%)

Associated with: dysgenesis of corpus callosum, large interhemispheric cyst

√ hole in sphenoid bone (seen on submentovertex film)
√ cranium bifidum = cranioschisis = "split cranium" (= skull defect) = smooth opening with well-defined sclerotic rim of cortical bone
√ hydrocephalus in 15–80% (from associated aqueductal stenosis, Arnold-Chiari malformation, Dandy-Walker cyst)
√ nonenhancing expansile homogeneous paracranial mass
√ mantle of cerebral tissue often difficult to image in encephalocele (except with MR)
√ intracranial communication often not visualized
√ metrizamide / radionuclide ventriculography diagnostic
√ microcephaly (20%)
√ polyhydramnios

DDx: (1) sonographic refraction artifact at skull edge
(2) clover leaf skull (temporal bone may be partially absent)

CEREBELLAR ASTROCYTOMA

2nd most frequent tumor of posterior fossa in children

Incidence: 10–20% of pediatric brain tumors

Histo: mostly grade I

Age: children > adults; no specific age peak; M:F = 1:1

Path:
(1) cystic lesion with tumor nodule ("mural nodule") in cyst wall (50%); (midline astrocytomas cystic in 50%, hemispheric astrocytomas cystic in 80%)
(2) solid mass with cystic (= necrotic) center (40–45%)
(3) solid tumor without necrosis (<10%)

- cerebellar signs: truncal ataxia, dysdiadochokinesia

Location: originating in midline with extension into cerebellar hemisphere (30%) > vermis > tonsils > brainstem

√ calcifications (20%): dense / faint / reticular / punctate / globular; mostly in solid variety
√ may develop extreme hydrocephalus (quite large when finally symptomatic)

CT:
√ round / oval cyst with density of cyst fluid > CSF
√ round / oval / plaquelike mural nodule with intense homogeneous enhancement
√ cyst wall slightly hyperdense + nonenhancing (= compressed cerebellar tissue)
√ uni- / multilocular cyst (= necrosis) with irregular enhancement of solid tumor portions
√ round / oval lobulated fairly well-defined iso- / hypodense solid tumor with hetero- / homogeneous enhancement

MR:
√ hypointense on T1WI + hyperintense on T2WI
√ enhancement of solid tumor portion

Angio: √ avascular

Prognosis:
malignant transformation exceedingly rare
— 40% 25-year survival rate for solid cerebellar astrocytoma
— 90% 25-year survival rate for cystic juvenile pilocytic astrocytoma

DDx of solid astrocytoma:
(1) Medulloblastoma (hyperdense mass, noncalcified)
(2) Ependymoma (fourth ventricle, 50% calcify)

DDx of cystic astrocytoma:
(1) Hemangioblastoma (lesion <5 cm)
(2) Arachnoid cyst
(3) Trapped 4th ventricle
(4) Megacisterna magna
(5) Dandy-Walker cyst

CEREBRITIS

= focal area of inflammation within brain substance

CT:
√ area of decreased density ± mass effect
√ no contrast enhancement (initially) / central or patchy enhancement (later)

MR:
√ focal area of increased intensity on T2WI

Cx: brain abscess

CHIARI MALFORMATION

Chiari I Malformation (adulthood)

= "cerebellar tonsillar ectopia" = herniation of cerebellar tonsils below a line connecting basion with opisthion (= foramen magnum)

◊ Frequently isolated hindbrain abnormality of little consequence without supratentorial anomalies!

Proposed causes:
(a) small posterior fossa
(b) disproportionate CSF absorption from subarachnoid spinal space
(c) cerebellar overgrowth

Associated with:
(1) syringohydromyelia (20–30%)
(2) hydrocephalus (25–44%)
(3) malformation of skull base + cervical spine:
(a) basilar impression (25%)
(b) craniovertebral fusion, eg, occipitalization of C1 (10%), incomplete ossification of C1-ring (5%)
(c) Klippel-Feil anomaly (10%)
(d) platybasia

◊ NOT associated with myelomeningocele!

• benign cerebellar ectopia <3 mm of no clinical consequence; 3–5 mm of uncertain significance; >5 mm clinical symptoms likely
• no symptoms in childhood (unless associated with hydrocephalus / syringomyelia)
• may have cranial nerve dysfunction / dissociated anesthesia of lower extremities in adulthood
√ downward displacement of cerebellar tonsils + medial part of the inferior lobes of the cerebellum 5 mm below the level of the foramen magnum
√ inferior pointing peglike / triangular tonsils
√ obliteration of cisterna magna
√ elongation of 4th ventricle, which remains in normal position
√ slight anterior angulation of lower brainstem

Chiari II Malformation (childhood)
= ARNOLD-CHIARI MALFORMATION
= most common and serious complex of anomalies secondary to a too small posterior fossa involving hindbrain, spine, mesoderm
HALLMARK is dysgenesis of hindbrain with
(1) caudally displaced 4th ventricle
(2) caudally displaced brainstem
(3) tonsillar + vermian herniation through foramen magnum
Associated with:
(a) spinal anomalies
(1) lumbar myelomeningocele (>95%)
(2) syringohydromyelia
(b) supratentorial anomalies
(1) dysgenesis of corpus callosum (80–85%)
(2) obstructive hydrocephalus (50–98%) following closure of myelomeningocele
(3) absence of septum pellucidum (40%)
(4) excessive cortical gyration (stenogyria = histologically normal cortex; polymicrogyria = histologically abnormal cortex)
NOT associated with basilar impression / C1-assimilation / Klippel-Feil deformity!
• newborn: respiratory distress, apneic spells, bradycardia, impaired swallowing, poor gag reflex, retrocollis, spasticity of upper extremities
• teenager: gradual loss of function + spasticity of lower extremities
Skull film:
√ Lückenschädel (most prominent near torcular herophili / vertex) in 85% = dysplasia of membranous skull disappearing by 6 months of age
√ scalloping of clivus + posterior aspect of petrous pyramids (from pressure of cerebellum) in 70–90% leading to shortening of IAC
√ small posterior fossa
√ enlarged foramen magnum + enlarged upper spinal canal secondary to molding in 75%
√ absent / hypoplastic posterior arch of C1 (70%)
@ Supratentorial
√ hydrocephalus (duct of Sylvius dysfunctional but probe patent); may not become evident until after repair of myelomeningocele (90%)
√ colpocephaly (= enlargement of occipital horns + atria) due to maldeveloped occipital lobes
√ hypoplasia / absence of splenium + rostrum of corpus callosum (80–90%)
√ "bat-wing" configuration of frontal horns on coronal views = frontal horns pointing inferiorly with blunt superolateral angle secondary to prominent impressions by enlarged caudate nucleus
√ "hourglass ventricle" = small biconcave 3rd ventricle secondary to large massa intermedia
√ interdigitation of medial cortical gyri (hypoplasia + fenestration of falx in up to 100%)
√ wide prepontine + supracerebellar cisterns
√ nonvisualization of aqueduct (in up to 70%)
√ stenogyria = multiple small closely spaced gyri at medial aspect of occipital lobe secondary to dysplasia (in up to 50%)
@ Cerebellum
√ "cerebellar peg" = protrusion of vermis + hemispheres through foramen magnum (90%) resulting in craniocaudal elongation of cerebellum
√ hypoplastic poorly differentiated cerebellum (poor visualization of folia on sagittal images) secondary to severe degeneration
√ elongated / obliterated vertically oriented thin-tubed 4th ventricle with narrowed AP diameter exiting below foramen magnum (40%)
√ obliteration of CPA cistern + cisterna magna by cerebellum growing around brainstem
√ dysplastic tentorium with wide U-shaped incisura inserting close to foramen magnum (95%)
√ "tectal beaking" = fusion of midbrain colliculi into a single beak pointing posteriorly and invaginating into cerebellum
√ V-shaped widened quadrigeminal plate cistern (due to hypoplasia of cingulate gyri)
√ "towering cerebellum" = "pseudomass" = cerebellar extension above incisura of tentorium
√ triple peak configuration = corners of cerebellum wrapped around brainstem pointing anteriorly + laterally (on axial images)
√ flattened superior portion of cerebellum secondary to temporoparietal herniation
√ vertical orientation of shortened straight sinus
@ Spinal cord
√ medulla + pons displaced into cervical canal
√ "cervicomedullary kink" = herniation of medulla posterior to spinal cord (up to 70%) at level of dentate ligaments
√ widened anterior subarachnoid space at level of brainstem + upper cervical spine (40%)
√ AP diameter of pons narrowed
√ upper cervical nerve roots ascend toward their exit foramina
√ syringohydromyelia
√ low-lying often tethered conus medullaris below L2

OB-US:
√ hydrocephalus

√ "banana sign" = cerebellum wrapped around posterior brainstem + obliteration of cisterna magna secondary to small posterior fossa + downward traction of spinal cord in Chiari II malformation

Chiari III Malformation

most severe rare abnormality; probably unrelated to type I and II Chiari malformation

√ low occipital / high cervical meningomyeloencephalocele

Prognosis: survival usually not beyond infancy

Chiari IV Malformation

extremely rare anomaly probably erroneously included as type of Chiari malformation

√ agenesis of cerebellum
√ hypoplasia of pons
√ small + funnel-shaped posterior fossa

CHOROID PLEXUS CYST

= cyst arising from folding of neuroepithelium with trapping of secretory products + desquamated cells

Incidence: 0.9–3.6% in sonographic population; 50% of autopsied brains

Histo: no epithelial lining, filled with clear fluid ± debris

May be associated with:

aneuploidy (76% with trisomy 18, 17% with trisomy 21, 7% with triploidy / Klinefelter syndrome)

◊ In absence of other anomalies 1% of fetuses with choroid plexus cysts will have trisomy 18!

◊ In presence of other anomalies 4% of fetuses with choroid plexus cysts will have trisomy 18!

◊ 40–71% of autopsied fetuses with trisomy 18 have choroid plexus cysts bilaterally >10 mm in diameter

◊ Risk of chromosomal abnormality not linked to size, bilaterality, gestational age at appearance / disappearance

• usually asymptomatic

Location: frequently at level of atrium; uni- / bilateral

√ single / multiple round anechoic cysts
√ ≥3 mm in size (average 4.5 mm, up to 25 mm)

Cx: hydrocephalus (if cyst large)

Prognosis: 90% disappear by 28th week; may persist; in 95% of no significance

OB-management:

a choroid plexus cyst should stimulate a thorough sonographic examination at >19 weeks; if no other sonographic abnormalities are identified, the yield of abnormal karyotype is low so that the risk of trisomy 18 (1:450–500) is lower than risk of fetal loss due to amniocentesis (approximately 1:200–300)

Risk of karyotype abnormality:

10 times with 1 additional defect
600 times with ≥2 additional defects

DDx: Choroid plexus pseudocyst in the inferolateral aspect of atrium (? corpus striatum) on oblique coronal plane, which elongates by turning transducer

CHOROID PLEXUS PAPILLOMA

Incidence: 0.5–0.6% of all intracranial tumors; 2–5% of brain tumors in childhood

Age: 20–40% <1 year of age; 86% <5 years of age; middle age; in 75% <2 years of age; M >> F

Path: large aggregation of choroidal fronds producing great quantities of CSF; occasionally found incidentally on postmortem examination

Pathophysiology: abnormal rate of CSF production of 1.0 mL/min (normal rate = 0.2 mL/min)

• signs of increased intracranial pressure

Location:
(a) glomus of choroid plexus in trigone of lateral ventricles, L > R (in children)
(b) 4th ventricle + cerebellopontine angle (in adults)
(c) 3rd ventricle (unusual)
(d) multiple in 7%

√ large mass with smooth lobulated border
√ small foci of calcifications (common)
√ engulfment of glomus of choroid plexus (distinctive feature)
√ asymmetric diffuse ventricular dilatation (CSF overproduction / decreased absorption secondary to obstruction of arachnoid granulations from repeated occult hemorrhage)
√ dilatation of temporal horn in atrial location (obstruction)
√ growth into surrounding white matter (occasionally, more common a feature of choroid plexus carcinoma)

CT:
√ iso- / mildly hyperdense with intense homogeneous enhancement on CECT

MR:
√ isointense / slightly hyperintense lesion on T1WI + slightly hypointense on T2WI relative to white matter
√ surrounded by hypointense signal on T1WI + hyperintense signal on T2WI (CSF)
√ intraventricular enhancing island of tumor on Gd-DTPA

US:
√ echogenic mass adjacent to normal choroid plexus

Angio:
√ supplied by anterior + posterior choroidal arteries

Cx: (1) transformation into malignant choroid plexus papilloma = choroid plexus carcinoma
(2) hydrocephalus (in children) secondary to increased intracranial pressure from CSF-overproduction

Rx: surgical removal (24% operative mortality) cures hydrocephalus

DDx: intraventricular meningioma, ependymoma, metastasis, cavernous angioma, xanthogranuloma, astrocytoma

COCKAYNE SYNDROME

= autosomal recessive diffuse demyelinating disease

Age: beginning at age 1

• dwarfism
• progressive physical + mental deterioration
• retinal atrophy + deafness

√ brain atrophy / microcephaly

√ calcifications in basal ganglia + cerebellum
√ skeletal changes superficially similar to progeria
DDx: Progeria

COLLOID CYST

Incidence: 2% of glial tumors of ependymal origin; 0.5–1% of CNS tumors
Histo: ciliated + columnar epithelium; mucin-secreting; squamous cells of ependymal origin; tough fibrous capsule
Age: young adults; M > F

- positional headaches (transient obstruction secondary to ball-valve mechanism at foramen of Monro)
- gait apraxia
- change in mental status ± dementia (related to increased intracranial pressure)
- papilledema (may become medical emergency with acute herniation)

Location: exclusively arising from inferior aspect of septum pellucidum protruding into anterior portion of 3rd ventricle between columns of fornix

√ ± sellar erosion
√ spherical iso- / hyperdense lesion on NCCT with smooth surface
√ fluid contents:
  (a) in 20% similar to CSF (= isodense)
  (b) in 80% mucinous fluid, proteinaceous debris, hemosiderin, desquamated cells (= hyperdense)
√ may show enhancement of border (draped choroid plexus / capsule)
√ 3rd ventricular enlargement (to accommodate cyst anteriorly)
√ asymmetric lateral ventricular enlargement (invariably)
√ occasionally widens septum pellucidum

MR:
  √ lesion hyperintense on T1WI + hyperintense on T2WI in 60% (related to large protein molecules / paramagnetic effect of magnesium, copper, iron in cyst)

DDx: meningioma, ependymoma of 3rd ventricle (rare) with enhancement

CORTICAL CONTUSION

= CEREBRAL CONTUSION = BRAIN CONTUSION
= traumatic injury to cortical surface of brain

Incidence: most common type of primary intraaxial lesion; in 21% of head trauma patients; children:adults = 2:1
Pathogenesis: capillary disruption leads to extravasation of whole blood, plasma (edema) and RBCs
Path: petechial hemorrhage (= admixture of blood with native tissue) followed by liquefaction + edema after 4–7 days, tissue necrosis
Mechanism: <u>linear</u> acceleration-deceleration forces / penetrating trauma

1. **Coup** (same side as impact)
   = small area of direct impact on stationary brain
   Associated with: skull fracture
2. **Contrecoup** (180° opposite to side of impact)
   = broad area of impact as a result of moving brain against stationary calvarium
   Associated with: fall

Location: multiple bilateral lesions;
— common: along anterior + lateral + inferior surfaces of <u>frontal lobe</u> (in orbitofrontal, inferior frontal, and rectal gyri above cribriform plate, planum sphenoidale, lesser sphenoid wing) and <u>temporal lobe</u> (just above petrous bone / posterior to greater sphenoid wing)
— less frequent: in parietal + occipital lobes, cerebellar hemispheres, vermis, cerebellar tonsils
— often bilateral / beneath an acute subdural hematoma

- confusion (mild initial impairment)
- focal cerebral dysfunction
- seizures, personality changes
- focal neurologic deficits (late changes)

CT (sensitive only to hemorrhage in acute phase):
  ◊ Look for scalp swelling to focus your attention on the location of the coup!
  √ "salt and pepper lesion" = mottled / speckled densities as focal / multiple (29%) poorly defined areas of low attenuation with irregular contour (edema) intermixed with a few tiny areas of increased density (petechial hemorrhage)
  √ diffuse cerebral hypodensity + swelling without hemorrhage in immediate posttraumatic period (common in children) due to hyperemia / ischemic edema
  √ some degree of contrast enhancement (leaking new capillaries)
  √ hemorrhage isodense after 2–3 weeks
  √ true extent of lesions becomes more evident with progression of edema + cell necrosis + mass effect over ensuing weeks

MR (best modality for initial detection of contusional edema + accurate portrayal of extent of lesions):
  √ hemorrhagic lesions (detected in 50% of all contusions):
    √ initially decreased intensity (deoxyhemoglobin of acute hemorrhage) surrounded by hyperintense edema on T2WI
    √ hyperintense on T1WI + T2WI in subacute phase (secondary to Met-Hb)
    √ hyperintense gliosis + hypointense hemosiderin on T2WI in chronic phase
  √ nonhemorrhagic lesions hypointense on T1WI + hyperintense on T2WI

Cx: (1) Progression to cerebral hematoma
  (2) Encephalomalacia (= scarred brain)
  (3) Porencephaly (= formation of cystic cavity lined with gliotic brain and communicating with ventricles / subarachnoid space)
  (4) Hydrocephalus as a result of adhesions caused by subarachnoid blood

CRANIOPHARYNGIOMA

Incidence: 3–4% of all intracranial neoplasms; 15% of supratentorial + 50% of suprasellar tumors in children; most common suprasellar mass

Origin: from epithelial rests along vestigial craniopharyngeal duct (Rathke cleft / pouch within intermediate lobe of pituitary gland)

Path: benign tumor originating from neuroepithelium in craniopharyngeal duct + primitive buccal epithelium

Histo: cystic (rich in liquid cholesterol) / complex / solid

Age: from birth–7th decade; bimodal age distribution: age peaks in 1st–2nd decade (75%) + in 5th decade (25%); M > F

- diabetes insipidus (compression of pituitary gland)
- growth retardation (compression of hypothalamus)
- bitemporal hemianopia (compression of optic nerve chiasm)
- headaches from hydrocephalus (compression of foramen of Monro / aqueduct of Sylvius)

Location:
(a) pituitary stalk / tuber cinereum
(b) suprasellar (20%)
(c) intrasellar (10%)
(d) intra- and suprasellar (70%)

Ectopic craniopharyngioma:
(e) floor of anterior 3rd ventricle (more common in adults)
(f) sphenoid bone

Skull films:
√ normal sella (25%)
√ enlarged J-shaped sella with truncated dorsum
√ thickening + increased density of lamina dura in floor of sella (10%)
√ extensive sellar destruction (75%)
√ curvilinear / flocculent / stippled calcifications / lamellar ossification; calcifications seen in youth in 70–90%, in adults in 30–40%

CT:
√ multilobulated inhomogeneous suprasellar mass
√ solid (15%) / mixed (30%) / cystic lesion (54–75%) [cystic appearance secondary to cholesterol, keratin, necrotic debris with higher density than CSF]
√ enhancement of solid lesion, peripheral enhancement of cystic lesion
√ marginal hyperdense lesion (calcification / ossification) in 70–90% in childhood tumors + 30–50% of adult tumors
√ ± obstructive hydrocephalus
√ extension into middle > anterior > posterior cranial fossa (25%)

MR (relatively ineffective in demonstrating calcifications):
√ mostly hyperintense, but also iso- / hypointense on T1WI (variable secondary to hemorrhage / cholesterol-containing proteinaceous fluid)
√ markedly hyperintense on T2WI
√ marginal enhancement of solid components with gadopentetate dimeglumine

Angio:
√ usually avascular
√ lateral displacement, elevation, narrowing of supraclinoid segment of ICA
√ posterior displacement of basilar artery

DDx: (1) Epidermoid (no contrast enhancement)
(2) Rathke cleft cyst (small intrasellar lesion)

CYSTICERCOSIS OF BRAIN

Larva of pork tapeworm *(Taenia solium)* frequently involving CNS, eyes, muscle, heart, fat tissue, skin

Route of Infection:
(1) Ingestion of ova by fecal-oral route via contaminated food / water or autoinfection; embryophore is dissolved by gastric acid and enzymes + oncosphere is liberated
(2) Ingestion of undercooked contaminated pork containing cysticerci; tapeworm develops in intestinal lumen + releases eggs

Organism:
embryos invade intestinal wall + enter circulation + disseminate in varies parts of body; embryo develops into a cysticercus (= complex wall surrounding a cavity containing vesicular fluid + scolex); following ingestion of cysticercus by definitive host a tapeworm develops within the intestinal tract

Incidence: most common parasitic infection involving CNS in developing countries; CNS involvement in up to 90%

Endemic to: Mexico, South America, Africa, eastern Europe, Asia, Indonesia

Location: meninges (39%) esp. in basal cisterns, parenchyma (20%), intraventricular (17%), mixed (23%), intraspinal (1%)
Seeding: through subarachnoid space + intraventricular system

A. LARVAL TISSUE INVASION STAGE
- asymptomatic

√ localized focus of edema on T2WI
√ nodular tissue enhancement

B. VESICULAR STAGE
= antigenetically inert, therefore without inflammatory reaction / circumferential edema
- asymptomatic

√ single / multiple thin-walled nonenhancing 4–20 mm spherical cysts:
√ center with clear fluid of CSF intensity
√ 2–3 mm mural nodule (= scolex) isointense with brain parenchyma

C. COLLOIDAL STAGE
= scolex dies and its metabolic breakdown (colloidal suspension) results in focal meningoencephalitis with breakdown of blood-brain barrier
- focal seizures (in endemic countries most common cause of adult-onset epilepsy)
- headache, signs of increased intracranial pressure

√ avid ring-enhancing capsule on T1WI
√ center hypointense to white matter and hyperintense to CSF on T1WI + markedly hyperintense on T2WI (due to proteinaceous nature of cyst fluid)

√ hypointense mural nodule on T2WI with strong homogeneous enhancement
√ with extensive white matter edema (DDx: metastasis without edema)

D. NODULAR-GRANULAR STAGE
= degeneration of cysticercus with mineralization
√ gradually subsiding perilesional edema
√ shrinkage of cyst becoming isointense with brain on T1WI + hypointense on T2WI
√ isoattenuating lesion with enhancement of thick nodular ring on CT

E. CALCIFIED STAGE
= complete involution of lesion with continued mineralization
• asymptomatic / posttreatment seizures
√ small focal calcifications; may appear within 8 months to 10 years after acute infection
√ "ricelike" muscle calcifications rarely visible

RADIOGRAPHIC TYPES
1. Parenchymal type
   √ multiple / solitary cystic lesions up to 6 cm in size:
      √ large cysts are usually multiloculated
   √ many terminate as calcified granulomata (larvae not dead unless completely calcified)
   √ encephalitic form may occur in children
2. **Subarachnoid** / **racemose neurocysticercosis**
   = infiltration of basal cisterns + sylvian fissures associated with local meningeal inflammation / fibrosis
   √ lucent cystic lesions up to several cm in basal cisterns (= racemose cysts) with variable enhancement, usually located in cerebellopontine angle / suprasellar cistern
   Cx: hydrocephalus; scattered infarctions (due to vasculitis of basal perforating vessels)
3. **Intraventricular neurocysticercosis**
   √ obstructive hydrocephalus caused by blockage within various portions of ventricular system from solitary / multiple cysts (OCCULT on CT!)
4. Mixed type (frequent)

CYTOMEGALOVIRUS INFECTION

= double-stranded DNA virus with replication inside cell nucleus causing a lytic productive / latent infection; member of Herpesviridae family (with varicella-zoster virus, Epstein-Barr virus, herpes simplex virus types 1 and 2)

◊ Most common intrauterine infection

Incidence: 0.4–2.4% of liveborn infants; 40,000 babies born each year with CMV infection

Transmission:
(a) horizontally by contact with saliva / urine or sexually
(b) vertically from mother to fetus transplacentally; spreads hematogenously throughout fetus
   ◊ Severe fetal morbidity if infected during first half of pregnancy!

Histo: necrotizing inflammatory process

Predilection: CMV has special affinity for metabolically active neuroblasts of germinal matrix

Prenatal screening:
antibodies in 30–60% of pregnant women;
primary CMV infection in 2.5% of pregnant women

Postnatal screening:
10% of neonates excrete virus;
1.6% of newborns shed CMV in urine / saliva

• asymptomatic + subclinical (90%)
• symptomatic at birth (5–10%):
   • sensorineural deafness, mental retardation, neurologic deficits, seizures
   • ocular abnormalities (15–50%): chorioretinitis, optic neuritis, optic atrophy, hypoplasia + coloboma of optic nerve, anterior uveitis, anophthalmia, microphthalmia, cataracts, cyclopia
   • jaundice, hemolytic anemia, thrombocytopenic purpura
   ◊ Leading cause of brain disease + hearing loss in children!
• symptomatic in adults (in up to 15%):
   • fever, pharyngitis, lymphadenopathy, polyarthritis

√ intrauterine growth retardation
√ hepatosplenomegaly (nontender)
√ ascites
√ hydrops
√ pneumonitis

@ CNS
   √ periventricular subependymal cysts (= focal areas of necrosis + glial reaction)
   √ intracranial calcifications:
      √ periventricular postinflammatory calcifications
      √ scattered calcifications in basal ganglia + thalami
      √ highly echogenic thickened walls of lenticulostriate vessels (= mineralized vasculopathy with deposition of amorphous basophilic material in arterial walls)
      √ calcifications throughout brain parenchyma
   √ ventricular dilatation (due to ventriculitis / obstruction by inflammatory exudate / brain atrophy)
   √ intraventricular septa
   √ microcephaly (due to encephaloclastic effect of virus / disturbance of cell proliferation resulting in brain atrophy)
   √ lissencephaly, cortical dysplasia / atrophy, heterotopia, polymicrogyria, schizencephaly (due to disturbed neuronal migration)
   √ severe diffuse hypoplasia / dysplasia of cerebellum

Dx: positive viral culture within first 2 weeks of life

Rx: no effective treatment for maternal infection

DDx: toxoplasmosis, teratoma, tuberous sclerosis, Sturge-Weber syndrome, venous sinus thrombosis

DANDY-WALKER MALFORMATION

= characterized by (1) enlarged posterior fossa with high position of tentorium (2) dys- / agenesis of cerebellar vermis (3) cystic dilatation of 4th ventricle filling nearly entire posterior fossa

Incidence: 12% of all congenital hydrocephaly

Path: defect in vermis connecting an ependyma-lined retrocerebellar cyst with 4th ventricle (PATHOGNOMONIC)

Cause: dysmorphogenesis of roof of 4th ventricle with failure to incorporate the area membranacea into developing choroid plexus; proposed originally as congenital atresia of foramina of **L**uschka (**l**ateral) + **M**agendie (**m**edian) not likely since foramina are not patent until 4th month

Associated anomalies:

— midline CNS anomalies (in >60%)
 (1) Dysgenesis of corpus callosum (20–25%), lipoma of corpus callosum
 (2) Holoprosencephaly (25%)
 (3) Malformation of cerebral gyri (dysplasia of cingulate gyrus) (25%)
 (4) Cerebellar heterotopia + malformation of cerebellar folia (25%)
 (5) Malformation of inferior olivary nucleus
 (6) Hamartoma of tuber cinereum
 (7) Syringomyelia
 (8) Cleft palate
 (9) Occipital encephalocele (<5%)

— other CNS anomalies:
 (1) Polymicrogyria / gray matter heterotopia (5–10%)
 (2) Schizencephaly
 (3) Lumbosacral meningocele

— non-CNS anomalies (25%)
 (1) Polydactyly, syndactyly
 (2) Klippel-Feil syndrome
 (3) Cornelia de Lange syndrome
 (4) Cleft palate
 (5) Facial angioma
 (6) Cardiac anomalies

Skull film:
- √ large skull secondary to hydrocephalus + dolichocephaly
- √ diastatic lambdoid suture
- √ disproportionately large expanded posterior fossa
- √ torcular herophili and lateral sinuses high above lambdoid angle = torcular-lambdoid inversion

CT / US / MR:
- √ absence / hypoplasia of cerebellar vermis: total (25%), partial (75%)
- √ superiorly displaced superior vermis cerebelli
- √ small + widely separated cerebellar hemispheres
- √ anterior + lateral displacement of ± hypoplastic cerebellar hemispheres
- √ large posterior fossa cyst with extension through foramen magnum = diverticulum of roofless 4th ventricle
- √ elevated insertion of tentorium cerebelli
- √ cerebellar hemispheres in apposition without intervening vermis following shunt procedure
- √ absence of falx cerebelli
- √ scalloping of petrous pyramids
- √ ventriculomegaly (in 72% open communication with 3rd ventricle; in 39% patent 4th ventricle; in 28% aqueductal stenosis; in 11% incisural obstruction); present prenatally in 30%, by 3 months of age in 75%
- √ anterior displacement of pons

Angio:
- √ high position of transverse sinus
- √ elevated great vein of Galen
- √ elevated posterior cerebral vessels
- √ anterosuperiorly displaced superior cerebellar arteries above the posterior cerebral arteries
- √ small / absent PICA with high tonsillar loop

Cx: trapping of cyst above tentorium = "keyhole configuration"

Prognosis: fetal demise in 66%; 22–50% mortality during 1st year of life

DDx:
 (1) Posterior fossa extra-axial cyst
 (2) Arachnoid cyst (normal 4th ventricle, patent foramina, intact vermis)
 (3) Isolated 4th ventricle
 (4) Megacisterna magna = giant cisterna magna (enlarged posterior fossa, enlarged cisterna magna, intact vermis, normal 4th ventricle)
 (5) Porencephaly

Dandy-Walker Variant

characterized by
 (1) variable hypoplasia of posteroinferior portion of vermis leading to communication between 4th ventricle and cisterna magna
 (2) cerebellar dysgenesis
 (3) cystic dilatation of 4th ventricle
 (4) NO enlargement of posterior fossa

◊ More common than Dandy-Walker malformation; accounts for 1/3 of all posterior fossa malformations

Cause: focal insult to developing cerebellum

Associated CNS anomalies:
agenesis of corpus callosum (21%), cerebral gyral malformation (21%), heterotopia, holoprosencephaly (10%), diencephalic cyst (10%), posterior fossa meningoencephalocele (10%)

Other associated anomalies:
polydactyly; cardiac, renal, facial anomalies; abnormal karyotype (29%)

- √ 4th ventricle smaller + better formed
- √ retrocerebellar cyst smaller
- √ communication between retrocerebellar cyst and subarachnoid space through a patent foramen of Magendie may be present
- √ posterior fossa smaller than in usual Dandy-Walker syndrome

OB-US:
- √ incomplete closure of vermis is normal until 18 weeks GA!

Dandy-Walker Complex

= continuum of anomalies, including Dandy-Walker malformation + Dandy-Walker variant + megacisterna magna, characterized by partial / complete dysgenesis of vermis cerebelli

Cause: broad insult to alar plate from a variety of abnormalities

Associated with:

A. Inherited genetic syndromes
 — autosomal recessive:
  1. Meckel-Gruber syndrome

2. Ellis-van Creveld syndrome
3. Walker-Warburg syndrome

— autosomal dominant:
1. X-linked cerebellar hypoplasia
2. Aicardi syndrome

B. Abnormal karyotype (33%)
1. Duplications of chromosomes 5p, 8p, 8q
2. Trisomies 9, 13, 18

C. Infection
1. Virus: CMV, rubella
2. Protozoan: toxoplasmosis

D. Teratogen: alcohol, sodium warfarin
E. Multifactorial

Pseudo-Dandy-Walker Malformation

= developing rhombencephalon during 1st trimester
√ fluid-filled space in posterior aspect of fetal head

DERMOID OF CNS

= pilosebaceous mass lined with skin appendages originating from inclusion of epithelial cells + skin appendages during closure of neural tube

Incidence: 1% of all intracranial tumors
Path: ectodermal + mesodermal lesion = squamous epithelium, mesodermal cells (hair follicles, sweat + sebaceous glands)
Age: <30 years (appears in adulthood secondary to slow growth); M < F

Location:
(a) spinal canal (most common): extra- / intramedullary in lumbosacral region
(b) posterior fossa within vermis / 4th ventricle (predilection for midline)
(c) posterior to superior orbital fissure, may be associated with bone defect

• bouts of chemical / bacterial meningitis possible
√ thick-walled inhomogeneous mass with focal areas of fat
√ mural / central calcifications / bone (possible)
√ may have sinus tract to skin surface (dermal sinus) if located in midline at occipital / nasofrontal region
√ fat-fluid level if cyst ruptures into ventricles, fat droplets in subarachnoid space
√ NO contrast enhancement

MR:
√ variointense on T1WI (hyperintense with contents of liquefied cholesterol products)
√ shortened T1 + T2 relaxation times (= fat)

DIFFUSE AXONAL INJURY

= WHITE MATTER SHEARING INJURY

Incidence: most common type of primary traumatic injury in patients with severe head trauma (48%)
Cause: high-velocity trauma (MVA) resulting in indirect injury due to rotational / angular (especially coronal) acceleration / deceleration forces (direct impact to head or fracture not required)

Pathogenesis:
cortex and deep structures move at different speed causing shearing stress of
(1) axons resulting in axonal tears followed by wallerian degeneration
(2) small white-matter vessels resulting in small petechial hemorrhages

Path: much of the injury is only microscopic
Histo: multiple axonal retraction balls (HALLMARK), numerous perivascular hemorrhages

• immediate severe impairment of consciousness at time of impact
• persistent vegetative state

Location (according to severity of trauma):
(a) lobar white matter at corticomedullary junction (67%): parasagittal region of frontal lobe + periventricular region of temporal lobe; occasionally in parietal + occipital lobes
(b) internal + external capsule / basal ganglia, corona radiata, cerebellar peduncles
(c) corpus callosum (21%): 3/4 of lesions at undersurface of posterior body + splenium
√ often associated with intraventricular hemorrhage
(d) brainstem: posterolateral quadrants of midbrain + upper pons; superior cerebellar peduncles especially vulnerable

√ sparing of cortex
√ 20% of lesions with small central areas of petechial hemorrhage

CT (negative in 30% of positive MR cases):
√ foci of decreased density (usually seen when >1.5 cm in size)

MR (most sensitive modality):
√ multiple small oval / round foci of decreased signal intensity on T1WI + increased signal on T2WI

Prognosis:
(1) poor due to sequelae (may go on to die without signs of high intracranial pressure)
(2) brain atrophy with enlargement of sulci + ventricles

DIFFUSE SCLEROSIS

sporadic, young adults, fulminant course
• dementia, deafness
√ low-attenuation regions in both hemispheres without symmetry

DURAL SINUS THROMBOSIS

= VENOUS SINUS THROMBOSIS

◊ The radiologist may be the first to suggest the diagnosis!

Cause:
A. Idiopathic = spontaneous (10–30%)
B. Septic causes (esp. in childhood):
mastoiditis, sub- / epidural empyema, meningitis, encephalitis, brain abscess, face + scalp cellulitis, septicemia
C. Aseptic causes:
(a) Tumor compressing sinuses: meningioma, blastic crisis of chronic myelogenous leukemia
(b) Trauma: fracture through sinus wall, cranial surgery, jugular vein catheterization
(c) Low-flow state: CHF, CHD, dehydration, shock

(d) Hypercoagulability: antiphospholipid syndrome, activated C protein resistance, pregnancy, peripartum state, oral contraceptives, polycythemia vera, idiopathic thrombocytosis, thrombocytopenia, sickle cell disease, cryofibrinogenemia, disseminated intravascular coagulopathy

(e) Chemotherapy: eg, ARA-C, asparaginase

D. Unusual causes:
Behçet disease. AIDS, ulcerative colitis, systemic lupus erythematosus, nephrotic syndrome

Associated with: CHD, antithrombin III deficiency, protein C resistance, protein S disease, antiphospholipid syndrome

Pathophysiology:
dural sinus thrombosis leads to venous congestion, brain edema, sulcal effacement, occasionally hydrocephalus (due to decreased CSF absorption)

- symptoms of increased intracranial pressure: headaches, nausea, vomiting, visual blurring
  often confused with: tension headaches, migraine
- drowsiness, decreased mentation, lethargy, obtundation
- stroke symptomatology, seizures
- fever

Location: superior sagittal > transverse > sigmoid > straight sinus

NCCT (usually subtle findings):
√ hyperattenuating material (clotted blood) in sagittal sinus / straight sinus / cerebral cortical veins = "cord sign" (20%)
√ compression of lateral ventricles in 32% (infarction / edema)
√ unilateral (2/3) / bilateral (1/3) parenchymal hemorrhage involving gray + white matter (20%)
√ subdural collection
√ stroke (often hemorrhagic)

CECT venography (30–40 sec delay):
√ "delta sign" / "empty triangle" = filling defect in straight sinus / superior sagittal sinus with outward bowing of sinus wall (in 25–70%)
False positive: subdural hematoma / empyema, arachnoid granulations
False negative: partial volume averaging, small thrombus, recanalized thrombus
√ enlargement of thrombosed vein near obstruction
√ shaggy irregular contour of veins (= small collateral veins enhance near the obstructed vein)
√ gyral enhancement in periphery of infarction (30–40%)
√ intense tentorial enhancement secondary to collaterals (rare)
√ dense transcortical medullary vein
Advantages over MRI: shorter exam time

MR:
√ replacement of flow void by abnormal signal intensity
(a) acute thrombosis (first few days)
√ clot isointense to gray matter on T1WI (and therefore easily missed) + hypointense on T2WI
√ low signal intensity rather than normal flow void on T1WI
(b) chronic thrombosis (when most cases are diagnosed)
√ hyperintense thrombus within sinus on T1WI (due to intra- and extracellular methemoglobin)
√ iso- / hyperintense thrombus on T2WI (due to extracellular methemoglobin)
N.B.: hypointense thrombus on T2WI (due to intracellular methemoglobin) may mimic flow void of a patent dural sinus
√ subcortical hemorrhagic infarcts (due to retrograde extension of thrombus)
√ wall-enhancement of thrombosed dural sinus

MR venography:
√ absence of flow-related enhancement
Pitfall: hyperintense thrombus on T1WI time-of-flight venography can simulate flow-related enhancement

Angio:
√ nonfilling of thrombosed sinus
√ filling of cortical veins, deep venous system, cavernous sinus
√ parasagittal hemorrhages (highly specific for superior sagittal sinus thrombosis) secondary to cortical venous infarction

Prognosis: high mortality
Rx: heparin (full recovery in 70%)

DYKE-DAVIDOFF-MASON SYNDROME

= CEREBRAL HEMIATROPHY = INFANTILE / CONGENITAL HEMIPLEGIA = SYNDROME OF HEMICONVULSIONS, HEMIPLEGIA, AND EPILEPSY
= unilateral cerebral atrophy with ipsilateral small skull

Cause: insult to immature brain resulting in neuronal loss + impaired brain growth:
(a) prenatal: congenital malformation, infection, vascular insult
(b) perinatal: birth trauma, anoxia, hypoxia, intracranial hemorrhage
(c) postnatal: trauma, tumor, infection, prolonged febrile seizures

Age: presents in adolescence

- seizures
- hemiparesis (typically spastic hemiplegia)
- mental retardation

√ unilateral thickening of skull
√ unilateral decrease in size of cranial fossa
√ unilateral overdevelopment of sinuses
√ contraction of a hemisphere / lobe
√ compensatory enlargement of adjacent ventricle + sulci with midline shift

DYSEMBRYOPLASTIC NEUROEPITHELIAL TUMOR

= benign tumor of neuroepithelial origin arising from cortical / deep gray matter

Origin: derived from secondary germinal layers; originally diagnosed as low-grade astrocytomas

Histo: specific glioneuronal element in a columnar pattern oriented perpendicular to cortical surface; admixture of astrocytes + oligodendroglial elements in association with "floating neurons" and mucinous degeneration; ±multinodular architecture

Age: usually <20 years; M > F

- medically refractory partial seizures
- neurologic deficits rare

Location: temporal (62%) / frontal (31%) lobe; caudate nucleus; cerebellum; pons

CT:

√ hypoattenuating mass ± calcifications
√ remodeling of inner table of skull

MR:

√ cortical mass without surrounding vasogenic edema:
√ hypointense on T1WI + hyperintense on T2WI
√ "soap bubble" / megagyrus appearance at cortical margin = enlargement of cortical surface
√ contrast enhancement (in 33%)

Prognosis: partial resection stops seizure activity; rarely recur

DDx: diffuse astrocytoma, ganglioglioma, oligodendroglioma

EMPTY SELLA SYNDROME

= extension of subarachnoid space into sella turcica, which becomes exposed to CSF pulsations secondary to defect in diaphragma sellae; characterized by normal / molded pituitary gland + normal or enlarged sella (empty sella = misnomer)

Incidence: 24% in autopsy study

A. PRIMARY EMPTY SELLA (anatomic spectrum)

Incidence: 10% of adult population; M:F = 1:4

Probable causes:

(1) pituitary enlargement followed by regression during pregnancy
(2) involution of a pituitary tumor
(3) congenital weakness of diaphragma sellae

◊ Occurs more frequently in patients with increased intracranial pressure

- usually asymptomatic
- increased risk for CSF rhinorrhea
- NO endocrine abnormalities

B. SECONDARY EMPTY SELLA

= postsurgical when diaphragma sellae has been disrupted

- visual disturbance
- headaches

√ slowly progressive symmetrical / asymmetrical (double floor) enlargement of sella
√ remodeled lamina dura remains mineralized
√ small rim of pituitary tissue displaced posteriorly + inferiorly
√ infundibulum sign = infundibulum extends to floor of sella

DDx: cystic tumor, large herniated 3rd ventricle (displaced infundibulum)

EMPYEMA OF BRAIN

Subdural Empyema

20% of all intracranial bacterial infections

Cause: paranasal sinusitis, otitis media, calvarial osteomyelitis, infection after craniotomy or ventricular shunt placement, penetrating wound, contamination of meningitis-induced subdural effusion

Location: frontal + inferior cranial space in close proximity to paranasal sinuses; 80% over convexity extending into interhemispheric fissure or posterior fossa

√ hypo- / isodense crescentic / lentiform zone adjacent to inner table
√ may show mass effect (sulcal effacement, ventricular compression, shift)
√ thin curvilinear rim of enhancement (7–10 days later) adjacent to brain
√ severe sinusitis / mastoiditis (may be most significant indicator)

Mortality: 30% (neurosurgical emergency)

Cx: venous thrombosis, infarction, seizures, hemiparesis, hemianopia, aphasia, brain abscess

DDx: subacute / chronic subdural hematoma

Epidural Empyema

Cause: same as above

- no neurologic deficits (dura minimizes pressure exerted on brain)

√ thick enhancing rim

ENCEPHALITIS

= term generally reserved for diffuse inflammatory process of viral etiology, most commonly arthropod-borne arboviruses (Eastern + Western equine encephalitis, California virus encephalitis, St. Louis encephalitis)

√ diffuse mild cerebral edema
√ small infarctions / hemorrhage (less frequent)
√ hyperintensity on T2WI in areas of cortical involvement

Herpes Simplex Encephalitis (HSE)

= most common cause of nonepidemic necrotizing meningoencephalitis in immunocompetent individuals in USA

◊ Neurologic emergency due to high morbidity + mortality

Organism: HSV type I (in adults); HSV type II (in neonates from transplacental infection)

- preceding viral syndrome
- mental status changes: confusion, disorientation, hallucination, personality change, aphasia
- low-grade fever, headache, seizures

Location: inferomedial temporal > frontal > parietal lobes; propensity for limbic system (olfactory tract, temporal lobes, cingulate gyrus, insular cortex); initially predominantly unilateral

√ mild patchy peripheral / gyral / cisternal enhancement (50%), may persist for several months

CT:
- √ may be negative in first 3 days
- √ poorly defined bilateral areas of mildly decreased attenuation in one / both temporal lobes + insulae
- √ spared putamen forms sharply defined concave / straight border (DDx: infarction, glioma)
- √ mild mass effect with compression of lateral ventricles + loss of sylvian fissure (brain edema)
- √ tendency for hemorrhage + rapid dissemination in brain

MR (study of choice, positive within 2 days):
- √ increased signal intensity on T2WI + mild to moderate hypointensity on T1WI
- √ increased signal on diffusion-weighted images (cytotoxic edema)
- √ small foci of hemorrhage (common)

NUC:
Agents: standard brain imaging (eg, Tc-99m DTPA), newer brain agents (eg, I-123 iodoamphetamine / Tc-99m HMPAO)
SPECT imaging improves sensitivity
- √ characteristic focal increase in activity in temporal lobes on brain scintigraphy (blood-brain barrier breakdown)

Dx: (1) identification of virus within CSF (using polymerase chain reaction technique)
(2) fluorescein antibody staining / viral culture from brain biopsy

Mortality: 30–70%
Rx: adenine arabinoside
DDx: (1) Infarction (involves either medial or lateral temporal lobe, almost exclusively unilateral)
(2) Low-grade glioma
(3) Abscess

Human Immunodeficiency Virus Encephalitis

often in combination with CMV encephalitis
Histo: microglial nodules + perivascular multinucleated giant cells accompanying gliosis of deep white + gray matter
- √ predominantly central CNS atrophy
- √ symmetric periventricular / diffuse white matter disease without mass effect (hypodense on CT, high intensity on T2WI)

Postinfectious Encephalitis

following exanthematous viral illness (measles, mumps, rubella, smallpox, chickenpox, , Epstein-Barr virus, varicella, pertussis) / vaccination

Acute Disseminated Encephalomyelitis (ADEM)

= POSTVIRAL LEUKOENCEPHALOPATHY
= autoimmune reaction against patient's white matter
- • 7–14 days / several weeks following an exanthematous viral infection / vaccination
- • confusion, headaches, fever
- • seizures, focal neurologic deficits

Histo: diffuse perivenous inflammatory process resulting in areas of demyelination

Location: subcortical white matter of both hemispheres asymmetrically

CT:
- √ multifocal hypodense white matter abnormalities
- √ sparing of cortical gray matter, occasionally deep gray matter involvement
- √ no additional lesions on follow-up exam

MR:
- √ focal areas of hyperintensity on T2WI
- √ may demonstrate contrast enhancement

Rx: corticosteroids result in dramatic improvement
Prognosis: complete resolution of neurologic deficits within 1 month (80–90%) / some permanent neurologic damage (10–20%)
DDx: simulating multiple sclerosis (rarely recurrent episodes as in multiple sclerosis)

Acute Hemorrhagic Leukoencephalitis

= fulminant myelinoclastic disease of CNS
= hyperacute form of acute disseminated encephalomyelitis
Cause: immunoreactive disease following prodromal illness (minor upper respiratory viral infection, ulcerative colitis)
Path: marked edema, brain softening
Histo: necrotizing angiitis of venules + capillaries within white matter with extravasation of PMNs + lymphocytes; fibrinoid necrosis of affected capillaries + surrounding tissues; confluent hemorrhages with ball-and-ring configuration due to diapedesis of RBCs
- • progressive coma, motor disturbance, speech difficulty, seizures
- • pyrexia, leukocytosis
- • pleocytosis, elevated protein in spinal fluid

Location: unilateral disease; parietal + posterior frontal white matter at level of centrum semiovale (sparing subcortical U-fibers + cortex) > basal ganglia, cerebellum, brainstem, spinal cord
- √ rapid development of profound mass effect resembling infarction
- √ multiple punctate white matter hemorrhages
- √ extensive hypoattenuation virtually confined to hemispheric white matter

Prognosis: usually results in death
DDx: (1) Herpes simplex encephalitis (cortical lesions in temporal + inferior frontal lobes + insular region, no imaging findings until 3–5 days after onset of significant symptoms)
(2) Tumefactive multiple sclerosis
(3) Osmotic demyelination
(4) Toxic encephalopathy: lipophilic solvent, methanol
(5) Hypertensive encephalopathy: eclampsia, thrombotic thrombocytopenic purpura

EPENDYMOMA

= in majority benign slow-growing neoplasm of mature well-differentiated ependymal cells lining the ventricles

Incidence: most commonly in children; 5–9% of all primary CNS neoplasms; 15% of posterior fossa tumors in children; 63% of spinal intramedullary gliomas

Histo: benign aggregates of ependymocytes in form of perivascular pseudorosettes; may have papillary pattern (difficult DDx from choroid plexus papilloma)

Age: (a) supratentorial: at any age (atrium / foramen of Monro)
(b) posterior fossa: <10 years; age peaks at 5 and 34 years; M:F = 0.8:1

Associated with: neurofibromatosis

• increased intracranial pressure (90%)

Location:
(a) infratentorial: floor of 4th ventricle (70% of all intracranial ependymomas)
(b) supratentorial: frontal > parietal > temporoparietal juxtaventricular region (uncommonly intraventricular), lateral ventricle, 3rd ventricle
(c) conus (40–65% of all spinal intramedullary gliomas)
in children: infratentorial in 70%, supratentorial in 30%

√ small cystic areas in 15–50% (central necrosis)
√ fine punctate multifocal calcifications (25–50%)
√ intratumoral hemorrhage (10%)
√ frequently grows into brain parenchyma extending to cortical surface (particularly in frontal + parietal lobes)
√ may invaginate into ventricles
√ expansion frequently through foramen of Luschka into cerebellopontine angle (15%) or through foramen of Magendie caudad into cisterna magna (up to 60%) (CHARACTERISTIC)
√ direct invasion of brainstem / cerebellum (30–40%)
√ insinuation around blood vessels + cranial nerves
√ communicating hydrocephalus (100%) secondary to protein exudate elaborated by tumor clogging resorption pathways

CT:
√ sharply marginated multilobulated iso- / slightly hyperdense 4th ventricular mass
√ thin well-defined low-attenuation halo (distended effaced 4th ventricle)
√ heterogeneous / moderately uniform enhancement of solid portions (80%)

MR:
√ low to intermediate heterogeneous signal intensity on T1WI
√ hypointense tumor margins on T1WI + T2WI in 64% (hemosiderin deposits)
√ foci of high-signal intensity on T2WI (= necrotic areas / cysts) + low signal intensity (= calcification / hemorrhage)
√ fluid-fluid level within cysts
√ homogeneous Gd-DTPA enhancement of tumor

Cx: subarachnoid dissemination via CSF (rare) (DDx: malignant ependymoma, ependymoblastoma)

Rx: surgery (difficult to resect due to adherence to surrounding brain) + radiation (partially radiosensitive) + chemotherapy

DDx of cerebellar ependymoma:
(1) Astrocytoma (hypodense, displaces 4th ventricle from midline, cystic lucency, intramedullary)
(2) Medulloblastoma (hyperdense, calcifications in only 10%)
(3) Trapped 4th ventricle (no contrast enhancement)

EPIDERMOID OF CNS

= EPIDERMOID [INCLUSION] CYST
= benign tumor with extremely slow linear growth resulting from desquamation of epithelial cells from tumor wall

Incidence: 0.2–1.8% of all primary intracranial neoplasms; most common congenital intracranial tumor

Etiology: inclusion of ectodermal epithelial tissue from pharyngeal pouch of Rathke / pluripotential cells during closure of neural tube in 5th week of fetal life (early inclusion results in midline lesion, later inclusion results in more lateral location)

Path: "pearly tumor" = well-defined solid lesion with glistening irregular nodular surface; soft flaky desquamated keratinaceous debris rich in cholesterol + triglycerides = PRIMARY / CONGENITAL CHOLESTEATOMA

Histo: tumor lined by simple stratified cuboidal squamous epithelium; surrounded by thin band of collagenous connective tissue; tumor center of lamellar appearance due to desquamation

Age: 10–60 years, peak age in 4th–5th decade; tumor slowly expands over decades by continued desquamation of the lining thus becoming symptomatic in adulthood; M:F = 1:1

• facial pain
• cranial nerve palsies from CP angle epidermoids (50%)
• hydrocephalus in suprasellar epidermoids
• chemical meningitis (secondary to leakage of tumor contents into subarachnoid space) in middle cranial fossa epidermoids

Site: midline / paramidline; intradural (90%) / extradural; transspatial growth (= extension from one into another intracranial space)

Location: (a) cerebellopontine angle (40%, account for 5% of CP angle tumors)
(b) suprasellar region, perimesencephalic cisterns (14%)
(c) in ventricles, brainstem, brain parenchyma
(d) skull vault

√ soft lesion conforming to + molding itself around brain surfaces
√ may intimately surround vessels + cranial nerves rather than displacing them (limited resectability)
√ little mass effect, no edema / hydrocephalus
√ NO contrast enhancement
√ may be associated with dermal sinus tract at occipital / nasofrontal region if midline in location

CT:
- √ typically lobulated round homogeneous mass with density similar to CSF (between water and –20 HU)
- √ occasionally hyperdense due to high protein content, saponification of keratinaceous debris, prior hemorrhage into cyst, ferrocalcium / iron-containing pigment, abundance of PMNs
- √ bony erosion with sharply defined well-corticated margins
- √ calcification (25%)
- √ peripheral enhancement (perilesional inflammation)

MR:
- √ lamellated onionskin appearance with septations (layer-on-layer accretion of desquamated material)
- √ "black epidermoid" = signal intensity similar to CSF: heterogeneously hypointense lesion on T1WI + hyperintense on T2WI (due to cholesterol in solid crystalline state + keratin within tumor + CSF within tumor interstices)
- √ "white epidermoid" (rare) = hyperintense on T1WI + isointense on T2WI due to presence of triglycerides + polyunsaturated fatty acids
- √ hypointense on T2WI (very rare) due to calcification, low hydration, viscous secretion, paramagnetic iron-containing pigment

Angio:
- √ avascular

Cisternography:
- √ papillary / frondlike surface with contrast material extending into tumor interstices

Rx: surgical resection (complicated by adherence to surrounding brain + cranial nerves, spillage of cyst contents with chemical meningitis, CSF seeding + implantation)

DDx: arachnoid cyst (smooth surface, earlier diffusion), cystic schwannoma, adenomatoid tumor, atypical meningioma, chondroma, chondrosarcoma, chordoma, calcified neurogenic tumor, teratoma, calcified astrocytoma, ganglioglioma

EPIDURAL HEMATOMA OF BRAIN

= EXTRADURAL HEMATOMA

= hematoma within potential space between naked inner table of skull + calvarial periosteum (inner dura layer), which is bound down firmly to cranium at sutural margins (= subperiosteal hematoma of inner table)

Incidence: 2% of all serious head injuries; in <1% of all children with cranial trauma; uncommon in infants

Cause: impact on skull causes laceration of periosteal layer of outer table + linear fracture; temporary inward displacement of fragments lacerates meningeal vessels and strips both dural layers from inner table while the inner layer (meningeal dura) remains intact; blood accumulates between naked inner table and dura

Age: more common in younger patients 20–40 years (dura more easily stripped away from skull)

Associated with:
(1) skull fracture in 75–85 –95% (best demonstrated on skull radiographs)
◊ Skull fractures frequently not visible in children ("ping-pong fracture")!
(2) subdural hemorrhage
(3) contusion

Source of bleeding:
(a) laceration of (middle) meningeal artery (high pressure) / meningeal vein (low pressure) adjacent to inner table from calvarial fracture (91%)
(b) disruption of dural venous sinuses (transverse / superior sagittal sinus) with low pressure + high flow due to diastatic fracture of lambdoid / coronal suture [major cause in younger children]
(c) avulsion of diploic veins / marrow sinusoids at points of calvarial perforations

Time of presentation: within first few days of injury (80%), 4–21 days (20%)

- transient loss of consciousness (= brief period of unconsciousness from concussion of brainstem)
- "lucid interval" (in <33%)
- delayed somnolence (24–96 hours after accident) due to accumulation of epidural hematoma:
  ◊ DANGEROUS because of focal mass effect + rapid onset (neurosurgical emergency unless small)!
- progressive deterioration of consciousness to coma
- focal neurologic signs: 3rd nerve palsy (sign of cerebral herniation), hemiparesis

◊ Most commonly clinically significant if located in temporoparietal region!

◊ Only a minority of skull fractures across the middle meningeal artery groove result in epidural hematomas!

Types:

I	acute epidural hematoma	(58%) from arterial bleeding
II	subacute hematoma	(31%)
III	chronic hematoma	(11%) from venous bleeding

Factors determining the rate of epidural expansion: injury to artery or vein, spasm of artery, containment of bleed through pseudoaneurysm or tamponade, decompression of hematoma into meningeal + diploic veins or through fracture into scalp

Location:
(a) in 66% temporoparietal (most often from laceration of middle meningeal artery)
(b) in 29% at frontal pole, parieto-occpital region, between occipital lobes, posterior fossa (most often from laceration of dural sinuses by fracture)
◊ NO crossing of sutures unless diastatic fracture of suture present!

CT:
- √ fracture line in area of epidural hematoma
- √ expanding biconvex (lenticular = elliptical) extra-axial fluid collection (most frequent) = under high pressure:
  - √ usually does not cross suture lines

√ separation of venous sinuses / falx from inner table of skull
◊ The ONLY hemorrhage displacing falx / venous sinuses away from inner table!

√ hematoma usually homogeneous:
√ fresh extravasated blood (30–50 HU) / coagulated blood (50–80 HU) in acute stage
√ rarely with hypoattenuated "swirl" (due to admixture of fresh blood into clotted blood in active bleeding)

√ mass effect ("compression cone effect") with effacement of gyri + sulci from:
— epidural hematoma (57%)
— hemorrhagic contusion (29%)
— cerebral edematous swelling (14%)

√ marked stretching of vessels
√ signs of arterial injury (rare): contrast extravasation, arteriovenous fistula, middle meningeal artery occlusion, formation of pseudoaneurysm

MR:
√ low intensity of fibrous dura mater allows differentiation of epidural from subdural blood in the late subacute phase (extracellular methemoglobin) with hyperintensity on T1WI + T2WI

Angio:
√ meningeal arteries displaced away from inner table of skull
√ pseudoaneurysm = extravasation of contrast material
√ arteriovenous fistula at fracture line

Cx: herniation, coma, death (15–30%)
Rx: after surgical evacuation return of ventricular system to midline
◊ Epidural hematoma at another site may be unmasked following surgical decompression!
DDx: Chronic subdural hematoma (may have similar biconvex shape, crosses suture lines, stops at falx, no associated skull fracture, no displaced dura on MRI)

GANGLION CELL TUMOR

Gangliocytoma

= rare benign tumor composed of mature ganglion cells
Prevalence: 0.1–0.5% of all brain tumors
Age: children + young adults
Associated with: dysplastic + malformed brain
Cause: ? dysplastic brain
Histo: purely neuronal tumor composed of abnormal mature ganglion cells without neoplastic glial cells (= no immunoreactivity for glial fibrillary acidic protein)
Location: floor of 3rd ventricle > temporal lobe > cerebellum > parieto-occiptal region > frontal lobe > spinal cord

CT:
√ hyperattenuating mass with little mass effect

MR:
√ iso- to hypointense on T1WI + T2WI
√ bright on proton density images

Dysplastic Cerebellar Gangliocytoma

= LHERMITTE-DUCLOS DISEASE
Age: young adults; average age of 34 years
Associated with: polydactyly, partial gigantism, leontiasis ossea, vascular malformation
Strong association with: Cowden disease (= autosomal dominant hamartoma syndrome characterized by mucocutaneous lesions, macrocephaly, hamartomas and neoplasia of breast, thyroid, colon, genitourinary organs, CNS)
Path: disruption of normal cerebellar laminar structure
Histo: hypertrophic ganglion cells expanding granular and molecular layers of cerebellar cortex + abnormally increased myelination in molecular layers; marked reduction in myelination of central white matter of cerebellar folia

• symptoms of increased intracranial pressure
• slowly progressive cerebellar syndrome (40%)
• megalencephaly (50%); mental retardation

CT:
√ hypo- / isoattenuating lesion
√ calcification uncommon
√ thinning of skull

MR:
√ striated cerebellum sign = laminated / lamellar mass of alternating bands of high + normal signal intensity on T2WI

Rx: decompresion of ventricles + resection of mass

Ganglioglioma

= uncommon slow-growing essentially benign tumor composed of glial + neuronal elements
Prevalence: 0.4–09.% of all intracranial neoplasms; 1–4% of all pediatric CNS neoplasms
Peak age: 10–20 years; in 80% <30 years of age; M > F
Histo: contain ganglion + glial elements: ganglion cells (neurons) arise from primitive neuroblasts + mature during growth; usually astrocytic glial cells predominate in various stages of neoplastic differentiation

• headaches
• medically refractory seizures:
◊ Most common cause of chronic temporal lobe epilepsy

Location: frequently above tentorium: in periphery of cerebral hemisphere [temporal (38%) / parietal (30%) / frontal (18%) lobes]; brainstem; cerebellum; pineal region; spinal cord; optic nerve; optic chiasm; ventricles; local involvement of subarachnoid space

√ circumscribed slow-growing mass:
√ solid (43%) / cystic (5%) / solid-cystic combination (52%)

√ calcifications (30%)
√ little associated mass effect / vasogenic edema

CT:
- √ hypoattenuating (38%) / mixed attenuation (32%) / isoattenuating (15%) / hyperattenuating (15%) mass
- √ ± remodeling of skull
- √ contrast enhancement (16–80%)
- ◊ Occasionally completely undetectable by CT

MR:
- √ variable (hypo- / isointense) nonspecific MR appearance on T1WI
- √ commonly at least one hyperintense region on T2WI
- √ nonenhancing / ringlike / homogeneously intense enhancement

Prognosis: favorable; malignant degeneration (6%)

Rx: gross total resection (with resolution of seizure activity in majority of patients)

Desmoplastic Infantile Ganglioglioma

= DESMOPLASTIC INFANTILE ASTROCYTOMA

= SUPERFICIAL CEREBRAL ASTROCYTOMA ATTACHED TO DURA

= uncommon variety of ganglioglioma exclusively in infants

Age: <18 months (vast majority); M:F = 2:1

Histo: spindle cell neoplasm with oval / elongated moderately pleomorphic nuclei + clusters of larger cells with large prominent eccentric nuclei and cytoplasm containing Nissl bodies

- rapidly increasing head circumference
- seizure activity (uncommon)

Location: frontal + parietal > temporal > occipital lobes

- √ exceptionally large heterogenous mass:
  - √ slightly hyperattenuating solid portion typically located along cortical margin
  - √ cystic components
- √ intense enhancement of solid component
- √ CHARACTERISTIC extension of enhancement to leptomeningeal margin (due to firm dural attachment)
- √ rare vasogenic edema
- √ NO calcification

Prognosis: good

Rx: surgical resection

Ganglioneuroma

= ganglion cells predominate over glial cells

GLIOBLASTOMA MULTIFORME

Most malignant form of all gliomas / astrocytomas; end stage of progressive severe anaplasia of preexisting Grade I / II astrocytoma (not from embryologic glioblasts)

Incidence: most common primary brain tumor; 50% of all intracranial tumors; 1–2% of all malignancies; 20,000 cases per year

Age: all ages; peak incidence at 65–75 years; M:F = 3:2; more frequently in whites

Genetics: Turcot syndrome, neurofibromatosis type 1, Li-Fraumeni syndrome (familial neoplasms in various organs based on abnormal p53 tumor-suppressor gene)

Path: multilobulated appearance; quite extensive vasogenic edema (transudation through structurally abnormal tumor vascular channels); deeply infiltrating neoplasm; hemorrhage; necrosis is essential for pathologic diagnosis (HALLMARK)

Histo: highly cellular, often bizarrely pleomorphic / undifferentiated multipolar astrocytes; common mitoses + prominent vascular endothelial proliferation; no capsule; pseudopalisading (= viable neoplastic cells forming an irregular border around necrotic debris as the tumor outgrows its blood supply)

Subtypes:
- (a) giant cell GBM = monstrocellular sarcoma
- (b) small cell GBM = gliosarcoma = Feigin tumor

Location:
- (a) hemispheric: white matter of centrum semiovale: frontal > temporal lobes; common in pons, thalamus, quadrigeminal region; relative sparing of basal ganglia + gray matter
  - *DDx:* solitary metastasis, tumefactive demyelinating lesion ("singular sclerosis"), atypical abscess
- (b) callosal: "butterfly glioma" may grow exophytically into ventricle
- (c) posterior fossa: pilocytic astrocytoma, brainstem astrocytoma
- (d) extraaxial: primary leptomeningeal glioblastomatosis
- (e) multifocal: in 2–5%

Spread:
- (a) direct extension along white matter tracts: corpus callosum (36%), corona radiata, cerebral peduncles, anterior commissure, arcuate fibers
  - √ readily crosses midline = "butterfly" glioma (clue: invasion of septum pellucidum)
  - √ frontal + temporal gliomas tend to invade basal ganglia
  - √ may invade pia, arachnoid and dura (mimicking meningioma)
- (b) subependymal carpet after reaching the surface of the ventricles
- (c) via CSF (<2%)
- (d) hematogenous (extremely rare)
  - √ osteoblastic bone lesion

NECT:
- √ inhomogeneous low-density mass with irregular shape + poorly defined margins (hypodense solid tumor / cavitary necrosis / tumor cyst / peritumoral "fingers of edema")
- √ considerable mass effect: compression + displacement of ventricles, cisterns, brain parenchyma
- √ iso- / hyperdense portions (hemorrhage) in 5%
- √ rarely calcifies (if coexistent with lower-grade glioma / after radio- or chemotherapy)

CECT:

Enhancement pattern: contrast enhancement due to breakdown of blood-brain barrier / neovascularity / areas of necrosis
- (a) diffuse homogeneous enhancement
- (b) heterogeneous enhancement

(c) ring pattern (occasionally enhancing mass within the ring)
(d) low-density lesion with contrast-fluid level (leakage of contrast)

√ almost always ring blush of variable thickness: multiscalloped ("garland"), round / ovoid; may be seen surrounding ventricles (subependymal spread); tumor usually extends beyond margins of enhancement
√ sedimentation level secondary to cellular debris / hemorrhage / accumulated contrast material in tumoral cyst

MR:
√ poorly defined lesion with some mass effect / vasogenic edema / heterogeneity
√ hemosiderin deposits (gradient echo images)
√ hemorrhage (hypointensity on T2WI and T2*-WI)
√ T1WI + gadolinium-DTPA enhancement separate tumor nodules from surrounding edema, central necrosis and cyst formation

Angio:
√ wildly irregular neovascularity + early draining veins
√ avascular lesion

PET:
√ increase in glucose utilization rate

Rx: surgery + radiation therapy + chemotherapy
Prognosis: 16–18 months postoperative survival (frequent tumor recurrence due to uncertainty during surgery about tumor margins)

Multifocal GBM

(1) Spread of primary GBM
(2) Multiple areas of malignant degeneration in diffuse low-grade astrocytoma ("gliomatosis cerebri")
(3) Inherited / acquired genetic abnormality

GLIOMA

= malignant tumors of glial cells growing along white matter tracts, tendency to increase in grade with time; may be multifocal

Incidence: 30–40% of all primary intracranial tumors; 50% of solitary supratentorial masses

√ contrast enhancement:
◊ Increases in proportion to degree of anaplasia
◊ Diminished intensity of enhancement with steroid therapy

CELL OF ORIGIN
1. Astrocyte .... Astrocytoma
2. Oligodendrocyte .... Oligodendroglioma
3. Ependyma .... Ependymoma
4. Medulloblast .... Medulloblastoma; (PNET = primitive neuroectodermal tumor)
5. Choroid plexus .... Choroid plexus papilloma

FREQUENCY OF INTRACRANIAL GLIOMAS

Glioblastoma multiforme	51%
Astrocytoma	25%
Ependymoma	6%
Oligodendroglioma	6%
Spongioblastoma polare	3%
Mixed gliomas	3%
Astroblastoma	2%

Age peak: middle adult life
Location: cerebral hemispheres; spinal cord; brainstem + cerebellum (in children)

Brainstem Glioma

Incidence: 1%; 12–15% of all pediatric brain tumors; 20–30% of infratentorial brain tumors in children
Histo: usually anaplastic astrocytoma / glioblastoma multiforme with infiltration along fiber tracts
Age: in children + young adults; peak age 3–13 years; M:F = 1:1

• become clinically apparent early before ventricular obstruction occurs
• ipsilateral progressive multiple cranial nerve palsies
• contralateral hemiparesis
• cerebellar dysfunction: ataxia, nystagmus
• eventually respiratory insufficiency

Location: pons > midbrain > medulla; often unilateral at medullopontine junction
◊ Medullary + mesencephalic gliomas are more benign than pontine gliomas!

Growth pattern:
(a) diffuse infiltration of brainstem with symmetric expansion + rostrocaudal spread into medulla / thalamus + spread to cerebellum
(b) focally exophytic growth into adjacent cisterns (cerebellopontine, prepontine, cisterna magna)

√ asymmetrically expanded brainstem
√ flattening + posterior displacement of 4th ventricle + aqueduct of Sylvius
√ compression of prepontine + interpeduncular cistern (in upward transtentorial herniation)
√ paradoxical widening of CP angle cistern with tumor extension into CP angle
√ paradoxical anterior displacement of 4th ventricle with tumor extension into cisterna magna

CT:
√ isodense / hypodense mass with indistinct margins
√ hyperdense foci (= hemorrhage) uncommon
√ absent / minimal / patchy contrast enhancement (50%)
√ ring enhancement in necrotic / cystic tumors (most aggressive)
√ prominent enhancement in exophytic lesion
√ hydrocephalus uncommon (because of early symptomatology)

MR: (better evaluation in subtle cases)
√ hypointense on T1WI + hyperintense on T2WI
√ often only subtle enhancement
√ ± engulfment of basilar artery

Angio:
√ anterior displacement of basilar artery + anterior pontomesencephalic vein
√ posterior displacement of precentral cerebellar vein

√ posterior displacement of posterior medullary + supratonsillar segments of PICA
√ lateral displacement of lateral medullary segment of PICA

Prognosis: 10–30% 5-year survival rate
Rx: radiation therapy
DDx: focal encephalitis, resolving hematoma, vascular malformation, tuberculoma, infarct, multiple sclerosis, metastasi, lymphoma

Hypothalamic / Chiasmatic Glioma

Point of origin often undeterminable: hypothalamic gliomas invade chiasm, chiasmatic gliomas invade hypothalamus

Incidence: 10–15% of supratentorial tumors in children
Age: 2–4 years; M:F = 1:1
Associated with: von Recklinghausen disease (20–50%)

- diminished visual acuity (50%) with optic atrophy
- diencephalic syndrome (in up to 20%): marked emaciation, pallor, unusual alertness, hyperactivity, euphoria
- obese child
- sexual precocity
- diabetes insipidus

√ obstructive hydrocephalus
√ suprasellar hypodense lobulated mass with dense inhomogeneous enhancement
√ hypointense on T1WI + hyperintense on T2WI
√ cyst formation, necrosis, calcifications render lesion inhomogeneous

DDx: hypothalamic hamartoma

GLOBOID CELL LEUKODYSTROPHY

= KRABBE DISEASE

Cause: deficiency of galactosylceramide beta-galactosidase resulting in cerebroside accumulation + destruction of oligodendrocytes
Dx: biochemical assay from white blood cells / skin fibroblasts
Age: 3–6 months

- restlessness + irritability
- marked spasticity
- optic atrophy
- hyperacusis

√ symmetric hyperdense lesions in thalami, caudate nuclei, corona radiata
√ decreased attenuation of white matter
√ brain atrophy with enlargement of ventricles

Prognosis: death within first few years of life

HALLERVORDEN-SPATZ DISEASE

= rare familial neurodegenerative metabolic disorder with abnormal iron retention in basal ganglia

Age: 2nd decade of life
Histo: hyperpigmentation + symmetrical destruction of globus pallidus + substantia nigra

- progressive gait impairment + rigidity of limbs
- slowing of voluntary movements, dysarthria
- choreoathetotic movement disorder
- progressive dementia

CT:
√ low- (= tissue destruction) / high-density (= dystrophic calcification) foci in globus pallidus

MR:
√ "eye-of-the-tiger" sign:
  √ initially hypointense globus pallidus on T2WI (= iron deposition)
  √ later central hyperintense foci on T2WI (= tissue destruction + gliosis)

HAMARTOMA OF CNS

rare tumor
(a) sporadic
(b) associated with tuberous sclerosis; may degenerate into giant cell astrocytoma

Age: 0–30 years
Location: temporal lobe, hamartoma of tuber cinereum, subependymal in tuberous sclerosis

√ cyst with little mass effect, possibly with focal calcifications
√ usually no enhancement

HEAD TRAUMA

= CNS TRAUMA

Incidence: 0.2–0.3% annually in United States are significant; peak at 550/100,000 people aged 15–24 years; second peak >50 years of age
Cause: motor vehicle accidents (51%), fall (21%), assault and violence (12%), sports and recreation (10%)
Classification:

A. Primary traumatic lesion
  (a) primary neuronal injury
    1. Cortical contusion
    2. Diffuse axonal injury
    3. Subcortical gray matter injury = injury to thalamus ± basal ganglia
    4. Primary brainstem injury
  (b) primary hemorrhages (from injury to a cerebral artery / vein / capillary)
    1. Subdural hematoma
    2. Epidural hematoma
    3. Intracerebral hematoma
    4. Diffuse hemorrhage (intraventricular, subarachnoid)
  (c) primary vascular injuries
    1. Carotid-cavernous fistula
    2. Arterial pseudoaneurysm
       Location: branches of ACA + MCA, intracavernous portion of ICA, pCom
    3. Arterial dissection / laceration / occlusion
    4. Dural sinus laceration / occlusion
  (d) traumatic pia-arachnoid injury
    1. Posttraumatic arachnoid cyst
    2. Subdural hygroma
  (e) cranial nerve injury

B. Secondary traumatic lesion
- deterioration of consciousness / new neurologic signs some time after initial injury

1. Major territorial arterial infarction
   Cause: prolonged transtentorial / subfalcine herniation pinching the artery against a rigid dural margin
   Location: PCA, ACA territory
2. Boundary + terminal zone infarction
3. Diffuse hypoxic injury
4. Diffuse brain swelling / edema
5. Pressure necrosis from brain herniation
   Cause: increased intracranial pressure
   Location: cingulate, uncal, parahippocampal gyri, cerebellar tonsils
6. Secondary "delayed" hemorrhage
7. Secondary brainstem injury (mechanical compression, secondary (Duret) hemorrhage in tegmentum of rostral pons + midbrain, infarction of median / paramedian perforating arteries, necrosis)
8. Other (eg, fatty embolism, infection)

- **Duret hemorrhage** = hemorrhage in lateral brainstem due to massive temporal lobe herniation
- **Kernahorn notch** = contusion of contralateral brainstem caused by pressure of free edge of tentorium

Pathomechanism:

A. Direct impact on brain due to fracture / skull distortion
√ scalp / skull abnormal
√ superficial neural damage localized to immediate vicinity of calvarial injury
1. Cortical laceration due to depressed fracture fragment
2. Epidural hematoma

B. Indirect injury irrespective of skull deformation
√ scalp / skull normal
(a) compression-rarefaction strain = change in cell volume without change in shape (rare)
(b) shear strain = change in shape without change in volume by
— rotational acceleration forces (more common)
√ bilateral multiple superficial / deep lesions possibly remote from the site of impact
1. Cortical contusion (brain surface)
2. Diffuse axonal injury (white matter)
3. Brainstem + deep gray matter nuclei
— linear acceleration forces (less common)
1. Subdural hematoma
2. Small superficial contusion

Prognosis: 10% fatal, 5–10% with residual deficits

Centripetal approach in search of injury:

A. Scalp
1. Scalp abrasion: not visible
2. Scalp laceration: air inclusion
3. Scalp contusion: salt-and-pepper densities

B. Subgaleal hematoma
Location: between periosteum of outer table and galea (= underneath scalp fat)

C. Skull fracture:
linear ~, stellate ~, depressed ~, basilar ~, eggshell ~

D. Epidural hematoma

E. Subdural hematoma

F. Subarachnoid hemorrhage

G. Brain injury
1. Contusion/ edema
2. Brain hematoma

H. Ventricular hemorrhage

Extracerebral Hemorrhage

1. Subdural hematoma
   in adults: dura inseparable from skull
2. Epidural hematoma
   in children: dura easily stripped away from skull
3. Subarachnoid hemorrhage
   common accompaniment to severe cerebral trauma

Intracerebral Hemorrhage

1. Hematoma
   = blood separating relatively normal neurons
   (a) shear-strain injury (most common)
   (b) blunt / penetrating trauma (bullet, ice pick, skull fracture fragment)
   Incidence: 2–16% of trauma victims
   Location: low frontal + anterior temporal white matter / basal ganglia (80–90%)
   - frequently no loss of consciousness
   - development may be delayed in 8% of head injuries

   √ well-defined homogeneously increased density
2. Cortical contusion
   = blood mixed with edematous brain
   √ poorly defined area of mixed high and low densities, may increase with time
3. Intraventricular hemorrhage
   = potential complication of any intracranial hemorrhage
   ◊ For earliest detection focus on occipital horns!

Other Posttraumatic Lesions

1. Pneumocephalus
2. Penetrating foreign body

Indications for radiographic skull series:
Only in conjunction with positive CT scan findings!
1. Evaluation of depressed skull fracture / fracture of base of the skull

Indications for CT:
1. Loss of consciousness (more than transient)
2. Altered mental status during observation
3. Focal neurologic signs
4. Clinically suspected basilar fracture
5. Depressed skull fracture (= outer table of fragment below level of inner table of calvarium)
6. Penetrating wound (eg, bullet)
7. Suspected acute subarachnoid hemorrhage, epidural / subdural / parenchymal hematoma

CT report must address:
- √ midline shift
- √ localized mass effect
- √ distortion / effacement of basal, perimesencephalic, suprasellar, quadrigeminal cisterns
- √ pressure on brainstem, brainstem abnormality
- √ hemorrhage / contusion: extraaxial, intraaxial, subarachnoid, intraventricular
- √ edema: generalized / localized
- √ hydrocephalus
- √ presence of foreign bodies, bullet, bone fragments, air
- √ base of skull, face, orbit
- √ scalp swelling

Indications for MR:
1. Postconcussive symptomatology
2. Diagnosis of small sub- / epidural hematoma
3. Suspected diffuse axonal (shearing) injury, cortical contusion, primary brainstem injury
4. Vascular damage (eg, pseudoaneurysm formation due to basilar skull fracture)

Sequelae of head injury:
1. Posttraumatic hydrocephalus (1/3)
   = obstruction of CSF pathways secondary to intracranial hemorrhage; develops within 3 months
2. Generalized cerebral atrophy (1/3)
   = result of ischemia + hypoxia
3. Encephalomalacia
   √ focal areas of decreased density, but usually higher density than CSF
4. Pseudoporencephaly
   = CSF-filled space communicating with ventricle / subarachnoid space from cystic degeneration
5. Subdural hygroma
6. Leptomeningeal cyst
   = progressive protrusion of leptomeninges through traumatic calvarial defect
7. Cerebrospinal fluid leak
   - rhinorrhea, otorrhea (indicating basilar fracture with meningeal tear)
8. Posttraumatic abscess
   secondary to (a) penetrating injury (b) basilar skull fracture (c) infection of traumatic hematoma
9. Parenchymal injury
   brain atrophy, residual hemoglobin degradation products, wallerian-type axonal degeneration, demyelination, cavitation, microglial scarring

Prognosis: up to 10% fatal; 5–10% with some degree of neurologic deficit

Mortality: 25/100,000 per year (traffic-related in 20–50%, gunshot 20–40%; falls)

HEMANGIOBLASTOMA OF CNS

= benign autosomal dominant tumor of vascular origin

Incidence: 1–2.5% of all intracranial neoplasms; most common primary infratentorial neoplasm in adults (10% of posterior fossa tumors)

Age: (a) adulthood (>80%): 20–50 years, average age of 33 years; M > F
(b) childhood (<20%): in von Hippel-Lindau disease (10–20%); girls

Associated with:
(a) von Hippel-Lindau disease (in 20%), may have multiple hemangioblastomas (only 20% of patients show other stigmata)
(b) pheochromocytoma (often familial)
(c) syringomyelia
(d) spinal cord hemangioblastomas

- headaches, ataxia, nausea, vomiting
- erythrocythemia in 20% (tumor elaborates stimulant)

Location: paravermian cerebellar hemisphere (85%) > spinal cord > cerebral hemisphere / brainstem; multiple lesions in 10%

- √ solid (1/3) / cystic / cystic + mural nodule
- √ solid portion often intensely hemorrhagic
- √ almost never calcifies

CT:
- √ cystic sharply marginated mass of CSF-density (2/3)
- √ peripheral mural nodule with homogeneous enhancement (50%)
- √ occasionally solid with intense homogeneous enhancement

MR:
- √ well-demarcated tumor mass moderately hypointense on T1WI + T2WI
- √ hyperintense areas on T1WI (= hemorrhage)
- √ hypointense areas on T1WI + hyperintense areas on T2WI (= cyst formation)
- √ intralesional vermiform areas of signal dropout (= high-velocity blood flow)
- √ heterogeneous enhancement on Gd-DTPA with nonenhancing foci of cyst formation + calcification + rapidly flowing blood
- √ perilesional Gd-DTPA enhancing areas of slow-flowing blood vessels feeding + draining the tumor
- √ peripheral hyperintense rim on T2WI (= edema)

Angio:
- √ densely stained tumor nidus within cyst ("contrast loading")
- √ staining of entire rim of cyst
- √ draining vein

Prognosis: >85% postsurgical 5-year survival rate

DDx: (1) Cystic astrocytoma (>5 cm, calcifications, larger nodule, thick-walled lesion, no angiographic contrast blush of mural nodule, no erythrocythemia)
(2) Arachnoid cyst (if mural nodule not visualized)
(3) Metastasis (more surrounding edema)

HEMATOMA OF BRAIN

= INTRACEREBRAL HEMATOMA

Etiology:

A. Very common
   1. Chronic hypertension (50%)
      Age: >60 years

Location: external capsule and basal ganglia (putamen in 65%) / thalamus (25%), pons (5%) + brainstem (10%), cerebellum (5%), cerebral hemisphere (5%)

2. Trauma
3. Aneurysm
4. Vascular malformation: AVM, cavernous hemangioma, venous angioma, capillary telangiectasia

B. Common
1. Hemorrhagic infarction = hemorrhagic transformation of stroke
2. Amyloid angiopathy (20%): elderly patients
3. Coagulopathy (5%): DIC, hemophilia, idiopathic thrombocytopenic purpura; aspirin, heparin, coumadin
4. Drug abuse (5%): amphetamines, cocaine, heroine
5. Bleeding into tumor
   (a) primary: GBM, ependymoma, oligodendroglioma, pituitary adenoma
   (b) metastatic: melanoma, choriocarcinoma, renal cancer, thyroid cancer, adenocarcinoma

C. Uncommon
1. Venous infarction
2. Eclampsia
3. Septic emboli
4. Vasculitis (especially fungal)
5. Encephalitis

Stages of Cerebral Hematomas

Progression: hematoma gradually "snowballs" in size, dissects along white matter tracts; may decompress into ventricular system / subarachnoid space

Resolution: resorption from outside toward the center; rate depends on size of hematoma (usually 1–6 weeks)

FALSE-NEGATIVE CT:
1. impaired clotting
2. anemia

√ iso- / hypodense stage

Hyperacute Cerebral Hemorrhage

Time period: <24 hours

Substrate: fresh oxygenated arterial blood contains 95% diamagnetic (= no unpaired electrons) intracellular oxyhemoglobin (Fe^{2+}) with higher water contents than white matter; oxyhemoglobin persists for 6–12 hours)

NCCT:
- √ homogeneous consolidated high-density lesion (50–70 HU) with irregular well-defined margins increasing in density during day 1–3 (hematoma attenuation dependent on hemoglobin concentration + rate of clot retraction)
- √ usually surrounded by low attenuation (edema, contusion) appearing within 24–48 hours
  (a) irregular shape in trauma
  (b) spherical + solitary in spontaneous hemorrhage
- √ less mass effect compared with neoplasms

MR (less sensitive than CT during first hours):
- √ little difference to normal brain parenchyma = center of hematoma iso- to hypointense on T1WI + minimally hyperintense on T2WI
- √ peripheral rim of hypointensity (= degraded blood products as clue for presence of hemorrhage)

Acute Cerebral Hematoma

Time period: 1–3 days

MR Appearance of Intracerebral Hematoma

Phase	*Age*	*Compartment*	*Hemoglobin*	*T1*	*T2*	*Comments*
Hyperacute	<24 hr	intracellular	oxyhemoglobin	iso	hyper	hyperacute bleed in <1 hr
						deoxygenation
Acute	1 – 3 d	intracellular	deoxyhemoglobin	**hypo**	**hypo**	within clotted intact hypoxic RBCs
		extracellular	deoxyhemoglobin	iso	iso	after lysis of RBCs
Subacute						oxidation
early	>3 d	intracellular	methemoglobin	**hyper**	**hypo**	within intact RBCs inside retracting clot
late	>7 d	extracellular	methemoglobin	**hyper**	**hyper**	after lysis of RBCs
Chronic	>14 d					
center		extracellular	hemichromes	iso	hyper	non–iron-containing heme pigments
rim		intracellular	hemosiderin	**hypo**	**hypo**	within macrophages, present for years
		fibrous tissue		hypo	hypo	
		edema		iso	hyper	

mnemonic: "DD-BD-BB-DD on T1/T2"

Dark-**D**ark	acute	0–2 days	deoxyhemoglobin
Bright-**D**ark	early subacute	3–7 days	intracellular methemoglobin
Bright-**B**right	late subacute	8–14 days	extracellular methemoglobin
Dark-**D**ark	chronic	>14 days	hemosiderin

Substrate: paramagnetic (= 4 unpaired electrons) intracellular deoxyhemoglobin (Fe^{2+}); deoxyhemoglobin persists for 3 days

MR:

√ slightly hypo- / isointense on T1WI (= paramagnetic deoxyhemoglobin within clotted intact hypoxic RBCs does not cause T1 shortening)

√ very hypointense on T2WI (progressive concentration of RBCs, blood clot retraction, and fibrin production shorten T2)

√ surrounding tissue isointense on T1WI / hyperintense on T2WI (edema)

Early Subacute Cerebral Hematoma

Time period: 3–7 days

Substrate: intracellular strongly paramagnetic (= 5 unpaired electrons) methemoglobin (Fe^{3+}) inhomogeneously distributed within cells

NCCT:

√ increase in size of hemorrhagic area over days / weeks

√ high-density lesion within 1st week; often with layering

MR:

√ very hyperintense on T1WI (= oxidation of deoxyhemoglobin to methemoglobin results in marked shortening of T1)

(a) beginning peripherally in parenchymal hematomas

(b) beginning centrally in partially thrombosed aneurysm (oxygen tension higher in lumen)

DDx: melanin, high-protein concentration, flow-related enhancement, gadolinium-based contrast agent

√ very hypointense on T2WI (= intracellular methemoglobin causes T2 shortening)

Late Subacute Cerebral Hematoma

Time period: 7–14 days

Substrate: extracellular strongly paramagnetic methemoglobin (homogeneously distributed)

NCCT:

√ gradual decrease in density from periphery inward (1–2 HU per day) during 2nd + 3rd week

CECT:

√ peripheral rim enhancement at inner border of perilesional lucency (1–6 weeks after injury) in 80% (secondary to blood-brain barrier breakdown / luxury perfusion / formation of hypervascular granulation tissue)

√ ring blush may be diminished by administration of corticosteroids

MR:

√ hyperintense on T1WI (= RBC lysis allows free passage of water molecules across cell membrane)

√ hyperintense on T2WI (= compartmentalization of methemoglobin is lost due to RBC lysis)

√ surrounding edema isointense on T1WI + hyperintense on T2WI

Chronic Cerebral Hematoma

Time period: >14 days

Substrate: superparamagnetic **ferritin** (= soluble + stored in intracellular compartment) and **hemosiderin** (= insoluble + stored in lysosomes) cause marked field inhomogeneities

NCCT:

√ isodense hematoma from 3rd–10th week with perilesional ring of lucency

CT:

√ hypodense phase (4–6 weeks) secondary to fluid uptake by osmosis

√ decreased density (3–6 months) / invisible

√ after 10 weeks lucent hematoma (encephalomalacia due to proteolysis and phagocytosis + surrounding atrophy) with ring blush (DDx: tumor)

MR:

√ rim slightly hypointense on T1WI + very hypointense on T2WI (= superparamagnetic hemosiderin + ferritin within macrophages); rim gradually increases over weeks in thickness, eventually fills in entire hematoma = HALLMARK

√ center hyperintense on T1WI + T2WI (= extracellular methemoglobin of lysed RBCs just inside the darker hemosiderin ring); present for months to 1 year

√ surrounding hyperintensity on T2WI (= edema + serum extruded from clot) with associated mass effect should resorb within 4–6 weeks (DDx: malignant hemorrhage)

Prognosis: (1) herniation (if 3–4 cm in size)
(2) death (if >5 cm in size)

Basal Ganglia Hematoma

= rupture of small distal microaneurysms in the lenticulostriate arteries in patients with poorly controlled systemic arterial hypertension

Cx: (1) Dissection into adjacent ventricles (2/3)
(2) Porencephaly
(3) Atrophy with ipsilateral ventricular dilatation

HETEROTOPIC GRAY MATTER

= collection of cortical neurons in an abnormal location secondary to arrest of migrating neuroblasts from ventricular walls to brain surface between 7–24 weeks of GA

Frequency: 3% of healthy population

May be associated with: agenesis of corpus callosum, aqueductal stenosis, microcephaly, schizencephaly

• seizures

Location:

(1) nodular form: usually symmetric bilaterally in subependymal region / periventricular white matter with predilection for posterior + anterior horns

(2) laminar form: deep / subcortical regions within white matter (less common)
√ single / multiple bilateral subependymal nodules along lateral ventricles
√ NO surrounding edema, isointense with gray matter on all sequences, no contrast enhancement
DDx: subependymal spread of neoplasm, subependymal hemorrhage, vascular malformation, tuberous sclerosis, intraventricular meningioma, neurofibromatosis

HOLOPROSENCEPHALY

= lack of cleavage / diverticulation of the forebrain (= prosencephalon) laterally (cerebral hemispheres), transversely (telencephalon, diencephalon), horizontally (optic + olfactory structures) as a consequence of arrested lateral ventricular growth in 6-week embryo; cortical brain tissue develops to cover the monoventricle and fuses in the midline; posterior part of the monoventricle becomes enlarged and saclike
◊ Septum pellucidum always absent!
Incidence: 1:16,000; M:F = 1:1
A. ALOBAR = no hemispheric development
B. SEMILOBAR = some hemispheric development
C. LOBAR = frontal and temporal lobation + small monoventricle
Associated with: polyhydramnios (60%), renal + cardiac anomalies; chromosomal anomalies (predominantly trisomy 13 + 18)
Associated borderline syndromes secondary to diencephalic malformation:
1. Anophthalmia
2. Microphthalmia
3. Aplasia of pituitary gland
4. Olfactogenital dysplasia
5. Septo-optic dysplasia

DDx:
(1) Severe hydrocephalus (roughly symmetrically thinned cortex)
(2) Dandy-Walker cyst (normal supratentorial ventricular system)
(3) Hydranencephaly (frontal + parietal cortex most severely affected)
(4) Agenesis of corpus callosum with midline cyst (lateral ventricles widely separated with pointed superolateral margin)

Alobar Holoprosencephaly

= extreme form in which the prosencephalon does not divide
• minimal motor activity, little sensory response (ineffective brain function); seizures
• severe facial anomalies ("the face predicts the brain"):
1. Normal face in 17%
2. Cyclopia (= midline single orbit); may have proboscis (= fleshy supraorbital prominence) + absent nose
3. Ethmocephaly = 2 hypoteloric orbits + proboscis between eyes and absence of nasal structures
4. Cebocephaly = 2 hypoteloric orbits + single nostril with small flattened nose + absent nasal septum
5. Median cleft lip + cleft palate + hypotelorism
6. Others: micrognathia, trigonocephaly (early closure of metopic suture), microphthalmia, microcephaly

√ thalami fused
√ protrusion of anteriorly placed fused thalami + basal ganglia into monoventricle
√ absence of: septum pellucidum, 3rd ventricle, falx cerebri, interhemispheric fissure, corpus callosum, fornix, optic tracts, olfactory bulb (= arrhinencephaly), internal cerebral veins, superior + inferior straight sagittal sinus, vein of Galen, tentorium, sylvian fissure, opercular cortex
√ crescent-shaped holoventricle = single large ventricle without occipital or temporal horns
√ large dorsal cyst occupying most of calvarium + widely communicating with single ventricle
√ "horseshoe" / "boomerang" configuration of brain = peripheral rim of cerebral cortex displaced rostrally (coronal plane)
(a) pancake configuration = cortex covers monoventricle to edge of dorsal cyst
(b) cup configuration = more cortex visible posteriorly
(c) ball configuration = complete covering of monoventricle without dorsal cyst

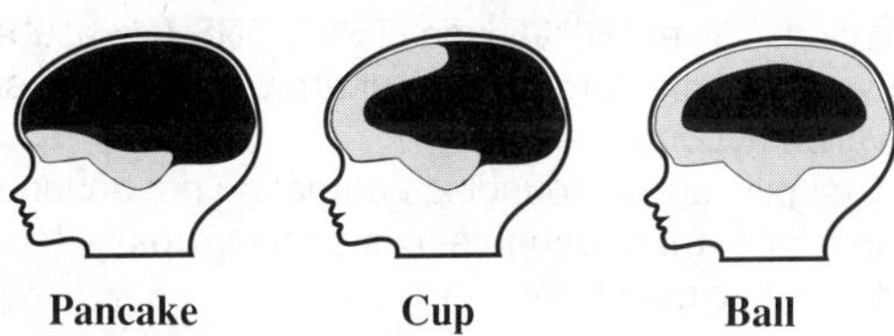

√ midbrain, brainstem, cerebellum structurally normal
√ pancakelike cerebrum in posterior cranium
√ cerebral mantle pachygyric
√ midline clefts in maxilla + palate
Prognosis: death within 1st year of life / stillborn
DDx: massive hydrocephalus, hydranencephaly

Semilobar Holoprosencephaly

= intermediate form with incomplete cleavage of prosencephalon (more midline differentiation + beginning of sagittal separation)
• mild facial anomalies: midline cleft lip + palate
• hypotelorism
• mental retardation
√ single ventricular chamber with partially formed occipital horns + rudimentary temporal horns
√ peripheral rim of brain tissue is several cm thick
√ partially fused thalami anteriorly situated + abnormally rotated resulting in small 3rd ventricle
√ absence of septum pellucidum + corpus callosum + olfactory bulb
√ rudimentary falx cerebri + interhemispheric fissure form caudally with partial separation of occipital lobes
√ incomplete hippocampal formation
Prognosis: infants survive frequently into adulthood

Lobar Holoprosencephaly
= mildest form with two cerebral hemispheres + two distinct lateral ventricles
◊ May be part of septo-optic dysplasia!
• usually not associated with facial anomalies except for hypotelorism
• mild to severe mental retardation, spasticity, athetoid movements
√ closely apposed bodies of lateral ventricles with distinct occipital + frontal horns
√ mild dilatation of lateral ventricles
√ colpocephaly
√ unseparated frontal horns of angular squared shape + flat roof (on coronal images) due to dysplastic frontal lobes
√ dysplastic anterior falx + interhemispheric fissure
√ absence of septum pellucidum + sylvian fissures
√ corpus callosum usually present
√ hippocampal formation nearly normal
√ basal ganglia + thalami may be fused / separated
√ pachygyria (= abnormally wide + plump gyri), lissencephaly (= o gyri)
Prognosis: survival into adulthood

HYDATID DISEASE OF BRAIN
= canine tapeworm (Echinococcus granulosus) in sheep- and cattle-grazing areas
Location: liver (60%), lung (25%), CNS (2%) subcortical
√ usually single, large round, sharply marginated smooth-walled hypodense cyst
√ no significant surrounding edema; no rim enhancement
√ development of daughter cysts (after rupture / following diagnostic puncture)

HYDRANENCEPHALY
= liquefaction necrosis of cerebral hemispheres replaced by a thin membranous sac of leptomeninges in outer layer + remnants of cortex and white matter in inner layer, filled with CSF + necrotic debris
Incidence: 0.2% of infant autopsies
Etiology: absence of supraclinoid ICA system (? vascular occlusion / infection with toxoplasmosis or CMV)
= ultimate form of porencephaly
• seizures; respiratory failure; generalized flaccidity
• decerebrate state with vegetative existence
√ normal skull size / macrocrania / microcrania
√ complete filling of hemicranium with membranous sac
√ absence of cortical mantle (inferomedial aspect of temporal lobe, inferior aspect of frontal lobe, occipital lobe may be identified in some patients)
√ brainstem usually atrophic
√ cerebellum almost always intact
√ thalamic, hypothalamic, mesencephalic structures usually preserved + project into cystic cavity
√ central brain tissue can be asymmetric
√ choroid plexus present
√ falx cerebri + tentorium cerebelli usually intact, may be deviated in asymmetric involvement, may be incomplete / absent

Prognosis: not compatible with prolonged extrauterine life (no intellectual improvement from shunting)
DDx: (1) Severe hydrocephalus (some identifiable cortex present)
(2) Alobar holoprosencephaly (facial midline anomalies)
(3) Schizencephaly (some spared cortical mantle)

HYDROCEPHALUS
= excess of CSF due to imbalance of CSF formation + absorption resulting in increased intraventricular pressure
Pathophysiology:
A. Overproduction (rare)
B. Impaired absorption
1. Blockage of CSF flow within ventricular system, cisterna magna, basilar cisterns, cerebral convexities
2. Blockage of arachnoid villi / lymphatic channels of cranial nerves, spinal nerves, adventitia of cerebral vessels

Compensated hydrocephalus = new equilibrium established at higher intracranial pressure due to opening of alternate pathways (arachnoid membrane / stroma of choroid plexus / extracellular space of cortical mantle = transependymal flow of CSF)

Skull film: signs of raised intracranial pressure
A. YOUNG INFANT / NEWBORN
√ increase in craniofacial ratio
√ bulging of anterior fontanel
√ sutural diastasis
√ macrocephaly + frontal bossing
√ "beaten brass" = "hammered silver" appearance = prominent digital impressions (wide range of normals in 4–10 years of age)
B. ADOLESCENT / ADULT (changes in sella turcica)
√ atrophy of anterior wall of dorsum sellae
√ shortening of the dorsum sellae producing pointed appearance
√ erosion / thinning / discontinuity of floor of sella
√ depression of floor of sella with bulging into sphenoid sinus
√ enlargement of sella turcica
DDx: osteoporotic sella (aging, excessive steroid hormone)

Signs favoring hydrocephalus over white matter atrophy:
√ commensurate dilatation of temporal horn with lateral ventricles (most reliable sign)
√ narrowing of ventricular angle (= angle between anterior / superior margins of frontal horns at level of foramen of Monro) due to concentric enlargement:
√ Mickey Mouse ears on axial scans
√ enlargement of frontal horn radius (= widest diameter of frontal horns taken at 90° angle to long axis of frontal horn):
√ rounding of frontal horn shape

√ enlargement of ventricular system disproportionate to enlargement of cortical sulci (due to compression of brain tissue against skull + consequent sulcal narrowing)
√ interstitial edema from transependymal flow of CSF:
  √ periventricular hypodensity
  √ rim of prolonged T1 + T2 relaxation times surrounding lateral ventricles
√ hydrocephalic distortion of ventricles + brain:
  √ atrial diverticulum = herniation of ventricular wall through choroidal fissure of ventricular trigone into supracerebellar + quadrigeminal cisterns
  √ dilatation of suprapineal recess expanding into posterior incisural space resulting in inferior displacement of pineal gland / shortening of tectum in rostral-caudal direction / elevation of vein of Galen
  √ enlargement of anterior recess of 3rd ventricle extending into suprasellar cistern

Obstructive Hydrocephalus

= obstruction to normal CSF flow + absorption

Communicating Hydrocephalus

= EXTRAVENTRICULAR HYDROCEPHALUS
= elevated intraventricular pressure secondary to blockade beyond the outlet of 4th ventricle within the subarachnoid pathways

Incidence: 38% of congenital hydrocephaly

Pathophysiology:
unimpeded CSF flow through ventricles; impeded CSF flow over convexities by adhesions / impeded reabsorption by arachnoid villi

Cause:
repetitive subarachnoid microhemorrhage (most common cause), immaturity of arachnoid villi, meningeal carcinomatosis (medulloblastoma, germinoma, leukemia, lymphoma, adenocarcinoma), purulent / tuberculous meningitis, subdural hematoma, craniosynostosis, achondroplasia, Hurler syndrome, venous obstruction (obliteration of superior sagittal sinus), absence of Pacchioni granulations

√ symmetric enlargement of lateral, 3rd, and often 4th ventricles
√ dilatation of subarachnoid cisterns
√ normal / effaced cerebral sulci
√ symmetric low attenuation of periventricular white matter (transependymal CSF flow)
√ delayed ascent of radionuclide tracer over convexities
√ persistence of radionuclide tracer in lateral ventricles for up to 48 hours

Changes after successful shunting:
  √ diminished size of ventricles + increased prominence of sulci
  √ cranial vault may thicken
    Cx: subdural hematoma (result from precipitous decompression)

Noncommunicating Hydrocephalus

= INTRAVENTRICULAR HYDROCEPHALUS
= blockade of CNS flow within the ventricular system with dilatation of ventricles proximal to obstruction

Pathogenesis: increased CSF pressure causes ependymal flattening with breakdown of CSF-brain barrier leading to myelin destruction + compression of cerebral mantle (brain damage)

Location:
(a) Lateral ventricular obstruction
  Cause: ependymoma, intraventricular glioma, meningioma
(b) Foramen of Monro obstruction
  Cause: 3rd ventricular colloid cyst, tuber, papilloma, meningioma, septum pellucidum cyst / glioma, fibrous membrane (post infection), giant cell astrocytoma
(c) Third ventricular obstruction
  Cause: large pituitary adenoma, teratoma, craniopharyngioma, glioma of 3rd ventricle, hypothalamic glioma
(d) Aqueductal obstruction
  Cause: Congenital web / atresia (often associated with Chiari malformation), fenestrated aqueduct, tumor of mesencephalon / pineal gland, tentorial meningioma, S/P intraventricular hemorrhage or infection
(e) Fourth ventricular obstruction
  Cause: Congenital obstruction, Chiari malformation, Dandy-Walker syndrome, inflammation (TB), tumor within 4th ventricle (ependymoma), extrinsic compression of 4th ventricle (astrocytoma, medulloblastoma, large CPA tumors, posterior fossa mass), isolated / trapped 4th ventricle

√ enlarged lateral ventricles (enlargement of occipital horns precedes enlargement of frontal horns)
√ effaced cerebral sulci
√ periventricular edema with indistinct margins (especially frontal horns)
√ radioisotope cisternography: no obstruction if tracer reaches ventricle
√ change in RI indicates increased intracranial pressure (ΔRI 47–132% versus 3–29% in normals)

Nonobstructive Hydrocephalus

= secondary to rapid CSF production

Cause: Choroid plexus papilloma

√ ventricle near papilloma enlarges
√ intense radionuclide uptake in papilloma
√ enlarged anterior / posterior choroidal artery and blush

Congenital Hydrocephalus

= multifactorial CNS malformation during the 3rd / 4th week after conception

Etiology:
(1) aqueductal stenosis (43%)
(2) communicating hydrocephalus (38%)
(3) Dandy-Walker syndrome (13%)
(4) other anatomic lesions (6%)
(a) Genetic factors: spina bifida, aqueductal stenosis (X-linked recessive trait with a 50% recurrence rate for male fetuses), congenital atresia of foramina of Luschka and Magendie (Dandy-Walker syndrome; autosomal recessive trait with 25% recurrence rate), cerebellar agenesis, cloverleaf skull, trisomy 13–18
(b) Nongenetic etiology: tumor compressing 3rd / 4th ventricle, obliteration of subarachnoid pathway due to infection (syphilis, CMV, rubella, toxoplasmosis), proliferation of fibrous tissue (Hurler syndrome), Chiari malformations, vein of Galen aneurysm, choroid plexus papilloma, vitamin A intoxication

Incidence: 0.3–1.8:1,000 pregnancies
Associated with:
(a) Intracranial anomalies (37%): hypoplasia of corpus callosum, encephalocele, arachnoid cyst, arteriovenous malformation
(b) extracranial anomalies (63%): spina bifida in 25–30% (with spina bifida hydrocephalus is present in 80%), renal agenesis, multicystic dysplastic kidney, VSD, tetralogy of Fallot, anal agenesis, malrotation of bowel, cleft lip / palate, Meckel syndrome, gonadal dysgenesis, arthrogryposis, sirenomelia
(c) chromosomal anomalies (11%): trisomy 18 + 21, mosaicism, balanced translocation

- elevated amniotic alpha-fetoprotein level

OB-US (assessment difficult prior to 20 weeks GA as ventricles ordinarily constitute a large portion of cranial vault):
√ "dangling choroid plexus sign":
√ choroid plexus not touching medial + lateral walls of lateral ventricles
√ downside choroid plexus falling away from medial wall + hanging from tela choroidea
√ upside choroid falling away from lateral wall
√ lateral width of ventricular atrium ≥10 mm (size usually constant between 16 weeks MA and term)
◊ 88% of fetuses with sonographically detected neural axis anomalies have atrial width >10 mm
√ BPD >95th percentile (usually not before 3rd trimester)
√ polyhydramnios (in 30%)

Recurrence rate: <4%
Mortality: (1) fetal death in 24%
(2) neonatal death in 17%
Prognosis: poor with
(1) associated anomalies
(2) shift of midline (porencephaly)
(3) head circumference >50 cm
(4) absence of cortex (hydranencephaly)
(5) cortical thickness <10 mm

Infantile Hydrocephalus

- ocular disturbances: paralysis of upward gaze, abducens nerve paresis, nystagmus, ptosis, diminished pupillary light response
- spasticity of lower extremities (from disproportionate stretching of paracentral corticospinal fibers)

Etiology:
mnemonic: "**A VP**-**S**hunt **C**an **D**ecompress **T**he **H**ydrocephalic **C**hild"
Aqueductal stenosis
Vein of Galen aneurysm
Postinfectious
Superior vena cava obstruction
Chiari II malformation
Dandy-Walker syndrome
Tumor
Hemorrhage
Choroid plexus papilloma

Doppler:
√ RI >0.8 (sign of increased ICP) in neonate:
√ RI of 0.84 ± 13% decreasing to 0.72 ± 11% after shunting
√ RI >0.65 (sign of increased ICP) in older children

Normal Pressure Hydrocephalus

= NPH = ADAM SYNDROME
= pressure gradient between ventricle + brain parenchyma in spite of normal CSF pressure
◊ Potentially treatable cause of dementia in elderly!

Cause: communicating hydrocephalus with incomplete arachnoidal obstruction from neonatal intraventricular hemorrhage, spontaneous subarachnoid hemorrhage, intracranial trauma, infection, surgery, carcinomatosis
mnemonic: "PAM the HAM"
Paget disease
Aneurysm
Meningitis
Hemorrhage (from trauma)
Achondroplasia
Mucopolysaccharidosis

Pathophysiology of CSF:
(?) brain pushed toward cranium from ventricular enlargement; brain unable to expand during systole thus compressing lateral + 3rd ventricles + expressing large CSF volume through aqueduct; reverse dynamic during diastole; "water-hammer" force of recurrent ventricular expansion damages periventricular tissues

Age: 50–70 years

- normal opening pressure at lumbar puncture
- dementia, gait apraxia, urinary incontinence
mnemonic: wacky, wobbly and wet

√ communicating hydrocephalus with prominent temporal horns
√ ventricles dilated out of proportion to any sulcal enlargement
√ upward bowing of corpus callosum
√ flattening of cortical gyri against inner table of calvarium (DDx: rounded gyri in generalized atrophy)

MR:
- √ pronounced aqueductal flow void (due to diminished compliance of normal pressure hydrocephalus)
- √ periventricular hyperintensity (due to transependymal CSF flow)

Rx: CSF shunting (only 50% improved)

HYPOTHALAMIC HAMARTOMA

= HAMARTOMA OF TUBER CINEREUM
= rare congenital malformation composed of normal neuronal tissue arising from posterior hypothalamus in region of tuber cinereum

Age: <2 years of age; M > F
Histo: heterotopic collection of neurons, astrocytes, oligodendroglial cells (closely resembling histologic pattern of tuber cinereum)

- • isosexual precocious puberty (due to LRH secretion)
- • gelastic seizures, hyperactivity
- • neurodevelopmental delay

Location: mamillary bodies / tuber cinereum of thalamus, rarely within hypothalamus itself

- √ well-defined round / oval mass projecting from base of brain into suprasellar / interpeduncular cistern
- √ attached to tuber cinereum / mamillary bodies by thin stalk (pedunculated)
- √ remain stable in size over time; up to 4 cm in diameter

CT:
- √ round homogeneous mass isodense with brain tissue
- √ NO enhancement

MR:
- √ well-defined round pedunculated mass suspended from tuber cinereum / mamillary bodies
- √ isointense on T1WI + iso- / slightly hyperintense on T2WI (imaging characteristics of gray matter)
- √ no gadolinium enhancement

IDIOPATHIC INTRACRANIAL HYPERTENSION

= PSEUDOTUMOR CEREBRI = BENIGN INTRACRANIAL HYPERTENSION (BIH)

secondary to
- (a) elevation in blood volume (85%)
- (b) decrease in regional cerebral blood flow with delayed CSF absorption (10%)

Etiology:
1. Sinovenous occlusive disease, SVC occlusion, obstruction of dural sinus, obstruction of both internal jugular veins
2. Dural AVM
3. S/P brain biopsy with edema
4. Endocrinopathies
5. Hypervitaminosis A
6. Hypocalcemia
7. Menstrual dysfunction, pregnancy, menarche, birth control pills
8. Drug therapy

Predilection for: obese young to middle-aged women

- • headache
- • papilledema
- • elevated opening pressures on lumbar puncture
- √ normal ventricular size / pinched ventricles
- √ increased volume of subarachnoid space

INFARCTION OF BRAIN

= brain cell death leading to coagulation necrosis

Cause: large vessel occlusion of ICA / MCA / PCA (50%) due to emboli from atherosclerotic stenosis, small-vessel lacunes (25%), cardiac cause (15%), blood disorder (5%), non-arteriosclerotic (5%)
◊ 33% of TIAs will lead to infarction!

Pathophysiology:
distal microstasis occurs within 2 minutes after occlusion of cerebral artery; regional cerebral blood flow is acutely decreased in area of infarction + remains depressed for several days at center of infarct; arterial circulation time may be prolonged in entire hemisphere; rapid development of vasodilatation due to hypoxia, hypercapnia, tissue acidosis; delayed filling + emptying of arterial channels in area of infarction (= arteriolar-capillary block) well into venous phase; by end of 1st week regional blood flow commonly increases to rates even above those required for metabolic needs (= hyperemic phase = luxury perfusion)

Detection rate by CT:
80% for cortex + mantle, 55% for basal ganglia, 54% for posterior fossa
◊ Positive correlation between degree of clinical deficit and CT sensitivity

CT sensitivity:

on day of ictus:	48%
1–2 days later:	59%
7–10 days later:	66%
10–11 days later:	74%

Location: cerebrum:cerebellum = 19:1
- (a) supratentorial
  - — cerebral mantle (70%) in territory of MCA (50%), PCA (10%), watershed between MCA + ACA (7%), ACA (4%)
  - — basal ganglia + internal capsule (20%)
- (b) infratentorial (10%)
  upper cerebellum (5%), lower cerebellum (3%), pons + medulla (2%)

Hyperacute Ischemic Infarction

Time period: <12 hours

CT (relatively insensitive + nonspecific):
- √ normal (in 10–60%)
- √ subtle decrease in attenuation within affected brain area:
  - √ loss of gray-white matter differentiation
  - √ insular ribbon sign = obscuration of lentiform nucleus due to decreased attenuation within insula (in 50–80% of MCA occlusions)
- √ early brain swelling:
  - √ hemispheric sulcal effacement
- √ "hyperdense middle cerebral artery sign" = acute intraluminal thrombus of 80 HU (due to extrusion of serum from thrombus) vs. 40 HU of flowing blood; transient phenomenon

Incidence: 35–50% of acute MCA occlusions
DDx: high hematocrit level, calcification of vessel wall
√ calcified intraluminal embolus (rare)

MR (routinely positive by 4–6 hours post ictus):
√ hyperintense signal on proton-density images + T2WI involving cortical gray matter
√ loss of normal intravascular flow voids (similar to hyperdense MCA sign)
√ stasis of contrast material within affected arteries
√ subtle parenchymal swelling with sulcal effacement due to cytotoxic edema (= increased intracellular water) can be seen by 2 hours post ictus (best on T1WI)
√ hyperintense signal from less signal loss (due to restricted water diffusibility) on diffusion-weighted images (MOST SENSITIVE, hyperintensity maintained for 7–10 days, which allows discrimination of acute from older infarcts)
√ ischemic penumbra = combination of perfusion + diffusion-weighted images allows identification of areas at risk for infarction

NUC:
◊ Newer imaging agents (eg, Tc-99m HM-PAO) may be positive within minutes of the event, while CT and MR are normal
√ hemispheric hypoperfusion throughout all phases
√ defect corresponding to nonperfused vascular territory
√ "flip-flop sign" in radionuclide angiogram (15%) = decreased uptake during arterial + capillary phase followed by increased uptake during venous phase
√ "luxury perfusion syndrome" (14%) = increased perfusion

Rx: recombinant tissue plasminogen activator (TPA)

Acute Ischemic Infarction

Histo: cortical cytotoxic edema (from loss of vascular autoregulation) followed by white matter vasogenic edema

Early Acute Ischemic Infarction

Time period: 12–24 hours

NCCT:
√ low-density basal ganglia
√ loss of differentiation between cortical gray matter and subjacent white matter:
  √ blurring of the clarity of internal capsule
  √ "insular ribbon sign" = hypodense extreme capsule no longer distinguishable from insular cortex
√ subtle sulcal effacement (8%)

CECT:
√ no iodine accumulation in affected cortical region
√ meningeal gyriform enhancement

MR:
√ subtle narrowing of sulci
√ blurring of gray-white matter junction on T2- and proton-density images
√ increase in thickness of cortex (= gyral swelling)
√ subtle low-signal intensity on T1WI, high-signal intensity on T2WI (masking of gyral infarcts on heavily T2WI due to sulcal CSF intensity)

MRA:
√ absence of flow for infarcts >2 cm in diameter

Late Acute Ischemic Infarction

Time period: 1–3–7 days

NCCT:
√ hypodense wedge-shaped lesion with base at cortex in a vascular distribution (in 70%) due to vasogenic + cytotoxic edema
√ mass effect (23–75%): sulcal effacement, transtentorial herniation, displaced subarachnoid cisterns + ventricles
√ "bland infarct" may be transformed into hemorrhagic infarct after 2–4 days (due to leakage of blood from ischemically damaged capillary endothelium following lysis of intraluminal clot + arterial reperfusion)

CECT:
√ decreased meningeal + intravascular contrast enhancement
√ increased parenchymal enhancement

MR:
√ intravascular enhancement sign (77%) = Gd-pentetate enhancement of cortical arterial vessels in area of brain injury after 1–3 days (due to slow arterial blood flow provided by collateral circulation via leptomeningeal anastomoses)
√ meningeal enhancement sign (33%) = Gd-pentetate enhancement of meninges adjacent to infarct after 2–6 days (due to meningeal inflammation)

Angio:
√ narrowed / occluded vessels supplying the area of infarction
√ delayed filling + emptying of involved vessels
√ early draining vein
√ luxury perfusion of infarcted area (rare) = loss of small vessel autoregulation due to local increase in pH

Subacute Ischemic Infarction

Time period: 7–30 days = paradoxical phase with resolution of edema + onset of coagulation necrosis

NCCT:
√ "fogging phenomenon" = low-density area less apparent
√ decrease of mass effect + ex vacuo dilatation of ventricles (in 57%)
√ ± transient calcification (especially in children)

CECT:
√ gyral blush + ring enhancement (breakdown of blood-brain barrier + luxury perfusion) for 2–8 weeks (in 65–80% within first 4 weeks)
√ no enhancement in 1/5 of patients

MR:

Histo: vasogenic edema (= increased extracellular water) due to disruption of blood-brain barrier

√ hypointense on T1WI, hyperintense on T2WI

√ intravascular + meningeal enhancement signs resolve toward end of 1st week

√ gyriform parenchymal Gd-pentetate enhancement

◊ Gyriform parenchymal enhancement permits differentiation of subacute from chronic infarction!

Chronic Ischemic Infarction

Time period: months to years (>30 days)

Histo: demyelination + gliosis complete (focal brain atrophy after 8 weeks)

√ cerebral atrophy + encephalomalacia + gliosis (HALLMARKS)

√ possible calcification (especially in children)

NCCT:

√ cystic foci of CSF density (= encephalomalacia) in vascular distribution

MR:

√ patchy region with increased intensity on T2WI

√ gliosis (hyperintense on T2WI) often surrounding encephalomalacic region

√ wallerian degeneration (= antegrade degeneration of axons secondary to neuronal injury) of corticospinal tracts in the wake of old large infarcts that involve the motor cortex

Hemorrhagic Infarction

Etiology: lysis of embolus / opening of collaterals / restoration of normal blood pressure following hypotension / hypertension / anticoagulation causes extravasation in reperfused ischemic brain

Incidence: 6% of clinically diagnosed brain infarcts, 20% of autopsied brain infarcts

Path: petechial hemorrhages in various degrees of coalescence

Location: corticomedullary junction

CT:

√ hyperdensity (56–76 HU) appearing within a previously imaged hypodense acute ischemic infarct = hemorrhagic transformation (in 50–72%)

False negative: hematoma isoattenuating if hematocrit <20%

MR:

√ hypointense area on T2WI within edema marking gyri = deoxyhemoglobin of acute hemorrhage

√ hyperintense area on T1WI = methemoglobin of subacute hematoma

Basal Ganglia Infarct

= occlusion of small penetrating arteries at base of brain (lenticulostriate / thalamoperforating arteries)

= lacunar infarct (infarcts <1 cm in size)

Cause:

(1) Embolism

(2) Hypoperfusionm

(3) Carbon monoxide poisoning

(4) Drowning

(5) Vasculopathy (hypertension, microvasculopathy, aging)

√ dense homogeneous enhancement outlining caudate nucleus, putamen, globus pallidus, thalamus

√ dense round nodular enhancement / peripheral ring enhancement

Laminar Necrosis

= ischemic changes affecting deep layers of the cortex (layers 3, 5, 6 very sensitive to oxygen deprivation)

MR:

(a) acute stage

√ linear cortical hyperintensity on T1WI

√ contrast enhancement

√ white matter edema on T2WI

(b) chronic stage

√ thin hypointense cortex

√ hyperintense white matter

√ enlargement of CSF spaces

Lacunar Infarction

= small deep infarcts in the distal distribution of penetrating vessels (lenticulostriate, thalamoperforating, pontine perforating arteries, recurrent artery of Heubner)

Cause: occlusion of small penetrating end arteries at base of brain due to fibrinoid degeneration

Predisposed: hypertensive / diabetic patients

Incidence: 20% of cerebral infarctions

Path: lacune = cavitated infarct resulting in small hole traversed by cobweblike fibrous strands

Histo: "microatheroma" = hyalinization + arteriolar sclerosis resulting in thickening of vessel wall + luminal narrowing

• pure motor / pure sensory stroke

• ataxic hemiparesis

Location: upper two-thirds of putamen > caudate > thalamus > pons > internal capsule

√ small discrete foci of hypodensity between 3 mm and 15 mm in size (most <1 cm in diameter)

√ higher in signal intensity than CSF (due to marginal gliosis)

√ unilateral pontine infarcts are sharply marginated at midline

TIA and RIND

√ hypodense small lesions located peripherally near / within cortex without enhancement

√ lesions detected in only 14%, contralateral lesion present in 14% (CT of marginal value)

INFECTION IN IMMUNOCOMPROMISED PATIENTS

Cause: underlying malignancy, collagen disease, cancer therapy, AIDS, immunosuppressive therapy in organ transplants

Organism: Toxoplasma, Nocardia, Aspergillus, Candida, Cryptococcus

√ poorly defined hypodense zones with rapid enlargement in size + number, particularly affecting basal ganglia + centrum semiovale (poorly localized + encapsulated infection with poor prognosis)

√ ring / nodular enhancement (sufficient immune defenses): Toxoplasma, Nocardia

√ enhancement may be blunted by steroid Rx

AIDS may be associated with:

thrombocytopenia, lymphoma, plasmacytoma, Kaposi sarcoma, progressive multifocal leukoencephalopathy

INIENCEPHALY

= complex developmental anomaly characterized by
- (1) exaggerated lordosis
- (2) rachischisis
- (3) imperfect formation of skull base at foramen magnum

M:F = 1:4

Associated with other anomalies in 84%:

anencephaly, encephalocele, hydrocephalus, cyclopia, absence of mandible, cleft lip / palate, diaphragmatic hernia, omphalocele, gastroschisis, single umbilical artery, CHD, polycystic kidney disease, arthrogryposis, clubfoot

√ dorsal flexion of head

√ abnormally short + deformed spine

Prognosis: almost uniformly fatal

DDx:
- (1) Anencephaly
- (2) Klippel-Feil syndrome
- (3) Cervical myelomeningocele

INTRAVENTRICULAR NEUROCYTOMA

= INTRAVENTRICULAR NEUROBLASTOMA

= benign primary neoplasm of lateral + 3rd ventricles

Incidence: unknown; tumor frequently mistaken for intraventricular oligodendroglioma

Age: 20–40 years

Histo: uniform round cells with central round nucleus + fine chromatin stippling ± perivascular pseudorosettes, focal microcalcifications (closely resembling oligodendroglioma but with neuronal differentiation into synapselike junctions)

Location: body ± frontal horn of lateral ventricle, may extend into 3rd ventricle

√ entirely intraventricular well-circumscribed tumor, coarsely calcified (69%), containing cystic spaces (85%)

√ mild to moderate contrast enhancement

√ attachment to septum pellucidum CHARACTERISTIC

√ ± hemorrhage into tumor / ventricle

√ hydrocephalus

√ peritumoral edema extremely uncommon

MR:

√ isointense relative to cortical gray matter on T1WI + T2WI with heterogeneous areas due to calcifications, cystic spaces, vascular flow voids (62%)

Rx: complete surgical resection

DDx:
- (1) Intraventricular oligodendroglioma (no hemorrhage)
- (2) Astrocytoma (peritumoral edema in 20%)
- (3) Meningioma (almost exclusively in trigone, >30 years of age)
- (4) Ependymoma (in + around 4th ventricle / trigone, in childhood)
- (5) Subependymoma (in + around 4th ventricle, young adults)
- (6) Choroid plexus papilloma (body + posterior horn of lateral ventricle, intense enhancement, younger patient)
- (7) Colloid cyst (anterior 3rd ventricle / foramen of Monro, calcifications uncommon)
- (8) Craniopharyngioma (extraventricular origin)
- (9) Teratoma + dermoid cyst (fat attenuation)

JAKOB-CREUTZFELDT DISEASE

= rare transmissible disease developing over weeks

Cause: "prion" = protein devoid of functional nucleic acid; ? slow-virus infection

Age: older adults

Histo: classified as "spongiform encephalopathy"

• rapidly progressive dementia, ataxia, myoclonus

√ hyperintense lesions in head of caudate nucleus + putamen, bilaterally on T2WI

√ NO gadolinium enhancement of lesions

√ NO white matter involvement

Prognosis: usually fatal within 1 year of onset

JOUBERT SYNDROME

• episodic hyperpnea

• abnormal eye movement

• ataxia, mental retardation

Path:
- (1) nearly total aplasia of cerebellar vermis
- (2) dysplasia + heterotopia of cerebellar nuclei
- (3) near total absence of pyramidal decussation
- (4) anomalies in structure of inferior olivary nuclei, descending trigeminal tract, solitary fascicle, dorsal column nuclei

√ 4th ventricle triangle-shaped at mid-level + bat-wing–shaped superiorly

√ cerebellar hemispheres appose one another in midline

√ superior cerebellar peduncles surrounded by CSF

LIPOMA

= congenital tumor developing within subarachnoid space as a result of abnormal differentiation of the meninx primitiva (which differentiates into pia mater, arachnoid, inner meningeal layer of dura mater)

Incidence: <1% of brain tumors

Age: presentation in childhood / adulthood

Associated with congenital anomalies:
- (a) in anterior location: various degrees of agenesis of corpus callosum (in 50–80%)
- (b) in posterior location (in <33%)

• asymptomatic in 50%

Location:
(usually in subarachnoid space) callosal cistern (25–50%), sylvian fissure, quadrigeminal cistern, chiasmatic cistern, interpeduncular cistern, CP angle cistern, cerebellomedullary cistern, tuber cinereum, choroid plexus of lateral ventricle

CT:
√ well-circumscribed mass with CT density of –100 HU
√ occasionally calcified rim (esp. in corpus callosum)
√ no enhancement

MR:
√ hyperintense mass on T1WI + less hyperintense on T2WI (CHARACTERISTIC)

Lipoma of Corpus Callosum

= congenital pericallosal tumor not actually involving the corpus callosum as a result of faulty disjunction of neuroectoderm from cutaneous ectoderm during process of neurulation

Incidence: approx. 30% of intracranial lipomas

Associated with:
(1) anomalies of corpus callosum (30% with small posterior lipoma, 90% with large anterior lipoma)
(2) frontal bone defect (frequent) = encephalocele
(3) cutaneous frontal lipoma

• in 50% symptomatic:
  • seizure disorders, mental retardation, dementia
  • emotional lability, headaches
  • hemiplegia

Plain film:
√ midline calcification with associated lucency of fat density

CT:
√ area of marked hypodensity immediately superior to lateral ventricles with possible extension inferiorly between ventricles / anteriorly into interhemispheric fissure
√ curvilinear peripheral / nodular central calcification within fibrous capsule (more common in anterior compared with posterior lipomas)

MR:
√ hyperintense midline mass superior + posterior to corpus callosum on T1WI
√ no callosal fibers dorsal to lipoma
√ branches of pericallosal artery frequently course through lipoma

DDx: dermoid (denser, extraaxial), teratoma

LISSENCEPHALY

= AGYRIA-PACHYGYRIA COMPLEX
= "smooth brain"
= most severe of neuronal migration anomalies; autosomal recessive disease with abnormal cortical stratification

agyria = absence of gyri on brain surface

pachygyria = focal / diffuse area of few broad flat gyri

A. COMPLETE LISSENCEPHALY = AGYRIA
most frequently parieto-occipital in location

B. INCOMPLETE LISSENCEPHALY
= areas of both agyria + pachygyria, pachygyric areas most frequently in frontal + temporal regions

Histo: thick gray + thin white matter with only four cortical layers I, III, V, VI (instead of six layers)

Often associated with:
(1) CNS anomalies: microcephaly, hydrocephalus, agenesis of corpus callosum, hypoplastic thalami
(2) micromelia, clubfoot, polydactyly, camptodactyly, syndactyly, duodenal atresia, micrognathia, omphalocele, hepatosplenomegaly, cardiac + renal anomalies

• micrencephaly
• severe mental retardation
• hypotonia + occasional myoclonic spasm
• early seizures refractory to medication

√ smooth thickened cortex with diminished white matter
√ figure-eight appearance of cerebrum on axial images due to shallow widened vertically oriented sylvian fissures
√ absent / shallow sulci and gyri (brain looks similar to that in fetuses <23 weeks GA)
√ middle cerebral arteries close to inner table of calvarium (absence of sulci)
√ small splenium + absent rostrum of corpus callosum
√ hypoplastic brainstem (lack of formation of corticospinal + corticobulbar tracts)
√ ventriculomegaly (atrium + occipital horns)
√ midline round calcification in area of septum pellucidum (CHARACTERISTIC)
√ polyhydramnios (50%)

Prognosis: death by age 2

DDx: polymicrogyria (= formation of multiple small gyri mimicking pachygyria on CT + MR, most common around sylvian fissures, broad thickened gyri with frequent gliosis subjacent to polymicrogyric cortex as the most important differentiating feature)

LYMPHOID HYPOPHYSITIS

= rare inflammatory autoimmune disorder with lymphocytic infiltration of pituitary gland

Associated with: thyrotoxicosis + hypopituitarism

Age: almost exclusively in early postpartum women

• headaches, vision loss, inability to lactate / to resume normal menses

√ enlarged homogeneously enhancing pituitary gland

Prognosis: spontaneous regression

Rx: steroids (reduction in pituitary size on follow-up)

LYMPHOMA

A. PRIMARY CNS LYMPHOMA (93%)
= RETICULUM CELL SARCOMA = HISTIOCYTIC LYMPHOMA = MICROGLIOMA

Risk: increased (350-fold) in immunocompromised patients: AIDS (6%), renal transplant, Wiskott-Aldrich syndrome, immunoglobulin deficiency A, rheumatoid arthritis, progressive multifocal leukoencephalopathy

Associated with: intraocular lymphoma

B. SECONDARY (7%) = SYSTEMIC LYMPHOMA
Type: NHL > Hodgkin disease
Location: tendency for dura mater + leptomeninges
• palsies of cranial nerves III, VI, VII
√ hydrocephalus

◊ Primary lymphoma is indistinguishable from secondary!
Clues: (1) multicentric involvement of deep hemispheres
(2) association with immunosuppression
(3) rapid regression with corticosteroids / radiation therapy = "ghost tumor"

Prevalence: 0.3–2% of all intracranial tumors; 7–15% of all primary brain tumors (equivalent to meningioma + low-grade astrocytoma); M > F
Peak age: 30–50 years; M:F = 2:1
Histo: atypical pleomorphic B-cells mixed with reactive T-cells infiltrate blood vessel walls + cluster within perivascular (Virchow-Robin) spaces simulating vasculitis
• symptoms of rapidly enlarging mass (60%)
• symptoms of encephalitis (<25%)
• stroke (7%)
• cranial nerve palsy, demyelinating disease
• personality changes, headaches, seizures
• cerebellar signs, motor dysfunction
• CSF cytology positive in 4–25–43%: elevated protein, mononuclear / blast / other lymphoma cells

Location: supratentorial:posterior fossa = 3–9:1; paramedian structures preferentially affected; white matter + corpus callosum (55%), deep central gray matter of basal ganglia + thalamus + hypothalamus (17%), posterior fossa + cerebellum (11%), spinal cord (1%); multicentricity in 11–47%
Site: tendency to abut ependyma + meninges (12–30%); "butterfly pattern" of frontal lobe lymphoma; dural involvement may mimic meningioma (rare)
Spread: typically infiltrating; may cross anatomic boundaries + midline, diffuse leptomeningeal spread; subependymal spread + ventricular encasement
√ commonly large discrete solitary lesion (57%)
◊ Large lesion suggests lymphoma!
√ small + symmetric multiple nodular lesions (43–81%)
√ diffusely infiltrating lesion with blurred margins
√ spontaneous regression (unique feature)

CT:
√ usually mildly hyperdense (33%) / occasionally isodense / low-density area (least common)
√ little mass effect with significant peritumoral edema
√ homogeneously dense + well-defined / irregular + patchy periventricular contrast enhancement
√ commonly thick-walled ring enhancement in immunocompetent patient

MR (superior to CT):
√ well-demarcated round / oval / gyral-shaped (rare) mass
√ relatively little mass effect for size
√ isointense / slightly hypointense relative to gray matter on T1WI
√ hypo- to isointense / hyperintense (less common) relative to gray matter on T2WI:
√ ring pattern (= central necrosis with densely cellular rim in hyperintense "sea of edema") typical in immunocompromised patients
√ intense ring-shaped contrast enhancement on T1WI
√ irregular sinuous / gyral-like contrast enhancement or homogeneous enhancement:
√ solid homogeneous enhancement in immunocompetent patient
√ irregular heterogeneous ringlike mass in immunocompromised patient
√ periventricular enhancement is highly SPECIFIC (DDx: CMV ependymitis)

Angio:
√ avascular mass / tumor neovascularity
√ focal blush in late arterial-to-capillary phase persisting well into venous phase
√ arterial encasement
√ dilated deep medullary veins

NUC:
√ increased uptake of C-11 methionine on PET
√ increased uptake of thallium-201 on SPECT

Prognosis: median survival of 45 days for AIDS patients; median survival of 3.3 months for immunocompetent patients; improved with radiation therapy (4.5–20 months) + chemotherapy

DDx:
A. Neoplastic disorders
(1) Glioma (may be bilateral with involvement of basal ganglia + corpus callosum, may show dense homogeneous enhancement with vascularity)
(2) Metastases (known primary, at gray-white matter junction)
(3) Primitive neuroectodermal tumor
(4) Meningioma
B. Infectious disease (multicentricity)
(1) Abscess, especially toxoplasmosis (large edema)
(2) Sarcoidosis
(3) Tuberculosis
C. Demyelinating disease
(1) Multiple sclerosis
(2) Progressive multifocal leukoencephalopathy

Spinal Epidural Lymphoma

(a) invasion of epidural space through intervertebral foramen from paravertebral lymph nodes
(b) destruction of bone with vertebral collapse (less common)
(c) direct involvement of CNS (rare)

Leukemia

CNS affected in 10% of patients with acute leukemia
√ enlargement of ventricles + sulci due to atrophy (31%)
√ sulcal / fissural / cisternal enhancement (meningeal infiltration) in 5%

Prognosis: 3–5 months survival if untreated

MEDULLOBLASTOMA

◊ Most malignant infratentorial neoplasm; most common neoplasm of posterior fossa in childhood (followed by cerebellar pilocytic astrocytoma)

Incidence: 15–20% of all pediatric intracranial tumors; 30–40% of all posterior fossa neoplasms in children; 2–10% of all intracranial gliomas

Origin: from external granular layer of inferior medullary velum (= roof of 4th ventricle)

Histo: completely undifferentiated cells (50%), desmoplastic variety (25%), glial / neuronal differentiation (25%)

Age: 40% within first 5 years of life; 75% in first decade; between ages 5 and 14 (2/3); between ages 15 and 35 (1/3); M:F = 2–4:1

- duration of symptoms <1 month prior to diagnosis: nausea, vomiting, headache, increasing head size, ataxia

Site: (a) vermis cerebelli + roof of 4th ventricle (younger age group) in 91%
(b) cerebellar hemisphere (older age group)

Size: usually >2 cm in diameter

√ well-defined vermian mass with widening of space between cerebellar tonsils
√ encroachment on 4th ventricle / aqueduct with hydrocephalus (85–95%)
√ shift / invagination of 4th ventricle
√ rapid growth with extension into cerebellar hemisphere / brainstem (more often in adults)
√ extension into cisterna magna + upper cervical cord, occasionally through foramina of Luschka into cerebellopontine angle cistern
√ mild / moderate surrounding edema (90%)

CT:

Classic features in 53%:
√ slightly hyperdense (70%) / isodense (20%) / mixed (10%) lesion
√ rapid intense homogeneous enhancement (97%) due to usually solid tumor

Atypical features:
√ cystic / necrotic areas (10–16%) with lack of enhancement
√ calcifications in 13%
√ hemorrhage in 3%
√ supratentorial extension

MR:
√ mixed / hypointense on T1WI
√ hypo- / iso- / hyperintense on T2WI
√ usually homogeneous Gd-DTPA enhancement with hypointense rim
√ cerebellar folia blurred

Cx: (1) Subarachnoid metastatic spread (30–100%) via CSF pathway to spinal cord + cauda equina ("drop metastases" in 40%), cerebral convexities, sylvian fissure, suprasellar cistern, retrograde into lateral + 3rd ventricle
√ continuous "frosting" of tumor on pia
(2) Metastases outside CNS (axial skeleton, lymph nodes, lung) after surgery

Rx: surgery + radiation therapy (extremely radiosensitive)

DDx of midline medulloblastoma:
ependymoma, astrocytoma (hypodense)

DDx of eccentric medulloblastoma:
astrocytoma, meningioma, acoustic neuroma

MENINGIOMA

Incidence: most common extraaxial tumor; 15–18% of intracranial tumors in adults; 1–2% of primary brain tumors in children; 33% of all incidental intracranial neoplasms

Origin: derived from meningothelial cells concentrated in arachnoid villi (= "arachnoid cap cells"), which penetrate the dura (villi are numerous in large dural sinuses, in smaller veins, along root sleeves of exiting cranial + spinal nerves, choroid plexus)

Histologic classification:

— benign behavior pattern
(a) fibroblastic type = fibrous type
interwoven bands of spindle cells + collagen + reticulin fibers
(b) transitional type = mixed type
features of meningothelial + fibroblastic forms

— aggressive imaging appearance
(c) meningothelial = syncytial type
forming a syncytium of closely packed cells with indistinct borders
(d) angioblastic / malignant type
probably hemangiopericytoma / hemangioblastoma arising from vascular pericytes

Age: peak incidence 45 years (range 35–70 years); rare <20 years (in children >50% malignant, M > F); M:F = 1:2 to 1:4

Associated with: neurofibromatosis type 2 (multiple meningiomas, occurrence in childhood), basal cell nevus syndrome

◊ 10% of patients with multiple meningiomas have type 2 neurofibromatosis!
◊ Most common radiation-induced CNS tumor with latency period of 19–35 years varying with dosage!

Types:

(1) **Globular meningioma** (most common):
compact rounded mass with invagination of brain; flat at base; contact to falx / tentorium / basal dura / convexity dura

(2) **Meningioma en plaque**:
pronounced hyperostosis of adjacent bone particularly along base of skull; difficult to distinguish hyperostosis from tumor cloaking the inner table (DDx: Paget disease, chronic osteomyelitis, fibrous dysplasia, metastasis)

(3) **Multicentric meningioma** (2–9%):
16% in autopsy series; tendency to localize to a single hemicranium; present clinically at earlier age; global / mixed; CSF seeding is exceptional; in 50% associated with neurofibromatosis type 2

Location:
A. Supratentorial (90%)
(a) convexity = lateral hemisphere (20–34%)
(b) parasagittal = medial hemisphere (18–22%): falcine meningioma (5%) below superior sagittal sinus, usually extending to both sides
(c) sphenoid ridge + middle cranial fossa (17–25%)
(d) frontobasal at olfactory groove (10%)
B. Infratentorial (9–15%)
(a) cerebellar convexity (5%)
(b) tentorium cerebelli (2–4%)
(c) cerebellopontine angle (2–4%)
(d) clivus (<1%)
C. Spine (12%)
Atypical location:
(a) cerebellopontine angle (<5%)
(b) optic nerve sheath (<2%)
(c) intraventricular (2–5%): 80% in lateral (L > R), 15% in 3rd, 5% in 4th ventricle; from infolding of meningeal tissue during formation of choroid plexus
◊ Most common trigonal intraventricular mass in adulthood!
(d) ectopic = extradural (<1%): intradiploic space, outer table of skull, scalp, paranasal sinus, parotid gland, parapharyngeal space, mediastinum, lung, adrenal gland
Plain film:
√ hyperostosis at site close to / within bone (exostosis, enostosis, sclerosis)
◊ Hyperostosis does NOT indicate tumor infiltration!
√ blistering at paranasal sinuses (ethmoid, sphenoid) ± sclerosis (= pneumosinus dilatans)
√ enlarged meningeal grooves (if location in vault), enlarged foramen spinosum
√ calcification (= psammoma bodies)
CT:
√ sharply demarcated well-circumscribed slowly growing mass
√ wide attachment to adjacent dura mater
√ "cortical buckling" of underlying brain
√ hyperdense (70–75% due to psammomatous calcifications) / isodense lesion on NECT
√ calcifications in circular / radial pattern in 20–25% (DDx: osteoma)
√ "intraosseous meningioma" = permeation of bone with intra- and extracerebral soft-tissue component (DDx: fibrous dysplasia)
√ hyperostosis of adjacent bone (18%)
√ intense uniform enhancement on CECT (absence of blood-brain barrier)
√ minimal peritumoral edema (in up to 75%): NO correlation between tumor size + amount of edema (DDx: intraaxial lesion)
√ cystic component: major in 2%, minor in 15%

MR (100% detection rate with gadolinium DTPA):
√ hypo- to isointense on T1WI + iso- to hyperintense on T2WI (intensity depends on amount of cellularity versus collagen elements):
√ tends to follow cortical signal intensity
√ homogeneous / heterogeneous texture (tumor vascularity, cystic changes, calcifications)
√ arcuate bowing of white matter + cortical effacement
√ tumor-brain interface of low-intensity vessels + high-intensity cerebrospinal cleft on T2WI
√ contrast enhancement for 3–60 minutes on T1WI as high as 148% over brain parenchyma
√ "dural tail" sign = curvilinear area of enhancement tapering off from the margin of tumor along dural surface in 60% (= dural tumor infiltration / reactive hypervascularity / reactive hyperplastic changes)
√ encasement + narrowing of vessels
Angio:
√ "mother-in-law" phenomenon (contrast material shows up early and stays late into venous phase)
√ "sunburst" / "spoke-wheel" pattern of tumor vascularity with hypervascular cloudlike stain
√ early draining vein (rare: perhaps in angioblastic meningioma)
√ en plaque meningioma is poorly vascularized
Vascular supply:
A. External carotid artery (almost always):
1. vault: middle meningeal artery
2. sphenoid plane + tuberculum: recurrent meningeal branch of ophthalmic a.
3. tentorium: meningeal branch of meningohypophyseal trunk of ICA
4. clivus + posterior fossa: vertebral artery / ascending pharyngeal artery
5. falx: partly middle meningeal artery + others
B. Internal carotid artery (rare):
1. intraventricular: choroidal vessels
Cx: local invasion of venous sinuses

ATYPICAL MENINGIOMA (15%)
1. Low attenuation area of necrosis, old hemorrhage, cyst formation, fat (DDx: malignant glioma, metastasis)
(a) **Cystic meningioma** (2–4%)
Frequency: 55–65% in 1st year of life; 10% in children
type I = intratumoral central / eccentric cyst (ischemic necrosis, microcystic degeneration, breakdown of hemorrhagic products); often associated with meningothelial / microcystic / atypical / malignant histologic subtypes
type II = extratumoral intraparenchymal cyst (arachnoid cyst / reactive gliosis / liquefactive necrosis of adjacent brain)
type III = trapped CSF (DDx: cystic / necrotic glioma)
(b) **Lipoblastic / xanthomatous meningioma** (5%) metaplastic change of meningothelial cells into adipocytes
2. Heterogeneous / ring enhancement (secondary to bland tumor infarction / necrosis in aggressive histologic variants / true cyst formation from benign fluid accumulation)

3. "En plaque" morphology
4. "Comma shape" = combination of semilunar component bounded by dural interface + spherical component growing beyond dural margin
5. Sarcomatous transformation with spread over hemisphere + invasion of cerebral parenchyma (leptomeningeal supply)
6. **Meningeal hemangiopericytoma**
   √ multilobulated contour
   √ narrow dural base / "mushroom" shape
   √ large intratumoral vascular signals
   √ bone erosion
   √ prominent peritumoral edema
   √ multiple irregular feeding vessels on angiogram

Sphenoid Wing Meningioma

1. Hyperostotic meningioma en plaque
   • slowly progressive unilateral painless exophthalmos
   • numbness in distribution of cranial nerve $V_1 + V_2$
   • headaches, seizures
2. Meningioma arising from middle third of sphenoid ridge
   • headaches, seizures
   √ compression of regional frontal + temporal lobes
3. Meningioma arising from clinoid process
   √ encasement of carotid + middle cerebral arteries
   √ compression of optic nerve + chiasm
4. Meningioma of planum sphenoidale
   √ subfrontal growth + posterior growth into sella turcica and clivus
   √ hyperostotic blistering of planum sphenoidale

Suprasellar Meningioma

Incidence: 10% of all intracranial meningiomas
Origin: from arachnoid + dura along tuberculum sellae / clinoids / diaphragma sellae / cavernous sinus with secondary extension into sella; NOT from within pituitary fossa

• hypothalamic / pituitary dysfunction (rare)
√ irregular hyperostosis = blistering adjacent to sinus (HALLMARK of meningiomas at planum sphenoidale / tuberculum sellae)
√ pneumatosis sphenoidale = increased pneumatization of sphenoid in area of anterior clinoids + dorsum sellae (DDx: normal variant)
√ broad base of attachment
√ intense homogeneous enhancement (may be impossible to differentiate from supraclinoid carotid aneurysm on CT)
√ blood supply: posterior ethmoidal branches of ophthalmic artery, branches of meningohypophyseal trunk

MR:
√ large mass isointense to gray matter on T1WI + T2WI
√ hyperintense flattened pituitary gland within floor of sella
√ marked homogeneous enhancement on T1WI

DDx: metastasis, glioma, lymphoma

MENINGITIS

= infection of the pia mater + arachnoid + adjacent CSF
1. Pachymeningitis: infection of dura mater
2. Leptomeningitis: infection of pia matter / arachnoid (most common) + CSF

• headaches, stiff neck
• confusion, disorientation
• positive CSF lab analysis

ROLE of CT and MR:
(1) to exclude parenchymal abscess, ventriculitis, localized empyema
(2) to evaluate paranasal sinuses / temporal bone as source of infection
(3) to monitor complications: hydrocephalus, subdural effusion, infarction

Purulent / Bacterial Meningitis

Cause: otitis media / sinusitis
Organism:
(a) adults: Meningococcus, Diplococcus pneumoniae, Haemophilus influenzae, Neisseria meningitidis, Staphylococcus aureus
(b) children: Escherichia coli, Citrobacter, β-hemolytic Streptococcus

• fever, headache, seizures
• altered consciousness, neck stiffness

NECT:
√ often normal
√ increased density in subarachnoid space (increased vascularity), esp. in children
√ small ventricles secondary to diffuse cerebral edema

CECT:
√ marked curvilinear meningeal enhancement over cerebrum (frontal + parietal lobes) and interhemispheric + sylvian fissures
√ obliteration of basal cisterns with enhancement (common)

MR (most sensitive modality):
√ no abnormality on nonenhanced MR in most cases
√ hyperintense obliterated basal cisterns on proton-density images + intermediate intensity on T1WI
√ hyperintense plaques on T2WI
√ leptomeningeal enhancement with Gd-DTPA (in chronic infection)

Cx:
(1) Cerebritis
(2) Ventriculitis = ependymitis (secondary to retrograde spread)
(3) Brain atrophy
(4) Brain infarction (arteritis, venous thrombosis)
(5) Subdural effusion [sterile subdural effusion secondary to H. influenzae meningitis (in children) may turn into subdural empyema]
(6) Hydrocephalus (cellular debris blocking foramen of Monro, aqueduct, 4th ventricular outlet / intraventricular septa / arachnoid adhesions)
(7) Cranial nerve dysfunction

Prognosis:
◊ Cerebral infarction + edema are predictive of poor outcome
◊ Enlargement of ventricles + subarachnoid spaces + subdural effusions have no predictive value

Mortality: 10% for H. influenza + meningococcus, 30% for pneumococcus (5th common cause of death in children between 1 and 4 years of age)

DDx: meningeal carcinomatosis

Granulomatous Meningitis

Histo: thick exudate, perivascular inflammation, granulation tissue + reactive fibrosis

(1) Tuberculous meningitis = basilar meningitis: part of generalized miliary tuberculosis / primary tuberculous infection

(2) Sarcoidosis (in 5% of sarcoidosis cases)
Histo: granulomatous infiltration of leptomeninges
√ nodular pattern (DDx from bacterial causes)
√ thick meningeal plaques over convexities (mimicking meningioma)
√ marked enhancement
√ may be associated with single / multiple intracerebral masses
Cx: cranial nerve palsy, hypothalamic-pituitary dysfunction, chronic meningitis

(3) Fungal meningitis: cryptococcosis, candidiasis, coccidioidomycosis (endemic), blastomycosis, mucormycosis (diabetics), nocardiosis, actinomycosis, aspergillosis (under chronic corticosteroid therapy)

• acute life-threatening process / chronic indolent disease

May be associated with: cerebritis, abscess formation

√ hydrocephalus

CT:
√ obliteration of basal cisterns, sylvian fissure, suprasellar cistern (isodense cisterns secondary to filling with debris)
√ intense contrast enhancement of gyri + involved subarachnoid spaces
√ calcification of meninges
√ decreased attenuation of white matter

MR:
√ high-signal intensity of basilar cisterns on T2WI
√ enhancement with gadopentetate dimeglumine

Cx: (1) Hydrocephalus (obliteration of basal cisterns; blocking of CSF flow + CSF absorption)
(2) Infarction (due to arteritis)

MESIAL TEMPORAL SCLEROSIS

Cause: long-standing temporal lobe epilepsy

Histo: marked neuronal loss throughout hippocampal subfields with relative sparing of the CA2 subfield

Mechanism for excitotoxicity-induced neuronal death: seizures cause excessive neuronal depolarization, which causes overproduction of excitory amino acid neurotransmitters, which cause excessive activation of N-methyl-D-aspartate receptors, which cause unregulated entry of Ca^{2+}, which causes neuronal swelling with cytotoxic edema

√ increased signal intensity + decreased volume of hippocampus compared to contralateral side on T2WI

Associated limbic system findings:
√ ipsilateral atrophy of fornix (55%)
√ ipsilateral atrophy of mamillary body (26%)

Associated extrahippocampal abnormalities:
√ increased signal intensity of anterior temporal lobe cortex (38%)
√ cerebral hemiatrophy (1%)

METACHROMATIC LEUKODYSTROPHY

= MLD = most common hereditary (autosomal recessive) leukodystrophy (dysmyelinating disorder)

Cause: deficiency of arylsulfatase A resulting in severe deficiency of myelin lipid sulfatide within macrophages + Schwann cells

Age of presentation: before age 3 (2/3), in adolescence (1/3)

A. LATE INFANTILE FORM
Age: 2nd year of life
• gait disorder + strabismus
• impairment of speech
• spasticity + tremor
• intellectual deterioration
Prognosis: death within 4 years of onset

B. JUVENILE FORM
Age: 5–7 years

C. ADULT FORM
• organic mental syndrome
• progressive corticospinal, corticobulbar, cerebellar, extrapyramidal signs

√ progressive loss of hemispheric brain tissue

CT:
√ symmetric low density of white matter adjacent to ventricles (esp. centrum ovale and frontal horns)
√ progressive atrophy
√ no contrast enhancement

MR:
√ progressive symmetrical areas of hypointensity on T1WI
√ hyperintensity on T2WI (increased water)

Prognosis: death within several years

METASTASES TO BRAIN

Incidence: 14–37% of all intracranial tumors
◊ Most common infratentorial mass in the adult

Metastatic primary:
Six tumors account for 95% of all brain metastases:
1. Bronchial carcinoma (47%): RARELY squamous cell carcinoma
2. Breast carcinoma (17%)

3. GI-tract tumors (15%): colon, rectum
4. Hypernephroma (10%)
5. Melanoma (8%)
6. Choriocarcinoma

In childhood:
1. Leukemia / lymphoma
2. Neuroblastoma

◊ Brain metastases from sarcomas are exceptionally rare!

Hemorrhagic Metastases to Brain (in 3–4%):
1. Malignant melanoma
2. Choriocarcinoma
3. Oat cell carcinoma of lung
4. Renal cell carcinoma
5. Thyroid carcinoma

√ hyperdense without contrast
√ hypervascular with contrast

mnemonic: "MATCH"
Melanoma
Anaplastic lung carcinoma
Thyroid carcinoma
Choriocarcinoma
Hypernephroma

Cystic Metastasis to Brain
1. Squamous cell carcinoma of lung
2. Adenocarcinoma of lung

Calcified Metastasis to Brain
1. Mucin-producing neoplasm: GI, breast
2. Cartilage- / bone-forming sarcoma
3. Effective radiochemotherapy

Location:
(a) corticomedullary junction of brain (most characteristic)
(b) subarachnoid space = carcinomatous meningitis (15%)
(c) subependymal spread (frequent in breast carcinoma)
(d) skull (5%)

N.B.: CORTICAL METASTASES
√ minimal / no edema
√ may not be identified on T2WI
√ contrast-enhancement essential for detection

Presentation:
— multiple lesions (2/3), single lesion (1/3)
— cerebral hemispheres (57%), cerebellum (29%), brainstem (32%)
— nodular deposits to dura are common

√ usually well-defined round masses:
√ multiple lesions of different sizes + locations
√ surrounding edema usually exceeds tumor volume

CT:
√ hypodense on NECT (unless hemorrhagic / hypercellular)
√ solid enhancement in small tumors / ringlike enhancement in large tumors

MR (combination of T2WI + contrast-enhanced T1WI offer greatest sensitivity):
√ hypointense on T1WI
√ hypointense mass relative to edema / variable intensity on T2WI (due to hemorrhage, necrosis, cyst formation):
√ hypointensity more pronounced in melanoma + mucinous adenocarcinoma (paramagnetic effect)
√ homogeneous / ring / nodular mixed enhancement after Gd-DTPA; often more than one metastatic focus identified in region of colliding edema
√ asymmetric enhancement of dura with dural spread
√ leptomeningeal enhancement (eg, in metastatic ependymoma)

DDx: glioma (indistinct border, less well defined, lesser amount of vasogenic edema)

Malignant Melanoma Metastatic to Brain
Prevalence: 39% at autopsy
◊ No clear consensus on contribution of paramagnetic effect of blood products versus melanin
1. Melanotic pattern (in 24–54%)
   √ hyperintense on T1WI + iso- / hypointense on T2WI
   Cause: free radicals in melanin + blood products
2. Amelanotic pattern (38%)
   √ hypo- / isointense on T1WI + hyper- / isointense on T2WI
3. Other patterns
   √ isointense on T1WI + hyperintense on T2WI

MICROCEPHALY
= clinical syndrome characterized by a head circumference below the normal range

Incidence: 1.6:1,000 or 1:6,200–1:8,500 births

Etiology:
(1) Undiagnosed intrauterine infection (toxoplasmosis, rubella, CMV, herpes, syphilis), toxic agents, drugs hypoxia, radiation, maternal phenylketonuria
(2) Premature craniosynostosis
(3) Chromosomal abnormalities (trisomies 13, 18, 21)
(4) Meckel-Gruber syndrome

Often associated with:
micrencephaly, macrogyria, pachygyria, atrophy of basal ganglia, decrease in dendritic arborization, holoprosencephaly

√ AC:HC discrepancy
√ head circumference <3 S.D. below the mean
√ apelike sloping of forehead
√ dilatation of lateral ventricles
√ poor growth of fetal cranium
√ intracranial contents may not be visible (rare)

Prognosis: normal to severe mental retardation (depending on degree of microcephaly)

MINERALIZING MICROANGIOPATHY
= RADIATION-INDUCED LEUKOENCEPHALOPATHY
= sequelae of radiotherapy combined with methotrexate therapy for leukemia

Incidence: in 25–30% after >9 months after treatment
Age: childhood
Cause: deposition of calcium within small vessels of previously irradiated brain parenchyma

- 85% without neurologic deficits

CT:
- √ thin reticular / serrated linear / punctate calcifications near corticomedullary junction, especially in basal ganglia + frontal and posterior parietal lobes
- √ symmetric low-attenuation process in white matter near corticomedullary area

MR:
- √ confluent diffuse periventricular distribution spreading peripherally with an irregular scalloped edge

MOYAMOYA DISEASE

= progressive obstructive / occlusive cerebral arteritis affecting distal ICA at bifurcation into its branches (anterior 2/3 of circle of Willis), usually involving both hemispheres

Etiology: unknown
Age: predominantly in children + young adults
Path: endothelial hyperplasia + fibrosis without associated inflammatory reaction

- headaches
- behavioral disturbances
- recurrent hemiparetic attacks

√ bilateral stenosis / occlusion of supraclinoid portion of internal carotid extending to proximal portions of middle + anterior cerebral arteries
√ large network of vessels in basal ganglia ("puff of smoke") + upper brainstem fed by basilar artery, anterior + middle cerebral arteries (dilatation of lenticulostriate + thalamoperforating arteries)
√ anastomoses between dural meningeal + leptomeningeal arteries

Cx: subarachnoid hemorrhage (occasionally)

Moyamoya Syndrome

Etiology: neurocutaneous syndromes (neurofibromatosis), bacterial meningitis, periarteritis nodosa, head trauma, tuberculosis, oral contraceptives, atherosclerosis, sickle cell anemia

MULTIPLE SCLEROSIS

= most frequent form of chronic inflammatory demyelinating disease of unknown etiology, which reduces the lipid content and brain volume; characterized by a relapsing + remitting course

Prevalence: 6:10,000 (higher frequency in cooler climates; increased incidence with positive family history)
Cause: ? viral / autoimmune mechanism
Peak age: 25–30 (range of 20–50) years; M:F = 2:3
Histo:
(a) acute stage: perivenular inflammation (at junctions of pial veins) with
— hypercellularity (= infiltration of lipid-laden macrophages + lymphocytes)
— well-demarcated demyelination (destruction of oligodendroglia with loss of myelin sheath)
— reactive astrocytosis (= gliosis), initially with preservation of axons (= denuded axons) resulting in scar (= white matter plaque)
(b) chronic stage: plaques advance to fibrillary gliosis with reduction in inflammatory component

Clinical forms: (a) relapsing remitting
(b) relapsing progressive
(c) chronic progressive

- waxing and waning course with
  - numbness, dysesthesia, burning sensations
  - signs of brain neoplasm: headaches, seizures, dizziness, nausea, weakness, altered mental status
  - ataxia, diplopia
  - optic neuritis = retrobulbar pain, central loss of vision, afferent pupillary defect (Marcus Gunn pupil)
  - trigeminal neuralgia (1–2%)
- <u>Schumacher criteria</u>:
  (1) CNS dysfunction
  (2) involvement of two / more parts of CNS
  (3) predominant white matter involvement
  (4) two / more episodes lasting >24 hours less than 1 month apart
  (5) slow stepwise progression of signs + symptoms
  (6) at onset 10–50 years of age
- <u>Rudick red flags</u> (suggests diagnosis other than MS):
  (1) no eye findings
  (2) no clinical remission
  (3) totally local disease
  (4) no sensory findings
  (5) no bladder involvement
  (6) no CSF abnormality

@ Brain
◊ Number + extent of plaques correlate with duration of disease + degree of cognitive impairment

Location:
subependymal periventricular location (along lateral aspects of atria + occipital horns), corpus callosum, internal capsule, centrum semiovale, corona radiata, optic nerves, chiasm, optic tract, brainstem (ventrolateral aspect of pons at 5th nerve root entry), cerebellar peduncles, cerebellum; rather symmetric involvement of cerebral hemispheres; subcortical U fibers NOT spared

√ lesion size of 1–25 (majority between 5 and 10) mm:
  √ large lesions may masquerade as brain tumors
√ lesions usually without mass effect / edema unless acute
√ ovoid lesions (86%) oriented with their long axis perpendicular to ventricular walls (due to perivenous demyelination; pathologically described as "Dawson fingers")
√ chronic plaques do not enhance (due to intact blood-brain barrier)

CT:
- √ normal CT scan (18%)
- √ nonspecific atrophy of brain (45%): enlarged ventricles, prominent sulci
- √ periventricular (near atria) multifocal nonconfluent lesions with distinct margins (location not always correlating well with symptoms)

(a) NECT: isodense / lucent
(b) CECT: transient enhancement during acute stage (active demyelination) for about 2 weeks; may require double dose of contrast; ultimately disappearance / permanent scar

MR (modality of choice; 95% specific):
√ well-marginated discrete foci of varying size with high-signal intensity on T2WI + proton density images (= loss of hydrophobic myelin produces increase in water content); hypointense on T1WI
√ Gd-DTPA enhancement of lesions on T1WI (up to 8 weeks following acute demyelination with breakdown of blood-brain barrier)
√ lesions on undersurface of corpus callosum (CHARACTERISTIC sagittal images)

@ Spinal cord
◊ Most common demyelinating process of spinal cord!
◊ In 12% without coexistent intracranial plaques!
• number + extent of plaques correlate with degree of disability

Location: predilection for cervical region
Site: eccentric involvement of dorsal + lateral elements abutting subarachnoid space
√ atrophic plaques oriented along spinal cord axis
√ length of plaque usually less than 2 vertebral body segments + width less than half of cross section
√ acute tumefactive MS = cord swelling + enhancement

DDx: (1) Cord tumor (follow-up after 6 weeks without decrease in size of lesion)
(2) Infection
(3) Acute transverse myelitis (after viral illness / vaccination)

Rx: steroids (inciting rapid decrease in size of lesions + loss of enhancement)

DDx:
(1) White matter ischemic disease (patients >50 years of age, lesions <5 mm, not infratentorial)
(2) Acute disseminated encephalomyelitis, subacute sclerosing panencephalitis (lesions of similar age)
(3) AIDS, CNS vasculitis, migraine, radiation injury, lymphoma, sarcoidosis, tuberculosis, systemic lupus erythematosus, cysticercosis, metastases, multifocal glioma, neurofibromatosis, contusions

MYELINOCLASTIC DIFFUSE SCLEROSIS

= SCHILDER DISEASE
= rare demyelinating disorder with episodic recurrence and remission

Age: children > adults; M:F = 1:1
Histo: selective confluent demyelination with relative axonal sparing, perivascular inflammatory infiltrate, reactive astrocytosis (indistinguishable from multiple sclerosis)

• hemiplegia, aphasia, ataxia, blindness
• swallowing difficulties, progressive dementia
• increased intracranial pressure

Location: centrum semiovale
√ large bilateral white matter lesions with mass effect
√ enhancement with IV contrast material

Rx: usually responsive to corticosteroids
DDx: (1) Acute disseminated encephalomyelitis (history of recent viral illness, monophasic course, lesions less confluent, no mass effect / enhancement)
(2) Adrenoleukodystrophy (bilaterally symmetric, confluent lesions, parietal location)
(3) Tumor, abscess, infarct

NEONATAL INTRACRANIAL HEMORRHAGE

Germinl Matrix Bleed

= GERMINAL MATRIX–RELATED HEMORRHAGE

Germinal matrix
= highly vascular gelatinous subependymal tissue adjacent to lateral ventricles in which the cells that compose the brain are generated; has its largest volume around 26 weeks GA; decreases in size with increasing fetal maturity; usually involutes by 32–34 weeks of gestation

Location: greatest portion of germinal matrix above caudate nucleus in floor of lateral ventricle, tapering as it sweeps from frontal horn posteriorly into temporal horn, roof of 3rd + 4th ventricle
Arterial supply: via Heubner artery from ACA, striate branches of MCA, anterior choroidal a., perforating branches from meningeal aa.
Capillary network: persisting immature vascular rete = large irregular endothelial-lined channels devoid of connective tissue support (collagen and muscle)
Venous drainage: terminal vv., choroidal v., thalamostriate v. course anteriorly + feed into internal cerebral v. which has a posterior course

Risk factors:
(1) prematurity
(2) low birth weight
(3) sex (M:F = 2:1)
(4) multiple gestations
(5) trauma at delivery
(6) prolonged labor
(7) hyperosmolarity
(8) hypocoagulation
(9) pneumothorax
(10) patent ductus arteriosus

Etiology: hypoxia with loss of autoregulation
Pathogenesis: rupture of friable vascular bed due to
(1) fluctuating cerebral blood flow in preterm infants with respiratory distress
(2) increase in cerebral blood flow with
(a) systemic hypertension (pneumothorax, REM sleep, handling, tracheal suctioning, ligation of PDA, seizures, instillation of mydriatics)
(b) rapid volume expansion (blood, colloid, hyperosmolar glucose / sodium bicarbonate)
(c) hypercarbia (RDS, asphyxia)

(3) increase in cerebral venous pressure with labor and delivery, asphyxia (= impairment in exchange of oxygen and carbon dioxide), respiratory disturbances
(4) decrease in cerebral blood flow with systemic hypotension followed by reperfusion
(5) platelet and coagulation disturbance

Incidence: in premature neonates <32 weeks of age; in 43% of infants <1,500 g (in 65% of 500–700 g infants, in 25% of 701–1,500 g infants) ; in up to 50% without prenatal care, in 5–10% with prenatal care

Location: region of the caudate nucleus and thalamostriate groove (= caudothalamic notch) remains metabolically active the longest; in 80–90% in infants <28 weeks of MA age

Time of onset: 36% on first day, 32% on second day, 18% on first 3 day of life; by 6th day 91% of all intracranial bleeds have occurred

GRADES (Papile classification)
I : subependymal hemorrhage confined to germinal matrix (GMH) on one / both sides
II : subependymal hemorrhage ruptured into nondilated ventricle (IVH)
III : intraventricular hemorrhage (IVH) with ventricular enlargement: (a) mild, (b) moderate, (c) severe
IV : extension of germinal matrix hemorrhage into brain parenchyma (IPH)

Serial scans: 5–10-day intervals

US (100% sensitivity + 91% specificity for lesions >5 mm; 27% sensitivity + 88% specificity for lesions ≤5 mm):

Germinal matrix hemorrhage (grade I)
√ well-defined ovoid area of increased echogenicity (= fibrin mesh within clot) inferolateral to floor of frontal horn ± body of lateral ventricle
√ bulbous enlargement of caudothalamic groove anterior to termination of choroid plexus
DDx: choroid plexus (attached to inferomedial aspect of ventricular floor, tapers toward caudothalamic groove, never anterior to foramen of Monro)
√ resolving bleed develops central sonolucency
√ outcome: (1) complete involution (2) thin echogenic scar (3) subependymal cyst

Mild intraventricular hemorrhage (grade II)
√ echogenic material filling a portion of lateral ventricles (acute phase) becoming sonolucent in a few weeks
√ clot may gravitate into occipital horns
√ vertical band of echogenicity between thalami on coronal scans (blood in 3rd ventricle)
√ irregular bulky choroid plexus (clot layered on surface of choroid plexus)
√ temporarily increased echogenicity of ventricular wall (= subependymal white halo between 7 days and 6 weeks after hemorrhagic event)

Extensive intraventricular hemorrhage (grade III)
√ intraventricular cast of blood distending the lateral ventricles
√ ± extension of hemorrhage into basal cisterns, cavum septi pellucidi
√ hemorrhage becomes progressively less echogenic
√ temporarily thickened echogenic walls of ventricles ("ventriculitis")

Intraparenchymal hemorrhage (grade IV)
Cause: (a) extension of hemorrhage originating from germinal matrix (unusual)
(b) separate hemorrhage within infarcted periventricular tissue (frequent)

Location: on side of largest amount of IVH, commonly lateral to frontal horns / in parietal lobe, rare in occipital lobe + thalamus
√ homogeneous highly echogenic intraparenchymal mass with irregular margins
√ central hypoechogenicity (liquefying hematoma after 10–14 days)
√ retracted clot settles to dependent position (3–4 weeks)
√ complete resolution by 8–10 weeks results in anechoic area (= porencephalic cyst)

CT:
Most sensitive + definite means to define site + extent of hemorrhage, especially in subdural hemorrhage, cerebral parenchymal hemorrhage, posterior fossa lesion
√ hyperdense bleed only visible up to 7 days before it becomes isodense

Cx:
(1) Posthemorrhagic hydrocephalus (30–70%)
◊ Severity of hydrocephalus directly proportional to size of original hemorrhage!
Cause:
(a) temporary blockage of arachnoid villi by particulate blood clot (within days), often transient with partial / total resolution
(b) obliterative fibrosing arachnoiditis often in cisterna magna (within weeks); frequently leads to permanent progressive ventricular dilatation (50%)
√ thickened echogenic ventricular walls
Time of onset: by 14 days (in 80%)
• delayed clinical signs because of compressible premature brain parenchyma
√ ventricular dilatation, particularly affecting the occipital horns (amount of compressible immature white matter is larger posteriorly)
DDx: ventriculomegaly secondary to periventricular cerebral atrophy (occurring slowly over several weeks)

(2) Cyst formation
  (a) cavitation of hemorrhage
  (b) unilocular subependymal cyst
  (c) unilocular porencephalic cyst
(3) Mental retardation, cerebral palsy
(4) Death in 25% (IVH most common cause of neonatal death)

Prognosis:
(1) Grade I + II: good with normal developmental scores (12–18% risk of handicap)

(2) Grade III + IV: 54% mortality; 30–40% risk of handicap (spastic diplegia, spastic quadriparesis, intellectual retardation)

Choroid Plexus Hemorrhage

affects primarily full-term infants
Cause: birth trauma, asphyxia, apnea, seizures
√ echogenicity of choroid plexus same as hemorrhage
√ nodularity of choroid plexus
√ enlargement of choroid plexus >12 mm in AP diameter
√ left-right asymmetry >5 mm
√ intraventricular hemorrhage without subependymal hemorrhage
Cx: intraventricular hemorrhage (25%)

Intracerebellar Hemorrhage

Cause:
  (a) full-term infant: traumatic delivery, intermittent positive pressure ventilation, coagulopathy
  (b) premature infant: subependymal germinal matrix hemorrhage up to 30 weeks gestation
Incidence: 16–21% of autopsies
√ echogenicity of vermis same as hemorrhage
√ echogenic mass in less echogenic cerebellar hemisphere (coronal scan most useful)
√ nonvisualization / deformity of 4th ventricle
√ asymmetry in thickness of paratentorial echogenicity is a sign of subarachnoid hemorrhage
Prognosis: poor + frequently fatal

Intraventricular Hemorrhage

Etiology:
  (a) germinal matrix hemorrhage ruptures through ependymal lining at multiple sites
  (b) bleeding from choroid plexus
Route of hemorrhage: blood dissipates throughout ventricular system + aqueduct of Sylvius, passes through foramina of 4th ventricle, collects in basilar cistern of posterior fossa
• seizures, dystonia, obtundation, intractable acidosis
• bulging anterior fontanel, drop in hematocrit, bloody / proteinaceous CSF
√ IVH usually cleared within 7–14 days
Cx: (1) Intracerebral hemorrhage
  (2) Hydrocephalus

Periventricular Leukoencephalopathy

Periventricular Leukomalacia

= PVL = perinatal hypoxic-ischemic encephalopathy
= principal ischemic lesion of the premature infant characterized by focal coagulation necrosis of deep white matter as a result of ischemic infarction involving the watershed (= arterial border) zones between central and peripheral vascularity
Vascular supply:
  (a) ventriculopetal branches penetrating cerebrum from pial surface are derived from MCA ± PCA ± ACA
  (b) ventriculofugal branches extending from ventricular surface are derived from choroidal arteries ± striate arteries
Incidence:
7–22% at autopsy (88% of infants between 900 and 2,200 g surviving beyond 6 days); in 34% of infants <1,500 g; in 59% of infants surviving longer than 1 week on assisted ventilation; only 28% detected by cranial sonography
Histo: edema, white matter necrosis, evolution of cysts + cavities / diminished myelin; nonhemorrhagic : hemorrhagic PVL = 3:1
Pathogenesis:
immature autoregulation of periventricular vessels secondary to deficient muscularis of arterioles limits vasodilation in response to hypoxemia + hypercapnia + hypotension of perinatal asphyxia (hypoxic-ischemic encephalopathy)
• "cerebral palsy" (in 6.5% of infants <1,800 g):
  • spastic diplegia (81%) > quadriparesis (necrosis of descending fibers from motor cortex)
  • choreoathetosis, ataxia
  • ± mental retardation
• severe visual / hearing impairment
• convulsive disorders
Location:
bilateral white matter subjacent to external angle of lateral ventricular trigones, involving particularly the centrum semiovale (frontal horn + body), optic (occipital horn), and acoustic (temporal horn) radiations
US (50% sensitivity + 87% specificity):
  Early changes (2 days to 2 weeks after insult)
  √ increased periventricular echogenicity (PVE) (DDx: echogenic periventricular halo / blush of fiber tracts in normal neonates, white matter gliosis, cortical infarction extending into deep white matter)
  √ bilateral often asymmetric zones, occasionally extending to cortex
  √ infrequently accompanied by IVH
  Late changes (1–3–6 weeks after development of echodensities):
  √ periventricular cystic PVL = cystic degeneration of ischemic areas (= multiple small never septated periventricular cysts in relationship to lateral ventricles; the larger the echodensities, the sooner the cyst formation)

√ brain atrophy secondary to thinning of periventricular white matter always at trigones, occasionally involving centrum semiovale
√ ventriculomegaly (after disappearance of cysts) with irregular outline of body + trigone of lateral ventricles
√ deep prominent sulci abutting the ventricles with little / no interposed white matter (DDx: schizencephaly)
√ enlarged interhemispheric fissure

CT (not sensitive in early phase):
√ periventricular hypodensity (DDx: immature brain with increased water + incomplete myelination)

MR (not sensitive in early phase):
√ hypointense areas on T1WI
√ hyperintense periventricular signals on T2WI in peritrigonal region
√ thinning of posterior body + splenium of corpus callosum (= degeneration of transcallosal fibers)

Prognosis:
major neurologic problem / death in up to 62%; PVL localized to frontal lobes show relative normal development; generalized PVL results in neurologic deficits in close to 100%

DDx: tissue damage from ventriculitis (sequelae of meningitis), metabolic disorders, in utero ischemia (eg, maternal cocaine abuse)

Periventricular Hemorrhagic Infarction

= hemorrhagic necrosis of periventricular white matter, usually large + asymmetric

Incidence: in 15–25% of infants with IVH

Pathogenesis:
(a) germinal matrix hemorrhage with intraventricular blood clot (in 80%)
(b) ischemic periventricular leukomalacia
lead to obstruction of terminal veins with sequence of venous congestion + thrombosis + infarction

Histo: perivascular hemorrhage of medullary veins near ventricular angle

Associated with: the most severe cases of intraventricular hemorrhage

Age: peak occurrence on 4th postnatal day

• spastic hemiparesis (affecting lower + upper extremities equally) / asymmetric quadriparesis (in 86% of survivors)

Location: lateral to external angle of lateral ventricle on side of more marked IVH: 67% unilateral; 33% bilateral but asymmetric

Early changes (hours to days after major IVH):
√ unilateral / asymmetric bilateral triangular "fan-shaped" echodensities
√ extension from frontal to parieto-occipital regions / localized (particularly in anterior portion of lesion)

Late changes:
√ single large cyst = porencephaly
√ bumpy ventricle / false accessory ventricle

Prognosis: 59% overall mortality with echodensities >1 cm; in 64% major intellectual deficits

Encephalomalacia

= more extensive brain damage than PVL; may include all of white matter in subcortex + cortex

Associated with:
(1) Neonatal asphyxia
(2) Vasospasm
(3) Inflammation of CNS

√ small ventricles (edema) with diffuse damage
√ increased parenchymal echogenicity making it difficult to define normal structures
√ decreased vascular pulsations
√ transcranial Doppler:
(a) group I (good prognosis)
√ normal flow profile, normal velocities, normal resistive index
(b) group II (guarded prognosis)
√ increase in peak-systolic + end-diastolic flow velocities + decreased resistive index
(c) group III (unfavorable prognosis)
√ reduced diastolic flow + decreased peak systolic and diastolic velocities + increased resistive index
√ ventricular enlargement + atrophy
√ extensive multicystic encephalomalacia with cysts often not communicating

NEUROBLASTOMA

Age at presentation: <2 years (50%); <4 years (75%); <8 years (90%); peak age <3 years

• abdominal mass (45%)
• neurologic signs (20%)
• bone pain / limp (20%)
• orbital ecchymosis / proptosis (12%)
• catecholamine production (95%) with paroxysmal episodes of flushing, tachycardia, hypertension, headaches, sweating, intractable diarrhea, acute cerebellar encephalopathy
• positive bone marrow aspiration (70%)

Location: adrenal gland (67%), chest (13%), neck (5%), intracranial (2%); commonly involvement of multiple skeletal sites

NUC (overall sensitivity of detection better than radiography):
CAVE: symmetric lytic neuroblastoma metastases occur frequently in metaphyseal areas where normal epiphyseal activity obscures lesions
√ purely lytic lesions may present as photopenic areas
√ soft-tissue uptake of Tc-99m phosphate in 60%
√ frequently Ga-67 uptake in primary site of neuroblastoma

Prognosis: 2-year survival (a) in 60% for age <1 year (b) in 20% for ages 1–2 years (c) in 10% for ages >2 years

A. PRIMARY CEREBRAL NEUROBLASTOMA (rare)
Age: childhood / early adolescence
√ large hypodense / mixed-density mass with well-defined margins

√ intratumoral coarse dense calcifications
√ central cystic / necrotic zones with hemorrhage
Cx: metastasizes via subarachnoid space to dura + calvarium

B. SECONDARY NEUROBLASTOMA (common)
metastatic to:
@ liver
@ skeleton
√ osteolysis with periosteal new-bone formation
√ sutural diastasis
√ hair-on-end appearance of skull
@ orbit:
√ unilateral proptosis
◊ Neuroblastoma usually not metastatic to brain!

Olfactory Neuroblastoma

= very malignant tumor arising from olfactory mucosa
Types:
1. Esthesioneuroepithelioma
2. Esthesioneurocytoma
3. Esthesioneuroblastoma

√ mass in superior nasal cavity with extension into ethmoid + maxillary sinuses
Cx: distant metastases in 20%

NEUROCUTANEOUS MELANOSIS

= rare sporadic congenital syndrome characterized by large multiple melanocytic nevi (in 5–15%) + melanotic lesions of CNS (in 40–60%)
Age: first 2 years of life (most); 2nd / 3rd decade (less commonly); M:F = 1:1
Cause: abnormal migration of melanocyte precursors, abnormal expression of melanin-producing genes within leptomeningeal cells, rapid proliferation of melanin-producing leptomeningeal cells
Histo: abnormal abundance of melanotic cells (which are normally found in basilar leptomeninges) with concomitant infiltration of perivascular spaces

• increased intracranial pressure
• seizures, ataxia, cranial nerve VI + VII palsies

√ high attenuation of melanin pigments on CT scan
√ hyperintense on T1WI, hypointense on T2WI (paramagnetic effect of oxygen-free radicals in melanin)
√ leptomeningeal melanosis = foci of abnormally thickened leptomeninges
Location: inferior surface of cerebellum; inferior surface of frontal, temporal, occipital lobes; ventral aspect of pons, cerebra; peduncles, upper cervical spinal cord
√ parenchymal melanosis (less common)
Location: cerebellum , anterior temporal lobes (esp. amygdala)
√ frankly hemorrhagic necrotic invasive mass with transformation into malignant melanoma
√ hydrocephalus
√ posterior fossa cyst
√ cerebellar hypoplasia
√ Dandy-Walker malformation
√ syringomyelia
√ intraspinal arachnoid cyst
√ intraspinal lipoma
Prognosis: rapid deterioration + death within 3 years of diagnosis due to development of malignant melanoma / complication of hydrocephalus

NEUROFIBROMATOSIS

= autosomal dominant inherited disorder, probably of neural crest origin affecting all 3 germ cell layers, capable of involving any organ system
Path: frequently combination of
(1) pure neurofibromas (= tumor of nerve sheath with involvement of nerve, nerve fibers run through mass)
(2) neurilemomas (= nerve fibers diverge and course over the surface of the tumor mass)
as
(a) localized neurofibroma (most common)
Location: dermis + subcutaneous tissue
= fibroma molluscum
(b) diffuse neurofibroma
(c) plexiform neurofibroma = tortuous tangles / fusiform enlargement of peripheral nerves (PATHOGNOMONIC of NF1)
◊ Often precedes development of cutaneous neurofibromas!
Histo: proliferation of fibroblasts + Schwann cells
◊ More frequent involvement of deep large nerves (sciatic nerve, brachial plexus) in NF1 in contradistinction to isolated neurofibromas without NF1!

Peripheral Neurofibromatosis (90%)

= NEUROFIBROMATOSIS TYPE 1 = NF1
= VON RECKLINGHAUSEN DISEASE
= dysplasia of mesodermal + neuroectodermal tissue with potential for diffuse systemic involvement; autosomal dominant with abnormalities localized to the pericentromeric region of chromosome **17** (site of tumor suppressor gene neurofibromin);
50% spontaneous mutants; variable expressivity
mnemonic: von Recklinghausen has **17** letters
Incidence: 1:2,000–4,000; M:F = 1:1; most common of phakomatoses
◊ One of the most common genetic diseases!
Predisposing factor:
advanced paternal age >35 years (2-fold increase in new mutations)
Diagnostic clinical criteria (at least two must be present):
(1) >6 café-au-lait spots >5 mm in greatest diameter (>15 mm in postpubertal individuals)
(2) ≥2 subcutaneous neurofibromas of any type / one plexiform neurofibroma
(3) axillary / inguinal freckling
(4) optic nerve glioma
(5) ≥2 Lisch nodules (= pigmented iris hamartomas)
(6) characteristic skeletal lesions (eg, sphenoid dysplasia / thinning of long bone cortex) ± pseudarthrosis

(7) first-degree relative (parent, sibling, child) with peripheral neurofibromatosis

CLASSIC TRIAD:
(1) Cutaneous lesions
(2) Skeletal deformity
◊ Musculoskeletal abnormalities predominate in NF1!
(3) Mental deficiency

May be associated with:
(1) MEA IIb (pheochromocytoma + medullary carcinoma of thyroid + multiple neuromas)
(2) CHD (10 fold increase): pulmonary valve stenosis, ASD, VSD, IHSS

A. CNS MANIFESTATIONS
@ Intracranial
1. Optic pathway glioma
isolated to single optic nerve ± extension to other optic nerve, chiasm, optic tracts
Histo: pilocytic astrocytoma with perineural / subarachnoid spread (optic nerve is embryologically part of hypothalamus and develops gliomas instead of schwannomas)
◊ In up to 30% of all neurofibromatosis patients
◊ 10% of all optic nerve gliomas are associated with neurofibromatosis
2. Cerebral gliomas
astrocytomas of tectum, brainstem, gliomatosis cerebri (= unusual confluence of astrocytomas)
3. Hydrocephalus
obstruction usually at aqueduct of Sylvius
Cause: benign aqueductal stenosis, glioma of tectum / tegmentum of mesencephalon
4. Vascular dysplasia
= occlusion / stenosis of distal internal carotid artery, proximal middle / anterior cerebral artery
√ moyamoya phenomenon (60–70%)
5. Neurofibromas (= arising from Schwann cells + fibroblasts) of cranial nerves III–XII (most commonly V + VIII)
◊ 30% of patients with solitary neurofibromas have NF1
◊ Virtually all patients with multiple neurofibromas have NF1
6. Craniofacial plexiform neurofibromas
= locally aggressive congenital lesion composed of tortuous cords of Schwann cells, neurons + collagen with progression along nerve of origin (usually small unidentified nerves)
Location: commonly orbital apex, superior orbital fissure
◊ Plexiform neurofibromas are PATHOGNOMONIC for NF1
7. CNS hamartomas (up to 75–90%)
= probably dysmyelinating lesions (may resolve)
Location: pons, basal ganglia (most commonly in globus pallidus), thalamus, cerebellar white matter
√ multiple foci of isointensity on T1WI + hyperintensity on T2WI without mass effect (= "unidentified bright objects")
8. Vacuolar / spongiotic myelinopathy (in 66%)
Location: basal ganglia (esp. in globus pallidus), cerebellum, internal capsule, brainstem
√ nonenhancing hyperintense foci on T2WI

@ Spinal cord
1. Paraspinal neurofibromas
√ tumors of varying sizes at nearly every level throughout the spinal canal
√ enlargement of neural foramina due to "dumbbell" neurofibroma of spinal nerves
√ fusiform / spherical mass:
√ low-attenuation mass (20–30 HU) in up to 73% due to cystic degeneration, xanthomatous features, confluent areas of hypocellularity, lipid-rich Schwann cells
√ areas of higher attenuation due to densely cellular components / collagen-rich regions
√ slightly hyperintense to muscle on T1WI, hyperintense periphery + hypointense core on T2WI
√ hypoechoic well-circumscribed cylindrical lesion
√ spinal cord displaced to contralateral side
2. Lateral / anterior intrathoracic meningocele
= diverticula of thecal sac extending through widened neural foramina / defects in vertebra
Cause: dysplasia of meninges focally stretched by CSF pulsations (due to pressure differences between thorax + subarachnoid space superimposed on bone vertebral defect)
Location: thoracic level (most common)
√ erosion of bony elements with marked posterior scalloping
√ widening of neural foramina (due to protrusion of spinal meninges)
DDx: mediastinal / lung abscess

B. SKELETAL MANIFESTATIONS (in 25–40%)
• dwarfism caused by scoliosis
@ Orbit
√ Harlequin appearance to orbit = partial absence of greater and lesser wing of sphenoid bone + orbital plate of frontal bone (failure of development of membranous bone)
√ hypoplasia + elevation of lesser wing of sphenoid
√ <u>defect in sphenoid bone</u> ± extension of middle cranial fossa structures into orbit
√ concentric enlargement of optic foramen (optic glioma)

√ enlargement of orbital margins + superior orbital fissure (plexiform neurofibroma of peripheral and sympathetic nerves within orbit / optic nerve glioma)
√ sclerosis in the vicinity of optic foramen (optic nerve sheath meningioma)
√ deformity + decreased size of ipsilateral ethmoid + maxillary sinus

@ Skull
√ macrocranium + macroencephaly
√ left-sided calvarial defect adjacent to lambdoid suture = parietal mastoid (rare)

@ Spine
√ sharply angled focal kyphoscoliosis (50%) in lower thoracic + lumbar spine; kyphosis predominates over scoliosis; incidence increases with age
Cause: abnormal development of vertebral bodies
√ hypoplasia of pedicles, transverse + spinous processes
√ posterior scalloping of vertebral bodies due to dural ectasia (secondary to weakened meninges allowing transmission of normal CSF pulsations)
√ dumbbell-shaped enlargement of neural foramina

@ Chest wall
√ numerous small well-defined subcutaneous neurofibromas
√ twisted "ribbonlike" ribs in upper thoracic segments due to bone dysplasia / multiple neurofibromas of intercostal nerves:
  √ localized cortical notches / depression of inferior margins of ribs
  (DDx: aortic coarctation)
√ chest wall mass invading / eroding / destroying adjacent ribs

@ Lung
• exertional dyspnea
√ intrathoracic lateral + anterior meningoceles
√ peripheral pulmonary nodule = pedunculated intercostal neurofibromas
√ progressive pulmonary interstitial fibrosis with lower lung field predominance (in up to 20%)
√ large thin-walled bullae with asymmetric upper lobe predominance

@ Mediastinum
◊ Neurogenic tumors account for 9% of primary mediastinal masses in adults + 30% in children
√ mediastinal masses:
  √ well-marginated smooth round / elliptic mass
  √ extensive fusiform / infiltrating mass
√ paravertebral neurofibromas

@ Appendicular skeleton
√ anterolateral bowing of lower half of tibia (most common) / fibula (frequent) / upper extremity (uncommon) secondary to deossification
√ pseudarthrosis after bowing fracture (particularly in tibia) in 1st year of life
√ atrophic thinned / absent fibulas
√ periosteal dysplasia = traumatic subperiosteal hemorrhage with abnormal easy detachment of periosteum from bone
√ subendosteal sclerosis
√ bone erosion from periosteal / soft-tissue neurofibromas
√ intramedullary longitudinal streaks of increased density
√ multiple nonossifying fibromas / fibroxanthomas
√ single / multiple cystic lesions within bone (? deossification / nonossifying fibroma)
√ focal gigantism = unilateral overgrowth of a limb bone; marked enlargement of a digit in a hand / foot (overgrowth of ossification center)

C. NEURAL CREST TUMORS
1. Pheochromocytoma: • hypertension in adults
2. Parathyroid adenomas: • hyperparathyroidism

D. VASCULAR LESIONS
Schwann cell proliferation within vessel wall
1. Cranial artery stenosis
2. Renal artery stenosis: very proximal, funnel-shaped (one of the most common causes of hypertension in childhood)
3. Renal artery aneurysm
4. Thoracic / abdominal aortic coarctation

E. GI TRACT MANIFESTATIONS (10–25%)
• pain, intestinal bleeding
• obstruction (simulating Hirschsprung disease with plexiform neurofibromas of colon)
Location: jejunum > stomach > ileum > duodenum; retroperitoneal / paraspinal
Associated with: increased prevalence of carcinoid tumors + GI stromal tumors
(a) solitary pattern = single neurofibroma, neuroma, ganglioneuroma, schwannoma
  √ subserosal / submucosal filling defect ("mucosal ganglioneurofibromatosis")
(b) plexiform pattern = regional enlargement of nerve root trunks
  √ mass effect on adjacent barium-filled loops
  √ multiple eccentric polypoid filling defects involving mesenteric side of small bowel
  √ mesenteric fat trapped within entangled network (15–30 HU) CHARACTERISTIC
  √ multiple leiomyomas ± ulcer
  Cx: intussusception

F. GENITOURINARY MANIFESTATIONS (rare)
1. Renal artery stenosis
  √ plexiform neurofibroma with vascular narrowing
2. Urinary bladder mass
  Origin: vesicoprostatic (male) / urethrovaginal plexus (female)
  • symptoms of urinary tract obstruction: frequency, urgency, incontinence, hematuria, abdominal pain
  √ solitary hypoechoic bladder wall mass
  √ diffuse bladder wall thickening; mass may surround uterus, vagina, sigmoid colon

G. OCULAR MANIFESTATIONS (6%)
- pulsatile exophthalmos / unilateral proptosis (herniation of subarachnoid space + temporal lobe into orbit)
- buphthalmos

1. Plexiform neurofibroma (most common)
2. Pigmented iris hamartomas <2 mm (Lisch nodules) in >90%, mostly bilateral; appear in childhood; asymptomatic
3. Optic glioma: in 12% of patients, in 4% bilateral; 75% in 1st decade
   √ extension into optic chiasm (up to 25%), optic tracts + optic radiation
   √ increased intensity on T2WI if chiasm + visual pathways involved
4. Perioptic meningioma
5. Choroidal hamartoma: in 50% of patients

H. SKIN MANIFESTATIONS
1. Café-au-lait spots
   of "coast of California" type (= smooth outline):
   ≥6 in number >5 mm in greatest diameter usually develop within 1st year of life / >15 mm in size in postpubertal individuals
   Histo: increased melanin pigment in basal epidermal layer
   DDx: tuberous sclerosis, fibrous dysplasia
   Location: axillary freckling (in 66%)
   Extent: often parallels disease severity
2. Cutaneous neurofibroma
   begin to appear around early childhood / puberty subsequent to detection of café-au-lait spots:
   (a) localized = **fibroma molluscum** = string of pearls along peripheral nerve
   - firm well-circumscribed movable tumor

   (b) plexiform neurofibroma = multilobulated tortuous entanglement / interdigitating network of tumor along a nerve + its branches
   - soft gritty often hyperpigmented tumor feeling like a "bag of worms" / braided ropes
   - may become very large hanging in a pendulous fashion associated with massive disfiguring enlargement of an extremity (= **elephantiasis neuromatosa**)

   √ ± osseous hypertrophy (due to chronic hyperemia)

   Rapid episodes of growth of neurofibromas: puberty, pregnancy, malignancy

Cx: malignant transformation to malignant neurofibromas + malignant schwannomas (2–5–29%), glioma, xanthomatous leukemia

Neurofibromatosis with Bilateral Acoustic Neuromas

= NEUROFIBROMATOSIS TYPE 2 = NF2 = CENTRAL NEUROFIBROMATOSIS
= rare autosomal dominant syndrome characterized by propensity for developing multiple schwannomas, meningiomas, and gliomas of ependymal derivation

mnemonic: "MISME"
Multiple **I**nherited **S**chwannomas
Meningiomas
Ependymomas

Incidence: 1:50,000 births
Etiology: deletion on the long arm of chromosome 22; in 50% new spontaneous mutation
◊ Neurofibromatosis **2** is located on chromosome **22**!
Symptomatic age: during 2nd / 3rd decade of life
Diagnostic criteria:
(1) bilateral 8th cranial nerve masses
(2) first-degree relative with unilateral 8th nerve mass, neurofibroma, meningioma, glioma (spinal ependymoma), schwannoma, juvenile posterior subcapsular lenticular opacity

- NO Lisch nodules, skeletal dysplasia, optic pathway glioma, vascular dysplasia, learning disability
- café-au-lait spots (<50%): pale, <5 in number
- cutaneous neurofibroma: minimal in size + number / absent

@ Intracranial
1. Bilateral acoustic schwannomas (*sine qua non*)
   Site: superior / inferior division of vestibular n.
   √ usually asymmetric in size
2. Schwannoma of other cranial nerves
   Frequency: trigeminal n. > facial n.
   ◊ Nerves without Schwann cells are excluded: olfactory nerve, optic nerve
3. Multiple meningiomas: intraventricular in choroid plexus of trigone, parasagittal, sphenoid ridge, olfactory groove, along intracranial nerves
4. Meningiomatosis = dura studded with innumerable small meningiomas
5. Glioma of ependymal derivation

@ Spinal
- symptoms of cord compression

A. Extramedullary
   1. Multiple paraspinal neurofibromas
   2. Meningioma of spinal cord (thoracic region)
B. Intramedullary
   1. Spinal cord ependymomas

NEUROMA

Prevalence: 8% of all intracranial tumors
Age: 20–50 years
- slow growth; not painful

Vestibular Schwannoma

= ACOUSTIC NEUROMA = ACOUSTIC SCHWANNOMA = NEURILEMMOMA
◊ Most common neoplasm of internal auditory canal / cerebellopontine angle!
Prevalence: 6–10% of all intracranial tumors; 85% of all intracranial neuromas; 60–90% of all cerebellopontine angle tumors
Age: (a) sporadic tumor: 35–60 years; M:F = 1:2
(b) type 2 neurofibromatosis: 2nd decade

Histo:
encapsulated neoplasm composed of proliferating fusiform Schwann cells with
(a) highly cellular dense regions (Antoni A) with reticulin + collagen, and
(b) loose areas with widely separated cells (Antoni B) in a reticulated myxoid matrix; common degenerative changes with cyst formation, vascular features, lipid-laden foam cells

May be associated with: central neurofibromatosis
◊ Solitary intracranial schwannoma is associated with type 2 neurofibromatosis in 5–25%!
◊ Bilateral acoustic schwannomas allow a presumptive diagnosis of type 2 neurofibromatosis!

• long history of slowly progressive unilateral sensorineural hearing loss affecting high-frequency sounds more severely (in 95%)
• tinnitus, pain
• diminished corneal reflex
• unsteadiness, vertigo, ataxia, dizziness (<10%)

Doubling time: 2 years

Location:
(a) arises from within internal auditory canal (IAC) in 80% / cochlea
(b) may arise in cerebellopontine angle cistern at opening of IAC (= porus acusticus) with intracanalicular extension in 5%

Site: (a) in 85% from the vestibular portion of 8th nerve (around vestibular ganglion of Scarpa / at the glial-Schwann cell junction) posterior to cochlear portion
(b) in 15% from the cochlear portion

√ round mass centered on long axis of IAC forming acute angles with dural surface of petrous bone
√ funnel-shaped component extending into IAC
√ IAC enlargement / erosion (70–90%)
√ widening / obliteration of ipsilateral cerebellopontine angle cistern
√ shift / asymmetry of 4th ventricle with hydrocephalus
√ degenerative changes (cystic areas ± hemorrhage) with tumors >2–3 cm

Plain film:
√ flaring porus acusticus
√ erosion of IAC: a difference in canal height of >2 mm is abnormal + indicates a schwannoma in 93%

CT:
√ isodense small / hypodense large solid tumor
√ cyst formation in tumor (= central necrosis in 15% of large tumors) / coexistent extramural arachnoid cyst adjacent to tumor
√ usually uniformly dense tumor enhancement with small tumors (50% may be missed without CECT) / ring enhancement with large tumors
√ NO calcification
√ intrathecal contrast / carbon dioxide insufflation (for tumors <5 mm)

MR (most sensitive test with Gd-DTPA enhancement):
√ iso- / slightly hypointense on T1WI relative to brain
√ intensely enhancing homogeneous mass / ringlike enhancement (if cystic) after Gd-DTPA
√ hyperintense on T2WI (DDx: meningioma remains hypo- / isointense)

Angio:
√ elevation + posterior displacement of anterior inferior cerebellar artery (AICA) on basal view
√ elevation of the superior cerebellar artery (large tumors)
√ displacement of basilar artery anteriorly / posteriorly + contralateral side
√ compression / posterior + lateral displacement of petrosal vein
√ posterior displacement of choroid point of PICA
√ vascular supply frequently from external carotid artery branches
√ rarely hypervascular tumor with tumor blush

DDx: ossifying hemangioma (bony spiculations)

Trigeminal Neuroma

= TRIGEMINAL SCHWANNOMA

Incidence: 2–5% of intracranial neuromas, 0.26% of all brain tumors

Origin: arising from gasserian ganglion within Meckel cave at the most anteromedial portion of the petrous pyramid / trigeminal nerve root

Age: 35– 60 years; M:F = 1:2

Symptoms of location in middle cranial fossa:
• facial paresthesia / hypesthesia
• exophthalmos, ophthalmoplegia

Symptoms of location in posterior cranial fossa:
• facial nerve palsy
• hearing impairment, tinnitus
• ataxia, nystagmus

Location: (in any segment of trigeminal nerve)
(a) middle cranial fossa (46%) = gasserian ganglion
(b) posterior cranial fossa (29%)
(c) in both fossae (25%)
(d) pterygoid fossa / paranasal sinuses (10%)

√ erosion of petrous tip
√ enlargement of contiguous fissures, foramina, canals
√ dumbbell / saddle-shaped mass (extension into middle cranial fossa + through tentorial incisura into posterior fossa)
√ isodense mass with dense inhomogeneous enhancement (tumor necrosis + cyst formation)
√ distortion of ipsilateral quadrigeminal cistern
√ displacement + cutoff of posterior 3rd ventricle
√ anterior displacement of temporal horn
√ angiographically avascular / hypervascular mass

OLIGODENDROGLIOMA

= uncommon form of slowly growing glioma; presenting with large size at time of diagnosis

Incidence: 2–10% of intracranial gliomas; 5–7% of all primary intracranial neoplasms

Histo: mixed glial cells (50%), astrocytic components (30%); hemorrhage + cyst formation infrequent

Age: 30–50 years; adult:child = 8:1

• seizures

Location: most commonly in cerebral hemispheres (propensity for periphery of frontal lobes) involving cortex + white matter, thalamus, corpus callosum; occasionally around / in ventricles ("subependymal oligodendroglioma") rare in cerebellum + spinal cord

√ large nodular clumps of calcifications (in 45% on plain film; in 70–90% on CT)

CT:
- √ round / oval hypodense lesion with mass effect (75%)
- √ commonly no / minimal tumor enhancement (75%), pronounced in high-grade tumors
- √ may be adherent to dura (mimicking meningiomas)
- √ ± erosion of inner table of skull
- √ cystic changes (uncommon)
- √ edema (in 50% of low-grade, in 80% of high-grade tumors)

MR:
- √ well-circumscribed heterogeneous hypo- / isointense lesion on T1WI + hyperintense foci on T2WI
- √ little edema / mass effect
- √ solid / peripheral / mixed moderate enhancement
- √ calcification may not be detected

Cx: malignant metaplasia + CSF seeding

Prognosis: 46% 10-year survival rate with low-grade; 20% 10-year survival rate with high-grade

DDx:
(1) Astrocytoma (no large calcifications)
(2) Ganglioglioma (in temporal lobes + deep cerebral tissues
(3) Ependymoma (enhancing tumor, often with internal bleeding producing fluid levels)
(4) Glioblastoma (infiltrating, enhancing, edema, no calcifications)

PARAGONIMIASIS OF BRAIN

= Oriental lung fluke (Paragonimus westermani) producing arachnoiditis, parenchymal granulomas, encapsulated abscesses

√ isodense / inhomogeneous masses surrounded by edema

√ ring enhancement

PELIZAEUS-MERZBACHER DISEASE

= rare X-linked sudanophilic leukodystrophy (5 types with different times of onset, rate of progression, genetic transmission)

Age: neonatal period

- bizarre pendular nystagmus + head shaking
- cerebellar ataxia
- slow psychomotor development

CT:
- √ hypodense white matter
- √ progressive white matter atrophy

MR:
- √ lack of myelination (appearance of newborn retained)
- √ hyperintense internal capsule, optic radiations, proximal corona radiata on T1WI
- √ near complete absence of hypointensity in supratentorial region on T2WI
- √ mild / moderate prominence of cortical sulci

Prognosis: death in adolescence / early adulthood

PICK DISEASE

= rare form of presenile dementia similar to Alzheimer disease; may be inherited with autosomal dominant mode; M < F

√ focal cortical atrophy of anterior frontal + anterior temporal lobes

√ dilatation of frontal + temporal horns of lateral ventricle

PINEAL CYST

= small nonneoplastic cyst of pineal gland

Incidence: 25–40% on autopsy, 4% on MRI

Types:
(a) developmental = persistence of ependymal-lined pineal diverticulum
(b) degenerative = glial-lined secondary cavitation within area of gliosis

- never associated with Parinaud syndrome
- rarely cause of hydrocephalus (compression / occlusion of aqueduct)
- may be symptomatic when large

√ ± calcification

CT:
- √ normal-sized gland (80%), slightly >1 cm in 20%, can be >2 cm in size
- √ isodense to CSF in surrounding cistern (infrequently noted)

MR:
- √ sharply marginated ovoid mass in pineal region
- √ slight impression on superior colliculi (sagittal image)
- √ isointense to CSF on T1WI + slightly hyperintense to CSF on T2WI (due to phase coherence in cysts but not in moving CSF)
- √ may have higher signal intensity than CSF due to high protein content
- √ contrast may diffuse from enhanced rim of residual pineal tissue into fluid center (no blood-brain barrier) on delayed sequence images

Prognosis: lack of growth over long time

PINEAL GERMINOMA

= DYSGERMINOMA = PINEALOMA = ATYPICAL TERATOMA (former inaccurate names)

◊ "pinealoma" = misnomer referring to any pineal mass

= malignant primitive germ cell neoplasm

Incidence: most common pineal tumor (>50% of all pineal tumors, 66% of pineal germ cell tumors)

Histo: identical to testicular seminoma + ovarian dysgerminoma, NO capsule facilitates invasion

Age: 10–25 years; M:F = 10:1 to 33:1

May be associated with: ectopic pinealoma = secondary focus in inferior portion of 3rd ventricle

- precocious puberty frequent in children <10 years of age
- **Parinaud syndrome** = paralysis of upward gaze (compression of mesencephalic tectum)

Location of germinomas: pineal gland (80%), suprasellar region (20%), basal ganglia, thalamus
√ displacement of calcified pineal gland
√ hydrocephalus (compression of aqueduct of Sylvius)
√ well-defined lesion restricted to pineal gland
√ may infiltrate quadrigeminal plate / thalamus
CT:
√ infiltrating variodense / frequently hyperdense homogeneous mass (attenuation usually similar to gray matter)
√ rarely psammomatous calcifications within tumor, but pineal calcifications in 100% (40% in normal population)
√ moderate / marked uniform contrast enhancement
MR:
√ round / lobular well-circumscribed relatively homogeneous mass isointense to gray matter:
√ intermediate intensity on T1WI
√ slightly hypointense mass on T2WI (occasionally)
√ strong Gd-DTPA enhancement
Cx: CSF seeding (frequent, CSF cytology more sensitive than imaging, contrast MR of entire neuroaxis)
Rx: combination of irradiation (very radiosensitive) + chemotherapy (Adriamycin®, cisplatin, cyclophosphamide)
Prognosis: 75% survival after radiation therapy alone

PINEAL TERATOCARCINOMA

= highly malignant variant of germ cell tumors
Types:
1. Choriocarcinoma
2. Embryonal cell carcinoma
3. Endodermal sinus tumor

Histo: arising from primitive germ cells, frequently containing more than one cell type
Age: <20 years; males
• Parinaud syndrome
• tumor markers elevated in serum + CSF
√ intratumoral hemorrhage (esp. choriocarcinoma)
√ invasion of adjacent structures
√ intense homogeneous contrast enhancement
Cx: seeding via CSF

PINEAL TERATOMA

= benign tumor containing one / all three germ cell layers (pineal region most common site of teratomas)
Incidence: 15% of all pineal masses (2nd most common tumor in pineal region)
Age: <20 years; M:F = 2:1 to 8:1
• Parinaud syndrome = paralysis of upward gaze (compression / infiltration of superior colliculi)
• hypothalamic symptoms
• headache
• somnolence (related to hydrocephalus)
Location: pineal, parapineal, suprasellar, 3rd ventricle
√ well-defined rounded / irregular lobulated extremely heterogenous mass of fat, cartilage, hair, linear / nodular calcifications + cysts
◊ Fat is absent in all other pineal tumors!
√ may show heterogeneous / rimlike contrast enhancement (limited to solid-tissue areas)
Angio:
√ elevation of internal cerebral vein
√ posterior displacement of precentral vein
CT:
√ heterogeneous mass with fat, calcification, cystic + solid areas
MR:
√ variegated appearance on all pulse sequences:
√ hyperintense areas of fat on T1WI with chemical shift artifact
Cx: chemical meningitis with spontaneous rupture

PINEAL CELL TUMORS

√ similar imaging appearance
√ peripherally displaced preexisting normal pineal calcification (= "exploded pineal pattern")

Pineoblastoma

= highly malignant tumor derived from primitive pineal parenchymal cells
Histo: unencapsulated highly cellular primitive small round cell tumor (similar to medulloblastoma, neuroblastoma, retinoblastoma)
Age: any age, more common in children; M < F
√ usually large mass
CT:
√ poorly marginated iso- / slightly hyperdense mass
√ may contain dense tumor calcifications
√ intense homogeneous contrast enhancement
MR:
√ iso- / moderately hypointense on T1WI + iso- / hyperintense on T2WI
√ dense homogeneous Gd-DTPA enhancement
Spread:
(1) direct extension posteriorly with invasion of cerebellar vermis + anteriorly into 3rd ventricle
(2) CSF seeding (frequent) along meninges / via ventricles

Pineocytoma

= rare slow-growing unencapsulated tumor composed of mature pineal parenchymal cells
Age: any age; M:F = 1:1
√ small tumor
CT:
√ well-marginated slightly hyperdense / isodense mass
√ dense focal tumor calcifications possible
√ well-defined marked homogeneous enhancement
MR:
√ intermediate intensity on T1WI + T2WI
√ may be isointense to CSF but containing trabeculations (DDx to pineal cyst)
√ mild to moderate Gd-DTPA enhancement
Cx: some metastasize via CSF

PITUITARY ADENOMA

= benign slow-growing neoplasm arising from adenohypophysis (= anterior lobe); most common tumor of adenohypophysis

Prevalence: 5–10–18% of all intracranial neoplasms

- pituitary hyperfunction / hypofunction / visual field defect

Former classification:

(a) Chromophobe adenoma (80%)
  associated with: hypopituitarism
  - elevation of prolactin, TSH, GH serum levels
  - √ greatest sella enlargement; calcified in 5%
    however: functioning microadenomas are part of chromophobe adenomas

(b) Acidophilic / eosinophilic enoma (15%)
  - increased secretion of GH (acromegaly), prolactin, TSH
  - √ tumor of intermediate size

(c) Basophilic adenoma (5%)
  - associated with ACTH secretion (Cushing syndrome), LH, FSH
  - √ small tumor

Plain film: (UNRELIABLE !)
- √ enlargement of sella + sloping of sella floor
- √ erosion of anterior + posterior clinoid processes
- √ erosion of dorsum sellae
- √ calcification in <10%
- √ may present with mass in nasopharynx

Functioning Pituitary Adenoma

Adenoma may secrete multiple hormones!

1. PROLACTINOMA (30%)
   most common of pituitary adenomas; approximately 50% of all cranial tumors at autopsy; M << F
   - prolactin levels do not closely correlate with tumor size
   - ◊ Any mass compressing the hypothalamus / pituitary stalk diminishes the tonic inhibitory effect of dopaminergic factors, which originate there, resulting in hyperprolactinemia!

   Female:
   Age: 15–44 years (during childbearing age)
   - infertility
   - amenorrhea
   - galactorrhea
   - elevated prolactin levels (normal <20 ng/mL)
   - ◊ >75% of patients with serum prolactin levels >200 ng/mL will show a pituitary tumor!

   Male:
   - headache
   - impotence + decreased libido
   - visual disturbance
   - √ characteristic lateral location, anteriorly / inferiorly; variable in size

   Rx: bromocriptine

2. CORTICOTROPHIC ADENOMA (14%)
   Function: ACTH-secreting tumor
   Age: 30–40 years; M:F = 1:3
   - Cushing disease
   - √ central location; posterior lobe; usually <5 mm in size
   - √ sampling of inferior petrosal sinuses (95% diagnostic accuracy compared with 65% for MRI)

   Rx: (1) suppression by high doses of dexamethasone of 8 mg/day
   (2) surgical resection difficult because ACTH adenomas usually require resection of an apparently normal gland (tumor small + usually not on surface)

3. SOMATOTROPHIC ADENOMA (14%)
   - gigantism, acromegaly, elevated GH >10 ng/mL, no rise in GH after administration of glucose / TRH

   Histo: (a) densely granulated type
   (b) sparsely granulated type: clinically more aggressive
   - √ hypodense region, may be less well-defined, variable size

4. GONADOTROPH CELL ADENOMA (7%)
   secretes follicle-stimulating hormone (FSH) / luteinizing hormone (LH)
   - √ slow-growing often extending beyond sella

5. THYROTROPH CELL ADENOMA (<1%)
   secretes thyroid-stimulating hormone (TSH)
   - √ often large + invasive pituitary adenoma

6. PLURIHORMONAL PITUITARY ADENOMA (>5%)

CECT (dynamic bolus injection):
- √ upward convexity of gland
- √ increased height >10 mm
- √ deviation of pituitary stalk
- √ floor erosion of sella
- √ gland asymmetry
- √ focal hypodensity (most specific for adenoma)
- √ shift of pituitary tuft / density change in region of adenoma

MR:
highest sensitivity on coronal nonenhanced T1WI (70%) + 3D FLASH sequence (69%) + combination of both (90%)
- ◊ 1/3 of lesions are missed with enhancement
- ◊ 1/3 of lesions are missed without enhancement
- √ focus of low signal intensity on T1WI
- √ focus of high-signal intensity on T2WI
- √ focal hypointensity within normally enhancing gland

DDx: simple pituitary cyst (= Rathke cleft cyst)

Nonfunctioning Pituitary Adenoma

1. NULL CELL ADENOMA
   = hormonally inactive pituitary tumor with no histologic / immunologic / ultrastructural markers to indicate its cellular derivation

   Prevalence: 17% of all pituitary tumors
   Age: older patient
   - √ slow-growing

2. ONCOCYTOMA
   Prevalence: 10% of all pituitary tumors
   - clinically + morphologically similar to null cell adenoma

Pituitary Macroadenoma

= tumor >10 mm in size

Incidence: 10% (70–80% of pituitary adenomas); M:F = 1:1

Age: 25–60 years

- symptoms of mass effect: hypopituitarism, bitemporal hemianopia (with superior extension), pituitary apoplexy, hydrocephalus, cranial nerve involvement (III, IV, VI)
- usually endocrinologically inactive

Extension into: suprasellar cistern / cavernous sinus / sphenoid sinus + nasopharynx (up to 67% are invasive)

√ occasionally tumor hemorrhage
√ lucent areas correspond to cysts / focal necrosis
√ invasion of cavernous sinus: encasement of carotid artery (surest sign)

CT:
√ tumor isodense to brain tissue
√ erosion of bone (eg, floor of sella)
√ calcifications infrequent

MR: (allows differentiation from aneurysm)
√ homogeneous enhancement

Cx:
(1) Obstructive hydrocephalus (at foramen of Monro)
(2) Encasement of carotid artery
(3) Pituitary apoplexy (rare)

DDx:
(1) Metastasis (more bone destruction, rapid growth)
(2) Pituitary abscess

Pituitary Microadenoma

= very small adenomas <10 mm

- usually become clinically apparent by hormone production (20–30% of all pituitary adenomas)

◊ Prolactin elevation (>25 ng/mL in females)
4–8 x normal: adenoma demonstrated in 71%
>8 x normal: adenoma demonstrated in 100%

- **incidentaloma** = nonfunctioning microadenoma / pituitary cyst

√ NO imaging features to distinguish between different types of adenomas

MRI:
√ small nonenhancing mass of hypointensity on pre- and postcontrast T1WI
√ occasionally isointense on precontrast images + hyperintense on postcontrast images
√ enhancement on delayed images
√ focal bulge on surface of gland
√ focal depression of sellar floor
√ deviation of pituitary stalk

PITUITARY APOPLEXY

Cause: massive hemorrhage into pituitary adenoma (especially in patients on bromocriptine for pituitary adenoma) / dramatic necrosis / sudden infarction of pituitary gland

◊ 25% of patients with pituitary hemorrhage will present with apoplexy!

Sheehan syndrome = postpartum infarction of anterior pituitary gland

- severe headache, nausea, vomiting
- hypertension
- stiff neck
- sudden visual-field defect, ophthalmoplegia
- obtundation (frequent)
- hypopituitarism (eg, secondary hypothyroidism)

◊ Area of destruction must be >70% to produce pituitary insufficiency!

√ enlargement of pituitary gland

NCCT:
√ increased density ± fluid level

MR:
√ bright signal from presence of hemoglobin on T1WI with persistence over hyperintensity on T2WI
√ intermediate signal intensity from deoxyhemoglobin on T1WI + T2WI

PORENCEPHALY

= focal cavity as a result of localized brain destruction

A. AGENETIC PORENCEPHALY
= Schizencephaly (= true porencephaly)

B. ENCEPHALOCLASTIC PORENCEPHALY
Time of injury: during first half of gestation
Histo: necrotic tissue completely reabsorbed without surrounding glial reaction (= liquefaction necrosis)
MR:
√ smooth-walled cavity filled with CSF on all pulse sequences (= porencephalic cyst)
√ lined by white matter

C. ENCEPHALOMALACIA
= Pseudoporencephaly = Acquired porencephaly
Cause: infectious, vascular
Time of injury: after end of 2nd trimester (brain has developed capacity for glial response)
Location: parasagittal watershed areas with sparing of periventricular region + ventricular wall

CT:
√ hypodense regions

MR:
√ hypointense on T1WI + hyperintense on T2WI
√ surrounding hyperintense rim on T2WI = gliosis)
√ glial septa coursing through cavity identified on T1WI + proton density images

US:
√ septations in cavity well visualized

PRIMITIVE NEUROECTODERMAL TUMOR

= PNET = PRIMARY CEREBRAL NEUROBLASTOMA

= group of very undifferentiated tumors arising from germinal matrix cells of primitive neural tube

Incidence: <5% of supratentorial neoplasms in children, 30% of posterior fossa tumors

Age: mainly in children <5 years of age; M:F = 1:1

Path: most undifferentiated form of malignant small cell neoplasms grouped with Ewing sarcoma, Askin tumor

Histo: highly cellular tumors composed of >90–95% of undifferentiated cells (histologically similar to medulloblastoma, pineoblastoma, peripheral neuroblastoma)

• signs of increased intracranial pressure / seizures

Location:
- (a) supratentorial: deep cerebral white matter (most commonly in frontal lobe), pineal gland, in thalamic + suprasellar territories (least frequently)
- (b) posterior fossa (= medulloblastoma)
- (c) outside CNS:
  - – chest wall, paraspinal region
  - – kidney

√ large (hemispheric) heterogenous mass with tendency for necrosis (65%), cyst formation, calcifications (71%), hemorrhage (10%)
√ thin rim of edema
√ mild / moderate enhancement of solid tumor portion

CT:
- √ solid tumor portions hyperdense (due to high nuclear to cytoplasmic ratio)

MR:
- √ mildly hypointense on T1WI + hyperintense on T2WI
- √ remarkably inhomogeneous due to cyst formation + necrosis
- √ areas of signal dropout due to calcifications
- √ hyperintense areas on T1WI + variable intensity (usually intermediate) on T2WI due to hemorrhage
- √ inhomogeneously moderately enhancing mass with tumor nodules + ringlike areas surrounding central necrosis after Gd-DTPA

Cx: meningeal + subarachnoid seeding (15–40%)

PROGRESSIVE MULTIFOCAL LEUKOENCEPHALOPATHY

= PML = rapidly progressive fatal demyelinating disease in patients with impaired immune system (chronic lymphocytic leukemia, lymphoma, Hodgkin disease, carcinomatosis, AIDS, tuberculosis, sarcoidosis, organ transplant)

Etiology: virus infection (probably latent papovavirus = JC virus)

Pathophysiology: destruction of oligodendrogliocytes leading to areas of demyelination + edema

Histo: intranuclear inclusion bodies within swollen oligodendrocytes (viral particles in nuclei), absence of significant perivenous inflammation

• progressive neurologic deficits, visual disturbances, dementia, ataxia, spasticity
• normal CSF fluid

Location: predilection for parieto-occipital region

Site: subcortical white matter spreading centrally

√ NO contrast enhancement

CT:
- √ multicentric confluent white matter lesions of low attenuation with scalloped borders along cortex
- √ NO mass effect

MR:
- √ patchy high-intensity lesions of white matter away from ependyma in asymmetric distribution on T2WI
- √ sparing of cortical gray matter

Prognosis: death usually within 6 months

DDx in early stages: primary CNS lymphoma

REYE SYNDROME

= hepatitis + encephalitis following viral upper respiratory tract infection with Hx of large doses of aspirin ingestion

Age: in children + young adults

• obtundation rapidly progressing to coma

√ initially (within 2–3 days) small ventricles
√ later progressive enlargement of lateral ventricles + sulci
√ markedly diminished attenuation of white matter

Mortality: 15–85% (from white matter edema + demyelination)

Dx: liver biopsy

REVERSIBLE POSTERIOR LEUKO-ENCEPHALOPATHY SYNDROME

= HYPERTENSIVE ENCEPHALOPATHY

◊ Emergency condition as patient may proceed to cerebral infarction and death if untreated!

Cause: acute rise in systemic blood pressure, preeclampsia or eclampsia, following immunosuppressive treatment with cyclosporine A, cisplatin, FK-501, tacrolimus

Pathophysiology: vasogenic edema due to loss of autoregulation (? due to decreased innervation of arteries by autonomic fibers)

Location: white matter of posterior half of brain

√ hypodense white matter on NECT
√ lesion hypointense on T1WI + hyperintense on T2WI
√ lesion isointense on diffusion-weighted images (due to a net effect of elevated diffusion coefficient from vasogenic edema + T2 shine-through effect)
√ no contrast enhancement

SARCOIDOSIS OF CNS

= inflammatory multisystem disease characterized by noncaseating granulomas

Incidence: CNS involvement in 1–8% (in up to 15% of autopsies)

Age: 20–40 years (more common in women + people of West African descent)

• cranial neuropathy (facial > acoustic > optic > trigeminal nerves) secondary to granulomatous infiltration + leptomeningeal fibrosis (50–75%)
• peripheral neuropathy + myopathy
• aseptic meningitis (20%)
• diffuse encephalopathy, dementia
• pituitary + hypothalamic dysfunction (eg, diabetes insipidus in 5–10%)
• generalized / focal seizures (herald poorer prognosis)
• multiple sclerosislike symptoms (from multifocal parenchymal involvement)
• prompt improvement following therapy with steroids

Location: leptomeninges, dura mater, subarachnoid space, peripheral nerves, brain parenchyma, ventricular system
◊ Affects meninges + cranial nerves more often than the brain!

@ Meningeal / ependymal invasion
√ diffuse meningeal enhancement (most common) / meningeal nodules (less common)
Site: particularly in basal cisterns (suprasellar, sellar, subfrontal regions) with extension to optic chiasm, hypothalamus, pituitary gland, cranial nerves where exiting brainstem
Cx: communicating / obstructive hydrocephalus is the most common finding (from arachnoiditis / adhesions)
DDx: carcinomatous / fungal / tuberculous meningitis
√ dense enhancement of falx + tentorium (granulomatous invasion of dura)
√ solitary / multiple dura-based mass
√ ependymal enhancement

@ Parenchymal disease (due to extension from meningeal / ventricular surfaces)
√ isodense / hyperdense homogeneously enhancing small single / multiple nodules (invasion of brain parenchyma via perivascular spaces of Virchow-Robin)
Site: periphery of parenchyma, intraspinal
Cx: stenosis / occlusion of blood vessels
√ small vessel ischemic change
√ lacunar infarction (especially brain stem + basal ganglia)
√ focal / widespread infarcts of peripheral gray matter / at gray-white matter junction (periarteritis)
√ reactive subcortical vasogenic edema

SCHIZENCEPHALY

= AGENETIC PORENCEPHALY = TRUE PORENCEPHALY
= "split brain"
= full-thickness CSF-filled parenchymal cleft lined by gray matter extending from subarachnoid space to subependyma of lateral ventricles

Frequency: 1:1,650
Cause: segmental developmental failure of cell migration to form cerebral cortex / vascular ischemia of portion of germinal matrix
Time of injury: 30–60 days of gestation
Often associated with: polymicrogyria, microcephaly, gray matter heterotopia
Types:
(a) clefts with fused lips
(may be missed in imaging planes parallel to the plane of cleft)
√ walls appose one another obliterating CSF space
(b) clefts with separated / open lips
√ CSF fills cleft from lateral ventricle to subarachnoid space

• seizure disorder
• mild / moderate developmental delay
• range of normal mentation to severe mental retardation
• blindness possible (optic nerve hypoplasia in 33%)

Location: most commonly near pre- and postcentral gyri (sylvian fissure); uni- / (mostly) bilateral; in middle cerebral artery distribution
√ polymicrogyria / pachygyria of cortex adjacent to cleft
√ full-thickness cleft through hemisphere with irregular margins
√ gray-matter lining of cleft (PATHOGNOMONIC) extending through entire hemisphere
√ bilateral often symmetric intracranial cysts, usually around sylvian fissure
√ asymmetrical dilatation of lateral ventricles with midline shift
√ wide separation of lateral ventricles + squaring of frontal lobes
√ absence of cavum septi pellucidi (80 - 90%) + corpus callosum

Prognosis: severe intellectual impairment, spastic tetraplegia, blindness
DDx: (1) Pseudoporencephaly = acquired porencephaly
= local parenchymal destruction secondary to vascular / infectious / traumatic insult (almost always unilateral)
(2) Arachnoid cyst
(3) Cystic tumor

SEPTO-OPTIC DYSPLASIA

= DeMORSIER SYNDROME
= rare anterior midline anomaly with (1) hypoplasia of optic nerves (2) hypoplasia / absence of septum pellucidum; often considered a mild form of lobar holoprosencephaly

M:F = 1:3
Cause: insult between 5–7th week of GA
Associated with: schizencephaly (50%)

• hypothalamic hypopituitarism (66%):
diabetes insipidus (in 50%), growth retardation (deficient secretion of growth hormone + thyroid stimulating hormone)
• diminished visual acuity (hypoplasia of optic discs), nystagmus, occasionally hypotelorism
• seizures, hypotonia

√ small optic canals
√ hypoplasia of optic nerves + chiasm + infundibulum
√ dilatation of chiasmatic + suprasellar cisterns
√ fused dilated boxlike frontal horns squared off dorsally + pointing inferiorly
√ bulbous dilatation of anterior recess of 3rd ventricle
√ hypoplastic / absent septum pellucidum
√ thin corpus callosum

SINUS PERICRANII

= subperiosteal venous angiomas adherent to skull and connected by anomalous diploic veins to a sinus / cortical vein

• soft painless scalp mass that reduces under compression

Location: frontal bone
√ calvarial thinning + defect

CT:
√ sessile sharply marginated homogeneous densely enhancing mass adjacent to outer table of skull, perforating it and connecting it with another similar structure beneath the inner table

Angio:
√ extracalvarial sinus may not opacify secondary to slow flow

SPONGIFORM LEUKOENCEPHALOPATHY

rare, hereditary

Age: >40 years

- deteriorating mental function

√ confluent areas of diminished attenuation

STURGE-WEBER-DIMITRI SYNDROME

= ENCEPHALOTRIGEMINAL ANGIOMATOSIS
= MENINGOFACIAL ANGIOMATOSIS
= vascular malformation with capillary venous angiomas involving face, choroid of eye, leptomeninges

Cause: persistence of transitory primordial sinusoidal plexus stage of vessel development; usually sporadic

- seizures (80%) in 1st year of life: usually focal involving the side of the body contralateral to nevus flammeus
- mental deficiency (>50%)
- increasing crossed hemiparesis (35–65%)
- hemiatrophy of body contralateral to facial nevus (secondary to hemiparesis)
- homonymous hemianopia

@ FACIAL MANIFESTATION
- congenital facial port-wine stain (nevus flammeus)

= telangiectasia of trigeminal region; usually 1st ± 2nd division of 5th nerve; usually unilateral
— V_1 associated with occipital lobe angiomatosis
— V_2 associated with parietal lobe angiomatosis
— V_3 associated with frontal lobe angiomatosis

@ CNS MANIFESTATION
√ leptomeningeal venous angiomas confined to pia mater

Location: parietal > occipital > frontal lobes

Angio:
√ capillary blush
√ abnormally large veins in subependymal + periventricular regions
√ abnormal deep medullary veins draining into internal cerebral vein (= venous shunt)
√ failure to opacify superficial cortical veins in calcified region (markedly slow blood flow / thrombosis of dysgenetic superficial veins)

√ cortical hemiatrophy beneath meningeal angioma due to anoxia (steal)
√ "tram track" gyriform cortical calcifications >2 years of age; in layers 2-3(-4-5) of opposing gyri underlying pial angiomatosis; bilateral in up to 20%

Location: temporo-parieto-occipital area, occasionally frontal, rare in posterior fossa

√ subjacent white matter hypodense on CT with slight prolongation of T1 + T2 relaxation times (gliosis)
√ choroid plexus enlargement ipsilateral to angiomatosis
√ ipsilateral thickening of skull + orbit (bone apposition as result of subdural hematoma secondary to brain atrophy)
√ elevation of sphenoid wing + petrous ridge
√ enlarged ipsilateral paranasal sinuses + mastoid air cells
√ thickened calvarium (= widening of diploic space)

@ ORBITAL MANIFESTATION (30%)

ipsilateral to nevus flammeus:
- congenital glaucoma (30%)

√ choroidal hemangioma (71%)
√ dilatation + tortuosity of conjunctival + episcleral + iris + retinal vessels
√ buphthalmos

Cx: retinal detachment

@ VISCERAL MANIFESTATION

localized / diffuse angiomatous malformation located in intestine, kidneys, spleen, ovaries, thyroid, pancreas, lungs

DDx: Klippel-Trenaunay syndrome, Wyburn-Mason syndrome

SUBARACHNOID HEMORRHAGE

Cause:

A. Spontaneous
(1) ruptured aneurysm (72%)
(2) AV malformation (10%)
(3) hypertensive hemorrhage
(4) hemorrhage from tumor
(5) embolic hemorrhagic infarction
(6) blood dyscrasia, anticoagulation therapy
(7) eclampsia
(8) intracranial infection
(9) spinal vascular malformation
(10) cryptogenic in 6% (negative 4-vessel angiography; seldom recurrent)

B. Trauma (common)

concomitant to cerebral contusion
(a) injury to leptomeningeal vessels at vertex
(b) rupture of major intracerebral vessels (less common)

Location: (a) focal, overlying site of contusion
(b) interhemispheric fissure, paralleling falx cerebri
(c) spread diffusely throughout subarachnoid space (rare in trauma)

Pathophysiology: irritation of meninges by blood + extra fluid volume increases intracranial pressure

- acute severe headache ("worst in life"), vomiting
- altered state of consciousness: drowsiness, sleepiness, stupor, restlessness, agitation, coma
- spectrophotometric analysis of CSF obtained by lumbar puncture

NCCT (60–90% accuracy of detection depending on time of scan; sensitivity depends on amount of blood; accuracy high within 4–5 days of onset):
◊ May occur in only two locations if subtle!
√ increased density in basal cisterns, superior cerebellar cistern, sylvian fissure, cortical sulci, intraventricular, intracerebral
√ along interhemispheric fissure = on lateral aspect irregular dentate pattern due to extension into paramedian sulci with rapid clearing after several days
√ cortical vein sign = visualization of cortical veins passing through extraaxial fluid collection

MR (relatively insensitive within first 48 hours):
√ deoxyhemoglobin effects not appreciable in acute phase (secondary to higher oxygen tension in CSF, counterbalancing effects of very long T2 of CSF, pulsatile flow effects of CSF)
√ low-signal intensity on brain surfaces in recurrent subarachnoid hemorrhages (hemosiderin deposition)

Prognosis: clinical course depends on amount of subarachnoid blood

Cx:
(1) Acute obstructive hydrocephalus (in <1 week) secondary to intraventricular hemorrhage / ependymitis obstructing aqueduct of Sylvius or outlet of 4th ventricle
(2) Delayed communicating hydrocephalus (after 1 week) secondary to fibroblastic proliferation in subarachnoid space and arachnoid villi interfering with CSF resorption
(3) Cerebral vasospasm + infarction (develops after 72 hours, at maximum between 5–17 days, amount of blood is prognostic parameter)
(4) Transtentorial herniation (cerebral hematoma, hydrocephalus, infarction, brain edema)

SUBDURAL HEMATOMA OF BRAIN

= accumulation of blood in potential space between pia-arachnoid membrane (leptomeninges) + dura mater (= "epiarachnoid space")

Incidence: in 5% of head trauma patients; in 15% of closed head injuries; in 65% of head injuries with prolonged interruption of consciousness

Age: accident-prone middle age; also in infants + elderly (large subarachnoid space with freedom to move in cerebral atrophy)

Cause: severe trauma, hemorrhagic diathesis

Source of blood:
(1) pial cortical arteries + veins: direct trauma = penetrating injury
(2) large contusions: direct / indirect trauma = "pulped brain"; occasionally in blood clotting disorder / during anticoagulation therapy
(3) torn bridging cortical veins: indirect due to sudden de-/acceleration; also with forceful coughing / sneezing / vomiting in elderly
Elderly predisposed: due to longer bridging veins in senile brain atrophy

◊ No consistent relationship to skull fractures!

Pathogenesis:
differential movement of brain + adherent cortical veins with respect to skull + attached dural sinuses tears the "bridging veins" (= subdural veins), which connect cerebral cortex to dural sinuses and travel through the subarachnoid and subdural space

Location: hematoma freely extending across suture lines, limited only by interhemispheric fissure and tentorium

• nonspecific headaches, nonlocalizing signs
• lethargy, confusion
• usually negative lumbar puncture
• low-voltage EEG

CT:
√ hyperdense 65–90 HU (<1 week) / isodense 20–40 HU (1–2 weeks) / hypodense 0–22 HU (3–4 weeks)
False-negative CT scan:
high-convexity location, beam-hardening artifact, volume averaging with high density of calvarium obscuring flat "en plaque" hematoma, too narrow window setting, isodense hematoma due to delay in imaging 10–20 days post injury / due to low hemoglobin content of blood / lack of clotting, CSF-dilution from associated arachnoid tear
◊ 38% of small subdural hematomas are missed!
Aids in detection of acute subdural hematoma:
√ thickening of ipsilateral portion of skull (hematoma of similar pixel brightness as bone)
√ "subdural window" setting = window level of 40 HU + window width of 400 HU
√ effacement of adjacent sulci
√ sulci not traceable to brain surface
√ ipsilateral ventricular compression / distortion
√ displacement of gray-white matter interface away from ipsilateral inner table
√ midline shift (often greater than width of subdural hematoma due to underlying brain contusion)
√ contrast enhancement of cortex but not of subdural hematoma
Aids in detection of bilateral subdural hematomas:
√ "parentheses" ventricles
√ ventricles too small for patient's age

MR: *see* HEMATOMA OF BRAIN

US (neonate):
√ linear / elliptical space between cranial vault + brain
√ flattened gyri + prominent sulci
√ ± distortion of ventricles, extension into interhemispheric space
Limitations:
(a) convexity hematoma may be obscured by pie-shaped display + loss of near-field resolution
◊ Use contralateral transtemporal approach!
(b) small loculations may be missed

Prognosis: poor (due to association with other lesions)

DDx: (1) Arachnoid cyst (extension into sylvian fissure)
(2) Subarachnoid hemorrhage (extension into sulci)

Acute Subdural Hematoma

Usually follows severe trauma, manifests within hours after injury

Time frame: <7 days old

Associated with: underlying brain injury (50%) with worse long-term prognosis than epidural hematoma, skull fracture (1%)

Location:

(a) over cerebral convexity, frequent extension into interhemispheric fissure, along tentorial margins, beneath temporal + occipital lobes; NO crossing of midline

(b) bilateral in 15–25% of adults (common in elderly) and in 80–85% in infants

√ extraaxial peripheral crescentic / convex fluid collection between skull and cerebral hemisphere usually with:

- √ concave inner margin (hematoma minimally pressing into brain substance)
- √ convex outer margin following normal contour of cranial vault
- √ hyperdense collection of 65–100 HU, hypodense if hematocrit <29%
- √ swirl sign = mixture of clotted and unclotted blood
- √ occasionally with blood-fluid level

√ after surgical evacuation: underlying parenchymal injury becomes more obvious

√ after healing: ventricular + sulcal enlargement

Cx: Arteriovenous fistula (meningeal artery + vein caught in fracture line)

Prognosis: may progress to subacute + chronic stage / may disappear spontaneously

Rx: evacuation, but with poor response (due to high uncontrollable intracranial pressure from associated injuries)

Mortality: 35–50% (higher number due to associated brain injury, mass effect, old age, bilateral lesions, rapid rate of hematoma accumulation, surgical evacuation >4 hours)

Interhemispheric Subdural Hematoma

Most common acute finding in child abuse (whiplash forces on large head with weak neck muscles)

- √ predominance for posterior portion of interhemispheric fissure
- √ crescentic shape with flat medial border
- √ unilateral increased attenuation with extension along course of tentorium
- √ anterior extension to level of genu of corpus callosum

Subdural Hemorrhage in Newborn

Cause: mechanical trauma during delivery (excessive vertical molding of head)

1. Posterior fossa hemorrhage
   (a) tentorial laceration with rupture of vein of Galen / straight sinus / transverse sinus
   (b) occipital osteodiastasis = separation of squamous portion from exoccipital portion of occipital bone
   √ high-density thickening of affected tentorial leaf extending down posterior to cerebellar hemisphere (better seen on coronal views)
   √ mildly echogenic subtentorial collection
   Cx: death from compression of brainstem, acute hydrocephalus
2. Supratentorial hemorrhage
   (a) laceration of falx near junction with tentorium with rupture of inferior sagittal sinus (less common than tentorial laceration)
   √ hematoma over corpus callosum in inferior aspect of interhemispheric fissure
   (b) convexity hematoma from rupture of superficial cortical veins
   √ usually unilateral subdural convexity hematoma accompanied by subarachnoid blood
   √ underlying cerebral contusion
   √ sonographic visualization of convexities difficult

Subacute Subdural Hematoma

Time frame: 7–22 days

CT:

√ isodense hematoma of 25–45 HU (1–3 weeks), may be recognizable by mass effect:

- √ effacement of cortical sulci
- √ deviation of lateral ventricle
- √ midline shift
- √ white matter buckling
- √ displacement of gray-white matter junction

√ contrast enhancement of inner membrane

AID in Dx: contrast enhancement defines cortical-subdural interface

MR (modality of choice in subacute stage):

√ high sensitivity for Met-Hb on T1WI (superior to CT during isodense phase for small subdural hematoma + for hematomas oriented in the CT scan plane, eg, tentorial subdural hematoma):

- √ hyperintense on T1WI

Chronic Subdural Hematoma

Time frame: >22 days old

Cause: mild unremembered head trauma ?

Pathogenesis: vessel fragility accounts for repeated episodes of rebleeding (in 10–30%) following minor injuries that tear fragile capillary bed within neomembrane surrounding subdural hematoma

Predisposing factors:

alcoholism, increased age, epilepsy, coagulopathy, prior placement of ventricular shunt

◊ >75% occur in patients >50 years of age!

Histo: hematoma enclosed by thick + vascular membrane, which forms <u>after 3–6 weeks</u>

- history of antecedent trauma often absent (25–48%)

• ill-defined neurologic signs + symptoms: cognitive deficit, behavioral abnormality, nonspecific headache
• progressive neurologic deficit
• low-voltage EEG, normal CSF
√ often biconvex lenticular = medially concave configuration, esp. after compartmentalization secondary to formation of fibrous septa
√ low-density lesion of 0–25 HU (= intermediate attenuation between CSF + brain):
  √ different attenuations within compartments
  √ sometimes as low as CSF
  √ high-density components of collection (after common rebleeding)
  √ fluid-sedimentation levels (sedimented fresh blood with proteinaceous fluid layered above)
√ displacement / absence of sulci, displacement of ventricles + parenchyma
√ No midline shift if bilateral (25%)
√ absent cortical vein sign = cortical veins seen along periphery of fluid collection without passing through it (1–4 weeks after injury)
DDx: Acute epidural hematoma (similar biconvex shape)

SUBDURAL HYGROMA

= localized CSF-fluid collection within subdural space; common in children
Cause: (a) result of chronic subdural hematoma
(b) traumatic tear in arachnoid with secondary ball valve mechanism
Age: most often in elderly + young children
Time of onset: 6–30 days following trauma
√ radiolucent crescent-shaped collection (as in acute subdural hematoma)
√ no evidence of blood products (DDx to subdural hematoma)
MR:
√ isointense to CSF / hyperintense to CSF on T1WI (increased protein content)
Prognosis: often spontaneous resorption
DDx: (1) Enlarged subarachnoid space
(2) Subdural empyema
(3) Subdural hematoma

TERATOMA OF CNS

Incidence: 0.5% of primary intracranial neoplasms; 2% of intracranial tumors before age 15
Histo: mostly benign, occasionally containing primitive elements + highly malignant
Location: pineal + parapineal region > floor of 3rd ventricle > posterior fossa > spine (associated with spina bifida)
√ heterogeneous midline lesion, occasionally homogeneous soft-tissue mass (DDx: astrocytoma)
√ contains fat + calcium
√ hydrocephalus (common)

TOXOPLASMOSIS OF BRAIN

Organism: obligate intracellular protozoan parasite Toxoplasma gondii, can live in any cell except for nonnucleated RBCs; felines are definite host
Infection: ingestion of undercooked meat containing cysts or sporulated oocysts / transplacental transmission of trophozoites; acquired through blood transfusion + organ transplantation
Prevalence of seropositivity:
11–16% of urban adults in United States;
up to 90% of European adults
Histo: inflammatory solid / cystic granulomas as a result of glial mesenchymal reaction surrounded by edea + microinfarcts due to vasculitis
Affected tissue:
@ Gray + white matter of brain
  ◊ Most common cause of focal CNS infection in patients with AIDS!
@ Retina: most common retinal infection in AIDS
@ Alveolar lining cells (4%):
mimics Pneumocystis carinii pneumonia
@ Heart (rare):
cardiac tamponade / biventricular failure
@ Skeletal muscle
• asymptomatic
• lymphadenopathy
• malaise, fever

A. AIDS INFECTION = toxoplasmic encephalitis
= reactivation of a chronic latent infection in >95%
Path: well-localized indolent granulomatous process / diffuse necrotizing encephalitis
• focal neurologic deficit of subacute onset (50–89%)
• seizures (15–25%)
• pseudotumor cerebri syndrome
Location: basal ganglia (75%), scattered throughout brain parenchyma at gray-white matter junction
√ multiple / solitary (up to 39%) lesions with nodular / thin-walled (common) ring enhancement
√ surrounding white matter edema
√ double-dose delayed CT scans with higher detection rate for multiple lesions (64–72%)
√ ± hemorrhage and calcifications after therapy
Dx: improvement on therapy with pyrimethamine + sulfadiazine within 1–2 weeks / biopsy
DDx: CNS lymphoma (particularly with single lesion)
  ◊ Multiple lesions suggest toxoplasmosis!

B. INTRAUTERINE INFECTION
Time of fetal infection: chances of transplacental transmission greater in late pregnancy
Screening: impractical due to high false-positive rate
• Toxoplasma gondii found in ventricular fluid
• chorioretinitis
• mental retardation
√ thickened vault, sutures apposed / overlapping
√ hydrocephalus with return to normal / persistence of large head size
√ intracerebral calcifications in posterior aspect of brain

√ multiple irregular, nodular / cystlike / curvilinear calcifications in periventricular area + thalamus + basal ganglia + choroid plexus (= necrotic foci); bilateral; 1–20 mm in size; increasing in number + size (usually not developed at time of birth)

OB-US (as early as 20 weeks MA):
- √ sonographic findings in only 36%
- √ evolving symmetric ventriculomegaly
- √ intracranial periventricular + hepatic densities
- √ increased thickness of placenta
- √ ascites
- ◊ Microcephaly is NOT a feature of toxoplasmosis!
  Dx: elevated toxospecific IgM levels in fetal blood

Dx: demonstration of elongated teardrop-shaped trophozoites in histologic sections of tissue

TUBERCULOSIS

Cranial Tuberculous Meningitis

Cause: rupture of initial subependymal / subpial focus of tuberculosis (Rich focus) from earlier hematogenous dissemination into CSF space

Predisposed: in AIDS patients + infants + small children (part of generalized miliary tuberculosis / primary tuberculous infection)

Location: basal cisterns, interhemispheric fissure, sylvian fissure, sulci of cerebral convexities

CT:
- √ iso- / hyperattenuating meninges relative to basal cisterns
- √ often homogeneous contrast enhancement extending into interhemispheric fissures + cortical surfaces

MR:
- √ normal at unenhanced SE (in early stage)
- √ distention of affected subarachnoid spaces with mild shortening on T1 + T2 relaxation times compared with CSF
- √ abnormal meningeal enhancement in basal cisterns (most pronounced) on gadolinium-enhanced T1WI (corresponds to gelatinous exudate)
- √ abnormal enhancement of choroid plexus + ependymal lining (rare)

Cx:
(1) Communicating hydrocephalus (most common) / obstructive hydrocephalus (rare)
(2) Ischemic infarcts of basal ganglia + internal capsule (due to vascular compression / occlusive panarteritis in basal cisterns); MCA distribution most frequent

DDx: infection (nontuberculous bacteria, virus, fungus, parasite), inflammatory disease (rheumatoid disease, sarcoidosis), neoplasia (meningiomatosis, CSF-seeding neoplasm)

Spinal Tuberculous Meningitis

MR:
- √ cerebrospinal fluid loculi with cord compression
- √ obliteration of spinal subarachnoid space:
  - √ loss of outline of spinal cord in cervicothoracic spine
  - √ matting of nerve roots in lumbar region
- √ nodular thick linear intradural enhancement of meninges

Cx: syringomyelia, syringobulbia

Tuberculoma of Brain

= result of granuloma formation within cerebral substance

Incidence: 0.15% of intracranial masses in Western countries, 30% in underdeveloped countries

Age: infant, small child, young adult

Associated with: tuberculous meningitis in 50%

• history of previous extracranial TB (in 60%)

Location: more common in posterior fossa (62%), cerebellar hemispheres (frontal + parietal lobes); may be associated with tuberculous meningitis

√ solitary (70%) / multiple (30–60%) lesions; may be multiloculated

NCCT:
- √ isodense (72%) / hyperdense rounded / lobulated lesions of 0.5–4 cm in diameter with mass effect (93%)
- √ moderate surrounding edema (72%) less marked than in pyogenic abscess
- √ central calcification (29%)

CECT:
- √ homogeneous enhancement
- √ ring blush (nearly all) with smooth / slightly shaggy margins + thick irregular wall around an isodense center (DDx: pyogenic abscess less thick + more regular)
- √ "target sign" = central calcification in isodense lesion + ring-blush (DDx: giant aneurysm)
- √ homogeneous blush in tuberculoma en plaque along dural plane (6%) (DDx: meningioma en plaque)

MR:
(a) noncaseating granuloma
- √ hypointense relative to brain on T1WI
- √ hyperintense on T2WI
- √ homogeneous nodular enhancement

(b) caseating granuloma
- √ isointense to markedly hyperintense on T2WI
- √ rim enhancement on T1WI
- – with a solid center
  - √ hypo- / isointense core on T1WI
  - √ iso- to hypointense core on T2WI
  - √ typically associated with surrounding edema
- – with necrotic center
  - √ hyperintense core on T2WI

DDx: other CNS infection (esp. toxoplasmosis, cysticercosis, fungus), lymphoma, atypical meningioma, radiation necrosis

TUBEROUS SCLEROSIS

= BOURNEVILLE DISEASE = EPIPLOIA

= neuroectodermal disorder characterized by hamartomatous tumors + malformations occurring in brain, kidney, lung, skin, heart with a spectrum of phenotypic expressions

CLASSIC TRIAD (Vogt, 1908) in only 30% of patients:
(1) Adenoma sebaceum
(2) Seizures
(3) Mental retardation
mnemonic: zits, fits, nitwits

Prevalence: 1:10,000 to 1:150,000 livebirths

Cause: autosomal dominant with low penetrance (frequent skips in generations); gene loci 9q34 and 16p13; spontaneous mutations in 50–80%

Dx: if >2 of the following signs present
(1) seizure
(2) calcified intraventricular tumor
(3) focal areas of increased attenuation in cerebral / cerebellar cortex
(4) wedge-shaped calcified cortical-subcortical lesions
(5) hypomelanotic cutaneous lesions
(6) shagreen patches
(7) multiple renal cysts
(8) cardiac rhabdomyoma
(9) pulmonary lymphangiomyomatosis
(10) immediate relative with tuberous sclerosis

Prognosis: 30% dead by age 5; 75% dead by age 20

@ CNS INVOVEMENT
- myoclonic sizures (80–100%): ofen first + most common sign of tuberous sclerosis with onset at 1st–2nd year, decreasing in frequency with age
- mental retardation (50–82%): mild to moderate (1/3) moderate to severe (2/3); progressive; observed in adulthood; common if onset of seizures before age 5 years

1. **Subependymal hamartomas**
   Location: along ventricular surface of caudate nucleus, on lamina of sulcus thalamo-striatus immediately posterior to foramen of Monro (most often), along frontal + temporal horns or 3rd + 4th ventricle (less commonly)
   √ multiple subependymal nodules of 1–12 mm:
      √ "candle drippings" appearance
   √ calcification with increasing age (in up to 88%)
   MR:
      √ subependymal nodules protruding into adjacent ventricle isointense with white matter
      √ iso- to hyperintense on T1WI + hyper- and hypointense on T2WI relative to gray and white matter
      √ minimal contrast enhancement (in up to 56%)
2. **Giant cell astrocytoma** (in 15%)
   = subependymal benign tumor with tendency for enlargement + growth into ventricle
   Incidence: 5–15%; M:F = 1:1
   Location: in the region of foramen of Monro
   √ hypo- / isodense well-demarcated rounded mass:
      √ 2–3 cm in diameter with interval growth
      √ partially calcified
      √ uniformly enhancing
      √ frequent extension into frontal horn / body of lateral ventricle
   √ hypo- / isointense on T1WI + hyperintense on TWI
   √ hydrocephalus (obstruction at foramen of Monro)
   Cx: degeneration into higher grade astrocytoma
3. **Cortical tubers** (in 56%)
   = CORTICAL / SUBCORTICAL HAMARTOMAS
   Histo: clusters of atypical glial cells surrounded by giant cells with frequent calcifications (if >2 years of age) = hamartomas
   Frequency: multiple (75%); bilateral (30%)
   √ large misshapen broadened gyri with central hypodense regions (due to abnormal myelination)
   √ masslike / curvilinear calcification of cortical tubers (in 15% <1 year of age, in 50% by age 10)
   MR:
      √ relaxation time similar to white matter (if uncalcified)
      √ multiple nodules hyperintense on T2WI + iso- to hypointense on T1WI (fibrillary gliosis / demyelination)
      √ enhancement extremely rare
4. **Heterotopic gray matter islands in white matter**
   Histo: grouping of bizarre and gigantic neuronal cells associated with gliosis + areas of demyelination
   Frequency: in up to 93%
   √ straight / curvilinear bands extending radially from ventricular wall
   √ wedge-shaped lesion with apex at ventricular wall
   √ conglomerate masses
   √ calcification of all / part of nodule
   √ may show contrast enhancement
   CT:
      √ hypodense well-defined regions within cerebral white matter
   MR:
      √ iso- to hypointense region on T1WI + well-defined hyperintense area on T2WI relative to normal white matter

DDx of CNS lesions:
(1) Intrauterine CMV / Toxoplasma infection (smaller lesions, brain atrophy, microcephaly)
(2) Basal ganglia calcification in hypoparathyroidism / Fahr disease (location)
(3) Sturge-Weber, calcified AVM (diffuse atrophy, not focal)
(4) Heterotopic gray matter (along medial ventricular wall, isodense, associated with agenesis of corpus callosum, Chiari malformation)

@ SKIN INVOLVEMENT
- Adenoma sebaceum (80–90%) = wartlike nodules of brownish red color averaging 4 mm in size with bimalar distribution ("butterfly rash")

Age: first discovered at age 1–5 years; family history in 30%

Path: small hamartomas from neural elements with blood vessel hyperplasia = angiofibromas

Location: nasolabial folds, eventually covers nose + middle of cheeks
- Shagreen rough skin patches (80%) = "pigskin" = "peau d'orange" = patches of fibrous hyperplasia; in intertriginous + lumbar location
- Ash leaf patches = hypopigmented macules shaped like ash / spearmint leaf on trunk + extremities (earliest manifestation in infancy); may be visible only under ultraviolet light
- Ungual fibromas (15–50%): sub- / periungual with erosion of distal tuft
- Café-au-lait spots: incidence similar to that in general population
  DDx: neurofibromatosis type 1, fibrous dysplasia

@ OCULAR INVOLVEMENT
- Phakoma (>5%) = whitish disk-shaped retinal hamartoma = astrocytic proliferation in / near optic disc, often multiple + usually in both eyes

√ small calcifications in region of optic nerve head
√ optic nerve glioma

@ RENAL INVOLVEMENT
- usually asymptomatic
- flank pain, hematuria
- renal failure in severe cases (5%); hypertension
  ◊ 75% of patients die from complications of renal failure by age 20

1. Angiomyolipoma (38–89%): usually multiple + bilateral; <1 cm in diameter
   Cx: spontaneous retroperitoneal hemorrhage (subcapsular / perinephrc) with shock
2. Multiple cysts of varying size in cortex + medulla mimicking adult polycystic kidney disease (15%)
   Path: cysts lined by columnar epithelium with foci of hyperplasia projecting into cyst lumen
   √ polycystic involvement in infants
3. Renal cell carcinoma (1–3%), bilateral in 40%: usually during adulthood
   ◊ Only 17 documented cases in literature by 1998

Recommendation:
US evaluation every 2–3 years before puberty + yearly thereafter to identify growing lesions

@ LUNG INVOLVEMENT (1%)
√ interstitial fibrosis in lower lung fields + miliary nodular pattern may progress to honeycomb lung (lymphangioleiomyomatosis = smooth muscle proliferation around blood vessels)
√ multiple bilateral small cysts in lung parenchyma
√ repeated episodes of spontaneous pneumothorax (50%)
√ chylothorax
√ cor pulmonale

@ HEART INVOLVEMENT
Prevalence: decreases with increasing age (due to spontaneous tumor regression + better survival of patients without cardiac tumor)
- congenital cardiomyopathy

√ circumscribed / diffuse subendocardial rhabdomyoma (in 5–30%) of ventricle (70%) / atrium (30%)
√ aortic aneurysm

@ BONE INVOLVEMENT
√ sclerotic calvarial patches (45%) = "bone islands" involving diploe + internal table; frontal + parietal location
√ thickening of diploe (long-term phenytoin therapy)
√ bone islands in pelvic brim, vertebrae, long bones
√ expansion + sclerosis of rib (may be isolated)
√ periosteal thickening of long bones
√ bone cysts with undulating periosteal reaction in distal phalanges (most common), metacarpals, metatarsals (DDx: sarcoid, neurofibromatosis)

@ OTHER VISCERAL INVOLVEMENT
1. Adenomas + lipomyomas of liver
2. Adenomas of pancreas
3. Tumors of spleen

@ VASCULAR INVOLVEMENT (rare)
√ thoracic + abdominal arterial aneurysms
Path: vascular dysplasia with intimal + medial abnormalities of large muscular + musculoelastic arteries

UNILATERAL MEGALENCEPHALY

= hamartomatous overgrowth of all / part of a cerebral hemisphere with neuronal migration defects
- intractable seizure disorder at early age, hemiplegia
- developmental delay

√ moderately / marked enlargement of hemisphere
√ ipsilateral ventriculomegaly proportionate to enlargement of affected hemisphere
√ straightened frontal horn of ipsilateral ventricle pointing anterolaterally
√ neuronal migration defects:
  √ polymicrogyria
  √ pachygyria
  √ heterotopia of gray matter
  √ white matter gliosis (low density in white matter on CT, prolonged T1 + T2 relaxation times on MR)

Rx: partial / complete hemispheric resection

VEIN OF GALEN ANEURYSM

= central AVM directly draining into secondarily enlarged vein of Galen (aneurysm is a misnomer)

Anatomical types:
- type 1 = AV fistula fed by enlarged arterial branches leading to dilatation of vein Galen + straight sinus + torcular herophili
- type 2 = angiomatous malformation involving basal ganglia + thalami ± midbrain draining into vein of Galen
- type 3 = transitional AVM with both features

Feeding vessels:
(a) posterior cerebral artery, posterior choroidal artery (90%)
(b) anterior cerebral artery + anterior choroidal artery
(c) middle cerebral artery + lenticulostriate + thalamic perforating arteries (least common)

Age at presentation: detectable in utero >30 weeks GA; M:F = 2:1

(a) neonatal pattern (0–1 month)
• high-output cardiac failure (36%) due to massive shunting
(b) infant pattern (1–12 months)
• macrocrania from obstructive hydrocephalus
• seizures
(c) adult pattern (>1 year)
• headaches ± intracranial hemorrhage
• ± hydrocephalus
• focal neurologic deficits (5%) due to steal of blood from surrounding structures
• cranial bruit

May be associated with: porencephaly, nonimmune hydrops

√ smoothly marginated midline mass posterior to indented 3rd ventricle
√ prominent serpiginous network in basal ganglia, thalami, midbrain
√ dilated straight + transverse sinus + torcular herophili
√ dilatation of lateral + 3rd ventricle (37%)

NCCT:
√ round well-circumscribed homogeneous slightly hyperdense mass in region of 3rd ventricular outlet
√ hyperdense intracerebral hematoma (ruptured AVM)
√ focal hypodense zones (ischemic changes)
√ rim calcification (14%)

CECT:
√ marked homogeneous enhancement of serpentine structures + vein of Galen + straight sinus

OB-US:
√ median tubular cystic space with high-velocity turbulent flow demonstrated by pulsed / color Doppler
√ brain infarction / leukomalacia (steal phenomenon with hypoperfusion)
√ cardiac enlargement (high-output heart failure)
√ dilated veins of head + neck
√ hydrocephalus (aqueductal obstruction / posthemorrhagic impairment of CSF absorption)

MR:
√ areas of signal void

Angio:
necessary to define vascular anatomy for surgical / endovascular intervention

Cx: subarachnoid hemorrhage
Rx: ligation, excision, embolization of vessels from transtorcular / transarterial approach
Prognosis: 56% overall mortality; 91% neonatal mortality
DDx: pineal tumor, arachnoid / colloid / porencephalic cyst

VENOUS ANGIOMA

= cluster of dilated medullary veins, which drain into an enlarged vein; bleed rarely

◊ Can be considered a normal variant!

Histo: venous channels without internal elastic lamina, separated by gliotic neural tissue that may calcify; probably representing persistent fetal venous system

√ no arterial vessels
√ "umbrella" configuration = multiple small radially oriented veins at periphery of lesion converging to a single larger vein

◊ Associated with increased incidence of cavernous angiomas which can bleed!

DDx: Sturge-Weber disease (diffuse pial angiomatosis with venous-type capillaries)

VENTRICULITIS

= EPENDYMITIS
= inflammation of ependymal lining of one / more ventricles

Cause: (1) rupture of periventricular abscess (thinner capsule wall medially)
(2) retrograde spread of infection from basal cisterns

CECT (necessary for diagnosis):
√ thin uniform enhancement of involved ependymal lining
√ often associated with intraventricular inflammatory exudate + septations

Cx: obstructive hydrocephalus (occlusion at foramen of Monro / aqueduct)
DDx: ependymal metastases, lymphoma, infiltrating glioma

VENTRICULOPERITONEAL SHUNT MALFUNCTION

◊ Peritoneum is an efficient site of absorption

Components: ventriculostomy catheter, pressure-sensitive valve + reservoir, barium-integrated silicone peritoneal catheter

• symptoms of increased intracranial pressure: seizures, headache, nausea, vomiting, lethargy, irritability
• abdominal pain, fever
• persistent bulging of anterior fontanel
• excessive rate of head growth
• slowed refill of shunt reservoir

Mechanical Shunt Failure

Cause: occlusion of catheter by choroid plexus / glial tissue, disconnection of tubes

√ sutural diastasis + increased size of cranial cavity
√ increasing ventricular size:
√ interval increase since last exam
√ enlargement of temporal horns (earliest finding)
√ preferential enlargement of temporal horns in infants
N.B.:
(1) no enlargement with scarring of ventricular walls
(2) marked ventricular dilatation does not necessarily indicate shunt malfunction
√ shuntogram (by scintigram / contrast radiography) determines site of obstruction
√ brain edema tracking along shunt + within interstices of centrum semiovale (with partial obstruction)
√ formation of white matter cyst surrounding ventricular catheter

Obstruction of VP Shunt

Location: ventricular end > peritoneal end

Cause: plugging of the catheter by brain parenchyma / choroid plexus / proteinaceous material / tumor cells; adhesions within peritoneum

Tc-99m albumin colloid (injected into shunt tubing proximal to reservoir):

√ no uptake within ventricles + normal peritoneal activity (= proximal obstruction)

Contrast study (injection of nonionic contrast material into shunt reservoir):

√ collection of contrast material at peritoneal end of shunt without spillage (= distal obstruction)

Disconnection & Breaks of VP Shunt

Location: connection of tubing to reservoir, at Y-connectors, areas of great mobility (neck)

DDx: pseudo-disconnection due to radiolucent tube components

Migration of VP Shunt

A. PROXIMAL CATHETER: into soft tissues of neck / unusual locations within CNS

B. DISTAL CATHETER: peritoneal cavity, thorax, abdominal wall, scrotum, perforation into GI tract

Leakage of VP Shunt

= CSF escape without complete break / disconnection

- palpable cystic mass

√ contrast verifies leak site

CSF Pseudocyst of VP Shunt

√ shunt tubing coiled in an abdominal soft-tissue mass

US / CT:

√ cyst surrounding catheter tip

Cx: bowel obstruction

Infection of VP Shunt

Incidence: 1–5–38%

Time of onset: within 2 months of shunt placement

- intermittent low-grade fever
- anemia, dehydration, hepatosplenomegaly
- stiff neck
- swelling + redness over shunting tract
- peritonitis

√ ventriculitis (= enlarged ventricles with irregular enhancing ventricular wall ± septations)

√ meningitis (= enhancement of cerebral cortical sulci)

Abdominal Complications of VP Shunt

1. Ascites
2. Pseudocyst formation
3. Perforation of viscus / abdominal wall
4. Intestinal obstruction
5. Metastases to peritoneum: germinoma, medulloblastoma, astrocytoma, glioblastoma

Subdural Hematoma / Hygroma of VP Shunt

Cause: precipitous drainage of markedly enlarged ventricles

Age: usually seen in children >3 years of age with relatively fixed head size

Prognosis: small hematomas resolve on their own

Granulomatous Lesion of VP Shunt

= rare granulomatous reaction adjacent to shunt tube within / near ventricle

√ irregular contrast-enhancing mass along course of shunt tube

Slit Ventricle Syndrome (0.9–3.3%)

= proximal shunt failure from ventricular collapse

Cause: overdrainage of CSF, intermittent shunt obstruction, decreased intracranial compliance, periventricular fibrosis, intracranial hypotension

Incidence: 0.9–3.3%

- intermittent / chronic headaches, vomiting, malaise
- slowed refill of shunt reservoir

√ small / slitlike ventricles

VISCERAL LARVA MIGRANS OF BRAIN

roundworm nematode (Toxocara canis)

√ small calcific nodules, especially in basal ganglia + periventricular

DDx: tuberous sclerosis

VON HIPPEL-LINDAU DISEASE

= vHL = RETINOCEREBELLAR ANGIOMATOSIS

= inherited neurocutaneous dysplasia complex; autosomal dominant (gene located on chromosome 3p25-p26) with 80–100% penetrance + variable delayed expressivity; grouped under hereditary phakomatosis (although the skin is not affected); in 20% familial

Prevalence: 1:35,000–1:50,000

Age at onset: 2nd–3rd decade; M:F = 1:1

Diagnostic criteria:

(a) >1 hemangioblastoma of CNS

(b) 1 hemangioblastoma + visceral manifestation

(c) 1 manifestation + known family history

Subclassification (NIH):

type I = renal + pancreatic cysts, high risk for renal cell carcinoma, NO pheochromocytoma

type IIA = pheochromocytoma, pancreatic islet cell tumor (typically without cysts)

type IIB = pheochromocytoma + renal + pancreatic disease

@ CNS MANIFESTATION

Age at presentation: 25–35 years

- signs of increased intracranial pressure: headache, vomiting
- vision changes: reactive retinal inflammation with exudate + hemorrhage, retinal detachment, glaucoma, cataract, uveitis, decreasing visual acuity, eye pain

- cerebellar symptoms: vertigo, dysdiadochokinesia, dysmetria, Romberg sign
- spinal cord symptoms (uncommon): loss of sensation, impaired proprioception

1. Retinal angiomatosis = **von Hippel tumor** (>50%)
   earliest manifestation of disease; multiple in up to 66%, bilateral in up to 50%
   Histo: hemangioblastoma of retina
   Dx: indirect ophthalmoscopy + fluorescein angiography
   √ small tumors rarely detected by imaging studies
   √ globe distortion
   √ thick calcified retinal density (calcified angioma-induced hematoma)
   US:
   √ small hyperechoic solid masses, most in temporal retina
   Cx: (1) repeated vitreous hemorrhage (frequent)
   (2) exudative retinal detachment posteriorly
2. Hemangioblastoma of CNS = **Lindau tumor** (40%)
   = benign nonglial neoplasm as the most commonly recognized manifestation of vHL disease
   Age: 15–40 years
   Site: cerebellum (65%), brainstem (20%), spinal cord (15%); multiple lesions in 10–15% (may be metachronous)
   ◊ 4–20% of single hemangioblastomas occur in von Hippel-Lindau disease!
   CT:
   √ large cystic lesion with 3–15-mm mural nodule (75%)
   √ solid enhancing lesion (10%)
   √ enhancing lesion with multiple cystic areas (15%)
   √ intense tumor blush / blushing mural nodule
   √ NO calcifications (DDx: cystic astrocytoma calcifies in 25%)
   MR (modality of choice):
   √ hypointense cystic component on T1WI (slightly hyperintense to CSF due to protein content); hyperintense on T2WI
   √ small tubular areas of flow void within mural nodule (= enlarged feeding + draining vessels); intense contrast enhancement of mural nodule
   √ slightly hypointense solid lesion on T1WI; hyperintense on T2WI; intense contrast enhancement
   Angio:
   √ intense staining of mural nodule ("mother-in-law phenomenon" = tumor blush comes early, stays late, very dense)
   √ presence of feeding vessels
   Prognosis: most frequent cause of morbidity and mortality; frequent recurrence after incomplete resection

@ LABYRINTH

1. Endolymphatic sac neoplasm
   = aggressive adenomatous tumor with mixed histologic features
   - sensorineural hearing loss

   Location: retrolabyrinthine temporal bone
   Site: endolymphatic sac
   √ aggressive lytic lesion containing intratumoral osseous spicules + areas of hemorrhage
   √ heterogeneous enhancement with hyperintense areas on T1WI + T2WI (due to hemorrhage)

@ HEART

1. Rhabdomyoma

@ KIDNEYS

- polycythemia due to elevated erythropoietin level (in 15% with hemangioblastoma, in 10% with renal cell carcinoma)

1. Cortical renal cysts (75%)
   multiple + bilateral (may be confused with adult polycystic kidney disease)
2. Renal cell carcinoma (20–45%)
   Age: 20–50 years
   √ multicentric in 87%, bilateral in 10–75%, may arise from cyst wall
   √ sensitivity: 35% for angiography, 37% for US, 45% for CT (due to inability to reliably distinguish between cystic RCC, cancer within cyst, atypical cyst)
   √ 50% metastatic at time of discovery
   Prognosis: RCC is cause of death in 30–50% as the second most frequent cause of mortality!
3. Renal adenoma
4. Renal hemangioma

@ ADRENAL pheochromocytoma (in up to 10–17%), bilateral in up to 40%; confined to certain families

@ EPIDIDYMIS

1. Cystadenoma of epididymis

@ PANCREAS

1. Pancreatic cystadenoma / cystadenocarcinoma
2. Pancreatic islet cell tumor
3. Pancreatic hemangioblastoma
4. Pancreatic cysts (in 30–50%); incidence in autopsies up to 72%

√ usually multiple and multilocular cysts in pancreatic body + tail
◊ Pancreatic cysts in a patient with a family history of von Hippel-Lindau disease are DIAGNOSTIC!

@ LIVER

1. Liver hemangioma
2. Adenoma

@ OTHERS

1. Paraganglioma
2. Cysts in virtually any organ: liver, spleen, adrenal, epididymis, omentum, mesentery, lung, bone

MULTIPLE ORGAN NEOPLASMS

@ Kidney : renal cell carcinoma (up to 40%), renal angioma (up to 45%)
@ Liver : adenoma, angioma
@ Pancreas : cystadenoma / adenocarcinoma
@ Epididymis : adenoma
@ Adrenal gland: pheochromocytoma

MULTIPLE ORGAN CYSTS

(1) Kidney (usually multiple cortical cysts in 75–100% at early age, most common abdominal manifestation)
(2) Pancreas (in 9–72% often numerous cysts; second most common affected abdominal organ)
(3) Others: liver, spleen, omentum, mesentery, epididymis, adrenals, lung, bone

DIFFERENTIAL DIAGNOSIS OF ORBITAL AND OCULAR DISORDERS

OPHTHALMOPLEGIA

Lesions of

1. Oculomotor nerve (III)
   innervates medial rectus, superior rectus, inferior rectus, inferior oblique muscle, pupilloconstrictor, levator palpebrae
2. Trochlear nerve (IV)
   innervates superior oblique muscle
3. Abducens nerve (VI)
   innervates lateral rectus muscle

ANOPIA

[numbers refer to drawing]

A. MONOCULAR DEFECTS
   1 = monocular blindness (optic nerve lesion in fracture of optic canal, amaurosis fugax)

B. BILATERAL HETERONYMOUS DEFECTS
   2 = bitemporal hemianopia (chiasmatic lesion)

C. BILATERAL HOMONYMOUS DEFECTS
   3 = homonymous hemianopia
   4 = upper right-sided quadrantanopia
   5 = central hemianoptic scotoma
   3,4,5 = most common type of hemianopia (CVA, brain tumor)

Monocular Blindness In Adulthood

1. Optic neuritis
2. Vascular ischemia
   (a) Amaurosis fugax = cholesterol emboli from internal carotid artery occluding central retinal artery and its branches
   (b) Occult cerebrovascular malformation affecting the optic nerve
3. Temporal arteritis
4. Malignant optic glioma of adulthood

ORBIT

Spectrum of Orbital Disorders

A. INFLAMMATORY DISEASE
   1. Tissue-specific inflammation:
      orbital cellulitis, optic neuritis, scleritis, myositis, Graves disease
   2. Panophthalmitis
   3. Pseudotumor of orbit

B. CYSTIC DISEASE
   1. Dermoid cyst
   2. Mucocele
   3. Retro-ocular cyst (developmental)

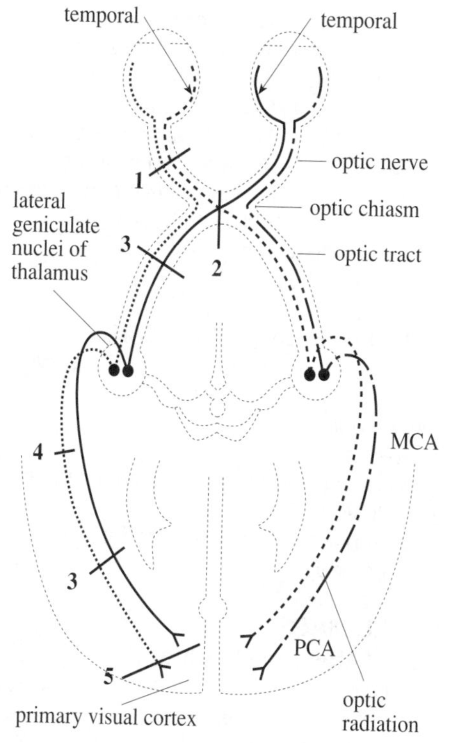

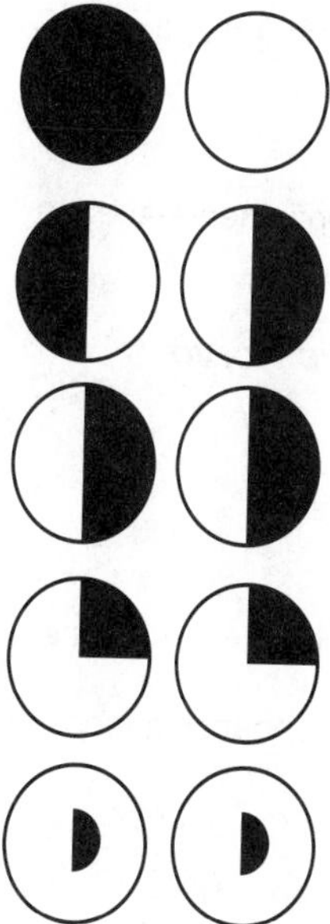

Types of Anopia

C. VASCULAR DISEASE
1. Cavernous angioma
2. Capillary angioma
3. Lymphangioma
4. Varix
5. Carotid-cavernous fistula

D. TUMORS
1. Rhabdomyosarcoma
2. Optic nerve glioma
3. Meningioma
4. Lymphoma
5. Metastasis

Intraconal Lesion

mnemonic: "**M**el **M**et **R**ita **M**ending **H**ems **O**n **P**oor **C**harlie's **G**rave"

Melanoma
Metastasis
Retinoblastoma
Meningioma
Hemangioma
Optic glioma
Pseudotumor
Cellulitis
Grave disease

Intraconal Lesion with Optic Nerve Involvement

1. Optic nerve glioma
2. Optic nerve sheath meningioma (10% of orbital neoplasm)
3. Optic neuritis
4. Inflammatory pseudotumor (may surround optic nerve)
5. Sarcoidosis
6. Intraorbital lymphoma (may surround optic nerve, older patient)
7. Elevated intracranial pressure
   = distension of optic sheath
   √ bilateral tortuous enlarged optic nerve-sheath complex

Intraconal Lesion without Optic Nerve Involvement

1. Cavernous hemangioma
2. Orbital varix
3. Carotid-cavernous fistula
4. Arteriovenous malformation
   least common of orbital vascular malformations (congenital, idiopathic, traumatic)
   √ irregularly shaped intensely enhancing mass of enlarged vessels
   √ associated with dilated superior / inferior ophthalmic vein
5. Hematoma
6. Lymphangioma
7. Neurilemoma
   √ commonly adjacent to superior orbital fissure, inferior to optic nerve
   √ local bone erosion

Extraconal Lesion

Extraconal-intraorbital Lesion

A. BENIGN TUMOR
1. Dermoid cyst
2. **Teratoma**
   <1% of all pediatric orbital tumors
   √ ± areas of fat, cartilage, bone
   √ expansion of bony orbit ± bone defect
3. Capillary hemangioma
4. Lymphangioma
5. Plexiform neurofibroma
6. Inflammatory orbital pseudotumor
7. Histiocytosis X
   lesion usually arises from bone

B. MALIGNANT TUMOR
1. Lymphoma / leukemia
2. Metastasis
3. Rhabdomyosarcoma

Extraconal-extraorbital Lesion

A. FROM SINUS
maxillary / sphenoid sinuses are rare locations of origin
1. Tumor: squamous cell carcinoma (80%), adenocarcinoma, adenoid cystic carcinoma, lymphoma
2. Paranasal sinusitis:
   most common cause of orbital infection;
   Origin: from ethmoid sinuses (in children), from frontal sinus (in adolescence)
   Organism: Staphylococcus, Streptococcus, Pneumococcus
   √ preseptal / orbital edema / cellulitis
   √ subperiosteal / orbital abscess
   √ mucormycosis (in diabetics) destroys bone + extends into cavernous sinus
   Cx: (1) epidural abscess (2) subdural empyema (3) cavernous sinus thrombosis (4) meningitis (5) cerebritis (6) brain abscess
3. Mucocele

B. FROM SKIN
1. Orbital cellulitis

C. FROM LACRIMAL GLAND
√ mass arising from superolateral aspect of orbit

mnemonic: "MOLD"
Metastasis
Others (rhabdomyosarcoma, lymphangioma, sinus lesion)
Lymphoma, **L**acrimal gland tumor
Dermoid

ORBITAL MASS

Orbital Mass in Childhood

1.	Dermoid cyst	46%
2.	Inflammatory lesion	16%
3.	Dermolipoma	7%
4.	Capillary hemangioma	4%
5.	Rhabdomyosarcoma	4%

6. Leukemia / lymphoma 2%
7. Optic nerve glioma 2%
8. Lymphangioma 2%
9. Cavernous hemangioma 1%

mnemonic: "LO VISHON"
Leukemia, **L**ymphoma
Optic nerve glioma
Vascular malformation: hemangioma, lymphangioma
Inflammation
Sarcoma: ie, rhabdomyosarcoma
Histiocytosis
Orbital pseudotumor, **O**steoma
Neuroblastoma

Primary Malignant Orbital Tumors

1. Retinoblastoma 86.0%
2. Rhabdomyosarcoma 8.1%
3. Uveal melanoma 2.3%
4. Sarcoma 1.7%

Secondary Malignant Orbital Tumors

1. Leukemia 36.7%
2. Sarcoma 14.3%
3. Hodgkin lymphoma 11.0%
4. Neuroblastoma 9.2%
5. Wilms tumor 6.7%
6. Non-Hodgkin lymphoma 5.6%
7. Histiocytosis 3.9%
8. Medulloblastoma 3.5%

Orbital Cystic Lesion

1. Abscess
2. Intraorbital hematoma
3. Dermoid cyst
4. Lacrimal cyst
5. Lymphangioma
6. Hydatid cyst

Orbital Vascular Tumors

1. Orbital varix
2. Arteriovenous malformation
3. Carotid-cavernous fistula
4. Hemangioma: capillary / cavernous
5. Blood cyst
6. Arterial malformation
7. Glomus tumor
8. Hemangiopericytoma

Mass in Superolateral Quadrant of Orbit

1. Lacrimal gland tumor
2. Dermoid cyst
3. Metastasis (breast, prostate, lung)
4. Lymphoma
5. Leukemic infiltration of lacrimal gland
6. Sarcoidosis
7. Wegener granulomatosis
8. Pseudotumor
9. Frontal sinus mucocele

Extraocular Muscle Enlargement

A. ENDOCRINE
   1. Graves disease (50%)
   2. Acromegaly
B. INFLAMMATION
   1. **Myositis**
      - rapid onset of proptosis, erythema of lids, conjunctival injection

      Location: single muscle (in adults); multiple muscles (in children)
      √ enlarged extraocular muscle
      √ positive response to steroids
   2. Orbital cellulitis
   3. Sjögren disease, Wegener granulomatosis, lethal midline granuloma, SLE
   4. Sarcoidosis
   5. Foreign-body reaction
C. TUMOR
   1. Pseudotumor
   2. Rhabdomyosarcoma
   3. Metastasis, lymphoma, leukemia
D. VASCULAR
   1. Spontaneous / traumatic hematoma
   2. Arteriovenous malformation
   3. Carotid-cavernous sinus fistula

GLOBE

Spectrum of Ocular Disorders

A. CONGENITAL
   1. Persistent hyperplastic primary vitreous
   2. Coats disease
   3. Coloboma
   4. Congenital cataract
B. VITREORETINAL
   1. Vitreous hemorrhage
   2. Retinal detachment
   3. Choroidal detachment
   4. Endophthalmitis
   5. Retinoschisis
   6. Retrolental fibroplasia
C. TUMOR
   1. Retinoblastoma
   2. Choroidal hemangioma
   3. Retinal angiomatosis
   4. Melanocytoma
   5. Choroidal osteoma
D. TRAUMA

Microphthalmia

= congenital underdevelopment / acquired diminution of globe

A. BILATERAL with cataract
   1. Congenital rubella
   2. Persistent hyperplastic vitreous
   3. Retinopathy of prematurity
   4. Retinal folds
   5. Lowe syndrome
      √ small globe + small orbit

EYE

B. UNILATERAL
1. Trauma / surgery / radiation therapy
2. Inflammation with disorganization of eye (phthisis bulbi)
√ shrunken calcified globe + normal orbit

Macrophthalmia

= enlargement of globe

A. WITHOUT INTRAOCULAR MASS
(a) generalized enlargement
1. Axial myopia (most common cause)
√ enlargement of globe in AP direction
√ ± thinning of sclera
2. Buphthalmos
3. Juvenile glaucoma
4. Connective tissue disorder: Marfan syndrome, Ehlers-Danlos syndrome, Weill-Marchesani syndrome (congenital mesodermal dysmorphodystrophy), homocystinuria
√ "wavy" contour of sclera

(b) focal enlargement
1. **Staphyloma**
= sacculation of posterior pole of globe (or berrylike protrusion of cornea)
Prevalence: increasing with size of globe
Cause: axial myopia (temporal side of optic disc / anteriorly / along equator), trauma, scleritis, necrotizing infection
√ focal bulge + thinning of sclera
Cx: advanced chorioretinal degeneration (77%), choroid retraction from optic disc, posterior vitreous detachment, choroidal hemorrhage, retinal detachment, cataract, glaucoma
2. Apparent enlargement due to contralateral microphthalmia

B. WITH INTRAOCULAR MASS
(rare cause for enlargement)
(a) with calcifications:
1. Retinoblastoma
(b) without calcifications:
1. Melanoma
2. Metastasis

Ocular Lesion

Intraocular Calcifications

1. Retinoblastoma (>50% of all cases)
2. Astrocytic hamartoma
3. **Choroidal osteoma**
= rare juxtapapillary tumor of mature bone
Age: young woman; may be bilateral
√ small flat very dense curvilinear mass aligned with choroidal margin of globe
DDx: calcified choroidal angioma
4. **Optic drusen**
= accretions of hyaline material on / near surface of optic disc; often familial
• headache, visual field defects
• pseudopapilledema
√ small flat / round calcification at junction of retina + optic nerve
√ bilateral in 75%
5. Scleral calcifications
(a) in systemic hypercalcemic states (HPT, hypervitaminosis D, sarcoidosis, secondary to chronic renal disease)
(b) in elderly: at insertion of extraocular muscles
6. Retrolental fibroplasia
7. **Phthisis bulbi**
secondary to trauma or infection
√ small contracted calcified disorganized nonfunctioning globe

mnemonic: "NMR CT"
Neurofibromatosis
Melanoma (hyperdense melanin)
Retinoblastoma
Choroidal osteoma
Tuberous sclerosis

Noncalcified Ocular Process

1. Uveal melanoma
2. Metastasis
86% of ocular lesions within globe; usually in vascular choroid
Origin: breast, lung, GI tract, GU tract, cutaneous melanoma, neuroblastoma
√ bilateral in 30%
3. Choroidal hemangioma
4. **Vitreous lymphoma**
√ diffuse ill-defined soft-tissue density
5. Developmental anomalies
(a) **Primary glaucoma** = enlargement of eye secondary to narrowing of Schlemm canal
(b) Coloboma
(c) Staphyloma

Vitreous Hemorrhage

Cause: trauma, surgical intervention, arterial hypertension, retinal detachment, ocular tumor, Coats disease
• visual loss frequent
US:
√ numerous irregular, poorly defined low-intensity echoes:
√ echogenic material moving freely within vitreous chamber during eye movement
√ voluminous hyperechoic fibrin clots not fixed to optic nerve (DDx to retinal detachment)
Prognosis: complete absorption / development of vitreous membranes (repetitive episodes)
Cx: retinal detachment (vitreous traction secondary to fibrovascular ingrowth following hemorrhage)

Dense Vitreous in Pediatric Age Group

1. Retinoblastoma
2. Persistent hyperplastic primary vitreous
3. Coats disease

4. Norrie disease
5. Retrolental fibroplasia
6. Sclerosing endophthalmitis

Leukokoria

= abnormal white / pinkish / yellowish pupillary light reflex [from Greek *leuko* = white and *koria* = pupil]

A. TUMOR
   1. Retinoblastoma (most common cause – 58%)
   2. Retinal astrocytic hamartoma (3%): associated with tuberous sclerosis + von Recklinghausen disease
   3. Medulloepithelioma (rare)

B. DEVELOPMENTAL
   1. Persistent hyperplastic primary vitreous (2nd most common cause – 28%)
   2. Coats disease (16%)
   3. Retrolental fibroplasia (3–5%)
   4. Coloboma of choroid / optic disc

C. INFECTION
   1. Uveitis
   2. Larval granulomatosis (16%)

D. DEGENERATIVE
   1. Posterior cataract

E. TRAUMA
   1. Retinopathy of prematurity (5%)
   2. Organized vitreous hemorrhage
   3. Long-standing retinal detachment

Leukokoria in Normal-sized Eye

A. CALCIFIED MASS
   1. Retinoblastoma
   2. Retinal astrocytoma

B. NONCALCIFIED MASS
   1. Toxocaral endophthalmitis
   2. Coats disease

Leukokoria with Microphthalmia

A. UNILATERAL
   1. Persistent hyperplastic primary vitreous (PHPV)

B. BILATERAL
   1. Retinopathy of prematurity
   2. Bilateral PHPV

OPTIC NERVE

Optic Nerve Enlargement

A. TUMOR:
   1. Optic nerve glioma
   2. Optic nerve sheath meningioma
   3. Infiltration by leukemia / lymphoma

B. FLUID:
   1. Perineural hematoma
   2. Papilledema of intracranial hypertension
   3. Patulous subarachnoid space

C. INFLAMMATION:
   1. Optic neuritis
   2. Sarcoidosis

√ fusiform thickening
= lens-shaped thickening of nerve-sheath complex
(a) with central lucency: meningioma
(b) without central lucency: optic nerve glioma

√ excrescentic thickening
= single / multiple nodules along nerve-sheath complex usually due to tumor

√ tubular enlargement
= uniform enlargement of nerve-sheath complex
(a) with central lucency: subarachnoid process (metastases, perineuritis, meningioma, perineural hemorrhage)
(b) without central lucency: papilledema, leukemia, lymphoma, sarcoid, optic nerve glioma

LACRIMAL GLAND

Lacrimal Gland Lesion

A. INFLAMMATION
   1. Dacryoadenitis
   2. **Mikulicz syndrome**
      = nonspecific enlargement of lacrimal + salivary glands
      Associated with: sarcoidosis, lymphoma, leukemia
   3. **Sjögren syndrome**
      = lymphocytic infiltration of lacrimal + salivary glands
      • decreased lacrimation, xerostomia
      Often associated with:
      rheumatoid arthritis, systemic lupus erythematosus, scleroderma, polymyositis
   4. Sarcoidosis

B. TUMOR
   (a) benign: granuloma, cyst, benign mixed tumor (= pleomorphic adenoma)
   (b) malignant: malignant mixed tumor (= pleomorphic adenocarcinoma), adenoid cystic carcinoma, lymphoma, metastasis (rare)

Lacrimal Gland Enlargement

mnemonic: "MELD"

Metastasis
Epithelial tumor
Lymphoid tumor
Dermoid

Bilateral Lacrimal Gland Masses

mnemonic: "LACS"

Lymphoma
And
Collagen-vascular disease
Sarcoidosis

EYE

ANATOMY OF ORBIT

ORBITAL CONNECTIONS

Superior Orbital Fissure

Boundaries *(Gray's Anatomy)*:
- — medial : sphenoid body
- — above : lesser wing of sphenoid = optic strut
- — below : greater wing of sphenoid
- — lateral : small segment of frontal bone

Contents:

(a) nerves:
- III oculomotor n.
- IV trochlear n.
- V_1 ophthalmic branch of trigeminal n.:
  - (a) lacrimal nerve
  - (b) frontal nerve
- VI abducens n.
- sympathetic filaments of internal carotid plexus

(b) veins: superior + inferior ophthalmic vein

(c) arteries:
1. meningeal branch of lacrimal artery
2. orbital branch of middle meningeal artery

Inferior Orbital Fissure

Location: between floor + lateral wall of orbit; connects with pterygopalatine + infratemporal fossa

Contents:

(a) nerves: infraorbital + zygomatic nn.
branches from pterygopalatine ganglion

(b) veins: connection between inferior orbital v. + pterygoid plexus

Optic Canal

completely formed by lesser wing of sphenoid

Contents:
- (a) nerve: optic nerve (I)
- (b) vessel: ophthalmic a.

NORMAL ORBIT MEASUREMENTS

Muscles
- medial rectus muscle .... 4.1 ± 0.5 mm
- inferior rectus muscle .... 4.9 ± 0.8 mm
- superior rectus muscle .... 3.8 ± 0.7 mm
- lateral rectus muscle .... 2.9 ± 0.6 mm
- superior oblique muscle .... 2.4 ± 0.4 mm

Superior ophthalmic vein
- axial CT .... 1.8 ± 0.5 mm
- coronal CT .... 2.7 ± 1.0 mm

Optic nerve sheath
- retrobulbar .... 5.5 ± 0.8 mm
- waist .... 4.2 ± 0.6 mm

Globe position
- behind interzygomatic line .... 9.9 ± 1.7 mm

ORBITAL COMPARTMENTS

the orbital septum + globe divide orbit into

A. ANTERIOR COMPARTMENT
lids, lacrimal apparatus, anterior soft tissues

B. POSTERIOR COMPARTMENT
= RETROBULBAR SPACE
the cone consisting of extraorbital muscles + envelope of fascia divides retrobulbar space into
- (a) intraconal space
- (b) extraconal space

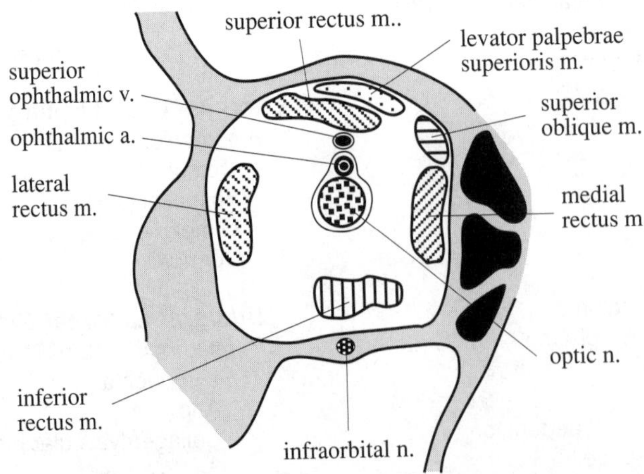

Coronal Orbital Tomogram through Midorbit

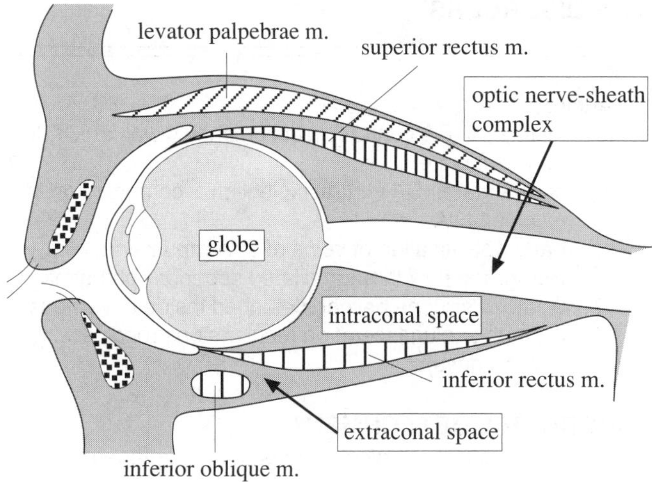

Orbital Spaces

globe: subdivided into anterior + posterior segments by lens

optic nerve-sheath complex: optic nerve surrounded by meningeal sheath as extension from cerebral meninges

intraconal space: orbital fat, ophthalmic a., superior ophthalmic v., nerves I, III, IV, V_1, VI

conus: incomplete fenestrated musculofascial system extending from bony orbit to anterior third of globe, consists of extraocular muscles + interconnecting fascia

extraconal space: between muscle cone + bony orbit containing fat, lacrimal gland, lacrimal sac, portion of superior ophthalmic v.

ORBITAL AND OCULAR DISORDERS

BUPHTHALMOS

= HYDROPHTHALMOS = MEGOPHTHALMOS
= diffuse enlargement of eye in children secondary to increased intraocular pressure

Cause:
1. Congenital / infantile glaucoma
2. Neurofibromatosis type 1: obstruction of canal of Schlemm by membranes / masses composed of aberrant mesodermal tissue
3. Sturge-Weber-Dimitri syndrome
4. Lowe (cerebrohepatorenal) syndrome
5. Ocular mesodermal dysplasia (eg, Axenfeld or Rieger anomalies)
6. Homocystinuria
7. Aniridia
8. Acquired glaucoma (rare)

Pathophysiology:
obstruction of canal of Schlemm located between cornea + iris leads to decreased resorption of aqueous humor (= anterior chamber fluid) with scleral distension
√ uniformly enlarged globe without mass of round / oval / bizarre shape

Rx: goniotomy (increases the angle of anterior chamber); trabeculotomy (lyses adhesions)

CAROTID-CAVERNOUS SINUS FISTULA

= abnormal communication between internal carotid artery + veins of cavernous sinus

Etiology:
(1) Trauma: laceration of ICA within cavernous sinus
  (a) usually secondary to basal skull fracture (cavernous ICA + small cavernous branches fixed to dura)
  (b) penetrating trauma
(2) Spontaneous: rupture of an intracavernous ICA aneurysm

Route of drainage:
(a) superior ophthalmic vein (common)
(b) contralateral cavernous sinus
(c) petrosal sinus
(d) cortical veins (rare)

• pulsating exophthalmos, chemosis, conjunctival edema
• persistent orbital bruit
• restricted extraocular movement
• decrease in vision due to increase in intraocular pressure (50%) = indication for emergent treatment

√ enlarged edematous extraocular muscles
√ dilatation of superior ophthalmic vein / facial veins / internal jugular vein
√ focal / diffuse enlargement of cavernous sinus
√ occasionally sellar erosion / enlargement
√ enlargement of superior orbital fissure (in chronic phase)

US + MR:
√ arterial flow in cavernous sinus + superior ophthalmic vein

Angio:
√ ipsilateral ICA contrast injection shows wall of ICA to be incomplete
√ contralateral ICA contrast injection + compression of involved ICA
√ early opacification of veins of cavernous sinus
√ retrograde flow through dilated superior ophthalmic v.

Rx: latex / silicone balloon detached inside cavernous sinus to plug laceration (ocular signs resolve within 7–10 days)

CHOROIDAL DETACHMENT

Cause: trauma, surgical intervention, spontaneous

US:
√ two convex lines projecting into the eye from periphery of globe + advancing to ciliary body with posterior fixation outside the optic disk (= macula)
√ minimal / no choroidal membrane mobility during eye movement

CHOROIDAL HEMANGIOMA

= vascular hamartoma

Age: 10–20 years (most common benign tumor in adults)
May be associated with: Sturge-Weber syndrome
Location: posterior pole temporal to optic disk (70%)

√ 0.5–3-mm small tumor
√ focal thickening of posterior wall of globe
√ enhancement similar to choroid
√ retinal detachment (frequent)

US:
√ hyperechoic homogeneous mass

DDx: melanoma (choroidal excavitation)

COATS DISEASE

= RETINAL TELANGIECTASIA
= Pseudoglioma = congenital idiopathic primary vascular malformation of the retina characterized by
(1) multiple abnormal telangiectatic retinal vessels
(2) lack of blood-retina barrier causing leakage of a lipoproteinaceous exudate into retina + subretinal space with secondary detachment of retina

Age: 6–8 years (but present at birth); M:F = 2:1

• strabismus
• may present with leukokoria (if retina massively detached) [16% of leukokoria cases]
• loss of vision, secondary glaucoma
• cholesterol crystals at funduscopy

Location: unilateral in 90%

Associated with: √ retinal detachment
√ slight microphthalmia

√ NO focal mass / calcification (HALLMARK)

US:
√ clumpy particulate echoes in subretinal space (due to cholesterol crystals suspended in fluid)

√ vitreous + subretinal hemorrhage (frequent)
DDx: unilateral noncalcifying retinoblastoma (before 3 years of age, no microphthalmia)

CT:
√ unilateral dense vitreous in normal-sized globe

MR:
√ hyperintense subretinal exudate on T1WI + T2WI (due to mixture of protein + lipid) / hypointense on T2WI (cholesterol crystals + membranous lipids)
√ abnormal enhancement of retina at ora serrata + of detached retinal leaves

DDx: (1) Persistent hyperplastic primary vitreous (thick tubular retrolental mass)
(2) Retinopathy of prematurity

Rx: photocoagulation / cryotherapy to obliterate telangiectasias (in early stages)

COLOBOMA

[*koloboun* , Greek = to mutilate]
= incomplete closure of embryonic choroidal fissure affecting eyelid / lens / iris / choroid / retina / macula; autosomal dominant trait with variable penetrance (30%) and expression; bilateral in 60%

Time of insult: 6th week of GA

May be associated with: encephalocele, agenesis of corpus callosum

Location: in 50% bilateral

√ cystic outpouching (= herniation) of vitreous at site of optic nerve attachment
√ small globe

DDx: microphthalmos with cyst = duplication cyst, axial (high) myopia

CONGENITAL CATARACT

= opacification of lens

Etiology: infection, hereditary

Location: frequently bilateral

US:
√ increase in thickness + echogenicity of posterior wall of lens ± intralenticular echoes

DACRYOADENITIS

= infection of lacrimal gland

Organism: staphylococci (most common), mumps, infectious mononucleosis, influenza

√ homogeneous enlargement of lacrimal gland
√ ± compression of globe

DERMOID CYST OF ORBIT

Most common benign orbital tumor in childhood (45% of all masses)

Age: 1st decade

Histo: contains keratin, hair, stratified epithelium + dermal appendages within thick capsule; usually arises in fetal cleavage planes (sutures)

Location: in anterior extraconal orbit, upper temporal quadrant (60%), upper nasal quadrant (25%)

√ well-defined cystic mass ± negative HU numbers
√ thick surrounding capsule
√ ± expansion / erosion of bony orbit

US:
√ encapsulated heterogeneous mass with variable cystic component

MR:
√ high signal intensity on T1WI + T2WI

EYE

ENDOPHTHALMITIS

Infectious Endophthalmitis

Organism: bacteria (rare in childhood, trauma, idiopathic), fungi, parasites

Cause:
(a) exogenous endophthalmitis: most commonly related to eye injury / surgery
(b) endogenous endophthalmitis: hematogenous spread from distant source of infection

US:
√ medium- to high-intensity echoes dispersed throughout vitreous (DDx: echoes in vitreous hemorrhage are more mobile)

CT:
√ increased attenuation of vitreous
√ uveal-scleral thickening
√ decreased attenuation of lens

Sclerosing Endophthalmitis

= TOXOCARA CANIS ENDOPHTHALMITIS
= granulomatous uveitis resulting in subretinal exudate, retinal detachment, organized vitreous

Age: 2–6–12 years

Mode of infection:
playing in soil contaminated by viable infective eggs from dog excrement (common in playgrounds)

Organism: helminthic nematode Toxocara canis causing visceral / ocular larva migrans (0.5 mm long, 20 μm wide); endemic throughout world; especially common in southeastern United States

Life cycle:
egg hatches into larva within intestines of definite host (dog) + develops into adult worm; alternatively dog may eat infective-stage larvae from intestines / viscera of other animals; in noncanine host larvae will not develop into adult worm, but burrow through intestinal wall and migrate to liver, lung, and other tissue including brain + eye

Pathophysiology:
migration through human tissue produces a severe eosinophilic reaction that becomes granulomatous; spreads hematogenously to temporal choroid

Path: retina elevated + distorted + partially replaced by an inflammatory mass containing abundant dense scar tissue; subjacent choroid infiltrated with chronic inflammatory cells including eosinophils; proteinaceous subretinal exudate

- red "hot" eye, photophobia, pain
- anterior chamber flare cells, keratic precipitates
- vitreous synechia
- vitreitis = accumulation of cellular debris in vitreous
- leukokoria (16% of cases of childhood leukokoria)
- fever, hepatomegaly, pneumonitis, convulsions
- peripheral blood eosinophilia

Location: usually unilateral
√ eye of normal size without calcifications
√ secondary retinal detachment
US:
 √ hypoechoic mass in peripheral fundus
 √ ± calcifications
CT:
 √ intravitreal mass
 √ focal uveoscleral thickening (granulomatous reaction around larva) with contrast enhancement
 √ increased density of vitreous cavity
MR:
 √ enhancing granuloma isointense to vitreous on T1WI
 √ mass usually hyperintense relative to vitreous on T2WI, occasionally hypointense (due to dense fibroconnective tissue)

Cx: retinal detachment (due to subretinal fluid / vitreoretinal traction), cataract
Dx: (1) Enzyme-linked immunosorbent assay (ELISA) on blood serum / vitreous aspirate
 (2) Histologic identification of organism
DDx: retinoblastoma

GRAVES DISEASE OF ORBIT

= THYROID OPHTHALMOPATHY = ENDOCRINE EXOPHTHALMOS
= increase in orbital pressure produces ischemia, edema, fibrosis of muscles

Etiology: produced by long-acting thyroid-stimulating factor (LATS); probably immunologic cross-reactivity against antigens shared by thyroid + orbital tissue
Age: adulthood; 5% younger than 15 years; M:F = 1:4
Histo: deposition of hygroscopic mucopolysaccharides + glycoprotein (early) + collagen (late); infiltration by mast cells and lymphocytes, edema, muscle fiber necrosis, lipomatosis, fatty degeneration
Time of onset: signs + symptoms usually develop within one year of the onset of hyperthyroidism

- proptosis
  ◊ Most common cause of uni- / bilateral proptosis in adult!
- lid lag = upper eyelid retraction
- periorbital swelling
- conjunctival injection
- restricted ocular motility (correlates with increase in mean muscle diameters)
- progressive optic neuropathy (5%)
- hyperthyroidism; euthyroidism (in 10–15%); severity of orbital involvement unrelated to degree of thyroid dysfunction

STAGING (Werner's modified classification):
 Stage I : eyelid retraction without symptoms
 Stage II : eyelid retraction with symptoms
 Stage III : proptosis >22 mm without diplopia
 Stage IV : proptosis >22 mm with diplopia
 Stage V : corneal ulceration
 Stage VI : loss of sight

Location:
 bilateral in 70–85%; single muscle in 10%; asymmetrical involvement in 10–30%; all muscles equally affected with similar proportional enlargements; superior muscle group most commonly when only single muscle involved [former notion: inferior > medial > superior rectus muscle + levator palpebrae > lateral rectus muscle]
 mnemonic: "I'M SLow"
  Inferior
  Medial
  Superior
  Lateral

√ proptosis = globe protrusion >21 mm anterior to interzygomatic line on axial scans at level of lens
√ swelling of muscles maximally in midportion (relative sparing of tendinous insertion at globe) = "Coke-bottle" sign
√ slight uveal-scleral thickening
√ apical crowding = orbital apex involved late (pressure on optic nerve)
√ dilatation of superior ophthalmic vein (compromised orbital venous drainage at orbital apex due to enlarged extraocular muscles)
√ increase in diameter of retrobulbar optic nerve sheath (dural distension due to accumulation of CSF in subarachnoid space with optic neuropathy)
√ increased density of orbital fat (late)
√ anterior displacement of lacrimal gland
√ intracranial fat herniation through superior ophthalmic fissure (best correlation with compressive neuropathy
MR:
 √ high signal intensity in enlarged eye muscles on T2WI (edema in acute inflammation)

Prognosis: in 90% spontaneous resolution within 3–36 months; in 10% decrease in visual acuity (corneal ulceration / optic neuropathy)
Rx: short- and long-term steroid therapy, cyclosporine, radiation, surgical decompression, correction of eyelid position
DDx: pseudotumor (usually includes tendon of eye muscles)

HEMANGIOMA OF ORBIT

◊ Most common benign orbital tumor

Location: 83–94% retrobulbar (intraconal)
√ sharply demarcated oval mass in superior-temporal portion of conus (2/3) often sparing orbital apex
√ displacement (not involvement) of optic nerve
√ expansion of bony orbit
√ uniform / inhomogeneous (when thrombosed) enhancement
√ small calcifications (phleboliths)
√ puddling of contrast material on angiography

US:
- √ well-defined encapsulated mass of intermediate echogenicity
- √ absent / poor predominantly venous flow

Capillary Hemangioma of Orbit

most common vascular tumor of orbit in children; 5–15% of all pediatric orbital masses

Age: first 2 weeks of life; 95% in <6 months of age; M < F

Histo: proliferation of endothelial cells with multiple capillaries

- • proptosis, chemosis (= edema) of eyelid + conjunctiva exaggerated by crying
- • associated with skin angioma (90%)

Location: anterior part of orbit, occasionally posterior

- √ mass with enhancement equal to / greater than orbital muscle
- √ poorly marginated (suggesting malignant cause)
- √ activity in radionuclide flow studies

US:
- √ poorly defined heterogeneous mass of intermediate echogenicity
- √ abundant internal flow decreasing with age

Prognosis: often increase in size for 6–10 months followed by spontaneous involution within 1–2 years

Cavernous Hemangioma of Orbit

Frequency: usually tumor of adulthood; 12–15% of all orbital masses; 1–2% of childhood orbital masses

Age: 20–40 years; F > M

Histo: large dilated venous channels with flattened endothelial cells surrounded by fibrous pseudocapsule

- • slowly progressive unilateral proptosis, diplopia, diminished visual acuity (optic nerve compression)

INFECTION OF ORBIT

Cause: bacterial infection extending from paranasal sinuses (especially ethmoid + frontal sinuses), face, eyelid, nose, teeth, lacrimal sac through thin lamina papyracea + valveless facial veins into orbit

Organism: staphylococci, streptococci, pneumococci

- • lid edema, ocular pain, ophthalmoplegia
- • fever, elevated WBC

Location: preseptal = periorbital soft tissue; subperiosteal; peripheral = extraconal fat; extraocular muscles; central = intraconal fat; optic nerve complex; globe; lacrimal gland

Cx: epidural abscess, subdural empyema, cavernous sinus thrombosis, cerebral abscess, osteomyelitis

Abscess of Orbit

Location: most commonly in subperiosteal space on medial wall

- √ subperiosteal fluid collection
- √ displacement of thickened periosteal membrane + increased enhancement
- √ displacement of adjacent fat + extraocular muscles

MR:
- √ hyperintensity on T1WI + T2WI

Cellulitis of Orbit

= acute bacterial infection, often extending from paranasal sinuses / eyelids

- • limitation of ocular movements
- • fever

Location: mostly confined to extraconal space

- √ proptosis
- √ scleral thickening
- √ enlargement + displacement of extraocular muscles (frequently medial rectus muscle)
- √ increased attenuation of retro-orbital fat + obliteration of fat planes
- √ opacification of ethmoid + maxillary sinuses (extension through thin lamina papyracea into orbit)
- √ subperiosteal abscess (with ethmoiditis)

MR:
- √ hypointense on T1WI + hyperintense on T2WI
- √ contrast-enhanced fat-suppressed images are most sensitive

US:
- √ diffuse hypoechoic area invading retrobulbar fat

Rx: antibiotics + corticosteroids

Cx: orbital abscess

DDx: cannot be differentiated from edema, chloroma, leukemic infiltrate

Preseptal Cellulitis

= fibrous orbital septum resists extension of infection into posterior compartment of orbit

- √ thickening of eyelids + septum
- √ swelling of anterior orbital tissues with increased density + obliteration of fat planes

Edema of Orbit

Location: usually confined to preseptal structures (eyelid, face); involvement of orbital structures (rare)

- √ swelling of eyelids / face
- √ increased attenuation of orbital fat + obliteration of fat planes
- √ displacement + enlargement of extraocular muscles

MR:
- √ hyperintensity on T2WI

LYMPHANGIOMA OF ORBIT

Incidence: 3.5:100,000; 1–2% of orbital childhood masses; 8% of expanding orbital lesions

Histo: dilated lymphatics, dysplastic venous vessels, smooth muscle, areas of hemorrhage

(a) simple / capillary lymphangioma
= lymphatic channels of capillary size

(b) cavernous lymphangioma
= dilated microscopic channels
(c) cystic hygroma
= macroscopic multilocular cystic mass

Age: 1st decade or later (mean age of 6 years)
- proptosis (sudden proptosis from spontaneous intratumoral hemorrhage = CARDINAL FEATURE; exacerbated during upper respiratory infections [rare])
- associated with lesions on lid, conjunctiva, cheek
- coincident lymphangiomatous cysts in oral mucosa

Location: usually medial to optic nerve with intra- and extraconal component, crossing anatomic boundaries (conal fascia / orbital septum); may involve conjunctiva + lid

√ poorly defined multilobulated inhomogeneous lesion
√ single / multiple cystlike areas with rim enhancement (after hemorrhage) = blood cyst = "chocolate cyst"
√ areas of enhancement (= venous channels) / ring enhancement (after hemorrhage)
√ rarely contains phleboliths (DDx: hemangioma, orbital varix)
√ mild to moderate enlargement of orbit

US:
√ area of predominantly cystic heterogeneous texture with infiltrative borders

MR:
√ may show hematoma of various duration within lesion

Prognosis: no involution, progression slows with termination of body growth
DDx: orbital varix

LYMPHOMA OF ORBIT

Usually presents without evidence of systemic disease; subsequent development of systemic disease frequent

Incidence: 3rd most common cause of proptosis after orbital pseudotumor + cavernous hemangioma; in 8% of leukemia; in 3–4% of lymphoma
Age: 50 years on average
Type: usually non-Hodgkin B-cell lymphoma; Burkitt lymphoma with orbit as primary manifestation; Hodgkin disease rare

- painless swelling of eyelid
- exophthalmos (late in course of disease)

Location: extraconal (especially lacrimal gland, anterior extraconal space, retrobulbar) > intraconal > optic nerve-sheath complex; may be bilateral

◊ Lacrimal gland is a common site for leukemic infiltrates!

Growth types:
(a) well-defined high-density mass (most commonly about lacrimal gland)
(b) diffuse infiltration (tends to involve entire intraconal region)

√ slight to moderate enhancement

US:
√ solitary / multiple hypoechoic homogeneous masses with infiltrative borders

METASTASIS TO ORBIT

Origin: only in 50% known; carcinoma of breast + lung (adults); neuroblastoma > Ewing sarcoma, leukemia, Wilms tumor (children)

Location: 12% intraorbital, 86% intraocular especially in posterior temporal portion of uvea (vascular layer between retina + sclera) near macula; may be bilateral

CT:
√ small areas of thickening + increased density
√ subretinal fluid

NORRIE DISEASE

= RETINAL DYSPLASIA
= X-linked recessive disease: ? inherited form of persistent hyperplastic primary vitreous

- seizures, mental retardation (50%)
- hearing loss, deafness by age 4 (30%)
- bilateral leukokoria + microphthalmia
- cataract, blindness (absence of retinal ganglion cells)

√ microphthalmia
√ dense vitreous with blood-fluid level
√ cone-shaped central retinal detachment
√ calcifications

OCULAR TRAUMA

Types: (a) Simple / complicated contusion with rupture of ocular wall
(b) Simple / perforating injury to the globe
(c) Foreign body

- clinical evaluation: testing of visual acuity, slit-lamp evaluation of cornea + anterior segment, intraocular pressure measurement, funduscopy

US (used if ocular media opaque due to vitreous hemorrhage / hyphema / traumatic cataract)

1. Hemorrhage
   (a) **vitreous hemorrhage** (53%)
   - visual loss frequent
   √ echogenic material moving freely within vitreous chamber during eye movement
   Cx: retinal detachment (vitreous traction secondary to fibrovascular ingrowth following hemorrhage)
   Rx: vitrectomy
   (b) **retrohyaloid hemorrhage** (2%)
   √ echogenic material remaining behind detached vitreous capsule during eye movement
   (c) hematoma in retro-ocular space
2. Retinal detachment
   (a) **total retinal detachment** (18%)
   √ slightly thick line of "V" shape with apex at optic disk
   √ retina remains bound down at ora serrata
   (b) **focal retinal detachment** (2%)
   √ elevated immobile line close to sclera at periphery of globe
4. **Vitreous detachment** (11%)
   √ thin undulate mobile line moving away from posterior aspect of globe during eye motion
5. Choroidal detachment (5%)

6. **Intraocular foreign body** (7%)
   US sensitivity: 95% for intraocular + 50% for intraorbital foreign body
   Cx: siderosis (if metallic); endophthalmitis
7. **Lens dislocation** (3%)
8. Thickening / rupture of ocular wall
9. Vascular complications
   (a) central renal artery occlusion
   (b) carotid-cavernous fistula
   (c) fistula of angular vein

OPTIC NERVE GLIOMA

= JUVENILE PILOCYTIC ASTROCYTOMA
= most common cause of optic nerve enlargement
Incidence: 1% of all intracranial tumors, 2% of childhood orbital masses; 80% of primary tumors of optic nerve
Histo: proliferation of well-differentiated astrocytes = low-grade glial neoplasm; most commonly pilocytic astrocytoma (in children) + glioblastoma (in adults)
Age: 1st decade (80%); peak age around 5 years; M < F
Associated with: neurofibromatosis in 10–50% (± bilateral optic gliomas)
◊ 15% of patients with neurofibromatosis have optic nerve gliomas!
• decreased visual acuity, minimal axial proptosis
√ tubular / fusiform / excrescentic well-circumscribed enlargement of optic nerve
√ posterior extension along optic tracts in 60–70% (indicates nonresectability)
√ calcifications (rare)
√ same attenuation as normal optic nerve; slight contrast enhancement
√ ipsilateral optic canal enlargement (90%) >3 mm / 1 mm difference compared with contralateral side
US:
√ well-defined homogeneous mass of medium echogenicity inseparable from optic nerve
MR: more sensitive than CT in detecting intracanalicular + intracranial extent
√ isointense to muscle on T1WI
√ hyperintense on T2WI
DDx: optic nerve sheath meningioma (no intracranial extension along optic pathway)

Malignant Optic Glioma of Adulthood

Incidence: extremely rare; 30 cases in this century
Mean age: 6th decade; M:F = 1.3:1.0
Histo: anaplastic astrocytoma / glioblastoma multiforme
• rapidly progressive monocular visual loss culminating in monocular blindness within a few weeks
• with retrograde tumor extension: contralateral temporal hemianopia, polyuria, polydipsia
√ focal / diffuse enlargement of optic nerve
√ hypo- to isointense on T1WI + hyperintense on T2WI
√ obliteration of subarachnoid space around affected portion of nerve
√ diffuse intense enhancement of optic nerve
√ thickening + abnormal enhancement of optic nerve sheath
Tumor extension: optic chiasm, hypothalamus, basal ganglia, brain stem, medial temporal lobes, leptomeninges, ependyma
Prognosis: <1-year survival despite aggressive therapy
DDx: (1) Optic neuritis (demyelinating plaques elsewhere)
(2) Perioptic meningioma (hypointense on T2WI, stippled calcifications, hyperostosis)
(3) Sarcoidosis, lymphoma, orbital pseudotumor (moderately / markedly hypointense on T2WI)

OPTIC NERVE SHEATH MENINGIOMA

= PERIOPTIC MENINGIOMA
Incidence: 10% of all intraorbital neoplasms; <2% of intracranial meningiomas
Age: middle-aged + elderly females; slightly more aggressive in children
Occasionally associated with: neurofibromatosis (usually in teenagers)
Primary origin: arising from arachnoid rests in the meningeal investiture of optic nerves in orbit / middle fossa
• progressive loss of visual acuity over months (optic atrophy), proptosis
√ ± enlargement of optic canal
√ tubular (most commonly) / fusiform / excrescentic thickening of optic nerve
√ sphenoid bone hyperostosis
√ frequently calcified (HIGHLY SUGGESTIVE)
US:
√ hypoechoic tumor with irregular border
CECT: enhancement is the rule
√ dense linear bands (axial view) as "tram tracks" / ringlike (coronal view) due to tumor enhancement around nonenhancing optic nerve
√ minimal extension into optic canal (not uncommon)
MR:
√ extrinsic soft-tissue mass surrounding optic nerve
√ hypointense to fat on T1WI

OPTIC NEURITIS

= nerve involvement by inflammation, degeneration, demyelination
Etiology: (1) multiple sclerosis (involves optic nerve in 1/3)
(2) inflammation secondary to ocular infection
(3) degeneration (toxic, metabolic, nutritional)
(4) ischemia
(5) meningitis / encephalitis
◊ 45–80% of patients develop multiple sclerosis within 15 years of their first episode of optic neuritis!
• ipsilateral orbital pain on eye movement
• sudden onset of unilateral loss of vision over several hours to several days
CT:
√ normal / mildly enlarged optic nerve + chiasm
√ may show enhancement

EYE

MR:
√ mild enlargement + enhancement of optic nerve well demonstrated on axial T1WI

Prognosis: spontaneous improvement of visual acuity within 1–2 weeks

PERSISTENT HYPERPLASTIC PRIMARY VITREOUS

= rare condition with persistence + proliferation of embryonic hyaloid vascular system of primary vitreous due to arrest of normal regression

May be associated with:
any severe ocular malformation / optic dysplasia / trisomy 13

◊ Bilaterality is a feature of a congenital syndrome (Norrie disease, Warburg disease)!

— Primary vitreous
= fibrillar ectodermal meshwork + mesodermal tissue consisting of embryonic hyaloid vascular system; appears during 1st month of life; extends between lens + retina; involutes by 6th month of gestation

— Hyaloid artery
= important source of intraocular nutrition until 8th month of gestation; arises from dorsal ophthalmic artery at 3rd week of gestation; grows anteriorly with branches supplying vitreous + posterior aspect of lens

— Secondary / adult vitreous
begins to form during 3rd gestational month; a watery mass of loose collagen fibers + hyaluronic acid gradually replaces primary vitreous, which is reduced to a small S-shaped remnant (hyaloid canal = Cloquet canal) and serves as lymph channel

• unilateral leukokoria (2nd most common cause) [2–3% of leukokoria cases]
• seizures, mental deficiency, hearing loss
• ± cataract
• ophthalmoscopy: S-shaped tubular mass extending between posterior surface of lens + region of optic nerve head; lens opacity may preclude diagnosis

√ microphthalmia = small hypoplastic globe
√ retinal detachment (due to vitreoretinal traction in 30%)

US:
√ hyperechoic band extending from posterior pole of globe to posterior surface of lens (= embryonic rest of primary vitreous)
√ central anechoic line (= persistent hyaloid artery) visible in cases of echogenic vitreous hemorrhage
√ hyperechoic band extending from papilla to ora serrata (= retinal detachment)

CT:
√ enhancing cone-shaped central retrolental density extending from lens through vitreous body to back of orbit, just lateral to optic nerve
√ small optic nerve
√ deformity of globe + lens
√ hyperdense vitreous (from previous hemorrhage)
√ fluid-fluid levels from breakdown of recurrent hemorrhage in subhyaloid (between vitreous + retina) / subretinal space (between sensory + pigment epithelium)
√ NO calcifications

MR:
√ hyperintense vitreous body on T1WI + T2WI from chronic blood degradation products (methemoglobin) / proteinaceous fluid
√ hypo- to isointense thin triangular band with base near optic disc and apex at posterior surface of lens
√ marked enhancement of fibrovascular mass within vitreous

Cx:
(1) Glaucoma, cataract from recurrent spontaneous intravitreal hemorrhage (due to friable vessels)
(2) Proliferation of embryonic tissue
(3) Retinal detachment from organizing hemorrhage / traction
(4) Hydrops / atrophy of globe + resorption of lens
(5) Phthisis bulbi (scarred shrunken eye)

PSEUDOTUMOR OF ORBIT

= IDIOPATHIC INFLAMMATORY PSEUDOTUMOR
= nongranulomatous inflammatory process affecting all intraorbital soft tissues

Etiology:
(a) cause not apparent at time of study: bacterial, viral, foreign body
(b) systemic disease presently not apparent: sarcoidosis, collagen, endocrine
(c) idiopathic: probably abnormal immune response

Incidence: 25% of all cases of unilateral exophthalmos; most common cause of an intraorbital mass lesion in adult

Age: young female

Histo: lymphocytic infiltrate

May be associated with:
Wegener granulomatosis, sarcoidosis, fibrosing mediastinitis, retroperitoneal fibrosis, thyroiditis, cholangitis, vasculitis, lymphoma

• unilateral painful ophthalmoplegia
• proptosis, chemosis, lid injection
• limitation of ocular movement

Location: retrobulbar fat (76%), extraocular muscle (57%), optic nerve (38%), uveal-scleral area (33%), lacrimal gland (5%)

(a) tumefactive type (common)
√ discrete / poorly defined intra- / extraconal mass = "pseudotumor" close to surface margin of globe

(b) myositic type (unusual)
√ enlargement of one / more extraocular muscles close to insertion in globe with ill-defined margins
√ typically involves muscles + tendon insertions (DDx to Graves disease with muscle involvement only)

√ increased density of retro-orbital fat (may involve anterior compartment)
√ thickening and enhancement of sclera near Tenon capsule

√ enlarged lacrimal gland
√ proptosis
MR:
√ lesion isointense to fat on T2WI
Prognosis:
(1) remitting / chronic + progressive course
(2) rapid dramatic + lasting response to steroid therapy
DDx: (1) Lymphoma (may be confused with lymphoma clinically, radiographically, pathologically)
(2) Thyroid ophthalmopathy (tapering of distal muscles, painless proptosis)
(3) Radiation therapy

RETINAL ASTROCYTOMA

= low-grade neoplasm / hamartoma arising from the nerve fiber layer of retina / optic nerve, usually associated with tuberous sclerosis
Etiology: tuberous sclerosis (53%); neurofibromatosis type 1 (14%); sporadic (33%)
Path: usually multiple + bilateral in tuberous sclerosis;
(1) small flat noncalcified semitranslucent lesion in posterior / peripheral retina
(2) "mulberry" lesion = raised white tumor in posterior retina with fine nodularity containing calcifications + cystic fluid accumulations
Histo: spindle-shaped fibrous astrocytes
• leukokoria (3% of all childhood cases of leukokoria)
• asymptomatic, progressive loss of vision
Location: retina near optic disc
√ retinal mass ± enhancement
√ typically unilateral (DDx to drusen)
Cx: (1) Central retinal vein occlusion + secondary hemorrhage
(2) Neovascular glaucoma
(3) Extensive tumor necrosis

RETINAL DETACHMENT

Cause: trauma, tumor, exudative / inflammatory process, scar
US:
√ curvilinear area of high echogenicity fixed at optic disk (= papilla) + extending to ora serrata
√ V-shaped (with total detachment)
√ in one quadrant only (partial detachment)
√ thick folded retina with loss of mobility (long-standing detachment)
√ subretinal space normal / occupied by blood, inflammation / tumor (depending on cause)
DDx: vitreous membranes, choroidal detachment (point of fixation not at papilla)

RETINOBLASTOMA

= rare malignant congenital intraocular tumor arising from primitive photoreceptor cells of retina (included in primitive neuroectodermal tumor group)

Types:
(A) Nonheritable form (66%)
(1) Sporadic postzygotic somatic mutation (subsequent generations unaffected)
Mean age at presentation: 23 months
√ unilateral disease
(2) Chromosomal anomaly
= monosomy 13 / deletions of 13q
Associated with: microcephaly, ear changes, facial dysmorphism, mental retardation, finger + toe abnormalities, malformation of genitalia
(B) Heritable form
(1) Heritable sporadic form (20–25%)
= sporadic germinal mutation (50% chance to occur in subsequent generations)
Mean age at presentation: 12 months
√ bilateral retinoblastomas in 66%
(2) Familial retinoblastoma (5–10%)
= autosomal dominant with abnormality of band 14 in chromosome 13 (95% penetrance)
Mean age at presentation: 8 months
√ usually 3 to 5 ocular tumors per eye
√ bilateral tumors in 66%
Risk of secondary nonocular malignancy: osteo~, chondro~, fibrosarcoma, malignant fibrous histiocytoma (20% risk within 10 years, >90% by 30 years of age)
Trilateral retinoblastoma (rare variant)
= bilateral retinoblastomas + neuroectodermal pineal tumor (pineoblastoma)
Quadrilateral retinoblastoma
= trilateral retinoblastoma + 4th focus in suprasellar cistern

Incidence: 1:15,000–34,000 livebirths; most common intraocular neoplasm in childhood; 1% of all pediatric malignancies
Age: mean age at presentation is 18 months; 98% in children <5 years of age; M:F = 1:1
Path: (1) Exophytic form = proliferation into subretinal space with detachment of retina + invasion of vascular choroid (hematogenous spread)
(2) Endophytic form = centripetal tumor invasion causing floating islands of tumor within semiliquid vitreous ± anterior chamber
(3) Diffuse form = thin en-plaque lesion extending along retina
Histo: (a) Flexner-Wintersteiner rosettes (in 50%)
= neuronal cells line up around an empty central zone filled with polysaccharides
◊ Very specific for retinoblastomas!
(b) Homer-Wright rosettes = neuronal cells line up around a central area containing a cobweb of filaments (also found in other primitive neuroectodermal tumors)
(c) "fleurettes" = flowerlike groupings of tumor cells that form photoreceptor elements (specific for retinal differentiation)

• "cat's eye" = leukokoria (whitish mass behind lens) in 60%
  ◊ About 50% of all childhood leukokoria are caused by retinoblastoma!
• decreased visual acuity, heterochromia iridis
• strabismus (crossed eyes), proptosis (less common)
• hyphema
• iris neovascularization, phthisis bulbi
• ocular pain from secondary angle-closure glaucoma

Location: posterolateral wall of globe (most commonly); 60% unilateral; 40% bilateral + frequently synchronous (90% bilateral in inherited forms)

√ normal ocular size

US:
  √ heterogeneous hyperechoic solid intraocular mass
  √ cystic appearance upon tumor necrosis
  √ secondary retinal detachment in all cases
  √ acoustic shadowing (in 75%)
  √ vitreous hemorrhage frequent

CT:
  √ solid smoothly marginated lobulated retrolental hyperdense mass in endophytic type (rarer exophytic type grows subretinally causing retinal detachment)
  √ partial punctate / nodular calcification (50–75–95%)
    ◊ Retinoblastoma is the most common cause of orbital calcifications!
  √ dense vitreous (common)
  √ extraocular extension (in 25%): optic nerve enlargement, abnormal soft tissue in orbit, intracranial extension
  √ contrast enhancement usual
  √ ± macrophthalmia

MR:
  √ iso- to mildly hyperintense tumor on T1WI relative to vitreous + moderate to marked enhancement
  √ distinctly hypointense on T2WI (similar to uveal melanoma)
  √ subretinal exudate usually hyperintense on T1WI + T2WI (proteinaceous fluid)

Cx: (1) Metastases to: meninges (via subarachnoid space), bone marrow, lung, liver, lymph nodes
(2) Radiation-induced sarcomas develop in 15–20%

Prognosis: spontaneous regression in 1%;
  √ calcifications = favorable prognostic sign
  √ contrast enhancement = poor prognostic sign

Mortality:
  (a) choroidal invasion: 65% if significant, 24% if slight
  (b) optic nerve invasion:
    <10% if not invaded
    15% if through lamina cribrosa
    44% if significantly posterior to lamina cribrosa
  (c) margin of resection not free of tumor: >65%

DDx: (1) Retinoma = retinocytoma (benign variant)
(2) Toxocara canis infection (no calcification)
(3) Retrolental fibroplasia (microphthalmia)
(4) Coats disease (subretinal exudation, no calcification)
(5) Norrie disease (retinal dysplasia)
(6) Persistent hyperplastic primary vitreous (hypoplastic globe, no calcification)

RETROLENTAL FIBROPLASIA

= RETINOPATHY OF PREMATURITY
= bilateral often asymmetric postnatal fibrovascular organization of vitreous humor, which usually leads to retinal detachment

Pathophysiology:
retinal vascularization occurs in 4th–9th months of fetal life progressing from the papilla to the periphery; vascularization is incomplete in premature neonates especially in temporal sectors

Predisposed: premature infants with respiratory distress syndrome requiring prolonged oxygen therapy

Severity directly related to:
  (1) degree of prematurity
  (2) birth weight
  (3) amount of oxygen used in therapy

• leukokoria in severe cases (traction retinal detachment, usually bilateral + temporal) [3–5% of all childhood leukokoria cases]
• Ophthalmoscopic stages:
  1st stage = arteriolar narrowing of most immature vessels at the border of the vascular-avascular retina (from spasm as a reaction to hyperoxygenation)
  2nd stage = dilatation + elongation + tortuosity of retinal vessels (after oxygen withdrawal)
  3rd stage = retinal neovascularization with growth into vitreous leads to vitreous hemorrhage
  4th stage = fibrosis with retraction of fibrovascular tissue + retinal detachment

√ bilateral microphthalmia ± retinal detachment

US:
  √ hyperechoic tracts extending from temporal side of periphery of retina to vitreous behind the lens

CT:
  √ dense vitreous bilaterally (neovascular ingrowth)
  √ ± dystrophic calcifications in choroid + lens (late stage)

MR:
  √ hyperintense vitreous on T1WI + T2WI (from chronic subretinal hemorrhage)
  √ hypointense retrolental mass (apposition of detached leaves of retina displaced from retinal pigment layer)

Prognosis:
  (1) spontaneous regression of vitreous neovascularization (85–95%) ± retinal detachment
  (2) progression to cicatricial stage characterized by formation of dense membrane of gray-white vascularized tissue in retrolental vitreous + retinal detachment + microphthalmia

DDx: (1) Retinoblastoma (calcifications in eye of normal size)

RHABDOMYOSARCOMA

Most common primary malignant orbital tumor in childhood
  ◊ 10% occur primarily in orbit
  ◊ 10% metastasize to / invade orbit

Incidence: 3–4% of all pediatric orbital masses

Histo: arising from undifferentiated mesenchyma of orbital soft tissues (not from striated muscle)
(1) embryonal type (75%)
(2) alveolar type (15%)
(3) pleomorphic type (10%)

Age at presentation: average 7 years; 90% by 16 years of age; M > F

Rarely associated with: neurofibromatosis

• rapidly progressive exophthalmos + proptosis of upper lid

Location: superior orbit / retrobulbar (71%), lid (22%), conjunctiva (7%)

√ large soft-tissue density mass with ill-defined margins (extraocular muscles not involved)
√ ± extension into preseptal space, adjacent sinus, nasal cavity, intracranial cavity with bony erosion
√ may show significant enhancement

US:
√ heterogeneous well-defined irregular mass of low to medium echogenicity

Metastases: lung, bone marrow, cervical lymph nodes (rare)

Prognosis: (1) 40% survival after exenteration
(2) 80–90% survival after radiation therapy (4,000–5,000 rad) + chemotherapy (vincristine, cyclophosphamide, Adriamycin®)

DDx: pseudotumor, lymphoma

UVEAL MELANOMA

Most common primary intraocular neoplasm in adult Caucasian

Age: 50–70 years

Location: choroid (85–93%) > ciliary body (4–9%) > iris (3–6%); almost always unilateral

• retinal detachment, vitreous hemorrhage
• astigmatism, glaucoma

US:
√ small flat hyperechoic solid mass

CT:
√ ill-defined hyperdense thickening of wall of globe with inward bulge

MR:
√ sharply circumscribed hyperintense lesion on T1WI (paramagnetic properties of melanin)

Metastases to: globe, optic nerve; liver, lung, subcutis

VARIX OF ORBIT

Etiology: (a) Congenital: venous malformation / venous wall weakness
(b) Acquired: intraorbital / intracranial AVM

• intermittent exophthalmos associated with straining
• frequent blindness

√ involvement of superior / inferior orbital vein; phleboliths rare
√ may produce bony erosion without sclerotic reaction
√ enlargement of mass during Valsalva maneuver / jugular vein compression
√ well-defined markedly enhancing mass
√ spontaneous thrombosis (common)

US:
√ anechoic tubular / oval structure ± thrombus
√ venous flow increasing with Valsalva

MR:
√ flow void (rapid flow) / flow-related enhancement (slow flow)

WARBURG DISEASE

= autosomal recessive syndrome characterized by
(1) bilateral persistent hyperplastic primary vitreous
(2) hydrocephalus, lissencephaly
(3) mental retardation

• bilateral leukokoria + microphthalmia

DIFFERENTIAL DIAGNOSIS OF EAR, NOSE, AND THROAT DISORDERS

FACIAL NERVE PARALYSIS

A. INTRACRANIAL SEGMENT
   (a) intraaxial
      brainstem glioma, metastasis, multiple sclerosis, cerebrovascular accident, hemorrhage
      • cranial nerve VI also involved
   (b) extraaxial
      CPA tumor (acoustic neuroma, meningioma, epidermoid), CPA inflammation (sarcoidosis, basilar meningitis), vertebrobasilar dolichoectasia, AVM, aneurysm
      • cranial nerve VIII also involved

B. INTRATEMPORAL SEGMENT
   fracture, cholesteatoma, paraganglioma, hemangioma, facial nerve schwannoma, metastasis, Bell palsy, otitis media
   • loss of lacrimation, hyperacusis, loss of taste

C. EXTRACRANIAL PAROTID SEGMENT
   forceps delivery, penetrating facial trauma, parotid surgery, parotid malignancy, malignant otitis externa
   • preservation of lacrimation, stapedius reflex, taste

EAR

Hearing Deficit

A. CONDUCTIVE HEARING LOSS
   • decrease in air conduction via EAC, tympanic membrane, ossicular chain, oval window (sound via headphones)
   • normal bone conduction (sound via bone oscillator)
      (a) trauma: incudostapedial / malleoincudal subluxation; incus dislocation; stapes dislocation; stapes / malleus fracture
      (b) destruction of ossicular chain: otitis media
      (c) restriction of ossicular chain: fenestral otosclerosis
   ◊ CT is the modality of choice!

B. SENSORINEURAL HEARING LOSS (most common)
   • elevated conduction thresholds for bone + air
   (a) sensory / **cochlear SNHL** = damage to cochlea / organ of Corti (less common)
      – bony labyrinth
         (1) demineralization: otosclerosis (otospongiosis), osteogenesis imperfecta, Paget disease, syphilis
         (2) congenital deformity: cochlear dys- / aplasia, Michel anomaly, Mondini dysplasia, enlarged vestibular aqueduct syndrome, X-linked sensorineural hearing loss
         (3) traumatic lesion: transverse fracture, perilymphatic fistula, cochlear concussion
         (4) destructive lesion: inflammatory lesion, neoplastic lesion
         ◊ CT is the modality of choice!
      – membranous labyrinth
         (1) enhancement: labyrinthitis, Cogan syndrome (early phase of autoimmune interstitial keratitis), intralabyrinthine schwannoma, site of postinflammatory perilymphatic fistula
         (2) obliteration: labyrinthitis ossificans, Cogan syndrome (late phase)
         (3) hemorrhage: trauma, labyrinthitis, coagulopathy, tumor fistulization
         (4) Ménière disease (vertigo + fluctuating sensory sensorineural hearing loss)
         ◊ MRI is the modality of choice!
   (b) neural / **retrocochlear SNHL** (more common)
      = abnormalities of neurons of spiral ganglion + central auditory pathways
      – IAC / cerebellopontine angle
         (1) neoplastic lesions: vestibular / trigeminal schwannoma (acoustic neuroma in 1%), meningioma, arachnoid cyst, epidermoid cyst, leptomeningeal carcinomatosis, lymphoma, lipoma, hemangioma
         (2) nonneoplastic lesion: sarcoidosis, meningitis, vascular loop, siderosis
      – intraaxial auditory pathway (brainstem, thalamus, temporal lobe)
         (1) ischemic lesion
         (2) neoplastic lesion
         (3) traumatic lesion
         (4) demyelinating lesion
      ◊ MRI is the modality of choice!

Pulsatile Tinnitus ± Vascular Tympanic Membrane

= perception of a rhythmic cardiac synchronous sound of ringing / buzzing / roaring

A. No abnormality (20%)

B. Congenital vascular variants (21%)
   1. Aberrant ICA
      = result of anastomosis of enlarged inferior tympanic artery with enlarged caroticotympanic artery when cervical ICA is underdeveloped
   2. Dehiscent jugular bulb
   3. High-riding nondehiscent jugular bulb (= jugular megabulb)
      √ high jugular bulb with diverticulum projecting cephalad into petrous temporal bone

C. Acquired vascular lesions (25%)
   1. Dural AVM
   2. Extracranial arteriovenous fistula
   3. High-grade stenotic vascular lesion: carotid artery atherosclerosis, fibromuscular dysplasia, carotid artery dissection
   4. Aneurysm involving horizontal segment of petrous ICA

D. Temporal bone tumors (31%)
   1. Paraganglioma (27%): glomus tympanicum, glomus jugulare
   2. Meningioma
   3. Hemangioma

E. Miscellaneous
   1. Cholesterol granuloma

Temporal Bone Sclerosis

1. Otosclerosis = otospongiosis
2. **Paget disease** = osteoporosis circumscripta
   • sensorineural / mixed hearing loss (cochlear involvement / stapes fixation in oval window)
   √ usually lytic changes beginning in petrous pyramid + progressing laterally; otic capsule last to be affected
   √ calvarial changes ± basilar impression
3. **Fibrous dysplasia**
   monostotic with temporal bone involvement
   • painless mastoid swelling
   • conductive hearing loss (from narrowing of EAC / middle ear)
   √ homogeneously dense thickened bone (fibro-osseous tissue less dense than calvarial bone)
   √ expanded bone with preserved cortex
   √ lytic lesions (less frequent)
   √ sparing of membranous labyrinth, facial nerve canal, IAC is the rule
4. Osteogenesis imperfecta
   √ changes similar to otosclerosis
   van der Hoeve syndrome = osteogenesis imperfecta + otosclerosis + blue sclera
5. Meningioma
6. Otosyphilis: labyrinthitis + osteitis
7. Metastasis
8. Ossifying fibroma
9. Osteosarcoma
10. Osteopetrosis

External Ear Masses

A. CONGENITAL
   1. Atresia

B. INFLAMMATORY
   1. Malignant external otitis
   2. **Keratosis obturans**
      bilateral process in association with chronic sinusitis + bronchiectasis
      Age: <40 years
   3. Cholesteatoma

C. BENIGN TUMOR
   1. **Exostosis** = surfer's ear
      Cause: irritation by cold water
      √ bony mass projecting into EAC; often multiple + bilateral
   2. **Osteoma**
      √ may invade adjacent bone; single in EAC / mastoid
   3. **Ceruminoma**
      from apocrine + sebaceous glands; bone erosion mimics malignancy

D. MALIGNANT TUMOR
   1. Squamous cell carcinoma
      • often long history of chronic suppurative otitis media = "malignant otitis"
   2. Basal cell carcinoma
   3. Melanoma, adenocarcinoma, adenoid cystic carcinoma
   4. Metastases
      (a) hematogenous: breast, prostate, lung, kidney, thyroid
      (b) direct spread: skin, parotid, nasopharynx, brain, meninges
      (c) systemic: leukemia, lymphoma, myeloma
   5. Histiocytosis X: in 15% of patients

Middle Ear Masses

A. CONGENITAL
   1. **Aberrant internal carotid artery**
      • vascular tympanic membrane
      • pulsatile tinnitus
      √ tubular soft-tissue density entering middle ear cavity posterolateral to cochlea, crossing mesotympanum along cochlear promontory, exiting anteromedial to become horizontal portion of carotid canal
      √ protrusion into middle ear without bony margin
   2. Dehiscent jugular bulb

B. INFLAMMATORY
   1. Cholesteatoma
   2. Cholesterol granuloma
   3. Granulation tissue
      √ linear strands partially opacifying middle ear cavity without bony erosion

C. BENIGN TUMOR
   1. Adenomatous tumor (mixed pattern type)
      √ intense enhancement
      √ no osseous destruction
   2. Glomus tumor (multiple in 10%; 8% malignant)
      (a) Glomus tympanicum: at cochlear promontory
         √ seldom erodes bone
      (b) Glomus jugulare: at jugular foramen
         √ invasion of middle ear from below
         √ destruction of bony roof of jugular fossa + bony spur separating vein from carotid artery
   3. Facial nerve schwannoma
      • persistent Bell palsy (in 5% caused by neurinoma)
      Location: intracanalicular > IAC
      √ tubular mass in enlarged / scalloped facial canal
   4. Ossifying hemangioma
   5. Choristoma = ectopic mature salivary tissue
   6. Endolymphatic sac tumor
      √ arises from region of vestibular aqueduct
   7. Meningioma

D. MALIGNANT TUMOR
   1. Squamous cell carcinoma
   2. Metastasis

3. Rhabdomyosarcoma
   Location: orbit > nasopharynx > ear
4. Adenocarcinoma (rare), adenoid cystic carcinoma

Mass on Promontory

[promontory = bone over basal turn of cochlea]
1. Glomus tympanicum
2. Congenital cholesteatoma
3. Aberrant carotid artery
4. Persistent stapedial artery

Inner Ear Masses

A. CONGENITAL
   1. Congenital / primary cholesteatoma = epidermoid tumor (3rd most common CPA tumor)

B. INFLAMMATION
   1. Cholesterol granuloma
   2. Petrous apex mucocele

C. TUMOR
   1. Glomus jugulare tumor
   2. Hemangioma, fibro-osseous lesion
   3. Metastasis
   4. Facial nerve neurinoma
   5. Large CPA tumors: acoustic neuroma, meningioma (2nd most common CPA tumor)

SINUSES

Opacification of Maxillary Sinus

A. WITHOUT BONE DESTRUCTION
   1. Sinus aplasia / hypoplasia
      Age: NOT routinely visualized at birth, by age 6 antral floor at level of middle turbinate, by age 15 of adult size
      Location: uni- / bilateral
      √ depression of orbital floor with enlargement of orbit
      √ lateral displacement of lateral wall of nasal fossa with large turbinate
   2. Maxillary dentigerous cyst
      usually containing a tooth / crown; without tooth = primordial dentigerous cyst
   3. Ameloblastoma
   4. Acute sinusitis
      √ air-fluid level

B. WITH BONE DESTRUCTION
   1. Maxillary sinus tumor
   2. Infection: aspergillosis, mucormycosis, TB, syphilis
   3. Wegener granulomatosis; lethal midline granuloma
   4. Blowout fracture

Paranasal Sinus Masses

1. Mucocele
   Cause: obstruction of a paranasal sinus
   √ ± bone remodeling / sinus expansion
2. Mucus retention cyst
   Cause: obstruction of small seromucinous gland
   Location: commonly in floor of maxilla
   √ smoothly marginated soft-tissue mass
3. Sinonasal polyp
4. Antrochoanal polyp
5. Inverting papilloma
6. Sinusitis
7. Carcinoma

Granulomatous Lesions of Sinuses

A. Chronic irritants
   1. Beryllium
   2. Chromate salts

B. Infection
   1. Tuberculosis
   2. Actinomycosis
   3. Rhinoscleroma
   4. Yaws
   5. Blastomycosis
   6. Leprosy
   7. Rhinosporidiosis
   8. Syphilis
   9. Leishmaniosis
   10. Glanders

C. Autoimmune disease
   1. Wegener granulomatosis

D. Lymphoma-like lesions
   1. Midline granuloma

E. Unclassified
   1. Sarcoidosis

Hyperdense Sinus Secretions

1. Inspissated secretions
2. Fungal sinusitis
3. Hemorrhage into sinus
4. Chronic sinusitis infected with bacteria (in particular in very long-standing disease / cystic fibrosis)

Opacified Sinus & Expansion / Destruction

mnemonic: "PLUMP FACIES"

Plasmacytoma
Lymphoma
Unknown etiology: Wegener granulomatosis
Mucocele
Polyp
Fibrous dysplasia, **F**ibroma (ossifying)
Aneurysmal bone cyst, **A**ngiofibroma
Cancer
Inverting papilloma
Esthesioneuroblastoma
Sarcoma: ie, rhabdomyosarcoma

NOSE

Nasal Vault Masses

A. BENIGN
   1. Sinonasal polyp
   2. Inverted papilloma
   3. Hemangioma
      • history of epistaxis
   4. Pyogenic granuloma
      √ pedunculated lobular mass
   5. Granuloma gravidarum
      = nasal hemangioma of pregnancy

ENT

6. Hemangiopericytoma
7. Juvenile nasopharyngeal angiofibroma
   √ arises in superior nasopharynx with extension into nose via posterior choana

B. MALIGNANT
1. Lymphoma
2. Melanoma
3. Vascular metastasis

Mass in Nasopharynx

mnemonic: "NASAL PIPE"

Nasopharyngeal carcinoma
Angiofibroma (juvenile)
Spine / skull fracture
Adenoids
Lymphoma
Polyp
Infection
Plasmacytoma
Extension of neoplasm (sphenoid / ethmoid sinus ca.)

Congenital Midline Nasal Mass

= result of faulty regression of embryologic dural diverticulum through foramen cecum + fonticulus frontalis (= nasofrontal fontanel) from the prenasal space

Frequency: 1:20,000 to 1:40,000 births

1. Dermoid cyst
2. Epidermoid cyst
3. Nasal glioma = nasal cerebral heterotopia
4. Nasal encephalocele
5. Hemangioma / lymphangioma
6. Dacryocystocele
7. Dacryocystitis

PHARYNX

Parapharyngeal Space Mass

A. BENIGN
1. Asymmetric pterygoid venous plexus
   √ racemose, enhancing area along medial border of lateral pterygoid muscle
2. Abscess
   Origin: pharyngitis (most common), dental infection, parotid calculus disease, penetrating trauma
3. Atypical second branchial cleft cyst
   Age: child / young adult
   • protruding parotid gland
   • bulging posterolateral pharyngeal wall
   √ cystic mass projecting from deep margin of faucial tonsil toward skull base
4. Pleomorphic adenoma of ectopic salivary tissue / of deep lobe of parotid gland (common)
5. Schwannoma, neurofibroma
   Origin: usually from cranial nerve X
   √ carotid artery pushed anteriorly
6. Paraganglioma
   √ posterior to carotid artery
   √ extremely vascular (numerous flow voids)
7. Lipoma

B. MALIGNANT
1. Squamous cell carcinoma
   √ direct extension from pharyngeal mucosal space
   √ vertical extension to skull base / hyoid bone
2. Salivary gland malignancy

Pharyngeal Mucosal Space Mass

1. Asymmetric fossa of Rosenmüller
   = lateral pharyngeal recess = asymmetry in amount of lymphoid tissue
2. Tonsillar abscess
   • sore throat, fever, painful swallowing
3. Postinflammatory retention cyst
   √ 1–2-cm well-circumscribed cystic mass
4. Postinflammatory calcification
   • remote history of severe pharyngitis
   √ multiple clumps of calcification
5. Benign mixed tumor
   • pedunculated mass arising from minor salivary glands
   √ oval / round well-circumscribed mass protruding into airway
6. Squamous cell carcinoma
   √ infiltrating mass with epicenter medial to + invading parapharyngeal space
   √ middle-ear fluid (eustachian tube malfunction)
   √ cervical adenopathy
7. Non-Hodgkin lymphoma
8. Minor salivary gland malignancy
9. Thornwaldt cyst

Masticator Space Mass

A BENIGN
1. Asymmetric accessory parotid gland
   Incidence: 21% of general population
   Location: usually on surface of masseter muscle
   √ prominent salivary gland tissue
2. Benign masseteric hypertrophy
   Cause: bruxism (= nocturnal gnashing of teeth)
   √ homogeneous enlargement of one / both masseters
3. Odontogenic abscess / mandibular cysts
   • bad dentition + trismus
4. Lymphangioma, hemangioma

B. MALIGNANT
1. Sarcoma (chondro-, osteo-, soft-tissue sarcoma, especially rhabdomyosarcoma in children)
   √ infiltrating mass with mandibular destruction
2. Malignant schwannoma
   √ tubular mass along cranial nerve V_3
3. Non-Hodgkin lymphoma
4. Infiltrating squamous cell carcinoma
   √ extending from pharyngeal mucosa
5. Salivary gland malignancy (mucoepidermoid carcinoma, adenoid cystic carcinoma)
   √ extending from parotid gland

N.B.: (1) check course of V_3 to foramen ovale for skull base extension to Meckel cave area + cavernous sinus
(2) check for extension to pterygopalatine fossa to infraorbital fissure into orbit

Carotid Space Mass
A. VASCULAR LESION
1. Ectatic common / internal carotid artery
2. Carotid artery aneurysm / pseudoaneurysm
3. Asymmetric internal jugular vein
4. Jugular vein thrombosis

B. BENIGN TUMOR
1. Paraganglioma (carotid body tumor + glomus jugulare + glomus vagale)
2. Schwannoma
√ displacement of carotid artery anteromedially + internal jugular vein posteriorly
√ well-encapsulated mass
3. Neurofibroma of cranial nerves IX, X, XI
4. Branchial cleft cyst

C. MALIGNANT TUMOR
1. Nodal metastasis from squamous cell carcinoma to interior jugular chain (common)
√ encasement of carotid artery = inoperable
2. Non-Hodgkin lymphoma

Retropharyngeal Space Mass
A. INFECTION
1. Reactive lymphadenopathy
√ nodes >10 mm in diameter
2. Abscess: √ bow-tie shape

B. BENIGN TUMOR
1. Hemangioma
2. Lipoma

C. MALIGNANT TUMOR
1. Metastasis to retropharyngeal nodes from nasopharyngeal squamous cell carcinoma, melanoma, thyroid carcinoma
N.B.: sentinel node of Rouviere (= lateral retropharyngeal node) is an early sign of nasopharyngeal cancer before primary mass becomes obvious
2. Non-Hodgkin lymphoma
3. Direct invasion by squamous cell carcinoma

Prevertebral Space Mass
A. PSEUDOTUMOR
1. Anterior disk herniation
2. Vertebral body osteophyte

B. INFLAMMATION
1. Vertebral body osteomyelitis
2. Abscess
√ extension from retropharyngeal space / osteomyelitis / diskitis / epidural abscess)

C. TUMOR
1. Chordoma
2. Vertebral body metastasis: lung, breast, prostate, non-Hodgkin lymphoma, myeloma

√ metastases to prevertebral space = inoperable

LARYNX
Vocal Cord Paralysis
1. Birth injury
2. Arnold-Chiari malformation
3. Intracranial tumor
4. Mediastinal mass / cyst
5. Vascular ring
6. Thyroidectomy
7. Malignancy

√ fixed vocal cords (fluoroscopy)

Epiglottic Enlargement
A. NORMAL VARIANT
1. Prominent normal epiglottis
2. Omega epiglottis

B. INFLAMMATION
1. Acute / chronic epiglottitis
2. Angioneurotic edema
3. Stevens-Johnson syndrome
4. Caustic ingestion
5. Radiation therapy

C. MASSES
1. Epiglottic cyst
2. Aryepiglottic cyst
3. Foreign body

Aryepiglottic Cyst
1. Retention cyst
2. Lymphangioma
3. Cystic hygroma
4. Thyroglossal cyst

• may be symptomatic at birth
√ well-defined mass in aryepiglottic fold

Laryngeal Neoplasms
A. SQUAMOUS CELL CARCINOMA (95–98%)
• endoscopically visible due to mucosal involvement

B. NON-SQUAMOUS CELL NEOPLASMS (2–5%)
malignant:benign = 1:1
(a) vasoformative tumor 33%
BENIGN
1. Hemangioma
2. Lymphangioma
3. Angiofibroma
4. Angiomatosis
5. Granuloma pyogenicum
6. Arteriovenous fistula
7. Phlebectasia, telangiectasia

MALIGNANT
1. Angiosarcoma (Kaposi sarcoma)
Location: epiglottis (most frequent)
√ intensely enhancing mass
2. Hemangiopericytoma

(b) chondrogenic tumor 20%
1. Chondroma
2. Chondrosarcoma
3. Osteosarcoma

ENT

(c) hematopoietic tumor 12%
1. Hodgkin / non-Hodgkin lymphoma / leukemia
2. Plasmacytoma
3. Pseudolymphoma

(d) salivary gland tumor 10%
1. Pleomorphic adenoma
2. Adenoid cystic carcinoma
3. Mucoepidermoid carcinoma
4. Adenocarcinoma

(e) fatty-tissue tumor 7%
1. Lipoma
2. Liposarcoma

(f) metastasis 7%
skin (melanoma) > kidney > breast > lung > prostate > colon > stomach > ovary

(g) neurogenic tumor 5%
(h) myogenic tumor 2%
(i) fibrohistiocytic tumor 2%

AIRWAYS

Inspiratory Stridor in Children

1. Croup
2. Congenital subglottic stenosis
3. Subglottic hemangioma
4. Airway foreign body
5. Esophageal foreign body
6. Epiglottitis

Airway Obstruction in Children

Nasopharyngeal Narrowing

(a) Congenital: Choanal atresia, choanal stenosis, encephalocele
(b) Inflammatory: Adenoidal enlargement, polyps
(c) Neoplastic: Juvenile angiofibroma, rhabdomyosarcoma, teratoma, neuroblastoma, lymphoepithelioma
(d) Traumatic: Foreign body, hematoma, rhinolith

Oropharyngeal Narrowing

(a) Congenital: Glossoptosis + micrognathia (Pierre Robin, Goldenhar, Treacher Collins syndrome), macroglossia (cretinism, Beckwith-Wiedemann syndrome)
(b) Inflammatory: Abscess, tonsillar hypertrophy
(c) Neoplastic: Lingular tumor / cyst
(d) Traumatic: Hematoma, foreign body

Retropharyngeal Narrowing

= potential space (normally <3/4 of AP diameter of adjacent cervical spine in infants / <3 mm in older children)
(a) Congenital: Branchial cleft cyst, ectopic thyroid
(b) Inflammatory: Retropharyngeal abscess
(c) Neoplastic: Cystic hygroma (originating in posterior cervical triangle with extension toward midline + into mediastinum), neuroblastoma, neurofibromatosis, hemangioma
(d) Traumatic: Hematoma, foreign body
(e) Metabolic: Hypothyroidism

Vallecular Narrowing

= valleys on each side of glossoepiglottic folds between base of tongue + epiglottis
(a) Congenital: Congenital cyst, ectopic thyroid, thyroglossal cyst
(b) Inflammatory: Abscess
(c) Neoplastic: Teratoma
(d) Traumatic: Foreign body, hematoma

Supraglottic Narrowing

= area between epiglottis and true vocal cords
(a) Congenital: Aryepiglottic fold cyst
(b) Inflammatory: Acute bacterial epiglottitis, angioneurotic edema
(c) Neoplastic: Retention cyst, cystic hygroma, neurofibroma
(d) Traumatic: Foreign body, hematoma, radiation, caustic ingestion
(e) Idiopathic: Laryngomalacia

Glottic Narrowing

= area of true vocal cords
(a) Congenital: Laryngeal atresia, laryngeal stenosis, laryngeal web (anterior commissure)
(b) Neoplastic: Laryngeal papillomatosis
(c) Neurogenic: Vocal cord paralysis (most common)
(d) Traumatic: Foreign body, hematoma

Subglottic Narrowing

= short segment between undersurface of true vocal cords + inferior margin of cricoid cartilage is the narrowest portion of child's airway
(a) Congenital: Congenital subglottic stenosis
(b) Inflammatory: Croup
(c) Neoplastic: Hemangioma, papillomatosis
(d) Traumatic: Acquired stenosis (result of prolonged endotracheal intubation in 5%), granuloma
(e) Idiopathic: Mucocele = mucous retention cyst (rare complication of prolonged endotracheal intubation)

NECK

Solid Neck Mass

Solid Neck Mass In Neonate

1. Cystic hygroma
2. Hemangioma
3. Neuroblastoma
4. Teratoma
5. Fibromatosis colli

Solid Neck Mass in Childhood

1. Lymphadenopathy
2. Fibromatosis colli

3. Aggressive fibromatosis
4. Malignancy: neuroblastoma (most common), lymphoma, embryonal rhabdomyosarcoma
5. Teratoma
6. Hemangioma
7. **Cervicothoracic lipoblastomatosis**
   (a) lipoblastoma = circumscribed encapsulated form (2/3)
   (b) lipoblastomatosis = diffuse infiltrative form (1/3)
   Histo: mature + immature fat cells
   √ regions of fat attenuation separated by septa
   √ NO enhancement
8. Lipoma
9. Thyroid mass / lingual thyroid
10. Parathyroid adenoma
11. Ectopic thymus

Lymph Node Enlargement of Neck

A. NORMAL LYMPH NODES
   √ few small oval hypoechoic
   √ ± central linear echogenicity (= invaginating hilar fat)
   √ larger in transverse than anteroposterior dimension
B. CERVICAL ADENITIS
   Location: posterior cervical triangle
   1. Tuberculous adenitis
      √ multichambered centrally hypoattenuating mass
      √ thick enhancing rim
      √ peripheral calcifications
C. MALIGNANT LYMPH NODES
   √ increased anteroposterior diameter
   √ prominent calcifications suggestive of medullary thyroid cancer
   √ axial diameter of >15 in jugulodigastric region / >11 mm elsewhere (in squamous cell carcinoma)
   CT:
   √ marginal enhancement
   √ central necrosis (regardless of size)
   √ fuzzy borders as sign of extracapsular extension

Low-density Nodes with Peripheral Enhancement

1. Tuberculosis
2. Metastatic malignancy
3. Lymphoma
4. Inflammatory conditions

Lymph Node Metastasis by Location

@ SUPRACLAVICULAR
head & neck, lung, breast, esophagus
@ INTERNAL JUGULAR
supraglottic larynx, esophagus, thyroid
@ MIDJUGULAR
tongue, pharynx, supraglottic larynx
@ JUGULODIGASTRIC
nasopharynx, oropharynx, tonsils, parotid gland, supraglottic larynx
@ SUBMANDIBULAR
skin, submandibular gland, base of tongue
@ POSTERIOR TRIANGLE
nasopharynx, base of tongue
@ LATERAL PHARYNGEAL
nasopharynx, oropharynx

Congenital Cystic Lesions of Neck

1. Thyroglossal duct cyst
   Location: anterior cervical triangle close to midline between foramen cecum + thyroid isthmus
2. Lymphangioma / cystic hygroma
   Location: mostly in posterior cervical triangle, occasionally in floor of mouth / tongue
3. Branchial cleft anomalies
   • often noted during upper respiratory infection
   (a) 2nd branchial cleft cyst
      Location: near angle of mandible anterior to sternocleidomastoid muscle
   (b) branchial cleft fistula
      Location: apex of piriform sinus to thyroid
4. Cervical dermoid / epidermoid cyst
   Location: floor of mouth
5. Cervical thymic cyst
6. **Parathyroid cyst**
   Age: 30–50 years
   • hormonally inactive
   √ noncolloidal cyst near lower pole of thyroid gland
7. **Cervical bronchogenic cyst**
   Cause: anomalous foregut development
   Histo: columnar ciliated pseudostratified epithelial lining
   M:F = 3:1
   • draining sinus in suprasternal notch / supraclavicular area
   √ cyst up to 6 cm in diameter
   √ indentation of trachea
8. Laryngocele

Air-containing Masses of Neck

1. Laryngocele
2. Tracheal diverticulum
   arising from anterior wall of trachea close to thyroid
3. Zenker diverticulum
4. Lateral pharyngeal diverticulum
   located in tonsillar fossa / vallecula / pyriform fossa

SALIVARY GLANDS

Parotid Gland Enlargement

A. LOCALIZED INFLAMMATION / INFECTION
   1. Chronic recurrent sialadenitis
   2. Sialosis
   3. Sarcoidosis
   4. Tuberculosis
   5. Cat-scratch fever
   6. Syphilis
   7. Parotid abscess secondary to acute bacterial (suppurative) sialadenitis

ENT

8. Reactive adenopathy
9. Parotitis: mumps (most common parotid disease in children), HIV

B. SYSTEMIC AUTOIMMUNE RELATED DISEASE
1. Sjögren disease (= myoepithelial sialadenitis)
2. Mikulicz disease

C. NEOPLASM
Frequency: 90–95% occur in parotid gland, 5% in submandibular + sublingual glands; only 1% of all pediatric tumors!

(a) benign tumor
1. Pleomorphic / monomorphic adenoma
2. Cystadenolymphoma (= Warthin tumor)
3. Benign lymphoepithelial cysts (AIDS)
4. Lipoma
5. Facial nerve neurofibroma
6. Oncocytoma
7. Parotid hemangioma
8. Angiolipoma

(b) primary malignant tumor
1. Mucoepidermoid carcinoma
2. Adenoid cystic carcinoma (= cylindroma)
3. Malignant mixed tumor
4. Adenocarcinoma
5. Acinus cell carcinoma
6. Rhabdomyosarcoma

(c) metastatic tumor
◊ Parotid gland undergoes late encapsulation, which leads to incorporation of lymph nodes!
1. Squamous cell carcinoma
2. Melanoma of periauricular region
3. Non-Hodgkin lymphoma
4. Thyroid carcinoma

D. LYMPHOPROLIFERATIVE DISORDER
1. Lymphoma / leukemia
2. Primary non-Hodgkin lymphoma (MALToma)

E. CONGENITAL
1. First branchial cleft cyst

Multiple Lesions of Parotid Gland

1. Warthin tumor
2. Metastases to lymph nodes: squamous cell carcinoma of skin, malignant melanoma, non-Hodgkin lymphoma
3. Benign lymphoepithelial cysts (AIDS)

THYROID

Congenital Dyshormonogenesis

1. Trapping defect
= defective cellular uptake of iodine into thyroid, salivary glands, gastric mucosa;
◊ High doses of inorganic iodine facilitate diffusion into thyroid permitting a normal rate of thyroid hormone synthesis
◊ Normal ratio of iodine concentrations for gastric juice:plasma = 20:1
√ nearly entire dose of administered radioiodine is excreted within 24 hours

2. Organification defect
= deficient peroxidase activity, which catalyzes the oxidation of iodide by H_2O_2 to form monoiodotyrosine (MIT) / diiodotyrosine (DIT)
• high serum TSH
• low serum T_4
• diffuse symmetric thyromegaly
√ high thyroidal uptake of radioiodine / pertechnetate
√ rapid I-131 turnover
√ positive perchlorate washout test
Pendred syndrome = autosomal recessive trait of deficient peroxidase regeneration characterized by hypothyroidism + goiter + nerve deafness

3. Deiodinase (dehalogenase) defect
= deficient deiodination of MIT / DIT to release iodide, which is reutilized to synthesize thyroid hormone production
• hypothyroidism
• identification of MIT + DIT in serum + urine following administration of I-131
• "intrinsic" iodine deficiency goiter
√ high thyroidal I-131 uptake
√ rapid intrathyroidal turnover of I-131

4. Thyroxin-binding globulin (TBG) deficiency
• abnormal T_4 transport
• low bound serum T_4 concentration
• euthyroid

5. End-organ resistance to thyroid hormone
• high serum T_4
• euthyroid / hypothyroid
• growth retardation
√ goiter
√ stippled epiphyses

Hyperthyroidism

= excess thyroid hormone
• tachycardia, weight loss, muscle weakness, anxiety, decreased temperature tolerance

1. Graves disease = toxic diffuse goiter (most common)
2. Toxic multinodular goiter
3. Solitary toxic adenoma
4. Iodine-induced hyperthyroidism = Jod-Basedow
5. Thyroiditis
(a) Hashimoto thyroiditis = chronic lymphocytic thyroiditis
(b) Subacute thyroiditis = de Quervain thyroiditis
(c) Painless thyroiditis
US:
√ decrease in overall echogenicity
√ discrete nodules (50%)
6. Thyrotoxicosis medicamentosa / factitia surreptitious self-administration of thyroid hormones
7. Struma ovarii
= ovarian teratoma containing thyroid tissue
8. Hydatidiform mole / choriocarcinoma / testicular trophoblastic carcinoma
= stimulation of thyroid by hCG

9. Pituitary hyperthyroidism = pituitary neoplasm
   • ± acromegaly
   • ± hyperprolactinemia
10. Thyroid carcinoma / hyperfunctioning metastases very rare (25 cases)

Radioiodine Therapy for Hyperthyroidism

Dose: (a) empiric: 15–30 mCi
(b) calculation (Y): 80–160 μCi/gram

Calculation:
Dose [mCi] = (gland weight [gram] x Y [μCi/gram]) divided by 24-hour uptake

Hypothyroidism

A. PRIMARY HYPOTHYROIDISM (most common)
   = thyroid's inability to produce sufficient thyroid hormone
   1. Agenesis of thyroid
   2. Congenital dyshormonogenesis
   3. Chronic thyroiditis
   4. Previous radioiodine therapy
   5. Ectopic thyroid (1:4,000)
B. SECONDARY HYPOTHYROIDISM
   = failure of anterior pituitary to release sufficient quantities of TSH
   1. Sheehan syndrome
   2. Head trauma
   3. Pituitary tumor (primary / secondary)
   4. Aneurysm
   5. Surgery
C. TERTIARY / HYPOTHALAMIC HYPOTHYROIDISM
   = failure of hypothalamus to produce sufficient amounts of TRH

Decreased / No Uptake of Radiotracer

A. BLOCKED TRAPPING FUNCTION
   1. Iodine load (most common)
      = dilution of tracer within flooded iodine pool (from administration of radiographic contrast / iodine-containing medication)
      ◊ Suppression usually lasts for 4 weeks!
   2. Exogenous thyroid hormone (replacement therapy)
      suppresses TSH release
B. BLOCKED ORGANIFICATION
   1. Antithyroid medication (propylthiouracil (PTU) / methimazole) / goitrogenic substances
   √ Tc-99m uptake not inhibited
C. DIFFUSE PARENCHYMAL DESTRUCTION
   1. Subacute / chronic thyroiditis
D. HYPOTHYROIDISM
   1. Congenital hypothyroidism
   2. Surgical / radioiodine ablation
   3. Thyroid ectopia (struma ovarii, intrathoracic goiter)

mnemonic: "H MITTE"
Hypothyroidism (congenital)
Medications: PTU, perchlorate, Cytomel, Synthroid, Lugol solution
Iodine overload (eg, after IVP)
Thyroid ablation (surgery, radioiodine)
Thyroiditis (subacute / chronic)
Ectopic thyroid hormone production

Increased Uptake of Radiotracer

mnemonic: "THRILLEr"
Thyroiditis (early Hashimoto)
Hyperthyroidism (diffuse / nodular)
Rebound after withdrawal of antithyroid medication
Iodine starvation
Low serum albumin
Lithium therapy
Enzyme defect

Prominent Pyramidal Lobe

= distal remnant of thyroid descent tract
1. Normal variant: present in 10%
2. Hyperthyroidism
3. Thyroiditis
4. S/P thyroid surgery

DDx: esophageal activity from salivary excretion (disappears after glass of water)

Thyroid Calcifications

= benign calcifications = stromal calcifications in adenoma
√ coarse calcifications with rough outline
√ alignment along periphery of lesion
√ irregular distribution

Psammoma Bodies

= microcalcifications (<1 mm) occur in 54% of thyroid neoplasms
√ seen on xeroradiography in 94%
1. Papillary carcinoma 61%
2. Follicular carcinoma 26%
3. Undifferentiated carcinoma 13%

Cystic Areas in Thyroid

15–25% of all thyroid nodules!

A. Anechoic fluid + smooth regular wall:
   1. Colloid accumulation in goiter = colloid-filled dilated macrofollicle
   2. Simple cyst (extremely uncommon)
B. Solid particles + irregular outline:
   1. Hemorrhagic colloid nodule
   2. Hemorrhagic adenoma (30%)
   3. Necrotic papillary cancer (15%)
   4. Liquefaction necrosis in adenoma / goiter
   5. Abscess
   6. Cystic parathyroid tumor

• bloody fluid = benign / malignant lesion
• clear amber fluid = benign lesion
◊ Cystic lesions often yield insufficient numbers of cells!

Thyroid Nodule

Incidence: (increasing with age)
- (a) 4–8% by palpation (>2 cm in 2%, 1–2 cm in 5%, <1 cm in 1%); M:F = 1:4
- (b) 50% by autopsy / thyroid US if clinically normal: multiple in 38%, solitary in 12% (occult small cancers found in 4%)

A. THYROID ADENOMA
1. Adenomatous nodule (42–77%)
2. Follicular adenoma (15–40%)
3. Ectopic parathyroid adenoma

B. INFLAMMATION / HEMORRHAGE
1. Inflammatory lymph node in subacute + chronic thyroiditis
2. Hemorrhage / hematoma: frequently associated with adenomas
3. Abscess

C. CARCINOMA (8–17%)
◊ Higher risk of malignancy if
— patient <20 and >60 years of age
— Hx of radiation therapy to neck / upper chest
— family Hx of thyroid cancer / MEN syndrome
— new nodule in long-standing goiter
1. Thyroid carcinoma
   (a) papillary carcinoma (70%)
   (b) follicular (15%)
   (c) medullary carcinoma (5–10%)
   (d) anaplastic carcinoma (5%)
   (e) thyroid lymphoma (5%)
2. Nonthyroidal neoplasm
   metastasis from breast, lung, kidney, malignant melanoma, Hodgkin disease
3. Hürthle cell carcinoma
   √ very thin hypoechoic halo
4. Carcinoma in situ
   √ echogenic area inside a goiter nodule

<u>Role of fine-needle aspiration biopsy (FNAB)</u>:
(large-needle biopsy has more complications with no increase in diagnostic yield)
◊ FNAB as initial test leads to a better selection of patients for surgery than any other test!
Diagnostic accuracy of 70–97%:
- (a) 70–80% negative
- (b) 10% positive specimens (3–6% false-positive rate often due to Hashimoto thyroiditis)
- (c) 10–20% indeterminate

Up to 20% nondiagnostic (too few cells) material

<u>Role of imaging:</u>
◊ Imaging cannot reliably distinguish malignant + benign nodules!
- (a) radionuclide scanning
  — useful in indeterminate cytology
  ◊ Hyperfunctioning nodule is almost always benign!
- (b) ultrasound
  — best method to determine volume of nodule
  — useful during follow-up to distinguish nodular growth from intranodular hemorrhage

Discordant Thyroid Nodule

= nodule hyperfunctioning on Tc-99m pertechnetate scan + hypofunctioning on I-131 scan, which indicates reduced organification capacity

Cause:
1. Malignancy : follicular / papillary carcinoma
2. Benign lesion : follicular adenoma / adenomatous hyperplasia
   (autonomous nontoxic nodules have accelerated iodine turnover and discharge radioiodine as hormone within 24 hours)

Hot Thyroid Nodule

Incidence: 8% of Tc-99m pertechnetate scans
1. Adenoma
   (a) Autonomous adenoma = TSH-independent
   • euthyroid (80%), thyrotoxicosis (20%)
   √ partial / total suppression of remainder of gland
   (b) Adenomatous hyperplasia = TSH-dependent secondary to defective thyroid hormone production
2. Thyroid carcinoma (extremely rare)
   √ discordant uptake

N.B.: any hot nodule on Tc-99m scan must be imaged with I-123 to differentiate between autonomous or cancerous lesion

Cold Thyroid Nodule

A. BENIGN TUMOR
1. Nonfunctioning adenoma
2. Cyst (11–20%)
3. Involutional nodule
4. Parathyroid tumor

B. INFLAMMATORY MASS
1. Focal thyroiditis
2. Granuloma
3. Abscess

C. MALIGNANT TUMOR
1. Carcinoma
2. Lymphoma
3. Metastasis

US features of cold nodule:
√ hypoechoic (71%)
√ isoechoic (22%)
√ mixed echogenicity (4%)
√ hyperechoic (3%)
√ cystic (rarely malignant)

◊ A palpable cold nodule in a patient with Graves disease has a high likelihood of malignancy (4%)!

mnemonic: "CATCH LAMP"
Colloid cyst
Adenoma (most common)
Thyroiditis
Carcinoma
Hematoma

Lymphoma, **L**ymph node
Abscess
Metastasis (kidney, breast)
Parathyroid

Probability of a cold nodule to represent thyroid cancer:

◊ Solitary cold nodules by scintigraphy are multinodular by US in 20–25%!

(a) 15–25% for solitary cold nodule

(b) 1–6% for multiple nodules (DDx: multinodular goiter)

(c) with history of neck irradiation in childhood
- — solitary nodule found in 70% (cancerous in 31%)
- — multiple nodules found in 25% (cancerous in 37%)
- — normal thyroid scan found in 5% (cancer detected in 20%)

ANATOMY AND FUNCTION OF NECK ORGANS

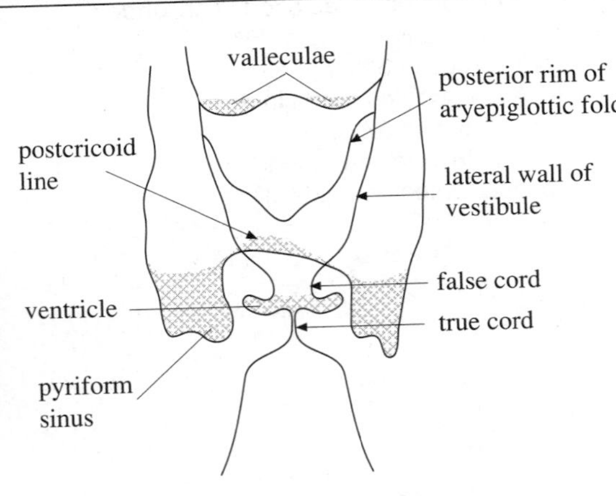

Frontal Laryngogram During Phonation

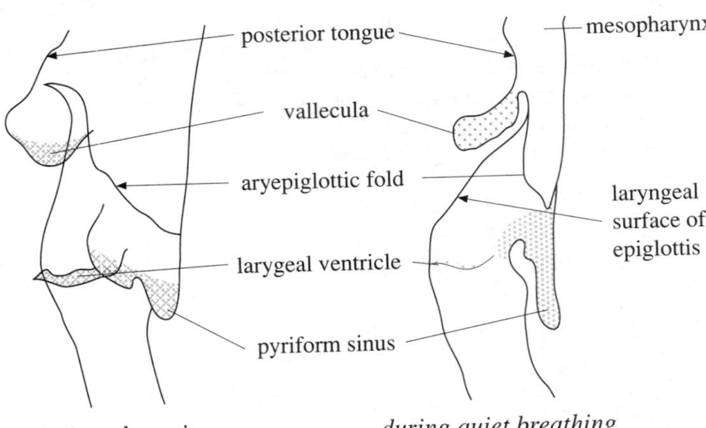

Lateral Laryngogram

PARANASAL SINUSES

Mucus production of 1 L/day; mucus blanket turns over every 20–30 minutes; irritants are propelled toward nasopharynx at a rate of 1 cm/minute

Maxillary Sinus

Size: 6–8 cm at birth
Walls: roof = floor of orbit; posterior wall abuts pterygopalatine fossa
Extension: 4–5 mm below level of nasal cavity by age 12
Ostium: maxillary ostium + infundibulum enter middle meatus within posterior aspect of hiatus semilunaris; additional ostia may be present
Plain film: present at birth; visible at 4–5 months; completely developed by 15 years of age
Variations: sinus hypoplasia in 9%; aplasia in 0.4%

Ethmoid Sinuses

Size: adult size by age 12; 3–18 air cells per side
Walls: roof = floor of anterior cranial fossa; lateral wall = lamina papyracea
Plain film: very small at birth; visible at 1 year of age; completely developed by puberty

(a) **anteromedial ethmoid air cells**
2–8 cells with a total area of 24 x 23 x 11 mm
Ostia: opening into anterior aspect of hiatus semilunaris of middle meatus (anterior group), opening into ethmoid bulla (middle group)

Agger nasi cells
= anteriormost ethmoid air cells in front of the attachment of middle turbinate to cribriform plate near the lacrimal duct
= anterior, lateral + inferior to frontoethmoidal recess = anteromedial margin of orbit
Prevalence: present in >90%

Ethmoidal bulla
= ethmoidal air cell above + posterior to infundibulum + hiatus semilunaris, located outside the lamina papyracea at the lateral wall of the middle meatus

Haller cells
= anterior ethmoid air cells inferolateral to ethmoidal bulla, on lateral wall of infundibulum, along inferior margin of orbit / roof of maxillary sinus, protruding into maxillary sinus
Prevalence: 10–45%

(b) **posterior ethmoid air cells**
1–8 cells, larger cells, total area smaller than that of anteromedial group
Location: behind the basal (= ground) lamella of the middle turbinate
Ostium: into superior meatus / supreme meatus, ultimately draining into sphenoethmoidal recess of nasal cavity

Onodi cell
= most posterior ethmoid air cell pneumatized into sphenoid bone ± surrounding the optic canal
Location: superolateral to sphenoid sinus

Frontal Sinus

Size: 28 x 24 x 20 mm in adults, rapid growth until the late teens
Walls: posterior wall = anterior cranial fossa; inferior wall = anterior portion of roof of orbit
Ostium: into frontal recess of middle meatus via frontoethmoidal recess (= nasofrontal duct)
Plain film: visible at age 6 years
Variations: sinus aplasia in up to 4% (in 90% with Down syndrome)

Sphenoid Sinus

Size: 20 x 23 x 17 mm in adults, small evagination of sphenoethmoidal recess at birth, invasion of sphenoid bone begins at age 5 years; aerated extensions into pterygoid plates (44%) + into clinoid processes (13%)

Walls: roof = floor of sella turcica; anterior wall shared with ethmoid sinuses; posterior wall = clivus; inferior wall = roof of nasopharynx

Ostium: 10 mm above sinus floor into sphenoethmoidal recess posterior to superior meatus at level of sphenopalatine foramen

Plain film: appears by 3 years of age; continues to grow posteriorly + inferiorly into the sella until adulthood

OSTIOMEATAL UNIT

= area of superomedial maxillary sinus + middle meatus as the common mucociliary drainage pathway of frontal maxillary, and anterior + middle ethmoid air cells into the nose

Coronal CT: visualized on two or three 3-mm-thick sections

Components:

1. Infundibulum
   = flattened conelike passage between inferomedial border of orbit / ethmoid bulla (laterally) + uncinate process (medially) + maxillary sinus (inferiorly) + hiatus semilunaris (superiorly)
2. Uncinate process
   = key bony structure in lateral nasal wall below hiatus semilunaris in middle meatus defines hiatus semilunaris together with adjacent ethmoid bulla
   √ pneumatized in <2.5% of patients
3. Ethmoid bulla
   √ located in cephalad recess of middle meatus
4. Hiatus semilunaris
   final segment for drainage of maxillary sinus; located just inferior to ethmoid bulla in middle meatus

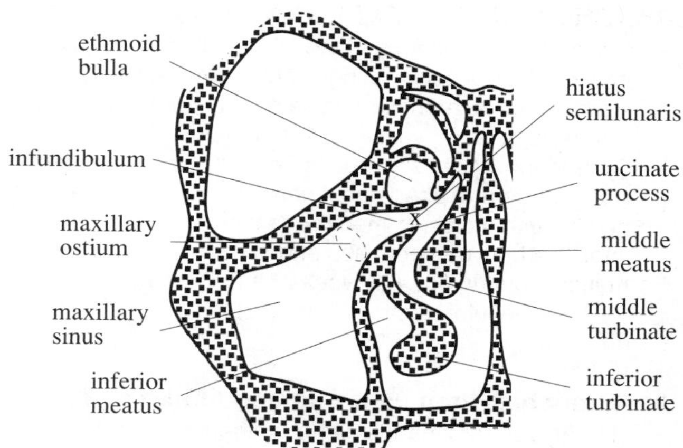

Coronal Scan of Ostiomeatal Unit

Ostia:

(1) multiple ostia from anterior ethmoid air cells (at its anterior aspect)

(2) maxillary ostium infundibulum (at its posterior aspect)

<u>Anatomic variations predisposing to ostiomeatal narrowing</u>:

1. Concha bullosa (4–15%) = aerated / pneumatized middle turbinate
2. Intralamellar cell = air cell within vertical portion of middle turbinate
3. Oversized ethmoid bulla
4. Haller cells
5. Uncinate process bulla
6. Bowed nasal septum
7. Paradoxical middle turbinate = convexity of turbinate directed toward lateral nasal wall (10–26%)
8. Deviation of uncinate process

◊ These conditions are not disease states per se!

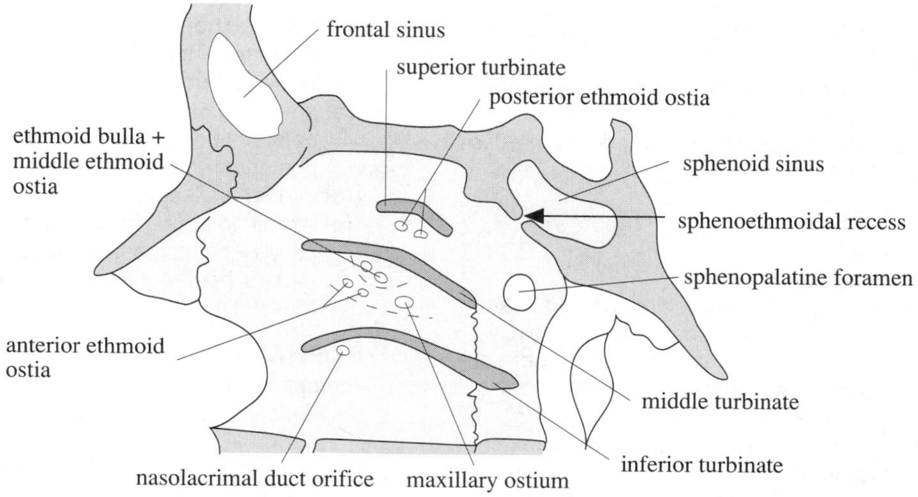

View of Lateral Nasal Wall (turbinates removed)

ENT

ENT

BRANCHIAL CLEFT DEVELOPMENT

— 6 paired branchial arches are responsible for formation of lower face + neck; recognizable by 4th week GA
— each branchial arch contains a central core of cartilage + muscle, a blood vessel, and a nerve
— 5 ectodermal "clefts" / grooves on outer aspect of neck + 5 endodermal pharyngeal pouches separate the 6 arches with a closing membrane located at the interface between pouches and clefts

Formation: during 4th–6th week of embryonic development

1st Branchial Arch = maxillomandibular arch

(a) large ventral / mandibular prominence
forms: mandible, incus, malleus, muscles of mastication
(b) small dorsal / maxillary prominence
forms: maxilla, zygoma, squamous portion of temporal bone, cheek, portions of external ear

nerve: mandibular division of trigeminal nerve
pouch forms: mastoid air cells + eustachian tube
cleft forms: external auditory canal + tympanic cavity

2nd Branchial Arch = hyoid arch

nerve: facial nerve
arch forms: thyroid gland, stapes, portions of external ear, muscles of facial expression
pouch forms: palatine tonsil + tonsillar fossa
cleft involutes completely by 9th fetal week; 2nd arch overgrows 2nd + 3rd + 4th clefts to form *cervical sinus* , which creates a tract that runs from supraclavicular area just lateral to carotid sheath, turns medially at mandibular angle between external + internal carotid artery, terminates in tonsillar fossa

3rd Branchial Arch

sinks into retrohyoid depression
nerve: glossopharyngeal nerve
arch forms: glossoepiglottic fold, superior constrictor m., internal carotid a., parts of hyoid bone
pouch forms:
(a) thymus gland, which descends into mediastinum by 9th fetal week
(b) inferior parathyroid glands passing down with the thymus

4th Branchial Arch

sunk into retrohyoid depression
nerve: superior laryngeal branch of vagus nerve
arch forms: epiglottis + aryepiglottic folds, thyroid cartilage, cricothyroid m., left component of aortic arch, right component of right proximal subclavian a.
pouch forms: superior parathyroid glands, apex of piriform fossa
cleft forms: ultimobranchial body, which provides parafollicular = "C" cells of thyroid

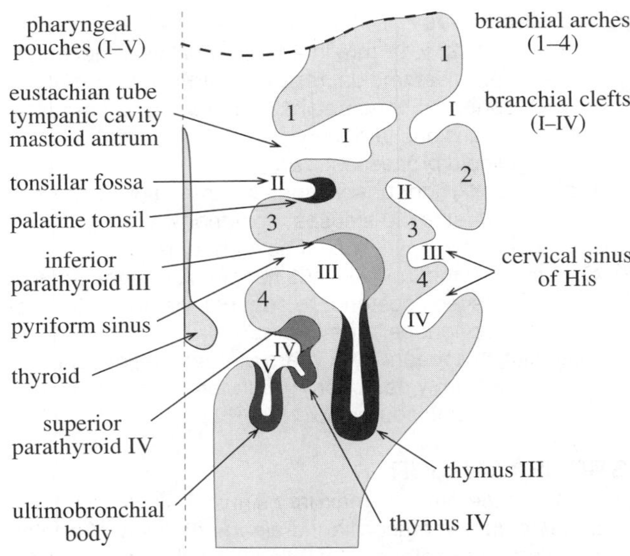

Branchial Apparatus

5th + 6th Branchial Arches

cannot be recognized externally
nerve: recurrent laryngeal branch of vagus nerve

ORAL CAVITY

comprises lip, upper + lower gingiva, buccal mucosa, hard palate, floor of mouth, anterior 2/3 of tongue

OROPHARYNX

consists of
(a) pharyngeal wall between nasopharynx + pharyngoepiglottic fold
(b) soft palate
(c) tonsillar region
(d) tongue base

Borders:
(a) superior: soft palate and Passavant ridge (= ridge of pharyngeal muscle that opposes the soft palate when soft palate is elevated)
(b) anterior: plane that joins the posterior border of soft palate, anterior tonsillar pillars, circumvallate papillae
(c) posterior: posterior pharyngeal wall
(d) inferior: vallecula
(e) lateral: tonsillar region consisting of anterior tonsillar pillar (= palatoglossus muscle) + palatine / faucial tonsil + posterior tonsillar pillar (= palatopharyngeus muscle)

HYPOPHARYNX

= compartment of aerodigestive tract between hyoid bone + inferior aspect of cricoid cartilage

1. Pyriform sinuses
   = two symmetric lateral stalactites of air hanging from hypopharynx behind larynx
   — inferior wall: level of cricoarytenoid joint

— anteromedial wall: lateral wall of aryepiglottic fold
— lateral wall: abuts posterior ala of thyroid cartilage
— posterior wall: most lateral aspect of posterior hypopharyngeal wall

2. Postcricoid area = pharyngoesophageal junction extends from level of arytenoid cartilages to inferior border of cricoid cartilage
   — anterior wall of hypopharynx = posterior wall of lower larynx = "party wall"
3. Posterior hypopharyngeal wall extends from level of valleculae to cricoarytenoid joints

LARYNX

Vertical length: 44 mm (males), 36 mm (females), at 4th–6th cervical vertebrae

A. SUPRAGLOTTIS
extends from tongue base + valleculae to laryngeal ventricle

1. Vestibule
   = airspace within supraglottic larynx
2. Epiglottis
   = leaf-shaped cartilage that functions as a lid to endolarynx
   (a) petiole = stem of epiglottis
   (b) thyroepiglottic ligament = connects petiole to thyroid cartilage inferiorly
   (c) hyoepiglottic ligament = connects epiglottis to hyoid bone anteriorly, covered by a mucosal fold between the valleculae (glossoepiglottic fold)
   (d) "free margin" = superior portion of epiglottis
3. False vocal cords
   = ventricular folds = inferior continuation of aryepiglottic folds = mucosal surface of ventricular ligaments; forming superior border of laryngeal ventricle
4. Arytenoid cartilages
5. Aryepiglottic folds
   = mucosal reflections between cephalad portion (= arytenoid processes) of arytenoid cartilage + inferolateral margin of epiglottis
   √ soft-tissue folds forming border between lateral pyriform sinuses + central laryngeal lumen
6. Laryngeal ventricle
   = fusiform fossa bounded by crescentic edge of false cords superiorly + straight margin of true cords inferiorly
   √ generally not visible on axial scans
7. Preepiglottic space
   √ low-density tissue between anterior margin of epiglottis + thyroid cartilage
8. Paralaryngeal space
   √ low-density tissue between true + false cords and thyroid cartilage
   √ continuous with preepiglottic space anteriorly + aryepiglottic folds superiorly

B. GLOTTIS

1. True vocal cords
   = extend from vocal process of arytenoid cartilage to anterior commissure

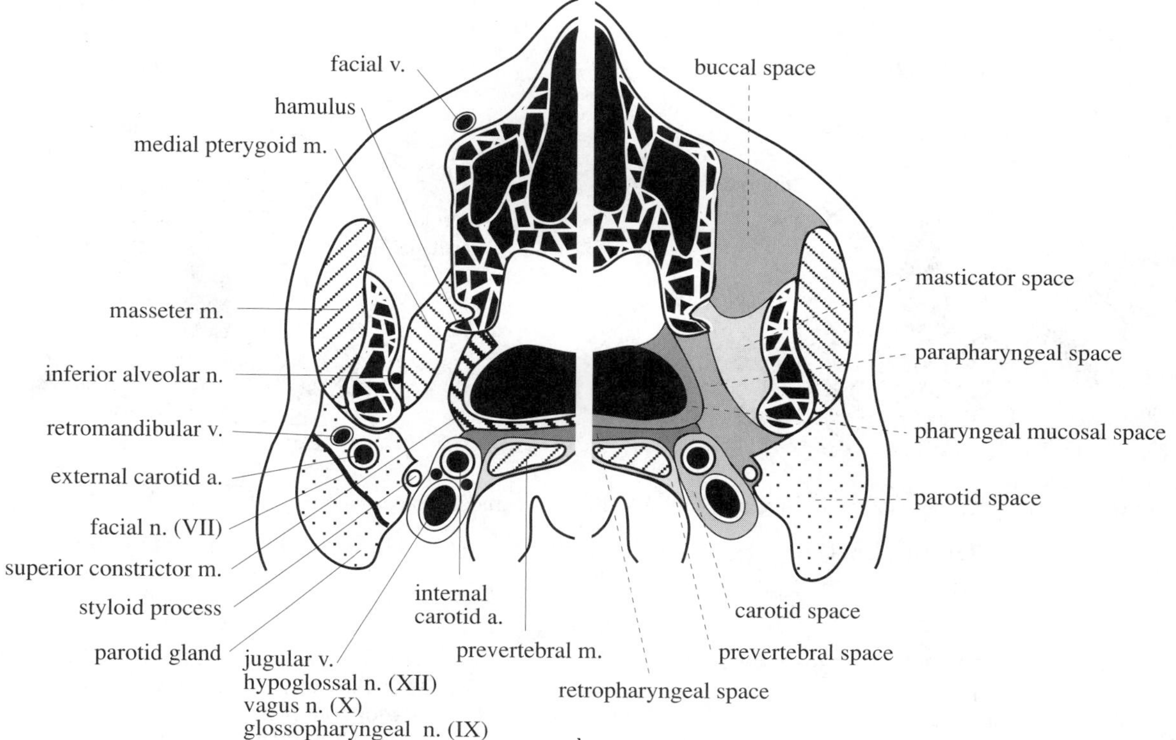

Transaxial Scan through Level of Lower Nasopharynx

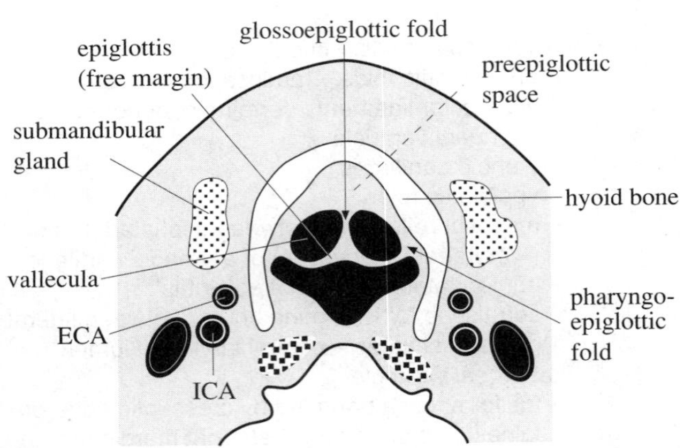

Hyoid Bone Level

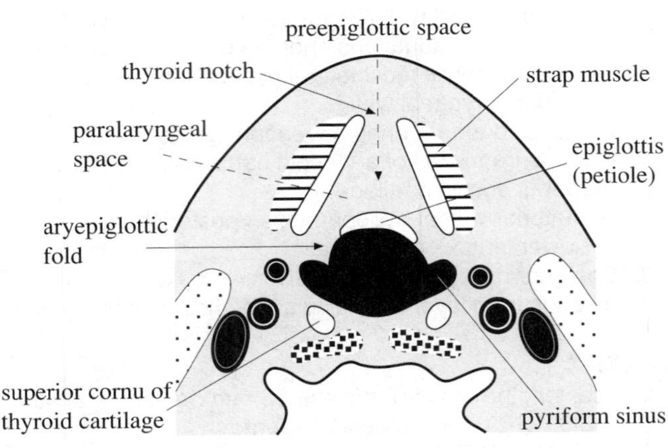

High Supraglottic Level

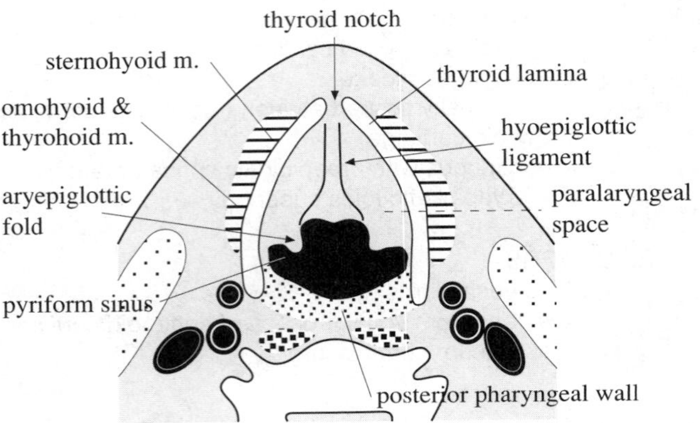

Mid Supraglottic Level

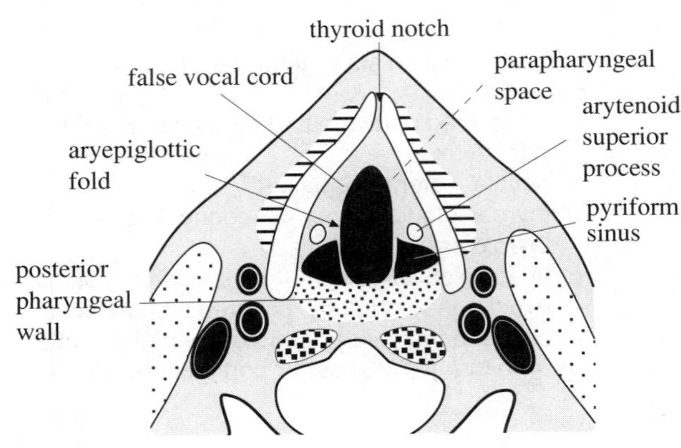

Low Supraglottic Level

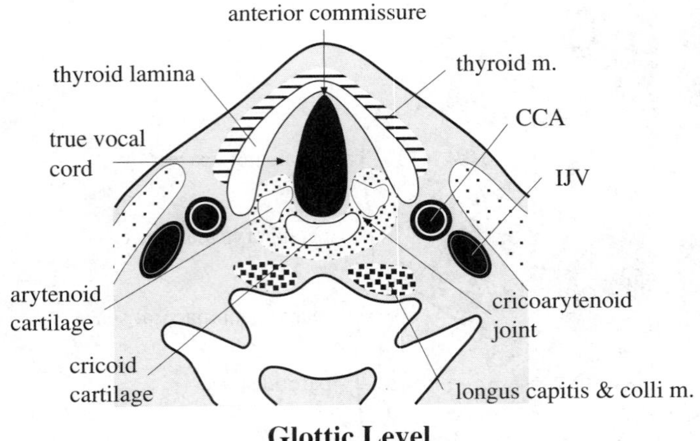

Glottic Level

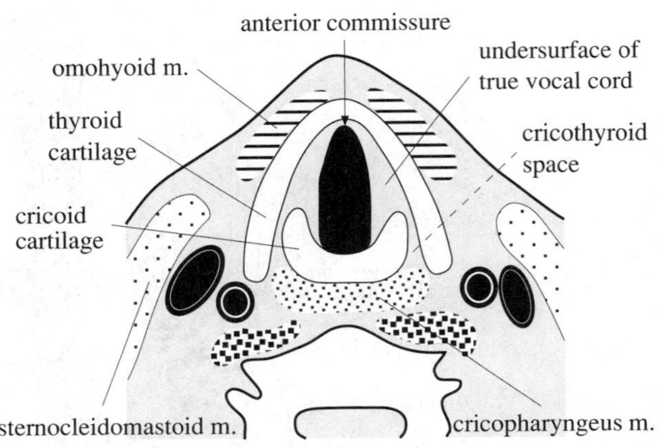

Undersurface of True Cord

√ vocal cords adduct during phonation of "E" / breath holding

2. Anterior commissure
   = midline laryngeal mucosa covering anterior portions of the true vocal cords where they abut the laryngeal surface of the thyroid cartilage

√ <1 mm soft tissue behind thyroid cartilage (during abduction of vocal cords with quiet breathing)

3. Posterior commissure
   = midline laryngeal mucosal surface between attachment of true vocal cords to the arytenoid cartilages

C. SUBGLOTTIS
extends from undersurface of true vocal cords to inferior surface of cricoid cartilage
1. Conus elasticus
= fibroelastic membrane extending from cricoid cartilage to medial margin of true vocal cords + forming lateral wall of subglottis

DEEP SPACES OF SUPRAHYOID HEAD & NECK

Masticator Space
= lateral to parapharyngeal space
Fascia:
superficial layer of deep cervical fascia encloses muscles of mastication
Contents:
muscles of mastication (medial + lateral pterygoid muscles, masseter, temporalis muscle)
ramus + body of mandible
cranial nerve V_3

Pharyngeal Mucosal Space
adenoids, faucial + lingual tonsils
superior + middle constrictor muscles
salpingopharyngeal muscle
levator palatini muscle
torus tubarius

Parapharyngeal Space
= triangular-shaped centrally located space; major vertical highway extending from skull base to hyoid
Fascial borders:
medial = middle layer of deep cervical fascia
lateral = superficial layer of deep cervical fascia
posterior = carotid sheath
Contents:
fat
internal maxillary artery
ascending pharyngeal artery
pharyngeal venous plexus
branches of cranial nerve V_3
Vectors: if parapharyngeal fat is effaced
anteriorly = lesion in masticator space
medially = lesion in pharyngeal mucosal space
laterally = lesion in parotid space
posteriorly = lesion in carotid space

Retropharyngeal Space
= potential space posterior to pharyngeal mucosal space + anterior to prevertebral space; major vertical highway from skull base to T4
Fascial borders:
mid + deep layers of cervical fascia;
alar fascia laterally
Contents:
fat
medial + lateral retropharyngeal nodes

Prevertebral Space
= major highway from skull base to T4; posterior to retropharyngeal space
Fascial borders:
(a) anterior compartment of deep cervical fascia: from one transverse process to the other anteriorly in front of longus colli muscle
(b) posterior compartment of deep cervical fascia: from transverse process posteriorly to spinous process
Contents:
prevertebral muscles (longus colli)
scalene muscles
vertebral artery + vein
brachial plexus
phrenic nerve

Carotid Space
Carotid fascia extends from skull base to aortic arch
Contents:
(a) below hyoid bone:
common carotid artery
internal jugular vein
cranial nerve X (vagus nerve)
cervical sympathetic plexus
(b) at level of nasopharynx:
internal carotid artery
internal jugular vein
cranial nerves IX–XII
internal jugular chain of nodes

Parotid Space
Contents:
parotid gland with Stenson duct
intraparotid lymph nodes
external carotid + internal maxillary arteries
retromandibular vein
facial nerve

Submandibular Space
Contents:
submandibular gland with Wharton duct
facial artery + vein
cranial nerve XII

TEMPORAL BONE
A. SQUAMOUS PORTION
= lateral wall of middle cranial fossa + floor of temporal fossa

B. MASTOID PORTION
1. Mastoid antrum
2. Aditus ad antrum
connects epitympanum (= attic) of middle ear cavity to mastoid antrum
3. Körner septum
= small bony projection extending inferiorly from roof of mastoid antrum as part of petrosquamosal suture between lateral + medial mastoid air cells

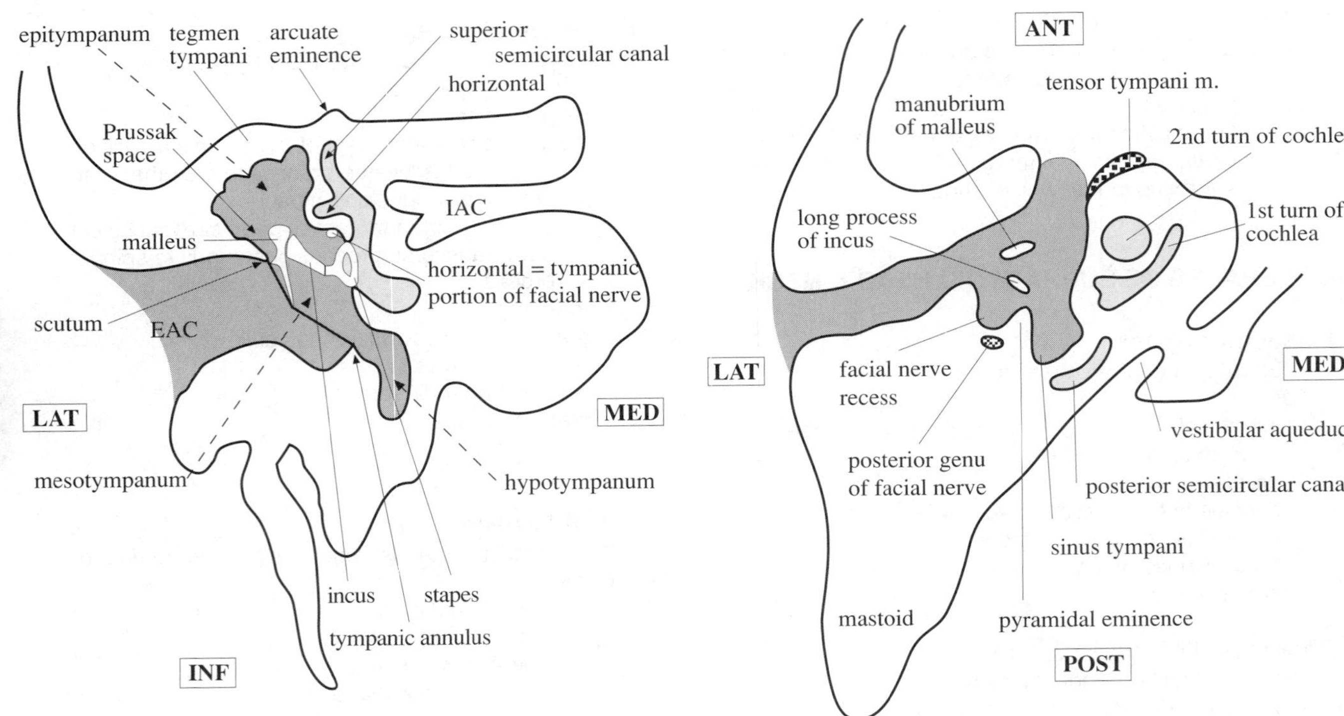

Coronal Tomogram of Temporal Bone

Axial Tomogram of Temporal Bone

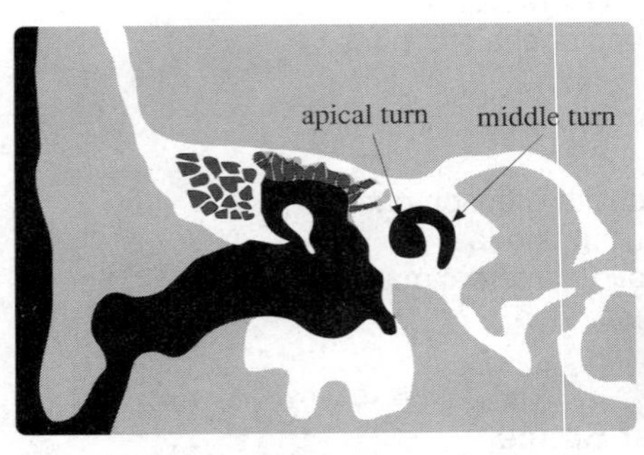

Most Anterior Scan through Cochlea

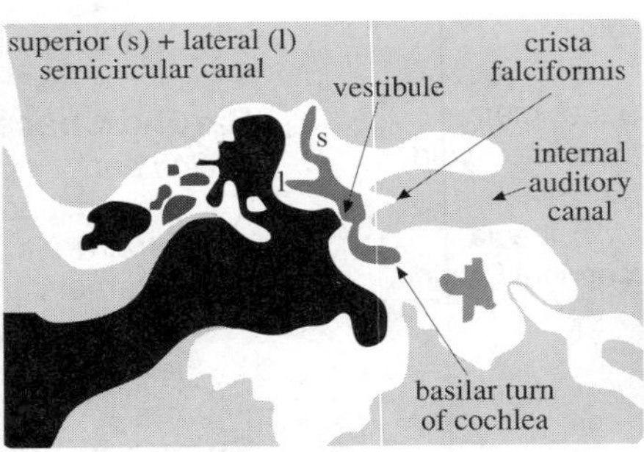

Scan at Vestibular Level

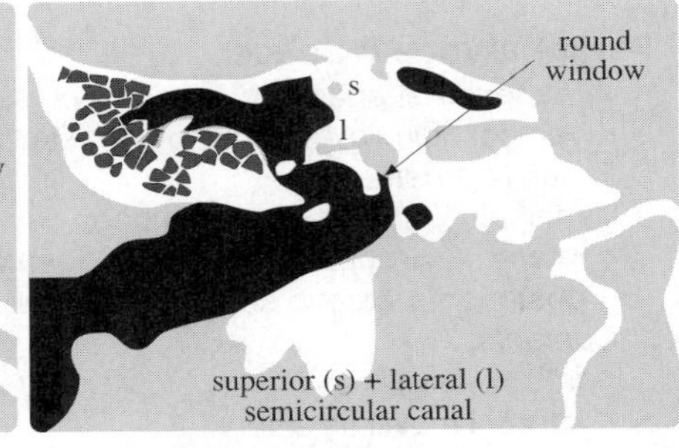

Most Posterior Scan through Round Window

Coronal Scan of Normal Right Ear

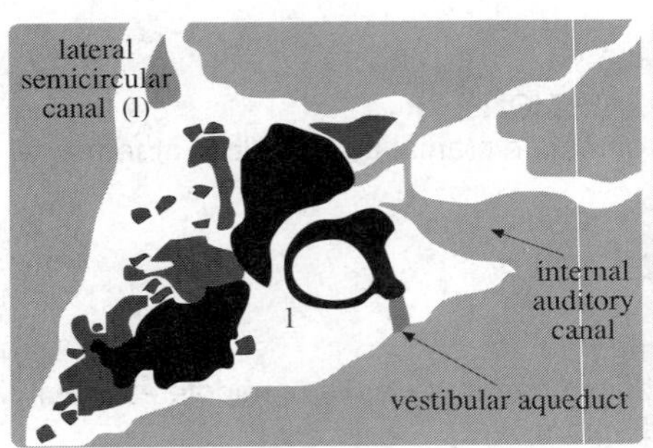

Most Superior Scan through Lateral Semicircular Canal

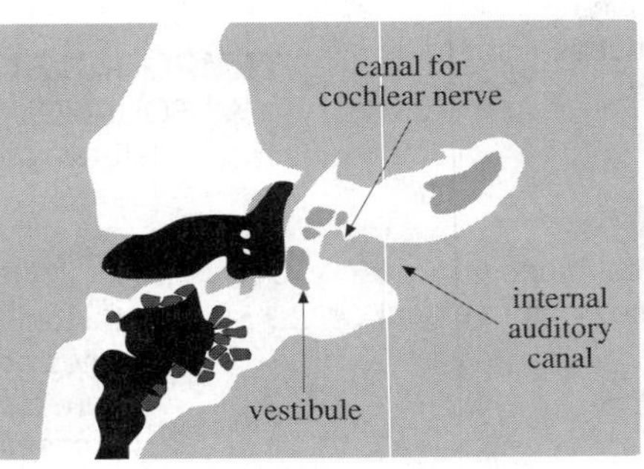

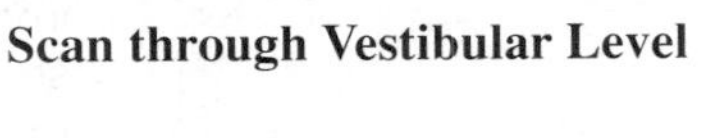

Scan through Vestibular Level

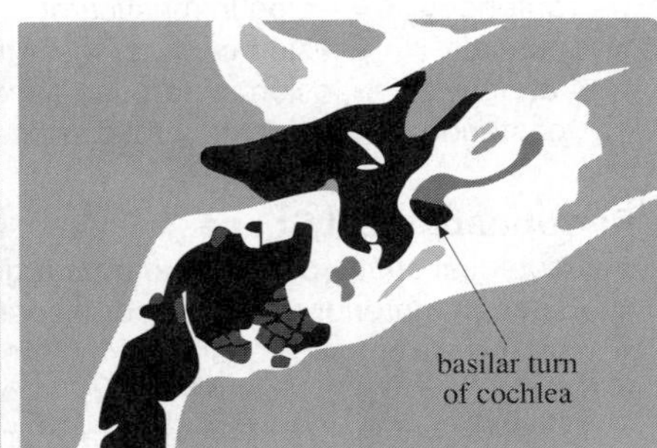

Most Inferior Scan through Basilar Turn of Cochlea

Axial Scan of Normal Right Ear

C. PETROUS PORTION = inner ear
1. Tegmen tympani
   = roof of tympanic cavity
2. Arcuate eminence
   = prominence of bone over superior semicircular canal
3. Internal auditory canal (IAC)
   (a) Porus acusticus internus
   = opening of internal auditory canal
   (b) Modiolus
   = entrance to cochlea
   (c) Crista falciformis
   = horizontal bony septum in IAC
4. Vestibular aqueduct
   = transmits endolymphatic duct
5. Cochlear aqueduct
   = transmits perilymphatic duct
6. Petrous apex
   = separated from clivus by petro-occipital fissure + foramen lacerum

D. TYMPANIC PORTION
1. External auditory canal (EAC)
   medial border formed by tympanic membrane, which attaches superiorly at scutum + inferiorly at tympanic annulus

E. STYLOID PORTION

MIDDLE EAR

Borders:
- anterior wall = carotid wall
- posterior wall = mastoid wall including
  (a) facial nerve recess for descending facial nerve
  (b) pyramidal eminence for stapedius muscle
  (c) sinus tympani (clinically blind spot)
- superior wall = tegmen tympani
- inferior wall = jugular wall
- lateral wall = tympanic membrane
- medial wall = labyrinthine wall

A. EPITYMPANUM
= tympanic cavity above the line drawn between the inferior tip of scutum + tympanic portion of facial nerve
Contents: malleus head, body + short process of incus, Prussak space (= area between incus + lateral wall of epitympanum)

B. MESOTYMPANUM
= tympanic cavity between inferior tip of scutum + line drawn parallel to inferior aspect of bony EAC
Contents: manubrium of malleus, long process of incus, stapes, tensor tympani muscle (innervated by V_3), stapedius muscle (innervated by VII)

C. HYPOTYMPANUM
= shallow trough in floor of middle ear

INNER EAR

1. Cochlea
   2 1/2 turns, basal first turn opens into round window posteriorly, encircles central bony axis of modiolus
2. Vestibule
   = largest part of membranous labyrinth with subunits of utricle + saccule (not separately visualized); separated from middle ear by oval window
3. Semicircular canals
   - superior semicircular canal forms convexity of arcuate eminence
   - posterior semicircular canal points posteriorly along line of petrous ridge
   - lateral / horizontal semicircular canal juts into epitympanum
4. Cochlear aqueduct
   contains 8-mm–long perilymphatic duct, extends from basal turn of cochlea to lateral border of jugular foramen paralleling IAC
   Function: regulates CSF + perilymphatic fluid pressure
5. Vestibular aqueduct
   encompasses endolymphatic duct, extends from vestibule to endolymphatic sac
   Function: equilibration of endolymphatic fluid pressure

PAROTID GLAND

Embryology:
glandular component arises from ingrowth of local proliferation of oral epithelium, which creates ducts by 10th week GA; secretions begin by 18th week GA
◊ Epithelial buds branch around divisions of facial nerve thus incorporating it into parotid parenchyma
◊ The only salivary gland to become encapsulated after development of lymphatic system resulting in intraglandular lymph nodes and lymph vessels

Location: wraps around mandibular angle (within parotid space)

Anatomic divisions:
(a) superficial lobe = main bulk of gland superficial and posterior to masseter muscle;
separated by facial nerve from:
(b) deep lobe = small extension of gland deep to angle of mandible
(c) accessory lobe (20%) = superficial and lateral to masseter muscle + anterior to superficial lobe draining directly into parotid duct

Drainage route: Stenson duct exiting above upper 2nd molar tooth

THYROID GLAND

CT values: 70–120 HU

THYROID HORMONES

Free hormone	: T_4	(0.03%)
	T_3	(0.4%)
Thyroxin-binding globulin (TBG)	: binds T_4	(70%)
	and T_3	(38%)

ENT

Thyroxin-binding prealbumin (TBPA): binds T_4 (10%) and T_3 (27%)
Albumin : binds T_4 (20%) and T_3 (35%)

A. ELEVATION OF TBG
  1. Pregnancy
  2. Estrogen administration
  3. Genetic trait

B. REDUCTION IN TBG
  1. Androgens
  2. Anabolic steroids
  3. Glucocorticoids
  4. Nephrotic syndrome
  5. Chronic hepatic disease

C. INHIBITION OF T_4 BINDING TO TBG: salicylates

PARATHYROID GLANDS

A. SUPERIOR PARATHYROID GLANDS
  Embryology: derived from 4th pharyngeal pouches, descending together with thyroid gland in close relationship to its posterolateral lobes
  Location: superior dorsal surface of thyroid gland / intrathyroidal

B. INFERIOR PARATHYROID GLANDS
  Embryology: derived from 3rd pharyngeal pouches migrating caudally with thymus
  Location: anywhere near / in thyroid, carotid bifurcation, lower neck, mediastinum

C. SUPERNUMERARY PARATHYROID GLANDS
  5th / 6th gland may occupy an ectopic site
  ◊ Up to 12 parathyroids may be present!

Embryology: parathyroid glands develop by 6 weeks GA + migrate into neck at 8 weeks

Size: 6 x 4 x 1 mm = 25–40 mg

Surgical success rates for finding parathyroid glands:
— 95% for initial cervical exploration
— 60% for repeat surgical exploration
Cause for failure: overlooking an adenoma, multiple abnormal glands, diffuse hyperplasia

Localization technique:
US (75% sensitivity), thallium-technetium subtraction scintigraphy, MR (88% sensitivity)

Duplex Identification

Criteria	*External Carotid Artery*	*Internal Carotid Artery*
Size	usually smaller than ICA	usually larger than ECA
Location	oriented medially + anteriorly toward face	oriented laterally + posteriorly toward mastoid process (*mnemonic:* **I**AC vis-à-vis ECA is positioned like hel**i**x vis-à-vis tragus of your ear)
Branches	gives off arterial branches (superior thyroidal a. as 1st branch)	NO arterial branches
Waveform	high-resistance flow pattern supplying capillary beds in skin + muscle √ forward systolic component √ early diastolic flow reversal occasionally followed by another forward component √ little / no flow in late diastole	low-resistance flow pattern supplying capillary bed in brain √ high-velocity forward systolic component √ sustained strong forward flow in diastole √ stagnant eddy with flow reversal opposite to flow divider in carotid bulb
Maneuver	oscillations on temporal tap maneuver	

EAR, NOSE, AND THROAT DISORDERS

ADENOID CYSTIC CARCINOMA

= CYLINDROMA

Incidence: 4–15% of all salivary gland tumors

Histo: (a) cribriform subtype, grade 1
(b) tubular subtype, grade 2
(c) solid / basaloid subtype, grade 3
◊ Perineural invasion is typical!

Age: 3rd–9th decade; maximum between 40 and 70 years; M = F

Location:
- @ Minor salivary glands (most common; 25–31% of malignant neoplasms in minor salivary glands)
  - ◊ Most common tumor of the minor salivary glands!
  - • nasal obstruction + swelling
  - Location: oral cavity > pharynx > nose > paranasal sinuses > trachea > larynx
- @ Submandibular gland (15% of tumors in this gland)
- @ Parotid gland (2–6% of tumors in this gland; arises from peripheral parotid ducts with propensity for perineural spread along facial nerve)
  - • hard mass + facial nerve pain / paralysis
  - √ infiltrating parotid mass

MR:
- √ hypo- to hyperintense (high signal corresponds to low cellularity with a better prognosis) on T2WI

Metastases to: lung, cervical lymph nodes, bone, liver, brain

Prognosis: slow growing but relentless malignant course with repeat recurrences; the greater the cellularity, the worse the prognosis (requires entire tumor); 60–69% 5-year survival rate; 40% 10-year survival rate

Rx: repeat surgical excision + radiation therapy

Laryngeal Adenoid Cystic Carcinoma

0.25–1% of all malignant laryngeal tumors

Histo: uniform small basaloid cells with large deeply staining ovoid nuclei arranged in anastomosing cords or islands

- • coughing attacks, wheezing, hemoptysis
- • paralysis of recurrent laryngeal nerve due to propensity to invade nerves (CHARACTERISTIC)
- • absent history of cigarette smoking

Location: subglottis at junction with trachea (80%)

- √ extensive submucosal tumor spread of entire larynx
- √ invasion of cricoid cartilage, thyroid + esophagus
- √ regional neck nodes hardly ever involved

ANGIOLIPOMA OF PAROTID GLAND

= benign nodular lesion similar to ordinary lipomas except for associated angiomatous proliferation

Age: rare before puberty

CT:
- √ circumscribed (more common) / infiltrating mass
- √ marked enhancement around fatty components

DDx: hemangioma with fatty degeneration

APICAL PETROSITIS

= PETROUS APICITIS

chronic > acute apicitis

Etiology: spread from middle ear + mastoid infection; requires presence of air cells in petrous apices (which is found in 30% of population)

Organism: Pseudomonas, Enterococcus

- • **Gradenigo syndrome** = otorrhea (otitis media) + retro-orbital pain (trigeminal pain) + 6th nerve palsy
- √ air cell opacification (fluid in ipsilateral middle ear + mastoid)
- √ bone destruction (osteomyelitis)

MR:
- √ enhancing mass about petrous tip

Cx: epidural abscess; cranial nerve palsy (abducens, trigeminal, vagus)

Mortality: up to 20% (prior to antibiotic era)

Rx: intravenous antibiotics, myringotomy, surgery

BRANCHIAL CLEFT ANOMALIES

= failure of involution of branchial clefts leads to branchial cleft cysts / fistula / sinus tracts

First Branchial Cleft Cyst (5–8%)

= PAROTID LYMPHOEPITHELIAL CYST

Residual embryonic tract begins near submandibular triangle + ascends through the parotid gland, terminates at junction of cartilaginous + bony external auditory canal

Incidence: 5–8% of all branchial cleft anomalies (rare)

Age: middle-aged women

- • enlarging mass near lower pole of parotid gland
- • recurrent parotid abscesses
- • ± facial nerve palsy
- • otorrhea (if cyst drains into EAC)

Pathologic classification (Work):

Type I duplication anomaly of membranous EAC; derived from ectoderm + lined with squamous epithelium; course parallel to EAC; medial to concha of ear; no skin appendages

Type II cyst arises from 1st branchial cleft containing ectoderm and mesoderm involving EAC + pinna; skin appendages (hair follicles, sweat and sebaceous glands)

- √ cystic mass within gland or immediate periparotid region (superficial to / deep to parotid gland)
- √ may extend into adjacent fat-containing parapharyngeal space ± connection to EAC

DDx: inflammatory parotid cyst, benign cystic parotid tumor, necrotic metastatic lymphadenopathy

Second Branchial Cleft Cyst (95%)

= incomplete obliteration of 2nd branchial cleft tract (cervical sinus of His) resulting in sinus tract / fistula / cyst (75%)

Incidence: 95% of all branchial cleft anomalies

Age: 10–40 years; M = F

Classification (Bailey):
- Type I — along anterior surface of sternocleidomastoid muscle, just deep to platysma
- Type II — along anterior surface of sternocleidomastoid muscle, lateral to carotid space, posterior to submandibular gland adhering to the great vessels (most common)
- Type III — extension medially between bifurcation of external and internal carotid arteries to lateral pharyngeal wall
- Type IV — within pharyngeal mucosal space

Path: 1–10-cm large thin-walled cyst, lined by stratified squamous epithelium overlying lymphoid tissue, filled with turbid yellowish fluid ± cholesterol crystals

• history of multiple parotid abscesses unresponsive to drainage + antibiotics
• otorrhea (if connected to external auditory canal)

Location:
anywhere along a line from the oropharyngeal tonsillar fossa to supraclavicular region of neck; classically at anteromedial border of sternocleidomastoid muscle + lateral to carotid space + at posterior margin of submandibular gland; may be in parapharyngeal space (after extension through stylomandibular tunnel + middle constrictor muscle)

√ oval / round cyst near mandibular angle
√ displacement of sternocleidomastoid muscle posteriorly, carotid artery + jugular vein posteromedially, submandibular gland anteriorly
√ cyst may enlarge after upper respiratory tract infection / injury

US:
√ compressible mass ± internal debris (due to hemorrhage / infection) obscuring its cystic nature
√ lack of internal flow

CT / MR:
√ "beak sign" = curved rim of tissue pointing medially between internal + external carotid arteries (PATHOGNOMONIC)
√ slight enhancement of capsule

DDx: necrotic neural tumor, cervical abscess, submandibular gland cyst, cystic lymphangioma, necrotic metastatic / inflammatory lymphadenopathy

Third Branchial Fistula / Cyst

= above superior laryngeal nerve
Incidence: extremely rare
Internal opening: piriform sinus anterior to fold formed by internal laryngeal nerve
Course: pierces thyrohyoid membrane, runs over hypoglossal nerve + under glossopharyngeal nerve, between internal + external carotid arteries, caudolateral / posterolateral to proximal internal + common carotid arteries
External opening: at base of neck anterior to sternocleidomastoid muscle
√ unilocular cystic mass within posterior cervical space

Fourth Branchial Fistula

= below superior laryngeal nerve
Incidence: extremely rare (R > L)
Internal opening: apex of piriform sinus
Course: between cricoid + thyroid cartilage, below cricothyroid muscle, caudal course between trachea + carotid vessels, deep to clavicle into mediastinum, looping forward below aorta (left side) / right subclavian artery (right side), ascending along ventral surface of common carotid artery, passing over hypoglossal nerve
External opening: at base of neck anterior to sternocleidomastoid muscle + anteroinferior to subclavian artery

• recurrent episodes of "suppurative thyroiditis'" / neck abscesses

Site: 90% on left side

CAROTID ARTERY ANEURYSM

= aneurysm of extracranial carotid artery
Etiology:
1. Trauma
2. Infection (mycotic aneurysm)
3. Congenital (very rare): manifestation of connective tissue disorder (Ehlers-Danlos, Marfan, Kawasaki, Mafucci syndrome)

CAROTID ARTERY STENOSIS

High-grade ICA stenosis is associated with increased risk for TIA, stroke, carotid occlusion, embolism arising from thrombi forming at site of narrowing

Increased risk for stroke:
(a) significant ICA stenosis (compromised blood flow)
Reduction of blood flow occurs at 50–60% diameter stenosis / 75% area stenosis
◊ 2% risk of stroke with nonsignificant stenosis
◊ 16% incidence of stroke with significant stenosis
◊ 2% incidence of subsequent stroke following endarterectomy
(b) intraplaque hemorrhage (embolic stroke)

Histo:
arteriosclerosis = generic term for all structural changes resulting in hardening of the arterial wall
1. Diffuse intimal thickening
   = growth of intima through migration of medial smooth muscle cells into subendothelial space through fenestrations in internal elastic lamella associated with increasing amounts of collagen, elastic fibers, glycosaminoglycans
   Age: beginning at birth slowly progressing to adult life
2. Atherosclerosis
   = intimal pool of necrotic, proteinaceous + fatty substances within hardened arterial wall
   Location: large + medium-sized elastic and muscular arteries

(a) fatty streak = superficial yellow-gray flat intimal lesion characterized by focal accumulation of subendothelial smooth muscle cells + lipid deposits
(b) fibrous plaque = whitish protruding lesion consisting of central core of lipid + cell debris surrounded by smooth muscle cells, collagen, elastic fibers, proteoglycans; a fibrous cap separates the lipid core (= atheroma) from the vessel lumen
(c) complicated lesion = fibrous plaque with degenerative changes such as calcification, plaque hemorrhage, intimal ulceration / rupture, mural thrombosis

Plaque hemorrhage from thin-walled blood vessels in vascularized plaque may cause ulceration, thrombosis + embolism, and luminal narrowing
◊ In 93% of symptomatic patients
◊ In 27% of asymptomatic patients

Plaque ulceration exposes thrombogenic subendothelial collagen + lipid-rich material
◊ Frequent in plaques occupying >85% of lumen
◊ 12.5% stroke incidence per year

3. Mönckeberg sclerosis = medial calcification
4. Hypertensive arteriosclerosis

Predilection sites of arterial stenosis:

	Incidence of lesions	
	Stenosis	Occlusion
Right ICA origin	33.8%	8.6%
Left ICA origin	34.1%	8.7%
Right vertebral artery origin	18.4%	4.8%
Left vertebral artery origin	22.3%	2.2%
Right carotid siphon	6.7%	9.0%
Left carotid siphon	6.6%	9.2%
Basilar artery	7.7%	0.8%
Right MCA	3.5%	2.2%
Left MCA	4.1%	2.1%

Decrease in Luminal Diameter vs. Cross-sectional Area

Decrease in Lumen Diameter	*Decrease in Cross-sectional Area*
20%	36%
40%	64%
60%	84%
80%	96%

Temporal course of carotid artery stenosis:
1. Stable stenosis (68%)
2. Progressive stenosis to >50% diameter reduction (25%)

Angiography:
@ Extracranial
√ smooth asymmetrical excrescence encroaching upon vessel lumen
√ crater / niche = ulceration
√ mound within base of crater = mural thrombus

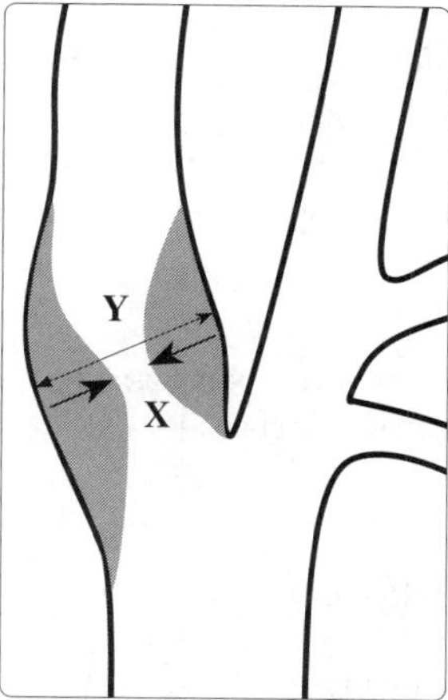

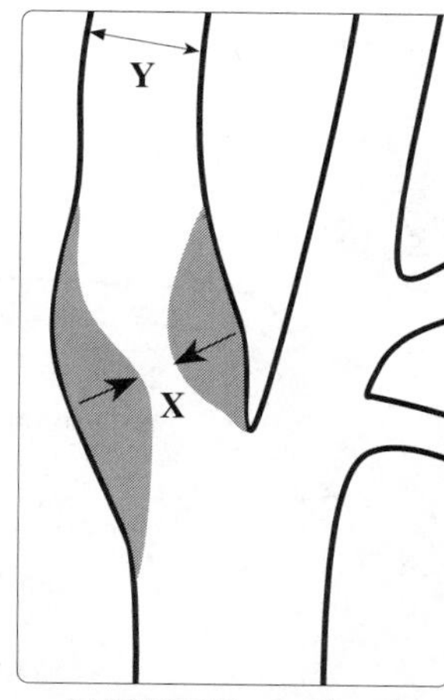

ECST method **NASCET method**

% Carotid Stenosis = (Y–X) / Y • 100

ECST = European Carotid Surgery Trial; NASCET = North American Symptomatic Carotid Endarterectomy Trial

√ Holman carotid slim sign = diffuse narrowing of entire ICA distal to high-grade stenosis due to decrease in perfusion pressure
√ occlusion of ICA

@ Intracranial
√ carotid siphon stenosis
√ retrograde flow in ophthalmic artery filled from ECA
√ small vessel occlusion
√ focal areas of slow flow
√ early draining vein = reactive hyperemia = "luxury perfusion" due to shunting between arterioles + venules surrounding an area of ischemia
√ ICA-MCA slow flow = delayed arrival + washout of ICA-MCA distribution in comparison to ECA

Carotid endarterectomy:
Benefit: 17% reduction of ipsilateral stroke at 2 years in patients with >70% carotid stenosis (NASCET = North American Symptomatic Carotid Endarterectomy Trial)
Risk: 1% mortality; 2% risk of intraoperative neurologic deficit

Carotid Duplex Ultrasound

Indications for carotid duplex US:
(1) Screening for suspected extracranial carotid disease
  (a) high-grade flow-limiting stenosis
  (b) low-grade stenosis with hemorrhage
(2) Nonhemispheric neurologic symptomatology
(3) History of transient ischemic attack / stroke
(4) Asymptomatic carotid bruit
(5) Retinal cholesterol embolus
(6) Preoperative evaluation before major cardiovascular surgery
(7) Intraoperative monitoring of vascular patency during endarterectomy

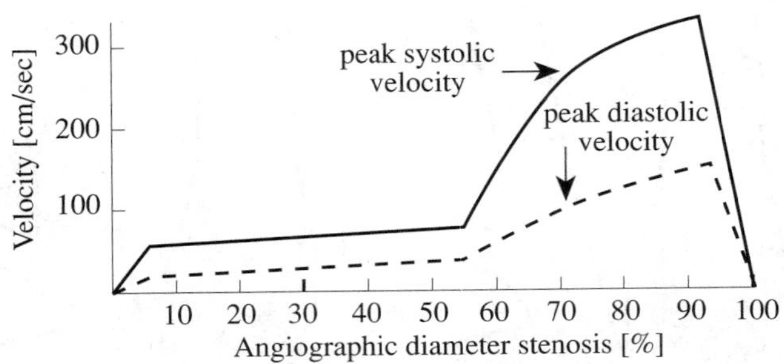

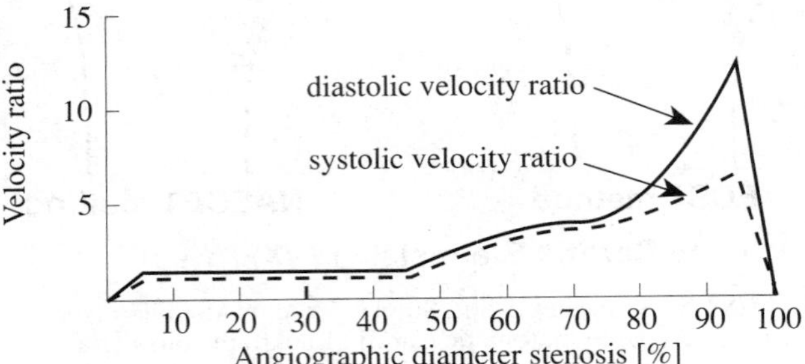

Doppler Parameters in Internal Carotid Artery Stenosis

(8) Sequential evaluation after endarterectomy
(9) Monitoring of known plaque during medical treatment

Grading of Carotid Stenosis

= severity of stenosis is primarily graded as a ratio of lumen diameter narrowing NOT reduction in cross sectional area

Limitations:

1. Calcifications >1 cm in length
   ◊ A jet associated with a >70% stenosis usually travels at least 1 cm downstream!
2. Contralateral high-grade stenosis
   = ipsilateral ICA functions as collateral with increased blood flow velocities
   ◊ Use velocity ratios to compensate for this effect!

Accuracy of duplex scans: (in comparison to arteriography for ICA lesions)
91–94% sensitivity, 85–99% specificity for >50% ICA diameter stenosis

Doppler Spectrum Analysis

Diameter Stenosis Classification	*(%)*	*ICA/CCA Peak Systolic Ratio*	*ICA/CCA Peak Diastolic Ratio*	*Peak Systolic Velocity (cm/sec)*	*Peak Systolic Velocity kHz†*	*Peak Diastolic Velocity (cm/sec)*	*Peak Diastolic Velocity kHz†*
Normal–mild	0–40	<1.5	<2.6	<110 > 25	<3.5	<40	<1.5
Moderate	41–59	<1.8	<2.6	>120	>3.5	<40	<1.5
Severe	60–79	>1.8	>2.6	>130	>5.0	>40	>1.5
Critical	80–99	>3.7	>5.5	>250	>8.0	>80–135	>4.5

† = based on 5-MHz pulsed Doppler carrier frequency at 60° flow angle (Blackshear)

Classification	(%)	Peak Systolic Ratio	Peak Diastolic Ratio	Peak Systolic Velocity (cm/sec)	Peak Systolic Velocity kHz	Peak Diastolic Velocity (cm/sec)	Peak Diastolic Velocity kHz
	0–39	<1.8	<2.4	<110		<40	
	40–59	<1.8	<2.4	<130		<40	
	60–79	>1.8	>2.4	>130		>40	
	80–99	>3.7	>5.5	>250		>100	
(Bluth)							

Classification	(%)	Peak Systolic Ratio	Peak Diastolic Ratio	Peak Systolic Velocity (cm/sec)	Peak Systolic Velocity kHz	Peak Diastolic Velocity (cm/sec)	Peak Diastolic Velocity kHz
	0–50	<2:1		<125		<40	
	50–75	>2:1		125–225		40–100	
	75–90	>3:1	>5:1	225–325		>100	
	>90	>4:1	>9:1	>325		>100	
	>95	resistive CCA	distortion	may be decreased		may be decreased	
(Gosink)							

Classification	(%)	Peak Systolic Ratio	Peak Diastolic Ratio	Peak Systolic Velocity (cm/sec)	Peak Systolic Velocity kHz	Peak Diastolic Velocity (cm/sec)	Peak Diastolic Velocity kHz
	1–15						
	16–49			(<125)	<4.0		
	50–79			(≥125)	≥4.0	(<140)	<4.5
(Fell)	80–99					(≥140)	≥4.5
(Strandness)	occlusion			no flow detected			

† = based on 5MHz pulsed Doppler carrier frequency at 60° flow angle (University of Washington)

Incorporating B-mode and Doppler spectrum analysis

A. NO LESION
  √ peak systolic velocity (PSV) < 125 cm/sec
  √ clear window under systole
  √ no spectral broadening
  √ no evidence of plaque

B. MINIMAL DISEASE
  = 0–15% diameter reduction
  √ PSV < 125 cm/sec
  √ clear window under systole
  √ minimal spectral broadening in deceleration phase of systole
  √ minimal plaque

C. MODERATE DISEASE
  = 16–49% diameter reduction
  √ peak systole <125 cm/sec
  √ no window under systole
  √ poststenotic spectral broadening throughout systole
  ◊ End-diastolic velocity (EDV) remains normal in <50% diameter reduction!
  √ moderate plaque

D. SEVERE DISEASE = HEMODYNAMICALLY SIGNIFICANT LESION
  (a) 50–59% stenosis
    √ PSV 120–130 cm/s
    √ EDV 30–40 cm/s
  (b) 60–79% stenosis
    √ PSV of 131–250 cm/s
    √ EDV of 40–100 cm/s
  (c) ≥60% stenosis
    √ end diastolic velocity of >80 cm/sec
  (d) 50–79% diameter reduction
    √ peak velocity ratio of ICA/CCA >1.5
    √ peak systole >125 cm/s
    √ marked poststenotic spectral broadening throughout cardiac cycle
  (e) **>70% stenosis** (benefit of endarterectomy documented in NASCET study)
    √ peak systole >230 cm/s
    √ end diastole >100 cm/s
    √ peak velocity ratio of ICA/CCA >4.0
    √ peak systolic velocity ICA ÷ end diastolic velocity CCA >15
  (f) 80–99% diameter reduction
    √ PSV of >250 cm/s
    √ EDV of >100 cm/s
    √ no window under systole
    √ poststenotic spectral broadening throughout systole
    √ "string sign" on color Doppler with slow-flow sensitivity setting

E. OCCLUDED VESSEL
  √ no signal in ICA on longitudinal / transverse images (color sensitivity + velocity scale must be set low enough to clearly discern flow signals within internal jugular vein)
  √ absence of diastolic flow in CCA (high impedance flow)
  √ diastolic flow reversal in CCA
  √ increased diastolic flow in ECA (if ECA assumes the role of primary supplier of blood to brain)
  √ increase in peak systolic velocities in contralateral ICA (due to collateral flow)

Limitations:
poor visualization due to calcification, tortuosity, increased depth of artery, "high" bifurcation

Common Carotid Waveform Analysis

A. DISTAL OBSTRUCTION
  √ high-pulsatility waveform (pulsatility changes occur only with >80% stenosis)
  √ reduced amplitude

B. PROXIMAL OBSTRUCTION
  √ low-amplitude damped waveform

Hemodynamic Variations of Carotid Artery Stenosis

A. MORPHOLOGY OF STENOSIS
  1. Degree of stenosis: velocities increase up to a luminal diameter of 1.0–1.5 mm
  2. Length of stenosis: peak velocities decrease with length of stenosis
  √ use the same angle + steering direction when following a patient for disease progression

B. PHYSIOLOGIC VARIABILITY
  ◊ A range of velocities may be encountered with a given degree of stenosis!
  ◊ ICA/CCA ratio obviates effects of physiologic variability!
  ◊ Compare left with right waveforms to avoid errors!
  ◊ Measure volume flow (more sensitive because of contralateral compensatory flow increase)

  Cause:
  1. Cardiac output
  2. Pulse rate
  3. Flow velocity: increased with obstruction in collateral vessels, decreased with proximal obstruction in same vessel
  4. Normal helical nature of blood flow with many different velocity vectors + nonaxial blood flow not detectable by color Duplex imaging
  5. Peripheral resistance
  6. Arterial compliance
  7. Hypertension
  8. Blood viscosity

Carotid Plaque

FORMATION THEORY
1. Stagnant eddy that rotates at outer vessel margin (opposite to the flow divider in area of flow separation + low shear stress) leads to net influx of fluid into subendothelial tissue with progressive deposition of lipids + smooth muscle cell proliferation
2. Increased likelihood of intraplaque hemorrhage (vascularization of plaque with fragile vessels derived from vasa vasorum / from lumen) + fissuring from a critical size on

◊ As the degree of stenosis increases, it is more likely that plaques become denser + more heterogeneous demonstrating an irregular surface!

PLAQUE DENSITY
1. Hypoechoic = low-echogenicity plaque
   = fibrofatty plaque / hemorrhage
   √ echogenicity less than sternocleidomastoid muscle
   √ flow void / flow disturbance on color Duplex
2. Isoechoic plaque
   = smooth muscle cell proliferation / laminar thrombus
   √ echogenicity equal to sternocleidomastoid muscle + lower than adventitia
3. Hyperechoic = moderately echogenic plaque
   = fibrous plaque
   √ echogenicity higher than sternocleidomastoid muscle + similar to adventitia
4. Calcification = strongly echogenic plaque
   √ acoustic shadow impairs visualization of intima

PLAQUE TEXTURE
1. Homogeneous plaque = stable plaque
   Histo: deposition of fatty streaks + fibrous tissue; rarely shows intraplaque hemorrhage / ulcerations
   Prognosis:
   ◊ Neurologic deficits develop in 4%
   ◊ Ipsilateral infarction on CT in 12%
   ◊ Ipsilateral symptoms develop in 22%
   ◊ Progressive stenosis develops in 18%
   √ homogeneous uniform echo pattern with smooth surface (acoustic impedance similar to blood)
2. Heterogeneous plaque
   = unstable plaque = mixture of high, medium, and low-level echoes with smooth / irregular surface; may fissure / tear resulting in intraplaque hemorrhage / ulceration + thrombus formation (embolus / increasing stenosis)
   B-mode ultrasound has 90–94% sensitivity, 75–88% specificity, 90% accuracy for intraplaque hemorrhage
   Histo: lipid-laden macrophages, monocytes, leukocytes, necrotic debris, cholesterol crystals, calcifications
   Prognosis:
   ◊ Neurologic deficits develop in 27%
   ◊ Ipsilateral infarction on CT in 24%
   ◊ Ipsilateral symptoms develop in 50%
   ◊ Progressive stenosis develops in 77%
   √ anechoic areas within plaque (= hemorrhage / lipid deposition / focal plaque degeneration)
   √ heterogeneous complex echo pattern

PLAQUE SURFACE CHARACTERISTICS
= US unreliable due to poor visualization of intima

Categories:
— smooth
— mildly irregular
— markedly irregular
— ulcerated

1. Intimal thickening
   Histo: fatty streaks
   √ wavy / irregular line paralleling vessel wall extending >1 mm into vessel lumen
2. Ulcerated plaque
   Accuracy: 60% sensitive, 60–70% specific
   ◊ The presence of intraplaque hemorrhage is much more common than normally appreciated
   ◊ Neither arteriography nor US has proved reliable!
   √ isolated crater of >2 mm within surface of plaque demonstrated on transverse + longitudinal images
   √ reversed flow vortices extending into plaque crater demonstrated by color Doppler
   √ proximal + distal undercutting of plaque
   √ anechoic area within plaque extending to surface

Errors In Duplex Ultrasound
1. Error in proper localization of stenosis (6%)
   Cause: ECA stenosis placed into ICA / carotid bifurcation or vice versa
2. Mistaking patent ECA branches for carotid bifurcation (4%)
   Cause: complete occlusion of ICA not recognized
   √ disparity in position of bifurcation
   √ no difference in pulsatility waveform
   √ high-resistance waveform in CCA
3. Interpreter error in estimating severity of stenosis (2.5%)
   usually overestimation, rarely underestimation
   √ absence of one / more components for diagnosis which are
   (a) significant elevation of peak velocity
   (b) poststenotic turbulence
   (c) extension of high velocity into diastole
4. Superimposition of ECA + ICA (2%)
   Cause: strict coronal orientation of ECA + ICA
   √ superimposition can be avoided by rotation of head to opposite side
5. Severe stenosis mistaken for occlusion
   minimal flow not detectable; angiogram necessary with delayed images
6. Weak signals misinterpreted as occlusion
7. Normal / weak signals in severe stenosis
   Cause: severe stenosis causes a decrease in blood flow + peak velocity with return to normal velocity levels
   √ high resistivity in CCA
8. Point of maximum frequency shift not identified
   Cause: extremely small lumen / short segment of stenosis
   √ unexplained (poststenotic) coarse turbulence
   √ ipsilateral ECA collateral flow
   √ abnormal CCA resistivity

9. Stenosis obscured by plaque / strong Doppler shift in overlying vessel
10. Inaccessible stenosis
    √ abnormal CCA resistivity
    √ abnormal oculoplethysmography
11. Unreliable velocity measurements
    (a) higher velocities: hypertension, severe bradycardia, obstructive contralateral carotid disease
    (b) lower velocities: arrhythmia, aortic valvular lesion, severe cardiomyopathy, proximal obstructive carotid lesion ("tandem lesion"), >95% ICA stenosis
    (c) aliasing = high velocities are displayed in reversed direction below zero baseline due to Doppler frequency exceeding half the pulse repetition frequency
    Remedy: shift zero baseline, increase pulse repetition frequency, increase Doppler angle, decrease transducer frequency, use continuous-wave Doppler probe

INDIRECT METHODS OF EVALUATION
1. Oculoplethysmography (OPG)
   = measurement of ophthalmic artery pressure + pulse arrival time by air calibrated system
   Contraindications: glaucoma, retinal detachment, recent eye surgery / trauma, lens implants
2. Periorbital bidirectional Doppler
   = insonation of frontal + supraorbital arteries to assess flow direction around orbit and to detect crossover flow through the circle of Willis (through contra- and ipsilateral compression)
3. Transcranial Doppler
   = insonation to establish flow direction in basal cerebral arteries through temporal bone (MCA, ACA, PCA, terminal portion of ICA), foramen magnum (both vertebral arteries, basilar artery), orbit (carotid siphon)
   ◊ Nondiagnostic in up to 35%!

CERVICAL DERMOID / EPIDERMOID CYST

Location: floor of mouth
(1) Cystic teratoma
  teratoma = neoplasm whose tissue is foreign to the part of the body from which the tumor arises
  (a) epidermoid cyst = epidermal inclusion cyst
      = lined by simple squamous epithelium without skin appendages
  (b) dermoid cyst
      = epithelial-lined cyst containing hair follicles + sebaceous + sweat glands
  (c) teratoid cyst
      = lined with squamous / respiratory epithelium containing derivatives of ectoderm + endoderm + mesoderm (skin appendages, nervous / GI / respiratory tissue)
(2) Nonteratomatous sequestration-type epithelial-lined cyst
  Location:
  — dorsum of nose in infants (most common)
  — midline anterior floor of mouth:
    (a) sublingual between mylohyoid muscle + tongue (DDx: inclusion cyst, ranula)
    (b) submental between platysma + mylohyoid muscle

CHOANAL ATRESIA

◊ Most common cause of neonatal nasal obstruction!
Frequency: 1:5,000 to 1:8,000 neonates; M < F
Etiology: failure of perforation of oronasal membrane, which normally perforates by 7th week EGA
◊ Associated with other anomalies in 50–75%: acrophalyngosyndactyly, amniotic band syndrome, malrotation of bowel, Crouzon syndrome, fetal alcohol syndrome, DiGeorge syndrome, Treacher-Collins syndrome, chromosome 18 / 12 anomalies, polydactyly, coloboma, facial cleft, CHD, TE fistula, craniosynostosis
Location: bilateral : unilateral atresia = 3:2
• respiratory distress in bilateral choanal atresia (relieved by crying in neonates who are obligate nose breathers during first 2–6 months)
• nasal stuffiness, rhinorrhea, infection in unilateral choanal atresia
Types:
  A. OSSEOUS / BONY SEPTATION (85–90%)
     Cause: incomplete canalization of choanae
  B. MEMBRANOUS SEPTATION (10–15%)
     Cause: incomplete resorption of epithelial plugs
  C. OSSEOMEMBRANOUS
CT (preceded by vigorous suctioning + administration of topical decongestant):
  √ narrowing of posterior choanae to a width of <3.4 mm (in children <2 years of age)
  √ inward bowing of posterior maxilla
  √ fusion / thickening of vomer
  √ bone / soft-tissue septum extending across the posterior choanae
Dx: nasal catheter cannot be advanced to beyond 32 mm
Cx: bilateral choanal atresia is life-threatening
Rx: endoscopic perforation, choanal reconstruction

CHOLESTEATOMA

= KERATOMA
= epithelium-lined sac filled with keratin debris leading to bone destruction by pressure + demineralizing enzymes

Primary Cholesteatoma (2%)

= CONGENITAL CHOLESTEATOMA = EPIDERMOID CYST
= derived from aberrant embryonic ectodermal rests in temporal bone (commonly petrous apex) / epidural space / meninges
• conductive hearing loss in child with NO history of middle ear inflammatory disease
• cholesteatoma seen through intact tympanic membrane
Associated with: EAC dysplasia

Location:
(a) epitympanum
(b) petrous pyramid: internal auditory canal first involved
(c) meninges: scooped out appearance of petrous ridge
(d) cerebellopontine angle: erosion of porus, shortening of posterior canal wall
(e) jugular fossa: erosion of posteroinferior aspect of petrous pyramid

Secondary Cholesteatoma (98%)

= INFLAMMATORY CHOLESTEATOMA = ACQUIRED EPIDERMOID

Cause:
ingrowth of squamous cell epithelium of EAC through tympanic membrane (= eardrum) secondary to
(a) repeated episodes of ear inflammation with invagination of posterosuperior retraction pocket
(b) marginal perforation of eardrum

Age: usually >40 years

• whitish pearly mass behind intact tympanic membrane (invasion of middle ear cavity and mastoid) diagnosed otoscopically in 95%
• facial paralysis (compression of nerve VII at geniculate ganglion)
• conductive hearing loss (compromise of nerve VIII in internal auditory canal / involvement of cochlea or labyrinth)
• severe vertigo (labyrinthine fistula)

Types:
1. **Pars flaccida cholesteatoma** = Primary acquired cholesteatoma = Attic cholesteatoma (most common)
   √ increasing width of attic
   √ initially destruction of lateral wall of attic, particularly the drum spur (scutum) with invasion of Prussak space
   √ extension posteriorly through aditus ad antrum into mastoid antrum
   √ destruction of Körner septum
2. **Pars tensa cholesteatoma** = Secondary acquired cholesteatoma (less frequent)
   √ displacement of auditory ossicles
   √ erosion of ossicular chain: first affecting long process of incus

√ nondependent homogeneous mass
√ perforation of tympanic membrane posterosuperiorly (pars flaccida = Shrapnell membrane)
√ poorly pneumatized mastoid (frequent association)
√ erosion of tegmen tympani (with more extensive cholesteatoma) producing an extradural mass
√ destruction of labyrinthine capsule (less common) involving the lateral semicircular canal first
√ erosion of facial canal

MRI:
√ iso- / hypointense relative to cortex on T1WI
√ no enhancement with Gd-DTPA (enhancement is related to granulation tissue)

Cx: (1) Intratemporal: ossicular destruction, facial nerve paralysis (1%), labyrinthine fistula, automastoidectomy, complete hearing loss
(2) Intracranial: meningitis, sigmoid sinus thrombosis, temporal lobe abscess, CSF rhinorrhea

DDx: chronic otitis media, granulation tissue = cholesterol granuloma, brain herniation through tegmen defect, neoplasm (rhabdomyosarcoma, squamous cell carcinoma)

CHOLESTEROL GRANULOMA

= CHOLESTEROL CYST
= acquired inflammatory lesion of petrous bone

Histo: cholesterol crystals surrounded by foreign-body giant cells; embedded in fibrous connective tissue with varying proportions of hemosiderin-laden macrophages, chronic inflammatory cells and blood vessels; brownish fluid contains cholesterol crystals + blood (= "chocolate cyst")

• blue (vascular) tympanic membrane without pulsatile tinnitus
√ ossicles remain intact

CT:
√ nonenhancing middle ear mass

MRI:
√ hyperintense signal on T1WI + T2WI secondary to methemoglobin (DDx to cholesteatoma, which is isointense to brain on T1WI)

CHRONIC RECURRENT SIALADENITIS

• painful periodic unilateral enlargement of parotid gland
• milky discharge may be expressed

Sialography:
√ Stensen duct irregularly enlarged / sausage-shaped
√ pruning of distal parotid ducts
√ ± calculi

CT:
√ diffusely enlarged dense gland
√ dilated Stensen duct ± calculi

Cx: Mucocele

COGAN SYNDROME

= AUTOIMMUNE INTERSTITIAL KERATITIS

MR:
√ membranous labyrinthine enhancement

CROUP

= ACUTE LARYNGOTRACHEOBRONCHITIS = ACUTE VIRAL SPASMODIC LARYNGITIS
= lower respiratory tract infection

Organism: parainfluenza, respiratory syncytial virus

Age: >6 months of age, peak incidence 2–3 years

• history of viral lower respiratory infection
• hoarse cry + "brassy" cough
• inspiratory difficulty with stridor
• fever
√ thickening of vocal cords
√ NORMAL epiglottis + aryepiglottic folds

√ "steeple sign" = subglottic "inverted V" = symmetrical funnel-shaped narrowing 1–1.5 cm below lower margins of pyriform sinuses on AP radiograph (loss of normal "shouldering" of air column caused by mucosal edema + external restriction by cricoid), accentuated on expiration, paradoxical inspiratory collapse, less pronounced during expiration
√ narrow + indistinct subglottic trachea on lateral radiograph
√ inspiratory ballooning of hypopharynx (nonspecific sign of any acute upper airway obstruction)
√ distension of cervical trachea on expiration
Prognosis: usually self-limiting

DACRYOCYSTOCELE

◊ 2nd most common cause of neonatal nasal obstruction (after choanal atresia)
Cause: obstruction of nasolacrimal duct (imperforate Hasner membrane distally, reason for proximal obstruction unknown)
• tense blue-gray mass at medial canthus / in nasal cavity
√ nasolacrimal duct dilatation
√ homogeneous well-defined mass of fluid attenuation
√ enhancement of thin wall
√ superior displacement of inferior turbinate bone
√ contralateral shift of nasal septum
Cx: dacryocystitis (postnatal infection with adjacent soft-tissue swelling + enhancement), periorbital cellulitis
Rx: duct massage, duct probing, prophylactic antibiotics

DERMOID CYST OF NECK

◊ 7% of all dermoid inclusion cysts occur in the head and neck
Age: 2nd–3rd decades; M = F
Path: circumscribed encapsulated lesions, covered by squamous epithelium, lumen filled with cheesy keratinaceous + sebaceous material
Histo: epithelial-lined cyst containing hair follicles + sebaceous glands + sweat glands
• slowly growing soft mobile mass in the suprahyoid midline (no movement with tongue protrusion!)
Location: lateral eye brow > floor of mouth (11%)
Site: (a) sublingual space (superior to mylohyoid muscle) = intraoral surgical approach (more frequent)
(b) submandibular (inferior to mylohyoid muscle) = external surgical approach
Size: few mm – up to 12 cm
√ thin-walled unilocular mass
CT:
√ homogeneous fluid material of 0–18 HU
√ heterogeneous mass (due to various germinal components)
√ fluid-fluid level (due to supernatant lipid)
√ "sack-of-marbles" appearance (= coalescence of fat) is PATHOGNOMONIC
√ rim enhancement frequent
MR:
√ hypointense / hyperintense (sebaceous fluid) / isointense relative to muscle on T1WI
√ hyperintense on T2WI + internally heterogeneous
Prognosis: malignant degeneration into squamous cell carcinoma in 5%
DDx: ranula

DISSECTION OF CERVICOCEPHALIC ARTERIES

= hematoma within media splitting off the vessel wall and causing a false lumen within media
Incidence: responsible for 5–20% of strokes in young and middle-aged adult
Location: cervical ICA (60%), vertebral artery (20%), both ICA + vertebral artery (10%); multiple simultaneous dissections (33%)
Site: (a) subintimal dissection = close to intima
(b) subadventitial dissection = close to adventitia
√ arterial narrowing / occlusion
√ intimal flap
√ pseudoaneurysm
√ embolic distal branch occlusion of intracranial artery
US (50% accuracy):
√ echogenic intimal flap
√ echogenic thrombus
√ dampened / high-resistance Doppler waveform
CECT:
√ narrowing / occlusion of contrast-filled artery
MR:
√ periarterial rim of hyperintense signal on T1WI + iso- to hyperintense on T2WI around flow void of artery (= intramural hematoma)
√ pseudoenlargement of external diameter of artery
Rx: early anticoagulant therapy (to prevent stroke)

Carotid Artery Dissection

◊ Twice as common as vertebral artery dissection!
Etiology:
A. SPONTANEOUS CAROTID DISSECTION
(1) nonrecalled minor / trivial trauma (frequent)
(2) primary arterial disease (rare): Marfan syndrome. fibromuscular dysplasia (in 15%), cystic medial necrosis, collagen vascular disease, homocystinuria
Associated with: hypertension (36%), smoking (47%), migraine (11%)
B. TRAUMATIC CAROTID DISSECTION (rare) blunt / penetrating trauma (automobile accident, boxing, accidental hanging, diagnostic carotid compression, manipulative therapy)
Associated with: fracture through carotid canal
Incidence: 2–5–20% of strokes in persons aged 40–60 years
Age: 18–76 years (66% between 35 and 50 years)
• unremitting unilateral anterior headache (86%), neck pain (25%)
• TIA / stroke (58%), amaurosis fugax (12%)
• oculosympathetic paresis = Horner syndrome (52%)
• bruit (48%)

ENT

ENT

Location: cervical ICA usually at level of C1-2 (60%) within a few cm of carotid bifurcation > supraclinoid segment of ICA; bilateral carotid dissections (15%)

Length: a few centimeters

Angiography:

√ string sign = elongated tapered irregular luminal stenosis extending to base of skull (76%)
√ abrupt luminal reconstitution at level of bony carotid canal (42%)
√ fingerlike / saccular aneurysm (40%), often in upper cervical / subcranial region
√ intimal flap (29%)
√ double-barrel lumen similar to aortic dissection (rare)
√ slow ICA-MCA flow
√ tapered "flamelike" / "radish taillike" occlusion (17%), often distal to carotid bulb

Cx: (1) Thromboemboli due to stenosis
(2) Subarachnoid hemorrhage (with intracranial location)
(3) Secondary aneurysm

Prognosis: complete / excellent recovery (8%) with normalization in a few months; worsening in 10%

Rx: best therapy not clear; anticoagulation (primary treatment), surgery, endovascular stent placement

Vertebral Artery Dissection

= hemorrhage into wall of vertebral artery

Prevalence: unknown; up to 15% of strokes in young adults

Etiology:
(a) traumatic stretching of artery over lateral mass of C2 during rotation of head (chiropractic manipulation, bowling, tennis, archery)
(b) spontaneous
Predisposed: fibromuscular dysplasia, Marfan syndrome, collagen vascular disease, homocystinuria

• headache: occipital (>50%), frontal (20%), orbital (20%)
• neck pain (30%)

Location: at level of C1/2 (65%); bilateral vertebral artery dissections (5%); site of direct trauma

MR (modality of choice):
√ decreased arterial lumen
√ diminished flow void
√ periarterial rim signal intensity changes with time (hemoglobin)

Angio:
√ tapering of artery / intimal flap / complete occlusion

Cx: stroke (in up to 95%) after hours / weeks

Prognosis: full recovery with some residual deficit (88%)

EPIGLOTTITIS

= ACUTE BACTERIAL EPIGLOTTITIS
= life-threatening infection with edema of epiglottis + aryepiglottic folds

Organism: Haemophilus influenzae type B, Pneumococcus, Streptococcus group A

Age: >3 years, peak incidence 6 years

• abrupt onset of respiratory distress with inspiratory stridor
• severe dysphagia

Location: purely supraglottic lesion; associated subglottic edema in 25%

Lateral radiograph should be taken in erect position only! (frontal view irrelevant)
√ enlargement of epiglottis + thickening of aryepiglottic folds
√ circumferential narrowing of subglottic portion of trachea during inspiration
√ ballooning of hypopharynx + pyriform sinuses
√ cervical kyphosis

Cx: Mortal danger of suffocation secondary to hazard of complete airway closure; patient needs to be accompanied by physician experienced in endotracheal intubation

EXTERNAL AUDITORY CANAL DYSPLASIA

Incidence: 1:10,000 births; family history in 14%

Etiology: (a) isolated (b) Trisomy 13, 18, 21 (c) Turner syndrome (d) Maternal rubella (e) Craniofacial dysostosis (f) Mandibulofacial dysostosis

SPECTRUM
1. Stenosis of EAC
2. Fibrous atresia of EAC
3. Bony atresia (in position of tympanic membrane)
4. Decreased pneumatization of mastoid (mastoid cells begin to form in 7th fetal month)
5. Decreased size / absence of tympanic cavity
6. Ossicular changes (rotation, fusion, absence)
7. Ectopic facial nerve = anteriorly displaced vertical (mastoid) portion of facial nerve canal
8. Decrease in number of cochlear turns / absence of cochlea
9. Dilatation of lateral semicircular canal

• bilateral in 29%; M:F = 6:4
• pinna deformity
• stenotic / absent auditory canal

Cx: congenital cholesteatoma (infrequent)

EXTRAMEDULLARY PLASMACYTOMA

Uncommon form; relatively benign course (dissemination may be found months / years later or not at all); questionable if precursor to multiple myeloma

Age : 35–40 years; M:F = 2:1

Location: air passages (50%) predominantly in upper nose and oral cavity; larynx; conjunctiva (37%); lymph nodes (3%)

• usually not associated with increased immunoglobulin titer or amyloid deposition

√ mass of one to several cm in size with well-defined lobulated border

Classification:
1. Medullary plasmacytoma
2. Multiple myeloma:
   (a) scattered involvement of bone
   (b) myelomatosis of bone
3. Extramedullary plasmacytoma

DDx:
(1) MULTIPLE MYELOMA
= malignant course with soft-tissue involvement in 50–73%:
(a) microscopic infiltration
(b) enlargement of organs
(c) formation of tumor mass (1/3)
- usually associated with protein abnormalities
- may have amyloid deposition

Age incidence: 50–85 years
◊ Tends to occur late in the course of the disease and indicates a poor prognosis (0–6% 5-year survival)

FIBROMATOSIS COLLI

= rare form of infantile fibromatosis that occurs solely in sternocleidomastoid muscle

Cause: in >90% associated with birth trauma during difficult delivery / forceps delivery

Pathology: compartment syndrome with pressure necrosis + secondary fibrosis of sternocleidomastoid m.

Age: 2nd to 4th weeks of life; M > F
- history of difficult delivery (forceps)
- firm soft-tissue mass in lower 1/3 of sternocleidomastoid muscle, which may grow over 2–4 additional weeks
- torticollis (14–20%) due to muscle contraction

Location: lower 1/3 of sternocleidomastoid muscle affecting sternal + clavicular heads of the muscle; usually unilateral (R > L)

√ focal / diffuse enlargement of sternocleidomastoid m.

US:
√ homogeneously enlarged sternocleidomastoid m. without a focal lesion
√ well- / ill-defined mass within sternocleidomastoid m.:
√ hypo- to iso- to hyperechoic mass depending on duration of disorder

MR:
√ diffuse abnormal high signal intensity (greater than that of fat) within muscle on T2WI

CT:
√ isoattenuating homogeneous muscle enlargement

Prognosis: gradual spontaneous regression by age 2 (in 66%) with / without treatment

Rx: (1) muscle stretching exercise (2) surgery in 10%

DDx:
(1) Neuroblastoma (heterogeneous solid mass with calcifications)
(2) Rhabdomyosarcoma
(3) Lymphoma (well-defined round /oval masses along cervical lymph node chain)
(4) Cystic hygroma (anechoic region with septations)
(5) Branchial cleft cyst
(6) Hematoma

GOITER

Adenomatous Goiter

= MULTINODULAR GOITER

US: (89% sensitivity, 84% specificity, 73% positive predictive value, 94% negative predictive value)
√ increased size + asymmetry of gland
√ multiple 1–4-cm solid nodules
√ areas of hemorrhage + necrosis
√ coarse calcifications may occur within adenoma (secondary to hemorrhage + necrosis)

Cx: compression of trachea

Diffuse Goiter

US:
√ increase in glandular size, R lobe > L lobe
√ NO focal textural changes
√ calcifications not associated with nodules

Iodine-deficiency Goiter

Not a significant problem in United States because of supplemental iodine in food

Etiology: chronic TSH stimulation
- low serum T_4

√ high I-131 uptake

Jod-Basedow Phenomenon (2%)

= development of thyrotoxicosis (= excessive amounts of T_4 synthesized + released) if normal dietary intake is resumed / iodinated contrast medium administered

Incidence: most common in individuals with long-standing multinodular goiter

Age: >50 years

√ multinodular goiter with in- / decreased uptake (depending on iodine pool)

Toxic Nodular Goiter

= PLUMMER DISEASE
= autonomous function of one / more thyroid adenomas

Peak age: 4–5th decade; M:F = 1:3
- elevated T_4
- suppressed TSH

√ nodular thyroid with hot nodule + suppression of remainder of gland
√ stimulation scan will disclose normal uptake in remainder of gland
√ increased radioiodine uptake by 24 hours of approximately 80%

Rx:
(1) I-131 treatment with empirical dose of 25–29 mCi (hypothyroidism in 5–30%)
(2) Surgery (hypothyroidism in 11%)
(3) Percutaneous ethanol injection (hypothyroidism in <1%, transient damage of recurrent laryngeal nerve in 4%)

Intrathoracic Goiter

= extension of cervical thyroid tissue / ectopic thyroid tissue (rare) into mediastinum

Incidence: 5% of resected mediastinal masses; most common cause of mediastinal masses; 2% of all goiters

- mostly asymptomatic
- symptoms of tracheal + esophageal + recurrent laryngeal nerve compression

Location:
(a) retrosternal (80%) = in front of trachea
(b) posterior descending (20%) = behind trachea but in front of esophagus, caudal extent limited by arch of azygos vein, exclusively on right side of trachea

√ continuity with cervical thyroid / lack of continuity (with narrow fibrous / vascular pedicle)
√ frequent focal calcifications

CT:
√ mass of high HU + well-defined margins
√ inhomogeneous texture with low-density areas (= degenerative cystic areas)
√ marked + prolonged enhancement

GRAVES DISEASE

= DIFFUSE TOXIC GOITER
= autoimmune disorder with thyroid-stimulating antibodies (LATS) producing hyperplasia + hypertrophy of thyroid gland

Peak age: 3rd–4th decade; M:F = 1:7

- elevated T_3 + T_4
- depressed TSH production
- dermopathy = pretibial myxedema (5%)
- ophthalmopathy = periorbital edema, lid retraction, ophthalmoplegia, proptosis, malignant exophthalmos

√ diffuse thyroid enlargement
√ uniformly increased uptake
√ incidental nodules superimposed on preexisting adenomatous goiter (5%)

US: (identical to diffuse goiter)
√ global enlargement of 2–3 x the normal size
√ normal / diffusely hypoechoic pattern
√ hyperemia on color Doppler

Rx: I-131 treatments (for adults):
Dose: 80–120 µCi/g of gland with 100% uptake (taking into account estimated weight of gland + measured radioactive iodine uptake for 24 hours)
Cx: 10–30% develop hypothyroidism within 1st year + 3%/year rate thereafter

HIV PAROTITIS

Histo: benign lymphoepithelial lesion consisting of an intranodal cyst lined with epithelial cells

US:
√ multiple hypoechoic / anechoic areas without posterior acoustic enhancement (70%)
√ anechoic cysts (30%)

CT / MR:
√ bilateral parotid gland enlargement with intraglandular cystic + solid masses
√ cervical lymphadenopathy + enlarged adenoids typically associated

Prognosis: parotid involvement is associated with a better prognosis in HIV-positive children!

HYPOPHARYNGEAL CARCINOMA

Histo: squamous cell carcinoma

May be associated with: Plummer-Vinson syndrome (= atrophic mucosa, achlorhydria, sideropenic anemia) affecting women in 90%

- sore throat, intolerance to hot / cold liquids (early signs)
- dysphagia, weight loss (late signs)
- cervical adenopathy (in 50% at presentation)

Stage:
T1 tumor limited to one subsite
T2 tumor involves >1 subsite / adjacent site without fixation of hemilarynx
T3 same as T2 with fixation of hemilarynx
T4 invasion of thyroid / cricoid cartilage / soft tissue of neck

Pyriform Sinus Carcinoma

Incidence: 60% of hypopharyngeal carcinomas

- may escape clinical detection if located at inferior tip; often origin of "cervical adenopathy with unknown primary" (next to primaries in lingual + faucial tonsils and nasopharynx)

√ invasion of posterior ala of thyroid cartilage, cricothyroid space, soft tissue of neck in T4 lesion

Prognosis: poor due to early soft-tissue invasion

Postcricoid Carcinoma

Incidence: 25% of hypopharyngeal carcinomas

√ difficult assessment due to varying thickness of inferior constrictor + prevertebral muscles

Prognosis: 25% 5-year survival (worst prognosis)

Posterior Pharyngeal Wall Carcinoma

Incidence: 15% of hypopharyngeal carcinomas

√ invasion of retropharyngeal space with extension into oro- and nasopharynx
√ retropharyngeal adenopathy

INVERTED PAPILLOMA

= INVERTING PAPILLOMA = ENDOPHYTIC PAPILLOMA = SQUAMOUS CELL PAPILLOMA = TRANSITIONAL CELL PAPILLOMA = CYLINDRICAL EPITHELIOMA = SCHNEIDERIAN PAPILLOMA

Incidence: 4% of all nasal neoplasms; most common of epithelial papillomas; commonly occurring after nasal surgery

Cause: unknown; association with human papillomavirus-11

Age: 40–60 years; M:F = 3–5:1

Path: vascular mass with prominent mucous cyst inclusions interspersed throughout epithelium

Histo: hyperplastic epithelium inverts into underlying stroma rather than in an exophytic direction; high intracellular glycogen content

◊ Squamous cell carcinoma coexistent in 5.5–27%!

Location: uniquely unilateral (bilateral in <5%)
(a) most often arising from the lateral nasal wall with extension into ethmoid / maxillary sinuses, at junction of antrum + ethmoid sinuses
(b) paranasal sinus (most frequently maxillary antrum)
(c) nasal septum (5.5–18%)
• unilateral nasal obstruction, epistaxis, postnasal drip, recurrent sinusitis, sinus headache
• distinctive absence of allergic history
√ commonly involves antrum + ethmoid sinus
√ widening of infundibulum / outflow tract of antrum
√ destruction of medial antral wall / lamina papyracea of orbit, anterior cranial fossa (pressure necrosis) in up to 30%
√ septum may be bowed to opposite side (NO invasion)
√ homogeneous enhancement
MR:
√ may have intermediate to low intensity on T2WI (DDx: squamous cell carcinoma, olfactory neuroblastoma, melanoma, small cell carcinoma)
Cx: (1) cellular atypia / squamous cell carcinoma (10%)
(2) recurrence rate of 15–78%
Rx: complete surgical extirpation (lateral rhinotomy with en bloc excision of lateral nasal wall)

JUVENILE ANGIOFIBROMA

= most common benign nasopharyngeal tumor, can grow to enormous size and locally invade vital structures
Incidence: 0.5% of all head and neck neoplasms
Age: teenagers (mean age of 15 years); almost exclusively in males
• recurrent + severe epistaxis (59%)
• nasal speech due to nasal obstruction (91%)
• facial deformity (less common)
Location: nasopharynx / posterior nares
Extension: posterolateral wall of nasal cavity; via pterygopalatine fossa into retroantral region / orbit / middle cranial fossa; laterally into infratemporal fossa
√ widening of pterygopalatine fossa (90%) with anterior bowing of posterior antral wall
√ invasion of sphenoid sinus (2/3) from tumor erosion through floor of sinus
√ widening of inferior + superior orbital fissures (spread into orbit via inferior orbital fissure + into middle cranial fossa via superior orbital fissure)
√ highly vascular nasopharyngeal mass (only enhances on CT scan immediately after bolus injection); supplied primarily by internal maxillary artery
MR:
√ intermediate signal intensity on T1WI with discrete punctate areas of hypointensity (secondary to highly vascular stroma)
NOTE: Biopsy contraindicated!

LABYRINTHITIS

Cause: viral infection (mumps, measles) > bacterial infection > syphilis, autoimmune, toxins
• sudden hearing loss, vertigo, tinnitus
MR: √ faint diffuse enhancement of labyrinth on T1WI (HALLMARK)

Ramsay-Hunt syndrome = herpes zoster oticus
• mucosal vesicles of external auditory canal
√ intracanalicular 8th nerve enhancement

Tympanogenic Labyrinthitis

Cause: agent enters through oval / round window in middle ear infection

Meningogenic Labyrinthitis

Cause: agent propagates along IAC / cochlear aqueduct in meningitis
Location: often bilateral

Labyrinthitis Ossificans

= LABYRINTHITIS OBLITERANS = SCLEROSING LABYRINTHITIS = CALCIFIC / OSSIFYING COCHLEITIS
Cause: suppurative infection (tympanogenic, meningogenic, hematogenic) in 90%, trauma, surgery, tumor, severe otosclerosis
Pathophysiology: progressive fibrosis + ossification of granulation tissue within labyrinth
• bi - / unilateral profound deafness
√ loss of normal fluid signal within labyrinth on T2WI (early in course of disease)
√ inner ear structures filled with bone

LARYNGEAL CARCINOMA

98% of all malignant laryngeal tumors; in 2% sarcomas
Risk factors: smoking, alcohol abuse, airborne irritants
Histo: squamous cell carcinoma
Suggestive of lymph node metastasis:
√ lymph node >1.5 cm in cross section
√ proximity to laryngeal mass
√ cluster of >3 lymph nodes 6–15 mm in size

Supraglottic Carcinoma

Incidence: 20–30% of all laryngeal cancers
Metastases: early to lymph nodes of deep cervical chain, in 25–55% at time of presentation
• symptomatic late in course of disease (often T3 / T4)
Stage:
T1 tumor confined to site of origin
T2 involvement of adjacent supraglottic site / glottis without cord fixation
T3 tumor limited to larynx with cord fixation or extension to postcricoid area / medial wall of pyriform sinus / preepiglottic space
T4 extension beyond larynx with involvement of oropharynx (base of tongue) / soft tissue of neck / thyroid cartilage

A. ANTERIOR COMPARTMENT
1. **Epiglottic carcinoma**
√ circumferential relatively symmetric growth
√ extension into preepiglottic space ± base of tongue ± paraglottic space
Prognosis: better than for tumors of posterolateral compartment

ENT

B. POSTEROLATERAL COMPARTMENT
1. **Aryepiglottic fold (marginal supraglottic) carcinoma**
   √ exophytic growth from medial surface of aryepiglottic fold
   √ growth into fixed portion of epiglottis + paraglottic (= paralaryngeal) space
2. **False vocal cord / laryngeal ventricle carcinoma**
   √ submucosal spread into paraglottic space
   √ ± destruction of thyroid cartilage
   √ ± involvement of true vocal cords
   Prognosis: poorer than for cancer of the anterior compartment

Glottic Carcinoma

Incidence: 50–60% of all laryngeal cancers
• early detection due to hoarseness
Stage:
T1 tumor confined to vocal cord with normal mobility
T2 supra- / subglottic extension ± impaired mobility
T3 fixation of true vocal cord
T4 destruction of thyroid cartilage / extension outside larynx
Patterns of tumor invasion:
(1) anterior extension into anterior commissure
   √ >1 mm thickness of anterior commissure
   √ invasion of contralateral vocal cord via anterior commissure
(2) posterior extension to arytenoid cartilage, posterior commissure, cricoarytenoid joint
(3) subglottic extension
   √ tumor >5 mm inferior to level of vocal cords
(4) deep lateral extension into paralaryngeal space
Prognosis: T1 carcinoma rarely metastasizes (0–2%) due to absence of lymphatics within true vocal cords

Subglottic Carcinoma

Incidence: 5% of all laryngeal cancers
• late detection due to minimal symptomatology
Stage:
T1 confined to subglottic area
T2 extension to vocal cords ± mobility
T3 tumor confined to larynx + cord fixation
T4 cartilage destruction / extension beyond larynx
Prognosis: poor due to early metastases to cervical lymph nodes (in 25% at presentation)

LARYNGEAL CHONDROSARCOMA

◊ The most common sarcoma of the larynx
Age: 50–70 years; M >> F
• lobulated submucosal mass
Location: posterior lamina of cricoid cartilage (50–70%), thyroid cartilage (20–35%)
√ coarse / stippled intratumoral calcifications
√ ± locally invasive
MR:
   √ very high signal intensity of tumor matrix on T2WI (corresponding to hyaline cartilage)
Rx: function-preserving laryngeal resection (local recurrence may be seen 10 years or more)
DDx: benign chondroma

LARYNGEAL HEMANGIOMA

Histo: cavernous / capillary type
• dark bluish red / pale red compressible swelling on endoscopy
√ strong contrast enhancement
CT:
   √ phleboliths (PATHOGNOMONIC for cavernous type)
MR:
   √ very high signal intensity on T2WI
DDx: paraganglioma, hypervascular metastasis (renal adenocarcinoma)

Infantile Laryngeal Hemangioma (10%)

= SUBGLOTTIC HEMANGIOMA
◊ Most common subglottic soft-tissue mass causing upper respiratory tract obstruction in neonates
Age: <6 months; M:F = 1:2
• crouplike symptoms (dyspnea, stridor) in neonatal period
• hemangiomas elsewhere (skin, mucosal membranes) in 50%
Location: subglottic region
√ eccentric thickening of subglottic portion of trachea (AP view)
√ arises from posterior wall below true cords (lateral view)
Rx: tracheostomy (waiting for spontaneous regression)

Adult Laryngeal Hemangioma

Location: supraglottic region (isolated); associated with extensive cervicofacial angiodysplasia
M > F
Rx: laser excision, cryotherapy, selective embolization

LARYNGEAL PAPILLOMATOSIS

= RECURRENT RESPIRATORY PAPILLOMATOSIS
◊ Squamous papilloma is the most common benign tumor of the larynx!
Etiology: human papilloma virus types 6 + 11 (Papova virus causing genital condyloma acuminatum)
Histo: core of vascular connective tissue covered by stratified squamous epithelium
Age of onset: 1–54 years; M:F = 1:1; bimodal distribution
(a) <10 years (diffuse involvement) = **juvenile laryngotracheal papillomatosis**; probably caused by transmission from mother to child during vaginal delivery
(b) 21–50 years (usually single papilloma)
• progressive hoarseness / aphonia
• repeated episodes of respiratory distress
• inspiratory stridor, asthmalike symptoms
• cough
• recurrent pneumonia

- hemoptysis

Location: (a) uvula, palate (b) vocal cord (c) subglottic extension (50–70%) (d) pulmonary involvement (1–6%)

√ thickened lumpy cords
√ bronchiectasis

Cx:

(1) **Tracheobronchial papillomatosis** (2–5%)
Cause: tracheostomy
Location: lower lobe + posterior predilection
√ solid pulmonary nodules in mid + posterior lung fields
√ 2–3 cm large thin-walled cavity with 2–4 mm thick nodular wall (foci of squamous papillomas enlarge centrifugally, undergo central necrosis, cavitate)
√ peripheral atelectasis + obstructive pneumonitis

(2) **Pulmonary papillomatosis**
from aerial dissemination (bronchoscopy, laryngoscopy, tracheal intubation) 10 years after initial diagnosis
√ irregularities of tracheal / bronchial walls
√ noncalcified granulomata progressing to cavitation

(3) Malignant transformation into invasive squamous cell carcinoma

Rx: CO_2 laser resection / surgical excision

LARYNGEAL PLASMACYTOMA

Age: 50–70 years; M >> F

Histo: large sheets of uniform cells indistinguishable from normal plasma cells; marked amyloid deposition (20%)

- pedunculated / slightly prominent mass that bleeds easily

Location: epiglottis, true + false vocal cords

CT:
√ large smoothly marginated homogeneous mass
√ no significant contrast enhancement

LARYNGOCELE

= dilated appendix / sacculus of the laryngeal ventricle extending beyond the superior border of the thyroid cartilage

Incidence: 1:2,500,000

Age: middle-aged men

Anatomy: laryngeal ventricle of Morgagni is a slitlike cavity between true + false cords; along the anterior third of its roof arises the small blind mucosa-lined laryngeal saccule of Hilton / laryngeal appendix; it extends superiorly between false vocal cord and aryepiglottic fold medially + thyroid cartilage laterally; the laryngeal appendix is relatively large in infancy; usually involutes by 6th year of life

Pathogenesis: chronic increase in intraglottic pressure

Cause: excessive coughing, shouting, playing wind instrument, blowing glass, obstruction of appendicular ostium (= secondary laryngocele) by chronic granulomatous disease / laryngeal neoplasm (15%)

N.B.: Almost 50% of laryngoceles detected with plain radiography contain a laryngeal carcinoma!

Histo: lined by pseudostratified columnar ciliated epithelium + mixture of submucosal serous and mucous glands

Types:

(a) internal (40%) = in parapharyngeal space confined within thyrohyoid membrane
(b) external (26%) = protrusion through thyrohyoid membrane at the point of insertion of the neurovascular bundle (superior laryngeal nerve + vessels) presenting as lateral neck mass near hyoid bone with normal size inside the membrane
(c) mixed (44%) = internal + external dilatation of saccule on both sides of thyrohyoid membrane

- visible in 10% of adults during phonation
- hoarseness / dysphagia / stridor (internal laryngocele)
- compressible anterior neck mass just below angle of mandible (external laryngocele)
- Bryce sign = gurgling / hissing sound on compression

Site: unilateral (80%), bilateral (23%)

√ sharply defined round / oval radiolucent area within paralaryngeal soft tissues
  √ increase in size during Valsalva maneuver
  √ decrease in size during compression
√ cystic mass that can be followed to level of ventricle
√ may be filled with fluid / contain air-fluid level
√ DIAGNOSTIC = connection between air sac + airway

Cx: infection (laryngopyocele) in 8–10%, formation of mucocele

DDx: laryngeal cyst (lined by squamous epithelium); lateral pharyngeal diverticulum (fills with barium)

LARYNGOMALACIA

= immaturity of cartilage; most common cause of stridor in neonate + young infant

- only cause of stridor to get worse at rest

√ hypercollapsible larynx during inspiration (supraglottic portion only)
√ backward bent of epiglottis + anterior kink of aryepiglottic folds during inspiration

Prognosis: transient (disappears by age 1 year)

LINGUAL THYROID

= solid embryonic rest of thyroid tissue, which remains ectopic along the tract of thyroglossal duct

Incidence: in 10% of autopsies (within tongue <3 mm); M << F

- may be only functioning thyroid tissue (70–80%)
- asymptomatic (usually)
- may enlarge causing dysphagia / dyspnea

Location: midline dorsum of tongue near foramen cecum (majority), thyroglossal duct, trachea

CT: √ small focus of intrinsic high attenuation

Cx: malignancy in 3% (papillary carcinoma)

LYMPHANGIOMA

= congenital lymphatic malformation

Incidence: 5.6% of all benign tumors of infancy + childhood

Age: present at birth in 50–65%, in 80–90% evident by age 2 (time of greatest lymphatic growth); M = F

Lymphatic development:
endothelial buds from veins in jugular region form confluent plexuses, which develop into rapidly enlarging bilateral juguloaxillary lymph sacs (7.5 weeks GA); these fused lymph sacs extend craniad and dorsolateral with extensive outgrowth of lymph vessels in all directions; connection with internal jugular vein at level of confluence with external jugular vein persists on the left side

Pathogenesis:
(1) early sequestration of embryonic lymphatic tissue with failure to join central lymphatic channels
(2) congenital obstruction of lymphatic drainage due to abnormal budding of lymph vessels (= loss of connection / noncommunication of primordial jugular lymphatic sac with jugular vein)

Classification (on basis of size of lymphatic spaces):
(1) Cystic lymphangioma = cystic hygroma
(2) Cavernous lymphangioma
= mildly dilated cavernous lymphatic spaces with cysts of intermediate size
Location: tongue, floor of mouth, salivary glands
√ penetration of contiguous structures
√ same signal intensities as cystic lymphangioma + fibrous stromal component of low intensity on T1WI + T2WI
(3) Capillary / simple lymphangioma (least common)
= capillary-sized lymphatic channels
Location: epidermis + dermis of proximal limbs
(4) Vasculolymphatic malformation
composed of lymphatic + vascular elements, eg, lymphangiohemangioma

Histo: endothelial-lined lymphatic channels containing serous / milky fluid + separated by connective tissue stroma

- asymptomatic (in majority) soft / semifirm mass
- ± dyspnea / dysphagia with encroachment upon trachea, pharynx, esophagus
- rapid increase in size (from infection / hemorrhage)

Location: anywhere in developing lymphatic system; mostly in posterior cervical triangle, occasionally in floor of mouth / tongue
(a) posterior triangle of neck (most common), with extension into mediastinum in 3–10%
  - visible at birth in 65%
  - clinically apparent by end of 2nd decade in 90%
(b) anterior mediastinum (<1%)
(c) axilla, chest wall, groin

Cx: infection, airway compromise, chylothorax, chylopericardium

Prognosis: spontaneous regression (10–15%)
Rx: surgical excision (treatment of choice but difficult since mass does not follow tissue planes) with recurrence rate of up to 15%

Cystic Hygroma

= CYSTIC LYMPHANGIOMA
= single / multiloculated fluid-filled cavities on either side of fetal neck + head (localized form) ± trunk (generalized form) as the most common form of lymphangioma developing within loose connective tissue

Incidence: 1:6,000 pregnancies
Path: multiple enormously dilated cystic lymphatic channels; varying between a few mm to >10 cm in diameter containing chylous fluid; separated by minimal intervening stroma; may invade adjacent soft tissues / muscle and surround vessels
Histo: cystic spaces lined by endothelial cells + supporting connective tissue stroma

Associated with:
(a) chromosomal abnormalities in 60–80% (in particular when detected in 2nd trimester)
  (1) Turner syndrome (45 XO, mosaic) in 40–80%
  (2) Trisomies 13, 18, 21, 13q, 18p, 22
  (3) Noonan syndrome
  (4) Distichiasis (= second row of hair behind eyelash) -lymphedema syndrome
  (5) Familial pterygium colli
  (6) Roberts, Cumming, Cowchock syndrome
  (7) Achondrogenesis type II
  (8) Lethal pterygium syndrome
(b) exposure to teratogens
  (1) Fetal alcohol syndrome
  (2) aminopterin
  (3) trimethadione

Types:
(1) Cystic hygroma with abnormal peripheral lymphatic system
  √ lymphangioma in posterior compartment of neck
  √ septations (indicate high probability for aneuploidy, development of hydrops, and perinatal death)
(2) Diffuse lymphangiectasia
  √ lymphangioma of chest + extremities
  √ peripheral lymphedema + nonimmune hydrops
(3) Isolated cystic hygroma
  (a) axillary lymph sac malformation
    √ lymphangioma restricted to axilla
  (b) jugular lymph sac malformation
    √ lymphangioma restricted to lateral neck
  (c) internal thoracic + paratracheal lymph sac malformation
    √ lymphangioma within mediastinum
  (d) combined lymph sac malformation
  (e) thoracic duct malformation
    √ thoracic duct cyst

- AF-AFP / MS-AFP may be elevated

Location: neck (frequently posterior cervical space) and lower portions of face (75–80%), mediastinum (3–10%, in 1/2 extension from neck), axilla (20%), chest wall (14%), face (10%), retroperitoneum (kidneys), abdominal viscera (colon, spleen, liver), groin, scrotum, skeleton

US:
- √ thin-walled fluid-filled structure with multiple septa of variable thickness + solid cyst wall components
- √ fluid-fluid level with layering hemorrhagic component
- √ isolated nuchal cysts
- √ webbed neck (= pterygium colli) following later communication with jugular veins
- √ nonimmune hydrops (43%)
- √ progressive peripheral edema
- √ fetal ascites
- √ oligo- / polyhydramnios / normal amount of fluid
- √ bradycardia

CT:
- √ poorly circumscribed multiloculated masses
- √ homogeneous attenuation of fluid values / higher (after infection)

MR:
- √ hyperintense on T2WI
- √ low to high signal intensity on T1WI (depending on protein content of fluid)
- √ may be hyperintense on T1WI (due to clotted blood / high chylous lipid content)
- √ ± fluid-fluid level (if hemorrhage present)

Cx: (1) Compression of airways / esophagus
(2) Slow growth / sudden enlargement (hemorrhage, inflammation)

Prognosis:
(1) Intrauterine demise (33%)
(2) Mortality of 100% with hydrops
(3) Spontaneous regression (10–15%)
◊ Favorable prognosis for localized lesions of anterior neck + axilla
◊ Only 2–3% of fetuses with posterior cystic hygroma become healthy living children!

DDx: twin sac of blighted ovum, cervical meningocele, encephalocele, cystic teratoma, nuchal edema, branchial cleft cyst, vascular malformation, lipoma, abscess

Pseudocystic Hygroma

= PSEUDOMEMBRANE
= anechoic space bordered by specular reflection on posterior aspect of fetal neck during 1st trimester

Cause: ? developing integument
- √ NO prominent posterior bulge / internal septations

MADELUNG DISEASE

= BENIGN SYMMETRICAL LIPOMATOSIS
= rare benign condition characterized by deposition of massive amounts of adipose tissue in neck, shoulders, upper chest

Cx: tracheal compression with respiratory compromise

MALIGNANT EXTERNAL OTITIS

= severe bacterial infection of the soft tissues + bones of base of skull

Organism: almost always Pseudomonas aeruginosa
Age: elderly
Predisposed: diabetes mellitus / immunocompromised

- • unrelenting otalgia, headache
- • purulent otorrhea unresponsive to topical antibiotics
- • may cause malfunction of nerves VII, IX, X, XI

Location: at bone-cartilage junction of EAC

Spread of infection:
(a) inferiorly into soft tissues inferior to temporal bone, parotid space, nasopharyngeal masticator space
(b) posteriorly into mastoid
(c) anteriorly into temporomandibular joint
(d) medially into petrous apex

CT:
- √ soft-tissue density in external auditory canal (100%)
- √ fluid in mastoid / middle ear (89%)
- √ disease around eustachian tube (64%)
- √ obliteration of fat planes beneath temporal bone (64%)
- √ involvement of parapharyngeal space (54%)
- √ masticator space disease (27%)
- √ mass effect in nasopharynx (54%)
- √ bone erosion of clivus (9%)
- √ intracranial extension (9%)

Cx: bone destruction, osteomyelitis, abscess
Prognosis: 20% recurrence rate
DDx: malignant neoplasm

MUCOCELE

= end stage of a chronically obstructed sinus

Incidence: most common lesion to cause expansion of paranasal sinus; increased incidence in cystic fibrosis
Etiology: obstructed paranasal sinus ostium
Path: expanded sinus cyst lined by mucosa with accumulated secretions and desquamations
Age: usually adulthood

- • history of chronic nasal polyposis + pansinusitis
- • commonly present with unilateral proptosis
- • decreased visual acuity, visual field defect
- • palpable mass in superomedial aspect of orbit (frontal mucocele)
- • intractable headaches

Location:
mnemonic: "fems"
frontal (60%) > **e**thmoid (30%) > **m**axillary (10%) > **s**phenoid (rare)

- √ soft-tissue density mass
- √ sinus cavity expansion (DDx: never in sinusitis)
- √ bone demineralization + remodeling at late stage but NO bone destruction (impossible DDx from neoplasm)
- √ surrounding zone of bone sclerosis / calcification of edges of mucocele (from chronic infection)
- √ macroscopic calcification in 5% (especially with superimposed fungal infection)
- √ uniform enhancement of thin rim

US:
- √ homogeneous hypoechoic mass

MR:
- √ signal intensity varies with state of hydration, protein content, hemorrhage, air content, calcification, fibrosis
- √ hypointense on T1WI + signal void on T2WI due to inspissated debris + fungus

ENT

√ peripheral enhancement pattern (DDx from solid enhancement pattern of neoplasms)

Cx: (1) protrusion into orbit displacing medial rectus muscle laterally
(2) expansion into subarachnoid space resulting in CSF leak
(3) mucopyocele = superimposed infection (rare)

DDx: paranasal sinus carcinoma, Aspergillus infection (enlargement of medial rectus muscle + optic nerve, focal / diffuse areas of increased attenuation), chronic infection, inverting papilloma

MUCOEPIDERMOID CARCINOMA

Path: arises from intercalated ducts of seromucinous glands

Histo: composed of a mixture of 3 cells: mucin-secreting cells + squamous cells + mucous cells; arranged in cords / sheets / cystic configuration

Prognosis: variable (well-encapsulated low-grade to infiltrating highly aggressive malignancy)

Rx: complete surgical removal

Parotid Mucoepidermoid Carcinoma

◊ Most common malignant lesion of parotid gland
◊ In children: up to 35% of all salivary gland tumors are malignant – 60% are mucoepidermoid carcinomas

- rock-hard mass
- pain / itching along course of facial nerve
- facial nerve paralysis

CT:
√ may contain cystic low-attenuating areas
√ focal calcifications (rare)

(a) low-grade lesion
√ well-circumscribed parotid mass
√ hypo- to isointense on T1WI
√ hyperintense on T2WI
Rx: wide local excision

(b) high-grade lesion
√ infiltrating poorly marginated, more solid, relatively homogeneous lesion with few cystic areas
Rx: wide block excision + radical neck dissection

Laryngeal Mucoepidermoid Carcinoma

Incidence: ~100 cases
M:F = 6:1
Location: epiglottis (most common)

NASAL GLIOMA

= misnomer (no neoplastic features) = NASAL CEREBRAL HETEROTOPIA
= rare developmental mass composed of dysplastic sequestered neurogenic tissue that has become isolated from the subarachnoid space

Age: usually identified at birth
Location: extranasal (60%); intranasal (30%); combination of intra- and extranasal (10%)
Site: unilateral right > left side

- no change in size during crying

√ may parallel the rate of brain growth
√ attached to middle turbinate bone / nasal septum
√ soft-tissue mass of glabella
√ attached to brain by stalk (10–30%)

MR:
√ iso- / hypointense relative to gray matter on T1WI
√ hyperintense on T2WI

OTIC CAPSULE DYSPLASIA

Cochlear Aplasia

= **Michel aplasia** = Michel anomaly = agenesis of osseous + membranous labyrinth (rare)

Cause: arrested development at 4 weeks GA

- total sensorineural hearing loss

√ region of otic capsule normally occupied by cochlea is replaced by dense labyrinthine + pneumatized bone
√ flat medial wall of middle ear (= undeveloped horizontal semicircular canal)
√ hypoplasia of internal auditory canal
√ dysplasia of vestibule = marked enlargement into region of lateral + superior semicircular canals

DDx: labyrinthitis obliterans (no loss of lateral convexity of medial wall of middle ear)

Single-cavity Cochlea

= saccular defect / cavity in otic capsule in the position normally occupied by cochlea without recognizable modiolus, osseous spiral lamina, interscalar septum

- profound hearing loss discovered in early childhood

May be associated with: recurrent bacterial meningitis, perilymphatic fistula of oval window

√ cystic cochlea (= developed basal turn, middle + apical turn occupy common nondeveloped space)

Insufficient Cochlear Turns

= normal basilar turn + varying degrees of hypoplasia of middle and apical turns

Mondini malformation

= absence of anterior 1 1/2 turns of cochlea often with preservation of the basilar turn

Cause: in utero insult at 7 weeks GA

Frequency: 2nd most common imaging finding in children with sensorineural hearing loss

- some high-frequency hearing preserved
- vertigo
- otorrhea, rhinorrhea, recurrent meningitis (perilymphatic fistula caused by absence / defect of stapes footplate)

√ absence of cochlear apex

May be associated with: deformity of vestibule + semicircular canals + vestibular aqueduct

Anomalies of Membranous Labyrinth

Scheibe dysplasia = abnormal cochlea + saccule
Alexander dysplasia = dysplasia of basal turn
√ normal CT findings

Small Internal Auditory Canal

= decrease in the diameter of IAC due to hypoplasia / aplasia of cochlear nerve (portion of cranial nerve VIII)
• total sensorineural hearing loss
√ hypoplastic anteroinferior quadrant of IAC

Large Vestibule

Associated with: underdeveloped lateral semicircular canal
• sensorineural hearing deficit (most common cause)
√ lateral semicircular canal smaller
√ vestibule extends further into lateral + superior aspects of otic capsule

Large Vestibular Aqueduct

= Enlarged vestibular aqueduct syndrome
Age: manifests around 3 years
Frequency: most common imaging abnormality detected in children with sensorineural hearing loss
• unilateral congenital deafness (commonly missed)
• vertigo, tinnitus (in 50%)
Location: bilateral in 50–66%
√ vestibular aqueduct >1.4–2 mm in diameter measured halfway between posterior petrous bone and common crus at level of vestibule
√ vestibular aqueduct larger than superior and posterior semicircular canals

OTOSCLEROSIS

= OTOSPONGIOSIS
= replacement of dense otic capsule by highly vascular spongy bone in active phase (misnomer) with restoration of density during reparative sclerotic phase
Etiology: unknown; frequently hereditary
Age: adolescent / young adult Caucasian; M:F = 1:2

A. STAPEDIAL = FENESTRAL OTOSCLEROSIS (80–90%)
Location: anterior oval window margin (= fissula ante fenestram); bilateral in 85%
• tinnitus early in course (2/3)
• progressive conductive hearing loss (stapes fixation in oval window)
√ oval window too wide (lytic phase)
√ new bone formation on anterior oval window margin ± posterior oval window margin ± round window
√ complete plugging of oval window = obliterative otosclerosis (in 2%)

B. COCHLEAR = RETROFENESTRAL OTOSCLEROSIS (10–20%)
Invariably associated with: fenestral otosclerosis
• progressive sensorineural hearing loss (involvement of otic capsule / cytotoxic enzyme diffusion into fluid of membranous labyrinth)
• Schwartze sign = reddish hue behind tympanic membrane when promontory involved
√ "double ring / double lucent" = lucent halo around cochlea (may appear as 3rd turn to cochlea) in early phase
√ bony proliferation in reparative sclerotic phase difficult to diagnose because of same density as cochlea

DDx: Paget disease, osteogenesis imperfecta, syphilis

PAPILLARY ENDOLYMPHATIC SAC TUMOR

= HEFFNER TUMOR
= adenomatous tumor of the temporal bone
Origin: epithelial lining of endolymphatic sac
Associated with: von Hippel-Lindau disease (may have bilateral papillary endolymphatic sac neoplasms)
• hearing loss, facial nerve palsy, vestibular dysfunction
√ solid + cystic components
√ surrounded by thin shell of reactive bone
√ may be hypervascular (supplied by branches of external carotid artery)
√ intratumoral calcifications = "bone sequestra" from destruction of petrous bone
√ contrast enhancement
MR:
√ speckled pattern of hyperintensity on T1WI (mimicking glomus tumor)
√ may contain blood products (hyperintense on T1WI + hypointense on T2WI)

DDx: paraganglioma, cystic and papillary adenocarcinoma, chondroid lesions (benign chondroma, low-grade chondrosarcoma, chondromyxoid fibroma), cholesterol granuloma, metastatic disease

PARAGANGLIOMA

= NONCHROMAFFIN PARAGANGLIOMA = GLOMUS TUMOR (describes the rich arborization of blood vessels and nerves) = CHEMODECTOMA (reflective of the chemoreceptor tissue of origin) = GLOMERULOCYTOMA = ENDOTHELIOMA = PERITHELIOMA = SYMPATHOBLASTOMA = FIBROANGIOMA = SYMPATHETIC NEVI
= rare neuroendocrine tumor arising from paraganglionic tissue found between base of skull and floor of pelvis; belong to amine-precursor-uptake decarboxylation (APUD) system characterized by cytoplasmic vesicles containing catecholamines
Paraganglion = collection of tissue of the extraadrenal neuroendocrine system, frequently located near nerves and vessels, with special chemoreceptor function
Origin: arises from nonchromaffin paraganglion cells of neuroectodermal origin; differs from adrenal medulla only in its nonchromaffin feature
Neuroendocrine system:
(a) Adrenal paraganglioma arising from adrenal medulla = pheochromocytoma
(b) Extraadrenal paraganglioma
1. Aorticosympathetic paraganglioma associated with sympathetic chain + retroperitoneal ganglia
2. Parasympathetic paraganglioma including branchiomeric chemodectoma, vagal + visceral autonomic paraganglioma

ENT

Glenner classification of extraadrenal paragangliomas:
(a) Branchiomeric distribution
1. Associated with great vessels of chest + neck including carotid body, glomus jugulare, glomus tympanicum

(b) Parasympathetic distribution
2. Associated with vagal nerve
3. Associated with aorticosympathetic chain in thoracolumbar region from aortic arch to urinary bladder, including organ of Zuckerkandl
4. Associated with visceral organs

Histo: acidophil-epithelioid cells in contact with endothelial cells of a vessel; storage of catecholamines (usually nonfunctioning); histologically similar to pheochromocytoma

Age: range of 6 months to 80 years; peak age in 5–6th decade; F:M = 4:1

Associated with: pheochromocytoma

- paroxysmal / permanent hypertension (due to secretion of vasopressor amines) with headache, pallor, perspiration, palpitations
- tumor may secrete catecholamine (= **functional paraganglioma**); proportion of hormonally active tumors high for pheochromocytomas, intermediate for aorticosympathetic paragangliomas, low for parasympathetic paragangliomas
- pheochromocytomas secrete norepinephrine + epinephrine, extraadrenal paragangliomas secrete only norepinephrine, some paragangliomas produce dopamine
- determination of free norepinephrine most sensitive with gas chromatography / high-pressure liquid chromatography (HPLC) performed on 24-hour urine specimens

Location of functioning paragangliomas:
(a) adrenal medulla (>80%)
(b) extraadrenal intraabdominal (8–16%)
(c) extraadrenal in head & neck (2–4%)

<u>Four primary sites in head & neck, chest</u>:
1. carotid body
2. jugular foramen
3. path of vagus nerve
4. middle ear

<u>Less common sites in head & neck</u>:
sella turcica, pineal gland, cavernous sinus, larynx (laryngeal branches of vagus nerve), orbit (ciliary ganglion of the eye), thyroid gland, nasopharynx, mandible, soft palate, face, cheek

(d) multiple paragangliomas in up to 20%, particularly in hereditary disorders (multiple endocrine neoplasia syndromes, neuroectodermal syndromes):
Synchronous multicentricity in 3–26%:
(a) autosomal dominant in 25–35%
(b) nonhereditary in <5%

Cx: malignant transformation in 2–10%

Carotid Body Tumor

Embryology:
derived from mesoderm of 3rd branchial arch + neural crest ectoderm cells, which differentiate into sympathogonia (= forerunner of paraganglionic cells)

◊ Chemodectoma is misnomer (not derived from chemoreceptor cells)!

Histo: nests of epithelioid cells ("Zellballen") with granular eosinophilic cytoplasm separated by trabeculated vascularized connective tissue
◊ Chromaffin-positive granules (= catecholamines) may be present

Function of carotid body:
5 x 3 x 2 mm carotid body regulates pulmonary ventilation through afferent input by way of glossopharyngeal nerve to the medullary reticular formation

<u>Chemoreceptor</u>: detects changes in arterial partial pressures of O_2 + CO_2 + pH

<u>Stimulus</u>: hypoxia > hypercapnia > acidosis

<u>Effect</u>: increase in respiratory rate + tidal volume; increase in sympathetic tone (heart rate, blood pressure, vasoconstriction, elevated catecholamines)

- painless pulsatile firm neck mass below the angle of the jaw, laterally mobile but vertically fixed

Location: within / outside adventitial layer of CCA at level of carotid bifurcation, commonly along posteromedial wall; bilateral in 5% with sporadic occurrence, in 32% with autosomal dominant transmission

√ enhancing oval mass with splaying of ICA + ECA above CCA bifurcation
√ no narrowing of ICA / ECA caliber

Extension: inferiorly to lower cranial nerves + pharynx; superiorly to skull base + intracranial cavity

Growth rate: about 5 mm/year

Cx: malignant transformation in 6% with metastases to regional lymph nodes, brachial plexus, cerebellum, lung, bone, pancreas, thyroid, kidney, breast

Glomus Tympanicum Tumor

Most common tumor in middle ear

- hearing loss, pulsatile tinnitus
- reddish purple mass behind tympanic membrane

Location: tympanic plexus on cochlear promontory of middle ear

CT (bone algorithm preferred):
√ globular soft-tissue mass abutting promontory
√ intense enhancement
√ usually small at presentation (early involvement of ossicles)
√ erosion + displacement of ossicles
√ inferior wall of middle ear cavity intact

Angio:
√ difficult to visualize because of small size

Glomus Jugulare Tumor

Most common tumor in jugular fossa with intracranial extension

<u>Glomus jugulotympanicum tumor</u> = large glomus jugulare tumor growing into the middle ear

Origin: adventitia of jugular vein

- tinnitus, hearing loss
- vascular tympanic membrane

Location: at dome of jugular bulb

√ soft-tissue mass in jugular bulb region / hypotympanum / middle ear space
√ intense enhancement
√ destruction of posteroinferior petrous pyramid + corticojugular spine of jugular foramen
√ destruction of ossicles (usually incus), otic capsule, posteromedial surface of petrous bone

MR:
√ "salt and pepper" appearance due to multiple small tumor vessels

Angio: (film entire neck for concurrent glomus tumors!)
√ hypervascular mass with persistent homogeneous reticular stain
√ invasion / occlusion of jugular bulb by thrombus / tumor
√ supplied by tympanic branch of ascending pharyngeal artery, meningeal branch of occipital artery, posterior auricular artery via stylomastoid branch, internal carotid artery, internal maxillary a.
√ arteriovenous shunting

Cx: malignant transformation with metastases to regional lymph nodes (in 2–4%)

Glomus Vagale Tumor

= PARAGANGLIA OF VAGUS NERVE = VAGAL BODY TUMOR

Histo: dispersed within perineurium / below nerve sheath / between nerve fiber fascicles; not organized into a compact mass

Location:
(1) within inferior ganglion (= ganglion nodosum), inferior to base of skull close to jugular foramen (most common location)
(2) within superior ganglion (= ganglion jugulare) within base of skull at level of jugular bulb
(3) elsewhere along course of vagus nerve

Inferior Nodose Paraganglion

√ spindle-shaped mass
√ compression of internal jugular vein
√ displacement of carotid vessels anteromedially
√ displacement of lateral pharyngeal wall medially
√ minimal destruction of skull base

Superior Jugular Paraganglion

√ dumbbell-shaped mass
√ may encase / displace ICA
√ extension:
(a) superiorly into posterior cranial fossa
± compression of brainstem
(b) inferiorly into infratemporal / parapharyngeal space (2/3)
(c) medially to involve arch of atlas
(d) laterally into middle ear structures
(e) posteriorly into mastoid air cells

Location in temporal bone:
(1) dome of jugular bulb
(2) mucosa of cochlear promontory related to tympanic branch of glossopharyngeal nerve (Jacobson nerve)
(3) auricular branch of vagus nerve (Arnold nerve)

- slow growing + asymptomatic

√ spherical / ovoid / spindle-shaped mass with sharp interfacing margins and homogeneous enhancement
√ highly vascular mass + neovascularity + intense tumor blush

Cx: malignant transformation with metastases in 15% to regional lymph nodes + lung (other paragangliomas in 10%)

ENT

PARANASAL SINUS CARCINOMA

Location: maxillary sinus (80%), nasal cavity (10%), ethmoid sinus (5–6%), frontal + sphenoid sinus (rare)

Maxillary Sinus Carcinoma

Incidence: 80% of all paranasal sinus carcinomas
Histo: squamous cell carcinoma (80%)
Age: >40 years in 95%; M:F = 2:1

- asymmetry of face, tumor in oral / nasal cavity

√ bone destruction (in 90%) predominates over expansion
√ nodal metastases in 10–18%

Nasopharyngeal Carcinoma

Incidence: 10% of paranasal sinus carcinomas; 0.25–0.5% of all malignant tumors in whites; M>F
Predisposed: Chinese population
Histo: squamous cell carcinoma (>85%), nonkeratinizing ca., undifferentiated ca.
Mean age: 40 years

- asymptomatic for a long time
- history of chronic sinusitis / nasal polyps (15%)
- unilateral nasal obstruction

Location: turbinates (50%) > septum > vestibule > posterior choanae > floor

Extension:
(a) lateral + superior: through sinus of Morgagni (= natural defect in superior portion of lateral nasopharyngeal wall) into cartilaginous portion of eustachian tube + levator veli palatini muscle
± masticator space and pre- and poststyloid parapharyngeal spaces
± involvement of levator + tensor veli palatini muscle, 3rd division of nerve V, petroclinoid fissure
± foramen lacerum of skull base encasing internal carotid artery
± cavernous sinus (along ICA / mandibular nerve / direct skull base invasion)
(b) anterior: posterior nasal cavity + pterygopalatine fossa
(c) inferior (1/3): submucosal spread along lateral pharyngeal wall + anterior and posterior tonsillar pillars

√ polypoid or papillary (2/3)
√ bone invasion (1/3)
MR:
√ signal intensity similar to that of adjacent mucosa

Ethmoid Sinus Carcinoma

Incidence: 5–6% of paranasal sinus carcinomas
Histo: squamous cell carcinoma (>90%), sarcoma, adenocarcinoma, adenoid cystic carcinoma; frequently secondarily involved from maxillary sinus carcinoma
• nasal obstruction, bloody discharge
• anosmia, broadening of nose

PAROTID HEMANGIOMA

Frequency: 90% of parotid gland tumors during 1st year of life; M < F
Histo: capillary type >> cavernous type (in older children)
• soft-tissue mass developing shortly after birth with progressive growth peaking at age 1–2 years
• gradual spontaneous regression usually complete by adolescence
US:
√ hypoechoic mass relative to parotid tissue
√ variable degree of abnormal flow
CT:
√ occasionally phleboliths
√ well-defined mass with uniform intense enhancement
MR:
√ low to intermediate signal intensity on short TR
√ bright signal intensity on long TR
√ flow voids due to prominent vasculature
Rx: surgery, sclerotherapy, laser ablation (therapy only with large size + encroachment on adjacent structures due to spontaneous regression)

PHARYNGEAL ABSCESS

Etiology: spread of infection from tonsils / pharynx
Age: children > adults
• trismus (most common presenting symptom) from involvement of pterygoid muscle
• sore throat
• low-grade fever
√ isodense / low-density mass with unsharp margins
√ rim enhancement
Cx: mycotic aneurysm of carotid artery (within 10 days)

PLASMA CELL GRANULOMA

= rare benign pseudotumor
Cause: ?hypersensitivity
Histo: polyclonal infiltration of normal plasma cells mixed with other inflammatory cells + nonnecrotizing epithelial cell granulomas
Location: lung, GI tract, salivary glands, larynx
√ large homogeneous submucosal mass
DDx: multiple myeloma, solitary plasmacytoma

PLEOMORPHIC ADENOMA

= BENIGN MIXED TUMOR OF PAROTIS
mnemonic: 80% in parotid gland
80% in superficial lobe
80% benign
Incidence: 80% of all benign parotid tumors; 3rd most common tumor in pediatric parotid gland (after hemangioma + lymphangioma)
Histo: mixture of epithelial + myoepithelial cells
Age: usually >50 years
• slow-growing hard painless lump in cheek
√ round / oval / lobulated sharply marginated mass
√ rarely dystrophic calcifications
√ variable, usually mild contrast enhancement
US:
√ hypo- to isoechoic mass
√ ± hyperechogenic shadowing foci of calcifications
CT:
√ homogeneous well-defined tumor (if small)
√ less well-defined with low-density center if large (mucoid matrix, hemnorrhage, necrosis)
MR:
√ hypointense on T1WI + hyperintense mass on T2WI
√ hyperintense areas in center (mucoid matrix)
Rx: facial nerve-sparing partial parotidectomy

RANULA

= mucus retention cyst due to obstruction of sublingual / adjacent minor salivary gland
(a) simple: confined to sublingual space
(b) diving: extends to below mylohyoid muscle into submandibular space

RAMSAY-HUNT SYNDROME

= HERPES ZOSTER OTICUS
• vesicles in mucosa of external auditory canal
√ intracanalicular 8th nerve enhancement

RETROPHARYNGEAL ABSCESS / HEMORRHAGE

Etiology: upper respiratory tract infection, tonsillar infection, perforating injury of pharynx / esophagus, suppuration of infected lymph node
Organism: Staphylococcus, mixed flora
Age: usually <1 year
• fever, neck stiffness, dysphagia
√ thickness of retropharyngeal space >3/4 of AP diameter of vertebral body
√ reversal of cervical lordosis
√ anterior displacement of airway
√ may contain gas and gas-fluid level

RHABDOMYOSARCOMA

Frequency:
5–10% of all malignant solid tumors in children <15 years of age (ranking 4th after CNS neoplasm, neuroblastoma, Wilms tumor); 3rd most common primary childhood malignancy of head + neck (following brain tumors + retinoblastomas); 10–25% of all sarcomas; annual incidence of 4.5:1,000,000 white + 1.3:1,000,000 black children

◊ Most common soft-tissue tumor in children!
Age: 2–5 years (peak prevalence); <10 years (70%); M:F = 2:1
Histo:
undifferentiated "blue cells" with scant cytoplasm + primitive-appearing nuclei; common perineural invasion
(a) embryonal rhabdomyosarcoma (>50%)
subtype: polypoidal form = sarcoma botryoides = grapelike
(b) alveolar rhabdomyosarcoma (worst prognosis)
(c) pleomorphic rhabdomyosarcoma (mostly in adults)
• cranial nerve palsy
Location: head + neck (28–36%), trigone + bladder neck (18–21%), orbit (10%), extremities (18–23%), trunk (7–8%), retroperitoneum (6–7%), perineum + anus (2%), other sites (7%)
Site: paranasal sinus, middle ear, nasopharyngeal musculature (1/3) especially in masticator space; most common primary extracranial tumor invading the cranial vault in childhood
Metastases: lymph nodes (50%), lung, bone
√ bulky nasopharyngeal mass
√ extension into cranial vault through fissures + foramina (up to 35%) usually involving cavernous sinus
√ bone destruction by direct invasion
√ uniform enhancement
CT:
√ heterogenous mass isodense to brain
√ expanded foramen / fissure
MR (imaging modality of choice):
√ signal intensity intermediate between muscle and fat on T1WI + hyperintense on T2WI
√ diffuse contrast enhancement
Prognosis: 12.5% 5-year survival

RHINOCEREBRAL MUCORMYCOSIS

= paranasal sinus infection caused by nonseptated fungi Rhizopus arrhizus and Rhizopus oryzae
Spread: fungus first involves nasal cavity, then extends into maxillary / ethmoid sinuses / orbits / intracranially along ophthalmic artery / cribriform plate (frontal sinuses are spared)
Predisposed:
(1) poorly controlled diabetes mellitus (2) chronic renal failure (3) cirrhosis (4) malnutrition (5) cancer
(6) prolonged antibiotic therapy (7) steroid therapy
(8) cytotoxic drug therapy (9) AIDS (10) extensive burns
• black crusting of nasal mucosa (in diabetics)
• small ischemic areas (invasion of arterioles + small arteries)
√ nodular thickening involving nasal septum + turbinates
√ mucoperiosteal thickening + clouding of ethmoids
√ focal areas of bone destruction
Cx: (1) blindness (2) cranial nerve palsy (3) hemiparesis
Prognosis: high mortality rate

SARCOIDOSIS

Blacks:Whites = 10:1
Location: eye, lacrimal glands, salivary glands (30%), larynx (5%), involvement of intra- and extraparotid lymph nodes (rare)
√ granulomas may enhance
√ enlargement of optic canal (optic neuritis)
√ thickening of larynx with enhancement of granulomas
√ multiple small granulomas of septum + turbinates

Heerfordt Syndrome

(1) Parotid enlargement
◊ May be the initial + only manifestation of sarcoid
• diffuse bilateral painless enlargement (10–30%)
• xerostomia
CT:
√ diffusely dense multiple noncavitating nodules within gland / enlargement of intraparotid lymph nodes
(2) Uveitis
(3) Facial nerve paralysis

SIALOSIS

= nontender noninflammatory recurrent enlargement of parotid gland
Cause: cirrhosis, alcoholism, diabetes, malnutrition, hormonal insufficiency (ovarian / pancreatic / thyroid), drugs (sulfisoxazole, phenylbutazone), radiation therapy
Histo: serous acinar hypertrophy + fatty replacement of gland
Sialography:
√ sparse peripheral ducts
CT:
√ enlarged / normal-sized gland
√ diffusely dense gland in end stage

SINONASAL POLYPOSIS

= benign sinonasal mucosal lesion
Incidence: in 25% of patients with allergic rhinitis; in 15% of patients with asthma
Cause: allergic rhinitis (atopic hypersensitivity), asthma, cystic fibrosis (child), Kartagener syndrome, nickel exposure, nonneoplastic hyperplasia of inflamed mucous membranes
Location: commonly maxillary antrum
√ rounded masses within nasal cavity enlarging sinus ostium
√ expansion of sinus
√ thinning of bony trabeculae ± erosive changes at anterior skull base
√ usually peripheral / occasionally solid heterogeneous enhancement
DDx: cancer, fungal infection

Antrochoanal Polyp

= benign antral polyp, which widens the sinus ostium and extends into nasal cavity; 5% of all nasal polyps
Age: teenagers + young adults

ENT

√ antral clouding
√ ipsilateral nasal mass
√ smooth mass enlarging the sinus ostium
√ NO sinus expansion

Angiomatous Polyp

= derivative of choanal polyp (following ischemia of polyp with secondary neovascularity along its surface)

DDx: juvenile angiofibroma (involvement of pterygopalatine fossa)

SINUSITIS

Incidence:
most common paranasal sinus problem; most common chronic disease diagnosed in United States (31,000,000 people affected each year); complicating common colds in 0.5% (3–4 colds/year in adults, 6–8 colds/year in children)

Pathogenesis:
mucosal congestion as a result of viral infection leads to apposition of mucosal surfaces resulting in retention of secretions with bacterial superinfection
(1) Obstruction of major ostia
  (a) middle meatus draining frontal, maxillary, anterior ethmoid sinus
  (b) sphenoethmoidal recess draining posterior ethmoid sphenoid sinus
(2) Ineffective mucociliary clearing secondary to contact of two mucosal surfaces

Predisposing anatomic variants:
(1) greater degree of nasal septal deviation
(2) horizontally oriented uncinate process
NOT concha bullosa, paradoxical turbinate, Haller cells, uncinate pneumatization

Location:
(1) Infundibular pattern (26%)
  = isolated obstruction of inferior infundibulum just above the maxillary sinus ostium
  √ limited maxillary sinus disease
(2) Ostiomeatal unit pattern (25%)
  √ middle meatus opacification
(3) Sphenoethmoidal recess obstruction (6%)
  √ sphenoid / posterior ethmoid sinus inflammation
(4) Sinonasal polyposis pattern
  √ enlargement of ostia, thinning of adjacent bone
  √ air-fluid levels

Plain films (Waters, Caldwell, lateral, submental vertex views):

1. **Acute sinusitis**
   √ air-fluid level [from retention of secretions secondary to mucosal swelling leading to ostial dysfunction] (54% sensitive, 92% specific in maxillary sinus)
   √ total opacification
   √ hyperintense secretions on T2WI (95% water content + 5% proteinaceous macromolecules)
2. **Chronic sinusitis**
   √ mucosal swelling >5 mm thick on Waters view (99% sensitive, 46% specific in maxillary sinus)
   √ bone remodeling + sclerosis (from osteitis)
   √ polyposis
   √ hyperattenuating lesion on NCCT (due to inspissated secretions / fungal disease)
   √ hypointense secretions on T1WI + T2WI due to inspissated material with chronic obstruction (DDx: air)

CT: to map bony anatomy for surgical planning

MR:
√ sinus thickening with high signal intensity on T2WI + low intensity on T1WI
√ near solid secretions with >28% protein concentration are hypointense on both T1WI + T2WI simulating air
√ rim gadolinium enhancement (DDx to neoplasms, which enhance centrally)

A. ALLERGIC SINUSITIS
Prevalence: 10% of population
√ involves multiple sinuses
√ bilaterally symmetric
√ uniform enhancement
√ sinonasal polyposis

B. BACTERIAL SINUSITIS
Organism:
(a) acute phase: Streptococcus pneumoniae + Haemophilus influenzae (>50%), beta-hemolytic streptococcus, Moraxella catarrhalis
(b) chronic phase: staphylococcus, streptococcus, corynebacteria, Bacteroides, fusobacteria
√ solitary antral disease (obstruction of sinus ostium)
√ uniform enhancement

C. MYCOTIC / FUNGAL SINUSITIS
Organism: Aspergillus fumigatus, mucormycosis, bipolaris, Drechslera, Curvularia, Candida
√ polypoid lesion / fungus ball (= extramucosal infection due to saprophytic growth on retained secretions, usually caused by Aspergillus)
√ infiltrating fungal sinusitis (in immune-competent host)
√ fulminant fungal sinusitis (aggressive infection in immune-compromised individual / diabetics)
CT:
  √ punctate calcifications (= calcium phosphate / calcium sulfonate deposition near mycelium)
MR:
  √ dark on T2WI secondary to high fungal mycelial iron, magnesium, manganese content from amino acid metabolism
  (DDx: inspissated secretions / polypoid disease)
Dx: failure to respond to antibiotic therapy

Cx:
(1) Mucous retention cyst (10%)
(2) Mucocele
(3) Orbital extension through neurovascular foramina, dehiscences, or thin bones: orbital cellulitis,
(4) Septic thrombophlebitis
(5) Intracranial extension: meningitis, epidural abscess, subdural empyema, venous sinus thrombosis, cerebral abscess

Rx: functional endoscopic sinus surgery (amputation of uncinate process, enlargement of infundibulum + maxillary ostium, creation of common channel for anterior ethmoid air cells, complete / partial ethmoidectomy)

SJÖGREN SYNDROME

= MYOEPITHELIAL SIALADENITIS
= autoimmune multisystem disorder (= collagen-vascular disease) characterized by inflammation + destruction of exocrine glands leading to dryness of mucous membranes affecting
(1) salivary + lacrimal glands
(2) mucosa + submucosa of pharynx
(3) tracheobronchial tree
(4) reticuloendothelial system
(5) joints

A. PRIMARY SJÖGREN SYNDROME
= autoimmune exocrinopathy
(a) recurrent parotitis in children
(b) SICCA SYNDROME = Mikulicz disease
= xerophthalmia + xerostomia

B. SECONDARY SJÖGREN SYNDROME
Associated with:
(a) connective tissue diseases
1. Rheumatoid arthritis (55%)
2. Systemic lupus erythematosus (2%)
3. Progressive systemic sclerosis (0.5%)
4. Psoriatic arthritis, primary biliary cirrhosis (0.5%)

(b) lymphoproliferative disorders
1. Lymphocytic interstitial pneumonitis (LIP)
2. Pseudolymphoma (25%)
3. Lymphoma (5%; 44 x increased risk): mostly B-cell lymphoma
4. Waldenström macroglobulinemia

Age: 35–70 (mean 57) years; M:F = 1:9
Path: benign lymphoepithelioma
Histo: lymphocytic infiltrate associated ductal dilatation, acinar atrophy, interstitial fibrosis (= parotid destruction)

- xerostomia (most common symptom) = atrophy of salivary + parotid glands leading to diminished saliva production and dryness of mouth + lips
- xerophthalmia = dryness of eyes
  = keratoconjunctivitis sicca = desiccation of cornea + conjunctiva
- xerorhinia = dryness of nose
- decreased sweating
- decreased vaginal secretions
- swelling of parotid gland:
  – recurrent acute episodes with tenderness; usually unilateral
  – chronic glandular enlargement with superimposed acute attacks of painless progressive swelling
- rheumatoid factor (positive in up to 95%)
- ANA (positive in up to 80%)
- mitochondrial antibodies (6%)

Location: lacrimal + salivary glands; mucous glands of conjunctivae, nasal cavity, pharynx, larynx, trachea, bronchi; extraglandular involvement in 5–10%

@ Chest
√ pulmonary fibrosis (10–14%, most common finding)
√ reticulonodular pattern (3–33–52%) involving lower lobes (= lymphocytic interstitial pneumonitis)
√ patchy consolidation
√ inspissated mucus
√ atelectasis
√ recurrent pneumonia
√ bilateral lower lobe bronchiectasis
√ acute focal / lipoid pneumonia (secondary to oils taken to combat dry mouth)
√ ± pleural effusion
HRCT:
√ bronchiectasis
√ bronchiolar inflammation
√ increased parenchymal lines

@ Parotid gland
Sialogram:
√ nonobstructive sialectasia (ducts + acini destroyed by lymphocytic infiltrates / infection)
Stage I : punctate contrast collection <1 mm
Stage II : globular contrast collection 1–2 mm
Stage III : cavitary contrast collection >2 mm
Stage IV : destruction of gland parenchyma
US:
√ enlarged heterogenous gland with punctate areas of increased echogenicity (= mucus-filled ducts)
√ multiple scattered cysts bilaterally (= sialectasis = cystic dilatation of intraparotid ducts + glands)
√ increased vascularity on color Doppler
MR:
√ inhomogeneous "honeycomb" / "salt and pepper" appearance (= areas of low intensity between nodular parenchyma of high signal intensity) on T2WI / Gd-enhanced T1WI

Cx: Salivary gland lymphoma (occurs in significant number of patients + follows an aggressive course)

SUBGLOTTIC STENOSIS

A. CONGENITAL SUBGLOTTIC STENOSIS
• crouplike symptoms, often self-limiting disease
Location: 1–2 cm below vocal cords
√ circumferential symmetrical narrowing of subglottic portion of trachea during inspiration
√ NO change in degree of narrowing with expiration

B. ACQUIRED SUBGLOTTIC STENOSIS
following prolonged endotracheal intubation (in 5%)

THORNWALDT CYST

= midline congenital pouch / cyst lined by ectoderm within nasopharyngeal mucosal space
Origin: persistent focal adhesion between notochord + ectoderm extending to the pharyngeal tubercle of the occipital bone
Incidence: 4% of autopsies
Peak age: 15–30 years

- asymptomatic incidental finding
- persistent nasopharyngeal drainage
- halitosis
- foul taste in mouth

Location: posterior roof of nasopharynx
√ smoothly marginated cystic mass of few mm to 3 cm in size
√ low density, not enhancing
√ NO bone erosion
Cx: infection of cyst
DDx: Rathke pouch (occurs in craniopharyngeal canal located anteriorly + cephalad to Thornwaldt cyst)

THYROGLOSSAL DUCT CYST

Incidence: most common congenital neck mass (70% of all congenital neck anomalies); 2nd most common benign neck mass after benign lymphadenopathy
Embryogenesis:
thyroglossal duct = duct along which thyroid gland descends to its final position from foramen cecum at base of tongue (in 3rd week GA) passing anterior to hyoid bone; duct makes a recurrent loop through / posterior to precursor of hyoid bone before finally descending; inferior end becomes pyramidal lobe of thyroid; thyroid reaches final location by 7 weeks GA; duct usually involutes by 8–10th week of fetal life
Histo: cyst lined by stratified squamous epithelium / ciliated pseudostratified columnar epithelium ± mucous glands; ectopic thyroid tissue in 5–62%
Age: <10 years in 50%; 2nd peak at 20–30 years; M=F

- enlarging painless midline neck mass
- cyst moves upward with tongue protrusion
- ± history of previous incision and drainage of an "abscess" in area of cyst

Location: suprahyoid (15%), at level of hyoid (20%), infrahyoid (65%)
Site: midline (75%), paramedian within 2 cm of midline frequently on left (25%)
Size: 1.5–3 cm (ranging from 0.5 to 6 cm)
√ midline cyst with occasional septation
√ infrahyoid cyst is embedded within strap muscle
 √ infrahyoid strap muscles beak over edge of cyst
US:
 √ anechoic cyst (42%) in midline
 √ hypoechoic mass with fine to coarse internal echoes (= proteinaceous material) + increased through transmission
Scintigraphy:
 √ uptake in functional thyroid tissue of thyroglossal duct cyst
CT:
 √ smooth well-circumscribed midline mass with thin wall
 √ homogeneous attenuation of 10–18 HU / occasionally higher (due to increased protein content)
 √ peripheral rim enhancement
MR:
 √ cyst hypointense on T1WI + hyperintense on T2WI
 √ nonenhancing rim (unless inflamed)
 √ thick irregular rim + variable signal intensity of fluid with inflammation
Cx: (1) infection
(2) thyroid carcinoma (1–4%): in 80% papillary ca.
(3) squamous cell carcinoma (even rarer)
Rx: Sistrunk procedure (= resection of central portion of hyoid bone + core of tissue following the expected course of entire thyroglossal duct) with a 2.6% recurrence rate
DDx: ectopic thyroid (no thyroid tissue in normal location)

THYROID ADENOMA

√ round / oval mass of low attenuation with enhancement

Adenomatous Nodule (42–77%)

= COLLOID NODULE = ADENOMATOUS HYPERPLASIA = DEGENERATIVE INVOLUTED NODULE
Cytology: abundant colloid + benign follicular cells with uniform slightly large nuclei, arranged in a honeycomb pattern (difficult DDx from follicular tumors)
√ often multiple nodules by US / scintigraphy / surgery
√ mostly hypofunctioning, rarely hyperfunctioning
√ solid form = incompletely encapsulated, poorly demarcated nodules merging with surrounding tissue
√ cystic form (= colloid cyst) = anechoic areas in nodule (hemorrhage / colloid degeneration
√ calcific deposits

Follicular Adenoma (15–40%)

= monoclonal tumor arising from follicular epithelium
Path: single lesion with well-developed fibrous capsule
Histo subtypes:
(a) Simple colloid (macrofollicular) adenoma: most common form
(b) Microfollicular (fetal) adenoma
(c) Embryonal (trabecular) adenoma
(d) Hürthle-cell (oxyphil / oncocytic) adenoma: large single polygonal cells with abundant granular cytoplasm + uniform eccentric nuclei + no colloid
(e) Atypical adenoma
(f) Adenoma with papillae
(g) Signet-ring adenoma
◊ 5% of microfollicular adenomas, 5% of Hürthle-cell adenomas, 25% of embryonal adenomas prove to be follicular cancers with careful study!
Functional status:
(1) Toxic adenoma
(2) Toxic multinodular goiter = hyperfunctioning adenoma within multinodular goiter; usually occurs in nodule >2.5 cm in size
(3) Nonfunctioning adenoma
√ mass with increased / decreased echogenicity
√ "halo sign" = complete hypoechoic ring with regular border surrounding isoechoic solid mass

THYROID CARCINOMA

Incidence: 13,000 new cancers/year in United States; clinically silent cancers in up to 35% at autopsy / surgery (usually papillary carcinomas of <1.0 cm in size)

Age: <30 years; M > F

Types (in order of worsening prognosis):
papillary (50–80%) > follicular (10–20%) > medullary (6–10%) > anaplastic

- history of neck irradiation
- rapid growth
- stone-hard nodule

√ hypoechoic / hypoattenuating mass
√ irregular ill-defined border without halo
√ NO hemorrhage / liquefaction necrosis
√ ancillary findings:
 √ lymphadenopathy
 √ destruction of adjacent structures
 √ loss of fat planes
 √ distant metastasis

RADIATION-INDUCED THYROID CANCER

Incidence increases with doses of thyroidal irradiation from 6.5–1,500 rad (higher doses are associated with hypothyroidism)

Peak occurrence: 5–30 (up to 50) years post irradiation

Thyroid abnormalities in 20%:
(a) in 14% adenomatous hyperplasia, follicular adenoma, colloid nodules, thyroiditis
(b) in 6% thyroid cancer

◊ Nondetectable microscopic foci of cancer in 25% of patients operated on for benign disease!
◊ In patients with multiple cold nodules frequency of cancer is 40%

DIAGNOSTIC WHOLE-BODY SCAN

Indication: to detect metastases of thyroid carcinoma after total thyroidectomy; preferred over bone scan (only detects 40%) for skeletal metastases

◊ Metastases not detectable in presence of normal functioning thyroid tissue because uptake is much less in metastases
◊ Tc-99m pertechnetate is useless because of high background activity + lack of organification
◊ False-negative I-131 scan in 24% secondary to nonfunctioning metastases

Technique:
(1) low iodine diet for 7 days = avoid iodized salt; milk and diary products; eggs; seafood; bread made with iodate dough conditioners; red food dyes; restaurant food; food containing iodized salt, sea salt, iodates, iodines, algin, alginates, agar agar
(2) T_4 replacement therapy discontinued for 6 weeks
(3) short-acting T_3 is administered for 4–6 weeks
(4) T_3 replacement therapy discontinued 10–14 days prior to whole-body scan
(5) measurement of TSH level to confirm adequate elevation (TSH >30–50 mIU/mL; administration of exogenous TSH not desirable because of uneven stimulation)
(6) oral administration of 0.6–5–10 mCi I-131
(7) whole-body scan after 24–48–72 hours (low background activity)

N.B.: posttherapy scan (1 week after therapeutic dose) identifies more lesions than diagnostic scan

Normal sites of accumulation: nasopharynx, salivary glands, stomach, colon, bladder, liver (I-131-labeled thyroxin produced by carcinoma is metabolized in liver), breasts in lactating women (breast feeding must be terminated after administration of I-131)

CONTRAINDICATED during pregnancy!

TREATMENT REGIMEN for follicular / papillary cancer:

(1) Surgery: total thyroidectomy + modified radical neck dissection
(2) Postoperative radioiodine treatment with I-131 if diagnostic scan positive (multiple treatments are usually necessary)
 ◊ Radioiodine therapy only appropriate for papillary / mixed / follicular thyroid carcinomas (NOT for medullary or anaplastic carcinomas)
 (a) **Ablation of thyroid tissue remnants**
  Time interval: 6 weeks after surgery
  - no thyroid hormone replacement for 3–4 weeks

  Calculated dose:
  = {(thyroid weight [g] x 80–120 μCi/g) π % uptake of I-123 by 24 hours} x 100
  Estimated dose:
  = 30–100 mCi I-131 orally
  » rescan after 3–7 days:
   √ no change from pre-ablation: on suppression therapy
   √ new foci (in up to 16%): consider therapy
   √ decreased uptake: may be due to "stunning"
 (b) **Treatment of metastases**
  Middle-of-the-road dose:
  » 100 mCi for residual neck activity
  » 150 mCi for regional lymph node metastases
  » 175 mCi for lung metastases
  » 200 mCi for bone metastases
  Tumor dose:
  150 mCi of I-131 with an uptake of 0.5% per gram of tumor tissue and a biologic half-life of 4 days will produce 25,000 rads to tumor
 ◊ Rapid turnover rates may exist in some metastases (lower dose advisable)
 ◊ Treatment of large tumors incomplete (range of beta radiation is a few mm)

Cx: radiation thyroiditis, radiation parotitis, GI symptoms (nausea, diarrhea), minimal bone marrow depression, leukemia (2%), anaplastic transformation (uncommon), lung fibrosis (with extensive pulmonary metastases and dose >200 mCi)

ENT

(3) Thyroid replacement therapy
exogenous thyroid hormone to suppress TSH stimulation of metastases
(4) External radiation therapy for anaplastic carcinoma + metastases without iodine uptake

FOLLOW-UP: thyroglobulin >50 ng/mL indicates functioning metastases following complete ablation of thyroid tissue

Papillary Carcinoma of Thyroid (60–70%)

Peak age: 5th decade; F > M
Histo: unencapsulated well-differentiated tumor
(a) purely papillary
(b) mixed with follicular elements (more common, especially under age 40)

Metastases:
(1) Lymphogenic spread to regional lymph nodes (40%, in children almost 90%)
(2) Hematogenous spread to lung (4%), bone (rare)

• carcinoma elaborates thyroglobulin

NUC:
√ tumor usually concentrates radioiodine (even some purely papillary tumors)

US:
√ tumor of decreased echogenicity
√ purely solid / complex mass with areas of necrosis, hemorrhage, cystic degeneration

X-ray:
√ punctate / linear psammomatous calcifications at tumor periphery

Rx: lobectomy + isthmectomy for papillary cancer <1.5 to 2.0 cm in size isolated to one lobe
Prognosis: 90% 10-year survival for occult + intrathyroidal cancer; 60% 10-year survival for extrathyroidal cancer; worse prognosis with increasing age

Follicular Carcinoma of Thyroid (20%)

Peak age: 5th decade; F > M
Histo: encapsulated well-differentiated tumor without papillary elements; in 25% multifocal; cytologically impossible to distinguish between well-differentiated follicular carcinoma + follicular adenoma (vascular invasion is only criteria)

Early hematogenous spread to:
(a) lung
(b) bone (30%): almost always osteolytic (more frequent than in papillary carcinoma)

• carcinoma elaborates thyroglobulin
√ psammoma bodies + stromal calcium deposits

NUC:
√ usually concentrates pertechnetate, but fails to accumulate I-123

US:
√ indistinguishable from benign follicular adenoma

Prognosis: slow growing; 90% 10-year survival with slight / equivocal angioinvasion; 35% 10-year survival with moderate / marked angioinvasion

Anaplastic Carcinoma of Thyroid (4–15%)

Age: 6th–7th decade; M:F = 1:1
√ intrathoracic extension in up to 50%
√ ± invasion of carotid a., internal jugular v., larynx

NUC:
√ NO radioiodine uptake

CT:
√ mass with inhomogeneous attenuation
√ areas of necrosis (74%)
√ calcifications (58%)
√ regional lymphadenopathy (74%)

Prognosis: 5% 5-year survival; average survival time of 6–12 months

Medullary Carcinoma of Thyroid (1–5–10%)

sporadic / familial
Histo: arises from parafollicular C-cells, associated with amyloid deposition in primary + metastatic sites
Mean age: 60 years for sporadic variety; in adolescence with MEN

May be associated with:
(1) MEN IIa = pheochromocytoma + parathyroid hyperplasia (Sipple syndrome)
(2) MEN IIb = without parathyroid component

Metastases: early spread to lymph nodes (50%), lung, liver, bone

• elevated calcitonin (from tumor production) stimulated by pentagastrin + calcium infusion
√ mass of 2–26 mm
√ granular calcifications within fibrous stroma / amyloid masses (50%)

NUC:
√ NO uptake by radioiodine / pertechnetate
√ frequently shows increased uptake of Tl-201

CT:
√ mass of low attenuation (no iodine concentration)

Prognosis:
90% 10-year survival without nodal metastases
42% 10-year survival with nodal metastases

Rx: total thyroidectomy + modified radical neck dissection

THYROIDITIS

Hashimoto Thyroiditis

= CHRONIC LYMPHOCYTIC THYROIDITIS

Most frequent cause of goitrous hypothyroidism in adults in the USA (iodine deficiency is the more common cause worldwide)

Etiology: autoimmune process with marked familial predisposition; antibodies are typically present; functional organification defect
Peak age: 4th–5th decade; M > F

• firm rubbery lobular goiter
• gradual painless enlargement
• thyrotoxicosis in early stage (4%)
• decreased thyroid reserve
• hypothyroidism at presentation (20%)
√ moderate enlargement of both lobes (18%)

NUC:
- √ low tracer uptake (occasionally increased) with poor visualization (4%)
- √ prominent pyramidal lobe
- √ positive perchlorate washout test
- √ patchy tracer distribution
- √ multiple (40%) / single cold defects (28%) / normal thyroid (8%)

US:
- √ initially heterogeneous diffusely decreased echogenicity + slight lobulation of contour
- √ marked hyperemia on color Doppler
- √ later densely echogenic (fibrosis) + acoustical shadows

Cx: hypothyroidism

DeQuervain Thyroiditis

= SUBACUTE THYROIDITIS

Etiology: probably viral

Histo: lymphocytic infiltration + granulomas + foreign body giant cells

Peak age: 2nd–5th decade; M:F = 1:5

- upper respiratory tract infection precedes onset of symptoms by 2–3 weeks
- painful tender gland + fever; only mild enlargement
- hyperthyroidism (50%) secondary to severe destruction
- short-lived hypothyroidism (25%) secondary to hormone depletion of gland

NUC:
- √ abnormally low radioiodine uptake with clinical and laboratory evidence of hyperthyroidism
- √ poor visualization of thyroid (initially)
- √ single / multiple hypofunctional areas (occasionally)
- √ increased uptake during phase of hypothyroidism (late event)

Cx: permanent hypothyroidism (rare)

Prognosis: usually full recovery

Painless Thyroiditis

Histo: resembles chronic lymphocytic thyroiditis
- clinical presentation similar to subacute thyroiditis
- NOT painful / tender

Acute Suppurative Thyroiditis

US:
- √ focal / diffuse enlargement; possibly abscess
- √ decreased echogenicity

WARTHIN TUMOR

= PAPILLARY CYSTADENOMA LYMPHOMATOSUM
= ADENOLYMPHOMA

Incidence: 2nd most common benign tumor of parotid gland; bilateral in 10%

Age: about 50 years; M > F

Origin: from heterotopic salivary gland tissue within parotid lymph nodes (direct result of incorporation of lymphatic elements + heterotopic salivary gland ductal epithelium within intraparotid + periparotid nodes during embryonic development

Histo: CHARACTERISTIC double layer of oncocytes (= epithelial cells) resting on a dense lymphoid stroma

- slow-growing painless mass

Location: often in tail of parotid gland

√ well-circumscribed single / multiple cystic / solid lesion in parotid region usually 3–4 cm in size
- ◊ Most common lesion to manifest as unilateral + multifocal masses
- ◊ Most common salivary neoplasm to manifest as multiple masses in one / both parotid glands

MR:
- √ hypointense compared with fat / surrounding parotid tissue on T2WI

NUC:
- √ increased uptake with Tc-99m, Tl-201, FDG

DDx: lymphoma, inflammatory disease

Rx: surgical resection

DIFFERENTIAL DIAGNOSIS OF CHEST DISORDERS

PULMONARY HEMORRHAGE

A. WITHOUT RENAL DISEASE
1. Bleeding diathesis: leukemia, hemophilia, disseminated intravascular coagulation (DIC)
2. Pulmonary embolism, thromboembolism
3. Blunt trauma: contusion
4. Idiopathic pulmonary hemosiderosis
5. Limited Wegener granulomatosis
6. Infectious diseases
7. Drugs: amphotericin B, mitomycin, high-dose cyclophosphamide, cytarabine (ara-C), D-penicillamine, anticoagulants, lymphangiography

B. WITH RENAL DISEASE
1. Goodpasture syndrome = anti-basement membrane antibody disease
2. Collagen vascular disease + systemic vasculitides: SLE, Wegener granulomatosis, polyarteritis nodosa, Henoch-Schönlein purpura, Behçet disease
3. Rapidly progressive glomerulonephritis ± immune complexes

C. HEMORRHAGIC PNEUMONIA
1. Bacteria: Legionnaires' disease
2. Viruses: CMV, herpes, Rocky Mountain spotted fever, infectious mononucleosis
3. Fungi: Aspergillosis, mucormycosis

D. BLEEDING METASTASIS: Choriocarcinoma

• acute respiratory distress
• hemoptysis (uncommon)

CXR:
√ bilateral heterogeneous + homogeneous opacities
√ focal consolidation (less common)

CT:
√ bilateral scattered / diffuse areas of ground-glass opacity

Hemoptysis

• frothy sputum, bright red blood, alkaline pH

Source: bronchial a. (most common), pulmonary a.

A. TUMOR
1. Carcinoma (35%)
2. Bronchial adenoma

B. BRONCHIAL WALL INJURY
1. Foreign body erosion
2. Bronchoscopy / biopsy

C. VASCULAR
1. COPD
2. Pulmonary embolus with infarction
3. Venous hypertension (most common): mitral stenosis
4. Arteriovenous malformation
5. Rupture of pulmonary artery aneurysm: TB, vasculitis, trauma, neoplasm, abscess, septic embolus, indwelling catheter

D. INFECTION (pneumonia)
1. Chronic bronchitis
2. Bronchiectasis, mouthful (15%)
3. Tuberculosis (Rasmussen aneurysm)
4. Aspergillosis
5. Abscess

◊ In 5–10% of patients no cause is found!
◊ The two most common identifiable causes are bronchial carcinoma + bronchiectasis!

DDx: hematemesis (containing food particles, dark blood, acid pH)

ASPIRATION

= intake of solid / liquid materials into the airways and lungs

Predisposing factors:
1. Alcoholism (most common in adults)
2. General anesthesia, loss of consciousness
3. Structural abnormalities of pharynx / esophagus (congenital / acquired tracheoesophageal + tracheopulmonary fistula), laryngectomy
4. Neuromuscular disorders
5. Deglutition abnormalities

Substrate:
(a) foreign bodies
(b) liquids
- gastric acid = Mendelson syndrome
- water = near drowning
- barium, water-soluble contrast material
- liquid paraffin / petroleum = acute exogenous lipoid pneumonia / fire-eater pneumonia
- mineral oil / cod liver oil = chronic exogenous lipoid pneumonia

(c) contaminated substances from oropharynx / GI tract

PULMONARY DISEASE ASSOCIATED WITH CIGARETTE SMOKING

1. Bronchogenic carcinoma
2. Chronic bronchitis
3. Centrilobular emphysema
4. Panacinar emphysema with alpha-1 antitrypsin deficiency
5. Respiratory bronchiolitis-associated interstitial lung disease
6. Pulmonary Langerhans cell histiocytosis

HYPERSENSITIVITY TO ORGANIC DUSTS

A. TRACHEOBRONCHIAL HYPERSENSITIVITY
large particles reaching the tracheobronchial mucosa (pollens, certain fungi, some animal / insect epithelial emanations)
1. Extrinsic asthma
2. Hypersensitivity aspergillosis
3. Bronchocentric granulomatosis
4. Byssinosis in cotton-wool workers

B. ALVEOLAR HYPERSENSITIVITY
= HYPERSENSITIVITY PNEUMONITIS
= EXTRINSIC ALLERGIC ALVEOLITIS
small particles of <5 μm reaching alveoli

DRUG-INDUCED PULMONARY DAMAGE

Histopathologic manifestations:

(a) Diffuse alveolar damage
bleomycin, busulfan, carmustine, mitomycin, cyclophosphamide, melphalan, gold salts
(b) Nonspecific interstitial pneumonia
amiodarone, methotrexate, carmustine, chlorambucil
(c) Bronchiolitis obliterans organizing pneumonia
bleomycin, gold salts, methotrexate, amiodarone, nitrofurantoin, penicillamine, sulfasalazine, cyclophosphamide
(d) Eosinophilic pneumonia
penicillamine, sulfasalazine, nitrofurantoin, nonsteroidal anti-inflammatory drugs, paraaminosalicylic acid
(e) Pulmonary hemorrhage
anticoagulants, amphotericin B, cytarabine (ara-C), penicillamine, cyclophosphamide

A. CYTOTOXIC DRUGS (most important group)

1. Cyclophosphamide
Use: variety of malignancies, Wegener granulomatosis, glomerulonephritis
Toxicity: after 2 weeks – 13 years (mean, 3.5 years), no relationship to dose / duration of therapy
Prognosis: good after discontinuation of therapy
√ diffuse alveolar damage (most common)
√ nonspecific interstitial pneumonia
√ BOOP (least common)
2. Busulfan = Myleran® (for CML)
Toxicity: dose-dependent, after 3–4 years on the drug in 1–10%
√ diffuse linear pattern (occasionally reticulonodular / nodular pattern)
√ partial / complete clearing after withdrawal of drug
DDx: Pneumocystis pneumonia, interstitial leukemic infiltrate
3. Nitrosoureas = carmustine (BCNU), lomustine (CCNU)
Use: CNS glioma, lymphoma, myeloma
Toxicity: in 50% after doses >1500 mg/m^2; sensitivity increased after radiation Rx
√ diffuse alveolar damage (most common)
√ nonspecific interstitial pneumonia:
  √ linear / finely nodular opacities (following treatment of 2–3 years)
√ high incidence of pneumothorax
4. Bleomycin
Use: squamous cell carcinoma of neck / cervix / vagina, Hodgkin lymphoma, testicular ca.
Toxicity: at doses >300 mg (in 3–6%); increased risk with age + radiation therapy + high oxygen concentrations
Prognosis: death from respiratory failure within 3 months of onset of symptoms
√ diffuse alveolar damage (most common)
√ nonspecific interstitial pneumonia / BOOP:
  √ subpleural linear / nodular opacities (5–30 mm) in lower lung zones occurring after 1–3 months following beginning of therapy
  DDx: metastases
5. Taxoid derivatives = paclitaxel, docetaxel, gemcitabine, topotecan, vinorelbine
Use: breast cancer, lung cancer, ovarian cancer

B. NONCYTOTOXIC DRUGS

1. Amiodarone
= triiodinated benzofuran
Use: refractory ventricular tachyarrhythmia
Toxicity: in 5–10%; risk increased with daily dose > 400 mg + in elderly
Prognosis: good after discontinuation of drug
• pulmonary insufficiency after 1–12 months in 14–18% on long-term therapy
√ nonspecific interstitial pneumonia (most common) + associated BOOP:
  √ alveolar + interstitial infiltrates (chronic presentation)
√ focal homogeneous peripheral consolidation (acute presentation):
  √ attenuation values of iodine (due to incorporation of amiodarone into type II pneumocytes)
√ pleural thickening (inflammation) adjacent to consolidation
√ associated high-attenuation of liver relative to spleen
2. Gold salts
Use: inflammatory arthritis
Toxicity: in 1% within 2–6 months
• mucocutaneous lesions (30%)
√ diffuse alveolar damage (common)
√ nonspecific interstitial pneumonia (common)
√ BOOP (less common)
3. Methotrexate, procarbazine
Use: lung cancer, breast cancer, head and neck epidermoid cancer, nonmetastatic osteosarcoma, advanced stage NHL, AML, recalcitrant psoriasis, severe rheumatoid arthritis, pemphigus)
Toxicity: in 5–10%; not dose-related
Prognosis: usually self-limited despite continuation of therapy
• blood eosinophilia (common)
√ nonspecific interstitial pneumonia (most common)
√ BOOP (less frequent)
√ linear / reticulonodular process (time delay of 12 days to 5 years, usually early)
√ acinar filling pattern (later)
√ transient hilar adenopathy + pleural effusion (on occasion)
DDx: Pneumocystis pneumonia

CHEST

4. Nitrofurantoin (Macrodantin®)
   Use: urinary tract infection
   Toxicity: rare
   • positive for ANA + LE cells
   (a) acute disorder within 2 weeks of administration:
      • fever, dyspnea, cough
      • peripheral eosinophilia (more common)
      Prognosis: prompt resolution after withdrawal from drug
      √ diffuse bilateral predominantly basal heterogenous opacities
   (b) chronic reaction with interstitial fibrosis (less common)
      • insidious onset of dyspnea + cough
      • may not be associated with peripheral eosinophilia
      √ nonspecific interstitial pneumonia (common)
         √ bilateral basilar interstitial opacities

C. OTHERS
1. Heroin, propoxyphene, methadone
   Toxicity: overdose followed by pulmonary edema in 30–40%
   √ bilateral widespread airspace consolidation
   √ aspiration pneumonia in 50–75%
2. Salicylates
   • asthma
   √ pulmonary edema (with chronic ingestion)
3. Intravenous contrast material
   √ pulmonary edema

DISORDERS WITH HEPATIC AND PULMONARY MANIFESTATIONS

1. α1-antitrypsin deficiency
2. Cystic fibrosis
3. Hereditary hemorrhagic telangiectasia
4. Autoimmune disease: primary biliary cirrhosis, rheumatoid arthritis, Hashimoto thyroiditis, Sjögren syndrome, scleroderma, sarcoidosis
5. Drugs with toxic effects on lung and liver: methotrexate, phenytoin, amiodarone

PULMONARY EDEMA

= abnormal accumulation of fluid in the extravascular compartments of the lung

Pathophysiology (Starling equation):
transcapillary flow dependent on
(1) hydrostatic pressure
(2) oncotic (= colloid osmotic) pressure
(3) capillary permeability (the *endothelial cells* are relatively impermeable to protein but remain permeable to water and solutes; the tight intercellular junctions of *alveolar epithelium* remain nearly impermeable to water and solutes)

$$Q_{filt} = K_{filt}\,(HP_{iv} - HP_{ev}) - t(OP_{iv} - OP_{ev})$$

Q_{filt} = amount of fluid filtered per unit area per unit time
HP_{iv} = intravascular hydrostatic pressure
HP_{ev} = extravascular hydrostatic pressure
OP_{iv} = intravascular oncotic pressure
OP_{ev} = extravascular oncotic pressure
K_{filt} = conductance of capillary wall = water resistance of capillary endothelial cell junction
t = oncotic reflection coefficient = permeability of capillary membrane to macromolecules

Cause: disturbed equilibrium of net flow F_{net} between fluid transudation / exudation Q_{filt} and lymphatic absorption Q_{lymph}

$$F_{net} = Q_{filt} - Q_{lymph}$$

1. Increased hydrostatic pressure edema:
   bat wing, asymmetric distribution, in acute asthma, postobstructive, in acute and chronic pulmonary embolism, in pulmonary venoocclusive disease, near drowning
2. Permeability edema with diffuse alveolar damage = ARDS
   ◊ Not caused / influenced by concurrent cardiac insufficiency!
3. Permeability edema without diffuse alveolar damage:
   heroin-induced, high-altitude, following administration of cytokines
4. Mixed edema due to increased hydrostatic pressure + permeability changes:
   neurogenic, reperfusion, reexpansion, air embolism, postpneumonectomy, lung reduction, after lung transplantation

A. INCREASED HYDROSTATIC PRESSURE EDEMA
   (a) cardiogenic (most common)
      = pulmonary venous hypertension
      Pulmonary capillary wedge pressure (PCWP):
         = reflects left atrial pressure and correlates well with radiologic features of CHF + pulmonary venous hypertension
         ◊ In acute CHF radiologic features are delayed in onset and resolution

PCWP [mm Hg]	*Findings*
5–12	normal
12–17	cephalization of pulmonary vessels (only in chronic conditions)
17–20	Kerley lines, subpleural effusions
>25	alveolar flooding edema

1. Heart disease: left ventricular failure, mitral valve disease, left atrial myxoma
2. Pulmonary venous disease: acute / chronic pulmonary embolism, primary venoocclusive disease, mediastinal fibrosis
3. Pericardial disease: pericardial effusion, constrictive pericarditis (extremely rare)
4. Drugs: antiarrhythmic drugs; drugs depressing myocardial contractility (beta-blocker)

√ flow inversion = "cephalization of pulmonary vessels" is only seen in longstanding left heart failure, never in pulmonary edema of renal failure / overhydration / low oncotic pressure

(b) noncardiogenic
1. Renal failure
2. IV fluid overload
3. Hyperosmolar fluid (eg, contrast medium)

(c) neurogenic
? sympathetic venoconstriction in cerebrovascular accident, head injury, CNS tumor, postictal state

B. DECREASED COLLOID OSMOTIC PRESSURE
1. Hypoproteinemia
2. Transfusion of crystalloid fluid
3. Rapid reexpansion of lung

C. INCREASED CAPILLARY PERMEABILITY
Endothelial injury from
(a) physical trauma: parenchymal contusion, radiation therapy
(b) aspiration injury:
1. Mendelson syndrome (gastric contents)
2. Near drowning in sea water / fresh water
3. Aspiration of hypertonic contrast media
(c) inhalation injury:
1. Nitrogen dioxide = silo-filler's disease
2. Smoke (pulmonary edema may be delayed by 24–48 hours)
3. Sulfur dioxide, hydrocarbons, carbon monoxide, beryllium, cadmium, silica, dinitrogen tetroxide, oxygen, chlorine, phosgene, ammonia, organophosphates
(d) injury via bloodstream
1. Vessel occlusion: shock (trauma, sepsis, ARDS) or emboli (air, fat, amniotic fluid, thrombus)
2. Circulating toxins: snake venom, paraquat
3. Drugs: heroin, morphine, methadone, aspirin, phenylbutazone, nitrofurantoin, chlorothiazide
4. Anaphylaxis: transfusion reaction, contrast medium reaction, penicillin
5. Hypoxia: high altitude, acute large airway obstruction

mnemonic: "ABCDEFGHI - PRN"
Aspiration
Burns
Chemicals
Drugs (heroin, nitrofurantoin, salicylates)
Exudative skin disorders
Fluid overload
Gram-negative shock
Heart failure
Intracranial condition
Polyarteritis nodosa
Renal disease
Near drowning

Atypical pulmonary edema = lung edema with an unusual radiologic appearance

Unusual form of pulmonary edema = lung edema from unusual causes

Interstitial Pulmonary Edema

= 1st phase of pressure edema with increase in quantity of extracellular fluid

Cause: increase in mean transmural arterial pressure of 15–25 mm Hg

√ early loss of definition of subsegmental + segmental vessels
√ mild enlargement of peribronchovascular spaces
√ appearance of Kerley lines
√ subpleural effusions
√ progressive blurring of vessels due to central migration of edema at lobar + hilar levels
√ small peripheral vessels difficult to identify due to a decrease in lung radiolucency
◊ Often marked dissociation between clinical signs + symptoms + roentgenographic evidence
◊ Nothing differentiates it from other interstitial lesions
◊ Does not necessarily develop before alveolar pulmonary edema
◊ NOT typical for bacterial pneumonia

Alveolar Flooding Edema

= 2nd phase of pressure edema

Cause: increase in mean transmural arterial pressure of >25 mm Hg ± pressure-induced damage to alveolar epithelium

√ tiny nodular / acinar areas of increased opacity
√ frank consolidation

Bat-Wing Edema (in <10%)

= central nongravitational distribution of alveolar edema

Cause: rapidly developing severe cardiac failure (acute mitral insufficiency associated with papillary muscle rupture, massive MI, valve leaflet destruction by septic endocarditis) or renal failure

√ lung cortex spared from fluid (due to pumping effect of respiration / contractile property of alveolar septa / mucopolysaccharide-filled perivascular matrix)

Asymmetric Distribution of Pressure Edema

Cause: morphologic lung changes in COPD, hemodynamics, patient position

√ lung apices spared (= lung emphysema in heavy smokers)
√ upper + middle portions of lung spared (= end-stage TB, sarcoidosis, asbestosis)
√ predominantly RUL involvement (= mitral regurgitation refluxes preferentially into right upper pulmonary vein)
√ anteroposterior gradient on CT in recumbent position
√ unilateral edema in lateral decubitus position

Pulmonary Edema with Acute Asthma

Cause: air trapping maintains a positive intraalveolar pressure and thus decreases hydrostatic pressure gradient

Pathogenesis: associated with severity of Müller maneuver

√ heterogenous edema (due to nonuniform airway obstruction)
√ peribronchial cuffing
√ ill-defined vessels
√ enlarged ill-defined hila
√ patency of narrowed airways maintained (due to high negative pleural pressure in forced inspiration)

Postobstructive Pulmonary Edema

Cause: following relief from an upper airway obstruction (impacted foreign body, laryngospasm, epiglottitis, strangulation)

Pathogenesis:
(a) forced inspiration causes a high negative intrathoracic pressure (Müller maneuver) and increases venous return
(b) obstruction creates high positive intrathoracic pressure that impairs development of edema

√ septal lines, peribronchial cuffing
√ central alveolar edema
√ normal heart size

Prognosis: resolution within 2–3 days

Edema with Pulmonary Embolism (<10%)

Cause: occlusion of pulmonary arterial bed causes redirection of blood flow and hypertension in uninvolved areas

√ areas of ground-glass attenuation
√ sharply demarcated from areas of transparency distal to occluded arteries
√ associated with dilated pulmonary arteries (70%)

Pulmonary Edema with Pulmonary Venoocclusive Disease

Cause: organized thrombi in small veins causes an increase in peripheral resistance and hydrostatic pressure

• rapidly progressive dyspnea, orthopnea
• ± hemoptysis
• normal / low pulmonary capillary wedge pressure

√ enlarged pulmonary arteries
√ diffuse interstitial edema + numerous Kerley lines
√ peribronchial cuffing
√ dilated right ventricle

Heroin-induced Pulmonary Edema

Hx: overdose of opiates (almost exclusively with heroin, rarely with cocaine / "crack")

Frequency: 15% of cases of heroin overdose

Pathophysiology: depression of medullary respiratory center leading to hypoxia + acidosis

√ widespread patchy bilateral airspace consolidations
√ ill-defined vessels + peribronchial cuffing
√ markedly asymmetric gravity-dependent distribution of edema (motionless recumbent position for hours / days)
√ resolution within 1 or 2 days in uncomplicated cases

Cx:
(1) extensive crush injuries with associated muscle damage and ensuing renal insufficiency (from motionless recumbency)
(2) aspiration of gastric contents

Prognosis: 10% mortality rate

Pulmonary Edema following Administration of Cytokines

(a) intravenous interleukin 2 (IL–2): enhances tumoricidal activity of natural killer cells in metastatic melanoma + RCC
(b) intraarterial tumor necrosis factor: increases production + release of IL–2

Frequency: in 75% of IL–2 therapy; in 20% of tumor necrosis factor therapy; in 25% of recombinant IL–2 therapy

Pathophysiology: permeability disruption of capillary endothelial cells

• 12 mm Hg increase in pulmonary capillary wedge pressure (direct toxic effect on myocardium)

√ pulmonary edema 1–5 days after start of therapy:
√ bilateral symmetric interstitial edema with thickened septal lines
√ peribronchial cuffing (75%)
√ small pleural effusions (40%)
√ no alveolar edema (unless associated cardiac insufficiency)

High-altitude Pulmonary Edema

Predisposed: young males after rapid ascent to >3,000 meters

Cause: prolonged exposure to low partial oxygen atmospheric pressure

Pathophysiology: acute persistent hypoxia with endothelial leakage

• prodromal acute mountain sickness
• dyspnea at rest, cough with frothy pink sputum
• neurologic disturbances (due to brain edema)
• arterial oxygen levels as low as 38%

√ central interstitial pulmonary edema
√ peribronchial cuffing
√ ill-defined vessels
√ patchy airspace consolidation

Neurogenic Pulmonary Edema

Frequency: in up to 50% of severe brain trauma, subarachnoid hemorrhage, stroke, status epilepticus

Pathophysiology: modification in neurovegetative pathways causes sudden increase in pressure in pulmonary venules with reduced venous outflow

CHEST

- dyspnea, tachypnea, cyanosis shortly after brain insult + rapid disappearance

√ bilateral inhomogeneous / homogeneous airspace consolidations, in 50% affecting predominantly the apices, disappearing within 1–2 days

Dx: by exclusion

DDx: fluid overload, postextubation edema

Reperfusion Pulmonary Edema

Frequency: in up to 90–100%

Cause: pulmonary thrombendarterectomy for massive pulmonary embolism / for webs and segmental stenosis

Pathophysiology: rapid increase in blood flow + pressure

- dyspnea, tachypnea, cough during the first 24–48 hours after reperfusion

√ pulmonary edema within 2 days after surgery:

√ heterogeneous airspace consolidations, predominantly in the areas distal to the recanalized vessels

√ random distribution in up to 50%

Reexpansion Pulmonary Edema

Cause: rapid reexpansion of a collapsed lung following evacuation of hydrothorax, hemothorax or pneumothorax

Pathophysiology: prolonged local hypoxic event, abrupt restoration of blood flow, sudden marked increase in intrapleural pressure, diffuse alveolar damage

- frank respiratory insufficiency: cough, dyspnea, tachypnea, tachycardia, frothy pink sputum
- may be asymptomatic

√ pulmonary edema within reexpanded entire lung within 1 hour (in 64%)

√ increase in severity within 24–48 hours with slow resolution over next 5–7 days

Prognosis: 20% mortality

Pulmonary Edema due to Air Embolism

Cause: usually iatrogenic complication (neurosurgical procedure in sitting position, placement / manipulation of central venous line), rare in open / closed chest trauma

Pathophysiology: embolized air bubbles cause mechanical obstruction of pulmonary microvasculature

- sudden onset of chest pain, tachypnea, dyspnea
- hypotension

√ air bubbles in right-sided cardiac chambers on echocardiography

√ interstitial edema

√ bilateral peripheral alveolar areas of increased opacity, predominantly at lung bases

Postpneumonectomy Pulmonary Edema

= life-threatening complication in the early postoperative period after pneumonectomy (rare in lobectomy or lung reduction surgery)

Frequency: 2.5–5%; R > L pneumonectomy

Risk factors: excessive administration of fluid during surgery, transfusion of fresh frozen plasma, arrhythmia, marked postsurgical diuresis, low serum colloidal osmotic pressure

Pathophysiology: increased capillary hydrostatic pressure, altered capillary permeability

- marked dyspnea during first 2–3 postop days

√ ARDS-like picture

Prognosis: very high mortality rate

Pulmonary Edema after Lung Transplantation

Frequency: in up to 97% during first 3 days after surgery

Pathophysiology: tissue hypoxia, disruption of pulmonary lymphatic drainage, lung denervation

√ progressive diffuse confluent areas of increased opacity, most pronounced on postop day 5

√ return to normal 2 weeks after surgery

Unilateral Pulmonary Edema

A. IPSILATERAL = on side of preexisting abnormality
   - (a) filling of airways
     1. Unilateral aspiration / pulmonary lavage
     2. Bronchial obstruction (drowned lung)
     3. Pulmonary contusion
   - (b) increased pulmonary venous pressure
     1. Unilateral venous obstruction
     2. Prolonged lateral decubitus position
   - (c) pulmonary arterial overload
     1. Systemic artery-to-pulmonary artery shunt (Waterston, Blalock-Taussig, Pott procedure)
     2. Rapid thoracentesis (rapid reexpansion)

B. CONTRALATERAL = opposite to side of abnormality
   - (a) pulmonary arterial obstruction
     1. Congenital absence / hypoplasia of pulmonary artery
     2. Unilateral arterial obstruction
     3. Pulmonary thromboembolism
   - (b) loss of lung parenchyma
     1. Swyer-James syndrome
     2. Unilateral emphysema
     3. Lobectomy
     4. Pleural disease

C. RIGHT UPPER LOBE
   PATHOGNOMONIC for mitral valve regurgitation

Pulmonary Edema with Cardiomegaly

1. Cardiogenic
2. Uremic (with cardiomegaly from pericardial effusion / hypertension)

CHEST

Pulmonary Edema without Cardiomegaly

mnemonic: "U DOPA"

Uremia
Drugs
Overhydration
Pulmonary hemorrhage
Acute myocardial infarction, **A**rrhythmia

Noncardiogenic Pulmonary Edema

mnemonic: "The alphabet"

ARDS, **A**lveolar proteinosis, **A**spiration, **A**naphylaxis
Bleeding diathesis, **B**lood transfusion reaction
CNS (increased pressure, trauma, surgery, CVA, cancer)
Drowning (near), **D**rug reaction
Embolus (fat, thrombus)
Fluid overload, **F**oreign-body inhalation
Glomerulonephritis, **G**oodpasture syndrome, Gastrografin aspiration
High altitude, **H**eroin, **H**ypoproteinemia
Inhalation (SO_2, smoke, CO, cadmium, silica)
-
Narcotics, **N**itrofurantoin
Oxygen toxicity
Pancreatitis
-
Rapid reexpansion of pneumothorax / removal of pleural effusion
-
Transfusion
Uremia

PNEUMONIA

"Classic" pneumonia pattern:

1. Lobar distribution : Streptococcus pneumoniae
2. Bulging fissure : Klebsiella
3. Pulmonary edema : Viral pneumonia, Pneumocystis pneumonia
4. Pneumatocele : Staphylococcus
5. Alveolar nodules : Varicella, bronchogenic spread of TB

Distribution:

A. SEGMENTAL / LOBAR
— Normal host: S. pneumoniae, Mycoplasma, virus
— Compromised host: S. pneumoniae

B. BRONCHOPNEUMONIA
— Normal host: Mycoplasma, virus, Streptococcus, Staphylococcus, S. pneumoniae
— Compromised host: Gram-negative, Streptococcus, Staphylococcus
— Nosocomial: Gram-negative, Pseudomonas, Klebsiella, Staphylococcus
— Immunosuppressed: Gram-negative, Staphylococcus, Nocardia, Legionella, Aspergillus, Phycomycetes

C. EXTENSIVE BILATERAL PNEUMONIA
— Normal host: virus (eg, influenza), Legionella
— Compromised host: candidiasis, Pneumocystis, tuberculosis

D. BILATERAL LOWER LOBE PNEUMONIA
— Normal host: anaerobic (aspiration)
— Compromised host: anaerobic (aspiration)

E. PERIPHERAL PNEUMONIA
— Noninfectious eosinophilic pneumonia

Transmission:

A. COMMUNITY-ACQUIRED PNEUMONIA
Organism: viruses, S. pneumoniae, Mycoplasma
Mortality: 10%

B. NOSOCOMIAL PNEUMONIA
(a) Gram-negative organism (>50%): Klebsiella pneumoniae, P. aeruginosa, E. coli, Enterobacter
(b) Gram-positive organism (10%): S. aureus, S. pneumoniae, H. influenzae

Complications:

1. Empyema
2. Pulmonary abscess
3. Cavitary necrosis
4. Pneumatocele
5. Pneumothorax
6. Pyopneumothorax
7. Bronchopleural fistula

CHEST

Bacterial Pneumonia

Lobar Pneumonia

= ALVEOLAR PNEUMONIA
= pathogens reach peripheral air space, incite exudation of watery edema into alveolar space, centrifugal spread via small airways, pores of Kohn + Lambert into adjacent lobules + segments
√ nonsegmental sublobar consolidation
√ round pneumonia (= uniform involvement of contiguous alveoli)
(a) Streptococcus pneumoniae
(b) Klebsiella pneumoniae (more aggressive); in immunocompromised + alcoholics
(c) any pneumonia in children
(d) atypical measles
√ expansion of lobe with bulging of fissures
√ lung necrosis with cavitation
√ lack of volume loss
DDx: Aspiration, pulmonary embolus

Lobular Pneumonia

= BRONCHOPNEUMONIA
= combination of interstitial + alveolar disease (injury starts in airways, involves bronchovascular bundle, spills into alveoli, which may contain edema fluid, blood, leukocytes, hyaline membranes, organisms)
Organisms:
(a) Staphylococcus aureus, Pseudomonas pneumoniae: thrombosis of lobular artery branches with necrosis + cavitation
(b) Streptococcus (pneumococcus), Klebsiella, Legionnaires' bacillus, Bacillus proteus, E. coli, anaerobes (Bacteroides + Clostridia), Nocardia, actinomycosis
(c) Mycoplasma
√ small fluffy ill-defined acinar nodules, which enlarge with time

√ lobar + segmental densities with volume loss from airway obstruction secondary to bronchial narrowing + mucus plugging

Atypical Bacterial Pneumonia

= bacterial infection with radiographic appearance of viral pneumonia

Organism:
(1) Mycoplasma
(2) Pertussis
(3) Chlamydia trachomatis

Viral Pneumonia

= infection of bronchi + peribronchial tissues

Pathophysiology:
tracheitis; bronchitis; bronchiolitis; peribronchial + interstitial septa infiltrates; injury to alveolar cells with hyaline membranes; necrosis of alveolar walls with blood, edema, fibrin, macrophages in alveoli

Organism:
(a) Influenza virus: cavitary lesion confirms superimposed infection
(b) Coxsackie virus, echovirus, reovirus
(c) Parainfluenzavirus
(d) Adenovirus
(e) RSV = respiratory syncytial virus (12%)
(f) Rhinovirus (43%)
(g) Cytomegalic inclusion virus: features suggestive of bronchopneumonia
(h) Varicella / herpes zoster: 10% of adults; 2–5 days after rash
(i) Rubeola (measles) = before / with onset of rash; following overt measles = giant cell pneumonia
(j) Mycoplasma (10%)

Path: necrosis of ciliated epithelial cells, goblet cells, bronchial mucous glands with frequent involvement of peribronchial tissues + interlobular septa

Age: most common cause of pneumonia in children under 5 years of age

Distribution: usually bilateral

√ "dirty chest" = peribronchial cuffing + opacification:
  √ parahilar peribronchial linear densities (bronchial wall thickening)
  √ interstitial pattern
√ hyperaeration + air trapping (due to bronchial + bronchiolar narrowing from edema + secretions)
√ segmental + subsegmental atelectasis (common)
√ airspace pattern (from hemorrhagic edema) in 50%
√ pleural effusion (20%)
√ hilar adenopathy (3%)
√ striking absence of pneumatoceles, lung abscess, pneumothorax
√ radiographic resolution lags 2–3 weeks behind clinical

Cx: (1) Bacterial superinfection (child becomes toxic after a week of sickness, peripheral consolidations + pleural effusion)
(2) Bronchiectasis
(3) Unilateral hyperlucent lung, bronchiolitis obliterans

◊ Atypical measles pneumonia does NOT show the typical radiographic findings of viral pneumonias!

Interstitial Pneumonia

Acute Interstitial Pneumonia

= NONBACTERIAL PNEUMONIA

◊ Initially predominantly affecting interstitial tissues

Organisms: viruses, Mycoplasma, Pneumocystis

• often subacute atypical pneumonia

√ diffuse interstitial process with peribronchial thickening
√ segmental / lobar densities (mucus plugging + damage of surfactant-producing type 2 alveolar cells)

Chronic Interstitial Pneumonia

= diverse group of inflammatory disorders that can progress to pulmonary fibrosis

Modified Liebow classification:
1. Usual interstitial pneumonia (UIP)
2. Desquamative interstitial pneumonia (DIP)
3. Bronchiolitis obliterans with organizing pneumonia (BOOP)

<u>added</u>:
4. Acute interstitial pneumonia = Hamman-Rich syndrome
5. Nonspecific interstitial pneumonitis
6. Respiratory bronchiolitis-associated interstitial lung disease

<u>no longer included</u>:
1. Lymphoid interstitial pneumonia (LIP)
   = potentially malignant lymphoproliferative disorder
2. Giant cell interstitial pneumonia (GIP)
   = manifestation of hard-metal pneumoconiosis

Gram-negative Pneumonia

In 50% cause of nosocomial necrotizing pneumonias (including staphylococcal pneumonia)

Predisposed: elderly, debilitated, diabetes, alcoholism, COPD, malignancy, bronchitis, Gram-positive pneumonia, treatment with antibiotics, respirator therapy

Organisms:
1. Klebsiella
2. Pseudomonas
3. E. coli
4. Proteus
5. Haemophilus
6. Legionella

√ airspace consolidation (Klebsiella)
√ spongy appearance (Pseudomonas)
√ affecting dependent lobes (poor cough reflex without clearing of bronchial tree)
√ bilateral
√ cavitation common

Cx: (1) Exudate / empyema
(2) Bronchopleural fistula

Mycotic Infections of Lung

A. IN HEALTHY SUBJECTS
  1. Histoplasmosis
  2. Coccidioidomycosis
  3. Blastomycosis

B. OPPORTUNISTIC INFECTION
  1. Aspergillosis
  2. Mucormycosis (phycomycosis)
  3. Candidiasis

Growth: (a) mycelial form
(b) yeast form (depending on environment)

Source of contamination:
(a) soil
(b) growth in moist areas (apart from Coccidioides)
(c) contaminated bird / bat excreta

Cavitating Pneumonia

1. Staphylococcus aureus
2. Haemophilus influenzae
3. S. pneumoniae

other Gram-negative organisms (eg, Klebsiella)

Cavitating Opportunistic Infections

A. FUNGAL INFECTIONS
  1. Aspergillosis
  2. Nocardiosis
  3. Mucormycosis (= phycomycosis)

B. SEPTIC EMBOLI
  1. Anaerobic organisms

C. STAPHYLOCOCCAL ABSCESS

D. TUBERCULOSIS (nummular form)

◊ Repeated infections in same patient are not necessarily due to same organism!

DDx: Metastatic disease in carcinoma / Hodgkin lymphoma

Pulmonary Infiltrates in Neonate

mnemonic: "I HEAR"

Infection (pneumonia)
Hemorrhage
Edema
Aspiration
Respiratory distress syndrome

Recurrent Pneumonia in Childhood

A. IMMUNE PROBLEM
  1. Immune deficiency
  2. Chronic granulomatous disease of childhood (males)
  3. Alpha 1-antitrypsin deficiency

B. ASPIRATION
  1. Gastroesophageal reflux
  2. H-type tracheoesophageal fistula
  3. Disorder of swallowing mechanism
  4. Esophageal obstruction, impacted esophageal foreign body

C. UNDERLYING LUNG DISEASE
  1. Sequestration
  2. Bronchopulmonary dysplasia
  3. Cystic fibrosis
  4. Atopic asthma
  5. Bronchiolitis obliterans
  6. Sinusitis
  7. Bronchiectasis
  8. Ciliary dysmotility syndromes
  9. Pulmonary foreign body

EOSINOPHILIC LUNG DISEASE

= PULMONARY INFILTRATION WITH BLOOD / TISSUE EOSINOPHILIA (PIE)

Classification:

1. IDIOPATHIC EOSINOPHILIC LUNG DISEASE
   (a) Transient pulmonary eosinophilia = Löffler syndrome
   • peripheral eosinophilia
   (b) Acute / chronic eosinophilic pneumonia
   • no peripheral eosinophilia
2. EOSINOPHILIC LUNG DISEASE OF SPECIFIC ETIOLOGY
   (a) drug induced: nitrofurantoin, penicillin, sulfonamides, ASA, tricyclic antidepressants, hydrochlorothiazide, cromolyn sodium, mephenesin
   (b) parasite induced: tropical eosinophilia (ascariasis, schistosomiasis), strongyloidiasis, ancylostomiasis (hookworm), filariasis, Toxocara canis (visceral larva migrans), Dirofilaria immitis, amebiasis (occasionally — in RLL + RML)
   (c) fungus induced: allergic bronchopulmonary aspergillosis, bronchocentric granulomatosis
   (d) Pulmonary eosinophilia with asthma
3. EOSINOPHILIC LUNG DISEASE ASSOCIATED WITH ANGITIS ± GRANULOMATOSIS
   (a) Wegener granulomatosis
   (b) Churg-Strauss syndrome
   (c) Lymphomatoid granulomatosis
   (d) Bronchocentric granulomatosis
   (e) Necrotizing sarcoid granulomatosis
   (f) Polyarteritis nodosa
   (g) Rheumatoid disease
   (h) Scleroderma
   (i) Dermatomyositis
   (j) Sjögren syndrome
   (k) CREST

CONGENITAL PULMONARY MALFORMATION

= SEQUESTRATION SPECTRUM

1. Congenital lobar emphysema
2. Bronchogenic cyst
3. Cystic adenomatoid malformation
4. Bronchopulmonary sequestration
5. Hypogenetic lung syndrome
6. Pulmonary arteriovenous malformation

NEONATAL LUNG DISEASE

Parenchymal Lung Disease on 1st Day of Life

◊ Radiographic findings overlap!

1. Transient tachypnea of newborn
2. Respiratory distress syndrome
3. Neonatal pneumonia

CHEST

4. Meconium aspiration syndrome
5. Premature with accelerated lung maturity (PALM)

Air Leaks in Neonatal Chest

1. Pulmonary interstitial emphysema
2. Pneumomediastinum
3. Pneumothorax
4. Gas below visceral pleura
   √ gas at lung base / against fissure
5. Pneumopericardium
6. Gas embolus to cardiac chambers / blood vessels

Mediastinal Shift & Abnormal Aeration in Neonate

A. SHIFT TOWARD LUCENT LUNG
   1. Diaphragmatic hernia
   2. Chylothorax
   3. Cystic adenomatoid malformation

B. SHIFT AWAY FROM LUCENT LUNG
   1. Congenital lobar emphysema
   2. Persistent localized pulmonary interstitial emphysema
   3. Obstruction of main-stem bronchus (by anomalous or dilated vessel / cardiac chamber)

Reticulogranular Densities in Neonate

1. Respiratory distress syndrome (90%): premature infant, inadequate surfactant
2. **Prematurity with accelerated lung maturity** (PALM)
   = IMMATURE LUNG SYNDROME: premature infant, normal surfactant (due to maternal steroid therapy / intrauterine stress)
   √ lung granularity, almost clear
   √ small thymus (stress / steroids)
3. Transient tachypnea of the newborn
4. Neonatal group-B streptococcal pneumonia
5. Idiopathic hypoglycemia
6. Congestive heart failure
7. Early pulmonary hemorrhage
8. Infant of diabetic mother

Hyperinflation in Newborn

√ level of inflation beyond 8th rib posteriorly
√ depressed configuration of hemidiaphragms best judged on LAT view

1. Fetal aspiration syndrome
2. Neonatal pneumonia
3. Pulmonary hemorrhage
4. Congenital heart disease
5. Transient tachypnea (mild)

Hyperinflation in Child

mnemonic: "BUMP FAD"

Bronchiectasis
Upper airway obstruction
Mucoviscidosis
Pneumonia (esp. staph)
Foreign body (ball-valve mechanism)
Asthma
Dehydration (diarrhea, acidosis)

ABNORMAL LUNG PATTERNS

1. Mass
   = any localized density not completely bordered by fissures / pleura
2. Consolidative (alveolar) pattern
   = commonly produced by filling of air spaces with fluid (transudate / exudate) / cells / other material, ALSO by alveolar collapse, airway obstruction, confluent interstitial thickening
   ground glass = hazy area of increased attenuation not obscuring bronchovascular structures
   consolidation = marked increase in attenuation with obliteration of underlying anatomic features
3. Interstitial pattern
4. Vascular pattern
   (a) increased vessel size: CHF, pulmonary arterial hypertension, shunt vascularity, lymphangitic carcinomatosis
   (b) decreased vessel size: emphysema, thromboembolism
5. Bronchial pattern
   √ wall thickening: bronchitis, asthma, bronchiectasis
   √ density without air bronchogram (= complete airway obstruction)
   √ lucency of air trapping (= partial airway obstruction with ball-valve mechanism)

DIFFUSE LUNG DISEASE ON HRCT

Patterns of Diffuse Lung Disease on HRCT

maximum resolution = 300 μm

1. **Linear densities** = septal thickening
   Cause: interstitial fluid / fibrosis / cellular infiltrates
   (a) smooth septal thickening: pulmonary edema, lymphangitic carcinomatosis
   (b) beaded septa / septal nodules: lymphangitic carcinomatosis
   (c) irregular septa imply fibrosis
   — distorted lobules: fibrosis
   — no architectural distortion of lobules: edema / infiltration
2. **Reticular densities**
   (a) predominantly subpleural small reticular elements of 6–10 mm in diameter with small cystic changes ("honeycombing")
   Associated with: interstitial fibrosis, lymphangioleiomyomatosis, amyloidosis
   (b) fine diffusely distributed network of 2–3-mm basic elements
   Associated with: miliary TB, reactions to methotrexate

   Distribution:
   — lower lung zones in subpleural areas: idiopathic pulmonary fibrosis, collagen vascular disease, asbestosis
   — mid lung zone / all lung zones: chronic extrinsic allergic alveolitis
   – mid + upper lung zones: sarcoidosis

3. **Nodules**
   (a) interstitial nodules
   lymphangitic carcinomatosis, sarcoidosis, histiocytosis X, silicosis, coal worker pneumoconiosis, tuberculosis, hypersensitivity pneumonitis, metastatic tumor, amyloidosis
   √ perihilar peribronchovascular, centrilobular, interlobular septa, subpleural nodules
   (b) airspace nodules
   lobular pneumonia, transbronchial spread of TB, bronchiolitis obliterans organizing pneumonia (BOOP), pulmonary edema
   √ ill-defined nodules, a few mm to 1 cm in size
   √ peribronchiolar + centrilobular
   Distribution:
   — along bronchoarterial bundles + interlobular septa + subpleural: sarcoidosis
   — upper zone: silicosis, coal-worker's pneumoconiosis
   — centrilobular: extrinsic allergic alveolitis
4. **Ground-glass attenuation**
   = hazy increase in lung opacity without obscuration of underlying vessels
   ◊ Often indicative of an acute, active, and potentially treatable process!
   Cause:
   (a) early interstitial lung disease = minimal alveolar wall thickening
   (b) alveolitis = minimal airspace filling
   √ areas of higher attenuation with nodular / centrilobular distribution
   √ pulmonary vessels uniform in size in areas of differing attenuation
   √ increase in lung attenuation in low- and high-attenuation areas on expiratory HRCT
   (c) edema = increased capillary blood volume
   (d) partial atelectasis = partial collapse of alveoli
   (e) normal during expiration
   Distribution:
   — peripheral in lower lung zones: DIP, UIP
   — mid + upper lung zones: sarcoidosis
   — "crazy paving" appearance: alveolar proteinosis
   — mosaic perfusion: chronic thromboembolism, bronchiolitis obliterans
5. **Consolidation**
   = increase in lung opacity with obscuration of underlying vessels ± air bronchograms
   — subpleural in mid + upper lung zones: chronic eosinophilic pneumonia
   — subpleural + peribronchial: BOOP
   — focal: bronchioloalveolar cell carcinoma, lymphoma
   — random: infection
6. **Cystic airspaces**
   = circumscribed air-containing lesions
   (a) with well-defined walls
   lymphangioleiomyomatosis, pulmonary Langerhans-cell granulomatosis, honeycomb lung, bronchiectasis
   (b) without well-defined walls
   centrilobular, panlobular (panacinar), paraseptal emphysema

HRCT of Bronchiolitis

[CT findings are nonspecific and must be interpreted in the appropriate clinical context]

Cause:
(a) infection via endobronchial spread:
   – bacterial (most common)
   – mycobacterial: classic TB, nonclassic M. avium-intracellulare ("Lady Windermere syndrome" commonly in RML + lingula)
   – viral: acute infectious bronchiolitis in infants and young children due to RSV, adenovirus, mycoplasma
   – parasitic
   – fungal
   ◊ Most common cause of tree-in-bud appearance
(b) aspiration of infected oral secretions / other irritant material / inert barium: mineral dust airway disease, extrinsic allergic alveolitis, chronic bronchitis
(c) immunologic deficiency or impaired host defense: cystic fibrosis, dyskinetic cilia syndrome
(d) cigarette smoking
   1. Respiratory bronchiolitis
(e) idiopathic
   1. Diffuse panbronchiolitis in Orientals
   2. Follicular bronchiolitis: rheumatoid arthritis, Sjögren syndrome
   3. Asthma
   4. Bronchiolitis obliterans
   5. Bronchiolitis obliterans with organizing pneumonia

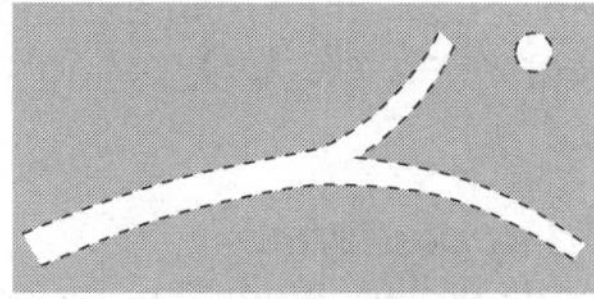

Normal Bronchiole
(<1 mm, not visible on CT)

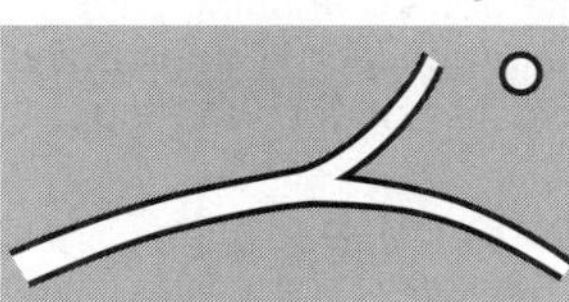

Thickened Bronchiolar Wall

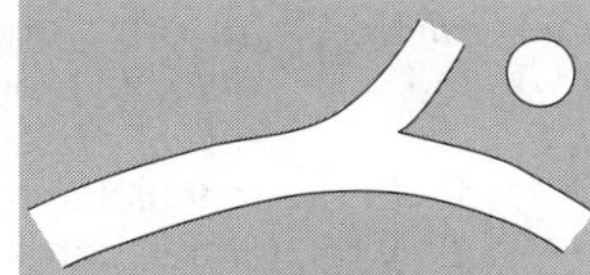

Dilated Bronchiole (>2 mm)

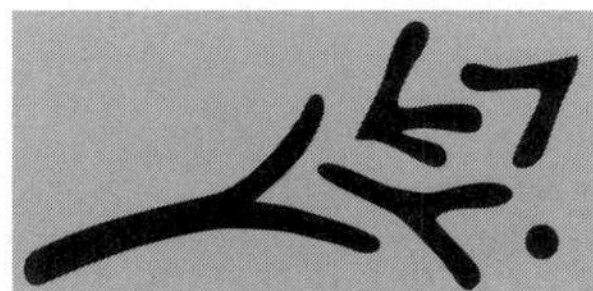

Bronchiolar Impaction

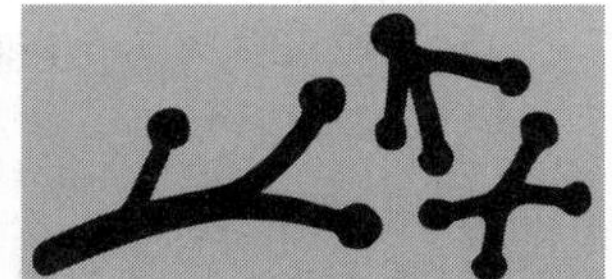

"Tree-in-bud" Appearance
= bronchiolar impaction + clubbing

Pattern of Bronchiolar Disease

CHEST

A. DIRECT SIGNS
- √ ringlike tubular structures in lung periphery
  Cause: wall thickening
- √ dilatation of bronchioles
  Cause: bronchiolectasis
- √ 2- to 4-mm nodules / branching linear structures in lung periphery
  Cause: bronchiolar luminal impaction with pus, mucus, granulomas, inflammatory exudate, fibrosis

B. INDIRECT SIGNS
- √ subsegmental atelectasis = wedge-shaped area of ground-glass attenuation
- √ air trapping = area of decreased attenuation from collateral air drift / ball-valve effect distal to occluded / stenotic airway more prominent on expiration:
  DDx: physiologic air trapping with a few lucent secondary pulmonary lobules
  - √ mosaic perfusion = scattered areas of air trapping
  - √ centrilobular emphysema = destruction of small airways + surrounding parenchyma in the center of the pulmonary lobule
- √ centrilobular airspace nodule = acinar nodule = <1 cm ill-defined nodule of ground-glass attenuation (from inflammation within alveolar space) less prominent on expiration
  Cause: extrinsic allergic alveolitis, sarcoidosis (perivenular nodules), pneumoconiosis (asbestosis, silicosis)

DDx: (1) Cystic lung disease (thin septum surrounds area of air attenuation, central vessel not present)
(2) Panlobular emphysema (distortion of vascular + septal architecture, bullae)

Tree-in-bud appearance

= small poorly defined centrilobular nodules + branching centrilobular areas of increased opacity occurring at multiple contiguous branching sites

Histo: severe bronchiolar impaction with clubbing of distal bronchioles analogous to "finger-in-glove" appearance

1. Endobronchial spread of active TB
2. Viral, fungal, parasitic infection
3. Allergic bronchopulmonary aspergillosis
4. Cystic fibrosis
5. Aspiration pneumonitis
6. Laryngotracheal papillomatosis

Mosaic Perfusion

= patchwork of normal and air-attenuated segments
- √ vessels in areas of low attenuation are smaller in 94% (due to differential blood flow)
- √ normal / dilated arteries in areas of hyperattenuation in 77%

Cause:
1. Air trapping
   - √ attenuation differences are accentuated on expiratory HRCT
2. Vascular obstruction
   - √ increase in lung attenuation in low- and high-attenuation areas on expiratory HRCT

ALVEOLAR (CONSOLIDATIVE) PATTERN

Classic appearance of airspace consolidation:
mnemonic: "A^2BC^3"
- √ **A**cinar rosettes: rounded poorly defined nodules in size of acini (6–10 mm), best seen at periphery of opacity
- √ **A**ir alveologram / bronchogram
- √ **B**utterfly / bat-wing distribution: perihilar / bibasilar
- √ **C**oalescent / confluent cloudlike ill-defined opacities
- √ **C**onsolidation in diffuse, perihilar / bibasilar, segmental / lobar, multifocal / lobular distribution
- √ **C**hanges occur rapidly (labile / fleeting)

HRCT:
- √ poorly marginated densities within primary lobule (up to 1 cm in size)
- √ rapid coalescence with neighboring lesions in segmental distribution
- √ predominantly central location with sparing of subpleural zones
- √ air bronchograms

Diffuse Airspace Disease

A. INFLAMMATORY EXUDATE = "PUS"
1. Lobar pneumonia
2. Bronchopneumonia: especially Gram-negative organisms
3. Unusual pneumonias
   (a) viral: extensive hemorrhagic edema especially in immunocompromised patients with hematologic malignancies + transplants
   (b) Pneumocystis
   (c) fungal: Aspergillus, Candida, Cryptococcus, Phycomycetes
   (d) tuberculosis
4. Aspiration

B. HEMORRHAGE = "BLOOD"
1. Trauma: contusion
2. Pulmonary embolism, thromboembolism
3. Bleeding diathesis: leukemia, hemophilia, anticoagulants, DIC
4. Vasculitis: Wegener granulomatosis, Goodpasture syndrome, SLE, mucormycosis, aspergillosis, Rocky Mountain spotted fever, infectious mononucleosis
5. Idiopathic pulmonary hemosiderosis
6. Bleeding metastases: choriocarcinoma

C. TRANSUDATE = "WATER"
1. Cardiac edema
2. Neurogenic edema
3. Hypoproteinemia
4. Fluid overload

5. Renal failure
6. Radiotherapy
7. Shock
8. Toxic inhalation
9. Drug reaction
10. Adult respiratory distress syndrome

D. SECRETIONS = "PROTEIN"
1. Alveolar proteinosis
2. Mucus plugging

E. MALIGNANCY = "CELLS"
1. Bronchioloalveolar cell carcinoma
2. Lymphoma

F. INTERSTITIAL DISEASE simulating airspace disease, eg, "alveolar sarcoid"

mnemonic: "AIRSPACED"

Aspiration
Inhalation, **I**nflammatory
Renal (uremia)
Sarcoidosis
Proteinosis (alveolar)
Alveolar cell carcinoma
Congestive (CHF)
Emboli
Drug reaction, **D**rowning

Diffuse Pulmonary Hemorrhage

√ nonspecific diffuse / bilateral multifocal air-space opacities

1. Wegener granulomatosis: c-ANCA, upper respiratory tract involvement, renal disease
2. Churg-Strauss syndrome
3. Systemic necrotizing vasculitis
4. Collagen-vascular disease
   (a) Systemic lupus erythematosus: granular pattern of immune complexes on tissue stains, noncaseating granulomas, malar rash
   (b) Rheumatoid arthritis
   (c) Seronegative juvenile rheumatoid arthritis
5. Goodpasture syndrome: antibasement membrane antibodies with a linear pattern on tissue stains
6. Immunoglobulin A nephropathy
7. Schönlein-Henoch purpura
8. Idiopathic pulmonary hemorrhage
9. Idiopathic glomerulonephritis

Air-space Opacification in Trauma

A. ACUTE PHASE
1. Pulmonary contusion = hemorrhage into alveoli
2. Pulmonary laceration = tear in lung parenchyma
   (a) spherical hematoma = filled with blood
   (b) traumatic pneumatocele = filled with air
3. Aspiration pneumonia
4. Atelectasis due to splinting / mucous plug
5. Pulmonary edema: cardiogenic / noncardiogenic

B. SUBACUTE PHASE (>24 hours) add
1. Fat embolism
2. Adult respiratory distress syndrome

Localized Airspace Disease

mnemonic: "4P's & TAIL"

Pneumonia
Pulmonary edema
Pulmonary contusion
Pulmonary interstitial edema
Tuberculosis
Alveolar cell carcinoma
Infant
Lymphoma

Acute Alveolar Infiltrate

mnemonic: "I 2 CHANGE FAST"

Infarct
Infection
Contusion
Hemorrhage
Aspiration
Near drowning
Goodpasture syndrome
Edema
Fungus
Allergic sensitivity
Shock lung
Tuberculosis

Chronic Alveolar Infiltrate

mnemonic: "STALLAG"

Sarcoidosis
Tuberculosis
Alveolar cell carcinoma
Lymphoma
Lipoid pneumonia
Alveolar proteinosis
Goodpasture syndrome

CT Angiogram Sign

= homogeneous low attenuation of lung consolidation, which allows vessels to be clearly seen

1. Lobar bronchioloalveolar cell carcinoma
2. Lobar pneumonia
3. Pulmonary lymphoma
4. Extrinsic lipid pneumonia
5. Pulmonary infarction
6. Pulmonary edema

INTERSTITIAL LUNG DISEASE

= thickening of lung interstices (= interlobular septa)

A. MAJOR LYMPHATIC TRUNKS
1. Lymphangitic carcinomatosis
2. Congenital pulmonary lymphangiectasia
3. Pulmonary edema
4. Alveolar proteinosis

B. PULMONARY VEINS (increased pulmonary venous pressure)
1. Left ventricular failure
2. Venous obstructive disease

C. SUPPORTING CONNECTIVE TISSUE NETWORK
   1. Interstitial edema
   2. Chronic interstitial pneumonia
   3. Pneumoconioses
   4. Collagen-vascular disease
   5. Interstitial fibrosis
   6. Amyloid
   7. Tumor infiltration within connective tissue
   8. Desmoplastic reaction to tumor

Path: stereotypical inflammatory response of alveolar wall to injury
(a) acute phase: fluid + inflammatory cells exude into alveolar space, mononuclear cells accumulate in edematous alveolar wall
(b) organizing phase: hyperplasia of type II pneumocytes attempt to regenerate alveolar epithelium, fibroblasts deposit collagen
(c) chronic stage: dense collagenous fibrous tissue remodels normal pulmonary architecture

Characterizing criteria:
(a) zonal distribution:
   – upper / lower lung zones
   – axial (core) / parenchymal (middle) / peripheral
(b) volume loss
(c) time course
(d) interstitial lung pattern

Classification scheme:
A. Interstitial pneumonias
   1. Usual interstitial pneumonia (UIP)
   2. Nonspecific interstitial pneumonia (NSIP)
   3. Acute interstitial pneumonia (AIP)
   4. Alveolar macrophage pneumonia (AMP) = desquamative interstitial pneumonia (DIP)
   5. Bronchiolitis obliterans organizing pneumonia
B. Diffuse infiltrative disease with granulomas
   1. Sarcoidosis
   2. Hypersensitivity pneumonitis
C. Lymphocytic interstitial pneumonia (LIP)
D. Pneumoconioses
E. Interstitial lung disease with cysts
   1. Langerhans cell histiocytosis
   2. Lymphangioleiomyomatosis
F. Interstitial lung disease with interlobular septal thickening
   1. Lymphangitic carcinomatosis
   2. Interstitial pulmonary edema
   3. Alveolar proteinosis
G. Eosinophilic syndrome
H. Pulmonary hemorrhage
I. Vasculitis

Interstitial Lung Pattern on CXR

1. LINEAR PATTERN
   (a) Kerley lines = septal lines
      = thickened connective septa
      Path: accumulation of fluid / tissue
      √ Kerley A lines = relatively long fine linear shadows in upper lungs, deep within lung parenchyma radiating from hila
      √ Kerley B lines = short horizontally oriented peripheral lines extending + perpendicular to pleura in costophrenic angles + retrosternal clear space
   (b) reticulations
      = innumerable interlacing linear opacities suggesting a mesh / network
      √ Kerley C lines = fine "spider web / lacelike" polygonal opacities distributed primarily in a peripheral / subpleural location
         Path: pulmonary fibrosis (lower lobes), hypersensitivity pneumonitis (upper lobes)
      √ thick linear opacities in a central / perihilar distribution
         Path: (a) dilated thick-walled bronchi of bronchiectasis, (b) cysts of lymphangioleiomyomatosis / tuberous sclerosis
2. NODULAR / MILIARY PATTERN
   = small well-defined innumerable uniform 3–5-mm nodules with even distribution
   Path: diffuse metastatic disease, infectious granulomatous disease (TB, fungal), noninfectious granulomatous disease (pneumoconioses, sarcoidosis, eosinophilic granuloma)
3. DESTRUCTIVE FORM = honeycomb lung

Thoracic Manifestations of Collagen Vascular Disease

	Ankylosing Spondylitis	*Dermatomyositis Polymyositis*	*Progressive Systemic Sclerosis*	*Rheumatoid Arthritis*	*Sjögren Syndrome*	*Systemic Lupus Erythematosus (SLE)*
Pulmonary fibrosis	occasional	common	frequent	frequent	occasional	occasional
Pleural disease	—	—	—	frequent	—	frequent
Diaphragm weakness	—	frequent	—	—	—	frequent
Aspiration pneumonia	—	frequent	frequent	—	—	—
Bronchiectasis	—	—	—	occasional	common	—
Apical fibrosis	frequent	—	—	—	—	—
Bronchiolitis obliterans	—	—	—	common	—	—
BOOP	—	common	—	common	—	—

Signs of Acute Interstitial Disease

√ peribronchial cuffing = thickened bronchial wall + peribronchial sheath (when viewed end on)
√ thickening of interlobular fissures
√ Kerley lines
√ perihilar haze = blurring of hilar shadows
√ blurring of pulmonary vascular markings
√ increased density at lung bases
√ small pleural effusions

Signs of Chronic Interstitial Disease

√ irregular visceral pleural surface
√ **reticulations**:
  √ fine reticulations = early potentially reversible / minimal irreversible alveolar septal abnormality
    (1) idiopathic pulmonary fibrosis (basilar predominance)
  √ coarse reticulations
    in 75% related to environmental disease, sarcoidosis, collagen-vascular disorders, chronic interstitial pneumonia
√ **nodularity**:
  in 90% related to infectious / noninfectious granulomatous process, metastatic malignancy, pneumoconioses, amyloidosis
√ **linearity**:
  (1) cardiogenic / noncardiogenic interstitial pulmonary edema
    √ symmetric linearity
  (2) lymphangitic malignancy
    √ asymmetric linearity
  (3) diffuse bronchial wall disorders (cystic fibrosis, bronchiectasis, hypersensitivity asthma)
√ **honeycombing** = usually subpleural clustered cystic air spaces <1 cm in diameter with thick well-defined walls set off against a background of increased lung density (end-stage lung)
◊ HRCT approximately 60% more sensitive than CXR

Distribution of Interstitial Disease

A. MIDLUNG / PERIHILAR DISEASE
  (a) Acute rapidly changing
    1. Pulmonary edema
    2. Pneumocystis pneumonitis
    3. Early extrinsic allergic alveolitis
  (b) Chronic slowly progressive
    1. Lymphangitic carcinomatosis
       often unilateral, associated with adenopathy, pleural effusion
B. PERIPHERAL LUNG DISEASE
  (a) Acute rapidly changing
    1. Interstitial pulmonary edema with Kerley B lines (most common)
    2. Active fibrosing alveolitis
  (b) Chronic slowly progressive
    1. Secondary pulmonary hemosiderosis
C. UPPER LUNG DISEASE
  (a) Chronic slowly progressive ± volume loss
    1. Postprimary TB (common)
    2. Silicosis (common)
  (b) Chronic slowly progressive with volume loss
    1. Sarcoidosis (common)
    2. Ankylosing spondylitis (rare)
    3. Sulfa drugs (rare)
  (c) Chronic slowly progressive without volume loss
    1. Extrinsic allergic alveolitis
    2. Eosinophilic granuloma
    3. Aspiration pneumonia
    4. Postradiation pneumonitis
    5. Recurrent Pneumocystis carinii pneumonia (PCP) in a patient receiving aerosolized pentamidine prophylaxis

mnemonic: "SHIRT CAP"
Sarcoidosis
Histoplasmosis
Idiopathic
Radiation therapy
Tuberculosis (postprimary)
Chronic extrinsic alveolitis
Ankylosing spondylitis
Progressive massive fibrosis

CHEST

Chronic Diffuse Infiltrative Lung Disease

= CHRONIC INTERSTITIAL LUNG DISEASE
  = GENERALIZED INTERSTITIAL LUNG DISEASE

Prevalence: up to 15% of pulmonary conditions
Cause: >200 described disorders;
  in only 25–30% known / established etiology;
  15–20 diseases comprise >90% of cases

• dyspnea (primary complaint)
• dry basilar rales / crackles that fail to clear with coughing

CXR:
  ◊ Difficult to characterize due to similar findings
  ◊ Differentiation into alveolar + interstitial disease is unreliable as "interstitial disease" invariably involves alveoli + vice versa
  √ ± nonspecific abnormality

mnemonic: "HIDE FACTS"
Hamman-Rich, **H**emosiderosis
Infection, **I**rradiation, **I**diopathic
Dust, **D**rugs
Eosinophilic granuloma, **E**dema
Fungal, **F**armer's lung
Aspiration (oil), **A**rthritis (rheumatoid, ankylosing spondylitis)
Collagen vascular disease
Tumor, **T**B, **T**uberous sclerosis
Sarcoidosis, **S**cleroderma

Zonal Predilection of Chronic Diffuse Lung Disease

CHRONIC DIFFUSE INFILTRATIVE LUNG DISEASE OF UPPER LUNG ZONE

= zone with higher oxygen tension and pH, but less efficient lymphatic drainage
  (a) inhalational disease
    1. Silicosis
    2. Coal worker pneumoconiosis

3. Extrinsic allergic alveolitis
4. Aspiration pneumonia

(b) granulomatous disease
1. Sarcoidosis
2. Langerhans cell histiocytosis (EG)
3. Postprimary TB (common)

(c) others
1. Cystic fibrosis
2. Ankylosing spondylitis
3. Chronic interstitial pneumonia
4. Sulfa drugs (rare)
5. Postradiation pneumonitis
6. Recurrent Pneumocystis carinii pneumonia (PCP) in a patient receiving aerosolized pentamidine prophylaxis

mnemonic: "CASSET"
Cystic fibrosis
Ankylosing spondylitis
Silicosis
Sarcoidosis
Eosinophilic granuloma
Tuberculosis, fungus

CHRONIC DIFFUSE INFILTRATIVE LUNG DISEASE OF LOWER LUNG ZONE

= zone with greater ventilation, perfusion, and lymphatic drainage

1. Idiopathic pulmonary fibrosis: usual interstitial pneumonia (common)
2. Lymphangitic carcinomatosis
3. Collagen vascular disease: scleroderma (common)
4. Asbestosis (posterior aspect of lung base)
5. Lymphangioleiomyomatosis
6. Chronic aspiration pneumonia with fibrosis (often regional + unilateral)

mnemonic: "BAD LASS RIF"
Bronchiectasis
Aspiration
Dermatomyositis
Lymphangitic spread
Asbestosis
Sarcoidosis
Scleroderma
Rheumatoid arthritis
Idiopathic pulmonary fibrosis
Furadantin

Compartmental Predilection of Chronic Diffuse Lung Disease

A. AXIAL COMPARTMENT
= peribronchial vascular bundles + lymphatics
1. Sarcoidosis
2. Lymphangitic carcinomatosis
3. Lymphoma

B. MIDDLE / PARENCHYMAL COMPARTMENT
= formed by alveolar walls
1. Sarcoidosis
2. Lymphangitic carcinomatosis
3. Chronic medications
4. Neurofibromatosis
5. Vasculitis
6. Silicosis

C. PERIPHERAL COMPARTMENT
= pleura with subpleural connective tissue, interlobular septa, pulmonary veins, lymphatics, walls of cortical alveoli
1. Sarcoidosis
2. Lymphangitic carcinomatosis
3. Idiopathic pulmonary fibrosis
4. Collagen vascular disease
5. Rheumatoid arthritis

Lung Volumes in Chronic Diffuse Lung Disease

CHRONIC DIFFUSE INFILTRATIVE LUNG DISEASE WITH NORMAL LUNG VOLUME
1. Sarcoidosis
2. Langerhans cell histiocytosis (in 66%)
3. Early stage

CHRONIC DIFFUSE INFILTRATIVE LUNG DISEASE WITH INCREASED LUNG VOLUME

mnemonic: "ELECT"
Emphysema with interstitial lung disease
Lymphangioleiomyomatosis
Eosinophilic granuloma (Langerhans) in 33%
Cystic fibrosis
Tuberous sclerosis

CHRONIC DIFFUSE INFILTRATIVE LUNG DISEASE WITH REDUCED LUNG VOLUME

due to fibrotic process
1. Systemic lupus erythematosus
2. Collagen vascular disease (eg, scleroderma, dermatomyositis, polymyositis)
3. Idiopathic pulmonary fibrosis
4. Chronic interstitial pneumonias
5. Asbestosis

Pleural Disease in Chronic Diffuse Lung Disease

CHRONIC DIFFUSE INFILTRATIVE LUNG DISEASE WITH PNEUMOTHORAX
1. Lymphangioleiomyomatosis
2. Langerhans cell histiocytosis
3. End-stage lung disease

CHRONIC DIFFUSE INFILTRATIVE LUNG DISEASE WITH PLEURAL EFFUSION
1. Lymphangioleiomyomatosis
2. Rheumatoid arthritis
3. Systemic lupus erythematosus
4. Mixed connective tissue disorder
5. Wegener granulomatosis
6. Lymphangitic carcinomatosis
7. Pulmonary edema

Chronic Diffuse Infiltrative Lung Disease with Pleural Thickening
1. Asbestosis
2. Collagen vascular disease

Lymphadenopathy in Chronic Diffuse Lung Disease
1. Silicosis
2. Sarcoidosis
3. Lymphoma
4. Lymphangitic carcinomatosis

Diffuse Fine Reticulations
Acute Diffuse Fine Reticulations
A. ACUTE INTERSTITIAL EDEMA
  1. Congestive heart failure
  2. Fluid overload
  3. Uremia
  4. Hypersensitivity

B. ACUTE INTERSTITIAL PNEUMONIA
  1. Viral pneumonia (Hantavirus, CMV)
  2. Mycoplasma pneumonia
  3. Pneumocystis carinii pneumonia

mnemonic: "HELP"
Hypersensitivity
Edema
Lymphoproliferative
Pneumonitis (viral)

Chronic Diffuse Fine Reticulations
A. VENOUS OBSTRUCTION
  1. Atherosclerotic heart disease
  2. Mitral stenosis
  3. Left atrial myxoma
  4. Pulmonary venoocclusive disease
  5. Sclerosing mediastinitis

B. LYMPHATIC OBSTRUCTION
  1. Lymphangiectasia (pediatric patient)
  2. Mediastinal mass (lymphoma)
  3. Lymphoma / leukemia
  4. Lymphangitic carcinomatosis: predominantly basilar distribution
    (a) bilateral (breast, stomach, colon, pancreas)
    (b) unilateral (lung tumor)
  5. Lymphocytic interstitial pneumonitis

C. INHALATIONAL DISEASE
  1. Silicosis: small nodules + reticulations
  2. Asbestosis: basilar distribution, pleural thickening + calcifications
  3. Hard metals
  4. Allergic alveolitis

D. GRANULOMATOUS DISEASE
  from a nodular to a reticular pattern if
    (a) nodules line up along bronchovascular bundles
    (b) interlobular septa show fibrotic changes
  1. Sarcoidosis: hilar + mediastinal adenopathy (may have disappeared)
  2. Eosinophilic granuloma: upper lobe distribution

E. CONNECTIVE-TISSUE DISEASE
  reticulations in late stages
  1. Rheumatoid lung
  2. Scleroderma
  3. Systemic lupus erythematosus

F. DRUG REACTIONS

G. IDIOPATHIC
  1. Usual interstitial pneumonitis (UIP)
  2. Desquamative interstitial pneumonitis (DIP)
  3. Tuberous sclerosis: smooth muscle proliferation
  4. Lymphangiomyomatosis
  5. Idiopathic pulmonary hemosiderosis
  6. Alveolar proteinosis (late complication)
  7. Amyloidosis
  8. Interstitial calcification (chronic renal failure)

mnemonic: "LIFE lines"
Lymphangitic spread
Inflammation / infection
Fibrosis
Edema

CHEST

Coarse Reticulations
= architectural destruction of interstitium = end-stage scarring of lung = interstitial pulmonary fibrosis = **honeycomb lung**

√ coarse reticular interstitial densities with intervening cystic spaces
√ rounded radiolucencies <1 cm in areas of increased lung density
√ small lung volume (decreased compliance)

Cx: (1) Intercurrent pneumothoraces
(2) Bronchogenic carcinoma = scar carcinoma

Cause:
A. INHALATIONAL DISEASE
  (a) Pneumoconioses
    1. Asbestosis: basilar distribution, shaggy heart, pleural thickening + calcifications
    2. Silicosis: upper lobe predominance, ± pleural thickening, ± hilar and mediastinal lymphadenopathy
    3. Berylliosis
  (b) Chemical inhalation (late)
    1. Silo-filler's disease (nitrogen dioxide)
    2. Sulfur dioxide, chlorine, phosgene, cadmium
  (c) Extrinsic allergic alveolitis (= hypersensitivity to organic dusts)
  (d) Oxygen toxicity
    sequelae of RDS therapy with oxygen
  (e) Chronic aspiration
    eg, mineral oil: localized process in medial basal segments / middle lobe

B. GRANULOMATOUS DISEASE
  1. Sarcoidosis
  2. Eosinophilic granuloma

C. COLLAGEN-VASCULAR DISEASE
  1. Rheumatoid lung
  2. Scleroderma
  3. Ankylosing spondylitis: upper lobes
  4. SLE: rarely produces honeycombing

D. IATROGENIC
   1. Drug hypersensitivity
   2. Radiotherapy
E. IDIOPATHIC
   1. Usual interstitial pneumonitis (UIP) honeycombing in 50%, severe volume loss in 45%
   2. Desquamative interstitial pneumonitis (DIP) honeycombing in 12.5%, severe volume loss in 23%
   3. Lymphangiomyomatosis
   4. Tuberous sclerosis (rare)
   5. Neurofibromatosis (rare)
   6. Pulmonary capillary hemangiomatosis (rare)

DDx: bronchiectasis, cavitary metastases (rare)

Reticulations & Pleural Effusion

A. ACUTE
   1. Edema
   2. Infection: viral, Mycoplasma (very rare)
B. CHRONIC
   1. Congestive heart failure
   2. Lymphangitic carcinomatosis
   3. Lymphoma / leukemia
   4. SLE
   5. Rheumatoid disease
   6. Lymphangiectasia
   7. Lymphangiomyomatosis
   8. Asbestosis

Reticulations & Hilar Adenopathy

1. Sarcoidosis
2. Silicosis
3. Lymphoma / leukemia
4. Lung primary: particularly oat cell carcinoma
5. Metastases: lymphatic obstruction / spread
6. Fungal disease
7. Tuberculosis
8. Viral pneumonia (rare combination)

Chronic Interstitial Disease Simulating Airspace Disease

A. REPLACEMENT OF LUNG ARCHITECTURE BY AN INTERSTITIAL PROCESS
   (a) neoplastic
      Hodgkin disease, histiocytic lymphoma
   (b) benign cellular infiltrate
      lymphocytic interstitial pneumonia, pseudolymphoma
   (c) granulomatous disease
      alveolar sarcoidosis
   (d) fibrosis
B. EXUDATIVE PHASE OF INTERSTITIAL PNEUMONIA
   1. UIP
   2. Adult respiratory distress syndrome
   3. Radiation pneumonitis
   4. Drug reaction
   5. Reaction to noxious gases
C. CELLULAR FILLING OF AIR SPACE
   1. Desquamative interstitial pneumonia
   2. Pneumocystis carinii pneumonia

Reticulonodular Lung Disease

mnemonic: "**P**lease **D**on't **E**at **S**tale **T**una **F**ish **S**andwiches **E**very **M**orning"

Pneumoconiosis
Drugs
Eosinophilic granuloma
Sarcoidosis
Tuberculosis
Fungal disease
Schistosomiasis
Exanthem (measles, chickenpox)
Metastases (thyroid)

Reticulonodular Pattern & Lower Lobe Predominance

mnemonic: "CIA"

Collagen vascular disease
Idiopathic
Asbestosis

Nodular Lung Disease

= round moderately well marginated opacity <3 cm in maximum diameter

A. GRANULOMATOUS LUNG DISEASE
   (a) infections: eg, tuberculosis
   (b) fungal disease: eg, histoplasmosis
   (c) silicosis
   (d) vasculitis: eg, Wegener granulomatosis
B. NEOPLASM
   (a) metastatic lung diseases: eg, thyroid cancer
   (b) lymphoma
   (c) bronchioloalveolar cell carcinoma
C. OTHER DISEASE
   (a) drug-induced: methotrexate
   (b) nongranulomatous vasculitis
   (c) sarcoidosis

Macronodular Lung Disease

√ nodules >5 mm in diameter

mnemonic: "GAMMA WARPS"

Granuloma (eosinophilic granuloma, fungus)
Abscess
Metastases
Multiple myeloma
AVM
Wegener granulomatosis
Amyloidosis
Rheumatoid lung
Parasites (Echinococcus, paragonimiasis)
Sarcoidosis

Micronodular Lung Disease

= discrete 3–5–7-mm small round focal opacity of at least soft-tissue attenuation

1. Granulomatous disease (miliary tuberculosis, histoplasmosis)
2. Hypersensitivity (organic dust)
3. Pneumoconiosis (inorganic dust, thesaurosis = prolonged hair spray exposure)
4. Sarcoidosis
5. Metastases (thyroid, melanoma)
6. Histiocytosis X
7. Chickenpox

DIFFUSE FINE NODULAR DISEASE & MILIARY NODULES

√ very small 1–4-mm sharply defined nodules of interstitial disease

(a) Inhalational disease
   1. Silicosis + coal worker's pneumoconiosis
   2. Berylliosis
   3. Siderosis
   4. Extrinsic allergic alveolitis (chronic phase)

(b) Granulomatous disease
   1. Eosinophilic granuloma
   2. Sarcoidosis (with current / previous adenopathy)

(c) Infectious disease
   1. Bacteria: salmonella, nocardiosis
   2. Tuberculosis
   3. Fungus: histoplasmosis, coccidioidomycosis, blastomycosis, aspergillosis (rare), cryptococcosis (rare)
   4. Virus: varicella (more common in adults), Mycoplasma pneumonia

(d) Metastases
   Thyroid carcinoma, melanoma, adenocarcinoma of breast, stomach, colon, pancreas

(e) Alveolar microlithiasis (rare)

(f) Bronchiolitis obliterans

(g) Gaucher disease

mnemonic: "TEMPEST"

Tuberculosis + fungal disease
Eosinophilic granuloma
Metastases (thyroid, lymphangitic carcinomatosis)
Pneumoconiosis, Parasites
Embolism of oily contrast
Sarcoidosis
Tuberous sclerosis

FINE NODULAR DISEASE IN AFEBRILE PATIENT

1. Inhalational disease
2. Eosinophilic granuloma
3. Sarcoidosis
4. Metastases
5. Fungal infection (late stage)
6. Miliary tuberculosis (rare)

FINE NODULAR DISEASE IN FEBRILE PATIENT

1. Tuberculosis
2. Fungal infection (early stage)
3. Pneumocystis
4. Viral pneumonia

End-stage Lung Disease

= evidence of honeycombing / cystic change / conglomerate fibrosis

A. DISTRIBUTION
   1. Usual interstitial pneumonia
      √ subpleural distribution + lower lobe predominance
   2. Asbestosis
      √ subpleural distribution + lower lobe predominance + pleural thickening
   3. Sarcoidosis
      √ subpleural honeycombing
      √ central cystic bronchiectasis
      √ conglomerate fibrosis
      √ peribronchovascular distribution
      √ upper lobe predominance
   4. Extrinsic allergic alveolitis
      √ diffuse random distribution + patchy areas of ground-glass attenuation

B. CYSTIC SPACES WITH WELL-DEFINED WALLS
   1. Langerhans cell histiocytosis
      √ upper lobe predominance
   2. Lymphangioleiomyomatosis
      √ no zonal predominance

C. CONGLOMERATE FIBROTIC MASSES
   1. Sarcoidosis
      √ peribronchovascular distribution
   2. Silicosis
      √ bronchi splayed around masses
   3. Talcosis
      √ areas of high attenuation (= talc deposits)

Honeycomb Lung

mnemonic: "SHIPS BOATS"

Sarcoidosis
Histiocytosis X
Idiopathic (UIP)
Pneumoconiosis
Scleroderma
Bleomycin, **B**usulfan
Oxygen toxicity
Arthritis (rheumatoid), **A**myloidosis, **A**llergic alveolitis
Tuberous sclerosis, **TB**
Storage disease (Gaucher)

PULMONARY NODULE / MASS

Solitary Nodule / Mass

Definition: any pulmonary / pleural sharply defined discrete nearly circular opacity

2–30 mm in diameter = nodule
>30 mm in diameter = mass (>90% prevalence of malignancy)

Incidence: 150,000 annually in USA
(a) roentgenographic survey of low-risk population: <5% of nodules are cancerous
(b) on surgical resection: 40% malignant tumors, 40% granulomas

A. INFLAMMATION / INFECTION
(a) infectious
1. Granuloma (most common lung mass): sarcoidosis (1/3), tuberculosis, histoplasmosis, coccidioidomycosis, nocardiosis, cryptococcosis, talc, Dirofilaria immitis (dog heartworm), gumma, atypical measles infection
2. Fluid-filled cavity: abscess, hydatid cyst, bronchiectatic cyst, bronchocele
3. Mass in preformed cavity: fungus ball, mucoid impaction
4. Rounded atelectasis
5. Inflammatory pseudotumor: fibroxanthoma, histiocytoma, plasma cell granuloma, sclerosing hemangioma
6. Paraffinoma = lipoid granuloma
7. Focal organizing pneumonia
8. Round pneumonia
(b) noninfectious
1. Rheumatoid arthritis
2. Wegener granulomatosis

B. MALIGNANT TUMORS (30–40%)
◊ A solitary pulmonary nodule is the initial radiographic finding in 20–30% of patients with lung cancer!
(a) Malignant primaries of lung
1. Bronchogenic carcinoma (66%, 2nd most common mass)
2. Primary pulmonary lymphoma
3. Primary sarcoma of lung
4. Plasmacytoma (primary / secondary)
5. Clear cell carcinoma, carcinoid, giant cell ca.
(b) Metastases (4th most common cause)
<u>in adults:</u> kidney, colon, ovary, testes
<u>in children:</u> Wilms tumor, osteogenic sarcoma, Ewing sarcoma, rhabdomyosarcoma

C. BENIGN TUMORS
(a) lung tissue : hamartoma (6%, 3rd most common lung mass), chondroma
(b) fat tissue : lipoma (usually pleural lesion)
(c) fibrous tissue : fibroma
(d) muscle tissue : leiomyoma
(e) neural tissue : schwannoma, neurofibroma, paraganglioma
(f) lymph tissue : intrapulmonary lymph node
(g) deposits : amyloid, splenosis, endometrioma, extramedullary hematopoiesis

D. VASCULAR
1. Arteriovenous malformation (AVM), hemangioma
2. Hematoma
3. Organizing infarct
4. Pulmonary venous varix
5. Pseudoaneurysm of pulmonary artery

E. DEVELOPMENTAL / CONGENITAL
1. Bronchogenic cyst (fluid-filled)
2. Pulmonary sequestration
3. Bronchial atresia

F. INHALATIONAL
1. Silicosis (conglomerate mass)
2. Mucoid impaction (allergic aspergillosis)

G. MIMICKING DENSITIES (20%)
(a) Pseudotumor
1. Fluid in fissure
2. Composite area of increased opacity
(b) Mediastinal mass
(c) Chest wall lesion
1. Nipple
2. Skin tumor: mole, neurofibroma, lipoma, keloid
3. Bone island, rib osteochondroma
4. Rib fracture / osteophyte
5. Pleural plaque / mass (mesothelioma)
(d) External object
1. Electrocardiographic lead attachment
2. Buttons, snaps

mnemonic: "**B**ig **S**olitary **P**ulmonary **M**asses **C**ommonly **A**ppear **H**opeless **A**nd **L**onely"
Bronchogenic carcinoma
Solitary metastasis, **S**equestration
Pseudotumor
Mesothelioma
Cyst (bronchogenic, neurenteric, echinococcal)
Adenoma, **A**rteriovenous malformation
Hamartoma, **H**istoplasmosis
Abscess, **A**ctinomycosis
Lymphoma

Morphologic Evaluation of Solitary Pulmonary Nodule

A. SIZE
◊ The smaller the nodule the more likely it is benign!
√ <20 mm nodule: in 80% benign
√ >30 mm nodule: likely malignant
N.B.: √ 15% of malignant nodules are <10 mm
√ 42% of malignant nodules are <20 mm
√ nodule >3 cm is suspect for malignancy

B. MARGIN / EDGE
√ smooth well-defined margin = likely benign
◊ Mostly benign, in 21% malignant
√ corona radiata = irregular spiculated margin
◊ In 89% malignant, in 55% benign
√ pleural tag
◊ In 25% malignant, in 9% benign

C. CONTOUR
√ sharply marginated lesions are benign in 79%
√ lobulated nodule implies
(a) organizing mass
(b) tumor with multiple cell types growing at different rates (malignancy, hamartoma)
◊ A lobulated contour frequently implies malignancy!

CHEST

◊ Lobulated growth occurs in 25% of benign nodules

√ vessel leading to mass: pulmonary varix, AVM

D. INTERNAL ATTENUATION

√ homogeneous attenuation in 55% of benign + 20% of malignant nodules

√ pseudocavitation (= small focal hypodense region) with air bronchogram suggest bronchioloalveolar cell carcinoma / lymphoma / resolving pneumonia

◊ Air bronchogram in <2 cm nodules: in 65% malignant, in 5% benign

√ bubblelike areas of low attenuation: bronchioloalveolar cell carcinoma (in 50%)

E. CAVITATION

√ a thin (≤4 mm) smooth wall is benign in 94%

√ a thick (>16 mm) irregular wall suggests a malignant nodule

F. INTRANODULAR FAT (–40 to –120 HU)

◊ Fat is a reliable indicator of a hamartoma!

√ fat density in up to 50% of hamartomas

G. INTRANODULAR CALCIUM

◊ HRCT is 10–20 times more sensitive than CXR!

√ >200 HU at CT densitometry indicates calcification within a nodule (66% sensitive, 98% specific for benign disease)

◊ 38–63% of benign nodules are not calcified!

√ diffuse amorphous, rarely punctate = malignant pattern

√ central, completely solid, laminated: granuloma of prior infection (TB / histoplasmosis)

√ popcornlike = chondroid calcification in a hamartoma in 5–50%

√ peripheral calcification: granuloma, tumor

Calcifying malignant lung tumors:
carcinoid (up to 33%), lung cancer (up to 6%), osteosarcoma, chondrosarcoma, metastatic mucinous adenocarcinoma

H. SATELLITE LESION

= nodule(s) in association with larger peripheral nodule

— in 99% due to inflammatory disease (often TB)

— in 1% due to primary lung cancer

Growth Rate Assessment of Indeterminate Solitary Pulmonary Nodule

= comparing size of nodule on current image with that on prior image

Best method:
early repeat HRCT (resolution in x and y planes of 0.3 mm) in 1–4 weeks for nodules >5 mm measuring volume / area / diameter of nodule

Doubling time (= time required to double in volume):

(a) for most malignant nodules: 30–400 days
= 26% increase in diameter
≈ 30 days: aggressive small cell cancer
≈ 90 days: squamous cell carcinoma
≈ 120 days: large cell carcinoma
≈ 150 days: aggressive adenocarcinoma
≈ 180 days: average adenocarcinoma

(b) for benign nodules: <30 and > 400 days
◊ Absence of growth over a 2-year period implies a doubling time of >730 days

Disadvantage:

(1) only 65% positive predictive value
— very slow growth:
hamartoma, bronchial carcinoid, inflammatory pseudotumor, granuloma, low-grade adenocarcinoma, metastases from renal cell carcinoma
— very rapid growth:
osteosarcoma, choriocarcinoma, testicular neoplasm, organizing infectious process, infarct (thromboembolism, Wegener granulomatosis)

(2) unreliable growth perception in nodules <10 mm: eg, a nodule with a doubling time of 6 months increases its diameter from 5 mm to only 6.25 mm remaining radiologically stable
better: volumetric growth assessment

√ decrease in size with time: benign lesion

◊ Bronchogenic carcinoma may show temporary decrease in size due to infarction - necrosis - fibrosis - retraction sequence!

CHEST

Clinical Assessment of Indeterminate Solitary Pulmonary Nodule

by patient age (prevalence of cancer <30 years is low), history of prior malignancy, presenting symptoms, smoking history

Management Strategies of Indeterminate Solitary Pulmonary Nodule

A. Bayesian Analysis

Likelihood ratio (LR) = probability of malignancy
= LR of 1.0 means a 50% chance of malignancy

Characteristic / Feature	Likelihood Ratio
spiculated margin	5.54
size >3 cm	5.23
>70 years of age	4.16
malignant growth rate	3.40
smoker	2.27
upper lobe location	1.22
size <10 mm	0.52
smooth margin	0.30
30–39 years of age	0.24
never smoked	0.19
20–29 years of age	0.05
benign calcification	0.01
benign growth rate	0.01

Odds of malignancy ($Odds_{ca}$) = sum of LR of radiologic features or patient characteristics

Probability of malignancy (pCa) = $Odds_{ca}$ / (1 + $Odds_{ca}$)

B. Decision Analysis
= cost-effective strategy for management decision determined by pCa

pCa <0.05 observation
pCa >0.05 and <0.6 biopsy
pCa ≥0.60 immediate surgical resection

C. Contrast-enhanced Thin-section CT
= degree of enhancement directly related to vascularity + likelihood of malignancy
• 300 mg/mL iodine at 2 mL/sec; total dose 420 mg/kg
• contiguous sections obtained every 30 seconds for 5 minutes
√ nodule enhancement of
(a) <15 HU suggests benign lesion
(b) >20 HU indicates malignancy
(98% sensitive, 73% specific, 85% accurate)

D. FDG Positron Emission Tomography
= increased glucose metabolism in tumors resulting in increased accumulation (= uptake and trapping of FDG-6-phosphate)
√ no uptake = benign nodule (92–100% sensitive, 52–100% specific, 94% accurate)
FN: carcinoid tumor, bronchioloalveolar carcinoma; malignant lesion <10 mm
Probability of malignancy: <5%
Precaution: radiographic follow-up at 3-month intervals
FP: active TB, histoplasmosis, rheumatoid nodule

E. Transthoracic Needle Aspiration Biopsy
95–100% sensitive for 10–15-mm malignancies; up to 91% sensitive for establishing a benign diagnosis
Cx: pneumothorax (5–30%) with chest tube placement in 15%; self-limiting hemorrhage

Benign Lung Tumor

A. CENTRAL LOCATION
1. Bronchial polyp
2. Bronchial papilloma
3. **Granular cell myoblastoma**
= cell of origin from neural crest
Age: middle-aged, esp. Black women
√ endobronchial lesion in major bronchi

B. PERIPHERAL LOCATION
1. Hamartoma
2. Leiomyoma
benign metastasizing leiomyoma, history of hysterectomy
3. Amyloid tumor
not associated with amyloid of other organs / rheumatoid arthritis / myeloma
4. Intrapulmonary lymph node
5. Arteriovenous malformation
6. Endometrioma, fibroma, neural tumor, chemodectoma

C. CENTRAL / PERIPHERAL
1. Lipoma:
(a) subpleural
(b) endobronchial

D. PSEUDOTUMOR
1. Fibroxanthoma / xanthogranuloma
2. Plasma cell granuloma
3. Sclerosing hemangioma
middle-aged woman, RML / RLL (most commonly), may be multiple
4. Pseudolymphoma
5. Round atelectasis
6. Pleural pseudotumor = accumulation of pleural fluid within interlobar fissure

Lung Tumor in Childhood

1. Metastatic (common)
2. Blastoma
3. Mucoepidermoid carcinoma
4. Bronchogenic carcinoma
5. Hemangiopericytoma
6. Rhabdomyosarcoma

Large Pulmonary Mass

mnemonic: "CAT PIES"
Carcinoma (large cell, squamous cell, cannon ball metastasis
Abscess
Toruloma (Cryptococcus)
Pseudotumor, **P**lasmacytoma
Inflammatory
Echinococcal disease
Sarcoma, **S**equestration

Cavitating Lung Nodule

A. NEOPLASM
(a) Lung primary:
1. Squamous cell carcinoma (10%)
2. Adenocarcinoma (9.5%)
3. Bronchioloalveolar carcinoma (rare)
4. Hodgkin disease (rare)

(b) Metastases (4% cavitate):
1. Squamous cell carcinoma (2/3)
nasopharynx (males), cervix (females), esophagus
2. Adenocarcinoma (colorectal)
3. Sarcoma: Ewing sarcoma, osteo-, myxo-, angiosarcoma
4. Melanoma
5. Seminoma, teratocarcinoma
6. Wilms tumor

B. COLLAGEN-VASCULAR DISEASE
1. Pulmonary angitis + granulomatosis
– Wegener granulomatosis + Wegener variant
2. Rheumatoid nodules + Caplan syndrome
3. SLE
4. Periarteritis nodosa (rare)

CHEST

C. GRANULOMATOUS DISEASE
   1. Histiocytosis X
   2. Sarcoidosis (rare)
D. VASCULAR DISEASE
   1. Pulmonary embolus with infarction
   2. Septic emboli (Staphylococcus aureus)
E. INFECTION
   1. Bacterial: pneumatoceles from staphylococcal / Gram-negative pneumonia
   2. Mycobacterial: TB
   3. Fungal: nocardiosis, cryptococcosis, coccidioidomycosis (in 10%), aspergillosis
   4. Parasitic: echinococcosis (multiple in 20–30%), paragonimiasis
F. TRAUMA
   1. Traumatic lung cyst (after hemorrhage)
   2. Hydrocarbon ingestion (lower lobes)
G. BRONCHOPULMONARY DISEASE
   1. Infected bulla
   2. Cystic bronchiectasis
   3. Communicating bronchogenic cyst

mnemonic: "CAVITY"
- **C**arcinoma (squamous cell), **C**ystic bronchiectasis
- **A**utoimmune disease (Wegener granulomatosis, rheumatoid lung)
- **V**ascular (bland / septic emboli)
- **I**nfection (abscess, fungal disease, TB, Echinococcus)
- **T**rauma
- **Y**oung = congenital (sequestration, diaphragmatic hernia, bronchogenic cyst)

Pulmonary Mass with Air Bronchogram
1. Bronchioloalveolar carcinoma
2. Lymphoma
3. Pseudolymphoma
4. Kaposi sarcoma
5. Blastomycosis

Air-crescent Sign
= air in a crescentic shape separating the outer wall of a nodule / mass from an inner sequestrum

A. INFECTION
   1. Invasive pulmonary aspergillosis
   2. Noninvasive mycetoma
   3. Echinococcal lung cyst
   4. Tuberculoma
   5. Rasmussen aneurysms (most are too small to be identified on CXR)
   6. Bacterial lung abscess ± pulmonary gangrene
B. CAVITATING NEOPLASM
   1. Primary / metastatic carcinoma / sarcoma
   2. Bronchial adenoma
   3. Cystic hamartoma
C. TRAUMA
   1. Pulmonary hematoma
D. THROMBOEMBOLISM

Shaggy Pulmonary Nodule
mnemonic: "**S**haggy **S**ue **M**ade **L**oving **A** **R**eally **W**ild **F**antasy **T**oday"
- **S**arcoidosis, alveolar type
- **S**eptic emboli
- **M**etastasis
- **L**ymphoma, **L**ung primary, **L**ymphomatoid granulomatosis
- **A**lveolar cell carcinoma
- **R**heumatoid lung
- **W**egener granulomatosis
- **F**ungus
- **T**uberculosis

Hemorrhagic Pulmonary Nodule
√ CT halo sign = central area of soft-tissue attenuation surrounded by a halo of ground-glass attenuation

Causes:

A. HEMORRHAGIC INFARCTION
   1. Early invasive aspergillosis
   2. Mucormycosis
   3. Hematogenous candidiasis
   4. Herpes simplex, CMV, varicella-zoster virus
B. VASCULITIS
   1. Wegener granulomatosis
C. FRAGILITY OF NEOVASCULAR TISSUE
   1. Metastatic angiosarcoma
   2. Metastatic choriocarcinoma
   3. Bronchioloalveolar carcinoma
   4. Lymphoma
   5. Kaposi sarcoma
D. BRONCHOARTERIAL FISTULA
   1. Coccidioidomycosis
   2. Tuberculoma associated with hemoptysis
E. TRAUMA
   1. Following lung biopsy

Multiple Pulmonary Nodules and Masses
√ homogeneous masses with sharp border
√ no air alveolo- / bronchogram

A. TUMORS
   (a) malignant
      1. Metastases: from breast, kidney, GI tract, uterus, ovary, testes, malignant melanoma, sarcoma, Wilms tumor
      2. Lymphoma (rare)
      3. Multiple primary bronchogenic carcinomas (synchronous in 1% of all lung cancers)
   (b) benign
      1. Hamartoma (rarely multiple)
      2. Benign metastasizing leiomyoma
      3. AV malformations
      4. Amyloidosis
B. VASCULAR LESIONS
   1. Thromboemboli with organizing infarcts
   2. Septic emboli with organized infarcts
C. COLLAGEN-VASCULAR DISEASE
   1. Wegener granulomatosis: vasculitis with organizing infarcts

2. Wegener variants
3. Rheumatoid nodules: tendency for periphery, occasionally cavitating

D. INFLAMMATORY GRANULOMAS
1. Fungal: coccidioidomycosis, histoplasmosis, cryptococcosis
2. Bacterial: nocardiosis, tuberculosis
3. Viral: atypical measles
4. Parasites: hydatid cysts, paragonimiasis
5. Sarcoidosis: large accumulation of interstitial granulomas
6. Inflammatory pseudotumors: fibrous histiocytoma, plasma cell granuloma, hyalinizing pulmonary nodules, pseudolymphoma

mnemonic: "SLAM DA PIG"
Sarcoidosis
Lymphoma
Alveolar proteinosis
Metastases
Drugs
Alveolar cell carcinoma
Pneumonias
Infarcts
Goodpasture syndrome

Multiple Cavitating Nodules / Masses

A. PULMONARY VASCULITIS
1. Wegener granulomatosis
2. Necrotizing sarcoid granulomatosis
3. Bronchocentric granulomatosis

B. METASTATIC DISEASE
particularly squamous histologic type

C. MULTIFOCAL INFECTION
1. Pseudomonas
2. Tuberculosis
3. Septic abscesses

D. MULTIPLE PULMONARY INFARCTS

E. BRONCHIECTASIS

F. NEOPLASMS
1. Lymphoma
2. Multicentric bronchioalveolar carcinoma

G. COLLAGEN-VASCULAR DISEASE
1. Rheumatoid nodules

H. GRANULOMATOUS DISEASE
1. Cystic form of sarcoidosis
2. Langerhans cell histiocytosis

Small Pulmonary Nodules

mnemonic: "MALTS"
Metastases (esp. thyroid)
Alveolar cell carcinoma
Lymphoma, **L**eukemia
TB
Sarcoid

Pulmonary Nodules & Pneumothorax

1. Osteosarcoma
2. Wilms tumor
3. Histiocytosis

Pleura-based Lung Nodule

√ ill-defined / sharply defined lesion mimicking a true pleural mass
√ associated linear densities in lung parenchyma

Cause:
1. Granuloma (fungus, tuberculosis)
2. Inflammatory pseudotumor
3. Metastasis
4. Rheumatoid nodule
5. Pancoast tumor
6. Lymphoma
7. Infarct: Hampton hump
8. Atelectatic pseudotumor

Intrathoracic Mass of Low Attenuation

A. CYSTS
1. Bronchogenic / neurenteric / pericardial cyst
2. Hydatid disease

B. FATTY SUBSTRATE
1. Hamartoma
2. Lipoma
3. Tuberculous lymph node
4. Lymphadenopathy in Whipple disease

C. NECROTIC MASSES
1. Resolving hematoma
2. Treated lymphoma
3. Metastases from ovary, stomach, testes

PNEUMOCONIOSIS

= tissue reaction to the presence of an accumulation of dust in the lungs

Path: 1. Fibrosis
(a) focal / nodular (silicosis)
(b) diffuse fibrosis (asbestosis)
2. Aggregates of particle-laden macrophages in inert dusts (iron, tin, barium)

Types:
1. Silicosis
2. Coal worker pneumoconiosis
3. Siderosis
4. Carbon black pneumoconiosis
= burning of natural gas + petroleum products (filler in rubber, plastics, phonograph records, inks, carbon paper, carbon electrodes)
√ fine reticulonodular pattern with lower zone predominance
5. Hard metal pneumoconiosis
= alloy of tungsten, carbon and cobalt (occasionally adding titanium, tantalum, nickel, chromium)
√ giant cell interstitial pneumonia, desquamative interstitial pneumonia, interstitial pneumonia
6. Asbestos-related disease

Pneumoconiosis Classification

according to ILO (International Labour Office)

A. TYPE OF OPACITIES
1. Silicosis, coal worker's pneumoconiosis
<u>nodular opacities</u>:
p = <1.5 mm

q = 1.5–3 mm
r = 3–10 mm

2.. Asbestosis
<u>linear opacities</u>:
s = fine
t = medium
u = coarse / blotchy

B. PROFUSION / SEVERITY
0 = normal
1 = slight
2 = moderate
3 = advanced
intermediate grading:
2/2 = definitely moderate profusion
2/3 = moderate, possibly advanced profusion

Pneumoconiosis with Mass

Anthracosilicosis with:

1. Granuloma (histoplasmosis, TB, sarcoidosis)
2. Bronchogenic carcinoma (incidence same as in general population)
3. Metastasis
4. Progressive massive fibrosis
5. Caplan syndrome (rheumatoid nodules)

PULMONARY CALCIFICATIONS

Multiple Pulmonary Calcifications

A. INFECTION
1. Histoplasmosis
2. Tuberculosis
3. Chickenpox pneumonia

B. INHALATIONAL DISEASE
1. Silicosis

C. MISCELLANEOUS
1. Hypercalcemia
2. Mitral stenosis
3. Alveolar microlithiasis

Calcified Pulmonary Nodules

mnemonic: "**HAM TV S**tation"
Histoplasmosis, **H**amartoma
Amyloid, **A**lveolar microlithiasis
Mitral stenosis, **M**etastasis (thyroid, osteosarcoma, mucinous carcinoma)
Tuberculosis
Varicella
Silicosis
◊ Central / laminated / popcorn / diffuse calcifications are characteristic of benign solitary lung nodules!

DENSE LUNG LESIONS

Ground-glass Attenuation

1. Desquamative interstitial pneumonia
2. Extrinsic allergic alveolitis
3. Sarcoidosis
4. Usual interstitial pneumonia
5. Alveolar proteinosis
6. Cryptogenic organizing pneumonia

Focal Area of Ground-glass Attenuation

1. Bronchioloalveolar cell carcinoma
2. Pulmonary infiltrate with eosinophilia syndrome
   (a) simple pulmonary eosinophilia
   (b) idiopathic hypereosinophilic syndrome
   (c) parasitic infection
3. Lymphoma
4. Hemorrhagic nodule

Opacification of Hemithorax

mnemonic: "FAT CHANCE"
Fibrothorax
Adenomatoid malformation
Trauma (ie, hematoma)
Collapse, **C**ardiomegaly
Hernia
Agenesis of lung
Neoplasm (ie, mesothelioma)
Consolidation
Effusion

CHEST

Atelectasis

Cause:

A. TUMOR
1. Bronchogenic carcinoma (2/3 of squamous cell carcinoma occur as endobronchial mass with persistent / recurrent atelectasis or recurrent pneumonia)
2. Bronchial carcinoid
3. Metastases: primary tumor of kidney, colon, rectum, breast, melanoma
4. Lymphoma (usually as a late presentation)
5. Lipoma, granular cell myoblastoma, amyloid tumor, fibroepithelial polyp

B. INFLAMMATION
1. Tuberculosis (endobronchial granuloma, broncholith, bronchial stenosis)
2. Right middle lobe syndrome (chronic right middle lobe atelectasis)
3. Sarcoidosis (endobronchial granuloma — rare)

C. MUCUS PLUG
1. Severe chest / abdominal pain (postoperative patient)
2. Respiratory depressant drug (morphine; CNS illness)
3. Chronic bronchitis / bronchiolitis obliterans
4. Asthma
5. Cystic fibrosis
6. Bronchopneumonia (peribronchial inflammation)

D. OTHER
1. Large left atrium (mitral stenosis + left lower lobe atelectasis)
2. Foreign body (aspiration of food, endotracheal intubation)
3. Broncholithiasis
4. Amyloidosis
5. Wegener granulomatosis
6. Bronchial transection

√ local increase in lung density
√ crowding of pulmonary vessels
√ bronchial rearrangement
√ displacement of fissures
√ displacement of hilus
√ mediastinal shift
√ elevation of hemidiaphragm
√ cardiac rotation
√ approximation of ribs
√ compensatory overinflation of normal lung

Types:

A. OBSTRUCTIVE ATELECTASIS

Resorptive Atelectasis

Pathophysiology:
sum of partial gas pressures in venous blood perfusing atelectatic region is less than atmospheric pressure, which is responsible for gradual resorption of air trapped distal to site of obstruction; continuing secretion into small airways leads to consolidation (postobstructive pneumonitis / bacterial infection)

Cause: bronchiolar obstruction by
1. Tumor
2. Stricture
3. Foreign body
4. Mucus plug
5. Bronchial rupture

• airless collapse within minutes to hours

MR:
√ high signal intensity on T2WI in atelectatic area

B. NONOBSTRUCTIVE ATELECTASIS

Pathophysiology:
pathway between bronchial system + alveoli is maintained because bronchi are less compliant than lung parenchyma + remain patent; secretions can be eliminated + convective airflow to distal bronchioles remains

• collapsed lung not completely airless (up to 40% residual air)

MR:
√ low-signal intensity on T2WI in atelectatic area

Passive Atelectasis

= pleural space-occupying process
1. Pneumothorax
2. Hydrothorax / hemothorax
3. Diaphragmatic hernia
4. Pleural masses: metastases, mesothelioma

Adhesive Atelectasis

= decrease in surfactant production
1. Respiratory distress syndrome of the newborn (hyaline membrane disease)
2. Pulmonary embolism: edema, hemorrhage, atelectasis
3. Intravenous injection of hydrocarbon

Cicatrizing Atelectasis

= parenchymal fibrosis causing decreased lung volume
1. Tuberculosis / histoplasmosis (upper lobes)
2. Silicosis (upper lobes)
3. Scleroderma (lower lobes)
4. Radiation pneumonitis (nonanatomical distribution)
5. Idiopathic pulmonary fibrosis

Discoid Atelectasis

mnemonic: "EPIC"
Embolus
Pneumonia
Inadequate inspiration
Carcinoma, obstructing

Rounded Atelectasis

Cause: any type of pleural inflammatory reaction (asbestos as leading cause)

Pathomechanism:
thickening of visceral pleura with progressive wrinkling + folding of subpleural lung

Location: posterobasal subpleural
√ round / lentiform mass incompletely surrounded by lung
√ increased attenuation in periphery of mass
√ pleural thickening n vicinity of mass
√ curving of vessels + bronchi toward mass
√ air bronchogram within mass
√ lesion may be stable / enlarge

Left Upper Lobe Collapse

PA view:
√ Luftsichel sign = sharply marginated paraaortic crescent of hyperlucency (= hyperexpanded superior segment of LLL extending toward lung apex + between aortic arch and atelectatic LUL)
√ hazy opacification of left hilum + cardiac border
√ elevation of left hilum
√ near horizontal course of left main bronchus
√ posterior + leftward rotation of heart

Lateral view:
√ retrosternal opacity
√ major fissure displaced anteriorly paralleling anterior chest wall

DDx: (1) Herniation of right lung across midline (leftward displacement of anterior junction line)
(2) Medial pneumothorax

Multifocal Ill-defined Densities

= densities 5–30 mm resulting in airspace filling

A. INFECTION
1. Bacterial bronchopneumonia
2. Fungal pneumonia: histoplasmosis, blastomycosis, actinomycosis, coccidioidomycosis, aspergillosis, cryptococcosis, mucormycosis, sporotrichosis
3. Viral pneumonia

4. Tuberculosis (primary infection)
5. Rocky Mountain spotted fever
6. Pneumocystis carinii

B. GRANULOMATOUS DISEASE
1. Sarcoidosis (alveolar form secondary to peribronchial granulomas)
2. Eosinophilic granuloma

C. VASCULAR
(a) thromboembolic disease
(b) septic emboli
(c) vasculitis
1. Wegener granulomatosis
2. Wegener variants: limited Wegener, lymphomatoid granulomatosis
3. Infectious vasculitis = invasion of pulmonary arteries: mucormycosis, invasive form of aspergillosis, Rocky Mountain spotted fever
4. Goodpasture syndrome
5. Scleroderma

D. NEOPLASTIC
1. Bronchioloalveolar cell carcinoma
= only primary lung tumor to produce multifocal ill-defined densities with air bronchograms
2. Alveolar type of lymphoma
= massive accumulation of tumor cells in interstitium with compression atelectasis + obstructive pneumonia
3. Metastases
(a) Choriocarcinoma: hemorrhage (however rare)
(b) Vascular tumors: malignant hemangiomas
4. Waldenström macroglobulinemia
5. Angioblastic lymphadenopathy
6. Mycosis fungoides
7. Amyloid tumor

E. IDIOPATHIC INTERSTITIAL DISEASE
1. Lymphocytic interstitial pneumonitis (LIP)
2. Desquamative interstitial pneumonitis (DIP)
3. Pseudolymphoma = localized form of LIP
4. Usual interstitial pneumonitis (UIP)

F. INHALATIONAL DISEASE
1. Allergic alveolitis: acute stage (eg, farmer's lung)
2. Silicosis
3. Eosinophilic pneumonia

G. DRUG REACTIONS

Diffuse Infiltrates in Immunocompromised Cancer Patient

mnemonic: "FOLD"

Failure (CHF)
Opportunistic infection
Lymphangitic tumor spread
Drug reaction

Segmental & Lobar Densities

A. PNEUMONIA
1. Lobar pneumonia
2. Lobular pneumonia
3. Acute interstitial pneumonia
4. Aspiration pneumonia
5. Primary tuberculosis

B. PULMONARY EMBOLISM
(rarely multiple / larger than subsegmental)

C. NEOPLASM
1. Obstructive pneumonia
2. Bronchioloalveolar cell carcinoma

D. ATELECTASIS

Chronic Infiltrates

Chronic Infiltrates in Childhood

mnemonic: "ABC'S"

Asthma, **A**gammaglobulinemia, **A**spiration
Bronchiectasis
Cystic fibrosis
Sequestration, intralobar

Chronic Multifocal Ill-defined Opacities

1. Organizing pneumonia
2. Granulomatous disease
3. Allergic alveolitis
4. Bronchioloalveolar cell carcinoma
5. Lymphoma

Chronic Diffuse Confluent Opacities

1. Alveolar proteinosis
2. Hemosiderosis
3. Sarcoidosis

Ill-defined Opacities with Holes

A. INFECTION
1. Necrotizing pneumonias:
Staphylococcus aureus, ß-hemolytic streptococcus, Klebsiella pneumoniae, E. coli, Proteus, Pseudomonas, anaerobes
2. Aspiration pneumonia:
mixed Gram-negative organisms
3. Septic emboli
4. Fungus:
histoplasmosis, blastomycosis, coccidioidomycosis, cryptococcosis
5. Tuberculosis

B. NEOPLASM
1. Primary lung carcinoma
2. Lymphoma (cavitates very rarely)

C. VASCULAR + COLLAGEN-VASCULAR DISEASE
1. Emboli with infarction
2. Wegener granulomatosis
3. Necrobiotic rheumatoid nodules

D. TRAUMA
1. Contusion with pneumatoceles

Recurrent Fleeting Infiltrates

1. Löffler disease
2. Bronchopulmonary aspergillosis / bronchocentric granulomatosis
3. Asthma
4. Subacute bacterial endocarditis with pulmonary emboli

Tubular Density

A. Mucoid impaction
B. Vascular malformation
   1. Arteriovenous malformation
   2. Pulmonary varix

Perihilar "Bat-wing" Infiltrates

mnemonic: "**P**lease, **P**lease, **P**lease, **S**tudy **L**ight, **D**on't **G**et **A**ll **U**ptight"

Pulmonary edema
Proteinosis
Periarteritis
Sarcoidosis
Lymphoma
Drugs
Goodpasture syndrome
Alveolar cell carcinoma
Uremia

Peripheral "Reverse Bat-wing" Infiltrates

mnemonic: "REDS"

Resolving pulmonary edema
Eosinophilic pneumonia
Desquamative interstitial pneumonia
Sarcoidosis

LUCENT LUNG LESIONS

Pulmonary Oligemia

Generalized Oligemia

= reduction in pulmonary blood volume

1. Aortic valve disease
   indicative of markedly diminished stroke volume + cardiac output
   √ LV enlargement
2. Overpenetration of film = artifact
3. Deep inspiration + Valsalva maneuver
4. Positive pressure ventilation

Regional Oligemia

A. DECREASE IN BLOOD VOLUME
   1. Pulmonary arterial hypoplasia
   2. Mitral valve disease
   3. Pulmonary embolism
   4. Flow inversion (= oligemic bases + hyperemic upper lobes in longstanding elevation of left heart pressure)
B. INCREASE IN AIR SPACES
   1. Swyer-James syndrome
   2. Regional emphysema
   3. Valvular air trapping

Hyperlucent Lung

Bilateral Hyperlucent Lung

A. FAULTY RADIOLOGIC TECHNIQUE
   1. Overpenetrated film
B. DECREASED SOFT TISSUES
   1. Thin body habitus
   2. Bilateral mastectomy
C. CARDIAC CAUSE of decreased pulmonary blood flow
   1. Right-to-left shunt:
      Tetralogy of Fallot (small proximal pulmonary vessels), pseudotruncus, truncus type IV, Ebstein malformation, tricuspid atresia
   2. Eisenmenger physiology of left-to-right shunt:
      ASD, VSD, PDA (dilated proximal pulmonary vessels)
D. PULMONARY CAUSE of decreased pulmonary blood flow
   (a) Decrease of vascular bed:
      1. Pulmonary embolism
         bilaterality is rare; localized areas of hyperlucency (Westermark sign)
   (b) Increase in air space:
      1. Air trapping (reversible changes):
         acute asthmatic attack, acute bronchiolitis (pediatric patient)
      2. Emphysema
      3. Bulla
      4. Bleb
      5. Interstitial emphysema

Unilateral Hyperlucent Lung

A. FAULTY RADIOLOGIC TECHNIQUE
   1. Rotation of patient
B. CHEST WALL DEFECT
   1. Mastectomy
   2. Absent pectoralis muscle (Poland syndrome)
C. INCREASED PULMONARY AIR SPACE with decreased pulmonary blood flow
   (a) Large airway obstruction with air trapping
      @ Bronchial compression:
        hilar mass (rare), cardiomegaly compressing LLL bronchus
      @ Endobronchial obstruction with air trapping (collateral air drift):
        foreign body, broncholith, bronchogenic carcinoma, carcinoid, bronchial mucocele
   (b) Small airway obstruction
      1. Bronchiolitis obliterans
      2. Swyer-James / Macleod syndrome
      3. Emphysema (particularly bullous emphysema)
      4. Emphysema + unilateral lung transplant
   (c) Pneumothorax (in supine patient)
D. PULMONARY VASCULAR CAUSE of decreased pulmonary blood flow
   1. Pulmonary artery hypoplasia
   2. Pulmonary embolism
   3. Congenital lobar emphysema
   4. Compensatory overaeration

Localized Lucent Lung Defect

A. CAVITY = tissue necrosis with bronchial drainage
   (a) Infection
      BACTERIAL PNEUMONIA
      1. Pyogenic infection = abscess = necrotizing pneumonia:

Staphylococcus, Klebsiella, Pseudomonas, anaerobes, β-hemolytic streptococcus, E. coli, mixed Gram-negative organisms
2. Aspiration pneumonia = gravitational pneumonia:
mixed Gram-negative organisms, anaerobes

GRANULOMATOUS INFECTION
1. Tuberculosis
cavitation indicates active infectious disease with risk for hematogenous / bronchogenic dissemination
2. Fungal infection:
nocardiosis (in immunocompromised), coccidioidomycosis (any lobe, desert Southwest), histoplasmosis, blastomycosis, mucormycosis, sporotrichosis, aspergillosis, cryptococcosis
√ very thin-walled cavities less likely to follow apical distribution of TB / histoplasmosis
3. Sarcoidosis (stage IV, upper lobe predominance)
4. Angioinvasive organism (septic lung infarction followed by cavity formation): Aspergillus, Mucorales, Candida, Torulosis, P. aeruginosa

PARASITIC INFESTATION: hydatid disease

(b) Neoplasm
PRIMARY LUNG TUMOR: 16% of peripheral lung cancers (in particular in squamous cell carcinoma (30%); also in bronchioloalveolar cell carcinoma

METASTASIS (usually multiple)
1. Squamous cell carcinoma (nasopharynx, esophagus, cervix) in 2/3
2. Adenocarcinoma (lung, breast, GI)
3. Osteosarcoma (rare)
4. Melanoma
5. Lymphoma (rare): with adenopathy; cavities often secondary to opportunistic infection with nocardiosis + cryptococcosis

(c) Vascular occlusion
1. Infarct (thromboembolic, septic)
2. Wegener granulomatosis
3. Rheumatoid arthritis

(d) Inhalational
1. Silicosis with coal worker's pneumoconiosis
— complicating tuberculosis
— ischemic necrosis of center of conglomerate mass (rare)

B. CYST
(a) Cystic bronchiectasis
1. Cystic fibrosis (more obvious in upper lobes)
2. Agammaglobulinemia (predisposed to recurrent bacterial infections)
3. Recurrent bacterial pneumonias
√ multiple thin-walled lucencies with air-fluid levels in lower lobes
4. Childhood infection: tuberculosis, pertussis
5. Allergic bronchopulmonary aspergillosis (in asthmatic patients)
√ involvement of proximal perihilar bronchi
6. Kartagener syndrome (ciliary dysmotility)

(b) Pneumatocele
1. Postinfectious pneumatocele
2. Traumatic pneumatocele: lung hematoma / hydrocarbon inhalation

(c) Congenital lesion (rare)
1. Multiple bronchogenic cysts
2. Intralobar sequestration: multicystic structure in lower lobes
3. Congenital cystic adenomatoid malformation (CCAM) type I
4. Diaphragmatic hernia (congenital / traumatic)

(d) Centrilobular / bullous emphysema
(e) Honeycomb lung

Multiple Lucent Lung Lesions

for details see causes of localized lucent lung defect

A. CAVITIES
(a) Infection
1. Bacterial pneumonia: cavitating pneumonia, lung abscess
2. Granulomatous infection: TB, sarcoidosis
3. Fungal infection: coccidioidomycosis
4. Parasitic infection: echinococcosis
5. Protozoan infection: pneumocystosis

(b) Neoplasm
(c) Vascular
1. Thromboembolic + septic infarcts
2. Wegener granulomatosis
3. Rheumatoid arthritis
4. Angioinvasive organism (septic lung infarction followed by cavity formation): Aspergillus, Mucorales, Candida, torulosis, P. aeruginosa

B. CYSTS
(a) Cystic bronchiectasis
1. Cystic fibrosis (more obvious in upper lobes)
2. Agammaglobulinemia (predisposed to recurrent bacterial infections)
3. Recurrent bacterial pneumonias
4. Tuberculosis
5. Allergic bronchopulmonary aspergillosis (in asthmatic patients)

(b) Pneumatoceles
(c) Congenital lesions (rare)
1. Multiple bronchogenic cysts
2. Intralobar sequestration:
multicystic structure in lower lobes
3. Congenital cystic adenomatoid malformation (CCAM) type I
4. Diaphragmatic hernia (congenital / traumatic)

(d) Centrilobular / bullous emphysema: blebs, bullae
(e) Tuberous sclerosis + lymphangiomyomatosis

(f) Honeycomb lung
(g) Juvenile pulmonary polyposis

Pulmonary Cyst

= round circumscribed space surrounded by an epithelial / fibrous wall of uniform / varied thickness containing air / liquid / semisolid / solid material

A. CONGENITAL CYST
1. Cystic adenomatoid malformation
2. Congenital lobar emphysema
3. Bronchial atresia
4. Bronchogenic cyst
5. Sequestration

B. ACQUIRED CYST
1. Pneumatocele (traumatic / infectious)
2. Pseudocyst (from interstitial emphysema)
3. Hydatid disease
4. **Bleb** = cystic air collection within visceral pleura; mostly apical with narrow neck; associated with spontaneous pneumothorax
5. **Bulla** = sharply demarcated dilated air space within lung parenchyma >1 cm in diameter with epithelialized wall <1 mm thick due to destruction of alveoli (= air cyst in localized / centrilobular / panlobular emphysema)
   • usually asymptomatic
   √ typically at lung apex
   √ slow progressive enlargement
   Cx: (1) Spontaneous pneumothorax
   (2) "Vanishing lung" = large area of localized emphysema causing atelectasis + dyspnea
   Rx: surgical resection if bulla >33% of hemithorax

Multiple Pulmonary Cysts

A. INFECTION
1. Tuberculosis
2. Pneumocystis carinii pneumonia in AIDS

B. VASCULAR-EMBOLIC
1. Cavitating septic emboli
   √ often seen at end of feeding vessel
2. Angioinvasive infection (invasive pulmonary aspergillosis, candida, P. aeruginosa)
3. Pulmonary vasculitis (Wegener granulomatosis)

C. DILATATION OF BRONCHI = bronchiectasis
   √ bronchial wall thickening

D. DISRUPTION OF ELASTIC FIBER NETWORK
1. Centrilobular emphysema
2. Panlobular emphysema
   √ lobular architecture preserved with bronchovascular bundle in central position, areas of lung destruction without arcuate contour
3. Lymphangiomyomatosis
   √ randomly scattered cysts in otherwise normal lung
4. Tuberous sclerosis
   √ associated skin abnormalities, mental retardation, epilepsy
5. Air-block disease (adult respiratory distress syndrome, asthma, bronchiolitis, viral / bacterial pneumonia)

E. REMODELING OF LUNG ARCHITECTURE
= honeycombing of idiopathic pulmonary fibrosis (= fibrosing alveolitis)
√ 3–10-mm small irregular thick-walled cystic air spaces usually of comparable diameter surrounded by abnormal lung parenchyma
√ predominantly peripheral + basilar distribution

F. MULTIFACTORIAL / UNKNOWN
1. Langerhans cell histiocytosis
   √ cysts with walls of variable thickness
   √ combination of nodules ± cavitation
   √ septal thickening
   √ predominant distribution in upper lung zones
2. Lymphocytic interstitial pneumonia
   √ thickening of interlobular septa + bronchovascular bundles
   √ enlarged mediastinal nodes
3. Klippel-Trenaunay syndrome
4. Juvenile tracheolaryngeal papillomatosis
5. Neurofibromatosis
   √ cystic air spaces predominantly apical

Cystlike Pulmonary Lesions

mnemonic: "C.C., I BAN WHIPS"

Coccidioidomycosis
Cystic adenomatoid malformation
Infection
Bronchogenic cyst, **B**ronchiectasis, **B**owel
Abscess
Neoplasm
Wegener granulomatosis
Hydatid cyst, **H**istiocytosis X
Infarction
Pneumatocele
Sequestration

Multiple Thin-walled Cavities

mnemonic: "BITCH"

Bullae + pneumatoceles
Infection (TB, cocci, staph)
Tumor (squamous cell carcinoma)
Cysts (traumatic, bronchogenic)
Hydrocarbon ingestion

Mass within Cavity

1. Mycetoma = aspergilloma
2. Tissue fragment within carcinoma
3. Necrotic lung within abscess
4. Disintegrating hydatid cyst
5. Intracavitary blood clot

MEDIASTINUM

Acute Mediastinal Widening

1. Rupture of aorta / brachiocephalic arteries
2. Venous hemorrhage: traumatic / iatrogenic (malpositioning of central venous line)
3. Congestive heart failure (venous dilatation)
4. Rupture of esophagus
5. Rupture of thoracic duct
6. Atelectasis abutting the mediastinum
7. Magnification + geometric distortion on supine radiograph (attempt at suspended full inspiration, no rotation, 10–15° caudal angulation of central beam)

Mediastinal Shift

= displacement of heart, trachea, aorta, hilar vessels

◊ Expiration film, lateral decubitus film (expanded lung down), fluoroscopy help to determine side of abnormality

A. DECREASED LUNG VOLUME
   1. Atelectasis
   2. Postoperative (lobectomy, pneumothorax)
   3. Hypoplastic lung / lobe
      √ small pulmonary artery + small hilum
      √ decreased peripheral pulmonary vasculature
      √ irregular reticular vascular pattern (bronchial origin) without converging on the hilum
   4. Bronchiolitis obliterans = Swyer-James syndrome

B. INCREASED LUNG VOLUME
   = **air trapping** = retention of excess gas in all / part of the lung, especially during expiration, as a result of (a) complete / partial airway obstruction, or (b) local abnormalities in pulmonary compliance

   @ Major bronchus
   1. Foreign body obstructing main-stem bronchus (common in children) with ball-valve mechanism + collateral air drift
      √ contralateral mediastinal shift increasing with expiration

   @ Emphysema
   1. Bullous emphysema (localized form)
      √ large avascular areas with thin lines
   2. Congenital lobar emphysema: only in infants
   3. Interstitial emphysema
      √ pattern of diffuse coarse lines;
      Cx of positive pressure ventilation therapy

   @ Cysts / masses
   1. Bronchogenic cyst: with bronchial connection + check-valve mechanism
   2. Cystic adenomatoid malformation
   3. Large mass (pulmonary, mediastinal)

C. PLEURAL SPACE ABNORMALITY
   1. Large unilateral pleural effusion:
      opaque hemithorax through empyema, congestive failure, metastases
   2. Tension pneumothorax:
      not always complete collapse of lung
   3. Large diaphragmatic hernia:
      usually detected in neonatal period
   4. Large mass

D. Partial absence of pericardium / pectus excavatum
   √ shift of heart without shift of trachea, aorta, or mediastinal border

Pneumomediastinum

Frequency: in 1% of patients with pneumothorax

Source of air:

A. INTRATHORACIC
   1. Trachea, major bronchi: blunt chest trauma
   2. Esophagus
   3. Lung
      (a) narrowed / plugged airways (most common)
          = air trapping in small airways as in asthma
      (b) straining against closed glottis: vomiting, parturition, weight-lifting
      (c) blunt chest trauma
      (d) alveolar rupture
   4. Pleural space

B. EXTRATHORACIC
   1. Head and neck: sinus fracture, dental extraction
   2. Intra- and retroperitoneum: perforation of hollow viscus

Pathophysiology:

after alveolar rupture air tracks along bronchovascular sheath + ruptures through fascial sheath at lung root into mediastinum and facial planes of the neck producing subcutaneous emphysema

√ subcutaneous emphysema
√ streaky lucencies of air in mediastinum (look at thoracic inlet on PA + retrosternal space on LAT film)
√ "ring around artery sign" = air surrounding intramediastinal segment of right pulmonary artery (LAT view)
√ "tubular artery sign" = air adjacent to major aortic branches, eg, left subclavian + left common carotid aa.
√ "continuous diaphragm" sign = air trapped posterior to pericardium produces lucency connecting both domes of hemidiaphragms (frontal view)
√ "double bronchial wall sign" = clear depiction of bronchial wall by air next to and within a bronchus
√ "V sign of Naclerio" / "extrapleural sign" = mediastinal air extending laterally between mediastinal pleura / lower thoracic aorta + diaphragm
√ "spinnaker sail" / "thymic sail" sign in children = air outlining the thymus
√ air in azygoesophageal recess
√ air in pulmonary ligament = triangular gas collection in low mid chest

DDx:

A. OTHER AIR COLLECTIONS
   medial / subpulmonary pneumothorax (simulating extrapleural sign); pneumoperitoneum (simulating extrapleural sign); pneumopericardium

B. MISTAKEN NORMAL ANATOMIC STRUCTURES
   superior aspect of major fissure (on lordotic view); anterior junction line; Mach band effect

Spontaneous Pneumomediastinum

Age: neonates (0.05-1%), 2nd–3rd decade

Cause:

1. Rupture of marginally situated alveoli from sudden / prolonged rise in intraalveolar pressure with subsequent dissection of air centrally along bronchovascular bundles to hila (interstitial emphysema) + rupture into mediastinum: Valsalva maneuver, status asthmaticus, aspiration pneumonia, hyaline membrane disease, measles, giant cell pneumonia, coughing, vomiting, strenuous exercise, parturition, diabetic acidosis, crack cocaine inhalation = free-basing (mixing solid cocaine salt with a solvent to render it "smokeable")
2. Tumor erosion of trachea / esophagus
3. Pneumoperitoneum / retropneumoperitoneum = extension from peritoneal / retroperitoneal / deep fascial planes of the neck

Traumatic Pneumomediastinum (rare)

Cause:

1. Pulmonary interstitial emphysema
   = disruption of marginal alveoli with gas traveling toward mediastinum due to positive pressure ventilation
2. Bronchial / tracheal rupture
   √ commonly associated with pneumothorax
3. Esophageal rupture: diabetic acidosis, alcoholic, Boerhaave syndrome
4. Iatrogenic - accidental
   neck / chest / abdominal surgery, subclavian vein catheterization, mediastinoscopy, bronchoscopy, gastroscopy, recto-sigmoido-colonoscopy, electrosurgery with intestinal gas explosion, positive pressure ventilation, intubation, barium enema

Mediastinal Fat

A. MEDIASTINAL LIPOMATOSIS

B. FAT HERNIATION
   = omental fat herniating into chest
   1. Foramen of Morgagni
      = cardiophrenic-angle mass, R >> L side
   2. Foramen of Bochdalek
      = costophrenic-angle mass, almost always on left
   3. Paraesophageal hernia = perigastric fat through phrenicoesophageal membrane

   CT:
   √ fat with fine linear densities (= omental vessels)

C. LIPOMA
   un- / encapsulated with variable amount of fibrous septa
   √ smooth + sharply defined boundaries
   DDx: Liposarcoma, lipoblastoma (infancy), fat-containing teratoma, thymolipoma (inhomogeneous, higher CT numbers, poor demarcation, ± invasion of surrounding structures)

D. MULTIPLE SYMMETRIC LIPOMATOSIS
   rare entity without involvement of anterior mediastinal / cardiophrenic / paraspinal areas
   √ compression of trachea
   √ periscapular lipomatous masses

Low-attenuation Mediastinal Mass

A. FLUID
   1. Foregut cyst
   2. Lymphocele
   3. Seroma
   4. Hematoma
   5. Abscess
   6. Hydatid disease

B. LYMPH NODE
   1. Tuberculous lymph nodes
   2. Metastasis from thyroid / testicular tumor
   3. Lymphoma: treated / untreated

C. PRIMARY NEOPLASM
   1. Neurogenic tumor
   2. Fat-containing neoplasm

Mediastinal Cyst

= 21% of all primary mediastinal tumors

@ Anterior mediastinum
   1. Thymic cyst
   2. Dermoid cyst
   3. Parathyroid cyst (uncommon as mediastinal mass)

@ Middle mediastinum
   1. Pericardial cyst
   2. Bronchogenic cyst

@ Posterior mediastinum
   1. Esophageal duplication cyst
   2. Neurenteric cyst
   3. **Thoracic duct cyst**
      rare, filled with chyle
      Etiology: degenerative / lymphangiomatous
   4. Transdiaphragmatic jejunal duplication
   5. Cystic hygroma
   6. **Lateral meningocele**
      = outpouching of leptomeninges through intervertebral foramen
      Etiology: in 75% neurofibromatosis
      √ spinal abnormalities (kyphoscoliosis, scalloping of dorsal vertebrae, enlargement of intervertebral foramen, pedicle erosion, thinning of ribs)
   7. Posttraumatic lymphocele
      = contained pleural / mediastinal lymph collection
      • history of prolonged chylous chest tube drainage
      Time of onset: several months after injury
   8. **Hydatid cyst**
      Location: paravertebral gutter
      √ erosion of ribs + vertebrae

Frequency of Developmental Mediastinal Cyst

1. Enterogenous cyst = Foregut cyst (45%):
   (a) Bronchogenic cyst (35%)
   (b) Esophageal duplication cyst (15%)
   (c) Neurenteric cyst (least common)
2. Pericardial cyst (30%)
3. Thymic cyst (10%)
4. Nonspecific mesothelial cyst (10%)
5. Cystic hygroma (5%)

Mediastinal Mass

(excluding hyperplastic thymus glands, granulomas, lymphoma, metastases)

1. Neurogenic tumors	(28%) :	malignant in 16%
2. Teratoid lesions	(19%) :	malignant in 15%
3. Enterogenous cysts	(16%)	
4. Thymomas	(13%) :	malignant in 46%
5. Pericardial cysts	(7%)	

A. BENIGN MEDIASTINAL MASS
   ◊ 66–75% of all mediastinal tumors are benign (in all age groups)
   ◊ 88% discovered incidentally on routine chest x-ray
B. MALIGNANT MEDIASTINAL MASS
   ◊ 57% found in association with symptoms (pain, cough, shortness of breath)
   ◊ 80% of malignant tumors are symptomatic

Cervicothoracic sign:
   √ posterior superior mediastinal masses are sharply outlined by apical lung
   √ anterior superior mediastinal masses extending into neck have unsharp borders

Thoracic Inlet Lesions

1. Thyroid mass
   1–3% of all thyroidectomies have a mediastinal component; 1/3 of goiters are intrathoracic
   Location: anterior (80%) / posterior (20%) mediastinum
   √ displacement of trachea posteriorly + laterally (anterior goiter)
   √ displacement of trachea anteriorly + esophagus posteriorly + laterally (posterior goiter)
   √ inhomogeneous density (cystic spaces, high-density iodine contents of >100 HU)
   √ focal calcifications (common)
   √ marked + prolonged contrast enhancement
   √ connection to thyroid gland
   √ vascular displacement + compression
   NUC (rarely helpful as thyroid tissue may be nonfunctioning):
      √ ± uptake on I-123 / I-131 scan (pertechnetate sufficient with modern gamma cameras, SPECT imaging may be helpful)
2. Cystic hygroma
   3–10% involve mediastinum; childhood
3. Lymphoma
4. Other tumors: adenoma, carcinoma, ectopic thymoma

Mass in Raider Triangle

Raider triangle = on LAT CXR formed by posterior wall of trachea + thoracic vertebrae + aortic arch
1. Aberrant right subclavian artery
2. Aberrant left subclavian a. with right aortic arch
3. Aneurysms
4. Posterior descending goiter
5. Enlarged lymph node
6. Esophageal mass / duplication cyst

Anterior Mediastinal Mass

mnemonic: "4 T's"
Thymoma
Teratoma
Thyroid tumor / goiter
Terrible lymphoma

A. SOLID THYMIC LESIONS
   1. Thymoma (benign, malignant): most common
   2. Normal thymus (neonate)
   3. Thymic hyperplasia (child)
   4. Thymic carcinoma
   5. Thymic carcinoid
   6. Thymolipoma
   7. Lymphoma
B. SOLID TERATOID LESIONS
   1. Teratoma
   2. Embryonal cell carcinoma
   3. Choriocarcinoma
   4. Seminoma
C. THYROID / PARATHYROID
   1. Substernal thyroid / intrathoracic goiter (10% of all mediastinal masses)
   2. Thyroid adenoma / carcinoma
   3. **Ectopic parathyroid adenoma**: ectopia in 1–3% (62–81% in anterior mediastinum / thymus, 30% within thyroid tissue, 8% in posterior superior mediastinum)
D. LYMPH NODES
   1. Lymphoma (Hodgkin, NHL): may arise in thymus, more common in young adults
   2. Metastases
   3. Benign lymph node hyperplasia
   4. Angioblastic lymphadenopathy
   5. Mediastinal lymphadenitis: sarcoidosis / granulomatous infection
E. CARDIOVASCULAR
   1. Tortuous brachiocephalic artery
   2. Aneurysm of ascending aorta
   3. Aneurysm of sinus of Valsalva
   4. Dilated SVC
   5. Cardiac tumor
   6. Epicardial fat-pad
F. CYSTS
   1. Cystic hygroma
   2. Bronchogenic cyst
   3. Extralobar sequestration
   4. Thymic cysts / dermoid cysts
   5. Pericardial cyst: (a) true cyst
      (b) pericardial diverticulum
   6. Pancreatic pseudocyst

G. OTHERS
1. Neural tumor (vagus, phrenic nerve)
2. Paraganglioma
3. Hemangioma / lymphangioma
4. Mesenchymal tumor (fibroma, lipoma)
5. Sternal tumors
   (a) metastases from breast, bronchus, kidney, thyroid
   (b) malignant primary (chondrosarcoma, myeloma, lymphoma)
   (c) benign primary (chondroma, aneurysmal bone cyst, giant cell tumor)
6. Primary lung / pleural tumor (invading mediastinum)
7. Mediastinal lipomatosis:
   (a) Cushing disease
   (b) Corticosteroid therapy
8. Morgagni hernia / localized eventration
9. Abscess

Middle Mediastinal Mass

mnemonic: "HABIT[5]"

Hernia, **H**ematoma
Aneurysm
Bronchogenic cyst / duplication cyst
Inflammation (sarcoidosis, histoplasmosis, coccidioidomycosis, primary TB in children)
Tumors - remember the 5 L's:
   Lung, especially oat cell carcinoma
   Lymphoma
   Leukemia
   Leiomyoma
   Lymph node hyperplasia

A. LYMPH NODES
◊ 90% of masses in the middle mediastinum are malignant
(a) Neoplastic adenopathy
   1. Lymphoma (Hodgkin:NHL = 2:1)
   2. Leukemia (in 25%): lymphocytic > granulocytic
   3. Metastasis (bronchus, lung, upper GI, prostate, kidney)
   4. Angioimmunoblastic lymphadenopathy
(b) Inflammatory adenopathy
   1. Tuberculosis / histoplasmosis (may lead to fibrosing mediastinitis)
   2. Blastomycosis (rare) / coccidioidomycosis
   3. Sarcoidosis (predominant involvement of paratracheal nodes)
   4. Viral pneumonia (particularly measles + cat-scratch fever)
   5. Infectious mononucleosis / pertussis pneumonia
   6. Amyloidosis
   7. Plague / tularemia
   8. Drug reaction
   9. Giant lymph node hyperplasia = Castleman disease
   10. Connective tissue disease (rheumatoid, SLE)
   11. Bacterial lung abscess
(c) Inhalational disease adenopathy
   1. Silicosis (eggshell calcification also in sarcoidosis + tuberculosis)
   2. Coal worker's pneumoconiosis
   3. Berylliosis

B. FOREGUT CYST
1. Bronchogenic / respiratory cyst: cartilage, respiratory epithelium
2. Enteric cyst = esophageal duplication cyst
3. Extralobar sequestration (anomalous feeding vessel)
4. Hiatal hernia
5. Esophageal diverticula: Zenker, traction, epiphrenic

C. PRIMARY TUMORS (infrequent)
1. Carcinoma of trachea
2. Bronchogenic carcinoma
3. Esophageal tumor: leiomyoma, carcinoma, leiomyosarcoma
4. Mesothelioma
5. Granular cell myoblastoma of trachea (rare)

D. VASCULAR LESIONS
1. Aneurysm of transverse aorta
2. Distended veins (SVC, azygos vein)
3. Hematoma

Subcarinal Space Lesion

1. Enlarged lymph nodes
2. Bronchogenic cyst
3. Pericardial effusion
4. Enlarged left atrium
5. Esophageal mass
6. Aortic aneurysm

Aorticopulmonary Window Mass

1. Adenopathy
2. Aneurysms: traumatic aortic pseudoaneurysm, pulmonary artery aneurysm, ductus Botalli aneurysm, bronchial artery aneurysm
4. Bronchogenic cyst
5. Tumor of tracheobronchial tree
6. Esophageal tumor
7. Neurogenic tumor
8. Mediastinal abscess

Widening of Paratracheal Space

Normal width: <5 mm
1. Dilated tortuous vessels (brachiocephalic artery, SVC, azygos vein)
2. Enlarged lymph node
3. Bronchogenic carcinoma
4. Mediastinal lipomatosis
5. Mediastinal hematoma
6. Bronchogenic cyst

Retrocardiac Space of Holzknecht Lesion

1. Hiatal hernia
2. Esophageal lesion
3. Left ventricular aneurysm

4. Pericardial cyst
5. Bronchogenic cyst
6. Aortic aneurysm
7. Vagal / phrenic nerve neurofibroma

Posterior Mediastinal Mass

A. NEOPLASM

NEUROGENIC TUMOR (largest group): 30% malignant

(a) Tumor of peripheral nerve origin
- more common in adulthood

√ 80% appear as round masses with sulcus
√ lower attenuation than muscle (in 73%)

1. Schwannoma = neurilemoma (32%): derived from sheath of Schwann without nerve cells
2. Neurofibroma (10%): contains Schwann cells + nerve cells, 3rd + 4th decade
3. Malignant schwannoma

(b) Tumor of sympathetic ganglia origin
- more common in childhood

√ 80% are elongated with tapered borders

1. Ganglioneuroma (23–38%): second most common tumor of posterior mediastinum after neurofibroma
2. Neuroblastoma (15%): highly malignant undifferentiated small round cell tumor originating in sympathetic ganglia, <10 years of age
3. Ganglioneuroblastoma (14%): both features, spontaneous maturation possible

(c) Tumors of paraganglia origin (rare)

1. Chemodectoma = paraganglioma (4%)
2. Pheochromocytoma

√ rib spreading, erosion, destruction
√ enlargement of neural foramina (dumbbell lesion)
√ scalloping of posterior aspect of vertebral body
√ scoliosis
CT: √ low-density soft-tissue mass (lipid contents)

SPINE TUMOR: metastases (eg, bronchogenic carcinoma, multiple myeloma), ABC, chordoma, chondrosarcoma, Ewing sarcoma

LYMPHOMA

INVASIVE THYMOMA

MESENCHYMAL TUMOR (fibroma, lipoma, leiomyoma)

HEMANGIOMA

LYMPHANGIOMA

THYROID TUMOR

B. INFLAMMATION / INFECTION

1. Infectious spondylitis: pyogenic, tuberculous, fungal
   √ destruction of endplates + disk space
   √ paravertebral soft-tissue mass
2. Mediastinitis
5. Pancreatic pseudocyst
3. Lymphoid hyperplasia
4. Sarcoidosis (in 2%, typically asymptomatic patient)

C. VASCULAR MASS

1. Aneurysm of descending aorta (curvilinear calcification; elderly)
2. Enlarged azygos + accessory hemiazygos vein
3. Esophageal varices
4. Congenital vascular anomalies: aberrant subclavian artery, double aortic arch, pulmonary sling, interruption of IVC with azygos / hemiazygos continuation

D. TRAUMA

1. Aortic aneurysm / pseudoaneurysm
2. Hematoma
3. Loculated hemothorax
4. Traumatic pseudomeningocele

E. FOREGUT CYST

√ cysts may demonstrate peripheral rimlike calcifications

1. Bronchogenic cyst
2. Enteric cyst
3. Neurenteric cyst
4. Extralobar sequestration

F. FATTY MASS

1. Bochdalek hernia
2. Mediastinal lipomatosis
3. Fat-containing tumors: lipoma, liposarcoma, teratoma (rare)

G. OTHER

1. Loculated pleural effusion
2. Pancreatic pseudocyst
3. Lateral meningocele (neurofibromatosis; enlarged neural foramen)
4. Extramedullary hematopoiesis: in chronic bone marrow deficiency; paraspinal area rich in RES-elements
   √ splenomegaly; widening of ribs
5. "Pseudomass" of the newborn

mnemonic: "BELLMAN"

Bochdalek hernia
Extramedullary hematopoiesis
Lymphadenopathy
Lymphangioma
Meningocele (lateral)
Aneurysm
Neurogenic tumor

Cardiophrenic-angle Mass

A. Lesion of pericardium

1. Pericardial cyst
2. Intrapericardiac bronchogenic cyst
3. Benign intrapericardiac neoplasm: teratoma, leiomyoma, hemangioma, lipoma
4. Malignant neoplasm: mesothelioma, metastasis (lung, breast, lymphoma, melanoma)

B. Cardiac lesion: aneurysm

C. Others: masses arising from lung, pleura, diaphragm, abdomen

CHEST

Right Cardiophrenic-angle Mass

A. Heart
1. Aneurysm (cardiac ventricle, sinus of Valsalva)
2. Dilated right atrium

B. Peri- / epicardium
1. **Epicardial fat-pad** / lipoma (most common cause)
√ triangular opacity in cardiophrenic angle less dense than heart
√ increase in size under corticosteroid treatment
2. Pericardial cyst

C. Diaphragm
1. Diaphragmatic hernia of Morgagni
2. Diaphragmatic lymph node (esp. in Hodgkin disease + breast cancer)

D. Anterior mediastinal mass
1. Thymolipoma

E. Primary lung mass

F. Paracardiac varices

G. Enlarged lymph node: lymphoma, metastasis (lung, breast, colon, ovary, melanoma)

Hypervascular Mediastinal Mass

1. Paraganglioma
2. Metastasis: typically renal cell carcinoma
3. Castleman disease
4. Hemangioma
5. Sarcoma
6. Tuberculosis
7. Sarcoidosis

Hilar Mass

A. LARGE PULMONARY ARTERIES
√ enlargement of main pulmonary artery
√ abrupt change in vessel caliber
√ enlarged pulmonary artery compared with bronchus (in same bronchovascular bundle)
√ cephalization
√ enlargement of right ventricle (RAO 45°, LAO 60°)

Cause:
1. Chronic obstructive disease (emphysema)
2. Chronic restrictive interstitial lung disease (idiopathic fibrosis, cystic fibrosis, rheumatoid arthritis, sarcoidosis)
3. Pulmonary embolic disease (acute massive / chronic)
4. Idiopathic pulmonary hypertension
5. Left-sided heart failure + mitral stenosis
6. Congenital heart disease with left-to-right shunt
(a) acyanotic: ASD, VSD, PDA
(b) cyanotic (admixture lesions): transposition of great vessels, truncus arteriosus

B. DUPLICATION CYST

C. UNILATERAL HILAR ADENOPATHY
(a) NEOPLASTIC
1. Bronchogenic carcinoma (most common)
2. Metastases (lack of mediastinal involvement exceptional)
3. Lymphoma

(b) INFLAMMATORY
1. Tuberculosis (primary) in 80%
2. Fungal infection: histoplasmosis, coccidioidomycosis, blastomycosis
3. Viral infections: atypical measles
4. Infectious mononucleosis
5. Drug reaction
6. Sarcoidosis (in 1–3%)
7. Bilateral lung abscess

mnemonic: "**F**at **H**ila **S**uck"
Fungus
Hodgkin disease
Squamous / oat cell carcinoma

D. BILATERAL HILAR ADENOPATHY
(a) NEOPLASTIC
1. Lymphoma (50% in Hodgkin disease)
2. Metastases
3. Leukemia
4. Primary bronchogenic carcinoma
5. Plasmacytoma

(b) INFLAMMATORY
1. Sarcoidosis (in 70–90%)
2. Silicosis
3. Histiocytosis X
4. Idiopathic pulmonary hemosiderosis
5. Chronic berylliosis

(c) INFECTIOUS
1. Rubella, ECHOvirus, varicella, mononucleosis

mnemonic: "**P**lease **H**elen **L**ick **M**y **P**opsicle **S**tick"
Primary TB
Histoplasmosis
Lymphoma
Metastases
Pneumoconiosis
Sarcoidosis

Eggshell Calcification of Nodes

A. PNEUMOCONIOSIS
1. Silicosis (5%)
2. Coal worker's pneumoconiosis (1.3–6%)
not seen in: asbestosis, berylliosis, talcosis, baritosis

B. SARCOIDOSIS (5%)

C. FUNGAL + BACTERILA INFECTION (rare):
1. Tuberculosis
2. Histoplasmosis
3. Coccidioidomycosis

D. FIBROSING MEDIASTINITIS

E. LYMPHOMA FOLLOWING RADIATION THERAPY

Enlargement of Azygos Vein

Normal azygos vein (on upright CXR): ≤7 mm

A. COLLATERAL CIRCULATION
1. Portal hypertension
2. SVC obstruction / compression below azygos vein
3. IVC obstruction / compression
4. Interrupted IVC with azygos continuation
5. Partial anomalous venous return (rare)

CHEST

6. Pregnancy
7. Hepatic vein occlusion

B. RIGHT ATRIAL HYPERTENSION
1. Right-sided heart failure
2. Constrictive pericarditis
3. Large pericardial effusion

THYMUS

Thymic Mass

1. Thymoma
2. Thymolipoma
3. Thymic cyst
4. Thymic carcinoid

Diffuse Thymic Enlargement

A. BENIGN
1. Thymic hyperplasia
2. Intrathymic hemorrhage
3. Hemangioma
4. Lymphangioma

B. MALIGNANT THYMIC INFILTRATION
• presence of adenopathy elsewhere
√ no pleural implants
1. Leukemia
2. Hodgkin / non-Hodgkin lymphoma
3. Langerhans cell histiocytosis

TRACHEA & BRONCHI

Tracheal Narrowing

A. ANTERIOR COMPRESSION
(a) Congenital
1. Congenital goiter
2. Innominate artery syndrome
• ablation of right radial pulse by rigid endoscopic pressure
√ posterior tracheal displacement
√ focal collapse of trachea at fluoroscopy
√ pulsatile indentation of anterior tracheal wall by innominate artery on MRI
Rx: surgical attachment of innominate artery to manubrium

(b) Inflammatory
1. Cervical / mediastinal abscess

(c) Neoplastic
1. Cervical / intrathoracic teratoma
√ amorphous calcifications + ossifications
2. Thymoma
3. Thyroid tumors
4. Lymphoma

(d) Traumatic: hematoma

B. POSTERIOR TRACHEAL COMPRESSION
(a) Congenital
1. Vascular ring
— complete: double aortic arch, right aortic arch
— incomplete: anomalous right subclavian a.
√ posterior indentation of esophagus + trachea
2. Pulmonary sling
= anomalous left pulmonary artery arising from right pulmonary artery, passing between trachea + esophagus en route to left lung
3. Bronchogenic cyst
most common between esophagus + trachea at level of carina

(b) inflammatory: abscess
(c) neoplastic: neurofibroma
(d) traumatic: esophageal foreign body, esophageal stricture, hematoma

C. INTRINSIC TRACHEAL CAUSES
(a) Congenital:
1. Congenital tracheal stenosis: generalized / segmental
= complete cartilaginous ring (instead of horseshoe shape)
2. Congenital tracheomalacia = immaturity of tracheal cartilage = chondromalacia
• expiratory stridor
√ tracheal collapse on expiration

(b) Neoplastic: papilloma, fibroma, hemangioma
(c) Traumatic: acquired stenosis (endotracheal + tracheostomy tubes), granuloma, acquired tracheomalacia (cartilage degeneration after inflammation, extrinsic pressure, bronchial neoplasia, TE fistula, foreign body)

Tracheal Tumor

• asthma symptomatology
• hoarseness, cough
• wheeze (inspiratory with extrathoracic lesion, expiratory with intrathoracic lesion)
• hemoptysis

A. MALIGNANT
1. Squamous-cell carcinoma (commonest primary)
◊ 50% of all malignant tracheal lesions
2. Adenoid cystic carcinoma = cylindroma
3. Carcinoid
4. Mucoepidermoid carcinoma
5. Metastasis from renal cell carcinoma, colon cancer, malignant melanoma
6. Lymphoma
7. Plasmacytoma

B. BENIGN TUMOR
1. Cartilaginous tumor (hamartoma)
2. Squamous cell papilloma
3. Fibroma / lipoma
4. Hemangioma
5. Granular cell myoblastoma

C. INFLAMMATION
1. Granulomatous disease: tuberculosis, sarcoidosis, Wegener granulomatosis
2. Inflammatory myoblastic pseudotumor
3. Amyloid tumor
4. Pseudotumor: inspissated mucus, foreign body

Endobronchial Tumor
1. Neuroendocrine tumor (typical / atypical carcinoid)
2. Mucoepidermoid carcinoma
3. Adenoid cystic carcinoma
4. Hamartoma
5. Leiomyoma
6. Myoblastoma
7. Mucous gland adenoma
8. Squamous cell carcinoma

Bronchial Obstruction
1. Foreign body: most commonly in young children
2. Granulomatous disease: due to granuloma formation in bronchial wall / extrinsic compression by adenopathy
3. Broncholiths = erosion of calcified nodes into bronchial lumen
4. Stenosis / atresia
5. Neoplasm
   (a) Bronchogenic carcinoma
   (b) Adenoid cystic carcinoma
   (c) Mucoepidermoid tumor
   (d) Hamartoma

mnemonic: "MEATFACE"
Mucus plug
Endobronchial granulomatous disease
Adenoma
Tuberculosis
Foreign body
Amyloid, **A**tresia (bronchial)
Cancer (primary)
Endobronchial metastasis

Mucoid Impaction
= BRONCHIAL MUCOCELE = BRONCHOCELE
= accumulation of inspissated secretions (mucus / pus / inflammatory products) within bronchial lumen; usually associated with bronchial dilatation

A. WITH BRONCHIAL OBSTRUCTION in the presence of collateral air drift
   1. Bronchial obstruction by neoplasm: bronchogenic carcinoma / adenoma
   2. Bronchial atresia

B. WITHOUT BRONCHIAL OBSTRUCTION
   1. Asthma (most frequent cause): esp. during acute attack or convalescent phase
   2. Fluid-filled bronchiectasis: history of childhood pneumonia; peripheral distribution
   3. Bronchopulmonary aspergillosis: central perihilar bronchiectasis
   4. Cystic fibrosis
   5. Chronic bronchitis

Signet-ring Sign
= cross section of usually thick-walled and dilated ringlike bronchus + branch of pulmonary artery as adjacent round soft-tissue opacity
1. Bronchiectasis
2. Multifocal bronchioloalveolar carcinoma
3. Metastatic adenocarcinoma

Bronchial Wall Thickening
◊ Apparent thickness of bronchial wall varies with lung window chosen on CT: a mean window that is too low can make the bronchial wall appear abnormal!

A. PERIBRONCHOVASCULAR
   1. Sarcoidosis
   2. Lymphangitic carcinomatosis
   3. Kaposi sarcoma
   4. Lymphoma
   5. Pulmonary edema

B. BRONCHIAL WALL
   1. Airway disease
   2. Relapsing polychondritis
   3. Wegener granulomatosis
   4. Amyloidosis

C. MUCOSAL INFECTION
   1. Croup
   2. Tuberculosis
   3. Fungal disease
   4. Aspergillosis

Broncholithiasis
1. Histoplasmosis
2. Tuberculosis
3. Cryptococcosis
4. Actinomycosis
5. Coccidioidomycosis

√ calcified lymph node within / adjacent to affected bronchus
√ bronchial obstruction: atelectasis, airspace disease, bronchiectasis, air trapping
√ absence of associated soft-tissue mass

PLEURA

Pneumothorax
= accumulation of air in the pleural space

Pathophysiology: disruption of visceral pleura / trauma to parietal pleura

• pleuritic back / shoulder pain, dyspnea (in 80–90%)

Etiology:

A. TRAUMATIC PNEUMOTHORAX
   (a) penetrating trauma
   (b) blunt trauma
      1. Rib fracture
      2. Increased intrathoracic pressure against closed glottis: lung contusion / laceration
      3. Bronchial fracture
         √ fallen lung sign = hilum of lung below expected level within chest cavity
         √ persistent pneumothorax with functioning chest tube
         √ mediastinal pneumothorax
   (c) iatrogenic
   tracheostomy, central venous catheter, PEEP ventilator (3–16%), thoracic irradiation

B. SPONTANEOUS PNEUMOTHORAX
   1. **Primary / idiopathic spontaneous pneumothorax** (80%)
   Cause: rupture of subpleural blebs in apical region of lung

Age: 20–40 years; M:F = 8:1; esp. in patients with tall asthenic stature; mostly in smokers
- chest pain (69%)
- dyspnea

Prognosis: recurrence in 30% on same side, in 10% on contralateral side
Rx: simple aspiration (in >50% success) / tube thoracostomy (in 90% effective)

2. Secondary spontaneous pneumothorax (20%):
   (a) Air-trapping disease: spasmodic asthma, diffuse emphysema, Langerhans cell histiocytosis, lymphangiomyomatosis, tuberous sclerosis, cystic fibrosis
   ◊ Chronic obstructive pulmonary disease is the most common predisposing disorder of secondary spontaneous pneumothorax
   (b) Pulmonary infections: lung abscess, necrotizing pneumonia, hydatid disease, pertussis, acute bacterial pneumonia, Staphylococcus aureus, Pneumocystis carinii pneumonia
   (c) Granulomatous disease: tuberculosis, coccidioidomycosis, sarcoidosis, berylliosis
   (d) Malignancy: primary lung cancer, lung metastases (esp. osteosarcoma, pancreas, adrenal, Wilms tumor)
   (e) Connective tissue disorder: scleroderma, rheumatoid disease, Marfan syndrome, Ehlers-Danlos syndrome
   (f) Pneumoconiosis: silicosis, berylliosis
   (g) Vascular disease: pulmonary infarction
   (h) **Catamenial** [*kata* , Greek = according to; *men* , Greek = month] **pneumothorax** = recurrent spontaneous pneumothorax during menstruation associated with endometriosis of the diaphragm; R >> L
   (i) Neonatal disease: meconium aspiration, respirator therapy for hyaline membrane disease
   (j) Cx of honeycomb lung: pulmonary fibrosis, cystic fibrosis, sarcoidosis, scleroderma, eosinophilic granuloma, interstitial pneumonitis, Langerhans cell histiocytosis, rheumatoid lung, idiopathic pulmonary hemosiderosis, pulmonary alveolar proteinosis, biliary cirrhosis

mnemonic: "THE CHEST SET"
Trauma
Honeycomb lung, **H**amman-Rich syndrome
Emphysema, **E**sophageal rupture
Chronic obstructive pulmonary disease
Hyaline membrane disease
Endometriosis
Spontaneous, **S**cleroderma
Tuberous sclerosis
Sarcoma (osteo-), **S**arcoidosis
Eosinophilic granuloma
Tuberculosis + fungus

Types:
1. Closed pneumothorax = intact thoracic cage
2. Open pneumothorax = "sucking" chest wound
3. **Tension pneumothorax**
   = accumulation of air within pleural space due to free ingress + limited egress of air
   Pathophysiology:
   intrapleural pressure exceeds atmospheric pressure in lung during expiration (check-valve mechanism)
   Frequency: in 3–5% of patients with spontaneous pneumothorax, higher in barotrauma
   √ displacement of mediastinum / anterior junction line
   √ deep sulcus sign = on frontal view larger lateral costodiaphragmatic recess than on opposite side
   √ diaphragmatic inversion
   √ total / subtotal lung collapse
   √ collapse of SVC / IVC / right heart border (decreased systemic venous return + decreased cardiac output)
   N.B.: Medical emergency!
4. **Tension hydropneumothorax**
   √ sharp delineation of visceral pleural by dense pleural space
   √ mediastinal shift to opposite side
   √ air-fluid level in pleural space on erect CXR

Pneumothorax size:
Average Interpleural Distance (AID) = (A + B + C) ÷ 3 [in cm] converts to percentage of pneumothorax
see nomogram in drawing

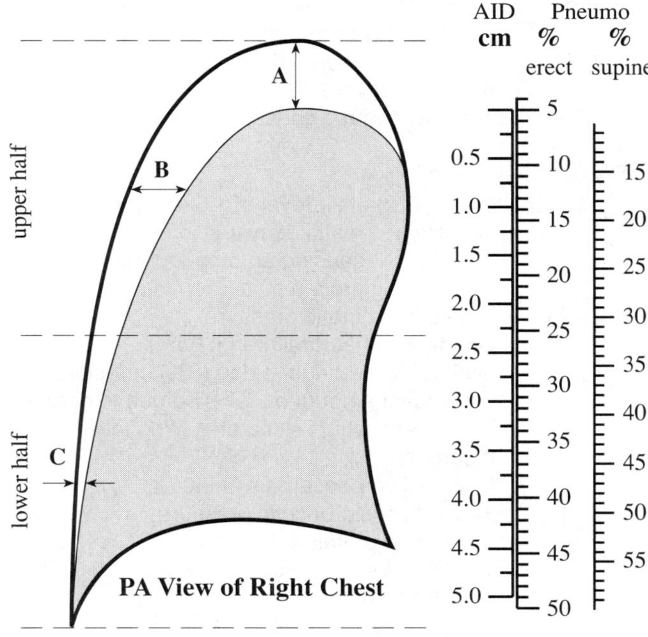

Estimate of Pneumothorax Size
A = maximum apical interpleural distance
B = interpleural distance at midpoint of upper half of lung
C = interpleural distance at midpoint of lower half of lung

CHEST

Radiographic signs in upright position:
√ white margin of visceral pleura separated from parietal pleura
DDx: skin fold, air trapped between chest wall soft tissues, hair braid)
√ absence of vascular markings beyond visceral pleural margin

Radiographic signs in supine position:
1. Anteromedial pneumothorax (earliest location)
   √ outline of medial diaphragm under cardiac silhouette
   √ sharp delineation of mediastinal contours (SVC, azygos vein, left subclavian artery, anterior junction line, superior pulmonary vein, heart border, IVC, deep anterior cardiophrenic sulcus, pericardial fat-pad)
2. Subpulmonic pneumothorax (second most common location)
   √ hyperlucent upper abdominal quadrant
   √ deep lateral costophrenic sulcus
   √ sharply outlined diaphragm in spite of parenchymal disease
   √ visualization of anterior costophrenic sulcus
   √ visualization of inferior surface of lung
3. Apicolateral pneumothorax (least common location)
   √ visualization of visceral pleural line
4. Posteromedial pneumothorax (in presence of lower lobe collapse)
   √ lucent triangle with vertex at hilum
   √ V-shaped base delineating costovertebral sulcus
5. Pneumothorax outlines pulmonary ligament

Prognosis: resorption of pneumothorax occurs at a rate of 1.25% per day (accelerated by increasing inspired oxygen concentrations)

Rx: A pneumothorax >35% usually requires management with a chest tube!

Pleural Effusion

A. TRANSUDATE (protein level of 1.5–2.5 g/dL)
   Pathophysiology: result of systemic abnormalities causing an outpouring of low-protein fluid
   (a) Increased hydrostatic pressure
      1. Congestive heart failure (in 65%)
         bilateral (88%); right-sided (8%); left-sided (4%); least amount on left side due to cardiac movement, which stimulates lymphatic resorption
      2. Constrictive pericarditis (in 60%)
   (b) Decreased colloid-oncotic pressure
      — decreased protein production
         1. Cirrhosis with ascites (in 6%):
            right-sided (67%)
      — protein loss / hypervolemia
         1. Nephrotic syndrome (21%), overhydration, glomerulonephritis (55%), peritoneal dialysis
         2. Hypothyroidism
   (c) Chylous effusion
      ◊ Most frequent cause of isolated pleural effusion in newborn with 15–25% mortality!
      • chylomicrons + lymphocytes in fluid

B. EXUDATE
   Pathophysiology: increased permeability of abnormal pleural capillaries with release of high-protein fluid into pleural space
   Criteria:
   • pleural fluid total protein / serum total protein ratio of >0.5
   • pleural fluid LDH / serum LDH ratio of >0.6
   • pleural fluid LDH >2/3 of upper limit of normal for serum LDH (upper limit for LDH ~200 IU)
   • pleural fluid specific gravity >1.016
   • protein level >3 g/dL
   √ effusion with septation / low-level echoes
   √ "split pleura" sign on CECT = thickened enhancing visceral + parietal pleura separated by fluid
   √ extrapleural fat thickening of >2 mm + increased attenuation (edema / inflammation)
   (a) Infection
      1. Empyema
         empyema necessitatis = chronic empyema attempting to decompress through chest wall (in TB, actinomycosis, aspergillosis, blastomycosis, nocardiosis)
      2. Parapneumonic effusion (in 40%)
         = any effusion associated with pneumonia / lung abscess / bronchiectasis without criteria for an empyema
      3. Tuberculosis (in 1%):
         high protein content (75 g/dL), lymphocytes >70%, positive culture (only in 20–25%)
      4. Fungi: Actinomyces, Nocardia
      5. Parasites: amebiasis (secondary to liver abscess in 15–20%), Echinococcus
      6. Mycoplasma, rickettsia (in 20%)
   (b) Malignant disease (in 60%)
      • positive cytologic results
      Pathogenesis:
      — pleural metastases (increased pleural permeability)
      — lymphatic obstruction (pleural vessels, mediastinal nodes, thoracic duct disruption)
      — bronchial obstruction (loss of volume + resorptive surface)
      — hypoproteinemia (secondary to tumor cachexia)
      Cause: lung cancer (26–49%), breast cancer (8–24%), lymphoma (10–28%, in 2/3 chylothorax), ovarian cancer (10%), malignant mesothelioma containing hyaluronic acid (5%)
      Rx: sclerosing agents: doxycycline, bleomycin, talc
   (c) Vascular
      Pulmonary emboli (in 15–30% of all embolic events): often serosanguinous

(d) Abdominal disease
1. Pancreatitis / pancreatic pseudocyst / pancreaticopleural fistula (in 2/3):
   √ usually left-sided pleural effusion
   • high amylase levels
2. Boerhaave syndrome: left-sided esophageal perforation
3. Subphrenic abscess
   √ pleural effusion (79%)
   √ elevation + restriction of diaphragmatic motion (95%)
   √ basilar platelike atelectasis / pneumonitis (79%)
4. Abdominal tumor with ascites
5. **Meigs-Salmon syndrome**
   = primary pelvic neoplasms (ovarian fibroma, thecoma, granulosa cell tumor, Brenner tumor, cystadenoma, adenocarcinoma, fibromyoma of uterus) cause pleural effusion in 2–3%; ascites + hydrothorax resolve with tumor removal
6. Endometriosis
7. Bile fistula

(e) Collagen-vascular disease
1. Rheumatoid arthritis (in 3%): unilateral; R > L (in 75%), recurrent alternating sides; pleural effusion relatively unchanged in size for months; predominantly in men; LOW GLUCOSE content of 20–50 mg/dL (in 70–80%) without increase following IV infusion of glucose (DDx: TB, metastatic disease, parapneumonic effusion)
2. SLE (in 15–74%) most common collagenosis to give pleural effusion, bilateral in 50%; L > R
   √ enlargement of cardiovascular silhouette (in 35–50%)
3. Wegener granulomatosis (in 50%)
4. Sjögren syndrome
5. Mixed connective tissue disease
6. Periarteritis nodosa
7. Postmyocardial infarct syndrome

(f) Traumatic
hemorrhagic, chylous, esophageal rupture, thoracic / abdominal surgery, intrapleural infusion = "infusothorax" (0.5%), radiation pneumonitis

(g) Miscellaneous
1. Sarcoidosis
2. Uremic pleuritis (in 20% of uremic patients)
3. Drug-induced effusion

CXR:
√ first 300 mL not visualized on PA view (collect in subpulmonic region first, then spill into posterior costophrenic sinus)
√ lateral decubitus views may detect as little as 25 mL
√ hemidiaphragm + costophrenic sinuses obscured
√ extension upward around posterior > lateral > anterior thoracic wall (mediastinal portion fixed by pulmonary ligament + hilum)
√ meniscus-shaped semicircular upper surface with lowest point in midaxillary line
√ associated collapse of ipsilateral lung

Massive pleural effusion:
   √ enlargement of ipsilateral hemithorax
   √ displacement of mediastinum to contralateral side
   √ severe depression / flattening / inversion of ipsilateral hemidiaphragm
   √ visible air bronchogram

Subpulmonic / subdiaphragmatic / infrapulmonary pleural effusion:
   √ peak of dome of pseudodiaphragm laterally positioned
   √ acutely angulated costophrenic angle
   √ increased distance between stomach bubble and lung
   √ blunted posterior costophrenic sulcus
   √ thin triangular paramediastinal opacity (mediastinal extension of pleural effusion)
   √ flattened pseudodiaphragmatic contour anterior to major fissure (on lateral CXR)

CT:
√ fluid outside diaphragm
√ fluid elevating crus of diaphragm
√ indistinct fluid-liver interface
√ fluid posteromedial to liver (= bare area of liver)

CAVE: "central oval" sign of ascites may be seen in subpulmonic effusion with inverted diaphragm

Unilateral Pleural Effusion

◊ The majority of massive unilateral pleural effusions are malignant (lymphoma, metastatic disease, primary lung cancer)!

1. Neoplasm
2. Infection: TB
3. Collagen vascular disease
4. Subdiaphragmatic disease
5. Pulmonary emboli
6. Trauma: fractured rib
7. Chylothorax

Left-sided Pleural Effusion

1. Spontaneous rupture of the esophagus
2. Dissecting aneurysm of the aorta
3. Traumatic rupture of aorta distal to left subclavian artery
4. Transection of distal thoracic duct
5. Pancreatitis: left-sided (68%), right-sided (10%), bilateral (22%)
6. Pancreatic + gastric neoplasm

Right-sided Pleural Effusion

1. Congestive heart failure
2. Transection of proximal thoracic duct
3. Pancreatitis

Pleural Effusion & Large Cardiac Silhouette

1. Congestive heart failure (most common)
   √ cardiomegaly
   √ prominence of upper lobe vessels + constriction of lower lobe vessels
   √ prominent hilar vessels
   √ interstitial edema (fine reticular pattern, Kerley lines, perihilar haze, peribronchial thickening)
   √ alveolar edema (perihilar confluent ill-defined densities, air bronchogram)
   √ "phantom tumor" = fluid localized to interlobar pleural fissure (in 78% in right horizontal fissure)
2. Pulmonary embolus + right heart enlargement
3. Myocarditis / pericarditis with pleuritis
   (a) viral infection
   (b) tuberculosis
   (c) rheumatic fever (poststreptococcal infection)
4. Tumor: metastatic, mesothelioma
5. Collagen-vascular disease
   (a) SLE (pleural + pericardial effusion)
   (b) rheumatoid arthritis

Pleural Effusion & Hilar Enlargement

1. Pulmonary embolus
2. Tumor
   (a) bronchogenic carcinoma
   (b) lymphoma
   (c) metastasis
3. Tuberculosis
4. Fungal infection (rare)
5. Sarcoidosis (very rare)

Pleural Effusion & Subsegmental Atelectasis

1. Postoperative (thoracotomy, splenectomy, renal surgery) secondary to thoracic splinting + mucous plugging of small airway
2. Pulmonary embolus
3. Abdominal mass
4. Ascites
5. Rib fractures

Pleural Effusion & Lobar Densities

1. Pneumonia with empyema
2. Pulmonary embolism
3. Neoplasm
   (a) bronchogenic carcinoma (common)
   (b) lymphoma
4. Tuberculosis

Hemothorax

A. TRAUMA
   1. Closed / penetrating injury
   2. Surgery
   3. Interventional procedures: thoracentesis, pleural biopsy, catheter placement
B. BLEEDING DIATHESIS
   1. Anticoagulant therapy
   2. Thrombocytopenia
   3. Factor deficiency
C. VASCULAR
   1. Pulmonary infarct
   2. Arteriovenous malformation
   3. Aortic dissection
   4. Leaking atherosclerotic aneurysm
D. MALIGNANCY
   1. Mesothelioma
   2. Lung cancer
   3. Metastasis
   4. Leukemia
E. OTHER
   1. Catamenial hemorrhage
   2. Extramedullary hematopoiesis

√ rapidly enlarging high-attenuation pleural effusion
√ heterogeneous attenuation
√ hyperattenuating areas of debris
√ fluid-hematocrit level

Solitary Pleural Mass

= density with incomplete margins and tapered superior + inferior borders

1. Loculated pleural effusion ("vanishing tumor")
2. Organized empyema
3. Metastasis
4. Local benign mesothelioma
5. Subpleural lipoma: may erode adjacent rib
6. Hematoma
7. Mesothelial cyst
8. Neural tumor: schwannoma, neurofibroma
9. Localized fibrous tumor of pleura
10. **Fibrin bodies**
    = 3–4 cm large tumorlike concentrations of fibrin forming in serofibrinous pleural effusions; usually near lung base

DDx: chest wall mass (rib destruction reliable sign of chest wall mass)

Multiple Pleural Densities

√ diffuse pleural thickening with lobulated borders

1. Loculated pleural effusion:
   infectious, hemorrhagic, neoplastic
2. Pleural plaques
3. Metastasis (most common cause)
   Origin: lung (40%), breast (20%), lymphoma (10%), melanoma, ovary, uterus, GI tract, pancreas, sarcoma
   ◊ Metastatic adenocarcinoma histologically similar to malignant mesothelioma!
4. Diffuse malignant mesothelioma
   almost always unilateral, associated with asbestos exposure
5. Invasive thymoma (rare)
   √ contiguous spread, invasion of pleura, spreads around lung
   √ NO pleural effusion
6. **Thoracic splenosis**
   = autotransplantation of splenic tissue to pleural space following thoracoabdominal trauma; discovered 10–30 years later

- asymptomatic / recurrent hemoptysis
- √ one or several nodules in left pleura / fissures measuring several mm to 6 cm
- √ positive Tc-99m–sulfur colloid scan, indium-111–labeled platelets, Tc-99m–labeled heat-damaged RBCs

mnemonic: "**M**ary **T**yler **M**oore **L**ikes **L**emon"
Metastases (especially adenocarcinoma)
Thymoma (malignant)
Malignant mesothelioma
Loculated pleural effusion
Lymphoma

Pleural Thickening

A. TRAUMA
1. **Fibrothorax** (most common cause)
   = organizing effusion / hemothorax / pyothorax
   √ dense fibrous layer of approx. 2 cm thickness; almost always on visceral pleura
   √ frequent calcification on inner aspect of pleural peel

B. INFECTION
1. Chronic empyema: over bases; history of pneumonia; parenchymal scars
2. Tuberculosis / histoplasmosis: lung apex; associated with apical cavity
3. Aspergilloma: in preexisting cavity concomitant with pleural thickening

C. COLLAGEN-VASCULAR DISEASE
1. Rheumatoid arthritis: pleural effusion fails to resolve

D. INHALATIONAL DISORDER
1. Asbestos exposure: lower lateral chest wall; basilar interstitial disease (<25%); thickening of parietal pleura with sparing of visceral pleura
2. Talcosis

E. NEOPLASM
1. Metastases: often nodular appearance; may be obscured by effusion
2. Diffuse malignant mesothelioma
3. Pancoast tumor

F. OTHER
1. **Pleural hyaloserositis**
   Path: hyaline sclerotic tissue = cartilagelike whitish sugar icing appearance (Zuckerguss) with occasional calcification
2. Mimicked by extrathoracic musculature, 1st + 2nd rib companion shadow, subpleural fat, focal scarring around old rib fractures

mnemonic: "TRINI"
Trauma (healed hemothorax)
Rheumatoid arthritis (collagen vascular disease)
Inhalation disease (asbestosis, talcosis)
Neoplasm
Infection

Apical Cap

1. Inflammatory process: TB, healed empyema
2. Postradiation fibrosis
3. Neoplasm
4. Vascular abnormality
5. Mediastinal hemorrhage
6. Mediastinal lipomatosis
7. Peripheral upper lobe collapse

Pleural Calcification

A. INFECTION
1. Healed empyema
2. Tuberculosis (and Rx for TB: pneumothorax / oleothorax), histoplasmosis

B. TRAUMA
1. Healed hemothorax = fibrothorax:
   - Hx of significant chest trauma
   - √ irregular plaques of calcium usually in visceral pleura
   - √ healed rib fracture
2. Radiation therapy

C. PNEUMOCONIOSIS
1. Asbestos-related pleural disease (most common):
   √ combination of basilar reticular interstitial disease (<1/3) + pleural thickening
   √ calcifications of parietal pleura frequently diagnostic (diaphragmatic surface of pleura, bilateral but asymmetric)
2. Talcosis: similar to asbestos-related disease
3. Bakelite
4. Muscovite mica

D. HYPERCALCEMIA
1. Pancreatitis
2. Secondary hyperparathyroidism of chronic renal failure / scleroderma

E. MISCELLANEOUS
1. Mineral oil aspiration
2. Pulmonary infarction

mnemonic: "TAFT"
Tuberculosis
Asbestosis
Fluid (effusion, empyema, hematoma)
Talc

DIAPHRAGM

Bilateral Diaphragmatic Elevation

A. Shallow inspiration (most frequent)
B. Abdominal causes
   Obesity, pregnancy, ascites, large abdominal mass
C. Pulmonary causes
   (1) Bilateral atelectasis
   (2) Restrictive pulmonary disease (SLE)
D. Neuromuscular disease
   (1) Myasthenia gravis
   (2) Amyotrophic lateral sclerosis

Unilateral Diaphragmatic Elevation

1. Subpulmonic pleural effusion
   √ dome of pseudodiaphragm migrates toward the costophrenic angle and flattens
2. Altered pulmonary volume
   (a) Atelectasis
      √ associated pulmonary density
   (b) Postoperative lobectomy / pneumonectomy
      √ rib defects, metallic sutures
   (c) Hypoplastic lung
      √ small hemithorax (more often on the right), crowding of ribs, mediastinal shift, absent / small pulmonary artery, frequently associated with dextrocardia + anomalous pulmonary venous return
3. Phrenic nerve paralysis
   (a) Primary lung tumor
   (b) Malignant mediastinal tumor
   (c) Iatrogenic
   (d) Idiopathic
   √ paradoxic motion on fluoroscopy (patient in lateral position sniffing)
4. Abdominal disease
   (a) Subphrenic abscess: history of surgery, accompanied by pleural effusion
   (b) Distended stomach / colon
   (c) Interposition of colon
   (d) Liver mass (tumor, echinococcal cyst, abscess)
5. Diaphragmatic hernia
6. Eventration of diaphragm
7. Traumatic rupture of diaphragm
   associated with rib fractures, pulmonary contusion, hemothorax
8. Diaphragmatic tumor
   Mesothelioma, fibroma, lipoma, lymphoma, metastases

CHEST WALL

Chest Wall Lesions

A. EXTERNAL
   1. Cutaneous lesion: moles, neurofibroma
   2. Nipples
   3. Artifact
B. NEOPLASTIC
   1. Mesenchymal tumor
      (a) Lipoma (common): growing between ribs presenting as intrathoracic + subcutaneous mass; CT diagnostic)
      (b) Muscle tumor, fibroma
   2. Neural tumor
      Schwannoma, neurofibroma (may erode ribs inferiorly with sclerotic bone reaction), neuroma, neuroblastoma
   3. Vascular tumor
      Hemangioma, lymphangioma, hemangiopericytoma, aneurysm, false aneurysm
   4. Bone tumor *(see also Rib lesion)*
C. TRAUMATIC
   1. Hematoma
   2. Rib fracture
D. INFECTIOUS
   cellulitis, pyomyositis, abscess, necrotizing fasciitis
   1. Actinomycosis (parenchymal infiltrate, pleural effusion, chest wall mass, rib destruction, cutaneous fistulas)
   2. Aspergillosis, nocardiosis, blastomycosis, tuberculosis (rare)
   3. Pyogenic: Staphylococcus, Klebsiella
E. CHEST WALL INVASION
   1. Peripheral lung cancer (eg, Pancoast tumor)
   2. Recurrent breast cancer
   3. Lymphomatous nodes

√ incomplete border sign (due to obtuse angle)
√ smooth tapering borders (tangential views)
√ tumor pedicle suggests a benign tumor

Lung Disease with Chest Wall Extension

A. Infectious
   1. Actinomycosis
   2. Nocardia
   3. Blastomycosis
   4. Tuberculosis
B. Malignant tumor
   1. Bronchogenic carcinoma
   2. Lymphoma
   3. Metastases
   4. Mesothelioma
   5. Breast carcinoma
   6. Internal mammary node
C. Benign tumor
   1. Capillary hemangioma of infancy
   2. Cavernous hemangioma
   3. Extrapleural lipoma
   4. Abscess
   5. Hematoma

Chest Wall Tumors in Children

Malignant Tumors of Chest Wall in Children

◊ More common than benign primary chest wall tumors!

1. Ewing sarcoma of rib (most common)
   (a) older child: rib involvement in 7%, predominant involvement of pelvis + lower extremity
   (b) child <10 years: rib involvement in 30%
   DDx: osteomyelitis, unusual-appearing fracture, callus, direct spread of lung infection
2. Rhabdomyosarcoma
   relatively common in children + adolescents
   √ sclerosis / destruction / scalloping of cortex (local extension to contiguous bone)
   √ may calcify
   Metastases to: lung, occasionally lymph nodes
   Prognosis: infiltrative growth with high risk of local recurrence

3. Metastasis
   (a) Neuroblastoma
      10% present as chest wall mass
      √ may calcify
   (b) Leukemia
4. **Askin tumor**
   = PRIMITIVE NEUROECTODERMAL TUMOR
   = uncommon tumor probably arising from intercostal nerves in young Caucasian females
   Path: neuroectodermal small cell tumor containing neuron-specific enolase (may also be found in neuroblastoma)
   √ rib destruction (occasionally arising from rib) in 25–63%
   √ malignant pleural effusion
   Metastases to: bone, CNS, liver, adrenal
   DDx: Ewing sarcoma, lymphoma, chest wall hamartoma in infancy
5. Chondro- / osteosarcoma
   quite rare in pediatric patients

Benign Tumors of Chest Wall in Children

A. OSSEOUS
   1. Aneurysmal bone cyst
   2. Chondroblastoma
   3. Enchondroma
   4. Osteoblastoma
   5. Osteochondroma
   6. Osteoid osteoma
   Often associated with systemic syndrome: neurofibromatosis, histiocytosis, osteochondromatosis
   √ cortical rib destruction + soft-tissue mass
B. SOFT TISSUE
   1. Lipoma
   2. Hemangioma
   3. Lymphangioma
   4. Teratoma

Pancoast Syndrome

= superior sulcus tumor invading brachial plexus + sympathetic stellate ganglion

CLINICAL TRIAD:
1. Ipsilateral arm pain
2. Muscle wasting of hand
3. Horner syndrome = enophthalmos, ptosis, miosis, anhidrosis

Cause: lung cancer (most common), breast cancer, multiple myeloma, metastases, lymphoma, mesothelioma

BEDSIDE CHEST RADIOGRAPHY

Unexpected findings: in 37–43%
Change in diagnostic approach / therapy: in 27%
Indications:
A. Apparatus position + complications
   1. Malposition of tracheal tube (12%)
      √ tube diameter should be 1/2 to 2/3 of tracheal lumen
   2. Malposition of central venous line (9%)
      • ideal position = origin of SVC = central to valves (= beyond upper margin of 1st rib)
   3. Malposition of nasogastric tube
      – esophageal malposition
      – bronchial intubation
      – esophageal perforation
      √ may not be on film if coiled in hypopharynx
   4. Swan-Ganz line (= balloon-directed line)
      Cx: pulmonary infarction, hemorrhage, pseudoaneurysm formation, malposition
   5. Thoracostomy tube
      √ break in radiopaque material (= most proximal side hole) should be intrathoracic
      √ intrafissural placement makes tube ineffective
B. Cardiopulmonary disease
   1. Pulmonary edema
      (a) cardiac (hydrostatic)
         √ usually cardiomegaly
         √ Kerley lines
         √ pleural effusion frequent
         √ central / diffuse lung opacity
         √ rapid onset + resolution
      (b) noncardiac (permeability)
         √ cardiomegaly rare
         √ Kerley lines absent
         √ pleural effusions unusual
         √ diffuse / peripheral lung opacity
         √ delayed onset + resolution
   2. Pleural effusion
      √ homogeneous density over lower lung
      √ fluid over apex / in fissures
      √ intrafissural pseudotumor
      √ not visible in 30%
   3. Atelectasis
      • most common CXR abnormality in ICU
      √ lobar / segmental versus platelike
      √ left lung base (most frequent)
      √ rapid temporal change possible
   4. Alveolar disease = pneumonia
      • in 10% of ICU patients, 60% with ARDS
      impossible DDx: ARDS, lobar atelectasis
   5. Air leak (in 4–15% of ventilated patients)
      √ anteromedial / subpulmonic location
   6. Lung trauma
   7. Thoracic bleeding
   8. Mediastinal disease

CHEST

FUNCTION AND ANATOMY OF LUNG

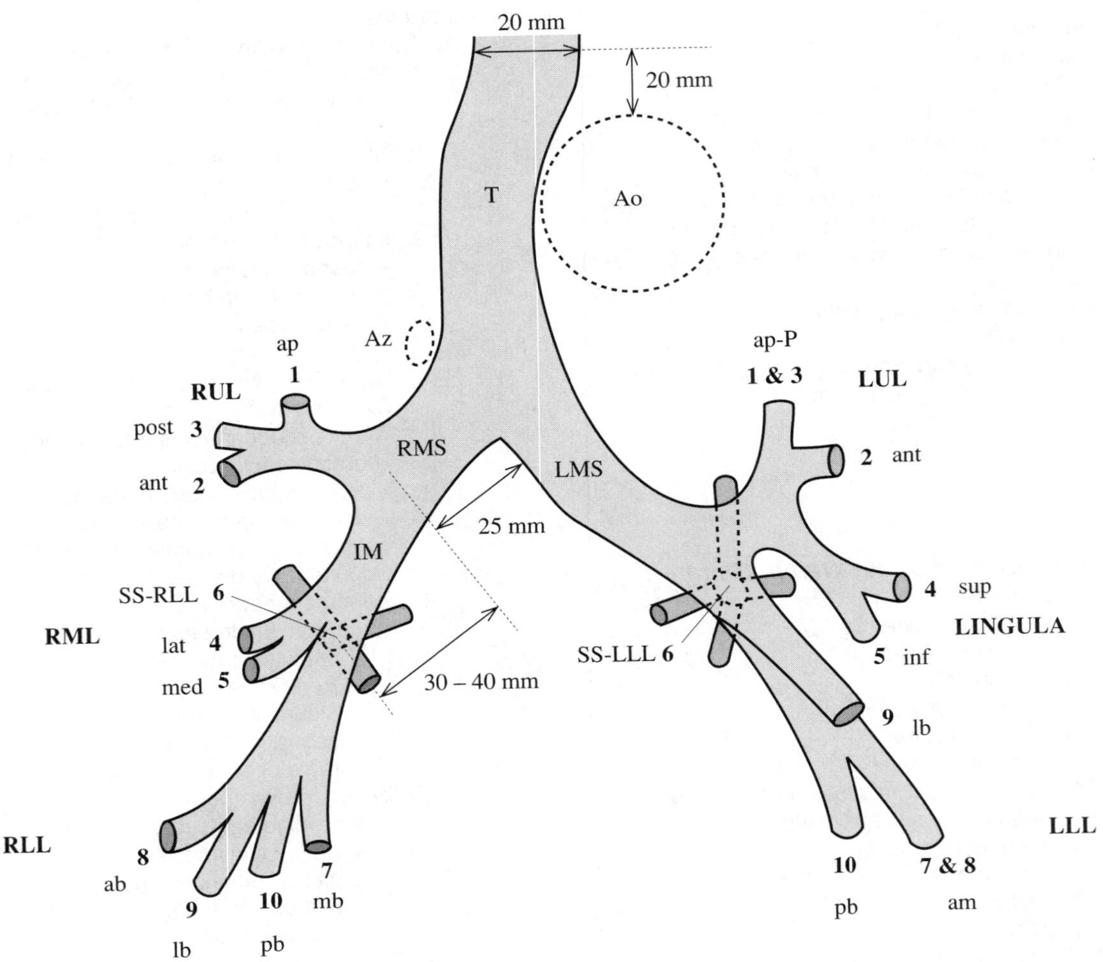

Bronchopulmonary Anatomy

Ao	=	aortic arch
Az	=	azygos vein
T	=	trachea (1st order bronchus)
SS-RLL	=	superior segment right lower lobe
RMS	=	right mainstem bronchus (2nd order bronchus)
LMS	=	left mainstem bronchus
IM	=	intermediate bronchus
SS-LLL	=	superior segment left lower lobe

RUL = right upper lobe
- 1 = apical
- 2 = anterior
- 3 = posterior

RML = right middle lobe
- 4 = lateral
- 5 = medial

RLL = right lower lobe
- 6 = superior
- 7 = mediobasal
- 8 = anterobasal
- 9 = laterobasal
- 10 = posterobasal

LUL = left upper lobe (3rd order bronchus)
- 1&3 = apicoposterior segment
- 2 = anterior (4th order bronchus)
- 4 = superior lingula
- 5 = inferior lingula

LLL = left lower lobe
- 6 = superior
- 7&8 = anteromedial
- 9 = laterobasal
- 10 = posterobasal

Order of lower lobe bronchi in frontal projection from lateral to medial:
mnemonic "ALPm" = **A**nterior-**L**ateral-**P**osterior-medial

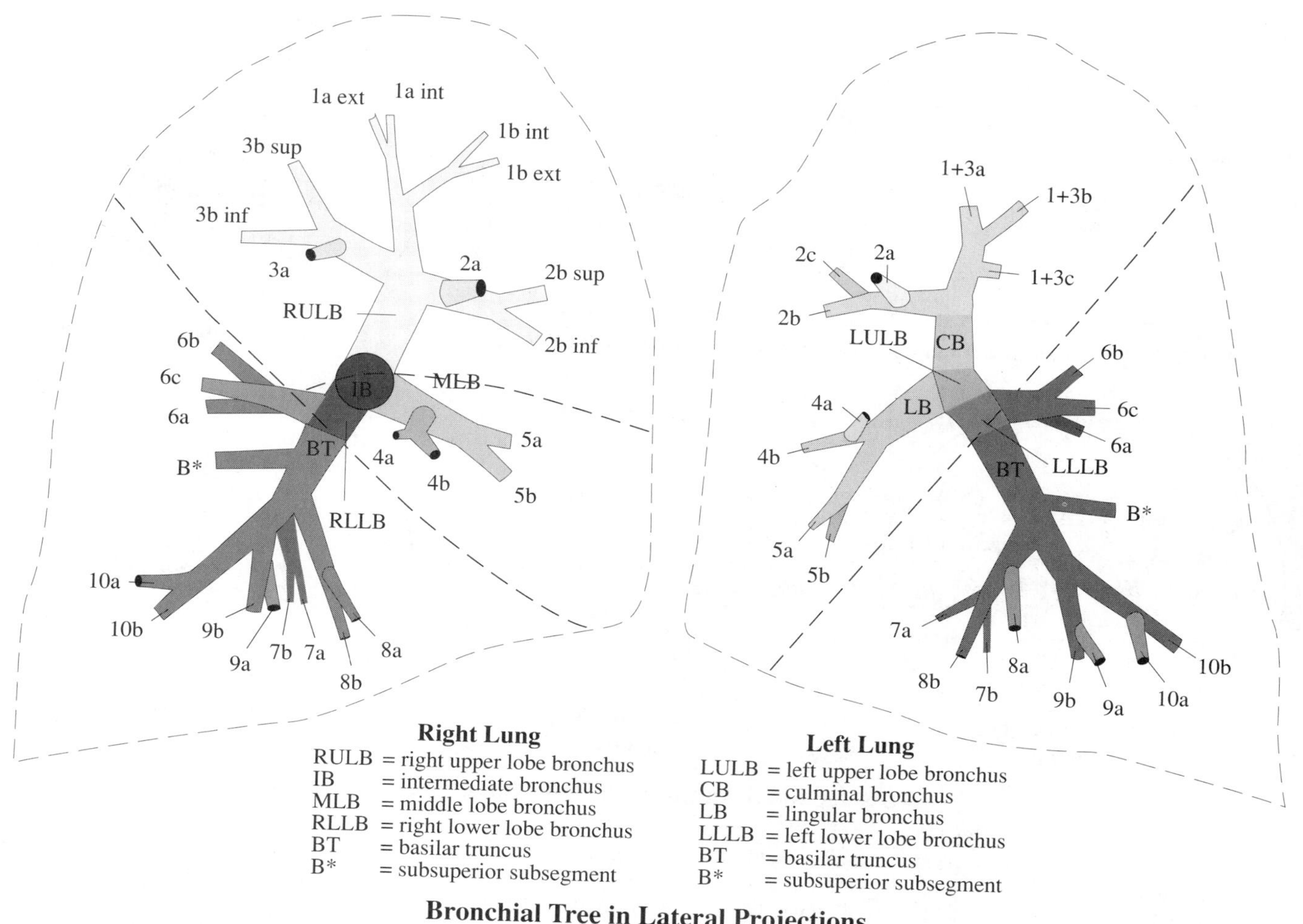

Bronchial Tree in Lateral Projections

AIRWAYS

Embryology of Airways

first 5 weeks GA	lung buds grow from ventral aspect of primitive foregut (from caudal end of laryngotracheal groove of primitive pharyngeal floor); *pulmonary agenesis*
5th week GA	trachea + esophagus separate
5–16 weeks	formation of tracheobronchial tree with bronchi, bronchioles, alveolar ducts, alveoli; *bronchogenic cyst* (= abnormal budding)*; pulmonary hypoplasia* (= fewer than expected bronchi)
16–24 weeks	dramatic increase in number + complexity of airspaces and blood vessels; *small airways + reduction in number and size of acini*

Anomalous Bronchial Division

Tracheal Bronchus

= bronchus of variable length arising from lower trachea

√ blind-ending pouch / aeration of a portion or all of the RUL

√ early origin of apicoposterior LUL bronchus (less common)

Accessory Cardiac Bronchus

= true supernumerary anomalous bronchus

M:F = 2.8:1

√ arises from medial wall of bronchus intermedius prior to origin of apical segmental RLL bronchus

√ caudal course toward pericardium

√ blind-ending pouch / ventilation of an accessory lobe

Paracardiac Bronchus

= normal bronchus arising from medial aspect of lower lobe

Prevalence: 5% of patients

Airway

= conducting branches for the transport of air; ~300,000 branching airways from trachea to bronchiole with an average of 23 airway generations

Definition:

bronchus	=	cartilage in wall
bronchiole	=	absence of cartilage (after 6 to 20 divisions of segmental bronchus)

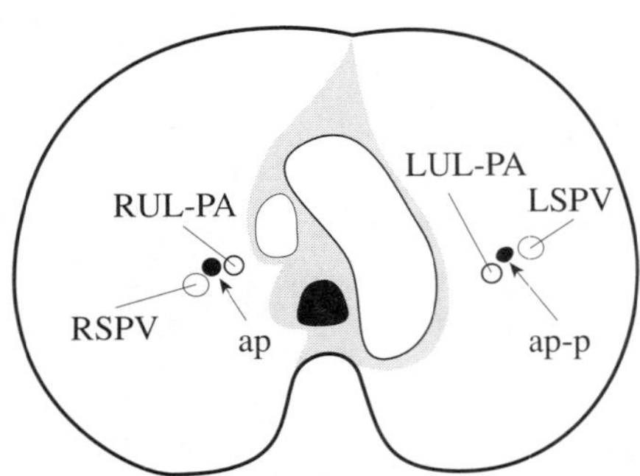

Level of Apical Segmental Bronchus

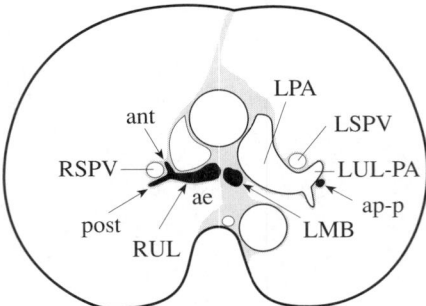

Level of Right Upper Lobe Bronchus

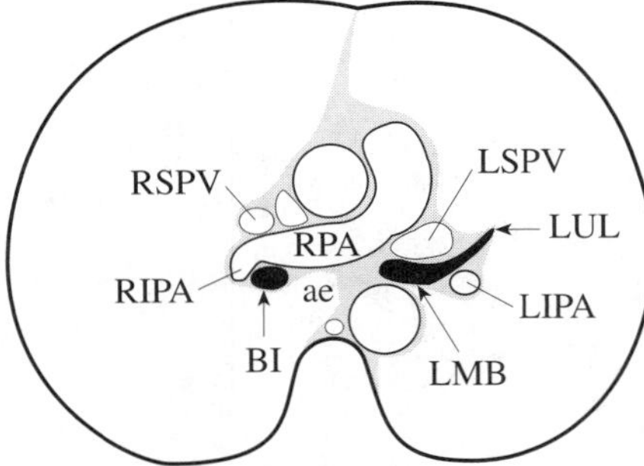

Level of Bronchus Intermedius

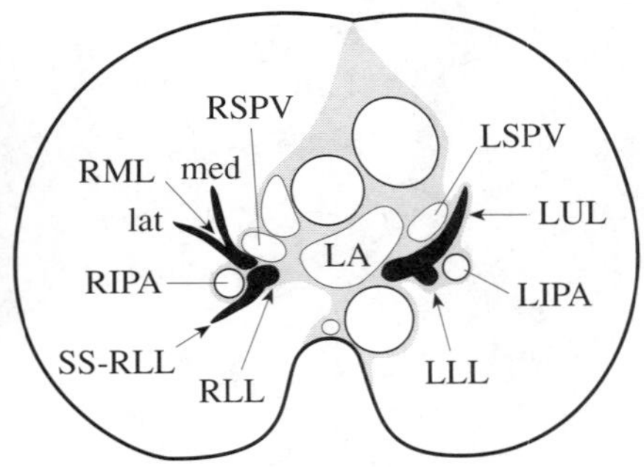

Level of Right Middle Lobe Bronchus

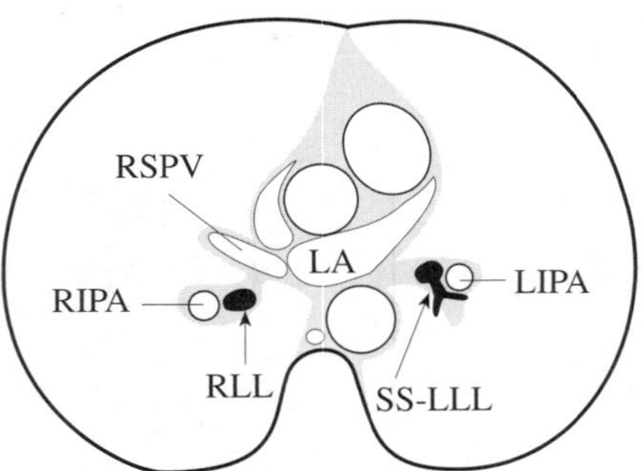

Level of Left Superior Segmental Bronchus

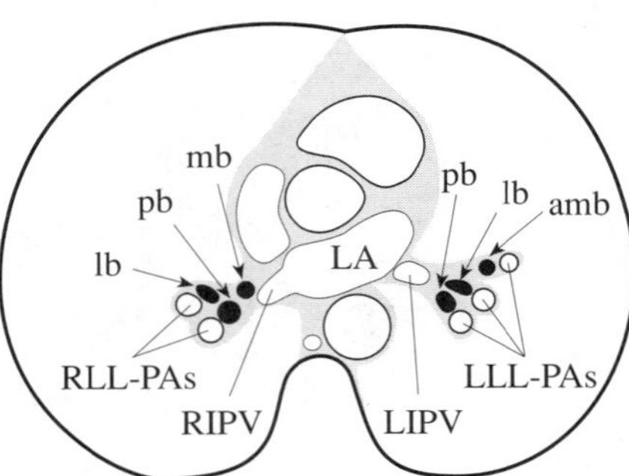

Level of Lower Lobe Bronchi

Cross-sectional Anatomy of Bronchovascular Divisions

Right

ant	= anterior RUL		pb	= posterobasal RLL
ap	= apical RUL		post	= posterior RUL
BI	= bronchus intermedius		RLL	= right lower lobe
lat	= lateral RML		RML	= right middle lobe
mb	= mediobasal RLL		RUL	= right upper lobe
med	= medial RML		s-RLL	= superior segment

Left

amb	= anteromediobasal LLL		ap-p	= apicoposterior LUL
lb	= laterobasal LLL		LLL	= left lower lobe
LMB	= left main bronchus		LUL	= left upper lobe
pb	= posterobasal LLL		s-LLL	= superior segment

ae = azygoesophageal recess

RIPV / LIPV = right / left inferior pulmonary vein
RPA / LPA = right / left pulmonary artery
RUL-PA / LUL-PA = right / left upper lobe pulmonary artery
RIPA / LIPA = right / left inferior pulmonary artery
RLL-PAs / LLL-PAs = right / left lower lobe pulmonary arteries
RSPV / LSPV = right / left superior pulmonary vein

— membranous bronchiole = purely air conducting
— respiratory bronchiole = containing alveoli in their walls
— lobular bronchiole = supplies secondary pulmonary lobule; may branch into 3 or more terminal bronchioles
— terminal bronchiole = last generation of purely conducting bronchioles; each supplying one acinus

small airways = diameter <2 mm = small cartilaginous bronchi + membranous and respiratory bronchioles; account for 25% of airway resistance

large airways = diameter >2 mm; account for 75% of airway resistance

HRCT of normal lung (window level –700 HU, window width 1,000–1,500):

√ –875 ± 18 HU at inspiration;
√ –620 ± 43 HU at expiration
√ 8th order bronchi visible = bronchi >2 mm in diameter
◊ Normal lobular bronchioles not visible!

Acinus

= functionally most important subunit of lung = all parenchymal tissue distal to one terminal bronchiole comprising 2–5 generations of respiratory bronchioles + alveolar ducts + alveolar sacs + alveoli

- gas exchange

√ radiologically not visible

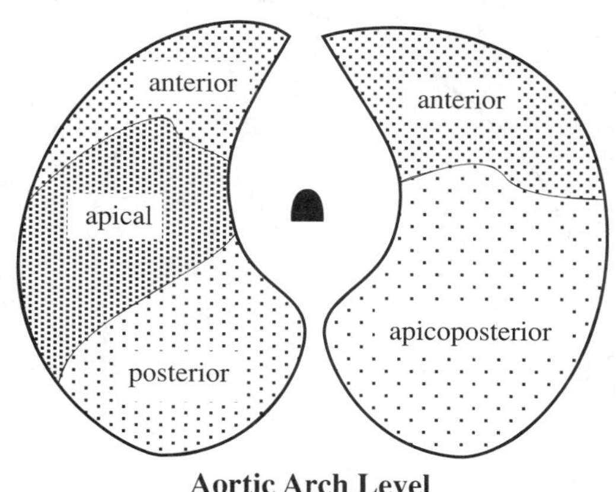

Aortic Arch Level

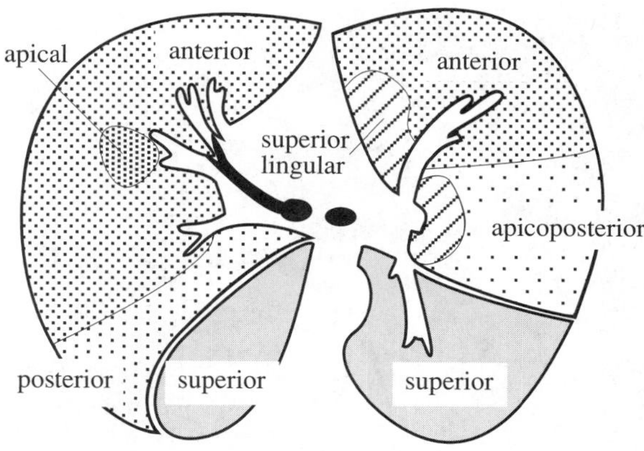

Left Pulmonary Artery Level

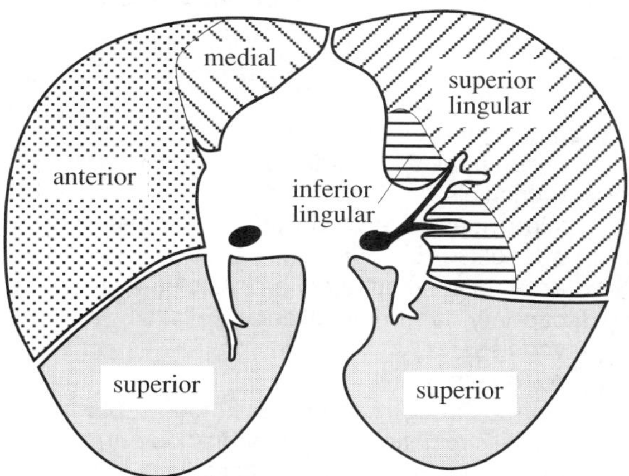

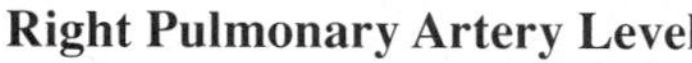
Right Pulmonary Artery Level

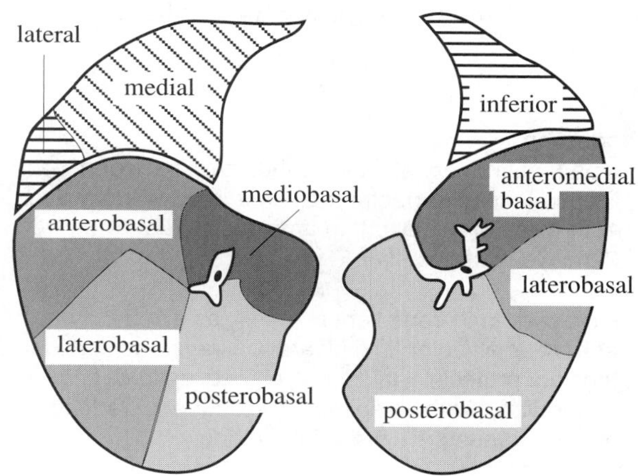

Cardiac Ventricular Level

Cross-sectional Anatomy of Lung Segments

[Primary Pulmonary Lobule]
= alveolar duct + air spaces connected with it

Secondary Pulmonary Lobule
= REID LOBULE
= smallest portion of lung surrounded by connective tissue septa = basic anatomic + functional pulmonary unit appearing as an irregular polyhedron; separated from each other by thin fibrous interlobular septa (100 μm); supplied by 3–5 terminal bronchioles; contains 3–24 acini

Size: 10–25 mm in diameter
- visible on surface of lung

Contents:
- — centrally = lobular core: branches of terminal bronchioles (0.1 mm wall thickness is below the resolution of HRCT) + pulmonary arterioles (1 mm)
- — peripherally (in interlobular septa): pulmonary vein + lymph vessels

HRCT:
- √ barely visible fine lines of increased attenuation in contact with pleura (= interlobular septa); best developed in subpleural areas of
  - — UL + ML: anterior + lateral + juxtamediastinal
  - — LL: anterior + diaphragmatic regions
- √ dotlike / linear / branching structures (= pulmonary arterioles) near center of secondary pulmonary lobule 3–5 mm from pleura

Surfactant
= surface-active material essential for normal pulmonary function

Substrate:
phospholipids (phosphatidylcholine, phosphatidylglycerol), other lipids, cholesterol, lung-specific proteins

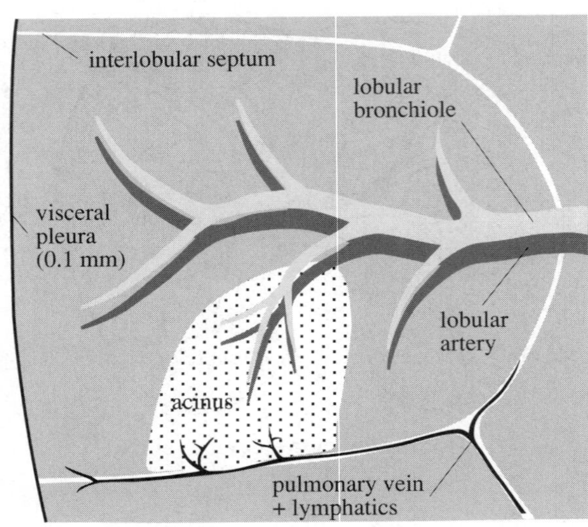

The Secondary Pulmonary Lobule

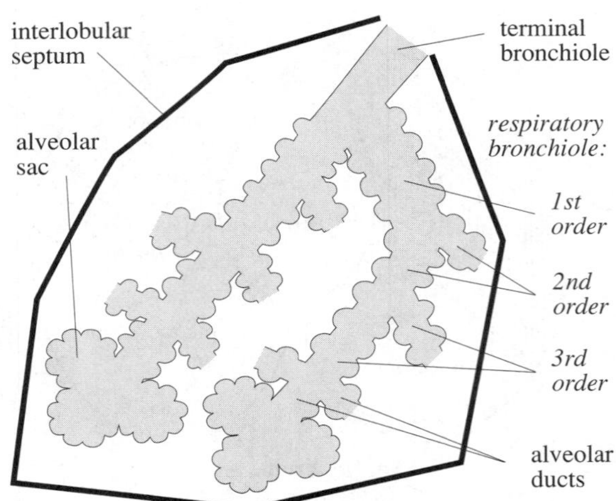

Terminal Airways within the Secondary Pulmonary Lobule

Production:
type II pulmonary alveoli synthesize + transport + secrete lung surfactant; earliest production around 18th week of gestation (in amniotic fluid by 22nd week of gestation)

Action:
increases lung compliance, stabilizes alveoli, enhances alveolar fluid clearance, reverses surface tension, protects against alveolar collapse during respiration, protects epithelial cell surface, reduces opening pressure + precapillary tone

Lung Interstitium

Division	*Components*
Axial	bronchovascular sheaths lymphatics
Middle (parenchymal)	alveolar wall (interalveolar septum)
Peripheral	pleura subpleural connective tissue interlobular septa (enclosing pulmonary veins, lymphatics, walls of cortical alveoli)

PULMONARY CIRCULATION

1. Primary pulmonary circulation
   pulmonary arteries travel along lobar + segmental bronchi down to subsegmental level matching caliber of airways
   (a) large elastic pulmonary arteries (500–>1,000 μm)
   accompany lobar + segmental bronchi matching caliber of airways
   (b) muscular arteries (50–1,000 μm)
   accompany subsegmental airways + terminal bronchioles
   √ provide active vasodilatation + constriction
   (c) arterioles (15–150μm)
   accompany respiratory bronchioles + alveolar ducts
   (d) capillary network in alveolar walls
   (e) venules
   (f) pulmonary veins
   course through interlobular fibrous septa
2. Bronchial circulation (1% of cardiac output)
   Origin: thoracic aorta, intercostal arteries (2 vessels for each lung)
   Supply: esophagus, trachea, visceral pleura, lymph nodes, extra- and intrapulmonary airways, bronchovascular + neural bundles, vasa vasorum of pulmonary circulation
   Course: tortuous path along peribronchial sheath of mainstem airway to terminal bronchioles
3. Anastomoses: through microvascular connections;
   √ bronchial blood flow may increase by 300% in the weeks following pulmonary artery embolization

LUNG FUNCTION

Lung Volumes & Capacities

1. Tidal volume (**TV**)
   = amount of gas moving in and out with each respiratory cycle
2. Residual volume (**RV**)
   = amount of gas remaining in the lung after a maximal expiration
3. Total lung capacity (**TLC**)
   = gas contained in lung at the end of a maximal inspiration
4. Vital capacity (**VC**)
   = amount of gas that can be expired after a maximal inspiration without force

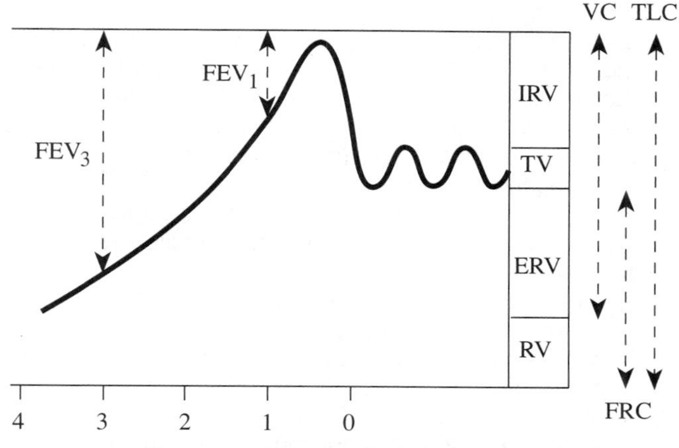

Lung Volumes and Capacities

5. Functional residual capacity (**FRC**)
   = volume of gas remaining in lungs at the end of a quiet expiration

Changes In Lung Volumes

A. DECREASED VC:
   1. Reduction in functioning lung tissue due to
      (a) space-occupying process (eg, pneumonia, infarction)
      (b) surgical removal of lung tissue
   2. Process reducing overall volume of the lungs (eg, diffuse pulmonary fibrosis)
   3. Inability to expand lungs due to
      (a) muscular weakness (eg, poliomyelitis)
      (b) increase in abdominal volume (eg, pregnancy)
      (c) pleural effusion

B. INCREASED FRC and RV:
   characteristic of air trapping and overinflation (eg, asthma, emphysema)
   Associated with: increased TLC
   √ normal level of inflation to 8 posterior ribs

C. DECREASED FRC and RV:
   1. Process reducing overall volume of lungs (eg, diffuse pulmonary fibrosis)
   2. Process that occupies volume within alveoli (eg, alveolar microlithiasis)
   3. Process that elevates diaphragm (eg, ascites, pregnancy), usually associated with decreased TLC

Flow Rates

A. Spirometric measurements:
   1. Forced expiratory volume (FEV)
      = amount of air expired during a certain period (usually 1 + 3 sec);
      Normal values: **FEV_1** = 83%; **FEV_3** = 97%
   2. Maximal midexpiratory flow rate (MMFR)
      = amount of gas expired during the middle half of forced expiratory volume curve (largely effort independent)
      Indicator of small airway resistance
   3. Flow-volume loop
      = gas flow is plotted against the actual volume of lung at which this flow is occurring
      Useful in identifying obstruction in large airways

B. Resistance in small airways
   Closing volume = lung volume at which dependent lung zones cease to ventilate because of airway closure in small airway disease or loss of lung elastic recoil
   - decrease in FEV, MMFR, MBC:
     (a) expiratory airway obstruction (reversible as in spasmodic asthma / irreversible as in emphysema)
     (b) respiratory muscle weakness

Diffusing Capacity

= rate of gas transfer across the alveolocapillary membrane in relation to a constant pressure difference across it; measured by the carbon monoxide diffusion method DL_{CO}.

Technique:
» patient inspires maximally a gas with a known small concentration of CO
» holds his/her breath for 10 seconds and then slowly expires to residual volume (RV)
» an aliquot of the end-expired (alveolar) gas is analyzed for amount of CO absorbed during breath

Measurement: in mL of CO absorbed/min/mm Hg
Reduction:
1. Ventilation / perfusion inequality: less CO is taken up by poorly ventilated or poorly perfused areas (eg, emphysema)
2. Reduction of total surface area (eg, emphysema, surgical resection)
3. Reduction in permeability from thickening of alveolar membrane (eg, cellular infiltration, edema, interstitial fibrosis)
4. Anemia with lack of hemoglobin

Arterial Blood Gas Abnormalities

- decreased pulmonary arterial O_2:
  1. Alveolar hypoventilation
  2. Impaired diffusion
  3. Abnormal ventilation/perfusion ratios
  4. Anatomic shunting

- elevated pulmonary arterial CO_2:
  1. Alveolar hypoventilation
  2. Impaired ventilation / perfusion ratios

V/Q Inequality

A. NORMAL
   (a) blood flow decreases rapidly from base to apex
   (b) ventilation decreases less rapidly from base to apex

◊ V/Q is low at base and high at apex
◊ Pulmonary arterial O_2 is substantially higher at apex
◊ Pulmonary arterial CO_2 is substantially higher at base

B. ABNORMAL
chiefly resulting from non- / underventilated lung regions (non- / underperfused regions do not result in blood gas disturbances)

Compliance

= relationship of the change in intrapleural pressure to the volume of gas that moves into the lungs

A. DECREASED COMPLIANCE
edema, fibrosis, granulomatous infiltration

B. INCREASED COMPLIANCE
emphysema (faulty elastic architecture)

√ height of diaphragm at TLC can provide some indication of lung compliance, particularly valuable in sequential roentgenograms for comparison in:
1. Diffuse interstitial pulmonary edema
2. Diffuse interstitial pulmonary fibrosis

MEDIASTINUM

Terminology: Spigelius (1578–1626): "Quod per medium stat" = what sits in the middle

A. SUPERIOR MEDIASTINAL COMPARTMENT
= thoracic inlet

B. INFERIOR MEDIASTINAL COMPARTMENT
(a) anterior mediastinum
= retrosternal region
(b) middle mediastinum
= visceral region
(c) posterior mediastinum
= contains esophagus, descending aorta, paraspinal region

THYMUS

Origin: residual thymic tissue in neck in 1.8–21%

Embryogenesis:
dorsal + ventral wings of 3rd (and possibly 4th) branchial pouch begin to form the primordia of the inferior parathyroid and thymic glands at 4th–5th week of gestation; both glands separate from pharyngeal wall + migrate caudally and medially with the thymus pulling the inferior parathyroid glands along the thymopharyngeal tract; thymic primordium fuses with its contralateral counterpart inferior to thyroid gland; thymic tail thins + disappears by 8th week

Thymic weight:
increases from birth to age 11–12 years (22 ± 13 g in neonate, 34 ± 15 g at puberty); ratio of thymic weight to body weight decreases with age (involution after puberty, total fatty replacement after age 60)
◊ Atrophies under stress (due to increase in endogenous steroids)

Extent: from manubrium to 4th costal cartilage; may bulge into neck / extend down to diaphragm

CXR:
√ prominent normal thymus visible in 50% of neonates + infants 0–2 years of age
√ notch sign = indentation at junction of thymus + heart
√ sail sign = triangular density extending from superior mediastinum, usually on right side
√ wave sign = rippled undulated lateral border due to indentation by ribs
√ shape changes with respiration + position
DDx: mediastinal mass, upper lobe pneumonia, atelectasis

CT:
√ measurement (perpendicular to axis of aortic arch): <18 mm before age 20; <13 mm after age 20
√ triangular shape like an arrowhead (62%), bilobed (32%), single lobe (6%)
√ muscular density of 30 HU (before puberty)
√ flat / concave borders with abundant fat (after puberty)
√ detected in 83% of subjects <50 years of age; in 17% of subjects >50 years of age

US (supra-, trans-, parasternal approach in infants):
√ homogeneous finely granular echotexture with some echogenic strands
√ mildly hypoechoic relative to liver, spleen, thyroid
√ smooth well-defined margin (due to fibrous capsule)
√ hypo- / avascular

Ectopic Thymus

√ solid mass
√ cystic mass (= endodermal-lined cavity of thymopharyngeal duct / cystic degeneration of Hassall corpuscles or glandular epithelium)

(1) Unilateral failure of thymic primordium to descend
√ neck mass of thymic tissue on one side of neck
√ ipsilateral absence of normal thymic lobe
√ parathyroid tissue within ectopic thymus

(2) Small rest of thymus left behind within thymopharyngeal tract during migration
√ neck mass
√ normally positioned bilobed thymus

(3) Atypical location: trachea, skull base, intrathyroidal

CHEST DISORDERS

ACUTE EOSINOPHILIC PNEUMONIA

Etiology: idiopathic (no evidence of infection / exposure to potential antigens) with abrupt increase in lung cytokines
Age: 32 ± 17 years; M > F
Histo: eosinophilic infiltrates + pulmonary edema (from release of eosinophilic granules altering vascular permeability)
- acute respiratory failure in previously healthy individuals
- markedly elevated levels of eosinophils in bronchoalveolar lavage fluid
- no peripheral eosinophilia
- acute febrile illness of 1–5 day's duration, myalgia

√ bilateral interstitial + air space opacities
√ pleural effusion
Rx: IV corticosteroids
Dx: bronchoscopy with bronchopulmonary lavage
DDx: chronic eosinophilic pneumonia (infiltrates with peripheral predominance)

AIDS

= ACQUIRED IMMUNE DEFICIENCY SYNDROME
= ultimately fatal disease characterized by HIV seropositivity, specific opportunistic infections, specific malignant neoplasms (Kaposi sarcoma, Burkitt lymphoma, primary lymphoma of brain)
= patient with CD4 cell count <200 cells/μL (normal range, 800–1,200 cells/μL)
Incidence: 2 million Americans are infected with HIV + 270,000 have AIDS (estimate in 1993); >50% develop pulmonary disease
Organism: human immunodeficiency virus (HIV) = human T-cell lymphotropic virus type III (HTLV III) = lymphadenopathy-associated virus (LAV)

Pathomechanism:
HIV retrovirus attaches to CD4 molecule on surface of T-helper lymphocytes + macrophages + microglial cells; after cellular invasion HIV genetic information is incorporated into cell's chromosomal DNA; virus remains dormant for weeks to years; after an unknown stimulus for viral replication CD4 lymphocytes are destroyed (normal range of 800–1,000 cells/mm^3) and others become infected leading to impairment of the immune system; CD4 lymphocyte number and function decreases (at an approximate rate of 50–80 cells/year)

AIDS-defining illness related to CD4 T-lymphocyte count [cells/μL]:
<400 extrapulmonary Mycobacterium tuberculosis, Kaposi sarcoma
<200 Candida albicans (thrush, hairy leukoplakia), Histoplasma capsulatum, Cryptosporidium species, Pneumocystis carinii pneumonia, non-Hodgkin lymphoma
<150 cerebral toxoplasmosis
<100 Cytomegalovirus, Herpes simplex virus, Mycobacterium avium complex (intestinal CMV + MAI infection)
<50 AIDS-related lymphoma
Prognosis: median survival with CD4 lymphocyte count <50 cells/mm^3 is 12 months
Transmission by: intimate sexual contact, exposure to contaminated blood / bloody body secretions
Groups at risk:
1. Homosexual males (74%)
2. IV drug abusers (16%)
3. Recipients of contaminated blood products (3%)
4. Sexual partner of drug abuser + bisexual man
5. Infants born to woman infected with AIDS virus

◊ HIV antibodies present in >50% of homosexuals + 90% of IV drug abusers!
◊ Rate of heterosexual transmission is increasing!

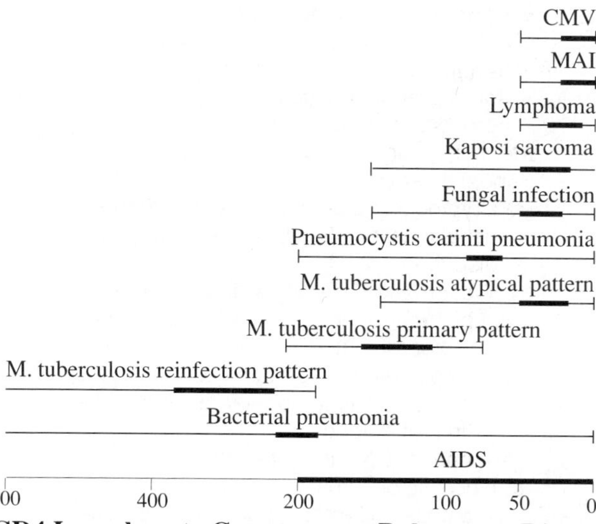

CD4 Lymphocyte Count versus Pulmonary Disease

Clinical classification:
group I acute HIV infection with seroconversion
group II asymptomatic HIV infection
group III persistent generalized lymphadenopathy
group IV other HIV disease
— subgroup A constitutional disease
— subgroup B neurologic disease
— subgroup C secondary infectious disease
— subgroup D secondary cancers
— subgroup E other conditions

AIDS-defining pulmonary conditions (CDC, 1987):
(1) Tracheal / bronchial / pulmonary candidiasis
(2) Pulmonary CMV infection
(3) Herpes simplex bronchitis / pneumonitis
(4) Kaposi sarcoma

(5) Immunoblastic / Burkitt lymphoma
(6) Pneumocystis carinii pneumonia

A. LYMPHADENOPATHY
Cause:
reactive follicular hyperplasia = HIV adenopathy (50%), AIDS-related lymphoma (20%), mycobacterial infection (17%), Kaposi sarcoma (10%), metastatic tumor, opportunistic infection with multiple organisms, drug reaction
Location: mediastinum, axilla, retrocrural

B. OPPORTUNISTIC INFECTION
accounts for majority of pulmonary disease
◊ Pulmonary infection is often the first AIDS-defining illness!
1. Pneumocystis carinii pneumonia (60–80%)
20–40% develop >1 episode during disease
• CD4+ T helper lymphocyte cell count ≤200/mm³
• subacute insidious onset with malaise, minimal cough
√ bilateral ground-glass infiltrates without effusion / adenopathy
√ bilateral perihilar interstitial infiltrates
√ diffuse bilateral alveolar infiltrates
√ frequently associated with pneumatoceles
√ apical predominance (in patients on prophylactic aerosolized pentamidine)
Mortality: in 25% fatal
2. Fungal disease (<5%)
(a) Cryptococcus neoformans pneumonia (2–15%) usually associated with brain / meningeal disease
√ segmental infiltrate + superimposed pulmonary nodules ± lymphadenopathy ± pleural effusion
(b) Histoplasma capsulatum
√ typically diffuse nodular / miliary pattern at time of diagnosis
√ normal CXR in up to 35%
(c) Coccidioides immitis
√ diffuse infiltrates + thin-walled cavities
(d) Candida albicans
(e) Aspergillus: less common + less invasive due to relative preservation of neutrophilic function
– invasive pulmonary aspergillosis
– chronic necrotizing aspergillosis
– necrotizing tracheobronchitis
– obstructing bronchopulmonary aspergillosis
3. Mycobacterial infection (10% per year):
(a) M. tuberculosis (increasing frequency):
◊ AIDS patients are 500 times more likely to become infected than general population!
√ postprimary TB pattern with upper-lobe cavitating infiltrate (CD4 lymphocyte count of 200–500 cells/mm³)
√ primary TB pattern with lung infiltrate / lung masses + hilar / mediastinal lymphadenopathy + pleural effusion (CD4 lymphocyte count of 50–200 cells/mm³)
√ atypical TB pattern with diffuse reticular / nodular infiltrates (CD4 lymphocyte count of <50 cells/mm³)
√ adenopathy of low attenuation with rim enhancement on CECT
(b) M. avium-intracellulare (5%)
• in patients with low CD4 lymphocyte count only
√ diffuse bilateral reticulonodular infiltrates
√ adenopathy, miliary disease
(c) M. kansasii and others
4. Bacterial pneumonia (5–30%):
(a) Haemophilus influenzae, Streptococcus pneumoniae, Staphylococcus aureus
√ frequently multilobar distribution
• bacteremia (common)
(b) Nocardia pneumonia (<5%)
usually occurs in cavitating pneumonia
√ segmental / lobar alveolar infiltrate ± cavitation ± ipsilateral pleural effusion
(c) Rhodococcus equii (aerobic, Gram negative)
√ cavitary pneumonia
(d) Bartonella henselae (Gram negative)
= bacillary angiomatosis
• cutaneous lesions
√ highly vascular small pulmonary nodules
√ dramatic enhancement of enlarged lymph nodes
5. CMV pneumonia
most frequent infection found at autopsy (49–81%), diagnosed before death in only 13–24%; high combined prevalence with Kaposi sarcoma
√ bilateral hazy infiltrates, focal nodules, masses
√ bronchiectasis / bronchial wall thickening
6. Toxoplasmosis
√ coarse interstitial / nodular pattern
√ focal areas of consolidation ± cavities
DDx: indistinguishable from PCP

C. TUMOR
1. Kaposi sarcoma (15%)
Location: lung involvement (20%) preceded by widespread skin + organ involvement
Site: peribronchovascular distribution (best appreciated on CT)
√ numerous fluffy ill-defined nodules / asymmetric clusters in a vague perihilar distribution
√ interlobular septal thickening
√ pleural effusion (30%)
√ lymphadenopathy (10–35%), late in disease
2. AIDS-related lymphoma of B-cell origin (2–5%)
primarily immunoblastic NHL / Burkitt lymphoma / non-Burkitt lymphoma; occasionally Hodgkin disease
Location: pulmonary involvement (8–15%), CNS, GI tract, liver, spleen, bone marrow
Site: primarily extranodal
√ pleural effusion (50%)
√ hilar / mediastinal adenopathy (25%); ± axillary / supraclavicular / cervical adenopathy
√ solitary / multiple well-defined pulmonary nodules (occasionally with doubling time of 4–6 weeks)

√ diffuse bilateral reticulonodular heterogeneous opacities
√ alveolar infiltrates
√ paraspinal masses

D. LYMPHOID INTERSTITIAL PNEUMONITIS
Age: in children <13 years of age

E. SEPTIC EMBOLI

F. PREMATURE DEVELOPMENT OF BULLAE (40%) with disposition to spontaneous pneumothorax

AIDS-related Complex (ARC)

= GENERALIZED LYMPHADENOPATHY SYNDROME
= prodromal phase of HIV seropositivity, generalized lymphadenopathy, CNS diseases other than those associated with AIDS

Time interval: approximately 10 years between seroconversion + clinical AIDS

• weight loss, malaise, diarrhea
• fever, night sweats, lymphadenopathy
• lymphopenia with selective decrease in helper T-cells

ADULT RESPIRATORY DISTRESS SYNDROME

= SHOCK LUNG = POSTTRAUMATIC PULMONARY INSUFFICIENCY = HEMORRHAGIC LUNG SYNDROME = RESPIRATOR LUNG = STIFF LUNG SYNDROME = PUMP LUNG = CONGESTIVE ATELECTASIS = OXYGEN TOXICITY
= severe unexpected life-threatening acute respiratory distress characterized by abrupt onset of marked dyspnea, increased respiratory effort, severe hypoxemia associated with widespread airspace consolidation

Etiology:
= most severe form of permeability edema associated with diffuse alveolar damage

A. PRIMARY = DIRECT INJURY
= ARDS due to underlying pulmonary disease
= exposure to chemical agents, infectious pathogens, gastric fluid, toxic gas
Associated with: pulmonary consolidation

B. SYSTEMIC CONDITION
= ARDS due to extrapulmonary disease
= systemic biochemical cascade creating oxidating agents, inflammatory mediators, enzymes during sepsis, pancreatitis, severe trauma, blood transfusion
Associated with: interstitial edema, alveolar collapse

Histo:
(a) up to 12 hours: fibrin + platelet microemboli
(b) 12–24 hours: interstitial edema
(c) 24–48 hours: capillary congestion, extensive interstitial + alveolar proteinaceous edema + hemorrhage, widespread microatelectasis, destruction of type I alveolar epithelial cells
(d) 5–7 days: extensive hyaline membrane formation, hypertrophy + hyperplasia of type II alveolar lining cells
(e) 7–14 days: extensive fibroblastic proliferation in interstitium + within alveoli, rapidly progressing collagen deposition + fibrosis; almost invariably associated with infection

Predisposed:
hemorrhagic / septic shock, massive trauma (pulmonary / general body), acute pancreatitis, aspiration of liquid gastric contents, heroine / methadone intoxication, massive viral pneumonia, traumatic fat embolism, near-drowning, conditions leading to pulmonary edema

mnemonic: "DICTIONARIES"
Disseminated intravascular coagulation
Infection
Caught drowning
Trauma
Inhalants: smoke, phosgene, NO_2
O$_2$ toxicity
Narcotics + other drugs
Aspiration
Radiation
Includes pancreatitis
Emboli: amniotic fluid, fat
Shock: septic, hemorrhagic, cardiogenic, anaphylactic

• initially few / no symptoms
• rapidly progressive dyspnea, tachypnea, cyanosis
• hypoxia unresponsive to oxygen therapy (due to arteriovenous shunting)
• no increase in pulmonary capillary pressure

Stages (often overlapping):

1st (exudative) stage
interstitial edema with high protein content rapidly filling the alveolar spaces
associated with hemorrhage + ensuing hyaline membrane formation
√ interstitial edema (with high protein content) initially
√ perihilar areas of increased opacity following rapidly
√ widespread alveolar consolidation with predominantly peripheral cortical distribution
√ air bronchogram
√ gravitational gradient (best seen on CT) due to dependent atelectasis
DDx: cardiogenic edema (cardiomegaly, apical vascular distribution, Kerley lines)

2nd (proliferative) stage
organization of fibrinous exudate
subsequent regeneration of alveolar lining + thickening of alveolar septa
√ inhomogeneous areas of ground-glass opacities

3rd (fibrotic) stage
varying degrees of scarring
√ subpleural and intrapulmonary cysts
Cx: pneumothorax

CXR:
√ NO cardiomegaly / pleural effusion
— up to 12 hours:
√ characteristic 12-hour delay between clinical onset of respiratory failure and CXR abnormalities

CHEST

— 12–24 hours:
√ patchy ill-defined opacities throughout both lungs
— 24–48 hours:
√ massive airspace consolidation of both lungs
— 5–7 days:
√ consolidation becomes inhomogeneous (resolution of alveolar edema)
√ local areas of consolidation (pneumonia)
— >7 days:
√ reticular / bubbly lung pattern (diffuse interstitial + airspace fibrosis)

Complication of continuous positive pressure ventilation (= **barotrauma**)
Path:
(a) rupture of alveoli along margins of interlobular septa + vascular structures (= parenchymal pseudocyst)
(b) air dissection along interlobular septa + perivascular spaces (= interstitial emphysema)
√ "pseudoclearing" of RDS
(c) interstitial air rupturing into pleural space (= pneumothorax) / into mediastinum (= pneumomediastinum) / into pericardial cavity (= pneumoperitoneum)
(d) interstitial air rupturing into peritoneal space (= pneumoperitoneum) pneumopericardium) / retroperitoneal space (=pneumoretroperitoneum)
(e) air dissecting into skin (= subcutaneous emphysema)
(f) air rupturing into vessel (= gas embolism)
√ mottled air opacities often outlining bronchovascular bundles
√ large subpleural cysts without definable wall usually at diaphragmatic + mediastinal surface compressing adjacent lung
Rx: mechanical ventilatory assistance with positive end-expiratory pressure (to increase oxygen diffusion)

ALPHA-1 ANTITRYPSIN DEFICIENCY

= rare autosomal recessive disorder
alpha-1 antitrypsin (glycoprotein) is to >90% synthesized in hepatocytes + released into serum
Gene: codominant gene expression on chromosome 14 with >100 genetic variants of the protein; most severe hepatopulmonary manifestations result from homozygous PiZZ phenotype
Action: proteolytic inhibitor of neutrophil elastase, trypsin, chymotrypsin, plasmin, thrombin, kallikrein, leukocytic + bacterial proteases; neutralizes circulating proteolytic enzymes
Mode of injury from deficiency:
PMNs + alveolar macrophages sequester into lung during recurrent bacterial infections + release neutrophil elastase, which acts unopposed + digests basement membrane
Age: early age of onset (20–30 years); M:F = 1:1
• rapid + progressive deterioration of lung function:
• dyspnea in 4th and 5th decade
◊ 20% of homozygotic individuals never develop clinically apparent emphysema
• chronic sputum production (50%)
√ severe panacinar emphysema with basilar predominance (due to gravitational distribution of pulmonary blood flow):
√ reduction in size + number of pulmonary vessels in lower lobes
√ redistribution of blood flow to unaffected upper lung zones
√ bullae at both lung bases
√ marked flattening of diaphragm
√ minimal diaphragmatic excursion
√ multilobar cystic bronchiectasis (40%)
√ hepatopulmonary syndrome
Cx: hepatic cirrhosis (in homozygotic individuals)
◊ Most common metabolic liver disease in children
Prognosis: 15–20-year decrease in longevity in smokers relative to nonsmokers

ALVEOLAR MICROLITHIASIS

= very rare disease of unknown etiology characterized by myriad of calcospherites (= tiny calculi) within alveoli
Age peak: 30–50 years; begins in early life; has been identified in utero; M:F = 1:1; in 50% familial (restricted to siblings)
• usually asymptomatic (70%)
• dyspnea on exertion (reduction in residual volume)
• cyanosis, clubbing of fingers
• striking discrepancy between striking radiographic findings and mild clinical symptoms
• NORMAL serum calcium + phosphorus levels
√ very fine, sharply defined, sandlike micronodulations (<1 mm)
√ diffuse involvement of both lungs
√ intense uptake on bone scan
Prognosis:
(a) late development of pulmonary insufficiency secondary to interstitial fibrosis
(b) disease may become arrested
(c) microliths may continue to form / enlarge
DDx: "mainline" pulmonary granulomatosis = IV abuse of talc-containing drugs such as methadone (rarely as numerous + scarring + loss of volume)

ALVEOLAR PROTEINOSIS

= PULMONARY ALVEOLAR PROTEINOSIS (PAP)
= accumulation of PAS-positive phospholipid material in alveoli (= surfactant)
Etiology: ?; associated with dust exposure (eg, silicoproteinosis is histologically identical to PAP), immunodeficiency, hematologic + lymphatic malignancies, AIDS, chemotherapy
Pathophysiology:
(a) overproduction of surfactant by granular pneumocytes
(b) defective clearance of surfactant by alveolar macrophages
Histo: alveoli filled with proteinaceous material (the ONLY pure airspace disease), normal interstitium

CHEST

Age peak: 30–50 years (age range 2–70 years); M:F = 3:1
• asymptomatic (10–20%)
• gradual onset of dyspnea + cough
• weight loss, weakness, hemoptysis
• defect in diffusing capacity
√ "bat-wing" consolidation of ground-glass pattern, predominant at bases
√ small acinar nodules + coalescence + consolidation
√ patchy peripheral / primarily unilateral infiltrates (rare)
√ reticular / reticulonodular / linear interstitial pattern with Kerley B lines (late stage)
√ slow clearing over weeks or months
√ slow progression (1/3), remaining stable (2/3)
√ NO adenopathy, NO cardiomegaly, NO pleural effusion
HRCT:
  √ patchy ground-glass opacity
  √ smooth septal thickening
Cx: infections (frequently secondary to poorly functioning macrophages + excellent culture medium): Nocardia asteroides (most common), mycobacterial, fungal, Pneumocystis, CMV
Prognosis:
highly variable course with clinical and radiologic episodes of exacerbation + remissions
(a) 50% improvement / recovery
(b) 30% death within several years under progression
Rx: bronchopulmonary lavage
DDx:
(a) during acute phase: pulmonary edema, diffuse pneumonia, ARDS
(b) in chronic stage:
1. Idiopathic pulmonary hemosiderosis (boys, symmetric involvement of mid + lower zones, progression to nodular + linear pattern)
2. Hemosiderosis (bleeding diathesis)
3. Pneumoconiosis
4. Hypersensitivity pneumonitis
5. Goodpasture syndrome (more rapid changes, renal disease)
6. Desquamative interstitial pneumonia ("ground-glass" appearance, primarily basilar + peripheral)
7. Pulmonary alveolar microlithiasis (widespread discrete intraalveolar calcifications primarily in lung bases, rare familial disease)
8. Sarcoidosis (usually with lymphadenopathy)
9. Lymphoma
10. Bronchioloalveolar cell carcinoma (more focal, slowly enlarging with time)

AMNIOTIC FLUID EMBOLISM

= most common cause of maternal peripartum death
• dyspnea
• shock during / after labor + delivery
Pathogenesis: amniotic debris enters maternal circulation resulting in:
(1) pulmonary embolization
(2) anaphylactoid reaction
(3) DIC
√ usually fatal before radiographs obtained
√ may demonstrate pulmonary edema

AMYLOIDOSIS

= disease characterized by an extracellular deposit of proteinaceous twisted ß-pleated sheet fibrils of great chemical diversity
Histo: protein (immunoglobulin) / polysaccharide complex; affinity for Congo red stain
@ Lung involvement
Incidence: 1° amyloidosis (in up to 70%), 2° amyloidosis (rare)
A. TRACHEOBRONCHIAL TYPE (most common)
• hemoptysis (most frequent complaint)
• stridor, cough, dyspnea, hoarseness, wheezing
√ multiple nodules protruding from wall of trachea / large bronchi
√ diffuse rigid narrowing of a long tracheal segment
√ prominent bronchovascular markings
√ destructive pneumonitis
B. NODULAR TYPE
Age: >60 years of age; M:F = 1:1
• usually asymptomatic
√ mediastinal / hilar adenopathy
√ solitary / multiple parenchymal nodules in a peripheral / subpleural location ± central calcification / ossification; slow growth over years
√ ± pleural effusion
DDx: metastatic disease, granulomatous disease, rheumatoid lung, sarcoidosis, mucoid impaction
C. DIFFUSE PARENCHYMAL TYPE (least common)
Age: >60 years of age
• usually asymptomatic with normal CXR
• cough + dyspnea with abnormal CXR
√ widespread small irregular densities (exclusively interstitial involvement) ± calcification
√ may become confluent ± honeycombing
DDx: idiopathic interstitial fibrosis, pneumoconiosis (especially asbestosis), rheumatoid lung, Langerhans cell histiocytosis, scleroderma

ASBESTOS-RELATED DISEASE

[*asbestos*, Greek = inextinguishable = several fibrous silicate minerals sharing the property of heat resistance]
Substances:
aspect (length-to-diameter) ratio effects carcinogenicity:
eg, aspect ratio of 32 = 8 μm long, 0.25 μm wide
– commercial amphiboles: crocidolite, amosite
– commercial serpentines (= nonamphiboles): chrysotile (the only mineral in the serpentine group accounting for >90% of asbestos used in the United States)
– noncommercial contaminating amphiboles: actinolite, anthophyllite, tremolite
(a) relatively benign:
(1) chrysotile (white asbestos) in Canada
(2) anthophyllite in Finland, North America
(3) tremolite

(b) relatively malignant:
(1) crocidolite (blue / black asbestos) in South Africa, Australia
(2) amosite (brown asbestos)
◊ Very fine fibers (crocidolite) associated with largest number of pleural disease!
◊ Asbestos fibers up to 100 μm in length

Occupational exposure:
(a) asbestos mining, milling, and processing
(b) insulation manufacturing, textile manufacturing, construction, shipbuilding, gaskets, brake linings

Asbestos-related Pleural Disease

1. Pleural Effusion (21%)
= earliest asbestos-related pleural abnormality, frequently followed by diffuse pleural thickening + rounded atelectasis
Prevalence: 3% (increases with increasing levels of asbestos exposure)
Latency period: 8–10 years after exposure
• **benign asbestos pleurisy:**
• may be associated with chest pain (1/3)
• usually small sterile, serous / hemorrhagic exudate
√ recurrent bilateral effusions
√ ± plaque formation
DDx: TB, mesothelioma

2. Focal Pleural Plaques (65%)
= hyalinized collagen in submesothelial layer of parietal pleura
Incidence: most common manifestation of exposure; 6% of general population will show plaques
Latency period: in 10% after 20 years; in 50% after 40 years
Histo: dense hypocellular undulating collagen fibers often arranged in a "basket weave" pattern ± focal / massive calcifications; may contain large numbers of asbestos fibers (almost exclusively chrysotile)
Location: bilateral + multifocal; posterolateral midportion of chest wall between 7–10th rib; aponeurotic portion of diaphragm; mediastinum; following rib contours; apices + costophrenic angles typically spared
Site: parietal pleura (visceral pleura typically spared)
• asymptomatic, no functional impairment
√ usually focal area of pleural thickening (<1 cm thick) with edges thicker than central portions of plaque; in 48% only finding; in 41% with parenchymal changes; stable over time
√ no hilar adenopathy
√ usually not calcified
DDx: chest wall fat, rib fractures, rib companion shadows

3. Pleural Calcification (21–25–60%)
◊ HALLMARK of asbestos exposure!
detected by radiography in 25%, by CT in 60%
Overall incidence: 20%
Latent period: >20 years to become visible; in 40% after 40 years
Histo: calcification starts in parietal pleura; calcium deposits may form within center of plaques
√ dense lines paralleling the chest wall, mediastinum, pericardium, diaphragm (bilateral diaphragmatic calcifications with clear costophrenic angles are (PATHOGNOMONIC)
√ advanced calcifications are leaflike with thick-rolled edges
DDx: talc exposure, hemothorax, empyema, therapeutic pneumothorax for TB (often unilateral, extensive sheetlike, on visceral pleura)

4. Diffuse Pleural Thickening (17%)
= smooth uninterrupted diffuse thickening of parietal pleura extending over at least 1/4 of chest wall (visceral pleura involved in 90%, but difficult to demonstrate)
• may cause restriction of pulmonary function
May be associated with: rounded atelectasis
√ bilateral process with "shaggy heart" appearance (20%)
√ smooth; difficult to assess when viewed en face
√ thickening of interlobar fissures
√ focally thickened diaphragm
√ obliterated costophrenic angles (minority of cases)
DDx: pleural thickening from parapneumonic effusion, hemothorax, connective tissue disease

Pulmonary Asbestosis

= (term asbestosis reserved for) chronic progressive diffuse interstitial fibrosis
Incidence: in 49–52% of industrial asbestos exposure
Latency period: 40–45 years; dose-effect relationship
Histo: interstitial fibrosis begins around respiratory bronchioles, then progresses to involve adjacent alveoli
Diagnostic criteria:
1. Reliable history of exposure
2. Appropriate time interval between exposure + detection
3. CXR evidence
4. Restrictive pattern of lung impairment
5. Abnormal diffusing capacity
6. Bilateral crackles at posterior lung bases, not cleared by cough

• dyspnea
• restrictive pulmonary function tests: progressive reduction of vital capacity + diffusing capacity
• asbestos bodies in bronchoalveolar lavage fluid
Location: most severe in lower posterior subpleural zones (concentration of asbestos fibers beneath visceral pleura)
√ small irregular linear opacities (NOT rounded as in coal / silica) progress from fine to coarse reticulation
√ confined to lung bases, progressing superiorly

√ septal lines (= fibrous thickening around secondary lobules)
√ "shaggy" heart border = obscuration secondary to parenchymal + pleural changes
√ ill-defined outline of diaphragm
√ honeycombing (uncommon)
√ rarely massive fibrosis, predominantly at lung bases without migration toward hilum (DDx from silicosis / CWP)
√ NO hilar adenopathy
√ Ga-67 uptake gives a quantitative index of inflammatory activity

HRCT:
- ◊ Obtain scan in prone position to differentiate from gravity-related physiologic phenomena
- √ thickened intralobular lines as initial finding (due to centrilobular peribronchiolar fibrosis):
  - √ multiple subpleural curvilinear branching lines ("subpleural pulmonary arcades") = dotlike reticulonodularities connected to the most peripheral branch of pulmonary artery
    Site: most prominent posteriorly parallel to and within 1 cm of pleura
- √ thickened interlobular septal lines (= interlobular fibrotic / edematous thickening):
  - √ reticulation = network of linear densities, usually posteriorly at lung bases
- √ parenchymal band = linear <5 cm long + several mm wide opacity, often extending to pleura, which may be thickened + retracted at site of contact
- √ patchy areas of ground-glass attenuation (= alveolar wall thickening due to fibrosis / edema)
- √ honeycombing = multiple cystic spaces <1 cm in diameter with thickened walls

DDx: idiopathic pulmonary fibrosis

Atelectatic Asbestos Pseudotumor

= ROUNDED ATELECTASIS = "FOLDED LUNG"
= infolding of redundant pleura accompanied by segmental / subsegmental atelectasis
◊ The most common of benign masses caused by asbestos exposure!

Location: posteromedial / posterolateral basal region of lower lobes (most common); frequently bilateral

√ 2.5–8 cm focal subpleural mass abutting a region of thickened pleura
√ size + shape show little progression, occasionally decrease in size

CT:
- √ rounded / lentiform / wedge-shaped peripheral mass
- √ pleural thickening ± calcification always present and frequently greatest near mass
- √ "crow's feet" = linear bands radiating from mass into lung parenchyma (54%)
- √ "vacuum cleaner" / "comet tail" sign
  = bronchovascular markings emanating from nodular subpleural mass + coursing toward ipsilateral hilum
- √ "Swiss cheese" air bronchogram (18%)
- √ partial interposition of lung between pleura + mass
- √ volume loss of affected lobe ± hyperlucency of adjacent lung

Lung Cancer in Asbestos-related Disease

Incidence: 20–25% of workers heavily exposed to asbestos

Occurrence related to:
- (a) cumulated dose of asbestos fibers
- (b) smoking (synergistic carcinogenic effect)
  - ◊ Increased risk by factor of up to 100 in smokers versus a factor of 5 in nonsmokers!
- (c) preexisting interstitial disease
- (d) occupational exposure to known carcinogen

Latency period: 25–35 years

Associated with: increased incidence of gastric carcinoma

Histo: bronchioloalveolar cell carcinoma (most common); bronchogenic carcinoma (adenocarcinoma + squamous cell)

Location: at lung base / in any location if associated with smoking

Malignant Mesothelioma

Risk: 10% over lifetime of an asbestos worker; household members of asbestos worker; residents near asbestos mines and plants

Latency period: 20–40 years

ASPERGILLOSIS

Organism:
Aspergillus fumigatus = intensely antigenic ubiquitous soil fungus existing as
- (a) conidiophores = reproductive form releasing thousands of spores
- (b) hyphae (= matured spores) characterized by 45° dichotomous branching pattern

Occurrence:
commonly in sputum of normal persons, ability to invade arteries + veins facilitating hematogenous dissemination

M:F = 3:1

Predisposed:
- (a) preexisting lung disease (tuberculosis, bronchiectasis)
- (b) impairment of immune system (alcoholism, advanced age, malnutrition, concurrent malignancy, poorly controlled diabetes, cirrhosis, sepsis)

- • positive precipitin test to Aspergillus antigen
- • elevated Aspergillus-specific IgE, IgG-ELISA, polymerase chain reaction identification

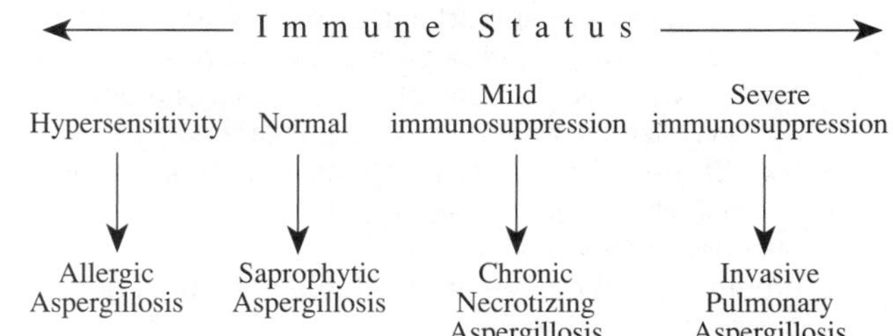

CHEST

Cx: dissemination to heart, brain, kidney, GI tract, liver, thyroid, spleen

◊ Sputum cultures are diagnostically unreliable because of normal (saprophytic) colonization of upper airways!

Noninvasive Aspergillosis

= SAPROPHYTIC ASPERGILLOSIS

= noninvasive colonization of preexisting cavity / cyst in immunologically normal patients with cavitary disease [tuberculosis, sarcoidosis (common), bronchiectasis, pulmonary fibrosis, abscess, lung trauma / surgery, ankylosing spondylitis, neurofibromatosis type 1, bullous emphysema, carcinoma]

- sputum blood-streaked / severe hemoptysis (45–95%)
- elevated serum precipitins level for Aspergillus (50%)

√ solid round gravity-dependent mass within preexisting spherical / ovoid thin-walled cavity (= Monad sign):

Histo: mycetoma = aspergilloma = **fungus ball** = masslike collection of intertwined hyphae matted together with fibrin, mucus, cellular debris colonizing a pulmonary cavity

√ air-crescent sign = crescent-shaped air space separating fungus ball from nondependent cavity wall

√ fungus ball may calcify in scattered / rimlike fashion

√ pleural thickening adjacent to preexisting cyst / cavity, commonly first sign before visualizing mycetoma

Dx: transthoracic needle biopsy / bronchial washings

DDx of other organisms causing fungus ball:
Candida albicans, Pseudallescheria boydii, Coccioides immitis, Nocardia, Actinomyces

Semiinvasive Aspergillosis

= CHRONIC NECROTIZING ASPERGILLOSIS

= chronic cavitary slowly progressive disease in patients with preexisting lung injury (COPD, radiation therapy), mild immune suppression, or debilitation (alcohol, diabetes)

- symptoms mimicking pulmonary tuberculosis

√ progressive consolidation (usually upper lobe)

√ development of air crescent and fungus ball

Dx: pathologic examination demonstrating local tissue invasion

Invasive Pulmonary Aspergillosis

= often fatal form in severely immunocompromised patients with absolute neutrophil count of <500

Predisposed: most commonly in lymphoma / leukemia patients with prolonged granulocytopenia, after organ transplantation

Path: endobronchial fungal proliferation followed by transbronchial vascular invasion eventually causes widespread hemorrhage + thrombosis of pulmonary arterioles + ischemic tissue necrosis + systemic dissemination; fungus ball = devitalized sequestrum of lung infiltrated by fungi

- Hx of series of bacterial infections + unremitting fever
- pleuritic chest pain (mimicking emboli)
- dyspnea, nonproductive cough
- progression of pulmonary infiltrates not responding to broad-spectrum antibiotics

(a) early signs

√ single / multiple ill-defined peripheral opacities

√ CT halo sign = single / multiple 1–3-cm peripheral nodules (= necrotic lung) with halo of ground-glass attenuation (= hemorrhagic edema)

√ patchy localized bronchopneumonia

(b) signs of progression

√ enlargement of nodules into diffuse bilateral consolidation

√ development into large wedge-shaped pleural-based lesions

√ air-crescent sign (in up to 50%) = cavitation of existing nodule (air crescent between retracting sequestered necrotic tissue and surrounding rim of hemorrhagic lung parenchyma) 1–3 weeks after granulocyte recovery

◊ has better prognosis than consolidation without cavitation (feature of resolution phase)

Prognosis: mortality rate of 30–90%

Dx: branching hyphae at tissue examination; sputum culture positive in only 10%

Rx: amphotericin B

Allergic Bronchopulmonary Aspergillosis

= hypersensitivity toward aspergilli in patients with long-standing asthma

Incidence: in 1–2% of patients with asthma, in 10% of patients with cystic fibrosis; most common + clinically important form

Age: mostly young patients (begins in childhood); may be undiagnosed for 10–20 years

A. ACUTE ALLERGIC BRONCHOPULMONARY ASPERGILLOSIS
Type I reaction = immediate hypersensitivity (IgE-mediated)
Histo: alveoli filled with eosinophils

B. CHRONIC ALLERGIC BRONCHOPULMONARY ASPERGILLOSIS
Type III reaction = delayed immune complex response = Arthus reaction (IgG-mediated)
Histo: bronchial damage secondary to Aspergillus antigen reacting with IgG antibodies, immune complexes activate complement leading to tissue injury

Pathophysiology:
inhaled spores are trapped in segmental bronchi of individuals with asthma, germinate, and form hyphae; immunologic response coupled with proteolytic enzymes causes pulmonary infiltrates + tissue damage + central bronchiectasis

Criteria:

(a) Primary diagnostic criteria:

acronym: ARTEPICS

Asthma (84–96%)

Roentgenographic transient or fixed pulmonary infiltrates

Test for A. fumigatus positive: immediate skin reaction

Eosinophilia in blood between 8% and 40%

Precipitating antibodies to A. fumigatus (70%)
IgE in serum elevated
Central bronchiectasis (late manifestation that proves diagnosis)
Serum-specific IgE and IgG A. fumigatus levels elevated

(b) Secondary diagnostic criteria (less common):
1. Aspergillus fumigatus mycelia in sputum
2. Expectoration of brown sputum plugs (54%)
3. Arthus reaction (= late skin reactivity with erythema + induration) to Aspergillus antigen

Staging:
I acute phase with all primary diagnostic criteria
II clearing of pulmonary infiltrates with declining IgE levels
III all criteria of stage I reappear after emission
IV corticosteroid dependency
V irreversible lung fibrosis

• flulike symptoms: fever, headache, malaise, weight loss, fleeting chest pain
√ migratory pneumonitis = transient recurrent "fleeting" alveolar patchy subsegmental / lobar infiltrates in upper lobes (50%), lower lobes (20%), middle lobe (7%), both lungs (65%); may persist for >6 months
√ central varicose / cystic bronchiectasis:
  √ "tramlike" bronchial walls (edema)
  √ 1–2-cm ring shadows (= bronchus on end) around hilum + upper lobes (HALLMARK)
  √ "finger-in-glove / toothpaste shadow" = V- or Y-shaped central mucus plugs in 2nd order bronchi of 2.5–6 cm in length remaining for months + growing in size
√ lobar consolidation (in 32%)
√ atelectasis (in 14%) with collateral air drift
√ cavitation (in 14%) secondary to postobstructive abscess
√ hyperinflation (due to bronchospasm)
√ pulmonary fibrosis + retraction
  √ hilar elevation due to lobar shrinkage
√ emphysema
√ NORMAL peripheral bronchi
√ UNUSUAL are aspergilloma in cavity (7%), empyema, pneumothorax

DDx: hypersensitivity pneumonitis or allergic asthma (no hyphae in sputum, normal levels of IgE + IgG to A. fumigatus), tuberculosis, lipoid pneumonia, Löffler syndrome, bronchogenic carcinoma

Pleural Aspergillosis

= Aspergillus empyema in patients with pulmonary tuberculosis, bacterial empyema, bronchopleural fistula
√ pleural thickening

ASPIRATION OF SOLID FOREIGN BODY

@ Childhood
Age: in 50% <3 years
Delay of diagnosis: within 2–3 days (usual); weeks to months (rare)
Source: in 85% vegetable origin (lentil, beans, peas, peanut, barley grass), broken fragments of teeth
Location: almost exclusively in lower lobes; R:L = 2:1
• varying degrees of cough
√ obstructive overinflation (68%) + reflex vasoconstriction
√ atelectasis (14–53%)
√ infiltrate (11%)
√ radiopaque foreign body (9%)
√ air trapping (expiratory / lateral decubitus film):
√ lobar / segmental overinflation

CT:
  √ low-attenuation intrabronchial material (SUGGESTIVE)

NUC:
  √ ventilation defect (initial breath) + retention (washout)

Cx: bronchiectasis (from long retention)
DDx: impacted esophageal foreign body

@ Adulthood (unusual)
• often clinically silent
• massive life-threatening hemoptysis
√ chronic volume loss of affected lobe
√ recurrent pneumonia
√ bronchiectasis
√ intrabronchial mass formation (= chronic inflammatory reaction around inhaled material)
√ centrally located mass + lobar / segmental collapse

Aspiration Bronchiolitis

= chronic inflammatory reaction to repeatedly aspirated foreign particles in the bronchioles
Predisposed: achalasia, Zenker diverticulum, esophageal carcinoma
Histo: resembling diffuse panbronchiolitis
• dysphagia, regurgitation, aspiration
√ moderate / marked dilatation of esophagus
√ lobar / segmental / disseminated small nodules

CT:
√ uni- / bilateral foci of branching areas of increased attenuation:
  √ tree-in-bud appearance
  √ mottled poorly defined opacified acinar areas

ASPIRATION PNEUMONIA

Predisposing conditions:
(1) CNS disorders / intoxication: alcoholism, mental retardation, seizure disorders, recent anesthesia
(2) Swallowing disorders: esophageal motility disturbances, head + neck surgery

• low-grade fever
• productive cough
• choking on swallowing

Location: gravity-dependent portions of lung, posterior segments of upper lobes + lower lobes in bedridden patients, frequently bilateral, right middle + lower lobe with sparing of left lung is common

CHEST

A. ACUTE ASPIRATION PNEUMONIA
Cause: gastric acid, food particles, anaerobic bacteria from GI tract provoke edema, hemorrhage, inflammatory cellular response, foreign-body reaction
Organism: Gram-negative bacteria; Pseudomonas aeruginosa, Actinomyces israelii
√ patchy bronchopneumonic pattern
√ lobar / segmental consolidation in dependent portion
√ necrotizing pneumonia
√ abscess formation

B. CHRONIC ASPIRATION PNEUMONIA
Cause: repeated aspiration of foreign material from GI tract over long time / mineral oil (eg, in laxatives)
Associated with: Zenker diverticulum, esophageal stenosis, achalasia, TE fistula, neuromuscular disturbances in swallowing
√ recurring segmental consolidation
√ progression to interstitial scarring (= localized honeycomb appearance)
√ bronchopneumonic infiltrates of variable location over months / years
√ residual peribronchial scarring
Upper GI:
√ abnormal swallowing / aspiration

Mendelson Syndrome

= aspiration of gastric acid with a pH <2.5
Associated with: vomiting, gastroesophageal reflux, achalasia, hiatal hernia
Pathophysiology:
acid rapidly disseminates throughout bronchial tree + lung parenchyma, incites a chemical pneumonitis within minutes; extent of injury from mild bronchiolitis to hemorrhagic pulmonary edema depends on pH + aspirated volume
Location: with patient in recumbent position: posterior segments of upper lobes + superior segments of lower lobes
√ bilateral perihilar ill-defined alveolar consolidations
√ multifocal patchy infiltrates
√ segmental / lobar consolidation localized to one / both lung bases
Prognosis: 30% mortality with massive aspiration; >50% with initial shock, apnea, secondary pneumonia, or ARDS

ASTHMA

= episodic reversible bronchoconstriction secondary to hypersensitivity to a variety of stimuli

A. INTRINSIC ASTHMA
Age: middle age
Pathogenesis:
probably autoimmune phenomenon caused by viral respiratory infection and often provoked by infection, exercise, pharmaceuticals; no environmental antigen

B. EXTRINSIC ASTHMA = ATOPIC ASTHMA
Pathogenesis:
secondary to antigens producing an immediate hypersensitivity response (type I); reagin sensitizes mast cells to release histamine followed by increased vascular permeability, edema, small muscle contraction; effects primarily bronchi causing airway obstruction
Nonoccupational allergens:
pollens, dog + cat fur, tamarind seed powder, castor bean, fungal spores, grain weevil
Occupational allergens:
(a) natural substances: wood dust, flour, grain, beans
(b) pharmaceuticals: antibiotics, ASA
(c) inorganic chemicals: nickel, platinum

Path: bronchial plugging with large amounts of viscid tenacious mucus (eosinophils, Charcot-Leyden crystals), edematous bronchial walls, hypertrophy of mucous glands + smooth muscle

ACUTE SIGNS:
- during asthmatic attack low values for FEV + MMFR and abnormal V/Q ratios
- increased resistance to airflow due to
  (a) smooth muscle contraction in airway walls
  (b) edema of airway wall caused by inflammation
  (c) mucus hypersecretion with airway plugging
- normal diffusing capacity

√ hyperexpansion of lungs = severe overinflation + air trapping:
  √ flattened diaphragmatic dome
  √ deepened retrosternal air space
√ peribronchial cuffing (inflammation of airway wall)
√ bronchial dilatation
√ localized areas of hypoattenuation

CHRONIC CHANGES:
Normal chest x-ray in 73%, findings of abnormalities depend on
(a) age of onset (<15 years of age in 31%; >30 years of age in none)
(b) severity of asthma
√ central ring shadows = bronchiectasis
√ scars (from recurrent infections)

Cx:
(1) Pneumonia (2 x as frequent as in nonasthmatics)
  √ peripheral pneumonic infiltrates (secondary to blocked airways)
(2) Atelectasis (5–15%) from mucoid impaction
(3) Pneumomediastinum (5%), pneumothorax, subcutaneous emphysema; predominantly in children
(4) Emphysema
(5) Allergic bronchopulmonary aspergillosis with central bronchiectasis

ATYPICAL MEASLES PNEUMONIA

= clinical syndrome in patients who have been previously inadequately immunized with killed rubeola vaccine and are subsequently exposed to the measles virus (= type III immune complex hypersensitivity); noted in children who have received live vaccine before 13 months of age

- 2- to 3-day prodrome of headache, fever, cough, malaise
- maculopapular rash beginning on wrists + ankles (sometimes absent)
- postinfectious migratory arthralgias
- history of exposure to measles

√ extensive nonsegmental consolidation, usually bilateral
√ hilar adenopathy (100%)
√ pleural effusion (0–70%)
√ nodular densities of 0.5–10 cm in diameter in peripheral location, may calcify and persist up to 30 months

BARITOSIS

= inhalation of nonfibrogenic barium sulfate

- asymptomatic
- normal pulmonary function (benign course)

√ bilateral nodular / patchy opacities, denser than bone (high atomic number)
√ similar to calcified nodules
√ NO cor pulmonale, NO hilar adenopathy
√ regression if patient removed from exposure

BEHÇET SYNDROME

= rare multisystem disease of unknown origin characterized by
(1) aphthous stomatitis
(2) genital ulceration
(3) iritis

- positive pathergy test = unusual hypersensitivity to pricking with formation of pustules at site of needle prick within 24–48 hours
- skin changes: erythema nodosum, folliculitis, papulopustular lesions
- arthritis, encephalitis
- epididymitis

@ Chest (5%)
√ multiple peripheral subpleural opacities (due to hemorrhage, necrotic pulmonary infarctions)
√ increased radiopacity near hila (pulmonary artery aneurysm)

@ Veins (25%)
√ large vein occlusion; may cause SVC syndrome
√ subcutaneous thrombophlebitis

@ Arteries
√ arterial occlusion / pulseless disease
√ aneurysm of large arteries (in 2%)

BERYLLIOSIS

= chronic granulomatous disorder as a result of beryllium-specific cell-mediated immune response (= delayed hypersensitivity reaction after exposure to acid salts from extraction of beryllium oxide)

Substance: one of the lightest metals (atomic weight 9), marked heat resistance, great hardness, fatigue resistance, no corrosion
Occupational exposure: fluorescent light bulb factories
Histo: noncaseating granulomas within interstitium + along vessels + in bronchial submucosa

- positive beryllium lymphocyte transformation test (blood test of T-lymphocyte response to beryllium)

A. ACUTE BERYLLIOSIS (25%)
√ pulmonary edema following an overwhelming exposure

B. CHRONIC BERYLLIOSIS
widespread systemic disease of liver, spleen, lymph nodes, kidney, myocardium, skin, skeletal muscle; removed from lungs + excreted via kidneys
Latent period: 5–15 years
√ fine nodularity (granulomas similar to sarcoidosis)
√ irregular opacities, particularly sparing apices + bases
√ hilar + mediastinal adenopathy (may calcify)
√ emphysema in upper lobes + interstitial fibrosis
√ pneumothorax in 10%
HRCT:
√ diffuse small parenchymal nodules (57%)
√ septal lines (50%)
√ patches of ground-glass attenuation (32%)
√ hilar adenopathy (21–35%), only in the presence of parenchymal abnormalities
√ bronchial wall thickening (46%)
√ pleural irregularities (25%)

DDx: (1) Nodular pulmonary sarcoidosis (indistinguishable)
(2) Asbestosis without hilar adenopathy

BLASTOMYCOSIS

= NORTH AMERICAN BLASTOMYCOSIS = GILCHRIST DISEASE = CHICAGO DISEASE
= rare systemic mixed pyogenic + granulomatous fungal infection

Organism: soil-born saprophytic dimorphic fungus Blastomyces dermatitidis, mycelial phase in soil + round thick-walled yeast form with broad-based budding in mammals
Geographic distribution:
worldwide; endemic in central + southeastern United States (Ohio + Mississippi river valleys, vicinity of Great Lakes), Africa, Canada (northern Ontario), Central + South America (acquired through activities in woods)
Age: several months of age to 80 years (peak between 25 and 50 years of age)
Mode of infection:
inhalation of fungal conidia (primary portal of entry); spread to extrapulmonary sites, eg, skin, bone (often direct extension from skin lesion resembling actinomycosis), joints
Predisposed: elderly, immunocompromised
Histo:
(a) exudative phase: accumulation of numerous neutrophils with infecting organism
(b) proliferative phase: proliferation of epithelioid granulomas + giant cells with central microabscesses containing neutrophils and yeast forms

- mouth ulcers
- fever, cough, weight loss, chest pain (majority)
- crusted verrucous lesions on exposed body areas

CHEST

@ Lung
- Clinical patterns following pulmonary infection:
  (a) severe pulmonary symptoms
  (b) asymptomatic pulmonary infection with spontaneous resolution
  (c) disseminated disease to single / multiple organs indolent for several years
  (d) extrapulmonary manifestation involving male GU system, skeleton, skin

√ segmental / lobar airspace disease in lower lobes in acute illness (26–61%)
√ solitary / multiple irregular nodular masses / satellite lesions in paramediastinal location
√ air bronchogram in area of consolidation / mass (87%)
√ interstitial disease
√ cavitation if communicating with airway (13%)
√ hilar / mediastinal lymph node enlargement (<25%)

@ Bone
√ marked destruction ± surrounding sclerosis
√ periosteal reaction in long bones, but not in short bones
√ multiple osseous lesions are frequent
√ vertebral bodies + intervertebral disks are destroyed (similar to tuberculosis)
√ psoas abscess
√ lytic skull lesions + soft-tissue abscess
√ usually monarticular arthritis: knee > ankle > elbow > wrist > hand

@ GU tract (20%): prostate, epididymis

Dx: (1) Culture of organism
(2) Silver stain microscopy of tissues

Prognosis: spontaneous resolution of acute disease in up to 4 weeks; disease may reactivate for up to 3 years

Rx: (1) Amphotericin B IV: 8–10 weeks for noncavitary + 10–12 weeks for cavitary lesions
(2) Ketoconazole

DDx: other pneumonias (ie, bacterial, tuberculous, fungal), pseudolymphoma, malignant neoplasm (ie, alveolar cell carcinoma, lymphoma, Kaposi sarcoma)

BLUNT CHEST TRAUMA

Incidence: 100,000 hospital admissions/year (in USA)
Cause: high-speed motor vehicle accidents (70%)
Type of injury:

1. Pneumothorax 69%
2. Lung contusion 67%
3. Rib fracture 66%
4. Hemothorax 28%
5. Flail chest.......................... 14%
6. Thoracic spine fracture 13%
7. Clavicle fracture 13%
8. Scapula fracture 8%
9. Sternal fracture 5%
10. Diaphragmatic injury 5%
11. Tracheobronchial tear 2%
12. Vascular injury 2%
13. Esophageal rupture 1%

BONE MARROW TRANSPLANTATION

= intravenous infusion of hematopoietic progenitor cells from patient's own marrow (autologous transplant) / HLA-matched donor (allogenic transplant) to reestablish marrow function after high-dose chemotherapy and total body irradiation for lymphoma, leukemia, anemia, multiple myeloma, congenital immunologic defects, solid tumors

Cx: pulmonary complications in 40–60%

Neutropenic Phase Pulmonary Complications

Time: 2–3 weeks after transplantation

1. Angioinvasive aspergillosis
   √ nodule surrounded by halo of ground-glass attenuation (= fungal infection spreading into lung parenchyma and surrounding area of hemorrhagic infarction)
   √ segmental / subsegmental consolidation (= pulmonary infarction)
   √ cavitation of nodule with air-crescent sign (during recovery phase with resolving neutropenia)
   √ <5-mm centrilobular nodules to 5-cm peribronchial consolidation (= airway invasion with surrounding zone of hemorrhage / organizing pneumonia)
2. Diffuse alveolar hemorrhage (20%)
   - hemosiderin-laden macrophages on lavage
   √ bilateral areas of ground-glass attenuation / consolidation
3. Pulmonary edema
   Cause: infusion of large volumes of fluid combined with cardiac + renal dysfunction
   √ prominent pulmonary vessels, interlobar septal thickening, ground-glass attenuation, pleural effusions
4. Drug toxicity
   Cause: bleomycin, busulfan, bischloronitrosurea (carmustine), methotrexate
   √ bilateral areas of ground-glass attenuation / consolidation / reticular attenuation (= fibrosis)

Early Phase Pulmonary Complications

Time: up to 100 days after transplantation

1. CMV pneumonia (23%)
   √ multiple small nodules + associated areas of consolidation + ground-glass attenuation (= hemorrhagic nodules)
2. Pneumocystis carinii pneumonia
   √ diffuse / predominantly perihilar / mosaic pattern of ground-glass attenuation with sparing of some secondary pulmonary lobules
3. Idiopathic interstitial pneumonia (12%)
   √ nonspecific findings (diagnosis of exclusion)

Late Phase Pulmonary Complications

Time: after 100 days post transplantation

1. Bronchiolitis obliterans (in up to 10%)
2. BOOP
3. Chronic graft-versus-host disease
   infections, chronic aspiration, bronchiolitis obliterans, lymphoid interstitial pneumonia

CHEST

BRONCHIAL ADENOMA

= misnomer secondary to locally invasive features, tendency for recurrence, and occasional metastasis to extrathoracic sites (10%) = low-grade malignancy

Path: arises from duct epithelium of bronchial mucous glands (predominant distribution of Kulchitsky cells at bifurcations of lobar bronchi)

Incidence: 6–10% of all primary lung tumors

Age: mean age of 35–45 years (range 12–60 years); 90% occur <50 years of age; most common primary lung tumor under age 16; M:F = 1:1; Whites:Blacks = 25:1

Types:

mnemonic: "CAMP"

Carcinoid	90%
Adenoid cystic carcinoma = Cylindroma	6%
Mucoepidermoid carcinoma	3%
Pleomorphic carcinoma	1%

Location: most commonly near / at bifurcation of lobar / segmental bronchi; central:peripheral = 4:1

— 48% on right : RLL (20%), RML (10%), RUL (7%), main right bronchus (8%), intermediate bronchus (3%)

— 32% on left : LLL (13%), LUL (12%), main left bronchus (6%), lingular bronchus (1%)

- hemoptysis (40–50%)
- atypical asthma
- persistent cough
- recurrent obstructive pneumonia
- asymptomatic (10%)

√ complete obstruction / air trapping in partial obstruction (rare) / nonobstructive (10–15%)
√ obstructive emphysema
√ recurrent postobstructive infection: pneumonitis, bronchiectasis, abscess
√ atelectasis / consolidation of a lung / lobe / segment (78%)
√ collateral air drift may prevent atelectasis
√ solitary round / oval slightly lobulated pulmonary nodule (19%) of 1–10 cm in size
√ hilar enlargement / mediastinal widening
= central endo- / exobronchial mass

CT:
√ well-marginated sharply defined mass
√ in close proximity to an adjacent bifurcation with splaying of bronchus
√ coarse peripheral calcifications in 1/3 (cartilaginous / bony transformation)
√ may exhibit marked homogeneous enhancement

Biopsy: risky secondary to high vascularity of tumor

Prognosis: 95% 5-year survival rate, 75% 15-year survival rate after resection

Carcinoid

= NEUROENDOCRINE CARCINOMA
= slow-growing low-grade malignant tumor

Incidence: 12–15% of all carcinoid tumors in the body; 1–4% of all bronchial neoplasms

Age peak: 5th decade (range of 2nd–9th decade); 4% occur in children + adolescents; M:F = 2:1; very uncommon in Blacks

Path:
originates from neurosecretory cells of bronchial mucosa (= Kulchitsky cells = argentaffine cells) just as small cell cancer; part of APUD (amine precursor uptake and decarboxylation) system = chromaffin paraganglioma, which produces serotonin, ACTH, norepinephrine, bombesin, calcitonin, ADH, bradykinin

Pathologic classification:
(KCC = **Kulchitsky cell carcinoma**)

KCC I = **classic carcinoid** (least aggressive);
= bronchial adenoma (misnomer)
= central location with endobronchial growth; usually <2.5 cm in size + well-defined; younger patient; M:F = 1:10; lymph node metastases in 3%

KCC II = **atypical carcinoid** (25% of carcinoid tumors); mass usually >2.5 cm with well-defined margins; older patient; M:F = 3:1; lymph node metastases in 40–50%; metastases to brain, liver, bone (in 30%)

KCC III = **small cell carcinoma** (most aggressive); mediastinal lymphadenopathy; ill-defined tumor margins

◊ Rarely cause for carcinoid syndrome or Cushing syndrome!

- recurrent unifocal pneumonitis, hemoptysis
- wheezing, persistent cough, dyspnea, chest pain
- carcinoid syndrome (rare)
- endobronchial exophytic mass at endoscopy

Location: 58–90% central in lobar / segmental bronchi, 10–42% peripheral; located in submucosa; endobronchial / along bronchial wall / exobronchial

√ polypoid tumor with average size of 2.2 cm
√ most extend through bronchial wall thus involving bronchial lumen + parenchyma (= collar button lesion)
√ calcification / ossification (26–33%): central carcinoid (43%), peripheral carcinoid (10%)
√ vascular tumor supplied by bronchial circulation
√ cavitation (rare)
√ segmental / lobar atelectasis
√ obstructive pneumonitis
√ bronchiectasis + pulmonary abscess

Malignant potential: low

Metastases:
(a) regional lymph nodes in 25%
(b) distantly in 5% (adrenal, liver, brain, skin, osteoblastic bone metastases)

Prognosis:
95% 5-year survival rate for classic carcinoids;
57–66% 5-year survival rate for atypical carcinoids

Cylindroma

= ADENOID CYSTIC CARCINOMA (7%)

Second most common primary tumor of trachea

Path: mixed serous + mucous glands; resembles salivary gland tumor

CHEST

Histo:
Grade 1: tubular + cribriform; no solid subtype
√ entirely intraluminal
Grade 2: tubular + cribriform; <20% solid subtype
√ predominantly intraluminal
Grade 3: solid subtype >20%
√ predominantly extraluminal
Age peak: 4th–5th decade
• typical Hx of refractory "asthma"
• hemoptysis, cough, stridor, wheezing
• dysphagia, hoarseness
√ endotracheal mass with extratracheal extension
Malignant potential:
more aggressive than carcinoid with propensity for local invasion + distant metastases (lung, bone, brain, liver) in 25%
Rx: tracheal resection + adjunctive radiotherapy
Prognosis: 8.3 years mean survival

Mucoepidermoid Carcinoma
Path: squamous cells + mucus-secreting columnar cells; resembles salivary gland tumor
√ may involve trachea = locally invasive tumor
√ sessile / polypoid endobronchial lesion

Pleomorphic Adenoma
= MIXED TYPE (extremely rare)

BRONCHIAL ATRESIA
= local obliteration of proximal lumen of a segmental bronchus
Proposed causes:
(a) local interruption of bronchial arterial perfusion >15 weeks GA (when bronchial branching is complete)
(b) tip of primitive bronchial bud separates from bud and continues to develop
Path: normal bronchial tree distal to obstruction patent and containing mucus plugs; alveoli distal to obstruction air-filled through collateral air drift
Associated with: lobar emphysema, cystic adenomatoid malformation
• minimal symptoms, apparent later in childhood (most by age 15) / adult life
Location: apicoposterior segment of LUL (>>RUL / ML)
√ decreased perfusion
√ overexpanded segment (collateral air drift with expiratory air-trapping)
√ fingerlike opacity lateral to hilum (= mucus plug distal to atretic lumen) is CHARACTERISTIC
OB-US (detected >24 weeks MA):
√ large echogenic fetal lung mass = fluid-filled lung distal to obstruction
√ dilated fluid-filled bronchus
Rx: no treatment because mostly asymptomatic
DDx: Congenital lobar emphysema (no mucus plug)

BRONCHIECTASIS
= localized mostly irreversible dilatation of bronchi often with thickening of the bronchial wall

Etiology:
A. Congenital
1. Structural defect of bronchi: bronchial atresia, Williams-Campbell syndrome
2. Abnormal mucociliary transport: Kartagener syndrome
3. Abnormal secretions: cystic fibrosis
B. Congenital / acquired immune deficiency (usually IgG deficiency): chronic granulomatous disease of childhood, alpha-1 antitrypsin deficiency
C. Postinfectious childhood pneumonias (after necrotizing viral / bacterial bronchitis): measles, whooping cough, Swyer-James syndrome, allergic bronchopulmonary aspergillosis, chronic granulomatous infection (TB)
D. Distal to bronchial obstruction (due to accumulation of secretions): neoplasm, inflammatory nodes, foreign body
E. Aspiration / inhalation: gastric contents / inhaled fumes (late complication)
F. "**Traction bronchiectasis**" (due to increased elastic recoil with bronchial dilatation + mechanical distortion of bronchi): advanced pulmonary fibrosis / radiation-induced lung injury
G. Increased inflationary pressure

Classification:
1. **Cylindrical / tubular / fusiform bronchiectasis**
= mildly and uniformly dilated bronchi (least severe type)
reversible if associated with pulmonary collapse
Path: 16 subdivisions of bronchi
√ square abrupt ending with lumen of uniform diameter and same width as parent bronchus
HRCT:
√ "tram lines" of nontapering air ways (horizontal course)
√ "signet-ring sign" (vertical course) = cross section of dilated bronchus + branch of pulmonary artery
√ Y- or V-shaped areas of attenuation = mucous plugs filling bronchiectatic segments
2. **Varicose bronchiectasis**
= moderately dilated and beaded bronchi (rare)
Associated with: Swyer-James syndrome
Path: 4–8 subdivisions of bronchi
√ beaded contour with normal pattern distally
3. **Saccular / cystic bronchiectasis**
= marked cystic dilatation (most severe type)
Associated with: severe bronchial infection
Path: <5 subdivisions of bronchi
√ progressive ballooning dilatation toward periphery with diameter of saccules >1 cm
√ irregular constrictions may be present
√ dilatation of bronchi on inspiration, collapse on expiration
√ contains variable amounts of pooled secretions
HRCT:
√ string of cysts = "string of pearls" (horizontal course) / cluster of cysts = "cluster of grapes"
√ air-fluid level (frequent)

Age: predominantly pediatric disease
- chronic cough, excess sputum production
- recurrent infection with expectoration of purulent sputum
- shortness of breath
- hemoptysis (50%)
- frequent exacerbations + resolutions (due to superimposed infections)

Associated with: obliterative + inflammatory bronchiolitis (in 85%)

Location: posterior basal segments of lower lobes, bilateral (50%), middle lobe / lingula (10%), central bronchiectasis in bronchopulmonary aspergillosis

CXR (37% sensitive):
- √ dilated air-filled bronchi
- √ bronchial wall thickening
- √ increased background density
- √ parenchymal volume loss:
  - √ crowding of lung markings (if associated with atelectasis)
  - √ increase in size of lung markings (retained secretions)
  - √ loss of definition of lung markings (peribronchial fibrosis)
- √ cystic spaces ± air-fluid levels <2 cm in diameter (dilated bronchi)
- √ honeycomb pattern (in severe cases)
- √ compensatory hyperinflation of uninvolved ipsilateral lung

HRCT (87–97% sensitive, 93–100% specific):
- √ lack of bronchial tapering (in 80% = most sensitive finding)
- √ bronchial wall thickening
- √ signet ring sign = internal diameter of bronchus larger than adjacent pulmonary artery (in 60%)
- √ bronchi visible within 1 cm of pleura (in 45%)
- √ mucus-filled dilated bronchi (in 6%)

Cx: frequent respiratory infections

DDx of CT appearance:
1. (1) Emphysematous blebs (no definable wall thickness, subpleural location)
2. (2) "Reversible bronchiectasis" = temporary dilatation during pneumonia with return to normal within 4–6 months

BRONCHIOLITIS OBLITERANS

= CONSTRICTIVE BRONCHIOLITIS = OBLITERATIVE BRONCHIOLITIS

= inflammation of bronchioles leading to (sometimes reversible) obstruction of bronchiolar lumen

Etiology:
- (1) Inhalation: 1–3 weeks after exposure to toxic fumes (isocyanates, phosgene, ammonia, sulfur dioxide, chlorine)
- (2) Postinfectious: Mycoplasma (children), virus (older individual); *see* Swyer-James syndrome
- (3) Drugs: bleomycin, gold salts, cyclophosphamide, methotrexate, penicillamine
- (4) Connective tissue disorder: rheumatoid arthritis, scleroderma, systemic lupus erythematosus
- (5) Chronic rejection: lung transplant, heart-lung transplant (30–50%)
- (6) Chronic graft-versus-host disease: bone marrow transplant
- (7) Cystic fibrosis (as a complication of repeated episodes of pulmonary infection)
- (8) Idiopathic (in immunocompetent patients)

Path: submucosal and peribronchiolar fibrosis
= irreversible fibrosis of small airway walls with narrowing / obliteration of airway lumina (respiratory bronchiole, alveolar duct, alveola) by granulation tissue of immature fibroblastic plugs (Masson bodies)

Peak age: 40–60 years; M:F = 1:1
- insidious onset of dyspnea over many months
- obstructive pulmonary function tests
- no response to antibiotics
- persistent nonproductive cough, fever
- √ normal CXR (in up to 40%)
- √ hyperinflated lungs = limited disease with connective tissue plugs in airways
- √ bilateral scattered heterogeneous + homogeneous opacities (typically peripheral in distribution; equally distributed between upper + lower lobes)
- √ bronchiectasis
- √ decreased vascularity (reflex vasoconstriction)

HRCT (paired expiration-inspiration images:
- √ "mosaic perfusion" of lobular air trapping (85–100%)
  = patchy areas of decreased lung attenuation alternating with areas of normal attenuation:
  - √ areas of decreased attenuation containing vessels of decreased caliber (due to alveolar hypoventilation + secondary vasoconstriction of alveoli distal to bronchiolar obstruction)
  - √ areas of increased attenuation containing vessels of increased caliber (uninvolved areas with compensatory increased perfusion)
- √ bronchial wall thickening (87%)
- √ bronchiectasis (66–80%)
- √ patchy air trapping on expiratory scans (due to collateral airdrift into postobstructive alveoli) = failure of volume / attenuation change between expiratory + inspiratory images
- √ poorly defined nodular areas of consolidation
- √ "tree-in-bud" appearance of bronchioles
  = centrilobular branching structures and nodules caused by peribronchiolar thickening + bronchiolectasis with secretions (the only direct, but uncommon sign)
- √ centrilobular ground-glass opacities

Rx: steroids may stop progression

DDx:
- (1) Bacterial / fungal pneumonia (response to antibiotics, positive cultures)
- (2) Chronic eosinophilic pneumonia (young female, eosinophilia in 2/3)
- (3) Usual interstitial pneumonia (irregular opacities, decreased lung volume)

CHEST

BRONCHIOLITIS OBLITERANS WITH ORGANIZING PNEUMONIA (BOOP)

= PROLIFERATIVE BRONCHIOLITIS = CRYPTOGENIC ORGANIZING PNEUMONITIS (COP)

Prevalence: 20–30% of all chronic infiltrative lung disease

Cause: postobstructive pneumonia, organizing adult respiratory distress syndrome, lung cancer, extrinsic allergic alveolitis, pulmonary manifestation of collagen vascular disease, pulmonary drug toxicity, silo filler disease, idiopathic (50%)

Path: granulation tissue polyps filling the lumina of alveolar ducts and respiratory bronchioles (bronchiolitis obliterans) + variable degree of infiltration of interstitium and alveoli with macrophages (organizing pneumonia)

◊ Bronchiolitis obliterans component not present in up to 1/3!

Histo: plugs of immature fibroblasts (Masson bodies) covered with low cuboidal epithelium, which may spread through collateral air drift pathways

Age: 40–70 years; M:F = 1:1

- clinical + functional + radiographic manifestation of organizing pneumonia
- nonproductive cough, dyspnea (1–4-month history), preceded by a brief flulike illness with sore throat (40%), low-grade fever, malaise (in 33%)
- late respiratory crackles
- restrictive pulmonary function tests + diminished diffusing capacity on pulmonary function tests
- unresponsive to broad-spectrum antibiotics
- no organism identified

Location: mainly mid + lower lung zones; often subpleural (50%) and peribronchiolar distribution (30–50%)

CXR:

frequently mixture of:

√ uni- / bilateral patchy alveolar airspace consolidation (25–73%), often subpleural
√ 3–5 mm nodules (up to 50%)
√ irregular linear opacities (15–42%)
√ unilateral focal / lobar consolidation (5–31%)
√ pleural thickening (13%)
√ cavitation / pleural effusion (<5%)

HRCT:

√ patchy airspace consolidation (80%)
  (a) bilateral in 90% involving all lung zones
  (b) subpleural / peribronchial distribution in 50–60%
√ patchy ground-glass opacities (due to alveolitis) in 60%
√ 3–5 mm centrilobular nodules (30–50%) due to organized pneumonia
√ air bronchograms = cylindrical bronchial dilatation in areas of airspace consolidation (36–70%)
√ pleural effusion (28–35%)
√ adenopathy (27%)

Rx: improvement with corticosteroid therapy (in 84% of patients with idiopathic form)

Prognosis: persistent abnormalities (30%); 10% mortality due to progressive / recurrent disease

Dx: tissue examination from open lung biopsy

BRONCHIOLOALVEOLAR CARCINOMA

= ALVEOLAR CELL CARCINOMA = BRONCHIOLAR CARCINOMA

Incidence: 1.5–6% of all primary lung cancers (increasing incidence to ? 20–25%)

Etiology: development from type II alveolar epithelial cells

Age: 40–70 years; M:F = 1:1 (strikingly high in women)

Path: peripheral neoplasm arising beyond a recognizable bronchus with tendency to spread locally using lung structure as a stroma (= **lepidic** growth)

Histo: subtype of well-differentiated adenocarcinoma; cuboidal / columnar cells grow along alveolar walls + septa without disrupting the lung architecture or pulmonary interstitium (serving as "scaffolding" for tumor growth)

Subtypes:

(a) mucinous (80%): mucin-secreting tall columnar peglike bronchiolar cells; more likely multicentric; 26% 5-year survival rate
(b) nonmucinous (20%): cuboidal type II alveolar pneumocytes with production of surfactant / nonciliated bronchiolar (Clara) cells; more localized + solitary; 72% 5-year survival rate

Risk factors: localized pulmonary fibrosis (tuberculous scarring, pulmonary infarct) in 27%, diffuse fibrotic disease (scleroderma), previous exogenous lipid pneumonia

- history of heavy smoking (25–50%)
- often asymptomatic (even with disseminated disease) with insidious onset
- pleuritic chest pain (due to peripheral location)
- cough (35–60%), hemoptysis (11%)
- bronchorrhea = abundant white mucoid / watery expectoration (5–27%); can produce hypovolemia + electrolyte depletion; unusual + late manifestation only with diffuse bronchioloalveolar carcinoma
- shortness of breath (15%)
- weight loss (13%), fever (8%)

Location: peripherally, beyond a recognizable bronchus

Spread: tracheobronchial dissemination = cells detach from primary tumor + attach to alveolar septa elsewhere in ipsi- / contralateral lung; lymphogenous + hematogenous dissemination

Metastases: involving almost any organ (in 50–60%); 33% of skeletal metastases are osteoblastic

A. LOCAL FORM (60–90%)

1. Ground-glass attenuation
   = early stage (due to lepidic growth pattern along alveolar septa with relative lack of acinar filling)
   √ ground-glass haziness
   √ bubblelike hyperlucencies / pseudocavitation
   √ airway dilatation
   √ lesion persists / progresses within 6–8 weeks
2. **Single mass** (43%)
   √ well-circumscribed focal mass in peripheral / subpleural location arising beyond a recognizable bronchus
   √ "open bronchus sign" = air bronchogram = tumor / mucus surrounding aerated bronchus ± narrowing / stretching / spreading of bronchi

√ "rabbit ears" / pleural tags / triangular strand / "tail sign" (55%) = linear strands extending from nodule to pleura (desmoplastic reaction / scarring granulomatous disease / pleural indrawing)
√ spiculated margin = sunburst appearance (73%)
√ solitary cavity due to central necrosis (7%)
◊ 2nd most common cell type associated with cavitation after squamous cell carcinoma
√ pseudocavitation (= dilatation of intact air spaces from desmoplastic reaction / bronchiectasis / focal emphysema) in 50–60%
√ heterogeneous attenuation (57%)
√ confined to single lobe
√ rarely evolving into diffuse form
√ slowly progressive growth on serial radiographs
√ NO atelectasis
√ negative FDG PET results in 55%
Prognosis: 70% surgical cure rate for tumor <3 cm; 4–15 years' survival time with single nodule

B. DIFFUSE FORM = Pneumonic form (10–40%)
1. **Diffuse consolidation** (30%)
√ acinar airspace consolidation + air bronchogram + poorly marginated borders
√ airspace consolidation may affect both lungs (mucus secretion)
√ ± cavitation within consolidation
√ "CT angiogram sign" = low-attenuation consolidation does not obscure vessels (mucin-producing subtype)
2. Lobar form
√ ± expansion of a lobe with bulging of interlobar fissures
3. **Multinodular form** (27%)
√ multiple bilateral poorly / well-defined nodules similar to metastatic disease
√ multiple poorly defined areas of ground-glass attenuation / consolidation

√ pleural effusion (8–10%)
Prognosis: worse with extensive consolidation / multifocal / bilateral disease; death within 3 years with diffuse disease

BRONCHOCENTRIC GRANULOMATOSIS

Age: 4th–7th decade
- asthma with underlying allergic bronchopulmonary aspergillosis (33–50%)
- fever, night sweats, cough, dyspnea, pleuritic chest pain
- seropositive arthritis (rare)
- ocular scleritis (rare)

Path: thick-walled ectatic bronchi + bronchioles containing viscous material of mucopurulent / caseous character
Histo: necrotizing granulomas surrounding small airways; pulmonary arteritis as a secondary phenomenon
(1) large masses of eosinophils in necrotic zones, associated with endobronchial mucus plugs, eosinophilic pneumonia, Charcot-Leyden crystals, fungal hyphae in granulomas (with asthma)
(2) polymorphonuclear cell infiltrate in necrotic zones (without asthma)

Location: unilateral (75%); upper lobe predominance
√ branching opacities / atelectasis (from mucoid impaction)
√ multiple / solitary nodules / masses
√ ill-defined parenchymal consolidation
√ ± cavitation
Rx: corticosteroid therapy

BRONCHOGENIC CARCINOMA

= LUNG CANCER = LUNG CARCINOMA

Most frequent cause of cancer deaths in males (35% of all cancer deaths) and females (21% of all cancer deaths); most common malignancy of men in the world; 6th leading cancer in women worldwide

Prevalence: in 1991 161,000 new cases; 143,000 deaths
Age at diagnosis: 55–60 years (range 40–80 years); M:F = 1.4:1

- asymptomatic (10–50%) usually with peripheral tumors
- symptoms of central tumors:
  - cough (75%), wheezing, pneumonia
  - hemoptysis (50%), dysphagia (2%)
- symptoms of peripheral tumors:
  - pleuritic / local chest pain, dyspnea, cough
  - Pancoast syndrome, superior vena cava syndrome
  - hoarseness
- symptoms of metastatic disease (CNS, bone, liver, adrenal gland)
- paraneoplastic syndromes:
  - cachexia of malignancy
  - clubbing + hypertrophic osteoarthropathy
  - nonbacterial thrombotic endocarditis
  - migratory thrombophlebitis
  - ectopic hormone production: hypercalcemia, syndrome of inappropriate secretion of antidiuretic hormone, Cushing syndrome, gynecomastia, acromegaly

Types:
1. **Adenocarcinoma** (50%)
◊ Most common cell type seen in women + nonsmokers!
Intermediate malignant potential (slow growth, high incidence of early metastases)
Doubling time: ~150–180 days
Histo: formation of glands / intracellular mucin
Subtype: bronchioloalveolar carcinoma
Location: almost invariably develops in periphery; frequently found in scars (tuberculosis, infarction, scleroderma, bronchiectasis) + in close relation to preexisting bullae
√ solitary peripheral subpleural mass (52%) / alveolar infiltrate / multiple nodules
√ may invade pleura + grow circumferentially around lung mimicking malignant mesothelioma
√ upper lobe distribution (69%)
√ air broncho- / bronchiologram on HRCT (65%)
√ calcification in periphery of mass (1%)
√ smooth margin / spiculated margin due to desmoplastic reaction with retraction of pleura

CHEST

2. **Squamous cell carcinoma** = **epidermoid carcinoma** (30–35%)
   ◊ Strongly associated with cigarette smoking
   Histo: mimics differentiation of the epidermis by producing keratin ("epidermoid carcinoma"); central necrosis is common
   Histogenesis: chronic inflammation with squamous metaplasia, progression to dysplasia + carcinoma in situ
   • positive sputum cytology
   ◊ Most common cell type diagnosed that is radiologically occult!
   • hypercalcemia from tumor-elaborated parathyroid hormonelike substance
   ◊ Slowest growth rate, lowest incidence of distant metastases
   Doubling time: ~90 days
   (a) Central location within main / lobar / segmental bronchus (2/3)
      √ large central mass ± cavitation
      √ distal atelectasis ± bulging fissure (due to mass)
      √ postobstructive pneumonia
         ◊ All cases of pneumonia in adults should be followed to complete radiologic resolution!
      √ airway obstruction with atelectasis (37%)
   (b) Solitary peripheral nodule (1/3)
      √ characteristic cavitation (in 7–10%)
         ◊ Squamous cell carcinoma is the most common cell type to cavitate!
      √ invasion of chest wall
         ◊ Squamous cell carcinoma is the most common cell type to cause Pancoast tumor!

3. **Small cell undifferentiated carcinoma** (15%)
   ◊ Strongly associated with cigarette smoking
   Rapid growth + high metastatic potential (early metastases in 60–80% at time of diagnosis); should be regarded as systemic disease regardless of stage; virtually never resectable
   Doubling time: ~30 days
   Path: arises from bronchial mucosa with growth in submucosa + subsequent invasion of peribronchial connective tissue
   Histo: small uniform oval cells with scant cytoplasm; nuclei with stippled chromatin; numerous mitoses + large areas of necrosis; in 20% coexistent with non-small cell histologic types (most frequently squamous cell)
   Subtype: oat cell cancer with hyperchromatic nuclei; ? related to Kulchitsky cell carcinomas
   • smooth-appearing mucosal surface endoscopically
   • ectopic hormone production: Cushing syndrome, inappropriate secretion of ADH
   ◊ Most common primary lung cancer causing superior vena caval obstruction (due to extrinsic compression / endoluminal thrombosis / invasion)!
   Location: 90% central within lobar / mainstem bronchus (primary tumor rarely visualized)
   √ typically large hilar / perihilar mass often associated with mediastinal widening (from adenopathy)
   √ extensive necrosis + hemorrhage
   √ small lung lesion (rare)
   Staging evaluation:
   CT of abdomen + head, bone scintigraphy, bilateral bone marrow biopsies
4. **Undifferentiated large cell carcinoma** (<5%)
   ◊ Strongly associated with smoking
   Intermediate malignant potential; rapid growth + early distant metastases
   Doubling time: ~120 days
   Histo: tumor cells with abundant cytoplasm + large nuclei + prominent nucleoli; diagnosed per exclusion due to lack of squamous / glandular / small cell differentiation
   Subtype: giant cell carcinoma with very aggressive behavior + poor prognosis
   √ large bulky usually peripheral mass >6 cm (50%)
   √ large area of necrosis
   √ pleural involvement
   √ large bronchus involved in central lesion (50%)

RISK FACTORS:
(1) cigarette smoking (squamous cell carcinoma + small cell carcinoma)
   — related to number of cigarettes smoked, depth of inhalation, age at which smoking began
   ◊ 85% of lung cancer deaths are attributable to cigarette smoking!
   ◊ Passive smoking may account for 25% of lung cancers in nonsmokers!
(2) radon gas: may be the 2nd leading cause for lung cancer with up to 20,000 deaths per year
(3) industrial exposure: asbestos, uranium, arsenic, chlormethyl ether
(4) concomitant disease: chronic pulmonary scar + pulmonary fibrosis
   Scar carcinoma
   7% of lung tumors; 1% of autopsies
   Origin: related to infarcts (>50%), tuberculosis scar (<25%)
   Histo: adenocarcinoma (72%), squamous cell carcinoma (18%)
   Location: upper lobes (75%)
   ◊ 45% of all peripheral cancers originate in scars!

PRESENTATION
√ solitary peripheral mass with corona radiata / pleural tail sign / satellite lesion
√ cavitation (16%): usually thick-walled with irregular inner surface; in 4/5 secondary to squamous cell carcinoma, followed by bronchioloalveolar carcinoma
√ central mass (38%): common in small cell carcinoma
√ unilateral hilar enlargement (secondary to primary tumor / enlarged lymph nodes)
Nodes on CT: 0–10 mm negative, 10–20 mm indeterminate, >20 mm positive

√ anterior + middle mediastinal widening (suggests small cell carcinoma)
√ segmental / lobar / lung atelectasis (37%) secondary to airway obstruction (particularly in squamous cell carcinoma)
√ "S sign of Golden" = incomplete lobar collapse with bulging contour produced by primary central tumor
√ rat tail termination of bronchus
√ bronchial cuff sign = focal / circumferential thickening of bronchial wall imaged end-on (early sign)
√ local hyperaeration (due to check-valve type endobronchial obstruction, best on expiratory view)
√ mucoid impaction of segmental / lobar bronchus (due to endobronchial obstruction)
√ persistent peripheral infiltrate (30%) = postobstructive pneumonitis
√ NO air bronchogram
√ pleural effusion (8–15%)
√ bone erosion of ribs / spine (9%)
√ involvement of main pulmonary artery (18%); lobar + segmental arteries (53%) may result in additional peripheral radiopacity (due to lung infarct)
√ calcification in 7% on CT (histologically in 14%) usually eccentric / finely stippled
(a) preexisting focus of calcium engulfed by tumor
(b) dystrophic calcium within tumor necrosis
(c) calcium deposit from secretory function of carcinoma (eg, mucinous adenocarcinoma)

Angio:
√ bronchogenic carcinoma supplied by bronchial arteries
√ distortion / stenosis / occlusion of pulmonary arterial circulation

MULTIPLE PRIMARY LUNG CANCERS

Incidence: 0.72–3.5%; in 1/3 synchronous, in 2/3 metachronous

◊ 10–32% of patients surviving resection of a lung cancer will develop a second primary!

Dx: biopsy mandatory for proper therapy because the tumor may have a different cell type

PARANEOPLASTIC MANIFESTATIONS

1. Carcinomatous neuromyopathy (4–15%)
2. Migratory thrombophlebitis
3. Hypertrophic pulmonary osteoarthropathy (3–5%)
4. Endocrine manifestations (15%) usually with small cell carcinoma: Cushing syndrome, inappropriate secretion of ADH, HPT, excessive gonadotropin secretion

LOCATION

60–80% arise in segmental bronchi
— central: small cell carcinoma, squamous cell carcinoma (sputum cytology positive in 70%); arises in central airway often at points of bronchial bifurcation, infiltrates circumferentially, extends along bronchial tree
— peripheral: adenocarcinoma, large cell carcinoma
— upper lobe: lower lobe = right lung:left lung = 3:2
— most common site: anterior segment of RUL
— **Pancoast tumor** (3%) = superior pulmonary sulcus tumor, frequently squamous cell carcinoma
 • atrophy of muscles of ipsilateral upper extremity due to lower brachial plexus involvement
 • Horner syndrome (enophthalmos, miosis, ptosis, anhidrosis) due to sympathetic chain + stellate ganglion involvement
 √ apical pleural thickening / mass
 √ ± soft-tissue invasion / bone destruction
— SVC obstruction (5%): often in small cell carcinoma

TNM STAGING

T1: <3 cm in diameter, surrounded by lung / visceral pleura
T2: >3 cm in diameter / invasion of visceral pleura / lobar atelectasis / obstructive pneumonitis / at least 2 cm from carina
T3: tumor of any size; less than 2 cm from carina / invasion of parietal pleura, chest wall, diaphragm, mediastinal pleura, pericardium; pleural effusion
T4: invasion of heart, great vessels, trachea, esophagus, vertebral body, carina / malignant effusion
N1: peribronchial / ipsilateral hilar nodes
N2: ipsilateral mediastinal nodes
N3: contralateral hilar / mediastinal nodes

STAGING FOR SMALL CELL LUNG CANCER

Limited disease:
1. Primary in one hemithorax
2. Ipsilateral hilar adenopathy
3. Ipsilateral supraclavicular adenopathy
4. Ipsi- and contralateral mediastinal adenopathy
5. Atelectasis
6. Paralysis of phrenic + laryngeal nerve
7. Small effusion without malignant cells

Extensive disease (60–80%):
1. Contralateral hilar adenopathy
2. Contralateral supraclavicular adenopathy
3. Chest wall infiltration
4. Carcinomatous pleural effusion
5. Lymphangitic carcinomatosis
6. Superior vena cava syndrome
7. Metastasis to contralateral lung
8. Extrathoracic metastases to bone (38%), liver (22–28%), bone marrow (17–23%), CNS (8–15%), retroperitoneum (11%), other lymph nodes

Prognosis: 7–11 months median survival; 15–20% 2-year disease-free survival rate

SPREAD

1. Direct local extension
2. Hematogenous (small cell carcinoma)
3. Lymphatic spread (squamous cell carcinoma); tumor in 10% of normal-sized lymph nodes
4. Transbronchial spread–least common

DISTANT METASTASES

@ Bone
(a) Marrow: in 40% at time of presentation

CHEST

(b) Gross lesions in 10–35%:
Location: vertebrae (70%), pelvis (40%), femora (25%)
√ osteolytic metastases (3/4)
√ osteoblastic metastases (1/4): in small cell carcinoma / adenocarcinoma
√ occult metastases in 36% of bone scans

@ Adrenals: in 37% at time of presentation
@ Brain: asymptomatic metastases on brain scan in 7% (30% at autopsy), in 2/3 multiple
@ Kidney, GI tract, liver, abdominal lymph nodes
@ Lung-to-lung metastases (in up to 10%, usually in late stage)

Cx:
(1) Diaphragmatic elevation (phrenic nerve paralysis)
(2) Hoarseness (laryngeal nerve involvement, left > right)
(3) SVC obstruction (5%): lung cancer is cause of all SVC obstructions in 90%
(4) Pleural effusion (10%): malignant, parapneumonic, lympho-obstructive
(5) Dysphagia: enlarged nodes, esophageal invasion
(6) Pericardial invasion: pericardial effusion, localized pericardial thickening / nodular masses

Prognosis: mean survival time <6 months; 10–15% overall 5-year survival; survival at 40 months: squamous cell 30% > large cell 16% > adenocarcinoma 15% > oat cell 1%

Rx:
(1) Surgical resection for non-small cell histologic types
Unresectable: involvement of heart, great vessels, trachea, esophagus, vertebral body, malignant pleural effusion
(2) Adjuvant chemotherapy + radiation therapy in extensive resectable disease
(3) Chemotherapy for small cell carcinoma + radiation therapy for bulky disease, CNS metastases, spinal cord compression, SVC obstruction

BRONCHOGENIC CYST

= budding / branching abnormality of ventral diverticulum of primitive foregut (ventral segment = tracheobronchial tree; dorsal segment = esophagus) between 26 and 40 days of embryogenesis

Incidence: most common intrathoracic foregut cyst (54–63% in surgical series)

Histo: thin-walled cyst filled with mucoid material, lined with columnar respiratory epithelium, mucous glands, cartilage, elastic tissue, smooth muscle

• contains mucus / clear or turbid fluid
√ sharply outlined round / oval mass
√ may contain air-fluid level

CT:
√ cyst contents of water density (50%) / higher density (50%)

OB-US:
√ single unilocular pulmonary cyst
√ echogenic distended lung obstructed by bronchogenic cyst

A. MEDIASTINAL BRONCHOGENIC CYST (86%)
Associated with: spinal abnormalities
M:F = 1:1
• usually asymptomatic
• stridor, dysphagia
Location: pericarinal (52%), paratracheal (19%), esophageal wall (14%), retrocardiac (9%); usually on right
√ rarely communicate with tracheal lumen
√ may show esophageal compression

B. INTRAPULMONARY BRONCHOGENIC CYST (14%)
M > F
• infection (75%)
• dyspnea, hemoptysis (most common)
Location: lower:upper lobe = 2:1; usually medial third
√ 36% will eventually contain air
DDx: solitary pulmonary nodule, cavitated neoplasm, cavitated pneumonia, lung abscess

BRONCHOPULMONARY DYSPLASIA

= RESPIRATOR LUNG
= complication of prolonged respirator therapy of intermittent PEEP with high oxygen concentration

Cause: oxygen toxicity + barotrauma
Pathogenesis: hypoxia + oxygen toxicity

— capillary wall damage, leakage of fluid into interstitium and pulmonary edema

Stage I (0–3 days):
Path: loss of ciliated cells + necrosis of bronchiolar mucosa
√ RDS pattern of hyaline membrane disease

Stage II (4–10 days):
Path: hyaline membranes, eosinophilic exudate, squamous metaplasia, interstitial edema
Associated with: congestive failure from PDA
√ complete opacification with air bronchogram

– fibrosis of interstitium + groups of emphysematous alveoli

Stage III (10–20 days):
Path: fewer hyaline membranes, persistent injury of alveolar epithelium, exudation of macrophages
√ "spongy" / "bubbly" coarse linear densities, esp. in upper lobes
√ hyperaeration of lung
√ lower lobe emphysema

Stage IV (after 1 month):
Path: septal wall thickening, dilated + tortuous lymphatics
√ same pattern as in stage IV
Prognosis: 40% mortality if not resolved by 1 month

• older child

Cx:
(1) Increased frequency of lower respiratory tract infections
(2) Cor pulmonale
(3) Focal atelectasis
(4) Asthmalike clinical picture
(5) Rib fractures, rickets, renal calcifications (from chronic furosemide therapy

(6) Cholelithiasis (hyperalimentation ± ? furosemide)
(7) Focal areas of tracheomalacia, tracheal stenosis, acquired lobar emphysema

Prognosis:
(1) Complete clearing over months / years (1/3)
(2) Retained linear densities in upper lobe emphysema (29%)

DDx:
(a) conditions present at birth:
(1) Diffuse neonatal pneumonia
(2) Meconium aspiration
(3) Total anomalous pulmonary venous return
(4) Congenital pulmonary lymphangiectasia
(b) conditions developing over time:
(1) Recurrent pneumonias with scarring (gastroesophageal reflux, TE fistula, immune deficiency, etc)
(2) Cystic fibrosis
(3) Idiopathic pulmonary fibrosis
(c) conditions not apparent at birth:
(1) Wilson-Mikity syndrome
(2) Pulmonary interstitial emphysema
(3) Patent ductus arteriosus (uncommon appearance)
(4) Overhydration
(5) Perinatally acquired viral infection (especially CMV)

BRONCHOPLEURAL FISTULA

= BRONCHOPULMONARY FISTULA
= communication between the bronchial system / lung parenchyma + pleural space

Cause:
(a) Trauma
1. Complication of resectional surgery (pneumonectomy, lobectomy, bullectomy)
2. Blunt / penetrating trauma
3. Barotrauma
(b) Lung necrosis
1. Putrid lung abscess
2. Necrotizing pneumonia: Klebsiella, H. influenzae, Staphylococcus, Streptococcus; tuberculosis; fungus; Pneumocystis
3. Infarction
(c) Airway disease
1. Bronchiectasis (very rare)
2. Emphysema complicated by pneumonia / pneumothorax
(d) Malignancy: lung carcinoma with postobstructive pneumonia / tumor necrosis following therapy

• large / persistent air leak
• acute / chronic empyema

HRCT:
√ direct visualization of bronchopleural fistula (in 50%)
√ peripheral air + fluid collection (indirect sign)

Dx: (1) Introduction of methylene blue into pleural space, in 65% dye appears in sputum
(2) Sinography
(3) Bronchography

Rx: tube thoracostomy, open drainage, decortication, thoracoplasty, muscle-pedicle closure, transbronchial occlusions

BRONCHOPULMONARY SEQUESTRATION

= congenital malformation consisting of
(1) nonfunctioning lung segment
(2) no communication with tracheobronchial tree
(3) systemic arterial supply

Incidence: 0.15–6.4% of all congenital pulmonary malformations; 1.1–1.8% of all pulmonary resections

√ usually >6 cm in size
√ round / oval, smooth, well-defined solid homogeneous mass near diaphragm with mass effect
√ occasionally fingerlike appendage posteriorly + medially (anomalous vessel)
√ contrast enhancement of sequestration at the same time as thoracic aorta on rapid sequential CT scans
√ multiple / single air-fluid levels if infected
√ surrounded by recurrent pulmonary consolidation in a lower lobe that never clears completely
√ may communicate with esophagus / stomach
◊ Pulmonary sequestration with communication to GI tract is termed **bronchopulmonary foregut malformation**!

DDx: bronchiectasis, lung abscess, empyema, bronchial atresia, congenital lobar emphysema, cystic adenomatoid malformation, intrapulmonary bronchogenic cyst, Swyer-James syndrome, pneumonia, arteriovenous fistula, primary / metastatic neoplasm, hernia of Bochdalek

Intralobar Sequestration (75–86%)

= enclosed by visceral pleura of affected pulmonary lobe but separated from bronchial tree

Etiology: controversial
(1) probably acquired in majority of patients
(2) early appearance of congenital accessory tracheobronchial bud leads to incorporation within one pleural investment

Path: chronic inflammation fibrosis: multiple irregular cordlike adhesions to mediastinum, diaphragm, parietal pleura; multiple cysts filled with fluid / thick gelatinous / purulent material; vascular sclerosis

Age at presentation: adulthood (50% >20 years); M:F = 1:1

Associated with congenital anomalies in 6–12%:
skeletal deformities (4%): scoliosis, rib + vertebral anomalies; esophagobronchial diverticula (4%); diaphragmatic hernia (3%); cardiac (including tetralogy of Fallot); renal: failure of ascent + rotation; cerebral anomalies; congenital pulmonary venolobar syndrome

• about 50% have symptoms by age 20; asymptomatic in 15%
• pain, repeated infection in same location (eg, recurrent acute lower lobe pneumonias)
• high-output congestive heart failure (in neonatal period) from L-to-L shunt

CHEST

• cough + sputum production, hemoptysis

Location: posterobasal segments, rarely upper lung / within fissure; L:R = 3:2

CXR:
- √ recurrent / persistent pneumonia localized to lower lobe
- √ cavitation and cysts ± fluid levels
  - ◊ Aeration of sequestered lung via Kohn pores / communication with tracheobronchial tree!

Bronchogram:
- √ NO communication of rudimentary bronchial system of sequestration with tracheobronchial tree (rare exceptions)

Angio:
- √ usually single large artery (mean diameter of 6 mm) coursing through inferior pulmonary ligament from
  - — distal thoracic aorta (73%)
  - — proximal abdominal aorta (22%)
  - — celiac / splenic artery
  - — intercostal artery (4%)
  - — anomalous branch of coronary artery
- √ multiple aa. in 16% (with vessel diameter of <3 mm)
- √ combined systemic + pulmonary arterial supply
- √ venous drainage via
  - — normal pulmonary veins to L atrium (in 95%)
  - — azygos / hemiazygos vv. / intercostal vv. / SVC into R atrium (in 5%)

CT:
- √ single / multiple thin-walled cysts containing fluid / mucus / pus / air-fluid level / air alone
- √ mucus-impacted ectatic bronchi (= fat density) in sequestered lung
- √ emphysema bordering normal lung (37%)
  = postobstructive hyperinflation of sequestered lung
- √ homogeneous / inhomogeneous soft-tissue mass with irregular borders
- √ irregular enhancement (rare)
- √ one / two anomalous systemic arteries arising from aorta (DDx: AVM, interrupted pulmonary artery, isolated anomaly, chronic infection / inflammation of lung or pleura, surgically created shunt)
- √ premature atherosclerosis of anomalous arteries
- ◊ Mucoid impaction of bronchus surrounded by hyperinflated lung is CHARACTERISTIC!

OB-US:
- √ spherical homogeneous highly echogenic mass
- √ anomalous systemic artery seen by color Doppler

Cx: massive spontaneous nontraumatic pleural hemorrhage, chronic inflammation, fibrosis

Bronchopulmonary Sequestrations

	Intralobar	*Extralobar*
Prevalence	75%	25%
Pleural investment	visceral pleura	own pleura
Venous drainage	pulmonary veins	systemic veins
Symptomatic	adulthood	first 6 months
Etiology	acquired	developmental
Congen. anomalies	15%	50%

DDx of mass: neurogenic tumor, lateral thoracic meningocele, extramedullary hematopoiesis, pleural tumor

DDx of cavity: lung abscess, necrotizing pneumonia, fungal / mycobacterial pneumonia, cavitating neoplasm, empyema

DDx of cysts: pulmonary abscess, empyema, bronchiectasis, emphysema, bronchogenic foregut cyst, pericardial cyst, eventration of diaphragm, congenital cystic malformation

Extralobar Sequestration (14–25%)

= accessory lobe with its own pleural sheath (= "Rokitansky lobe"), which prevents collateral air drift resulting in an airless round mass

Etiology: development of an anomalous accessory / supernumerary tracheobronchial foregut bud

Path: single ovoid / rounded / pyramidal airless lesion between 0.5 and 15 cm (generally 3 to 6 cm) in size

Histo: resembles normal lung with diffuse dilatation of bronchioles + alveolar ducts + alveoli; dilatation of subpleural + peribronchiolar lymph vessels; covered by mesothelial layer overlying fibrous connective tissue; congenital cystic adenomatoid malformation type II is present in 15–25%

Incidence: 0.5–6% of all congenital lung lesions

Age: neonatal presentation; 61% within first 6 months of life; occasionally in utero; M:F = 4:1

Associated with congenital anomalies in 15–65%:
- @ Lung: congenital diaphragmatic hernia (20–30%), eventration / diaphragmatic paralysis (up to 60%), cystic adenomatoid malformation (15–25%), lobar emphysema, bronchogenic cyst, pectus excavatum, congenital pulmonary venolobar syndrome
  - ◊ May coexist / form part of spectrum with CAM
- @ Heart: anomalous pulmonary venous return, cardiac / pericardial anomalies (8%)
- @ GI tract: epiphrenic diverticula (2%), TE fistula (1.5%), duplication of GI tract, ectopic pancreas
- @ Others: renal anomaly, vertebral anomaly

• respiratory distress + cyanosis + CHF in newborn (due to shunting of blood)
• feeding difficulties
• asymptomatic (rarely becomes infected) in 10%

Location: L:R = 4:1; typically within pleural space in posterior costodiaphragmatic sulcus between diaphragm + lower lobe (63–77%); mediastinum; within pericardium; within / below diaphragm (5–15%)

- √ airless (NO communication with bronchial tree); in presence of air connection with GI tract is inferred
- √ may contain cystic areas
- √ mediastinal shift (if large)

Angio (diagnostic):
- √ arterial supply from
  - — aorta as single / several small branches (80%)

— splenic, gastric, subclavian, intercostal branches (15%)
— pulmonary artery (5%)
√ venous drainage via
— systemic veins (80%) to R heart (IVC, azygos, hemiazygos, SVC, portal vein)
— pulmonary vein (25%)

CXR:
√ single well-defined homogeneous triangular mass (most commonly located adjacent to posterior medial hemidiaphragm)
√ NO air bronchograms
√ small "bump" on hemidiaphragm / inferior paravertebral region
√ opaque hemithorax ± ipsilateral pleural effusion (if sequestration large)
√ ± air-fluid level

CT:
√ homogeneous well-circumscribed soft-tissue density mass (no bronchial communication)

NUC (radionuclide angiography):
√ lack of perfusion during pulmonary phase followed by rapid perfusion in systemic phase

DDx: intrathoracic kidney, scimitar syndrome (with systemic supply to affected lung), hepatic herniation through diaphragm

OB-US:
◊ The vast majority in fetuses are extralobar!
√ conical / triangular homogeneous highly echogenic mass (many interfaces from multiple microscopically dilated structures)
√ color duplex may demonstrate vascular supply
√ polyhydramnios (? esophageal compression, excessive fluid secretion by sequestration)
√ fetal hydrops (? venous compression):
  √ edema, ascites
  √ hydrothorax (obstructed lymphatics + veins in torsed sequestration)

DDx for chest lesion:
congenital cystic adenomatoid malformation, neuroblastoma, teratoma, diaphragmatic hernia

DDx for infradiaphragmatic lesion:
neuroblastoma, teratoma, adrenal hemorrhage, mesoblastic nephroma, foregut duplication

Cx: infection (in cases of communication with bronchus / GI tract)

Rx: resection (delineation of vascular supply helpful)

Prognosis: favorable (worse if pulmonary hypoplasia present); decreases in size / disappears in up to 65% before birth

Esophageal / Gastric Lung

= rare variant of pulmonary sequestration

Age: infancy (as it is symptomatic)

• cough related to feeding
• recurrent pulmonary infections
√ communication of bronchial tree of sequestered lung with esophagus / stomach

CANDIDIASIS

Organism: ubiquitous human saprophyte (Candida albicans most commonly) characterized by blastospheres (yeasts) admixed with hyphae / pseudohyphae (conventional stains)

At risk: patient with lymphoreticular malignancy

Entry: (a) aspiration
(b) hematogenous dissemination from GI tract / infected central venous catheter

• prolonged fever despite broad-spectrum antibacterial coverage
• cough, hemoptysis
√ patchy airspace consolidation in lower lobe distribution
√ interstitial pattern
√ diffuse micro- / macronodular disease
√ pleural effusion (25%)

CARDIOPULMONARY SCHISTOSOMIASIS

= form of parasitic embolism

Organism: Schistosoma mansoni (endemic in Middle East, Africa, Atlantic coast of South America, Caribbean; S. japonicum and S. haematobium (less commonly)

At risk: >5 years of continuous ova secretion

Prerequisite: portal hypertension with periportal hepatic fibrosis

Cycle: eggs travel as emboli via portosystemic collateral pathways to lodge in pulmonary muscular arteries and arterioles (50–150 μm in diameter)

Pathogenesis:
trapped eggs are antigenic and incite an obliterative endarteritis (due to delayed host hypersensitivity)

Path: intra- and perivascular granulomas, intimal hyperplasia, medial hypertrophy, concentric collagen deposition and fibrosis of vessel walls; localized alveolitis with eosinophilic infiltration; pulmonary infarction

Age: 25–35 (range of 1–93) years

• gradually worsening hepatosplenomegaly
• dyspnea, cough, chest pain
• severe hypoxemia, cyanosis, digital clubbing

CXR:
√ cardiomegaly
√ central pulmonary arterial enlargement
√ tiny scattered lung nodules occasionally

HRCT:
√ nodules, interstitial thickening
√ patchy ground-glass attenuation
√ dilatation of right atrium + right ventricle + central pulmonary arteries

Cx: cor pulmonale (2–33%)

Rx: praziquantel, oxamniquine

CASTLEMAN DISEASE

= ANGIOFOLLICULAR LYMPH NODE HYPERPLASIA = BENIGN GIANT LYMPH NODE HYPERPLASIA = ANGIOMATOUS LYMPHOID HAMARTOMA = LYMPHOID HAMARTOMA
= diverse group of rare lymphoproliferative disorders of differing histopathologic properties + biologic behavior

Histo:
(a) hyaline-vascular Castleman disease (76–91%) lymph node hyperplasia, hyalinization with involuted germinal centers penetrated by capillaries, prominent capillary proliferation with endothelial hyperplasia in interfollicular areas
(b) plasma cell Castleman disease (4–9–24%) sheets of plasma cells between normal / enlarged follicles; relatively few capillaries

Localized / Unicentric Angiofollicular Lymph Node Hyperplasia

Cause: chronic viral antigenic stimulation with reactive lymphoid hyperplasia / developmental growth disturbance of lymphoid tissue
Age: all age groups (peak in 4th decade); M:F = 1:4
Histo: mostly hyaline-vascular cell type
Location: middle mediastinum + hila, cervical lymph nodes, mesenteric + retroperitoneal lymph nodes
Morphologic types:
(a) solitary well-circumscribed mass without associated adenopathy (50%)
(b) dominant mass displacing / surrounding / invading contiguous structures + lymphadenopathy (40%)
(c) multiple enlarged lymph nodes confined to one mediastinal compartment (10%)

- asymptomatic in 58–97%
- cough, dyspnea, hemoptysis
- lassitude, weight loss, fever
- growth retardation
- elevated sedimentation rate
- IgG, IgM, IgA hypergammaglobulinemia (50%)
- refractory microcytic anemia

Size: up to 16 cm in diameter
CT:
√ sharply marginated smooth / lobulated mass of muscle density
√ spotty coarse central calcifications (5–10%)
√ enhancing rim (vascular capsule)
√ intense enhancement almost equal to aorta (in hyalin-vascular type)
√ slight enhancement (in plasma cell type)
√ pleural effusion (uncommon)
MR:
√ heterogeneous mass hyperintense compared with muscle on T1WI
√ markedly hyperintense on T2WI
√ flow voids of feeding vessels surrounding mass
Angio:
√ hypervascular mass with intense homogeneous blush (hyalin-vascular type)
√ enlarged feeding vessels arising from bronchial / internal mammary / intercostal arteries
√ some hypervascularity (plasma cell type)
DDx: indistinguishable from lymphoma
Prognosis: treatment ~100% curative
Rx: (1) Complete surgical resection
(2) Radiation + steroid therapy

Disseminated / Generalized / Multicentric Angiofollicular Lymph Node Hyperplasia

= potentially malignant lymphoproliferative disorder
Cause: disordered immunoregulation with polyclonal plasma cells from viral infection with uncontrolled B-cell proliferation + interleukin-6 dysregulation
Mean age: 40–60 years; M:F = 2:1
Histo: mostly plasma cell type (66%) with infiltration of nodes by sheets of mature plasma cells
Associated with:
(a) hyperplasia without neuropathy
- fatigue, anorexia, skin lesions, CNS disorders

(b) hyperplasia with POEMS (polyneuropathy, organomegaly, endocrinopathy, monoclonal proteinemia, skin changes) syndrome
- skin lesions: hypertrichosis, hirsutism, sclerodermatous thickening, hyperpigmentation, hemangiomas
- distal symmetric sensorimotor neuropathy (50%)
- papilledema, pseudotumor cerebri (66%)
- monoclonal IgG (75%)

(c) osteosclerotic myeloma, Kaposi sarcoma, AIDS
√ 1–6 cm large homogeneous lymph nodes in multiple mediastinal compartments
√ variable mild contrast enhancement
√ peripheral multicentric adenopathy
√ hepatosplenomegaly
√ salivary gland enlargement
√ ascites
√ lymphocytic interstitial pneumonitis (LIP):
√ ± ill-defined centrilobular nodules
√ ground-glass attenuation
√ air-space consolidation
√ cysts (due to partial airway obstruction by peribronchial + peribronchiolar LIP)
√ thickening of bronchovascular bundles
Rx: surgical resection, irradiation, systemic chemotherapy + corticosteroids
Prognosis: mean survival of 24–33 months

CHEMICAL PNEUMONITIS

= inhalation of noxious chemical substances
(a) organic: organophosphates, paraquat, polyvinyl chloride, polymer fumes, smoke
(b) nonorganic: ammonia, hydrogen sulfide, nitrogen oxide, sulfur dioxide
(c) metal: cadmium, mercury, nickel, vanadium

Carbamates

= agricultural insecticides functioning as cholinesterase inhibitor (similar to organophosphates) but with poor penetration into CNS
√ pulmonary edema with respiratory failure

Paraquat

= agricultural herbicide
Exposure: often intentional ingestion

CHEST

Pathophysiology: rapid accumulation in lungs with production of superoxide radicals damaging pulmonary cells

CXR (wide radiographic variation):
- √ no abnormality
- √ increased interstitial / granular opacities
- √ pulmonary edema
- √ pneumomediastinum

HRCT:
- √ bilateral diffuse areas of ground-glass attenuation evolving into consolidation with bronchiectasis, irregular lines, traction bronchiectasis of interstitial fibrosis

Hydrogen Sulfide

= irritant + chemical asphyxiant gas

Industries: coal mines, tanneries, petroleum manufacturing plants, geothermal power plants, aircraft factories, sewer works, rubber works

Effect: toxic for respiratory (large quantities cause inhibition of medullary respiratory center) + neurologic systems

- • smell of rotten eggs
- • "knockdown" = brief loss of consciousness due to bronchial hyperpresponsiveness
- • determination of urine thiosulfate levels (to monitor occupational exposure)
- √ pulmonary edema

Ammonia

= highly soluble corrosive gas acts as a mucosal irritant

Industries: production of explosives, petroleum, agricultural fertilizer, plastics

√ pulmonary edema

Prognosis: complete recovery; bronchiectasis

+ bronchiolitis obliterans may develop

Hydrocarbon

Exposure: ingestion / aspiration (eg, accidental poisoning in children; fire-eating performers)

Path: (a) acute phase: intraalveolar, intrabronchial, peribronchial, interstitial accumulation of inflammatory cells + edema
(b) chronic phase (1–2 weeks after initial onset): proliferative bronchiolitis, parenchymal fibrosis, pneumatocele formation

- √ uni- / bilateral consolidation, well-defined nodules
- √ pneumatoceles (from coalescing areas of bronchiolar necrosis / partial obstruction of bronchial lumen)

Mercury

Exposure: inhalation of mercury vapor

Industries: electrolysis, manufacture of thermometers, cleaning of boilers, smelting silver from dental amalgam containing mercury

Pathophysiology: acute chemical bronchiolitis + pneumonitis followed by diffuse alveolar damage with hyaline membrane formation

- • pulmonary function impairment
- √ perivascular haziness + fine reticular opacities
- √ pulmonary interstitial fibrosis

Prognosis: acute inhalation poisoning usually fatal

CHRONIC EOSINOPHILIC PNEUMONIA

= numerous eosinophils, macrophages, histiocytes, lymphocytes, PMNs within lung interstitium + alveolar sacs

Etiology: unknown

Age: middle-age; M < F

- • common history of atopia (may occur during therapeutic desensitization procedure)
- • adult onset asthma (wheezing)
- • high fever, malaise, dyspnea (DDx to Löffler syndrome)
- • peripheral blood eosinophilia (with rare exceptions)
- √ homogeneous alveolar lung infiltrates with distribution at lung periphery = "photographic negative" of pulmonary edema (best seen on CT)
- √ frequently bilateral nonsegmental
- √ unchanged for many days / weeks (DDx to Löffler syndrome)
- √ fast regression of infiltrates under steroids

Rx: dramatic response to steroid therapy (within 3–10 days)

CHRONIC MEDIASTINITIS

Etiology:
(1) Granulomatous infection: histoplasmosis (most frequent), tuberculosis, actinomycosis, Nocardia
(2) Mediastinal granuloma
(3) Fibrosing mediastinitis
(4) Radiation therapy

Mediastinal Granuloma

= relatively benign massive coalescent adenitis with caseating / noncaseating lesions

Cause: primary lymph node infection (commonly tuberculosis / histoplasmosis)

Histo: thin fibrous capsule surrounding granulomatous lesion

√ lymphadenopathy

DDx: fibrosing mediastinitis (infiltrative, rare)

Fibrosing Mediastinitis

= SCLEROSING MEDIASTINITIS = MEDIASTINAL COLLAGENOSIS = MEDIASTINAL FIBROSIS

= uncommon benign disorder characterized by proliferation of dense fibrous tissue within mediastinum

Cause: abnormal host immune response to Histoplasma capsulatum antigen (organisms recovered in 50%); autoimmune disease, methysergide-induced

CHEST

May be associated with: retroperitoneal fibrosis, orbital pseudotumor, Riedel struma
Path: ill-defined soft-tissue mass with minimal / no apparent granulomatous foci
Histo: abundant paucicellular fibrous tissue infiltrating + obliterating adipose tissue
Age: 2nd–5th decade of life; M = F
- symptoms of central airway obstruction:
  - cough (41%), dyspnea (32%)
- symptoms of pulmonary venous occlusion:
  - "pseudo-mitral stenosis syndrome" = progressive exertional dyspnea, hemoptysis (31%)
  - cor pulmonale (secondary to pulmonary arterial hypertension caused by compression of pulmonary arteries / veins)
- dysphagia (2%)
- superior vena cava syndrome (6–39%)
- low left atrial pressure + widely differential elevation of pulmonary capillary wedge pressures

Location: middle mediastinum (subcarinal + paratracheal regions) and hila
Site: right > left side of mediastinum
CXR:
√ nonspecific widening of mediastinum:
  √ distortion of normally recognizable interfaces
  √ lobulated (in 86% calcified) paratracheal / hilar mass
√ typically unilateral pulmonary arterial obstruction:
  √ enlargement of main pulmonary artery + right heart
  √ diminution in size + quantity of vessels
  √ localized regional oligemia
√ pulmonary venous obstruction:
  √ peribronchial cuffing, septal thickening
  √ ipsilateral Kerley B lines
  √ pulmonary infarct
√ central airway narrowing:
  √ segmental / lobar atelectasis
  √ recurrent pneumonia
UGI:
√ circumferential narrowing / long-segment stricture of esophagus at junction of upper + middle thirds
√ "downhill" esophageal varices
CT:
√ focal mass (82%):
  √ calcified in 63%; in right paratracheal / subcarinal / hilar location
√ diffusely infiltrative process (18%):
  √ soft-tissue attenuation, no calcification
  √ obliteration of normal mediastinal fat planes
  √ encasement / invasion of adjacent structures mediastinal + hilar nodal masses with coarse calcifications
√ wedge-shaped peripheral consolidation of venous / arterial infarction
MR:
√ heterogenous infiltrative mass of intermediate signal intensity on T1WI
√ mixture of regions of increased + markedly decreased signal intensity on T2WI
NUC:
√ unilateral decreased / absent perfusion with normal ventilation (in focal hilar fibrosis)
√ large segmental / smaller subsegmental unmatched perfusion defects
√ ventilation defects in lobar / segmental occlusion
Angio (with therapeutic intent):
√ unilateral / asymmetric narrowing of central pulmonary arteries / distal arterial cutoffs
√ funnel-like pulmonary vein stenosis / obstruction / focal dilatation near left atrium
Cx: (1) Compression of SVC (64%) + pulmonary veins (4%)
(2) Chronic obstructive pneumonia (narrowing of trachea / central bronchi) in 5%
(3) Esophageal stenosis (3%)
(4) Pulmonary infarcts + fibrosis (narrowing of pulmonary artery)
(5) Prominent intercostal arteries (narrowing of pulmonary artery)
Rx: resection, ketoconazole, steroid therapy (limited success)
DDx: (1) Bronchogenic carcinoma
(2) Lymphoma
(3) Metastatic carcinoma
(4) Mediastinal sarcoma

CHURG-STRAUSS SYNDROME

= ALLERGIC ANGITIS AND GRANULOMATOSIS
= variant of polyarteritis nodosa in asthmatic patients
CLASSIC TRIAD:
(1) Allergic rhinitis or asthma (phase 1)
(2) Peripheral blood + tissue eosinophilia with Löffler syndrome (phase 2)
(3) Systemic small-vessel granulomatous vasculitis (phase 3), usually develops within 3 years of onset of asthma

Etiology: ? hypersensitivity response to an inhaled agent
Age: 20–40 (mean 28) years; M:F = 1:1
Path: (1) necrotizing vasculitis
(2) eosinophilic tissue infiltration
  (a) eosinophilic pneumonia
  (b) eosinophilic gastroenteritis
(3) extravascular "allergic" granulomas / eosinophilic abscesses
- allergic rhinitis, sinus pain, headaches, asthma
- fever, malaise, gastrointestinal symptoms, arthralgias
- eosinophilia (almost 100%): peripheral eosinophilia in >30%
- p-ANCA (perinuclear antineutrophil cytoplasmic autoantibodies) in 70%
- elevated rheumatoid factor in 52%

√ vascular aneurysms + thrombosis
@ Lung: intraalveolar hemorrhage
  √ normal CXR (25%)
  √ often transient peripheral widespread nonsegmental air-space opacities without zonal predominance
  √ diffuse miliary nodules:
    √ nodules may coalesce up to 2 cm (rare)
    √ cavitation is atypical (and suggests infection)

CHEST

√ eosinophilic pleural effusions (29%)
HRCT:
√ consolidation / ground-glass attenuation (59%)
√ pulmonary nodules
√ interlobar septal thickening
√ bronchial wall thickening
@ GI tract (20%): ulceration, hemorrhage, perforation
• diarrhea, bleeding, obstruction
√ mesenteric vasculitis
√ bowel wall infiltration by eosinophils
@ Heart (up to 47%): coronary vasculitis, myocarditis, pericardial tamponade (accounting for 50% of deaths)
◊ Higher frequency of cardiac involvement than Wegener granulomatosis
@ CNS: diffuse neuritis, mononeuritis multiplex, cerebral hemorrhage
@ Skin: palpable purpura
@ Kidney:
• renal artery-induced hypertension, hematuria
√ glomerulonephritis
◊ Less frequent + less severe renal disease compared with Wegener granulomatosis + microscopic polyangitis

Prognosis: 85% 5-year survival; death from cardiac / intraabdominal complications, cerebral hemorrhage, renal failure, status asthmaticus
Rx: corticosteroids, cyclophosphamide

CHYLOTHORAX

= leakage of chyle (= lymph containing chylomicrons = suspended fat) from thoracic duct or its branches into pleural space secondary to obstruction / disruption of thoracic duct (in 2%)

*Route of **thoracic duct**:*
Origin: arises from cisterna chyli anterior to L1/2 (10–15 mm in diameter and 5–7 cm long)
Course: enters thorax through aortic hiatus; ascends in right prevertebral location (between azygos vein + descending aorta); swings to left at T4–6 posterior to esophagus; ascends for a short distance along right of aorta; crosses behind aortic arch; runs ventrally at T3 between left common carotid artery + left subclavian artery
Termination: 3–5 cm above clavicle at venous angle (= junction of left subclavian + internal jugular veins)
Variation: two (33%) or more (in up to 50%) main ducts each consisting of up to 8 separate channels

Etiology:
A. Developmental defects
1. Thoracic duct atresia
2. Lymphangiectasia
3. Lymphangioma
4. Lymphangiomatosis (rare): mediastinal / thoracic cystic hygroma of neck growing into mediastinum
5. Lymphangioleiomyomatosis ± tuberous sclerosis

B. Trauma
1. Closed / penetrating chest trauma / birth trauma (25%): latent period of 10 days
2. Surgery (2nd most common cause): esophagectomy / cardiovascular surgery, esp. coarctation repair (0.5%), retroperitoneal surgery, neck surgery
3. Subclavian venous catheter

C. Neoplasm (54%)
1. Lymphoma (most common cause)
2. Metastatic cancer

D. Fibrosing conditions
1. Mediastinitis
2. Tuberculosis
3. Filariasis (rare)

E. Obstruction of central venous system / thoracic duct
F. Idiopathic / cryptogenic (15%): most common cause in neonatal period
G. Transdiaphragmatic passage of chylous ascites

Age: in full-term infants; may be present in utero; M:F = 2:1
Incidence: 1:10,000 deliveries
May be associated with:
Trisomy 21, TE-fistula, extralobar lung sequestration, congenital pulmonary lymphangiectasia

• high in neutral fat + fatty acid (low in cholesterol):
• triglyceride level >110 mg/dL
• milky viscoid fluid (chylomicrons) after ingestion of milk / formula and clear during fasting
√ usually unilateral loculated pleural effusion
(a) right chylothorax due to duct disruption inferior to T5–6 (more common)
(b) left-sided chylothorax if duct disrupted above T5–6
√ low attenuation (fat) / high attenuation (protein content)
√ ± leakage of lymphangiographic contrast
√ polyhydramnios (? result of esophageal compression)

Cx: (1) Pulmonary hypoplasia
(2) Hydrops (congestive heart failure secondary to impaired venous return)

Rx: (1) Thoracentesis (leading to loss of calories, lymphocytopenia, hypogammaglobulinemia)
(2) Total parenteral nutrition
(3) Thoracic duct ligation (if drainage exceeds 1,500 mL/day for adults or 100 mL/yr-age/day for children >5 years of age; drainage >14 days)
(4) Pleuroperitoneal shunt; tetracycline pleurodesis; mediastinal radiation; intrapleural fibrin glue; pleurectomy

COAL WORKER'S PNEUMOCONIOSIS

= CWP = ANTHRACOSIS = ANTHRACOSILICOSIS
= coal dust inhalation taken up by alveolar macrophages, in part cleared by mucociliary action (particle size >5 μm), in part deposited around bronchioles + alveoli, coal dust in itself is inert, but admixed silica is fibrogenic

Simple CWP

= aggregates of coal dust = coal macules (usually <3 mm)
NO progression in absence of further exposure

Histo: development of reticulin fibers associated with bronchiolar dilatation (focal emphysema) + bronchiolar artery stenosis (decreased capillary perfusion)

- poor correlation between symptoms, physiologic findings + roentgenogram

√ small round 1–5-mm opacities, frequently in upper lobes (radiographically only seen through superposition after an exposure of >10 years)

√ nodularity correlates with amount of collagen (NOT amount of coal dust)

Cx: (1) Chronic obstructive bronchitis
(2) Focal emphysema
(3) Cor pulmonale

COCCIDIOIDOMYCOSIS

Organism: dimorphic soil fungus Coccidioides immitis; arthrospores in desert soil spread by wind aerosolized in dry dust; highly infectious

Geographic distribution:
endemic in southwest desert of USA (San Joaquin Valley, central southern Arizona, western Texas, southern New Mexico) + northern Mexico + in parts of Central + South America; similar to histoplasmosis

Mode of infection: deposited in alveoli after inhalation + maturation into large thick-walled spherules with release of hundreds of endospores

Dx: (1) Culture of organism
(2) Spherules in pathologic material (demonstrated with Gomori-methenamine silver stain)
(3) Positive skin test
(4) Complement fixation titer

Primary Coccidioidomycosis

= ACUTE RESPIRATORY COCCIDIOIDOMYCOSIS

- 60–80% asymptomatic
- "valley fever" = influenza-like symptoms
- desert rheumatism (33%) most commonly in ankle
- rash, erythema nodosum / multiforme (5–20%)

√ segmental / lobar consolidation
√ patchy infiltrates mainly in lower lobes (46–80%) frequently subpleural + abutting fissures
√ peribronchial thickening
√ hilar adenopathy (20%)
√ pleural effusion (10%)

Chronic Respiratory Coccidioidomycosis

Prevalence: 5% of infected patients

- symptoms of postprimary tuberculosis
- hemoptysis in 50%

√ one / several well-defined nodules (= coccidioidomycoma) of 5–30 mm in size (in 5%)
√ persistent / progressive consolidation
√ "grape skin" thin-walled cavities (in 10–15%), in 90% solitary, 70% in anterior segment of upper lobes (DDx: TB), 3% rupture into pleural space due to subpleural location (pneumothorax / empyema / persistent bronchopleural fistula)
√ bronchiectasis
√ mediastinal adenopathy (10–20%)

Disseminated Coccidioidomycosis (in 1%)

= secondary phase of hematogenous spread to meninges, bones, skin, lymph nodes, subcutaneous tissue, joints (except GI tract)

- skin granulomas / abscesses

√ micronodular "miliary" lung pattern
√ pericardial effusion

CONGENITAL LOBAR EMPHYSEMA

= progressive overdistension of one / multiple lobes

M:F = 3 :1

Etiology:
(a) deficiency / dysplasia / immaturity of bronchial cartilage
(b) endobronchial obstruction (mucosal fold / web, prolonged endotracheal intubation, inflammatory exudate, inspissated mucus)
(c) bronchial compression (PDA, aberrant left pulmonary artery, pulmonary artery dilatation)
(d) polyalveolar / macroalveolar hyperplasia

Associated with: CHD in 15% (PDA, VSD)

- respiratory distress (90%) + progressive cyanosis within first 6 months of life

Location: LUL (42–43%), RML (32–35%), RUL (20%), two lobes (5%)

√ hazy masslike opacity immediately following birth (delayed clearance of lung fluid in emphysematous lobe over 1–14 days)
√ air trapping
√ hyperlucent expanded lobe (after clearing of fluid)
√ compression collapse of adjacent lobes
√ contralateral mediastinal shift
√ widely separated vascular markings

Mortality: 10%

Rx: surgical resection

CONGENITAL LYMPHANGIECTASIA

1. PRIMARY PULMONARY LYMPHANGIECTASIA (2/3)
   = abnormal development of lungs between 14–20th week of GA characterized by anomalous dilatation of pulmonary lymph vessels

   Path: subpleural cysts, ectatic tortuous lymph channels in pleura, interlobular septa + along bronchoarterial bundles; NO obstruction

   Age: usually manifest at birth; 50% stillborn; M = F

   May be associated with: total anomalous pulmonary venous return, hypoplastic left heart, Noonan syndrome

   - respiratory distress within few hours of birth

   Site: diffuse involvement of both lungs, occasionally only in one / two lobes (with good prognosis)

   √ marked prominence of coarse interstitial markings (simulating interstitial edema)
   √ hyperinflation
   √ scattered radiolucent areas (dilated airways)
   √ patchy areas of pneumonia + atelectasis
   √ pneumothorax

Prognosis: in diffuse form invariably fatal at <2 months of age

2. GENERALIZED LYMPHANGIECTASIA
   = DIFFUSE LYMPHANGIOMA
   = proliferation of mainly lymphatic vascular spaces with relentless systemic progression
   Age: children, young adults
   Location: widespread visceral + skeletal involvement
   √ diffuse pulmonary interstitial disease
   √ chylous effusions in pleural + pericardial spaces
   √ ± lytic bone lesions
   √ lymphangiographic pooling of contrast material in dilated lymphatic channels / lymph nodes
3. LOCALIZED LYMPHANGIOMA
   = rare benign usually cystic lesion
   Histo: collection of dilated + proliferated lymph vessels (? hamartoma / benign neoplasm / focal sequestration of ectatic lymph tissue)
   Age: first 3 years of life; M = F
   • asymptomatic (33%)
   • dyspnea (from tracheal compression)
   Location: neck (80%), mediastinum, axilla, extremity
   √ discrete featureless mass
   √ may have chylous / pleural effusion
   √ may have lytic lesion in contiguous skeleton
   Prognosis: propensity for local recurrence
   DDx: hemangioma
4. SECONDARY LYMPHANGIECTASIA
   Secondary to elevated pulmonary venous pressure in CHD (TAPVR)

CONGENITAL PULMONARY VENOLOBAR SYNDROME

= unique form of lung hypoplasia / aplasia affecting one / more lobes in a constellation of distinctly different congenital anomalies of the thorax that often occur together; M:F = 1:1.4

A. MAJOR COMPONENTS
   1. Hypogenetic lung (69%): lobar agenesis / aplasia / hypoplasia
   2. Partial anomalous pulmonary venous return (31%) = scimitar syndrome
   3. Absence of pulmonary artery (14%)
   4. Pulmonary sequestration (24%)
   5. Systemic arterialization of lung without sequestration (10%)
   6. Absence / interruption of inferior vena cava (7%)
   7. Duplication of diaphragm = accessory diaphragm (7%)
      = thin membrane in right hemithorax fused anteriorly with the diaphragm coursing posterosuperiorly to join with the posterior chest wall + trapping all / part of RML / RLL
      √ accessory fissurelike oblique line above right posterior costophrenic sinus (if trapped lung is aerated)
      √ solid mass along posterior right hemidiaphragm (if trapped lung is unaerated)
      CT:
      √ ovoid area of increased density in posterior right hemithorax (= dome of accessory diaphragm)
B. MINOR COMPONENTS
   1. Tracheal trifurcation (extremely rare): 2 mainstem bronchi supply the right lung
   2. Eventration of diaphragm
   3. Partial absence of diaphragm
   4. Phrenic cyst
   5. Horseshoe lung
   6. Esophageal / gastric lung
   7. Anomalous superior vena cava
   8. Absence of left pericardium

◊ The most constant components of the syndrome are hypogenetic lung + PAPVR!

Associated with:
(1) Vascular anomalies: hypoplastic artery, anomalous venous return, systemic arterial supply
(2) Anomalies of hemidiaphragm on affected side:
   √ retrosternal band on lateral CXR due to mediastinal rotation
   √ phrenic cyst
   √ diaphragmatic hernia
   √ accessory hemidiaphragm
(3) Hemivertebrae + scoliosis
(4) CHD (25–50%): secundum-type ASD, VSD, tetralogy of Fallot, PDA, coarctation of aorta, hypoplastic left heart, double-outlet right ventricle, double-chambered right atrium, endocardial cushion defect, persistent left SVC, pulmonary stenosis

• asymptomatic (40%)
• may have dyspnea / recurrent infections

Location: right-sided predominance; M:F = 1.0:1.4
√ hypoplasia / aplasia of one / more lobes of the lung with errors of lobation (bilateral left bronchial branching pattern / horseshoe lung)
√ "scimitar vein" (90%) = partial anomalous pulmonary venous return (commonly infradiaphragmatic into IVC / portal vein / hepatic vein / R atrium), on CXR seen only in 1/3
√ systemic arterial supply to abnormal segment may be present from thoracic aorta (bronchial, intercostal, transpleural) or abdominal aorta (celiac artery, transdiaphragmatic)
√ reticular densities (enlarged bronchial / transpleural arterial collaterals)
√ small hilus (absent / small pulmonary artery)
√ small right hemithorax + mediastinal shift
√ haziness of right heart border
√ cardiac dextroposition (in right lung hypoplasia)
√ anomalies of bony thorax / thoracic soft tissues
√ absent inferior vena cava
√ rib hypoplasia / malsegmentation
√ rib notching

CT:
√ small hemithorax + mediastinal shift
√ abnormalities of bronchial branching
√ anomalously located pulmonary fissure
√ discontinuity of hemidiaphragm
√ pulmonary arterial hypoplasia

CHEST

√ hyparterial right bronchus (instead of eparterial)
√ one / more vessels increasing in diameter toward diaphragm
√ rind of subpleural fatty tissue in affected hemithorax
√ lack of normal venous confluence of right lung

DDx: meandering pulmonary vein, dextrocardia, hypoplastic lung, Swyer-James syndrome

COSTOCHONDRITIS

= musculoskeletal infection

Incidence: increased with IV drug abuse

Agents: Staphylococcus epidermidis, Streptococcus pneumoniae, Candida albicans, Aspergillus

CT:
√ soft-tissue swelling
√ cartilage fragmentation, bone destruction
√ low-attenuation cartilage
√ focal peripheral cartilaginous calcification

Rx: surgical excision

CHEST

CRYPTOCOCCOSIS

= TORULOSIS = EUROPEAN BLASTOMYCOSIS

Organism: encapsulated unimorphic yeastlike fungus Cryptococcus neoformans; spherical single-budding yeast cell with thick capsule, stains with India ink; often in soil contaminated with pigeon excreta

Histo: granulomatous lesion with caseous necrotic center

Predisposed: opportunistic invader in diabetics + immunocompromised patients

• low-grade meningitis (affinity to CNS); M:F = 4:1

@ Lung
√ well-circumscribed mass (40%) of 2–10 cm in diameter, usually peripheral location
√ lobar / segmental consolidation (35%)
√ cavitation (15%)
√ hilar / mediastinal adenopathy (12%)
√ calcifications (extremely rare)
√ interstitial pneumonia (rare, in AIDS patients)

@ Musculoskeletal
√ osteomyelitis (5–10%)
√ arthritis (rare, usually from extension of osteomyelitis)

CYSTIC ADENOMATOID MALFORMATION

= CAM = congenital cystic abnormality of the lung characterized by an intralobar mass of disorganized pulmonary tissue communicating with bronchial tree + having normal vascular supply + drainage but delayed clearance of fetal lung fluid

Incidence: 25% of congenital lung disorders; 95% of congenital cystic lung lesions

Cause: arrest of normal bronchoalveolar differentiation between 5th–7th week of gestation with overgrowth of terminal bronchioles

Path: proliferation of bronchial structures at the expense of alveolar saccular development, modified by intercommunicating cysts of various size (adenomatoid overgrowth of terminal bronchioles, proliferation of smooth muscle in cyst wall, absence of cartilage)

TYPE I (50%):
Histo: single / multiple large cyst(s) >20 mm lined by ciliated pseudostratified columnar epithelium, mucus-producing cells in 1/3
Prognosis: excellent following resection

TYPE II (40%):
Histo: multiple cysts 5–12 mm lined by ciliated cuboidal / columnar epithelium
Prognosis: poor secondary to associated abnormalities

TYPE III (10%):
Histo: solitary large bulky firm mass of bronchuslike structures lined by ciliated cuboidal epithelium with 3–5-mm small microcysts
Prognosis: poor secondary to pulmonary hypoplasia / hydrops

In 25% associated with: cardiac malformation, pectus excavatum, renal agenesis, prune-belly syndrome, jejunal atresia, chromosomal anomaly, bronchopulmonary sequestration

Age of detection: children, neonates, fetus; M:F = 1:1

• respiratory distress + severe cyanosis in first week of life (66%) / within first year of life (90%) due to compression of normal lung + airways
• superimposed chronic recurrent infection (10%) after first year of life

Location: equal frequency in all lobes (middle lobe rarely affected); more than one lobe involved in 20%; mostly unilateral without side preference

CXR:
√ almost always unilateral expansile mass with well-defined margins (80%) (due to retained fetal lung fluid / type III lesion)
√ multiple air- / occasionally fluid-filled cysts
√ compression of adjacent lung
√ contralateral shift of mediastinum (87%)
√ hypoplastic ipsilateral lung
√ proper position of abdominal viscera
√ spontaneous pneumothorax (late sign)

CT:
◊ Postnatally becoming obstructed and filled with air
√ solitary / multiple fluid or air-fluid filled cysts with thin walls
√ surrounding focal emphysematous changes

OB-US:
√ single large cyst / multiple large cysts of 2–10 cm in diameter (Type I)
√ multiple small cysts of 5–12 mm in diameter (type II)
√ large homogeneously hyperechoic mass compared with liver (type III)
√ contralateral mediastinal shift (89%)
√ polyhydramnios (25–75%, ? from compression of esophagus or increased fluid production by abnormal lung) / normal fluid (28%) / oligohydramnios (6%)

√ fetal ascites (62–71%)
√ fetal hydrops in 33–81% (decreased venous return from compression of heart / vena cava)
Risk of recurrence: none
Cx: ipsi- / bilateral pulmonary hypoplasia
Prognosis: 50% premature, 25% stillborn
◊ Polyhydramnios, ascites, hydrops indicate a poor outcome!
◊ CAM becomes smaller in fetuses in many cases and occasionally almost disappears by birth!
DDx: (1) Congenital lobar emphysema
(2) Diaphragmatic hernia
(3) Bronchogenic cyst (small solitary cyst near midline)
(4) Neurenteric cyst
(5) Bronchial atresia
(6) Bronchopulmonary sequestration (less frequently associated with polyhydramnios / hydrops)
(7) Mediastinal / pericardial teratoma

CYSTIC FIBROSIS

= MUCOVISCIDOSIS = FIBROCYSTIC DISEASE
= autosomal recessive multisystem disease characterized by mucous plugging of exocrine glands secondary to
(a) dysfunction of exocrine glands forming a thick tenacious material obstructing conducting system
(b) reduced mucociliary transport
Incidence: 1:2,000–1:2,500 livebirths; almost exclusively in Caucasians (5% carry a CF mutant gene allele); unusual in Blacks (1:17,000), Orientals, Polynesians
◊ The most common inherited disease among Caucasian Americans!
Cause: cystic fibrosis transmembrane regulator gene (CFTR) on long arm of chromosome 7 builds a defective ion transport protein for an epithelial chloride channel; abnormal transmembrane conductance for Cl^- decreases osmotic forces and thus luminal water; >230 different gene mutations (in 70% ΔF_{508})
Screening (for 6 most common mutations of CF gene): carrier detection rate of 85% of Northern Europeans, 90% of Ashkenazi Jews, 50% of American Blacks
Age at diagnosis: 1st year of life (70%), by age 4 years (80%), by age 12 years (90%); mean age of 2.9 years; M:F = 1:1
• elevated concentrations of sodium + chloride (>40 mmol/L for infants) in sweat
• decreased urinary PABA excretion
• infertility in males
• increased susceptibility to infection by Staphylococcus aureus + Pseudomonas aeruginosa
Prognosis: median survival of 28 years; pulmonary complications are the most predominant cause of morbidity and death (90%)

@ Lung
• chronic cough
• recurrent pulmonary infections (reduced mucociliary clearance encourages Pseudomonas colonization)
• progressive respiratory insufficiency due to obstructive lung disease
Location: predilection for apical + posterior segments of upper lobes
√ "fingerlike" mucus plugging (mucoid impaction in dilated bronchi) within 1st month of life
√ subsegmental / segmental / lobar atelectasis with right upper lobe predominance (10%)
√ progressive cylindrical / cystic bronchiectasis (in 100% at >6 months of age) ± air-fluid levels due to prolonged mucus plugging preponderant in upper lobes
√ parahilar linear densities + peribronchial cuffing
√ focal peripheral / generalized hyperinflation secondary to collateral air drift into blocked airways)
√ hilar adenopathy
√ large pulmonary arteries (pulmonary arterial hypertension)
√ recurrent local pneumonitis (initiated by staphylococcus / Haemophilus influenza, succeeded by Pseudomonas)
√ allergic bronchopulmonary aspergillosis (with bronchial dilatation + mucoid impaction)

CT:
√ cylindrical (varicose / cystic) bronchiectasis
√ peribronchial thickening
√ bronchiectatic cyst (= bronchus directly leading into sacculation) in 56%
√ interstitial cysts in 32%
√ emphysematous bulla (= peripheral air space with long pleural attachment + without communication to bronchus) in 12%
√ periseptal emphysema
√ mucus plugs = tubular structures ± branching pattern
√ subsegmental / segmental collapse / consolidations

NUC:
√ matched patchy areas of decreased ventilation + perfusion

Cx: (1) Pneumothorax (rupture of bulla / bleb), common + recurrent
(2) Hemoptysis (parasitized bronchial arteries connect to pulmonary arteries + veins resulting in AV fistulae)
(3) Cor pulmonale
(4) Hypertrophic pulmonary osteoarthropathy (rare)
Cause of death: massive mucus plugging (95%)
Rx: intratracheal instillation of aerosolized adenoviral + liposomal vector-CFTR gene preparations

@ GI tract (85–90%)
• chronic obstipation
• failure to thrive
√ gastroesophageal reflux (21–27%) due to transient inappropriate lower esophageal sphincter relaxation
√ meconium plug syndrome (25%, most common cause of colonic obstruction in the infant)
√ distal intestinal obstruction syndrome (10–15–47%) = meconium ileus equivalent syndrome (in older child / young adult)

√ meconium ileus (10–16% at birth)
  ◊ Earliest clinical manifestation of cystic fibrosis!
√ fibrosing colonopathy = stricture of right colon with longitudinal shortening secondary to high-dose lipase supplementation
√ thickened nodular duodenal mucosal folds (due to unbuffered gastric acid, production of abnormal mucus, Brunner gland hypertrophy)
√ mild generalized small bowel dilatation with diffuse distortion + thickening of mucosal folds (at times involving colon + rectum)
√ large distended colon with mottled appearance (retained bulky dry stool)
√ pneumatosis intestinalis of colon (5%) from air block phenomena of obstructive pulmonary disease
√ "microcolon" = colon of normal length but diminished caliber
√ "jejunization of colon" = coarse redundant + hyperplastic colonic mucosa (distended crypt goblet cells)
√ Crohn disease
√ appendicitis
√ rectal prolapse between 6 months and 3 years in untreated patients (18–23%)

Cx: gastrointestinal perforation with meconium peritonitis (50%), volvulus of dilated segments, bowel atresia, intussusception at an average age of 10 years (1%)

@ Liver
√ steatosis (30%) due to untreated malabsorption, dietary deficiencies, hepatic dysfunction, medications (= initial manifestation in infants)
√ focal (40%) / multilobular (5–12%) biliary cirrhosis from inspissated bile:
  • signs of portal hypertension in multilobular form (clinically in 4–6%, autoptic in up to 50%)
√ portal hypertension (in 1% of biliary cirrhosis) + hepatosplenomegaly + hypersplenism

@ Biliary tree
Histo: mucus-containing cysts in gallbladder wall
• cholestasis (secondary to CBD obstruction)
• symptoms of gallbladder disease (3.6%)
√ sludge (33%)
√ cholelithiasis (12–24%): mostly cholesterol stones due to (1) interrupted enterohepatic circulation after ileal resection / (2) ileal dysfunction in distal intestinal obstruction syndrome
√ gallbladder atony
√ microgallbladder (25% at autopsy)
√ thickened trabeculated gallbladder wall
√ subepithelial cysts of gallbladder wall
√ atresia / stenosis of cystic duct

@ Pancreas
Pathophysiology: duct obstruction from inspissated secretions (= protein plugs) as a result of precipitation of relatively insoluble proteins
Path: progressive ductectasia, pancreatic atrophy, increased pancreatic lobulation, fibrosis due to recurrent acute pancreatitis, replacement by fat
Histo: dilatation of acini and ducts + cyst formation
• steatorrhea + malabsorption + fat intolerance due to exocrine pancreatic insufficiency in 80–90% without affecting endocrine function (only after 98% of pancreas is damaged)
  ◊ Cystic fibrosis is the most common cause of exocrine pancreatic insufficiency in patients <30 years of age!
• abdominal pain, bloating, flatulence, failure to thrive
• diabetes mellitus (secondary to pancreatic fibrosis) increasing with age (in 1% of children + 13% of adults):
  • glucose intolerance in 30–50%
  • 1–2% require insulin therapy
• acute pancreatitis (clinically rare)
√ diffuse pancreatic atrophy without fatty replacement
√ lipomatous pseudohypertrophy of pancreas
√ generalized increased echogenicity (70–100%)
√ complete / partial fatty replacement (–90 to –120 HU)
√ calcific chronic pancreatitis
√ **pancreatic cystosis** = microscopic / 1–3-mm small cysts replacing pancreas (common), occasionally macroscopic cysts up to 12 cm

@ Skull
√ sinusitis with opacification of well-developed maxillary, ethmoid, sphenoid sinuses
√ hypoplastic frontal sinuses

OB-US:
√ hyperechogenic bowel (in up to 60–70% of fetuses affected with cystic fibrosis)

Prognosis: median survival of 28 years; 2.3 deaths/100 patients from cardiorespiratory causes (78%), hepatic disease (4%)

DIAPHRAGMATIC HERNIA

Congenital Diaphragmatic Hernia

= absence of closure of the pleuroperitoneal fold by 9th week of gestational age

Embryology:
ventral component of diaphragm formed by septum transversum during 3rd–5th week GA; gradually extends posteriorly to envelop esophagus + great vessels; fuses with foregut mesentery to form the posteromedial portions of the diaphragm by 8th week GA; lateral margins of diaphragm develop from muscles of the thoracic wall; the posterolaterally located pleuroperitoneal foramina (Bochdalek) close last

Incidence: 1: 2,200–3,000 livebirths (0.04%); M:F = 2:1; most common intrathoracic fetal anomaly
  ◊ Delayed onset following group B streptococcal infection!

Etiology:
(1) delayed fusion of diaphragm (spontaneous self-correction may occur) / premature return of bowel from its herniated position within the umbilical coelom

(2) insult that inhibits / delays normal migration of the gut + closure of the diaphragm between 8th and 12th week of embryogenesis

Classification (Wiseman):

I. herniation early during bronchial branching leading to severe bilateral pulmonary hypoplasia; uniformly fatal

II. herniation during distal bronchial branching leading to unilateral pulmonary hypoplasia; survival possible

III. herniation late in pregnancy with compression of otherwise normal lung; excellent prognosis

IV. postnatal herniation with compression of otherwise normal lung; excellent prognosis

Associated anomalies in 20% of liveborn and in 90% of stillborn fetuses:

1. CNS (28%): neural tube defects
2. Gastrointestinal (20%): particularly malrotation, oral cleft, omphalocele
3. Cardiovascular (9–23%)
4. Genitourinary (15%)
5. Chromosomal abnormalities (4%): trisomy 18 + 21
6. Spinal defects
7. IUGR (with concurrent major abnormality in 90%)

Location: L:R = 5–9:1

◊ Right-sided hernias are frequently fatal!

(1) **Bochdalek hernia** (85–90%)

= posterolateral defect caused by maldevelopment / defective fusion of the cephalic fold of the pleuroperitoneal membranes

Incidence: 1:2,200–12,500 livebirths

Location: left (80%), right (15%), bilateral (5%)

Herniated organs:

(a) on left: omental fat (6%), bowel, spleen, left lobe of liver, stomach (rare), kidney, pancreas

(b) on right: part of liver, gallbladder, small bowel, kidney

mnemonic: "4 B's"

Bochdalek
Back (posterior location)
Babies (age at presentation)
Big (usually large)

(2) **Morgagni hernia** (1–2%)

= anteromedial parasternal defect (space of Larrey) caused by maldevelopment of septum transversum; R > L

Incidence: 1:100,000

Herniated organs: omental fat, transverse colon, liver

Often associated with:

chromosomal abnormality, mental retardation, heart defects, pericardial deficiency

(a) abdominal viscera / fat may herniate into pericardial sac

(b) heart may herniate into upper abdomen

mnemonic: "4 M's"

Morgani
Middle (anterior + central location)
Mature (tend to present in older children)
Minuscule (usually small)

(3) Septum transversum defect = defect in central tendon

(4) Hiatal hernia = congenitally large esophageal orifice

(5) **Eventration** (5%) = upward displacement of abdominal contents secondary to a congenitally thin hypoplastic diaphragm

Unilateral eventration may be associated with:
Beckwith-Wiedemann syndrome, trisomy 13, trisomy 15, trisomy 18

Bilateral eventration may be associated with:
toxoplasmosis, CMV, arthrogryposis

Location: anteromedial on right, total involvement on left side; R:L = 5:1

√ small diaphragmatic excursions
√ often lobulated diaphragmatic contour

• respiratory distress in neonatal period (life-threatening deficiency of small airways + alveoli)
• scaphoid abdomen

Herniated organs:
small bowel (90%), stomach (60%), large bowel (56%), spleen (54%), pancreas (24%), kidney (12%), adrenal gland, liver, gallbladder

√ bowel loops in chest
√ contralateral shift of mediastinum + heart
√ complete (1–2%) / partial absence of diaphragm
√ absence of stomach, small bowel in abdomen
√ passage of nasogastric tube under fluoroscopic control entering intrathoracic stomach
√ incomplete rotation + anomalous mesenteric attachment of bowel

OB-US (diagnosis possible by 18 weeks GA):

√ solid / multicystic / complex chest mass
√ mediastinal shift
√ nonvisualization of fetal stomach below diaphragm
√ fetal stomach at level of fetal heart
√ peristalsis of bowel within fetal chest (inconsistent)
√ paradoxical motion of diaphragm with fetal breathing (defect in diaphragm sonographically not visible)
√ scaphoid fetal abdomen with reduced abdominal circumference
√ herniated liver frequently surrounded by ascites
√ polyhydramnios (common, due to partial esophageal obstruction or heart failure) / normal fluid volume / oligohydramnios
√ swallowed fetal intestinal contrast appears in chest (CT amniography confirms diagnosis)

Cx: (1) Bilateral pulmonary hypoplasia
(2) Persistent fetal circulation (postsurgical pulmonary hypertension)

Prognosis: (1) Stillbirth (35–50%)
(2) Neonatal death (35%)

◊ Survival is determined by size of defect + time of entry + associated anomalies (34% survival rate if isolated, 7% with associated anomalies)

Indicators for poor prognosis:
large intrathoracic mass with marked mediastinal shift, IUGR, polyhydramnios, hydrops fetalis, detection <25 weeks MA, intrathoracic liver, dilated intrathoracic stomach, other malformations

Mortality: in 10% death before surgery;
40–50% operative mortality;
(a) stomach intrathoracic vs. intraabdominal = 60% vs. 6%
(b) polyhydramnios vs. normal amniotic fluid = 89% vs. 45%

DDx: congenital adenomatoid malformation, mediastinal cyst (bronchogenic, neurenteric, thymic)

Traumatic Diaphragmatic Hernia

= DIAPHRAGMATIC RUPTURE

Prevalence: 0.8–1.6% of all blunt trauma; 5% of all diaphragmatic hernias, but 90% of all strangulated diaphragmatic hernias

Etiology of traumatic rupture of diaphragm:
(a) blunt trauma (5–50%) due to marked increase in intraabdominal pressure: motor vehicle accident (>90%), fall from height, bout of hyperemesis; L:R = 3:1, bilateral rupture in <3.6%
(b) penetrating trauma (50%): knife, bullet, repair of hiatus hernia
◊ Usually <1 cm in diameter; detected at surgery

Herniation of organs (32–58%) in order of frequency: stomach, colon, small bowel, omentum, spleen, kidney, pancreas

- may be asymptomatic for months / years following trauma, onset of symptoms may be so long delayed that traumatic event is forgotten
- virtually all become ultimately symptomatic, most in <3 years
- **Bergqvist triad**:
  (1) rib fractures (2) fracture of spine / pelvis
  (3) traumatic rupture of diaphragm

Location: 77–90–98% on left side; posterolateral portion of diaphragm medial to spleen in a radial orientation; medial central tendon with intrapericardial hernia (3.4%)

Size: most tears are >10 cm in length

CXR:
◊ The first posttraumatic CXR is abnormal in 46–77% but nonspecific!
◊ Positive intrathoracic pressure from ventilation may delay herniation!
◊ Serial CXRs may show progressive changes!
√ nonvisualization of diaphragmatic contour
√ elevated asymmetric / irregular contour of hemidiaphragm
Cave: cephalad margin of bowel may simulate an elevated diaphragm (look for haustra)
√ herniation of air-filled viscus: stomach, colon
√ shift of mediastinum + lung to opposite side
√ lower lobe mass / consolidation (herniated solid organ / omentum / airless bowel loop)
√ inhomogeneous mass with air-fluid level in left hemithorax
√ mushroomlike mass of herniated liver in right hemithorax
√ "collar sign" = hourglass constriction of afferent + efferent bowel loops at orifice
√ hydrothorax / hemothorax indicates strangulation
√ fractures of lower left ribs
√ abnormal U-shaped course of nasogastric tube above suspected level of hemidiaphragm
N.B.: tube first dips below diaphragm (rent spares esophageal hiatus with gastroesophageal junction remaining in its normal position)
√ location of diaphragm may be documented by
1. gas-filled bowel constricted at site of diaphragmatic laceration
2. barium study

CT (61% sensitive, 87% specific):
◊ Best detected on reformatted SAG + COR images!
Associated with: abdominal + pelvic injury in 90–94%
√ abrupt discontinuity of hemidiaphragm (73–82%)
√ herniation of omentum / bowel / abdominal organs into thorax (55%)
√ visualization of peritoneal fat / abdominal viscera lateral to lung or diaphragm / posterior to crus of hemidiaphragm
√ "collar sign" = waistlike constriction of viscera at level of diaphragm (27%)
√ "absent diaphragm sign" = failure to see diaphragm
√ concurrent pneumothorax, pneumoperitoneum, hemothorax, hemoperitoneum

MR:
√ interruption of hypointense band of diaphragmatic muscle outlined by hyperintense abdominal + mediastinal fat

Associated injuries:
√ fractures of lower ribs / pelvis (42%)
√ intraabdominal injuries (72%):
√ perforation of hollow viscus
√ rupture of spleen

Reasons for diagnostic misses:
(1) left-sided defect covered by omentum
(2) right-sided defect sealed by liver
(3) positive pressure ventilation
(4) associated injuries mask tear: atelectasis, pleural effusion, lung contusion, phrenic nerve paralysis

Cx: life-threatening strangulation of bowel / stomach occurs in majority
◊ 90% of strangulated hernias are traumatic!

Prognosis: 30% mortality in unrecognized cases

DDx: eventration; diaphragmatic paralysis; normal variant of acquired diaphragmatic discontinuity posteriorly related to congenital Bochdalek hernia (6–11%)

EMPHYSEMA

= group of pulmonary diseases characterized by permanently enlarged air spaces distal to terminal bronchioles accompanied by destruction of alveolar walls + local elastic fiber network

◊ The clinical term "chronic obstructive pulmonary disease (COPD)" should not be used in image interpretation! It encompasses: asthma, chronic bronchitis, emphysema!

Prevalence: 1.65 million people in USA

CHEST

Cause: imbalance in elastase-antielastase system (due to increase in elastase activity in smokers / α_1-antiprotease deficiency) causing proteolytic destruction of elastin resulting in alveolar wall destruction

• dyspnea on exertion
• irreversible expiratory airflow obstruction (due to decreased elastic recoil from parenchymal destruction)
• decreased carbon monoxide diffusing capacity

CXR (moderately sensitive, highly specific):
√ hyperinflated lung (most reliable sign):
  √ low hemidiaphragm (= at / below 7th anterior rib)
  √ flat hemidiaphragm (= <1.5 cm distance between line connecting the costo- and cardiophrenic angles + top of midhemidiaphragm)
  √ retrosternal air space >2.5 cm
  √ "barrel chest" = enlarged anteroposterior chest diameter
√ saber-sheath trachea
√ pulmonary vascular pruning + distortion (± pulmonary arterial hypertension)
√ right-heart enlargement
√ bullae

HRCT:
√ well-defined areas of abnormally decreased attenuation without definable wall (<–910 HU)

Rx: lung volume reduction surgery

Centrilobular Emphysema

= CENTRIACINAR EMPHYSEMA = PROXIMAL ACINAR EMPHYSEMA
= emphysematous change selectively affecting the acinus at the level of 1st + 2nd generations of respiratory bronchioles (most common form)

Path: normal + emphysematous alveolar spaces adjacent to each other

Histo: enlargement of respiratory bronchioles + destruction of centrilobular alveolar septa in the center of the secondary pulmonary lobule; CHARACTERISTICALLY surrounded by normal lung; distal alveoli spared; severity of destruction varies from lobule to lobule

Predisposed: smokers (in up to 50%), coal workers

Cause: excess protease with smoking (elastase is contained in neutrophils + macrophages found in abundance in lung of smokers)

• blue bloater

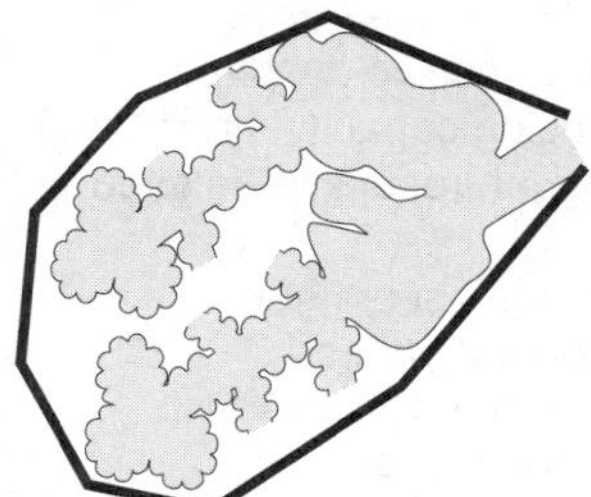

Centrilobar Emphysema

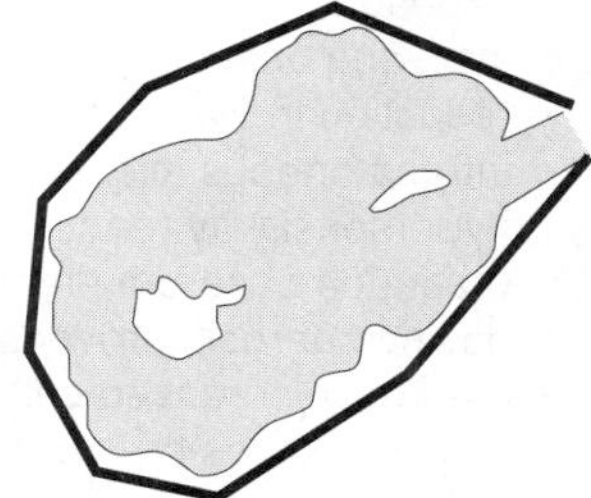

Panacinar Emphysema

Site: apical and posterior segments of upper lobe + superior segment of lower lobe (relatively greater ventilation-perfusion ratio in upper lobes favors deposition of particulate matter and release of elastase in upper lungs)

CXR (80% sensitivity for moderate / severe stages):
√ irregular scattered area of radiolucency (best appreciated if lung opacified by edema / pneumonia / hemorrhage) = area of bullae, arterial depletion + increased markings
√ hyperinflated lung

HRCT:
√ "emphysematous spaces" (= focal area of air attenuation) >1 cm in diameter with central dot / line (representing the centrilobular artery of secondary pulmonary lobule) without definable wall and surrounded by normal lung
√ pulmonary vascular distortion + pruning with lack of juxtaposition of normal lung (advanced stage)

Panacinar Emphysema

= PANLOBULAR EMPHYSEMA = DIFFUSE EMPHYSEMA = GENERALIZED EMPHYSEMA
= emphysematous change involving the entire acinus
= uniform nonselective destruction of all air spaces throughout both lungs (rare)

Path: uniform enlargement of acini from respiratory bronchioles to terminal alveoli (from center to periphery of secondary pulmonary lobule) secondary to destruction of lung distal to terminal bronchiole

Cause: autosomal recessive alpha-1 antitrypsin deficiency in 10–15% (proteolytic enzymes carried by leukocytes in blood gradually destroy lung unless inactivated by alpha-1 protease inhibitor)

Age: 6th–7th decade (3rd–4th decade in smokers)

• pink puffer

Site: affects whole lung, but more severe at lung bases (due to greater blood flow)

CXR:
√ hyperinflated lung
√ decreased pulmonary vascular markings
√ lung destruction extremely uniform

HRCT:
√ diffuse simplification of lung architecture with pulmonary septal and vascular distortion + pruning (difficult to detect early, ie, prior to considerable lung destruction for lack of adjacent normal lung)
√ paucity of vessels
√ bullae

Paracicatricial Emphysema

= PERIFOCAL / IRREGULAR EMPHYSEMA
= airspace enlargement + lung destruction developing adjacent to areas of pulmonary scarring

Usual cause: granulomatous inflammation, organized pneumonia, pulmonary infarction

Path: no consistent relationship to any portion of secondary lobule / acinus; frequently associated with bronchiolectasis producing "honeycomb lung"
- little functional significance

CXR (rarely detectable):
√ fine curvilinear reticular opacities + interposed radiolucent areas

HRCT:
√ low-attenuation areas adjacent to areas of fibrosis (diagnosable only in the absence of other forms of emphysema)

Paraseptal Emphysema
= DISTAL ACINAR / LOCALIZED / LINEAR EMPHYSEMA
= focal enlargement + destruction of air spaces in one site in otherwise normal lung

Path: predominant involvement of alveolar ducts + sacs

Site: characteristically within subpleural lung and adjacent to interlobular septa + vessels

CXR:
√ area of lucency, frequently sharply demarcated from normal lung
√ bands of radiopacity (residual vessels / interstitium) may be present

HRCT:
√ peripheral low-attenuation area with remainder of lung normal

Cx: spontaneous pneumothorax; bullae formation

EMPYEMA
= parapneumonic effusion characterized by presence of pus ± positive culture

Organism: S. aureus, Gram-negative + anaerobic bacteria
- positive Gram stain
- positive culture (anaerobic bacteria most frequent)

Stage

I *exudative phase* = inflammation of visceral pleura results in increased capillary permeability with weeping of proteinaceous fluid into pleural space = sterile exudate
- pH **>7.20**
- glucose >40 mg/dL (2.2 mmol/L)
- LDH <1,000 IU/L

II *fibrinopurulent phase* = accumulation of inflammatory cells and neutrophils within pleural space + fibrin deposition on pleural surfaces
— early stage II empyema
- WBCs $>5x10^9/mm^3$, but no gross pus
- pH between **7.0 and 7.2**
- glucose level >40 mg/dL
- LDH <1,000 IU/L

— late stage II empyema
- gross pus (WBC $>15,000/cm^3$) = frank pus
- pH **<7.0**
- glucose level **<40 mg/dL**
- LDH **>1,000** IU/L

Cx: multiloculation
Rx: chest tube drainage

III *organizing phase* = recruitment of fibroblasts + capillaries results in deposition of collagen + granulation tissue on pleural surfaces = pleural fibrosis = "pleural peel / pleural rind"
Cx: limited expansion of lung
Rx: decortication (with persistent sepsis despite appropriate antibiotic Rx + drainage / persistent thick pleural rind trapping underlying lung)

CT:
√ thickening of parietal pleura in 60% on NECT, in 86% on CECT
√ increased thickness + density of paraspinal subcostal tissue (inflammation of extrapleural fat)
√ curvilinear enhancement of chest wall boundary in 96% (inflammatory hyperemia of pleura)
√ "split pleura" sign = pleural fluid between enhancing thickened parietal + visceral pleura
√ gas bubbles in pleural space (gas-forming organism / bronchopleural fistula)

DDx: simple / complicated parapneumonic effusion (negative Gram + culture stain), malignant effusion after sclerotherapy, malignant invasion of chest wall, mesothelioma, pleural tuberculosis, reactive mesothelial hyperplasia, pleural effusion of rheumatoid disease

EXTRINSIC ALLERGIC ALVEOLITIS
= HYPERSENSITIVITY PNEUMONITIS
= characterized by an inappropriate host response to inhaled organic allergens that are often related to patient's occupation

Cause: inhalation of organic dust (= particulate organism / protein complex) typically of 1–2 μm (always <5 μm) particle size deposited in distal airspaces of lung acting as antigen for a type III + type IV immune reaction

Histo: diffuse predominantly mononuclear cell inflammation of bronchioles (bronchiolitis) + pulmonary parenchyma (alveolitis); ill-defined granulomas of <1 mm in diameter
- asymptomatic (10–40%)
- recurrent episodes of fever, chills, dry cough, dyspnea following exposure after 6-hour interval
- resolution of episodic symptoms after cessation of exposure, abate spontaneously over 1–2 days
- insidious onset of gradually progressive dyspnea
- reduction in vital capacity, diffusing capacity, arterial PO_2
- intracutaneous injection of antigen results in delayed hypersensitivity reaction
- presence of serum precipitins against antigen
- positive aerosol provocation inhalation test
- markedly increased cell count with often >50% T-lymphocytes on bronchoalveolar lavage

Location: predominantly midlung zones, occasionally lower lung zones, rarely upper lung zones

Specific antigens for immune complex disease (type III = Arthus reaction):

1. **Farmer's lung** from moldy hay (Thermoactinomyces vulgaris or Micropolyspora faeni)
2. Hypersensitivity pneumonitis from forced-air equipment = **Pandora's pneumoniti**s with heating / humidifying / air conditioning systems (thermophilic actinomycetes)
3. **Bird-fancier's lung**, pigeon breeder's lung from protein in bird serum / excrements / feathers
4. **Mushroom worker's lung** from mushroom compost (Thermoactinomyces vulgaris or Micropolyspora faeni)
5. **Bagassosis** from moldy sugar cane in sugar mill (contamination with Thermoactinomyces sacchari / vulgaris and Micropolyspora faeni)
6. **Malt worker's lung** from malt dust (Aspergillus clavatus)
7. **Maple bark disease** from moldy maple bark in saw mill (Cryptostroma corticale)
8. **Suberosis** from moldy cork dust (Penicillium frequentans)
9. **Sequoiosis** from redwood dust (Graphium species)

Thermophilic actinomycetes
= bacteria <1 μm in diameter with morphologic characteristics of fungi; found in soil, grains, compost, fresh water, forced-air heating, cooling system, humidifier, air-conditioning system

Isocyanates
used for large-scale production of polyurethane polymers in the manufacture of flexible / rigid foams, elastomers, adhesives, surface coating)
◊ Principal cause of occupational asthma!

Rx: mask, filter, industrial hygiene, alterations in forced-air ventilatory system, change in patient's habits / occupation / environment

Acute Extrinsic Allergic Alveolitis

= heavy exposure to inciting antigen in domestic, occupational, atmospheric environment

Histo: filling of air spaces by polymorph neutrophils + lymphocytes

Onset of symptoms after exposure: 4–8 hours

- fever, chills, malaise, chest tightness, cough, dyspnea
- scanty mucoid expectoration
- frontal headache, arthralgia (common)

√ No CXR abnormalities in 30–95%
√ diffuse acinar consolidative pattern (edema + exudate filling alveoli) resolving within a few days
√ lymph node enlargement (unusual, more common with recurrence)

HRCT:
√ small + medium rounded opacities (large active granulomas)
√ diffuse dense airspace consolidation (confluent collections of intraalveolar histiocytes, interstitial + intraalveolar edema)

Dx: classical presentation of a known exposure history + typical symptoms + detection of serum precipitins to suspected antigen

Subacute Extrinsic Allergic Alveolitis

= less intense but continuous exposure to inhaled antigens, usually in domestic environment

Histo: predominantly interstitial lymphocytic infiltrate, poorly defined granulomas, cellular bronchiolitis

Onset of symptoms after exposure: weeks – months

- recurrent respiratory / systemic symptoms:
  - breathlessness upon exertion, fever + cough
  - weight loss, muscle + joint pain

√ changes may be completely reversible if present less than 1 year
√ interstitial nodular / reticulonodular pattern

HRCT:
√ poorly defined centrilobular micronodules <5 mm (cellular bronchiolitis + small granulomas)
√ widespread patchy / diffuse ground-glass attenuation in 52% (obstructive pneumonitis, filling of alveoli by large mononuclear cell infiltrates)
√ areas of decreased attenuation + mosaic perfusion (86%)

Chronic Extrinsic Allergic Alveolitis

= prolonged insidious dust exposure

Onset of symptoms after exposure: months – years

- insidious progressive exertional dyspnea indistinguishable from idiopathic pulmonary fibrosis

Histo: proliferation of epithelial cells + predominantly peribronchiolar interstitial fibrosis

Location: usually in mid zones, relative sparing of lung apices + costophrenic sulci

√ irregular linear opacities (fibrosis)
√ loss of lung volume (cicatrization atelectasis)
√ pleural effusion (rare)
√ lymph node enlargement may occur

CT:
√ fibrosis of middle + lower lung zones with relative sparing of lung bases:
√ intralobular interstitial thickening
√ irregular interlobular septal thickening
√ honeycombing
√ traction bronchiectasis
√ focal air trapping / diffuse emphysema
√ coexistent subacute changes (due to continuing exposure)

FAT EMBOLISM

= obstruction of pulmonary vessels by fat globules followed by chemical pneumonitis from unsaturated plasma fatty acids producing hemorrhage / edema

Incidence: in necropsy series in 67–97% of patients with major skeletal trauma; however, symptomatic fat embolism syndrome in <10% (M > F)

Onset: 24–72 hours after trauma

- dyspnea (progressive pulmonary insufficiency)
- fever
- systemic hypoxemia
- mentation changes: headaches, confusion

- petechiae (50%) from coagulopathy (release of tissue thromboplastin)

√ initial chest film usually negative (normal up to 72 hours)
√ platelike atelectasis
√ bilateral diffuse alveolar infiltrates
√ consolidation (may progress to ARDS)

NUC:
- √ mottled peripheral perfusion defects (1–4 days after injury), later enlarging secondary to pneumonic infiltrates

FOCAL ORGANIZING PNEUMONIA

= unresolving pneumonia / pneumonia with incomplete resolution beyond 8 weeks

Prevalence: 5–10% of all pneumonias (87% of pneumonias resolve within 4 weeks, 12% within 4–8 weeks)

Predisposing factors: ? age, diabetes mellitus, chronic bronchitis, overuse of antibiotics

Histo: organization of intraalveolar exudate + thickening of alveolar septa / chronic inflammatory change of bronchial mucosa + obstructive lesion in bronchioles with organization

- cough, sputum, fever, hemoptysis (in 1/4)

√ ill-defined localized parenchymal abnormality with irregular margin
√ decrease in size of mass within 3–4 weeks

HRCT:
- √ flat / ovoid lesion with irregular margin in subpleural location / along bronchovascular bundle
- √ ± satellite lesions (44%) + air bronchogram (22%)

FRACTURE OF TRACHEA / BRONCHUS

= TRACHEOBRONCHIAL TEAR

Cause: blunt chest trauma (in 1.5%)

- delayed diagnosis is common

Location: (a) mainstem bronchus within 2.5 cm of carina (80%); R > L
(b) just above carina (20%)

Associated injuries:
- √ fracture of first 3 ribs (53–91%), rare in children
- √ fracture of clavicle, sternum, scapula (40%)

√ pneumothorax (70%)
√ increasing mediastinal ± subcutaneous emphysema
√ absence of pleural effusion
√ "fallen lung sign" = collapsed lung droops to dependent position peripherally (loss of anchoring support in bronchial transection)
√ inadequate reexpansion of lung despite adequate placement of one / more chest tubes (due to large size of air leak)
√ elevation of hyoid bone above level of C3 vertebral body / elevation of greater cornu to <2 cm from angle of mandible (on LAT radiograph of spine) due to infrahyoid muscle rupture + unopposed action of suprahyoid mm.
√ atelectasis (may be late development)

CT:
- √ focal peribronchial collections of air
- √ discontinuity / irregularity of bronchial wall
- √ abnormal position of endotracheal tube:
  - √ overdistension of tube cuff
  - √ protrusion of tube wall beyond expected margins of trachea
  - √ extraluminal position of tip of tube

Prognosis: 30% mortality (in 15% within 1 hour)

Long-term Cx: airway stenosis / bronchomalacia; recurrent atelectasis / pneumonia

GIANT CELL INTERSTITIAL PNEUMONIA

◊ Almost pathognomonic for hard metal pneumoconiosis

√ diffuse micronodular pattern
√ reticular pattern; in advanced disease coarse and accompanied by small cystic spaces
√ ± lymph node enlargement

HRCT:
- √ bilateral areas of ground-glass attenuation
- √ areas of consolidation
- √ extensive reticulations
- √ traction bronchiectasis

GOODPASTURE SYNDROME

= ANTI-GLOMERULAR BASEMENT MEMBRANE ANTIBODY DISEASE

= autoimmune disease characterized by
(1) glomerulonephritis
(2) circulating antibodies against glomerular + alveolar basement membrane
(3) pulmonary hemorrhage

Pathogenesis:
cytotoxic antibody-mediated disease = type II hypersensitivity; alveolar basement membrane becomes antigenic (perhaps viral etiology); IgG / IgM antibody with complement activation causes cell destruction + pulmonary hemorrhage, leads to hemosiderin deposition and pulmonary fibrosis

Age peak: 26 years (range 17–78 years); M:F = 7:1

- iron-deficiency anemia
- hepatosplenomegaly
- systemic hypertension

@ Lung
- preceding upper respiratory infection (in 2/3) + renal disease
- mild hemoptysis (72%) with hemosiderin-laden macrophages in sputum, commonly precedes the clinical manifestations of renal disease by several months
- cough, mild dyspnea, basilar rales
- √ extensive bilateral air-space consolidation:
  - √ symmetric consolidation of perihilar area + lung bases with sparing of lung apices
  - √ air bronchogram
  - √ consolidation replaced by interstitial pattern within 2–3 days (due to organization of hemorrhage resulting in interlobular septal thickening)
- √ hilar lymph nodes may be enlarged during acute episodes

@ Kidney
- glomerulonephritis with IgG deposits in characteristic linear pattern in glomeruli
- hematuria

Prognosis: death within 3 years (average 6 months) because of renal failure
Rx: cytotoxic chemotherapy, plasmapheresis, bilateral nephrectomy
DDx: idiopathic pulmonary hemosiderosis

GRANULOMA OF LUNG

Cause:
A. Sarcoidosis
B. Non-sarcoid granulomatous disease
 (a) infectious
  – bacterial: TB, gumma
  – opportunistic: cryptococcosis
  – parasitic: Dirofilaria immitis (dog heartworm)
  – fungal: histoplasmosis, coccidioidomycosis, nocardiosis
 (b) noninfectious
  – foreign body: talc, beryllium, algae, pollen, cellulose, lipids, abuse of nasally inhaled drugs, aspiration of medication
  – angiocentric lymphoproliferative disease
  – vasculitides
  – extrinsic allergic alveolitis
  – Langerhans cell histiocytosis
  – pulmonary hyalinizing granuloma
  – peribronchial granuloma
  – chronic granulomatous disease of childhood

Histo: epithelial cells, lymphocytes, macrophages, giant cells of Langhans type
Frequency: constitutes the majority of solitary pulmonary nodules
- nonproductive cough
- shortness of breath
- spontaneous pneumothorax

CXR:
 ◊ CXR detection requires multiple granulomas / clusters of granulomas (individual granuloma too small)!
 √ central nidus of calcification in a laminated / diffuse pattern
 √ absence of growth for at least 2 years

CT (most effective in nodules ≤3 cm of diameter with smooth discrete margins):
 √ 50–60% of pulmonary nodules demonstrate unsuspected calcification by CT

DDx: carcinoma (in 10% eccentric calcification in preexisting scar / nearby granuloma / true intrinsic stippled calcification in larger lesion)

HAMARTOMA OF CHEST WALL

= MESENCHYMOMA (incorrect as it implies neoplasm)
= focal overgrowth of normal skeletal elements with a benign self-limited course; extremely rare
Age: 1st year of life
√ moderate / large extrapleural well-circumscribed mass affecting one / more ribs
√ ribs near center of mass partially / completely destroyed
√ ribs at periphery deformed / eroded
√ significant amount of calcification / ossification (DDx: aneurysmal bone cyst)
√ mass compresses underlying lung
Rx: resection curative

HAMARTOMA OF LUNG

= most common benign tumor of the lung
Incidence: 0.25% in population (autopsy); 6–8% of all solitary pulmonary neoplasms; 77% of all benign lung tumors
Etiology:
 1. Congenital malformation of a displaced bronchial anlage
 2. Hyperplasia of normal structures
 3. Cartilaginous neoplasm
 4. Response to inflammation

Path: solitary mass composed of tissues normally found in this location in abnormal quantity, mixture, and arrangement
Histo: columnar, cuboidal, ciliated epithelium, fat (in 50%), bone, cartilage (predominates), muscle, vessels, fibrous tissue, calcifications, plasma cells originating in fibrous connective tissue beneath mucous membrane of bronchial wall
Age peak: 5th + 6th decade; M:F = 2:1 – 3:1
May be associated with:
 Carney triad (pulmonary chondromatous lesion, gastric leiomyosarcoma, functioning extraadrenal paraganglioma); pulmonary hamartoma syndrome
- mostly asymptomatic
- hemoptysis (rare)
- cough, vague chest pain, fever (with postobstructive pneumonitis)

Location: 2/3 peripheral; endobronchial in 3–10–20%; multiplicity (rare)
√ round smooth lobulated mass <4 cm (averages 2.5 cm)
√ calcification in 15–20% (almost pathognomonic if of chondroid "popcorn" type)
√ fat density in 50% (DIAGNOSTIC)
√ cavitation (extremely rare)
√ growth patterns: slow / rapid / stable with later growth
√ usually diameter increase by 1.5 mm/year doubling in size every 14 years

HRCT:
 √ fat density detectable in 34% (–80 to –120 HU)
 √ calcium + fat detectable in 19%

Transthoracic needle biopsy: 85% diagnostic accuracy
DDx: lipoid pneumonia (ill-defined mass / lung infiltrate); granulomatous disease, carcinoid tumor; metastatic mucinous adenocarcinoma, amyloidoma

HEREDITARY HEMORRHAGIC TELANGIECTASIA

= RENDU-OSLER-WEBER SYNDROME
= group of autosomal dominant inherited disorders that result in a variety of systemic fibrovascular dysplasias affecting mucous membranes, skin, lung, brain, GI tract:
 (1) telangiectasias
 (2) arteriovenous malformations (AV hemangiomas)
 (3) aneurysms

Etiology: gene that encodes transforming growth factor binding protein

Path: direct connections between arteries + veins with absence of capillaries (telangiectases are small AVMs)
  (a) small telangiectasis = focal dilatation of postcapillary venules with prominent stress fibers in pericytes along luminal borders
  (b) fully developed telangiectasis = markedly dilated + convoluted venules with excessive layers of smooth muscle without elastic fibers directly connecting to dilated arterioles

• frequent bleeding into mucous membranes, skin, lungs, genitourinary system, gastrointestinal system (due to vascular weakness)

@ Nose (telangiectasis of nasal mucosa)
  • recurrent epistaxis (32–85%): more severe over time in 66%; begins by age 10, present by age 21 in most cases; up to 45 episodes per month

@ Skin
  • telangiectases = small red vascular blemishes
  Age: present in most cases by age 40; increase in number + size with age
  Location: lips, tongue, palate, fingers, face, conjunctiva, trunk, arms, nail beds

@ Lung (5–15%)
  ◊ 5–15% of patients with hereditary hemorrhagic telangiectasia have pulmonary AVMs
  ◊ Up to 60% of patients with pulmonary AVMs have hereditary hemorrhagic telangiectasia
  see PULMONARY ARTERIAL MALFORMATION

@ CNS (cerebral or spinal AVMs)
  • subarachnoid hemorrhage
  • seizure; paraparesis (less common)
  • headache

@ GI tract (stomach, duodenum, small bowel, colon) occasionally associated with AVMs / angiodysplasia
  • recurrent GI bleeding (in 5th–6th decade)

@ Liver (8–31%)
  √ hepatomegaly
  √ presence of multiple AVMs (between hepatic artery branches + branches of hepatic / portal veins:
    √ simultaneous enhancement of hepatic arteries + veins
    √ multiple transient peripheral wedge-shaped areas of hepatic enhancement on hepatic arterial phase
  √ widened tortuous hepatic arteries
  √ dilatation of hepatic veins
  √ diffuse mottled capillary blush on angio
  Cx: atypical cirrhosis, portal hypertension, variceal GI hemorrhage, ascites, encephalopathy

Cx: (1) congestive heart failure (due to AV shunting)
  (2) cerebral abscess (from paradoxical emboli)

HISTOPLASMOSIS

Prevalence: nearly 100% in endemic area; up to 30% in Central + South America, Puerto Rico, West Africa, Southeast Asia

Organism: Histoplasma capsulatum = dimorphic fungus; worldwide most often in temperate climates; widespread in soil enriched by bird droppings of central North America (endemic in Ohio, Mississippi, St. Lawrence River valley; exists as a spore in soil + transforms into yeast form at normal body temperatures

Infection: inhalation of wind-borne spores (microconidia of 2–6 μm, macroconidia of 6–14 μm), which germinate within alveoli releasing yeast forms, which are phagocytized but not killed by macrophages; invasion of pulmonary lymphatics with spread to hilar + mediastinal lymph nodes; hematogenous dissemination of parasitized macrophages throughout reticuloendothelial system (spleen!)

Path: spores incite formation of epithelioid granulomas, necrosis, calcification

Dx: (1) Culture (sputum, lung tissue, urine, bone marrow, lymph node)
  (2) Identification of yeast forms stained with PAS / Gomori methenamine silver
  (3) Complement fixation test (absolute titer of 1:64 or 4-fold rise in convalescent titer suggest active / recent infection)
  (4) Serum immunodiffusion: agar gel diffusion test (H precipitin band)

Rx: ketoconazole

Pulmonary Histoplasmosis

A. ACUTE HISTOPLASMOSIS
  • mostly asymptomatic and self-limiting illness (in 99.5%)
  • fever, cough, malaise simulating viral upper respiratory infection 3 weeks after massive inoculum / in debilitated patients (infants, elderly)
  • positive skin test for histoplasmosis
  √ generalized lymphadenopathy
  √ bilateral nonsegmental bronchopneumonic pattern with tendency to clear in one area + appear in another
  √ multiple nodules changing into hundreds of punctate calcifications (usually >4 mm) after 9–24 months
  √ "target lesion" = central calcification is PATHOGNOMONIC
  √ hilar / mediastinal lymph node enlargement (DDx: acute viral / bacterial pneumonia)
  √ "popcorn" calcification of mediastinal lymph nodes >10 mm
  √ >5 splenic calcifications (40%)
  CT:
    √ paratracheal / subcarinal mass with regions of low attenuation (necrosis) + enhancing septa

B. CHRONIC HISTOPLASMOSIS (0.03%)
  Predisposed: individuals with chronic obstructive pulmonary disease
  Age: adult middle-aged white men
  Pathophysiology: hyperimmune reaction

- cough, low-grade fever, night sweats simulating postprimary tuberculosis
- √ segmental wedge-shaped peripheral consolidation of moth-eaten appearance from scattered foci of emphysematous lung
- √ fibrosis in apical posterior segments of upper lobes (indistinguishable from postprimary TB) adjacent to emphysematous blebs

C. DISSEMINATED HISTOPLASMOSIS
Predisposed: impaired T-cell immunity; AIDS
Prevalence: 1:50,000 exposed individuals
Pathophysiology: progression of exogenous infection / reactivation of latent focus

- acute rapidly fatal infection:
  - fever, weight loss, anorexia, malaise
  - cough (<50%)
  - abdominal pain, nausea, vomiting, diarrhea
- chronic intermittent illness:
  - low-grade fever, weight loss, fatigue
  - adrenal insufficiency
- √ normal CXR (>50%)
- √ miliary / diffuse reticulonodular pattern rapidly progressing to diffuse airspace opacification
- √ hilar + mediastinal adenopathy
- √ hepatosplenomegaly

Cx: arthritis (most often knee), tenosynovitis, osteomyelitis

D. DELAYED MANIFESTATIONS

- √ **histoplasmoma** (= continued growth of primary focus at 0.5–2.8 mm/year) adjacent to pleura + typically with laminated calcific rings;
  in 20% associated with: mediastinal granulomas
- √ broncholithiasis
- √ **mediastinal granuloma** (more common)
  = direct infection of mediastinal lymph nodes
  Histo: involved nodes with varying degrees of central caseation ± calcification
  - usually asymptomatic

  Location: subcarinal / right paratracheal / hilar lymph nodes
  - √ widened mediastinum (enlarged nodes + veins)
  - √ lobulated mass of low-density lymph nodes 3–10 cm in thickness surrounded by a 2–5-mm thick fibrous capsule crisscrossed by irregularly shaped septa (CHARACTERISTIC)
  - √ displacement of SVC / esophagus
- √ fibrosing mediastinitis (less common)
- ◊ Organism recovered in only 50%!

HODGKIN DISEASE

= disease of T cells
Incidence: 0.75% of all cancers diagnosed each year; 40% of all lymphomas
Age: bimodal peaks at age 25–30 years and 75–80 years
Histo: Reed-Sternberg cell = binucleate cell with prominent centrally located nucleolus

(1) Lymphocyte predominance (5%)
= abundance of normal-appearing lymphocytes + relative paucity of abnormal cells
- often diagnosed in younger people <35 years
- systemic symptoms are uncommon
- frequently in early stage + localized disease

Prognosis: most favorable natural history

(2) Nodular sclerosis (78%)
= lymph nodes traversed by broad bands of birefringent collagen separating nodules, which consist of normal lymphocytes, eosinophils, plasma cells, and histiocytes
- 1/3 with systemic symptoms
- √ typically localized anterior mediastinal involvement

Prognosis: good

(3) Mixed cellularity (17%)
= diffuse effacement of lymph nodes with lymphocytes, eosinophils, plasma cells + relative abundance of atypical mononuclear and Reed-Sternberg cells; more commonly advanced stage at presentation and older age
- √ more commonly abdominal than mediastinal

Prognosis: less favorable

(4) Lymphocyte depletion (1%)
= paucity of normal-appearing lymphocytes + abundance of abnormal mononuclear and Reed-Sternberg cells; least common subtype with worst prognosis
Age: older patients
- systemic symptoms
- √ disseminated advanced stage

Prognosis: rapidly fatal

Ann Arbor Staging Classification:
Stage I = limited to one / two contiguous anatomic regions on same side of diaphragm
Stage II = >2 anatomic regions / two noncontiguous regions on same side of diaphragm
Stage III = on both sides of diaphragm, not extending beyond lymph nodes, spleen (Stage III_S), Waldeyer's ring
III_E = with extralymphatic organ / site
Stage IV = organ involvement (bone marrow, bone, lung, pleura, liver, kidney, GI tract, skin) ± lymph node involvement
E = extralymphatic site
S = splenic involvement
Substage A = absence of systemic symptoms
Substage B = fever, night sweats, pruritus, ≥10% weight loss in past 6 months

- painless lymphadenopathy
- alcohol-induced pain
- unexplained fevers, night sweats, weight loss
- generalized pruritus

@ CHEST
At presentation: 67% with intrathoracic disease
Sites of lymphoid aggregates:
1. Lymph nodes in mediastinum
2. Lymph nodes at bifurcation of 1st + 2nd order bronchi

CHEST

3. Encapsulated lymphoid collections on thoracic surface deep to parietal pleura
4. Unencapsulated nodules at points of divisions of more distally situated bronchi, bronchioles, and pulmonary vessels
5. Unencapsulated lymphoid aggregates within peribronchial connective tissue
6. Small accumulations of lymphocytes in interlobular septa + lymphatic channels

A. INTRAPULMONARY MANIFESTATIONS

Frequency: 6–11%; in 4.3% bilateral (more frequent in recurrent disease)

◊ Most commonly in nodular sclerosing type
◊ Subsequent to hilar adenopathy in ipsilateral lung

1. Bronchovascular form (most common type of involvement)
   √ coarse reticulonodular pattern contiguous with mediastinum = direct extension from mediastinal nodes along lymphatics
   √ nodular parenchymal lesions
   √ miliary nodules
   √ endobronchial involvement
   √ lobar atelectasis secondary to endobronchial obstruction (rare)
   √ cavitation secondary to necrosis (rare)
2. Subpleural form
   √ circumscribed subpleural masses
   √ pleural effusion (20–50%) from lymphatic obstruction
3. Massive pneumonic form (68%)
   √ diffuse nonsegmental infiltrate (pneumonic type)
   √ massive lobar infiltrates (30%)
   √ homogeneous confluent infiltrates with shaggy borders
   √ air bronchogram
4. Nodular form
   √ multiple nodules <1 cm in diameter (DDx: metastatic disease)

DDx in treated patients:
relapse, infection, radiation pneumonitis, drug-induced lung disease

B. EXTRAPULMONARY MANIFESTATIONS

1. Mediastinal + hilar lymphadenopathy
   Most common manifestation, present in 90–99%, in thorax commonly multiple lymph node groups involved
   Location:
   anterior mediastinal + retrosternal nodes commonly involved (DDx: sarcoidosis); confined to anterior mediastinum in 40%; 20% with mediastinal nodes have hilar lymphadenopathy also; hilar lymph nodes involved bilaterally in 50%
   Spread from anterior mediastinum to:
   other mediastinal locations, pleura, pericardium, chest wall
   ◊ Involvement of multiple lymph node groups in 95%!
   √ CXR: on initial film adenopathy identified in 50%
   √ necrotic lymph nodes (commonly nodular sclerosing type)
   √ lymph nodes may calcify following radiation / chemotherapy
2. Pleural effusion (13%)
   ◊ Not of prognostic significance
   Prognosis: usually resolves following treatment
3. Pleural masses + plaques
   (a) sternal erosion
   (b) invasion of anterior chest wall

Cx:

1. Superimposed infection
   √ consolidation with bulging borders: necrotizing bacterial pneumonia
   √ multiple nodular foci: aspergillosis + nocardiosis

Comparison of Histologic Classifications of Non-Hodgkin Lymphoma

International Working Formulation	*Rappaport Classification*
Low grade	
A. Small lymphocytic	Well-differentiated lymphocytic
B. Follicular, predominantly small cleaved cell	Nodular, poorly differentiated lymphocytic
C. Follicular, mixed small and large cell	Nodular, mixed
Intermediate grade	
D. Follicular, predominantly large cell	Nodular, histiocytic
E. Diffuse, small cleaved cell	Diffuse, poorly differentiated lymphocytic
F. Diffuse, mixed small and large cell	Diffuse, mixed
G. Diffuse, large cell, cleaved or noncleaved	...
High grade	
H. Diffuse large cell, immunoblastic	...
I. Small, noncleaved cell	...
J. Lymphoblastic	Undifferentiated

CHEST

√ bilateral diffuse consolidation: Pneumocystis carinii
√ rapidly developing cavitation within consolidation: anaerobes / fungus
Dx: by culture, sputum cytology, lung biopsy
2. Drug toxicity

EXTRANODAL HODGKIN DISEASE (15–30%)
@ BONE (5–20%)
◊ During course of disease 5–32% will develop bone marrow involvement
At presentation: 1–4%; indicative of widespread aggressive disease with poor prognosis
Location: dorsolumbar spine > pelvis > ribs > femora > sternum
√ solitary (33%) / polyostotic (66%) lesions:
√ usually wide ill-defined lesion edge / sclerotic margin
√ lamellated / "sunburst" periosteal reaction
√ predominantly osteolytic with blurred borders; rarely sclerotic / mixed lytic-sclerotic
√ fractures occur rarely at presentation
√ vertebral osteolysis with collapse / patchy sclerosis / "ivory vertebra" / mixed lytic + blastic lesion
√ gouge defect of anterior vertebral body margin (due to erosion by lymph nodes)
√ osteolysis of sternum (due to its proximity to thoracic lymph ducts)
@ HEAD & NECK (<1%)
• nasopharyngeal biopsy positive in 20%
√ thyroid mass as secondary involvement (2%)
@ CNS (uncommon)
Frequency: secondary hematogenous involvement in 0.2–0.5%
Location: supratentorial cerebral cortex + meninges in inferior aspect of brain (most frequent)
√ leptomeningeal + choroid plexus masses
√ white matter mass, typically periventricular / basal ganglionic / cerebellar
√ paraneoplastic cerebellar atrophy
√ epidural mass with spinal cord compression (in 3–7.6%) from extension of paraspinal nodes through intervertebral neural foramen:
√ concomitant vertebral bone involvement (32–42%)
@ THYMUS (30–56%)
◊ Considered a "lymph node" in staging
√ remains enlarged after treatment in 33% (due to recurrent disease / rebound hyperplasia / persistence of thymic cysts)
@ CHEST WALL (6.4%)
√ infiltration of parasternal soft tissues by direct extension from internal mammary nodes
√ mass beneath / between pectoralis muscles (rare)
@ HEART (7.5% at autopsy)
√ pericardial effusion (with large mediastinal mass)
√ invasion of pericardium + SVC
√ pericardial nodular mass
@ LIVER (6–20%)
◊ Primary involvement very rare
Associated with: splenic disease (almost invariable)
√ discrete nodules (10%) = miliary lesions of <10 mm
√ diffuse disease (87%) = patchy irregular infiltrates in portal areas
@ SPLEEN
◊ Considered a "nodal organ"
Frequency: 30–40% at staging laparotomy
√ diffuse involvement (not detectable by imaging) ± splenomegaly
√ hypoechoic hypoattenuating nodules with reduced contrast enhancement
MR:
√ hypo- / isointense nodules on T1WI + hyperintense on T2WI
√ reduced enhancement compared with normal spleen
DDx: reactive splenomegaly (in 30%)
@ PANCREAS (extremely rare)
◊ Secondary to contiguous lymph node disease
@ GI TRACT (10–15%)
@ Esophagus (extremely rare):
√ esophageal nodules / irregular narrowing
@ Stomach (9% of all intestinal lymphomas):
√ narrow rigid obstructive lesion (DDx: scirrhous carcinoma)
√ wall thickening + smoothly lobulated outer border
@ Small intestine:
• spruelike symptoms, steatorrhea
√ abundance of desmoplastic reaction (DDx from NHL)
√ infiltrating (60%); polypoid (26%); ulcerated (14%)
Prognosis: poorer 5-year survival rate than with other forms of the disease
@ GU TRACT (extremely rare)
√ perirenal / renal masses (due to invasion from surrounding nodes)
Cx: increased risk for other malignancies from aggressive therapy (acute leukemia, NHL, radiation-induced sarcoma)

HYDATID DISEASE

= LUNG ECHINOCOCCOSIS
◊ Most common site of secondary involvement in children + 2nd most frequent site in adults
Source: hematogenous spread from liver lesion
Frequency: 15–25% of hydatid disease
• asymptomatic
• eosinophilia (<25%)
• sudden cough attacks, hemoptysis, chest pain, fever
• expectoration of cyst fluid / membranes / scolices
• positive Casoni skin test in 60%
• hypersensitivity reaction (if cyst rupture occurs)
Location: lower lobes in 60%; bilateral in 20%
√ solitary (70–75%) / multiple (25–30%) sharply circumscribed spherical / ovoid masses
√ size of 1–20 cm in diameter (16–20 weeks doubling time)

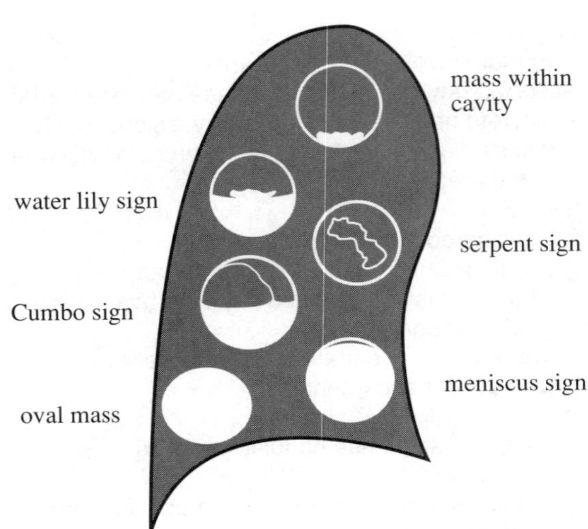

Presentations of Lung Echinococcosis on Upright Chest Radiograph

√ cyst communication with bronchial tree:
 √ "meniscus sign", "double arch sign," "moon sign," "crescent sign" (5%) = thin radiolucent crescent in uppermost part of cyst (due to rupture of pericyst with air dissecting between pericyst + laminated membrane)
 √ air-fluid level = rupture of all cyst walls with air entering the endocyst
 √ Cumbo sign = air-fluid level inside endocyst + air between pericyst and endocyst with an "onion peel" appearance
 √ serpent sign = collapsed membranes inside cyst outlined by air (after expectoration of cyst contents)
 √ "water lily sign," "sign of the Camalotte" = completely collapsed crumpled cyst membrane floating on the cyst fluid
 √ mass within cavity = crumpled membranes fall to most dependent portion of cavity after complete expectoration of cyst fluid
 √ hydropneumothorax
√ calcification of cyst wall (0.7%)
√ rib + vertebral erosion (rare)
√ mediastinal cyst: posterior (65%), anterior (26%), middle (9%) mediastinum

Cx: bacterial infection (after cyst rupture)

HYPOGENETIC LUNG SYNDROME

= collective name for congenital underdevelopment of one / more lobes of a lung separated into 3 forms:

1. **Pulmonary agenesis**
   = complete absence of a lobe + its bronchus
   CT:
   √ missing bronchus + lobe(s)
2. **Pulmonary aplasia**
   = rudimentary bronchus ending in blind pouch + absence of parenchyma + vessels
   Incidence: 1:10,000; R:L = 1:1
   CT:
   √ absence of ipsilateral pulmonary artery
   √ bronchus terminates in dilated blind pouch
   √ absence of ipsilateral pulmonary tissue
3. **Pulmonary hypoplasia** (38%)
   = completely formed but congenitally small bronchus with rudimentary parenchyma + small vessels
   Developmental causes:
   resulting in intrauterine compression of chest
   (a) Idiopathic (rare)
   (b) Extrathoracic compression (= Potter syndrome)
      1. Oligohydramnios (renal agenesis, bilateral cystic renal disease, obstructive uropathy, premature rupture of membranes)
      2. Fetal ascites
   (c) Thoracic cage compression
      1. Thoracic bone dysplasia (Jeune, thanatophoric dystrophy, Ellis-van Creveld, severe achondroplasia)
      2. Muscular disease
   (d) Intrathoracic compression
      1. Diaphragmatic defect
      2. Excess pleural fluid
      3. Large intrathoracic cyst / tumor
   CT:
   √ small bronchus + lobe

◊ Hypogenetic lung is the most constant component of **congenital pulmonary venolobar syndrome**!

May be associated with: congenital tracheal stenosis, bronchitis, bronchiectasis

Location: R:L = 3:1; RML (65%) > RUL (40%) > RLL (20%) > LUL (20%) > LLL (15%); multiple lobes (45%)

• usually asymptomatic (in isolated hypogenetic lung)
• exertional dyspnea
√ small ipsilateral hemithorax + elevated hemidiaphragm
√ diminished pulmonary vascularity on involved side
√ small hilum on involved side (absent / small pulmonary artery)
√ mediastinum + heart shifted toward involved side
√ indistinct cardiomediastinal border on involved side
√ diminished radiolucency on involved side
√ large ipsilateral apical cap + blunted costophrenic angle
√ broad retrosternal band of opacity (LAT view)

Horseshoe Lung

= uncommon variant of hypogenetic lung syndrome in which RLL crosses midline between esophagus and heart + fuses with opposite lung
√ oblique fissure in left lower hemithorax (if both lungs separated by pleural layers)
√ pulmonary vessels + bronchi crossing midline

IDIOPATHIC INTERSTITIAL PNEUMONIA

Acute Interstitial Pneumonia

= AIP = [ACCELERATED INTERSTITIAL PNEUMONIA]
= DIFFUSE ALVEOLAR DAMAGE = IDIOPATHIC ARDS
= ACUTE DIFFUSE INTERSTITIAL FIBROSIS = HAMMAN-RICH SYNDROME

= rapidly progressive fulminant disease of unknown etiology that usually occurs in previously healthy subjects + produces diffuse alveolar damage

Path: temporally homogeneous organizing diffuse alveolar damage; little mature collagen deposition / architectural distortion / honeycombing (as opposed to UIP)

Histo: (a) acute exudative phase: thickening of alveolar wall due to alveolar / interstitial edema + inflammatory cells; extensive alveolar damage with hyaline membrane formation (most prominent in 1st week after lung injury)
(b) marked interstitial fibroblast proliferation with stabilizing nonprogressive scarring

Mean age: 50 years; M = F

• prodromal viral upper respiratory infection: cough, fever
• rapidly increasing dyspnea + acute respiratory failure
• requires ventilation within days to 1–4 weeks
• decreased diffusing capacity for carbon monoxide

Location: mainly lower lung zones

Site: predominantly central / subpleural (in 22%)

CXR:
√ progressive extensive bilateral hetero- / homogeneous airspace opacification: symmetric, bilateral, basilar

CT:
√ diffuse extensive bilateral airspace consolidation (in 67%) with basal predominance (similar to ARDS)
√ patchy (67%) / diffuse (38%) bilateral ground-glass opacities
√ anteroposterior lung attenuation gradient
√ marked architectural distortion + honeycomb lung if fibrosis progressive

Dx: negative bacterial / viral / fungal cultures; no inhalational exposure to noxious agents; no pulmonary drug toxicity

Prognosis: death within 1–6 months (60–90%); recovery in 12%

Subacute Interstitial Pneumonia

BOOP *see* BRONCHIOLITIS OBLITERANS

Nonspecific Interstitial Pneumonia with Fibrosis

= NONCLASSIFIABLE INTERSTITIAL PNEUMONIA
= interstitial pneumonia that cannot be classified as UIP / DIP / acute interstitial pneumonia / BOOP

Histo: temporal uniformity of
(a) cellular interstitial infiltrate with little / no fibrosis (48%)
(b) inflammation + fibrosis (38%)
(c) dense fibrosis dominant (14%);
occasionally intraalveolar accumulation of macrophages + focal areas of bronchiolitis obliterans organizing pneumonia

Cause: collagen vascular disease (16%), inhalational exposure to noxious agents (17%), recent surgery / severe pneumonia / ARDS (8%)

Mean age: 46 years; M < F

• dyspnea + dry cough (1-week to 5-year history)
• low-grade fever, malaise
• decreased diffusing capacity for carbon monoxide

Location: no zonal predominance

√ normal CXR in 14%
√ bibasilar irregular linear opacities + diffuse heterogeneous airspace consolidation
√ normal / slightly decreased lung volume

CT:
√ bilateral areas of scattered ground-glass opacities (100%)
√ bibasilar airspace consolidation (71%)
√ irregular linear opacities (29%)
√ bronchial dilatation in areas of consolidation (71%)
√ mediastinal lymphadenopathy (29%)
√ NO honeycombing

Prognosis: 11% overall mortality

Rx: corticosteroids (clinical + functional + radiographic improvement in 50–86%)

DDx: usual interstitial pneumonia (irregular reticular pattern + honeycombing involving subpleural + lower lung zones

Respiratory Bronchiolitis-Interstitial Lung Disease

= interstitial pneumonia of smokers in which respiratory bronchiolitis is associated with limited peribronchiolar interstitial inflammation; ? early manifestation of DIP

Mean age: 36 years; M = F

Cause: heavy cigarette smoking

Histo: accumulation of brown-pigmented macrophages in respiratory bronchioles + surrounding air spaces

• mild dyspnea + cough
• pulmonary function test: mixed restrictive + obstructive

√ normal CXR (21%)
√ diffuse bibasilar small linear + nodular opacities (71%)
√ bibasilar atelectasis (12%)
√ bronchial wall thickening

CT:
√ scattered ground-glass opacities (66%)
√ centrilobular micronodules
√ centrilobular emphysema

Prognosis: excellent (after cessation of smoking / corticoid therapy) without progression to end-stage lung fibrosis

Chronic Interstitial Pneumonia

= ORGANIZING INTERSTITIAL PNEUMONIA = CHRONIC DIFFUSE SCLEROSING ALVEOLITIS

Usual Interstitial Pneumonia

= UIP = IDIOPATHIC PULMONARY FIBROSIS (IPF)
= MURAL TYPE OF FIBROSING ALVEOLITIS
= CRYPTOGENIC FIBROSING ALVEOLITIS
= commonest (90%) form of idiopathic interstitial pneumonia (may represent late stage of DIP)

Etiology: 50% idiopathic; 25% familial; drug exposure (bleomycin, cyclophosphamide (Cytoxan®), busulfan, nitrofurantoin); 20–30% associated with collagen vascular disease / immunologic disorder (mostly rheumatoid arthritis)

Pathophysiology:
repetitive episodes of lung injury to the alveolar wall causing alveoli to flood with proteinaceous fluid + cellular debris; incomplete lysis of intraalveolar fibrin; type II pneumocytes regenerate over the intraalveolar collagen incorporating the fibrous tissue into alveolar septa (= injury-inflammation-fibrosis sequence)

Mean age: 64 years; M>F

Path: simultaneous presence of inflammatory cell infiltration + fibrotic alveolar walls + honeycombing + areas of normal lung tissue (= temporal variegation)

Histo: proteinaceous exudate in interstitium + hyaline membrane formation in alveoli; necrosis of alveolar lining cells followed by cellular infiltration of mono- and lymphocytes + regeneration of alveolar lining; intraalveolar histiocytes; proliferation of fibroblasts + deposition of collagen fibers + smooth muscle proliferation; progressive disorganization of pulmonary architecture

- progressive dyspnea, dry cough, fatigue (over 1–3 years)
- "Velcro" rales = crepitations
- clubbing of fingers (83%)
- lymphocytosis on bronchoalveolar lavage (marker of alveolitis)
- pulmonary function tests: restrictive defects + decreased diffusing capacity for carbon monoxide

√ occasionally ground-glass pattern in early stage of alveolitis (alveolar wall injury, interstitial edema, proteinaceous exudate, hyaline membranes, infiltrate of monocytes + lymphocytes) in 15–62%
√ bilateral diffuse linear / small irregular reticulations (100%); basilar (85%) + peripheral (59%)
√ reticulonodular pattern = superimposition of linear opacities
√ heart border "shaggy"
√ honeycombing = numerous cystic spaces (up to 74%)
√ elevated diaphragm = progressive loss of lung volume (45–75%)
√ 1.5–3-mm diffusely distributed nodules (15–29%)
√ pleural effusion (4–6%), pleural thickening (6%)
√ pneumothorax in 7% (in late stages)
√ normal CXR (2–8%)

HRCT (88% sensitive):
Location: lung bases (68–80%)
Site: predominantly subpleural regions (79%)
√ patchy distribution with areas of normal parenchyma, active alveolitis, early + late fibrosis present at the same time (HALLMARK)
√ irregular linear intralobular opacities (82%) with architectural distortion of secondary pulmonary lobule
√ interlobular septal thickening (10%)
√ subpleural areas of honeycombing with cystic spaces outlined by thick fibrous walls (up to 96%)
√ subpleural lines (= fibrosis / functional atelectasis)
√ small peripheral convoluted cysts (= traction bronchiectasis) in 50%
√ ground-glass opacities (= diffuse inflammatory mononuclear cell infiltrates of active disease + fibroblast proliferation) in 65–76%

Cx: bronchogenic carcinoma (more frequent occurrence)

Rx: response to steroids in only 10–15%

Prognosis: average survival of 3–6 years; 45% 5-year mortality rate (overall 87%); no recovery

Desquamative Interstitial Pneumonia

= DIP = DESQUAMATIVE TYPE OF FIBROSING ALVEOLITIS = ALVEOLAR MACROPHAGE PNEUMONIA
= second commonest (although rare) form of interstitial pneumonia with more benign course than UIP, may be self-limited disease or lead to UIP

Mean age: 42 years (approximately 8 years younger than in UIP); M > F

Path: focal filling of alveolar spaces with foamy histiocytes + relative preservation of lung architecture + mild fibrosis (temporally uniform)

Histo: alveoli lined by large cuboidal cells + filled with heavy accumulation of mononuclear cells (macrophages, NOT desquamated alveolar cells); relative preservation of alveolar anatomy; histologic uniformity from field to field

Predisposed: smokers (history in up to 90%)

- asymptomatic
- weight loss
- dyspnea + nonproductive cough (for 6–12 months)
- clubbing of fingers
- mild pulmonary function abnormalities

√ normal chest x-ray (3–22%)
√ ground-glass alveolar pattern sparing costophrenic angles (25–33%), diffuse ground-glass opacities (15%)
√ linear irregular opacities (60%), bilateral + basilar (46–73%)
√ lung nodules (15%)
√ honeycombing (13%)
√ preserved lung volume

HRCT:
Location: mainly middle + lower lung zones (73%); bilateral + symmetric (86%)
Site: predominantly subpleural distribution (59%)
√ patchy ground-glass attenuation
√ irregular linear opacities (= fibrosis) + architectural distortion (50%)
√ honeycombing + traction bronchiectasis (32%)
√ fibrosis of lower lung zones in late stage

Prognosis: better response to corticosteroid Rx than UIP (in 60–80%); median survival of 12 years; 5% 5-year mortality rate (overall 16–27%); 70% 10–year survival

IDIOPATHIC PULMONARY FIBROSIS

= clinical syndrome

Age: 50–70 years; M > F

- dry cough, exertional dyspnea
- "Velcro-type" inspiratory crackles
- digital clubbing (25–50%)
- restrictive pulmonary function tests
- decreased total lung capacity + functional residual capacity + residual volume
- reduced diffusing capacity for carbon monoxide

CXR:

√ decreased lung volume, progressive over time
√ bibasilar subpleural reticulations
√ honeycombing (30%)
√ bibasilar ground-glass appearance (uncommon)
√ small nodules (<10–15%)

HRCT:

√ patchy bibasilar subpleural reticular (= irregular linear) opacities (= intralobular, interstitial thickening)
√ traction bronchiectasis
√ honeycombing (90%)
√ ground-glass opacities (occasionally)
√ discrete nodules (occasionally)
√ mild mediastinal lymph node enlargement (common)

Rx: corticosteroids, immunosuppressive / cytotoxic agents (<10% respond); lung transplantation

Prognosis: 30–50% 5-year survival

IDIOPATHIC PULMONARY HEMOSIDEROSIS

= IPH = probable autoimmune process with clinical + radiologic remissions + exacerbations characterized by eosinophilia + mastocytosis, immunoallergic reaction, pulmonary hemorrhage, iron deficiency anemia

Age: (a) Chronic form: most commonly <10 years of age
(b) Acute form (rare): in adults; M:F = 2:1

- iron deficiency anemia
- clubbing of fingers
- hepatosplenomegaly (25%)
- bilirubinemia
- recurrent episodes of severe hemoptysis

√ bilateral patchy alveolar-filling pattern (= blood in alveoli); initially for 2–3 days with return to normal in 10–12 days unless episode repeated
√ reticular pattern (= deposition of hemosiderin in interstitial space) later
√ moderate fibrosis after repeated episodes
√ hilar lymph nodes may be enlarged during acute episodes

Prognosis: death within 2–20 years (average survival 3 years)

DDx: SECONDARY PULMONARY HEMOSIDEROSIS caused by mitral valve disease
√ septal lines (NOT in idiopathic form)
√ lung ossifications (NOT in idiopathic form)

INFLAMMATORY MYOBLASTIC PSEUDOTUMOR

= PLASMA CELL GRANULOMA = INFLAMMATORY PSEUDOTUMOR = (FIBROUS) HISTIOCYTOMA = XANTHOMA = XANTHOFIBROMA = XANTHOGRANULOMA = SCLEROSING HEMANGIOMA

Prevalence: <1% of all tumors of lung + airways

Histo: composed of variable portions of plasma cells, lymphocytes, fibroblasts, blood vessels; foamy histiocytes + multinucleated giant cells + spindle cells (70% of tumor) grouped in CHARACTERISTIC pinwheel / whorled pattern

Age: young patient

- asymptomatic
- airway obstruction (symptoms often attributed to asthma / pneumonia)

Location: lung > bronchus / trachea > pleura

√ smoothly marginated mass in trachea

Rx: surgical excision

KARTAGENER SYNDROME

= IMMOTILE / DYSMOTILE CILIA SYNDROME

Incidence: 1:40,00; high familial incidence

Etiology: abnormal mucociliary function secondary to generalized deficiency of dynein arms of cilia affecting respiratory epithelium, auditory epithelium, sperm

Triad: (1) Situs inversus (in 50%)
◊ 50% of patients with immotile cilia syndrome have situs inversus!
◊ Kartagener syndrome is present in 20% of patients with situs inversus!
(2) Nasal polyposis with chronic sinusitis
(3) Bronchiectasis

- deafness
- infertility (abnormal sperm tails)

Associated anomalies:
transposition of great vessels, tri- / bilocular heart, pyloric stenosis, postcricoid web, epispadia

KLEBSIELLA PNEUMONIA

Most common cause of Gram-negative pneumonias; community acquired

Incidence: responsible for 5% of adult pneumonias

Organism: Friedländer bacillus = encapsulated, nonmotile, Gram-negative rod

Predisposed: elderly, debilitated, alcoholic, chronic lung disease, malignancy

- bacteremia in 25%

√ propensity for posterior portion of upper lobe / superior portion of lower lobe
√ dense lobar consolidation
√ bulging of fissure (large amounts of inflammatory exudate) CHARACTERISTIC but unusual
√ empyema (one of the most common causes)
√ patchy bronchopneumonia may be present
√ uni- / multilocular cavities (50%) appearing within 4 days
√ pulmonary gangrene = infarcted tissue (rare)

Cx: meningitis, pericarditis

Prognosis: mortality rate 25–50%

CHEST

DDx: Acute pneumococcal pneumonia (bulging of fissures, abscess + cavity formation, pleural effusion / empyema frequent)

LANGERHANS CELL HISTIOCYTOSIS

= LCH = EOSINOPHILIC GRANULOMA = HISTIOCYTOSIS X = LANGERHANS CELL GRANULOMATOSIS

= group of disorders characterized by abnormal clonal proliferation of the Langerhans cell (from the monocyte-macrophage cell line) resulting in granulomatous infiltration of lungs, bone, skin, lymph nodes, liver, spleen, brain, kidneys, endocrine glands

Age: most frequently in 3rd–4th decade (range 3 months to 69 years); M:F = 4:1; Caucasians >> Blacks

Histo:
granuloma containing Langerhans cells, foamy histiocytes, lymphocytes, plasma cells, eosinophils
Langerhans cell:
— dendritic antigen-presenting cell found in basal layer of skin + in liver (Kupffer cell), lymph nodes, spleen, bone marrow, lung
— contains unique mostly rod-shaped cytoplasmatic inclusion bodies known as Birbeck granules (identifiable only with electron microscopy)

@ Pulmonary Langerhans Cell Histiocytosis

Pathogenesis:
heavy cigarette smoking in young men with accumulation + activation of Langerhans cells (90% smokers) as a result of excess neuroendocrine cell hyperplasia + secretion of bombazine-like peptides

Path:
multifocal granulomatous infiltration centered on walls of bronchioles (= bronchiolitis) often extending into surrounding alveolar interstitium with subsequent bronchiolar destruction leading to thick-walled cysts presumably caused by check-valve bronchial obstruction + pneumothorax (no necrosis); in end-stage disease foci of LCG are replaced by fibroblasts forming CHARACTERISTIC stellate "starfish" scars with central remnants of persisting inflammatory cells

◊ CXR abnormalities more severe than clinical symptoms + pulmonary function tests!

• asymptomatic (up to 25%)
• nonproductive cough (75%)
• combination of obstructive + restrictive pulmonary function: presenting with pneumothorax in 15%
• fatigue, weight loss, fever (15–30%)
• dyspnea (40%)
• chest pain (25%) from pneumothorax / eosinophilic granuloma in rib
• diabetes insipidus (10–25%)
• lymphocytosis with predominance of T-suppressor cells on bronchoalveolar lavage (DDx: excess of T-helper cells in sarcoidosis)

Location: usually bilaterally symmetric, upper lobe predominance, sparing of costophrenic angles

Evolutionary sequence:
nodule – cavitated nodule – thick-walled cyst – thin-walled cyst (secondary to progressive enlargement + air trapping of original cavitary nodule)

√ ill-defined / stellate nodules 1–10 mm (granuloma stage):
 √ diffuse fine reticular / reticulonodular pattern (cellular infiltrate)
 √ cavitation of large nodules (rare)
√ "honeycomb lung" = multiple 1–5-cm cysts + subpleural blebs (fibrotic stage)
√ increased lung volumes in 1/3 (most other fibrotic lung diseases have decreased lung volumes!)
√ pleural effusion (8%), hilar adenopathy (unusual)
√ thymic enlargement

HRCT (combination virtually diagnostic):
 √ complex / branching thin-walled cysts <5 mm in size equally distributed in central + peripheral lung zones
 √ centrilobular peribronchiolar nodules
 √ intervening lung appears normal

DDx for nodules:
sarcoidosis, hypersensitivity pneumonitis, berylliosis, TB, atypical TB, metastases, silicosis, coal worker's pneumoconiosis

DDx for cysts:
emphysema, bronchiectasis, idiopathic pulmonary fibrosis, lymphangiomyomatosis

Cx:
1. Recurrent pneumothorax in 25% (from rupture of subpleural cysts) CHARACTERISTIC
2. Pulmonary hypertension
3. Superimposed Aspergillus fumigatus infection

Prognosis: poor with multisystem disease + organ dysfunction (especially with skin lesions);
(a) complete / partial regression (13–55%)
(b) stable (33%)
(c) rapid progression (7–21%) to air-flow obstruction + impaired diffusing capacity + respiratory failure

Mortality: 2–25%

Rx: cessation of smoking, chemotherapy (vincristine sulfate, prednisone, methotrexate, 6-mercaptopurine)

DDx: sarcoidosis (equal sex distribution, always multisystem disease, not related to smoking, erythema nodosum, bilateral hilar lymphadenopathy, lung cavitation + pneumothorax rare, epithelioid cells)

LEGIONELLA PNEUMONIA

= LEGIONNAIRES' DISEASE

Organism: Legionella pneumophila, 1–2 μm, aerobic, Gram-negative bacillus, weakly acid-fast, silver-impregnation stain

Predisposed: middle-aged / elderly, immunosuppressed, alcoholism, chronic obstructive lung disease, diabetes, cancer, cardiovascular disease, chronic renal failure, transplant recipients
Transmission: direct inhalation (air conditioning systems)
Prevalence: 6% of community-acquired pneumonias
Histo: leukocytoclastic fibrinopurulent pneumonia with histiocytes in intraalveolar exudate
• fever
• absence of sputum / lack of purulence (22–75%)
Clue: involvement of other organs with
 • diarrhea (0–25%), myalgia, toxic encephalopathy
 • liver + renal disease
 • hyponatremia (20%)
 • elevated serum transaminase / transpeptidase levels
 • lack of quick response to penicillin / cephalosporin / aminoglycoside
Concomitant infection (in 5–10%):
Streptococcus pneumoniae, Chlamydia pneumoniae, Mycobacterium tuberculosis, Pneumocystis carinii
Location: unilateral / bilateral (less frequent); lobar / segmental
√ patchy bronchopneumonia (= multifocal consolidation)
√ moderate volume of pleural effusion (6–30–63%)
√ cavitation (rare)
Cx: progressive respiratory failure (most common cause of death; 6% mortality in healthy patients)
Rx: erythromycin

LIPOID PNEUMONIA

Acute Exogenous Lipoid Pneumonia

= FIRE-EATER PNEUMONIA
Material: liquid paraffin, petroleum (hydrocarbons)
Cause: accidental poisoning in children, fire-eaters
√ ill-defined nodular areas of increased radiopacity
√ pneumatoceles / thin-walled collections of air

Chronic Exogenous Lipoid Pneumonia

Etiology: aspiration / inhalation of fatlike material
Types of oils:
(a) vegetable oil: sesame oil used in medical suspensions for the treatment of constipation
(b) animal oil: cod liver oil (commonly given to children); squalene = derivative of shark liver oil (folk remedy in some Asian countries); milk
(c) mineral oil (most common): as liquid paraffin in nose drops (taken at bedtime) / oral laxatives
 = inert pure hydrocarbon that does not initiate cough reflex
Predisposed: elderly, debilitated, neuromuscular disease, swallowing abnormalities (eg, scleroderma)
Path: pool of oil emulsified by lung lipase + surrounded by giant cell foreign body reaction (mineral oil aspiration) / necrotizing hemorrhagic bronchopneumonia (higher content of free fatty acid in animal fat aspiration)
◊ The degree + type of tissue reaction depend on the frequency of aspiration + chemical character of the oil
Histo: numerous lipid-laden macrophages distending alveolar walls + interstitium, accumulation of lipid material, inflammatory cellular infiltration, variable amount of fibrosis
• mostly asymptomatic
• fever, constitutional symptoms
• lipid-laden macrophages in sputum / lavage fluid
• oil droplets in bronchial washing / needle aspirate
Location: predilection for RML + lower lobes
√ homogeneous segmental airspace consolidation (most common)
√ interstitial reticulonodular pattern (rare)
√ paraffinoma = circumscribed peripheral mass (granulomatous reaction + fibrosis often causing stellate appearance)
√ slow progression / no change
CT:
 √ diffuse ground-glass opacity of centri- / panlobular distribution (= acinar pattern) + thickening of interlobular septa as earliest finding
 √ airspace consolidation (filling of alveoli with exudate + inflammatory cells) at 1 week
 √ return to ground-glass opacity (due to expectoration + lymphatic drainage of lipid droplets and inflammatory cells) at 2–4 weeks
 √ volume loss + fibrosis of interlobular septa and pleura at 14–16 weeks
 √ mass of low-attenuation approaching that of subcutaneous fat (–150 to 50 HU)
Dx: bronchoalveolar lavage, transbronchial biopsy

LÖFFLER SYNDROME

= disorder of unknown etiology characterized by local areas of transient parenchymal consolidation associated with blood eosinophilia
Path: interstitial + alveolar edema containing a large number of lymphocytes
• no / mild symptoms
• eosinophilia
• history of atopia
√ single / multiple areas of homogeneous ill-defined consolidation
√ uni- or bilateral, nonsegmental distribution, predominantly in lung periphery
√ transient + shifting in nature (changes within one to several days)
Prognosis: may undergo spontaneous remission

LUNG TRANSPLANT

Indications:
emphysema, cystic fibrosis, CHD, idiopathic pulmonary fibrosis, alpha-1 antitrypsin deficiency, primary pulmonary hypertension, sarcoidosis, pneumoconiosis, malignancy
Survival rate: 90% 1-month survival, 70% 1-year survival

Acute Rejection of Lung Transplant

Incidence: 60–80% with 2–3 significant episodes in first 3 months

Histo: mononuclear cell infiltrate around arteries, veins, bronchioles, alveolar septa with alveolar edema (initially) + fibrinous exudate (later)

Time of onset: first episode 5–10 days after transplantation; occasionally by 48 hours

• drop in arterial oxygen pressure WITHOUT infection / airway obstruction / fluid overload
• pyrexia, fatigue, decreased exercise tolerance
√ heterogeneous opacities in perihilar areas
√ ground-glass attenuation on HRCT
√ new increasing pleural effusion + septal thickening (most common, 90% specific, 68% sensitive) WITHOUT concomitant signs of LV dysfunction (increase in cardiac size / vascular pedicle width / vascular redistribution)
√ subpleural edema, peribronchial cuffing, airspace disease

Dx: (1) Transbronchial biopsy
(2) Rapid improvement of radiologic abnormalities after treatment with IV bolus of corticosteroids for 3 days

Rx: methylprednisolone, polyclonal T-cell antibody (antithymocyte globulin), monoclonal antibodies (CD3, OKT3), lymphoid irradiation

Anastomotic Complications of Lung Transplant

1. Airway dehiscence (2–8%)
   √ presence of extraluminal air collections at anastomotic site (80%)
2. Airway stricture
   DDx: telescoped anastomosis
   Rx: laser resection, balloon bronchoplasty
3. Vascular stenosis
4. Diaphragmatic hernia from omentopexy
   Procedure: omental pedicle is harvested at time of transplantation through a small diaphragmatic incision + wrapped around anastomosis to prevent dehiscence

Chronic Rejection of Lung Transplant

Prevalence: 24%

Path: obliterative bronchiolitis (36%), interstitial pneumonitis, rejection-mediated vasculopathy

Time of onset: 3–75 months after transplantation

• persistent coughing and wheezing
• slowly worsening exertional dyspnea
√ increased / diminished lung volumes
√ central + peripheral bronchiectasis
√ localized airspace disease
√ partial lobar atelectasis
√ thin irregular areas of increased opacity
√ pleural thickening
√ diminished peripheral lung markings
√ nodular / reticular opacities associated with peribronchial thickening

Hyperacute Rejection of Lung Transplant

= rejection in cases of an immunoglobulin G donor-specific HLA antibody positive crossmatch

Path: acute diffuse alveolar damage

Posttransplantation Infection

Cause: immunosuppression, reduced mucociliary clearance, interruption of lymphatic drainage, direct contact of transplant with environment via airways

A. INFECTION OF LUNG TRANSPLANT
   Prevalence: 35–50%; major cause of morbidity + mortality in early postoperative period
   Cause: ? absent cough reflex, impaired mucociliary transport in denervated lung
   Organism: bacteria (23%) > CMV > Aspergillus > Pneumocystis
   (1) within 1st month: Gram-negative bacteria, fungi (candidiasis, aspergillosis)
   (2) after 1st month: CMV, Pneumocystis carinii, bacteria, fungi
   • fever, leukocytosis
   √ lobar / multilobar consolidation (due to bacterial > fungal pathogens)
   √ diffuse heterogeneous / ground-glass opacities (due to viral / disseminated fungal pathogens)
   √ nodular opacities (due to fungal / unusual bacterial pathogens / CMV / septic emboli)
   Cx: may progress rapidly to respiratory failure + death
   Dx: transbronchial / open biopsy (80% accurate)
B. EXTRAPULMONARY INFECTION
   thoracotomy wound infection, bacteremia, sepsis, empyema, central venous line infection

Posttransplantation Lymphoproliferative Disease

Incidence: 4%

Histo: spectrum from benign polyclonal proliferation of lymphoid tissue to non-Hodgkin lymphoma

Associated with: Epstein-Barr virus

Time of onset: 1 month to several years; related to immunosuppressive regimen

√ solitary / multiple discrete nodules
√ mediastinal / hilar lymphadenopathy

Reperfusion Edema

= REIMPLANTATION RESPONSE
= infiltrate appearing within 48 hours after transplantation unrelated to fluid overload, LV failure, infection, atelectasis, or rejection; diagnosed by exclusion

Pathogenesis: permeability edema due to lymphatic disruption, pulmonary denervation, organ ischemia, trauma

Histo: fluid accumulation in interstitium consistent with noncardiogenic pulmonary edema

Time course: manifests within 24 hours, peaks at 2nd–4th postoperative day, resolves at variable rate ranging from days to 1–2 weeks to months

• increasing hypoxia before extubation; poor correlation between radiographic severity + physiologic parameters

Location: perihilar areas + basal regions

√ perihilar haze / rapid uni- or bilateral heterogeneously dense interstitial and/or airspace disease

Dx: per exclusion (radiographic changes not due to LV failure, hyperacute rejection, fluid overload, infection, atelectasis)

LYMPHANGIOMYOMATOSIS

= LAM = LYMPHANGIOLEIOMYOMATOSIS

= rare disorder characterized by

(1) gradually progressive diffuse interstitial lung disease

(2) recurrent chylous pleural effusions

(3) recurrent pneumothoraces

Etiology: unknown, ? forme fruste of tuberous sclerosis

Age: 17–50 years, exclusively in women of childbearing age

Histo: proliferation of atypical smooth muscle in pulmonary lymphatic vessels, blood vessels, and airways

Pathogenesis:
proliferated smooth muscle obstructs (a) bronchioles (trapping of air, overinflation, formation of cysts, pneumothorax), (b) venules (pulmonary edema, hemorrhage, hemosiderosis), (c) lymphatics (thickening of lymphatics, chylothorax)

May be associated with: Tuberous sclerosis (lung involvement in 1%)

• progressive exertional dyspnea + cough
• disease aggravated by pregnancy + oral contraceptives
• hemoptysis (30–40%), chyloptysis
• radiologic-physiologic discrepancy = severe airflow obstruction (reduced FEV_1, reduced ratio of FEV_1 / FVC%) despite relatively normal findings on CXR
• near normal FVC and TLC
• combination of restrictive + obstructive ventilatory defects: hypoxia, markedly impaired DL_{CO}%
• positive immunohistochemical staining of LAM cells with HMB-45 (monoclonal antibody for melanocytic lesion)

√ <u>classic signs</u>:
  √ coarse reticular interstitial pattern (caused by summation of multiple cyst walls)
  √ recurrent large chylothorax (20–50–75%)
  √ recurrent pneumothorax (40-50% at presentation; in 80% during course of disease)
√ normal / increased lung volume
  ◊ The only interstitial lung disease to develop increase in lung volume!
√ Kerley B lines
√ pulmonary cysts (visible if >1 cm) + honeycombing
√ occasionally chylous ascites
√ mediastinal + retroperitoneal adenopathy (from smooth muscle proliferation)

HRCT:
  √ numerous randomly scattered thin-walled (<2 mm) cysts of various sizes (0.5–6 cm) surrounded by normal lung parenchyma (? due to air trapping distal to small airways narrowed by smooth muscle proliferation / destruction of collagen + elastin in the interstitium from metalloproteinases elaborated by LAM cells)
  √ bronchovascular bundles at periphery of cyst walls
  √ consolidations (due to hemorrhage following destruction of pulmonary microvasculature)
  √ pericardial effusion
  √ dilated thoracic duct
  √ precarinal + retrocrural lymph nodes

NUC (V/Q scan):
  √ "speckling" = well-defined hot spots on ventilation scan (presumably due to accumulation of coalescing droplets of DTPA aerosol trapped in peripheral cysts) in 66%

@ Abdomen
  • bloating, increased abdominal girth, abdominal pain
  • perineal swelling, chylous vaginal discharge
  √ lymphadenopathy of up to 4 cm (33%):
    Histo: replacement of lymph node with smooth muscle
    √ central hypoattenuating areas of –72 to +50 HU (due to chylous lymph collections / fat)
  √ **lymphangioleiomyoma** (20%) = well-defined lobulated complex lymphatic mass:
    √ volumes of 10–1,500 mL
    √ hypoattenuating center of 3–25 HU
    Path: smooth muscle proliferation in walls of lymphatics resulting in lymphatic dilatation + mural thickening
    Location: retroperitoneum > pelvis > chest > neck
  √ low-density ascites (10%) of –10 to +21 HU (due to rupture of overdistended lymph cysts)
  √ dilatation of thoracic duct (10%)
  √ fatty liver masses (5%): AML / lipoma

@ Kidneys
  • flank pain, hematuria
  √ angiomyolipoma (50%):
    √ occasionally lacking fat
    √ multiplicity in <20%
  √ simple cysts (occasionally large enough to lead to renal insufficiency)

Dx: open / transbronchial lung biopsy

Prognosis: 8.5-year survival rate of 38–78%; death within 10 years from progressive pulmonary insufficiency

DDx:
(1) Tuberous sclerosis (cortical tubers, subependymal nodules, retinal hamartomas, facial angiofibromas, periungual fibromas, mental retardation, epilepsy, multiple renal AML in 40–80%)

CHEST

(2) Histiocytosis (cysts in upper 2/3 of lung with sparing of costophrenic angles, cyst walls more variable in thickness, pulmonary nodules + cavitation, septal thickening)
(3) Emphysema (imperceptible cyst walls, cysts may be segmentally distributed, lobular architecture preserved with bronchovascular bundle in central position, areas of lung destruction without arcuate contour)
(4) Idiopathic pulmonary fibrosis = fibrosing alveolitis (small irregular thick-walled cysts + predominantly peripheral interstitial thickening)
(5) Bronchiectasis (bronchial wall thickening)
(6) Neurofibromatosis (cystic air spaces predominantly in apical location)

LYMPHANGITIC CARCINOMATOSIS

= INTERSTITIAL CARCINOMA
= tumor cell accumulation within connective tissue (bronchovascular bundles, interlobular septa, subpleural space, pulmonary lymphatics) from tumor embolization of blood vessels followed by lymphatic obstruction, interstitial edema, and collagen deposition (fibrosis from desmoplastic reaction when tumor cells extend into adjacent pulmonary parenchyma)

Incidence: 7% of all pulmonary metastases
Tumor origin: bronchogenic carcinoma, carcinoma of breast (56%), stomach (46%), thyroid, pancreas, larynx, cervix
mnemonic: "**C**ertain **C**ancers **S**pread **B**y **P**lugging **T**he **L**ymphatics"
Cervix
Colon
Stomach
Breast
Pancreas
Thyroid
Larynx

Path: (1) interstitial edema, (2) interstitial fibrotic changes, (3) lymphatic dilatation, (4) tumor cells within connective tissue planes

• dyspnea (often preceding radiographic abnormalities)
• rarely dry cough + hemoptysis

Location: bilateral; unilateral if secondary to lung primary
CXR (accuracy 23%):
√ normal chest radiograph
√ reticular densities
√ coarsened bronchovascular markings
√ Kerley A + B lines
√ small lung volume
√ hilar adenopathy (20–50%)

HRCT:
√ well-defined smoothly thickened polygonal reticular network of 10–25 mm in diameter (= thickened interlobular septa)
√ irregular / nodular = "beaded" thickening of interlobular septa
√ central dot within secondary pulmonary lobule = thickened centrilobular bronchovascular bundle
√ subpleural thickening
√ pleural effusion (30–50%)
√ hilar / mediastinal lymphadenopathy (30–50%)

Prognosis: death within 1 year
DDx: (1) Fibrosing alveolitis (peripheral predominance)
(2) Extrinsic allergic alveolitis (no polygonal structures, pleural changes rare)
(3) Sarcoidosis (nodules of irregular outline more frequent in upper lobes, polygonal structures uncommon)

LYMPHOID INTERSTITIAL PNEUMONIA

= LYMPHOCYTIC INTERSTITIAL PNEUMONITIS = LIP
= benign lymphoproliferative disorder characterized by diffuse interstitial lymphocytic infiltration (probably immunologic disorder) with highly variable course

Histo: extensive infiltration of bronchovascular bundles, interlobular septa, and pleura by polyclonal mature small lymphocytes + plasma cells; many cases reclassified as lymphoma
Associated with: Sjögren syndrome, autoimmune thyroid disease, AIDS, Castleman disease, systemic lupus erythematosus, myasthenia gravis, pernicious anemia, chronic active hepatitis

◊ Indicative of AIDS when present in child under 13 years of age!

• dyspnea + cough
• cyanosis + clubbing (50%)
• enlargement of salivary glands (20%)
• NO lymphocytosis or history of atopia
• monoclonal gammopathy (usually IgM)

Distribution: bilateral, involving all lung zones
√ fine reticular changes in both lungs
√ reticulonodular pattern
√ resembling airspace disease (in severe form)

CT:
√ ill-defined centrilobular nodules (100%)
√ ground-glass attenuation (100%)
√ thickening of bronchovascular bundles + interlobular septa (in majority)
√ subpleural small nodules (in majority)
√ airspace consolidation
√ cysts (due to partial airway obstruction by peribronchial + peribronchiolar LIP) in 68%
√ mediastinal lymph node enlargement (50%)

Prognosis:
(a) recovery / slowly improving / stable disease
(b) progressive disease (in 33%)

Rx: responsive to steroids
DDx: Hypersensitivity pneumonitis (ground-glass attenuation, small centrilobular nodules, NOT cystic airspaces / thickening of interlobular septa or bronchovascular bundles)

Localized form = PSEUDOLYMPHOMA

LYMPHOMA

◊ 7th leading cause of death from cancer in United States
Pathogenesis: ? viral cause

HD: contiguous spread requires scanning of abnormal area only
NHL: noncontiguous spread requires scanning of chest, abdomen, pelvis
@ Thorax
◊ Hodgkin disease more common in thorax than NHL at presentation (HD in 85%, NHL in 45%)
1. Lymphadenopathy
anterior mediastinal, pretracheal, hilar, subcarinal, axillary, periesophageal, paracardiac, superior diaphragmatic internal mammary lymph nodes
— anterior mediastinum: nodular sclerosing type of HD (75%); M < F
— posterior mediastinum: NHL
2. Lung parenchyma involvement (HD in 12%, NHL in 4%)
3. Pleural + subpleural lymphoma (up to 30%)
@ Abdomen
1. Periaortic adenopathy .... HD in 25%
NHL in 49%
2. Mesenteric adenopathy .... HD in 4%
NHL in 51%
3. Liver involvement .... HD in 8%
NHL in 14%
√ hepatomegaly with involvement .... HD in <30%
NHL in 57%
HD: commonly diffuse infiltrating process
NHL: diffuse infiltrating / discrete tumor nodules
4. Splenic involvement .... HD in 37%
NHL in 41%
HD: most common site of abdominal involvement
NHL: 3rd most common site of abdominal involvement; may be initial manifestation in large cell NHL
◊ Staging laparotomy necessary as 2/3 of tumor nodules <1 cm in size
5. Gastrointestinal involvement
in 10% of patients with abdominal lymphoma (uncommon in HD, common in histiocytic NHL); NHL accounts for 80% of all gastric lymphomas
6. Renal involvement
late manifestation, most commonly in NHL
7. Adrenal involvement
more common in NHL
8. Extranodal involvement
more frequent with histologically diffuse forms of NHL

LYMPHOMATOID GRANULOMATOSIS

= angiocentric + angiodestructive lymphoproliferative + granulomatous disease
Age: 7–85 (mean of 48) years; M:F = 2:1
Path: multiple sharply marginated masses adjacent to a bronchus causing obstructive pneumonitis
Histo: angiocentric infiltrate of atypical lymphoid cells (of B-cell lineage containing Epstein-Barr virus) with vascular invasion + destruction; necrotic lung parenchyma in higher grade lesions; giant cells absent (DDx to Wegener granulomatosis)
• malaise, weight loss (35%)
• no specific serum markers
◊ Less commonly found in lymph nodes, bone marrow, spleen
◊ Involvement of upper respiratory tract + sinuses is very unusual
@ Lung (100%)
• fever (60%), cough (56%), dyspnea (29%)
√ normal CXR
√ diffuse reticulonodular opacities (= granulomas)
√ large masslike opacities (= granulomas + pulmonary infarcts)
√ multiple bilateral nodules in middle + lower lobes (80%)
√ unilateral involvement (21%)
√ small pleural effusions (40%)
√ hilar lymphadenopathy (25%)
CT:
√ peripheral subpleural 0.6–8 cm large nodules / masses
√ central cavitation (30%)
√ reticular / nodular airspace opacities (10–43%)
@ Skin (39–53%)
• nodules, ulcers, maculopapular rash (20–39%)
@ CNS (37–53%)
• neurologic complaints (21%)
@ Kidneys (32–40%)
Cx: lymphoma (12–47%)
Mortality: in 53–90% from sepsis, respiratory failure, pulmonary embolism, massive hemoptysis, CNS lesions

LYMPHOPROLIFERATIVE DISEASE AFTER TRANSPLANTATION

= abnormal proliferation of lymphoid cells in immunocompromised organ transplant recipients in a spectrum ranging from mild lymphoid hyperplasia to malignant lymphoma
Incidence: 2% of all allograft recipients:
bone marrow transplantation 0.6%
renal graft transplantation 1–5%
cardiac transplantation 1.8–20%
liver transplantation 2%
lung transplantation 6.2–9.4%
Pathophysiology of B-cell (in 86%) origin:
1. infection of B lymphocytes with EBV (Epstein-Barr virus) causes increased proliferation of B cells (= polyclonal B-cell expansion)
2. loss of protective immune control by T cells allows for uncontrolled proliferation of EBV-infected B lymphocytes (= oligoclonal B-cell expansion)
3. genetic mutation transforms some B cells into malignant cells
◊ 14% of posttransplantation LPD is of T-cell origin
Time of onset: 2–5 months (mean) after bone marrow, lung, heart-lung transplantation;
23–32 months (mean) after kidney, heart, liver transplantation
◊ Under cyclosporine / OKT3 within 1 month

CHEST

Unique features:
(a) predilection for extranodal sites
(b) varied morphologic appearance
(c) strong / probably causal association with EBV infection
(d) frequent absence of immunophenotypic / genotypic evidence of monoclonality
(e) poor response to cytolytic chemotherapy / irradiation
• illness resembling infectious mononucleosis = pharyngitis, fever, lymphadenopathy, hepatosplenomegaly
@ any site, including CNS, lymph nodes, thorax, GI tract, or allograft
@ Chest
√ well-circumscribed nodules ± low-attenuation center
√ patchy air space consolidation
√ mediastinal / hilar lymphadenopathy
@ Liver
√ focal hepatic mass in orthotopic liver transplant
√ periportal adenopathy

MECONIUM ASPIRATION SYNDROME

= most common cause of neonatal respiratory distress in full term / postmature infants (hyaline membrane disease most common cause in premature infants)

Etiology: fetal circulatory accidents / placental insufficiency / postmaturity result in perinatal hypoxia + fetal distress with meconium defecated in utero

Pathogenesis: severe hypoxemia induces gasping reflex with inhalation of tenacious meconium that produces medium and small airway obstruction + chemical pneumonitis

Incidence: 10% of all deliveries have meconium-stained amniotic fluid, 1% of all deliveries have respiratory distress

• cyanosis (rare)
• **persistent fetal circulation syndrome** = neonatal pulmonary hypertension (secondary to thick-walled pulmonary arterioles) + R-to-L shunt through PDA and foramen ovale + severe cyanosis
Rx: extracorporeal membrane oxygenation (major indication besides diaphragmatic hernia + neonatal pneumonia)
√ large infant
√ bilateral diffuse grossly patchy opacities (atelectasis + consolidation)
√ hyperinflation with areas of emphysema (air trapping)
√ spontaneous pneumothorax + pneumomediastinum (25–40%) requiring no therapy
√ small pleural effusions (10–20%)
√ NO air bronchograms
√ rapid clearing usually within 48 hours

Cx: morbidity from anoxic brain damage is high

MEDIASTINAL LIPOMATOSIS

= excess unencapsulated fat deposition

Etiology:
(a) exogenous steroids (average daily dose of >30 mg prednisone):
(1) chronic renal disease, renal transplant (5%)
(2) collagen vascular disease, vasculitis
(3) hemolytic anemia
(4) asthma
(5) dermatitis
(6) Crohn disease
(7) myasthenia gravis
(b) endogenous steroid elevation:
(1) adrenal tumor
(2) pituitary tumor / hyperplasia = Cushing disease
(3) ectopic ACTH-production (carcinoma of the lung)
(c) obesity
• moon facies
• buffalo hump
• supraclavicular + episternal fat

Location: upper mediastinum (common), cardiophrenic angles + paraspinal areas (less common)

√ upper mediastinal widening
√ paraspinal widening
√ increase in epicardial fat-pads
√ symmetric slightly lobulated extrapleural deposits extending from apex to 9th rib laterally

OTHER FEATURES:
√ osteoporosis
√ fractures
√ aseptic necrosis
√ increased rectosacral distance

MESOTHELIOMA

Benign Mesothelioma

= LOCALIZED FIBROUS MESOTHELIOMA = LOCALIZED FIBROUS TUMOR OF THE PLEURA = SOLITARY FIBROUS TUMOR OF PLEURA = BENIGN LOCALIZED MESOTHELIOMA = BENIGN PLEURAL FIBROMA = FIBROSING MESOTHELIOMA = PLEURAL FIBROMYXOMA

Incidence: <5% of all pleural tumors

◊ No recognized association with asbestos exposure!

Age: 3rd–8th decade; mean age of 50–60 years; M:F = 1:1

Path: usually solitary mass arising from visceral pleura in 80% + parietal pleura in 20%

Histo: tumor originates from submesothelial fibroblasts, lined by layer of mesothelial cells
(a) relatively acellular fibrous tissue
(b) rounded spindle-shaped densely packed cells
(c) resembling hemangiopericytoma of lung

• asymptomatic in 50%
• cough, fever, dyspnea, chest pain (larger mass)
• digital clubbing (rare) + hypertrophic pulmonary osteoarthropathy in 20–35%
• episodic hypoglycemia (4%)
√ sharply circumscribed spherical / ovoid lobular mass of 2–30 cm in diameter located near lung periphery / adjacent to pleural surface / within fissure
√ sessile with smooth tapered margin (common) / pedunculated with obtuse angle toward chest wall (rare, benign feature)
√ tumor may change in shape + location upon alteration of patient's position (if pedunculated)

√ areas of hemorrhage / necrosis may be present (favors malignancy)
√ ipsilateral pleural effusion (rare) containing hyaluronic acid
CT:
√ substantial contrast enhancement
√ heterogeneous enhancement due to myxoid degeneration + hemorrhage
MR:
√ hypointense on T1WI + hyperintense on T2WI
Cx: malignant degeneration in 37%
DDx: metastatic deposit
Rx: excision is curative (recurrence rate lower for pedunculated versus nodular tumor)

Malignant Mesothelioma

= DIFFUSE MALIGNANT MESOTHELIOMA
= uncommon fatal neoplasm of serosal lining of pleural cavity, peritoneum, or both
◊ Most common primary neoplasm of pleura!
Prevalence: 7–13:1,000,000 persons/year; 2,000–3,000 cases/year in USA
Etiology: asbestos exposure (13–100%); zeolite (nonasbestos mineral fiber); chronic inflammation (TB, empyema); irradiation
Carcinogenic potential:
proportional to aspect ratio (= length-to-diameter) of fiber and durability in human tissue:
crocidolite > amosite > chrysotile > actinolite, anthophyllite, tremolite
◊ Occupational exposure of asbestos found in only 40–80% of all cases!
◊ 5–10% of asbestos workers will develop mesothelioma in their lifetime (risk factor of 30 compared with general population)
◊ No relation to duration / degree of exposure or smoking history
Latency period: 20–35–45 years (earlier than asbestosis; later than asbestos-related lung cancer)
Peak age: 50–70 years (66%); M:F = 2–4–6:1
Path: multiple tumor masses involving predominantly the parietal pleura + to a lesser degree the visceral pleura; progression to thick sheetlike / confluent masses resulting in lung encasement
Histo: (a) epithelioid (60%), (b) sarcomatoid (15%), (c) biphasic (25%); intracellular asbestos fibers in 25%
Associated with: peritoneal mesothelioma; hypertrophic osteoarthropathy (10%)
Staging (Boutin modification of Butchart staging)
IA confined to ipsilateral parietal / diaphragmatic pleura
IB + visceral pleura, lung , pericardium
II invasion of chest wall / mediastinum (esophagus, heart, contralateral pleura) or metastases to thoracic lymph nodes
III penetration of diaphragm with peritoneal involvement or metastases to extrathoracic lymph nodes
IV distant hematogenous metastases
Stage at presentation: II in 50%, III in 28%, I in 18%, IV in 4%
• nonpleuritic (56%) / pleuritic chest pain (6%)
• dyspnea (53%)
• fever + chills + sweats (30%)
• weakness, fatigue, malaise (30%)
• cough (24%), weight loss (22%), anorexia (10%)
• expectoration of asbestos bodies (= fusiform segmented rodlike structures = iron-protein deposition on asbestos fibers [a subset of ferruginous bodies])
Spread:
(a) contiguous: chest wall, mediastinum, contralateral chest, pericardium, diaphragm, peritoneal cavity; lymphatics, blood, lung
(b) lymphatic: hilar + mediastinal (40%), celiac (8%), axillary + supraclavicular (1%), cervical nodes
(c) hematogenous: lung, liver, kidney, adrenal gland
√ extensive irregular lobulated bulky pleural-based masses typically >5 cm / pleural thickening (60%)
√ exudative / hemorrhagic unilateral pleural effusion (30–60–80%) without mediastinal shift ("frozen hemithorax" = fixation by pleural rind of neoplastic tissue); effusion contains hyaluronic acid in 80–100%; bilateral effusions (in 10%)
√ distinct pleural mass without effusion (<25%)
√ associated pleural plaques in 50% = HALLMARK of asbestos exposure
√ pleural calcifications (20%)
√ circumferential encasement = involvement of all pleural surfaces (mediastinum, pericardium, fissures) as late manifestation
√ extension into interlobar fissures (40–86%)
√ superficial invasion of underlying lung (primarily as extension into interlobular septa)
√ rib destruction in 20% (in advanced disease)
√ ascites (peritoneum involved in 35%)
CT:
√ pleural thickening (92%)
√ thickening of interlobar fissure (86%)
√ pleural effusion (74%)
√ contraction of affected hemithorax (42%):
√ ipsilateral mediastinal shift
√ narrowed intercostal spaces
√ elevation of ipsilateral hemidiaphragm
√ calcified pleural plaques (20%)
MR (best modality to determine resectability):
√ minimally hyperintense relative to muscle on T1WI
√ moderately hyperintense relative to muscle on T2WI
Metastases to:
ipsilateral lung (60%), hilar + mediastinal nodes, contralateral lung + pleura (rare), extension through chest wall + diaphragm
Prognosis: 10% of occupationally exposed individuals die of mesothelioma (in 50% pleural + in 50% peritoneal mesothelioma); mean survival time of 5–11 months
DDx: pleural fibrosis from infection (TB, fungal, actinomycosis), fibrothorax, empyema, metastatic adenocarcinoma (differentiation impossible)

Dx: video-assisted thoracoscopic surgery (postprocedural radiation therapy of all entry ports for tumor seeding of needle track [21%])

METASTASIS TO LUNG

Pulmonary metastases occur in 30% of all malignancies; mostly hematogenous

Age: >50 years (in 87%)

FREQUENCY:

	Origin of pulmonary mets		*Probability of pulmonary mets*	
1.	Breast	22%	Kidney	in 75%
2.	Kidney	11%	Osteosarcoma	in 75%
3.	Head and neck	10%	Choriocarcinoma	in 75%
4.	Colorectal	9%	Thyroid	in 65%
5.	Uterus	6%	Melanoma	in 60%
6.	Pancreas	5%	Breast	in 55%
7.	Ovary	5%	Prostate	in 40%
8.	Prostate	4%	Head and neck	in 30%
9.	Stomach	4%	Esophagus	in 20%

Incidence of pulmonary metastases:

mnemonic: "CHEST"

Choriocarcinoma	60%
Hypernephroma / Wilms tumor	30 / 20%
Ewing sarcoma	18%
Sarcoma (rhabdomyo- / osteosarcoma)	21 / 15%
Testicular tumor	12%

√ multiple nodules (in 75%) of varying sizes (most typical), 82% subpleural

√ fine micronodular pattern: highly vascular tumor (renal cell, breast, thyroid, prostate carcinoma, bone sarcoma, choriocarcinoma)

√ pneumothorax (2%): especially in children with sarcoma + frequently with osteosarcoma (due to bronchopleural fistula caused by subpleural metastasis)

CT:

√ noncalcified multiple (>10) round lesions >2.5 cm likely to be metastatic

√ connection to pulmonary arterial branches (75%)

Solitary Metastatic Lung Nodule

◊ A solitary lung nodule represents a primary lung tumor in 62% in patients with known Hx of neoplasm

◊ 0.4–5–9% of all solitary nodules are metastatic; most likely origin: colon carcinoma (30–40%), melanoma, osteosarcoma, renal cell carcinoma, bladder cancer, testicular tumor, breast carcinoma

Calcifying Lung Metastases (<1%)

mnemonic: "BOTTOM"

Breast
Osteo- / chondrosarcoma
Thyroid (papillary)
Testicular
Ovarian
Mucinous adenocarcinoma (colon)

\+ others: synovial sarcoma, giant cell tumor of bone, lung metastases following radiation / chemotherapy

Cavitating Lung Metastases

Frequency: 4% (compared with 9% in primary bronchogenic carcinoma)

Histo: squamous cell carcinoma (10%), adenocarcinoma (9.5%)

mnemonic: "**S**quamous **C**ell **M**etastases **T**end to **C**avitate"

Squamous cell carcinoma, **S**arcoma
Colon
Melanoma
Transitional cell carcinoma
Cervix, during **C**hemotherapy

Hemorrhagic Lung Metastases

CT: √ ill-defined nodules with fuzzy margin + halo sign (= surrounding ground-glass opacity)

1. Angiocarcinoma
2. Choriocarcinoma
3. Renal cell carcinoma
4. Melanoma
5. Thyroid carcinoma

Endobronchial Metastasis

Frequency: 1%

√ subsegmental / segmental atelectasis or atelectasis of entire unilateral lung

√ round endobronchial lesion on CT

1. Bronchogenic carcinoma
2. Lymphoma
3. Renal cell carcinoma
4. Breast cancer
5. Colorectal carcinoma

Lung Metastases in Childhood

mnemonic: "ROWE"

Rhabdomyosarcoma
Osteosarcoma
Wilms tumor
Ewing sarcoma

Metastases with Airspace Pattern

= lepidic growth along intact alveolar walls similar to bronchioloalveolar carcinoma mimicking pneumonia

√ airspace nodules

√ consolidation with air bronchogram

√ focal /extensive ground-glass opacities

1. Adenocarcinoma of GI tract (10%)
2. Adenocarcinoma of breast / ovary

Sterilized Metastasis

= persistence of metastatic nodule without significant change in size after adequate chemotherapy

Histo: necrotic nodule ± fibrosis without viable tumor cells

1. Choriocarcinoma
2. Testicular cancer
   √ growing teratoma syndrome = conversion to a benign mature teratoma
   √ pulmonary lacunae (= transformation into thin-walled cavity) may persist for years

Metastasis of Benign Tumor to Lung
1. Leiomyoma of uterus
2. Hydatidiform mole of uterus
3. Giant cell tumor of bone
4. Chondroblastoma
5. Pleomorphic adenoma of salivary gland
6. Meningioma

METASTASIS TO PLEURA
1. Lung (36%)
2. Breast (25%)
3. Lymphoma (10%)
4. Ovary (5%)
5. Stomach (2%)

MYCOPLASMA PNEUMONIA
= PRIMARY ATYPICAL PNEUMONIA (PAP)

◊ Varied radiographic + clinical picture!

Commonest cause of community-acquired nonbacterial pneumonia with a mild course (only 2% require hospitalization), usually lasts 2–3 weeks; only 10% of infected subjects develop pneumonia

Incidence: 10–33% of all pneumonias; autumn peak

Organism: Eaton agent = pleuropneumonia-like organism (PPLO) = 350 μm long pleomorphic Mycoplasma pneumoniae with lack of cell wall

Spread: direct contact / aerosol

Age: most common in ages 5–20 years (esp. in closed populations

Histo: peribronchial mononuclear cell infiltrates (similar to viral lower respiratory infection)

- incubation period: 1–2 weeks
- gradual onset beginning with pharyngitis, headache, myalgia (rhinorrhea + nasal congestion uncommon)
- mild symptoms of dry cough + low fever, malaise, otitis
- sputum with PMNs but few bacteria
- mild leukocytosis (20%)
- most common respiratory cause of cold agglutinin production (60%)

◊ Severity of radiologic findings discrepant to mild clinical condition!

◊ Pulmonary infiltrates show a significant lag time

√ focal reticular <u>interstitial infiltrate</u>:
  √ unilobar from hilum into lower lobe as earliest change (52%), bilobar (10%)
  √ parahilar peribronchial opacification (12%)
  √ atelectasis (29%)

√ <u>alveolar infiltrates</u>:
  √ patchy inhomogeneous unilateral (L > R) airspace consolidation in segmental lower lobe in 50%, bilateral in 10–40%

√ small pleural effusions in 20%

√ hilar adenopathy (7–22%)

Rx: erythromycin, azithromycin, tetracycline

Cx: ? as an autoimmune response
  (1) Acute disseminated encephalomyelitis
  (2) Cerebral arteriovenous occlusion
  (3) Erythema nodosum, erythema multiforme, Stevens-Johnson syndrome
  (4) pulmonary: Swyer-James syndrome, pulmonary fibrosis, bronchiolitis obliterans, ARDS

Prognosis: 20% with recurrent symptoms of pharyngitis + bronchitis ± infiltrations

DDx: viral infection of lower respiratory tract, pertussis, chlamydia (indistinguishable)

NEAR DROWNING
= asphyxiation due to water inhalation followed by survival for a minimum of 24 hours

Stage 1:
  (a) acute laryngospasm after inhalation of a small amount of water
    √ no roentgenographic abnormality
  (b) prolonged laryngospasm = "dry drowning" due to negative pressure edema arising from a prolonged episode of the Müller maneuver as in postobstructive pulmonary edema
    √ Kerley lines, peribronchial cuffing
    √ patchy perihilar alveolar airspace consolidation
    Prognosis: resolution within 24–48 hours (under therapy)

Stage 2:
  = laryngospasm + swallowing of water into the stomach

Stage 3:
  (a) persistent laryngospasm with dry drowning (10–15%)
    √ pressure edema
  (b) aspiration of water after hypoxia-induced relaxation of laryngospasm (85–90%)
    √ permeability edema (due to hypoxia + diffuse alveolar damage)
    Cx: ARDS, aspiration of gastric fluid, infection by fresh-water saprophytic bacteria

1. Sea-water drowning
   - hemoconcentration, hypovolemia
2. Fresh-water drowning
   - hemodilution, hypervolemia
   - hemolysis
3. Secondary drowning
   (a) pneumonia due to toxic debris
   (b) progressive pulmonary edema
4. Dry drowning (20–40%)
   = laryngeal spasm prevents water from entering
   √ no roentgenographic abnormality

Similarities of all 4 types:
- hypoxemia
- metabolic acidosis

√ central extensive fluffy areas of increased opacity (alveolar edema indistinguishable from other types):
  √ tendency for opacities to coalesce

√ hyaline membrane formation = considerable loss of protein from blood

Cx: pneumonia (due to aspirated bacteria / fungi / mycobacteria)

NECROTIZING SARCOID GRANULOMATOSIS

Etiology: ? variant of sarcoidosis
Age: 3rd –7th decade (mean age, 49 years); M:F = 1:2.2
Path: pleural + subpleural + peribronchovascular scattered nodules / conglomerate masses ± central cavitation
Histo: confluent noncaseating granulomas, extensive necrosis, vasculitis of muscular pulmonary arteries + veins with frequently total vascular occlusion, bronchiolar obstruction, bronchiolitis obliterans, obstructive pneumonitis

- asymptomatic (15–40%)
- cough, chest pain, dyspnea, fever, weight loss, fatigue
- uveitis, hypothalamic insufficiency (13%)

◊ Almost exclusively affects lungs
√ multiple bilateral subpleural + peribronchovascular pulmonary nodules
√ numerous ill-defined parenchymal opacities
√ ± cavitation
√ hilar lymphadenopathy (8–79%)
√ pleural thickening
◊ No upper airway disease / glomerulonephritis / systemic vasculitis

Rx: corticosteroid therapy alone
DDx: sarcoidosis (high prevalence of mediastinal + hilar lymphadenopathy, little propensity for cavitation)

NEONATAL PNEUMONIA

Pathogenesis:
(a) in utero infection (ascending from premature rupture of membranes or prolonged labor / transplacental route) = major risk factor
(b) aspiration of infected vaginal secretions during delivery
(c) infection after birth

Organism:
(1) Group B streptococcus (GBS) = most common cause: in low–birth-weight premature infants; 50% mortality
√ pulmonary opacities (87%):
√ appearance identical to RDS (in 52%)
√ appearance suggesting retained lung fluid / focal infiltrates (35%)
√ normal CXR (13%)
√ cardiomegaly (common)
√ pleural effusions (in 2/3, but RARE in RDS)
Associated with: delayed onset of diaphragmatic hernia (evidenced by clinical deterioration)
Prognosis: often lethal
(2) Pneumococci: RDS-like
(3) Listeria: RDS-like
(4) Candida: progressive consolidation + cavitation
(5) Chlamydia trachomatis: bronchopneumonic pattern
(6) others: H. influenzae, Staphylococcus aureus, E. coli, CMV, pneumocystis

- afebrile
- lower ventilatory pressure requirements

√ bilateral focal / diffuse areas of opacities (may initially appear similar to fetal aspiration syndrome)
√ hyperaeration
√ may cause lobar atelectasis
√ may cause pneumothorax / pneumomediastinum
√ pleural effusion (exceedingly rare)

NOCARDIOSIS

Organism: Gram-positive acid-fast bacterium resembling fungus
Predisposed: immunocompromised
√ multiple poorly / well-defined nodules ± cavitation
√ lobar consolidation
√ empyema without sinus tracts
√ SVC obstruction (rare)

NON-HODGKIN LYMPHOMA

= NHL = disease of B cells
Incidence: 3% of all newly diagnosed cancers; 3rd most common cancer in childhood (behind leukemia + CNS neoplasms); 4 times more common than Hodgkin disease
Predisposed: (40–100 times greater risk) congenital immunodeficiency syndromes, organ transplant patients undergoing immunosuppression, patients with HIV infection, collagen vascular diseases
Age: all ages; median age of 55 years; M:F = 1.4:1

- chest / shoulder pain, dyspnea, dysphagia
- CHF, hypotension, SVC syndrome

Modified Rappaport Classification:
= categorization according to histologic distribution of lymphomatous cells
A. Nodular form = organized in clusters
1. Poorly differentiated lymphocytic (PDL)
2. Mixed lymphocytic / histiocytic (mixed cell)
3. Large cell (histiocytic)
B. Diffuse form = distortion of tissue architecture
1. Well-differentiated lymphocytic (WDL)
2. Intermediate-differentiated lymphocytic (IDL)
3. Poorly differentiated lymphocytic (PDL)
4. Mixed lymphocytic / histiocytic large cell (histiocytic) (DLCL); undifferentiated Burkitt lymphoma; undifferentiated non-Burkitt lymphoma (pleiomorphic); lymphoblastic (LBL); unclassified

Luke and Collins Classification:
= categorization by morphologic characteristics of cell + cell of origin (T cell, B cell, non-B, non-T cell)
Working Formulation Classification (Kiel / Lennert):
= categorization by grade
A. Low grade
1. Small lymphocytic (3.6%)
median age 61 years, 59% 5-year survival
2. Follicular, small cleaved cell (22.5%)
median age 54 years, 70% 5-year survival
3. Follicular, mixed (7.7%)
median age 56 years, 50% 5-year survival

B. Intermediate grade
   1. Follicular, large cell (3.8%)
      median age 55 years, 45% 5-year survival
   2. Diffuse, small cleaved cell (6.9%)
      median age 58 years, 33% 5-year survival
   3. Diffuse, mixed (6.7%)
      median age 58 years, 38% 5-year survival
   4. Diffuse, large cell (19.7%)
      median age 57 years, 35% 5-year survival

C. High grade
   1. Large cell, immunoblastic (7.9%)
      median age 51 years, 32% 5-year survival
   2. Lymphoblastic (4.2%)
      median age 17 years, 26% 5-year survival
   3. Small noncleaved cell (5%)
      median age 30 years, 23% 5-year survival

D. Miscellaneous (12%)
   composite, mycosis fungoides, histiocytic, extramedullary plasmacytoma

Staging: same Ann Arbor system as for Hodgkin disease

Extranodal involvement:
- @ GI tract:
  stomach (3%), small bowel (5%), large bowel (2%), pancreas (0.7%), peritoneal nodules + ascites (1.4%)
- @ Chest (40–50%):
  lung (6%), pleural fluid (3.3%), pericardial fluid (0.7%), heart (0.2%)
  - √ hilar + mediastinal adenopathy (DDx: sarcoidosis; anterior nodes favor lymphoma)
    - ◊ Nodes frequently not involved!
  - √ isolated lymph nodes may enhance (DDx: Castleman disease)
  - √ lung nodules + air bronchograms
  - √ pleural effusion

  Prognosis: unfavorable
- @ GU tract (10%):
  kidneys (6%), testes (1.2%), ovaries (1.8%), uterus (1.2%)
- @ Bone (3.8%)
- @ CNS (2.4%)
- @ Breast (1.2%)
- @ Skin (6.4%)
- @ Head and neck (1.7%)
- @ Liver (14%)
- @ Spleen (41%)

Nodal involvement:
- @ Paraaortic lymph nodes (49%)
- @ Mesenteric lymph nodes (51%):
  predominantly in middle mediastinum, cardiophrenic angle
  - ◊ Single lymph node involvement is often the only manifestation of intrathoracic disease!
- @ Splenic hilar lymph nodes (53%)
  - ◊ Lymphography 89% sensitive + 86% specific

Non-Hodgkin Lymphoma in Childhood

Incidence: 3rd most common childhood malignancy (after leukemia + CNS tumors); 7% of all malignancies in children <15 years of age

Origin: B or T cell (in 90%) located outside marrow; (rarely) non-B and non-T cells located within bone marrow

Age: median age of 10 years; <15 years of age (most common); unusual <5 years of age; M > F

- chest pain, back pain, cough, dyspnea
- fever, anorexia, weight loss
- ± peripheral blood + bone marrow involvement (particularly in lymphoblastic NHL):
  with lymphoblastic bone marrow involvement of <25% patient is classified as having lymphoma

Staging (St. Jude):

I single extranodal tumor / single anatomic area

II (a) single extranodal tumor + regional nodes
   (b) ≥2 nodal areas on same side of diaphragm
   (c) 2 single extranodal tumors ± nodes on same side of diaphragm
   (d) primary gastrointestinal tract tumor ± nodes

III (a) 2 single extranodal tumors on opposite sides of diaphragm
   (b) ≥2 nodal areas on both sides of the diaphragm
   (c) primary intrathoracic tumors (mediastinum, pleura, thymus)
   (d) extensive primary intraabdominal disease
   (e) paraspinal / epidural tumor

IV any of the above + initial CNS / bone marrow involvement

Differences between Adult and Childhood NHL

Characteristics	*Adult NHL*	*Childhood NHL*
Primary site	nodal	extranodal
Histology	50% follicular, 50% diffuse	diffuse
Grade	low, intermediate, high	high
Histologic subtype	many	three
Sex predilection	none	70% male

Prognosis: 80% cure rate with multiple-agent chemotherapy

DDx: (1) Acute lymphocytic leukemia (>25% lymphoblasts within bone marrow)
(2) Hodgkin disease (contiguous spread, nodes are site of origin)

1. **Undifferentiated / small noncleaved NHL** (39%);
   Path: non-Burkitt lymphoma; Burkitt lymphoma
   - abdominal mass ± ascites
   - pain similar to appendicitis / intussusception

   Primary site: abdomen (distal ileum, cecum, appendix); ovaries
   Common site: mesenteric, inguinal, iliac nodes; CNS; bone marrow; kidney

CHEST

Rare site: orbit, supradiaphragmatic paraspinal region, mediastinum, paranasal sinuses, bone, testes, pulmonary parenchyma
Cx: "leukemic transformation" (= extensive bone marrow involvement)

2. **Lymphoblastic (T-cell) NHL** (28%)
Primary site: mediastinum (66%)
Common site: neck, thymus, liver, spleen, CNS, bone marrow, gonads
Rare site: subdiaphragmatic (ileum, cecum, kidney, mesentery, retroperitoneum), orbit, paranasal sinus, thyroid, parotid
• respiratory distress, dysphagia
• SVC syndrome, pericardial tamponade

3. **Large cell (histiocytic) NHL** (26%)
Origin: B cell, T cells (small percentage)
Location: nodal + extranodal
Primary site: variable (Waldeyer ring, Peyer patches)
Common site: peripheral lymph nodes, lung, bone, brain, skin
Rare site: hard palate, esophagus, trachea

NONTUBERCULOUS MYCOBACTERIAL INFECTION OF LUNG

= ATYPICAL TUBERCULOSIS

Organisms:
M. kansasii: lung infection in subjects with good immune status
M. marinum: "swimming pool granuloma"
M. ulcerans: "Buruli ulcer" in tropical areas
M. scrofulaceum: cervical lymphadenitis in infants
M. avium intracellulare: esp. in AIDS

Organism causing pulmonary disease (Runyon classification):
ubiquitous organisms as part of normal environmental flora

1. Photochromogens
M. kansasii, M. simiae, M. asiaticum
• colonies turn yellow with exposure to light
◊ 70–80% of individuals from rural areas test positive on PPD-B (= antigen from M. kansasii)!
2. Scotochromogens
M. scrofulaceum, M. xenopi, M. szulgai, M. gordonae
• yellow colonies turn orange with exposure to light
3. Nonchromogens
M. avium-intracellulare, M. malmoense, M. terrae
• white / beige colonies without color change
4. Rapid growers
M. fortuitum-chelonei
• appear in culture in 3–5 days (all other groups appear in culture in 2–4 weeks)

Histo: lesions indistinguishable from M. tuberculosis
Source: soil, water, dairy products, bird droppings
Infection: inhalation of aerosolized water droplets (M. avium-intracellulare complex), food aspiration in patients with achalasia (M. fortuitum-chelonei), GI tract (in AIDS)

• cough (60–100%), hemoptysis (15–20%)
• asthma, dyspnea
• fever distinctly uncommon (10–13%)
• weakness + weight loss (up to 50%)
• weekly positive tuberculin skin test

A. CLASSICAL FORM
Age: 6th–7th decade, in Whites (80–90%), M > F
Predisposing factors:
COPD (25–72%), previous TB (20–24%), interstitial lung disease (6%), smoking >30 pack-years (46%), alcohol abuse (40%), cardiovascular disease (36%), chronic liver disease (32%), previous gastrectomy (18%)
Location: apical + anterior segments of upper lobes
√ chronic fibronodular / fibroproductive apical opacities (indistinguishable from reactivation TB)
√ cavitation in 80–95%
√ apical pleural thickening in 37–56%
√ additional patchy nodular alveolar opacities (due to bronchogenic spread) in ipsi- / contralateral lung in 40–70%
√ adenopathy (0–4%)
√ pleural effusion (5–20%)
√ typically NO hilar elevation

B. NONCLASSICAL FORM (20–30%)
Age: 7th–8th decade, 86% in Whites; M:F = 1:4
Predisposing factors: NONE
Location: predominantly in middle lobe + lingula
√ multiple bilateral nodular opacities throughout both lungs in random distribution
√ irregular curvilinear interstitial opacities (resembling bronchiectasis)

C. ASYMPTOMATIC GRANULOMAS
√ cluster of similar-sized nodules

D. ACHALASIA-RELATED INFECTION
with M. fortuitum-chelonei

E. DISSEMINATED DISEASE
in immunocompromised patients: AIDS, transplant patients, lymphoproliferative disorders (esp. hairy cell leukemia), steroid + immunosuppressive therapy

CT:
√ multifocal bronchiectasis (79–94%), esp. middle lobe + lingula
√ centrilobular nodules of varying sizes, usually <1 cm (= micronodules) in 76–97%
√ bronchial wall thickening (97%)
√ airspace disease (76%)
√ cavitation (21%), esp. in upper lobes
√ interlobular septal thickening (12%)

◊ Unfavorable response to antituberculous therapy is suspicious for atypical TB!

DDx: M. tuberculosis (bronchiectasis less common + less extensive), bronchiolitis obliterans, sarcoidosis, fungal disease

PANBRONCHIOLITIS

= inflammatory lung disease, prevalent in Orientals but rare in Europeans + North Americans

Pathogenesis: unknown

HRCT:
- √ centrilobular branching structures (segments of bronchiolectasis filled with secretions) + nodules surrounding respiratory bronchioles
- √ mosaic perfusion
- √ air trapping
- √ bronchial dilatation

DDx: bronchiolitis obliterans

PARAGONIMIASIS OF LUNG

= parasitic disease caused by trematode Paragonimus (usually P. westermani = lung fluke) endemic to certain areas of East + Southeast Asia (China, Korea, Japan, Thailand, Laos, Philippines, India)

Infection: ingestion of raw / incompletely cooked freshwater crab / crayfish infected with metacercaria; larva exists in small intestine + penetrates the intestinal wall + enters peritoneal cavity; larva penetrates diaphragm + pleura to enter the lung

Cycle: from the final host (tiger, cat, dog, fox, weasel, opossum, human) eggs of worm pass to the outside with blood-streaked sputum; in fresh water ciliated embryos (miracidia) develop; they become tailed larvae (cercariae) after invading a fresh-water snail; when the infected snail is eaten by a crustacean, their tails detach and they become 300 μm encysted larvae (metacercariae)

@ CNS
- • meningoencephalitis (in 25%)
- √ shell-like / soap–bubble-like calcifications of varying size (~50%)

CXR (pulmonary lesions in 83%, pulmonary + pleural lesions in 44%, pleural lesions in 17%):

early findings (lesions occur 3–8 weeks after ingestion):
- √ uni- / bilateral pneumo- / hydropneumothorax (17%)
- √ uni- / bilateral pleural effusion (3–54%)
- √ focal patchy migrating airspace consolidation (= worm migration causing focal hemorrhagic pneumonia) (45%)
- √ lobar / segmental collapse (airway obstruction from egg granuloma / intrusion of worm)
- √ 2–4-mm thick and 2–7-cm long linear opacities abutting the pleura (41%) due to worm migration track

late findings:
- √ lung cyst (cyst formation from infarction after arteriolar / venous obstruction by worm or egg; expansion of small airway by intraluminal parasite):
  - √ thick-walled cyst (due to fibrosis)
  - √ "eclipse effect" = eccentric thickening of cyst wall (due to intracystic one / two worms)
  - √ thin-walled cyst (when cyst connected to airway)
- √ 10–15-mm nodules + masslike consolidation (24%) (due to cyst initially masked by pericystic airspace consolidation ± cyst filled with chocolate-colored necrotic fluid)
- √ bronchiectasis (35%)

DDx: tuberculosis (nodular slowly changing lesion, residual fibrosis after treatment, no subpleural linear opacities)

PERICARDIAL CYST

Etiology:
(1) defect in embryogenesis of coelomic cavities
(2) sequelae of pericarditis

Histo: lined by single layer of mesothelial cells

Age: 30–40 years; M:F = 3:2
- • asymptomatic (50%)

Location: (a) cardiophrenic angle (75%), R:L = 3:1 / 3:2, 25% higher; may extend into major fissure
(b) mediastinum (rare)
- √ sharply marginated round / ovoid / triangular mass usually 3–8 cm (range 1–28 cm) in diameter
- √ change in size + shape with respiration / body position
- √ attenuation values of 20–40 HU, occasionally higher

PNEUMATOCELE

= cystic air collection within lung parenchyma due to obstructive overinflation

= regional obstructive emphysema

◊ Does not indicate destruction of lung parenchyma
◊ Occurs during healing phase
◊ Appears to enlarge while patient improves
◊ Frequently multiple

Developmental theories:
(1) small bronchioles undergo severe distension secondary to check-valve endobronchial / peribronchial obstruction
(2) focus of necrotic lung evacuates through a bronchus narrowed by edema / inflammation; airspace subsequently enlarges due to check-valve mechanism from enlarging pneumatocele / inflammatory exudate
(3) air from ruptured alveoli / bronchioles dissects along interstitial interlobular tissue and accumulates between visceral pleura and lung parenchyma
= subpleural emphysematous bulla
= subpleural air cyst

A. PNEUMATOCELE ASSOCIATED WITH INFECTION
Organism: pneumococci, E. coli, Klebsiella, Staphylococcus (in childhood)
- √ appears within 1st week, disappears within 6 weeks
- √ thin-walled + completely air-filled cavity
- √ ± air-fluid level + wall thickening (during infection)
- √ pneumothorax
- √ spontaneous resolution (in most)

B. TRAUMATIC PNEUMATOCELE = PNEUMATOCYST
Cause:
(a) air trapped within area of pulmonary laceration is initially obscured by surrounding contusion (hematoma); pneumatocyst appears within hours after blunt chest trauma
(b) intensive inflammatory response from hydrocarbon (furniture polish, kerosene) inhalation / ingestion
- √ single / multiple pneumatoceles
- √ spontaneous resolution over several weeks to months

C. "PULVERIZED LUNG"
Cause: severe chest trauma
- √ multiple 5–10-mm air cysts in an area of airspace opacification

PNEUMOCOCCAL PNEUMONIA

Most common Gram-positive pneumonia
90% community-acquired, 10% nosocomial

Incidence: 15% of all adulthood pneumonias, uncommon in child; peaks in winter + early spring; increased during influenza epidemics

Organism: Streptococcus pneumoniae (formerly Diplococcus pneumoniae), Gram-positive, in pairs / chains, encapsulated, capsular polysaccharide responsible for virulence + serotyping

Susceptible: elderly, debilitated, alcoholics, CHF, COPD, multiple myeloma, hypogammaglobulinemia, functional / surgical asplenia

- rusty blood-streaked sputum
- left-shift leukocytosis
- impaired pulmonary function

Location: usually involves one lobe only; bias for lower lobes + posterior segments of upper lobes (bacteria flow under gravitational influence to most dependent portions as in aspiration)

√ extensive airspace consolidation abutting against visceral pleura (lobar / beyond confines of one lobe through pores of Kohn) CHARACTERISTIC
√ slight expansion of involved lobes
√ prominent air bronchograms (20%)
√ patchy bronchopneumonic pattern (in some)
√ pleural effusion (parapneumonic transudate) uncommon with antibiotic therapy
√ cavitation (rare, with type III)

Variations (modified by bronchopulmonary disease, eg, chronic bronchitis, emphysema):
 √ bronchopneumonia-like pattern
 √ effusion may be only presentation (esp. in COPD)
 √ empyema (with persistent fever)
 — in children:
  √ round pneumonia = sharply defined round lesion

Prognosis: prompt response to antibiotics (if without complications); 5% mortality rate

Dx: blood culture (positive in 30%)

Cx: meningitis, endocarditis, septic arthritis, empyema (now rarely seen)

PNEUMOCYSTOSIS

= PNEUMOCYSTIS CARINII PNEUMONIA

◊ Most common cause of interstitial pneumonia in immunocompromised patients, which quickly leads to airspace disease

Organism:
ubiquitous obligate extracellular protozoan / fungus Pneumocystis carinii
(a) trophozoite develops into a cyst
(b) cyst produces up to eight daughter sporozoites, which are released at maturity + develop into trophozoites

Pathomechanism:
trophozoite attaches to cell membrane of type I alveolar pneumocytes with subsequent cell death + leakage of proteinaceous fluid into alveolar space

Predisposed:
(1) debilitated premature infants, children with hypogammaglobulinemia (12%)
(2) AIDS (60–80%)
(3) other immunocompromised patients: congenital immunodeficiency syndrome, lymphoproliferative disorders, organ transplant recipients (renal transplant patients in 10%), patients on long-term corticosteroid therapy (nephrotic syndrome, collagen vascular disease), patients on cytotoxic drugs [under therapy for leukemia (40%), lymphoma (16%)]

◊ Often associated with simultaneous infection by CMV, Mycobacterium avium-intracellulare, herpes simplex

- severe dyspnea + cyanosis over 3–5 days
- subacute insidious onset of malaise + minimal cough (frequent in AIDS patients)
- respiratory failure (5–30%)
- WBC slightly elevated (PMNs)
- lymphopenia (50%) heralds poor prognosis

√ normal CXR in 10–39%
√ bilateral diffuse symmetric finely granular / reticular interstitial / airspace infiltrates (in 80%) with perihilar + basilar distribution (CHARACTERISTIC central location)
√ response to therapy within 5–7 days
√ rapid progression to diffuse alveolar homogeneous consolidation (DDx: pulmonary edema)
√ air bronchogram
√ fine / coarse linear / reticular pattern = thickened coarse interstitial lung markings (in healing phase)
√ pleural effusion + hilar lymphadenopathy (uncommon)
√ <u>atypical pattern</u> (in 5%):
 √ isolated lobar disease / focal parenchymal opacities
 √ lung nodules ± cavitation
 √ hilar / mediastinal lymphadenopathy
 √ thin- / thick-walled regular / irregular cysts / cavities with predilection for upper lobes + subpleural regions
√ <u>effect of prophylactic use of aerosolized pentamidine</u>:
 √ redistribution of infection to upper lobes
 √ cystic lung disease
 √ spontaneous pneumothorax, frequently bilateral (6–7%)
 √ disseminated extrapulmonary disease (1%)
 √ punctate / rimlike calcifications in enlarged lymph nodes + abdominal viscera

CT:
 √ patchwork pattern (56%)
  = bilateral asymmetric patchy mosaic appearance with sparing of segments / subsegments of pulmonary lobe
 √ ground-glass pattern (26%)
  = bilateral diffuse airspace disease (fluid + inflammatory cells in alveolar space) in symmetric distribution
 √ interstitial pattern (18%)
  = bilateral symmetric / asymmetric, linear / reticular markings (thickening of lobular septa)
 √ air-filled spaces (38%):
  (a) pneumatoceles = thin-walled spaces without lobar predilection resolving within 6 months
  (b) subpleural bullae (due to premature emphysema)

(c) thin-walled cysts (? check-valve obstruction of small airways from aerosolized pentamidine)
(d) necrosis of PCP granuloma

√ pneumothorax (13%)
√ lymphadenopathy (18%)
√ pleural effusion (18%)
√ pulmonary nodules
usually due to malignancy (leukemia, lymphoma, Kaposi sarcoma, metastasis) / septic emboli
√ pulmonary cavities
usually due to superimposed fungal / mycobacterial infection

NUC:
√ bilateral and diffuse Ga-67 uptake without mediastinal involvement prior to roentgenographic changes
DDx: TB / MAI infection (with mediastinal involvement)

Dx: (1) sputum collection, (2) bronchoscopy with lavage, (3) transbronchial / transthoracic / open lung Bx
Prognosis: rapid fulminant disease; death within 2 weeks
Rx: co-trimoxazole IV, nebulized pentamidine

PNEUMONECTOMY CHEST

Early signs (within 24 hours):
√ partial filling of thorax
√ ipsilateral mediastinal shift + diaphragmatic elevation
Late signs (after 2 months):
√ complete obliteration of space
N.B.: Depression of diaphragm / shift of mediastinum to contralateral side indicates a bronchopleural fistula / empyema / hemorrhage!

POSTOBSTRUCTIVE PNEUMONIA

= chronic inflammatory disease distal to bronchial obstruction
Cause:
1. Bronchogenic carcinoma (most commonly)
2. Bronchial adenoma
3. Granular cell myoblastoma (almost always tracheal lesion)
4. Bronchostenosis

Histo: "golden pneumonia" = cholesterol pneumonia endogenous lipid pneumonia = mixture of edema, atelectasis, round cell infiltration, bronchiectasis, liberation of lipid material from alveolar pneumocytes secondary to inflammatory reaction
√ frequently associated with some degree of atelectasis
√ persists unchanged for weeks
√ recurrent pneumonia in same region after antibiotic treatment

PROGRESSIVE MASSIVE FIBROSIS

= (PMF) = COMPLICATED PNEUMOCONIOSIS
= CONGLOMERATE ANTHRACOSILICOSIS
May develop / progress after cessation of dust exposure
Path: avascular amorphous central mass of insoluble proteins stabilized by cross-links + ill-defined bundles of coarse hyalinized collagen at periphery
Location: almost exclusively restricted to posterior segment of upper lobe / superior segment of lower lobe
√ large >1 cm opacities initially in middle + upper lung zones at periphery of lung
√ discoid contour (44%) = mass flat from front to back (thin opacity on lateral view, large opacity on PA view), medial border often ill-defined, lateral borders sharp + parallel to rib cage
√ migration toward hila starting at lung periphery; bilateral symmetry
√ apparent decrease in nodularity (incorporation of nodules from surroundings)
√ cavitation (occasionally) due to ischemic necrosis / superimposed TB infection
√ bullous scar emphysema
√ pulmonary hypertension

PSEUDOLYMPHOMA

= reactive benign lesion = localized form of lymphocytic interstitial pneumonitis (LIP); no progression to lymphoma
Histo: aggregates of plasma cells, reticulin cells, large + small lymphocytes with preserved lymphoid architecture resembling lymphoma histologically without lymph node involvement
Associated with: Sjögren syndrome
• mostly asymptomatic
√ well-demarcated dense infiltrate
√ infiltrate typically in central location extending to visceral pleura
√ prominent air bronchogram
√ NO lymphadenopathy
Prognosis: occasionally progression to non-Hodgkin lymphoma
Rx: most patients respond well to steroids initially

PSEUDOMONAS PNEUMONIA

= most dreaded nosocomial infection because of resistance to antibiotics in patients with debilitating diseases on multiple antibiotics + corticosteroids; rare in community
Organism: Pseudomonas aeruginosa, Gram-negative
• bradycardia
• temperature with morning peaks
√ widespread patchy bronchopneumonia (secondary to bacteremia; unlike other Gram-negative pneumonias)
√ predilection for lower lobes
√ extensive bilateral consolidation
√ "spongelike pattern" with multiple nodules >2 cm (= extensive necrosis with formation of multiple abscesses)
√ small pleural effusions

PULMONARY ARTERIAL MALFORMATION

= PAVM = PULMONARY ARTERIOVENOUS ANEURYSM
= PULMONARY ARTERIOVENOUS FISTULA = PULMONARY ANGIOMA = PULMONARY TELANGIECTASIA

= abnormal vascular communication between pulmonary artery and vein (95%) or systemic artery and pulmonary vein (5%)

Etiology:
(a) congenital defect of capillary structure (common)
(b) acquired in cirrhosis (hepatogenic pulmonary angiodysplasia), cancer, trauma, surgery, actinomycosis, schistosomiasis, TB (Rasmussen aneurysm)

Path: hemangioma of cavernous type

Pathophysiology:
low-resistance extracardiac R-to-L shunt (which may result in paradoxical embolism); quantification with Tc-99m–labeled albumin microspheres by measuring fraction of dose reaching kidneys

Age: 3rd–4th decade; manifest in adult life, 10% in childhood

Occurrence:
(a) isolated abnormality (40%)
(b) multiple (in 1/3)
associated with Rendu-Osler-Weber syndrome (in 30–60–88%) = hereditary hemorrhagic telangiectasia
◊ 15–50% of patients with Rendu-Osler-Weber disease have pulmonary AVMs!

Types:
1. Simple type (79%)
= single feeding artery empties into a bulbous nonseptated aneurysmal segment with a single draining vein
2. Complex type (21%)
= more than one feeding artery empties into septated aneurysmal segment with more than one draining vein

- asymptomatic in 56% (until 3rd–4th decade) if AVM single and <2 cm
- orthodeoxia (= increased hypoxemia with PaO_2 <85 mm Hg in erect position due to gravitational shift of pulmonary blood flow to base of lung)
- cyanosis with normal-sized heart (R-to-L shunt) in 25–50%, clubbing
- bruit over lesion (increased during inspiration)
- dyspnea on exertion (60–71%)
- hemoptysis (10–15%)
- palpitation, chest pain
- No CHF

Location: lower lobes (65–70%) > middle lobe > upper lobes; bilateral (8–20%); medial third of lung

√ sharply defined, lobulated oval / round mass (90%) of 1 to several cm in size ("coin lesion")
√ cordlike bands from mass to hilum (feeding artery + draining veins)
√ in 2/3 single lesion, in 1/3 multiple lesions
√ enlargement with advancing age
√ change in size with Valsalva / Mueller maneuver / erect vs. recumbent position (decrease with Valsalva maneuver)
√ phleboliths (occasionally)
√ increased pulsations of hilar vessels

CT (98% detection rate):
√ homogeneous circumscribed noncalcified nodule / serpiginous mass up to several cm in diameter
√ vascular connection of mass with enlarged feeding artery + draining vein
√ sequential enhancement of feeding artery + aneurysmal part + efferent vein on dynamic CT

MR (if contraindication to contrast material / if flow slow due to partial thrombosis / for follow-up):
√ signal void on standard spin echo / high signal intensity on GRASS images

Angio (mostly obviated by MR / CT unless surgery or embolization contemplated):
◊ 100% sensitive for detection of vessels >2 mm

Cx: CNS symptoms are commonly the initial manifestation
(1) Cerebrovascular accident: stroke (18%), transient ischemic attack (37%) secondary to paradoxical bland emboli
(2) Brain abscess (5–9%) secondary to loss of pulmonary filter function for septic emboli
(3) Hemoptysis (13%) secondary to rupture of PAVM into bronchus, most common presenting symptom
(4) Hemothorax (9%) secondary to rupture of subpleural PAVM
(5) Polycythemia

Prognosis: 26% morbidity, 11% mortality
Recommendation: screening of first-degree relatives
DDx: solitary / multiple pulmonary nodules
Rx: embolization with coils / detachable balloons

PULMONARY CAPILLARY HEMANGIOMATOSIS

= bilateral pulmonary disease behaving like a low-grade nonmetastatic vascular neoplasm with slowly progressive pulmonary hypertension

Histo: sheets of thin-walled capillary blood vessels infiltrating pulmonary interstitium + invading pulmonary vessels, bronchioles, and pleura

Pathomechanism of pulmonary hypertension:
(a) venoocclusive phenomenon secondary to invasion of small pulmonary veins
(b) progressive vascular obliteration secondary to in situ thrombosis + infarction
(c) pulmonary scar formation secondary to recurrent pulmonary hemorrhage

Age: 20–40 years

- dyspnea on exertion
- cor pulmonale: jugular venous distension, pedal edema, ECG signs of RV failure (DDx: pulmonary venoocclusive disease)
- elevated PA pressures + normal pulmonary wedge pressure
- hemoptysis + pleuritic chest pain in 1/3 (DDx: pulmonary thromboembolic disease)

CXR:
√ diffuse reticulonodular pattern
√ focal areas of interstitial fibrosis (recurrent episodes of pulmonary hemorrhage + thrombotic infarction)

CT:
√ thickening + nodularity of inter- and intralobular septa + walls of pulmonary veins
√ areas of ground-glass attenuation (= increased perfusion to extensive proliferating hemangiomatous tissue)

Angio:
√ combination of increased flow (to hemangiomatous areas) + decreased flow (to regions of thrombosis, infarction, and scarring)

Prognosis: death after 2–12-year interval from onset of symptoms

Rx: bilateral lung transplantation

DDx: (1) Pulmonary venoocclusive disease
(2) Idiopathic interstitial fibrosis
(3) Primary pulmonary hypertension (no increase in lung markings)
(4) Pulmonary hemangiomatosis (only in children, cavernous hemangiomas involving several organs)

PULMONARY CONTUSION

= most common manifestation of blunt chest trauma, esp. deceleration trauma

Path: exudation of edema + blood into airspace + interstitium

Time of onset: apparent within 6 hours after trauma

• clinically inapparent
• hemoptysis (50%)

Location: posterior (in 60%)

Site: directly deep to site of impact / contrecoup

√ irregular patchy / diffuse homogeneous extensive consolidation (CT is more sensitive)
√ opacity may enlarge for 48–72 hours
√ rapid resolution beginning 24–48 hours, complete within 2–10 days
√ overlying rib fractures (frequent)

CT:
√ nonsegmental coarse ill-defined crescentic (50%) / amorphous (45%) opacification of lung parenchyma without cavitation
√ "subpleural sparing" = 1–2-mm rim of uniformly nonopacified subpleural portion of lung

Cx: pneumothorax

DDx: fat embolism (1–2 days after injury)

PULMONARY INFARCTION

= ischemic coagulative necrosis of lung parenchyma

Frequency: rare (due to protective effect of collateral blood flow from bronchial circulation)

Path: dark necrotic material (with faint ghostlike structures of lung tissue remaining evident on histology) surrounded by a narrow rim of hyperemia + inflammation

Cause: pulmonary artery occlusion (medium- to small-sized vessel)

Pathogenesis:
increased vascular permeability (ischemic capillary endothelial injury) + reperfusion via bronchial circulation causes intraalveolar extravasation of blood cells in a confined area with possible progression to infarction

Co-condition to progress to infarction:
CHF, high embolic burden, underlying malignancy, diminished bronchial flow (due to shock, hypotension, chronically impaired circulation), vasodilator use, elevated pulmonary venous pressure, interstitial edema

Prognosis: replacement by vascular fibrous tissue folding into a collagenous platelike mass producing pleural retraction

PULMONARY INTERSTITIAL EMPHYSEMA

= PIE = complication of respirator therapy with PEEP

Pathogenesis:
gas escapes from overdistended alveolus, dissects into perivascular sheath surrounding arteries, veins, and lymphatics, tracks into mediastinum forming clusters of blebs

• sudden deterioration in patient's condition during respiratory therapy

√ elongated lucencies following distribution of bronchovascular tree
√ pseudocysts = circular densities caused by subpleural blebs
√ bilateral, symmetrical distribution
√ lobar overdistension (occasionally)

Cx: (1) pneumomediastinum, pneumothorax, subcutaneous emphysema, pneumopericardium, intracardiac air, pneumoperitoneum, pneumatosis intestinalis
(2) **air-block phenomenon** = buildup of pressure in mediastinum / pericardial tamponade impeding blood flow in low-pressure pulmonary veins causing diminished blood return to heart (obstruction esp. during expiration); particularly common in neonatal period
√ microcardia

PULMONARY LYMPHANGIOMATOSIS

= increased number of communicating lymphatic channels

√ smooth thickening of bronchovascular bundles + interlobular septa

CT:
√ diffuse increased attenuation of mediastinal fat
√ mild perihilar infiltration
√ pleural effusion
√ pleural thickening

PULMONARY MAINLINE GRANULOMATOSIS

= PULMONARY TALCOSIS

= pulmonary microembolism in drug addicts due to chronic IV injection of suspensions prepared from crushed tablet compounds (talc is a common insoluble additive)

Drugs: amphetamines, methylphenidate hydrochloride ("West coast"), tripelen amine ("blue velvet"), methadone hydrochloride, dilaudid, meperidine, pentazocine, propylhexedrine, hydromorphone hydrochloride

Pathogenesis: talc (= magnesium silicate) particles incite a pronounced granulomatous foreign-body reaction + subsequent fibrosis in perivascular distribution

Path: multiple scattered whitish nodules of 0.3–3 mm converging into gritty fibrotic masses in central + upper lungs measuring several cm

Histo: widespread granulomas packed with doubly refractile talc particles expanding the walls of muscular pulmonary arteries and arterioles + perivascular connective tissue + alveolar septa

- talc retinopathy (80%) = small glistening crystals
- angiothrombotic pulmonary hypertension + cor pulmonale

Early changes:
- √ widespread micronodularity of "pinpoint" size (1–2–3 mm) with perihilar / basilar predominance
- √ well-defined nodules predominantly in middle zones

Late changes:
- √ loss of lung volume of upper lobes + hilar elevation + hyperlucency at lung bases
- √ indistinctly marginated coalescent opacities similar to progressive massive fibrosis (DDx: in silicosis slightly further away from pulmonary hila + distinct margin)

Cx: mycotic pulmonary artery aneurysm; right-sided endocarditis with septic emboli; chronic respiratory failure; emphysema; systemic talc breakthrough to liver + spleen + kidneys + retina

DDx of late changes:
(1) Progressive massive fibrosis of silicosis / coal worker's pneumoconiosis
(2) Chronic sarcoidosis

Dx: lung biopsy

PULMONARY THROMBOEMBOLIC DISEASE

= PULMONARY EMBOLISM (PE)

Prevalence: 630,000 Americans/year with missed / delayed diagnosis in 400,000, causing death in 120,000; diagnosed in 1% of all hospitalized patients; in 12–64% at autopsy; in 9–56% of patients with deep venous thrombosis

Age: 60% >60 years of age

Cause: deep vein thrombosis (DVT) of extremities / pelvis (>90%), right atrial neoplasia / thrombus, thrombogenic intravenous catheters, endocarditis of tricuspid / pulmonic valves

Time of onset: PE usually occurs within first 5–7 days of thrombus formation

Predisposing factors:
primary thrombophlebitis (39%), immobilization (32%), recent surgery (31%), venous insufficiency (25%), recent fracture (15%), myocardial infarction (12%), malignancy (8%), CHF (5%), no predisposition (6%)

Pathophysiology: A clot from the deep veins of the leg breaks off + fragments in right side of heart + showers lung with emboli varying in size

◊ On average >6–8 vessels are embolized!

Class 1 = <20% of pulmonary arteries occluded
- asymptomatic
- normal arterial blood gas levels
- normal pulmonary + systemic hemodynamics

Class 2 = 20–30% of pulmonary arteries occlude
- anxiety, hyperventilation
- arterial PO_2 <80 torr
- PCO_2 <35 torr

Class 3 = 30–50% of pulmonary arteries occluded
- dyspnea, collapse
- arterial PO_2 <65 torr
- arterial PCO_2 <30 torr
- elevated central venous pressure

Class 4 = >50% of pulmonary arteries occluded
- shock, dyspnea
- arterial PO_2 <50 torr
- arterial PCO_2 <30 torr
- elevated central venous pressure
- mean PA pressure >20 mm Hg
- systolic blood pressure <100 mm Hg

◊ Clinical presentation is protean + nonspecific!
◊ False-positive clinical diagnosis in 62%

- Classic triad (<33%):
  (1) hemoptysis (25–34%) (2) pleural friction rub (3) thrombophlebitis
- symptoms (nonfatal PE versus fatal PE):
  - pleuritic chest pain (88% vs. 10%)
  - acute dyspnea (84% vs. 59%)
  - apprehension (59% vs. 17%)
  - cough (53% vs. 3%)
  - hemoptysis (30% vs. 3%)
  - sweats (27% vs. 9%)
  - syncope (13% vs. 27%)
- signs (nonfatal PE versus fatal PE):
  - respiratory rate >16 (92% vs. 66%)
  - rales due to loss of surfactant (58% vs. 42%)
  - tachycardia >100 bpm (44% vs. 54%)
  - temperature >37.8°C (43% vs. 30%)
  - diaphoresis (36% vs. 10%)
  - heart gallop (34% vs. 10%)
  - phlebitis (32% vs. 7%)
  - heart murmur (23%)
  - cyanosis (19% vs. 12%)
  - ECG changes (83%), mostly nonspecific: P-pulmonale, right-axis deviation, right bundle branch block, classic $S_1Q_3T_3$ pattern
  - elevated levels of fibrinopeptide-A (FPA) = small peptide split off of fibrinogen during fibrin generation
  - positive D-dimer assay (generated during clot lysis)

Location of PE: bilateral emboli (in 45%), RT lung only (36%), LT lung only (18%); multiple emboli [3–6 on average] in 65%

Distribution: RUL (16%), RML (9%), RLL (25%), LUL (14%), LLL (26%)

Site: central = segmental / larger (in 58%);
peripheral = subsegmental / smaller (in 42%);
in subsegmental branches exclusively (in 30%)

◊ Emboli are occlusive in 40%!

RESOLUTION OF PE
(through fibrinolysis + fragmentation):
in 8% by 24 hours, in 56% by 14 days, in 68% by 6 weeks, in 77% by 7 months; complete in 65%, incomplete in 39% by 11 months, partial in 23%, no resolution in 12%
◊ Resolution less favorable with increasing age + cardiac disease
◊ Resolution improved with urokinase > heparin within first week (after 1 year 80% for both)

A. EMBOLISM WITHOUT INFARCTION (90%)
Histo: hemorrhage + edema

B. EMBOLISM WITH INFARCTION (10–60%)
= any opacity developing as a result of thromboembolic disease; more likely to develop in presence of cardiopulmonary disease with obstruction of pulmonary venous outflow (diagnosed in retrospect)
Histo: (1) incomplete infarction = reversible transient hemorrhagic congestion / edema usually resolving over several days to weeks
(2) complete infarction = hemorrhagic infarction with necrosis of lung parenchyma remaining permanently

CXR (33% sensitive, 59% specific):
◊ Abnormal nonspecific CXR in 84%; a normal CXR has a negative predictive value of only 74%!
√ general findings (patients with PE vs. no PE):
√ atelectasis / infiltrate (68% vs. 48%)
√ pleural effusion (48% vs. 31%)
√ pleural opacity (35% vs. 21%)
√ elevated diaphragm (24% vs. 19%)
√ decreased vascularity (21% vs. 12%)
√ prominent pulmonary artery (17% vs. 28%)
√ cardiomegaly (12% vs. 11%)
√ pulmonary edema (4% vs. 13%)
√ local findings:
√ Westermark sign = area of oligemia (due to vasoconstriction distal to embolus) in 2–7%
√ Fleischner sign = local widening of artery by impaction of embolus (due to distension by clot / pulmonary hypertension developing secondary to peripheral embolization)
√ "knuckle sign" = abrupt tapering of an occluded vessel distally
√ Fleischner lines = long-line shadows (fibrotic scar) from invagination of pleura at the base of the collapse resulting in pseudofissure
√ Hampton hump = segmentally distributed pleura-based shallow wedge-shaped consolidation with base against pleural surface + convex medial border:
√ NO air-bronchogram (hemorrhage into alveoli)
√ ± cavitation
√ "melting sign" = within few days to weeks regression from periphery toward center
√ subsequent nodular / linear scar
√ thoracentesis: bloody (65%), predominantly PMNs (61%), exudate (65%)

NECT (purpose):
√ depiction of acute changes of PE:
√ atelectasis / linear bands (100%)
√ pleural effusion (87%)
√ consolidation (57%)
√ ground-glass opacification (57%)
√ Hampton's hump (50%)
√ dilated central / segmental pulmonary artery
√ depiction of chronic changes of PE *(see below)*
√ chest findings leading to alternative diagnosis
√ localization of volume-of-interest for CECT

CECT (53–88–100% sensitive, 78–94–100% specific):
◊ Helical CT equal to angio in detection of emboli within proximal arteries of ≤5th / 6th generation
◊ Subsegmental intraluminal filling defects (in 2–30%) usually not detectable!
◊ Detection poor in middle lobe + lingular branches (in 18%)!
N.B.: evaluate the vessel adjacent to a bronchus
√ partial central filling defect in pulmonary artery:
√ peripheral rimlike contrast enhancement
√ "railway track" sign = thromboembolus floating freely within lumen
√ partial marginal filling defect in pulmonary artery:
√ mural filling defect of low attenuation
√ complete filling defect of low attenuation occupying entire arterial section
Pseudo-filling defects:
(1) Breathing artifact in tachypneic patient
(2) Too short / long scanning delay
(3) Unilateral increase in vascular resistance
(4) R-to-L shunt
Technical failure rate: 3–4% due to severe dyspnea

NUC (VQ scan = guide for angiographic evaluation) interpreted in reference to Biello or PIOPED criteria:
√ low- / intermediate-probability scans (in 73%): additional studies recommended
◊ 25–30% disagreement between expert readers in interpreting intermediate- and low-probability V/Q scans
√ high-probability scan: in 12% normal angiogram
N.B.: V/Q abnormalities vary over time due to autoregulation (hypoxic vasoconstriction, hypercapneic bronchoconstriction) and resolution

Angio (>95% sensitive + specific):
Indication:
(1) Indeterminate NUC scan (angio within 24 hours)
(2) Mismatch between interpretation + clinical findings
(3) Significant risk for anticoagulation + high probability for PE
(4) Prior to intervention: pulmonary embolectomy, caval ligation, caval filter placement
(5) Patients too ill to undergo V/Q scan
Technique: AP & ipsilateral posterior oblique projection
√ intraluminal defect (94%)
√ abrupt termination of pulmonary arterial branch
√ pruning + attenuation of branches
√ wedge-shaped parenchymal hypovascularity

√ absence of draining vein in affected segment
√ tortuous arterial collaterals

Risks in pulmonary angiography:
(1) left bundle branch block: requires temporary pacing wire prior to right heart catheterization
(2) marginal cardiac function: therapy must be available to treat frank pulmonary edema
(3) Right ventricular end diastolic pressure >20 mm Hg: selective catheterization with occlusion balloon

Cx of pulmonary angiography (1–2%):
arrhythmia, endocardial injury, cardiac perforation, cardiac arrest, contrast reaction

Mortality rate of pulmonary angiography: 0.2–0.5%

False-negative rate:
1–4–9% due to difficulty in visualizing subsegmental emboli (with only 30% interobserver agreement about presence of subsegmental emboli)

Acute Thromboembolic Pulmonary Arterial Hypertension

◊ Hypertension disappears as emboli lyse
- sudden onset of chest pain
- acute dyspnea
- hemoptysis occasionally

Mortality:
3:1,000 surgical procedures; 200,000 deaths in 1975; 7–10% of all autopsies (death within first hour of PE in most patients); 26–30% if untreated; 3–10% if treated; fatal if >60% of pulmonary bed obstructed; healthy patients may survive obstruction of 50–60% of vascular bed

Rx:
1. Heparin IV: 10,000–15,000 units as initial dose; 8,000–10,000 units/hour during diagnostic evaluation; continued for 10–14 days
2. Streptokinase: better results with massive PE
3. Urokinase: slightly better than streptokinase
4. Coumadin: maintained for at least 3 months (15% complication rate)

Chronic Thromboembolic Pulmonary Arterial Hypertension

= CHRONIC THROMBOEMBOLIC DISEASE

Frequency: 1–5% of patients with acute pulmonary thromboembolism

At risk: underlying malignancy, cardiovascular disease, pulmonary disease; M < F

Path: fibrous webs and bands (= organized thromboemboli), often with overlying recent thrombosis

Pathogenesis:
patent pulmonary arteries develop medial hypertrophy + intimal thickening + atherosclerotic plaques in response to pressure elevation; bronchial arteries may dilate + form extensive collateral pathways to minimize areas of lung infarction

- may be clinically silent / asymptomatic for years ("honeymoon period")
- history of previous embolic episodes
- recurrent acute / gradual progressive exertional dyspnea (DDx: interstitial lung disease)
- chronic nonproductive cough, atypical chest pain
- tachycardia, syncope
- elevated pulmonary arterial pressure (36–78 mm Hg), normal pulmonary capillary wedge pressure
- high right atrial pressures, reduced cardiac output
- lupus anticoagulant (11–24%)

CXR:
√ prominence of right side of heart
√ asymmetric enlargement of central pulmonary arteries
√ oligemic vascularity in patchy distribution
√ triangular / rounded opacity + adjacent pleural thickening (from pulmonary infarction)
√ patchy bilateral perihilar alveolar opacities of "reperfusion edema" after thrombendarterectomy

CT (77% sensitive):
√ cardiac changes:
  √ hypertrophy + enlargement of RA + RV
√ vascular abnormalities:
  √ main pulmonary artery diameter >28.6 mm
  √ complete filling defect at level of stenosed pulmonary artery
  √ calcified clot
  √ eccentric mural arterial irregularities / nodules
  √ arterial stenosis / web
  √ evidence of recanalization
  √ abrupt narrowing / cutoff of distal lobar / segmental branches
  √ decrease in caliber of small branches + narrowing of peripheral pulmonary vessels
  √ collateral systemic supply of occluded pulmonary arterial bed:
    √ bronchial artery dilatation + tortuosity (77%) within mediastinum
√ parenchymal abnormalities:
  √ wedge-shaped pleura-based parenchymal bands with tip pointing to hila, often multiple, esp. involving lower lung (70%) = infarcted tissue replaced by scar
  √ mosaic perfusion on HRCT:
    √ scattered geometric areas of low attenuation in 55% (due to oligemia) associated with vessels of small cross-sectional diameter
    √ regional sharply demarcated areas of high attenuation (perfused lung on background of oligemic / nonperfused lung)
    [DDx: primary pulmonary hypertension (more diffuse pattern of mosaic perfusion)]
√ cylindric bronchial dilatation of segmental / subsegmental bronchi (64%) adjacent to stenotic / obstructed pulmonary arterial segment

MR (lowest sensitivity):
√ discrete fixed areas of low-to-medium signal intensity on T1WI
Disadvantage: slow flow in central vessels may obscure embolic fixed signal

NUC:
√ V/Q scan characteristically of high probability

Angio (highest specificity):
- √ webs, bands
- √ stenotic / absent arterial segments
- √ pouchlike filling defects
- √ abrupt cutoffs often confined to 1 / 2 lung segments
- √ unilateral occlusion / hypoperfusion
- √ selective bronchial arteriography shows dilated bronchial artery collaterals (up to 30% of systemic blood flow) filling pulmonary arteries downstream from sites of occlusion
- √ markedly elevated pulmonary artery pressure

Prognosis: 30% 5-year survival with a mean PA pressure of 30 mm Hg

Rx: thrombendarterectomy (7–40% operative mortality); supplemental warfarin anticoagulation therapy ± vasodilators

Tumor Embolism

◊ Diagnosis frequently missed until postmortem exam!

Frequency: 2–26% of patients with known malignancy

Primary: gastric carcinoma (most common), breast, prostate, lung, hepatocellular, ovarian, osteosarcoma, lymphoma, choriocarcinoma
◊ Right atrial myxoma + RCC tend to embolize to large central + segmental pulmonary arteries!

Pathogenesis: tumor cells form emboli in vena cava subsequently occlude small muscular pulmonary arteries + arterioles

Histo: intravascular malignant cells, acute and organizing platelet-fibrin thrombi, small artery intimal fibrosis, adjacent intralymphatic tumor

- • progressive dyspnea, cough, pleuritic chest pain
- • hemoptysis, syncope
- • hypoxemia <50 mm Hg

CXR:
- √ enlarged central pulmonary arteries
- √ cardiomegaly
- √ ill-defined nodular / confluent peripheral parenchymal opacities (with multiple pulmonary infarcts)

CT:
- √ subpleural linear + wedge-shaped opacities (at sites of pulmonary infarctions)
- √ companion manifestations: lymphadenopathy, pulmonary venous hypertension, lymphangitic carcinomatosis

CECT:
- √ filling defects in main pulmonary artery branches
- √ multifocal beading + dilatation of subsegmental pulmonary arteries

NUC:
- √ multiple small subsegmental unmatched perfusion defects on V/Q scan

Angio:
- √ delayed arterial phase
- √ filling defects / occlusions of subsegmental arterial branches
- √ arterial wall irregularities
- √ peripheral pruning of smaller arteries

Cx: subacute cor pulmonale (heralds death within 4–12 weeks)

Mercury Embolism

Cause: accidental / suicidal IV injection

Pathomechanism: intravascular mercury becomes encased in thrombus or migrates into pulmonary interstitium / alveolar spaces resulting in significant granulomatous response

- √ high-density fine-caliber branching structures in symmetric distribution
- √ mercury collection within apex of right ventricle

PULMONARY VENOUS VARIX

= abnormal tortuosity + dilatation of pulmonary vein just before entrance into left atrium

Etiology: congenital / associated with pulmonary venous hypertension

- • usually asymptomatic; may cause hemoptysis

Location: medial third of either lung below hila close to left atrium

- √ well-defined lobulated round / oval mass
- √ change in size during Valsalva / Mueller maneuver
- √ opacification at same time as LA (on CECT)

Risk: (1) death upon rupture during worsening heart failure
(2) source of cerebral emboli

DDx: pulmonary arteriovenous fistula

RADIATION PNEUMONITIS

= damage to lungs after radiation therapy depends on:
- (a) irradiated lung volume (most important):
  - • asymptomatic in <25% of lung volume
- (b) radiation dose (almost always exceeds critical value for tumoricidal doses):
  - – pneumonitis unusual if <20 Gy given in 2–3 weeks
  - – pneumonitis common if >60 Gy given in 5–6 weeks
  - – significantly increased risk for pneumonitis if daily dose fraction > 2.67 Gy
- (c) fractionation of dose
- (d) concurrent / later chemotherapy

Pathologic phases:
- (1) Exudative phase = edema fluid + hyaline membranes
- (2) Organizing / proliferative phase
- (3) Fibrotic phase = interstitial fibrosis

Time of onset: usually 4–6 months after treatment

Location: confined to radiation portals

1. ACUTE RADIATION PNEUMONITIS

Onset: within 4–8 (1–12) weeks after radiation Rx

Path: depletion of surfactant (1 week to 1 month later), plasma exudation, desquamation of alveolar + bronchial cells

- • asymptomatic (majority)
- • nonproductive cough, shortness of breath, weakness, fever (insidious onset)
- • acute respiratory failure (rare)
- √ changes usually within portal entry fields
- √ patchy / confluent consolidation, may persist up to 1 month (exudative reaction)

CHEST

√ atelectasis + air bronchogram
√ spontaneous pneumothorax (rare)
CT:
√ homogeneous slight hazy increase in attenuation obscuring vessel outlines (2–4 months after Rx)
√ coalescing patchy consolidations (1–12 months after therapy) not conforming to shape of portals
√ nonuniform discrete consolidation (most common; 3 months to 10 years after therapy) forming sharp edge, which conforms to treatment portals
Prognosis: recovery / progression to death / fibrosis
Rx: steroids

2. CHRONIC RADIATION DAMAGE
Onset: 9–12 (6–24) months after radiation therapy; stabilized by 1–2 years after therapy
Histo: permanent damage of endothelial + type I alveolar cells
May be associated with:
(1) thymic cyst
(2) calcified lymph nodes (in Hodgkin disease)
(3) pericarditis + effusion (within 3 years)
√ severe loss of volume
√ dense fibrous strands from hilum to periphery
√ thickening of pleura
√ pericardial effusion
CT:
√ solid consolidation with parenchymal distortion (due to radiation fibrosis + atelectasis)
√ traction bronchiectasis
√ mediastinal shift
√ pleural thickening

RESPIRATORY DISTRESS SYNDROME OF NEWBORN

= RDS = HYALINE MEMBRANE DISEASE
= acute pulmonary disorder characterized by generalized atelectasis, intrapulmonary shunting, ventilation-perfusion abnormalities, reduced lung compliance

Cause: immature surfactant production (usually begins at 18–20 weeks of gestational age) leads to increased alveolar surface tension + decreased alveolar distensibility causing acinar atelectasis (persistent collapse of alveoli) + dilatation of terminal airways
Histo: uniformly collapsed alveoli + variable distension of alveolar ducts + terminal bronchioles; lined by fibrin ("hyaline membranes") 2° to protein seepage from damaged hypoxic capillaries
Predisposed: perinatal asphyxia, cesarean section, infants of diabetic mothers, premature infants (<1,000 g in 66%; 1,000 g in 50%; 1,500 g in 16%; 2,000 g in 5%; 2,500 g in 1%)
Onset: <2–5 hours after birth, increasing in severity from 24 to 48 hours, gradual improvement after 48–72 hours; M:F = 1.8:1

- abnormal retraction of chest wall
- cyanosis (carbon dioxide retention)
- expiratory grunting
- increased respiratory rate

√ diffuse granularity of reticulogranular pattern (coincides with onset of clinical signs) = visualization of distended terminal bronchioles + alveolar ducts against a background of alveolar atelectasis
√ prominent air bronchograms (distension of compliant airways)
√ hypoaeration with loss of lung volume (counteracted by respirator therapy)
√ bilateral + symmetrical distribution
Prognosis: spontaneous clearing within 7–10 days (mild course in untreated survivors); death in 18%
Rx: exogenous surfactant intratracheally results in rapid clearing of RDS
DDx:
(1) Diffuse pneumonia accompanying sepsis
(2) Retained fetal lung fluid (first few hours)
(3) Pulmonary hemorrhage
(4) Pulmonary venous congestion (eg, TAPVR, pulmonary vein atresia, hypoplastic left heart)
(5) Premature with accelerated lung maturity (PALM baby)

ACUTE & SUBACUTE COMPLICATIONS OF RDS
(a) Persistent patency of ductus arteriosus (PDA) oxygen stimulus is missing to close duct; gradual decrease in pulmonary resistance (by end of 1st week) leads to significant L-to-R shunt
(b) Barotrauma with air-block phenomena
(c) Hemorrhage
1. Pulmonary hemorrhage
2. Cerebral hemorrhage
(d) Focal atelectasis (usually from mucus plug)
(e) Persisting fetal circulation
(f) Myocardial ischemia
(g) Diffuse opacity
1. Worsening RDS (first 1–2 days only)
2. Congestive heart failure (PDA, fluid overload)
3. Pulmonary hemorrhage
4. Superimposed pneumonitis
5. Massive aspiration
6. Stage II bronchopulmonary dysplasia
7. "Weaning effect" from removal of endotracheal tube / diminished ventilator pressure
8. Extracorporeal membrane oxygenation
(h) Disseminated intravascular coagulopathy
(i) Necrotizing enterocolitis
(j) Acute renal failure
(k) Metabolic disturbance (eg, hyperbilirubinemia, hypocalcemia)

CHRONIC COMPLICATIONS OF RDS
1. Bronchopulmonary dysplasia (10–20%)
2. Subglottic stenosis (intubation)
3. Localized interstitial emphysema
4. Hyperinflation
5. Retrolental fibroplasia
6. Malnutrition, rickets
7. Lobar emphysema
8. Delayed onset of diaphragmatic hernia
9. Recurrent inspiratory tract infections

RETAINED FETAL LUNG FLUID

= NEONATAL WET LUNG DISEASE = TRANSIENT RESPIRATORY DISTRESS OF THE NEWBORN
= TRANSIENT TACHYPNEA OF THE NEWBORN

Incidence: 6%; most common cause of respiratory distress in newborn

Cause: cesarean section, precipitous delivery, breech delivery, prematurity, maternal diabetes

Pathophysiology:
delayed resorption of fetal lung fluid (normal clearance occurs through capillaries (40%), lymphatics (30%), thoracic compression during vaginal delivery (30%); stiff lungs cause labored ventilation until fluid is cleared

Onset: within 6 hours of life; peaks at 1st day of life

- increasing respiratory rates during first 2–6 hours of life
- intercostal + sternal retraction
- normal blood gases during hyperoxygenation

√ linear opacities + perivascular haze + thickened fissures + interlobular septal thickening (interstitial edema):
 √ symmetric perihilar radiating congestion
√ mild hyperaeration
√ mild cardiomegaly
√ small amount of pleural fluid

Prognosis: resolving within 1–2–4 days (retrospective diagnosis)

DDx: (1) Normal (during first several hours of life)
(2) Diffuse pneumonitis / sepsis
(3) Mild meconium aspiration syndrome
(4) Alveolar phase of RDS
(5) “Drowned newborn syndrome” = clear amniotic fluid aspiration
(6) Pulmonary venous congestion (eg, left heart failure, overhydration, placental transfusion)
(7) Pulmonary hemorrhage
(8) Hyperviscosity syndrome = thick blood
(9) Immature lung syndrome = premature with accelerated lung maturity (PALM baby)

RHEUMATOID LUNG

= autoimmune disease of unknown pathogenesis

Prevalence: 2–54% of patients with rheumatoid arthritis; M:F = 5:1 (although incidence of rheumatoid arthritis: M < F)

- rheumatoid arthritis

Stage 1: multifocal ill-defined alveolar infiltrates
Stage 2: fine interstitial reticulations (histio- and lymphocytes)
Stage 3: honeycombing

A. PLEURAL DISEASE (most frequent thoracic manifestation)
 - Hx of pleurisy (21%)

 Associated with: pericarditis, subcutaneous nodules

 √ pleural effusion (3%) with little change over months:
  √ unilateral (92%), may be loculated
  √ most often without other pulmonary changes
  - M:F = 9:1
  - usually late in the disease, but may antedate rheumatoid arthritis
  - exudate (with protein content >4 g/dL)
  - low in sugar content (<30 mg/dL) without rise during glucose infusion (75%)
  - low WBC high in lymphocytes
  - positive for rheumatoid factor, LDH, RA cells

 √ pleural thickening, usually bilateral

B. DIFFUSE INTERSTITIAL FIBROSIS (30%)

 Prevalence: 2–9% of patients with rheumatoid arthritis

 - restrictive ventilatory defect

 Location: lower lobe predominance

 Histo: deposition of IgM in alveolar septa (DDx to IPF)

 √ punctate / nodular densities (mononuclear cell infiltrates in early stage)
 √ reticulonodular densities
 √ medium to coarse reticulations (mature fibrous tissue in later stage):
  √ irregular interlobular septal thickening on HRCT, predominantly in periphery of lower lung zones
 √ honeycomb lung (uncommon in late stage) with progressive volume loss

C. NECROBIOTIC NODULES (rare)

 = well-circumscribed nodular mass in lung, pleura, pericardium identical to subcutaneous nodules associated with advanced rheumatoid arthritis

 Path: central zone of eosinophilic fibrinoid necrosis surrounded by palisading fibroblasts; nodule often centered on necrotic inflamed blood vessel (? vasculitis as initial lesion)

 - subcutaneous nodules (same histology)

 Associated with: interstitial lung disease

 √ well-circumscribed usually multiple nodules of 3–70 mm in size
 √ commonly located in lung periphery
 √ cavitation with thick symmetric walls + smooth inner lining (in 50%)
 √ NO calcification

D. CAPLAN SYNDROME

 = RHEUMATOID PNEUMOCONIOSIS
 = pneumoconiosis + rheumatoid arthritis in coal workers with rheumatoid disease;
 = hypersensitivity reaction to irritating dust particles in lungs of rheumatoid patients

 Incidence: 2–6% of all men affected by pneumoconioses (exclusively in Wales)

 Path: disintegrating macrophages deposit a pigmented ring of dust surrounding the central necrotic core + zone of fibroblasts palisading the zone of necrosis

 ◊ NOT necessarily evidence of long-standing pneumoconiosis

 - concomitant with joint manifestation (most frequent) / may precede arthritis by several years
 - concomitant with systemic rheumatoid nodules

 √ rapidly developing well-defined nodules of 5–50 mm in size with a tendency to appear in crops predominantly in upper lobes + in periphery of lung
 √ nodules may remain unchanged / increase in number / calcify / result in thick-walled cavities
 √ background of pneumoconiosis

CHEST

√ pleural effusion (may occur)

E. BRONCHIAL ABNORMALITIES (30%)
 √ bronchiectasis
 √ bronchiolitis obliterans (may be transient + regardless of penicillamine / gold therapy):
  √ mosaic pattern (= areas of decreased attenuation + vascularity) on end-inspiratory HRCT
  √ air trapping on end-expiratory HRCT
 √ bronchiolitis obliterans organizing pneumonia (BOOP):
  √ bilateral air-space consolidation in peripheral / peribronchial distribution
 √ follicular bronchiolitis (in 66%):
  √ small centrilobular nodules with patchy areas of ground-glass attenuation

F. PULMONARY ARTERITIS
 = fibroelastoid intimal proliferation of pulmonary arteries
 • pulmonary arterial hypertension + cor pulmonale

G. CARDIAC ENLARGEMENT
 (pericarditis + carditis / congestive heart failure)

H. BONE ABNORMALITIES ON CXR
 √ erosive arthritis of acromioclavicular joint, sternoclavicular joint, shoulder joint:
  √ resorption of distal end of clavicles
 √ ankylosis of vertebral facet joints
 √ vertebral body collapse due to steroid use

ROUND PNEUMONIA

= NUMMULAR PNEUMONIA
= fairly spherical pneumonia caused by pyogenic organisms

Organism: Haemophilus influenzae, Streptococcus, Pneumococcus

Age: children >> adults

• cough, chest pain, fever

Location: always posterior, usually in lower lobes

√ spherical infiltrate with slightly fluffy borders + air bronchogram
√ triangular infiltrate abutting a pleural surface (usually seen on lateral view)
√ rapid change in size and shape

SARCOIDOSIS

= BOECK SARCOID [*sarkos* , Greek = flesh; *sarcoid* = sarcoma-like; Caesar Boeck describes skin lesions in 1899]
= immunologically mediated multisystem granulomatous disease of unknown etiology with variable presentation, progression, and prognosis

Prevalence: 10–40:100,000 in USA

Age peak: 20–40 years; M:F = 1:3 (more common in women + people of West African descent); American Blacks:American Whites = 10:1 (rare in African / South American Blacks); more common in blood group A

Epidemiology:
found with varying frequency in every country in the world; higher prevalence in temperate climates compared to tropical regions (<10/100,000)

Immunology:
unknown antigen activates alveolar macrophages, which release
— interleukin-1 (T-cell activator)
— fibronectin (fibroblast chemotactic factor)
— alveolar macrophage-derived growth factor (stimulates fibrosis)

and activates T lymphocytes, which release
— interleukin-2 (stimulates growth of T-helper / cytolytic cells)
— immune interferon (polyclonal B-cell activator)
— monocyte chemotactic factor (attracts circulating monocytes and stimulates granuloma formation)

Histo: alveolitis (earliest changes); noncaseating epithelioid granulomas [composed of lymphocytes, peripheral fibroblasts, multinucleated giant cells] with occasional minimal central necrosis
 Location: along course of lymphatic vessels: subpleural, septal, perivascular, peribronchial
 DDx: indistinguishable from granulomas of berylliosis, treated TB, leprosy, fungal disease, hypersensitivity pneumonitis, Crohn disease, primary biliary cirrhosis

• angiotensin-converting enzyme (ACE) elevated in 70% [ACE is a product of macrophages and an indicator for the granuloma burden of the body]
 DDx: tuberculosis, leprosy, histoplasmosis, berylliosis, cirrhosis, hyperthyroidism, diabetes
• hypercalcemia + hypercalciuria in 2–15% [result of hydroxylation of 1,25-dihydroxy vitamin D in macrophages leading to increased intestinal resorption of calcium]
• Kveim-Siltzbach test (positive in 70%) = intracutaneous injection of 0.1–0.2 mL of a previously validated saline suspension of human sarcoid spleen / lymph nodes, rarely used
• functional pulmonary impairment (even with NO radiographic abnormality):
 — reduced VC + FRC + TLC [from generalized reduction in lung volume]
 — low lung compliance [from diffuse interstitial disease]
 — obstructive airway disease [from endobronchial lesions, peribronchial fibrosis]

Dx: based on a combination of clinical + radiological + histologic features after exclusion of other infectious / inflammatory entities

A. ACUTE FORM = **Löfgren Syndrome** (17%)
 • fever + malaise + bilateral hilar adenopathy
 • erythema nodosum
 • arthralgia of large joints
 • (occasionally) uveitis + parotitis

B. CHRONIC FORM
 • asymptomatic (50%)
 • fever, malaise, weight loss
 • dry cough + shortness of breath (25%)
 • hemoptysis in 4% (from endobronchial lesion / vascular erosion / cavitation)

Stage at presentation:

0	normal chest radiograph	5%
I	hilar + mediastinal lymphadenopathy only	50%
II	lymphadenopathy + parenchymal disease	30%
III	diffuse parenchymal disease only	15%
IV	pulmonary fibrosis	20%

Prognosis:
- 80% spontaneous remission of stage 1 + 2 disease
- 75% complete resolution of hilar adenopathy
- 33% complete resolution of parenchymal disease
- 30% improve significantly
- 20% irreversible pulmonary fibrosis (may persist unchanged for >15 years)
- 10% mortality (cor pulmonale / CNS / lung fibrosis / liver cirrhosis)
- 25% relapse (in 50% detected by CXR)

@ Thoracic disease (90%)
- mild symptoms in spite of extensive radiographic changes (DIAGNOSTICALLY SIGNIFICANT)

— adenopathy alone (43%)
— adenopathy + parenchymal disease (41%)
— parenchymal disease alone (16%)

Associated with: tuberculosis in up to 13%

√ intrathoracic lymphadenopathy (>85%):
Location:
(a) "1-2-3 sign" = Garland triad = symmetric bilateral hilar nodes + right paratracheal and aortopulmonary window nodes (75–95%)
(b) isolated unilateral hilar enlargement (1–8%)
(c) mediastinal nodes are regularly enlarged on CT

Prognosis: adenopathy commonly decreases as parenchymal disease gets worse; subsequent parenchymal disease in 32%; adenopathy does not develop subsequent to parenchymal disease

√ eggshell calcification of lymph nodes (in 3% after 5 years, in 20% after 10 years)

√ parenchymal disease (60%); without adenopathy in 16–20%:
◊ Parenchymal granulomas are invariably present on open lung biopsy!
Site: predominantly mid-zone involvement
√ reticulonodular pattern (46%)
√ acinar pattern (20%) = ill-defined 6–7-mm nodules / coalescent opacities
√ "alveolar / acinar sarcoidosis" (2–10%) = multiple nodules >10–50 mm (= coalescence of numerous interstitial granulomas):
√ indistinct margins
√ ± air bronchogram
√ ± cavitation of occasional nodule
√ progressive fibrosis with upper lobe retraction + bullae (20%)
√ irreversible fibrotic changes of end-stage lung disease (11–20%)

√ airway disease:
√ tracheal stenosis
√ bronchial stenosis (extrinsic compression by large lymph nodes / endobronchial granulomas)
√ bronchiectasis (scarring / fibrosis)

HRCT:
√ irregular septal thickening
√ perilymphatic nodules (= small nodules along bronchoarterial bundles and veins, in subpleural + interlobular septal lymphatics representing epithelioid cell granulomas)
√ traction bronchiectasis (TYPICAL)
√ ground-glass opacity (in alveolitis)
√ bullae in honeycombing
√ irregular / nodular bronchial wall thickening
√ air trapping

Atypical manifestations (25%):
√ pleural effusion (2%) = exudate with predominance of lymphocytes, effusion clears in 2–3 months
√ focal pleural thickening
√ solitary / multiple pulmonary nodules
√ cavitation of nodules (0.6%)
√ isolated hilar / mediastinal nodal enlargement
√ bronchostenosis (2%) with lobar / segmental atelectasis
√ pulmonary arterial hypertension (periarterial granulomatosis without extensive pulmonary fibrosis)

Cx: √ pneumothorax secondary to chronic lung fibrosis (rare)
√ cardiomegaly from cor pulmonale (rare)
√ aspergilloma formation in apical bulla (in >50% of stage IV disease)

Diagnostic criteria:
(1) compatible clinical + radiologic picture
(2) noncaseous epithelioid granulomas on bronchial / transbronchial biopsy (diagnostic results in 60–95% and 80–95% respectively)
(3) negative results of special stains / cultures for other entities

ASSESSMENT OF ACTIVITY
(1) ACE titer (= angiotensin I converting enzyme)
(2) Bronchoalveolar lavage: 20–50% lymphocytes with number of T-suppressor lymphocytes 4–20 times above normal
(3) Gallium scan
√ uptake in lymph nodes + lung parenchyma + salivary glands (correlates with alveolitis + disease activity); monitor of therapeutic response (indicator of macrophage activity)

◊ Extrathoracic manifestations without intrathoracic involvement occur in <10%!

@ Abdominal disease
- strikingly elevated ACE levels in 91%

@ Liver (pathologic involvement in 24–59%):
√ homogeneous hepatomegaly (18–29%)
√ 2–5-mm nodular lesions in liver and spleen in 5–15% (= coalescent granulomata) occurring within 5 years of diagnosis
√ abdominal adenopathy (mean size of 2.6 cm)

CHEST

MR:
√ heterogeneous / nodular hepatic texture and periportal high signal intensity on T2WI
@ Spleen (pathologic involvement in 24–59%)
√ splenomegaly (20–33%)
√ scattered nodular lesions (18%)
@ Lymphadenopathy (10–31%)
• frequently associated with thoracic adenopathy
√ mean lymph node size of 2.6 cm
@ Pancreas
√ mass + pain mimicking pancreatic carcinoma
@ Gastrointestinal disease:
Location: anywhere from esophagus to rectum
@ Stomach (60 cases)
√ polypoid / nodular mass
√ ± ulcer (simulating peptic ulcer disease)
√ diffuse fold thickening
√ circumferential narrowing + loss of antral compliance (resembling scirrhous carcinoma)
@ Esophagus
√ plaquelike lesions, narrowing, aperistalsis
@ Colon
√ annular involvement (tends to be focal) with obstruction
@ Genitourinary disease (0.2–5%):
@ Kidney
√ renal calculi
@ Scrotum (0.5%)
√ hyperechoic lesions of epididymis + testis
@ Skin disease (10–30%)
• erythema nodosum = multiple bilateral tender erythematous nodules mostly on anterior aspect of lower extremities:
• often associated with fever + arthralgia
√ hilar lymph node enlargement
• lupus pernio = indurated bluish purple elevations mainly on nose + digits
• skin plaques / scars
@ Peripheral lymph node enlargement (30%)
@ Muscle (25%): myopathy
@ Myocardium (6–25%): ventricular arrhythmia, heart block, cardiomyopathy, congestive failure, angina, ventricular aneurysm
@ Bone (6–15–20%):
√ densely sclerotic lesions in spine, pelvis, ribs
√ lesions of distal + middle phalanges of hand + foot:
• pain and swelling
√ lytic lesion with lacelike trabecular pattern
√ sharply marginated cystlike area of rarefaction
@ Eyes (5–25%): uveitis, photophobia, blurred vision, glaucoma (rare)
@ CNS (9%): hypothalamus, basal granulomatous meningitis, facial nerve palsy
@ Salivary gland (4%): bilateral parotid enlargement

SEPTIC PULMONARY EMBOLI

= lodgment of an infected thrombus in a pulmonary artery
Organism: S. aureus, Streptococcus
Predisposed: IV drug abusers, alcoholism, immunodeficiency, CHD, dermal infection (cellulitis, carbuncles)
Source:
(a) infected venous catheter / pacemaker wires, arteriovenous shunts for hemodialysis, drug abuse producing septic thrombophlebitis (eg, heroin addicts), pelvic thrombophlebitis, peritonsillar abscess, osteomyelitis
(b) tricuspid valve endocarditis (most common cause in IV drug abusers)
Age: majority <40 years
• sepsis, cough, dyspnea, chest pain
• shaking chills, high fever, severe sinus tachycardia
Location: predilection for lung bases
√ multiple nondescript pulmonary infiltrates (initially)
√ migratory infiltrates (old ones heal, new ones appear)
√ cavitation (frequent), usually thin-walled
√ pleural effusion (rare)
CT (more sensitive than CXR):
√ multiple peripheral parenchymal nodules ± cavitation / air bronchogram (83%)
√ wedge-shaped subpleural lesion with apex of lesion directed toward pulmonary hilum (50%)
√ feeding vessel sign = pulmonary artery leading to nodule (67%)
√ cavitation (50%), esp. in staphylococcal emboli
√ air bronchogram within pulmonary nodule (28%)
Cx: empyema (39%)

SIDEROSIS

= inert iron oxide / metallic iron deposits
Path: iron phagocytosed by macrophages in alveoli / respiratory bronchioles, elimination from lung by lymphatic circulation
Occupational exposure:
electric arc welding, oxyacetylene torch workers (iron oxide in fumes), mining + processing of iron ores, cutting / burning of iron + steel, foundry workers, grinders, fettlers, silver polishers (jewelry industry)
√ diffuse fine reticulonodular opacities (may disappear after exposure discontinued)
√ small round opacities (indistinguishable from silica / coal)
√ NO secondary fibrosis + NO hilar adenopathy (unless mixed dust inhalation as in **siderosilicosis** / **silicosiderosis** = mixed-dust pneumoconiosis)
HRCT:
√ widespread poorly defined centrilobular micronodules
√ branching linear structures
√ extensive ground-glass attenuation without zonal predominance
DDx: silicosis (nodular opacities more dense + profuse)

SILICOSIS

= inhalation of silicon dioxide; most prevalent silicosis of progressive nature after termination of exposure; similar to CWP (because of silica component in CWP)
Substance: crystalline silica (quartz); one of the most widespread elements on earth

Occupational exposure:
tunneling, mining, quarrying, stone cutting, polishing, glass manufacturing, foundry work, sandblasting, pottery, brick lining, boiler scaling, vitreous enameling, ceramic industry
Dust deposition: dependent on
(a) airflow: deposition of 1–5-µm particles predominantly around respiratory bronchioles in a centrilobular location within secondary pulmonary lobule
(b) lymphatic clearance: related to pulmonary arterial pressure (gravity-related vertical gradient) + blood flow (higher blood flow through LUL) + passive milking of lymphatics by respiratory motion (lateral > anterior > posterior chest wall)
Path: small particles engulfed by macrophages; liberation of silica results in cell death; 2–3-mm nodules with layers of laminated connective tissue around smaller vessels
Cx: predisposes to tuberculosis
DDx: coal worker pneumoconiosis (identical radiographs)

Acute Silicosis
= SILICOPROTEINOSIS
= heavy exposure to respirable free silica in enclosed space with minimal / no protection of airways
Histo: proliferation of type II pneumatocytes + profuse surfactant production
Exposure time: as short as 6–8 months
Associated with: increased risk to develop autoimmune disease
Distribution: lung periphery
Distribution: predominantly lower lung zones; bilateral
√ diffuse airspace / ground-glass disease
√ air bronchograms
HRCT:
√ patchy ground-glass opacities
√ fine intralobular reticulations (= "crazy paving")
Cx: infection with TB + atypical mycobacteria
Prognosis: often rapidly progressive with death from respiratory failure
DDx: alveolar proteinosis

Chronic Simple Silicosis
At least 10–20 years of dust exposure before appearance of roentgenographic abnormality
Location: upper + posterior lung zones
√ small 2–5 (range, 1–10)-mm rounded opacities
√ may calcify centrally in 5–10% (rather typical for silicosis)
√ hilar + mediastinal lymphadenopathy, may calcify in 5% ("eggshell pattern")
√ ± reticulonodular pattern
HRCT:
√ nodules of 3–10 mm in size
√ thickened intra- and interlobular lines
√ subpleural curvilinear lines (peribronchiolar fibrosis)
√ ground-glass pattern = mild thickening of alveolar wall + interlobular septa (fibrosis / edema)
√ parenchymal fibrous bands
√ multiple subpleural nodules
√ "pseudoplaques" = aggregate of subpleural nodules
√ traction bronchiectasis
√ honeycombing

Complicated Silicosis
= PROGRESSIVE MASSIVE FIBROSIS
= appearance of large opacities >1 cm in diameter
Location: midzone / periphery of upper lung migrating toward hila
Distribution: often bilateral symmetric + nonsegmental
√ conglomerate sausage-shaped masses with ill-defined margins (in advanced stages)
√ compensatory emphysema in unaffected portion between mass + pleura
√ slow change over years
√ may calcify + cavitate (ischemic necrosis)

Silicotuberculosis
Doubtful synergistic relationship between silicosis + tuberculosis
√ little change over years with intermittently positive sputa

Caplan Syndrome
More common in coal worker's pneumoconiosis

STAPHYLOCOCCAL PNEUMONIA
Most common cause of bronchopneumonia
(a) common nosocomial infection (patients on antibiotic drugs most susceptible)
(b) accounts for 5% of community-acquired pneumonias (esp. in infants + elderly)
◊ Secondary invader to influenza (commonest cause of death during influenza epidemics)
Organism: Staphylococcus aureus = Gram-positive, appears in clusters, coagulase-producing
√ rapid spread through lungs
√ empyema (esp. in children)
√ pneumothorax, pyopneumothorax
√ abscess formation
√ bronchopleural fistula
A. in CHILDREN:
√ rapidly developing lobar / multilobar consolidation
√ pleural effusion (90%)
√ pneumatocele (40–60%)
B. in ADULTS:
√ patchy often confluent bronchopneumonia of segmental distribution, bilateral in >60%
√ segmental collapse (air bronchograms absent)
√ late development of thick-walled lung abscess (25–75%)
√ pleural effusion / empyema (50%) (DDx from other pneumonias)
Cx: meningitis, metastatic abscess to brain / kidneys, acute endocarditis

STREPTOCOCCAL PNEUMONIA
Incidence: 1–5% of bacterial pneumonias (rarely seen); most common in winter months

Organism: Group A ß-hemolytic streptococcus
= Streptococcus pyogenes, Gram-positive cocci appearing in chains
Predisposed: newborns, following infection with measles
Associated with: delayed onset of diaphragmatic hernia (in newborns)
- rarely follows tonsillitis + pharyngitis

√ patchy bronchopneumonia
√ lower lobe predominance (similar to staphylococcus)
√ empyema

Cx: (1) Residual pleural thickening (15%)
(2) Bronchiectasis
(3) Lung abscess
(4) Glomerulonephritis

SWYER-JAMES SYNDROME

= MACLEOD SYNDROME = UNILATERAL LOBAR EMPHYSEMA
= IDIOPATHIC UNILATERAL HYPERLUCENT LUNG
= chronic complication of bronchiolitis

Etiology: acute viral bronchiolitis in infancy / early childhood (adenovirus, RSV) preventing normal development of lung
Path: variant of postinfectious constrictive bronchiolitis with acute obliterative bronchiolitis, bronchiectasis, distal airspace destruction (developing in 7–30 months)
- asymptomatic
- cough, dyspnea on exertion, hemoptysis
- history of recurrent lower respiratory tract infections during childhood

Location: one / both lungs (usually entire lung, occasionally lobar / subsegmental)
√ hyperlucency of one lung
√ diminished number + size of pulmonary vessels:
  √ small ipsilateral hilum (diminuted hilar vessels + attenuated arteries)
√ small hemithorax with decreased / normal volume (collateral air drift)
√ air trapping during expiration
  DDx: no air trapping with proximal interruption of pulmonary artery (no hilum), hypogenetic lung syndrome, pulmonary embolus
√ mild cylindrical bronchiectasis with paucity of bronchial subdivisions (cutoff at 4th–5th generation = "pruned tree" bronchogram)

HRCT (most useful modality):
  √ bilateral areas of decreased attenuation:
    √ areas of normal lung attenuation within hypoattenuating lung
    √ air trapping within hypoattenuating lung
    √ bronchiectasis
  √ diminished size of pulmonary vessels in hyperlucent areas

Angio:
  √ "pruned tree" appearance

NUC (V/Q scan):
  √ matched defects of perfusion + ventilation (with delayed washout) in hyperlucent regions

Bronchography:
  √ dilated bronchi with sharply terminating segments

DDx: pulmonary artery atresia (uncommon in adults), localized bullous emphysema (deviation of vessels), bronchial obstruction

SYSTEMIC LUPUS ERYTHEMATOSUS

= SLE = most prevalent of the potentially grave connective tissue diseases characterized by involvement of vascular system, skin, serous + synovial membranes

Prevalence: 1:2,000; Blacks:Caucasians = 3:1; increased risk in relatives
Cause: local deposition of antigen-antibody complexes / antibodies inducing necrotizing vasculitis (type III immune complex phenomenon) of the small blood vessels
Age: 16–41 years; M:F = 1:10 (women of childbearing age)
Diagnostic criteria:
(1) malar rash
(2) discoid rash
(3) photosensitivity
(4) oral ulcers
(5) arthritis
(6) serositis
(7) antinuclear antibodies
(8) renal disease
(9) neurologic disease
(10) hematologic disease
(11) immunologic disorder

- fatigue, malaise, anorexia, fever, weight loss
- clinically heterogeneous due to different types of serum antibodies
- antinuclear DNA antibodies (87%)
- hypergammaglobulinemia (77%)
- LE cells (= antigen-antibody complexes engulfed by PMNs) in 78%
- chronic false-positive Wassermann test for syphilis (24%)
- Sjögren syndrome (frequent)
- anemia (78%)
- leukopenia (66%)
- thrombocytopenia (19%)

@ Skin changes (81%)
  - "butterfly rash" (= facial erythema), discoid lupus erythematosus, alopecia, photosensitivity
  - Raynaud phenomenon (15%)

@ Thoracic involvement (30–70%)
  ◊ Affects respiratory system more commonly than any other connective tissue disease
  - dyspnea, pleuritic chest pain (35%)
  - respiratory dysfunction (>50%): single-breath diffusing capacity for carbon monoxide most sensitive indicator

  (a) Pulmonary disease
    Cause: chronic antibody damage to alveolar-capillary membrane
    √ parenchymal opacification:
      √ pneumonia (most common) due to bacteria / opportunistic organism
      √ lung hemorrhage
      √ pulmonary edema

√ lupus pneumonitis (acute form) = poorly defined patchy areas of increased density peripherally at lung bases (alveolar pattern) secondary to infection / uremia in 10%
√ cavitating nodules (vasculitis)
√ pulmonary fibrosis (30%):
√ interstitial reticulations in lung periphery of lower lung fields (chronic form) in 3%
√ fleeting platelike atelectasis in both bases (? infarction due to vasculitis)
√ progressive loss of lung volume:
√ elevated sluggish diaphragms (due to diaphragmatic dysfunction)
√ hilar + mediastinal lymphadenopathy (extremely rare)

(b) Pleural disease (50%)
√ recurrent uni- / bilateral pleural effusions (70%) from pleuritis
√ pleural thickening

(c) Cardiovascular disease
√ pericardial effusion (from pericarditis)
√ cardiomegaly (primary lupus cardiomyopathy)

@ Joints
• arthralgia (95%)
√ nonerosive arthritis of hands (characteristic) without deformity
√ tumoral calcinosis

@ Kidney
Prevalence: kidneys involved in 100% with renal disease developing in 30–50%
Histo: focal membranoproliferative glomerulonephritis
• renal failure (fibrinoid thickening of basement membrane)
√ aneurysms in interlobular + arcuate arteries (similar to but less frequent than polyarteritis nodosa)
√ normal / decreased renal size
√ hydronephrosis (due to detrusor muscle spasm with vesicoureteral reflux / fibrosis of ureterovesical junction)

US:
√ kidney enlarged (early) / diminutive (late stage)
√ increased parenchymal echogenicity

CT:
√ multiple linear hypoattenuating bands (due to vasculitis)

Cx: (1) Nephrotic syndrome (common)
(2) Renal vein thrombosis (in 33%)

Prognosis: end-stage renal disease is common cause of death

@ GI tract (in up to 50%)
• buccal erosions / ulcerations
• GI tract bleeding
√ mesenteric ischemia: colitis, pseudoobstruction, ileus, thumbprinting, luminal narrowing
√ motility disorder of lower esophagus (similar to scleroderma)
√ esophagitis ± ulcers
√ gastritis
√ nodularity of folds
√ pneumatosis intestinalis, perforation
√ painful ascites
√ hepatomegaly, hepatitis, cirrhosis
√ splenomegaly

Prognosis: 60–90% 10-year survival; death from renal failure / sepsis / CNS involvement / myocardial infarction

Drug-induced Lupus Erythematosus (DIL)

• temporary phenomenon

Agents: procainamide, hydralazine, isoniazid, phenytoin account for 90%

√ pulmonary + pleural disease more common than in SLE

TALCOSIS

= prolonged inhalation of magnesium silicate dust containing amphibole fibers (tremolite and anthophyllite) and silica

Talcosis resembles:

(1) Asbestosis (indistinguishable)
√ massive and bizarre pleural plaques
√ may encase lung with calcification

(2) Silicosis
√ small rounded + large opacities
√ fibrogenic process (NO regression after removal of patient from exposure)

TERATOID TUMOR OF MEDIASTINUM

= MEDIASTINAL GERM CELL TUMOR [= TERATOMA]

◊ The anterior mediastinum is the most common extragonadal site of primary germ cell tumors (1–3% of all germ cell tumors)!

Pathogenesis: "misplaced" multipotential primitive germ cells during migration from yolk endoderm to gonad

Incidence:
— adults: 15% of anterior mediastinal tumors
— children: 24% of anterior mediastinal tumors
◊ 16–28% of all mediastinal cysts!
◊ Occurs in same frequency as the usually larger thymoma!
◊ 1/3 of primary neoplasms in this area are in children

Classes: (1) Mature teratoma (solid)
(2) Cystic teratoma (dermoid cyst)
(3) Immature teratoma
(4) Malignant teratoma (teratocarcinoma)
(5) Mixed teratoma

Location: mediastinum is 3rd most common site for teratoid lesions (after gonadal + sacrococcygeal location); 5% of all teratomas occur in mediastinum, mostly anterosuperiorly (in only 1% posteriorly)

√ often inseparable from thymus gland

A. BENIGN TERATOID TUMOR (75–86%)
= MATURE TERATOMA
= most common histologic type
1. Epidermoid (52%) = ectodermal derivatives
2. Dermoid (27%) = ecto- + mesodermal derivatives

CHEST

3. Teratoma (21%) = ecto- + meso- + endodermal derivatives
Path: spherical lobulated well-encapsulated tumor; typically multi- / unilocular cystic cavities with clear / yellow / brown liquid
Histo:
(a) ectoderm: skin, sebaceous material, hair, cysts lined by squamous epithelium
(b) mesoderm: bone, cartilage, muscle
(c) endoderm: GI + respiratory tissue, mucus glands
◊ Tumor capsule commonly has remnants of thymic tissue!
◊ Cyst formation is typical (usually lined by mucus-secreting tall epithelial cells)!
Age: young adults / children; M = F
• asymptomatic (in up to 53%)
• cough, dyspnea, chest pain, pulmonary infection, respiratory distress (due to compression by large tumor)
Location:
(a) anterior superior mediastinum near thymus / within thymic parenchyma
(b) posterior mediastinum (rare = 3–8%)
√ rounded mass bulging into right / left hemithorax sharply demarcated against adjacent lung
√ variations in density (may all be present):
√ fat-fluid level (rare but SPECIFIC)
√ water density
√ homogeneous soft-tissue density (indistinguishable from lymphoma / thymoma)
√ curvilinear peripheral / central calcification (20–43%, 4 x more common in benign lesions) in tumor wall / substance, ossification in mature bone
√ visualization of tooth (PATHOGNOMONIC)
√ often inseparable from thymic gland
√ enhancement of rim / tissue septa
Prognosis: approx. 100% 5-year survival rate
Rx: complete surgical excision

B. MALIGNANT TERATOID TUMOR (14–20%)
Histo: similar to mature teratoma but with primitive / immature tissue elements; commonly neural tissue arranged in rosettes / primitive tubules
◊ <u>Teratocarcinoma / malignant teratoma</u> = identical to teratoma with components of seminoma, endodermal sinus tumor, embryonal carcinoma, choriocarcinoma, sarcoma, carcinoma
1. **Seminoma** = germinoma = dysgerminoma
◊ 2nd most common mediastinal germ cell tumor!
◊ Most common primary malignant germ cell tumor of mediastinum!
Incidence: 2–6% of all mediastinal tumors; 5–13% of all malignant mediastinal tumors
Age: 3rd–4th decade; M >> F; white
Histo: uniform polyhedral / round cells arranged in sheets or forming small lobules separated by fibrous septa; varying amounts of mature lymphocytes
Path: large unencapsulated well-circumscribed mass
• asymptomatic (20–30%)
• chest pain / pressure, shortness of breath, weight loss, hoarseness, dysphagia, fever
• SVC obstruction (10%)
• elevated serum levels of hCG (7–18%)
• elevated serum levels of LDH (80%) correlate with tumor burden + rate of tumor growth
Metastases: to regional lymph nodes, lung, bone, liver
√ large bulky well-marginated lobulated mass
√ usually NO calcification
√ homogeneous soft-tissue density with slight enhancement
Prognosis: 75–100% 5-year survival rate; death from distant metastases
Rx: surgery + radiation therapy (very radiosensitive) ± cisplatin
2. **Nonseminomatous malignant germ cell tumor**
(a) embryonic tissue
(1) <u>Embryonal carcinoma</u>
(b) extraembryonic tissue
(1) <u>Yolk sac</u> = <u>endodermal sinus tumor</u>
(2) <u>Choriocarcinoma</u> (least frequent)
(c) combination = mixed germ cell tumor
Path: large unencapsulated heterogeneous soft-tissue mass with tendency for invasion of adjacent structures
Age: during 2nd–4th decade M:F = 9:1; in children M = F
Associated with: Klinefelter syndrome (in 20%), hematologic malignancy
• chest pain, dyspnea, cough, weight loss, fever, SVC syndrome (90–100%)
• elevated serum level of α-fetoprotein (80%) with endodermal sinus tumor / embryonal carcinoma
• elevated serum level of LDH (60%)
• elevated serum level of hCG (30%) [DDx: lung cancer; hepatocellular carcinoma; adenocarcinoma of pancreas, colon, stomach]
Metastases to: lung, liver
√ large tumor of heterogeneous texture with central hemorrhage / necrosis
√ well circumscribed / with irregular margins
√ enhancement of tumor periphery
√ lobulation suggests malignancy
√ invasion of mediastinal structures (SVC obstruction is ominous)
√ pleural / pericardial effusion (from local invasion)
◊ Absence of primary testicular tumor / retroperitoneal mass proves primary!
Rx: cisplatin-based chemotherapy + tumor resection
Prognosis: 50% long-term survivors
Cx:
(1) Hemorrhage
(2) Pneumothorax (from bronchial obstruction with air trapping + alveolar rupture)
(3) Respiratory distress (rapid increase in size from fluid production) with compression of trachea / SVC (SVC syndrome)

(4) Fistula formation to aorta, SVC, esophagus
(5) Rupture into bronchus (expectoration of oily substance / trichoptysis in 5–14%, lipoid pneumonia)
(6) Rupture into pericardium (pericardial effusion), pleural cavity (pleural effusion)

DDx: thymoma

THORACIC PARAGANGLIOMA

= CHEMODECTOMA
= rare neural tumor arising from paraganglionic tissue

Age: 3rd–5th decade; M:F = 1:1
Path: extremely vascular well-marginated / irregular mass that may adhere to / envelop / invade adjacent mediastinal structures (bronchus, spinal canal)
Histo: anastomosing cords of granule-storing chief cells arranged in a trabecular pattern; identical appearance for benign and malignant tumors

May be associated with:
syn- / metachronous adrenal / extrathoracic paragangliomas; multiple endocrine neoplasia type 2; bronchial carcinoid tumor

• asymptomatic
• dyspnea, cough, chest pain, hemoptysis, neurologic deficits, SVC syndrome (if tumor large)
• signs of excessive catecholamine production: hypertension, headache, tachycardia, palpitations, tremor

Location: base of heart + great vessels (adjacent to pericardium / heart, within interatrial septum / left atrial wall); paravertebral sulci

CT:
√ sharply marginated 5–7-cm middle / posterior mediastinal mass
√ hypodense areas due to extensive cystic degeneration / hemorrhage
√ exuberant enhancement

MR:
√ heterogeneous intermediate signal intensity with areas of signal void from flowing blood on T1WI
√ high signal intensity on T2WI

NUC (I-123 / I-131 metaiodobenzylguanidine):
√ useful for localization as relatively specific

Angio (may precipitate cardiovascular crisis):
√ marked hypervascularity, multiple feeding vessels
√ homogeneous capillary blush

Rx: surgical excision with preoperative administration of α- or β-blockers (hypertensive crisis, tachycardia, dysrhythmia during manipulation)

THYMIC CYST

Pathogenesis:
(1) Congenital cyst (persistent tubular remnants of 3rd pharyngeal pouch = thymopharyngeal duct, develops during 5th–8th week of gestation)
(2) Acquired reactive multilocular cysts = progressive cystic degeneration of thymic (Hassall) corpuscles + thymic epithelial reticulum induced by an inflammatory process: eg, HIV
(3) Neoplastic cyst (cystic teratoma, cystic degeneration within a thymoma), S/P radiation therapy for Hodgkin disease

◊ No association with myasthenia gravis / neoplasia!

Incidence: very uncommon lesion; 1–2% of mediastinal masses
Age: 2/3 in 1st decade; 1/3 in 2nd + 3rd decades; M>F
Path: unilocular thin-walled cyst with thymic tissue
Histo: squamous / cuboidal / respiratory epithelium in cyst wall; lobulated lymphoid tissue in cyst wall containing Hassall corpuscles; cholesterol crystals; small foci of thyroid / parathyroid tissue

• commonly asymptomatic slowly enlarging painless mass
• hoarseness, dysphagia, stridor, respiratory distress in newborns
• sudden symptomatic enlargement with Valsalva maneuver / hemorrhage / recent viral infection

Location:
(a) adjacent to carotid sheath from angle of mandible to thoracic inlet (along path of thymopharyngeal duct) parallel to sternocleidomastoid muscle; L > R
(b) anterior mediastinum

√ unilocular cyst with thin walls containing clear fluid / multilocular cyst with thick walls containing turbid fluid or gelatinous material
√ direct extension / fibrous cord along migratory tract of thymic tissue into mediastinum in 50%: through thyrohyoid membrane into pyriform sinus
√ may show partial wall calcification (rare)
√ low-density fluid (0–10 HU), may be higher depending on cyst contents

US:
√ typically anechoic

DDx: branchial cleft cysts (no thymic tissue), benign thymoma, teratoma, dermoid cyst, Hodgkin disease, non-Hodgkin lymphoma, pleural fibroma

THYMIC HYPERPLASIA

◊ Most common anterior mediastinal mass in pediatric age group through puberty

Age: particularly in young individual
Histo: numerous active lymphoid germinal centers
Etiology:
1. Hyperthyroidism (most common), Graves disease, treatment of primary hypothyroidism, idiopathic thyromegaly
2. Rebound hyperplasia in children recovering from severe illness (eg, from burns), after treatment for Cushing disorder, after chemotherapy
   √ thymus may regrow more than 50% (transient overgrowth, reducible with steroids)
3. Myasthenia gravis (65%)
4. Acromegaly
5. Addison disease

√ normal thymus visible in 50% of neonates 0–2 years of age
√ notch sign = indentation at junction of thymus + heart
√ sail sign = triangular density extending from superior mediastinum

CHEST

√ wave sign = rippled border due to indentation by ribs
√ shape changes with respiration + position

THYMOLIPOMA

Incidence: 2–9% of thymic tumors
Age: 3–60 years (mean age of 22 years); M:F = 1:1
Path: lobulated pliable encapsulated tumor capable of growing to large size (in 68% >500 g, in 20% >2,000 g, the largest >16 kg)
Histo: benign adult adipose tissue interspersed with areas of normal / hyperplastic / atrophic thymus tissue (thymic tissue <33% of tumor mass)
• chest pain, dyspnea, cough (in 50%)
√ large lesions slump inferiorly from anterior mediastinum toward diaphragm
√ may drape around heart enlarging cardiac silhouette on frontal view
√ apparent elevation of diaphragm on lateral view
√ NO compression / invasion of adjacent structures
DDx: mediastinal lipoma (most common of intrathoracic fatty tumors), liposarcoma

THYMOMA

◊ Most common primary neoplasm of anterior superior mediastinum
Age: majority >40 years; 70% occur in 5th–6th decade; less frequent in young adults, rare in children; M:F = 1:1
Associated with: parathymic syndromes (40%) such as
- **Myasthenia gravis**:
  = autoimmune disorder characterized by antibodies against acetylcholine receptors of the postjunctional muscle membrane:
  - progressive weakness, fatigue
  - fatigability of skeletal muscles innervated by cranial nerves, eg, ptosis, diplopia, dysphagia, dysarthria, drooling, difficulty with chewing
  - elevated serum level of anti-acetylcholine receptor antibodies

  ◊ 10–15–25% of patients with myasthenia gravis have a thymoma (in 65% due to thymic hyperplasia)
  ◊ 7–30–54% of patients with thymoma have myasthenia gravis; removal of thymic tumor often results in symptomatic improvement; myasthenia gravis may develop after surgical thymoma excision
  Rx: edrophonium chloride
- Pure red cell aplasia = aregenerative anemia
  = almost total absence of marrow erythroblasts + blood reticulocytes resulting in severe normochromic normocytic anemia
  ◊ 50% of patients with red cell aplasia have thymoma
  ◊ 5% of patients with thymoma develop red cell aplasia
- Acquired hypogammaglobulinemia
  ◊ 10% of patients with hypogammaglobulinemia have thymoma
  ◊ 6% of patients with thymoma have hypogammaglobulinemia
- Paraneoplastic syndromes occur with thymic carcinoid (10%): eg, Cushing syndrome (ACTH production)

• chest pain, dyspnea, cough (33%)

Path:
round / ovoid slow-growing primary epithelial neoplasm with smooth / lobulated surface divided into lobules by fibrous septa; areas of hemorrhage + necrosis may form cysts
(a) encapsulated = thick fibrous capsule ± calcifications
(b) locally invasive = microscopic foci outside capsule
(c) metastasizing = benign cytologic appearance with pleural + pulmonary parenchymal seeding
(d) thymic carcinoma

Histo:
(a) biphasic thymoma (most common)
= epithelial + lymphoid elements in equal amounts
(b) predominantly lymphocytic thymoma
= >2/3 of cells are lymphocytic
(c) predominantly epithelial thymoma
= >2/3 of cells are epithelial
◊ Prognosis unrelated to cell type!

• asymptomatic (50% discovered incidentally)
• signs of mediastinal compression (25–30%): cough, dyspnea, chest pain, respiratory infection, hoarseness (recurrent laryngeal n.), dysphagia
• signs of tumor invasion (rare): SVC syndrome

Location: any anterior mediastinal location between thoracic inlet and cardiophrenic angle; rare in neck, other mediastinal compartments, lung parenchyma, or tracheobronchial tree
Size: 1–10 cm (up to 34 cm)

Noninvasive [Benign] Thymoma

Age peak: 5th–6th decade, almost all are >25 years of age
√ oval / round lobulated sharply demarcated asymmetric homogeneous mass of soft-tissue density (equal to muscle), usually on one side of the midline
√ abnormally wide mediastinum
√ displacement of heart + great vessels posteriorly

CT:
√ homogeneous soft-tissue mass with smooth / lobulated border partially / completely outlined by fat
√ homogeneous enhancement
√ areas of decreased attenuation (fibrosis, cysts, hemorrhage, necrosis)
√ amorphous, flocculent central / curvilinear peripheral calcification (5–25%)

MRI:
√ isointense to skeletal muscle on T1WI
√ increased signal intensity (approaching that of fat) on T2WI
√ fluid characteristics of cysts with high water content

Invasive [Malignant] Thymoma

◊ Malignancy defined according to extent of invasion into adjacent mediastinal fat + fascia!
Frequency: in 30–35% of thymomas
Stage I : intact capsule
Stage II : pericapsular growth into mediastinal fat
Stage III : invasion of surrounding organs such as lung, pericardium, SVC, aorta

Stage IVa : dissemination within thoracic cavity (metastases to pleura + lung in 6%)
Stage IVb : distant metastases (liver, bone, lymph nodes, kidneys, brain)

√ heterogeneous attenuation
√ spread by contiguity along pleural reflections, extension along aorta reaching posterior mediastinum / crus of diaphragm / retroperitoneum (transdiaphragmatic tumor extension)
√ irregular interface with lung
√ unilateral diffuse nodular pleural thickening / pleural masses encasing lung circumferentially
√ vascular encroachment
√ pleural effusion UNCOMMON

DDx: malignant mesothelioma, lymphoma, thymic carcinoma / malignant germ cell tumor (older male, no diffuse pleural seeding), peripheral lung carcinoma (no dominant mediastinal mass), metastatic disease (not unilateral)

Rx: radical excision ± adjuvant radiation therapy
Prognosis: 5-year survival of 93% for stage I, 86% for stage II, 70% for stage III, 50% for stage IV; 2–12% rate of recurrence for resected encapsulated thymomas

TORSION OF LUNG

= rare complication of severe chest trauma
Incidence: rare (<30 cases)
Age: almost invariably in children
Cause: compression of lower thorax, tear on inferior pulmonary ligament, completeness of fissures
Mechanism: compression of lower thorax with lung twisted through 180°; usually in presence of a large amount of pleural air / fluid
Associated with:
surgery (lobectomy), trauma, diaphragmatic hernia, pneumonia, pneumothorax, bronchus-obstructing tumor
Histo: ± hemorrhagic infarction + excessive air trapping

√ collapsed / consolidated lobe in unusual position + configuration:
  √ hilar displacement of atelectatic-appearing lobe in an inappropriate direction
  √ change in position of opacified lobe on sequential radiographs
√ alteration in normal course of pulmonary vasculature:
  √ main lower lobe artery sweeping upward toward apex
√ rapid opacification of an ipsilateral lobe from edema + hemorrhage into airspaces secondary to infarction (DDx: pleural effusion)
√ bronchial cutoff / distortion
√ lobar air trapping
√ lower lung vessels diminutive

TRACHEOBRONCHOMEGALY

= MOUNIER-KUHN SYNDROME
= primary atrophy / dysplasia of supporting structures of trachea + major bronchi with abrupt transition to normal bronchi at 4th–5th division

Incidence: 0.5–1.5%
Age: discovered in 3rd–5th decade

• cough with copious sputum
• shortness of breath on exertion
• long history of recurrent pneumonias

May be associated with: Ehlers-Danlos syndrome

√ marked dilatation of trachea (>29 mm), right (>20 mm) + left (>15 mm) mainstem bronchi
√ sacculated outline / diverticulosis of trachea on lateral CXR (= protrusion of mucous membrane between rings of trachea)
√ may have emphysema, bullae in perihilar region

TRACHEOBRONCHOPATHIA OSTEOCHONDROPLASTICA

= rare benign disease characterized by multiple submucosal cartilaginous / osseous nodules projecting into tracheobronchial lumen
Cause: unknown; may be due to chronic inflammation, degenerative process, irritation by oxygen / chemical, metabolic disturbance, amyloidosis, tuberculosis, syphilis, heredity (high prevalence in Finland)
Pathogenetic theories:
(1) Ecchondrosis / exostosis of cartilage rings
(2) Cartilaginous / osseous metaplasia of internal elastic fibrous membrane of trachea
Path: foci of submucosal hyaline cartilage with areas of lamellar bone
Histo: adipose tissue + calcified areas with foci of bone marrow; thinned normal overlying mucosa with inflammation + hemorrhage
Average age: 50 years (11–78 years); M:F = 3:1

• usually asymptomatic (incidentally diagnosed)
• dyspnea, productive cough, hoarseness, hemoptysis, fever, recurrent pneumonia

Location: distal 2/3 of trachea, larynx, lobar / segmental bronchi, entire length of trachea; spares posterior membrane of trachea

CXR:
  √ scalloped / linear opacities surrounding + narrowing the trachea (best on lateral view)
CT:
  √ deformed thickened narrowed tracheal wall
  √ irregularly spaced 1–3-mm calcific submucosal nodules of trachea + bronchi (similar to plaques)

Dx: bronchoscopy
DDx: relapsing polychondritis, tracheobronchial amyloidosis (does not spare posterior membranous wall of trachea), sarcoidosis, papillomatosis, tracheobronchomalacia

TRAUMATIC LUNG CYST

Age: children + young adults are particularly prone
√ thin-walled air-filled cavity (50%) ± air-fluid level preceded by homogeneous well-circumscribed mass (hematoma)

√ oval / spherical lesion of 2–14 cm in diameter
√ single / multiple lesions; uni- or multilocular
√ usually subpleural under point of maximal injury
√ persistent up to 4 months + progressive decrease in size (apparent within 6 weeks)

TUBERCULOSIS

Prevalence: 10 million people worldwide, active TB develops in 5–10% of those exposed
Organism: Mycobacterium = acid-fast aerobic rods staining red with carbol-fuchsin; M. tuberculosis (95%), atypical types increasing: M. avium-intracellulare, M. kansasii, M. fortuitum
Susceptible: infants, pubertal adolescents, elderly, alcoholics, Blacks, diabetics, silicosis, measles, AIDS (30–40% infected with HIV), sarcoidosis (in up to 13%)
At risk: immunocompromised, minorities, poor, alcoholics, immigrants from 3rd world countries, prisoners, the aged, nursing home residents, homeless
Pathologic phases:
(a) exudative reaction (initial reaction, present for 1 month)
(b) caseous necrosis (after 2–10 weeks with onset of hypersensitivity)
(c) hyalinization = invasion of fibroblasts (granuloma formation in 1–3 weeks)
(d) calcification / ossification
(e) chronic destructive form in 10% (<1 year of age, adolescents, young adults)
Spread: regional lymph nodes, hematogenous dissemination, pleura, pericardium, upper lumbar vertebrae
Mortality: 1:100,000
• Positive PPD tuberculin test: 3 weeks after infection
• Negative PPD test:
1. Overwhelming tuberculous infection (miliary TB)
2. Sarcoidosis
3. Corticosteroid therapy
4. Pregnancy
5. Infection with atypical Mycobacterium
Former Rx: plombage with insertion of plastic packs, Lucite balls, polythene spheres; oleothorax = injection of oil / paraffin

ENDOBRONCHIAL (ACINAR) TUBERCULOSIS
◊ Most common complication of tuberculous cavitation with active organisms spreading via airways following caseous necrosis of bronchial wall
Path: ulceration of bronchial mucosa followed by fibrosis leads to
(a) bronchial stenosis (lobar consolidation)
(b) bronchiectasis
(c) acinar nodules reflecting airway spread
HRCT:
√ airspace nodules
√ "tree-in-bud" appearance = small poorly defined centrilobular nodules + branching centrilobular areas of increased opacity (= severe bronchiolar impaction with clubbing of distal bronchioles) occurring at multiple contiguous branching sites
√ bronchiectasis

TUBERCULOMA
= manifestation of primary / postprimary TB
√ round / oval smooth sharply defined mass
√ 0.5–4 cm in diameter remaining stable for a long time
√ lobulated mass (25%)
√ satellite lesions (80%)
√ may calcify

CAVITARY TUBERCULOSIS
= hallmark of reactivation tuberculosis
= semisolid caseous material is expelled into bronchial tree after lysis
√ moderately thick-walled cavity with smooth inner surface
Cx:
(1) Dissemination to other bronchial segments
√ multiple small acinar shadows remote from massive consolidation
(2) Colonization with Aspergillus
√ aspergilloma

Primary Pulmonary Tuberculosis

Mode of infection: inhalation of infected airborne droplets
Age: most common form in infants + childhood; increasingly encountered in adults (23–34% of all adult cases)
• asymptomatic (91%)
• symptomatic (5–10%)
√ one / more areas of homogeneous dense well-defined airspace consolidation of 1–7 cm in diameter in 25–50–78% (requires several weeks for complete clearing with antituberculous therapy):
√ absent response to antibiotic Rx for "pneumonia"
Location: middle lobe, lower lobes, anterior segment of upper lobes
√ fine discrete nodular areas of increased opacity
DDx: varicella pneumonia, histoplasmosis, metastases, sarcoidosis, pneumoconiosis, hemosiderosis
√ in children: massive hilar (60%) / paratracheal (40%) / subcarinal lymphadenopathy, in 80% on right side; in adults: mediastinal lymphadenopathy in 5–35–48%
DDx of Lnn: metastases, histoplasmosis
√ atelectasis (8–18%), esp. in right lung (anterior segment of upper lobe / medial segment of middle lobe) secondary to
(a) endobronchial tuberculosis
(b) bronchial / tracheal compression by enlarged lymph nodes (68%)

CHEST

√ pleural effusion (10% in childhood, 23–38% in adulthood) most commonly 3–7 months after initial exposure (from subpleural foci rupturing into pleural space)
√ pneumonic reaction (mid or lower lung zones) with segmental / lobar consolidation
√ calcified lung lesion (17%) / parenchymal scar <5 mm = **Ghon lesion**
√ calcified lymph node (36%) in hilus / mediastinum
√ **Ranke complex** = Ghon lesion + calcified lymph node (22%)
√ **Simon focus** = healed site of primary infection in lung apex

CT:
- √ tuberculous adenopathy may demonstrate necrotic center with low attenuation after enhancement

Outcome of primary infection:
1. Immunity prevents multiplication of organism (containment of initial infection by delayed hypersensitivity response + granuloma formation in 1–3 weeks)
2. Progressive primary TB (inadequate immune mechanism with local progression) in 10%, most common in older children / teenagers
3. Miliary tuberculosis (uncontrolled massive hematogenous dissemination overwhelming host defense system)
4. Postprimary TB = reactivation TB (reactivation of dormant organisms after asymptomatic years)

Prognosis: 3.6% mortality rate
Cx: (1) Bronchopleural fistula + empyema
(2) Fibrosing mediastinitis

Postprimary Pulmonary Tuberculosis

= REACTIVATION TB = RECRUDESCENT TB
= infection under the influence of acquired hypersensitivity and immunity secondary to longevity of bacillus + impairment of cellular immunity

Incidence: 1% per year in persons with normal immunity, up to 10% in persons with deficient T-cell immunity
Age: predominantly in adolescence + adulthood
Etiology:
(a) reactivation of focus acquired in childhood (90%)
(b) continuation of initial infection
= progressive primary tuberculosis (rare)
(c) initial infection in individual vaccinated with BCG

Path: foci of caseous necrosis with surrounding edema, hemorrhage, mononuclear cell infiltration; formation of tubercles = accumulation of epithelioid cells + Langhans giant cells; bronchial perforation leads to intrabronchial dissemination (19–21%)

Site: 85% in apical + posterior segments of upper lobe, 10% in superior segment of lower lobe, 5% in mixed locations (anterior + contiguous segments of upper lobe); R > L (*DDx:* histoplasmosis tends to affect anterior segment)

Local Exudative Tuberculosis

√ patchy / confluent ill-defined areas of acinar consolidation (87–91%), commonly involving two / more segments (earliest finding)
√ thin-walled cavitation with smooth inner surface (present in more advanced disease):
- √ cavity under tension (air influx + obstructed efflux)
- √ air-fluid level is strong evidence for superimposed bacterial / fungal infection
- √ air-crescent sign = mobile intracavitary mycetoma

√ accentuated drainage markings toward ipsilateral hilum
√ acinar nodular pattern (20%) due to bronchogenic spread
√ pleural effusion (18%)

CT:
- √ micronodules in centrilobular location (62%)
  = solid caseation material in / surrounding the terminal / respiratory bronchioles
- √ interlobular septal thickening (34–54%)
  = increase in lymphatic flow as inflammatory response / impaired lymphatic drainage due to hilar lymphadenopathy

Local Fibroproductive Tuberculosis

@ Parenchymal disease:
- √ sharply circumscribed irregular + angular masslike fibrotic lesion (in up to 7%)
- √ thick-walled irregular cavitation (HALLMARK) secondary to expulsion of caseous necrosis into airways, esp. in apical / posterior segments of upper lobes (rare in children, in up to 45–51% in adults), often multiple (high likelihood of activity)
- √ reticular pulmonary scars
- √ cicatrization atelectasis = volume loss in affected lobe

@ Airway involvement:
- √ bronchial stenosis::
  - √ persistent segmental / lobar collapse
  - √ lobar hyperinflation
  - √ obstructive pneumonia
  - √ mucoid impaction
- √ traction bronchiectasis in apical / posterior segments of upper lobes

@ Pleural extension:
- √ pleural thickening
- √ apical cap = pleural rind = thickening of layer of extrapleural fat (3–25 mm) + pleural thickening (1–3 mm)
- √ air-fluid level in pleural space = bronchopleural fistula
- √ rim-enhancing / calcified soft-tissue mass of chest wall with destruction of bone / costal cartilage
- √ fistulization to skin

@ Lymphadenopathy:
- √ tuberculous lymphadenitis = enlarged nodes with central areas of low attenuation

√ calcified hilar / mediastinal nodes:
  - broncholithiasis = erosion into adjacent airway

√ Rasmussen aneurysm = aneurysm of terminal branches of pulmonary artery within wall of TB cavity secondary to inflammatory necrosis of the vessel wall (4% at autopsies of cavitary TB):
  √ central cavity near hilum
  √ enlargement of central solid component of cavity
  √ opacification of pseudoaneurysm on CT / angio

Miliary Pulmonary Tuberculosis

= massive hematogenous dissemination of organisms any time after primary infection

Cause:
(1) severe immunodepression during postprimary state of infection
(2) impaired defenses during primary infection = PROGRESSIVE PRIMARY TB

Incidence: 2–3.5% of TB infections

√ chronic focus often not identifiable
√ radiographically recognizable after 6 weeks post hematogenous dissemination
√ generalized granulomatous interstitial small foci of pinpoint to 2–3 mm size
√ rapid complete clearing with appropriate therapy

HRCT (earlier detection than CXR):
√ diffusely scattered discrete 1–2-mm nodules

Cx: dissemination via bloodstream affecting lymph nodes, liver, spleen, skeleton, kidneys, adrenals, prostate, seminal vesicles, epididymis, fallopian tubes, endometrium, meninges

UNILATERAL PULMONARY AGENESIS

= one-sided lack of primitive mesenchyme

Associated with:
anomalies in 60% (higher if right lung involved): PDA, anomalies of great vessels, tetralogy of Fallot (left-sided pulmonary agenesis), bronchogenic cyst, congenital diaphragmatic hernia, bone anomalies

- may be asymptomatic
- respiratory infections

√ complete opacity of hemithorax
√ ipsilateral absence of pulmonary artery + vein
√ absent ipsilateral mainstem bronchus
√ symmetrical chest cage with approximation of ribs
√ overdistension of contralateral lung
√ ipsilateral shift of mediastinum + diaphragm

VARICELLA-ZOSTER PNEUMONIA

Incidence: 14% overall; 50% in hospitalized adults

Age: >19 years (90%); 3rd–5th decade (75%); contrasts with low incidence of varicella in this age group

- vesicular rash

√ patchy diffuse airspace consolidation
√ tendency for coalescence near hila + lung bases
√ widespread nodules (30%) representing scarring
√ tiny 2–3-mm calcifications widespread throughout both lungs (2%)

Cx: unilateral diaphragmatic paralysis

Prognosis: 11% mortality rate

WEGENER GRANULOMATOSIS

= probable autoimmune disease characterized by systemic necrotizing granulomatous destructive angitis

Path: peribronchial necrotizing granulomas + vasculitis not intimately related to arteries

Mean age of onset: 40 years (range of all ages); M:F = 2:1

CLASSIC TRIAD:
(1) respiratory tract granulomatous inflammation
(2) systemic small-vessel vasculitis
(3) necrotizing glomerulonephritis

- The most common presenting symptoms are those of upper respiratory tract involvement (in up to 67%):
  - rhinitis, sinusitis, otitis media

@ Pulmonary disease (94%)
  - stridor (from tracheal inflammation + sclerosis)
  - intractable cough, occasionally with hemoptysis
  - fever, chest pain, dyspnea

  Path: vasculitis of medium-sized and small pulmonary arteries + veins + capillaries, geographic necrosis, granulomatous inflammation

  √ bilateral interstitial reticulonodular opacities, most prominent at lung bases (earliest stage)
  √ widely distributed irregular masses / nodules of varying sizes (5 mm to 10 cm), especially in lower lung fields (69%) usually sparing apices:
    √ usually multiple masses, solitary in up to 25%
    √ cavitation of nodules with thick wall + irregular shaggy inner lining (25–50%)
  √ bilateral multifocal patchy air-space opacities (in up to 50%):
    √ acute airspace pneumonia
    √ intraalveolar pulmonary hemorrhage
  √ smooth / nodular thickening of subglottic / tracheal / bronchial wall producing stenosis with oligemia + emphysema + lobar / segmental atelectasis (60%)
  √ pleural effusion (usually exudative) in 10–25–50%
  √ focal pleural thickening
  √ hilar / mediastinal lymphadenopathy (very unusual)
  √ interstitial pulmonary edema ± cardiomegaly (from renal / cardiac involvement)

  CT:
    √ nodules in peribronchovascular distribution:
      √ central cavitation in nodules >2 cm in diameter
      √ feeding vessels entering nodules (= angiocentric distribution)
    √ pleural-based wedge-shaped lesions (= infarcts)
    √ CT halo sign (= rim of ground-glass attenuation surrounding a pulmonary lesion) due to angiocentric parenchymal microinfarction (nonspecific)
    √ focal / elongated segments of tracheobronchial stenosis ± intra- and extraluminal soft-tissue masses / thickening

Cx: (1) Dangerous airway stenosis (15% of adults, 50% of children)
(2) Massive life-threatening pulmonary hemorrhage
(3) Spontaneous pneumothorax (rare)

@ Renal disease (85%)
focal glomerulonephritis in 20% at presentation, as disease progresses in 83%
Histo: focal necrosis, crescent formation, paucity/ absence of immunoglobulin deposits

@ Paranasal sinuses (91%)
Location: maxillary antra most frequently
- sinus pain, purulent sinus drainage, rhinorrhea
- √ thickening of mucous membranes of paranasal sinuses

@ Nasopharynx (64%)
- epistaxis from nasal mucosal ulceration
- necrosis of nasal septum
- saddle nose deformity
- √ progressive destruction of nasal cartilage + bone (DDx: relapsing polychondritis)
- √ granulomatous masses filling nasal cavities

@ Other organ involvement:
(a) Joints (67%): migratory polyarthropathy
(b) Ear (61%): otitis media
(c) Eye (58%): ocular inflammation, proptosis
(d) Skin + muscle (45%): inflammatory nodular skin lesions, cutaneous purpura
(e) Heart + pericardium (12–28%):
coronary vasculitis, pancarditis, valvular lesions
Cx: acute pericarditis, dilated congestive cardiomyopathy, acute valvular insufficiency with pulmonary edema, cardiac arrest due to ventricular arrhythmia, myocardial infarction
(f) CNS (22%): central / peripheral neuritis
(g) Splenic disease
(h) GI tract (10%):
- abdominal pain, diarrhea, blood loss
- √ ischemia, inflammation, ulceration, perforation

Cx: (1) Hypertension
(2) Uremia
(3) Facial nerve paralysis

Dx: (1) c-ANCA (cytoplasmic pattern of antineutrophil cytoplasmic autoantibodies): 96% sensitive for generalized disease, 99% specific
(2) Lung / renal biopsy

Prognosis: death within 2 years from renal (83%) / respiratory failure; 90–95% mean 5-year survival under treatment

Rx: corticosteroids, cytotoxic drugs (cyclophosphamide), renal transplantation; 93% remission with therapy

DDx: Churg-Strauss (asthma, 47% cardiac involvement, less severe renal + sinus disease, p-ANCA)

Limited Wegener Granulomatosis

= Wegener granulomatosis largely confined to lung WITHOUT renal / upper airway involvement
Dx: c-ANCA (96% sensitive, 99% specific)
M < F
Prognosis: more favorable than classical Wegener's

Midline Granuloma

= mutilating granulomatous + neoplastic lesions limited to nose + paranasal sinuses with very poor prognosis; considered a variant of Wegener granulomatosis WITHOUT the typical granulomatous + cellular components

WILLIAMS-CAMPBELL SYNDROME

= congenital bronchial cartilage deficiency in the 4th–6th bronchial generation either diffuse or restricted to focal area

HRCT:
- √ cystic bronchiectasis distal to 3rd bronchial generation
- √ emphysematous lung distal to bronchiectasis
- √ inspiratory ballooning + expiratory collapse of dilated segments

CHEST

WILSON-MIKITY SYNDROME

= PULMONARY DYSMATURITY
= similarity to bronchopulmonary dysplasia in normal preterm infants breathing room air; rarely encountered anymore

Predisposed: premature infants <1,500 g who are initially well
- gradual onset of respiratory distress between 10 and 14 days
- √ hyperinflation
- √ reticular pattern radiating from both hila
- √ small bubbly lucencies throughout both lungs (identical to bronchopulmonary dysplasia)

Prognosis: resolution over 12 months
DDx: perinatally-acquired infection (especially CMV)

ZYGOMYCOSIS

= PHYCOMYCOSIS
= group of severe opportunistic sinonasal + pulmonary disease caused by a variety of Phycomycetes (soil fungi)

Organism: ubiquitous Mucor (most common), Rhizopus, Absidia with broad nonseptated hyphae of irregular branching pattern
At risk: immunoincompetent host with
1. lymphoproliferative malignancies and leukemia
2. acidotic diabetes mellitus
3. immunosuppression through steroids, antibiotics immunosuppressive drugs (rare)

Entry: inhalation / aspiration from sinonasal colonization
Path: angioinvasive behavior similar to aspergillosis

A. RHINOCEREBRAL FORM
= involvement of paranasal sinuses (frontal sinus usually spared) with extension into:
(a) orbit = orbital cellulitis
(b) base of skull = meningoencephalitis + cerebritis

B. PULMONARY FORM
- √ segmental homogeneous consolidation
- √ cavitary consolidation + air-crescent sign
- √ nodules (from arterial thrombi + infarction)
- √ rapidly progressive (often fatal) pneumonia

Dx: culture of fungus from biopsy specimen / demonstration within pathologic material

DDx: aspergillosis

DIFFERENTIAL DIAGNOSIS OF BREAST DISORDERS

VARIATIONS IN BREAST DEVELOPMENT

Unilateral Breast Development
may exist 2 years before other breast becomes palpable

Premature Thelarche
= breast development <8 years of age

Cause:
(1) isolated idiopathic = mostly subtle overfunction of pituitary-ovarian axis
- NO growth spurt / advanced bone age / menses

(2) central precocious puberty
√ enlargement of uterus + ovaries

√ uni- / bilateral normal breast tissue

Congenital Anomalies
1. Polythelia
= more than normal number of nipples
2. Polymastia
= more than normal number of breasts
3. Amastia
= absence of mammary glands

BREAST DENSITY

Asymmetric Breast Density
A. BENIGN
1. Postsurgical scarring
2. Noniatrogenic trauma
3. Postinflammatory fibrosis
4. Radial scar
5. Ectopic breast tissue
6. Asymmetric breast development
7. Simple cyst
8. Fibrocystic conditions: fibrosis / sclerosing adenosis
9. Hormonal therapy: replacement, contraceptives

B. MALIGNANT
1. Invasive ductal carcinoma: desmoplastic reaction
2. Invasive lobular carcinoma
3. Tubular carcinoma
4. Primary lymphoma of breast

C. IMAGING PROBLEMS
1. Superimposed normal fibroglandular tissue
2. Lesion obscured by overlapping dense parenchyma
3. Lesion outside field of view

Breast Imaging Reporting and Data System (BI-RADS) Categories
◊ Additional image evaluation may be necessary: off-angle / spot compression mammographic views; ultrasound
◊ Unexplained abnormalities warrant biopsy

Asymmetric Breast Tissue
= greater volume / density in one breast compared with corresponding area in contralateral breast

Density in One Projection
= density seen on only one standard mammographic view

Architectural Distortion
= focal area of distorted breast tissue (spiculations with common focal point / focal retraction / tethering) without definable central mass

Focal Asymmetric Density
= focal asymmetric density seen on two mammographic views but not identified as a true mass

Diffuse Increase in Breast Density
√ generalized increased density
√ skin thickening
√ reticular pattern in subcutis

A. CANCER
1. "Inflammatory" breast cancer
2. Diffuse primary noninflammatory breast cancer
3. Diffuse metastatic breast cancer
4. Lymphoma / leukemia
due to obstructive lymphedema of breast

B. INFECTIOUS MASTITIS
usually in lactating breast

C. RADIATION
(a) diffuse exudative edema within weeks after beginning of radiation therapy
(b) indurational fibrosis months after radiation therapy

D. EDEMA
1. Lymphatic obstruction: extensive axillary / intrathoracic lymphadenopathy, mediastinal / anterior chest wall tumor, axillary surgery
2. Generalized body edema: congestive heart failure (breast edema may be unilateral if patient in lateral decubitus position), hypoalbuminemia (renal disease, liver cirrhosis), fluid overload

E. HEMORRHAGE
1. Posttraumatic
2. Anticoagulation therapy
3. Bleeding diathesis

F. ACCIDENTAL INFUSION OF FLUID
into subcutaneous tissue

OVAL-SHAPED BREAST LESIONS

Mammographic Evaluation of Breast Masses
True mass or pseudomass?

A. SIZE
— well-defined nodules <1.0 cm are of low risk for cancer

— "most likely benign" nodules approaching 1 cm should be considered for ultrasound / aspiration / biopsy

B. SHAPE
— increase in probability of malignancy: architectural distortion > irregular > lobulated > oval > round

C. MARGIN (most important factor)
— well-circumscribed mass with sharp abrupt transition from surrounding tissue is almost always benign
— "halo" sign of apparent lucency = optical illusion of Mach effect + true radiolucent halo is almost always (92%) benign but not pathognomonic for benignity
— microlobulated margin worrisome for cancer
— obscured margin may represent infiltrative cancer
— irregular ill-defined margin has a high probability of malignancy
— spiculated margin due to
(a) fibrous projections extending from main cancer mass
(b) previous surgery
(c) sclerosing duct hyperplasia (radial scar)

D. LOCATION
— intramammary lymph node typically in upper outer quadrant (in 5% of all mammograms)
— large hamartoma + abscess common in retro- / periareolar location
— sebaceous cyst in subcutaneous tissue

E. X-RAY ATTENUATION = DENSITY
— fat-containing lesions are never malignant
— high-density mass suspicious for carcinoma (higher density than equal volume of fibroglandular tissue due to fibrosis)

F. NUMBER
— multiplicity of identical lesions decreases risk

G. INTERVAL CHANGE
— enlarging mass needs biopsy

H. PATIENT RISK FACTORS
— increasing age increases risk for malignancy
— positive family history
— history of previous abnormal breast biopsy
— history of extramammary malignancy

Well-circumscribed Breast Mass

◊ Well-defined nonpalpable lesions have a 4% risk of malignancy!

A. BENIGN
1. Cyst (45%)
2. Fibroadenoma
3. Sclerosing adenoma
4. Intraductal papilloma (intracystic / solid)
5. Galactocele
6. Sebaceous cyst
7. Pseudoangiomatous stromal hyperplasia

B. MALIGNANT
1. Medullary carcinoma
2. Mucinous carcinoma
3. Intracystic papillary carcinoma
4. Invasive ductal cancer not otherwise specified (rare)
5. Pathologic intramammary lymph node
6. Metastases to breast: melanoma, lymphoma / leukemia, lung cancer, hypernephroma

Well-circumscribed De Novo Mass in Woman >40 Years of Age

1. Cyst
2. Papilloma
3. Carcinoma
4. Sarcoma (rare)
5. Fibroadenoma (exceedingly rare)
6. Metastasis (extremely rare)

Fat-containing Breast Lesion

◊ Fat contained within a lesion proves benignity!

1. Lipoma
2. Galactocele
   = fluid with high lipid content (last phase)
   • during / shortly after lactation
3. Traumatic lipid cyst = fat necrosis = oil cyst
   • site of prior surgery / trauma
4. Focal collection of normal breast fat

Mixed Fat- and Water-density Lesion

1. Intramammary lymph node
2. Galactocele
3. Hamartoma = lipofibroadenoma = fibroadenolipoma
4. Small superficial hematoma

Breast Lesion with Halo Sign

A. HIGH-DENSITY LESION
= vessels + parenchymal elements not visible in superimposed lesion
1. Cyst
2. Sebaceous cyst
3. Wart

B. LOW-DENSITY LESION
= vessels + parenchyma seen superimposed on lesion
1. Fibroadenoma
2. Galactocele
3. Cystosarcoma phylloides

Stellate / Spiculated Breast Lesion

= mass / architectural distortion characterized by thin lines radiating from its margins

Risk of malignancy:
— 75% for nonpalpable spiculated masses
— 32% for nonpalpable irregular masses

A. PSEUDOSTELLATE STRUCTURE
= SUMMATION SHADOWS
caused by fortuitous superimposition of normal fibrous + glandular structures; unveiled by rolled views, spot compression views ± microfocus magnification technique

B. "BLACK STAR"
   √ groups of fine fibrous strands bunched together
   √ circular / oval lucencies within center
   √ change in appearance on different views
   1. Radial scar = sclerosing duct hyperplasia
   2. Sclerosing adenosis
   3. Posttraumatic fat necrosis

C. "WHITE STAR"
   √ individual straight dense spicules
   √ central solid tumor mass
   √ little change in different views
   (a) malignant lesions
      1. Invasive ductal carcinoma = scirrhous carcinoma
         = desmoplastic reaction + secondary retraction of surrounding structures
         • clinical dimensions larger than mammographic size
         √ distinct central tumor mass with irregular margins
         √ length of spicules increase with tumor size
         √ localized skin thickening / retraction when spiculae extend to skin
         √ commonly associated with malignant-type calcifications
      2. Infiltrating lobular carcinoma
      3. Tubular carcinoma
      4. Ductal carcinoma in situ
   (b) benign lesions
      1. Postoperative scar
         • correlation with history + site of biopsy
         √ scar diminishes in size + density over time
      2. Postoperative hematoma
         • clinical information
         √ short-term mammographic follow-up confirms complete resolution
      3. Breast abscess
         • clinical information
         √ high-density lesion with flamelike contour
      4. Hyalinized fibroadenoma with fibrosis
         √ changing pattern with different projections
         √ may be accompanied by typical coarse calcifications of fibroadenomas
      5. Granular cell myoblastoma
      6. Fibromatosis
      7. Extra-abdominal desmoid

mnemonic: "STARFASH"
Summation shadow
Tumor (malignant)
Abscess
Radial scar
Fibroadenoma (hyalinized), **F**at necrosis
Adenosis (sclerosing)
Scar (postoperative)
Hematoma (postoperative)

Tumor-mimicking Lesions

1. "Phantom breast tumor" = simulated mass
   (a) asymmetric density
      √ scalloped concave breast contour
      √ interspersed fatty elements
   (b) summation artifact = chance overlap of normal glandular breast structures
      √ failure to visualize "tumor" on more than one view
2. Silicone injections
3. Skin lesions
   (a) Dermal nevus
      √ sharp halo / fissured appearance
   (b) Skin calcifications
      √ lucent center (clue)
      √ superficial location (tangential views)
   (c) Sebaceous / epithelial inclusion cyst
   (d) Neurofibromatosis
   (e) Biopsy scar
4. Lymphedema
5. Lymph nodes
   Frequency: 5.4% for intramammary nodes
   Location: axilla, subcutaneous tissue of axillary tail, lateral portion of pectoralis muscle, intramammary (typically in upper outer quadrant)
   √ ovoid / bean-shaped mass(es) with fatty notch representing hilum
   √ central zone of radiolucency (fatty replacement of center) surrounded by "crescent" rim of cortex
   √ usually <1.5 cm (up to 4 cm) in size
   √ well-circumscribed with slightly lobulated margin
   US:
      √ reniform hypoechoic rim with echogenic center
      √ echogenic hilum for entry and exit of vessels
6. Hemangioma

BREAST

Solid Breast Lesion by Ultrasound

Malignant Sonographic Characteristics

(according to data from A.T. Stavros)

US Characteristic	*Sens.*	*Specif.*	*PPV*	*Rel. risk*
Spiculation	36.0	99.4	91.8	5.5
Taller than wide	41.6	98.1	81.2	4.9
Angular margins	83.2	92.0	67.5	4.0
Acoustic shadowing	48.8	94.7	64.9	3.9
Branch pattern	29.6	96.6	64.0	3.8
Markedly hypoechoic	68.8	60.1	60.1	3.6
Calcifications	27.2	96.3	59.6	3.6
Duct extension	24.8	95.2	50.8	3.0
Microlobulation	75.2	83.8	48.2	2.9

◊ Approximately 5 malignant features are found per cancer. The combination of 5 findings increases the sensitivity to 98.4%!
√ spiculation = alternating straight lines radiating perpendicularly from surface of nodule
   (a) hypoechoic relative to echogenic fibrous tissue
   (b) hyperechoic relative to surrounding fat
√ taller-than-wide lesion = AP dimension greater than craniocaudal / transverse dimension
√ angular margin = contour of junction between hypo- or isoechoic solid nodule and surrounding tissue at acute / obtuse / 90° angles

√ acoustic shadowing behind all / part of nodule (= fibroelastic host response to scirrhous cancer)
√ central part of solid lesion very hypoechoic with respect to fat
√ punctate echogenic calcifications within hypoechoic mass (acoustic shadowing commonly not present)
√ radial extension / branch pattern (= intraductal component of breast cancer)
√ microlobulation = many small lobulations at surface of solid nodule

Benign Sonographic Characteristics

√ absence of any malignant characteristics
◊ A single malignant feature prohibits classification of a nodule as benign!
√ marked hyperechogenic well-circumscribed nodule compared with fat = normal stromal fibrous tissue (may represent a palpable pseudomass / fibrous ridge)
√ smooth well-circumscribed ellipsoid shape
√ 2–3 smooth well-circumscribed gentle lobulations
√ thin echogenic capsule
√ kidney-shaped lesion = intramammary lymph node
◊ If specific benign features are not found the lesion is classified as indeterminate!

(according to data from A.T. Stavros)

US Characteristic	*Sens.*	*Specif.*	*NPV*	*Rel. risk*
Hyperechoic	100.0	7.4	100.0	0.00
≤3 lobulations	99.2	19.4	99.2	0.05
Ellipsoid shape	97.6	51.2	99.1	0.05
Thin echogenic capsule	95.2	76.0	98.8	0.07

BREAST CALCIFICATIONS

Indicative of focally active process; often requiring biopsy
◊ 75–80% of biopsied clusters of calcifications represent a benign process
◊ 10–30% of microcalcifications in asymptomatic patients are associated with cancers

Composition: hydroxyapatite / tricalcium phosphate / calcium oxalate

Results of breast biopsies for microcalcification:
(without any other mammographic findings)
(a) benign lesions (80%)
1. Mastopathy without proliferation 44%
2. Mastopathy with proliferation 28%
3. Fibroadenoma 4%
4. Solitary papilloma 2%
5. Miscellaneous 2%

(b) malignant lesions (20%)
1. Lobular carcinoma in situ 10%
in 8% no spatial relationship to LCIS
2. Infiltrating carcinoma 6%
3. Ductal carcinoma in situ 4%

◊ A positive biopsy rate of >35% is desirable goal!

A. LOCATION
(a) intramammary
1. **Ductal microcalcifications**
√ 0.1–0.3 mm in size, irregular, sometimes mixed linear + punctate
Occurrence: secretory disease, epithelial hyperplasia, atypical ductal hyperplasia, intraductal carcinoma
2. **Lobular microcalcifications**
√ smooth round, similar in size + density
Occurrence:
cystic hyperplasia, adenosis, sclerosing adenosis, atypical lobular hyperplasia, lobular carcinoma in situ, cancerization of lobules (= retrograde migration of ductal carcinoma to involve lobules), ductal carcinoma obstructing egress of lobular contents

N.B.: lobular and ductal microcalcifications occur frequently in fibrocystic disease + breast cancer!

(b) extramammary: arterial wall, duct wall, fibroadenoma, oil cyst, skin, etc.

B. SIZE
√ malignant calcifications usually <0.5 mm; rarely >1.0 mm

C. NUMBER
√ <4–5 calcifications per 1 cm^2 have a low probability for malignancy

D. MORPHOLOGY
(a) benign
1. Smooth round calcifications: formed in dilated acini of lobules
2. Solid / lucent-centered spheres: usually due to fat necrosis
3. Crescent-shaped calcifications that are concave on horizontal beam lateral projection = sedimented milk of calcium at bottom of cyst
4. Lucent-centered calcifications: around accumulated debris within ducts / in skin
5. Solid rod-shaped calcifications / lucent-centered tubular calcifications: formed within / around normal / ectatic ducts
6. Eggshell calcifications in rim of breast cysts
7. Calcifications with parallel track appearance = vascular calcifications

(b) malignant
= calcified cellular secretions / necrotic cancer cells within ducts
√ calcifications of
– vermicular form
– varying in size
– linear / branching shape

E. DISTRIBUTION
1. Clustered heterogeneous calcifications: adenosis, peripheral duct papilloma, hyperplasia, cancer
2. Segmental calcifications within single duct network: suspect for multifocal cancer within lobe
3. Regional / diffusely scattered calcifications with random distribution throughout large volumes of breast: almost always benign

F. TIME COURSE
malignant calcifications can remain stable for >5 years!

G. DENSITY

Malignant Calcifications

1. **Granular calcifications** = resembling fine grains of salt
   √ amorphous, dotlike / elongated, fragmented
   √ grouped very closely together
   √ irregular in form, size, and density
2. **Casting calcifications** = fragmented cast of calcifications within ducts
   √ variable in size + length
   √ great variation in density within individual particles + among adjacent particles
   √ jagged irregular contour
   √ ± Y-shaped branching pattern
   √ clustered (>5 per focus within an area of 1 cm^2)

Benign Calcifications

1. **Lobular calcifications =** arise within a spherical cavity of cystic hyperplasia, sclerosing adenosis, atypical lobular hyperplasia
   √ sharply outlined, homogeneous, solid, spherical "pearl-like"
   √ little variation in size
   √ numerous + scattered
   √ associated with considerable fibrosis
   (a) adenosis
      √ diffuse calcifications involving both breasts symmetrically
   (b) periductal fibrosis
      √ diffuse / grouped calcifications + irregular borders, simulating malignant process
2. Sedimented milk of calcium
   Frequency: 4%
   √ multiple, bilateral, scattered / occasionally clustered calcifications within microcysts
   √ smudge-like particles at bottom of cyst on vertical beam
   √ crescent-shaped on horizontal projection = "teacup-like"
3. Plasma cell mastitis = periductal mastitis
   √ sharply marginated calcifications of uniform density = intraductal form
   √ sharply marginated hollow calcifications = periductal form
4. Peripheral eggshell calcifications
   (a) with radiolucent lesion
      — liponecrosis micro- / macrocystica calcificans (= fatty acids precipitate as calcium soaps at capsular surface) as calcified fat necrosis / calcified hematoma
      ◊ May mimic malignant calcifications!
   (b) with radiopaque lesion
      — degenerated fibroadenoma
      — macrocyst
      √ high uniform density in periphery
      √ usually subcutaneous
      √ no associated fibrosis
5. Papilloma
   √ solitary raspberry configuration in size of duct
   √ central / retroareolar
6. Degenerated fibroadenoma
   √ bizarre, coarse, sharply outlined, "popcornlike" very dense calcification within dense mass (= central myxoid degeneration)
   √ eggshell type calcification (= subcapsular myxoid degeneration)
7. Arterial calcifications
   √ parallel lines of calcifications
8. Dermal calcifications
   Site: sebaceous glands
   √ hollow radiolucent center
   √ polygonal shape
   √ peripheral location (may project deep within breast even on 2 views at 90° angles)
   √ linear orientation when caught in tangent
   √ same size as skin pores
   Proof: superficial marking technique
9. Metastatic calcifications
   Cause: 2° hyperparathyroidism (in up to 68%)

NIPPLE & SKIN

Nipple Retraction

1. Positional
2. Relative to inflammation / edema of periareolar tissue
3. Congenital
4. Acquired (carcinoma, ductal ectasia)

Nipple Discharge

Prevalence: 7.4 % of breast surgeries
Classification:

A. PROVOKED
   postovulatory state, duct ectasia, medication, stimulation by exercise, breast self-examination, sexual manipulation
B. SPONTANEOUS
   (a) physiologic: pregnancy, lactation, galactorrhea, duct ectasia
   (b) pathologic: benign / malignant neoplasm, galactorrhea due to hyperprolactinemia from a pituitary adenoma
C. UNILATERAL
   ◊ Unilateral spontaneous discharge is significant + requires investigation!
D. BILATERAL
   ◊ Expressed bilateral multipore blood-negative discharge is physiologic and benign!

Type of discharge:

A. LACTATING BREAST: galactorrhea
B. NONLACTATING BREAST:
   (a) normal:
      1. milky
      2. multicolored sticky (blue, green, gray, brown, black)
   (b) abnormal:
      3. purulent: antibiotics, incision, drainage

BREAST

(c) surgically significant (in 14.3% cancerous)
4. clear / watery: cancer in 33%
5. bloody / sanguineous: cancer 28%,
6. pink / serosanguineous: cancer in 13%
7. yellow / serous: cancer in 6%
◊ The most common cause of bloody and serosanguineous discharge is intraductal papilloma!
◊ Exfoliative cytology not helpful (true positive in only 11%, false negative in 18%)

Site of origin:
A. Lobules + terminal duct lobular unit:
1. Galactorrhea
2. Fibrocystic changes
B. Larger lactiferous ducts (collecting duct, segmental duct, subsegmental duct)
1. Solitary papilloma
2. Papillary carcinoma
3. Duct ectasia

Galactography / ductography:
injection of 0.2–0.3 mL of water-soluble contrast material (Conray 60®, Isovue®) through straight blunt 27-gauge pediatric sialography cannula (0.4–0.6 mm outer diameter) / 30-gauge cannula / Jabczenski cannula (tip bent 90°)
Results of positive galactography:
papilloma (48%), benign conditions (42%), intraductal carcinoma (10%)

Contraindications to ductography:
history of severe allergy to iodinated contrast material, inability of patient to cooperate (debilitating anxiety, mental disorder), history of prior nipple surgery

DDx of intraductal defects:
gas bubble, clot, inspissated secretions, solitary intraductal papilloma, epithelial hyperplastic lesion, duct carcinoma

Galactographic Filling Defect		
	Single	*Multiple*
Multiple papilloma	5.6%	14.0%
Cancer	0.05%	9.7%

Secretory Disease
1. Retained lactiferous secretions
result of incomplete / prolonged involution of lactiferous ducts
√ branching pattern of fat density in dense breast (high lipid content)
2. Prolonged inspissation of secretion + intraductal debris
= Mammary duct ectasia
√ duct dilatation
√ calcifications with linear orientation toward subareolar area a few mm long: rod-shaped / sausage-shaped / spherical with hollow center
3. Galactocele
4. Plasma cell mastitis

Skin Thickening of Breast
Normal skin thickness: 0.8–3 mm; may exceed 3 mm in inframammary region
A. LOCALIZED SKIN THICKENING
1. Trauma (prior biopsy)
2. Carcinoma
3. Abscess
4. Nonsuppurative mastitis
5. Dermatologic conditions
B. GENERALIZED SKIN THICKENING
◊ Skin is thickened initially and to the greatest extent in the lower dependent portion of breast!
√ overall increased density with coarse reticular pattern (= dilated lymph vessels + interstitial fluid triggering fibrosis)
(a) Axillary lymphatic obstruction
1. Primary breast cancer
— advanced breast cancer
— invasive comedocarcinoma in large area
◊ Primary breast cancer not necessarily seen due to small size / hidden location (axillary tail, behind nipple)!
2. Primary malignant lymphatic disease (eg, lymphoma)
(b) Intradermal + intramammary obstruction of lymph channels
1. Lymphatic spread of breast cancer from contralateral side
2. Inflammatory breast carcinoma = diffusely invasive ductal carcinoma
(c) Mediastinal lymphatic blockage
1. Sarcoidosis
2. Hodgkin disease
3. Advanced bronchial / esophageal carcinoma
4. Actinomycosis
(d) Advanced gynecologic malignancies from thoracoepigastric collaterals
1. Ovarian cancer
2. Uterine cancer
(e) Inflammation
1. Acute mastitis
2. Retromamillary abscess
3. Fat necrosis
4. Radiation therapy
5. Reduction mammoplasty
(f) Right heart failure
may be unilateral (R > L) / migrating with change in patient position (to avoid decubitus ulcer)
(g) Nephrotic syndrome, anasarca
1. Dialysis
2. Renal transplant
(h) Subcutaneous extravasation of pleural fluid following thoracentesis

Lymphadenopathy

Radiographic features of normal lymph nodes:

- • nonpalpable
- √ mass of low to moderate density
- √ sharply defined
- √ round to oval
- √ radiolucent fatty hilus (visible in 78%)
- √ <1 cm within breast tissue, <1.5 cm within axilla

Intramammary Lymphadenopathy

= adenopathy >1 cm surrounded by breast tissue

N.B.: nodes located high within axillary tail (= tail of Spence) are mammographically difficult to differentiate from inferior axillary lymph nodes

Axillary Lymphadenopathy

= solid node >1.5 cm in size without fatty hilum

N.B.: lymph nodes of up to 3 cm may be normal if largely replaced by fat

A. MALIGNANT
1. Metastasis from breast cancer in 26%
   ◊ Primary breast lesion may not be found in 33% of cases!
2. Metastases from non-breast primary (lung, melanoma, thyroid, GI tract, ovary)
3. Lymphoproliferative disease: lymphoma / chronic lymphocytic leukemia (17%)
   ◊ Bilateral axillary lymphadenopathy is suggestive of lymphoproliferative disease!

B. BENIGN
1. Nonspecific benign lymphadenopathy (29%)
2. Reactive nodal hyperplasia (breast infection / abscess / biopsy)
3. Collagen vascular disease: rheumatoid arthritis, systemic lupus erythematosus
4. Granulomatous disease: sarcoidosis
5. Psoriasis
6. HIV-related adenopathy
7. Silicone adenopathy

Radiographic features suspicious for malignancy:

- √ size increase of >100% over baseline
- √ size >3.3 cm
- √ change in shape
- √ spiculation of margins
- √ intranodal microcalcifications (without history of gold therapy)
- √ loss of radiolucent center / hilar notch
- √ increase in density

MAMMOGRAPHY REPORTS

Breast Imaging Reporting and Data System (BIRD)

N = negative
there is nothing to comment on; breasts are symmetrical without masses, architectural disturbances / suspicious calcifications

B = benign finding
confidently labeled, eg, calcified fibroadenoma, multiple secretory calcifications, fat-containing lesion such as oil cyst, lipoma, galactocele, mixed-density hamartoma, intramammary lymph node, implant

P = probably benign finding – short interval follow-up
high probability of benign with radiologist's preference to establish its stability

S = suspicious abnormality – consider biopsy
lesion without characteristic morphology of cancer but definite probability of being malignant

M = highly suggestive of malignancy
biopsy is mandatory

Lexicon Descriptors for Reporting (ACR)

A. MASS

size	
shape	circular, oval, lobulated, irregular
margins	circumscribed, lobulated, obscured, indistinct, speculated
location	based on face of clock + depth in breast
associated findings	skin changes, calcifications, nipple retraction, trabecular thickening
attenuation	relative to an equal volume of breast tissue: high density, isodense, low density, fat density

B. CALCIFICATIONS

type	skin, vascular, coarse, rodlike, eggshell, punctate, pleomorphic
number	
size	
distribution	clustered, linear, segmental, regional, scattered, multiple groups
associated findings	skin changes, nipple retraction, architectural distortion, trabecular thickening

BREAST

BREAST ANATOMY AND MAMMOGRAPHIC TECHNIQUE

BREAST DEVELOPMENT

Embryology

"Milk line" develops from ectodermal elements + extends from axillary region to groin; lack of regression leads to development of accessory breast tissue / accessory nipples

Tanner Stages

Stage I (prepubertal)
- nipple elevates
- √ ill-defined hyperechoic retroareolar tissue

Stage II

Cause: estrogen for ductal + progesterone for lobuloalveolar development
- palpable subareolar bud = **thelarche** begins with onset of puberty (mean age, 9.8 years)
- breast tissue + nipple arise as a single mound of tissue
- √ hyperechoic retroareolar nodule
- √ central star-shaped / linear hypoechoic area (simple branched ducts)

Stage III
- enlargement + elevation of single mound
- √ hyperechoic glandular tissue extending away from retroareolar area
- √ central spider-shaped hypoechoic area

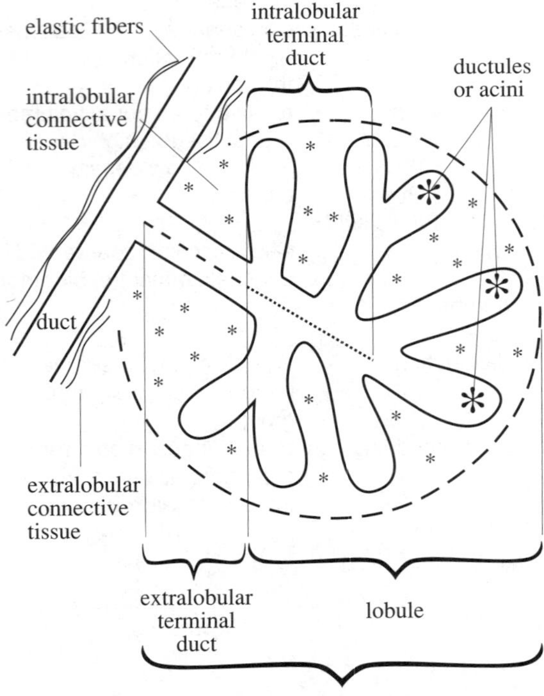

Terminal Ductal Lobular Unit

Stage IV (areolar mounding)
- secondary mound develops (very transient) with nipple + areola projecting above the breast tissue
- √ hyperechoic periareolar fibroglandular tissue
- √ prominent central hypoechoic nodule

Stage V (mature breast)
- regression of areola forming a smooth contour with the rest of the breast tissue
- √ hyperechoic glandular tissue
- √ increased subcutaneous adipose tissue anteriorly
- √ NO hypoechoic central nodule

BREAST ANATOMY

Lobes

15–20 lobes disposed radially around nipple, each lobe has a main lactiferous duct of 2.0–4,5 mm converging at the nipple with an opening in the central portion of nipple

Main duct: branches dichotomously eventually forming terminal ductal lobular units

Histo: epithelial cells, myoepithelial cells surrounded by extralobular connective tissue with elastic fibers

Terminal Duct Lobular Unit (TDLU)

(1) Extralobular terminal duct
  Histo: lined by columnar cells + prominent coat of elastic fibers + outer layer of myoepithelium

(2) Lobule
  (a) intralobular terminal duct
    Histo: lined by 2 layers of cuboidal cells + outer layer of myoepithelium
  (b) ductules / acini
  (c) intralobular connective tissue

Size: 1–8 mm (most 1–2 mm) in diameter

Change:
  (a) reproductive age: cyclic proliferation (up to time of ovulation) + cyclic involution (during menstruation)
  (b) post menopause: regression with fatty replacement

Significance:
TDLU is site of fibroadenoma, epithelial cyst, apocrine metaplasia, adenosis (= proliferation of ductules + lobules), epitheliosis (= proliferation of mammary epithelial cells within preexisting ducts + lobules), ductal + lobular carcinoma in situ, infiltrating ductal + lobular carcinoma

Components of Normal Breast Parenchyma

1. Nodular densities surrounded by fat
   (a) 1–2 mm = normal lobules
   (b) 3–9 mm = adenosis
2. Linear densities
   = ducts and their branches + surrounding elastic tissue
3. Structureless ground-glass density
   = stroma / fibrosis with concave contours

Parenchymal Breast Pattern (László Tabár)

Pattern I

named QDY = quasi dysplasia (for Wolfe classification)

√ concave contour from Cooper's ligaments
√ evenly scattered 1–2 mm nodular densities (= normal terminal ductal lobular units)
√ oval-shaped / circular lucent areas (= fatty replacement)

Pattern II

similar to N1 (Wolfe)

√ total fatty replacement
√ NO nodular densities

Pattern III

similar to P1 (Wolfe)

√ normal parenchyma occupying <25% of breast volume in retroareolar location

Pattern IV = adenosis pattern

similar to P2 (Wolfe)

Cause: hypertrophy + hyperplasia of acini within lobules

Histo: small ovoid proliferating cells with rare mitoses

√ scattered 3–7 mm nodular densities (= enlarged terminal ductal lobular units) = adenosis
√ thick linear densities (= periductal elastic tissue proliferation with fibrosis) = fibroadenosis
√ no change with increasing age (genetically determined)

Pattern V

similar to DY (Wolfe)

√ uniformly dense parenchyma with smooth contour (= extensive fibrosis)

MAMMOGRAPHIC FILM READING TECHNIQUE

1. Compare with earlier films
2. Scan "forbidden" areas
   (a) "Milky Way" = 2–3 cm wide area parallel with the edge of the pectoral muscle on MLO projection
   (b) "No man's land" = fatty replaced area between posterior border of parenchyma + chest wall on CC projection
   (c) Medial half of breast on CC view
3. Look for increased retroareolar density
4. Look for parenchymal contour retraction
5. Look for architectural distortion
6. Look for straight lines superimposed on normal scalloped contour
7. Compare left with right side
8. Don't stop looking after one lesion is found

MAMMOGRAPHIC TECHNIQUE

BEAM QUALITY

Molybdenum target material with characteristic emission peaks of 17.9 + 19.5 keV (lower average energy than tungsten)

FOCAL SPOT

0.1–0.4 mm (0.1 mm for magnification views)

TUBE OUTPUT

80–100 mA

EXPOSURE

(a) without grid: 25 kV (optimum between contrast + penetration), exposure time of 1.0 seconds
(b) with grid: 26–27 kV; exposure time of 2.3 seconds
(c) microfocus magnification: 26–27 kV; 1.5–2.0 times magnification with 16–30 cm air gap
(d) specimen radiography: 22–24 kV

FILTER

(a) beryllium window (absorbs less radiation than glass tube)
(b) molybdenum filter (0.03 mm): allows more of lower energy radiation to reach breast

BREAST

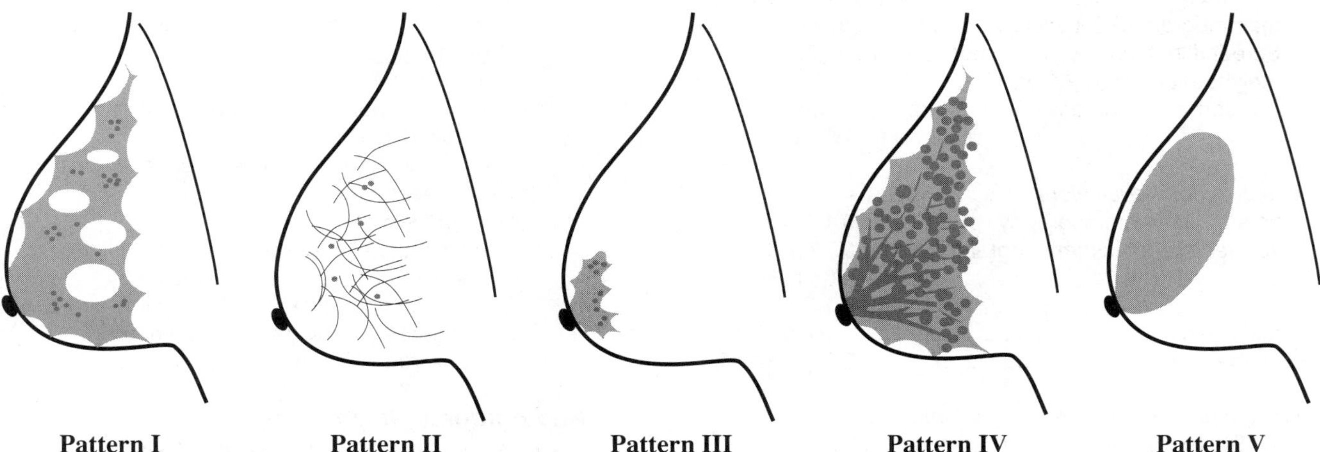

Parenchymal Breast Pattern

REDUCTION OF SCATTER RADIATION
(1) adequate compression (also improves contrast + decreases radiation dose)
(2) beam collimation to <8–10 cm
(3) air gap with microfocus magnification
(greater spatial resolution, 2–3-fold increase in radiation exposure)
(4) Moving grid
grid if compressed breast >5 cm / very dense breast (facilitates perception, 2–3-fold increase in radiation exposure)

SCREEN-FILM COMBINATION
(1) Intensifying screen phosphor
single screen systems
(2) Film-screen contact
(3) Mammography film with minimal base fog, sufficient maximum density + contrast

FILM PROCESSING
(1) Processing time of 3 minutes (42–45 seconds in developing fluid) superior to 90-second processor for double-emulsion film (which creates underdevelopment + compensatory higher radiation exposure)
(2) Developing temperature of 35°C (95°F)
(3) Developing fluid replenishment rate:
450–500 mL replenisher per square meter of film

QUALITY CONTROL
(1) Processor (daily)
with sensito- / densitometric measurements
(a) base fog <0.16–0.17
(b) maximum density >3.50
(c) contrast >1.9–2.0
(2) X-ray unit (semiannually)
(a) beam quality
(b) phototimer

Average glandular dose:
<0.6 mGy per breast for nonmagnification film-screen mammogram (ACR accreditation requirement)
Screen/film technique (molybdenum target; 0.03 mm molybdenum filter, 28 kVp):
mean absorbed dose: 0.05 rad for CC view
0.06 rad for LAT view

Effective dose equivalent H_E:

screen-film mammography	0.11 mSv
xeroradiographic mammography	0.78 mSv
chest	0.05 mSv
skull	0.15 mSv
abdomen	1.40 mSv
lumbar spine	2.20 mSv

Advantages of magnification mammography
1. Sharpness effect = increased resolution
2. Noise effect = noise reduced by a factor equal to the degree of magnification
3. Air-gap effect = increased contrast by reduction in scattered radiation
4. Visual effect = improved perception and analysis of small detail

Factors Affecting Mammographic Image Quality

Radiographic Sharpness
= subjective impression of distinctness / perceptibility of structure boundary / edge
1. **Radiographic contrast**
= magnitude of optical density difference between structure of interest + surroundings influenced by
(a) subject contrast
= ratio of x-ray intensity transmitted through one part of the breast to that transmitted through a more absorbing adjacent part; affected by
— absorption differences in the breast (thickness, density, atomic number)
— radiation quality (target material, kilovoltage, filtration)
— scattered radiation (beam limitation, grid, compression)
(b) receptor contrast
= component of radiographic contrast that determines how the x-ray intensity pattern will be related to the optical density pattern in the mammogram
affected by
— film type
— processing (chemicals, temperature, time, agitation)
— photographic density
— fog (storage, safelight, light leaks)
2. **Radiographic blurring**
= lateral spreading of a structural boundary (= distance over which the optical density between the structure and its surroundings changes)
(a) motion
reduced by compression + short exposure time
(b) geometric blurring
affected by
— focal spot: size, shape, intensity distribution
— focus-object distance (= cone length)
— object-image distance
(c) receptor blurring
= light diffusion (= spreading of the light emitted by the screen) affected by
— phosphor thickness + particle size
— light-absorbing dyes + pigments
— screen-film contact

Radiographic Noise
= unwanted fluctuation in optical density
1. **Radiographic mottle**
= optical density variations consist of

(a) receptor graininess
= optical density variation from random distribution of finite number of silver halide grains

(b) quantum mottle (principal contributor to mottle)
= variation in optical density from random spatial distribution of x-ray quanta absorbed in image receptor

affected by
— film speed + contrast
— screen absorption + conversion efficiency
— light diffusion
— radiation quality

(c) structure mottle
= optical density fluctuation from nonuniformity in the structure of the image receptor (eg, phosphor layer of intensifying screen)

2. **Artifacts**
= unwanted optical density variations in the form of blemishes on the mammogram

(a) improper film handling (static, crimp marks, fingerprints, scratches)
(b) improper exposure (fog)
(c) improper processing (streaks, spots, scratches)
(d) dirt + stains

BREAST DISORDERS

BREAST CANCER

Incidence: 1.5–4.5 cases per 1,000 women per year
Origin: terminal ductal lobular unit

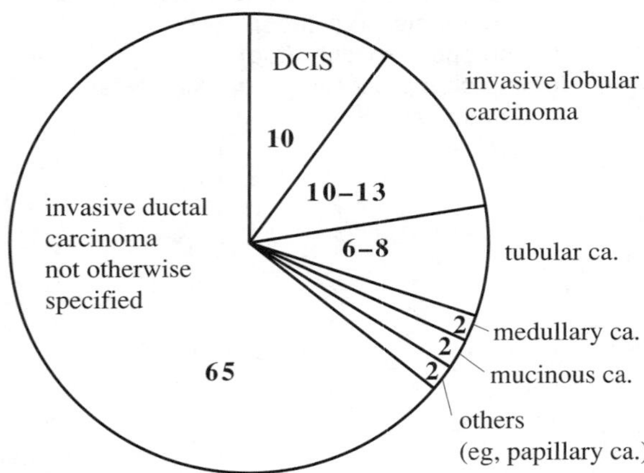

Distribution of Breast Cancers in Screening Population
(numbers are percentages)

A. NONINVASIVE BREAST CANCER (15%)
= malignant transformation of epithelial cells lining mammary ducts + lobules confined within boundaries of basement membrane
Rx: few data are available to provide insight into proper treatment

1. **Ductal carcinoma in situ** (DCIS)
= intraductal carcinoma
Incidence: 10–25–40% in screening population; 70% of noninvasive carcinomas
Age: most >55 years
Histo: heterogeneous group of malignancies originating within extralobular terminal duct + without invasion of basement membrane
<u>Subgroups</u>: comedocarcinoma, non-comedocarcinomas (solid, micropapillary, cribriform)
• may persist for years without palpable abnormality (in screening population)
• palpable mass / Paget disease of nipple / nipple discharge (in symptomatic patients)
◊ 50% of DCIS are >5 cm in size
◊ Histologic size of DCIS is independent of histologic subgroup
◊ Almost all "comedo" type DCIS contain significant microcalcifications
◊ DCIS often involves the nipple + subareolar ducts
Spectrum of mammographic findings:
√ calcifications only (72%)
√ soft-tissue abnormality + calcification (12%)
√ soft-tissue abnormality only (10%)
√ nonvisible (6%)
MR (40–100% sensitive):
√ linear contrast enhancement
Prognosis: 20–50% develop invasive disease 5–10 years after initial diagnosis of DCIS
Rx: (1) Simple / modified mastectomy: cure rate of almost 100%
(2) Local excision alone: 25% rate of recurrence within 26 months in immediate vicinity of biopsy site
(3) Local excision + radiotherapy: 2–17% rate of recurrence
Treatment problems:
1. Occult invasion in 5–20% of patients
2. Multifocality (= >1 focus in same quadrant of breast)
3. Multicentricity (= >1 focus in different quadrants of breast) in 14% of lesions <25 mm, in 100% of lesions >50 mm
4. Axillary metastases in 1–2%

(a) *high nuclear grade DCIS* ("**comedo type**")
Prevalence: 60% of all DCIS
Precursor: none; one stage development
Path: "comedo" = pluglike appearance of necrotic material that can be expressed from the cut surface
Characteristics:
– nuclear grade: large / intermediate nuclei, <u>numerous mitoses</u>, aneuploidy
– growth pattern: predominantly <u>solid cell proliferation</u>; atypically micropapillary / cribriform
– necrosis: extensive (HALLMARK)
– calcifications (90%): dystrophic / amorphous within necrosis in center of dilated ductal system outlining most of the lobe in classic solid growth pattern
• estrogen- + progesterone-receptor negative
• overexpression of c-erb B-2 oncogene product and P53 suppressor gene mutation
• often symptomatic lesion with nipple discharge
√ ductal system enlarged to 300–350 μm
√ linear / branching pattern of calcifications scattered in a large part of lobe / whole lobe
√ large solid high-density casting calcifications (fragmented, coalesced, irregular) in solid growth pattern
√ "snake skin–like" / "birch tree flowerlike" <u>dotted casting calcifications</u> within necrosis of micropapillary / cribriform growth pattern
√ palpable dominant mass without calcifications (very unusual)
√ nipple discharge (rare)

Prognosis: higher recurrence rate than noncomedo-group

(b) *low nuclear grade DCIS* ("**noncomedo** type")
Prevalence: 40% of all DCIS
Precursor lesion:
atypical ductal hyperplasia (ADH) with slight / moderate / severe atypia
◊ 52–56% of ADH at core biopsy are associated with malignancy at excision!
Characteristics:
- nuclear grade: monomorphic small round nuclei, few / no mitoses
- growth pattern: predominantly micropapillary / cribriform; atypically solid cell proliferation (often coexist)
- necrosis: not present in classic micropapillary / cribriform growth pattern
- calcifications (50%): laminated / psammoma-like due to active secretion by malignant cells into duct lumen

√ fine granular "cotton ball" calcifications in micropapillary / cribriform growth pattern
√ coarse granular "crushed stone" / "broken needle tip" / "arrowhead" calcifications in less common solid growth pattern
◊ Size of "noncomedo" DCIS often underestimated mammographically (? due to lower density of calcifications at periphery of lesion)!
√ palpable dominant mass without calcifications (intracystic papillary carcinoma, multifocal papillary carcinoma in situ)
√ nonpalpable asymmetric density with architectural distortion
√ occasionally serous / bloody nipple discharge + ductal filling defects on galactography
Risk of recurrence: 2%
Prognosis: 30% eventually develop into invasive cancer
Dx: surgical biopsy
◊ Core needle biopsy could result in diagnosis of only proliferative breast disease that is usually intermixed!

2. **Lobular carcinoma in situ** (LCIS)
= arises in epithelium of blunt ducts of mammary lobules
Incidence: 0.8–3.6% in screening population; 3–6 % of all breast malignancies; 25% of noninvasive carcinomas; high incidence during reproductive age but decreasing with age
Age: most 40–54 years (earlier than DCIS / invasive tumors)
Histo: monomorphous small cell population filling + expanding ductules of the lobule
◊ Synchronous invasive cancer in 5%!
• not palpable
√ mammographically occult
√ may atypically present as a noncalcified mass (in 7%), calcifications + mass (in 10%), asymmetric opacity (2%)
◊ High frequency of multicentricity (70%) + bilaterality (30%)!
Dx: incidental microscopic finding depending on accident of biopsy (performed for unrelated reasons + findings)
Prognosis:
20–30% develop invasive ductal > lobular carcinoma within 20 years after initial diagnosis
◊ 1% per year lifetime risk for invasive malignancy
◊ LCIS serves as a marker of increased risk for developing invasive carcinoma in either breast!
Rx: recommendations range from observation (with follow-up examinations every 3–6 months + annual mammograms) to unilateral / bilateral simple mastectomy

3. **Intracystic papillary carcinoma in situ** (0.5–2%)
= rare variant of noncomedo DCIS
Age: usually older postmenopausal woman; peak prevalence between 34 and 52 years
Histo: papillary fronds within the wall of a cystically dilated duct
• well-circumscribed + freely movable
• aspiration yields straw-colored / dark red / brown fluid (due to ruptured capillaries in cyst wall / necrosis of tumor cells); reaccumulation of fluid within 3–4 weeks
• fluid cytology negative for cancer in 80%
√ mean tumor size of 1.9 cm (range 0.4–7.5 cm) due to fast growth (from accumulation of fluid + proliferation of neoplastic cells)
√ intracystic mass on pneumocystography
√ solid intracystic mass on US
√ round benign appearing mass with sharply circumscribed lobulated borders on mammography
Rx: lumpectomy
Prognosis: 10-year survival of 100%; 10-year disease-free survival rate of 91%
DDx for mammogram: mucinous / medullary ca., hematoma, metastasis

B. INVASIVE BREAST CANCER (85%)
MR:
√ peripheral / rim enhancement

1. **Infiltrating / invasive ductal carcinoma** (65%) of no special type / otherwise not specified (NOS)
10% false-negative ratio
Histo:
grade I = well-differentiated
grade II = moderately differentiated
grade III = poorly differentiated
• palpable in 70%
• larger by palpation than on mammogram
√ spiculated mass (36%) is PRINCIPAL FINDING
√ malignant calcifications (45–60%)

BREAST

2. **Infiltrating / invasive lobular carcinoma** (5–10%)
= neoplasm arising from terminal ductules of breast lobules
◊ 2nd most common type of breast cancer; 30–50% of patients will develop a second primary in same / opposite breast within 20 years
◊ Most frequently missed breast cancer (difficult to detect mammographically + clinically) with 19–43% false-negative rate (occult in dense breast)
Median age: 45–56 years; 2% of all ILC occur in women <35 years
Path: multicentricity + bilaterality (in up to 1/3); tendency to grow around ducts, vessels, and lobules without destruction of anatomic structures (targetoid growth); no substantial connective tissue reaction
Histo: 20% grade I, 64% grade II, 16% grade III
Metastases: GI tract, gynecologic organs, peritoneum, retroperitoneum, carcinomatous meningitis
• palpable in 69%:
  • area of subtle skin thickening / induration
  • large hard mass / fine nodularity
√ architectural distortion (= retraction of normal glandular tissue with thickening + disturbance of fibrous septa) in 18–30% is MOST COMMON MAMMOGRAPHIC FINDING
Histo: straight single file of uniform small cells with round oval nuclei ("Indian files") growing around ducts resulting in subtle changes in architecture
√ irregular spiculated mass >1 cm (16–28%)
√ poorly defined mass ± spicules <1 cm (22%)
√ asymmetric opacity (= ill-defined area of increased opacity without central tumor nidus) in 8–19%
√ round / ovoid mass with regular borders (1%)
√ microcalcifications (0–24%)
√ retraction of skin (25%) + nipple (26%)
√ skin thickening
◊ May be evident on ONLY one standard view CC > ML > MLO view)!
N.B.: difficulties in early diagnosis result in disproportionate potential for malpractice suits!

3. **Tubular carcinoma** (6–8%)
= well-differentiated form of ductal carcinoma
(a) low grade: bilateral in 1:3
(b) high grade: bilateral in 1:300
Associated with: lobular carcinoma in situ in 40%
Mean age: 40–49 years
• positive family history in 40%
• nonpalpable
√ high-opacity nodule with spiculated margins
√ <17 mm in diameter; mean diameter of 8 mm
DDx: radial scar

4. **Medullary carcinoma** (2%)
= SOLID CIRCUMSCRIBED CARCINOMA
◊ Fastest growing breast cancer!
Path: well-circumscribed mass with nodular architecture + lobulated contour; central necrosis is common in larger tumors; reminiscent of medullary cavity of bone
Histo: intense lymphoplasmocytic reaction (reflecting host resistance); propensity for syncytial growth; no glands
Incidence: 11% of breast cancers in women <35 years of age; 40–50% of medullary cancers in women <50 years of age
Mean age: 46–54 years
• softer than average breast cancer
√ well-defined round / oval noncalcified uniformly dense mass (hemorrhage) with lobulated margin
√ may have partial / complete halo sign
US:
  √ hypoechoic mass with some degree of through transmission
  √ distinct / indistinct margins
  √ large central cystic component
DDx: fibroadenoma
Prognosis: 92% 10-year survival rate

5. **Mucinous / colloid carcinoma** (1.5–2%)
Path:
(a) *pure form:* aggregates of tumor cells surrounded by abundant pools of extracellular mucin (gelatinous / colloid fluid)
(b) *mixed form:* contains areas of infiltrating ductal carcinoma not surrounded by mucin
Age: 1% in women <35 years; 7% of carcinomas in women >75 years
• slow growth rate of pure form
• "swish" / "crush" sensation during palpation
• 60% estrogen-receptor positive
√ well-circumscribed usually lobulated mass of round / ovoid shape
√ pleomorphic clustered / clumped amorphous / punctate calcifications (rare)
√ may enlarge fast (through mucin production)
√ solid mass on US
Prognosis: favorable

6. **Papillary carcinoma** (1–2–4%)
= rare ductal carcinoma forming papillary structures
N.B.: Do not confuse with micropapillary / cribriform growth pattern of ductal carcinoma
Histo: multilayered papillary projections extending from vascularized stalks; no myoepithelial layer (as in benign lesions); neurosecretory granules + positive CEA-reactivity in 85% (absent in benign lesions)
Types:
(a) multiple intraductal carcinomas with papillary configuration
(b) Intracystic papillary carcinoma
= in situ malignancy
(c) invasive carcinoma with papillary growth pattern (microscopic frond formation)

Age: 25–89 (mean 50–60) years; peak age of 40–75 years
• palpable mass (67%)
• nipple discharge (22–35%) often tinged with blood
• rich in estrogen and progesterone receptors
Location: single nodule in central portion of breast; multiple nodules extending from subareolar area to periphery of breast
√ multinodular pattern (55%) = lobulated mass / cluster of well-defined contiguous nodules
√ solitary well-circumscribed round / ovoid nodule with average diameter of 2–3 cm
√ usually confined to single quadrant
√ associated microcalcifications in 60%
√ multiple filling defects / disruption of an irregular duct segment / complete obstruction of duct system at galactography
US:
√ solid hypoechoic mass with lobulated smooth margins + acoustic enhancement
√ ± blood flow on color Doppler
Prognosis: 90% 5-year survival after simple mastectomy + axillary node dissection
DDx: solitary central duct papilloma; multiple peripheral benign papillomas

C. PAGET DISEASE OF THE NIPPLE (5%)

D. INFLAMMATORY BREAST CARCINOMA
= tumor emboli within dermal lymphatics (angiolymphatic spread)
Prevalence: 1–4% of breast cancers
Age: 52 years (on average)
Histo: infiltrating ductal carcinoma
Location: L > R breast; bilaterality in 30–55%
• rapid symptomatic development over 1/3 of breast surface:
  • palpable tumor (63%)
  • erythema of skin (13–64%)
  • peau d'orange edema of skin (13%)
  • nipple retraction (13%)
• palpable axillary adenopathy (up to 91%)
√ tumor mass ± malignant-type calcifications
√ diffusely increased breast density
√ stromal coarsening (50%)
√ thickening of Cooper ligaments
√ extensive skin thickening (71%)
Dx: skin biopsy
Prognosis: 2% 5-year survival; median survival time of 7 months (untreated) + 18 months (after radical mastectomy)
DDx: breast abscess

Epidemiology of Breast Cancer

Incidence:
2–5 breast cancers/1,000 women; in USA >142,000 new cases per year (of which 25,000 are in situ); 25% of all female malignancies
◊ One of 9 women will develop breast cancer during her life!
Age: 0.3–2% in women <30 years of age;
15% in women <40 years of age;
85% in women >30 years of age
Mortality: 43,000 deaths per year
◊ Death rate has remained stable for past 60 years!

Risk Factors (increasing risk):

A. DEMOGRAPHIC FACTORS
• increasing age (66% of cancers in women >50 years):

Age	*Prevalence of Cancer*	
25	5:100,000	1:19,608
40	80:100,000	1:1,250
45	1075:100,000	1:93
50	180:100,000	1:555
55	3030:100,000	1:33
60	240:100,000	1:416

Relative Risk Compared with Woman of Age 60:

30 years of age	0.07	60 years of age	1.00
35 years of age	0.19	70 years of age	1.27
40 years of age	0.35	80 years of age	1.45
50 years of age	0.71		

Predictive Values of Radiographic Signs for Malignancy

1. Classic mammographic findings of malignancy + palpable abnormality 100%
(only 3% of cancers present this way)
2. Classic mammographic findings of malignancy + NO palpable finding 74%
(only 6% of cancers present this way)
3. Indeterminate mammographic features + palpable mass 11%
4. Indeterminate mass + no palpable finding 5%
5. Mammographically benign mass 2%
6. Asymmetric density (mass questionable) + clinical finding 4%
7. Asymmetric density (mass questionable) + NO clinical finding 0%
8. Microcalcifications + clinical abnormality 25%
9. Microcalcifications + NO clinical abnormality 21%
(>3 punctate irregular microcalcifications in area <1 cm^2)
10. Vein dilatation 0%
11. Skin thickening 0%
12. Duct dilatation 0%

- Jewish women + nuns
- upper > lower social class
- unmarried > married women
- Whites > Blacks after age 40

B. REPRODUCTIVE VARIABLES

- nulliparous > parous:

Relative Risk Compared with Nulliparous:

age at 1st pregnancy	<19 years	0.5
age at 1st pregnancy	20–30 years	—
age at 1st pregnancy	30–34 years	1.0
age at 1st pregnancy	>35 years	>1.0

- first full-term pregnancy after age 35: 2 x risk
- low parity > high parity
- early age at menarche (<12 years): relative risk compared with onset of regular ovulatory cycle:

	Menarche <12	*Menarche >12*
immediately	3.7	1.6
1–4 years	2.3	1.6

- late age at menopause: relative risk compared with menopause before age 44 years:
  - natural menopause >55 years of age 2.0
- early bilateral oophorectomy: relative risk compared with menopause between ages 45–49 years:
  - artificial menopause at 50–54 years 1.34
  - artificial menopause before age 45 0.77

C. MULTIPLE PRIMARY CANCERS

- 4–5 x increase in risk for cancer in contralateral breast
- increased risk after ovarian + endometrial cancer

D. FAMILY HISTORY

- breast cancer in first-degree relative
  Relative risk compared with negative family Hx:
  - (+) for mother 1.8
  - (+) for sister 2.5
  - (+) for mother + sister 5.6
- 25% of patients with carcinoma have a positive family history
- carcinoma tends to affect successive generations approx. 10 years earlier

E. BENIGN BREAST DISEASE

- 2–4 x increased risk with atypical hyperplasia: relative risk compared with no biopsy:

benign breast disease in all patients	1.5
nonproliferative disease	0.9
proliferative disease without atypia	1.6
fibroadenoma + hyperplasia	3.5
atypical duct hyperplasia (ADH)	
no family history of breast cancer	4.4
family history of breast cancer	8.9

F. MAMMOGRAPHIC FEATURES

- prominent duct pattern + extremely dense breasts according to Wolfe classification N1 (0.14%), P1 (0.52%), P2 (1.95%), DY (5.22%)

G. RADIATION EXPOSURE

excess risk of 3.5–6 cases per 1,000,000 women per year per rad after a minimum latent period of 10 years (atomic bomb, fluoroscopy during treatment of tuberculosis, irradiation for postpartum mastitis)

H. GEOGRAPHY

- Western + industrialized nations (highest incidence)
- Asia, Latin America, Africa (decreased risk)

Breast Cancer Evaluation

A. PRIMARY = LOCALIZING SIGNS OF BREAST CANCER

1. Dominant mass seen on two views with
   (a) *spiculation* = stellate / star-burst appearance (= fine linear strands of tumor extension + desmoplastic response); "scirrhus" caused by:
      (1) infiltrating ductal carcinoma (75% of all invasive cancers)
      (2) invasive lobular carcinoma (occasionally)
      √ mass feels larger than its mammographic / sonographic size
      DDx: prior biopsy / trauma / infection
   (b) *smooth border*
      (1) intracystic carcinoma (rare): subareolar area; bloody aspiration
      (2) medullary carcinoma: soft tumor
      (3) mucinous / colloid carcinoma: soft tumor
      (4) papillary carcinoma
      √ "telltale" signs: lobulation, small comet tail, flattening of one side of the lesion, slight irregularity
      √ halo sign (= Mach band) may be present
      DDx: cyst (sonographic evaluation)
   (c) *lobulation*
      Appearance similar to fibroadenoma (only characteristic calcifications may exclude malignancy)
      ◊ The likelihood of malignancy increases with number of lobulations
      • clinical size of mass > radiographic size (Le Borgne's law)
2. Asymmetric density = star-shaped lesion
   √ distinct central tumor mass with volumetric rather than planar appearance (additional coned compression views!)
   √ denser relative to other areas (= vessels + trabeculae cannot be seen within high-density lesion)
   √ fat does not traverse density
   √ corona of spicules

BREAST

√ in any quadrant (but fatty replacement occurs last in upper outer quadrant)
DDx: postsurgical fibrosis, traumatic fat necrosis, sclerosing duct hyperplasia

3. Microcalcifications
Associated with malignant mass by mammogram in 40%, pathologically with special stains in 60%, on specimen radiography in 86%
◊ 20% of clustered microcalcifications represent a malignant process!
(a) *shape:* fragmented, irregular contour, polymorphic, casting rod-shaped without polarity, Y-shaped branching pattern, granular "salt and pepper" pattern, reticular pattern
(b) *density:* various densities
(c) *size:* 100–300 μm (usually); rarely up to 2 mm
(d) *distribution:* tight cluster over an area of 1 cm^2 or less is most suggestive; coursing along ductal system seen in ductal carcinoma with comedo elements

4. Architectural distortion
due to desmoplastic reaction
√ ragged irregular border
DDx: postsurgical fibrosis

5. Interval change
(a) neodensity = de novo developing density (in 6% malignant)
(b) enlarging mass (malignant in 10–15%)

6. Enlarged single duct
(low probability for cancer in asymptomatic woman with normal breast palpation)
√ solitary dilated duct >3 cm long
DDx: inspissated debris / blood, papilloma

7. Diffuse increase in density (late finding)
Cause: (1) plugging of dermal lymphatics with tumor cells
(2) less flattening of sclerotic + fibrous elements of neoplasm in comparison with more compressible fibroglandular breast tissue

B. SECONDARY = NONLOCALIZING SIGNS OF BREAST CANCER

1. Asymmetric thickening
2. Asymmetric ducts, especially if discontinuous with subareolar area
3. Skin changes
(a) retraction = dimpling of skin
from desmoplastic reaction causing shortening of Cooper ligaments / direct extension of tumor to skin
DDx: trauma, biopsy, abscess, burns
(b) skin thickening secondary to blocked lymphatic drainage / tumor in lymphatics
• peau d'orange
DDx: normal in inframammary region
4. Nipple / areolar abnormalities
(a) retraction / flattening of nipple
DDx: normal variant
(b) Paget disease = eczematoid appearance of nipple + areola in ductal carcinoma
√ associated with ductal calcifications toward the nipple
DDx: nipple eczema
(c) nipple discharge
• spontaneous persistent discharge
• need not be bloody
DDx: lactational discharge
5. Abnormal veins
venous diameter ratio of >1.4:1 in 75% of cancers; late sign + thus not very important
6. Axillary nodes (sign of advanced / occult cancer)
√ >1.5 cm without fatty center
DDx: reactive hyperplasia

LOCATION OF BREAST MASSES
benign + malignant masses are of similar distribution
@ upper outer quadrant (54%)
@ upper inner quadrant (14%)
@ lower outer quadrant (10%)
@ lower inner quadrant (7%)
@ retroareolar (15%)
◊ Mediolateral oblique view is important part of screening because it includes largest portion of breast tissue + considers most common location of cancers!

Metastatic Breast Cancer

@ Axillary lymph adenopathy
Incidence: 40–74%
Risk for positive nodes: 30% if primary >1 cm, 15% if primary <1 cm
@ Bone
@ Liver
Incidence: 48–60%
US: √ hypoechoic (83%) / hyperechoic (17%) masses

Screening of Asymptomatic Patients

Definition of screening (World Health Organization):
A screening test must
(a) be adequately sensitive and specific
(b) be reproducible in its results
(c) identify previously undiagnosed disease
(d) be affordable
(e) be acceptable to the public
(f) include follow-up services

Guidelines of American Cancer Society, American College of Radiology, American Medical Association, National Cancer Institute:

1. Breast self-examination to begin at age 20
2. Breast examination by physician every 3 years between 20–40 years, in yearly intervals after age 40
3. Baseline mammogram between age 35–40; follow-up screening based upon parenchymal pattern + family history
4. Initial screening at 30 years if patient has first-degree relative with breast cancer in premenopausal years; follow-up screening based upon parenchymal pattern

BREAST

5. Mammography at yearly intervals after age 40
6. All women who have had prior breast cancer require annual follow-up

Additional recommendations:

1. Screening at 2-year intervals for women >70 years
2. Baseline mammogram 10 years earlier than age of mother / sister when their cancer was diagnosed

Rate of detected abnormalities
30 abnormalities in 1,000 screening mammograms:
20–23 benign lesions
7–10 cancers

Acceptable recall rate for screening examination:
10% for initial prevalence screening;
5% for subsequent incidence screening

Interval cancers:
10–20% of cancers surface between annual screenings

Value of Screening Mammography

Indication:
decrease in cancer mortality through earlier detection + intervention when tumor size small + lymph nodes negative; tumor grade of no prognostic significance in tumors <10 mm in size

1. Health Insurance Plan (HIP) 1963–1969
randomized controlled study of 62,000 women aged 40–64
   - 25–30% reduction in mortality in women >50 years (followed for 18 years)
   - 25% reduction in mortality in women 40–49 years (followed for 18 years); no significant effect at 5- and 10-year follow-up
   - 19% of cancers found by mammography alone
   - 61% of cancers found at physical examination
   - effectiveness of screening <50 years of age is uncertain
2. Breast Cancer Detection Demonstration Project (BCDDP) 1973–1980
4,443 cancers found in 283,000 asymptomatic volunteers
   - 41.6% of cancers found by mammography alone (77% with negative nodes)
   - 8.7% of cancers found by physical examination alone
   - 59% of noninfiltrating cancers found by mammography alone
   - 25% of cancers were intraductal (vs. 5% in previous series)
   - 21% of cancers found in women aged 40–49 years (mammography alone detected 35.4%)
   - 51% of cancers found with both mammography + physical examination
3. Two-county Swedish trial 1977–1990
randomized controlled study of 78,000 women in study group + 56,700 in control group aged 40–74 years
(a) single MLO mammogram at 2-year intervals for women <50 years of age
(b) single MLO mammogram at 3-year intervals for women ≥50 years of age
   - 40% reduction in mortality at 7 years in women 50–74 years
   - 0% reduction in mortality at 7 years in women 40–49 years
4. Metaanalysis of combined results of 5 Swedish trials for women aged 39–49
   - 29% reduction in breast cancer mortality with screening mammograms offered at intervals from 18 to 28 months

OCCULT VERSUS PALPABLE CANCERS
27% are occult cancers (NO age difference)
Positive axillary nodes: occult cancers (19%); palpable cancers (44%)
10-year survival: occult cancers (65%); palpable cancers (25%)

Role of Mammography

Overall detection rate:
58–69%; 8% if <1 cm in size

Mammographic accuracy:
88% correctly diagnosed by radiologist
27% detected only by mammography
8% misinterpretations
4% not detected
15–30% positive predictive value (national average): 25% PPV for women in 5th decade; 50% PPV for women in 8th decade

Mammographically Missed Cancers

False-negative screening mammogram = pathologic diagnosis of breast cancer within 1 year after negative mammogram with the following types of misses:
(a) lesion could not be seen in retrospect (25–33%) = "acute cancer" = cancer surfacing in screening interval
(b) cancer undetected by first reader but correctly identified by second reader (14%)
(c) visible in retrospect on prior mammogram (61%)

Incidence: approx. 4–15–34% of all cancers; approx. 3 cancers:2,000 mammograms; 5–15–22% of palpable breast cancers

◊ A second reader will detect an additional 5–15% of cancers!

Cause:

1. Interpretation error (52%):
(a) benign appearance (18%): medullary carcinoma, colloid carcinoma, intracystic papillary carcinoma, some infiltrating ductal carcinomas
(b) present on previous mammogram (17%)
(c) seen on one view only (9%)
(d) site of previous biopsy (8%)
2. Observer error (30–43%):
(a) overlooked
(b) presence of an obvious finding leads to overlooking of a more subtle lesion = "satisfied search" phenomenon

BREAST

(c) no knowledge of clinical finding
(d) rushed interpretation
(e) heavy caseload
(f) extraneous distraction
(g) eye fatigue
(h) inexperience

3. Technical error (5%):
   (a) inadequate radiographic technique: improper positioning, inadequate compression, under- / overexposed image, poor screen-film contact, geometric motion blurring
   (b) failure to image region of interest
   (c) suboptimal viewing conditions: inadequate luminance of view boxes, extraneous view box light, high ambient room light
4. Tumor biology:
   (a) small tumor size
   (b) failure to incite desmoplastic reaction (eg, invasive lobular carcinoma)
   (c) limitations of screen-film mammography in physically dense breasts
   (d) no associated microcalcifications (approx. 50% of cancers)
   (e) developing soft-tissue radiopacity
   (f) stability of mammographic findings
      ◊ Malignant calcifications may be stable for up to 63 months
      ◊ A mass may not change for up to 4.5 years

Location of missed cancers:
retroglandular area (33%), lateral parenchyma (31%), central (18%), medial (13%), subareolar (4%)

Radiation-induced Breast Carcinoma

◊ Lifetime risk with cumulative carcinogenic effect related to age!
(a) women age <35: 7.5 additional cancers per 1 million irradiated women per year per rad
(b) women age >35: 3.5 additional cancers per 1 million irradiated women per year per rad

Role of Breast Ultrasound

Indications:
◊ Ultrasound is no screening tool!
A. TARGETED EXAM
   (1) Initial study of palpable lump in patient <30 years of age / pregnant / lactating
      ◊ Ultrasound will not add useful information in an area that contains only fatty tissue on a mammogram!
   (2) Characterization of mammographic / palpable mass as fluid-filled / solid
      ◊ Ultrasound will add useful information if there is water-density tissue in the area of palpable abnormality!
      ◊ Differentiation of cystic from solid lesion is the principal role of ultrasound!
   (3) additional evaluation of nonpalpable abnormality with uncertain mammographic diagnosis
   (4) search for focal lesion as cause for mammographic asymmetric density
   (5) confirmation of lesion seen in one mammographic projection only
B. WHOLE-BREAST EXAM
   (1) Breast secretions
   (2) Suspected leaks from silicone implant
   (3) Follow-up of multiple known mammographic / sonographic lesions
   (4) Radiographically dense breast with strong family history of breast cancer
   (5) Metastases thought to be of breast origin, but with negative clinical + mammographic exam
   (6) Mammography not possible: "radiophobic" patient, bedridden patient, after mastectomy
C. INTERVENTIONAL PROCEDURE
   (1) Ultrasound-guided cyst aspiration
   (2) Ultrasound-guided core biopsy
   (3) Ultrasound-guided ductography, if
      (a) secretions cannot be expressed
      (b) duct cannot be cannulated

Accuracy: 98% accuracy for cysts; 99% accuracy for solid masses; small carcinomas have the least characteristic features

Role of Breast MRI

Indications: ambiguous mammographic findings; positive clinical examination + negative mammographic/sonographic findings; staging prior to excisional biopsy; assessment of residual disease after excision; axillary node malignancy with unknown primary site
Sensitivity: 72–93–100%
MR:
√ rapid increase in signal intensity after contrast injection reaching a markedly higher amplitude than parenchymal tissue, followed by a plateau + early washout
   DDx: fibroadenoma in premenopausal patient, ductal hyperplasia ± atypia, lobular neoplasia, inflammatory disease, scar <6 months old in nonirradiated breast, scar <18 months old in irradiated breast, fibrocystic change (apocrine metaplasia, sclerosing adenosis)
√ intense early rim / peripheral enhancement (± central necrosis)
√ malignant mass margination

Role of Stereotactic Biopsy

Indications: obviously malignant nonpalpable lesion, indeterminate likely benign lesion, anxiety over lesion
Types: well-defined solid mass, indistinct / spiculated mass, clustered microcalcifications
Advantage: single-stage surgical procedure

Problematic: 3–5-mm small lesion, fine scattered microcalcifications, indistinct density, area of architectural distortion

Excision:
radial scar suspected (in up to 28% associated with tubular carcinoma), lesion close to chest wall, lesion in axillary tail, very superficial lesion, atypia / atypical hyperplasia (in 49–61% associated with malignancy), carcinoma in situ (in 9–20% associated with invasion), branching microcalcifications suggestive of DCIS with comedo necrosis

Sensitivity: 85–99% with core needle biopsy (100% specific), 68–93% with fine-needle aspiration (88–100% specific)

Miss rate: 3–8% for stereotactic biopsy, 3% for surgery

BREAST CYST

Incidence: most common single cause of breast lumps between 35 and 55 years of age

Age: any; most common in later reproductive years + around menopause

Histo: cyst wall lined by single layer of
(a) flattened epithelial cells; cyst fluid with Na^+/K^+ ratio ≥3
(b) epithelial cells with apocrine metaplasia (secretory function); cyst fluid with Na^+/K^+ ratio <3

Cause: fluid cannot be absorbed due to obstruction of extralobular terminal duct by fibrosis / intraductal epithelial proliferation

• size changes over time

Simple Breast Cyst

√ well-defined flattened oval / round (if under pressure) mammographic mass + surrounding halo (DDx: well-defined solid mass)
√ solitary / multiple
√ needle aspiration of fluid (proof) + postaspiration mammogram as new baseline

US (98–100% accuracy):
◊ Correlate with palpation / mammogram as to size, shape, location, surrounding tissue density!
√ spherical / ovoid lesion with anechoic center
√ well-circumscribed thin echogenic capsule
√ posterior acoustic enhancement (may be difficult to demonstrate in small / deeply situated cysts)
√ thin edge shadows
√ occasionally multilocular ± thin septations / cluster of cysts

PNEUMOCYSTOGRAPHY (for symptomatic cysts):
√ air remains mammographically detectable for up to 3 weeks
√ therapeutic effect of air insufflation (equal to 60–70% of aspirated fluid volume): no cyst recurrence in 85–94% (40–45% cyst recurrence without air insufflation)

Complex Breast Cyst

= any cyst that does not meet criteria of simple cyst

Cause: fibrocystic changes (vast majority), infection, malignancy (extremely rare)
◊ 0.3% of all breast cancers are intracystic

◊ Patients with apocrine cysts are at greater risk to develop breast cancer!
√ uniformly thick wall + tenderness = inflammation / infection
√ diffuse low-level internal echoes (= "foam" cyst)
(a) with mobility upon increase in power output = subcellular material like protein globs, floating cholesterol crystals, cellular debris
(b) without mobility upon increase in power output = cells like foamy macrophages, apocrine metaplasia, epithelial cells, pus, blood
√ fluid-debris level
Rx: aspiration to rule out blood / pus
√ thick septation / eccentric wall thickening further characterized by protruding ill-defined outer margin, convex microlobulated inner margin ("mural nodule"), nonmobile mass with coarse heterogeneous echotexture, CD flow within thickening
Rx: treated like solid nodule
√ spongelike cluster of microcysts
Rx: treated like solid nodule

Rx: complete aspiration (assures benign cause), core needle biopsy (if partially / nonaspiratable)

DDx: artifactual scatter in superficial / deep small cysts, fibroadenoma, papilloma, carcinoma

CYST ASPIRATION
• inspection of cyst fluid:
(a) normal: turbid greenish / grayish / black fluid
(b) abnormal: straw-colored clear fluid / dark blood
√ needle moves within nonaspiratable complex cyst
√ fluid without blood should be discarded
√ bloody fluid should be examined cytologically

CARCINOMA OF MALE BREAST

Incidence: 0.2%; 1,400 new cases/year with 300 deaths;
◊ 3.7% of male breast carcinomas occur in men with Klinefelter syndrome!

Peak age: 60–69 years

At risk: (males with increased estrogen levels)
1. Klinefelter syndrome (20-fold risk over normals): XXY chromosomes
2. Liver disease: cirrhosis, schistosomiasis, malnutrition
3. Radiation therapy to chest
4. Occupational heat exposure (diminished testicular function)
5. Testicular atrophy: injury, mumps-orchitis, undescended testis
6. Jewish background
7. Family history

◊ Gynecomastia is NOT a risk factor!

Histo: infiltrating ductal carcinoma

• firm painless retroareolar / upper-outer-quadrant mass
• breast swelling, bloody nipple discharge, retraction

Location: L > R breast; bilaterality is uncommon

√ resembles scirrhous carcinoma of female breast
√ usually located eccentrically

√ calcifications fewer + more scattered + more round + larger
√ enlarged axillary nodes (in 50% at time of presentation)
√ metastases to pleura, lung, bone, liver
Delay in diagnosis from onset of symptoms: 6–18 months
Rx: surgery, hormonal manipulation (85% estrogen receptor and 75% progesterone receptor positive)
Prognosis: 5-year survival rate for stage 1 = 82–100%, for stage 2 = 44–77%, for stage 3 = 16–45%, for stage 4 = 4–8% (same as for women!)
DDx: breast abscess, gynecomastia, epidermal inclusion cyst

CHRONIC ABSCESS OF BREAST

= COLD ABSCESS usually seen in lactating women
• fever, pain, increased WBC (clinical diagnosis)
• rapid response to antibiotics
Location: most commonly in central / subareolar area
√ ill-defined mass of increased density with flamelike contour
√ secondary changes common: architectural distortion, nipple + areolar retraction, lymphedema, skin thickening, pathologic axillary nodes
√ liquefied center can be aspirated
US:
√ anechoic / nearly anechoic area with posterior enhancement

CYSTOSARCOMA PHYLLOIDES

= GIANT FIBROADENOMA = ADENOSARCOMA
= PHYLLODE TUMOR
= usually benign giant form of intracanalicular fibroadenoma
Incidence: 1: 6,300 examinations; 0.3–1.5% of all breast tumors; 3% of all fibroadenomas
Age: 5th–6th decade (mean age of 45 years, occasionally in women <20 years of age
Histo: similar to fibroadenoma but with increased cellularity + pleomorphism (wide variations in size, shape, differentiation) of its stromal elements; fibroepithelial tumor with leaflike (phylloides) growth pattern = branching projections of tissue into cystic cavities; cavernous structures contain mucus; cystic degeneration + hemorrhage
• rapidly enlarging breast mass; periods of remission
• sense of fullness
• huge, firm, mobile, discrete, lobulated, smooth mass
• discoloration of skin, wide veins, shining skin
√ large noncalcified mass with smooth polylobulated margins mimicking fibroadenoma
√ rapid growth to large size (>6–8 cm), may fill entire breast
US:
√ fluid-filled clefts in large tumors
Prognosis: limited invasion frequently seen; 15–20% recurrence rate if not completely excised
Cx: in 5–10% degeneration into malignant fibrous histiocytoma / fibrosarcoma / liposarcoma / chondrosarcoma / osteosarcoma with local invasion + hematogenous metastases to lung, pleura, bone (axillary metastases quite rare)

DERMATOPATHIC LYMPHADENOPATHY

= benign reactive lymphadenopathy within breast associated with cutaneous rashes
Cause: exfoliative dermatitis, erythroderma, psoriasis, atopic dermatitis, skin infection)
Histo: follicular pattern retained, germinal centers enlarged, enlarged paracortical area with pale-staining cells (lymphocytes, Langerhans cells, interdigitating reticulum cells)
• mobile nontender firm subcutaneous nodules
Location: often bilateral
Site: predominantly upper outer quadrant
√ regional subcentimeter masses with central / peripheral radiolucent notches

EPIDERMAL INCLUSION CYST

= benign cutaneous / subcutaneous lesion
Cause: congenital, metaplasia, trauma (needle biopsy, reduction mammoplasty), obstructed hair follicle
Path: cyst filled with keratin
Histo: stratified squamous epithelium
• smooth round nodule attached to skin with blackened pore, movable against underlying tissue
√ circumscribed round / oval iso- / high-density mass of 0.8–10.0 cm in diameter
√ may contain heterogeneous microcalcifications
US:
√ circumscribed hypoechoic solid mass extending into dermis
DDx: sebaceous cyst (epithelial cysts containing sebaceous glands)

FAT NECROSIS OF BREAST

= TRAUMATIC LIPID CYST = OIL CYST
= aseptic saponification of fat by tissue lipase after local destruction of fat cells with release of lipids + hemorrhage + fibrotic proliferation
Etiology: direct external trauma (seat belt injury), breast biopsy, reduction mammoplasty, implant removal, breast reconstruction, irradiation, nodular panniculitis (Weber-Christian disease), ductal ectasia of chronic mastitis
Incidence: 0.5% of breast biopsies
At risk: middle-aged obese women with fatty pendulous breasts
Histo: cavity with oily material surrounded by "foam cells" (= lipid-laden macrophages)
• history of trauma in 40% (eg, prior surgery, radiation >6 months ago, reduction mammoplasty, lumpectomy)
• usually clinically occult
• firm, slightly fixed tender / painless mass
• skin retraction (50%)
• yellowish fatty fluid on aspiration
Location: anywhere; more common in superficial periareolar region; near biopsy site / surgical scar
√ ill-defined irregular spiculated dense mass (indistinguishable from carcinoma if associated with distortion, skin thickening, retraction)

√ well-circumscribed mass with translucent areas at center (= homogeneous fat density of oil cyst) surrounded by thin pseudocapsule (in old lesions)
√ calcifies in 4–7% (= **liponecrosis macrocystica calcificans**):
  √ occasionally curvilinear / eggshell calcification in wall
√ fine spicules of low density vary with projection
√ localized skin thickening / retraction possible
US:
  √ hypo- / anechoic mass with ill- / well-defined margins ± acoustic shadowing
  √ complex cyst with mural nodules / echogenic bands

Weber-Christian Disease

= nonsuppurative panniculitis with recurrent bouts of inflammation = areas of fat necrosis, involving subcutaneous fat + fat within internal organs
• accompanied by fever + nodules over trunk and limbs

FIBROADENOMA

= ADULT-TYPE FIBROADENOMA
= estrogen-induced benign tumor originating from TDLU; forms during adolescence; pregnancy + lactation are growth stimulants; regression after menopause (mucoid degeneration, hyalinization, involution of epithelial components, calcification)

Incidence: 3rd most common type of breast lesion after fibrocystic disease + carcinoma; most common benign solid tumor in women of childbearing age

Age: mean age of 30 years (range 13–80 years); median age 25 years; most common breast tumor under age 25 years

Hormonal influence:
slight enlargement at end of menstrual cycle + during pregnancy; regresses after menopause; may occur in postmenopausal women receiving estrogen replacement therapy

Histo: mixture of proliferated fibrous stroma + epithelial ductal structures
 (a) intracanalicular fibroadenoma compressing ducts
 (b) pericanalicular fibroadenoma without duct compression
 (c) combination

• firm, smooth, sometimes lobulated, freely movable mass
• in 35% not palpable
• NO skin fixation
• rarely tender / painful
• clinical size = radiographic size

Size: 1–5 cm (in 60%); multiple in 15–25%; bilateral in 4%

√ circular / oval-shaped lesion of low density
√ nodular / lobulated contour when larger (areas with different growth rates)
√ smooth, discrete margins (indistinguishable from cysts when small)
√ often with "halo" sign
√ smoothly contoured calcifications of high + fairly equal density in 3% due to necrosis from regressive changes in older patients:
 (a) peripheral subcapsular myxoid degeneration
  √ peripheral marginal ringlike calcifications
 (b) central myxoid degeneration
  √ "popcorn" type of calcification (PATHOGNOMONIC)
 (c) calcifications within ductal elements
  √ pleomorphic linear ± branching pattern
 ◊ Calcifications enlarge as soft-tissue component regresses!

US:
 √ round (3%) / oval mass (96%) with length-to-depth ratio of >1.4 (in carcinomas usually <1.4)
 √ hypoechoic similar to fat lobules (80–96%) / hyperechoic / mixed pattern / anechoic / isoechoic compared with adjacent fibroglandular tissue
 √ homogeneous (48–89%) / inhomogeneous (12–52%) texture
 √ regular (57%) / lobulated (15–31%) / irregular (6–58%) contour
 √ "hump and dip" sign = small focal contour bulge immediately contiguous with a small sulcus (57%)
 √ intratumoral bright echoes (10%) = macrocalcifications
 √ posterior acoustic enhancement (17–25%) / acoustic shadow without calcifications (9–11%)
 √ echogenic halo (capsule) with lateral shadowing

MR:
 √ internal septations

Juvenile / Giant / Cellular Fibroadenoma

= fibroadenoma >5 cm in diameter / weighing >500 g

Cause: hyperplasia + distortion of normal breast lobules secondary to hormonal imbalances between estradiol + progesterone levels

Age: any (mostly in adolescent girls)

Histo: more glandular + more stromal cellularity than adult type of fibroadenoma; ductal epithelial hyperplasia

• rapidly enlarging well-circumscribed nontender mass
• dilated superficial veins, stretched skin
√ discrete mass with rounded borders

DDx: medullary / mucinous / papillary carcinoma / carcinoma within fibroadenoma

FIBROCYSTIC CHANGES

= MAZOPLASIA = MASTITIS FIBROSA CYSTICA = CHRONIC CYSTIC MASTITIS = CYSTIC DISEASE = GENERALIZED BREAST HYPERPLASIA = DESQUAMATED EPITHELIAL HYPERPLASIA = FIBROADENOMATOSIS = MAMMARY DYSPLASIA = SCHIMMELBUSCH DISEASE = FIBROUS MASTITIS = MAMMARY PROLIFERATIVE DISEASE

◊ Not a disease since found in 72% of screening population >55 years of age
◊ The College of American Pathologists suggests use of the term "fibrocystic changes / condition" in mammography reports!

Incidence: most common diffuse breast disorder; in 51% of 3,000 autopsies

Age: 35–55 years

Etiology: exaggeration of normal cyclical proliferation + involution of the breast with production + incomplete absorption of fluid by apocrine cells

- asymptomatic in macrocystic disease
- fullness, tenderness, pain in microcystic disease
- palpable nodules + thickening
- symptoms occur with ovulation; regression with pregnancy + menopause

Histo:
(1) overgrowth of fibrous connective tissue = stromal fibrosis, fibroadenoma
(2) cystic dilatation of ducts + cyst formation (in 100% microscopic, in 20% macroscopic)
(3) hyperplasia of ducts + lobules + acini = adenosis; ductal papillomatosis

√ individual round / ovoid cysts with discrete smooth margins
√ lobulated multilocular cyst
√ enlarged nodular pattern (= fluid-distended lobules + extensive extralobular fibrous connective tissue overgrowth)
√ "teacup-like" curvilinear thin calcifications with horizontal beam + low-density round calcifications in craniocaudal projection = milk of calcium (4%)
√ "oyster pearl–like" / psammoma-like calcifications

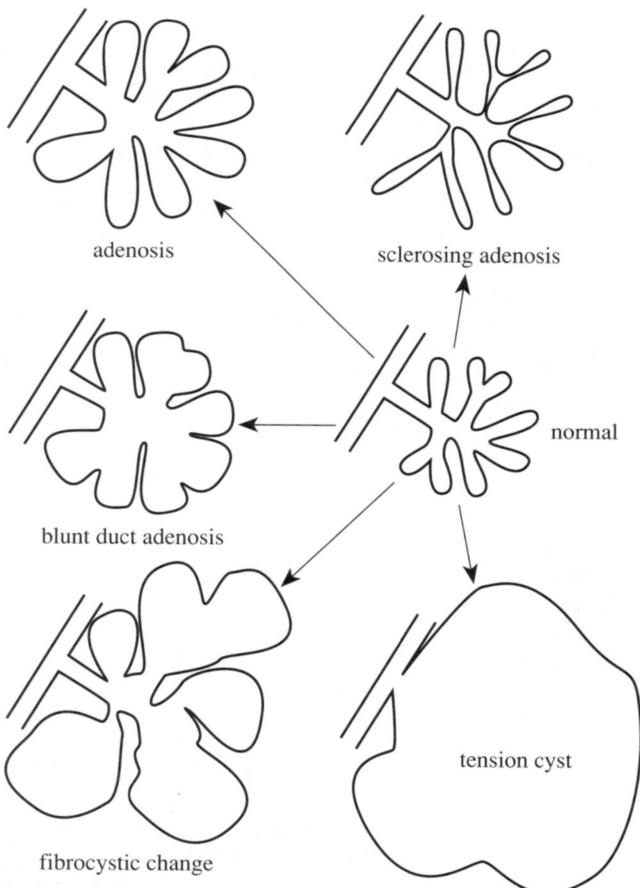

Benign Diseases of the Terminal Ductal Lobular Unit

√ "involutional type" calcifications = very fine punctate calcifications evenly distributed within one / more lobes against a fatty background (from mild degree of hyperplasia in subsequently atrophied glandular tissue)

US:
√ ductal pattern, ductectasia, cysts, ill-defined focal lesions

Risk for Invasive Breast Carcinoma

A. NO INCREASED RISK
   1. Nonproliferative lesions: adenosis, florid adenosis, apocrine metaplasia without atypia, macro- / microcysts, duct ectasia, fibrosis, mild hyperplasia (more than 2 but not more than 4 epithelial cells deep), mastitis, periductal mastitis, squamous metaplasia
   2. Fibroadenoma
B. SLIGHTLY INCREASED RISK (1.5–2 times):
   1. Moderate + florid solid / papillary hyperplasia
   2. Papilloma with fibrovascular core
   3. Sclerosing adenosis
C. MODERATELY INCREASED RISK (5 times): Ductal / lobular atypical hyperplasia (borderline lesion with some features of carcinoma in situ)
D. HIGH RISK (8–11 times):
   1. Atypical hyperplasia + family history of breast cancer
   2. Ductal / lobular carcinoma in situ

Adenosis

Path: lobulocentric lesion derived from TDLU with distortion and effacement of underlying lobules

Histo: epithelial and myoepithelial proliferation of ductules + lobules with nuclear pleomorphism + increase in cell size

√ increase in size of TDLUs to 3–7 mm
√ "snowflake pattern" of widespread ill-defined nodular densities
√ adenosis lobules are sonographically iso- to mildly hypoechoic compared with fat
√ calcifications less common + extensive than in sclerosing adenosis

Sclerosing Adenosis

Path: myoepithelial proliferation + reactive stromal fibrosis

Histo: stromal sclerosis involving >50% of all TDLUs, which become elongated + distorted + compressed by sclerosis

DDx: tubular carcinoma (absence of basement membrane + myoepithelial cells); radial scar (more extensive fibrosis + central fibrocollagenous scar)

- palpable mass (rare) = "adenosis tumor"

Rarely associated with: lobular carcinoma in situ > ductal carcinoma in situ

◊ Sclerosing adenosis is not a risk factor / precursor of breast cancer!

BREAST

√ calcifications in 50%
(a) focal form
√ focal cluster of microcalcifications
√ focally dense breast appearing as a nodule / spiculated lesion
(b) diffuse form
√ adenosis + diffusely scattered calcifications (calcifications in cystically dilated acinar structure)
√ diffusely dense breast
DDx: other spiculated lesions

Fibrosis

√ round / oval clustered microcalcifications with smooth contours + associated fine granular calcifications filling lobules

Atypical Lobular Hyperplasia

= proliferation of round cells of LCIS type growing along terminal ducts in permeative fashion (pagetoid growth) between benign epithelium + basal myoepithelium BUT NOT completely obliterating terminal ductal lumina / distending lobules (as in lobular carcinoma in situ)
√ no mammographic correlate

Atypical Ductal Hyperplasia

= low-grade intraductal proliferation with partial / incompletely developed features of noncomedo DCIS
√ frequent calcifications

Intraductal Papillomatosis

= hyperplastic polypoid lesions within a duct
Age: perimenopausal
• spontaneous bloody / serous / serosanguinous nipple discharge (most common cause of nipple discharge)
√ small retroareolar opacity (= dilated duct) extending 2–3 cm into breast
√ intraluminal filling defect on galactography

FIBROUS NODULE OF THE BREAST

= FIBROUS DISEASE OF THE BREAST = FIBROUS DISEASE = FIBROSIS OF THE BREAST = FIBROUS MASTOPATHY = FIBROUS TUMOR OF THE BREAST
Frequency: 3–4% of benign masses; 8% of surgical breast specimens
Histo: focally dense collagenous stroma surrounding atrophic epithelium; NONSPECIFIC
Age: 20–50 years; only 8% postmenopausal
• palpable / nonpalpable mass: edge merges into surrounding dense tissue
Location: unilateral (80–85%) / bilateral (15–20%)
√ circumscribed (55%) / indistinct (32%) margin
√ suggestive of malignancy (11%): irregular shape, spiculated margin, posterior acoustic shadowing
DDx: fibroadenoma, malignancy

GALACTOCELE

= retention of fatty material in areas of cystic duct dilatation appearing during / shortly after lactation
Cause: ? abrupt suppression of lactation / obstructed milk duct
Age: occurs during / shortly after lactation
• thick inspissated milky fluid (colostrum)
Location: retroareolar area
√ large radiopaque lesion of water density (1st phase)
√ smaller lesion of mixed density + fat-water level with horizontal beam (2nd phase)
√ small radiolucent lesion resembling lipoma
√ ± fluid-calcium level
US:
√ complex mass
Dx: aspiration of milky fluid

GRANULAR CELL TUMOR

= GRANULAR CELL MYOBLASTOMA OF BREAST
= benign tumor, occasionally locally invasive + metastasizing
Origin: ? Schwann cell, smooth muscle, or undifferentiated mesenchymal cell
Prevalence: 1:1,000 primary breast carcinomas
Age: 20–59 (mean 35) years; more common in Blacks
Histo: rounded groups of large cells with small dark regular nuclei + abundant eosinophilic granular cytoplasm; not immunoreactive to cytokeratin + epithelial membrane antigen BUT to S-100 protein
DDx: carcinoma, lymphoma, metastasis
◊ Fine-needle aspirate may be difficult to interpret!
Location: tongue, skin, bronchial wall, subcutaneous breast tissue (6–8%)
Site: more commonly <u>other than</u> upper outer quadrant
• asymmetric lump with slow growth, hardness, skin fixation / retraction, ulceration
• often fixed to pectoralis fascia
√ well-circumscribed spiculated mass 1–3 cm in diameter
√ stellate extensions (tumor insinuating itself into surrounding breast tissue)
√ may exhibit acoustic shadow
Rx: wide local excision

GYNECOMASTIA

= excessive development of breast in male
Cause:
(1) Hormonal
(a) neonate: influence from maternal estrogens crossing placenta
(b) puberty: high estradiol levels
Incidence: in up to 60–75% of healthy boys
Age: 1 year after onset of puberty (13–14 years)
Prognosis: subsides within 1–2 years
(c) older men: decline in serum testosterone levels
(d) hypogonadism (Klinefelter syndrome, anorchism, acquired testicular failure (eg, testicular neoplasm)
(e) tumors: adrenal carcinoma, pituitary adenoma, testicular tumor, hyperthyroidism

(2) Systemic disorders
advanced alcoholic cirrhosis, hemodialysis in chronic renal failure, chronic pulmonary disease (emphysema, TB), malnutrition
(3) Drug-induced
anabolic steroids, estrogen treatment for prostate cancer, digitalis, cimetidine, thiazide, spironolactone, reserpine, isoniazid, ergotamine, marijuana
(4) Neoplasm: hepatoma (with estrogen production)
(5) Idiopathic

mnemonic: "CODES"
Cirrhosis
Obesity
Digitalis
Estrogen
Spironolactone

Incidence: 85% of all male breast masses
Age: neonatal period, adolescent boys (40%), men >50 years (32%)
Histo: increased number of ducts, proliferation of duct epithelium, periductal edema, fibroplastic stroma, adipose tissue
• palpable firm mass >2 cm in subareolar region
Location: bilateral (63%), left-sided (27%), right-sided (10%)
√ mild prominence of subareolar ducts in flame-shaped distribution (focal type)
√ homogeneously dense breast (diffuse type)
DDx: pseudogynecomastia (= fatty proliferation in obesity)

HAMARTOMA OF BREAST

= FIBROADENOLIPOMA = LIPOFIBROADENOMA
= ADENOLIPOMA
Incidence: 2–16:10,000 mammograms
Mean age: 45 (27–88) years
Histo: normal / dysplastic mammary tissue composed of dense fibrous tissue + variable amount of fat, delineated from surrounding tissue without a true capsule
• soft, often nonpalpable (60%)
Location: retroareolar (30%), upper outer quadrant (35%)
√ round / ovoid well-circumscribed mass usually > 3 cm
√ mixed density with mottled center (secondary to fat) = "slice of sausage" pattern
√ thin smooth pseudocapsule (= thin layer of surrounding fibrous tissue)
√ peripheral radiolucent zone
√ may contain calcifications
DDx: liposarcoma, Cowden disease

HEMATOMA OF BREAST

Cause: (1) surgery / biopsy (most common)
(2) blunt trauma
(3) coagulopathy (leukemia, thrombocytopenia)
(4) anticoagulant therapy
√ well-defined ovoid mass (= hemorrhagic cyst)
√ ill-defined mass with diffuse increased density (edema + hemorrhage)
√ adjacent skin thickening / prominence of reticular structures
√ regression within several weeks leaving (a) no trace, (b) architectural distortion, (c) incomplete resolution
√ calcifications (occasionally)
US:
√ hypoechoic mass with internal echoes

JUVENILE PAPILLOMATOSIS

Path: many aggregated cysts with interspersed dense stroma
Histo: cysts lined by flat duct epithelium / epithelium with apocrine metaplasia, sclerosing adenosis, duct stasis; marked papillary hyperplasia of duct epithelium with often extreme atypia
Mean age: 23 years (range of 12–48 years)
• localized palpable tumor
• family history of breast cancer in 28% (affected first-degree relative in 8%; in one / more relatives in 28%)
Prognosis: development of synchronous (4%) / metachronous (4%) breast cancer after 8–9 years.
DDx: fibroadenoma

LACTATING ADENOMA

= newly discovered painless mass during 3rd trimester of pregnancy / in lactating woman
Etiology: ? variant of fibroadenoma / tubular adenoma / lobular hyperplasia or de novo neoplasm
Path: well-circumscribed yellow spherical mass with lobulated surface + rubbery firm texture and without capsule
Histo: secretory lobules lined by granular and foamy to vacuolated cytoplasm + separated by delicate connective tissue
• firm freely movable painless mass
√ homogeneously hypoechoic / isoechoic mass
√ posterior acoustic enhancement (most) / shadowing
√ fibrous septa
Prognosis: regression after completion of breast feeding
DDx: breast carcinoma (1:1,300–1:6,200 pregnancies)

LIPOMA OF BREAST

= usually solitary asymptomatic slow-growing lesion
Mean age: 45 years + postmenopause
• soft, freely movable, well delineated
√ usually >2 cm
√ radiolucent lesion easily seen in dense breast; almost invisible in fatty breast
√ discrete thin radiopaque line (= capsule), seen in most of its circumference
√ displacement of adjacent breast parenchyma
√ calcification with fat necrosis (extremely rare)
DDx: fat lobule surrounded by trabeculae / suspensory ligaments

LYMPHOMA OF BREAST

A. Primary Lymphoma
= extranodal lymphoma of the breast without prior history of lymphoma / leukemia

Prevalence: 0.12–0.53% of all breast malignancies; 2.2% of all extranodal lymphomas
- asymptomatic

B. Secondary Lymphoma
◊ One of the most common type of metastatic lesions in the breast!
- fever, pain

Histo: B-cell NHL (majority), Hodgkin disease, leukemia (CLL), plasmacytoma
Age: 50–60 years; M < F
Location: right-sided predominance; 13% bilateral
√ well / incompletely circumscribed round / oval lobulated mass / masses
√ infiltrate with poorly defined borders
√ NO calcifications / spiculations
√ skin thickening + trabecular edema
√ bilateral axillary adenopathy in 30–50%
US:
√ oval / round homo- / heterogeneously hypoechoic mass / masses
√ sharply defined / poorly defined borders
√ posterior acoustic shadowing / enhancement
Prognosis: 3.4% 5-year disease-free survival for all stages; 50% remission rate with aggressive chemotherapy
Recurrence: mostly in contralateral breast / other distant sites
DDx: circumscribed breast carcinoma, fibroadenoma, phylloides tumor, metastatic disease

Pseudolymphoma
= lymphoreticular lesion as an overwhelming response to trauma

MAMMARY DUCT ECTASIA
= PLASMA CELL MASTITIS = VARICOCELE TUMOR OF BREAST = MASTITIS OBLITERANS = COMEDOMASTITIS = PERIDUCTAL MASTITIS = SECRETORY DISEASE OF BREAST
= rare aseptic inflammation of subareolar area
Pathogenesis (speculative):
(1) Stasis of intraductal secretion leads to duct dilatation + leakage of inspissated material into parenchyma giving rise to an aseptic chemical mastitis (periductal mastitis); the extravasated material is rich in fatty acids = nontraumatic fat necrosis
(2) Periductal inflammation causes damage to elastic lamina of duct wall resulting in duct dilatation

Histo: ductal ectasia, heavily calcified ductal secretions; infiltration of plasma cells + giant cells + eosinophils
Mean age: 54 years
- often asymptomatic
- breast pain, nipple discharge, nipple retraction, mamillary fistula, subareolar breast mass

Location: subareolar, often bilateral + symmetric; may be unilateral + focal
√ dense triangular mass with apex toward nipple
√ distended ducts connecting to nipple
√ periphery blending with normal tissue
√ multiple often bilateral dense round / oval calcifications with lucent center + polarity (= orientation toward nipple)
(a) periductal
√ oval / elongated calcified ring around dilated ducts with very dense periphery (surrounding deposits of fibrosis + fat necrosis)
(b) intraductal
√ fairly uniform linear, often "needle-shaped" calcifications of wide caliber, occasionally branching (within ducts / confined to duct walls)
√ nipple retraction / skin thickening may occur
Sequelae: cholesterol granuloma
DDx: breast cancer

MAMMOPLASTY
= COSMETIC BREAST SURGERY

Augmentation Mammoplasty
Most frequently performed plastic surgery in USA
Frequency: 150,000 procedures in 1993 (80% for cosmetic reasons, 20% for reconstruction); 2 million American women have breast implants (estimate)

Methods:
1. Injection augmentation (no longer practiced): paraffin, silicone, fat from liposuction
Cx: tissue necrosis resulting in dense, hard, tender breast masses; lymphadenopathy; infection; granuloma formation (= siliconoma)
2. Implants
(a) spongelike masses of Ivalon, Etrheron, Teflon
(b) Silicone elastomer (silastic) smooth / textured shell containing silicone gel / saline: >100 varieties
— single lumen of polymerized methyl polysiloxane with smooth / textured outer silicone shell / polyurethane coating
— double lumen with inner core of silicone + outer chamber of saline
— triple lumen
(c) expandable implant ± intraluminal valves = saline injection into port with gradual tissue expansion for breast reconstruction
Location: retroglandular / subpectoral
3. Autogenous tissue transplantation (for breast reconstruction) with musculocutaneous flaps: transverse rectus abdominis muscle (TRAM), latissimus dorsi, tensor fascia lata, gluteus maximus

Mammographic technique for implants:
1. Two standard views (CC and MLO views) for most posterior breast tissue
◊ 22–83% of fibroglandular breast tissue obscured by implant depending on size of breast + location of implant + degree of capsular contraction on standard views!

BREAST

◊ The false-negative rate of mammography increases from 10–20% to 41% in patients with implants!

2. Two Eklund (= implant displacement) views (CC and 90° LAT views) for compression views of anterior breast tissue = "push-back" view = breast tissue pulled anteriorly in front of implant while implant is pushed posteriorly + superiorly thus excluding most of the implant

Cx of silicone-gel–filled implant:

1. Capsular fibrosis, calcification, contracture (15–50%): more frequent with retroglandular implants
   - distortion of breast contour with hard capsule
   - √ crenulated contour (US helpful)
   - √ capsular calcifications at periphery of prosthesis
   - √ fibrous capsule delineated by US (unleaked silicone is echolucent)
2. Implant migration
   Cause: overdistension of implant pocket at surgery
3. Rupture of prosthesis
   Prevalence: >50% after 12 years
   - change in contour / location of implant
   - flattening of implant
   - breast pain
   - √ extracapsular silicone in 11–23% (97% specific, 5% sensitive)
4. "Gel bleed" = leakage of silicone through semiporous but intact barrier shell made of silicone elastomer
5. Localized pain / paresthesia
6. ? development of autoimmune disorders (eg, scleroderma, lupus erythematosus)
7. Infection / hematoma formation

Intracapsular Rupture (more common)

= broken implant casing with silicone leakage contained by intact fibrous capsule

Mammo (11–23% sensitive, 89–98% specific):

√ bulging / peaking of implant contour

US (59–70% sensitive, 57–92% specific, 49% accurate):

√ "stepladder" sign = series of parallel horizontal echogenic straight / curvilinear lines inside implant (= collapsed implant shell floating within silicone gel)

√ heterogeneous aggregates of low- to medium-level echogenicity (65% sensitive, 57% specific)

N.B.: visualization of internal lumen within anechoic space in double-lumen implants can be confused on US with intracapsular rupture

MR (81–94% sensitive, 93–97% specific, 84% accurate):

√ "linguine" sign = multiple hypointense wavy lines within implant (= pieces of free-floating collapsed envelope surrounded by silicone gel)

√ "inverted teardrop" / "noose" / "keyhole" / "lariat (= lasso)" sign = loop-shaped hypointense structure contiguous with implant envelope (= small focal invagination of shell with silicone on either side)

√ = infolded polyurethane coat of a single lumen prosthesis

√ hypointense subcapsular lines paralleling the fibrous capsule (= minimally displaced ruptured shell as early sign) (DDx: phase-encoding artifact caused by motion)

Extracapsular Rupture

= extrusion + migration of silicone droplets through tear in both implant + overlying fibrous capsule

- palpable breast masses

US:

√ "snowstorm" / "echogenic noise" pattern
= markedly hyperechoic nodule with well-defined anterior + indistinct echogenic noise posteriorly (= free silicone droplets mixed with breast tissue)

√ highly echogenic area with acoustic shadowing

√ hypoechoic masses almost indistinguishable from cysts + usually surrounded by echogenic noise (= large to medium-sized collections of free silicone) with low-level internal echoes

MR:

√ discrete hypointense foci on fat-suppressed T1WI + hyperintense signal on water-suppressed T2WI in continuity with / separate from implant

Mammography:

√ lobular / spherical dense area of opacities adjacent to / separate from silicone implant

√ rim calcifications

EXTRACAPSULAR SPREAD OF SILICONE

Source: gel bleed, implant rupture (11–23%) more common with thinner shell + older implants

- silicone lymphadenopathy
- paresthesia of arm (from nerve impingement secondary to fibrosis surrounding silicone migrated to axilla / brachial plexus)
- silicone nipple discharge (rare)
- migration to arm (+ constrictive neuropathy of radial nerve), subcutaneous tissue of lower abdominal wall, inguinal canal

√ migration to ipsilateral chest wall + axillary nodes

√ silicone droplets in breast

√ granuloma formation (siliconoma) + fibrosis

Reduction Mammoplasty

√ swirled architectural distortion (in inferior breast best seen on mediolateral view)

√ postsurgical distortion

√ residual isolated islands of breast tissue

√ fat necrosis

√ dystrophic calcifications

√ asymmetric tissue oriented in nonanatomic distribution

BREAST

MASTITIS

- tender swollen red breast (DDx: inflammatory carcinoma)
- enlarged painful axillary lymph nodes
- ± febrile, elevated ESR, leukocytosis

√ diffuse increased density
√ diffuse skin thickening
√ swelling of breast
√ enlarged axillary lymph nodes
√ rapid resolution under antibiotic therapy

Puerperal Mastitis

= LACTATIONAL MASTITIS
= usually interstitial infection during lactational period
(a) through infected nipple cracks
(b) hematogenous
(c) ascending via ducts = galactophoritis

Organism: Staphylococcus, Streptococcus
Rx: incision + drainage

Nonpuerperal Mastitis

1. Infected cyst
2. Purulent mastitis with abscess formation
3. Plasma cell mastitis
4. Nonspecific mastitis

Granulomatous Mastitis

1. Foreign-body granuloma
2. Specific disease (TB, sarcoidosis, leprosy, syphilis, actinomycosis, typhus)
3. Parasitic disease (hydatid disease, cysticercosis, filariasis, schistosomiasis)

METASTASES TO BREAST

Incidence: 1%
Mean age: 43 years
Primaries: leukemia / lymphoma > malignant melanoma > ovarian carcinoma > lung cancer > sarcoma
◊ In up to 40% no known history of primary cancer!
in children: rhabdomyosarcoma, leukemia, non-Hodgkin lymphoma

√ solitary mass (85%), esp. in upper outer quadrant
√ multiple masses
√ skin adherence (25%) ± skin thickening
√ axillary node involvement (40%)

PAGET DISEASE OF THE NIPPLE

[Sir James Paget (1814-1899), surgeon and pathologist at St. Bartholomew's Hospital, London, England; first described in 1874]
= uncommon manifestation of breast cancer characterized by infiltration of the nipple epidermis by adenocarcinoma

Prevalence: 2–3% of all breast cancers

- nipple changes (32%): erythema, scaling, erosion, ulceration, retraction of nipple and areola:
  ◊ Median delay of correct diagnosis by 6–11 months as features suggest a benign diagnosis of eczema!
  - nipple changes + palpable mass / thickening of breast (45%)
- palpable mass / thickening of breast only (14%)
- ± bloody nipple discharge + itching

Histo: Paget cell = large pleomorphic cells with pale cytoplasm arising in main secretory ducts and migrating into epidermis; histologically and biologically similar to comedocarcinoma

Associated with:
extensive invasive / in situ ductal carcinoma limited to one duct in subareolar area / remote + multicentric

√ negative mammogram in 50%
√ nipple / areolar / skin thickening
√ nipple retraction
√ dilated duct
√ linearly distributed subareolar / diffuse malignant microcalcifications
√ discrete retroareolar soft-tissue mass / masses

Dx: cytologic smear of a weeping nipple secretion / excisional biopsy of a nipple lesion
Prognosis: survival rate with palpable mass similar to infiltrating duct carcinoma; 85–90% 10-year survival rate without palpable mass; positive axillary nodes in 0–13%

PAPILLOMA OF BREAST

= usually benign proliferation of ductal epithelial tissue

Age: 30–77 years (juvenile papillomatosis = 20–26 years); may occur in men
Histo: hyperplastic proliferation of ductal epithelium; lesion may be pedunculated / broad-based; connective tissue stalk covered by epithelial cells proliferating in the form of apocrine metaplasia / solid hyperplasia may cause duct obstruction + distension to form an intracystic papilloma
DDx: invasive papillary carcinoma

Central Solitary Papilloma

Location: subareolar within major duct
NOT premalignant

- spontaneous usually bloody / serous (9–48%) / clear nipple discharge (52–88–100%):
  ◊ Most common cause of serous / sanguineous nipple discharge!
- "trigger point" = nipple discharge produced upon compression of area with papilloma
- intermittent mass disappearing with discharge

√ negative mammogram / intraductal nodules in subareolar area
√ asymmetrically dilated single duct
√ subareolar amorphous coarse calcifications
√ dilated duct with obstructing / distorting intraluminal filling defect on ductography (= galactography)

Cx: 0–5–14% frequency of carcinoma development

Peripheral Multiple Papillomas

Location: within terminal ductal lobular unit; bilateral in up to 14%

In 10–38% associated with:
atypical ductal hyperplasia, lobular carcinoma in situ, papillary + cribriform intraductal cancers, radial scar

- nipple discharge (20%)
- √ round / oval / slightly lobulated well-circumscribed nodules
- √ segmental distribution with dilated ducts extending from beneath the nipple (20%)
- √ may be associated with coarse microcalcifications

Cx: 5% frequency of carcinoma development; increased risk dependent on degree of cellular atypia

Prognosis: in 24% recurrence after surgical treatment

PSEUDOANGIOMATOUS STROMAL HYPERPLASIA

= benign proliferative lesions of mammary stroma in a spectrum from focal incidental findings to clinically + mammographically evident breast masses

Histo: (a) incidental focal microscopic finding in 23% of all breast specimens
(b) tumoral form (rare)

Tumoral Form of Pseudoangiomatous Stromal Hyperplasia

Age: 4–5th decade (range 14–67 years)

Histo: proliferating myofibroblasts creating slit-like spaces positive for CD34 + muscle actin; similar in appearance to low-grade angiosarcoma

- single circumscribed palpable mass
- √ well-circumscribed 5–6 (range, 1–12)-cm mass
- √ growth over time ± recurrence after excisional biopsy

US:
- √ hypoechoic solid mass with slightly heterogeneous echotexture
- √ ± small cystic component

DDx: fibroadenoma, phylloides tumor

RADIAL SCAR

= SCLEROSING DUCT HYPERPLASIA = INDURATIVE MASTOPATHY = FOCAL FIBROUS DISEASE = BENIGN SCLEROSING DUCTAL PROLIFERATION = INFILTRATING EPITHELIOSIS = NONENCAPSULATED SCLEROSING LESION

= benign proliferative breast lesion (malignant potential is controversial) unrelated to prior surgery / trauma

Incidence: 0.1–2.0/1,000 screening mammograms; in 2–16% of mastectomy specimens

Cause: ? localized inflammatory reaction, ? chronic ischemia with slow infarction

Path: "scar" = sclerotic center composed of acellular connective tissue (= fibrosis) and elastin deposits (= elastosis); entrapped ductules with intact myoepithelial layer in sclerotic core; corona of distorted ducts + lobules composed of benign proliferations (sclerosing adenosis, ductal hyperplasia, cyst formation, papillomatosis)

In up to 50% associated with:
tubular carcinoma, comedo carcinoma, invasive lobular carcinoma + contralateral breast cancer

◊ Avoid frozen section, core needle biopsy, fine-needle aspiration!

- rarely palpable
- √ mean diameter of 0.33 cm (range, 0.1–0.6 cm)
- √ typically no central mass (BUT: irregular noncalcified mass often with architectural distortion)
- √ variable appearance in different projections (= radial scars are typically planar in configuration)
- √ oval / circular translucent areas at center
- √ very thin long spicules, clumped together centrally
- √ radiolucent linear structures (= fat) paralleling spicules ("black star" appearance)
- √ no skin thickening / retraction

Rx: surgical excision required for definite diagnosis

DDx: carcinoma, postsurgical scar, fat necrosis, fibromatosis, granular cell myoblastoma

SARCOMA OF BREAST

Incidence: 1% of malignant mammary lesions

Age: 45–55 years

Histo: fibrosarcoma, rhabdomyosarcoma, osteogenic sarcoma, mixed malignant tumor of the breast, malignant fibrosarcoma and carcinoma, liposarcoma

- rapid growth
- √ smooth / lobulated large dense mass
- √ well-defined outline
- √ palpated size similar to mammographic size

BREAST

Angiosarcoma

= highly malignant vascular breast tumor

Incidence: 200 cases in world literature; 0.04% of all malignant breast tumors; 8% of all breast sarcomas

Age: 3rd–4th decade of life

Histo: hyperchromatic endothelial cells; network of communicating vascular spaces
stage I: cells with large nucleoli
stage II: endothelial lining displaying tufting + intraluminal papillary projections
stage III: mitoses, necrosis, marked hemorrhage

Metastasis: hematogenous spread to lung, skin, subcutaneous tissue, bone, liver, brain, ovary; NOT lymphatic

- rapidly enlarging painless immobile breast mass
- √ skin thickening + nipple retraction
- √ large solitary mass with ill-defined nonspiculated border

US:
- √ well-defined multilobulated hypoechoic mass with hyperechoic areas (from hemorrhage)

Prognosis: 1.9–2.1 years mean survival; 14% overall 3-year survival rate

Rx: simple mastectomy without axillary lymph node dissection

DDx: phylloides tumor, lactating breast, juvenile hypertrophy
◊ Frequently misdiagnosed as lymphangioma / hemangioma!

DIFFERENTIAL DIAGNOSIS OF CARDIOVASCULAR DISORDERS

CONGENITAL HEART DISEASE

Approach to Congenital Heart Disease

	Acyanotic √ enlarged main pulmonary artery	*Cyanotic* √ concave main pulmonary artery
Increased PBF + increased C/T ratio	*L-R shunts* VSD ASD PDA ECD PAPVR	*Admixture lesions = bidirectional shunts = T-lesions* Transposition Truncus arteriosus TAPVR Tricuspid atresia (without RVOT obstruction) "Tingles" (single ventricle / atrium)
Normal PBF + normal C/T ratio + pulmonary venous hypertension	*LV outflow obstruction* AS Coarctation Interrupted aortic arch Hypoplastic left heart *LV inflow obstruction* Obstructed TAPVR Cor triatriatum Pulmonary vein atresia Congenital MV stenosis *Muscle disease* Cardiomyopathy Myocarditis Anomalous LCA	
Decreased PBF + normal C/T ratio		*R-to-L shunts* *+ nonrestrictive intracardiac shunt* Tetralogy of Fallot Tricuspid atresia (with PS + nonrestrictive ASD) Pulmonary atresia + nonrestrictive VSD
+ increased C/T ratio		*+ restrictive intracardiac shunt* Pulmonary atresia + ASD without VSD PS with ASD / patent foramen ovale Tricuspid atresia + PS + restrictive ASD Trilogy of Fallot Ebstein anomaly Congenital tricuspid insufficiency

Incidence of CHD in Liveborn Infants

Overall incidence: 8–9:1000 livebirths

◊ Most common CHD: mitral valve prolapse (5–20%), bicuspid aortic valve (2%) [usually not recognized before late infancy / childhood]

◊ ASD + VSD + PDA account for 45% of all CHD

◊ 12 lesions account for 89% of all CHD

Ventricular septal defect	30.3%
Patent ductus arteriosus	8.6%
Pulmonary stenosis	7.4%
Septum secundum defect	6.7%
Coarctation of aorta	5.7%
Aortic stenosis	5.2%
Tetralogy of Fallot	5.1%
Transposition	4.7%
Endocardial cushion defect	3.2%
Hypoplastic right ventricle	2.2%
Hypoplastic left heart	1.3%
TAPVR	1.1%
Truncus arteriosus	1.0%
Single ventricle	0.3%
Double outlet right ventricle	0.2%

High-risk pregnancy:
(1) Previous sibling with CHD: 2– 5%
(2) Previous 2 siblings with CHD: 10–15%
(3) One parent with CHD: 2–10%

Most common causes for CHF + PVH in neonate:
1. Left ventricular failure due to outflow obstruction
2. Obstruction of pulmonary venous return

CHD Presenting in 1st Year of Life

1. VSD
2. d-transposition of great vessels
3. Tetralogy of Fallot
4. Isolated coarctation
5. Patent ductus arteriosus
6. Hypoplastic left heart syndrome

CHD with Relatively Long Life

Congenital lesions compatible with a relative long life are:
1. Mild tetralogy: mild pulmonic stenosis + small VSD
2. Valvular pulmonic stenosis: with relatively normal pulmonary circulation
3. Transposition of great vessels: some degree of pulmonic stenosis + large VSD
4. Truncus arteriosus: delicate balance between systemic + pulmonary circulation
5. Truncus arteriosus type IV: large systemic collaterals
6. Tricuspid atresia + transposition + pulmonic stenosis
7. Eisenmenger complex
8. Ebstein anomaly
9. Corrected transposition without intracardiac shunt

Juxtaposition of Atrial Appendages

1. Tricuspid atresia with transposition
2. Complete transposition
3. Corrected transposition of great arteries
4. DORV

Continuous Heart Murmur

1. PDA
2. AP window
3. Ruptured sinus of Valsalva aneurysm
4. Hemitruncus
5. Coronary arteriovenous fistula

Syndromes with CHD

5 p – (Cri-du-chat) Syndrome

Incidence of CHD: 20%

DiGeorge Syndrome

= congenital absence of thymus + parathyroid glands
1. Conotruncal malformation
2. Interrupted aortic arch

Down Syndrome = MONGOLISM = TRISOMY 21

1. Endocardial cushion defect (25%)
2. Membranous VSD
3. Ostium primum ASD
4. AV communis
5. Cleft mitral valve
6. PDA
7. 11 rib pairs (25%)
8. Hypersegmented manubrium (90%)

Ellis-van Creveld Syndrome

Incidence of CHD: 50%
• polydactyly
√ single atrium

Holt-Oram Syndrome

= UPPER LIMB-CARDIAC SYNDROME
Incidence of CHD: 50%
1. ASD
2. VSD
3. Valvular pulmonary stenosis
4. Radial dysplasia

Presenting Age in CHD

Age	*Severe PVH*	*PVH + Shunt Vascularity*
0–2 days	Hypoplastic left heart Aortic atresia TAPVR below diaphragm Myocardiopathy in IDM	Hypoplastic left heart TAPVR above diaphragm Complete transposition
3–7 days	PDA in preterm infant	
7–14 days	CoA + VSD / PDA Aortic valve stenosis Peripheral AVM Endocardial fibroelastosis Anomalous left coronary artery	Coarctation of aorta (CoA) Peripheral AVM

HEART

Hurler Syndrome
Cardiomyopathy

Ivemark Syndrome
Incidence of CHD: 100%
- asplenia

√ complex cardiac anomalies

Klippel-Feil Syndrome
Incidence of CHD: 5%
1. Atrial septal defect
2. Coarctation

Marfan Syndrome = ARACHNODACTYLY
1. Aortic sinus dilatation
2. Aortic aneurysm
3. Aortic insufficiency
4. Pulmonary aneurysm

Noonan Syndrome
1. Pulmonary stenosis
2. ASD
3. Hypertrophic cardiomyopathy

Osteogenesis Imperfecta
1. Aortic valve insufficiency
2. Mitral valve insufficiency
3. Pulmonic valve insufficiency

Postrubella Syndrome
- low birth weight
- deafness
- cataracts
- mental retardation

1. Peripheral pulmonic stenosis
2. Valvular pulmonic stenosis
3. Supravalvular aortic stenosis
4. PDA

Trisomy 13–15
VSD, tetralogy of Fallot, DORV

Trisomy 16–18
VSD, PDA, DORV

Turner Syndrome (XO) = OVARIAN DYSGENESIS
Incidence of CHD: 35%
1. Coarctation of the aorta (in 15%)
2. Bicuspid aortic valve
3. Dissecting aneurysm of aorta

Williams Syndrome = IDIOPATHIC HYPERCALCEMIA
- peculiar elfinlike facies
- mental + physical retardation
- hypercalcemia (not in all patients)

1. Supravalvular aortic stenosis (33%)
2. ASD, VSD
3. Valvular + peripheral pulmonary artery stenosis
4. Aortic hypoplasia, stenoses of more peripheral arteries

SHUNT EVALUATION
Evaluation of L-to-R Shunts
A. AGE
- — Infants:
  - (1) Isolated VSD
  - (2) VSD with CoA / PDA / AV canal
  - (3) PDA
  - (4) Ostium primum
- — Children / adults:
  - (1) ASD
  - (2) Partial AV canal with competent mitral valve
  - (3) VSD / PDA with high pulmonary resistance
  - (4) PDA without murmur

B. SEX
99% chance for ASD / PDA in female patient

C. CHEST WALL ANALYSIS
- √ 11 pair of ribs + hypersegmented manubrium: Down syndrome
- √ pectus excavatum + straight back syndrome + funnel chest: prolapsing mitral valve
- √ rib notching

D. CARDIAC SILHOUETTE
- √ absent pulmonary trunk: corrected transposition with VSD; pink tetralogy
- √ left-sided ascending aorta: corrected transposition with VSD
- √ tortuous descending aorta: aortic valve incompetence + ASD
- √ huge heart: persistent complete AV canal (PCAVC); VSD + PDA; VSD + mitral valve incompetence
- √ enlarged left atrium: intact atrial septum; mitral regurgitation (endocardial cushion defect, prolapsing mitral valve + ASD)

Differential Diagnosis of L-R Shunts

	RA	*RV*	*PA*	*LA*	*LV*	*Prox. Ao*
ASD	↑	↑	↑	↔	↔	↔
VSD	↔	↑	↑	↑	↑	↔
PDA	↔	↔	↑	↑	↑	often ↑

Shunt with Normal Left Atrium
A. PRECARDIAC SHUNT
1. Anomalous pulmonary venous connection

B. INTRACARDIAC SHUNT
1. ASD (8%)
2. VSD (25%)

C. POSTCARDIAC SHUNT
1. PDA (12%)

Aortic Size in Shunts
A. EXTRACARDIAC SHUNTS

√ aorta enlarged + hyperpulsatile
1. PDA

HEART

B. PRE- AND INTRACARDIAC SHUNTS
√ aorta small but not hypoplastic
1. Anomalous pulmonary venous return
2. ASD
3. VSD
4. Common AV canal

CYANOTIC HEART DISEASE

Chemical cyanosis = $PaO_2 \leq 94\%$
Clinical cyanosis = $PaO_2 \leq 85\%$
◊ Decrease in hemoglobin delays detectability!
Most common cause of cyanosis
— in newborn: transposition of great vessels
— in child: tetralogy of Fallot!
N.B.: tricuspid atresia = the great mimicker

Increased Pulmonary Blood Flow with Cyanosis

= ADMIXTURE LESIONS = bidirectional shunt with 2 components:
(a) mixing of saturated blood (L-R shunt) and unsaturated blood (R-L shunt)
(b) NO obstruction to pulmonary blood flow

Evaluation process:
√ cardiomegaly
√ increased pulmonary blood flow
√ concave main pulmonary artery:
√ PA segment absent = transposition
√ PA segment present:
(a) L atrium normal (= extracardiac shunt) = TAPVR
(b) L atrium enlarged (= intracardiac shunt) = truncus arteriosus

N.B.: Overcirculation + cyanosis = complete transposition until proven otherwise!

ADMIXTURE LESIONS = T-LESIONS
mnemonic: "5 T's + CAD"
Transposition of great vessels = complete TGV ± VSD
◊ Most common cause for cyanosis in neonate
Tricuspid atresia with or without transposition + VSD
◊ 2nd most common cause for cyanosis in neonate
Truncus arteriosus
Total anomalous pulmonary venous return (TAPVR) above diaphragm:
(a) supracardiac
(b) cardiac (coronary sinus / right atrium)
"**T**ingle" = single ventricle
Common atrium
Aortic atresia
Double-outlet right ventricle (DORV type I) / Taussig-Bing anomaly (DORV type II)

Clues:
√ skeletal anomalies: Ellis-van Creveld syndrome (truncus / common atrium)
√ polysplenia: common atrium
√ R aortic arch: persistent truncus arteriosus
√ ductus infundibulum: aortic atresia
√ pulmonary trunk seen: supracardiac TAPVR; DORV; tricuspid atresia; common atrium
√ ascending aorta with leftward convexity: single ventricle
√ dilated azygos vein: common atrium + polysplenia + interrupted IVC; TAPVR to azygos vein
√ left-sided SVC: vertical vein of TAPVR
√ "waterfall" right hilum: single ventricle + transposition
√ large left atrium (rules out TAPVR)
√ prominent L heart border: single ventricle with inverted rudimentary R ventricle; levoposition of right atrial appendage (tricuspid atresia + transposition)
√ age of onset ≤2 days: aortic atresia

Decreased Pulmonary Blood Flow with Cyanosis

= two components of
(a) impedance of blood flow through right heart due to obstruction / atresia at pulmonary valve / infundibulum
(b) R-to-L shunt

• pulmonary circulation maintained through systemic arteries / PDA

√ normal / decreased pulmonary blood flow
√ concave main pulmonary artery
√ cardiomegaly
√ restrictive intracardiac R-to-L shunt

mnemonic: "P2 TETT"
Pulmonic stenosis with ASD
Pulmonic atresia
Tetralogy of Fallot
Ebstein anomaly
Tricuspid atresia with pulmonic stenosis
Transposition of great vessels with pulmonic stenosis

A. SHUNT AT VENTRICULAR LEVEL
1. Tetralogy of Fallot
2. Tetralogy physiology (associated with pulmonary obstruction):
— complete / corrected transposition
— single ventricle
— DORV
— tricuspid atresia (PS in 75%)
— asplenia syndrome

√ prominent aorta with L / R aortic arch; inapparent pulmonary trunk
√ NORMAL R atrium (without tricuspid regurgitation)
√ NORMAL-sized heart (secondary to escape mechanism into aorta)

Clues:
1. Skeletal anomaly (eg, scoliosis): tetralogy (90%)
2. Hepatic symmetry: asplenia
3. Right aortic arch: tetralogy, complete transposition, tricuspid atresia
4. Aberrant right subclavian artery: tetralogy
5. Leftward convexity of ascending aorta: single ventricle with inverted right rudimentary ventricle, corrected transposition, asplenia, JAA (tricuspid valve atresia)

HEART

B. SHUNT AT ATRIAL LEVEL
mnemonic: "PET"
1. **P**ulmonary stenosis / atresia with intact ventricular septum
2. **E**bstein malformation + Uhl anomaly
3. **T**ricuspid atresia (ASD in 100%)

√ moderate to severe cardiomegaly
√ R atrial dilatation
√ R ventricular enlargement (secondary to massive tricuspid incompetence)
√ inapparent aorta
√ left aortic arch

Pulmonary Venous Hypertension with Cyanosis

(a) during 1st week of life
1. Hypoplastic left heart syndrome
   √ marked cardiomegaly
2. TAPVR below diaphragm
   √ normal cardiac size

(b) during 2nd week of life
3. Aortic coarctation
4. Aortic atresia

(c) during 4–6th week of life
5. Critical aortic stenosis
6. Endocardial fibroelastosis
7. Anomalous origin of LCA
8. Atresia of common pulmonary vein

ACYANOTIC HEART DISEASE

Increased Pulmonary Blood Flow without Cyanosis

= indicates L-R shunt with increased pulmonary blood flow (shunt volume >40%)

A. WITH LEFT ATRIAL ENLARGEMENT
indicates shunt distal to mitral valve = increased volume without escape defect
1. VSD (25%): small aorta in intracardiac shunt
2. PDA (12%): aorta + pulmonary artery of equal size in extracardiac shunt
3. Ruptured sinus of Valsalva aneurysm (rare)
4. Coronary arteriovenous fistula (very rare)
5. Aortopulmonary window (extremely rare)

B. WITH NORMAL LEFT ATRIUM
indicates shunt proximal to mitral valve = volume increased with escape mechanism through defect
1. ASD (8%)
2. Partial anomalous pulmonary venous return (PAPVR) + sinus venosus ASD
3. Endocardial cushion defect (ECD) (4%)

Normal Pulmonary Blood Flow without Cyanosis

A. OBSTRUCTIVE LESION
1. Right ventricular outflow obstruction
   (a) at level of pulmonary valve: subvalvular / valvular / supravalvular pulmonic stenosis
   (b) at level of peripheral pulmonary arteries: peripheral pulmonary stenosis
2. Left ventricular inflow obstruction
   (a) at level of peripheral pulmonary veins: pulmonary vein stenosis / atresia
   (b) at level of left atrium: cor triatriatum
   (c) at level of mitral valve: supravalvular mitral stenosis, congenital mitral stenosis / atresia, "parachute" mitral valve
1. Left ventricular outflow obstruction
   (a) at level of aortic valve: anatomic subaortic stenosis, functional subaortic stenosis (IHSS), valvular aortic stenosis, hypoplastic left heart, supravalvular aortic stenosis
   (b) at level of aorta: interruption of aortic arch, coarctation of aorta

B. CARDIOMYOPATHY
1. Endocardial fibroelastosis
2. Hypertrophic cardiomyopathy
3. Glycogen storage disease

C. HYPERDYNAMIC STATE
1. Noncardiac AVM (cerebral AVM, vein of Galen aneurysm, large pulmonary AVM, hemangioendothelioma of liver)
2. Thyrotoxicosis
3. Anemia
4. Pregnancy

D. MYOCARDIAL ISCHEMIA
1. Anomalous left coronary artery
2. Coronary artery disease (CAD)

PULMONARY VASCULARITY

Normal Pulmonary Vasculature

A. VASCULAR DISTRIBUTION
√ pulmonary vessels within upper perihilum approximate 1/3 of total vascularity
√ pulmonary vessels within lower perihilum approximate 2/3 of total vascularity

B. VASCULAR TAPERING
√ pulmonary vessels taper near transition of middle 1/3 to outer 1/3 of lung

C. VASCULAR CALIBER
√ straight / slightly concave main pulmonary artery contour (mild convexity is normal in young females)
√ pulmonary trunk measures <4.5 cm (leftward distance from vertical line at carina to most lateral aspect of main pulmonary artery contour)
√ right interlobar / intermediate pulmonary artery measures 10–15 mm in males and 9–14 mm in females on PA radiographs
√ pulmonary vessel size <1–2 mm in extreme lung periphery
√ arteries within 1st anterior intercostal space measure ≤3 mm

Normal Pulmonary Vascularity & Normal-sized Heart

mnemonic: "MAN"
Myocardial ischemia
Afterload (= pressure overload problems)
Normal

HEART

Increased Pulmonary Vasculature

A. OVERCIRCULATION
 = shunt vascularity = arterial + venous overcirculation
 (a) congenital heart disease (most common)
  (1) L-R shunts
  (2) Admixture cyanotic lesions
 (b) high-flow syndromes
  (1) Thyrotoxicosis
  (2) Anemia
  (3) Pregnancy
  (4) Peripheral arteriovenous fistula
 √ diameter of right descending pulmonary artery larger than trachea just above aortic knob
 √ increased size of veins + arteries with size larger than accompanying bronchus (= "kissing cousin" sign), best seen just above hila on AP view
 √ enlarged hilar vessels (lateral view)
 √ visualization of vessels below 10th posterior rib

B. PULMONARY VENOUS HYPERTENSION
 √ redistribution of flow (not seen in younger children)
 √ indistinctness of vessels with Kerley lines (= interstitial edema)
 √ fine reticulated pattern
 √ alveolar edema

C. PRECAPILLARY HYPERTENSION
 √ enlarged main + right and left pulmonary arteries
 √ abrupt tapering of pulmonary arteries

D. PROMINENT SYSTEMIC / AORTOPULMONARY COLLATERALS
 1. Tetralogy of Fallot with pulmonary atresia (= pseudotruncus)
 2. VSD + pulmonary atresia (single ventricle, complete transposition, corrected transposition)
 3. Pulmonary-systemic collaterals
 √ coarse vascular pattern with irregular branching arteries (from aorta / subclavian arteries)
 √ small central vessels despite apparent increase in vascularity

Decreased Pulmonary Vascularity

= obstruction to pulmonary flow
√ vessels reduced in size and number
√ hyperlucent lungs
√ small pulmonary artery segment + hilar vessels

PULMONARY ARTERY

Invisible Main Pulmonary Artery

A. UNDERDEVELOPED = RVOT OBSTRUCTION
 1. Tetralogy of Fallot
 2. Hypoplastic right heart syndrome (tricuspid / pulmonary atresia)

B. MISPLACED PULMONARY ARTERY
 1. Complete transposition of great vessels
 2. Persistent truncus arteriosus

Unequal Pulmonary Blood Flow

1. Tetralogy of Fallot
 √ diminished flow on left side (hypoplastic / stenotic pulmonary artery in 40%)
2. Persistent truncus arteriosus (esp. type IV)
 √ diminished / increased blood flow to either lung
3. Pulmonary valvular stenosis
 √ increased flow to left lung secondary to jet phenomenon

Dilatation of Pulmonary Trunk

1. Idiopathic dilatation of pulmonary artery
2. Pulmonic valve stenosis
 √ poststenotic dilatation of trunk + left pulmonary a.
3. Pulmonary regurgitation
 (a) severe pulmonic valve insufficiency
 (b) absence of pulmonic valve (may be associated with tetralogy)
4. Congenital L-to-R shunts
5. Pulmonary arterial hypertension
6. Aneurysm: mycotic / traumatic

Pulmonary Artery-Bronchus Ratios

= ratio of diameters of end-on segmental pulmonary artery + accompanying end-on bronchus

A. ERECT CHEST FILM
 1. Normal (effect of gravity):
  upper lung zone .... 0.85 ± 0.15
  lower lung zone .... 1.34 ± 0.25
 2. Equalized / balanced redistribution pattern:
  upper lung zone .... 1.62 ± 0.31
  lower lung zone .... 1.56 ± 0.28
  Cause: systemic volume overload
 3. Cephalized redistribution pattern:
  upper lung zone .... 1.50 ± 0.25
  lower lung zone .... 0.87 ± 0.20
  Cause: hydrostatic cardiogenic edema

B. SUPINE CHEST FILM
 1. Normal (gravitational effect lost):
  upper lung zone .... 1.01 ± 0.13
  lower lung zone .... 1.05 ± 0.13
 2. Decompensated CHF (inverted pattern / plethora pattern):
  upper lung zone .... 1.49 ± 0.31
  lower lung zone .... 0.96 ± 0.31

PULMONARY HYPERTENSION

= sustained pulmonary arterial pressure in systole >25 mm Hg at rest / >30 mm Hg during exercise (in diastole >15 mm Hg, mean pressure >20 mm Hg) secondary to reduction in cross-sectional area of the pulmonary vascular bed with concomitant increase in pulmonary vascular resistance

Cx: central arterial thrombosis, premature atherosclerosis of central elastic + muscular pulmonary arteries, aneurysmal dissection of pulmonary arteries, hypertrophy + dilatation of right side of heart

Dx: clinical assessment of hemodynamic parameters, medical history, histologic findings

Pulmonary Arterial Hypertension

= PAH = precapillary pulmonary hypertension
= changes limited to arterial side of pulmonary circulation

Pathogenesis:

A. HYPERKINETIC CAUSES
  1. L-to-R shunt
  2. High cardiac output states: thyrotoxicosis, chronic anemia

B. OBLITERATIVE CAUSES
  (a) vascular = precapillary pulmonary hypertension:
    1. Primary plexogenic pulmonary arteriopathy = Primary pulmonary hypertension (PPH)
    2. Arteritis (eg, Takayasu)
    3. Embolization
      – chronic thromboembolic disease
      – tumor
        √ lymphangitic carcinomatosis
      – parasites, eg, schistosomiasis
        √ hepatosplenomegaly
      – talc crystals
        √ micronodular opacities
        √ perihilar fibrotic masses
    4. Persistent fetal circulation
    5. Pulmonary capillary hemangiomatosis
  (b) pleuropulmonic disease
    1. Chronic interstitial lung disease
      = **cor pulmonale**:
      COPD, emphysema, chronic bronchitis, asthma, bronchiectasis, malignant infiltrate, granulomatous disease, cystic fibrosis, end-stage fibrotic lung, S/P lung resection, idiopathic hemosiderosis, alveolar proteinosis, alveolar microlithiasis
    2. Pleural disease + chest deformity: fibrothorax, thoracoplasty, kyphoscoliosis
  (c) vasoconstrictive
    1. Chronic alveolar hypoxia
      = hypoxic pulmonary arterial hyperperfusion: chronic high altitude, sleep apnea, chronic hypercapnea due to hypoventilation from neuromuscular disease / obesity
    2. Portopulmonary hypertension (rare)

C. Chronic pulmonary venous hypertension

√ main pulmonary artery diameter >29 mm (69% sensitive, 100% specific)
√ "pruning" of peripheral pulmonary arteries
  = disproportionate increase in caliber of central fibrous arteries + decrease in caliber of smaller muscular arteries (from sustained increase in flow by a factor of >2)
√ mosaic perfusion
√ normal-sized heart / right heart enlargement
√ NO increase of pulsations in middle third of lung
√ complications:
  √ dilatation of bronchial arteries
  √ subpleural pulmonary infarcts (with elevated pulmonary venous pressure / underlying malignancy)
  √ calcified plaques of central pulmonary arteries (PATHOGNOMONIC)
  √ dissection / massive thrombosis of central pulmonary arteries

Cor Pulmonale

mnemonic: "TICCS BEV"

Thoracic deformity
Idiopathic
Chronic pulmonary embolism
COPD
Shunt (ASD, VSD, etc)
Bronchiectasis
Emphysema
Vasculitis

Pulmonary Venous Hypertension

= INCREASED VENOUS PULMONARY PRESSURE
= VENOUS CONGESTION
= postcapillary pulmonary hypertension = primary findings located within pulmonary venous circulation between capillary bed + left atrium

Dx: uniform / widely variable elevation of pulmonary capillary wedge pressure (PCWP) >15 mm Hg

Cause:

A. LEFT VENTRICULAR INFLOW TRACT OBSTRUCTION
  √ normal-sized heart with right ventricular hypertrophy
  √ prominent pulmonary trunk

Evaluation of Pulmonary Vasculature

	Normal	*PAH*	*PVH*	*Overload*
Distribution (UL:LL)	1:2	1:2	1:1 or 1:2	1:1
Vessel tapering	middle:outer third	variably pruned	outer third	outer third
Vascular caliber		increased	increased	increased
Artery-bronchus ratio				
upper lung zone	0.85 ± 0.15		1.50 ± 0.25	1.62 ± 0.31
lower lung zone	1.34 ± 0.25		0.87 ± 0.20	1.56 ± 0.28
Vascular margins	sharp	sharp	obscured	obscured

HEART

@ proximal to mitral valve:
√ normal-sized left atrium
— pulmonary veins
1. TAPVR below the diaphragm
2. Primary pulmonary venoocclusive disease (PVOD)
3. Stenosis of individual pulmonary veins
4. Atresia of common pulmonary vein
— mediastinum
1. Fibrosing mediastinitis (may also affect precapillary vessels)
2. Constrictive pericarditis
— left atrium
1. Cor triatriatum
2. Left atrial mass: tumor, clot
3. Supravalvular ring of left atrium

@ at mitral valve level = mitral valve stenosis
√ enlarged left atrium
1. Rheumatic mitral valve stenosis ± regurgitation (99%)
√ enlarged left atrial appendage
2. Congenital mitral valve stenosis
3. Parachute mitral valve (= single bulky papillary muscle)

B. LEFT VENTRICULAR FAILURE
(a) ABNORMAL PRELOAD with secondary mitral valve incompetence (= volume overload)
1. Aortic valve regurgitation
2. Eisenmenger syndrome (= R-to-L shunt in VSD)
3. High-output failure:
noncardiac AVM (cerebral AVM, vein of Galen aneurysm, large pulmonary AVM, hemangioendothelioma of liver, iatrogenic), thyrotoxicosis, anemia, pregnancy
(b) ABNORMAL AFTERLOAD
(= pressure overload)
= LV outflow tract obstruction
1. Hypoplastic left heart syndrome
2. Aortic stenosis (supravalvular, valvular, anatomic subaortic)
3. Interrupted aortic arch
4. Coarctation of the aorta
(c) DISORDERS OF CONTRACTION AND RELAXATION
1. Endocardial fibroelastosis
2. Glycogen storage disease (Pompe disease)
3. Cardiac aneurysm
4. Cardiomyopathy
(a) congestive (alcohol)
(b) hypertrophic obstructive cardiomyopathy (HOCM), particularly in IDM
— asymmetric septal hypertrophy (ASH)
— idiopathic hypertrophic subaortic stenosis (IHSS)
(d) MYOCARDIAL ISCHEMIA
1. Anomalous left coronary artery
2. Coronary artery disease (CAD)

Histo:
(a) primary changes: venous medial hypertrophy + intimal proliferation, marked thickening of venous internal elastic lamina
(b) secondary changes: capillary bed congestion with adjacent vascular proliferation, interlobular septal and pleural edema + fibrosis, lymphatic dilatation, alveolar hemosiderosis, paraseptal venous infarcts adjacent to complete venous occlusion

Cx: secondary pulmonary arterial hypertension
√ equalization of pulmonary vascularity (PCWP 13–15 mm Hg)
√ cephalization of pulmonary vascularity (PCWP 16–18 mm Hg)
√ interstitial pulmonary edema (PCWP 19–24 mm Hg)
= fluid within peribronchovascular connective tissue:
√ peribronchial thickening / cuffing
√ indistinct vessel margins
√ Kerley B lines = short horizontal reticulations within lateral subpleural lung bases
√ Kerley A lines = 3–4-cm-long lines of interlobular septal thickening radiating from hila to mid and upper lung zones
√ perihilar haze = hilar interstitial edema
√ thickened pleural fissures / pseudoeffusion = fluid within subpleural connective tissue
√ alveolar pulmonary edema (PCWP ≥25 mm Hg)
= bilateral perihilar and basilar airspace opacification
√ small pleural effusions

ABNORMAL HEART SIZE

Cardiothoracic Ratio

= ratio of cardiac diameter (measured as the sum of the most rightward + leftward margins from the midline) to inner thoracic margin at its largest diameter

<0.45	normal
0.45—0.55	mild cardiomegaly
>0.55	moderate / severe cardiomegaly

Vascular Pedicle Width

= distance on a horizontal line between (1) point where right mainstem bronchus + SVC cross and (2) point where left subclavian artery crosses horizontal line

48 ± 5 mm	normal
>53 mm	in 60% of cardiogenic edema, in 85% of volume overload

Abnormal Heart Chamber Dimensions

A. LEFT VENTRICULAR VOLUME OVERLOAD
1. VSD
2. PDA
3. Mitral incompetence
4. Aortic incompetence

B. LEFT VENTRICULAR HYPERTROPHY
1. Coarctation
2. Aortic stenosis

C. RIGHT VENTRICULAR VOLUME OVERLOAD
1. ASD
2. Partial APVR / total APVR
3. Tricuspid insufficiency

4. Pulmonary insufficiency
5. Congenital / acquired absence of pericardium
[6. Ebstein anomaly] – not truly RV

D. RIGHT VENTRICULAR HYPERTROPHY
1. Pulmonary valve stenosis
2. Pulmonary hypertension
3. Tetralogy of Fallot
4. VSD

E. FIXED SUBVALVULAR AORTIC STENOSIS

F. HYPOPLASTIC LEFT / RIGHT VENTRICLE, COMMON VENTRICLE

G. CONGESTIVE CARDIOMYOPATHY

Right Atrial Enlargement

◊ RA enlarges in rightward + posterior direction

PA CXR:
- √ >5.5 cm from midline to most lateral RA margin
- √ >2.5 cm from right vertebral margin
- √ >50% vertical height of RA compared with cardiovascular mediastinal height (from top of aortic arch to base of heart)

LAT CXR:
- √ double density on left side of heart

Right Ventricular Enlargement

◊ RV enlarges in anterior, superior + leftward direction causing levorotation of heart

PA CXR:
- √ straightening / convexity of left upper cardiac contour
- √ upturned cardiac apex
- √ left upper cardiac margin parallels left mainstem bronchus
- √ increased distance between left upper cardiac margin + left mainstem bronchus
- √ small appearance of rotated aortic arch + SVC
- √ large appearance of main pulmonary artery

LAT CXR:
- √ prominent convexity of anterior heart border >1/3 distance from anterior cardiophrenic sulcus to sternal angle

Left Atrial Enlargement

◊ LA enlarges in multiple directions

PA CXR:
- √ right retrocardiac double density
- √ >7.0 (female) / 7.5 (male) cm distance between midpoint of undersurface of left mainstem bronchus + right lateral LA shadow
- √ >75° splaying of carina with horizontal orientation of distal left mainstem bronchus
- √ enlargement of left atrial appendage
  ± calcifications (in 90% due to rheumatic heart disease)

LAT CXR:
- √ increased convexity of posterosuperior cardiac margin
- √ posterosuperior atrial convexity crosses vertical plane formed by tracheal midline + upper lobe bronchus
- √ posterior displacement of LUL bronchus

Left Ventricular Enlargement

◊ LV enlarges in posterior, inferior + leftward direction

PA CXR:
- √ leftward displacement of downturned cardiac apex = left ventricular configuration
- √ compression of left hemidiaphragm + gastric bubble

LAT CXR:
- √ increased convexity of posteroinferior cardiac margin
- √ posterior cardiac margin projects >1.8 cm posterior to IVC measured at a point 2 cm above intersection of IVC with right hemidiaphragm (Hofman-Rigler rule)

Cardiomegaly in Newborn

A. NONCARDIOGENIC
(a) metabolic:
1. Ion imbalance in serum levels of sodium, potassium, and calcium
2. Hypoglycemia

(b) decreased ventilation
1. Asphyxia
2. Transient tachypnea
3. Perinatal brain damage

(c) erythrocyte function
1. Anemia
2. Erythrocythemia

(d) endocrine
1. Glycogen storage disease
2. Thyroid disease: hypo- / hyperthyroidism

(e) infant of diabetic mother

(f) arteriovenous fistula
1. Vein of Galen aneurysm
2. Hepatic angioma
3. Chorioangioma

B. CARDIOGENIC
1. Arrhythmia
2. Myo- / pericarditis
3. Cardiac tumor
4. Myocardial infarction
5. Congenital heart disease

Neonatal Cardiac Failure

A. LEFT-SIDED OBSTRUCTIVE LESIONS
1. Segmental hypoplasia of aorta
2. Critical coarctation of the aorta
3. Aortic valve stenosis
4. Asymmetrical septal hypertrophy / hypertrophic obstructive cardiomyopathy
5. Mitral valve stenosis
6. Cor triatriatum

B. VOLUME OVERLOAD
1. Congenital mitral valve incompetence
2. Corrected transposition with left (= tricuspid) AV valve incompetence
3. Congenital tricuspid insufficiency
4. Ostium primum ASD

C. MYOCARDIAL DYSFUNCTION / ISCHEMIA
   1. Nonobstructive cardiomyopathy
   2. Anomalous origin of LCA from pulmonary trunk
   3. Primary endocardial fibroelastosis
   4. Glycogen storage disease (Pompe disease)
   5. Myocarditis

D. NONCARDIAC LESIONS
   1. AV fistulas: hemangioendothelioma of liver, AV fistula of brain, vein of Galen aneurysm, large pulmonary AV fistula
   2. Transient tachypnea of the newborn
   3. Intraventricular / subarachnoid hemorrhage
   4. Neonatal hypoglycemia (low birth weight, infants of diabetic mothers)
   5. Thyrotoxicosis (transplacental passage of LATS hormone)

Congestive Heart Failure & Cardiomegaly

mnemonic: "Ma McCae & Co."

Myocardial infarction
anemia
Malformation
cardiomyopathy
Coronary artery disease
aortic insufficiency
effusion
Coarctation

Congenital Cardiomyopathy

mnemonic: "CAVE GI"

Cystic medial necrosis of coronary arteries
Aberrant left coronary artery / **A**bsent coronary a.
Viral myocarditis
Endocardial fibroelastosis
Glycogen storage disease (Pompe)
Infant of diabetic mother / **I**schemia

ACQUIRED HEART DISEASE

√ LA enlargement = MV disease
√ dilated ascending aorta = aortic valve disease
√ RA enlargement = tricuspid valve disease

Pressure Overload

1. Systemic hypertension
2. Aortic stenosis
3. Mitral stenosis

Decreased Compliance

1. Myocardial infarction
2. Hypertrophic cardiomyopathy
3. Restrictive cardiomyopathy

Volume Overload

1. Aortic insufficiency
2. Mitral insufficiency
3. Tricuspid insufficiency

AORTA

Enlarged Aorta

PA CXR:
√ aortic knob >4.0 cm measured from indented trachea to most lateral margin of aorta
√ right convex contour above RA margin + lateral displacement of SVC (= dilatation of ascending aorta)

A. INCREASED VOLUME LOAD
   1. Aortic insufficiency
   2. PDA

B. POSTSTENOTIC DILATATION
   1. Valvular aortic stenosis

C. INCREASED INTRALUMINAL PRESSURE
   1. Coarctation
   2. Systemic hypertension

Approach to Acquired Heart Disease

	Mild–Moderate Cardiomegaly	*Moderate–Severe Cardiomegaly*
C/T ratio	0.45–0.55	>0.55
LA enlargement	*pressure overload* mitral stenosis *decreased LV compliance* hypertrophic cardiomyopathy restrictive cardiomyopathy	*volume overload* mitral insufficiency
Ascending aortic enlargement	*pressure overload* aortic stenosis	*volume overload* aortic insufficiency
Normal LA + aorta	*myocardial* acute infarction hypertrophic cardiomyopathy restrictive cardiomyopathy *pericardial* constrictive pericarditis	*myocardial* dilated cardiomyopathy ischemic cardiomyopathy *pericardial* pericardial effusion

D. MURAL WEAKNESS / INFECTION
   1. Cystic media necrosis: Marfan / Ehlers-Danlos syndrome
   2. Congenital aneurysm
   3. Syphilitic aortitis
   4. Mycotic aneurysm
   5. Atherosclerotic aneurysm (compromised vasa vasorum)

E. LACERATION OF AORTIC WALL
   1. Traumatic aneurysm
   2. Dissecting hematoma

Aortic Wall Thickening

1. Intramural hematoma
   = aortic dissection without intimal tear
2. Aortitis
   segments of aortic arch + branch vessels
3. Atherosclerotic plaque
   √ irregular narrowing of aortic lumen
4. Adherent thrombus

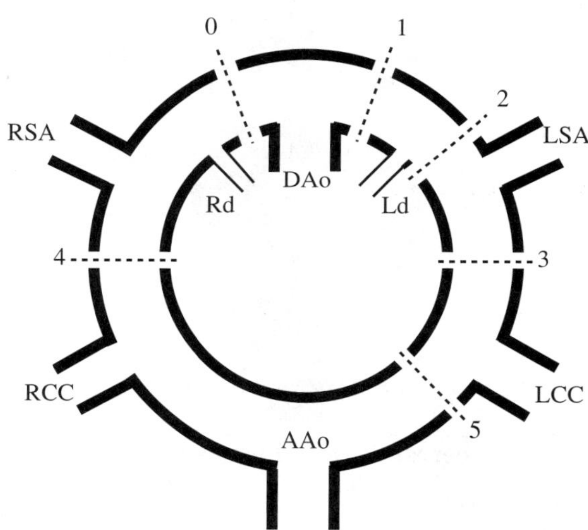

Edwards' Hypothetical Aortic Arch Development

RSA = right subclavian a.	AAo = ascending aorta
LSA = left subclavian a.	DAo = descending aorta
RCC = right common carotid a.	Rd = right ductus
LCC = left common carotid a.	Ld = left ductus

0 = normal left aortic arch
1 = right aortic arch with mirror-image branching; ductus from pulmonary a. to left brachiocephalic / subclavian a. = no vascular ring
2 = right aortic arch with mirror-image branching; ductus from pulmonary a. to descending aorta = complete vascular ring
3 = right aortic arch with aberrant left subclavian a.; ductus from pulmonary a. to descending aorta (most common complete vascular ring)
4 = left aortic arch with aberrant right subclavian a.
5 = right aortic arch with aberrant left brachiocephalic artery; ductus from pulmonary a. to descending aorta (very uncommon)
2 + 3 = right aortic arch with isolated left subclavian a. (very uncommon)

Aortic Calcifications

Intimal Calcification

Cause: part of atherosclerotic plaque
Associated with: inflammatory cells, lipid, vascular smooth muscle cells
Site: within perimeter of internal elastic lamina
√ discrete punctate lesion of radiograph

Medial Calcification

Cause: aging, diabetes, end-stage renal disease, neuropathy, genetic syndromes
Associated with: elastin + vascular smooth muscle cells
√ linear deposit along elastic lamellae resembling railroad tracks (when severe)

Double Aortic Arch

most common + serious type of a complete vascular ring; usually isolated condition
Embryology: failure of regression of either arch
Incidence: 55% of all vascular rings
Age: usually detected in infancy
- usually asymptomatic
- stridor, dyspnea, recurrent pneumonia
- dysphagia (less common than respiratory symptoms, more common after starting baby on solids)

Location: descending aorta in 75% on left, in 25% on right side; smaller arch anterior in 80%; right arch larger + more cephalad than left in 80%
√ two separate arches arise from single ascending aorta
√ each arch joins to form a common descending aorta
√ trachea in midline:
  √ impressions may be present on both sides of trachea: usually R > L (in older children)
  √ trachea narrowed and displaced posteriorly with small anterior impression

Esophagogram:
  √ broad horizontal posterior indentation at the level of 3rd / 4th thoracic vertebra (by right arch crossing obliquely to join left arch)
  √ bilateral esophageal indentations with a reversed S-shaped configuration (= right indentation higher than left)

CT:
  √ "four-artery sign" = each arch gives rise to 2 dorsal subclavian + 2 ventral carotid arteries evenly spaced around trachea on section cephalad to aortic arch

DDx: right arch with aberrant left subclavian artery (indistinguishable by esophagogram when dominant arch on right side)

Right Aortic Arch

Incidence: 1–2%
Embryology: persistence of right aortic arch and right descending aorta + regression of left aortic arch

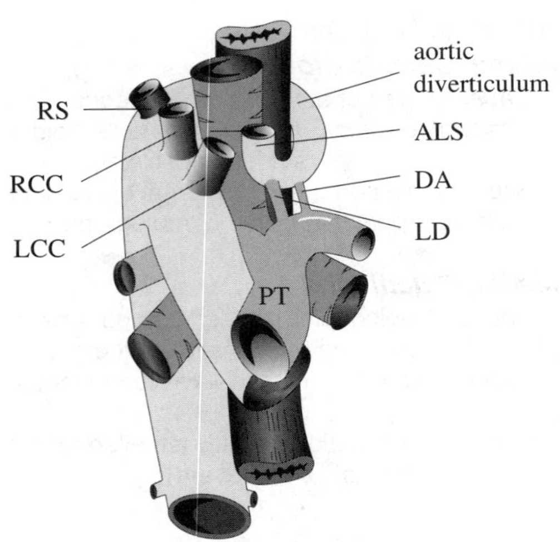

Right Aortic Arch with Aberrant Left Subclavian Artery

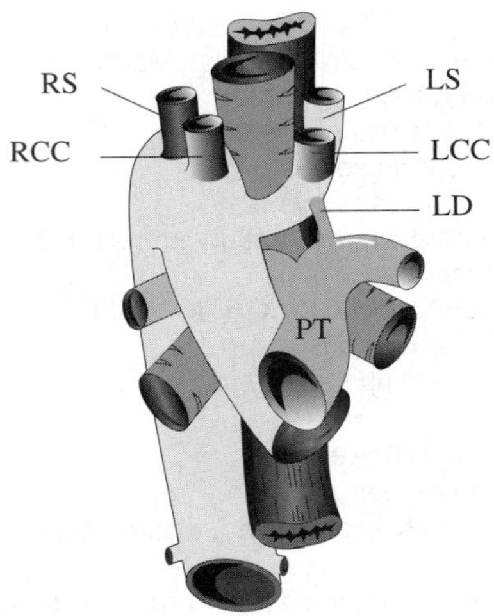

Right Aortic Arch with Mirror-image Branching

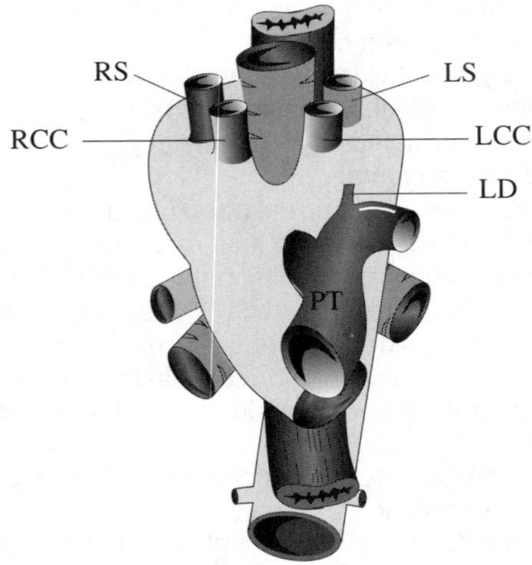

Double Aortic Arch

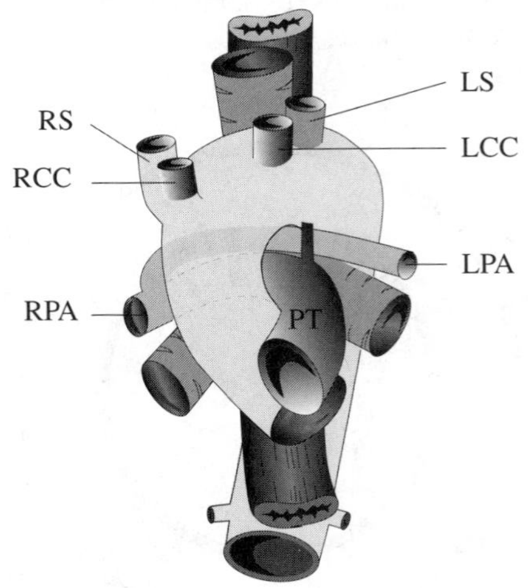

Aberrant Left Pulmonary Artery

ALS = aberrant left subclavian a.
LPA = left pulmonary a.
RS = right subclavian a.
LS = left subclavian a.
PT = pulmonary trunk
LCC = left common carotid a.
RCC = right common carotid a.
LD = left ductus arteriosus
RPA = right pulmonary a.

Course: to right of trachea + esophagus, over right mainstem bronchus; crosses lower thoracic spine; passes through left hemidiaphragm

INCIDENCE OF RIGHT AORTIC ARCH IN CONGENITAL HEART DISEASE

1. Truncus arteriosus 35%
2. Pulmonary atresia 25%
3. Tetralogy of Fallot 20%
4. Tricuspid atresia.............. 15%
5. DORV................................ 12%
6. TGV...................................... 8%
7. Large VSD 2%

Rare anomalies:

1. Corrected transposition
2. Pseudotruncus
3. Asplenia
4. Pink tetralogy

Right Aortic Arch with Aberrant Left Subclavian Artery

= RAA with ALSA
= interruption of embryonic left arch between left CCA and left subclavian artery
◊ Most common type of right aortic arch anomaly
◊ 2nd most common cause of vascular ring after double aortic arch

Incidence: 1:2,500; 35–72% of right aortic arch anomalies

Associated with: congenital heart disease in 5–12%:

1. Tetralogy of Fallot (2/3 = 8%)
2. ASD ± VSD (1/4 = 3%)
3. Coarctation (1/12 = 1%)

- usually asymptomatic (loose ring around trachea + esophagus)
- may be symptomatic in infancy / early childhood provoked by bronchitis + tracheal edema

- may be symptomatic in adulthood provoked by torsion of aorta

√ left common carotid artery is first branch of ascending aorta
√ left subclavian artery arises from descending aorta via the remnant of the left dorsal aortic root
√ bulbous configuration of origin of LSA (= remnant of embryonic left arch) = retroesophageal aortic diverticulum = diverticulum of Kommerell (N.B.: originally described as diverticular outpouching at origin of right subclavian artery with left aortic arch):
  √ small rounded density left lateral to trachea
  √ impression on left side of esophagus simulating a double aortic arch (by aortic diverticulum or ductus / ligamentum arteriosum)
√ vascular ring (= left ductus extends from aortic diverticulum to left pulmonary artery):
  √ impression on tracheal air shadow (by right aortic arch)
  √ right esophageal indentation (by right aortic arch)
  √ masslike density silhouetting top of aortic arch just posterior to trachea on LAT CXR (by aberrant left subclavian artery)
  √ broad posterior impression on esophagus (left subclavian artery / aortic diverticulum)
  √ small anterior impression on trachea (by left common carotid artery)
  √ descending aorta on right side

Right Aortic Arch with Mirror-image Branching

2nd most common aortic arch anomaly: 24–60%
= interruption of embryonic left arch between left subclavian artery and descending aorta; dorsal to left ductus arteriosus

(a) Type 1 = interruption of left aortic arch distal to ductus arteriosus (common)
Associated with: cyanotic CHD in 98%:
1. Tetralogy of Fallot (87%)
2. Multiple defects (7.5%)
3. Truncus arteriosus (2–6%)
4. Transposition (1–10%)
5. Tricuspid atresia (5%)
6. ASD ± VSD (0.5%)

◊ 25% of patients with tetralogy have right aortic arch!
◊ 37% of patients with truncus arteriosus have right aortic arch!

√ NO vascular ring, NO retroesophageal component
√ NO structure posterior to trachea
√ R arch impression on tracheal air shadow
√ NORMAL barium swallow

(b) Type 2 = interruption of left aortic arch proximal to ductus arteriosus (rare)
true vascular ring (if duct persists);
rarely associated with CHD

Right Aortic Arch with Isolated Left Subclavian Artery

◊ 3rd most common right aortic arch anomaly: 2%
= interruption of embryonic left arch between
(a) left CCA and left subclavian artery and
(b) left ductus and descending aorta
resulting in a connection of left subclavian artery with left pulmonary artery

Associated with: tetralogy of Fallot

√ left common carotid artery arises as the first branch
√ left subclavian artery attaches to left pulmonary artery through PDA
√ NO vascular ring, NO retroesophageal component

- congenital subclavian steal syndrome

Right Aortic Arch with Aberrant Left Brachiocephalic Artery

Similar in appearance to R aortic arch + aberrant L subclavian artery

Left Aortic Arch

Left Aortic Arch with Aberrant Right Subclavian Artery

= right subclavian artery arises as 4th branch from proximal descending aorta

Incidence: 0.4–2.3% of population; in 37% of Down syndrome children with CHD;
◊ Most common congenital aortic arch anomaly!

Associated with: (1) Absent recurrent pharyngeal n.
(2) CHD in 10–15%

Course: (a) behind esophagus (80%)
(b) between esophagus + trachea (15%)
(c) anterior to trachea (5%)

- asymptomatic / dysphagia lusoria (rare)

√ soft-tissue opacity crossing the esophagus obliquely upward toward the right shoulder (PATHOGNOMONIC)
√ masslike opacity in right paratracheal region
√ rounded opacity arising from superior aortic margin posterior to trachea + esophagus on LAT CXR
√ dilated origin of aberrant right subclavian artery (in up to 60%) = **diverticulum of Kommerell**
= remnant of embryonic right arch
√ unilateral L-sided rib notching (if aberrant right subclavian artery arises distal to coarctation)

Anomalous Innominate Artery Compression Syndrome

= origin of R innominate artery to the left of trachea coursing to the right
√ anterior tracheal compression

- ablation of right radial pulse by rigid endoscopic pressure

√ posterior tracheal displacement
√ focal collapse of trachea at fluoroscopy
√ pulsatile indentation of anterior tracheal wall by innominate artery on MRI

HEART

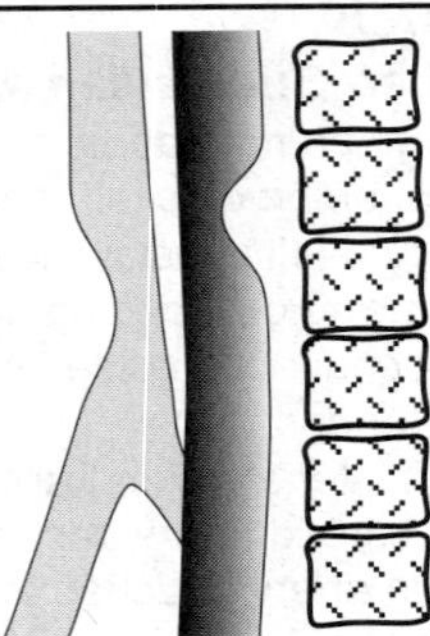

A. Anterior tracheal indentation + large posterior esophageal impression:
1. Double aortic arch
2. Right aortic arch with aberrant left subclavian + left ductus / ligamentum arteriosus
3. Left aortic arch with aberrant right subclavian + right ductus / ligamentum (extremely rare)

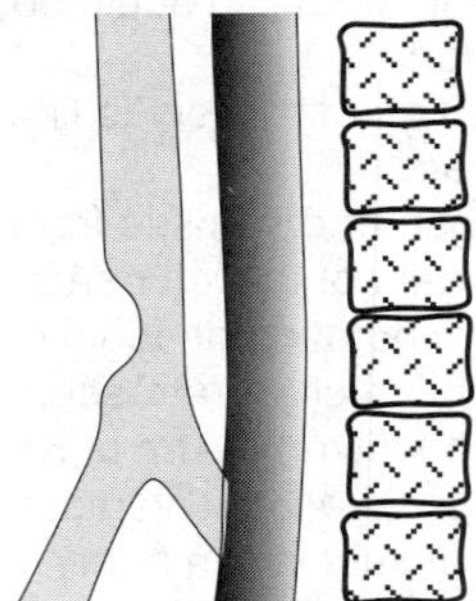

B. Anterior tracheal indentation
1. Compression by innominate artery with origin more distal along aortic arch
2. Compression by left common carotid artery with origin more proximal on arch
3. Common origin of innominate and left common carotid artery

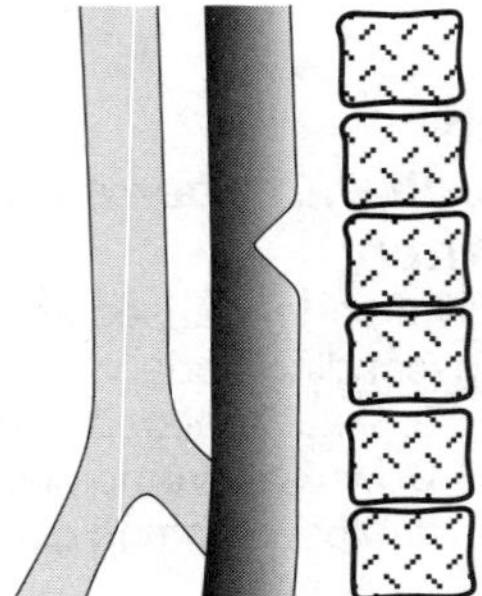

C. Small posterior esophageal impression
- dysphagia lusoria (lusorius, *Latin* = playful)
1. Left aortic arch with aberrant right subclavian artery
2. Right aortic arch with aberrant left subclavian

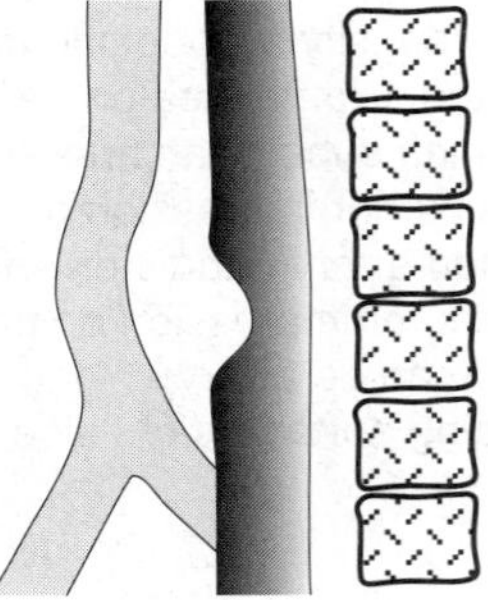

D. Posterior tracheal indentation + anterior esophageal impression
1. Aberrant left pulmonary artery

Pattern of Vascular Compression of Esophagus and Trachea

Rx: surgical attachment of innominate artery to manubrium

Vascular Rings

= anomaly characterized by encirclement of trachea + esophagus by aortic arch + branches

A. USUALLY SYMPTOMATIC LESIONS
- chronic stridor, wheezing, recurrent pneumonia
- dysphagia, failure to thrive

1. Double aortic arch with R descending aorta + L ductus arteriosus
2. R aortic arch with R descending aorta + aberrant L subclavian artery + persistent L ductus / ligamentum arteriosum

   N.B.: left obliterated ductus arteriosus (= **ligament of Botallo**) passes from L pulmonary a. to descending aorta / L subclavian a.

   - symptoms + radiographic findings identical to double aortic arch

   √ indentation on right lateral esophageal wall (by aortic arch)
   √ impression on the anterolateral esophageal wall (by ligament of Botallo)
   √ origin of L subclavian artery frequently dilated
3. L arch with L descending aorta + R ductus / ligamentum
4. Aberrant L pulmonary artery = "pulmonary sling"

Frequency of CXR findings:
- frontal CXR:
  - √ right aortic arch (85%)
  - √ focal indentation of distal trachea (73%)
- lateral CXR:
  - √ anterior tracheal bowing (92%)
  - √ increased retrotracheal opacity (79%)
  - √ focal tracheal narrowing (77%)

B. OCCASIONALLY SYMPTOMATIC LESIONS
1. Anomalous R innominate artery
2. Anomalous L common carotid artery / common trunk

3. R aortic arch with L descending aorta + L ductus / ligamentum

C. USUALLY ASYMPTOMATIC LESIONS
1. L aortic arch + aberrant R subclavian artery
2. L aortic arch with R descending aorta
3. R aortic arch with R descending aorta + mirror-image branching
4. R aortic arch with R descending aorta + aberrant L subclavian artery
5. R aortic arch with R descending aorta + isolation of L subclavian artery
6. R aortic arch with L descending aorta + L ductus / ligamentum

Aortic Stenosis

A. ACQUIRED
1. Takayasu aortitis
2. Radiation aortitis
3. Aortic dissection
4. Infected aortic aneurysm with abscess
5. Pseudoaneurysm from laceration
6. Atherosclerosis (rare)
7. Syphilitic aortitis (rare)

B. CONGENITAL
1. Williams syndrome
2. Neurofibromatosis
3. Rubella
4. Mucopolysaccharidosis
5. Hypoplastic left heart syndrome

Abnormal Left Ventricular Outflow Tract

LVOT = area between IVS + aML from aortic valve cusps to mitral valve leaflets

1. Membranous subaortic stenosis
   = crescent-shaped fibrous membrane extending across LVOT + inserting at aML
   √ diffuse narrowing of LVOT
   √ abnormal linear echoes in LVOT space (occasionally)
2. Prolapsing aortic valve vegetation
3. Narrowed LVOT (<20 mm)
   (a) Long-segment subaortic stenosis
      √ aortic valve closure in early systole with coarse fluttering
      √ high-frequency flutter of mitral valve in diastole (aortic regurgitation)
      √ symmetric LV hypertrophy
   (b) ASH / IHSS
      √ asymmetrically thickened septum bulging into LV + LVOT
      √ systolic anterior motion of aML (SAM)
   (c) Mitral stenosis
   (d) Endocardial cushion defect

SITUS

= "position / site / location" referring to the position of the atria and viscera relative to the midline
(a) systemic / right atrium
   √ has a broad-based appendage
   √ receives blood from IVC
   √ has terminal crest + coarse pectinate muscles
(b) pulmonary / left atrium
   √ has a small narrow appendage
   √ receives blood from pulmonary veins

A. SITUS SOLITUS = normal / usual situs
- on right side: √ systemic atrium
  √ trilobed lung
  √ liver
  √ gallbladder
  √ IVC
- on left side: √ pulmonary atrium
  √ bilobed lung
  √ stomach
  √ single spleen
  √ aorta

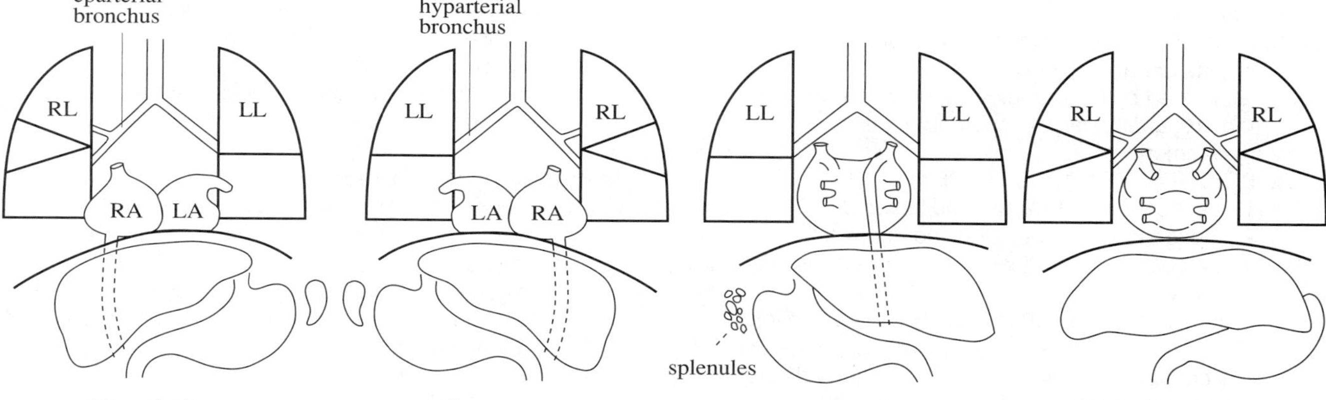

Situs Solitus

Situs Inversus anterior view

Left Isomerism posterior view

Right Isomerism posterior view

Situs Anomalies

Associated with:
(a) levocardia : 0.6–0.8% chance for CHD
(b) dextrocardia : 95% chance for CHD

B. SITUS INVERSUS
= mirror-image arrangement of situs solitus
Frequency: 0.01%
- on left side: √ systemic atrium
√ trilobed lung
√ liver
√ gallbladder
√ IVC
- on right side: √ pulmonary atrium
√ bilobed lung
√ stomach
√ single spleen
√ aorta

Associated with:
(a) dextrocardia = situs inversus totalis (usual variant): 3–5% chance for CHD, eg, Kartagener syndrome (in 20%)
(b) levocardia (extremely rare): 95% chance for CHD

C. SITUS AMBIGUUS = HETEROTAXIA
= visceral malposition + dysmorphism associated with indeterminate atrial arrangement
Subclassification:
1. Asplenia syndrome = double right-sidedness
= right isomerism = Ivemark syndrome
√ both lungs have 3 lobes
√ eparterial bronchi = main bronchus passes superior to ipsilateral main pulmonary artery
2. Polysplenia syndrome = double left-sidedness
= left isomerism
√ both lungs have 2 lobes
√ hyparterial bronchi = main bronchus passes inferior to ipsilateral main pulmonary artery

Associated with: CHD in 50–100%

Cardiac Malposition

(a) location of heart other than within left hemothorax in situs solitus
(b) location of heart within left hemithorax when other organs are ambiguous

◊ Determined by base-apex axis; no assumption is made regarding cardiac chamber / vessel arrangement

A. POSITION OF CARDIAC APEX
1. Levocardia = apex directed leftward
2. Dextrocardia = apex directed rightward
3. Mesocardia = vertical / midline heart (usually with situs solitus)

√ atrial septum characteristically bowed into left atrium in cardiac situs solitus with dextrocardia + cardiac situs inversus with levocardia (DDx: juxtapositioned atrial appendages)

B. CARDIAC DISPLACEMENT
by extracardiac factors (eg, lung hypoplasia, pulmonary mass)
1. Dextroposition
suggests hypoplasia of ipsilateral pulmonary artery (PAPVR implies scimitar syndrome)
2. Levoposition
3. Mesoposition

C. CARDIAC INVERSION
= alteration of normal relationship of chambers
1. D-bulboventricular loop
2. L-bulboventricular loop

D. TRANSPOSITION
= alteration of anterior-posterior relationship of great vessels

CARDIAC TUMOR

Prevalence: 0.001–0.03% (autopsy series)

◊ Rare often asymptomatic tumors until very large!

- symptoms of cardiopulmonary diseases:
  - congestive heart failure: dyspnea, orthopnea, peripheral edema, paroxysmal nocturnal dyspnea
  - palpitations, heart murmur
  - cough, chest pain
- symptoms caused by peripheral emboli to cerebral / systemic / coronary circulation:
  - syncope
- weight loss, fever, malaise

Location: intracavitary (obstruction, emboli), intramural (arrhythmia), pericardial (tamponade)

CXR:
√ cardiomegaly, pericardial effusion
√ signs of CHF
√ abnormal cardiac contour
√ pleural effusion

Benign Heart Tumor in Adults

◊ More common than malignant neoplasms

1. Myxoma (most common primary cardiac tumor; 50% of all primary cardiac tumors)
2. Papillary fibroelastoma (10% of all primary cardiac tumors; most common valvular tumor)
3. Lipoma
4. Hydatid cyst (uncommon):
√ localized bulge of left cardiac contour
√ curvilinear / spotty calcifications (resembling myocardial aneurysm)
Cx: may rupture into cardiac chamber / pericardium

Malignant Heart Tumors

Prevalence: 25% of all cardiac tumors in adults
10% of all cardiac tumors in children

1. Sarcoma:
◊ Majority of primary malignant cardiac neoplasms!
◊ 2nd most common primary cardiac neoplasm
2. Rhabdomyosarcoma
◊ Most common primary in children
3. Metastatic disease
(a) to peri- / epicardium
lung > breast > lymphoma > leukemia (most commonly)

(b) myocardium: malignant melanoma; secondary extension to myocardium from epicardium
(c) endocardial / intracavitary (in only 5%)
◊ 20–1000 times more frequent than primary tumor!
4. Lymphoma (rare)
5. Malignant teratoma
6. Multiple cardiac myxomas

Congenital Cardiac Tumor

Incidence: 1:10,000
1. Rhabdomyoma (58%): usually multiple masses
2. Teratoma (20%): intrapericardiac, extracardiac
√ multicystic mass
3. Fibroma (12%): intramural
may be associated with: Gorlin syndrome
Location: free LV wall / interventricular septum
√ may be pedunculated
√ calcification and cystic degeneration centrally
√ tendency for slow growth
Cx: fetal hydrops secondary to obstruction, pericardial effusion, fetal arrhythmia, fetal death
4. Hemangioma (arise from RT atrium, pericardial effusion, skin hemangiomas), lymphangioma, neurofibroma, myxoma, mesothelioma:
√ mass-occupying lesion impinging upon cardiac cavities

Cardiac Tumor by Location

A. ENDOCARDIAL / INTRACAVITARY
1. Myxoma
2. Thrombus
3. Myofibroblastic sarcomas (MFH, leiomyosarcoma, fibrosarcoma, myxosarcoma)

B. VALVULAR
1. Papillary fibroelastoma
2. Vegetations
3. Thrombus
4. Myxoma

C. MYOCARDIAL / INTRAMURAL
1. Rhabdomyoma: multifocal, high signal on T2WI
2. Fibroma: always solitary, calcifications, cystic degeneration, low signal on T2WI

D. ENDO- / MYO- / EPICARDIAL
1. Lipoma
2. Sarcoma
3. Primary cardiac lymphoma: right heart, multifocal, extension into pericardium

CARDIAC CALCIFICATIONS

Detected by:
fluoroscopy (at low-beam energies ≤75 kVp is 57% sensitive) < digital subtraction fluoroscopy < conventional CT < ultrafast CT (96% sensitive)

@ Coronary arteries

@ Cardiac valves
◊ Valvar calcification means stenosis — its amount is proportionate to degree and duration of stenosis!

1. **Aortic valve**
• usually indicates significant aortic stenosis
Cause:
congenital bicuspid valve (70–85%) > atherosclerotic degeneration > rheumatic aortic stenosis (rare), syphilis, ankylosing spondylitis
Location: above + anterior to a line connecting carina + anterior costophrenic angle (lateral view)
(a) Congenital bicuspid aortic valvular stenosis
• calcium first detected at an average age of 28 years
◊ In patients <30 years aortic valve calcifications are mostly due to a bicuspid aortic valve!
√ usually extensive cluster of heavy dense calcific deposits assuming a nodular contour
√ poststenotic dilatation of ascending aorta
(b) Isolated rheumatic aortic stenosis
• calcium first detected at an average age of 47 years
◊ In patients 30–60 years of age aortic valve calcification suggests rheumatic valve disease!
√ cluster of heavy dense calcific deposits without bicuspid contour
(c) Degenerative aortic stenosis
• calcium first detected at an average age of 54 years
◊ In patients >65 years aortic valve calcification in 90% due to atherosclerosis!
√ curvilinear shape of calcium outlining tricuspid leaflets
√ diffuse dilatation + tortuosity of aorta (NO poststenotic dilatation)
2. **Mitral valve leaflet**
Cause: rheumatic heart disease (virtually always), mitral valve prolapse
Location: inferior to a line connecting carina + anterior costophrenic angle (on lateral view)
• calcium first detected in early thirties when patients become overtly symptomatic
√ delicate calcification similar to coronary arteries (DDx: calcium in RCA / LCX)
√ superior-to-inferior motion
3. **Pulmonic valve**
Cause: tetralogy of Fallot, pulmonary stenosis, atrial septal defect
√ calcific pattern similar to calcified mitral valve
4. **Tricuspid valve** (extremely rare)
Cause: rheumatic heart disease, septal defect, tricuspid valve defect, infective endocarditis

@ Annulus
= valve rings serve as fibrous skeleton of the heart for attachment of myocardial fibers + cardiac valves
1. **Mitral annulus**
Cause: degenerative (physiologic in elderly)
Age: >65 years
May be associated with: mitral valve prolapse
Commonly associated with: aortic valve calcium

HEART

√ dense bandlike calcification starting at posterior aspect + progressing laterally frequently forming a "reversed C" / "O" / "U" / "J"

Cx: mitral insufficiency (due to impaired anterior mitral leaflet), atrial fibrillation, heart block (due to infiltration into posterior wall conduction pathway)

2. **Aortic annulus**
   √ usually in combination with degenerative aortic valve calcification
3. **Tricuspid annulus**
   Associated with: long-standing RV hypertension
   Location: right AV groove
   √ bandlike C-shaped configuration

@ Pericardium
Cause: idiopathic pericarditis, rheumatoid arthritis (5%), tuberculosis, viral, chronic renal failure, radiotherapy of mediastinum
Location: calcification over less pulsatile right-sided chambers along diaphragmatic surface, atrioventricular grooves, pulmonary trunk
◊ 50% of patients with constrictive pericarditis show pericardial calcifications!
Cx: constrictive pericarditis

@ Myocardium
Cause: infarction, aneurysm, rheumatic fever, myocarditis
Frequency: in 8% post myocardial infarction; M > F
Location: apex / anterolateral wall of LV (coincides with LAD vascular distribution + typical location of LV aneurysms)
√ thin curvilinear contour outlines the aneurysm
√ shaggy laminated calcification suggests calcification of associated mural thrombus
√ coarse amorphous calcifications are caused by trauma, cardioversion, infection, endocardial fibrosis

@ Interventricular septum
Location: triangular fibrous area between mitral + tricuspid annuli (= trigona fibrosa) representing the basal segment of interventricular septum, closely related to bundle of His
Always associated with:
heavy calcification of mitral annulus / aortic valve
Cx: heart block

@ Left atrial wall
Cause: rheumatic mitral valve disease
(a) diffuse form
- patient usually in bilateral CHF + atrial fibrillation

√ diffuse sheetlike calcification starting in the appendage sparing posterolateral wall on right side
Cx: mural thrombus formation + emboli

(b) localized form
√ nodular calcific scar in posterior wall (= McCallum patch) due to injury from a forceful jet in mitral valve insufficiency

@ Cardiac tumor
atrial myxoma (in 10% calcified), rhabdomyoma, fibroma, angioma, osteosarcoma, osteoclastoma

@ Endocardium
Cause: cardiac aneurysm, thrombus, endocardial fibroelastosis

@ Pulmonary artery
Cause: severe precapillary pulmonary arterial hypertension, syphilis

@ Ductus arteriosus
(a) in adults: indicates patency of ductus with associated long-standing precapillary pulmonary hypertension
(b) in children: ductus likely closed
√ calcium deposition in ligament of Botallo

Coronary Artery Calcification

◊ The amount of coronary calcification correlates with the extent of atherosclerosis!
◊ The absence of calcification implies the absence of angiographically significant coronary vessel narrowing!

Cause: (1) arteriosclerosis of intima
(2) Mönckeberg medial sclerosis (exceedingly rare)

Histo: calcified subintimal plaques

Pathophysiology:
injury to endothelium allows circulating histiocytes to lodge in vessel wall where they are transformed into macrophages; these accumulate lipids ("fatty streaks" beneath surface endothelium); lipids calcify; the thin fibrous cap overlying lipid deposits may rupture allowing circulating blood to mount a thrombogenic reaction resulting in narrowing of lumen
◊ Calcium is deposited as calcium hydroxyapatite in hemorrhagic areas within atheromatous plaques!

Location: "coronary artery calcification triangle"
= triangular area along mid left heart border, spine, and shoulder of LV containing left main coronary artery, proximal portions of LAD + LCX calcifications at autopsy: LAD (93%), LCX (77%), left main CA (70%), RCA (69%)

CXR (detection rate up to 42%):
◊ Indicating more severe coronary artery disease
√ parallel calcified lines (lateral view)

Fluoroscopy: (promoted as inexpensive screening test)
(a) asymptomatic population
— calcifications in 34% in asymptomatic male individuals
— in 35% of patients with calcifications exercise test will be positive (without calcifications only in 4% positive)
— calcifications indicate >50% stenosis with 72–76% sensitivity, 78% specificity); frequency of coronary artery calcifications with normal angiogram increases with age; predictive values in population <50 years as good as exercise stress test

(b) symptomatic population
— in 54% of symptomatic patients with ischemic heart disease
◊ In symptomatic patients 94% specificity for obstructive disease (>75% stenosis) of at least one of the three major vessels!

HEART

CT:
(a) electron beam: threshold of +130 HU
(b) spiral CT: threshold of +90 HU

Clinical outcome:
(a) for coronary calcifications detected at fluoroscopy: 5.4% event risk at 1 year (vs. 2.1% without calcification)
(b) for electron beam CT a calcification score of ≥100 is highly predictive to identify patients with events

Prognosis: 58% 5-year survival rate with and 87% without calcifications

PERICARDIUM

Pericardial Effusion

= pericardial fluid >50 mL

Etiology:

A. SEROUS FLUID = transudate
congestive heart failure, hypoalbuminemia, irradiation

B. BLOOD = hemopericardium
(a) iatrogenic: cardiac surgery / catheterization, anticoagulants, chemotherapy
(b) trauma: penetrating / nonpenetrating
(c) acute myocardial infarction / rupture
(d) rupture of ascending aorta / pulmonary trunk
(e) coagulopathy
(f) neoplasm: mesothelioma, sarcoma, teratoma, fibroma, angioma, metastasis (lung, breast, lymphoma, leukemia, melanoma)

C. LYMPH
neoplasm, congenital, cardiothoracic surgery, obstruction of hilum / SVC

D. FIBRIN = exudate
(a) infection: viral, pyogenic, TB
(b) uremia: 18% in acute uremia; 51% in chronic uremia; dialysis patient
(c) collagen disease: rheumatoid arthritis, SLE, acute rheumatic fever
(d) hypersensitivity

mnemonic: "CUM TAPPIT RV"
Collagen vascular disease
Uremia
Metastasis
Trauma
Acute myocardial infarction
Purulent infection
Post MI syndrome
Idiopathic
Tuberculosis
Rheumatoid arthritis
Virus

CXR:
√ normal with fluid <250 mL / in acute pericarditis
√ "water bottle configuration" = symmetrically enlarged cardiac silhouette
√ loss of retrosternal clear space
√ "fat-pad sign" = separation of retrosternal from epicardial fat line >2 mm (15%)
√ rapidly appearing cardiomegaly + normal pulmonary vascularity
√ "differential density sign" = increase in lucency at heart margin secondary to slight difference in contrast between pericardial fluid + heart muscle
√ diminished cardiac pulsations

ECHO:
√ separation of epi- and pericardial echoes extending into diastole (rarely behind LA)
√ volume estimates by M-mode:
(a) separation only posteriorly = <300 mL
(b) separation throughout cardiac cycle = 300–500 mL
(c) plus anterior separation = >1000 mL

Pneumopericardium

Etiology: shearing mechanism of injury of the heart during blunt trauma

Path: tear in fibrous pericardium, usually along the course of the phrenic nerve, allows pneumomediastinal air to enter

√ thick shaggy soft-tissue density of fibrous pericardium separated by air from cardiac density
√ air limited to distribution of pericardial reflection

Pericardial Tumor

1. Pericardial teratoma: benign tumor of infants + children
2. Pericardial mesothelioma: malignant tumor of adulthood

DDx: pericardial invasion (sarcoma, lymphoma)

VENA CAVA

Vena cava anomalies

Circumaortic Left Renal Vein

Prevalence: 1.5–8.7%

Etiology: persistence of anterior intersubcardinal + posterior intersupracardinal anastomosis

√ venous collar encircling aorta
√ superior left renal vein crosses aorta anteriorly
√ inferior left renal vein receives left gonadal vein + crosses aorta posteriorly 1–2 cm below the superior left renal vein

Significance: preoperative plan for nephrectomy

Duplicated IVC

= DOUBLE IVC

Prevalence: 0.2–3%

Etiology: persistence of both supracardinal veins

√ small / equal-sized left IVC formed by left iliac vein
√ crossover to right IVC via left renal vein / or more inferiorly
√ crossover usually anterior / rarely posterior to aorta

Significance: recurrent pulmonary embolism after IVC filter placement

DDx: left gonadal v./ a., inferior mesenteric v.

DOUBLE IVC WITH RETROAORTIC RIGHT RENAL VEIN AND AZYGOS CONTINUATION OF IVC

Etiology: persistence of left supracardinal v. and dorsal limb of renal collar + regression of ventral limb + failure of formation of right subcardinal-hepatic anastomosis

DOUBLE IVC WITH RETROAORTIC RIGHT RENAL VEIN AND HEMIAZYGOS CONTINUATION OF IVC

Etiology: persistence of left lumbar + thoracic supracardinal v. + left suprasubcardinal anastomosis + failure of formation of right subcardinal-hepatic anastomosis

√ right IVC and right renal vein join the left IVC and continue cephalad as the hemiazygos vein
√ hemiazygos vein follows alternative pathways:
  (a) crosses posterior to aorta at T8/9 and joins the rudimentary azygos vein
  (b) continues cephalad + joins coronary vein via persistent left SVC
  (c) accessory hemiazygos continuation to left brachiocephalic vein
√ hepatic segment of IVC drains into right atrium

Interrupted IVC with Azygos / Hemiazygos Continuation

see AZYGOS CONTINUATION

Left IVC

= TRANSPOSITION OF IVC = SOLITARY LEFT IVC

Prevalence: 0.2–0.5%

Etiology: persistence of left + regression of right supracardinal vein

√ left IVC usually joins left renal vein
√ crossover as left renal vein usually anterior / rarely posterior to aorta

DDx: left-sided paraaortic adenopathy

Significance: difficult transjugular access to infrarenal IVC filter placement

Persistent Left SVC

= BILATERAL SVCs

Prevalence: 0.3% of general population; 4.3–11% of patients with CHD

Etiology: failure of regression of left anterior + common cardinal veins + left sinus horn

May be associated with: ASD, azygos continuation of IVC

Course: lateral to aortic arch, anterior to left hilum

√ left SVC drains into enlarged coronary sinus (common)
√ left SVC drains into LA (rare) creating a R-to-L shunt (increased prevalence of CHD)
√ hemiazygos arch formed by left superior intercostal vein + persistent left SVC (20%)
√ absent / small left brachiocephalic vein (65%)
√ absence of right SVC (10–18%)
√ anastomosis between right + left anterior cardinal veins (in 35%)

Retroaortic Left Renal Vein

Prevalence: 1.8–2.1%

Etiology: persistence of posterior intersupracardinal anastomosis + regression of anterior intersubcardinal anastomosis

√ crossover usually below / occasionally at level of right renal vein

IVC Obstruction

A. INTRINSIC OBSTRUCTION
  (a) neoplastic (most frequent)
    1. Renal cell carcinoma (in 10%), Wilms tumor
    2. Adrenal carcinoma, pheochromocytoma
    3. Pancreatic carcinoma, hepatic adenocarcinoma
    4. Metastatic disease to retroperitoneal lymph nodes (carcinoma of ovary, cervix, prostate)
  (b) nonneoplastic
    1. Idiopathic
    2. Proximally extending thrombus from femoroiliac veins
    3. Systemic disorders: coagulopathy, Budd-Chiari syndrome, dehydration, infection (pelvic inflammatory disease), sepsis, CHF
    4. Postoperative / traumatic phlebitis, ligation, plication, clip, cava filter, severe exertion
B. INTRINSIC CAVAL DISEASE
  (a) neoplastic
    1. Leiomyoma, leiomyosarcoma, endothelioma
  (b) nonneoplastic
    1. Congenital membrane
C. EXTRINSIC COMPRESSION
  (a) neoplastic
    1. Retroperitoneal lymphadenopathy (adults) due to metastatic disease, lymphoma, granulomatous disease (TB)
    2. Renal + adrenal tumors (children)
    3. Hepatic masses
    4. Pancreatic tumor
    5. Tumor-induced desmoplastic reaction (eg, metastatic carcinoid)
  (b) nonneoplastic
    1. Hepatomegaly
    2. Tortuous aorta / aortic aneurysm
    3. Retroperitoneal hematoma
    4. Massive ascites
    5. Retroperitoneal fibrosis
D. FUNCTIONAL OBSTRUCTION
  1. Pregnant uterus
  2. Valsalva maneuver
  3. Straining / crying (in children)
  4. Supine position with large abdominal mass
E. COLLATERAL PATHWAYS
  1. Deep pathway: ascending lumbar veins to azygos vein (right) + hemiazygos vein (left) + intravertebral, paraspinal, extravertebral plexus (Batson plexus)
  2. Intermediate pathway: via periureteric plexus + left gonadal vein to renal vein

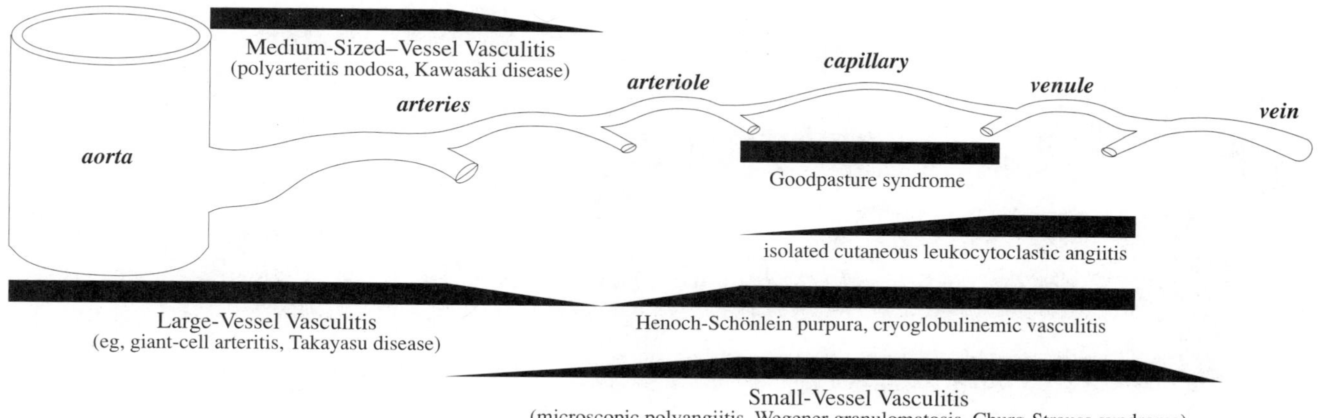

Noninfectious Vasculitides

3. Superficial pathway: external iliac vein to inferior epigastric vein + superior epigastric vein + internal mammary vein into subclavian vein
4. Portal pathway: retrograde flow through internal iliac vein + hemorrhoidal plexus into inferior mesenteric vein + splenic vein into portal vein

VASCULITIS

= inflammation and necrosis of vessel wall

A. LARGE-VESSEL VASCULITIS
   1. Giant cell (temporal) arteritis
   2. Takayasu disease

B. MEDIUM-SIZED–VESSEL VASCULITIS
   1. Polyarteritis nodosa
   2. Kawasaki disease
   3. Drug-induced vasculitis:
      – methamphetamine
      – cocaine: neurovascular, cardiovascular complications, aortic dissection, venous thrombosis, mesenteric artery thrombosis, renal infarction

C. SMALL-VESSEL VASCULITIS
   (a) ANCA-associated small-vessel vasculitis (= antineutrophil cytoplasmic autoantibodies)
      1. Wegener granulomatosis
      2. Churg-Strauss syndrome
      3. Microscopic polyangitis
   (b) immune-complex small-vessel vasculitis
      1. Henoch-Schönlein purpura
      2. Essential cryoglobulinemic vasculitis
      3. Cutaneous leukocytoclastic angitis
      others: lupus, rheumatoid, Sjögren, Behçet, Goodpasture, serum sickness, drug-induced, hypocomplementemic urticaria
   (c) inflammatory bowel disease vasculitis

Multiple Aneurysms

1. Polyarteritis nodosa
2. Rheumatoid vasculitis
3. Systemic lupus erythematosus
4. Churg-Strauss syndrome

CARDIAC SURGERY

Surgical Procedures

A. AORTICOPULMONARY WINDOW SHUNT
   = side-to-side anastomosis between ascending aorta and left pulmonary artery (reversible procedure)
   ◊ Tetralogy of Fallot

B. BLALOCK-HANLON PROCEDURE
   = surgical creation of ASD
   ◊ Complete transposition

C. BLALOCK-TAUSSIG SHUNT
   = end-to-side anastomosis of subclavian artery to pulmonary artery, performed ipsilateral to innominate artery / opposite to aortic arch
   Modified Blalock-Taussig shunt uses synthetic graft material such as polytetrafluoroethylene (Gore-Tex®) in an end-to-side anastomosis between subclavian artery + ipsilateral branch of pulmonary artery
   ◊ Tetralogy of Fallot, tricuspid atresia with pulmonic stenosis

D. FONTAN PROCEDURE
   (1) external conduit from right atrium to pulmonary trunk (= venous return enters pulmonary artery directly)
   (2) closure of ASD: floor constructed from flap of atrial wall and roof from piece of prosthetic material
   ◊ Tricuspid atresia

E. GLENN SHUNT
   = end-to-side shunt between distal end of right pulmonary artery and SVC; reserved for patients with cardiac defects in which total correction is not anticipated
   ◊ Tricuspid atresia

F. NORWOOD PROCEDURE
   (1) construction of "neoaorta" from aortic arch + descending aorta + main pulmonary artery supplying coronary and systemic circulation
   (2) communication between RV as systemic ventricle and systemic circulation

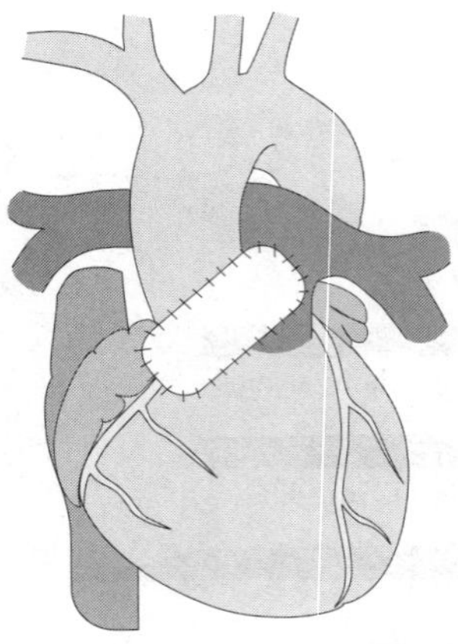
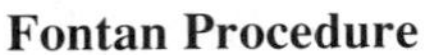

Fontan Procedure

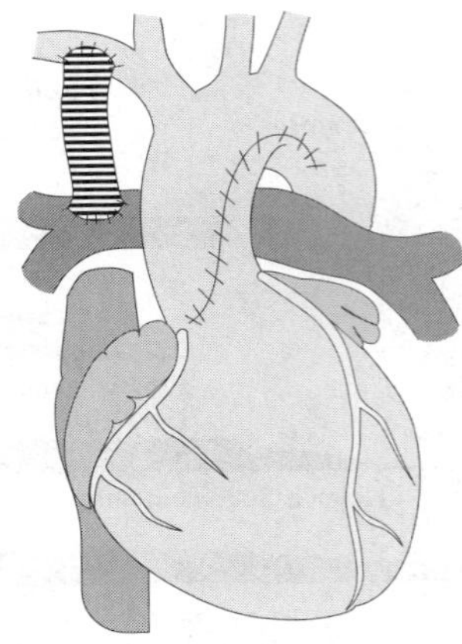

Norwood Procedure

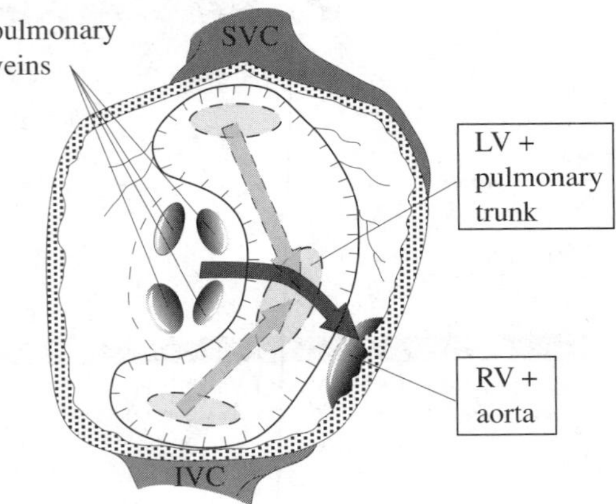

Mustard Procedure
(lateral view into opened right atrium)

(3) shunt between innominate artery + main pulmonary artery to control pulmonary arterial blood flow
(4) excision of distal ductus arteriosus + atrial septum to prevent pulmonary venous hypertension
◊ Hypoplastic left heart syndrome

G. POTT SHUNT
= side-to-side anastomosis between descending aorta + left pulmonary artery
◊ Tetralogy of Fallot

H. MUSTARD PROCEDURE
(a) removal of atrial septum
(b) pericardial baffle placed into common atrium such that systemic venous blood is rerouted into left ventricle and pulmonary venous return into right ventricle and aorta
◊ Complete transposition

I. RASHKIND PROCEDURE = balloon atrial septostomy
◊ Complete transposition

J. RASTELLI PROCEDURE
external conduit (Dacron) with porcine valve connecting RV to pulmonary trunk
◊ Transposition

K. WATERSTON-COOLEY SHUNT
= side-to-side anastomosis between ascending aorta and right pulmonary artery;
(a) extrapericardial (WATERSTON)
(b) intrapericardial (COOLEY)
◊ Tetralogy of Fallot

Postoperative Thoracic Deformity

A. ON RIGHT SIDE
1. Systemic-PA shunt: Blalock-Taussig shunt, Waterston-Cooley shunt, Glenn shunt, central conduit shunt
2. Atrial septectomy: Blalock-Hanlon procedure
3. VSD repair: through RA
4. Mitral valve commissurotomy

B. ON LEFT SIDE
1. PDA
2. Coarctation
3. PA banding
4. Mitral valve commissurotomy
5. Systemic-PA shunt: Blalock-Taussig shunt, Pott shunt

Heart Valve Prosthesis

1. Starr-Edwards
√ caged ball
◊ Predictable performance from large long-term experience
2. Bjørk-Shiley / Lillehei-Kaster / St. Jude
√ tilting disk
◊ Excellent hemodynamics, very low profile, durable
3. Hancock / Carpentier-Edwards (= porcine xenograft) Ionescu-Shiley (= bovine xenograft)
◊ Low incidence of thromboembolism, no hemolysis, central flow, inaudible

PULSUS ALTERNANS

= alternating arterial pulse height with regular cardiac rhythm
1. Intrinsic myocardial abnormality
severe left ventricular dysfunction (CHF, aortic valvular disease, hypothermia, hypocalcemia, hyperbaric stress, ischemia)
2. Alternating end-diastolic volumes
abnormalities in venous filling + return (obstructed venous return, IVC balloon

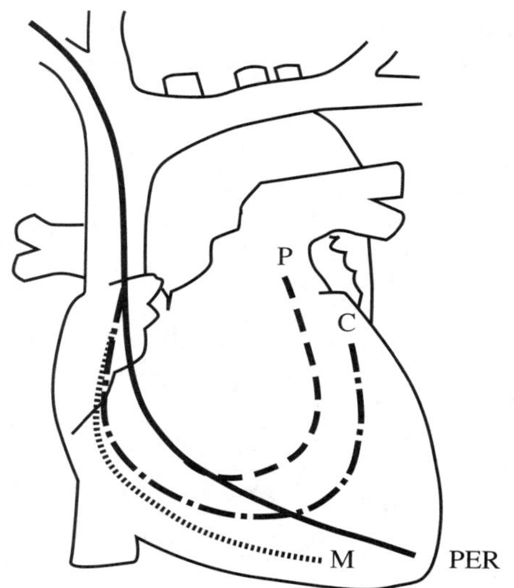

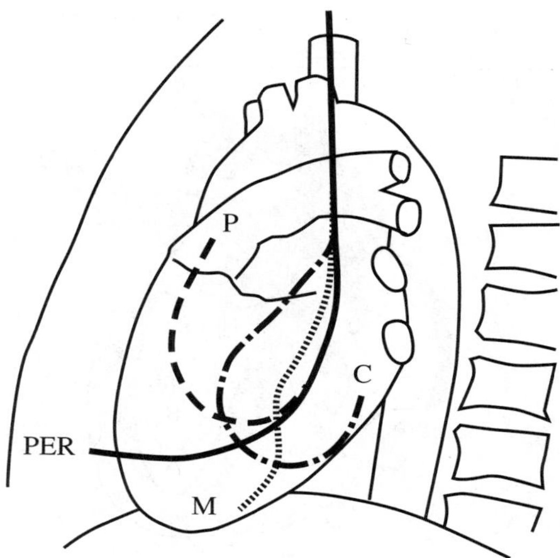

Central Venous Line Position

C = coronary sinus, M = middle cardiac vein, P = main pulmonary artery, PER = perforation

CARDIOVASCULAR ANATOMY AND ECHOCARDIOGRAPHY

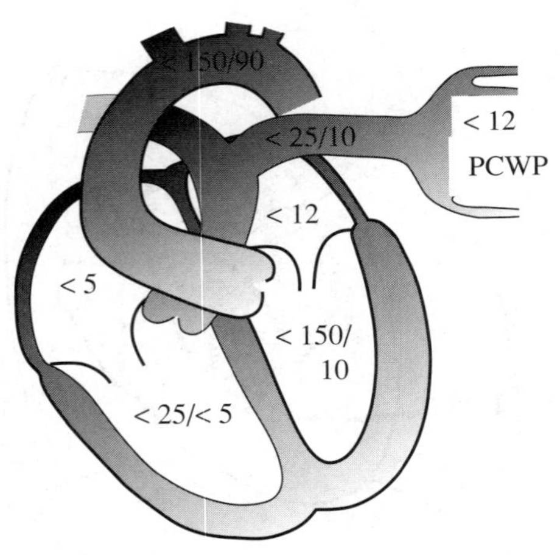

Normal Blood Pressures
PCWP = pulmonary capillary wedge pressure

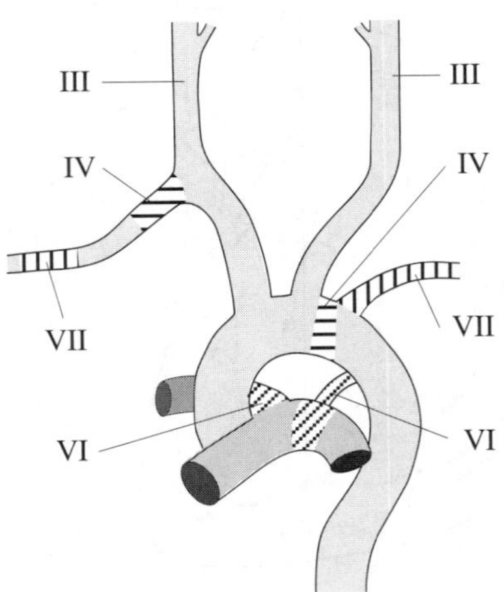

Development of Major Blood Vessels
numbers refer to embryologic aortic arches
most portions of aortic arches I, II, V regress

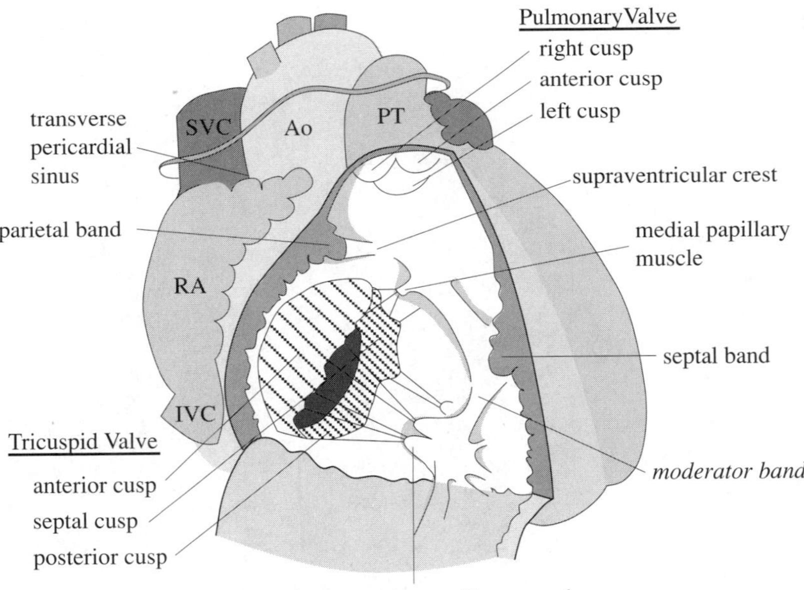

Right Ventricle Viewed from Front

Demarcation between posteroinferior inflow portion and anterosuperior outflow portion by prominent muscular bands forming an almost circular orifice

- parietal band
- crista supraventricularis
- septomarginal trabeculae (= septal band + moderator band)

Anterior papillary muscle originates from moderator band!

Ao = aorta IVC = inferior vena cava PT = pulmonic trunk
RA = right atrium SVC = superior vena cava

HEART

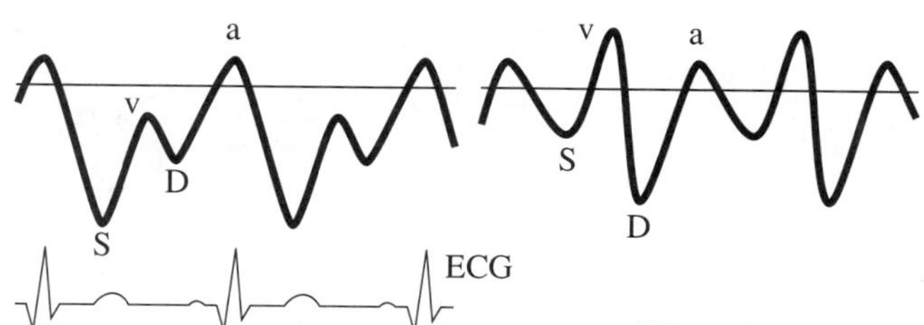

Normal Hepatic Waveform

Type 1
Tricuspid Regurgitation

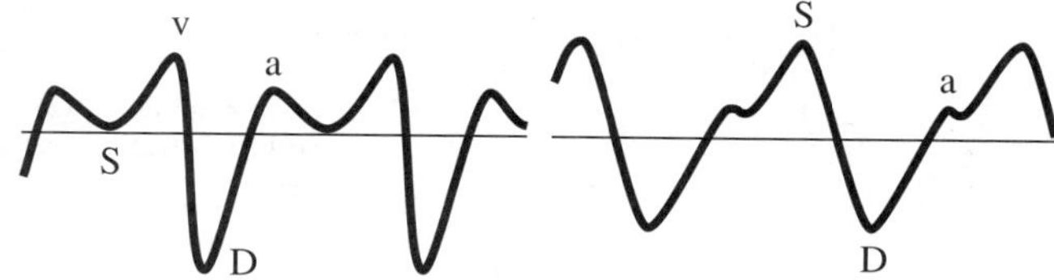

Type 2
Tricuspid Regurgitation

Type 3
Tricuspid Regurgitation

Doppler Waveforms of Hepatic Veins

S wave = systolic wave resulting from negative RA pressure caused by atrial relaxation + movement of tricuspid anulus toward cardiac apex

v wave = resulting from elevated RA pressure caused by RA overfilling against a closed tricuspid valve; occurs in <50% of patients

D wave = diastolic wave resulting from negative RA pressure caused by opening of tricuspid valve + blood flow from RA into RV; equal to / smaller than S wave

a-wave = resulting from elevated RA pressure caused by RA contraction; in 66% of patients

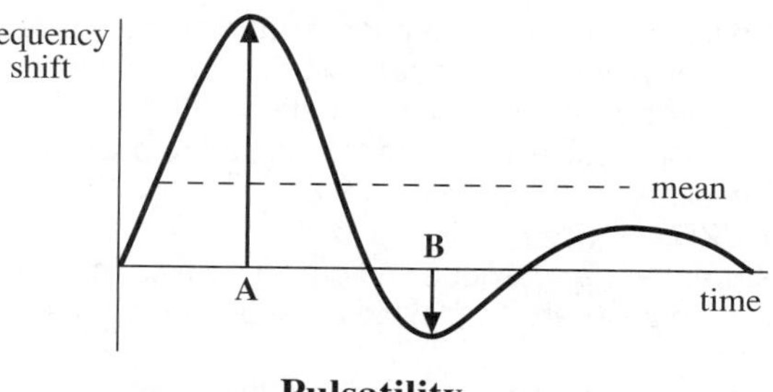

Pulsatility

PULSATILITY

= assessment of vascular resistance (increased resistance reduces diastolic flow)

◊ Can be assessed in vessels too small / tortuous to be imaged (Doppler angle unnecessary)!

◊ Index should be calculated for each of several cardiac cycles (5 heartbeats adequate) an average value taken

S = A = maximal systolic shift
D = B = end-diastolic frequency shift

1. Full pulsatility index of Gosling (PI_F) = $1/A_0^2\ SA_i^2$
2. Simplified pulsatility index (PI) = (S - D)/mean
3. Resistance index (RI) = Pourcelot index = (S - D)/S or 1 - (D/S)
4. Stuart index = A/B ratio = S/D ratio
5. B/A ratio = B(100%)/A

HEART VALVE POSITIONS

PA CXR:

reference line = oblique line drawn from distal left mainstem bronchus to right cardiophrenic angle

√ aortic valve resides in profile superior to this line overlying the thoracic spine

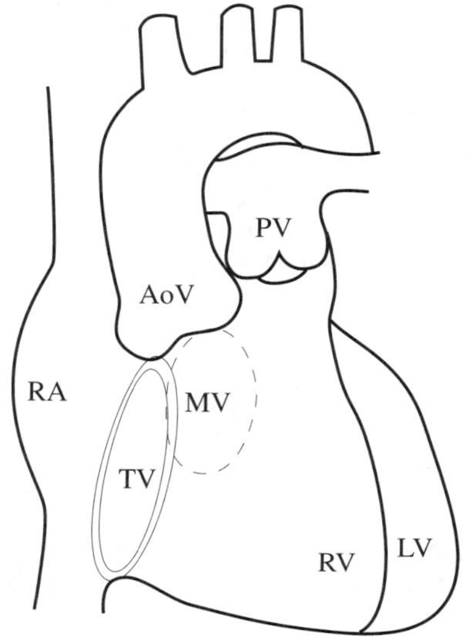

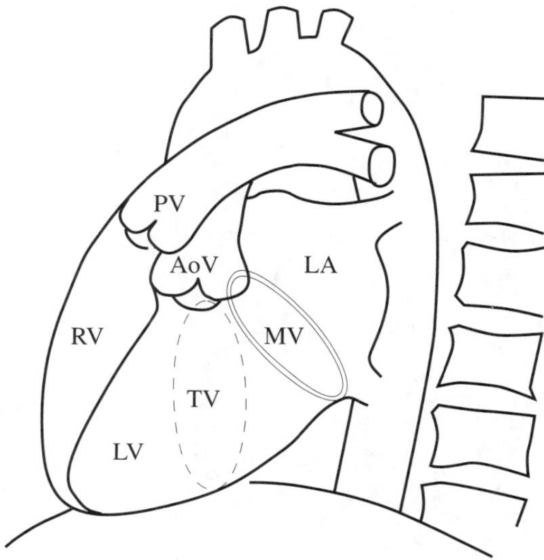

Heart Valve Positions
AoV = aortic valve, LA = left atrium, LV = left ventricle, MV = mitral valve, PV = pulmonic valve, RA = right atrium, RV = right ventricle, TV = tricuspid valve

√ pulmonic valve just inferior to left mainstem bronchus
√ mitral valve resides inferior to this line centrally located within cardiac silhouette
√ tricuspid valve inferior to this line more basilar and midline

LAT CXR:
reference line = oblique line drawn from carina / right pulmonary artery shadow to anterior cardiophrenic sulcus
√ aortic valve resides superior to this line
√ pulmonic valve anterior + superior to aortic valve
√ mitral valve resides inferoposteriorly to this line
√ tricuspid valve inferior to this line anteriorly

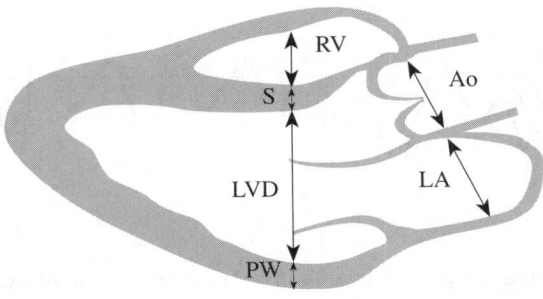

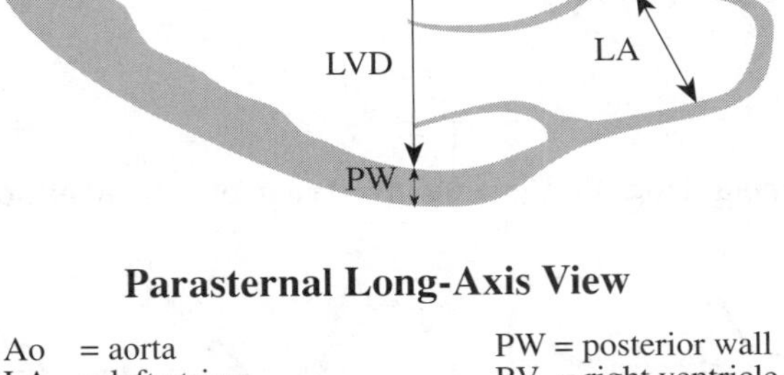

Parasternal Long-Axis View

Ao = aorta
LA = left atrium
LVD = left ventricular diameter
PW = posterior wall
RV = right ventricle
S = septum

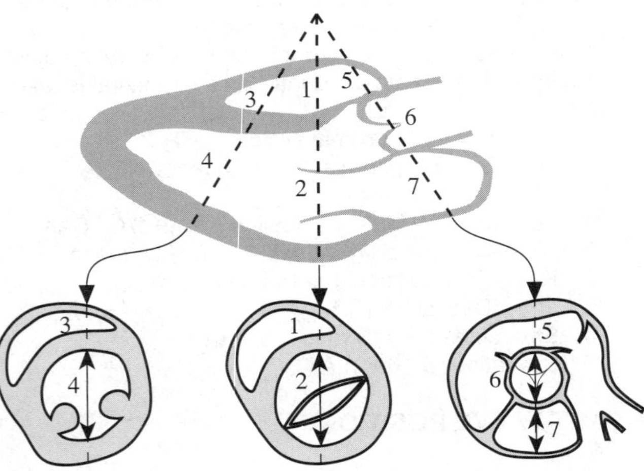

Parasternal Long- And Short-Axis

1, 3, 5 = RV dimension
6 = aortic root
7 = LA
2 = LV dimension at mitral level
4 = LV dimension at papillary muscle level

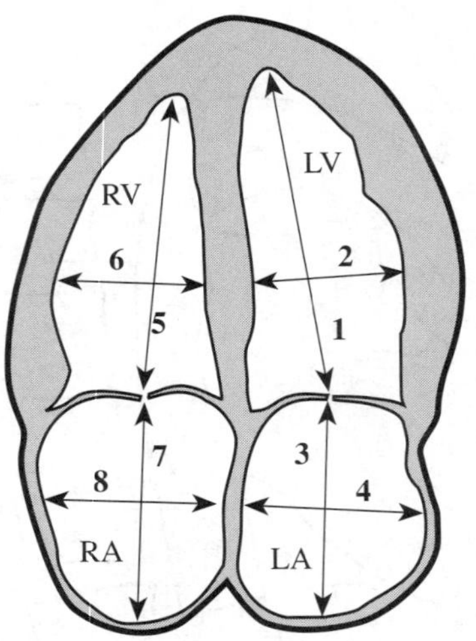

Apical 4-Chamber View

1 = LV long axis
2 = LV short axis
3 = LA major axis
4 = LA minor axis
5 = RV long axis
6 = RV short axis
7 = RA major axis
8 = RA minor axis

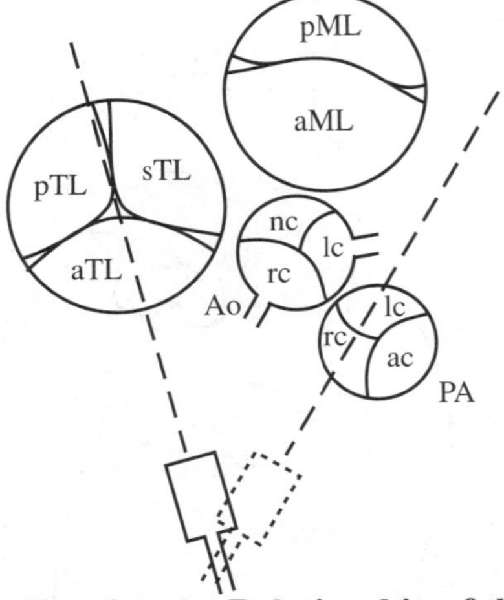

Diagram Showing the Relationship of the Four Cardiac Valves in Cross Section

aTL, pTL, sTL = anterior, posterior, septal tricuspid valve leaflets
aML, pML = anterior, posterior mitral valve leaflets
rc, lc, nc (Ao) = right, left, noncoronary cusps of aorta
rc, lc, ac (PA) = right, left, anterior cusps of pulmonary artery

HEART

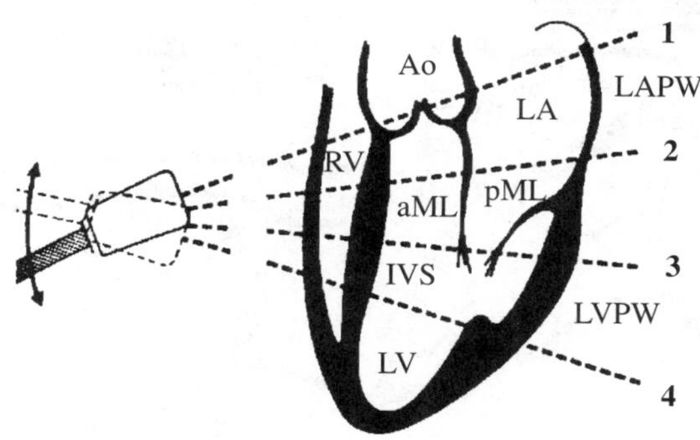

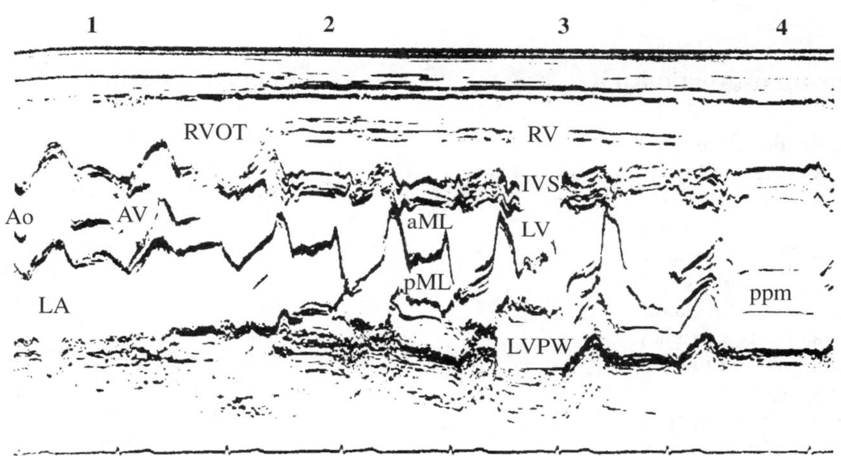

Sweep of Transducer from Aorta toward Apex

Area 1: recognized by parallel motion of both aortic walls (a) toward the transducer during systole, (b) away from the transducer during diastole. Left atrial posterior wall (LAPW) does not move because of mediastinal attachment by pulmonary veins.
Aortic valve cusps (right coronary + noncoronary / left cusps) are positioned in middle of aorta during diastole, open abruptly during systole at onset of ventricular ejection in a "box-like" fashion.
Aortic + LA dimension are similar in most cases.

Area 2: Aortic-septal continuity = anterior aortic wall becomes interventricular septum
Aortic-mitral continuity = posterior aortic wall becomes anterior mitral valve leaflet
Mitral valve with typical "M" configuration during diastole; motion of aML toward transducer during systole secondary to movement of whole mitral valve apparatus

Area 3: posterior mitral valve leaflet (pML) = reciprocal "W-shaped" configuration; left ventricular posterior wall (LVPW) shows anterior motion during systole.

Area 4: Chordae tendineae in continuity with mitral valve leaflets merge with a thick posterior band of echoes representing the posteromedial papillary muscle (ppm).

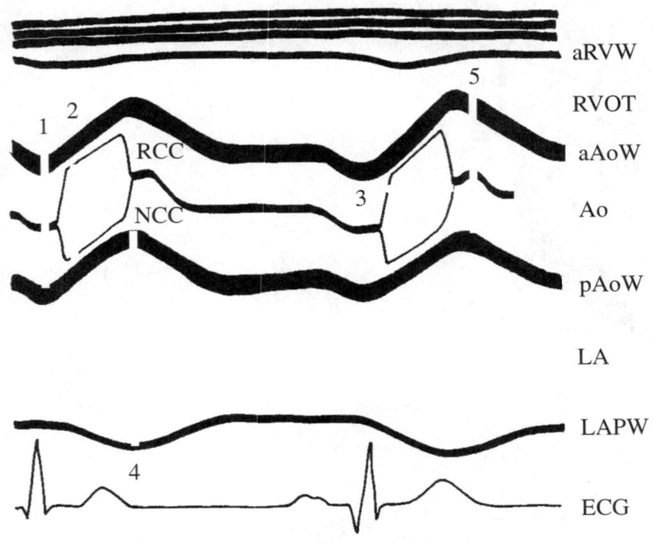

Echocardiogram of Aortic Root

1 = **aortic root dimension**, measured at end-diastole at R-wave of ECG .... 2.1–4.3 cm
increased in: aneurysm of aorta, aortic insufficiency

2 = **aortic cusp separation**: .... 1.7–2.5 cm
decreased in: aortic stenosis, low stroke volume
increased in: aortic insufficiency

3 = **left ventricular ejection time**

4 = **left atrial diameter**, measured at moment of mitral valve opening .... 2.3–4.4 cm

5 = **eccentricity index of aortic valve cusps** = ratio of anterior to posterior dimension (rarely used) .... <1.3

4 ÷ 1 = **ratio of LA-to-aortic root dimension** 0.87–1.11

aRVW = anterior right ventricular wall
RVOT = right ventricular outflow tract
aAoW = anterior aortic wall
Ao = aorta
pAoW = posterior aortic wall
LA = left atrium
LAPW = left atrial posterior wall
NCC = noncoronary cusp
RCC = right coronary cusp
ECG = electrocardiogram

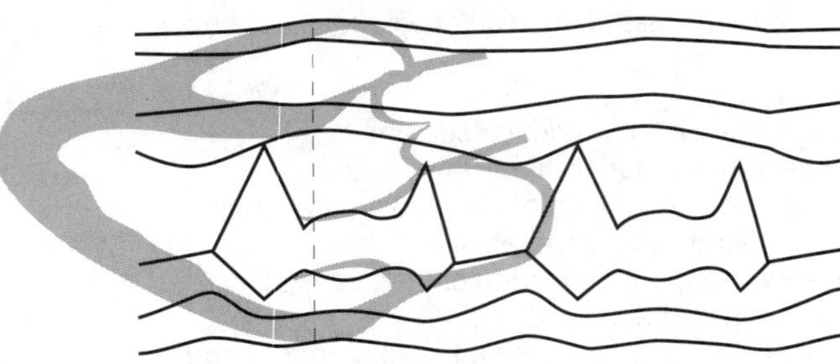

Mitral Valve in Mid-Diastole

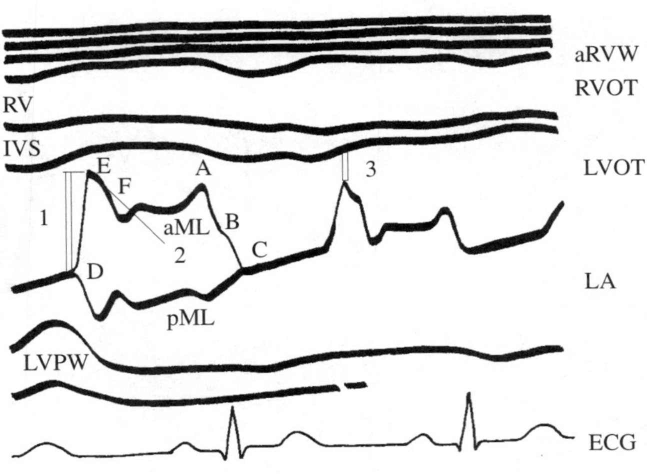

Echocardiogram of Mitral Valve

1 = **mitral valve excursion** = opening amplitude of anterior leaflet of mitral valve (DE amplitude) .... 2–3 cm
decreased in: nonpliable MV stenosis, low cardiac output, low compliance of LV
increased in: MV prolapse, high flow through MV

2 = **E to F slope** = early diastolic posterior motion of anterior leaflet ...... 7–15 cm/sec
decreased in: mitral valve stenosis, low compliance of LV

3 = **septal-mitral valve distance** = E point septal separation .... 2.9–4.1 mm
decreased in: ostium primum ASD, IHSS
increased in: dilated LV

RV = right ventricle
IVS = interventricular septum
LVPW = left ventricular posterior wall
aML = anterior mitral valve leaflet
pML = posterior mitral valve leaflet
aRVW = anterior right ventricular wall
RVOT = right ventricular outflow tract
LVOT = left ventricular outflow tract
LA = left atrium
ECG = electrocardiogram
A = point of atrial contraction
C = closure point
DE = opening secondary to passive ventricular filling
CD = systole with steady anterior drift of coapted leaflets (passive movement secondary to movement of entire heart toward chest wall)

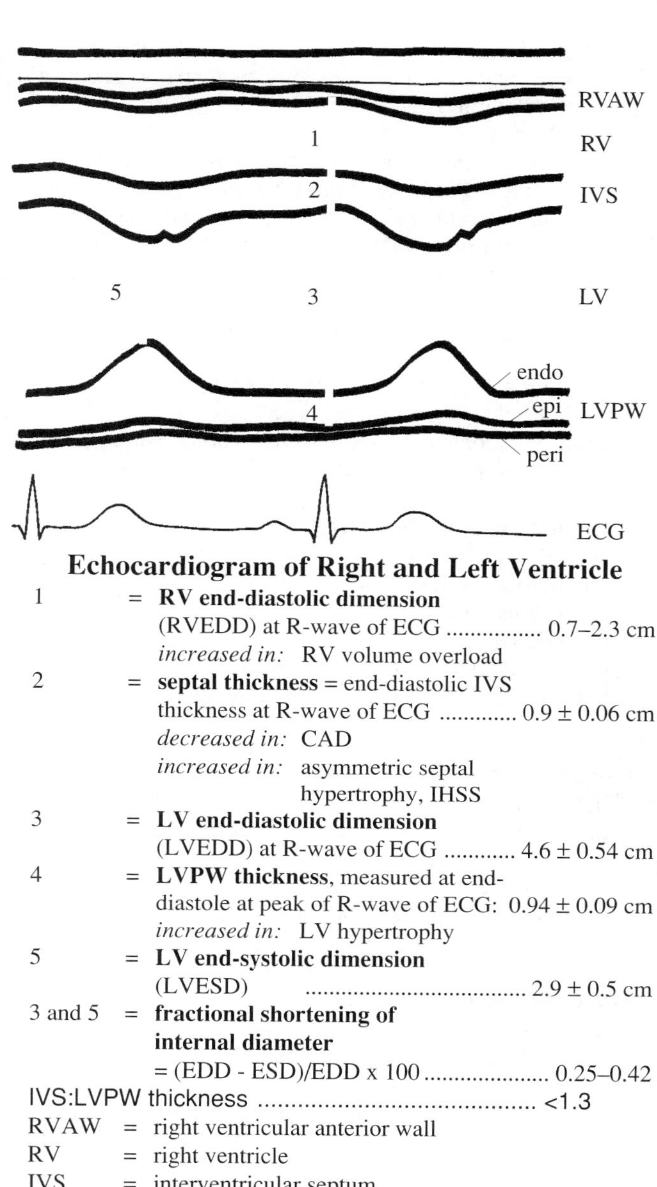

Echocardiogram of Right and Left Ventricle

1 = **RV end-diastolic dimension** (RVEDD) at R-wave of ECG .... 0.7–2.3 cm
increased in: RV volume overload

2 = **septal thickness** = end-diastolic IVS thickness at R-wave of ECG .... 0.9 ± 0.06 cm
decreased in: CAD
increased in: asymmetric septal hypertrophy, IHSS

3 = **LV end-diastolic dimension** (LVEDD) at R-wave of ECG .... 4.6 ± 0.54 cm

4 = **LVPW thickness**, measured at end-diastole at peak of R-wave of ECG: 0.94 ± 0.09 cm
increased in: LV hypertrophy

5 = **LV end-systolic dimension** (LVESD) .... 2.9 ± 0.5 cm

3 and 5 = **fractional shortening of internal diameter**
= (EDD - ESD)/EDD x 100 .... 0.25–0.42

IVS:LVPW thickness .... <1.3

RVAW = right ventricular anterior wall
RV = right ventricle
IVS = interventricular septum
LV = left ventricle
LVPW = left ventricular posterior wall
endo = endocardium
epi = epicardium
peri = pericardium

Fractional shortening (FS) = [(end-diastolic size - systolic size) / end-diastolic size] x 100
— for LV = 25–42%
— for IVS = 28–62%
— for LVPW = 36–70%

AORTIC ARCH BRANCHING PATTERNS

1. "Standard" branching pattern (65–75%) brachiocephalic trunk, left CCA, left subclavian artery
2. Common origin of brachiocephalic trunk + left CCA (13%)
3. Bovine aortic arch (9%)
   = origin of left CCA from brachiocephalic trunk
4. Vertebral artery (usually left) arising from aortic arch (3%)
5. Left and right brachiocephalic trunks (1%)
6. Aberrant right subclavian artery as the last branch of the aortic arch (<1%)

Cervical Aortic Arch

Associated with: right aortic arch (in 2/3)
- pulsatile neck mass
- upper airway obstruction
- dysphagia

√ mediastinal widening
√ absence of normal aortic knob
√ aortic arch near lung apex
√ tracheal displacement to opposite side + anteriorly
√ apparent cutoff of tracheal air column (secondary to crossing of descending aorta to side opposite of arch)

DDx: carotid aneurysm

AORTIC ISTHMUS VARIANTS

Aortic Isthmus

= narrowing of the aorta in newborn between left subclavian artery and ductus arteriosus

Age: up to 2 months of age

Prognosis: aortic isthmus disappears due to cessation of flow through ductus arteriosus + increased flow through narrowed region

Aortic Spindle (16%)

= congenital narrowing of the aorta at the ligamentum arteriosum with distal fusiform dilatation

Ductus Diverticulum

= localized bulge along anteromedial aspect of aortic isthmus

Origin: remnant of enlarged mouth of ductus arteriosus / result of traction from ligamentum arteriosum

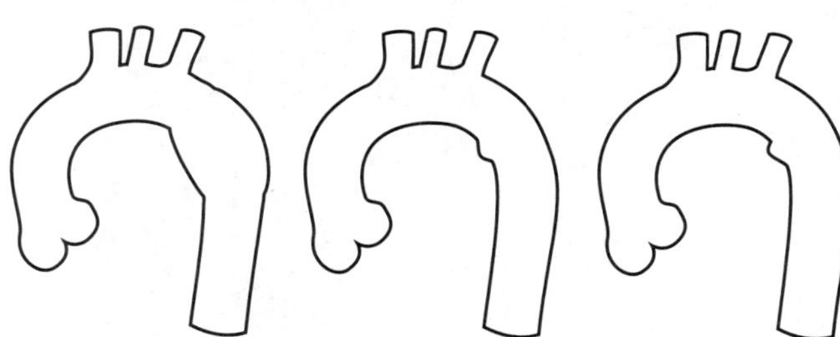

Aortic Spindle | **Classical Ductus Diverticulum** | **Atypical Ductus Diverticulum**

Normal Aortic Arch in 45° LAO Projection

HEART

Frequency: in 33% of infants, in 9% of adults
√ focal bulge with smooth uninterrupted margins
  √ gently sloping symmetric shoulders (classic ductus diverticulum)
  √ shorter steeper slope superiorly + more gentle slope inferiorly (atypical ductus diverticulum)
DDx: posttraumatic false aneurysm

Prominent bronchial-intercostal trunk

CORONARY ARTERIES

Anatomy of Coronary Arteries

RIGHT CORONARY ARTERY (RCA)
travels within right atrioventricular sulcus, rounds the acute margin of heart
- **Conus artery** (CB) = 1st branch from RCA (in 50% directly from aorta) to supply RVOT
- **Sinoatrial node artery** (SANA) = 2nd branch from RCA (in >50%)
- **Acute / RV marginal branches** (M1, M2, etc) have an anterior course
- **Posterior descending artery** (PDA) originates from RCA near crux or from a distal acute marginal branch, supplies posterior third of ventricular septum + diaphragmatic segment of LV, gives blood supply to posteromedial papillary muscle
- **Atrioventricular node artery** (AVNA) small branch to AV node
- **Posterolateral segment arteries** (PLSA) supply posterolateral wall of LV

LEFT CORONARY ARTERY (LCA)
- **Left main coronary artery** (LM) 0.5–2.0 cm short stem before bi- / trifurcation

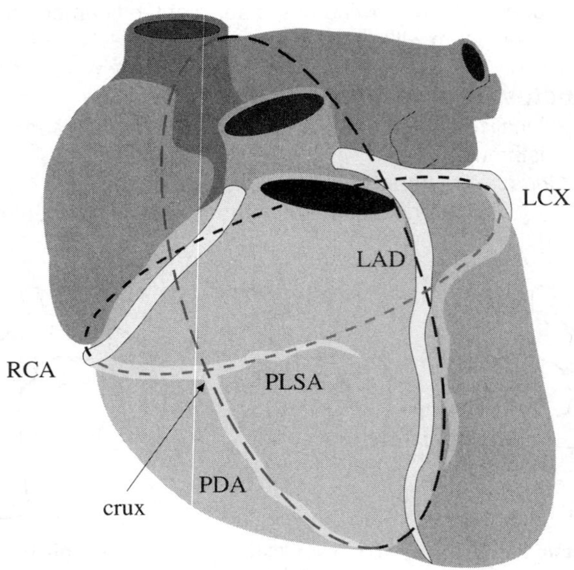

AP View of Heart and Coronary Arteries
(abbreviations in text)

Left anterior descending (LAD) travels within anterior interventricular groove, gives blood supply to anterolateral papillary muscle
- *Diagonal branches* (D1, D2, etc) arise from LAD and course over anterolateral wall of LV
  N.B.: **D**iagonals from LA**D**
- *Septal branches* (S) for interventricular septum

Left circumflex artery (LCX) travels within left atrioventricular sulcus, terminates at obtuse margin of heart
- *Obtuse marginal branches* (OM1,OM2, etc) for lateral wall of LV
- *Left atrial circumflex artery* (LACX) for atrium

Crux = junction of posterior atrioventricular sulcus + posterior interventricular groove

Coronary Artery Territory

septum = LAD
anterior wall = LAD
lateral wall = LCX
posterior wall = RCA
inferior / diaphragmatic wall = RCA
apex + inferolateral wall = watershed areas

Coronary Artery Dominance

determined by the origin of the posterior descending artery (PD), which supplies the inferior portion of LV:
— from RCA in 85%
— from LCX in 10%
— RCA + LCA = codominance / balanced supply (5%)

Coronary Arteriography

Contrast agents:
1. Monomeric ionic contrast material:
   (a) negative inotropic = depression of myocardial contractility due to hyperosmolality of sodium + decrease in total calcium
   (b) peripheral vasodilatation
2. Meglumine diatrizoate (contains small quantities of sodium citrate + EDTA)
3. Nonionic contrast material = slight increase in LV contractility

Dose: 3–10 mL
Mortality: 0.05%
Risk factors associated with death:
1. Multiple ventricular premature contractions
2. Congestive heart failure
3. Systemic hypertension
4. Severe triple-vessel coronary artery disease (highest risk)
5. LV ejection fraction <30%
6. Left main coronary artery stenosis

Clues for projection:
45–70° LAO:
√ ribs slanting to left side of image
√ catheter in descending aorta on right side of image

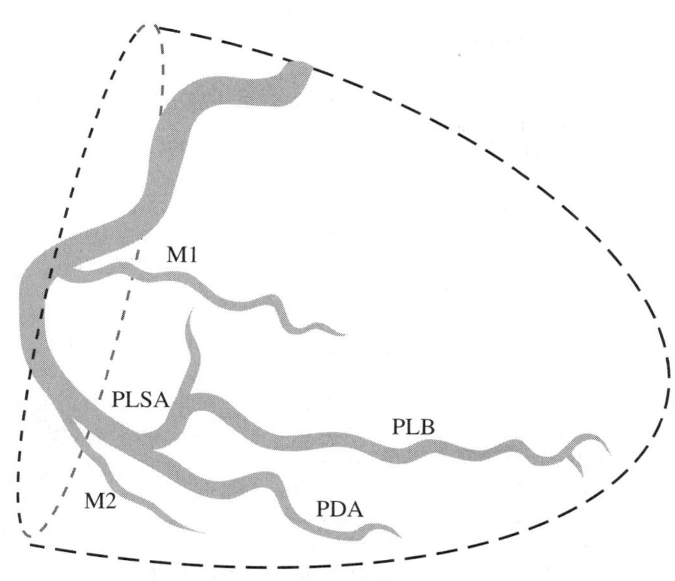

Right Coronary Artery in RAO View

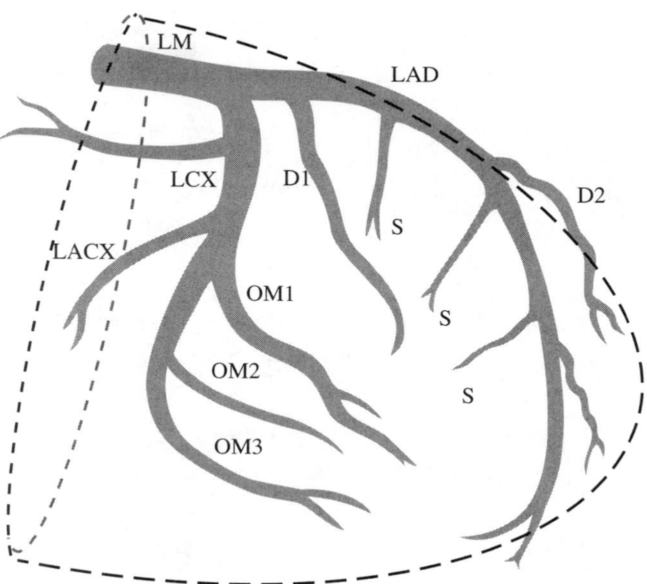

Left Coronary Artery in RAO View

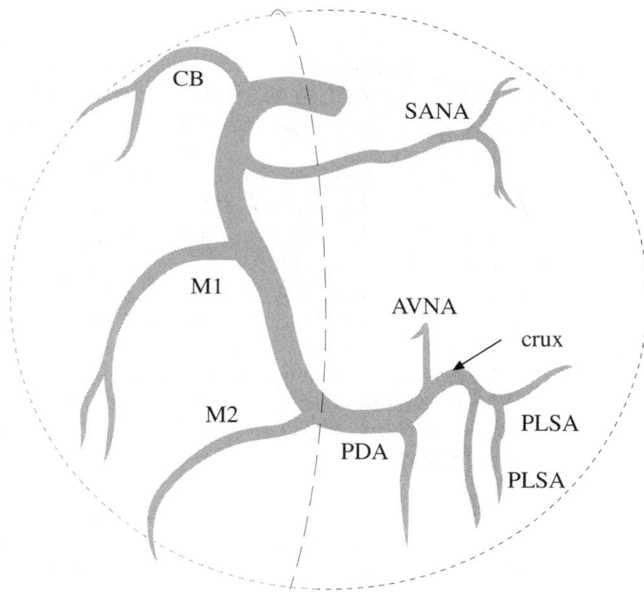

Right Coronary Artery in LAO View

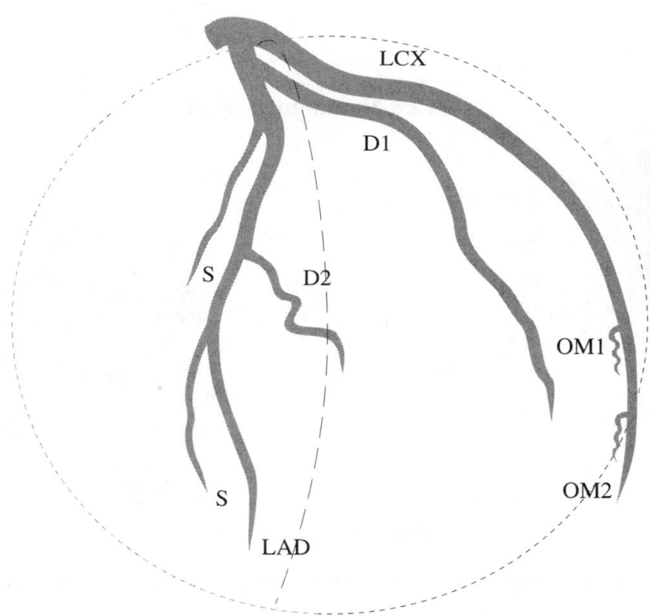

Left Coronary Artery in Caudocranial LAO

Right and Left Coronary Artery Angiograms

AVNA = atrioventricular node artery
CB = conus branch artery
D1 = 1st diagonal artery
D2 = 2nd diagonal artery
LACX = left atrial circumflex artery
LM = left main coronary artery
LAD = left anterior descending artery
LCX = left circumflex artery
M1 = 1st acute marginal branch artery
M2 = 2nd acute marginal branch artery
OM1 = 1st obtuse marginal artery
OM2 = 2nd obtuse marginal artery
PDA = posterior descending artery
PLB = posterolateral branch artery

HEART

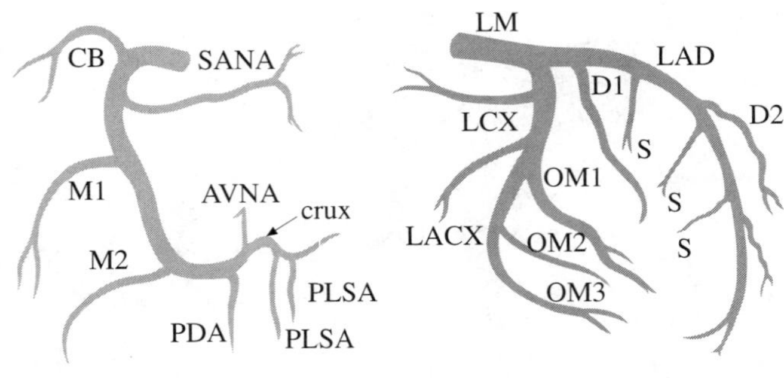

30° LAO view RAO view

Right Dominant System

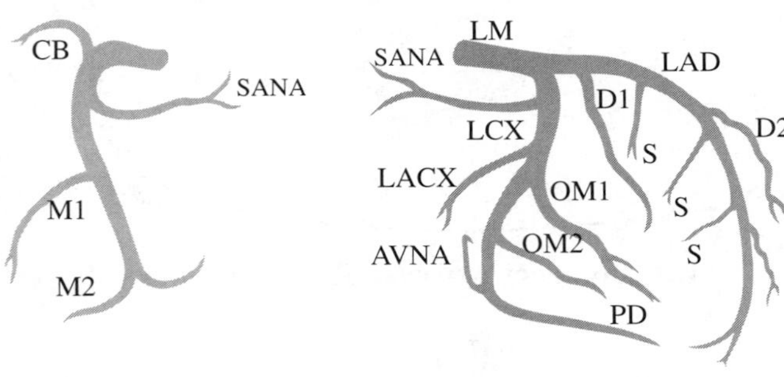

LAO view RAO view

Left Dominant System

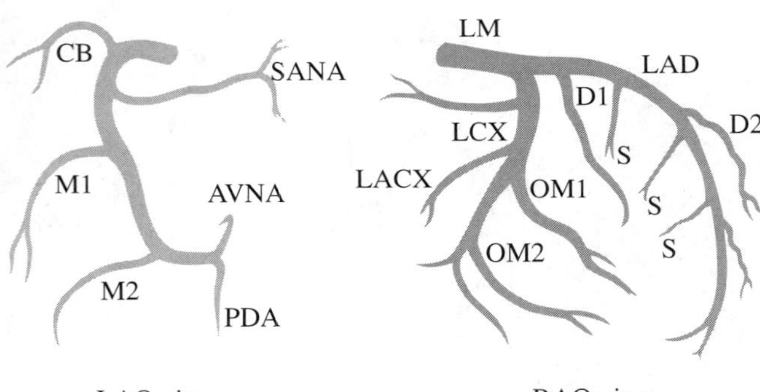

LAO view RAO view

Balanced Circulation

Coronary Artery Angiograms of Varying Dominance

AVNA = atrioventricular node artery
CB = conus branch artery
D1 = 1st diagonal artery
D2 = 2nd diagonal artery
LACX = left atrial circumflex artery
LM = left main coronary artery
LAD = left anterior descending artery
LCX = left circumflex artery
M1 = 1st acute marginal branch artery
M2 = 2nd acute marginal branch artery
OM1 = 1st obtuse marginal artery
OM2 = 2nd obtuse marginal artery
PDA = posterior descending artery
PLB = posterolateral branch artery
PLSA = posterolateral segment artery
S = septal branches
SANA = sinoatrial node artery

15–30° RAO:
- √ ribs slanting to right side of image
- √ catheter in descending aorta on left side of image

Technique:

◊ 20–30° of cranial / caudal angulation variably used

Catheter in left coronary orifice:
- (a) LAO + caudocranial angulation: proximal 1/3 of LAD + origin of first diagonal branch
- (b) LAO + craniocaudal angulation = "spider view": LCA, proximal LCX, first marginal / diagonal branches
- (c) RAO + craniocaudal angulation: proximal third of LCX + origin of its branches
- (d) RAO + caudocranial angulation: separation of LAD from diagonal branches

Catheter in right coronary artery orifice: LAO ± RAO

False-negative interpretation:
1. (1) eccentric lesion in 75%
2. (2) foreshortening of vessel
3. (3) overlap of other vessels remedied by angulated projections: improved diagnosis (50%), upgrade to more significant stenosis (30%), lesion unmasked (20%)

Coronary Artery Collaterals

A. INTRACORONARY COLLATERALS
= filling of a distal portion of an occluded vessel from the proximal portion
√ tortuous course outside the normal path

B. INTERCORONARY COLLATERALS
= between different coronary arteries / between branches of the same artery
Location: on epicardial surface, in atrial / ventricular septum, in myocardium

1. Proximal RCA to distal RCA
   - (a) by way of acute marginal branches
   - (b) from sinoatrial node artery (SANA) to atrioventricular node artery (AVNA) = Kugel collateral
2. RCA to LAD
   - (a) between PDA and LAD through ventricular septum / around apex
   - (b) conus artery (1st branch of RCA) to proximal part of LAD
   - (c) acute marginals of RCA to right ventricular branches of LAD
3. Distal RCA to distal LCX
   - (a) posterolateral segment artery of RCA to distal LCX (in AV groove)
   - (b) AVNA of RCA to LCX (through atrial wall)
   - (c) posterolateral branch of RCA to obtuse marginal branches of LCX (over left posterolateral ventricular wall)
4. Proximal LAD to distal LAD
   - (a) proximal diagonal to distal diagonal artery of LAD
   - (b) proximal diagonal to LAD directly
5. LAD to obtuse marginal of LCX

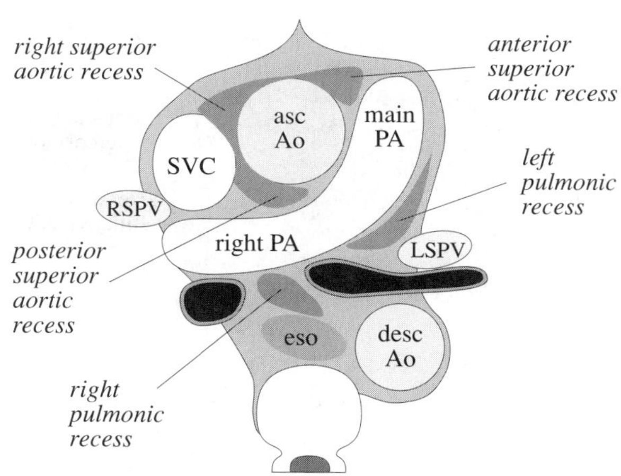

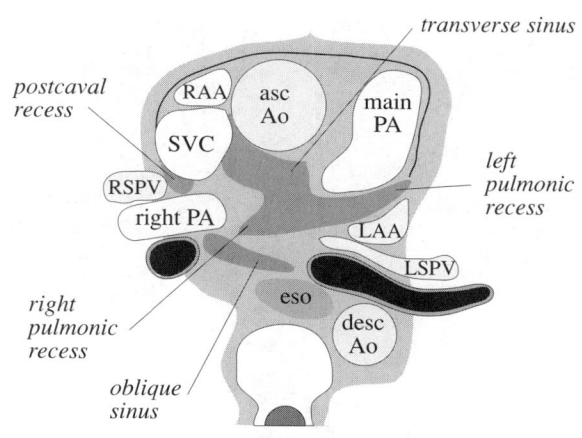

At Level of Pulmonary Artery

transverse sinus
postcaval recess
RAA
asc Ao
main PA
SVC
left pulmonic recess
RSPV
right PA
LAA
LSPV
eso
right pulmonic recess
desc Ao
oblique sinus

Below Level of Right Pulmonary Artery

Pericardial Sinuses & Recesses

asc Ao = ascending aorta
desc Ao = descending aorta
eso = esophagus
main PA = main pulmonary artery
right PA = right pulmonary artery
SVC = superior vena cava
LSPV = left superior pulmonary vein
RSPV = right superior pulmonary vein
RAA = right atrial appendage
LAA = left atrial appendage

PERICARDIUM

A. FIBROUS PERICARDIUM
   = outer fibrous layer
B. SEROUS PERICARDIUM
   = inner serous sac forming the pericardial cavity
   √ contains 20–25 mL of serous fluid
   (a) inner visceral layer = **epicardium**
      • intimately connected to heart + epicardial fat
   (b) outer parietal layer
      • lines fibrous pericardium

Pericardial Sinuses and Recesses

= extensions of pericardial cavity

A. Recesses of pericardial cavity proper
   1. Postcaval recess (23%*)
      √ behind and right lateral to SVC
   2. Right pulmonic vein recess (29%*)
      √ behind and right lateral to SVC
   3. Left pulmonic vein recess (60%*)
      √ behind and right lateral to SVC
B. Transverse sinus
   √ posterior to ascending aorta and pulmonary trunk + above left atrium (95%*)
   1. Superior aortic recess
      √ along ascending aorta; may be divided into anterior, posterior, right lateral portion
      DDx: aortic dissection on NECT
   2. Left pulmonic recess
      √ below left pulmonary artery + posterolateral to proximal right pulmonary artery
   3. Right pulmonic recess
      √ below right pulmonary artery + above left atrium
   4. Inferior aortic recess
      √ between ascending aorta + inferior SVC / right atrium
      √ extending down to level of aortic valve
C. Oblique sinus (89%*)
   √ behind left atrium + anterior to esophagus
   √ separated from transverse sinus by double reflection of pericardium (and fat) between right + left superior pulmonic veins
   1. Posterior pericardial recess (67%*)
      √ behind distal right pulmonary artery + medial to bronchus intermedius

DDx: lymph nodes, esophageal / thymic process, vascular abnormality, pericardial cyst / tumor

* = percentages give depiction on HRCT

EMBRYOGENESIS OF VENA CAVA

Time of development: 6–8th week of embryonic life

Origin:

A. Vitelline (omphalomesenteric) venous system: blood from yolk sac to sinus venosus
B. Umbilical venous system
   blood from chorionic villi to sinus venosus via ductus venosus
C. Intraembryonic cardinal venous system
   continuous appearance + regression of 3 paired embryonic veins
   (1) Cardinal veins
      join to form common cardinal vein, which enters left + right sinus horns
      (a) anterior cardinal veins
         drain the cranial region
      (b) posterior cardinal veins
         drain body of embryo + mesonephros + anterior extremities
         Location: dorsolateral part of urogenital fold
   (2) Subcardinal veins
      drain urogenital system of metanephros + suprarenal glands
      Location: ventromedial to posterior cardinal veins + ventrolateral to aorta

HEART

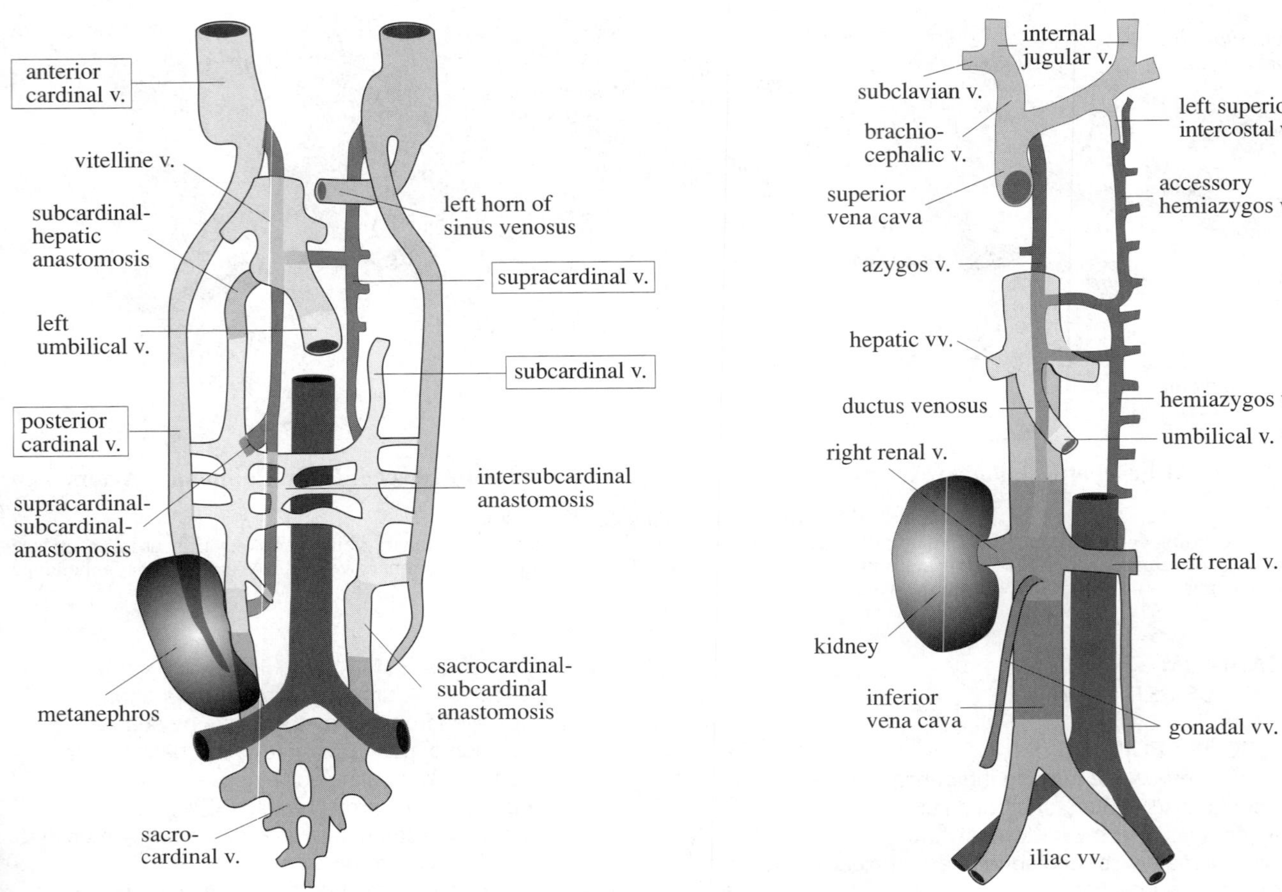

Development of the Major Venous System

vitelline vein ⇒ hepatic segment of IVC; right subcardinal-hepatic anastomosis ⇒ suprarenal segment of IVC
right supracardinal-subcardinal anastomosis ⇒ renal segment of IVC; right abdominal supracardinal vein ⇒ infrarenal segment of IVC
thoracic supracardinal veins ⇒ azygos and hemiazygos veins

- Intersubcardinal anastomoses form anterior to aorta below superior mesenteric artery and connect left + right subcardinal veins

(3) Supracardinal veins
drain body wall via intercostal veins
Location: dorsomedial to posterior cardinal vein + dorsolateral to aorta

- CRANIAL
  (a) azygos vein on the right
  drains 4–11 right intercostal veins
  (b) portion of superior intercostal vein
  drains 2–3 left intercostal veins
  (c) accessory hemiazygos
  drains 4–7 left intercostal veins
  (d) hemiazygos vein
  drains left 8–11 intercostal veins
- CAUDAL: lumbar veins

Inferior Vena Cava

1. Hepatic = posthepatic segment
   Origin: terminal part of right vitelline vein
2. Suprarenal segment
   Origin: subcardinal-hepatic anastomosis
3. Renal segment
   Origin: part of right subcardinal vein + supracardinal-subcardinal anastomoses
4. Infrarenal segment
   Origin: right supracardinal / sacrocardinal vein

VENOUS SYSTEM OF LOWER EXTREMITY

Deep Veins of Lower Extremity

3 paired stem veins of the calf accompany the arteries as venae commitantes + anastomose freely with each other:

1. **Anterior tibial veins**
   draining blood from dorsum of foot, running within extensor compartment of lower leg close to interosseous membrane
2. **Posterior tibial veins**
   formed by confluence of superficial + deep plantar veins behind ankle joint

3. **Peroneal veins**
   directly behind + medial to fibula
4. Calf veins
   (a) **Soleal muscle veins**
   baggy valveless veins in soleus muscle (= sinusoidal veins); draining into posterior tibial + peroneal veins or lower part of popliteal vein
   (b) **Gastrocnemius veins**
   thin straight veins with valves; draining into lower + upper parts of popliteal vein
5. **Popliteal vein**
   formed by stem veins of lower leg
6. **Femoral / superficial femoral vein**
   continuation of popliteal vein; receives deep femoral vein about 9 cm below inguinal ligament
7. **Deep femoral vein**
   draining together with superficial femoral vein into common femoral vein; may connect to popliteal vein (38%)
8. **Common femoral vein**
   formed by confluence of deep + superficial femoral vein; becomes external iliac vein as it passes beneath inguinal ligament

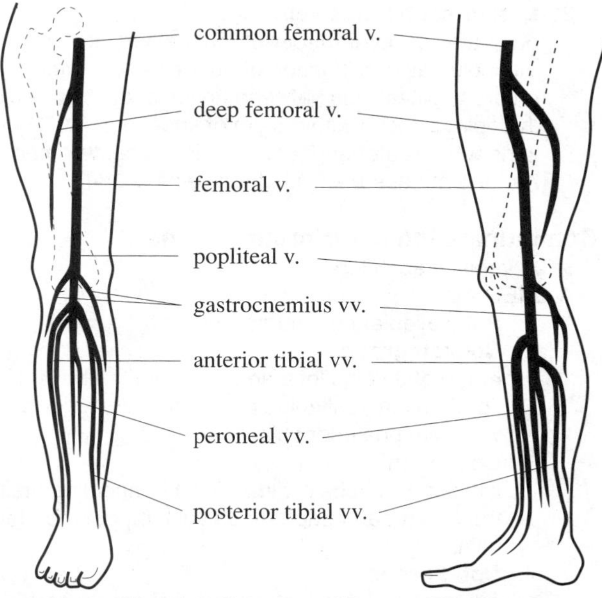

Deep Venous System of Lower Extremity

Superficial Veins of Lower Extremity

1. **Greater saphenous vein**
   formed by union of veins from medial side of sole of foot with medial dorsal veins; ascends in front of medial malleolus; passes behind medial condyles of tibia + femur
   (a) Posterior arch vein
   connected to deep venous system by communicating veins
   (b) **Anterior superficial tibial vein**
   (c) **Posteromedial superficial thigh vein**
   often connects with upper part of lesser saphenous vein
   (d) **Anterolateral superficial thigh vein**
   (e) Tributaries in fossa ovalis
   — superficial inferior epigastric vein
   — superficial external pudendal vein
   — superficial circumflex iliac vein

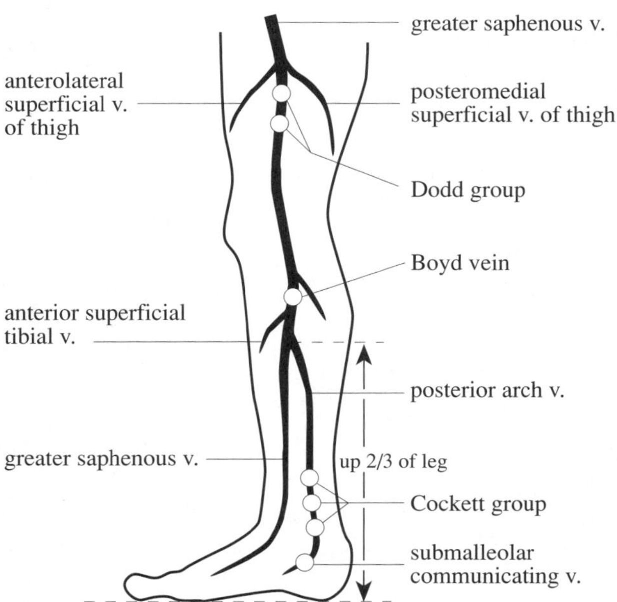

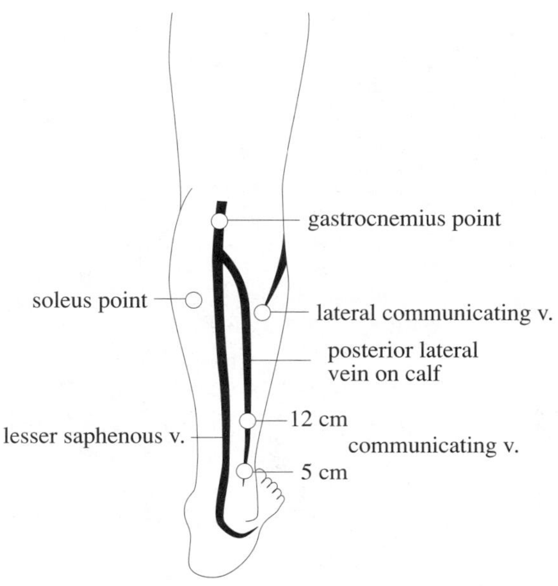

Superficial Venous System of Lower Extremity

2. **Lesser saphenous vein**
originates at outer border of foot behind lateral malleolus as continuation of dorsal venous arch; enters popliteal vein between heads of gastrocnemius in popliteal fossa within 8 cm of knee joint (60%) or joins with greater saphenous vein via posteromedial / anterolateral superficial thigh veins (20%)

Communicating = Perforating Veins

>100 veins in each leg

A. MEDIAL
1. Submalleolar communicating vein
2. **Cockett group**
group of 3 veins located 7, 12, 18 cm above the tip of medial malleolus connecting posterior arch vein with posterior tibial vein
3. **Boyd vein**
located 10 cm below knee joint connecting main trunk of greater saphenous vein to posterior tibial veins
4. **Dodd group**
group of 1 or 2 veins passing through Hunter canal (= subsartorial canal) to join greater saphenous vein with superficial femoral vein

B. LATERAL
1. **Lateral communicating vein**
located from just above lateral malleolus to junction of lower-to-mid thirds of calf connecting lesser saphenous vein with peroneal veins
2. **Posterior mid-calf communicating veins**
located posteriorly 5 + 12 cm above os calcis joining lesser saphenous vein to peroneal veins
3. **Soleal + gastrocnemius points**
joining short saphenous vein to soleal / gastrocnemius veins

CONTENTS OF FEMORAL TRIANGLE

mnemonic: "NAVEL" (from lateral to medial)

Nerve
Artery
Vein
Empty space
Lymphatics

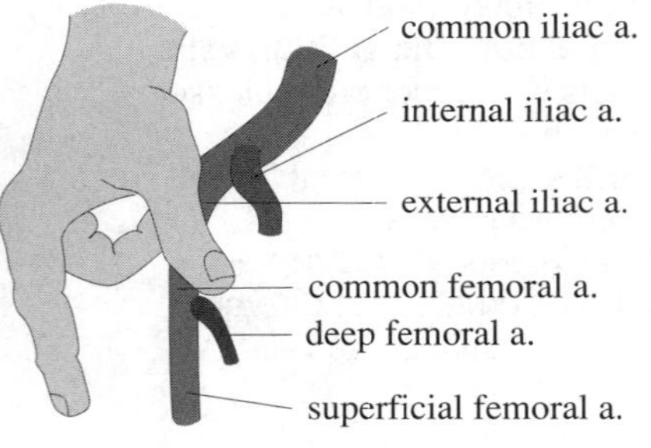

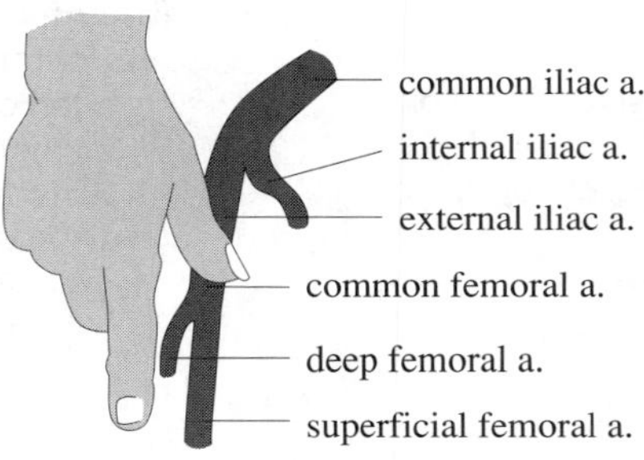

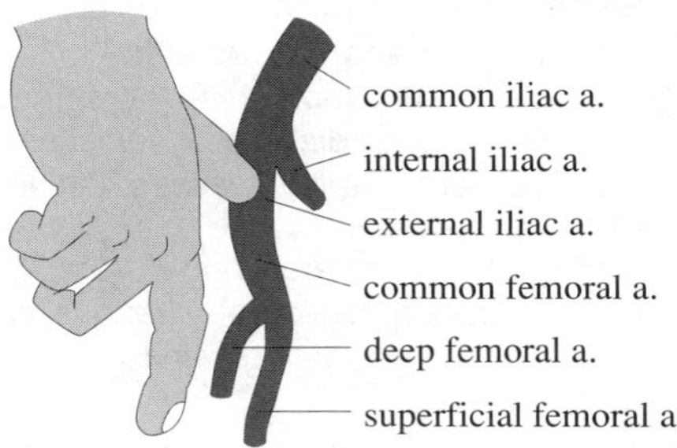

Pelvic Arterial Anatomy (right side)

CARDIOVASCULAR DISORDERS

ABERRANT LEFT PULMONARY ARTERY

= PULMONARY ARTERY SLING

Embryology: failure of development / obliteration of left 6th aortic arch (= vascular pedicle for left lung); left lung parenchyma maintains a connection with right lung leading to development of a collateral branch of the right pulmonary artery to supply the left lung

Site: left PA passes above right mainstem bronchus + between trachea and esophagus on its way to left lung

Age at presentation: neonate / infant / child

Associated with:

(1) "napkin-ring trachea" = absent pars membranacea (50%)

(2) PDA (most common), ASD, persistent left SVC

- stridor (most common), wheezing, apneic spells, cyanosis
- respiratory infection
- feeding problems

√ deviation of trachea to left
√ "inverted-T" appearance of mainstem bronchi = horizontal course secondary to lower origin of right mainstem bronchus
√ anterior bowing of right mainstem bronchus
√ "carrot-shaped trachea" = narrowing of tracheal diameter in caudad direction resulting in functional tracheal stenosis
√ obstructive emphysema / atelectasis of RUL + LUL
√ low left hilum
√ separation of trachea + esophagus at hilum by soft-tissue mass
√ anterior indentation on esophagram

AMYLOIDOSIS

= extracellular deposits of insoluble fibrillar protein

- asymptomatic / CHF (restrictive cardiomyopathy), arrhythmia

CXR:
√ normal / generalized cardiomegaly
√ pulmonary congestion
√ pulmonary deposits of amyloid

NUC:
√ striking uptake of Tc-99m pyrophosphate greater than bone (50–90%)

ECHO:
√ granular sparkling appearance of myocardium
√ LV wall thickening
√ decreased LV systolic + diastolic function

ANOMALOUS LEFT CORONARY ARTERY

= left coronary artery arises from pulmonary trunk (left sinus of Valsalva)

Hemodynamics:

with postnatal fall in pulmonary arterial pressure perfusion of LCA drops (ischemic left coronary bed), collateral circulation from RCA with flow reversal in LCA

— adequate collateral circulation = lifesaving
— inadequate collateral circulation = myocardial infarction
— large collateral circulation = L-to-R shunt with volume overload of heart

- episodes of sweating, ashen color (angina symptomatology)
- ECG: anterolateral infarction
- continuous murmur (if collaterals large)

√ dilatation of LV
√ enlargement of LA
√ normal pulmonary vascularity / redistribution

Rx:

(1) Ligation of LCA at its origin from pulmonary trunk
(2) Ligation of LCA + graft of left subclavian artery to LCA
(3) Creation of an AP window + baffle from AP window to ostium of LCA

DDx: endocardial fibroelastosis, viral cardiomyopathy (NO shocklike symptoms)

ANOMALOUS PULMONARY VENOUS RETURN

Total Anomalous Pulmonary Venous Return

= TAPVR = admixture lesion because of the combination of cyanosis + increased pulmonary vascularity (L-to-R and R-to-L shunt)

Embryology: anomalous connection between pulmonary veins and systemic veins secondary to embryologic failure of the common pulmonary vein to join the posterior wall of the left atrium

Prevalence: 2% of CHD

Age: symptomatic in 1st year of life

- cyanosis

Hemodynamics:

obstruction along the pulmonary venous pathway

RA	↔	RV	↔	Main PA	↔
Pulm vessels		↑			
LA	↔	LV	↔	Ao	↔

Associated with:

ASD / patent foramen ovale (necessary for survival), bronchopulmonary sequestration, pulmonary arteriovenous malformation, cystic adenomatoid malformation

Overall prognosis: 75% mortality rate within 1 year of birth if untreated

Supradiaphragmatic TAPVR

Type I = SUPRACARDIAC TAPVR (52%)
= drainage into left brachiocephalic vein / right + left persistent SVC / azygos vein; <10% obstructed

HEART

Type II = CARDIAC TAPVR (30%)
= drainage into coronary sinus (80%) / RA

Hemodynamics:
- — functional L-to-R shunt from pulmonary veins to right atrium
- — increased pulmonary blood flow (= overcirculation)
- — ASD restores oxygenated blood to left side
- — normal systemic venous pressure with increased flow through widened SVC
- — after birth CHF secondary to
  - (a) mixture of systemic + pulmonary venous blood in RA
  - (b) volume overload of RV

- • cyanosis
- • neck veins undistended (shunt level distally)
- • R ventricular heave (= increased contact of enlarged RV with sternum)
- • systolic ejection murmur (large shunt volume)

√ overall heart size notably normal:
- √ slightly enlarged RV (= volume overload with time)
- √ normal / enlarged RA
- √ normal LA (= ASD acts as escape valve)

√ dilated SVC + left vertical vein:
- √ "figure of 8" / "snowman" configuration of cardiac silhouette (= dilated SVC + left vertical vein)
- √ pretracheal density on lateral film (= left vertical vein)

√ increased pulmonary blood flow (= overcirculation)
√ absent connection of pulmonary veins to LA

Sub- / Infradiaphragmatic TAPVR (12%)

= type III
= drainage into portal vein / IVC / ductus venosus / left gastric vein with constriction of descending pulmonary vein by diaphragm en route through esophageal hiatus leading to pulmonary venous hypertension + RV pressure overload; >90% obstructed

- • intense cyanosis + respiratory distress (R-to-L shunt through ASD)

Prognosis: death within a few days of life
Associated with: asplenia syndrome (80%), polysplenia

√ unique appearance of pulmonary edema + pulmonary venous congestion with normal-sized heart (DDx: hyaline membrane disease)
√ low anterior indentation on barium-filled esophagus

Mixed Type of TAPVR (6%)

= type IV
= with various connections to R side of heart (6%)

Partial Anomalous Pulmonary Venous Return

= PAPVR
May occur in isolation
N.B.: venous return almost never obstructed!
Prevalence: 0.3–0.5% of patients with CHD

May be associated with:
(1) Atrial septal defect (25%)
- (a) RUL pulmonary vein enters SVC / RA (2/3)
  frequently associated with: sinus venosus type ASD (90%)
  √ RUL vein courses in a horizontal direction
- (b) LUL pulmonary vein enters brachiocephalic vein (1/3)
  frequently associated with: ostium secundum type ASD (10–15%)
  √ vertical mediastinal density lateral to aortic knob extending upward and medially with smooth curvilinear border (DDx: persistent left SVC)

(2) Hypogenetic lung as a component of congenital pulmonary venolobar syndrome
= SCIMITAR SYNDROME
= part / all of the hypogenetic lung is drained by an anomalous vein

Anomalous vein drains into:
- — IVC below right hemidiaphragm (33%)
- — suprahepatic portion of IVC (22%)
- — hepatic veins
- — portal vein (11%)
- — azygos vein
- — coronary sinus
- — right atrium (22%)
- — left atrium = "meandering pulmonary vein"
  ◊ Drainage into suprahepatic portion of IVC / right atrium may be a clue for interruption of intrahepatic portion of IVC!

May be associated with: systemic arterialization of the lung without sequestration
Location: almost exclusively on right side
√ tubular structure paralleling the right heart border in the configuration of a Turkish sword = "scimitar" (PA view)

- • acyanotic
- • ASD symptomatology

√ radiographic findings similar to ASD
√ anomalous course of draining vein
√ enlargement of draining site: SVC, IVC, azygos vein

CECT:
√ nodular / tubular opacity (= anomalous vein), which opacifies in phase with pulmonary vein

AORTIC ANEURYSM

Cause:
1. Atherosclerosis (73–80–90%): descending aorta
2. Traumatic (15–20%): following transection; descending aorta
3. Congenital (2%): aortic sinus, post coarctation, ductus diverticulum
4. Syphilis (19%): ascending aorta + arch
5. Mycotic = bacterial dissection; anywhere
6. Cystic media necrosis (Marfan / Ehlers-Danlos syndrome, annuloaortic ectasia): ascending aorta

7. Inflammation of media + adventitia:
   Takayasu arteritis, giant cell arteritis, relapsing polychondritis, rheumatic fever, rheumatoid arthritis, ankylosing spondylitis, Reiter syndrome, psoriasis, ulcerative colitis, systemic lupus erythematosus, scleroderma, Behçet disease, radiation
8. Increased pressure:
   systemic hypertension, aortic valve stenosis
9. Abnormal volume load: severe aortic regurgitation

TRUE ANEURYSM
= permanent dilatation of all layers of weakened but intact wall

FALSE ANEURYSM
= focal perforation with all layers of wall disrupted; escaped blood contained by adventitia / perivascular connective tissue + organized blood

FUSIFORM ANEURYSM (80%)
= circumferential involvement

SACCULAR ANEURYSM
= involvement of portion of wall

Abdominal Aortic Aneurysm (AAA)

◊ There is no consensus regarding the definition of an atherosclerotic AAA!

= focal widening >3 cm (ultrasound literature); twice the size of normal aorta / >4 cm [Bergan, Ann Surg 1984]

Normal size of abdominal aorta >50 years of age:
12–19 mm in women; 14–21 mm in men

Prevalence: 1.4–8.2% in unselected population; in 6% >80 years of age; in 6–20% of patients with signs of atherosclerotic disease; M > F; Whites:Blacks = 3:1

Cause: ? genetic (10-fold increase in risk as first-degree relative of patient with AAA); structural defect of aortic wall caused by increased proteolysis; copper deficiency

Risk factors: male sex, age >75 years, white race, prior vascular disease, hypertension, cigarette smoking, family history, hypercholesterolemia

Age: >60 years; M:F = 5–9:1

Associated with:
(a) visceral + renal artery aneurysm (2%)
(b) isolated iliac + femoral artery aneurysm (16%): common iliac (89%), internal iliac (10%), external iliac (1%)
(c) stenosis / occlusion of celiac trunk / SMA (22%)
(d) stenosis of renal artery (22–30%)
(e) occlusion of inferior mesenteric artery (80%)
(f) occlusion of lumbar arteries (78%)

Growth rate of aneurysm of 3–6 cm in diameter:
0.39 cm / year

- asymptomatic (30%)
- abdominal mass (26%)
- abdominal pain (37%)

◊ Imaging should provide information about
(a) the proximal extent of the aneurysm, which determines the site of clamping of the aorta (origin of renal arteries)
(b) the course of the left renal vein (retroaortic?)!

Location: infrarenal (91–95%) with extension into iliac arteries (66–70%)

Plain film: √ mural calcification (75–86%)

US: √ >98% accuracy in size measurement

NCCT:
√ perianeurysmal fibrosis (10%), may cause ureteral obstruction
√ "crescent sign" = peripheral high-attenuating crescent in aneurysm wall (= acute intramural hematoma) = **sign of impending rupture**

CECT:
(a) ruptured aneurysm
√ anterior displacement of kidney
√ extravasation of contrast material
√ fluid collection / hematoma within posterior pararenal + perirenal spaces
√ free intraperitoneal fluid
√ perirenal "cobwebs"
(b) contained leak
√ laminated mural calcification
√ periaortic mass of mixed / soft-tissue density
√ lateral "draping" of aneurysm around vertebral body
√ focal discontinuity of calcifications (unreliable)
√ indistinct aortic wall (unreliable)

Angio (AP + LAT filming):
√ focally widened aortic lumen >3 cm
√ apparent normal size of lumen secondary to mural thrombus (11%)
√ mural clot (80%)
√ slow antegrade flow of contrast medium

Contained rupture = extraluminal hematoma / cavity
√ absent parenchymal stain = avascular halo
√ displacement + stretching of aortic branches

Cx:
(1) Rupture (25%)
(a) into retroperitoneum: commonly on left
(b) into GI tract: massive GI hemorrhage
(c) into IVC: rapid cardiac decompensation
Incidence: aneurysm <4 cm in 10%, 4–5 cm in 23%, 5–7 cm in 25%, 7–10 cm in 46%, >10 cm in 60%
- sudden severe abdominal pain ± radiating into back
- faintness, syncope, hypotension

Prognosis: 64–94% die before reaching hospital
Increased risk: size >6 cm, growth >5 mm / 6 months, pain + tenderness
◊ The exact moment of rupture is unpredictable!
◊ Cause of death in 1.3% of men >65 years!
(2) Peripheral embolization
(3) Infection
(4) Spontaneous occlusion of aorta

Prognosis: 17% 5-year survival without surgery, 50–60% 5-year survival with surgery

Rx: surgery recommended if >5 cm in diameter; 4–5% surgical mortality for nonruptured, 30–80% for ruptured aneurysm

Postoperative Cx:
(1) Left colonic ischemia (1.6%) with 10% mortality
(2) Renal failure (14%)
(3) 0–8% mortality rate for elective surgery

Atherosclerotic Aneurysm

Incidence: leading cause of thoracic aortic aneurysm
Histo: diseased intima with secondary degeneration + fibrous replacement of media; ultimately wall of aneurysm composed of acellular + avascular connective tissue
Pathophysiology:
progressive weakening of media results in vessel dilatation + increased tension of vessel wall (law of Laplace = tensile stress varies with product of blood pressure and radius of vessel); compromise of mural vascular nutrition (vasa vasorum) causes further degeneration + progressive dilatation
Age: elderly; M > F
Location: distal abdominal aorta > iliac a. > popliteal a. > common femoral a. > aortic + descending thoracic aorta > carotid a.
Site: (1) infrarenal aorta (associated with thoracic aneurysm in 29%)
(2) descending thoracic aorta distal to left subclavian artery
(3) thoracoabdominal
√ fusiform (80%), saccular (20%)
Cx: rupture (cause of death in 50%): usually unrestrained + fatal in thoracic location

HEART

Degenerative Aneurysm

= medial degeneration
Most common cause of aneurysm in ascending aorta
Cause: (1) genetically transmitted metabolic disorder: Marfan syndrome, Ehlers-Danlos syndrome
(2) acquired: result of repetitive aortic injury + repair associated with aging

Inflammatory Aortic Aneurysm

= defined as triad of
(1) thickened wall of aneurysm
(2) extensive perianeurysmal + retroperitoneal fibrosis
(3) dense adhesions of adjacent abdominal organs
Frequency: 3–10% of all AAAs; M:F = 6:1 to 30:1
Mean age: 62–68 years
- abdominal / back pain
- weight loss + anorexia (20–41%)
- elevated ESR (40–88%)
- tender pulsatile abdominal mass (15–30%)

Comorbidities: arterial hypertension (34–69%), arterial occlusive disease (10–47%), diabetes mellitus (3–13%), coronary artery disease (33–55%)
Size: usually small at presentation because of early symptomatology
CT:
√ rind of homogeneous soft-tissue density surrounding aorta anteriorly + laterally
√ contrast enhancement (DDx from hematoma)
√ entrapment of ureters (10–21%)
US:
√ sonolucent halo around aorta
Cx: enlargement + rupture (lower rate than in noninflammatory aneurysm)

Mycotic Aneurysm

Incidence: 2.6% of all abdominal aneurysms
A. PRIMARY MYCOTIC ANEURYSM (rare)
unassociated with any demonstrable intravascular inflammatory process
B. SECONDARY MYCOTIC ANEURYSM
= aneurysm due to nonsyphilitic infection
Predisposing factors:
(1) IV drug abuse, (2) bacterial endocarditis (12%), (3) immunocompromise (malignancy, alcoholism, steroids, chemotherapy, autoimmune disease, diabetes), (4) atherosclerosis, (5) aortic trauma caused by accidents / aortic valve surgery / coronary artery bypass surgery / arterial catheterization
Mechanism:
(a) septicemia with abscess formation via vasa vasorum
(b) septicemia with abscess formation via vessel lumen
(c) direct extension of contiguous infection
(d) preexisting intima laceration (trauma, atherosclerosis, coarctation)

Organism: S. aureus (53%), Salmonella (33-50%), nonhemolytic Streptococcus, Pneumococcus, Gonococcus, Mycobacterium (contiguous spread from spine / lymph nodes)
Histo: loss of intima + destruction of internal elastic lamella; varying degrees of destruction of muscularis of media + adventitia
- frequently insidious, fever
- positive blood culture in 50%

Site: ascending aorta > abdominal visceral artery > intracranial artery > lower / upper extremity artery
√ true aneurysm (majority)
√ saccular structure arising eccentrically from aortic wall with rapid enlargement
√ interrupted ring of aortic wall calcification
√ periaortic gas collection
√ adjacent vertebral osteomyelitis
√ adjacent reactive lymph node enlargement
Cx: (1) Life-threatening rupture + hemorrhage (75%)
(2) Uncontrolled sepsis if untreated
Prognosis: 67% overall mortality

Syphilitic Aneurysm

Spectrum:
1. Uncomplicated syphilitic aortitis
2. Syphilitic aortic aneurysm (mostly saccular)
3. Syphilitic aortic vasculitis (aortic regurgitation)

Incidence: 12% of patients with untreated syphilis
Onset: 10–30 years after initial spirochete infection
Histo: chronic inflammation of aortic adventitia + media beginning at vasa vasorum + leading to obstruction of vasa vasorum followed by nutritional impairment of media + loss of elastic fibers + smooth muscle fibers
• positive venereal disease research laboratory (VDRL) test
• positive microhemagglutination assay - Treponema pallidum (MHA-TP) test
Location: ascending aorta (36%), aortic arch (34%), proximal descending aorta (25%), distal descending aorta (5%), aortic sinuses (<1%)
√ asymmetric enlargement of aortic sinuses (DDx to medial degeneration with symmetric enlargement)
√ saccular (75%) / fusiform (25%) aneurysm
√ pencil-thin dystrophic aortic wall calcification (up to 40%) most severe in ascending aorta, frequently obscured by thick coarse irregular calcifications of secondary atherosclerosis
Prognosis: death in 2%, rupture in up to 40%; death within months of onset of symptoms if untreated

Thoracic Aortic Aneurysm
Most common vascular cause of mediastinal mass!
◊ 10% of mediastinal masses are of vascular origin!
Average diameter of thoracic aorta (<4–5 cm wide):
— aortic root: 3.6 cm
— ascending aorta 1 cm proximal to arch: 3.5 cm
— proximal descending aorta: 2.6 cm
— middle descending aorta: 2.5 cm
— distal descending aorta: 2.4 cm
Associated with: hypertension, coronary artery disease, abdominal aneurysm
Mean age: 65 years; M:F = 3:1
• substernal / back / shoulder pain (26%)
• SVC syndrome (venous compression)
• dysphagia (esophageal compression)
• stridor, dyspnea (tracheobronchial compression)
• hoarseness (recurrent laryngeal nerve compression)
√ mediastinal mass with proximity to aorta
√ wide tortuous aorta
√ curvilinear peripheral calcifications (75%)
√ circumferential / crescentic mural thrombus
√ Angio: may show normal caliber secondary to mural thrombus
Cx: (1) Rupture into mediastinum, pericardium, either pleural sac, extrapleural space
√ high-attenuation fluid
(2) Aortobronchopulmonary fistula
√ consolidation of lung adjacent to aneurysm
◊ Most aneurysms rupture when >10 cm in size
Prognosis: 1-year survival 57%, 3-year survival 26%, 5-year survival 19% (60% die from ruptured aneurysm, 40% die from other causes)
Rx: operative repair considered if >6 cm in diameter
Surgical mortality: 10%

Traumatic Aortic Pseudoaneurysm
= CHRONIC AORTIC PSEUDOANEURYSM
◊ 2nd most common form of thoracic aortic aneurysm
◊ Most common type occurring in young patients
Incidence: 2.5% of patients who survive initial trauma of acute aortic transection
√ usually calcified
√ may contain thrombus
Cx: (1) progressive enlargement
(2) rupture (even years after insult)

Complications of Endovascular Stent-Graft Repair
1. Endoleak (2–45%)
= leakage into the aneurysm outside stent-graft
Type 1 = incomplete fixation of stent-graft to aortic wall at the proximal / distal attachment site
Type 2 = retrograde flow via parent artery (eg, lumbar / inferior mesenteric artery)
Type 3 = emdograft defect with disruption of either metallic support / fabric
Prognosis: enlargement of leak, aneurysm rupture
2. Graft kinking
Cause: diminishing diameter of aneurysm after stent-graft implantation also decreases length of aneurysm
Associated with: distal migration of stent-graft
3. Graft infection
√ interval development of perigraft soft-tissue attenuation / air
Rx: antibiotics + total excision of infected graft
4. Graft thrombosis (3–19%)
= intraluminal circular / semicircular thrombus
Prognosis: spontaneous shrinkage, development of complete thrombosis
5. Graft occlusion
6. Shower embolism (4–17%)
Cause: mural thrombus dispersed by delivery system
Prognosis: perioperative death
7. Colon necrosis
Cause: occlusion of inferior mesenteric artery by stent-graft
8. Aortic dissection
Cause: retrograde injury by delivery system

AORTIC DISSECTION
= spontaneous longitudinal separation of aortic intima + adventitia by circulating blood having gained access to the media of the aortic wall splitting it in two
Path: (a) transverse tear in weakened intima (95–97%)
(b) no intimal tear (3–5–13%) = INTRAMURAL HEMATOMA OF AORTA
Pathogenesis:
intimal tear results from combination of following factors:
(1) media degeneration decreases cohesiveness within aortic wall
(2) persistent aortic motion secondary to a beating heart stresses the aortic wall
(3) hydrodynamic forces accentuated by hypertension

Incidence: 3:1,000 (more common than all ruptures of thoracic + abdominal aorta combined); 1:205 autopsies; 2,000 cases/year in USA
Peak age: 60 years (range 13–87 years); M:F = 3:1
Predisposed: (cystic medial necrosis / disease of aortic wall)

◊ Starts in fusiform aneurysms in 28%
◊ Does not occur in aneurysms <5 cm in diameter

1. Hypertension (60–90%)
2. Marfan syndrome (16%)
3. Ehlers-Danlos syndrome
4. Relapsing polychondritis
5. Valvular aortic stenosis
6. Turner syndrome
7. Behçet disease
8. Coarctation
9. Bicuspid aortic valve
10. S/P prosthetic valve
11. Trauma (rare)
12. Catheterization
13. Pregnancy
14. Aortitis (eg, SLE)
15. Cocaine abuse

NOT syphilis

◊ In women 50% of dissections occur during pregnancy!

- sharp tearing intractable anterior / posterior chest pain (75–95%) radiating to jaw, neck, low back (DDx: myocardial infarction)
- murmur ± bruit (65%) from aortic regurgitation
- asymmetric peripheral pulses + blood pressures (59%)
- absent femoral pulses (25%), reappearing after reentry
- pulse deficit: in up to 50% of type A dissection, in 16% of type B dissection
- hemodynamic shock (25%)
- neurologic deficits (25%): hemiplegia, paraparesis (due to compromise of anterior spinal artery of Adamkiewicz)
- persistent oliguria
- congestive heart failure (rare) due to acute aortic insufficiency
- recurrent arrhythmias / right bundle branch block
- signs of pericardial tamponade: clouded sensorium, extreme restlessness, dyspnea, distended neck veins

Types:

DeBakey type I (29–34%) = ascending aorta + portion distal to arch
DeBakey type II (12–21%) = ascending aorta only
DeBakey type III (50%) = descending aorta only
  subtype IIIA = up to diaphragm
  subtype IIIB = below diaphragm

Stanford type A (60–70%) = ascending aorta ± arch in first 4 cm in 90%
Stanford type B (30–40%) = descending aorta only
mnemonic: **A** **a**ffects **a**scending aorta and **a**rch;
B **b**egins **b**eyond **b**rachiocephalic vessels;
I = II + III

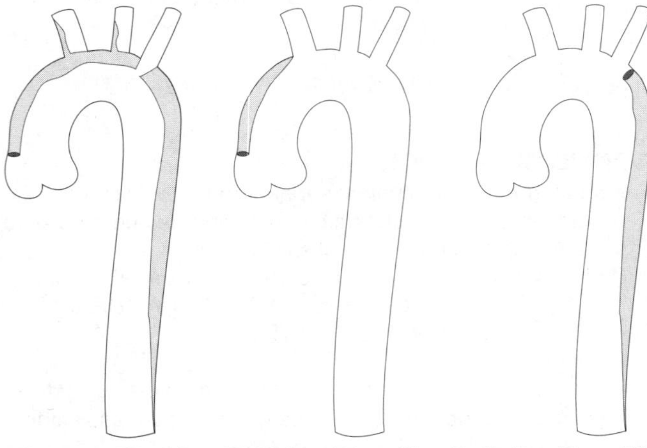

Aortic Dissection

Clinical classification:
(1) Acute aortic dissection: <2 weeks old
(2) Chronic aortic dissection: >2 weeks old

Location of dissection (following helical flow pattern):
— on anterior + right lateral wall of ascending aorta just distal to aortic valve (65%)
— on superior + posterior wall of transverse aortic arch (10%)
— on posterior + left lateral wall of upper descending aorta distal to left subclavian artery (20%)
— more distal aorta (5%) usually terminating in left iliac artery (80%) / right iliac artery (10%) [involvement of left renal artery in 50%]
◊ An exit / distal tear / reentry occurs in 10%!

Atypical configurations of intimal flap:
√ circumferential intimal flap due to dissection of entire intima
√ filiform intimal flap creating an extremely narrow true lumen (± ischemic complications)
√ mural calcification of false lumen (in chronic dissection)
√ three-channel aorta (= Mercedes-Benz sign) due to two false channels
√ intimointimal intussusception

CXR (best assessment from comparison with serial films):
√ normal CXR in 25%
√ "calcification sign" = inward displacement of atherosclerotic plaque by >4–10 mm from outer aortic contour (7%), can only be applied to contour of descending aorta secondary to projection, may be misleading in presence of periaortic soft-tissue mass / hematoma
√ disparity in size between ascending + descending aorta
√ irregular wavy contour / indistinct outline of aorta
√ widening of superior mediastinum to >8 cm due to hemorrhage / enlarging false channel (40–80%)
√ cardiac enlargement (LV hypertrophy / hemopericardium)
√ left pleural effusion (27%)
√ atelectasis of lower lobe
√ rightward displacement of trachea / endotracheal tube

ECHO:
(a) transthoracic US: 59–85% sensitive + 63–96% specific for type A dissection; poorer for type B

HEART

(b) transesophageal US: up to 99% sensitive + 77–97% specific
(c) intravascular in conjunction with aortography to differentiate true from false lumen
√ intimal flap (seen in more than one view)
√ pericardial fluid
√ aortic insufficiency
False-positives: reverberation echoes from aneurysmal ascending aorta / calcified atheromatous plaque, postoperative periaortic hematoma

Angio (86–88% sensitive, 75–94% specific):
◊ Aortography 1st choice for final confirmation + staging because of contrast limitation!
Superior to any other technique in demonstrating
— entry + reentry points (in 50%)
— branch vessel involvement + coronary arteries
— aortic insufficiency
√ visualization of intimal / medial flap (75–79%) = linear radiolucency within opacified aorta
√ "double barrel aorta" (87%) = opacification of two aortic lumens
√ abnormal catheter position outside anticipated aortic course
√ compression of true lumen by false channel (72–85%)
√ aortic valvular regurgitation (30%)
√ increase in aortic wall thickness >6–10 mm
√ obstruction of aortic branches: left renal artery (25–30%)
√ ulcerlike projections caused by truncated branches
√ slower blood flow in false lumen
False-negative: complete thrombosis of false channel (10%), intimal flap not tangential to x-ray beam
False-positive: thickening of aortic wall due to aneurysm, aortitis, adjacent neoplasm / hemorrhage

CECT (87–94% sensitive, 87–100% specific):
within 4 hours (if patient responds rapidly to medical Rx); detection as accurate as angio with single-level dynamic scanning
√ crescentic high-attenuation clot within false lumen
√ internally displaced intimal calcification (DDx: calcification of thrombus on luminal surface or within)
√ intimal flap separating two aortic channels (may be seen without contrast in anemic patients)
False-negative: inadequate contrast opacification, thrombosed lumen misinterpreted as aortic aneurysm with mural thrombus
False-positive: perivenous streaks secondary to beam hardening + motion, cardiac / aortic motion artifacts, opacified normal sinus of Valsalva, normal pericardial recess mistaken for thrombus, mural thrombus in a fusiform aortic aneurysm, periaortic fibrosis, anemia with apparent high attenuation of aortic wall

MR (95–100% sensitive, 90–100% specific):
√ intimal flap of medium intensity outlined by signal voids of rapidly flowing blood
√ intimal flap more difficult to detect in presence of slow flow / thrombus
√ "cobwebs" (= bands of medial elastic lamellae spanning the junction of the dissecting septum with the outer wall of the false lumen) mark the false lumen in 80%

Cx: (1) Retrograde dissection (in Stanford type A)
(a) aortic insufficiency
(b) occlusion of coronary artery (8%)
(c) internal rupture into RV, LA, vena cava, pulmonary artery producing large L-to-R shunt
(2) Occlusion / transient obstruction of major aortic branches (in up to 27%)
(a) static obstruction
√ flap enters branch-vessel origin
(b) dynamic obstruction = flap spares branch-vessel origin but covers it like a curtain
√ collapsed true lumen outlined by a C-shaped flap envelope which is concave toward false lumen (ischemic configuration)
(3) External rupture of aorta into pleural cavity / pericardial sac: 70% mortality (= most common cause of death within 24 hours)
(4) Development of aneurysm (15%) of the true / false lumen
◊ Organs may receive their blood supply through either the true or false lumen or both!

Rx:
(1) Reducing peak systolic pressure to 120–70 mm Hg (adequate alone for type III = B, which rarely progresses proximally): death from rupture of aortic aneurysm in 46% of hypertensive + 17% of normotensive patients
Survival rate: 40–70% (with medical / surgical management)
(2) Immediate surgical graft reinforcement of aortic wall (Type I, II = A) preventing rupture + progressive aortic valve insufficiency
Nonsurgical survival rate: <10%
Postsurgical mortality: 10–35%
Cx: myocardial infarction, stroke, respiratory insufficiency, pulmonary embolism, aortic rupture, pseudoaneurysm, graft infection

Prognosis without Rx:
immediate death (3%); death within: 1 day (20–30%), 1 week (50–62%), 3 weeks (60%), 1 month (75%), 3 months (80%), 1 year (80–95%)

Prognosis with Rx:
5–10% mortality rate following timely surgery; 40% 10-year survival rate after leaving hospital

DDx: penetrating ulcer of thoracic aorta (= atherosclerotic lesion of mid-descending aorta with ulceration extending through intima into aortic media)

Intramural Aortic Hematoma (3–13%)

= aortic dissection without rupture of intima
Cause: hemorrhage of vasa vasorum
• signs + symptoms identical to classic dissection
NECT:
√ cuff / crescent of high attenuation
√ displacement of intimal calcification

HEART

CECT:
- √ mural region of low attenuation with smooth border maintaining a constant circumferential relationship with aortic wall

Aortography: not useful!

Cx: ulcerlike projection with progression to open dissection / saccular or fusiform aneurysm

Rx: (1) emergency surgical repair for type A hematoma (probably represents early stage of classic aortic dissection)
(2) observation for type B hematoma (may heal completely)

DDx:
(1) Acutely thrombosed false lumen of dissection (tendency to spiral longitudinally around aorta)
(2) Atheromatous mural thrombus (irregular internal border)
(3) Focal periaortic soft-tissue mass (irregular external border)
(a) idiopathic periaortic fibrosis
(b) periaortic lymphoma

AORTIC PROSTHETIC GRAFT INFECTION

Incidence: 1.3–6% of prosthetic graft procedures

Classification:
(1) PERIGRAFT INFECTION (2–6%)
- fever, chills, leukocytosis
- groin swelling, heat, tenderness, pulsatile mass, draining sinus tract

(2) AORTOENTERIC FISTULA (0.6–2%)
- acute / chronic GI bleeding (may be occult)
- sepsis

- may be temporally remote (up to 10 years): median time of 3 years to manifestation (70% occur after 1st year)
- intracavitary signs: malaise, back pain, fever, elevated sedimentation rate, hydronephrosis, ischemia from clotted graft

Normal postoperative course:
- √ ring of fat attenuation in early postoperative period <5 mm between aneurysm wall and graft
- ◊ Complete resolution of hematoma by 3 months
- ◊ Disappearance of ectopic gas complete by 4–7 weeks

CT (94% sensitive, 85% specific, 91% accurate):
- √ perigraft fluid
- √ perigraft soft-tissue attenuation with indistinctness of graft margins
- √ ectopic gas (fistulous communication with bowel / gas-producing organism)
- √ pseudoaneurysm (25%)
- √ focal bowel wall thickening (indicates fistula)
- √ >5 mm soft tissue between graft + surrounding wrap (beyond 7th postoperative week)
- √ focal discontinuity of calcified aneurysmal wrap

False positives:
perigraft hematoma in early postoperative period, pseudoaneurysm (in 15–20%)

NUC:
- √ uptake of Tc-99m hexametazine labeled leukocytes (drawbacks: not performed quickly, hepatobiliary excretion)

Prognosis: 17–75% mortality; 30–50% morbidity

Dx: positive culture from needle aspirate (incubation period should be up to 14 days as organisms may be slow-growing)

AORTIC REGURGITATION

= AORTIC INSUFFICIENCY

Cause:

A. INTRINSIC AORTIC VALVE DISEASE
1. Congenital bicuspid valve
2. Rheumatic endocarditis
3. Bacterial endocarditis (perforation / prolapse of cusp)
4. Myxomatous valve associated with cystic medial necrosis
5. Aortic valve prolapse
6. Prosthetic valve: mechanical break, thrombosis, paravalvular leak

B. PRIMARY DISEASE OF ASCENDING AORTA
(a) Dilatation of aortic annulus
1. Syphilitic aortitis
2. Rheumatoid arthritis
3. Rheumatoid variants:
— Ankylosing spondylitis (5–10%)
— Reiter disease
— Psoriatic arthritis
4. Relapsing polychondritis
5. Familial connective tissue disease:
mnemonic: "HOME"
— **H**omocystinuria
— **O**steogenesis imperfecta
— **M**arfan syndrome
— **E**hlers-Danlos syndrome

(b) Laceration = aortic dissection
1. Deceleration trauma
2. Hypertension

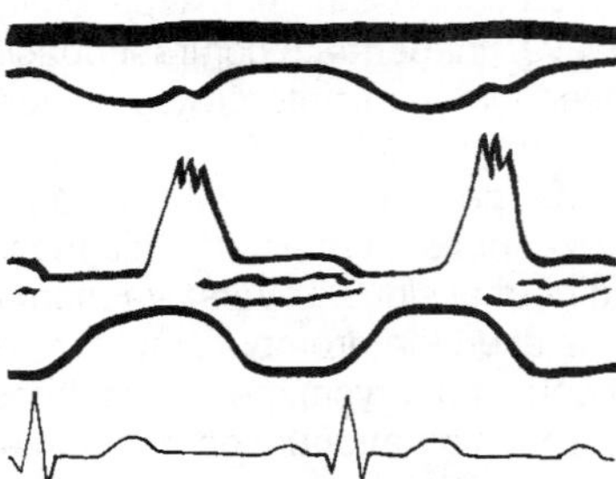

Mitral Valve in Severe Aortic Regurgitation

The valve is almost completely closed before onset of ventricular systole. Atrial contraction has little effect in reopening the valve. Complete closure occurs with ventricular systole. A high-velocity flutter of aML is present in diastole.

HEART

Pathogenesis: progressive enlargement of diastolic + systolic LV dimensions result in increase in myocardial fiber length + increase in stroke volume; decompensation occurs if critical limit of fiber length is reached

- "water-hammer pulse" = twin-peaked pulse
- systolic ejection murmur + high-pitched diastolic murmur
- Austin Flint murmur = soft mid-diastolic or presystolic bruit

√ LV enlargement (cardiothoracic ratio >0.55) + initially normal pulmonary vascularity (DDx: congestive cardiomyopathy, pericardial effusion)
√ normal aorta (in intrinsic valve disease)
√ dilatation of aorta (in systemic disease):
  √ ± calcification of ascending aorta (in aortic wall disease)
  √ ± enlarged aortic arch + tortuous descending aorta
√ increased pulsations along entire aorta

ECHO:
  √ aortic root dilatation
  √ high frequency flutter of aML (occasionally pML) during first 2/3 of diastole (CHARACTERISTIC)
  √ high frequency diastolic flutter of IVS (uncommon)
  √ diastolic flutter of aortic valve (SPECIFIC, but rare)
  √ premature aortic valve opening (high diastolic LV pressure)
  √ decreased MV opening (aML pushed posteriorly by regurgitant aortic jet)
  √ premature closure of mitral valve (high diastolic LV pressure produces MV closure before beginning of systole in severe acute aortic insufficiency)
  √ LV dilatation + large amplitude of LV wall motion (volume overload, increased ejection fraction):

End-systolic LV diameter	Action
<50 mm	yearly follow-up
50–54 mm	4- to 6-month follow-up
>55 mm	valve replacement

Doppler:
  √ slope of peak diastolic to end-diastolic velocity decrease >3 m/sec^2 in severe aortic regurgitation
  √ area of color Doppler regurgitant flow
  √ ratio of width of regurgitant beam to width of aortic root is good predictor of severity (color Doppler)

AORTIC RUPTURE

= blood leakage through aortic wall

1. Spontaneous rupture of aortic aneurysm
   Pathogenesis: small clefts occur at a fragile site within inner thrombus gradually expanding to outer layer of thrombus with gradual seepage of flowing blood into mural thrombus and aneurysmal wall
   CT:
   √ high-attenuation crescent sign (71%)
2. Spontaneous rupture of descending thoracic aorta
   Predisposed: hypertension and atherosclerosis, NO preformed aneurysm!
   Pathogenesis: pressure atrophy of media due to overlying intimal atheromatous plaque causing localized ballooning of aortic wall prior to perforation
3. Traumatic rupture / transection of thoracic aorta
   Cause: blunt trauma to thoracic aorta

AORTIC STENOSIS

Aortic valve area decreased to <0.8 cm^2 = 0.4 cm^2/m^2 BSA (normal 2.5–3.5 cm^2)

A. ACQUIRED AORTIC STENOSIS
   1. Rheumatic valvulitis (almost invariably associated with mitral valve disease)
   2. Fibrocalcific senile aortic stenosis (degenerative)
B. CONGENITAL AORTIC STENOSIS (most common)
   = most frequent CHD associated with IUGR
   1. Subvalvular AS (15–30%)
   2. Valvular AS (60–70%): degeneration of bicuspid valve most common cause
   3. Supravalvular AS (rare)

Pathogenesis: increased gradient across valve produces LV hypertrophy and diminished LV compliance; increased muscle mass may outstrip coronary blood supply (subendocardial myocardial ischemia with angina); LV decompensation leads to LV dilatation + pulmonary venous congestion

- asymptomatic for many years
- angina, syncope, heart failure
- systolic murmur
- carotid pulsus parvus et tardus

Valvular Aortic Stenoses

	Congenital	*Rheumatic*	*Degenerative*
Clinically apparent	<30 years	30–60 years	>65 years
Valve calcifications			
first appearance	25 years	47 years	54 years
pattern	nodular / bicuspid	nodular	nodular / tricuspid
on CXR	>90% (40–65 years)	<10%	>90% (>65 years)
Aortic ectasia	ascending Ao	ascending Ao	entire Ao

HEART

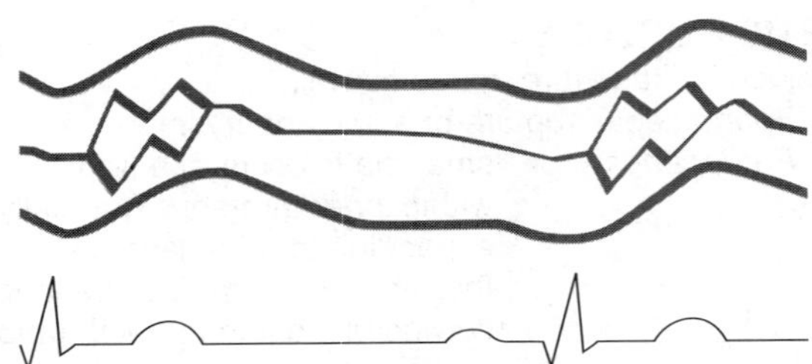

Aortic Valve in Hypertrophic Subaortic Stenosis
during midsystole the aortic valve closes secondary to subvalvular obstruction

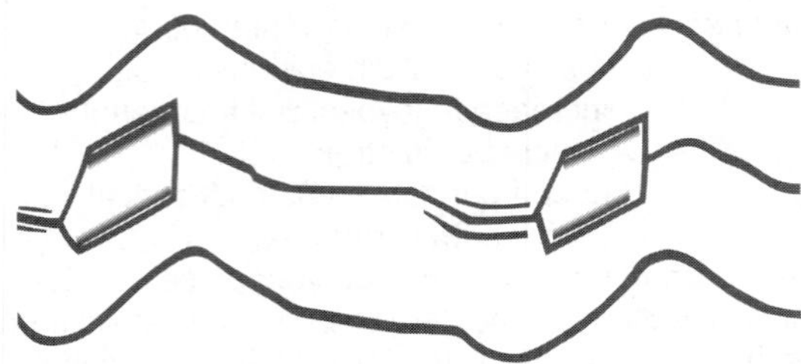

Aortic Valvular Stenosis
decreased separation of thickened deformed leaflets

- diminished aortic component of 2nd heart sound
- sudden death in severe stenosis (20%) after exercise (diminished flow in coronary arteries causes ventricular dysrhythmias + fibrillation)

√ poststenotic dilatation of ascending aorta (in 90% of acquired, in 70% of congenital AS)
√ normal-sized / enlarged LV (small LV chamber with thick walls)
@ in adults >30 years
 √ calcification of aortic valve (best seen on RAO); indicates gradient >50 mm Hg
 √ discrete enlargement of ascending aorta (NO correlation with severity of stenosis)
 √ calcification of mitral annulus
 √ "left ventricular configuration" = concavity along mid left lateral heart border + increased convexity along lower left lateral heart border
@ in children / young adults
 √ prominent ascending aorta
 √ left ventricular heart configuration
@ in infancy:
 √ left ventricular stress syndrome
ECHO:
 √ thickened + calcified aortic valve with multiple dense cusp echoes throughout cardiac cycle (right > noncoronary > left coronary cusp)
 √ decreased separation of leaflets in systole with reduced opening orifice (13–14 mm = mild AS; 8–12 mm = moderate AS; <8 mm = severe AS)
 √ ± doming in systole
 √ dilated aortic root
 √ increased thickness of LV wall (= concentric LV hypertrophy)
 √ hyperdynamic contraction of LV (in compensated state)
 √ decreased mitral EF slope (reduced LV compliance)
 √ LA enlargement
 √ increased aortic valve gradient (Doppler)
 √ decreased aortic valve area (unreliable)
 DDx: calcification of aortic annulus in elderly / calcified coronary artery ostium (thickened cusp echoes only in diastole)
Prognosis: depends on symptomatology (angina, syncope, CHF)

Subvalvular Aortic Stenosis

= SUBAORTIC STENOSIS
(a) Anatomic / fixed subaortic stenosis
 Associated with: cardiac defects in 50% (usually VSD)
 Type I : thin 1–2-mm membranous diaphragmatic stenosis, usually located within 2 cm or less of valve annulus
 Type II : thick collarlike stenosis
 Type III : irregular fibromuscular stenosis
 Type IV : "tunnel subaortic stenosis" = fixed tunnel-like narrowing of LVOT = excessive thickening of only upper ventricular septum with normal mitral valve motion
(b) Functional / dynamic subaortic stenosis
 1. Asymmetric septal hypertrophy (ASH)
 2. Idiopathic hypertrophic subaortic stenosis (IHSS)
 3. Hypertrophic obstructive cardiomyopathy (HOCM) may occur in infants of diabetic mothers

√ no dilatation of ascending aorta
√ asymmetrically thicker ventricular septum than free wall of LV (95%)
√ normal / small left + right ventricular cavities (95%)
√ lucent subaortic filling defect in systole
√ focal convexity of left upper-mid cardiac margin = anterior aspect of ventricular septum (rare)
ECHO:
 √ coarse systolic flutter of valve cusps
 √ opening of leaflets followed by rapid inward move in mid systole, leaflets may remain in partially closed position through latter portion of systole (to appose borders of the flow jet)
 √ systolic anterior motion of mitral valve
Cx: mitral regurgitation (secondary to abnormal position of anterolateral papillary muscle preventing complete closure of MV in systole)

Valvular Aortic Stenosis

= fusion of commissures between cusps
Degree: mild: >0.7 cm^2; moderate: 0.5–0.7 cm^2; severe: <0.5 cm^2

Congenital types:
(a) bicuspid / unicuspid (in 95%): in 1–2% of population; M > F; commonly associated with coarctation of the aorta
(b) tricuspid (5%)
(c) dysplastic thickened aortic cusps
√ valvular calcifications (in 60% of patients >24 years of age)

@ IN INFANT with critical aortic stenosis:
- intractable CHF in first days / weeks of life with severe dyspnea
- may simulate neonatal sepsis

Associated with: L-to-R shunts (ASD, VSD)
√ marked cardiomegaly (thickened wall of LV)
√ pulmonary venous hypertension
√ decreased ejection fraction
√ doming of thickened valve cusps
√ dilated ascending aorta
Rx: emergency surgical dilatation

@ IN CHILD:
- asymptomatic until late in life

√ normal pulmonary vascularity
√ LV configuration with normal size of heart
√ large posterior noncoronary cusp, smaller fused right + left cusps
√ doming of thickened valve cusps
√ eccentric jet of contrast
√ poststenotic dilatation of ascending aorta

ECHO:
√ increase in echoes from thickened deformed leaflets (maximal during diastole)
√ decrease in leaflet separation

Supravalvular Aortic Stenosis

Types:
(a) localized hourglass narrowing just above aortic sinuses
(b) discrete fibrous membrane above sinuses of Valsalva
(c) diffuse tubular hypoplasia of ascending aorta + branching arteries

Associated with: peripheral PS, valvular + discrete subvalvular AS, Marfan syndrome, Williams syndrome, infantile hypercalcemia syndrome

√ small ascending thoracic aorta
√ dilatation + tortuosity of coronary arteries (may undergo early atherosclerotic degeneration secondary to high pressure)

ECHO:
√ narrowing of supravalvular aortic area (normal root diameter: 20–37 mm)
√ normal movement of cusps

AORTOPULMONIC WINDOW

= defect in septation process characterized by large round / oval communication between left wall of ascending aorta + right wall of pulmonary trunk

- clinically resembles PDA

CXR:
√ shunt vascularity
√ cardiomegaly (LA + LV enlarged)
√ diminutive aortic knob
√ prominent pulmonary trunk

Angio (left ventriculogram / aortogram in AP / LAO projection):
√ defect several mm above aortic valve
√ pulmonary valve identified (DDx to truncus arteriosus)

ARTERIOSCLEROSIS OBLITERANS

= ASO = HARDENING OF THE ARTERIES

Prevalence: 2.4 million people in USA; in 1978 12% of autopsies had ASO as leading cause of death (excluding MI)

Etiology: unknown

Contributing factors:
aging, diabetes (16–44%), hypertension, atherosclerosis
Effect of hyperlipidemia:
(a) High-density lipoproteins (HDL) have a protective effect: carry 25% of blood cholesterol
(b) Low-density lipoproteins (LDL): carry 60% of blood cholesterol

Histo: deposition of lipids, blood products, carbohydrates, begins as disruption of intimal surface; fatty streaks (as early as childhood); fibrous plaques (as early as 3rd decade); thrombosis, ulceration, calcification, aneurysm

Age: 50–70 years; M > F (after menopause)

Clinical classification:
(1) intermittent claudication = ischemic symptoms with exercise: calf, thigh, hip, buttock
(2) ischemic symptoms at rest (indicative of multisegment disease)

- cramping / burning / aching pain
- cold extremity
- paresthesia
- trophic changes: hair loss, thickened nails
- ulcer, gangrene
- decreased / absent pulses

Location: medium + large arteries; frequently at bifurcations; most frequent:
— superficial femoral artery in adductor canal (diabetics + nondiabetics)
— aortoiliac segment (nondiabetics)
— tibioperoneal trunk (diabetics)

Prognosis:
accelerated by diabetes (34% will require amputation), hypertension, lipoprotein abnormalities, heart disease (decreased cardiac output resulting in increased blood viscosity from polycythemia), chronic addiction to tobacco (11.4% will require amputation), intermittent claudication (5–7% require amputation if nondiabetic = 1–2% per year), ischemic ulcer / rest pain (19.6% require amputation)

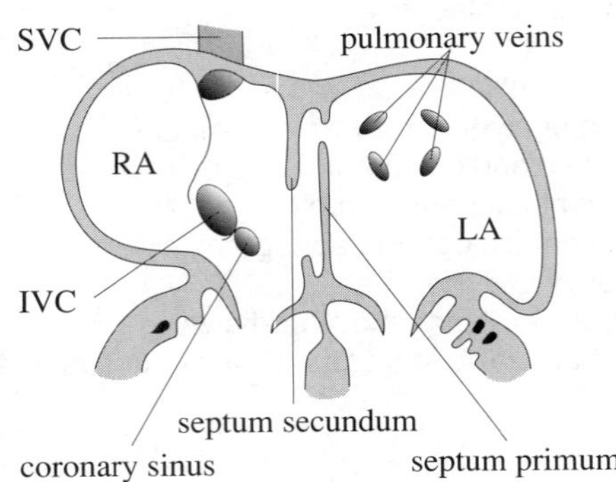

Normal Newborn Heart

Atrial septum consists of two components
(a) right side: septum secundum (muscular, firm) with posterior opening = foramen ovale
(b) left side: septum primum (fibrous, thin) with anterior opening = ostium secundum

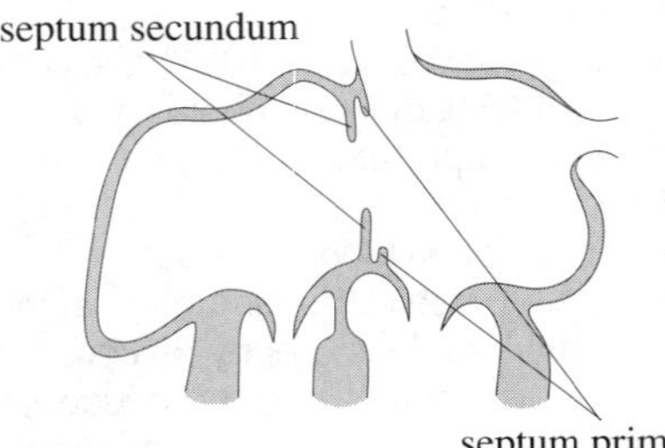

Ostium Secundum Defect

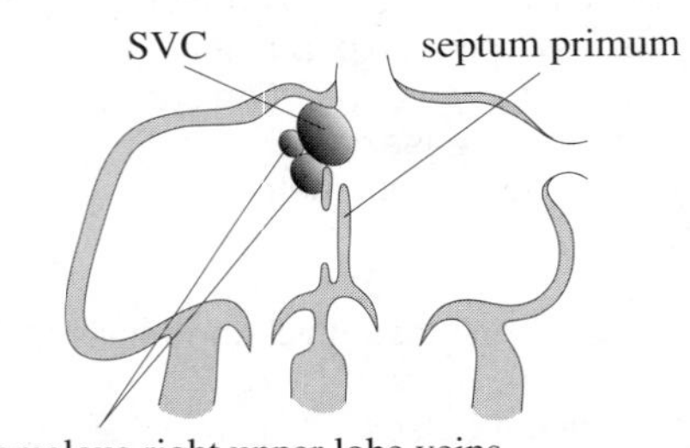

Sinus Venosus Defect

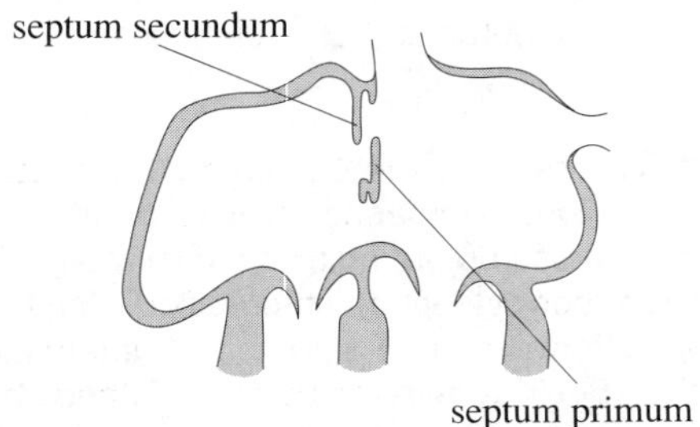

Ostium Primum Defect

ATRIAL SEPTAL DEFECT

◊ Most common congenital cardiac defect in adults >20 years of age!

Incidence: 8–14% of all CHD; M:F = 1:4

Age: presentation frequently > age 40 secondary to benign course
- (a) mildly symptomatic (60%): dyspnea, fatigue, palpitations
- (b) severely symptomatic (30%): cyanosis, heart failure

Embryology:
1. Septum primum = at 4th week membrane grows from dorsal atrial wall toward endocardial cushions
2. Ostium primum = temporary orifice between septum primum + endocardial cushions close to AV valves; it becomes obliterated by 5th week
3. Ostium secundum = multiple small coalescing fenestrations in center of septum primum
4. Septum secundum = membrane developing on right side of septum primum + covering part of ostium secundum
5. Foramen ovale = orifice limited by septum secundum + septum primum
6. Foramen ovale flap = lower edge of septum primum (patent in 6%, probe-patent in 25%); not considered an ASD

A. OSTIUM SECUNDUM ASD (60–70%)
   = exaggerated resorptive process of septum primum leads to absence / fenestration of the foramen ovale flap (Chiari network)
   Location: in the center of the atrial chamber at fossa ovalis
   Size: large defect of 1–3 cm in diameter
   May be associated with:
   prolapsing mitral valve (20–30%), pulmonary valve stenosis, tricuspid atresia, TAPVR, hypoplastic left heart, interrupted aortic arch

B. OSTIUM PRIMUM ASD (30%)
   = defect of atrioventricular endocardial cushion
   Location: lower end of septum inferior to fossa ovalis (at outlet portion of atrial septum)
   Almost always associated with:
   endocardial cushion defects, cleft mitral valve, anterior fascicular block

C. SINUS VENOSUS ASD (5%)
   = defect of the superior inlet portion of the atrial septum
   Location: superior to fossa ovalis near entrance of superior vena cava (SVC straddles ASD)
   Associated with: partial anomalous pulmonary venous return in 90% (RUL pulmonary veins connect to SVC / right atrium), Holt-Oram syndrome, Ellis-van Creveld syndrome

D. LUTEMBACHER SYNDROME = ASD + mitral stenosis

Hemodynamics:
no hemodynamic perturbance in the fetus; after birth physiologic increase in LA pressure creates a L-to-R shunt (shunt volume may be 3–4 times that of systemic blood flow) with volume overload of RV leading to RV dilatation, right heart failure, pulmonary hypertension; diastolic pressure differences in atria determine direction of shunt; pulmonary pressure remains normal for decades before Eisenmenger syndrome sets in; pulmonary hypertension in young adulthood (6%)

RA	↑	RV	↑	Main PA	↑
Pulm vessels		↑			
LA	↔	LV	↔	Ao	↓/↔

- repeated respiratory infections
- feeding difficulties
- arrhythmias
- thromboembolism
- asymptomatic; occasionally discovered by routine CXR
- right ventricular heave
- fixed splitting of second heart sound with accentuation of pulmonary component (ejection murmur grade II/VI) heard at 2nd left intercostal space along PA
- ECG: right axis deviation + some degree of right bundle branch block
- exertional dyspnea after development of pulmonary arterial hypertension (= Eisenmenger syndrome)
- cyanosis may occur (shunt reversal to R-to-L shunt), typically during 3rd–4th decade
- right heart failure in patients >40 years

CXR:
√ normal (if shunt <2 x systemic blood flow)
√ overcirculation = increase in pulmonary blood flow (if pulmonary-to-systemic blood flow ≥2:1)
√ cardiomegaly:
  √ heart small compared with pulmonary vascularity = closing shunt
  √ heart large compared with pulmonary vascularity = intercurrent myocardial / aortic disease
√ loss of visualization of SVC (= clockwise rotation of heart due to RV hypertrophy)
√ small appearing aorta with normal aortic knob
√ normal size of LA after shunt reversal (due to immediate decompression into RA) in Eisenmenger syndrome:
  √ enlargement of PA + central pulmonary arteries
  √ RV enlargement
√ "hilar dance" = increased pulsations of central pulmonary arteries (DDx: other L-to-R shunts)

ECHO:
√ paradoxical interventricular septal motion (due to volume overload of RV)
√ direct visualization of ASD (= lack of echoes of atrial septum) in subcostal view
√ diastolic blood flow from interatrial septum crossing RA + tricuspid valve observed by color Doppler

Angio:
√ RA fills with contrast shortly after LA is opacified (on levophase of pulmonary angio in AP or LAO projection)
√ injection into RUL pulmonary vein to visualize exact size + location of ASD (LAO 45° + C-C 45°)

Prognosis:
(1) Mortality: 0.6% in 1st decade; 0.7% in 2nd decade; 2.7% in 3rd decade; 4.5% in 4th decade; 5.4% in 5th decade; 7.5% in 6th decade; median age of death is 37 years
(2) Spontaneous closure: 22% in infants <1 year; 33% between ages 1 and 2 years; 3% in children >4 years

Cx: (1) Tricuspid insufficiency (secondary to dilatation of AV ring)
(2) Mitral valve prolapse
(3) Atrial fibrillation (in 20% 1st presenting symptom in patients > age 40)

Rx: (if vascular changes still reversible = resistance of pulmonary-to-systemic system ≤0.7); 1% surgical mortality
1. Surgical patch closure
2. Rashkind foam + stainless steel prosthesis

BENEFICIAL ASD
= secundum type ASD serves an essential compensatory function in:
1. Tricuspid atresia
   RA blood reaches pulmonary vessels via ASD + PDA; improvement through Rashkind procedure
2. TAPVR
   significant shunt volume only available through ASD (VSD / PDA much less reliable)
3. Hypoplastic left heart
   systemic circulation maintained via RV with oxygenated blood from LA through ASD into RA

AZYGOS CONTINUATION OF IVC

= INTERRUPTED IVC WITH AZYGOS / HEMIAZYGOS CONTINUATION = ABSENCE OF THE HEPATIC SEGMENT OF THE IVC WITH AZYGOS CONTINUATION

Prevalence: 0.6%

Etiology: formation failure of right subcardinal-hepatic anastomosis with atrophy of right subcardinal vein + shunting of blood from supracardinal-subcardinal anastomosis to cranial portion of supracardinal vein (= retrocrural azygos vein)

May be associated with:
polysplenia syndrome (more common), asplenia syndrome (rare), indeterminate situs (= situs ambiguus), persistent left SVC, dextrocardia, transposed abdominal viscera, duplicated IVC, retroaortic left renal vein, congenital pulmonary venolobar syndrome

√ absence of hepatic ± infrahepatic IVC:
  √ drainage of hepatic veins into right atrium via supra- / posthepatic segment of IVC (N.B.: IVC shadow present on LAT CXR!)
√ drainage of iliac + renal veins via azygos / hemiazygos vein:
  √ right renal artery crosses anterior to "IVC" on US

HEART

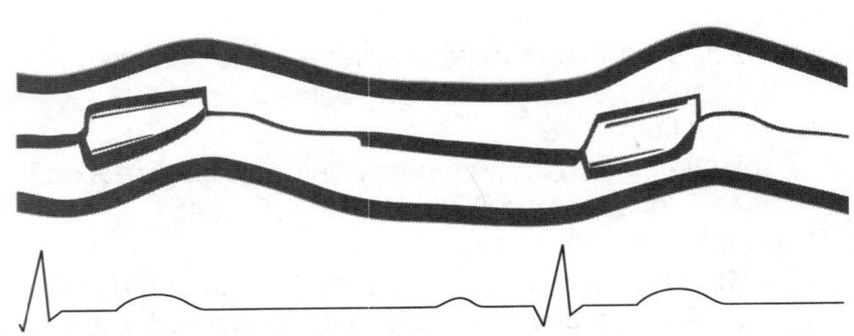

Aortic Valve Endocarditis

√ both gonadal veins drain into ipsilateral renal vein (since postcardinal-subcardinal anastomosis does not contribute to formation of IVC)

CXR:
- √ enlargement of azygos arch to >7 mm
- √ widening of right paraspinal stripe contiguous with azygos arch (= enlarged paraspinal + retrocrural azygos veins)
- √ widening of left paraspinal stripe (= enlarged hemiazygos vein)

DDx: right-sided paratracheal mass with retrocrural adenopathy

BACTERIAL ENDOCARDITIS

Predisposed:
1. Rheumatic valve disease
2. Mitral valve prolapse with mitral regurgitation
3. Aortic stenosis, mitral stenosis, aortic regurgitation, mitral regurgitation
4. Most CHD (VSD, TOF) except ostium secundum ASD
5. Previous endocarditis
6. Drug addicts:
   endocarditis of tricuspid valve causes multiple septic pulmonary emboli
7. Bicuspid aortic valve:
   responsible for 50% of aortic valvular bacterial endocarditis
8. Prosthetic valve:
   4% incidence of bacterial endocarditis
   - √ exaggerated valve motion (= disintegration of suture line + regurgitation)

Valve Vegetations

ECHO:
- √ usually discrete focal echodensities with sharp edges; may show fuzzy / shaggy nonuniform thickening of cusps (vegetations) in systole + diastole
- √ may appear as shaggy echoes that prolapse when the valve is closed (DDx to mitral valve prolapse)

BUERGER DISEASE

= THROMBANGITIS OBLITERANS

= idiopathic recurrent segmental obliterative vasculitis of small + medium-sized peripheral arteries + veins (panangitis)

Incidence: <1% of all chronic vascular diseases; more common in Israel, Orient, India

Etiology: unknown

Histo:
- (a) acute stage: multiple microabscesses within fresh / organizing thrombus; all layers of vessel wall inflamed but intact; internal elastic lamina may be damaged; multinucleated giant cells within microabscesses (PATHOGNOMONIC)
- (b) subacute stage: thrombus organization with little residual inflammation
- (c) chronic stage: lumen filled with organized recanalized thrombus, fibrosis of adventitia binds together artery, vein, and nerve

Associated with: cigarette smoking (95%)

- • instep claudication ± distal ulceration (symptoms abate on cessation of smoking + return on its resumption)
- • Raynaud phenomenon (33%)

Location: legs (80%), arms (10–20%)

Site: starts in palmar + plantar vessels with proximal progression

- √ superficial + deep migratory thrombophlebitis (20–33%)
- √ arterial occlusions, tapered narrowing of arteries
- √ abundant corkscrew-shaped collaterals
- √ direct collateral following the path of the original artery (Martorell sign) in 80%
- √ skip lesions = multiple segments involved with portions of arterial wall remaining unaffected
- √ absence of generalized arteriosclerosis / arterial calcifications (90%)

BLUNT TRAUMA TO THORACIC AORTA

= AORTIC LACERATION

= laceration that disrupts the physical integrity of >1 structural layers of the aorta

Cause: rapid deceleration (high-speed MVA >48 km/h with unrestrained driver or ejected passenger, fall from height >3 m) / crushing chest injury

Pathomechanism: horizontal / vertical deceleration, hydrostatic force, osseous pinch

Length of tear: circumferential tear (in majority)

Site:
- (a) Aortic isthmus just distal to left subclavian artery (88–95%): brachiocephalic arteries + ligamentum arteriosum fix aorta in this region
- (b) Aortic arch with avulsion of brachiocephalic trunk (4.5%)
- (c) Ascending aorta immediately above aortic valve (5–9%)
  Cx: aortic valve rupture, coronary artery laceration, hemopericardium + cardiac tamponade; NO mediastinal hematoma
- (d) Diaphragmatic hiatus (1–3%)
- ◊ Most often posteriorly (in noncircumferential tear)

Extent of laceration:
1. Incomplete rupture (15%)
   ◊ Aorta goes on to rupture completely within 24 hours in 50% of patients!

— INTIMA
  (a) intimal hemorrhage without tear
  (b) transverse laceration of intima with hemorrhage (= **intimal tear / flap** = **traumatic aortic dissection**)
— MEDIA
  tear into media with subadventitial accumulation of blood (40–60%)
— ADVENTITIA
  (a) periaortic hemorrhage ± aortic injury
  (b) traumatic false aneurysm = involves intima + media + adventitia with locally contained hematoma

2. Complete rupture (85%) = transmural extension of laceration = **aortic transection** = **traumatic aortic rupture**
   • exsanguination before reaching a hospital

Acute Thoracic Aortic Injury

Prevalence: 10–16–20% of all fatalities in high-speed deceleration accidents

• severe chest pain: precordial (ascending aorta), neck-jaw (aortic arch), interscapular (descending thoracic aorta)
• anterior chest wall contusion, dyspnea, dysphagia
• blood pressure changes:
  • unexplained hypotension
  • scapulothoracic syndrome = decreased / absent upper extremity pulses
  • acute coarctation syndrome = decreased / absent lower extremity + normal upper extremity pulses with upper extremity hypertension + systolic murmur in 2nd left parasternal interspace

CXR:
◊ A normal anteroposterior upright CXR virtually excludes acute thoracic aortic injury (96–98% negative predictive value)!
N.B.: There are no plain CXR findings of aortic injury (since aortic integrity is maintained by intact adventitia)! The sources of <u>mediastinal hematoma</u> are frequently the azygos, hemiazygos, internal thoracic, paraspinal and intercostal vessels!
  ◊ Aortic injury is the cause of mediastinal hematoma in only 12.5%!
√ normal admission CXR in 28% (radiographic signs may not develop until 6–36 hours): supine CXR is very inaccurate for mediastinal widening
<u>Most specific signs</u>:
  √ deviation of nasogastric / endotracheal tube to the right of T3-T4 spinous process (12–100% sensitive, 80–95% specific)
  √ depression of left mainstem bronchus anteroinferiorly >40° below the horizontal + toward right (53%)
√ mediastinal widening >8 cm at level of origin of left subclavian artery (present in 75–92%; 53–93–100% sensitive, 1–34–60% specific):
  √ mediastinal width to chest width >0.25
  √ indistinct aortic contour at arch / descending aorta (53–100% sensitive, 21–55% specific)
  √ obscuration of aortopulmonary window (40–100% sensitive, 56–83% specific)
  √ widened left paraspinal "stripe" >5 mm (12–83% sensitive, 89–97% specific)
  √ thickening of right paratracheal stripe >4–5 mm (= hematoma between pleura + trachea)
  √ left / right "apical pleural cap" sign in 37% (= extrapleural hematoma along brachiocephalic vessels)
  √ tracheal compression + displacement toward right (61%)
  √ rapidly accumulating commonly left-sided hemothorax without evident rib fracture (break in mediastinal pleura)
  √ fractures of 1st + 2nd rib (17%)
  mnemonic: "BAD MEAT"
    Bronchus depression (left main)
    Aortic silhouette shaggy
    Death in 80–90%
    Mediastinal widening
    Enteric (nasogastric) tube displacement
    Apical cap
    Tracheal shift

NECT screening (55–100% sensitive, 65–87% specific):
  √ obliteration of aorta-fat interface with increased attenuation (= mediastinal hematoma)
  DDx: residual thymic tissue, periaortic atelectasis, pleural effusion adjacent to descending aorta, volume averaging of pulmonary artery
  ◊ A negative CT examination for mediastinal hemorrhage has an almost 100% NPV for aortic injury!
  ◊ All patients with periaortic / middle / superior mediastinal hemorrhage require aortography! Save your contrast for that study!
  False positive:
  residual thymic tissue, atelectatic lung, pericardial recess, patient motion, streak artifacts, partial volume effect with pulmonary artery

CECT (100% sensitive; 81% specific; 0–39% false positive; 0.7% false negative):
  Technique: 100–150 mL at 2 mL/sec with 20–30 second scanning delay
  Advantages:
    (a) negative findings will obviate invasive angio
    (b) unsuspected injuries are discovered
    (c) saves health care dollars
  Disadvantages:
    (a) CT delays the definitive aortography + surgery
    (b) two contrast studies are needed in the frequent cases of mediastinal hemorrhage
    (c) few data exist on accuracy of CT for branch vessel injury
  √ intraluminal area of low attenuation:
    √ linear = intimal flap
    √ polypoid = clot

√ contour deformity of inner aortic wall = intramural hematoma
√ aortic pseudoaneurysm
√ pseudocoarctation = abrupt tapering of the diameter of the descending aorta compared with the ascending aorta
√ extravasation of contrast material (rare)
False positive:
linear motion artifact (aortic valve leaflets, wall of ascending aorta), volume averaging, prominent periaortic bronchial / mediastinal vessels, prominent atheroma, small ductus diverticulum

Transesophageal echocardiography
(in 2–15% technically unsuccessful, 57–63% sensitive, 84–91% specific):
√ intimal flap
√ intraluminal thick stripes
√ pseudoaneurysm
√ aortic occlusion (= pseudocoarctation)
√ fusiform aneurysm
√ aortic wall hematoma

Aortography (almost 100% sensitive, 98% specific):
Technique: LAO + RAO projection; high-flow pigtail catheter; 50 mL at 35 mL/sec
True positive:
In 17–20% of patients with mediastinal hematoma angio demonstrates acute traumatic aortic injury!
False negative:
◊ Small transverse intimal tears may be missed!
√ resistance in advancing guide wire
√ intimal irregularity, linear defect, filling defect = intimal flap = posttraumatic dissection (5–10%)
√ intramural injury:
√ thickening of aortic wall
√ posttraumatic coarctation
√ transmural laceration:
√ contained extravasation = traumatic false aneurysm
√ free extravasation = aortic rupture
DDx: ductus diverticulum (in 10% of normals), aortic spindle, infundibula of brachiocephalic arterial branches; volume averaging with left brachiocephalic vein / left superior intercostal vein / right bronchial arteries (vs. intimal flap); artifact from physiologic streaming / mixing of contrast material; atherosclerotic aortic ulceration; atheromatous plaque; syphilitic aortic aneurysm

Recommendations for work-up:
(1) Normal well-defined mediastinal contours on CXR: no further imaging
(2) Unstable patient + unequivocally abnormal CXR / strong clinical evidence of aortic injury: angiography / emergency surgery
(3) Stable patient
(a) with unequivocally abnormal CXR: CT of chest + head + abdomen (while waiting for angiographic examination)
(b) with equivocal CXR: screening CT of chest
(c) abnormal chest CT: angiography for confirmation / surgery

Prognosis:
(1) 80–90% fatal at scene of trauma
(2) 10–20% reach hospital (due to formation of periaortic hematoma + false aneurysm contained by adventitia ± surrounding connective tissue)
(a) without intervention: 30% dead within 6 hours; 40–50% dead within 24 hours, 90% dead within 4 months; chronic false aneurysm may develop in 2–5% at isthmus / descending aorta
(b) with surgical repair: 60–70% survive; surgical mortality rate of 9–44% varies with degree of hemodynamic instability + severity of associated injuries + magnitude of aortic laceration
Cx: postoperative paraplegia (9%) due to aortic cross clamping >30 minutes

Chronic Posttraumatic Aortic Pseudoaneurysm

= aneurysm existing for >3 months (amount of wall fibroplasia following rupture usually not sufficient to prevent subsequent rupture until at least 3 months after initial traumatic episode)
Incidence: 2–5% of patients surviving aortic transection >24–48 hours
• symptom-free period of months to years (in 11% >10 years)
• delayed clinical symptoms (42% within 5 years, 85% within 20 years): chest pain, back pain, dyspnea, cough, hoarseness, dysphagia, systolic murmur
Location: descending aorta at level of lig. arteriosum filling the aorticopulmonary window (most commonly)
√ well-defined rounded mass in left paramediastinal region
√ ± inferior displacement of left mainstem bronchus
Cx: CHF, partial obstruction of aortic lumen, bacterial endocarditis, aortoesophageal fistula, aortic dissection, obstruction of tracheobronchial tree, systemic emboli
Prognosis: enlargement + eventual rupture;
10-year survival rate: 85% with surgical repair, 66% without surgical repair

CARDIAC FIBROMA

= FIBROMATOSIS = FIBROUS HAMARTOMA = FIBROELASTIC HAMARTOMA
= congenital neoplasm / hamartoma of the heart
Incidence: 100 cases reported; 2nd most common benign cardiac neoplasm of childhood (after rhabdomyoma)
Age: 0–56 years (mean age, 13 years); 33% in children <1 year of age / in utero; 15% in adolescents + adults
Increased prevalence in: Gorlin (= basal cell nevus) syndrome
• heart failure, cardiac murmur (33%), arrhythmia
• NO embolism; asymptomatic (33%)

HEART

Path: 2–10-cm large single round bulging well-circumscribed tumor within ventricular myocardium; foci of calcification / ossification (50%)
Histo: collection of fibroblasts interspersed among large amounts of collagen; numerous elastic fibers (>50%); NO foci of cystic change / hemorrhage / necrosis
Location: ventricular septum > left ventricular free wall
√ cardiomegaly
√ focal cardiac bulge (with tumor in free ventricular wall)
√ ± pericardial effusion
ECHO:
- √ noncontractile echogenic heterogeneous solid mass:
  - √ mean diameter >5 cm; may obliterate cardiac chamber
  - √ multifocal dystrophic central tumor calcifications
- √ affected myocardium hypokinetic

DDx: focal hypertrophic cardiomyopathy, hypertrophy of ventricular septum

CT:
- √ homogeneous mural mass of soft-issue attenuation
- √ sharply marginated / infiltrative
- √ calcifications (25%)
- √ variable enhancement

MR:
- √ iso- / hyperintense homogeneous discrete mural mass / myocardial thickening on T1WI
- √ hypointense on T2WI
- √ no / little hetero- or homogeneous enhancement

Prognosis:
(1) sudden death (due to invasion / compression of cardiac conduction system resulting in arrhythmia)
◊ 2nd most common primary cardiac tumor associated with sudden death (after endodermal heterotopia of AV node)
(2) may remain stable in size for years / regress
Rx: surgical excision / partial resection
DDx in infants: rhabdomyoma (multiple masses)
DDx in children: rhabdomyosarcoma (no calcification, cystic or necrotic tumor, invasion of pulmonary veins or pericardial space)

CARDIAC HEMANGIOMA

= rare benign vascular tumor of the heart
Prevalence: 5–10% of benign cardiac tumors
Association: Kasabach-Merritt syndrome (multiple systemic hemangiomas, recurrent thrombocytopenia, consumptive coagulopathy)
Path: predominantly intramural spongy mass / well-circumscribed endocardial-based soft mass growing into pericardial space; may contain fat
Histo: capillary (= smaller capillary-like vessels); cavernous (= multiple thin-walled dilated vessels); arteriovenous (= thick-walled dysplastic arteries + veins + capillaries)
- asymptomatic
- dyspnea on exertion, chest pain, right-sided CHF
- arrhythmia, syncope, pericarditis, sudden death

√ ± pericardial effusion
US:
- √ hyperechoic mass

CT:
- √ heterogeneous intensely enhancing mass

MR:
- √ intermediate intensity on T1WI + hyperintense on T2WI

Angio:
- √ vascular blush in capillary + arteriovenous type
- √ no enhancement for cavernous type

Prognosis: spontaneous regression possible
Rx: surgical resection (for symptomatic lesion)

CARDIAC LIPOMA

= very rare benign neoplasm
Incidence: 60 reported cases
Age: typically in adults
- mostly symptomatic
- dyspnea (in intracavitary lipoma secondary to blood flow obstruction, in pericardial lipoma secondary to displacement of lung)
- arrhythmia (involvement of conduction system)

Path: encapsulated spherical / elliptical solitary mass, often very large (up to 4,800 g) by the time the come to clinical attention; multiple lipomas in CHD, tuberous sclerosis
Histo: mature adipocytes surrounded by capsule
Location:
(a) broad-based from epicardial surface growing into pericardial space
(b) broad-based from endocardial surface growing into cardiac chamber
(c) interatrial septum
√ cardiomegaly, globular-shaped heart
√ echogenic / hypoechoic broad-based nonmobile mass
√ round mass with smooth contour
√ homogeneous mass of ≤ -50 HU in cardiac chamber / pericardial space
√ homogeneous mass of increased signal intensity ± a few thin septations on T1WI:
- √ decreasing intensity with fat saturation

√ no enhancement
Rx: surgical resection
DDx: lipomatous hypertrophy of interatrial septum (infiltrative, at level of fossa ovalis with sparing of fossa ovalis, >2 cm thick in transverse dimension, composed of brown fat, not a true neoplasm, associated with advanced age + obesity)

CARDIAC PARAGANGLIOMA

= extremely rare, usually benign sporadic neoplasm arising from intrinsic cardiac sympathetic paraganglial (chromaffin) cells
Incidence: <50 cases
Age: 18–85 (mean, 40) years
- catecholamine-producing tumor (in the majority):
  - headache, arterial hypertension, palpitations, flushing
  - elevated levels of urinary norepinephrine, vanillylmandelic acid, total metanephrine
  - elevated levels of plasma norepinephrine, epinephrine

HEART

Associated with:
(a) additional paragangliomas (in 20%) in carotid body, adrenal gland, bladder, paraaortic
(b) metastases to bone (in 5%)
Path: 2–14 cm large encapsulated / poorly circumscribed and infiltrative highly vascular mass; necrotic in 60%
Histo: monomorphic tumor composed of nests of paraganglial cells (= "Zellballen") surrounded by sustentacular cells

Location: posterior wall of left atrium > roof of left atrium > atrial cavity > interatrial septum > ventricle
Site : epicardial surface of the base of the heart with tendency to involve coronary arteries
CXR:
√ middle mediastinal mass splaying carina simulating left atrial enlargement (for typically located tumor)
ECHO:
√ large echogenic left atrial mass
√ compression of SVC, encasement of coronary aa.
DDx: myxoma (broad base of attachment, softer)
NUC (I-131 or I-123 MIBG):
√ for total body imaging with a sensitivity of 90%
NECT:
√ circumscribed / ill-defined heterogeneous mass:
√ hypoattenuating
√ isoattenuating to cardiac structures (may be missed)
√ ± tumor calcifications
√ ± extracardiac extension
CECT:
◊ Premedicate patient with alpha- and beta-blockers as contrast material can trigger a hypertensive crisis!
√ markedly enhancing mass adherent to / involving left atrium / anterior to aortic root
√ central area of low attenuation (in 50%) from necrosis
MR:
√ mass iso- / hypointense to myocardium on T1WI
√ very hyperintense mass on T2WI
√ intense often heterogeneous enhancement

CARDIAC SARCOMAS

◊ Majority of primary malignant cardiac neoplasms!
◊ 2nd most common primary cardiac neoplasm
Mean age: 41 years; extremely rare in infants + children
(a) right-sided heart inflow obstruction
1. Angiosarcoma (37%): tumor in right atrium
(b) mitral valve obstruction (tumor in left atrium)
2. Undifferentiated sarcoma (24%)
3. Malignant fibrous histiocytoma (11–24%)
4. Leiomyosarcoma (8–9%): tends to invade pulmonary veins + mitral valve
Age: 5–10 years earlier than other sarcomas
5. Primary cardiac osteogenic sarcoma (3–9%)
DDx: myxoma (at fossa ovalis)
• dyspnea, pericardial tamponade, arrhythmia, syncope, peripheral edema, sudden death
• embolic phenomena, chest pain, pneumonia, fever
√ cardiomegaly
√ CHF
√ pleural effusion, pericardial effusion
√ focal cardiac mass
√ pulmonary consolidation
Metastatic to: lung, lymph nodes, bone, liver, brain, bowel, spleen, adrenal gland, pleura, diaphragm, kidney, thyroid, skin
Prognosis: mean survival of 3 month to 1 year

Angiosarcoma (37%)

Frequency: most common cardiac sarcoma
Age: typically in middle-aged men
Path: frequently hemorrhagic + necrotic mass, often adherent to pericardium
Histo: endothelial cells lining ill-defined vascular spaces
• right-sided heart failure, tamponade
• fever, weight loss
• bloody fluid on pericardiocentesis (rarely with malignant cells)
Metastases at presentation: in 66–89%
Location: right atrial free wall + involvement of pericardium (80%)
(a) well-defined mass protruding into a cardiac chamber
√ usually originating from right atrium with sparing of atrial septum
√ areas of central necrosis communicating with cardiac chamber
√ low-attenuation mass on CT
√ heterogeneous contrast enhancement
√ heterogeneous MR signal:
√ "cauliflower appearance" = local nodular hyperintense areas interspersed within areas of intermediate signal intensity on T1WI + T2WI
(b) diffusely infiltrative mass extending along epicardial surface
√ obliterated pericardial space (hemorrhage + necrotic tumor debris)
√ "sunray appearance" = linear contrast enhancement along vascular lakes on MR
Prognosis: 12–30 months survival

Undifferentiated Sarcoma (24%)

= PLEOMORPHIC SARCOMA = ROUND CELL SARCOMA = SPINDLE CELL SARCOMA
Age: 45 years (neonates to elderly)
• pulmonary congestion
Location: left atrium
√ large irregular hypodense intracavitary mass
√ polypoid mass isointense to myocardium
√ thickening / irregularity of myocardium (due to tumor infiltration)
√ tendency to involve valves
√ hemorrhagic mass replacing the pericardium (similar to angiosarcoma)

CARDIAC TAMPONADE

= significant compression of heart by fluid contained within pericardial sac resulting in impaired diastolic filling of ventricles

Cause: *see* PERICARDIAL EFFUSION
• tachycardia
• pulsus paradoxus = exaggeration of normal pattern = drop in systolic arterial pressure >10 mm Hg during inspiration (secondary to increase in right heart filling during inspiration at the expense of left heart filling)
• elevated central venous pressure with distended neck veins
• falling blood pressure
• distant heart sounds / friction rub
• ECG: reduced voltage, ST elevation, PR depression, nonspecific T-wave abnormalities
√ normal lung fields + normal pulmonary vascularity
√ rapid enlargement of heart size
√ distension of SVC, IVC, hepatic + renal veins
√ periportal edema
√ hepatomegaly
Doppler-US:
√ episodes of high-velocity hepatopetal flow separated by long intervals of minimal flow
ECHO:
√ diastolic collapse of RV
√ cyclical collapse of either atrium
Rx: pericardiocentesis / pericardial drainage

CARDIAC THROMBUS

A. Left Atrial Thrombus
Associated with: mitral valve disease
• atrial fibrillation
Site: atrial appendage
√ atrial dilatation
√ irregular / lobulated border
√ microcavitations
√ laminated appearance
B. Left Ventricular Thrombus
Site: region of ventricular dyskinesia / aneurysm (from prior myocardial infarction)
√ homogeneous attenuation on CT
√ heterogeneous signal on SE MR images
√ low-signal intensity on GRE MR images
DDx: myxoma (heterogeneous texture on CT)

CARDIOMYOPATHY

Dilated and Ischemic Cardiomyopathy

= CONGESTIVE CARDIOMYOPATHY
Etiology:
1. Idiopathic
2. Myocarditis: viruses, bacteria
3. Alcoholism
4. Pregnancy / post partum
5. Endocardial fibroelastosis = thickened endocardium + reduced contractility
6. Infants of diabetic mothers
7. Inborn error of metabolism: glycogenosis, mucolipidosis, mucopolysaccharidosis
8. Coronary artery disease: myocardial infarction, anomalous origin of left coronary artery, coronary calcinosis
9. Muscular dystrophies

• tendency for CHF when EF <40%
√ global 4-chamber enlargement
√ poor ventricular contractility
√ LA enlargement without enlargement of LA appendage
√ bilateral atrioventricular valve insufficiency
ECHO:
√ enlarged LV with global hypokinesis
√ IVS and LVPW of equal thickness with decreased amplitude of motion
√ low-profile / "miniaturized" mitral valve
√ mildly enlarged LA (elevated end-diastolic LV pressure)
√ enlarged hypokinetic right ventricle

Hypertrophic Cardiomyopathy

= OBSTRUCTIVE CARDIOMYOPATHY
= characterized by nondilated hypertrophy of left ventricle in the absence of cardiac / systemic disease that would cause LV hypertrophy
1. SYMMETRIC / CONCENTRIC HYPERTROPHY (2–20%)
(a) midventricular
(b) diffuse
(c) apical
2. ASYMMETRIC SEPTAL HYPERTROPHY (ASH)
= IDIOPATHIC HYPERTROPHIC SUBAORTIC STENOSIS (IHSS) = SUBAORTIC STENOSIS
= HYPERTROPHIC OBSTRUCTIVE CARDIOMYOPATHY
= basal septum of LV disproportionately thickened
3. APICAL HYPERTROPHY (2–3%)
= myocardial wall thickening confined to apical portion of LV
• usually clinically benign
• giant inverted T wave
Left ventriculography:
√ spade-shaped deformity of LV cavity
Hemodynamics:
— LV hypertrophy leads to subaortic stenosis, abnormal diastolic function, myocardial ischemia
— rapid blood flow through narrow outflow tract causes the anterior leaflet of mitral valve to displace anteriorly toward septum during systole (Venturi effect)
— mitral regurgitation (from displaced MV leaflet)

Etiology: autosomal dominant transmission
• exertional angina + dyspnea, fatigue
• syncope, arrhythmia, sudden death
√ normal heart size
√ LA enlargement with mitral insufficiency (in 30%)
√ prominent left midheart border (septal hypertrophy)
√ ± mild pulmonary venous hypertension
ECHO (modality of choice):
√ IVS >14 mm thick; posterolateral wall >11 mm thick; IVS:LVPW thickness >1.3:1
√ systolic anterior motion of mitral valve (SAM) causing narrowed LVOT in systole
√ midsystolic closure of aortic valve
√ increased LVOT gradient with late systolic peaking on Doppler

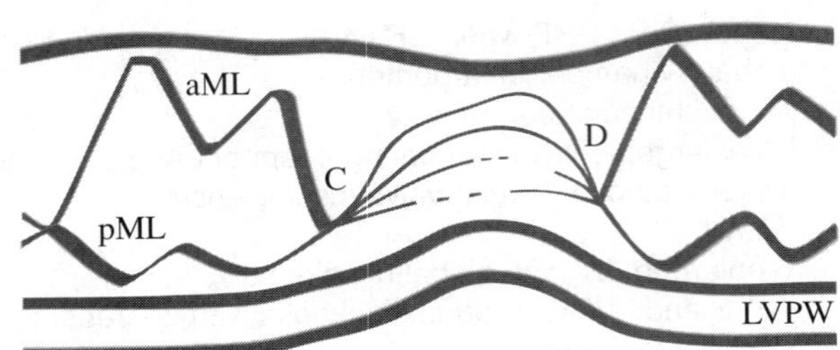

Systolic Anterior Motion (SAM) of MV in IHSS
mitral valve leaflets move abruptly toward septum at a rate greater than the endocardium of the posterior wall; responsible for obstruction to blood ejected from LV (for abbreviations see page 594)

Restrictive Cardiomyopathy

Etiology: (a) idiopathic: endomyocardial fibroelastosis
(a) infiltrative disease: amyloidosis, glycogen, hemochromatosis, sarcoidosis
(b) constrictive pericarditis

√ varying degrees of pulmonary venous hypertension
√ ± LA enlargement

CHRONIC VENOUS STASIS DISEASE

= CHRONIC VENOUS INSUFFICIENCY
= insufficiency / incompetence of venous valves in deep venous system of lower extremity

Cause:
(a) postphlebitic valvular incompetence: destruction of valve apparatus results in short thickened valves secondary to scar formation
(b) primary valvular incompetence: shallow elongated redundant valve cusps prevent effective closure

Associated with: incompetent venous valves in the calf (secondary to pressure dilatation from stasis in deep venous system) leading to superficial vein varicosities

- edema, induration (= fluid exudation from increased capillary pressure)
- ulceration (from minor trauma + decreased diffusion of oxygen secondary to fibrin deposits around capillaries)
- skin hyperpigmentation (= breakdown products of exudated RBCs)
- aching pain

√ venous reflux on descending venography with Valsalva
(a) 82% in deep venous system alone
(b) 2% in saphenous vein alone
(c) 16% in both
bilateral in 75%

Grade:
1 = minimal incompetence = to level of upper thigh
2 = mild incompetence = to level of lower thigh
3 = moderate incompetence = to level of knee
4 = severe incompetence = to level of calf veins

COARCTATION OF AORTA

= localized obstruction at the junction of aortic arch and descending aorta secondary to a fibrous ridge protruding into aortic lumen
M:F = 4:1; rare in Blacks

A. LOCALIZED COARCTATION
= ADULT / POSTDUCTAL / JUXTADUCTAL TYPE [former classification]
= short discrete narrowing close to ligamentum arteriosum (most common type)
◊ Coexistent cardiac anomalies uncommon!
Location: most frequent in juxtaductal portion of arch
- incidental finding late in life
- ductus usually closed

√ shelflike lesion at any point along the aortic arch
√ narrow isthmus above the lesion
√ poststenotic aortic dilatation distally

B. TUBULAR HYPOPLASIA
= INFANTILE / PREDUCTAL / DIFFUSE TYPE [former classification]
= hypoplasia of long segment of aortic arch after origin of innominate artery
◊ Coexistent cardiac anomalies common!
- CHF in neonatal period (in 50%)

√ patent ductus arteriosus

Hemodynamics:
fetus : no significant change because only 10% of cardiac output flows through aortic isthmus
neonate : determined by how rapidly the ductus closes; without concurrent VSD overload of LV leads to CHF in 2nd / 3rd week of life

Collateral circulation: via subclavian artery and its branches:
— intercostals — internal mammary
— anterior spinal artery — scapular artery
— lateral thoracic — transverse cervical artery

Associated in 50% with:
1. Bicuspid aortic valve (in 25–50%), which may result in calcific aortic valve stenosis (after 25 years of age) + bacterial endocarditis
2. Intracardiac malformations:
PDA (33%), VSD (15%), aortic stenosis, aortic insufficiency, ASD, TGV, ostium primum defect, truncus arteriosus, double-outlet right ventricle
3. Noncardiac malformations (13%):
Turner syndrome (13–15%)
4. Cerebral berry aneurysms
5. Mycotic aneurysm distal to CoA

Prognosis: 11% mortality prior to 6 months of age
Rx: ages 3–5 years are ideal time for operation (late enough to avoid restenosis + early enough before irreversible hypertension occurs); surgical correction past 1 year of age decreases operative mortality drastically; 3–11% perioperative mortality

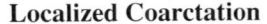

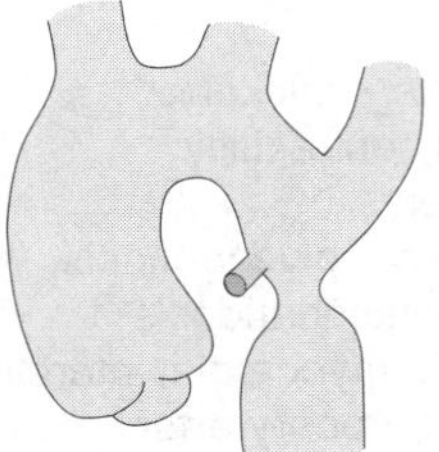
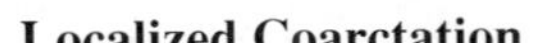
Localized Coarctation

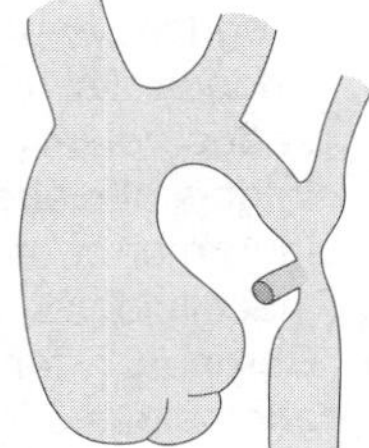
Tubular Hypoplasia

Procedures:

1. Resection + end-to-end anastomosis
2. Patch angioplasty
3. Subclavian flap (Waldhausen procedure) using left subclavian artery as a flap

Postsurgical Cx:

1. Residual coarctation (in 32%)
2. Subsequent obstruction (rare)
3. Mesenteric arteritis: 2–3 days after surgery secondary to paradoxical hypertension from increased plasma renin
   • abdominal pain, loss of bowel control
4. Chronic persistent hypertension

Symptomatic CoA

◊ Second most common cause of CHF in neonate (after hypoplastic left heart)

Time: (a) toward the end of 1st week of life in "critical stenosis"
(b) more commonly presents in older child

• lower extremity cyanosis (in tubular hypoplasia)
• left ventricular failure (usually toward end of 1st week of life)

√ generalized cardiomegaly
√ increased pulmonary vascularity (L-to-R shunt through PDA / VSD)
√ pulmonary venous hypertension / edema
√ "figure 3 sign" hidden by thymus

Asymptomatic CoA

• headaches (from hypertension)
• claudication (from hypoperfusion)

√ "figure 3 sign" = indentation of left lateral margin of aortic arch in the region of aortic-pulmonic window (at site of coarctation and poststenotic dilatation)
√ "reverse 3 sign" on barium esophagram
√ elevated left ventricular apex (secondary to left ventricular hypertrophy)
√ scalloped contouring of soft-tissues posterior to sternum (= dilated tortuous internal mammary arteries) on LAT CXR (in 28%)
√ dilatation of brachiocephalic vessels + aorta proximal to stenosis
√ obscuration of superior margin of aortic arch
√ inferior rib notching (in 75%; mostly in adults over age 20; unusual before age 6)
Location: ribs 3–9 (most pronounced in 3rd + 4th ribs, less pronounced in lower ribs); 1st + 2nd rib do not participate because they have arteries originating from subclavian a.
Site: central + lateral thirds of posterior rib
(a) bilateral
(b) unilateral on left side: left aortic arch with aberrant right subclavian artery below CoA
(c) unilateral on right side: right aortic arch with anomalous left subclavian artery below CoA

CONGENITAL ABSENCE OF PULMONARY VALVE

Massive regurgitation between pulmonary artery and RV

In 90% associated with: VSD, tetralogy of Fallot (50%)

• cyanosis (not in immediate newborn period)
• repeated episodes of respiratory distress
• continuous murmur
• ECG: right ventricular hypertrophy

√ prominent main, right, and left pulmonary artery
√ RV dilatation (increased stroke volume)
√ partial obstruction of right / left mainstem bronchus (compression by vessel)
√ right-sided aorta (33%)

CONGESTIVE HEART FAILURE

= increase in circulating blood volume with diminishing cardiac function leads to elevation of microvascular pressure of lung

Incidence: most common cause of interstitial + airspace edema of lungs

Cause:
(a) back pressure from LV: long-standing systemic hypertension, aortic valve disease, coronary artery disease, cardiomyopathy, myocardial infarction
(b) obstruction proximal to LV: mitral valve disease, LA myxoma, cor triatriatum

Histo:
(a) Interstitial phase: fluid in loose connective tissue around conducting airways and vessels + engorgement of lymphatics
(b) Alveolar phase: increase in alveolar wall thickness
(c) Alveolar airspace phase: alveoli filled with fluid + loss of alveolar volume; pulmonary fibrosis upon organization of intra-alveolar fibrin (if chronic)

√ large heart

1. **Interstitial pulmonary edema** (invariably precedes alveolar edema)
   • NO abnormal physical finding
   • hypoxemia (ventilation-perfusion inequality)
   √ loss of sharp definition of vascular markings
   √ thickening of interlobular septa (pulmonary venous wedge pressure 17–20 mm Hg)
   √ poorly defined increased bronchial wall thickness
   √ thickening of interlobar fissures (due to fluid in subpleural connective tissue layer)
2. **Airspace edema**
   Cause: acute LA pressure elevation with volume of capillary filtration exceeding that of lymphatic drainage
   • severe dyspnea / orthopnea
   • tachypnea + cyanosis
   • dry cough / copious frothy sputum
   • hypoxemia (vascular shunting)
   √ poorly defined patchy acinar opacities
   √ coalescence of acinar consolidation, particularly in medial third of lung
   √ butterfly / bat-wing distribution of consolidation (= consolidated hilum + uninvolved lung cortex)

3. **Flow inversion**
   Cause: chronic elevation of LA pressure (as in left heart failure / mitral valve disease)
   Pathophysiology:
   long-standing elevation of LA pressure causes an increase in atriovenous reflux; initially the increased LA pressure is met with an increased tonus of the LA wall (= absence of atrial enlargement in acute left heart failure); eventually LA enlarges inciting a protective atrial-pulmonary-vascular reflex vasospasm, which narrows the lower lobe vessels and decreases atriovenous reflux
   √ basal oligemia
   √ hyperemia of upper lobes
   N.B.: flow inversion is never seen in pulmonary edema of renal failure / overhydration / low oncotic pressure
4. **Generalized oligemia**
   Cause: aortic valvular disease

CONSTRICTIVE PERICARDITIS

= fibrous thickening of pericardium interfering with filling of ventricular chambers through restriction of heart motion

Age: 30–50 years; M:F = 3:1

Etiology:

A. IDIOPATHIC
B. INFECTIOUS / INFLAMMATORY
   1. Viral (Coxsackie B)
   2. Tuberculosis (formerly most common)
   3. Rheumatoid arthritis
C. TRAUMATIC
   1. Cardiac surgery (most common)
   2. Radiotherapy to mediastinum
D. UREMIA = chronic renal failure
E. NEOPLASTIC = tumor invasion

Causes of acute pericarditis:
mnemonic: "MUSIC"
Myocardial infarction (acute)
Uremia
Surgery (cardiac)
Infection
Cancer

• dyspnea
• abdominal enlargement (ascites + hepatomegaly)
• peripheral edema
• pericardial knock sound = loud early-diastolic sound
• neck vein distension
• Kussmaul sign = failure of venous pressure to fall with inspiration
• prominent X and Y descent on venous pressure curve

√ linear / plaquelike pericardial calcifications (50–70%): predominantly over RV, posterior surface of LV, in atrioventricular groove
√ dilatation of SVC (77%), azygos vein (69%)
√ small atria; occasionally compensatory dilatation of nonconstricted portions, eg, LA enlargement (20%)
√ normal / small-sized heart (enlargement only due to preexisting disease)
√ normal pulmonary vascularity / pulmonary venous hypertension (43%)
√ straightening of heart borders:
  √ straight / concave on right side
  √ squared on left side
  √ pericardial tenting
√ increase in ejection fraction (small EDV)
√ pleural effusion (34% bilateral, 26% right PE)

CT:
  √ epicardium = visceral pericardium >2 mm thick
  √ dilatation of SVC + IVC
  √ reflux of contrast into coronary sinus
  √ flattening of right ventricle + curvature of interventricular septum toward left
  √ pleural effusion + ascites

ECHO (nonspecific features):
  √ thickening of pericardium
  √ rapid early filling motion followed by flat posterior wall motion during diastasis period (= period between early rapid filling and atrial contraction)

Cx: protein-losing enteropathy (increased pressure in IVC + portal vein)

DDx: cardiac tamponade, restrictive cardiomyopathy (eg, amyloid)

CORONARY ARTERY FISTULA

= single / multiple fistulous connections between a coronary artery (R > L) and other heart structures

Abnormal communication with (>90% right heart):
RV > RA > pulmonary trunk > coronary sinus > SVC

Hemodynamics: L-to-R shunt; pulmonary:systemic blood flow = <1.5:1 (usually)

√ may have normal CXR (in small shunts)
√ cardiomegaly + shunt vascularity (in large shunts)

Angio:
  √ dilated tortuous coronary a. with anomalous connection

COR TRIATRIATUM

= rare congenital anomaly in which a fibromuscular septum with a single stenotic / fenestrated / large opening separates the embryologic common pulmonary vein from the left atrium:
(1) proximal / accessory chamber lies posteriorly receiving pulmonary veins
(2) distal / true atrial chamber lies anteriorly connected to left atrial appendage + emptying into LV through mitral valve

Etiology: failure of common pulmonary vein to incorporate normally into left atrium

Associated with: ASD, PDA, anomalous pulmonary venous drainage, left SVC, VSD, tetralogy of Fallot, atrioventricular canal

• dyspnea, heart failure, failure to thrive
• clinically similar to mitral valve stenosis

√ pulmonary venous distention + interstitial edema + dilatation of pulmonary trunk and pulmonary arteries (in severe obstruction)
√ enlarged RA + RV
√ mild enlargement of LA

HEART

Angio:
√ dividing membrane on levophase of pulmonary arteriogram

Prognosis (if untreated):
usually fatal within first 2 years of life; 50% 2-year survival; 20% 20-year survival

Rx: surgical excision of obstructing membrane

DEEP VEIN THROMBOSIS

= DVT

Incidence: 140,000–250,000 new cases per year in United States with an estimated sole / major cause of 50,000–200,000 deaths per year (15% of in-hospital deaths); 6–7 million stasis skin changes; in 0.5% cause of skin ulcers

Pathogenetic factors:
1. Hypercoagulability
2. Decreased blood flow / stasis
3. Intimal injury
4. Decreased fibrinolytic potential of veins
5. Platelet aggregation

Risk factors:
1. Surgery, esp. on legs / pelvis: orthopedic (45–50%) especially total hip replacement >50%), gynecologic (7–35%), neurosurgery (18–20%), urologic (15–35%), general surgery (20–25%)
2. Severe trauma
3. Prolonged immobilization: hemiplegic extremity, paraplegia + quadriplegia, casting / orthopedic appliances
4. Malignancy (risk factor 2.5) = Trousseau syndrome
5. Obesity (risk factor 1.5)
6. Diabetes
7. Pregnancy (risk factor 5.5) and for 8–12 weeks postpartum
8. Medication: birth control pills, estrogen replacement, tamoxifen (risk factor 3.2)
9. Decreased cardiac function: congestive heart failure, myocardial infarction (20–50%; risk factor 3.5)
10. Age >40 years (risk factor 2.2)
11. Varicose veins
12. Previous DVT (risk factor 2.5)
13. Patients with blood group A > blood group 0
14. Polycythemia
15. Smoking

Pathologic terminology:
"organized thrombus" = transition to a vascularized lesion of connective tissue adherent to vessel wall
"recanalized thrombus" = vascular channel network within an organized clot reducing it to septations of collagen and elastic fibers often lined by endothelium

Location:
1. Dorsal veins of calf (± ascending thrombosis)
2. Iliofemoral veins (± descending thrombosis)
3. Peripheral + iliofemoral veins simultaneously
4. rare: internal iliac v., ovarian v., ascending lumbar vv.

L:R = 7:3 due to compression of left common iliac v. by left common iliac a. (arterial pulsations lead to chronic endothelial injury with formation of intraluminal spur, which is present in 22% of autopsies + in 90% of patients with DVT)

- Local symptoms due to obstruction / phlebitis usually only when (a) thrombus occlusive, (b) clot extends into popliteal / more proximal vein (14–78% sensitivity, 4–21% specificity):
  - warmth
  - swelling (measurement of circumference)
  - blanching of skin (phlegmasia dolens alba) / blue leg with complete obstruction (phlegmasia cerulea dolens)
  - deep crampy pain in affected extremity, worse in erect position, improved while walking
  - tenderness along course of affected vein
  - Homans sign = calf pain with dorsal flexion of foot
  - Payr sign = pain upon compression of sole of foot
  - ◊ 2/3 of deep vein thromboses are clinically silent:
    - ◊ DVT diagnosed ante mortem in <30%
    - ◊ Only 10–33% of patients with fatal PE are symptomatic for DVT
  - ◊ Clinically suspected DVT accurate in only 26–45%:
    - ◊ DVT symptomatology due to other causes in 15–35% of patients
  - ◊ Negative bilateral venograms in 30% of patients with angiographically detected pulmonary emboli (big bang theory = clot embolizes in toto to the lung leaving no residual in vein)

Venography (89% sensitivity, 97% specificity):
false negative in 11%, false positive in 5%;
study aborted / nondiagnostic in 5%
Risk: postvenography phlebitis (1–2%), contrast reaction, contrast material-induced skin slough, nephropathy
√ intraluminal filling defect constant on all images
√ nonfilling of calf veins
√ inadequate filling of common femoral vein + external + common iliac veins

B-Mode US (88–100% sensitivity, 92–100% specificity, >90% accuracy for DVT in thigh and popliteal veins):
√ lack of complete luminal collapse with venous compression (DDx: deformity + scarring from prior DVT; technical difficulties in adductor canal + distal deep femoral vein)
√ visualization of clot within vein (DDx: slow flowing blood; machine noise)
√ <75% increase in diameter of common femoral vein during Valsalva
√ venous diameter at least twice that of adjacent artery suggests thrombus <10 days old

Doppler US:
√ absence of spontaneity (= any waveform recording), not reliable in peripheral veins

√ continuous venous signal = absence of phasicity (= no cyclic variation in flow velocity with respiration, ie, decrease in expiration + increase in inspiration) is suspicious for proximal obstruction
√ attenuation / absence of augmentation (= no increase in flow velocity with distal compression) indicates venous occlusion / compression in intervening venous segments
√ pulsatile venous flow is a sign of congestive heart failure / pericardial effusion / cardiac tamponade / pulmonary embolism with pulmonary hypertension

Venous Occlusion Plethysmography :
— 87–95–100% sensitivity, 92–100% specificity for above-knee DVT
— 17–33% sensitivity for below-knee DVT
= temporary obstruction of venous outflow by pneumatic cuff around mid-thigh inflated above venous pressure leads to progressive increase in blood volume in lower leg; upon release of cuff limb quickly returns to resting volume with prompt venous runoff; limb blood volume changes are measured by *impedance plethysmography* in which a weak alternating current is passed through the leg; the electrical resistance varies inversely with blood volume; the current strength is held constant and voltage changes directly reflect blood volume changes

√ initial rise in venous volume (= venous capacitance) diminished
√ delay in venous outflow = "fall" measured at 3 seconds
False positives (6%): severe cardiopulmonary disease, pelvic mass, reduced arterial inflow
False negatives: calf vein thrombosis, small thrombus

I-125–Labeled Fibrinogen:
— 90% sensitive for calf vein thrombus
— 60–80% sensitive for femoral vein thrombus
— insensitive for thrombus in upper thigh / pelvis
Risk: results not available for several days, transmission of viral infection
False positives: hematoma, inflammation, wound, old small thrombus isolated in common femoral / iliac vein

Cx:
(1) Pulmonary embolism (50%): in 90% from lower extremity / pelvis; in 60% with proximal "free-floating" / "widow-maker" thrombus; occurs usually between 2nd to 4th (7th) day of thrombosis
Source of pulmonary emboli:
multiple sites (1/3), cryptogenic in 50%;
(a) lower extremity (46%)
(b) inferior vena cava (19%)
(c) pelvic veins (16%)
(d) mural heart thrombus (4.5%)
(e) upper extremity (2%)
Likelihood of pulmonary embolism:
77% for iliac veins, 35–67% for femoropopliteal vein, 0–46% for calf veins
(2) Postphlebitic syndrome (PPS) in 20% of cases with DVT (= recanalization to a smaller lumen, focal wall changes) due to valvular incompetence
(3) Phlegmasia cerulea / alba dolens (= severely impaired venous drainage resulting in gangrene)

Prognosis: tibial / peroneal venous thrombi resolve spontaneously in 40%, stabilize in 40%, propagate into popliteal vein in 20%
Prophylaxis: intermittent compression of legs, heparin, warfarin
Rx:
(1) Heparin IV
(2) Systemic anticoagulation (warfarin) for ≥3 months decreases risk of recurrent DVT in initial 3 months from 50% to 3% + fatal pulmonary embolism from 30% to 8%; necessity for anticoagulation in DVT of calf veins is controversial
(3) Caval filter (10–15%) in patients with contraindication / complication from anticoagulation or progression of DVT / PE despite adequate anticoagulation
DDx: pseudothrombophlebitis (= signs + symptoms of DVT produced by popliteal cyst / traumatic hematoma)

DOUBLE-OUTLET RIGHT VENTRICLE
= DORV = TAUSSIG-BING HEART
= most of the aorta + pulmonary artery arise from the RV secondary to maldevelopment of conotruncus
Type 1 = aorta posterior to pulmonary artery + spiraling course (most frequent)
Type 2 = Taussig-Bing heart = aorta posterior to pulmonary artery + parallel course
Type 3 = aorta anterior to pulmonary artery + parallel course
Hemodynamics:
fetus : no CHF in utero (in absence of obstructing other anomalies)
neonate : ventricular work overload leads to CHF
Associated with: VSD (100%), pulmonary stenosis (50%), PDA
√ aorta overriding the interventricular septum with predominant connection to RV
√ aorta posterior / parallel / anterior to pulmonary artery
√ LV enlargement (volume overload)

DUCTUS ARTERIOSUS ANEURYSM
= fusiform aneurysm of ductus arteriosus, usually patent toward aorta + completely / incompletely occluded toward pulmonary artery
Incidence: <100 cases
Classification:
(a) according to age: infantile, childhood, adult type
(b) according to cause: congenital, infectious, traumatic
Pathogenesis: ? delay in closure, ? myxoid degeneration of ductus wall, ? abnormal elastic fibers

Age: most <2 months of age
• dyspnea, tachypnea, hoarseness
√ pulmonary artery displaced anteromedially
√ distal aortic arch displaced laterally
CXR:
√ left-sided upper mediastinal mass in aorticopulmonary window
√ tracheal displacement to right + anteriorly / posteriorly
√ consolidation of adjacent lung (compression, fibrosis, hemorrhage)
CT: √ contrast-enhancing mass in classic location
ECHO: √ cystic mass with pulsatile flow
Cx: rupture, dissection, infection, thromboembolic disease, phrenic nerve compression
Prognosis: usually fatal (without prompt surgery)

EBSTEIN ANOMALY

= downward displacement of septal + posterior leaflets of dysplastic tricuspid valve with ventricular division into
(a) a large superior atrialized portion (incorporating part of the RV into the RA) and
(b) a small inferior functional chamber with shortened chordae tendineae
Etiology: chronic maternal lithium intake (10%)
Hemodynamics:
tricuspid valve insufficiency leads to tricuspid regurgitation ("ping-pong" volume) + severely dilated RA; RA dilatation stretches interatrial septum causing incompetence of foramen ovale (R-to-L shunt)

RA	↑	RV	↓	Main PA	↔
Pulm. vessels		↔/↓			
LA	↔	LV	↔	Ao	↔

Associated with: PDA, ASD (R-to-L shunt)
• ± cyanosis in neonatal period (depending on degree of R-to-L shunt): may improve / disappear postnatally with decrease in pulmonary arterial pressure
• CHF in utero / in neonate (in 50%)
• systolic murmur (tricuspid insufficiency)
• Wolff-Parkinson-White syndrome (10%) = paroxysmal supraventricular tachycardia / right bundle branch block (responsible for sudden death)
Cause: conduction system develops during formation of tricuspid valve adjacent to it
√ "boxlike / funnel-like" cardiomegaly (enlargement of RA + RV)
√ extreme RA enlargement (secondary to insufficient tricuspid valve)
√ IVC + azygos dilatation (secondary to tricuspid regurgitation)
√ hypoplastic aorta + pulmonary trunk (the ONLY cyanotic CHD to have this feature)
√ normal LA
√ calcification of tricuspid valve may occur
ECHO:
√ large "sail-like" tricuspid valve structure within dilated right heart
√ tricuspid regurgitation identified by Doppler ultrasound
Prognosis: 50% infant mortality; 13% operative mortality; survival into adulthood if valve functions normally

Rx:
1. Digitalis + diuretics
2. Tricuspid valve prosthesis

EISENMENGER COMPLEX

= EISENMENGER DEFECT
= (1) high VSD ± overriding aorta with hypoplastic crista supraventricularis
(2) RV hypertrophy
and as consequence of increased pulmonary blood flow:
(3) dilatation of pulmonary artery + branches
(4) intimal thickening + sclerosis of small pulmonary arteries + arterioles
• cyanosis appears in 2nd + 3rd decade with shunt reversal

EISENMENGER SYNDROME

= EISENMENGER REACTION
= development of high pulmonary vascular resistance after many years of increased pulmonary blood flow secondary to L-to-R shunt (ASD, PDA, VSD), which leads to a bidirectional (= balanced) shunt and ultimately to R-to-L shunt
Etiology:
pulmonary microscopic vessels undergo reactive muscular hypertrophy, endothelial thickening, in situ thrombosis, tortuosity + obliteration; once initiated, pulmonary hypertension accelerates the vascular reaction, thus increasing pulmonary hypertension in a vicious cycle with RV failure + death
Path: adaptive anastomotic pathways connect plexiform lesions of pulmonary arterial vessels to bronchial arteries supplying terminal bronchioles + vasa vasorum of pulmonary arteries
Pathologic classification of severity (Heath & Edwards):
Grade I = medial hypertrophy of muscular pulmonary arteries and arterioles
• potentially reversible
Grade II = grade I + intimal proliferation in small muscular arteries and arterioles
• potentially reversible
Grade III = grade II + intimal laminar fibrosis + progressive vessel obliteration
• borderline for reversibility
Grade IV = occlusion of vessels with progressive aneurysmal dilatation of small arteries nearby
• irreversible
Grade V = tortuous "glomeruloid" channels within proliferation of endothelial cells (= plexiform + angiomatoid lesions)
• irreversible
Grade VI = thrombosis + necrotizing arteritis
• irreversible

CXR:
√ pronounced dilatation of central pulmonary arteries (pulmonary trunk, main pulmonary artery, intermediate branches)
√ pruning of peripheral pulmonary arteries

HEART

√ enlargement of RV + RA (proportionate to volume overload)
√ LA + LV return to normal size (with decrease of L-to-R shunt due to markedly elevated pulmonary vascular resistance)
√ normal pulmonary veins (unless superimposed cardiac volume overload):
  √ pulmonary veins NOT distended (NO increase in pulmonary blood flow)
  √ NO redistribution of pulmonary veins (normal venous pressure)

CT:
√ linear calcification + thrombus in central pulmonary arteries
√ mural calcification / aneurysmal dilatation of ductus arteriosus (in cases of patent ductus arteriosus)

Dx: measurement of pulmonary artery pressure + flow via catheter

ENDOCARDIAL CUSHION DEFECT

= ECD = ATRIOVENTRICULAR SEPTAL DEFECT
= PERSISTENT OSTIUM ATRIOVENTRICULARE COMMUNE
= PERSISTENT COMMON ATRIOVENTRICULAR CANAL
= persistence of primitive atrioventricular canal + anomalies of AV valves

A. INCOMPLETE / PARTIAL ECD
= (1) Ostium primum ASD
  (2) Cleft in anterior mitral valve leaflet / trileaflet
  (3) Accessory short chordae tendineae arising from anterior MV leaflet insert directly into crest of deficient ventricular septum

√ left atrioventricular valve usually has 3 leaflets with a wide cleft between anterior + septal leaflet
√ "gooseneck" deformity secondary to downward attachment of anterior MV leaflet close to interventricular septum by accessory chordae tendineae
√ communication between LA–RA or LV–RA, occasionally LV–RV
√ right atrioventricular valve usually normal

B. TRANSITIONAL / INTERMEDIATE ATRIOVENTRICULAR CANAL (uncommon)
= (1) Ostium primum ASD
  (2) High membranous VSD
  (3) Wide clefts in septal leaflets of both AV valves
  (4) Bridging tissue between anterior + posterior common leaflet of both AV valves

C. COMPLETE ECD = AV COMMUNIS = COMMON AV CANAL
= (1) Ostium primum ASD above
  (2) Posterior inlet VSD below
  (3) One AV valve common to RV + LV with 5–6 leaflets
    (a) anterior common "bridging" leaflet
    (b) two lateral leaflets
    (c) posterior common "bridging" leaflet

Type 1 = chordae tendineae of anterior bridging leaflet attached to both sides of ventricular septum
Type 2 = chordae tendineae of anterior leaflet attached medially to anomalous papillary muscle within RV, but unattached to septum
Type 3 = free-floating anterior leaflet with chordae attachments to septum; only type becoming symptomatic in infancy!

Associated with:
(1) Down syndrome:
  in 25% of trisomy 21 an ECD is present;
  in 45% of ECD trisomy 21 is present
(2) Asplenia, polysplenia

√ common atrioventricular orifice
√ oval septal defect consisting of a low ASD + high VSD
√ atrial septum secundum usually spared ("common atrium" if absent)
√ frequently associated with mesocardia / dextrocardia

Hemodynamics:
fetus : atrioventricular valves frequently incompetent leading to regurgitation + CHF
neonate : L-to-R shunt after decrease of pulmonary vascular resistance resulting in pulmonary hypertension

• incomplete right bundle branch block (distortion of conduction tissue)
• left-anterior hemiblock

CXR:
◊ Radiographic findings similar to ASD, but more marked
√ increased pulmonary vascularity (= shunt vascularity)
√ redistribution of pulmonary blood flow (mitral regurgitation)
√ enlarged pulmonary artery
√ diminutive aorta (secondary to L-to-R shunt)
√ cardiac enlargement out of proportion to pulmonary vascularity (L-to-R shunt + mitral insufficiency)
√ enlarged RV + LV
√ enlarged RA (LV blood shunted to RA)
√ normal-sized LA (secondary to ASD)

ECHO:
√ visualization of ASD + VSD + valve + site of insertion of chordae tendineae
√ paradoxical anterior septal motion (secondary to ASD)
√ atrioventricular insufficiency + shunts identified by Doppler ultrasound

Angio:
AP projection:
  √ gooseneck deformity of LVOT (in diastole)
  √ cleft in anterior leaflet of mitral valve (in systole)
  √ mitral regurgitation
Hepatoclavicular projection in 45° LAO + C-C 45° (= 4-chamber view):
  √ best view to demonstrate LV-RA shunt
  √ best view to demonstrate VSD (inflow tract + posterior portion of interventricular septum in profile)

LAT projection:
√ irregular appearance of superior segment of anterior mitral valve leaflet over LVOT

Prognosis: 54% survival rate at 6 months, 35% at 12 months, 15% at 24 months, 4% at 5 years; 91% long-term survival with primary intracardiac repair, 4–17% operative mortality

ENDOCARDIAL FIBROELASTOSIS

= diffuse endocardial thickening of LV + LA from deposition of collagen + elastic tissue

Etiology:
(1) ? viral infection
(2) Secondary endocardial fibroelastosis
= subendocardial ischemia in critical LVOT obstruction: aortic stenosis, coarctation, hypoplastic left heart syndrome

• sudden onset of CHF during first 6 months of life
√ mitral insufficiency:
(a) involvement of valve leaflets
(b) shortening + thickening of chordae tendineae
(c) distortion + fixation of papillary muscles
√ enlarged LV = dilatation of hypertrophied LV from mitral regurgitation
√ restricted LV motion
√ enlarged LA
√ pulmonary venous congestion + pulmonary edema
√ LLL atelectasis (= compression of left lower lobe bronchus by enlarged LA)

Prognosis: mortality almost 100% by 2 years of age

FIBROMUSCULAR DYSPLASIA

= nonatherosclerotic angiopathy of unknown pathogenesis

Incidence: <1% of cerebral angiographies; 1,100 patients reported (by 1982)

Age: children + young adults <30–40 years; 2/3 >50 years; M:F = 1:3 to 1:9

• hypertension
• progressive renal insufficiency

Location:

@ Cephalic arteries:
cervical + intracranial ICA (85%), extracranial carotid artery (30%), vertebral artery (7%); both anterior + posterior circulation (8%); bilateral (60–65%)
Associated with: brain ischemia (up to 50%), intracranial aneurysms (up to 30%), intracranial tumors (30%), bruits, trauma

@ Abdominal aorta:
renal artery (60%), other aortic branches (in 1–2%: celiac a., hepatic a., splenic a., mesenteric a., iliac a.)
◊ Simultaneous involvement of renal / muscular arteries in 3%

1. INTIMAL FIBROPLASIA (1–2%)
= intimal hyperplasia
• progressive
Path: circumferential / eccentric fibrous tissue between intima + internal elastic lamina
Age: children + young adults; M:F = 1:1
Site: main renal artery + major segmental branches; often bilateral
√ narrow annular radiolucent band
√ poststenotic fusiform dilatation
Cx: dissection

2. MEDIAL FIBROPLASIA (60–85%)
= fibromuscular hyperplasia = medial fibroplasia with microaneurysm
Age: 20–50 years; typically affects women
Path: multiple fibromuscular ridges + severe mural thinning with loss of smooth muscle + internal elastic lamina
Site: mid + distal renal artery + branches; usually bilateral
√ "string-of-beads" sign = alternating areas of stenoses (weblike constrictions) + aneurysms (which exceed the normal diameter of the artery)
√ single tubular focal stenosis

3. MEDIAL HYPERPLASIA (5–15%)
= FIBROMUSCULAR HYPERPLASIA
Path: smooth muscle + fibrous tissue hyperplasia within arterial media
Site: main renal artery and branches
√ long smooth concentric tubular narrowing
DDx: Takayasu arteritis, sclerosing arteritis, vessel spasm, arterial hypoplasia

4. PERIMEDIAL FIBROPLASIA (20%)
= SUBADVENTITIAL FIBROPLASIA
Age: young females
Path: fibroplasia of outer 1/2 of media replacing external elastic lamina
Site: distal (mostly right) main renal artery
√ long irregular stenosis
√ beading = NO aneurysm formation (diameter of beads not wider than normal diameter of artery)

5. MEDIAL DISSECTION (5–10%)
Path: new channel in outer 1/3 of media within external elastic lamina
Site: main renal artery + branches
√ false channel, aneurysm

6. ADVENTITIAL FIBROPLASIA (<1%)
= SUBADVENTITIAL HYPERPLASIA
Path: adventitial + periarterial proliferation in fibrofatty tissue
Site: main renal artery, large branches
√ long segmental stenosis

7. ATYPICAL FIBROMUSCULAR DYSPLASIA
(= ? variant of intimal fibroplasia)
√ web = smooth / corrugated mass involving only one wall of vessel + projecting into lumen
DDx: atherosclerotic disease, posttraumatic aneurysm

VARIANT: **Segmental mediolytic arteriopathy**
= rare noninflammatory disease of small + medium arteries
Histo: focal segmental disruption of medial smooth muscle cells with mediolysis
√ string-of-beads appearance
√ irregular stenoses + aneurysms

HEART

Heterotaxy Syndromes

	Asplenia = bilateral R sidedness	*Polysplenia* = bilateral L sidedness
Clinical		
Presenting age	newborn / infant	infant / adult
Sex predominance	male	female
Cyanosis	severe	usually absent
Heart disease	severe	moderate / none (5–10%)
Howell-Jolly / Heinz bodies	present	absent
Spleen scan	no spleen	multiple small spleens
Characteristic ECG	none	abnormal P-wave vector
Prognosis	poor	good
Mortality	high	low
Plain radiograph		
Lung vascularity	decreased	normal / increased
Aortic arch	right / left	right / left
Cardiac apex	right / left / midline	right / left
Bronchi	bilateral eparterial	bilateral hyparterial
Minor fissure	possibly bilateral	none / normal
Stomach	midline / right / left	right / left
Liver	symmetrical / R / L	in various positions
Malrotation of bowel	yes (microgastria)	yes
Cardiography		
Coronary sinus	usually absent	sometimes absent
Atrial septum	common atrium (100%)	ASD (84%)
AV valve	atresia / common valve	normal / abnormal MV
Single ventricle	44%	infrequent
IVS	VSD	VSD common
Great vessels	d- / l-transposition (72%)	normal relationship
Pulmonary stenosis	the rule	frequent
Pulmonary veins	TAPVR	PAPVR (42%) TAPVR (6%)
Single coronary artery	19%	
SVC	bilateral (53%)	bilateral (33%)
IVC-aorta relationship	same side of spine	normal
IVC	normal	interrupted (84%) / normal
Azygos vein	inapparent	continuation R / L

Cx: dissection (in 3%), macroaneurysm formation, intramural hemorrhage

Prognosis: tends to remain stable / minimal progression of lesions in 20% causing decline in renal function

Rx:
(1) Resection of diseased segment with end-to-end anastomosis
(2) Replacement by autogenous vein graft, excision + repair by patch angioplasty
(3) Transluminal balloon angioplasty (90% success rate with very low restenosis rate)

FLAIL MITRAL VALVE

Cause:
(1) ruptured chordae tendineae in rheumatic heart disease, ischemic heart disease, bacterial endocarditis
(2) rupture of head of papillary muscle in acute myocardial infarction, chest trauma

Location: chordae to leaflet from posteromedial papillary muscle (single vessel blood supply)

√ deep holosystolic posterior movement
√ random anarchic motion pattern of flail parts in diastole
√ excessively large amplitude of opening of aML

HETEROTAXY SYNDROME

[*hetero* , Greek = different; *taxis* , Greek = arrangement]

= CARDIOSPLENIC SYNDROMES

= situs ambiguus with a spectrum of various congenital truncal abnormalities + frequently cardiac malformations from asplenia to polysplenia

Embryology:
primary defect in lateralization with disruption of complete separation of cardiac chambers during 20–30 days of gestation

Inheritance: multifactorial (autosomal dominant, autosomal recessive, X-linked recessive)

HEART

Individualized approach of classification:
describes all critical structures by analyzing
(a) position of atria
(b) position of venous drainage below diaphragm relative to midline
(c) position of aorta relative to midline
(d) position of the stomach + presence of malrotation
(e) position of liver + gallbladder
(f) position of cardiac apex
(g) presence, appearance, and number of spleens
(h) presence of bi- / trilobed lungs

Asplenia Syndrome

= BILATERAL RIGHT-SIDEDNESS = RIGHT ISOMERISM
= IVEMARK SYNDROME

Incidence: 1:1,750–1:40,000 livebirths; M > F

Associated with:
(a) CHD (in 50%):
TAPVR (almost 100%), endocardial cushion defect (85%), single ventricle (51%), TGA (58%), pulmonary stenosis / atresia (70%), dextrocardia (42%), mesocardia, VSD, ASD, absent coronary sinus, common atrium, common hepatic vein
(b) GI anomalies:
Partial / total situs inversus, annular pancreas, agenesis of gallbladder, ectopic liver, esophageal varices, duplication + hypoplasia of stomach, Hirschsprung disease, hindgut duplication, imperforate anus
(c) GU anomalies (15%):
Horseshoe kidney, double collecting system, hydroureter, cystic kidney, fused / horseshoe adrenal, absent left adrenal, bilobed urinary bladder, bicornuate uterus
(d) Cleft lip / palate, scoliosis, single umbilical artery, lumbar myelomeningocele

• cyanosis in neonatal period / infancy (if severe cyanotic CHD)
• severe respiratory distress
• Howell-Jolly bodies = RBC inclusions in patients with absent spleen

√ cardiac apex discordant from stomach + liver
√ absent spleen (risk of sepsis)

@ Lung
√ bilateral trilobed lungs = bilateral minor fissures (SPECIFIC)
√ bilateral eparterial bronchi (MR / tomogram)
= pulmonary arteries inferior to bronchi on PA view + projecting anterior to trachea on LAT view
√ diminished pulmonary vascularity / pulmonary venous hypertension (TAPVR below diaphragm)

@ Heart & great vessels
√ bilateral systemic / right atria with broad-based appendages
√ ipsilaterality of abdominal aorta + IVC
= juxtaposed "piggybacked" IVC (aorta usually posterior) (MOST RELIABLE INDICATOR)
√ bilateral SVC

@ Abdomen
√ absent spleen
√ centrally located "bridging" liver = hepatic symmetry
√ stomach on right / left side / in central position and small (microgastria)

Prognosis: up to 80% mortality by end of 1st year of life

Polysplenia Syndrome

= BILATERAL LEFT-SIDEDNESS = LEFT ISOMERISM

Age: presentation in infancy / adulthood; M < F

Associated with:
(a) CHD (>50%):
APVR (70%), dextrocardia (37%), ASD (37%), ECCD (43–65%), pulmonic valvular stenosis (23%), TGA (13–17%), DORV (13–20%)
• no / mild CHD in most patients
(b) GI abnormalities:
esophageal atresia, TE fistula, gastric duplication, preduodenal portal vein, duodenal webs + atresia, short bowel, mobile cecum, malrotation, semiannular pancreas, biliary atresia, absent gallbladder
(c) GU anomalies (15%):
renal agenesis, renal cysts, ovarian cysts
(d) Vertebral anomalies, common celiac trunk–SMA

• CHF (due to L-to-R shunt)
• heart murmur, occasional cyanosis
• leftward / superiorly directed P-wave vector
• heart block (due to ECCD)
• extrahepatic biliary obstruction

√ absence of IVC (on LAT CXR)
√ large azygos vein (on AP CXR) may mimic aortic arch

@ Lung
√ bilateral morphologic left lungs (55–68%), normal (18%), bilateral R-sided lungs (7%)
√ bilateral hyparterial bronchi (= arteries projecting superior to bronchi on PA view + posterior to tracheobronchial tree on LAT view)
√ normal / increased pulmonary vascularity
√ absence of middle lobe fissure

@ Heart & great vessels
√ bilateral pulmonary / left atria + pointed, tubular, narrow-based appendages
√ cardiac apex on R / in midline
√ bilateral SVC (50%)
√ interruption of hepatic segment of IVC with azygos / hemiazygos continuation in 65–70% (MOST CONSISTENT FINDING)

@ Abdominal heterotaxy (56%)
√ presence of ≥2 spleens (usually two major + indefinite number of splenules) located on both sides of the mesogastrium (esp. greater curvature of stomach)
√ centrally located liver = hepatic symmetry
√ absence of gallbladder (50%)
√ stomach always on same side of spleen(s)
√ malrotation of bowel (80%)
√ preduodenal portal vein

OB-US:
√ absence of intrahepatic IVC

HEART

√ aorta anterior to spine in midline
√ "double vessel" sign = 2 vessels of similar size in paraspinous location posterior to heart = aorta + azygos vein on left / right side of spine

Prognosis: 50% mortality by 4 months;
75% mortality by 5 years;
90% mortality by midadolescence

HYPOPLASTIC LEFT HEART SYNDROME

= SHONE SYNDROME = AORTIC ATRESIA
= underdevelopment of left side of heart characterized by
(a) hypoplastic / atretic aortic valve
(b) hypoplastic / atretic mitral valve
(c) hypoplastic LV (due to endocardial fibroelastosis)
(d) hypoplastic ascending aorta
(e) normally related great vessels

Prevalence: 0.2 / 1,000 live births; M:F = 2:1
◊ 4th most common cardiac malformation manifesting in 1st year of life (after VSD, TGV, tetralogy of Fallot)
◊ Most common cause of CHF in neonate
◊ Responsible for 25% of all cardiac deaths in 1st week of life

Hemodynamics:
pulmonary venous blood in LA faces an atretic / stenotic MV (= pulmonary venous outflow obstruction) and is diverted to RA through herniated foramen ovale / ASD (L-to-R shunt); RV supplies (a) pulmonary artery, (b) ductus arteriosus, (c) descending aorta (antegrade flow), (d) aortic arch + ascending aorta + coronary circulation (retrograde flow) leading to RV work overload + CHF

Associated malformations:
coarctation of aorta, PDA, patent foramen ovale, dilated pulmonary artery, VSD, dilated RA, enlarged RV, double-outlet right ventricle, endocardial fibroelastosis

• severe CHF (RV volume + pressure overload):
  • characteristically presents within first few hours of life
• ashen gray color / dusky complexion (systemic underperfusion due to inadequate atrial L-to-R shunt)
• myocardial ischemia (decreased perfusion of aorta [= "common coronary artery"] + coronary arteries):
  • cardiogenic shock, metabolic acidosis (when ductus arteriosus closes)

CXR:
√ hypoplastic / normal / enlarged cardiac silhouette:
  √ prominent right atrial border
  √ ± absence of left ventricular silhouette
  √ ± thymic atrophy
√ interstitial + alveolar pulmonary edema (due to pulmonary venous hypertension with severely restrictive interatrial communication in 80%)
√ normal pulmonary vasculature (with wide nonrestrictive interatrial communication in 20%)

OB-US (may be missed <22 weeks GA):
√ small left ventricular cavity (apex of LV and RV should be at same level)
√ hypoplastic ascending aorta
√ aortic coarctation (in 80%)
√ diastolic flow reversal in narrow ascending aorta is DIAGNOSTIC

ECHO:
√ normal / enlarged LA
√ slitlike / small / normal LV
√ enlarged RA
√ herniation + prolapse of foramen ovale flap into RA
√ hypoplastic ascending aorta (<5 mm = aortic atresia)
√ absent / grossly distorted mitral valve echoes

Angio:
√ retrograde flow in ascending aorta + aortic arch + coronary arteries via PDA
√ stringlike ascending aorta <6 mm in diameter
√ massive enlargement of RV + RVOT

Prognosis: almost 100% fatal by 6 weeks
Time of diagnosis: 32% pre-, 65% 1–4 days postnatally
Rx: (1) Prostaglandin E1 (patency of ductus arteriosus)
(2) Hypoventilation (increase in CO_2 maintains high pulmonary vascular resistance)
(3) Nitroprusside IV (decreases systemic vascular resistance)
(4) Norwood procedure = palliative attempt
(5) Cardiac transplant

HYPOPLASTIC RIGHT VENTRICLE

= PULMONARY ATRESIA WITH INTACT VENTRICULAR SEPTUM
= underdeveloped right ventricle due to pulmonary atresia in the presence of an intact interventricular septum

Type I = small RV secondary to competent tricuspid valve (more common)
Type II = normal / large RV secondary to incompetent tricuspid valve

Hemodynamics:
fetus : L-to-R atrial shunt through foramen ovale; retrograde flow through ductus arteriosus into pulmonary vascular bed
neonate : closure of ductus results in cyanosis, acidosis, death

√ small right ventricular cavity (apex of RV + LV should be at same level)
√ atresia of pulmonary valve
√ hypoplastic proximal pulmonary artery
√ secundum atrial septal defect (frequently associated)

Rx: prostaglandin E1 infusion + valvotomy + systemic-pulmonary artery shunt

IDIOPATHIC DILATATION OF PULMONARY ARTERY

= CONGENITAL ANEURYSM OF PULMONARY ARTERY

Age: adolescence; M < F
• systolic ejection murmur (in most cases)
√ dilated main pulmonary artery
√ normal peripheral pulmonary vascularity
√ normal pulmonary arterial pulsations
√ NO lateralization of pulmonary flow

Dx per exclusion:
1. Absence of shunts, CHD, acquired disease
2. Normal RV pressure
3. No significant pressure gradient across pulmonic valve

DDx: (1) Marfan syndrome
(2) Takayasu arteritis

INTERRUPTION OF AORTIC ARCH

= rare congenital anomaly as a common cause of death in the neonatal period

Trilogy: (1) Interrupted aortic arch
(2) VSD
(3) PDA (pulmonary blood supplies lower part of body)

Associated with (in 1/3):
1. Bicuspid aortic valve
2. Muscular subaortic stenosis
3. ASD
4. Truncus arteriosus
5. Transposition
6. Complete anomalous pulmonary venous return

• presents with CHF

Location:
Type A: distal to left subclavian artery (42%)
Type B: between left CCA and subclavian artery (53%) associated with: DiGeorge syndrome
Type C: between innominate and left CCA (4%)

√ dilatation of right atrium + ventricle
√ dilatation of pulmonary artery
√ ascending aorta much smaller than pulmonary artery
√ arch formed by pulmonary artery + ductus arteriosus gives the appearance of a low aortic arch
√ aortic knob absent
√ trachea in midline
√ NO esophageal impression
√ retrosternal clear space increased (small size of ascending aorta)
√ increased pulmonary vascularity (L-to-R shunt)

Prognosis: 76% dead at end of 1st month

INTERRUPTION OF PULMONARY ARTERY

= pulmonary trunk continues only as one large artery to one lung while systemic aortic collaterals supply the other side

Associated with: CHD (particularly if interruption on left side):
1. Tetralogy of Fallot
2. Scimitar syndrome = congenital pulmonary venolobar syndrome
3. PDA, VSD
4. Pulmonary hypertension

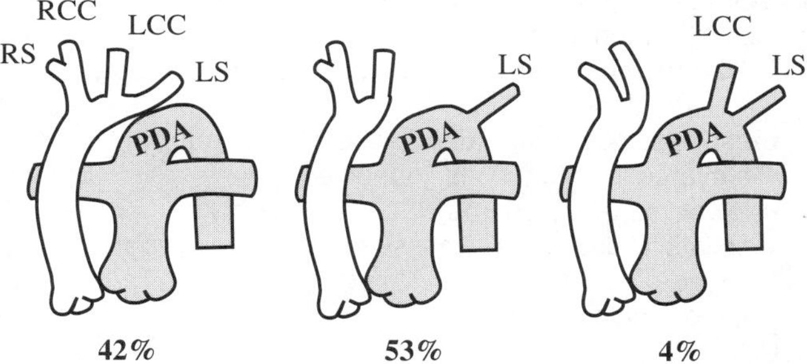

Interruption of Aortic Arch
LCC = left common carotid artery, LS = left subclavian artery,
RCC = right common carotid artery, RS = right subclavian artery,
PDA = patent ductus arteriosus

Collateral supply:
1. Arteries arising from arch + ascending aorta
2. Bronchial vessels
3. Intercostal vessels
4. Branches from subclavian artery

Location: usually opposite from aortic arch; R + L pulmonary artery equally involved

CXR:
√ hypoplastic ipsilateral lung
√ mediastinal shift toward involved lung
√ hemidiaphragm may be elevated
√ small hyperlucent ipsilateral chest with narrowed intercostal spaces
√ "comma-shaped" small distorted hilar shadow
√ asymmetry of pulmonary vascularity
√ normal respiratory motion (normal aeration of hypoplastic lung)

NUC: √ absent perfusion with normal aeration
Angio: √ absent pulmonary artery

Rx: surgical anastomosis between proximal + distal pulmonary artery (to prevent progressive pulmonary hypertension with dyspnea, cyanosis, hemoptysis, death)

DDx: (1) Hemitruncus
(2) Swyer-James syndrome (ipsilateral air trapping, reduced ventilation + perfusion)

INTRAVENOUS DRUG ABUSE

Complications secondary to:
(a) direct toxic effects of drugs or drug combinations (eg, heroin + cocaine / Talwin)
(b) direct toxic effects of adulterants [eg, heroin is mixed ("cut") with quinine, baking soda, sawdust]
(c) septic preparation
(d) injection technique
(e) choice of injection site (eg, "groin hit" into femoral vein; "pocket shot" into jugular, subclavian, brachiocephalic vein)

A. Cardiovascular complications
1. Arterial pseudoaneurysm
may be followed by rupture with exsanguination / loss of limb
2. Arteriovenous fistula
3. Arterial occlusion
(a) at injection site due to intimal damage, thrombosis, spasm
(b) distal to injection site due to embolization, spasm
4. Venous thrombosis
5. Intravenous migration of needle to heart / lungs
6. Embolization of infectious agent / foreign body / air through inadvertent arterial injection ("hit the pink")
7. Endocarditis (most commonly S. aureus)

B. Soft-tissue complications
1. Hematoma / abscess
2. Foreign bodies
3. Lymphadenopathy
4. Cellulitis

HEART

C. Skeletal complications
  1. Osteomyelitis
    (a) direct contamination: eg, pubic bone ("groin hit") / clavicle ("pocket shot")
    (b) hematogenous: spine most commonly affected
  2. Septic arthritis: spine, sacroiliac, sternoclavicular, symphysis pubis, acromioclavicular, hip, knee, wrist
D. Pleuropulmonary complications
  1. Pneumothorax ("pocket shot")
  2. Hemo- / pyothorax
  3. Septic pulmonary emboli
E. Gastrointestinal complications
  1. Severe colonic ileus
  2. Colonic pseudoobstruction
  3. Necrotizing enterocolitis
  4. Liver abscess
F. Genitourinary complications
  1. Focal / segmental glomerulosclerosis (heroin abuser)
  2. Amyloidosis
G. CNS complications
  1. Spinal epidural abscess in 5–18% (from vertebral osteomyelitis)
  2. Cord compression (from collapsed vertebral body)
  3. Cerebral infarction (from subacute bacterial endocarditis, toxic effect of drug, spasm, intimal damage from "pocket shot")
  4. Intracranial hemorrhage (from trauma, hypertension, injection of anticholinergic drugs, vasculitis, rupture of mycotic aneurysm)
  5. Meningitis, cerebral abscess

HEART

ISCHEMIC HEART DISEASE

= CORONARY ARTERY DISEASE (CAD)

Incidence: 1.5 million/year; leading cause of death in industrial nations
Morbidity: 28.7 cases per 1,000 men per year
Mortality: 3.1 deaths per 1,000 men per year

Noninvasive testing:
  1. Noninvasive testing is of marginal benefit when disease prevalence is <0.2 / >0.7
  2. Concordant thallium-201 and stress ECG are greater predictors of disease probability than either one used alone and/or when discordant
  3. Sequential thallium-201 and stress ECG are most useful to establish the diagnosis of CAD when pretest prevalence is intermediate + test results are concordant

CXR:
  √ often normal
  √ coronary artery calcification
  √ pulmonary venous hypertension following acute infarction (40%)
  √ LV aneurysm

ECHO:
  √ region of dilatation with disturbance of wall movement
    (1) Akinesis = no wall motion
    (2) Hypokinesis = reduced wall motion
    (3) Dyskinesis = paradoxical systolic expansion
    (4) Asynchrony = disturbed temporal sequence of contraction

Coronary angiography: 1.2 million procedures per year

KAWASAKI SYNDROME

= MUCOCUTANEOUS LYMPH NODE SYNDROME
= acute febrile multisystem vasculitis of unknown cause involving large + medium-sized + small arteries with a predilection for the coronary arteries

Incidence: average of 1.1:100,000 population per year
Histo: panvasculitis
Age: <5 years of age (in 85%); peak age of 1–2 years; M:F = 1.5:1
Associated with: polyarthritis (30–50%), aseptic meningitis (25%), hepatitis (5–10%), pneumonitis (5–10%)

• fever >5 days
• mucosal reddening (injected fissured lips, injected pharynx, strawberry tongue) in 99%
• nonpurulent cervical lymphadenopathy (82%)
• maculopapular rash on extensor surfaces (99%)
• bilateral nonpurulent conjunctivitis (96%)
• erythema of palms + soles with desquamation (88%)

@ Cardiovascular system (1/3)
  1. Coronary artery abnormality (15–25%)
    √ coronary artery aneurysm: LCA (2/3), RCA (1/3); proximal segment in 70%; 48% regress, 37% diminish in size
    √ coronary artery stenosis (39%) due to thrombus formation in aneurysm + intimal thickening
    √ coronary artery occlusion (8%) in aneurysms >9 mm
  2. Myocarditis (25%)
  3. Pericarditis
  4. Valvulitis
  5. Atrioventricular conduction disturbance

√ intestinal pseudoobstruction
√ transient gallbladder hydrops

Prognosis: 0.4–3% mortality (from myocardial infarction / myocarditis with congestive heart failure / rupture of coronary artery aneurysm)
Rx: aspirin (100 mg/kg per day) + gamma globulin
DDx: infantile polyarteritis

LEIOMYOSARCOMA OF IVC

most common intravascular venous tumor

Path: growth patterns: extravascular, intravascular, combined

• shortness of breath (decreased cardiac return)
• elevated liver functions, jaundice
• lower-extremity edema

√ collateral pathways bypassing IVC: hemiazygos, azygos
√ tumor extension from IVC into right atrium

US:
  √ blood flow in IVC / hepatic veins may be absent / reversed / turbulent (depending on degree of obstruction)
  √ tumor vascularity (DDx from thrombus)

CT:
√ contrast enhancement of tumor
Cx: Budd-Chiari syndrome (from sudden / gradual occlusion of hepatic veins / IVC / both)
DDx of tumor extension into right atrium:
renal cell carcinoma, hepatocellular carcinoma

LYMPHOMA OF HEART

Secondary Cardiac Lymphoma

Incidence: in 16–28% on autopsy; pericardial involvement more frequent; more common in immunocompromised patients

Primary Cardiac Lymphoma

= lymphoma that involves only heart / pericardium at time of diagnosis (extremely rare)
Age: 13–90 (mean, 60) years
Predisposed: immunocompromised patients, esp. AIDS
Path: multiple firm nodules; contiguous invasion of pericardium
Histo: typically NHL: well-differentiated B-cell lymphoma, follicular center cell lymphoma, diffuse large cell lymphoma, undifferentiated Burkitt-like lymphoma
• unresponsive rapidly progressive heart failure
• arrhythmia, cardiac tamponade, SVC syndrome
• chest pain
Location: RA > RV > LV > LA > atrial septum > ventricular septum; >1 chamber (75%)
CXR:
√ cardiomegaly
√ signs of CHF
√ massive pericardial effusion
ECHO:
√ hypoechoic myocardial masses in RA / RV
√ pericardial effusion
CT:
√ hypo- / isoattenuating masses relative to myocardium
√ heterogeneous enhancement of masses
MR:
√ poorly marginated heterogeneous lesions of iso- to hypointensity relative to myocardium on T1WI
√ lesions isointense to myocardium on T2WI
√ heterogeneous enhancement with gadolinium
Dx: positive cytology in pericardial fluid (in 67%); exploratory thoracotomy with biopsy of cardiac tissue
Prognosis: very poor

MICROSCOPIC POLYANGITIS

= MICROSCOPIC POLYARTERITIS = HYPERSENSITIVITY VASCULITIS = LEUKOCYTOCLASTIC VASCULITIS
= pauci-immune necrotizing small-vessel angitis without granulomatous inflammation
Path: necrotizing arteritis identical to polyarteritis nodosa but in vessels smaller than arteries (= arterioles, venules and capillaries)
Trigger: drugs (eg, penicillin), microorganisms, heterologous proteins, tumor antigens
• hemoptysis, hematuria, proteinuria
• abdominal pain, GI bleeding, muscle pain + weakness
• ANCA (antineutrophil cytoplasmic autoantibodies) in >80%
• negative serologic tests for hepatitis B
Location: skin, mucous membranes, lung, brain, heart, GI tract, kidney, muscle
◊ Most common cause of the pulmonary-renal syndrome!
√ pulmonary infiltrates (due to capillaritis)
√ glomerulonephritis (90%)
Rx: removal of offending agent

MITRAL REGURGITATION

= MITRAL INSUFFICIENCY
Cause:
A. ACUTE
1. Spontaneous rupture of chordae tendineae
2. Myocardial infarction with involvement of papillary muscle (posteromedial > anterolateral papillary muscle)
3. Bacterial endocarditis
4. Periprosthetic valve leak

B. CHRONIC
1. Acute rheumatic fever
(a) isolated: frequently seen in children
(b) uncommon in adults (mostly combined with stenosis)
2. Mitral valve prolapse syndrome
3. Atrial myxoma
4. Coronary artery disease
5. Idiopathic hypertrophic subaortic stenosis (IHSS)
6. Myxomatous degeneration of mitral valve: eg, Marfan syndrome
7. Mitral annulus calcification
8. Functional / secondary (from dilatation of mitral ring in any condition with severe dilatation of LV)
9. Congenital heart disease: short / abnormally inserted chordae tendineae; persistent ostium primum ASD with cleft mitral valve, corrected transposition with Ebstein-like anomaly

Hemodynamics:
backward flow of blood from LV into LA during LV systole; increased volume of blood under elevated pressure causes dilatation of LA; marked increase in LV diastolic volume with little increase in LV diastolic pressure (= increase in preload without increase in afterload = elevated ejection fraction)

A. ACUTE MITRAL REGURGITATION
√ pulmonary venous hypertension with engorged pulmonary vessels and cephalization (less than with mitral stenosis)
√ symmetric interstitial / alveolar pulmonary edema:
√ asymmetric right upper lobe edema (9%) due to preferential flow of regurgitant jet into pulmonary vein of RUL (PATHOGNOMONIC)
√ limited cardiac enlargement

HEART

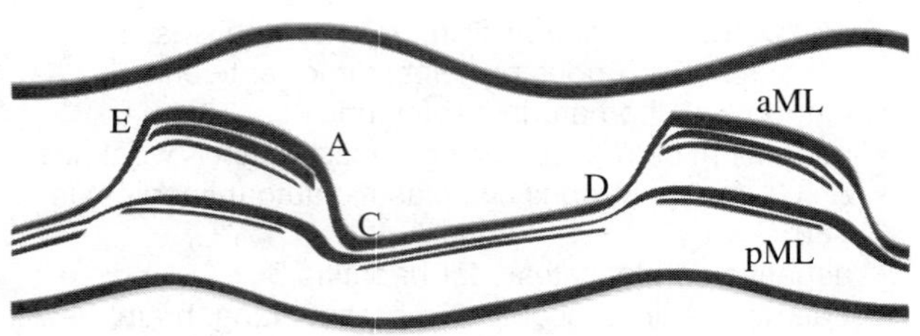

Classic Mitral Valve Stenosis
(for abbreviations see page 594)

B. CHRONIC MITRAL REGURGITATION
- √ enlarged heart
- √ massive LA:
  - √ LA posterior wall calcification (McCallum patch)
  - √ enlarged LA appendage (with history of previous rheumatic heart disease)
- √ mitral annular calcification (frequent)
- √ marked LV enlargement (cardiothoracic ratio >0.55) + LV failure

ECHO:
- √ LV volume overload:
  - √ normal-sized / enlarged LV
  - √ increased septal + posterior wall motion
- √ increased EF slope
- √ early closure of aortic valve (LV stroke volume partially lost to LA)
- √ LA enlargement (in chronic MV insufficiency)
- √ bulging of interatrial septum to the right during systole
- √ Doppler is only diagnostic tool + allows assessment of severity

MITRAL STENOSIS

Cause: rheumatic heart disease (5–15 years after initial episode of rheumatic fever); carcinoid syndrome; eosinophilic endocarditis; rheumatoid arthritis; SLE; mass obstructing LV inflow (tumor, atrial myxoma, thrombus); congenital

M:F = 1:8

Hemodynamics:
rise in left atrial + pulmonary vascular pressure throughout systole and into diastole; compensatory dilation of LA + pulmonary venous hypertension; development of medial hypertrophy + intimal sclerosis in pulmonary arterioles leads to postcapillary pulmonary arterial hypertension; RV hypertrophy; tricuspid regurgitation; RV dilatation; right heart failure

May be associated with: ASD = Lutembacher syndrome (in 0.6%) causing L-to-R shunt

- • history of rheumatic fever (in 50%)
- • dyspnea on exertion, orthopnea, paroxysmal nocturnal dyspnea
- • atrial fibrillation
- • systemic embolization from thrombosis of atrial appendage

Stages (according to degree of pulmonary venous hypertension):
- Stage 1 : loss of hilar angle, redistribution
- Stage 2 : interstitial edema
- Stage 3 : alveolar edema
- Stage 4 : hemosiderin deposits + ossification

@ Left heart
- √ enlarged LA ± wall calcification:
  - √ "double density" seen through right upper cardiac border (AP view)
  - √ bulge of superior posterior cardiac border below carina (lateral view)
  - √ splaying of mainstem bronchi
  - √ esophagus displaced toward right + posteriorly
  - √ dilated left atrial appendage (not present with retracting clot), in 90% associated with rheumatic heart disease
    - ◊ Dilatation of left atrial appendage + calcification = rheumatic heart disease!
- √ calcification of valve leaflets in 60% of severe MS, usually >50 years of age (DDx: calcification of mitral annulus)
- √ normal / undersized LV
- √ small aorta (due to decrease of forward cardiac output)

@ Right heart
- √ prominent pulmonary artery segment (precapillary hypertension)
- √ hypertrophy of RV

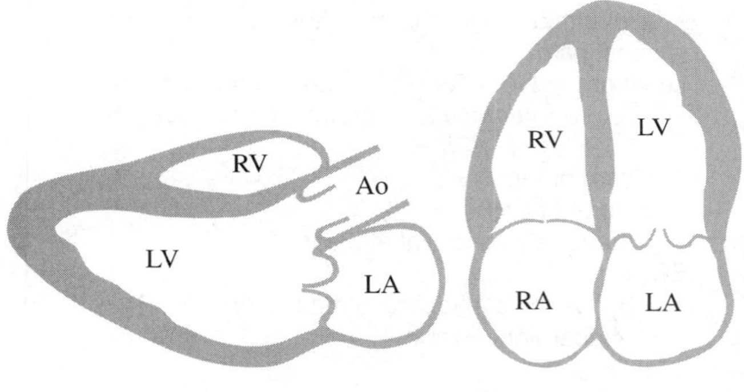

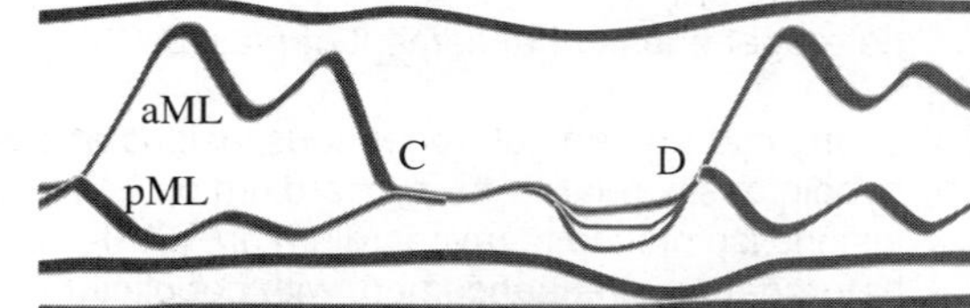

Midsystolic Mitral Valve Prolapse

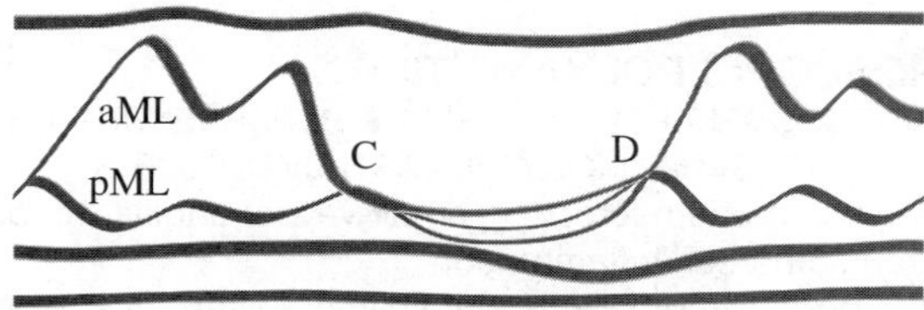

Holosystolic Mitral Valve Prolapse

√ dilatation of RV (tricuspid insufficiency / pulmonary hypertension)
√ increase in cardiothoracic ratio
√ diminution of retrosternal clear space
√ IVC pushed backward (lateral view)

@ Lung
√ pulmonary vascular cephalization = redistribution of pulmonary blood flow to upper lobes (postcapillary pressure 16–19 mm Hg)
√ interstitial pulmonary edema (postcapillary pressure 20–25 mm Hg)
DDx: interstitial fibrosis / deposition of hemosiderin-laden macrophages (= "brown induration") of chronic mitral valve stenosis
√ alveolar edema (postcapillary pressure 25–30 mm Hg)
DDx: diffuse alveolar hemorrhage = diffuse confluent acinar / ground-glass areas of increased opacity sparing the lung periphery (= "window frame" effect)
√ pulmonary hemosiderosis:
√ 1–3 mm ill-defined nodules
√ fine / coarse reticular areas of increased opacity with bias for middle and lower lungs
√ pulmonary ossification (3–13%) = densely calcified 1–3–5 mm nodules (± trabeculae) mainly in middle and lower lungs

ECHO:
√ thickening of leaflets toward free edge (fibrosis, calcification)
√ flattening of EF slope = MV remains open throughout diastole due to persistently high LA pressure (crude index of severity of MV stenosis)
√ diastolic anterior tracking of pML in 80% (secondary to diastolic anterior pull by larger + more mobile aML)
√ diastolic doming of MV leaflets
√ commissure fusion = increased echodensity + decreased leaflet motion at level of commissure
√ area reduction of MV orifice: normal within 4–6 cm^2; mild narrowing with <2 cm^2; severe narrowing with <1 cm^2 (reproducible to within 0.3 cm^2)
√ shortening + fibrosis of chordae tendineae
√ abnormal septal motion = early diastolic dip of IVS due to rapid filling of RV (in severe MV stenosis)
√ slowed LV filling pattern of small LV
√ dilatation of LA (>5 cm increases risk of atrial fibrillation + left atrial thrombus)
√ DE opening amplitude reduced to <20 mm indicating loss of valve pliability (DDx: low cardiac output state)
√ absent A-wave common (atrial fibrillation)
√ increase in valve gradient + pressure halftime on Doppler

Rx: (1) Commissurotomy if valves pliable + calcium absent + MV regurgitation absent
(2) Valve replacement for symptomatic patients with severely stenotic valves

DDx:
(1) Pseudomitral stenosis in decreased LV compliance (decreased EF slope, normal leaflet thickness + motion)
(2) Rheumatic mitral insufficiency (indistinguishable findings + evidence of LV volume overload)
(3) LA myxoma (mass behind MV + in LA)
(4) Low cardiac output (apparent small valve orifice)

LUTEMBACHER SYNDROME = rheumatic mitral valve stenosis + ASD

MITRAL VALVE PROLAPSE

Incidence: 2–6% of general population; 5–20% of young women; ? autosomal dominant inheritance
Age: commonly 14–30 years
Cause:
(1) "Floppy mitral valve" = elongation of cusps + chordae leading to redundant valve tissue, which prolapses into LA during systole
Associated with:
(a) Skeletal abnormalities: scoliosis, straightening of thoracic spine, narrow anteroposterior chest dimension, pectus excavatum deformity of sternum
(b) Barlow syndrome = straight back syndrome
(c) Marfan syndrome
(d) Tricuspid valve prolapse
(e) Long-standing ASD
(f) Autosomal dominant polycystic kidney disease
(2) Secondary MV prolapse:
papillary muscle dysfunction, rupture of chordae tendineae, rheumatic mitral insufficiency, primary pulmonary hypertension, ostium secundum ASD

• arrhythmias, palpitation, chest pain, light-headedness, syncope
• responsible for midsystolic click + late systolic murmur (when associated with mitral regurgitation)

√ LA not enlarged (unless associated with significant mitral regurgitation)

ECHO:
√ interruption of CD line with bulge toward left atrium:
√ abrupt midsystolic posterior buckling of both leaflets (classic pattern)
√ "hammocklike" pansystolic posterior bowing of both leaflets
√ multiple scallops on mitral valve leaflets (short-axis parasternal view)
√ valve leaflets may appear thickened (myxomatous degeneration + valve redundancy)
√ mitral valve leaflets passing >2 mm posterior to plane of mitral annulus (apical 4-chamber view)
√ hyperactive atrioventricular groove
√ mitral annulus may be dilated >4.7 cm^2

DDx: (1) Pericardial effusion (systolic posterior displacement of MV leaflets + entire heart)
(2) Bacterial endocarditis (mimicked by locally thickened + redundant leaflets)

MYOCARDIAL INFARCTION

Incidence: 1,500,000 per year in USA resulting in 500,000 deaths (50% occur in asymptomatic individuals)

• atrioventricular block (common with inferior wall infarction as AV nodal branch originates from RCA); complete heart block has worse prognosis because it indicates a large area of infarction

CXR:
- √ normal-sized heart (84–95%) in acute phase if previously normal
- √ cardiomegaly: high incidence of congestive heart failure with anterior wall infarction, multiple myocardial infarctions, double- and triple-vessel CAD, LV aneurysm

CECT:
- √ perfusion defect within 60–90 seconds after bolus injection
- √ delayed enhancement of infarcted tissue peaking at 10–15 minutes (due to accumulation of iodine in ischemic cells), size of enhanced area correlates well with size of infarct

Cx: (myocardium is prone to rupture during 3rd–14th day post infarction)

A. LEFT VENTRICULAR FAILURE (60–70%)
- • "cardiac shock" = systolic pressure <90 mm Hg
- ◊ Signs of pulmonary venous hypertension are a good predictor of mortality (>30% if present, <10% if absent)
- √ progressive enlargement of heart
- √ haziness + indistinctness of pulmonary arteries
- √ increase in size of right descending pulmonary artery >17 mm
- √ pleural effusion
- √ septal lines
- √ perihilar ± peripheral parenchymal clouding
- √ alveolar pulmonary edema

Mortality: 30–50% with mild LV failure; 44% with pulmonary edema; 80–100% with cardiogenic shock; 8% in absence of LV failure

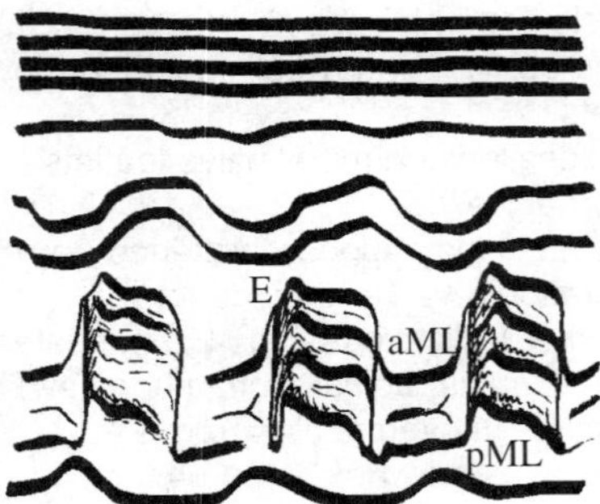

Atrial Myxoma Prolapsing into Mitral Valve Orifice

Note the interval between the opening of aML and pML and the moment that the tumor reaches its maximal anterior excursion at point E when a slight additional opening of the aML results; aML stays open during entire diastole as a result of obstruction to left atrial emptying.

B. ANEURYSM (12–15% of survivors)

C. MYOCARDIAL RUPTURE (3.3%)
- • occurs usually on 3rd–5th day post MI
- √ enlargement of heart (slow leakage of blood into pericardium)

Prognosis: cause of death in 13% of all infarctions; almost 100% mortality

D. RUPTURE OF PAPILLARY MUSCLE (1%)
from infarction of posteromedial papillary muscle in inferior MI (common) / anterolateral papillary muscle in anterolateral MI (uncommon)
- • sudden onset of massive mitral insufficiency
- • unresponsive to medical management
- √ abrupt onset of severe persistent pulmonary edema
- √ asymmetric PVH in right upper lobe
- √ minimal LV enlargement / normal-sized heart
- √ NO dilatation of LA (immediate decompression into pulmonary veins)

Prognosis: 70% mortality within 24 hours; 80–90% within 2 weeks

E. RUPTURE OF INTERVENTRICULAR SEPTUM (0.5–2%)
- • occurs usually within 4–21 days with rapid onset of L-to-R shunt
- • Swan-Ganz catheterization: increase in oxygen content of RV, capillary wedge pressure may be within normal limits
- √ right-sided cardiac enlargement
- √ engorgement of pulmonary vasculature:
  - √ asymmetric PVH of right upper lobe
- √ NO pulmonary edema (DDx to ruptured papillary muscle)

Prognosis: 24% mortality within 24 hours; 87% within 2 months; >90% in 1 year

F. DRESSLER SYNDROME (<4%)
= POSTMYOCARDIAL INFARCTION SYNDROME

Etiology: autoimmune reaction

Onset: 2–3 weeks (range 1 week–several months) following infarction
- • relapses occur as late as 2 years after initial episode
- • fever
- √ pericarditis + pericardial effusion
- √ pleuritis + pleural effusion
- √ pneumonitis

Right Ventricular Infarction

- ◊ Right ventricle involved in 33% of left inferior myocardial infarction
- √ decreased RV ejection fraction
- √ accumulation of Tc-99m pyrophosphate

Prognosis: in 50% RV ejection fraction returns to normal within 10 days

Cx:
(1) cardiogenic shock (unusual)
(2) elevation of RA pressure
(3) decrease of pulmonary artery pressure

MYXOMA

= most common benign primary cardiac tumor (true neoplasm) in adults, 40–50% of all cardiac tumors

HEART

Age: 11–82 (mean 50) years; 90% of patients are between ages 30 and 60 years; M:F = 1:1.7 to 1:4
Classification: sporadic (most frequent); familial type (mean age of 24 years); complex type = Carney syndrome
Path: (a) gelatinous, friable, papillary / villous pedunculated tumor
(b) round / lobular smooth sessile tumor (25%) with firm surface
◊ No infiltration of underlying tissues!
Histo: composed of myxoma cells (= ovoid nucleus with inconspicuous / large nucleoli + abundant eosinophilic cytoplasm)) forming rings / syncytia / cords; hypocellular amorphous acid mucopolysaccharide matrix in areas without fibrosis; covered by a monolayer of endothelial cells (= endocardial tumor)
Size: 0.6–12 (mean, 5.7) cm

- short history + rapid progression
- dyspnea, chest pain
- constitutional symptoms (30%):
  - fever, myalgia, arthralgia, weight loss, lethargy
  - leukocytosis, anemia, elevated ESR, petechiae
  - hypergammaglobulinemia
- positional symptoms (ie, change with position) due to hemodynamic obstruction:
  - arrhythmia (20%), heart murmur
  - congestive heart failure (valve obstruction)
  - syncope
- embolization (30–40%) to CNS, coronary artery, aorta, kidney, spleen, extremities, pulmonary artery (caused by tumor fragments / accumulated thrombus)

Location: left atrium (75–80%); right atrium (10–20%); ventricle (5%); biatrial (with growth through fossa ovalis)
Site: attached to interatrial septum by small stalk in fossa ovalis (75%) / to wall of cardiac chambers / to valve surfaces; may protrude into ventricle causing partial obstruction of atrioventricular valve
√ small myxomas produce no CXR findings
√ cardiomegaly
√ atrial obstruction (mimicking valvular stenosis)
√ persistent defect in atrium / diastolic defect in ventricle

A. LEFT ATRIAL MYXOMA (75–80%)
with obstruction of mitral valve:
√ pulmonary venous hypertension:
  √ pulmonary vascular redistribution
  √ interstitial edema
√ enlargement of LA
√ NO enlargement of atrial appendage
√ ossific lung nodules
Cx: systemic emboli (27%) in 50% to CNS (stroke / "mycotic" aneurysm)

B. RIGHT ATRIAL MYXOMA (10–20%)
with obstruction of tricuspid valve:
√ tumor calcification: R > L
√ enlargement of RA
√ prominent SVC, IVC, azygos vein
√ decreased pulmonary vascularity
√ pleural effusion (occasionally)
Cx: pulmonary emboli

ECHO: (2D-ECHO is study of choice)
√ tumor attached by narrow stalk
√ tumor mobility:
  √ prolapse across AV valve during diastole
√ tumor distensibility
√ hyperechoic spherical mass:
  √ internal hypoechoic areas (= hemorrhage, necrosis)
  √ speckled echogenic foci (= calcifications)
  √ frondlike surface projections
Doppler:
  √ valvular regurgitation
M-mode findings of only historical interest:
  √ dense echoes appearing posterior to aML soon after onset of diastole
  √ pML obscured
  √ tumor echoes can be traced into LA
  √ dilated LA
  √ reduced E-F slope

CT:
√ well-defined spherical / ovoid intraluminal filling defect
√ lobular / smooth surface contour
√ tumor attenuation lower than unopacified blood (due to gelatinous component)
√ heterogeneous texture (due to hemorrhage, necrosis, cyst formation, fibrosis, calcification [16%], ossification)

MR:
√ iso- / hypointense on T1WI relative to myocardium
√ heterogeneous contrast enhancement (secondary to necrotic areas)
√ markedly hyperintense on T2WI
√ areas of decreased signal intensity (calcifications, hemosiderin deposits)

Rx: urgent surgical excision ± valvuloplasty / valve replacement
Prognosis: 5–14% recurrence rate (multifocal myxomas)
DDx: (1) Thrombus (most commonly in LA + LV)
(2) Other cardiac tumors: sarcoma, malignant mesenchymoma, metastasis, papillary fibroelastoma (also arises from narrow stalk)

Carney Complex

= COMPLEX MYOMA
= autosomal-dominant inherited disorder
Prevalence: 7% of all myxomas; 150 patients identified since 1985 worldwide
Age: younger than patients with sporadic myxoma

- endocrine overactivity:
  - Cushing syndrome
  - sexual precocity
  - acromegaly

(1) Cardiac myxomas: multifocal (66%), outside left atrium, recurring at an increased rate after resection
(2) Hyperpigmented skin lesions: lentigines, ephelides, blue nevi

HEART

(3) Myxoid fibroadenoma of the breast
(4) Psammomatous melanotic schwannoma
(5) Pituitary adenoma
(6) Testicular tumor: large calcifying Sertoli cell tumor
(7) Primary pigmented nodular adrenocortical hyperplasia
N.B.: not related to Carney triad (pulmonary hamartomas, extraadrenal paragangliomas, gastric leiomyosarcoma)

PAPILLARY FIBROELASTOMA

= FIBROELEASTIC PAPILLOMA = PAPILLOMA / MYXOMA / FIBROMA OF VALVES = GIANT LAMBL EXCRESCENCE = MYXOFIBROMA = HYALINE FIBROMA

= benign endocardial papilloma predominantly affecting cardiac valves

Prevalence: 25% of all cardiac valvular tumors (most common valvular tumor); 10% of all primary cardiac tumors (2nd most common primary benign cardiac neoplasm after myxoma)

Mean age: 60 years; M:F = 1:1

Cause: ? reactive process, ? hamartoma

- mostly asymptomatic (incidental finding at autopsy, surgery, echocardiography, cardiac catheterization)
- chest pain, dyspnea, embolic events (TIA / stroke from thrombi collecting on tumor)
- NO valvular dysfunction

Path: gelatinous mass with "sea anemone" appearance due to multiple delicate branching papillary fronds attached to endocardium by short pedicle

Histo: avascular papilloma composed of fibrous core + lined by a single layer of endothelium; scattered smooth muscle cells within papillary projections

Location: aortic (29%) > mitral (25%) > tricuspid (17%) > pulmonary valve (13%); nonvalvular endocardial surface of atrium / ventricle (16%)

Size: <1 cm in diameter (may be as large as 5 cm)

ECHO:
√ <1.5 cm homogeneous mobile pedunculated mass:
  √ elongated strandlike projection / well-defined head
  √ CHARACTERISTIC stippled edge with a "shimmer / vibration" at interface between tumor and surrounding blood (DDx: amorphous thrombus)
  √ flutters / prolapses with cardiac motion
√ turbulent blood flow

Rx: surgical excision ± leaflet repair / valve replacement

PATENT DUCTUS ARTERIOSUS

= PDA = persistence of left 6th aortic arch, which connects the left pulmonary artery with the descending aorta beyond the origin of the left subclavian artery

Incidence: 9% of all CHD; M:F = 1:2

Associated with: prematurity, birth asphyxia, high-altitude births, rubella syndrome, coarctation, VSD, trisomy 18 + 21

Normal ductus physiology in mature infant:
increase in arterial oxygen pressure leads to constriction + closure of duct
◊ Functional closure due to muscular contraction within 10–15–48 hours
◊ Anatomic closure due to subintimal fibrosis + thrombosis: in 35% by 2 weeks; in 90% by 2 months; in 99% by 1 year

Hemodynamics of PDA:
increased volume of blood flows from aorta through PDA + pulmonary artery into lungs and then to left side of heart

RA	↔	RV	↔	Main PA	↑
Pulm. vessels		↑			
LA	↔/↑	LV	↔/↑	Ao	↑

- mostly asymptomatic
- congestive heart failure (rare) usually by 3 months of age if L-to-R shunt large
- continuous murmur
- bounding peripheral pulses (intraaortic pressure runoff through PDA)

CXR (mimics VSD):
√ enlarged pulmonary artery segment
√ increase of pulmonary vasculature; less flow directed to LUL
√ enlarged ascending aorta + aortic arch (thymus may obscure this)
√ LA + LV enlargement
√ enlarged RV (only with pulmonary hypertension)
√ prominent ductus infundibulum (diverticulum) = prominence between aortic knob + pulmonary artery segment
√ obscured aortopulmonary window
√ "railroad track" = calcified ductus arteriosus

ECHO:
√ LA:Ao ratio ≥1.2:1 (signalizes significant L-to-R shunt)

Angio:
√ catheter course from RA to RV, main pulmonary artery, PDA, descending aorta
√ communication from aorta (distal to left subclavian artery) to left pulmonary artery on AP / LAT / LAO aortogram

PDA in Premature Infant

premature infant not subject to medial muscular hypertrophy of small pulmonary artery branches (which occurs in normal infants subsequent to progressive hypoxia in 3rd trimester)

- CHF
  Cause:
  (a) pulmonary artery pressure remains low without opposing any L-to-R shunts (PDA / VSD)
  (b) ductus arteriosus remains open secondary to hypoxia in RDS

√ recurrence of alveolar airspace filling after resolution of RDS
√ granular pattern of hyaline membrane disease becomes more opaque
√ enlargement of heart (masked by positive pressure ventilation)

Rx:
(a) Medical therapy:
  (1) supportive oxygen, diuretics, digitalis
  (2) avoid fluid overload (not to increase shunt volume)

HEART

(3) antiprostaglandins = indomethacin opposes prostaglandins, which are potent duct dilators
(b) Surgical ligation

Beneficial PDA

= compensatory effect of PDA in:

1. Tetralogy of Fallot
   cyanosis usually occurs during closure of duct shortly after birth
2. Eisenmenger pulmonary hypertension
   PDA acts as escape valve shunting blood to descending aorta
3. Interrupted aortic arch
   supply of lower extremity via PDA

Nonbeneficial PDA

in L-to-R shunts (VSD, aortopulmonic window) a PDA increases shunt volume

PENETRATING AORTIC ULCER

= PENETRATING ATHEROSCLEROTIC ULCER OF THE AORTA
= atheromatous plaque characterized by ulceration that penetrates the internal elastic lamina

Pathophysiology:
atheromatous intimal plaque progresses to a deep atheromatous ulcer that penetrates the elastic lamina + extends into media; hemorrhage within media causes a communicating "double-barreled" / thrombosed aortic dissection; stretching of aortic wall leads to formation of a saccular aortic aneurysm; aortic dissection / aneurysm may rupture

• may present with back pain

Location: middle / distal third of descending thoracic aorta; occasionally abdominal aorta

√ extensive atherosclerotic disease + ectasia
√ lack of compression of the aortic lumen

CECT:
√ focally ulcerated plaque
√ adjacent subintimal hematoma (differentiation from intraluminal thrombus / atherosclerotic plaque not possible):
√ displacement of frequently calcified intima inwardly
√ thickening / enhancement of adjacent aortic wall

MR:
√ deeply ulcerated aortic plaque
√ subacute hematoma in aortic wall of high signal intensity on T1WI + T2WI (methemoglobin) either localized or mimicking type 3 dissection

Angio:
√ ulcerated atherosclerotic plaque
√ aortic wall thickening

Cx: (1) Aortic dissection (controversial)
(2) Saccular false aneurysm due to incomplete rupture
(3) Spontaneous complete aortic rupture (40% risk compared with 7% risk in aortic dissection)

DDx: (1) Aortic dissection (intimal flap, patent false lumen)
(2) Atheroma / chronic intramural thrombus (low signal intensity on T1WI + T2WI)

PERICARDIAL DEFECT

= failure of pericardial development secondary to premature atrophy of the left duct of Cuvier (cardinal vein), which fails to nourish the left pleuropericardial membrane

Frequency: 1:13,000; M:F = 3:1
Age at detection: newborn to 81 years (mean 21 years)

Location:
A. PARTIAL ABSENCE (91%)
(a) complete absence on left side (35%)
(b) foraminal defect on left side (35%)
(c) diaphragmatic pericardial aplasia (17%)
(d) foraminal defect on right side (4%)
B. TOTAL BILATERAL ABSENCE (9%)

In 30% associated with:
(1) Bronchogenic cyst (30%)
(2) VSD, PDA, mitral stenosis
(3) Diaphragmatic hernia, sequestration

• mostly asymptomatic
• palpitations, tachycardia, dyspnea, dizziness, syncope
• positional discomfort while lying on left side
• nonspecific intermittent chest pain (lack of pericardial cushioning, torsion of great vessels, tension on pleuropericardial adhesions, pressure on coronary arteries by rim of pericardial defect)
• ECG: right axis deviation, right bundle branch block

√ size:
— small foraminal defect = no abnormality
— large defect = herniation of cardiac structures / lung
— complete absence = levoposition of heart

√ absence of left pericardial fat-pad
√ levoposition of heart with lack of visualization of right heart border
√ prominence / focal bulge in the area of RVOT, main pulmonary artery, left atrial appendage
√ sharp margination + elongation of left heart border
√ insinuation of lung between heart + left hemidiaphragm
√ insinuation of lung between aortic knob + pulmonary a.
√ increased distance between heart + sternum secondary to absence of sternopericardial ligament (cross-table lateral projection)
√ pneumopericardium following pneumothorax
√ NO tracheal deviation

Cx: cardiac strangulation
Rx: foraminal defect requires surgery because of (a) herniation + strangulation of left atrial appendage, (b) herniation of LA / LV
(1) Closure of defect with pleural flap
(2) Resection of pericardium

PERICARDIAL MESOTHELIOMA

= malignant primary neoplasm arising from mesothelial cells of the pericardium

Incidence: <1% of all mesotheliomas; 50% of all primary pericardial tumors
Age: 2–78 (mean, 46) years; M:F = 2:1

HEART

Path: multiple coalescing pericardial masses with obliteration of pericardial space; myocardial invasion is rare
Histo: biphasic tumor composed of epithelial areas forming tubulopapillary structures (resembling carcinoma) and spindled areas (resembling sarcoma)
• chest pain, cough, dyspnea, palpitations
• signs of pericarditis, cardiac tamponade
√ irregular diffuse pericardial thickening
√ cardiac encasement by soft-tissue masses
√ pericardial effusion
CXR:
√ cardiac enlargement with irregular contour
√ diffuse mediastinal enlargement
Rx: palliative surgery + radiation therapy
Prognosis: 6–12-month survival after diagnosis

PERICARDIAL TERATOMA

= benign germ cell neoplasm
Age: infants + children
Histo: derivatives of all 3 germ cell layers (neuroglia, cartilage, skeletal muscle, liver, intestine, pancreas, glandular tissue)
Location: within pericardial sac connected to a great vessel via a pedicle; intramyocardial (rare)
• respiratory distress, cyanosis (due to pericardial tamponade + compression of SVC, RA, aortic root, PA)
CXR:
√ enlarged cardiomediastinal silhouette
√ formed calcified teeth
US:
√ intrapericardial heterogeneous complex multilocular cystic mass:
√ intrinsic echogenic foci (= calcifications)
√ pericardial effusion
√ fetal hydrops (ascites, pleural effusion, subcutaneous edema, polyhydramnios)
MR:
√ large mass of heterogeneous signal intensity
Rx: emergent pericardiocentesis (life-threatening lesion); urgent surgical excision
Prognosis: good

PERSISTENT FETAL CIRCULATION

= PERSISTENT PULMONARY HYPERTENSION OF THE NEWBORN
= delay in transition from intra- to extrauterine pulmonary circulation
Cause: primary disorder related to birth asphyxia, concurrent parenchymal lung disease (meconium aspiration, pneumonia, pulmonary hemorrhage, hyaline membrane disease, pulmonary hypoplasia), concurrent cardiovascular disease, hypoxic myocardial injury, hyperviscosity syndromes)
• labile PO_2
√ structurally normal heart

POLYARTERITIS NODOSA

= PERIARTERITIS NODOSA = PAN
= systemic fibrinoid necrotizing inflammation of medium-sized + small muscular arteries <u>without</u> glomerulonephritis or vasculitis in arterioles, capillaries, venules
Frequency: 4–9 cases/million/year (rare); 70 per million/year in patients with hepatitis B; M:F = 2:1
Etiology: ? deposition of immune complexes
Age: 18–81 (mean age, 55) years
Path: focal panmural necrotizing vasculitis; mucoid degeneration + fibrinoid necrosis begins within media; absence of vasculitis in vessels other than arteries (DDx: necrotizing angitis, mycotic aneurysm)
Histo: polymorphonuclear cell infiltrate in all layers of arterial wall + perivascular tissue (acute phase), mononuclear cell infiltrate, intimal proliferation, thrombosis, perivascular inflammation (chronic stage)
Associated with: hepatitis B + HIV antigenemia
• low-grade fever, malaise, abdominal pain, weight loss
• elevated ESR, thrombocytosis, anemia
• positive for hepatitis B surface antigen (up to 30%)
• positive perinuclear ANCA titers

Location: all organs may be involved, kidney (70–90%), heart (65%), liver (50–60%), spleen (45%), pancreas (25–35%), GI tract, CNS (cerebrovascular accident, seizure), skin

@ Kidney (involved in 70–80–90%)
• painless hematuria
√ irregular nephrogram
√ radiolucent cortical areas
√ prolonged washout of contrast material
√ multiple small intrarenal microaneurysms (at bifurcation of interlobar / arcuate arteries)
√ aneurysms may disappear (thrombosis) or appear in new locations
√ arterial narrowing + thrombosis (chronic stage / healing stage)
√ multiple small cortical infarcts
CECT:
√ lobulated renal contour + irregular thinning (due to prior cortical infarcts)
√ multiple hypoattenuating bands (arterial occlusion)
Cx: intrarenal / subcapsular / perinephric hemorrhage (rupture of aneurysm)
@ Chest (involved in 70%)
• CHF, myocardial infarction
√ cardiac enlargement / pericardial effusion (14%)
√ pleural effusion (14%)
√ pulmonary venous engorgement (21%)
√ massive pulmonary edema (4%)
√ linear densities / platelike atelectasis (10%)
√ wedge-shaped / round peripheral infiltrates of nonsegmental distribution (14%) (simulating thromboembolic disease with infarction)
√ cavitation may occur
√ interstitial lower lung field pneumonitis

@ Liver (50–66%)
√ prolonged washout of contrast material (due to increase in peripheral hepatic arterial resistance + hepatic infarcts
@ GI tract (50–70%)
Location: small intestine > mesentery > colon
• abdominal pain, nausea, vomiting (66%)
√ ulcer formation, GI bleeding (6%)
√ bowel perforation (5%), intestinal infarction (1.4%)
@ Skeletal muscle (39%)
• myalgia, arthralgia (50%), limb claudication
√ aneurysms of lumbar + intercostal arteries (19%)
√ lower extremity ischemia (16%)
@ Skin (20%)
• palpable purpura, infection, ischemic ulcer
• tender subcutaneous nodules (15%)
• peripheral neuropathy (= mononeuritis multiplex)

Angiography (61–89% sensitive, 90% specific, 55% PPV, 98% NPV, 80% true-positive rate):
√ multiple (>10) aneurysms of small + medium-sized arteries typically at branching points as a result of pannecrosis of the internal elastic lamina in 50–60% (HALLMARK):
√ 1–5 mm saccular aneurysms in 60–75%
√ fusiform aneurysms / arterial ectasia
◊ Aneurysms are found in 12–94% of patients with polyarteritis nodosa
√ luminal irregularities (in up to 90%)
√ stenoses of arteries
√ arterial occlusions + organ infarcts (98%)
DDx: rheumatoid vasculitis, drug abuse, systemic lupus erythematosus, Churg-Strauss syndrome

Dx: angiography, tissue biopsy
Cx: renin-mediated hypertension, renal failure, hemorrhage secondary to aneurysm rupture (9%), organ infarction due to vessel thrombosis, gangrene of fingers / toes
Prognosis: clinical course lasts several months to >1 year; relapse in 40% with median interval of 33 months; 13% 5-year survival rate if untreated
Rx: immunosuppression with corticosteroids + cyclophosphamide (increases 5-year survival rate to 48–90%)

POPLITEAL ARTERY ENTRAPMENT SYNDROME

= popliteal artery classically winding medially and then inferiorly to the tendinous insertion of the medial head of the gastrocnemius
Incidence: 35 cases in American surgical literature; bilateral in up to 66%
Cause: anomalous development and course of medial head of gastrocnemius muscle, which attaches to medial femoral condyle after development of primitive popliteal artery in 20-mm embryo slinging around lateral aspect of popliteal a.
Pathophysiology:
flow unimpeded when muscle relaxed; increased arterial angulation with muscle contraction (early); progressive intimal hyperplasia ("atheroma" = misnomer) due to microtrauma in area of repeated arterial compression; ultimately occlusion / thrombosis within aneurysm (late)
Age: <35 years in 68%; age peaks at 17 and 47 years; M:F = 9:1
• slowly progressive intermittent unilateral calf claudication (early) esp. during periods of prolonged standing
• acute ischemia of leg with permanent occlusion of popliteal a. (late)
√ posterior tibial pulse obliterated during active plantar flexion against resistance
√ PVR has 40% false-positive results
√ ankle-arm index reduced during active muscle contraction
√ Doppler waveforms of posterior tibial a. diminished during muscle contractions
Angio (biplanar views with hyperextended knee):
√ medial deviation of artery (29%), popliteal stenosis (11%), poststenotic dilatation (8%)
Dx:
√ arteriography with typical medial deviation of popliteal a. before + after gastrocnemius contraction
√ popliteal a. thrombosis / occlusion
Cx: popliteal a. aneurysm
DDx: cystic adventitial disease of popliteal a., arterial embolism, premature arteriosclerosis, popliteal aneurysm with thrombosis, popliteal a. trauma, popliteal a. thrombosis, Buerger disease, spinal cord stenosis (= neurogenic claudication)

PRIMARY PULMONARY HYPERTENSION

= PLEXOGENIC PULMONARY ARTERIOPATHY
Diagnosis per exclusion:
clinically unexplained progressive pulmonary arterial hypertension without evidence for thromboembolic disease / pulmonary venoocclusive disease
At risk: portal hypertension (with / without liver disease), collagen vascular disease, HIV infection, aminorex fumarate (appetite suppressant) ingestion
Histo: plexiform + angiomatoid lesions = tortuous channels within "glomeruloid" proliferation of endothelial cells (75%); acute + organizing thrombi (50%)
Age: 3rd decade; M:F = 1:3
• progressive dyspnea (60%)
• easy fatigability, syncope, angina
• hyperventilation, hemoptysis
• Raynaud phenomenon
√ right ventricular enlargement (dilatation + hypertrophy)
√ dilatation of central pulmonary arteries
CXR:
√ prominent central pulmonary arteries:
√ enlarged pulmonary trunk
√ right descending pulmonary artery >25 mm wide

√ pulmonary vascularity:
   √ oligemia + rapidly tapering vessels
   √ overcirculation + vascular distension

CT:
√ enlargement of central pulmonary arteries:
   √ diameter of main pulmonary artery > 29 mm (87% sensitive, 89% specific) measured at scan plane of bifurcation at right angle to its long axis just lateral to ascending aorta
   √ segmental artery-to-bronchus ratio >1:1
   √ pulmonary artery-to-aorta ratio (rPA) >1
√ abruptly diminished caliber of peripheral pulmonary vessels (at outer to medial third of lung mantle)

HRCT:
√ mosaic pattern of lung attenuation (due to regional variations in lung perfusion):
   √ hyperdense areas contain large caliber vessels
   √ hypodense areas contain small caliber vessels

MR:
√ reversal of interventricular septal curvature
√ direct linear correlation between mean pulmonary artery pressure (PAP) and ratio of main pulmonary artery caliber to descending aorta (MPA/AO)
√ abnormal intravascular signal (due to slow arterial flow) in 92% on gated SE images

NUC:
√ normal / low-probability V/Q scans

Angio:
√ symmetrically enlarged central arteries
√ diffuse pattern of abruptly tapering + pruned subsegmental vessels
√ filamentous / "corkscrew" peripheral arteries
√ subpleural collaterals (occasionally)

Prognosis: death in 2–5 years

Rx: vasodilators, calcium channel blockers, diuretics, anticoagulants; lung / heart-lung transplantation

PSEUDOCOARCTATION

= AORTIC KINKING
= elongated redundant thoracic aorta with acute kink / anterior buckling just distal to origin of left subclavian artery at lig. arteriosum
= variant of coarctation without a pressure gradient

Age: 12–64 years

Associated with:
hypertension, bicuspid aortic valve, PDA, VSD, aortic / subaortic stenosis, single ventricle, ASD, anomalies of aortic arch branches

• asymptomatic
• ejection murmur
• NO pressure gradient across the buckled segment

√ anteromedial deviation of aorta
√ "chimney-shaped" high aortic arch (in children)
√ rounded / oval soft-tissue mass in left paratracheal region + superior to presumed normally positioned aortic arch [secondary to elongation of ascending aorta + aortic arch] (in adults)
√ anterior displacement of esophagus
√ NO rib notching / dilatation of brachiocephalic arteries / LV enlargement / poststenotic dilatation

Angio:
√ high position of aortic arch
√ "figure 3 sign" = notch in descending aorta at attachment of short ligamentum arteriosum

DDx: true coarctation, aneurysm, mediastinal mass

PULMONARY ARTERY PSEUDOANEURYSM

= tear / disruption of layers of vessel wall with extravasation of blood contained by adventitia / clot / compressed surrounding tissue

Cause:
A. TRAUMA
   1. Improper placement of Swan-Ganz catheter
   2. Blunt / penetrating trauma
B. INFECTION: mycotic, syphilitic, mycobacterial
C. VASCULAR ABNORMALITY: cystic medial necrosis, Behçet disease, Marfan syndrome
D. OTHER: septic emboli, neoplasm

• hemoptysis (= leakage of blood into bronchial tree)

CXR:
√ stable / increasing focal lung mass

CT:
√ enhancing round lung mass isointense to central pulmonary artery

Cx: 100% mortality with rupture

PULMONARY ATRESIA

= CONGENITAL ABSENCE OF PULMONARY ARTERY
= atretic pulmonary valve with underdeveloped pulmonary artery distally

May be associated with: hypogenetic lung

CXR:
√ small hemithorax of normal radiodensity
√ mediastinal shift to affected side
√ elevation of ipsilateral diaphragm
√ reticular network of vessels on affected side (due to systemic collateral circulation from bronchial arteries)
√ rib notching from prominence of intercostal arteries (due to large transpleural collateral vessels)

OB-US:
√ small / enlarged / normal right ventricle
√ progressive atrial enlargement (tricuspid regurgitation)
√ flow reversal in ductus arteriosus + main pulmonary artery (most reliable)

Pulmonary Atresia with Intact Interventricular Septum

Associated with: ASD (R-to-L shunt)

Type I : no remaining RV, no tricuspid regurgitation
   √ moderately enlarged RA (depending on size of ASD)

Type II : normal RV with tricuspid regurgitation
   √ massive enlargement of RA

√ cardiomegaly (LV, RA)
√ concave / small pulmonary artery segment
√ diminished pulmonary vascularity

HEART

PULMONARY VENOOCCLUSIVE DISEASE

= fibrous narrowing of intrapulmonary veins; the postcapillary counterpart of primary pulmonary hypertension

Cause: idiopathic (rare condition); venous thrombosis initiated by infection / toxic exposure / immune complex deposition

May be associated with:
pregnancy, transplantation, drug toxicity (carmustine, bleomycin, mitomycin)

Hemodynamics:
- elevated pressure in right atrium + pulmonary artery
- decreased cardiac output
- normal / variably elevated capillary wedge pressures
- normal pressure in left atrium + left ventricle (excludes cardiac disease as the cause for venous hypertension)

Age: children (33%), adolescents; M:F = 1:1

Histo:
(a) specific changes: webs, recanalized thrombus (in up to 95%), intimal fibrosis of pulmonary veins; "capillary hemangiomatosis" = sheets and nodular collections of thin-walled capillaries invading pulmonary arteries + veins + bronchioles + pleura
(b) nonspecific changes of venous hypertension: venous medial hypertrophy, septal edema + fibrosis, paraseptal venous infarction, interstitial + pleural lymphatic dilatation, intraalveolar hemosiderin-laden macrophages

- progressive dyspnea, hemoptysis
- antecedent flulike symptoms

CXR:
√ pulmonary arterial hypertension
√ diffuse interstitial pulmonary edema
√ normal-sized left atrium
√ mediastinal lymphadenopathy

CT:
√ markedly small central pulmonary veins
√ central and gravity-dependent parenchymal ground-glass attenuation
√ smoothly thickened interlobular septa
√ pleural effusions
√ normal-sized left atrium
√ centrilobular nodules

NUC:
√ patchy distribution of Tc-99m MAA (of "upstream" pulmonary arterial hypertension)

Angio:
√ enlarged right ventricle + central pulmonary arteries
√ prolonged parenchymal phase enhancement
√ delayed filling of normal pulmonary veins
√ normal to small left atrium

Prognosis: death within 3 years (no effective therapy)

Cx: potentially fatal pulmonary edema following administration of vasodilators for presumed precapillary pulmonary hypertension

Dx: often missed initially (clinical presentation + radiographic findings mimic interstitial lung disease)

PULMONIC STENOSIS

Frequency: pulmonary artery stenosis without VSD in 8% of all CHD

Embryology: infundibulum formed from proximal portion of bulbis cordis; pulmonary valves develop in 6–9th week from outgrowth of 3 tubercles

- mostly asymptomatic
- cyanosis / heart failure
- loud systolic ejection murmur

√ systolic doming of pulmonary valve (= incomplete opening)
√ normal / diminished / increased pulmonary vascularity (depending on presence + nature of associated malformations)
√ enlarged pulmonary trunk + left pulmonary artery (poststenotic dilatation)
√ prominent left pulmonary artery + normal right pulmonary artery
√ hypertrophy of RV with reduced size of RV chamber:
  √ elevation of cardiac apex
  √ increased convexity of anterior cardiac border on LAO
  √ diminution of retrosternal clear space
√ cor pulmonale
√ mild enlargement of LA (reason unknown)
√ calcification of pulmonary valves in older adults (rare)

Prognosis: death at mean age of 21 years if untreated

Subvalvular Pulmonic Stenosis

A. INFUNDIBULAR PULMONIC STENOSIS
typically in tetralogy of Fallot

B. SUBINFUNDIBULAR PULMONIC STENOSIS
= hypertrophied anomalous muscle bundles crossing portions of RV
Associated with: VSD (73–85%)
(a) low type: courses diagonally from low anterior septal side to crista posteriorly
(b) high type: horizontal defect across RV below infundibulum

√ no dilatation of PA because of dissipation of RV force through elongated area of obstruction

Valvular Pulmonic Stenosis

1. CLASSIC / TYPICAL PULMONIC VALVE STENOSIS (95%)
   = commissural fusion of pulmonary cusps
   Age of presentation: childhood
   - pulmonic click
   - ECG: hypertrophy of RV
   √ thin mobile <u>dome-shaped</u> valve
   √ jet of contrast through small central orifice
   √ dilated main + left pulmonary artery
   Rx: balloon valvuloplasty
2. DYSPLASTIC PULMONIC VALVE STENOSIS (5%)
   = thickened redundant distorted cusps, immobile secondary to myxomatous tissue
   - NO click
   √ NO poststenotic dilatation
   Rx: surgical resection of redundant valve tissue

Hemodynamics: obstruction of RV systolic ejection with pressure burden on RV

HEART

RA	↔/↑	RV	↑	Main PA	↑
Pulm. vessels		↔		LPA	↑
LA	↔	LV	↔	Ao	↔

CXR:
√ normal pulmonary vascularity
√ normal-sized heart

Angio:
√ increase in trabecular pattern of RV
√ hypertrophied crista supraventricularis (lateral projection)

Supravalvular Pulmonic Stenosis

60% of all pulmonic valve stenoses

Site of narrowing: pulmonary trunk, pulmonary bifurcation, one / both main pulmonary arteries, lobar pulmonary artery, segmental pulmonary artery

Shape of narrowing:
(a) localized with poststenotic dilatation
(b) long tubular hypoplasia

May be associated with:
(1) Valvular pulmonic stenosis, supravalvular aortic stenosis, VSD, PDA, systemic arterial stenoses
(2) Familial peripheral pulmonic stenoses + supravalvular aortic stenosis
(3) Williams-Beuren syndrome: PS, supravalvular AS, peculiar facies
(4) Ehlers-Danlos syndrome
(5) Postrubella syndrome: peripheral pulmonic stenoses, valvular pulmonic stenosis, PDA, low birth weight, deafness, cataract, mental retardation
(6) Tetralogy of Fallot / critical valvular pulmonic stenosis

Peripheral Pulmonary Artery Stenosis

Frequency: 5% of all pulmonary artery stenoses with an intact ventricular septum

RAYNAUD SYNDROME

= episodic digital ischemia in response to cold / emotional stimuli

Pathogenesis:
(1) increase in vasoconstrictor tone
(2) low blood pressure
(3) slight increase in blood viscosity
(4) immunologic factors (4–81%)
(5) cold provocation

- exaggerated response of digit to cold / emotional stress:
  - numbness + loss of tactile perception
  - demarcated pallor / cyanosis
- hyperemic throbbing during rewarming
- sclerodactyly
- small painful ulcers at tip of digit

Raynaud Disease

= PRIMARY VASOSPASM = SPASTIC FORM OF RAYNAUD SYNDROME
= exaggerated cold-induced constriction of smooth muscle cells in otherwise normal artery

Cause: ? acquired adrenoreceptor hypersensitivity

May be associated with: reflex sympathetic dystrophy, early stages of autoimmune disorders

Age: most common in young women

- usually affects all fingers of both hands equally

√ normal segmental arm + digit pressures at room temperature
√ peaked digit volume pulse = rapid rise in systole, anacrotic notch just before the peak, dicrotic notch high on the downslope

PPG:
√ flat-line tracing at low temperatures (10°–22°C) with sudden reappearance of normal waveform at 24–26°C = "threshold phenomenon"

Raynaud Phenomenon

= SECONDARY VASOSPASM WITH OBSTRUCTION
= OBSTRUCTIVE FORM OF RAYNAUD SYNDROME
= digital artery occlusion due to stenotic process in normally constricting artery / associated with an abnormally high blood viscosity

Cause:
1. Atherosclerosis (most frequent)
   (a) embolization from an upstream lesion
   (b) occlusion of major arteries supplying arm
2. Arterial trauma
3. End stage of many autoimmune disorders: eg, scleroderma, rheumatoid arthritis, systemic lupus erythematosus
4. Takayasu disease
5. Buerger disease
6. Drug intoxication (ergot, methysergide)
7. Dysproteinemia
8. Primary pulmonary hypertension
9. Myxedema

- normal vasoconstrictive response to cold

√ reduced segmental arm + digit pressures at room temperature

PPG (76% sensitivity, 92% specificity):
√ flat-line / barely detectable tracing at low temperature with gradual increase of amplitude upon rewarming

Hand magnification angiography:
1. Baseline angiogram with ambient temperature
2. Stress angiogram immediately following immersion of hand in ice water for 20 seconds

RHABDOMYOMA OF HEART

= benign myocardial hamartoma

Prevalence: most common cardiac tumor in infancy + childhood (up to 90%)

Age: usually discovered <1 year of age

Path: well-circumscribed intramural lobulated nodule / multiple <1 mm nodules (= rhabdomyomatosis)

Histo: "spider cells" = enlarged vacuolated cells with high glycogen content + central nucleus surrounded by clear cytoplasm and radial extensions

Associated with: tuberous sclerosis (in 50–86%); congenital heart disease

- asymptomatic (incidental detection at prenatal US / screening)
- murmur, arrhythmia
- heart failure (secondary to obstruction of outflow tract / reduction of enddiastolic volume / decreased contractility)
- supraventricular tachycardia (accessory conductive pathways within tumor)

Location: usually multiple; ventricular wall with intramural growth + tendency to involve interventricular septum; atrial wall (rare)

Size: up to 10 cm in diameter (average 3–4 cm)

US (good for small intramural lesions):

√ fetal nonimmune hydrops
√ solid echogenic sessile mass ± intracavitary component bulging into ventricular outflow tract / atrioventricular valve
√ diffuse myocardial thickening (with multiple small lesions)

MR (complimentary to US):

√ tumor isointense on T1WI + hyperintense to myocardium on T2WI

Prognosis: may regress spontaneously in patients <4 years of age

Rx: surgical excision for life-threatening symptoms

DDx: fibroma (solitary centrally calcified + cystic tumor, in ventricular myocardium, associated with Gorlin syndrome), teratoma (single intrapericardial multicystic mass), hemangioma (arise from RT atrium, pericardial effusion, skin hemangiomas)

SINGLE VENTRICLE

= UNIVENTRICULAR HEART = DOUBLE INLET SINGLE VENTRICLE

= failure of development of interventricular septum ± absence of one atrioventricular valve (mitral / tricuspid atresia) ± aortic / pulmonic stenosis

Associated with: TGV or DORV

- conduction defect (aberrant anatomy of conduction system)

√ two atrioventricular valves connected to a main ventricular chamber
√ the single ventricle may be a LV (85%) / RV / undetermined
√ a second rudimentary ventricular chamber may be present, which is located anteriorly (in left univentricle) / posteriorly (in right univentricle):
 √ rudimentary chamber ± connection to one great artery
√ may be associated with tricuspid / mitral atresia

SINUS OF VALSALVA ANEURYSM

= deficiency between aortic media + annulus fibrosis of aortic valve resulting in distension + eventual aneurysm formation

Age: puberty to 30 years of age

Site: right sinus / noncoronary sinus (>90%)

◊ Right sinus usually ruptures into RV, occasionally into RA
◊ Noncoronary sinus ruptures into RA

- sudden retrosternal pain, dyspnea, continuous murmur

√ shunt vascularity
√ cardiomegaly
√ prominent ascending aorta

SPLENIC ARTERY ANEURYSM

= most frequent of visceral artery aneurysms

Etiology: medial degeneration with superimposed atherosclerosis, congenital, mycotic, pancreatitis, trauma, portal hypertension (7–10% of cases due to high flow rate)

Predisposed: women with ≥2 pregnancies (88%)

May be associated with: fibromuscular disease (in 20%)

M:F = 1:2

- usually asymptomatic
- pain, GI bleeding

Location: intra- / extrasplenic

√ calcified wall of aneurysm (2/3)

Cx: rupture of aneurysm (6–9%, higher during pregnancy) especially if >1.5 cm in diameter

Mortality: up to 76%

DDx: renal artery aneurysm, tortuous splenic artery

SUBCLAVIAN STEAL SYNDROME

= stenosis / obstruction of subclavian artery near its origin with flow reversal in ipsilateral vertebral artery at the expense of the cerebral circulation

Incidence: 2.5% of all extracranial arterial occlusions

Etiology:

(a) congenital: interruption of aortic arch, preductal infantile coarctation, hypoplasia of left aortic arch, hypoplasia / atresia / stenosis of an anomalous left subclavian artery with right aortic arch, coarctation with aberrant subclavian artery arising distal to the coarctation

(b) acquired: atherosclerosis (94%), dissecting aneurysm, chest trauma, embolism, tumor thrombosis, inflammatory arteritis (Takayasu, syphilitic), ligation of subclavian artery in Blalock-Taussig shunt, complication of coarctation repair, radiation fibrosis

Age: average 59–61 years; M:F = 3:1; Whites:Blacks = 8:2

Associated with: additional lesions of extracranial arteries in 81%

- lower systolic blood pressure by >20–40 mm Hg on affected side
- delayed weak / absent pulse in ipsilateral extremity
- signs of vertebrobasilar insufficiency (40%):
  - syncopal episodes initiated by exercising the ischemic arm
  - headaches, nausea, vertigo, ataxia
  - mono-, hemi-, para-, quadriparesis, paralysis
  - diplopia, dysphagia, dysarthria, paresthesias around mouth
  - uni- / bilateral homonymous hemianopia

- signs of brachial insufficiency (3–10%):
  - intermittent / constant pain in affected arm precipitated by increased activity of that arm
  - paresthesia, weakness, coolness, numbness, burning in fingers + hand
  - fingertip necrosis

Location: L:R = 3:1

Color Doppler:

√ reversal of vertebral artery flow, augmented by reactive hyperemia (blood pressure cuff inflated above systolic pressure for 5 minutes) / arm exercise

Angio:

√ subclavian stenosis / occlusion (aortic arch injection)

√ reversal of vertebral artery flow (selective injection of contralateral subclavian / vertebral artery)

CAVE: "false steal" = transient retrograde flow in contralateral vertebral artery caused by high-pressure injection

Rx: bypass surgery, PTA (good long-term results)

Partial Subclavian Steal Syndrome

= retrograde flow in systole + antegrade flow in diastole

Occult Subclavian Steal Syndrome

= reverse flow seen only after provocative maneuvers, ie, ipsilateral arm exercise of 5 minutes / 5 minutes inflation of sphygmomanometer > systolic blood pressure levels

SUPERIOR VENA CAVA SYNDROME

= obstruction of SVC with development of collateral pathways

Etiology:

(a) Malignant lesion (80–90%)
1. Bronchogenic carcinoma (>50%)
2. Lymphoma

(b) Benign lesion
1. Granulomatous mediastinitis (usually histoplasmosis, sarcoidosis, TB)
2. Substernal goiter
3. Ascending aortic aneurysm
4. Pacer wires / central venous catheters (23%)
5. Constrictive pericarditis

Collateral routes:
1. Esophageal venous plexus = "downhill varices" (predominantly upper 2/3)
2. Azygos + hemiazygos veins
3. Accessory hemiazygos + superior intercostal veins = "aortic nipple" (visualization in normal population in 5%)
4. Lateral thoracic veins + umbilical vein
5. Vertebral veins

- head and neck edema (70%)
- cutaneous enlarged venous collaterals
- headache, dizziness, syncope
- with benign etiology: slower onset + progression, both sexes, 25–40 years of age
- with malignancy: rapid progression within weeks, mostly males, 40–60 years of age
- proptosis, tearing
- dyspnea, cyanosis, chest pain
- hematemesis (11%)

√ superior mediastinal widening (64%)

√ encasement / compression / occlusion of SVC

√ dilated cervical + superficial thoracic veins (80%)

√ SVC thrombus

NUC:

√ increased tracer uptake in quadrate lobe + posterior aspect of medial segment of left lobe (umbilical pathway toward liver when injected in upper extremity)

SYPHILITIC AORTITIS

= LUETIC AORTITIS

Incidence: in 10–15% of untreated patients (accounts for death in 1/3)

Path: periaortitis (via lymphatics), mesaortitis (via vasa vasorum) = primarily disease of media leading to secondary injury of intima, which predisposes the intima to premature calcific atherosclerosis

Age: between 40 and 65 years

Site: ascending aorta (36%), aortic arch (24%), descending aorta (5%), sinus of Valsalva (1%), pulmonary artery

√ thick aortic wall (fibrous + inflammatory tissue)

√ saccular (75%) / fusiform (25%) dilatation of ascending aorta

√ small saccular aneurysms often protrude from fusiform aneurysm

√ fine pencil-like calcifications of intima (15–20%) in ascending aorta, late in disease

Cx: (1) stenosis of coronary ostia (intimal thickening)
(2) aortic regurgitation (syphilitic valvulitis), rare

DDx: degenerative calcification of ascending aorta (older population, no aneurysm, no aortic regurgitation)

TAKAYASU ARTERITIS

= PULSELESS DISEASE = AORTITIS SYNDROME
= AORTOARTERITIS = IDIOPATHIC MEDIAL AORTOPATHY
= AORTIC ARCH SYNDROME

= granulomatous inflammation of unknown pathogenesis affecting segments of aorta + major aortic branches + pulmonary arteries limited to persons usually <50 years of age

◊ The only form of aortitis that produces stenosis / occlusion of the aorta!

Etiology: probably cell-mediated inflammation

Incidence: 2.6 new cases/million/year;
2.2% (at autopsy)

Age: 12–66 years; M:F = 1:8; especially in Orientals

Histo: (a) Acute stage: granulomatous infiltrative process focused on elastic fibers of media of arterial wall consisting of multinucleated giant cells, lymphocytes, histiocytes, plasma cells

(b) Fibrotic stage (weeks to years): progressive fibrosis of vessel wall resulting in constriction from intimal proliferation / thrombotic occlusion / aneurysm formation (from extensive destruction of elastic fibers in the media); ultimately leads to fibrosis of intima + adventitia

◊ Morphologically indistinguishable from temporal arteritis!

- prepulseless / systemic phase of a few months to a year = nonspecific systemic signs + symptoms of fever, night sweats, weakness, weight loss, myalgia, arthralgia
  - ◊ Mean interval of 8 years between onset of symptoms and diagnosis
- pulseless phase = signs + symptoms of ischemia of limb (claudication, pulse deficit, bruits) + renovascular hypertension
- erythrocyte sedimentation rate (ESR) >20 mm/hour in 80%

Location:

Type I : classic pulseless type = brachiocephalic trunk + carotid arteries + subclavian arteries

Type II : combination of type I + III

Type III : atypical coarctation type = thoracic and abdominal aorta distal to arch + its major branches

Type IV : dilated type = extensive dilatation of the length of the aorta + its branches

Commonly involved: left subclavian artery (<50%), left common carotid artery (20%), brachiocephalic trunk, renal arteries, celiac trunk, superior mesenteric artery, pulmonary arteries (>50%)

Infrequently involved: axillary, brachial, vertebral, iliac arteries (usually bilaterally), coronary arteries

Angiography:

difficult catheterization / risk of ischemic complications (increase in coagulation)

√ arterial wall thickening + contrast enhancement

√ full-thickness calcification (chronic disease)

√ mural thrombi

@ Aorta

√ long + diffuse / short + segmental irregular stenosis / occlusion of major branches of aorta near their origins

√ stenotic lesions of descending thoracic aorta > abdominal aorta

√ frequent skipped lesions

√ abundant collateralization (late phase)

√ aneurysmal dilatation of ascending aorta + arch = diffusely dilated lumen with irregular contours

√ fusiform / saccular aortic aneurysms (10–15%) (common in descending thoracic + abdominal aorta)

@ Brachiocephalic arteries

√ multisegmented dilatation of carotid artery producing segmental septa

√ diffuse homogeneous circumferential thickening of vessel wall in proximal common carotid artery

√ increase in flow velocity + turbulence

√ distal CCA, ICA, ECA spared with dampened waveforms

@ Pulmonary arteries (50–80%)

√ dilatation of pulmonary trunk (19%)

√ nodular thrombi (3%)

√ "pruned tree" appearance of pulmonary arteries (66%)

√ systemic-pulmonary artery shunts

CXR:

√ widened supracardiac shadow >3.0 cm

√ wavy / scalloped appearance of lateral margin of descending aorta

√ aortic calcification (15%) commonly in aortic arch + descending aorta

√ focal decrease of pulmonary vascularity

Cx: (1) Cerebrovascular accidents

(2) Heart failure due to aortic regurgitation

DDx: atherosclerosis, temporal arteritis (CCA not involved), fibromuscular dysplasia (in ICA not CCA), idiopathic carotid dissection (ICA), syphilitic aortitis (calcification of ascending aorta)

Rx: steroids, angioplasty after decline of active inflammation

TEMPORAL ARTERITIS

= CRANIAL / GRANULOMATOUS ARTERITIS

= POLYMYALGIA RHEUMATICA = GIANT CELL ARTERITIS (poor choice because Takayasu disease is also a giant cell arteritis)

= systemic granulomatous vasculitis limited to persons usually >50 years of age

Incidence: 1.7 new cases/million/year

Histo:

(a) acute stage: granulomatous infiltrative process focused on elastic fibers of arterial wall consisting of multinucleated giant cells, lymphocytes, histiocytes, plasma cells

(b) fibrotic stage (weeks to years): progressive fibrosis of vessel wall resulting in constriction from intimal proliferation / thrombotic occlusion / aneurysm formation

◊ Morphologically indistinguishable from Takayasu arteritis!

Age peak: 65–75 years; M:F = 1:3

- prodromal phase of flulike illness of 1–3 weeks:
  - malaise, low-grade fever, weight loss, myalgia
  - unilateral headache (50–90%)
- chronic stage:
  - jaw claudication (while chewing + talking)
  - palpable tender temporal artery
  - neuroophthalmic manifestations: visual impairment / diplopia / blindness
  - polymyalgia rheumatica (50%) = intense myalgia of shoulder + hip girdles
- erythrocyte sedimentation rate (ESR) of 40–140 mm/hour (HALLMARK)

Location: any artery of the body; mainly medium-sized branches of aortic arch (10%), external carotid artery branches (particularly temporal artery); extracranial arteries below neck (9%): subclavian > axillary > brachial > profunda femoris > forearm > calf; commonly bilateral + symmetric

HEART

√ long smooth stenotic arterial segments with skip areas
√ smooth tapered occlusions with abundance of collateral supply
√ absence of atherosclerotic changes
√ aortic root dilatation + aortic valve insufficiency

Dx: biopsy of palpable temporal artery

Prognosis: disease may be self-limiting (1–2 years); 10% mortality within 2–3 years

TETRALOGY OF FALLOT

= underdevelopment of pulmonary infundibulum secondary to unequal partitioning of the conotruncus

Frequency: 8% of all CHD; most common CHD with cyanosis after 1 year of life

TETRAD:

1. Obstruction of right ventricular outflow tract: usually of pulmonary infundibulum, occasionally of pulmonic valve
2. Large VSD immediately below aortic valve
3. Right ventricular hypertrophy secondary to elevated RV systolic pressure
4. Overriding aorta straddling the VSD and receiving blood from both ventricles

Embryology:

abnormal spiraling caudad growth of truncoconal ridges in 3rd–4th week causing unequal partitioning of the conotruncus into a small underdeveloped anteromedial pulmonary infundibulum + large posterolateral LV outflow tract

Hemodynamics:

fetus : pulmonary blood flow supplied by retrograde flow through ductus arteriosus with absence of RV hypertrophy / IUGR

neonate : R-to-L shunt bypassing pulmonary circulation with decrease in systemic oxygen saturation (cyanosis); pressure overload + hypertrophy of RV secondary to pulmonic-infundibular stenosis

RA	↔/↑	RV	↑	Main PA	↓
Pulm. vessels		↓		LPA	↑
LA	↔	LV	↔	Ao	↑

Associated with:

1. Bicuspid pulmonic valve (40%)
2. Stenosis of left pulmonary artery (40%)
3. Right aortic arch (25%)
4. TE fistula
5. Down syndrome
6. Forked ribs, scoliosis
7. Anomalies of coronary arteries in 10% (single RCA / LAD from RCA)

- cyanosis by 3–4 months of age (concealed at birth by PDA)
- dyspnea on exertion, clubbing of fingers and toes
- "squatting position" when fatigued (increases pulmonary blood flow)
- "episodic spells" = loss of consciousness
- polycythemia, lowered PO_2 values, systolic murmur in pulmonic area

√ coeur en sabot (boot-shaped heart) = enlargement of right ventricle
√ pronounced concavity in region of pulmonary artery trunk (small / absent PA)
√ marked reduction in caliber + number of pulmonary vessels:
  √ asymmetric pulmonary vascularity
  √ reticular pattern with horizontal course usually in periphery (= prominent collateral circulation of bronchial vessels + pleuropulmonary connections)
√ enlarged aorta
√ right-sided aortic arch in 25%

OB-US:
  √ dilated aorta overriding the interventricular septum
  √ usually perimembranous VSD
  √ mildly stenotic RV outflow tract
  √ NO RV hypertrophy in midtrimester

ECHO:
  √ discontinuity between anterior aortic wall + interventricular septum (= overriding of the aorta)
  √ small left atrium
  √ RV hypertrophy with small right ventricular outflow tract
  √ widening of the aorta
  √ thickening of right ventricular wall + interventricular septum

Prognosis: spontaneous survival without surgical correction in 50% up to age 7; in 10% up to age 21

Rx: surgery in early childhood

(a) palliative
   1. Blalock-Taussig shunt = end-to-side anastomosis of subclavian to pulmonary artery opposite aortic arch (64% survival rate at 15 years, 55% at 20 years)
   2. Pott operation on left = anastomosis of left PA with descending aorta
   3. Waterston-Cooley procedure = anastomosis between ascending aorta + right pulmonary artery
   4. Central shunt = Rastelli procedure = tubular synthetic graft between ascending aorta + pulmonary artery

(b) corrective open cardiac surgery = VSD-closure + reconstruction of RV outflow tract by excision of obstructing tissue (82% survival rate at 15 years)

Operative mortality: 3–10%

Pink Tetralogy

= infundibular hypertrophy in VSD (3%)

Pentalogy of Fallot

= tetralogy + ASD

Trilogy of Fallot (infantile presentation)

(1) severe pulmonic valvular stenosis
(2) hypertrophy of RV
(3) ASD with R-to-L shunt (increased pressure in RA forces foramen ovale open)

HEART

THORACIC OUTLET SYNDROME

= compression of nerves, veins, and arteries between chest and arm

Cause:

A. CONGENITAL
1. Cervical rib
2. Scalenus minimus muscle (rare) extending from transverse process of 7th cervical vertebra to 1st rib with insertion between brachial plexus + subclavian artery
3. Anterior scalene muscle = scalenus anticus syndrome (most common) = wide / abnormal insertion / hypertrophy of muscle
4. Anomalous 1st rib = unusually straight course with narrowing of costoclavicular space

B. ACQUIRED
1. Muscular body habitus = arterial compression in pectoralis minor tunnel
2. Slender body habitus with long neck, sagging shoulders
3. Fracture of clavicle / 1st rib (34%) with nonanatomic alignment / exuberant callus
4. Supraclavicular tumor / lymphadenopathy

- pain in forearm + hand that increases upon elevation of arm
- paresthesias of hand + fingers (numbness, "pins and needles") in 95%
- decreased skin temperature, discoloration of hand
- intermittent claudication of fingers (from ischemia)
- hyperabduction maneuver with obliteration of radial pulse (34%)
- Raynaud phenomenon (40%): episodic constriction of small vessels
- supraclavicular bruit (15–30%)

Bidirectional Doppler:
1. Adson maneuver (for scalenus anticus muscle) = hold deep inspiration while neck is fully extended + head turned toward ipsilateral and opposite side

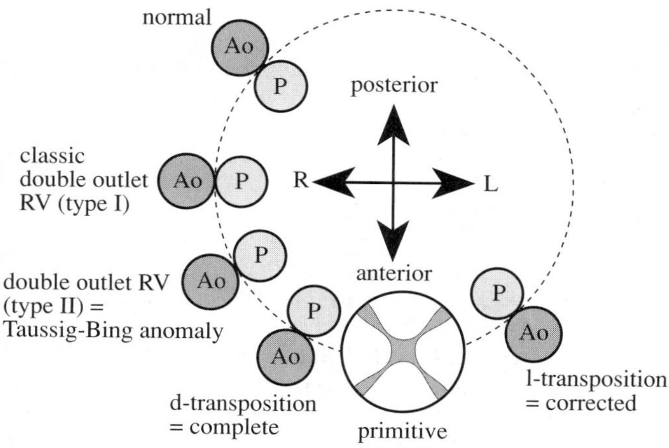

Variations of Transpositions

2. Costoclavicular maneuver (compression between clavicle + 1st rib) = exaggerated military position with shoulders drawn back and downward
3. Hyperabduction maneuver (compression by humeral head / pectoralis minor muscle) = extremity monitored through range of 180° abduction

√ complete cessation of flow in one position

Photoplethysmography:
1. Photo pulse transducer secured to palmar surface of one fingertip of each hand
2. Arterial pulsations recorded with arm in
   (a) neutral position
   (b) extended 90° to side
   (c) 180° over the head
   (d) in "military" position with arms at 90° + shoulders pressed back

√ complete disappearance of pulse in one position

Angio:
√ abnormal course of distal subclavian artery
√ focal stenosis / occlusion
√ poststenotic dilatation of distal subclavian artery
√ aneurysm
√ stress test: bandlike / concentric constriction
√ mural thrombus ± distal embolization
√ venous thrombosis / obstruction

DDx: Cervical disk disease, radiculopathy, spinal cord tumor, trauma to brachial plexus, arthritis, carpal tunnel syndrome, Pancoast tumor, peripheral arterial occlusive disease, aneurysm, causalgia, thromboembolism, Raynaud disease, vasculitis

TRANSPOSITION OF GREAT ARTERIES

Complete Transposition of Great Arteries

= TGA = D-TRANSPOSITION

= great vessels originate from inappropriate ventricle:
(1) aorta originating from RV with an infundibulum
(2) pulmonary artery originating from LV
(3) normal position of atria + ventricles

Embryology:
failure of the aorticopulmonary septum (= truncoconal ridges) to follow a spiral course

Incidence: 10% of all CHD

VARIATIONS:
1. Complete TGA + intact interventricular septum
2. Complete TGA + VSD: CHF due to VSD
3. Complete TGA + VSD + PS: PS prevents CHF = longest survival

Hemodynamics:
fetus : no hemodynamic compromise with normal birth weight
neonate : mixing of the 2 independent circulations necessary for survival

Admixture of blood from both circulations via:
(1) PDA (carries aortic blood into pulmonary artery) + patent foramen ovale (allows saturated blood to enter RA from LA)
Prognosis: worst when PDA closes
(2) VSD (in 50%)

HEART

RA	↑	RV	↑	Main PA	↔
Pulm. vessels		↑			
LA	↔	LV	↔	Ao	↔

- cyanosis (most common cause for cyanosis in neonate) 2nd most common cause of cyanosis after tetralogy of Fallot
- symptomatic 1–2 weeks following birth

CXR:
- √ "egg-on-its-side" appearance of heart = narrow superior mediastinum secondary to hypoplastic thymus + hyperaeration + abnormal relationship of great vessels
- √ cardiac enlargement beginning 2 weeks after birth
- √ right heart enlargement
- √ enlargement of LA (with VSD)
- √ absent pulmonary trunk (99%) = PA located posteriorly in midline
- √ increased pulmonary blood flow (if not associated with PS)
- √ midline aorta (30%) / ascending aorta with convexity to the right
- √ right aortic arch in 3% (difficult assessment due to midline position + small size)

OB-US:
- √ great arteries arise from ventricles in a parallel fashion
- √ aorta anterior + to right of pulmonary artery (in 60%; rarely side by side)

Prognosis: overall 70% survival rate at 1 week, 50% at 1 month, 11% at 1 year by natural history

Rx:
- (1) Prostaglandin E1 administration to maintain ductal patency
- (2) Rashkind procedure = balloon septostomy to create ASD
- (3) Blalock-Hanlon procedure = surgical creation of ASD
- (4) Mustard operation (corrective) = removal of atrial septum + creation of intraatrial baffle directing the pulmonary venous return to RV + systemic venous return to LV; 79% 1-year survival rate; 64–89% 5-year survival

Corrected Transposition of Great Arteries

= CONGENITALLY CORRECTED TRANSPOSITION
= L-TRANSPOSITION

= anomalous looping of the bulboventricular loop (= primordial ventricles) associated with lack of spiral rotation of conotruncal septum characterized by
- (1) Transposition of great arteries
- (2) Inversion of ventricles (LV on right side, RV on left side):
  - (a) RA connected to morphologic LV
  - (b) LA connected to morphologic RV
- (3) AV valves + coronary arteries follow their corresponding ventricles

Hemodynamics: functionally corrected abnormality

Associated with:
- (1) usually perimembranous VSD (in >50%)
- (2) pulmonic stenosis (in 50%)
- (3) anomaly of left (= tricuspid) atrioventricular valves (Ebstein-like)
- (4) dextrocardia (high incidence)

- NO cyanosis
- atrioventricular block (malalignment of atrial + ventricular septa)

CXR:
- √ abnormal convexity / straightening in upper portion of left heart border (ascending aorta arising from inverted RV)
- √ inapparent aortic knob + descending aorta (overlying spine)
- √ inapparent pulmonary trunk (rightward posterior position) = PREMIER SIGN
- √ humped contour of lower left heart border with elevation above diaphragm (anatomic RV)
- √ apical notch (= septal notch)
- √ increased pulmonary blood flow (if shunt present)
- √ pulmonary venous hypertension (if left-sided AV valve incompetent)
- √ LA enlargement

Angio:
- √ original LV on right side: smooth-walled, cylinder- / cone-shaped with high recess emptying into aorta (= venous ventricle)
- √ original RV on left side: bulbous, triangular shape, trabeculated chamber with infundibular outflow tract into pulmonary trunk (= arterial ventricle)

OB-US:
- √ great arteries arise from ventricles in a parallel fashion
- √ aortic valve separated from tricuspid valve by a complete infundibulum
- √ fibrous continuity between pulmonic valve + mitral valve

Prognosis: (unfavorable secondary to additional cardiac defects) 40% 1-year survival rate, 30% 10-year survival rate

TRICUSPID ATRESIA

2nd most common cause of pronounced neonatal cyanosis (after transposition) characterized by
- (1) absent tricuspid valve
- (2) ASD
- (3) small VSD (in most patients)

Frequency: 1.5% of all CHD

Embryology: imbalanced tissue proliferation + resorption results in absence of valvular tissue

1. TRICUSPID ATRESIA WITHOUT TRANSPOSITION (80%)
   (a) without PS, (b) with PS, (c) with pulmonary atresia
2. TRICUSPID ATRESIA WITH TRANSPOSITION
   (a) without PS, (b) with PS [most favorable combination], (c) with pulmonary atresia

◊ Usually small VSD + PS (75%) restrict pulmonary blood flow

HEART

Hemodynamics:
absent tricuspid valve forces blood from an enlarged RA through an ASD into LA (R-to-L shunt); pulmonary blood flow limited by pulmonary valvular stenosis

RA	↑	RV	↓	Main PA	↓
Pulm. vessels		↓			
LA	↑	LV	↑	Ao	↑

- progressive cyanosis from birth on, increasing with crying = OUTSTANDING FEATURE (inverse relationship between degree of cyanosis + volume of pulmonary blood flow)
- pansystolic murmur (VSD)
- ECG: left-axis deviation

CXR (typical cardiac contour):
√ heart size ranging from normal to moderately enlarged (depending on volume of pulmonary blood flow and size of RA)
√ left rounded contour = enlargement + hypertrophy of LV
√ right rounded contour = enlarged RA
√ flat / concave pulmonary segment
√ normal / decreased pulmonary vascularity
√ typical flattening of right heart border with transposition (in 15%)

Prognosis: may survive well into early adulthood
Rx:
(1) Blalock-Taussig procedure (if pulmonary blood flow decreased in infancy)
(2) Glenn procedure = shunt between IVC + right PA (if total correction not anticipated)
(3) Fontan procedure = external conduit from RA to pulmonary trunk + closure of ASD (if pulmonary vascular disease has not developed)

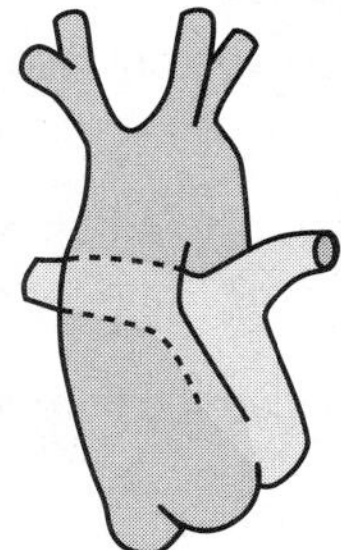
Type I

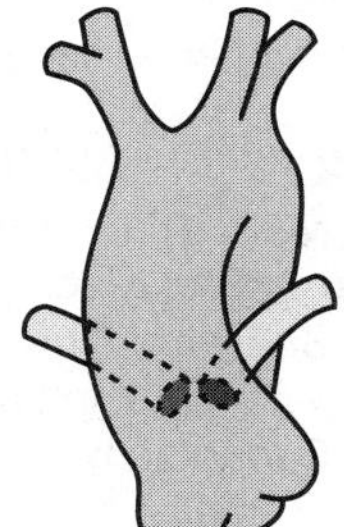
Type II

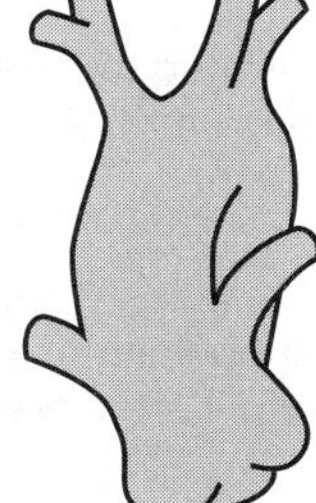
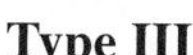
Type III

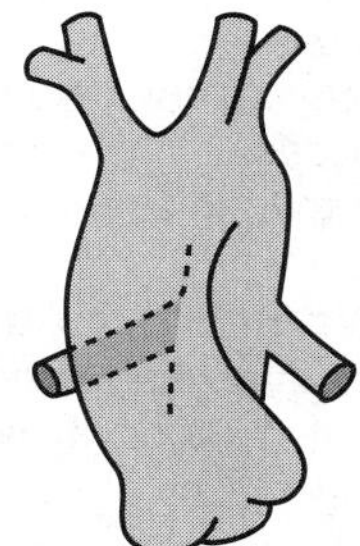
Type IV

Variations in Truncus Arteriosus

TRICUSPID INSUFFICIENCY

Cause:
1. Right ventricular failure (most common)
2. Carcinoid syndrome
3. Bacterial endocarditis
4. Rheumatic heart disease
5. Congenital heart disease: Ebstein anomaly, atrioventricular cushion defect

√ normal / reduced pulmonary vascularity
√ cardiomegaly
√ RA + RV enlargement
√ distension of IVC > SVC

TROUSSEAU SYNDROME

= PARANEOPLASTIC THROMBOEMBOLISM
Incidence: 1–11%; higher in terminally ill cancer patients
Tumors: mucin-secreting adenocarcinoma of GI tract and pancreas (most common), lung, breast, ovary, prostate
Pathogenesis: (?)
(a) tumors activate coagulation + depress anticoagulant function
(b) cancer cells cause injury to endothelial lining, activate platelets + coagulation

Type of lesion: (1) Venous thrombosis
(2) Arterial thromboembolism
(3) Nonbacterial thrombotic endocarditis

◊ Patients with thromboembolism have an increased incidence of occult malignancy!

Prevalent criteria:
— absence of apparent cause for thromboembolism
— age >50 years
— multiple sites of venous thrombosis
— simultaneous venous + arterial thromboembolism
— resistance to oral anticoagulant therapy
— associated other paraneoplastic syndromes
— regression of thromboembolism with successful treatment of cancer

- disorders of consciousness (cerebral emboli)
- muscular pain + weakness (emboli to skeletal muscle)
- decompensated disseminated intravascular coagulation

√ deep vein thrombosis
√ pulmonary embolism
√ nonbacterial thrombotic endocarditis (echocardiography)

Rx: (1) Heparin (more successful than warfarin)
(2) Greenfield filter

TRUNCUS ARTERIOSUS

= PERSISTENT TRUNCUS ARTERIOSUS = SINGLE OUTLET OF THE HEART
= failure of septation of the conotruncus characterized by
(1) one great artery arising from the heart giving rise to the coronary, pulmonary, and systemic arteries, and straddling a
(2) large VSD

Incidence: 2% of all CHD
Types:
Type I (50%) = main PA + aorta arise from common truncal valve

Type II (25%) = both pulmonary arteries arise from back of trunk
Type III (10%) = both pulmonary arteries arise from side of trunk
Type IV = "pseudotruncus" = absence of pulmonary arteries; pulmonary supply from systemic collaterals arising from descending aorta
Subtype A = infundibular VSD present
Subtype B = VSD absent

Associated with:
(1) Right aortic arch (in 35%)
◊ right aortic arch + cyanosis + shunt vascularity = TRUNCUS
(2) Forked ribs

Hemodynamics:
admixture lesion (R-to-L and L-to-R shunt across VSD) with volume of pulmonary blood flow inversely related to degree of pulmonary vascular resistance
fetus : CHF only with incompetent valve secondary to massive regurgitation from truncus to ventricles
neonate : L-to-R shunt after decrease in pulmonary resistance (massive diversion of flow to pulmonary district) leads to CHF (ventricular overload) / pulmonary hypertension with time

RA	↔	RV	↑	Trunk	↑
Pulm. vessels		↑			
LA	↔	LV	↑		

- moderate cyanosis (degree inversely related to volume of pulmonary blood flow), apparent with crying
- severe CHF within first days / months of life (in large R-to-L shunt)
- systolic murmur (similar to VSD)
- early diastolic murmur (with truncal insufficiency)
- wide pulse pressure

CXR:
√ cardiomegaly:
√ increased volume of both ventricles
√ enlarged LA (50%) secondary to increased pulmonary blood flow
√ wide mediastinum due to large "aortic shadow" = truncus arteriosus
√ "waterfall / hilar comma sign" = elevated right hilum (30%); elevated left hilum (10%)
√ concave pulmonary segment (50%) (type I has left convex pulmonary segment)
√ markedly increased pulmonary blood flow, may be asymmetric

ECHO:
√ single arterial vessel overriding the interventricular septum (DDx: tetralogy of Fallot)
√ frequently dysplastic single semilunar valve with 3–6 leaflets (most commonly 3 leaflets)
√ truncal valve may be stenotic
√ truncal valve insufficiency with age (in 25%)

Prognosis: 40% 6-months survival rate, 20% 1-year survival rate

Rx: Rastelli procedure (30% no longer operable at 4 years of age) = (a) artificial valve placed high in RVOT and attached via a Dacron graft to main pulmonary artery (b) closure of VSD

Hemitruncus

= rare anomaly characterized by
(a) one pulmonary artery (commonly right PA) arising from trunk
(b) one pulmonary artery arising from RV / supplied by systemic collaterals

Associated with: PDA (80%), VSD, tetralogy (usually isolated to left PA)

- acyanotic

Pseudotruncus Arteriosus

= TRUNCUS TYPE IV
= severe form of tetralogy of Fallot with atresia of the pulmonary trunk; entire pulmonary circulation through bronchial collateral arteries (NOT a form of truncus arteriosus in its true sense); characterized by
(1) pulmonary atresia
(2) VSD with R-to-L shunt
(3) RV hypertrophy

Associated with: right aortic arch in 50%

- cyanosis

√ concavity in area of pulmonary segment
√ commalike abnormal appearance of pulmonary artery
√ absent normal right and left pulmonary artery (lateral chest film)
√ esophageal indentation posteriorly (due to large systemic collaterals)
√ prominent hilar + intrapulmonary vessels (= systemic collaterals)
√ "coeur en sabot" = RV enlargement
√ prominent ascending aorta with hyperpulsations

VENTRICULAR ANEURYSM

A. CONGENITAL LEFT VENTRICULAR ANEURYSM
rare, young Black adult
(1) Submitral type:
√ bulge at left middle / upper cardiac border
(2) Subaortic type:
√ small + not visualized
√ heart greatly enlarged (from aortic insufficiency)

B. ACQUIRED LEFT VENTRICULAR ANEURYSM
= complication of myocardial infarction, Chagas disease
- may be asymptomatic + well tolerated for years
- occasionally associated with persistent heart failure, arrhythmia, peripheral embolization

True Ventricular Aneurysm

= circumscribed noncontractile outpouching of ventricular cavity with broad mouth + localized dyskinesis

Cause: sequelae of transmural myocardial infarction

Location:
(a) left anterior + anteroapical: readily detected (anterior + LAO views)

(b) inferior + inferoposterior: less readily detected (steep LAO + LPO views)

Detection rate: 50% by fluoroscopy; 96% by radionuclide ventriculography; frequently not visible on CXR

√ localized bulge of heart contour = "squared-off" appearance of mid left lateral margin of heart border
√ localized paradoxical expansion during systole (CHARACTERISTIC)
√ rim of calcium in fibrotic wall (chronic), rare
√ akinetic / severely hypokinetic segment
√ left ventriculography in LAO, RAO is diagnostic
√ wide communication with heart chamber (no neck)

Cx: wall thrombus with embolization

Prognosis: rarely ruptures

Pseudoaneurysm of Ventricle

= FALSE ANEURYSM = left ventricular rupture contained by fused layers of visceral + parietal pericardium / extracardiac tissue

(a) cardiac rupture with localized hematoma contained by adherent pericardium; typically in the presence of pericarditis

(b) subacute rupture with gradual / episodic bleeding

Etiology: trauma, myocardial infarction

Location: typically at posterolateral / diaphragmatic wall of LV

√ left retrocardiac double density
√ diameter of mouth smaller than the largest diameter of the globular aneurysm
√ delayed filling

Cx: high risk of delayed rupture (infrequent in true aneurysms)

VENTRICULAR SEPTAL DEFECT

Most common CHD (25–30%):

(a) isolated in 20%

(b) with other cardiac anomalies in 5% (PDA, coarctation of aorta)

◊ Acyanotic L-to-R shunt + right aortic arch (in 2–5%) = VSD

Embryology:

single ventricular chamber divides into two by fusion of membranous portion of ventricular septum + endocardial cushions + bulbis cordis (= proximal part of truncus arteriosus) between 4–8th week

1. MEMBRANOUS = PERIMEMBRANOUS VSD (75–80%)

   Location: posterior + inferior to crista supraventricularis near commissure between right and posterior (= noncoronary) aortic valve cusps

   May be associated with:

   small aneurysms of membranous septum commonly leading to decrease in size of membranous VSD (their presence does not necessarily predict eventual complete closure)

2. SUPRACRISTAL = CONAL VSD (5–8%)

   ◊ Crista supraventricularis = inverted U-shaped muscular ridge posterior + inferior to pulmonary valve

   (a) RV view = VSD just beneath pulmonary valve with valve forming part of superior margin of defect

   (b) LV view = VSD just below commissure between R + L aortic valve cusps

   Cx: right aortic valve cusp may herniate into VSD (= aortic insufficiency)

3. MUSCULAR VSD (5–10%)

   May consist of multiple VSDs; bordered entirely by myocardium

   Location: (a) inlet portion
   (b) trabecular portion
   (c) infundibular / outlet portion

4. ATRIOVENTRICULAR CANAL TYPE
   = ENDOCARDIAL CUSHION TYPE
   = POSTERIOR VSD (5–10%)

   Location: adjacent to septal + anterior leaflet of mitral valve; rare as isolated defect

Hemodynamics:

small bidirectional shunt during fetal life (similar pressures in RV + LV); after birth pulmonary arterial pressure decreases + systemic arterial pressure increases with development of L-to-R shunt

Classification:

<u>"Maladie de Roger"</u>

= small restrictive VSD with defect <1 cm; little / no hemodynamic significance with normal pulmonary artery pressure, normal pulmonary vascular resistance

• asymptomatic
• holosystolic heart murmur at 4th left rib interspace
√ normal plain film

Prognosis: spontaneous closure

<u>Moderate Shunt</u>

VSD defect <75% of aortic diameter (1–1.5 cm); systolic LV pressure > systolic RV pressure; intermediate pulmonary artery pressure; normal pulmonary vascular resistance

Heart size	↑	Main PA	↔ to ↑
Pulm. vessels	↔ to ↑	LA	↑

• respiratory infections, mild dyspnea
√ slight prominence of pulmonary vessels (45% shunt)
√ slight enlargement of LA

Prognosis: spontaneous closure in large percentage

<u>Nonrestrictive Large Shunt</u>

VSD defect >75% of aortic diameter; systolic LV pressure = systolic RV pressure (pulmonary vascular disease + hypertension increases RV pressure); pulmonary artery pressure approaching systemic levels; slightly increased pulmonary vascular resistance; pulmonary blood flow 2–4 x systemic flow;

Heart size	↑	Main PA	↑
Pulm. vessels	↑	LA	↑

HEART

- bouts of respiratory infections
- feeding problems, failure to thrive
- CHF soon after birth (due to RV overload)

√ prominent pulmonary segment + vessels (= shunt vascularity)
√ calcification of pulmonary arteries
= PATHOGNOMONIC for pulmonary arterial hypertension
√ enlargement of LA + LV
√ normal / small thoracic aorta

Eisenmenger syndrome

large VSD eventually leads to shunt reversal (R-to-L shunt) due to irreversible increase in pulmonary vascular resistance (= intima + medial hyperplasia) when pulmonary vascular resistance >0.75 of systemic vascular resistance

RA	↑	RV	↑	Main PA	↑
Pulm. vessels		↓/↑			
LA	↑ to ↔	LV	↑ to ↔	Ao	↑ to ↔

Frequency: 10% of large VSDs by 2 years of age

- cyanotic, but less symptomatic; CHF rare

√ eventual decrease of pulmonary vessel caliber
√ eventual decrease in size of LA + LV

NATURAL HISTORY OF VSD causing reduction in pulmonary blood flow:

1. Spontaneous closure
   in 40% within first 2 years of life; 60% by 5 years (65% with muscular VSD, 25% with membranous VSD); with large VSD in 10%; with small VSD in 50%
2. RVOT obstruction
   infundibular hypertrophy in 3% = pink tetrad
3. Prolapse of right aortic valve cusp
   = aortic valve insufficiency

CXR (with increase in size of VSD):
√ variable appearance due to variations in defect size
√ enlargement of LA
√ enlargement of pulmonary artery segment
√ enlargement of LV
√ RV hypertrophy
√ increase in pulmonary blood flow (if >45% of pulmonary blood flow from systemic circulation)
√ Eisenmenger reaction

ECHO:
√ prolapse of aortic valve cusp (in supracristal VSD)
√ deformity of aortic cusp (in membranous VSD)
√ lack of echoes in region of interventricular septum with sharp edges (DDx: artifactual dropout with sound beam parallel to septum); muscular VSD difficult to see
√ LA enlargement

Angio:
Projections:
(a) LAO 60° C-C 20° for membranous + anterior muscular VSD
(b) LAO 45° C-C 45° (hepatoclavicular) for posterior endocardial cushion + posterior muscular VSD
(c) RAO for supracristal VSD + assessment of RVOT
√ RVOT / pulmonary valve fill without filling of RV chamber (in supracristal VSD)

Rx:
(a) large VSD + left heart failure at 3 months of age: aim is to delay closure until child is 18 months of age; pulmonary-to-systemic blood flow >2:1 requires surgery before pulmonary hypertension becomes manifest
1. Digitalis + diuretics
2. Pulmonary artery banding
3. Patching of VSD: surgical approach through RA / through RV for supracristal VSD

(b) small VSDs without increase in pulmonary arterial pressure are followed

LIVER, BILE DUCTS, PANCREAS, AND SPLEEN

DIFFERENTIAL DIAGNOSIS OF HEPATIC, BILIARY, PANCREATIC, AND SPLENIC DISORDERS

RIGHT UPPER QUADRANT PAIN

A. BILE DUCTS
1. Biliary colic / bile duct obstruction
2. Acute cholecystitis / cholangitis

B. LIVER
1. Acute hepatitis: alcoholic, viral, drug-related, toxic
2. Hepatic abscess
3. Hepatic tumor: metastases, hepatocellular carcinoma, hemangioma, focal nodular hyperplasia, hepatic adenoma
4. Hemorrhagic cyst
5. Hepatic congestion: acute hepatic congestion, Budd-Chiari syndrome
6. Perihepatitis from gonococcal / chlamydial infection (Fitz-Hugh-Curtis syndrome)

C. PANCREAS
1. Acute pancreatitis

D. INTESTINES
1. Acute appendicitis
2. Peripyloric ulcer
3. Small bowel obstruction
4. Irritable bowel
5. Colitis / ileitis
6. Intestinal tumor

E. LUNG
1. Pneumonia
2. Pulmonary infarction

F. KIDNEY
1. Acute pyelonephritis
2. Ureteral calculus
3. Renal / perirenal abscess
4. Renal infarction
5. Renal tumor

G. OTHERS
1. Costochondritis
2. Herpes zoster

LIVER

Diffuse Liver Disease

1. Fatty liver
2. Cirrhosis
3. Hepatitis
4. Hemochromatosis
5. Glycogen storage disease
6. Budd-Chiari syndrome

Diffuse Hepatic Enlargement

A. METABOLIC
1. Fatty infiltration
2. Amyloid
3. Wilson disease
4. Gaucher disease
5. Von Gierke disease
6. Niemann-Pick disease
7. Weber-Christian disease
8. Galactosemia

B. MALIGNANCY
1. Lymphoma
2. Diffuse metastases
3. Diffuse HCC
4. Angiosarcoma

C. INFLAMMATION / INFECTION
1. Hepatitis
2. Mononucleosis
3. Miliary TB, histoplasmosis, sarcoid
4. Malaria
5. Syphilis
6. Leptospirosis
7. Chronic granulomatous disease of childhood
8. Sarcoidosis

D. VASCULAR
1. Passive congestion

E. OTHERS
1. Early cirrhosis
2. Polycystic liver disease

Increased Liver Attenuation

Abnormal deposits of substances with high atomic numbers

A. IRON
- (a) diffuse iron accumulation
  1. Genetic / primary hemochromatosis
  2. Erythropoietic hemochromatosis
  3. Bantu siderosis
  4. Transfusional iron overload
- (b) focal iron accumulation
  1. Hemorrhagic metastases: choriocarcinoma, melanoma
  2. Hepatic adenoma
  3. Siderotic regenerative nodules of cirrhosis
     ◊ An iron-poor focus within a siderotic nodule on T2WI suggests HCC!
  4. Focal hemochromatosis

B. COPPER
Wilson disease = hepatolenticular degeneration = increased copper deposits in liver + basal ganglia

C. IODINE
Amiodarone (= antiarrhythmic drug with 37% iodine by weight)
√ 95–145 HU (range of normal for liver 30–70 HU)

D. GOLD
Colloidal form of gold for therapy of rheumatoid arthritis

E. THOROTRAST
Alpha-emitter with atomic number of 90

F. THALLIUM
Accidental / suicidal ingestion of rodenticides (lethal dose is 0.2–1.0 gram)

G. ACUTE MASSIVE PROTEIN DEPOSITS

H. GLYCOGEN STORAGE DISEASE

mnemonic: "GG CHAT"
Gold therapy
Glycogen storage disease
Cyclophosphamide
Hemochromatosis / hemosiderosis
Amiodarone
Thorotrast

Generalized Increase In Liver Echogenicity

1. Fatty liver
2. Steatohepatitis
3. Cirrhosis (fibrosis + fatty liver)
4. Chronic hepatitis
5. Vacuolar degeneration

Liver Mass

◊ Hepatic masses account only for 5–6% of all intraabdominal masses in children!

Primary Benign Liver Tumor

A. EPITHELIAL TUMORS
  (a) hepatocellular
    1. Regenerative nodules
    2. Adenomatous hyperplastic nodules
    3. Focal nodular hyperplasia
    4. Hepatic adenoma
  (b) cholangiocellular
    1. Bile duct hamartoma / adenoma
    2. Biliary cystadenoma
    3. Papillary adenoma
B. MESENCHYMAL TUMORS
  (a) tumor of adipose tissue
    1. Hepatic lipoma
    2. Hepatic myelolipoma
    3. Hepatic angiomyolipoma
  (b) tumor of muscle tissue
    1. Leiomyoma
  (c) tumor of blood vessels
    1. Infantile hemangioendothelioma
    2. Hemangioma
    3. Peliosis hepatis
  (d) mesothelial tumor
    1. Benign mesothelioma
C. MIXED TISSUE TUMOR
  1. Mesenchymal hamartoma
  2. Benign teratoma
D. MISCELLANEOUS
  1. Adrenal rest tumor
  2. Pancreatic rest

Primary Malignant Liver Tumor

◊ Hepatic malignancies are the most common GI malignancy in children, but account for <2% of all pediatric malignancies!

A. EPITHELIAL TUMOR
  (a) hepatocellular
    1. Hepatoblastoma (7%)
    2. Hepatocellular carcinoma (75%)
  (b) cholangiocellular (6%)
    1. Cholangiocarcinoma
    2. Biliary cystadenocarcinoma
B. MESENCHYMAL TUMOR
  (a) tumor of blood vessels
    1. Angiosarcoma
    2. Epithelioid hemangioendothelioma
    3. Kaposi sarcoma
  (b) other tumor
    1. Embryonal sarcoma
    2. Fibrosarcoma
C. TUMOR OF MUSCLE TISSUE
  1. Leiomyosarcoma
  2. Embryonal rhabdomyosarcoma of the biliary tree
D. MISCELLANEOUS
  1. Carcinosarcoma
  2. Teratoma
  3. Yolk sac tumor
  4. Carcinoid
  5. Squamous carcinoma
  6. Primary lymphoma

Solitary Liver Lesion

A. BENIGN TUMOR
  1. Cavernous hemangioma
  2. Adenoma
  3. Focal nodular hyperplasia
B. INFECTION
  1. Pyogenic abscess
  2. Echinococcal cyst
  3. Inflammatory pseudotumor
C. TRAUMA
  1. Hematoma
  2. Traumatic cyst
D. MALIGNANT TUMOR
  1. Primary tumor
  2. Metastasis
E. OTHER
  1. Fatty change
  2. Simple cyst

Solitary Echogenic Liver Mass

mnemonic: "**H**yperechoic **F**ocal **M**asses **A**ffecting the **L**iver"
Hematoma, **H**epatoma, **H**emangioma, **H**emochromatosis
Fatty infiltration, **F**ocal nodular hyperplasia, **F**ibrosis
Metastasis
Adenoma
Lipoma

Liver Mass Surrounded by Echogenic Rim

1. Metastasis: esp., cystic islet cell tumor
2. Adenoma
3. Hemangioma

LIVER

Multiple Liver Lesions

A. BENIGN TUMOR
   1. Cavernous hemangioma
   2. Adenoma
   3. Regenerating hepatic nodules
   4. Multiple bile duct hamartoma

B. INFECTION
   1. Multiple abscesses
   2. Mycobacterial + fungal infection
   3. Inflammatory pseudotumors

C. CONGENITAL
   1. Polycystic disease
   2. Caroli disease

D. MALIGNANCY
   1. Metastases (most common malignant liver tumor)
   2. Multifocal hepatoma
   3. Lymphoma

E. OTHER
   1. Sarcoidosis
   2. Simple cysts
   3. Langerhans cell histiocytosis (echogenic nodules)

Bull's-eye Lesions of Liver

1. Candidiasis (in immunocompromised)
2. Metastases
3. Lymphoma, leukemia
4. Sarcoidosis
5. Septic emboli
6. Other opportunistic infections
7. Kaposi sarcoma

Miliary hepatosplenic lesions

1. Tuberculosis
2. Metastases
3. Fungal infections
4. Sarcoidosis
5. Lymphoma

Cystic Liver Lesion

A. NONNEOPLASTIC
   1. Congenital hepatic cyst
   2. Hematoma
   3. Echinococcal cyst
   4. Abscess
   5. Cystic liver disease
   6. Autosomal dominant polycystic disease

B. NEOPLASTIC
   1. Mesenchymal hamartoma
   2. Undifferentiated sarcoma (embryonal sarcoma)
   3. Malignant mesenchymoma
   4. Biliary cystadenoma / cystadenocarcinoma
      ◊ <5% of intrahepatic cysts are of biliary origin!
   5. Lymphangioma
   6. Necrotic neoplasm
   7. Cystic metastasis (ovarian / gastric carcinoma)

Vascular "Scar" Tumor of Liver

1. Focal nodular hyperplasia
2. Hepatic adenoma
3. Giant cavernous hemangioma
4. Fibrolamellar carcinoma of liver
5. Well-differentiated hepatocellular carcinoma
6. Hypervascular metastasis
7. Intrahepatic cholangiocarcinoma

Liver Mass with Capsular Retraction

1. Cholangiocarcinoma
2. Fibrolamellar carcinoma

or any hepatic malignancy

Low-density Mass in Porta Hepatis

1. Choledochal cyst
2. Hepatic cyst
3. Pancreatic pseudocyst
4. Enteric duplication
5. Hepatic artery aneurysm
6. Biloma
7. Embryonal rhabdomyosarcoma of biliary tree

Low-density Hepatic Mass with Enhancement

1. Hepatoma
2. Hypervascular metastases (lesions that may be obscured after contrast injection: pheochromocytoma, carcinoid, melanoma)
3. Cavernous hemangioma
4. Focal nodular hyperplasia with central fibrous scar
5. Hepatic adenoma

Fat-containing Liver Mass

1. Hepatoma
2. Angiomyolipoma

Hyperintense Liver Mass on T1WI

1. Focal fat deposit
2. High protein content
3. Hemorrhage (methemoglobin)
4. Melanoma metastasis
5. Paramagnetic contrast agents + iodized oil

Hypervascular Liver Mass

√ detected during hepatic arterial phase

A. PRIMARY
   1. Hepatocellular carcinoma
   2. Hemangioma
   3. Focal nodular hyperplasia
   4. Hepatic adenoma

B. METASTASES
   1. Neuroendocrine tumors: islet cell, carcinoid
   2. Renal cell carcinoma
   3. Breast carcinoma

Hepatic Calcification

A. INFECTION (most common cause)
   1. Granulomatous disease: tuberculosis (48%), histoplasmosis, brucellosis, coccidioidomycosis
      √ calcium involves entire lesion

2. Echinococcal cyst (in 10–20%)
   √ curvilinear / ring calcification
3. CMV, toxoplasmosis, Pneumocystis carinii
4. Chronic granulomatous disease of childhood
5. Old pyogenic / amebic abscess
6. Schistosomiasis, cysticercosis, filariasis, paragonimiasis, Armillifer infection, dracunculiasis
7. Syphilitic gumma

B. VASCULAR
1. Hepatic artery aneurysm
2. Portal vein thrombosis
3. Hematoma

C. BILIARY
1. Intrahepatic calculi
2. Ascariasis, clonorchiasis

D. BENIGN TUMORS
1. Congenital cyst
2. Cavernous hemangioma
   √ large coarse centrally located calcification (in 10–20%)
3. Hepatocellular adenoma
4. Capsule of regenerating nodules
5. Infantile hemangioendothelioma

E. PRIMARY MALIGNANT TUMOR
1. Fibrolamellar carcinoma (calcified in 15–25%)
2. Hepatocellular carcinoma
3. Hepatoblastoma (10–20%)
4. Intrahepatic cholangiocarcinoma (in 18%)
   √ calcification accompanied by desmoplastic reaction
5. Epithelioid hemangioendothelioma
6. Cystadenocarcinoma

F. METASTATIC TUMOR
1. Mucin-producing neoplasm: carcinoma of colon, breast, stomach
2. Ovarian carcinoma (psammomatous bodies)
3. Melanoma, thyroid carcinoma, pleural mesothelioma, chondro- and osteosarcoma, carcinoid, leiomyosarcoma, neuroblastoma

mnemonic: "4H TAG MAP"
Hepatoma
Hemochromatosis
Hemangioma
Hydatid disease
Thorotrast
Abscess
Granulomas (healed)
Metastases
Absent mnemonic
Porcelain gallbladder

Spontaneous Hepatic Hemorrhage
1. Hepatocellular carcinoma
2. Hepatocellular adenoma
3. Focal nodular hyperplasia
4. Hepatic hemangioma
5. Hepatic metastases: lung, RCC, melanoma
6. HELLP syndrome
7. Amyloidosis
8. Peliosis hepatis
9. Angiomyolipoma

LIVER CIRCULATION

Transient Hepatic Parenchymal Enhancement
= HYPERPERFUSION ABNORMALITIES OF LIVER
= areas of early enhancement on arterial-dominant phase due to decreased portal blood flow / formation of intrahepatic arterioportal shunts / increased aberrant drainage through hepatic veins

A. LOBAR / SEGMENTAL
1. Portal vein obstruction:
portal vein thrombosis, tumor invasion, surgical ligation
2. Cirrhosis with arterioportal shunt
3. Hypervascular gallbladder disease

B. SUBSEGMENTAL
1. Obstruction of peripheral portal branches
2. Percutaneous needle biopsy + drainage procedure / ethanol ablation
3. Acute cholecystitis + cholangitis

C. SUBCAPSULAR
(a) due to peripheral parenchymal compression
   1. Rib compression
   2. Perihepatic peritoneal implants
   3. Pseudomyxoma peritonei
   4. Perihepatic fluid collections
(b) idiopathic / unexplained

D. PSEUDOLESIONS
= systemic venous blood flow draining into hepatic sinusoids
1. Accessory cystic vein of gallbladder fossa
2. Aberrant right gastric vein
3. Capsular veins

E. RETICULAR-MOSAIC PATTERN
1. Cirrhosis
2. Hereditary hemorrhagic telangiectasia
3. Hepatic vein obstruction

Arterioportal Shunt
= organic / functional communication between high-pressure hepatic arterial branch + low-pressure portal venous system

Cause:

A. Primary hepatic neoplasm
1. Hepatocellular carcinoma
2. Hemangioma
3. Cholangiocarcinoma

B. Metastatic tumor

C. Hepatic trauma
1. Blunt abdominal trauma
2. Iatrogenic: biopsy, percutaneous abscess drainage, percutaneous biliary drainage, ethanol injection

D. Cirrhosis

E. Rupture of hepatic artery pseudoaneurysm

F. Congenital malformation

Routes:
1. Macroscopic fistula
2. Transsinusoidal = between microscopic interlobular arteriole + portal venule
3. Transvasal = via tumor thrombus
4. Transtumoral = via draining vein from a hypervascular tumor
5. Transplexal / peribiliary = via capillary network surrounding bile ducts

Pathophysiology:
shunted contrast material enhances a focal area of liver parenchyma before adjacent parenchyma is enhanced via the usual splanchnic route

CECT (in hepatic arterial phase):
- √ pseudolesion = transient peripheral wedge-shaped hepatic parenchymal enhancement:
  - √ small shunt may resemble nodular lesion
  - √ lesion disappears in portal venous phase
- √ enhancement of portal vein branch ± main portal vein from periphery without enhancement of splenic vein / superior mesenteric vein

Hepatic Artery Enlargement

1. Cirrhosis (compensatory response to decreased portal venous flow)
2. Intrahepatic arteriovenous shunting
   (a) vascular neoplasm
   (b) hepatic artery-portal vein fistula
   Cause: biopsy, trauma
   - √ turbulent high-velocity low-resistance flow
   - √ soft-tissue bruit (= random assignment of color in perivascular soft tissue due to tissue vibration)
   - √ arterialized frequently retrograde flow in portal vein
3. Hereditary hemorrhagic telangiectasia
   - √ large tortuous feeding arteries with high velocity + aliased flow
   - √ multiple dilated vessels (representing AVMs)
   - √ large draining veins
   - √ areas of fatty change + fibrosis
4. Chronic active hepatitis

Dampening of Hepatic Vein Doppler Waveform

= dampened oscillations of hepatic veins resembling portal vein flow due to "shielding" of hepatic veins from activity of right atrium

= "portalization" of hepatic vein flow pattern

A. Increased liver tissue stiffness
   1. Liver cirrhosis
   2. Various parenchymal abnormalities of liver
B. Intrinsic / extrinsic venous obstruction
   1. Budd-Chiari syndrome
   2. Inferior vena cava obstruction
   3. Extrinsic compression of hepatic veins

Pulsatile Portal Vein

= waveform pulsatility with >2/3 change from peak to minimal velocity

1. Congestive heart failure
2. Hepatic artery-portal vein fistula
3. Arteriovenous shunt in cirrhosis
4. Portal-to-hepatic vein fistula

Portal Venous Gas

◊ Should be considered a life-threatening event and sign of bowel infarction + gangrene until proved otherwise!

Etiology:

A. INTESTINAL NECROSIS (in 74% of adults)
   1. Bowel infarction secondary to arterial and venous occlusions (vascular accidents, superior mesenteric artery syndrome)
   2. Ulcerative colitis
   3. Necrotizing enterocolitis associated with mesenteric arterial thrombosis
   4. Perforated gastric ulcer
B. GI OBSTRUCTION
   1. Small bowel obstruction (duodenal atresia)
   2. Imperforate anus
   3. Esophageal atresia
C. MISCELLANEOUS
   1. Hemorrhagic pancreatitis
   2. Sigmoid diverticulitis
   3. Intraabdominal abscess
   4. Pneumonia
   5. Iatrogenic injection of air during endoscopy
   6. Dead fetus
   7. Diabetes, diarrhea

mnemonic: "BE NICE"
BE (air embolism during double contrast barium enema)
Necrotizing enterocolitis
Infarction (mesenteric)
Catheterization of umbilical vein
Erythroblastosis fetalis

Pathogenesis:
1. Intestinal wall alteration permitting passage of intraluminal air into intestinal venules:
   (a) ulceration of gastric, duodenal, bowel wall
   (b) sloughing of epithelial lining
   (c) enhanced mucosal permeability
   eg, intestinal ischemia with bowel necrosis (most common), perforated gastric carcinoma / ulcer, inflammatory bowel disease (Crohn disease, ulcerative colitis)
   Prognosis: 75–90% mortality rate within 1 week of diagnosis
2. Bowel distension with elevated intraluminal pressure causes minimal mucosal disruption + permits passage of intraluminal air into veins:
   (a) iatrogenic dilatation of hollow viscus (gastrostomy, sclerotherapy, ERCP, colonoscopy, barium enema)
   (b) spontaneous paralytic ileus, mechanical obstruction, acute gastric dilatation

(c) blunt trauma (<1%) with acute pressure changes
(d) barotrauma
Prognosis: surgery often not indicated
3. Intraabdominal sepsis
(a) ? gas from septicemia in branches of mesenteric veins / portal vein (pylephlebitis)
(b) ? increased intraluminal fermentation of carbohydrates due to bacterial overgrowth
(c) ? mesocolic abscess causing inframesocolic perforation dissecting between peritoneal leaflets
eg, diverticulitis, intra- or retroperitoneal abscess / gangrene, TB
4. Idiopathic (15%)
eg, organ transplantation (liver [18%], kidney, bone marrow), pulmonary disease (chronic obstructive pulmonary disease, bronchopneumonia, asthma), drugs (steroids, cytostatics), seizure

Composition of colonic gas:
methane, carbon dioxide, oxygen, nitrogen, hydrogen

Plain film:
◊ Substantial amount necessary for detection
√ branching linear gas densities:
√ in periphery of liver extending to within 2 cm of liver capsule
√ predominantly within more anteriorly located left lobe of liver
√ pneumatosis of intestinal wall

CT:
◊ Small amount of gas detectable
√ tubular areas of decreased attenuation in periphery of liver
√ gas in superior / inferior mesenteric veins
√ gas in small mesenteric veins at mesenteric border of bowel

US:
◊ Small amount of gas detectable
√ intensely hyperechoic foci within lumen of portal vein + liver parenchyma

Doppler:
√ tall sharp bidirectional spikes (overloading of Doppler receiver from strong reflection of gas bubble in bloodstream) superimposed on normal portal vein spectrum

DDx: pneumobilia (located centrally within bile ducts close to liver hilum + within left lobe of liver)

GALLBLADDER

Nonvisualization of Gallbladder on OCG

Peak opacification of gallbladder: 14–19 hours (13–35% of dose excreted in urine)

A. EXTRABILIARY CAUSES
1. Failure to ingest contrast
2. Fasting
3. Failure to reach absorptive surface of bowel
(a) vomiting, nasogastric suction
(b) esophageal / gastric obstruction
(c) hiatal, umbilical, inguinal hernias
(d) Zenker, epiphrenic, gastric, duodenal, jejunal diverticulum
(e) gastric ulcer, gastrocolic fistula
(f) malabsorption, diarrhea
(g) postoperative ileus, severe trauma
(h) inflammation: acute pancreatitis, acute peritonitis
4. Deficiency of bile salts
Crohn disease, surgical resection of terminal ileum, liver disease, cholestyramine therapy, abnormal communication between biliary system and gastrointestinal tract

B. INTRINSIC GALLBLADDER DISEASE
1. Cholecystectomy
2. Anomalous position
3. Obstruction of cystic duct
4. Chronic cholecystitis

Oral Cholecystogram (OCG)

Dose: 6 x 0.5 g tablets 2 hours after evening meal

A. PATIENT SELECTION
• bilirubin <5 mg% (not necessary if due to hemolysis)
◊ Contraindicated in serious liver disease!
◊ Relative contraindications in peritonitis, postoperative ileus, acute pancreatitis!

B. TOXICITY
1. Nausea + vomiting (also noted in 29% on placebo)
2. Immediate anaphylactic response
3. Delayed hypotensive reaction (increased risk in cirrhosis)
4. Renal failure
5. Precipitation of hyperthyroidism

Nonvisualization of Gallbladder on US

1. Status post cholecystectomy
2. Obscured by costal margin
3. Anomalous position (intrahepatic, subphrenic)
4. Gallbladder carcinoma replacing gallbladder
5. Perforation of gallbladder
6. Congenital absence
7. Contracted gallbladder
(a) nonfasting status without stones
(b) in fasting status with stones
√ wall-echo-shadow (WES triad) interfaces

Shadowing in Gallbladder Fossa

1. WES (wall-echo-shadow) triad
2. Gas in duodenum / colon obscuring gallbladder
3. Porcelain gallbladder
4. Emphysematous cholecystitis
5. Cholecystoenteric fistula
6. Status post ERCP with retrograde air injection

High-density Bile

1. Hemorrhagic cholecystitis
2. Hemobilia

LIVER

3. Prior contrast administration
   (a) vicarious excretion of urographic agent
   (b) cholecystopaque
4. Milk of calcium bile

Displaced Gallbladder

A. NORMAL IMPRESSION
   by duodenum / colon (positional change)
B. HEPATIC MASS
   hepatoma, hemangioma, regenerating nodule, metastases, intrahepatic cyst, polycystic liver, hydatid disease, hepar lobatum (tertiary syphilis), granuloma, abscess
C. EXTRAHEPATIC MASS
   1. Retroperitoneal tumor (renal, adrenal)
   2. Polycystic kidney
   3. Lymphoma
   4. Lymph node metastasis to porta hepatis
   5. Pancreatic pseudocyst

Alteration in Gallbladder Size

Enlarged Gallbladder

= CHOLECYSTOMEGALY = HYDROPS OF GALLBLADDER

Size:
- (a) infants <1 year: >3 cm in length
- (b) children: >7 cm in length
- (c) adults: >4 x 10 cm

A. OBSTRUCTION
   1. Cystic duct obstruction (40%)
      (a) Hydrops: chronic cystic duct obstruction + distension with clear sterile mucus (white bile)
      (b) Empyema: acute / chronic obstruction with superinfection of bile
   2. Cholelithiasis causing obstruction (37%)
   3. Cholecystitis with cholelithiasis (11%)
   4. Courvoisier phenomenon (10%) = secondary to neoplastic process in pancreas / duodenal papilla / ampulla of Vater / common bile duct
   5. Pancreatitis
   6. Infection: leptospirosis, ascariasis, typhoid fever, scarlet fever, familial Mediterranean fever
B. UNOBSTRUCTED (mostly neuropathic)
   1. S/P vagotomy
   2. Diabetes mellitus
   3. Alcoholism
   4. Appendicitis (in children)
   5. Narcotic analgesia
   6. WDHA syndrome
   7. Hyperalimentation
   8. Acromegaly
   9. Kawasaki syndrome
   10. Anticholinergics
   11. Bedridden patient with prolonged illness
   12. AIDS (in 18%)
   13. Dehydration
   14. Prolonged fasting
   15. Total parenteral nutrition
   16. Sepsis
C. NORMAL (2%)

Small Gallbladder

1. Chronic cholecystitis
2. Cystic fibrosis: in 25% of patients
3. Congenital hypoplasia / multiseptated gallbladder
4. Postprandial
5. Intrahepatic cholestasis (viral, drug-related)

Gallbladder Wall Thickening

Diffuse Gallbladder Wall Thickening

= anterior wall of gallbladder >3 mm

A. INTRINSIC
   1. Acute cholecystitis
   2. Chronic cholecystitis (10–25%)
   3. Xanthogranulomatous cholecystitis
   4. Hyperplastic cholecystosis (in 91% diffuse)
   5. Gallbladder perforation
   6. Sepsis
   7. Gallbladder carcinoma (in 41% diffuse)
   8. AIDS cholangiopathy (average of 9 mm in up to 55%)
   9. Sclerosing cholangitis
   10. Gallbladder varices
   11. Chemoinfusion of hepatic artery (ischemia)
B. EXTRINSIC
   1. Hepatitis (in 80%)
   2. Hypoalbuminemia
   3. Renal failure
   4. Right heart failure
   5. Systemic venous hypertension
   6. Hepatic venous obstruction
   7. Ascites
   8. Multiple myeloma
   9. Portal node lymphatic obstruction
   10. Cirrhosis
   11. Acute myelogenous leukemia
   12. Brucellosis
   13. Graft-versus-host disease
C. PHYSIOLOGIC
   = contracted gallbladder after eating

Focal Gallbladder Wall Thickening

A. METABOLIC
   1. Metachromatic sulfatides
   2. Hyperplastic cholecystoses
B. BENIGN TUMOR
   1. Adenoma: glandular elements (0.2%)
   2. Papilloma: fingerlike projections (0.2%)
   3. Villous hyperplasia
   4. Fibroadenoma
   5. Cystadenoma: ? premalignant
   6. Neurinoma, hemangioma
   7. Carcinoid tumor
C. MALIGNANT TUMOR
   1. Carcinoma of gallbladder: adenocarcinoma / squamous cell carcinoma (in 59% focal)
   2. Leiomyosarcoma
   3. Metastases: from malignant melanoma (15%), lung, kidney, esophagus, breast, carcinoid, Kaposi sarcoma, lymphoma, leukemia

D. INFLAMMATION / INFECTION
   1. Inflammatory polyp: in chronic cholecystitis
   2. Parasitic granuloma: Ascaris lumbricoides, Paragonimus westermani, Clonorchis, filariasis, Schistosoma, Fasciola
   3. Intramural epithelial cyst / mucinous retention cyst
   4. Xanthogranulomatous cholecystitis (in 9% focal)

E. WALL-ADHERENT GALLSTONE = embedded stone

F. HETEROTOPIC MUCOSA
   1. Ectopic pancreatic tissue
   2. Ectopic gastric glands
   3. Ectopic intestinal glands
   4. Ectopic hepatic tissue
   5. Ectopic prostatic tissue

Filling Defects of Gallbladder

Fixed Filling Defects of Gallbladder

mnemonic: "PANTS"

Polyp
Adenomyomatosis
Neurinoma
Tumor, primary / secondary
Stone, wall-adherent

Mobile Intraluminal Mass in Gallbladder

1. Tumefactive sludge
2. Blood clot
3. Nonshadowing stone

Comet-tail Artifact in Liver and Gallbladder

A. LIVER
   1. Foreign metallic body (eg, surgical clip)
   2. Intrahepatic calcification
   3. Pneumobilia
   4. Multiple bile duct hamartoma = von Meyenburg complex

B. GALLBLADDER
   1. Rokitansky-Aschoff sinus
   2. Intramural stone
   3. Cholesterolosis of gallbladder

Echogenic Fat in Hepatoduodenal Ligament

= sign of pericholecystic inflammation

1. Cholecystitis
2. Perforated duodenal ulcer
3. Pancreatitis
4. Diverticulitis

BILE DUCTS

Hemobilia

1. Iatrogenic trauma: percutaneous needle biopsy, transhepatic cholangiography / biliary drainage / portography
2. Blunt / penetrating trauma
3. Rupture of aneurysm / pseudoaneurysm

Gas in Biliary Tree = Pneumobilia

mnemonic: "I GET UP"

Incompetent sphincter of Oddi (after sphincterotomy / passage of a gallstone)
Gallstone ileus
Emphysematous cholecystitis (actually in gallbladder)
Trauma
Ulcer (duodenal ulcer perforating into CBD)
Postoperative (eg, cholecystoenterostomy)

√ gas outlines choledochus ± gallbladder
√ peripheral branches of bile ducts not filled

Obstructive Jaundice in Adult

Etiology:

A. BENIGN DISEASE (76%)
   1. Traumatic / postoperative stricture (44%)
   2. Calculi (21%)
   3. Chronic pancreatitis (8%)
   4. Sclerosing cholangitis (1%)
   5. Recurrent pyogenic cholangitis
   6. Parasitic disease (ascariasis)
   7. Liver cysts
   8. Aortic aneurysm
   9. Papillary stenosis

B. MALIGNANCY (24%)
   1. Pancreatic carcinoma (18%)
   2. Ampullary / duodenal carcinoma (8%)
   3. Cholangiocarcinoma (3%)
   4. Metastatic disease (2%)
      from stomach, pancreas, lung, breast, colon, lymphoma

Level and cause of obstruction:

A. INTRAPANCREATIC
   1. Choledocholithiasis
      ◊ Most common cause of biliary obstruction (in 15% of patients with cholelithiasis)!
   2. Chronic pancreatitis
   3. Pancreatic carcinoma

B. SUPRAPANCREATIC (5%)
   = between pancreas + porta hepatis
   1. Cholangiocarcinoma
   2. Metastatic adenopathy

C. PORTA HEPATIS (5%)
   1. Klatskin tumor
   2. Spread from adjacent tumor (GB, liver)
   3. Surgical stricture

D. INTRAHEPATIC
   1. Cystadenoma, cystadenocarcinoma
   2. Mirizzi syndrome
   3. Caroli disease
   4. Cholangitis: recurrent pyogenic cholangitis, sclerosing cholangitis, AIDS cholangitis

Incidence of infected bile in bile duct obstruction:

(a) incomplete / partial obstruction in 64%
(b) complete obstruction in 10%
◊ Infection twice as high with biliary calculi than with malignant obstruction!

Organism: E. coli (21%), Klebsiella (21%), enterococci (18%), Proteus (15%)

Test Sensitivity for Common Bile Duct Obstruction:

1. Intravenous cholangiography
   depends on level of bilirubin: <1 mg/dL in 92%; <2 mg/dL in 82%; <3 mg/dL in 40%; >4 mg/dL in <10%
   False-negative rate: 45%
   Cx: adverse reactions in 4–10%
2. US
   88–90% sensitivity for dilatation of CBD
   ◊ In 27–95% correct level of obstruction determined by US
   ◊ In 23–81% correct cause of obstruction determined by US
   √ CBD >4–6 mm / 10% of patient's age in years
   √ increase in CBD size after fatty meal
   √ "Swiss cheese sign" = abundance of fluid-filled structures on liver sections
   √ intrahepatic "double channel" / "shotgun" sign = two parallel tubular structures composed of portal vein + dilated intrahepatic bile ducts
   √ intrahepatic bile duct >2 mm / >40% of adjacent portal vein branch
   False-negative: not dilated in acute obstruction (in 70%), sclerosing cholangitis, intermittent obstruction from choledocholithiasis
   False-positive: dilated hepatic artery in cirrhosis / portal hypertension / hepatic neoplasm, patients after cholecystectomy
3. CT
   100% visualization in tumorous obstruction, 60% in nontumorous obstruction
4. NUC
   √ delayed / nonvisualization of biliary system (93% specificity)
   √ vicarious excretion of tracer through kidneys
   DDx: Hepatocellular dysfunction (delayed clearance of cardiac blood pool)

Hyperbilirubinemia in Infants

= UNCONJUGATED HYPERBILIRUBINEMIA

A. PHYSIOLOGIC
   Frequency: in 60% of full-term infants, in 80% of preterm infants
   Course: increase by day 2–3, peak by day 5–7 (up to 12 mg/dL in full-term babies, up to 14 mg/dL in premature infants)
   ◊ Breast-fed babies may have an elevated bilirubin level until the end of 2nd week of life!

B. NONPHYSIOLOGIC
   - onset of jaundice within first 24 hours
   - persistent / new-onset jaundice in infants 2 weeks of age
   - rise of serum bilirubin >5 mg/dL per 24 hours
   - direct bilirubin level >1 mg/dL

Neonatal Obstructive Jaundice

= severe persistent jaundice in a child beyond 3–4 weeks of age

Cause:

A. INFECTION
   (a) bacterial: E. coli, Listeria monocytogenes
   (b) viral: TORCH, Coxsackie virus, echovirus, adenovirus

B. METABOLIC
   (a) inherited: alpha-1 antitrypsin deficiency, cystic fibrosis, galactosemia, hereditary tyrosinemia
   (b) acquired: inspissated bile syndrome = "bile plug" syndrome (= cholestasis due to erythroblastosis); cholestasis due to total parenteral nutrition; choledocholithiasis

C. BILIARY TRACT ABNORMALITIES
   (a) extrahepatic: biliary obstruction / hypoplasia / atresia, choledochal cyst, spontaneous perforation of bile duct
   (b) intrahepatic: ductular hypoplasia / atresia

D. IDIOPATHIC NEONATAL HEPATITIS

◊ The 3 most common causes of jaundice in neonates are hepatitis, biliary atresia, and choledochal cyst!
mnemonic: "CAN"
Choledochal cyst
Atresia
Neonatal hepatitis

NUC–imaging regimen:

(1) Premedication with phenobarbital (5 mg/kg/day) over 5 days to induce hepatic microsomal enzymes, which enhance uptake and excretion of certain compounds and increase bile flow
(2) IDA scintigraphy (50 μCi/kg; minimum of 1 mCi)
(3) Imaging at 5-minute intervals for 1 hour + at 2, 4, 6, 8, 24 hours

Jaundice in Older Children

A. DISEASE OF HEPATOCYTES
   (a) hepatitis
      1. Acute hepatitis: infection, toxic agents, drugs
      2. Chronic hepatitis
   (b) metabolic
      1. Wilson disease
      2. Cystic fibrosis
      3. Glycogen storage disease
      4. Tyrosinemia
      5. Alpha-1 antitrypsin deficiency

B. OBSTRUCTION
   (a) malignant neoplasm
      1. Hepatoblastoma
      2. Hepatocellular carcinoma

3. Sarcomas: angiosarcoma, lymphosarcoma, rhabdomyosarcoma of bile ducts, undifferentiated embryonal sarcoma
4. Metastatic disease: neuroblastoma, Wilms tumor, leukemia/lymphoma

(b) benign neoplasm
1. Infantile hemangioendothelioma
2. Mesenchymal hamartoma

(c) benign stricture
(d) cholelithiasis / choledocholithiasis (uncommon)

Large Nonobstructed CBD

1. Passage of stone (return to normal after days to weeks)
2. Common duct surgery (return to normal in 30–50 days)
3. Postcholecystectomy dilatation (in up to 16%)
4. Intestinal hypomotility
5. Normal variant (aging)

Fatty-meal sonography (to differentiate from obstruction with 74% sensitivity, 100% specificity)

Method: peroral Lipomul (1.5 mL/kg) followed by 100 mL of water [cholecystokinin causes contraction of gallbladder, relaxation of sphincter of Oddi, increase in bile secretion], CBD measured before and 45 / 60 minutes after stimulation

√ little change / decrease in size = normal response
√ increase in size >2 mm = partial obstruction

Filling Defect in Bile Ducts

A. ARTIFACT
1. Pseudocalculus
(a) contracted sphincter of Boyden + Oddi with smooth arcuate contour
(b) bridge of tissue between cystic duct + CHD
(c) underfilling of cystic duct during ERCP
(d) admixture defect at cystic duct junction
2. Air bubble: confirmed by positional changes
3. Blood clot: spheroid configuration, spontaneous resolution with time

B. BILIARY CALCULI

C. MIRIZZI SYNDROME

D. NEOPLASM
(a) malignant
1. Cholangiocarcinoma: irregular stricture, intraluminal polypoid mass
2. Metastatic tumor (GI tract, pancreas, breast, melanoma, lymphoma)
3. Others: ampullary carcinoma, hepatoma, hamartoma, carcinoid, embryonal rhabdomyosarcoma of biliary tree

(b) benign
1. Papilloma (most common benign neoplasm)
Histo: vascular connective tissue covered by single layer of columnar epithelium
2. Adenoma
Histo: epithelial glandular tissue surrounded by fibrous tissue
3. Fibroma, lipoma, neuroma
4. Granular cell myoblastoma (= Schwann-cell–derived biliary tumor) in young black woman

E. PARASITES
1. Ascaris lumbricoides: long linear filling defect / discrete mass if coiled
2. Liver fluke (Clonorchis sinensis, Fasciola hepatica): intrahepatic epithelial hyperplasia, periductal fibrosis, cholangitis, liver abscess, hepatic duct stones, common duct obstruction
3. Schistosoma japonicum: portal vein infection
3. Hydatid cyst: after erosion into biliary tree

Echogenic Material in Bile Ducts

1. Calculi
2. Gas
3. Blood
4. Tumor
5. Parasites

Bile Duct Narrowing

A. BENIGN STRICTURE (44%)
(a) trauma
1. Postoperative stricture (95–99%) associated with cholecystectomy
2. Blunt / penetrating trauma
3. Hepatic artery embolization
4. Infusion of chemotherapeutic agents

(b) inflammation
1. Sclerosing cholangitis
2. Recurrent pyogenic cholangitis
3. Acute / chronic pancreatitis
4. Pancreatic pseudocyst
5. Perforated duodenal ulcer
6. Erosion by biliary calculus
7. Gallstones + cholecystitis
8. Abscess
9. Radiation therapy
10. Papillary stenosis
11. Acquired immunodeficiency syndrome

(c) congenital
1. Choledochal cyst

B. MALIGNANT STRICTURE
1. Pancreatic carcinoma
2. Ampullary carcinoma
3. Cholangiocarcinoma
4. Compression by enlarged lymph node
5. Metastasis

Multifocal Intrahepatic Bile Duct Strictures

1. Primary sclerosing cholangitis
2. Ascending cholangitis due to stricture / stone / bile duct anomaly
3. Oriental cholangiohepatitis
4. AIDS-related cholangitis
5. Ischemia
(a) floxuridine treatment
(b) hepatic arterial thrombosis (in liver transplant)

6. Neoplasm
   (a) cholangiocarcinoma
   (b) metastases
7. Previous bile surgery
8. Congenital biliary anomalies

Papillary Stenosis

Etiology:

A. PRIMARY PAPILLARY STENOSIS (10%)
   1. Congenital malformation of papilla
   2. Sequelae of acute / chronic inflammation
   3. Adenomyosis

B. SECONDARY PAPILLARY STENOSIS (90%)
   1. Mechanical trauma of stone passage (choledocholithiasis in 64%; cholecystolithiasis in 26%)
   2. Functional stenosis: associated with pancreas divisum, history of pancreatitis
   3. Reflex spasm = papillary dyskinesia
   4. Scar from previous surgical manipulation
   5. Periampullary neoplasm

√ prestenotic dilatation of CBD
√ increase in pancreatic duct diameter (83%)
√ long smooth narrowing / beak (fibrotic stenosis)
√ prolonged bile-to-bowel transit time >45 minutes on Tc-IDA scintigraphy

Periampullary Tumor

1. Pancreatic carcinoma (85%)
2. Cholangiocarcinoma of distal common bile duct (6%)
3. Ampullary tumor (4%)
4. Duodenal wall tumor
   adenocarcinoma, adenoma, carcinoid, smooth muscle tumor

Double-Duct Sign

= dilatation of common bile duct + pancreatic duct

1. Ampullary tumor (most common)
2. Other periampullary tumor
3. Papillary stenosis
4. Stone impacted in ampulla of Vater

Congenital Biliary Cysts

(Todani classification)

I. Choledochal cyst (77–87%)
   - IA cystic dilatation of CBD
   - IB focal segmental dilatation of CBD
   - IC fusiform dilatation of CBD

II. Diverticulum of extrahepatic ducts (1.2–3%) originating from CBD / CHD
   √ neck of diverticulum open / closed

III. Choledochocele (1.4–6%)

IV. Multiple segmental bile duct cysts
   - IVA multiple intra- and extrahepatic biliary cysts + saccular dilatation of CBD (19%)
   - IVB multiple extrahepatic biliary cysts + normal intrahepatic bile ducts (rare)

V. Caroli disease = intrahepatic biliary cysts

PANCREAS

Congenital Pancreatic Anomalies

1. Pancreas divisum
2. Annular pancreas
3. Agenesis of dorsal pancreas
   May be associated with:
   abnormal situs, polysplenia, intestinal malrotation

Pancreatic Calcification

1. CHRONIC PANCREATITIS
   Numerous irregular stippled calcifications of varying size; predominantly intraductal
   (a) Alcoholic pancreatitis (in 20–50%):
      √ calcifications limited to head / tail in 25%
   (b) Biliary pancreatitis (in 2%)
   (c) Hereditary pancreatitis (in 35–60%):
      √ round calcifications throughout gland
   (d) Idiopathic pancreatitis
   (e) Pancreatic pseudocyst
2. NEOPLASM
   (a) Microcystic adenoma (in 33%):
      √ "sunburst" appearance of calcifications
   (b) Macrocystic cystadenoma In 15%):
      √ amorphous peripheral calcifications

LIVER

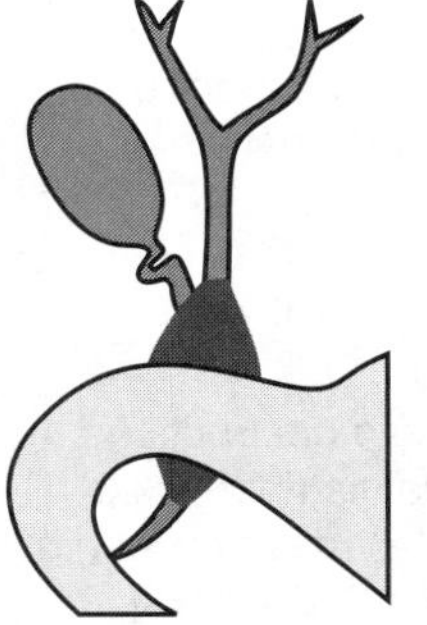
Type I
Choledochal Cyst

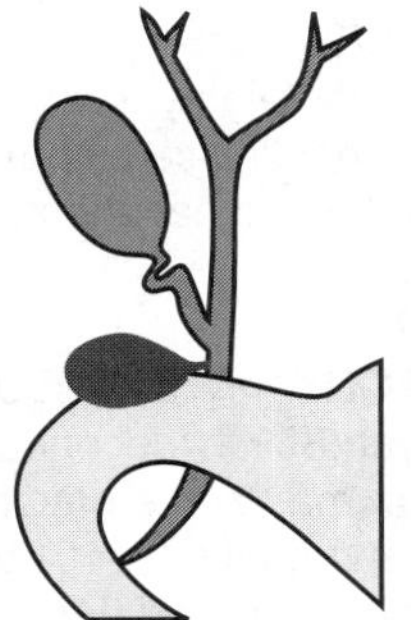
Type II
Diverticulum

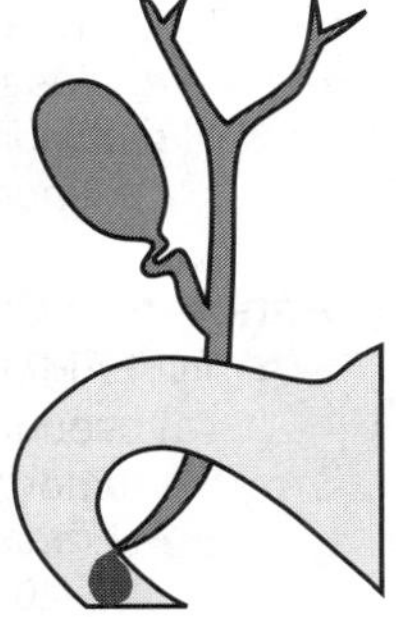
Type III
Choledochocele

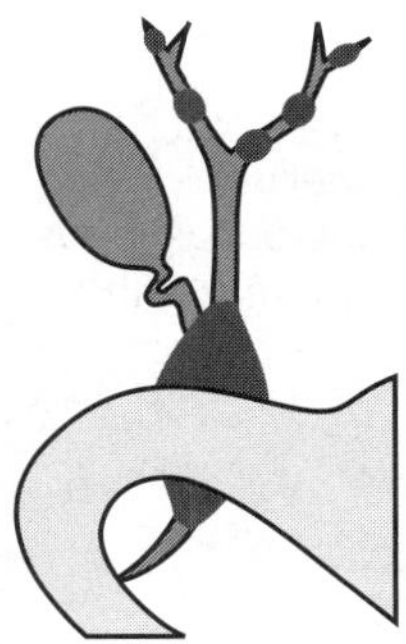
Type IVa
Saccular Dilatation of CBD + Intrahepatic Ducts

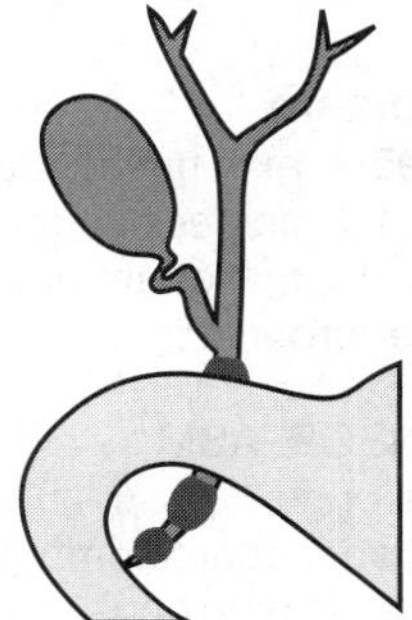
Type IVb
Saccular Dilatation of CBD

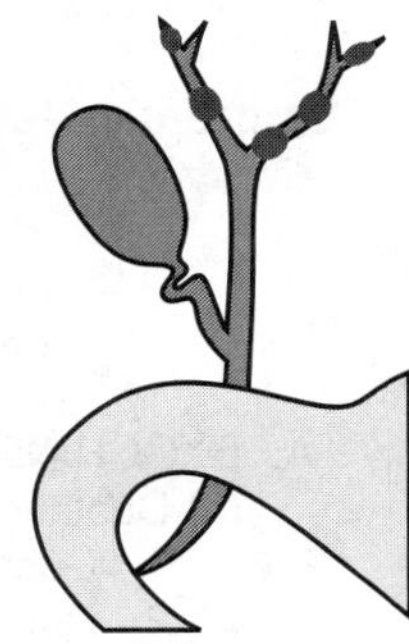
Type V
Caroli Disease

Classification of Congenital Biliary Cysts

(c) Adenocarcinoma (in 2%): with "sunburst" pattern
(d) Cavernous lymphangioma / hemangioma:
√ multiple phleboliths
(e) Metastases from colon cancer
3. INTRAPARENCHYMAL HEMORRHAGE
(a) Old hematoma / abscess / infarction
(b) Rupture of intrapancreatic aneurysm
4. HYPERPARATHYROIDISM (in 20%):
◊ 50% of patients develop chronic pancreatitis + concomitant nephrocalcinosis
◊ Indistinguishable from alcoholic pancreatitis
5. CYSTIC FIBROSIS
Fine granular calcifications imply advanced pancreatic fibrosis
6. HEMOCHROMATOSIS
7. KWASHIORKOR = juvenile tropical pancreatitis
◊ Indistinguishable from alcoholic pancreatitis

Atrophy of Pancreas

1. Main pancreatic duct obstruction
2. Cystic fibrosis
◊ Most common cause in childhood!
3. Schwachman-Diamond syndrome
4. **Johanson-Blizzard syndrome** (= pancreatic insufficiency, nasal alar hypoplasia, absence of permanent teeth, short stature, congenital deafness)
5. Hemochromatosis
6. Viral infection
7. Malnutrition
8. Cushing syndrome, steroid therapy, obesity

Pancreatic Mass

A. NEOPLASTIC
1. Adenocarcinoma
2. Islet cell tumor
3. Cystadenoma / -carcinoma
4. Solid and papillary neoplasm
5. Lymphoma

B. INFLAMMATORY
1. Acute pancreatitis
2. Pseudocyst
3. Pancreatic abscess

Pancreatic Neoplasm

Origin: — in 99% exocrine ductal epithelium
— in 1% acinar portion of pancreatic glands
— in 0.1% malignant ampullary tumor with better prognosis

A. EXOCRINE NEOPLASM
(a) Ductal cell origin
1. Ductal adenocarcinoma (90%)
2. Ductectatic mucinous tumor
= mucin-hypersecreting carcinoma
3. Cystic neoplasm (10–15%)
— serous microcystic neoplasm
— mucinous macrocystic neoplasm
4. Solid and papillary epithelial neoplasm (rare)
5. Cystic changes of von Hippel-Lindau disease

(b) Acinar cell origin
1. Acinar cell carcinoma (1%)
2. Adenoma

(c) Indeterminate origin
1. Pancreatoblastoma = infantile pancreatic carcinoma
2. Dermoid cyst

B. ENDOCRINE NEOPLASM
(a) Nonfunctioning islet cell tumor
(b) Functioning islet cell tumor
1. Insulinoma (β cells)
2. Glucagonoma
3. Gastrinoma (δ cells)
4. Somatostatinoma
5. VIPoma (WDHA syndrome)
6. "PP-oma" = pancreatic polypeptide
7. Carcinoid

C. NONEPITHELIAL ORIGIN
(a) Primary tumor
1. Primary lymphoma
<1% of pancreatic neoplasms
2. Primitive neuroectodermal tumor
3. Rhabdomyosarcoma

(b) Metastases
1. Secondary lymphoma:
√ large homogeneous solid mass, infrequently with central cystic area
√ peripancreatic nodal masses
√ peripancreatic vessels displaced + stretched
2. Primitive neuroectodermal tumor
3. Kaposi sarcoma
4. Renal cell carcinoma
5. Melanoma
6. Lung cancer
7. Breast cancer
8. Ovarian cancer
9. Hepatocellular carcinoma
10. Sarcoma

Hypervascular Pancreatic Tumors

A. PRIMARY
Islet cell tumor, microcystic adenoma, solid and papillary epithelial neoplasm

B. METASTASES from
angiosarcoma, leiomyosarcoma, melanoma, carcinoid, renal cell carcinoma, adrenal carcinoma, thyroid carcinoma

Pancreatic Cyst

A. INFLAMMATORY / INFECTIOUS
(a) pseudocyst (85%): secondary to obstructive tumor / trauma / acute pancreatitis (in 2–4%), chronic pancreatitis (in 10–15%) [develop within 10–20 days, consolidated after 6–8 weeks]
(b) acquired cyst:
1. Retention cyst (= exudate within bursa omentalis from acute pancreatitis)
2. Parasitic cyst: Echinococcus multilocularis, amebiasis
3. Pancreatic abscess

B. CONGENITAL (rare)
  (a) solitary true cyst
  (b) multiple true cysts (when associated with cystic disease of the liver / other organs):
    1. Autosomal dominant polycystic kidney disease (hepatic cysts in 90% at autopsy)
       √ nearly always associated with renal cysts
    2. Von Hippel-Lindau disease (pancreatic cysts in 72% at autopsy; in only 25% on CT)
    3. Cystic fibrosis

C. NEOPLASTIC
  (a) cystic pancreatic neoplasm (5–15%): <5% of all pancreatic tumors
    1. Serous cystadenoma = microcystic adenoma
    2. Mucinous cystic tumors
       — peripheral branch-duct tumor = mucinous cystadenoma / cystadenocarcinoma (= macrocystic adenoma)
       — main duct tumor = intraductal papillary mucinous adenoma / adenocarcinoma
    3. Solid and papillary epithelioid neoplasm
    4. Cystic islet cell tumor (rare)
    5. Pancreatic sarcoma (extremely rare)
  (b) cystic metastases (3–12% at autopsy): renal cell carcinoma, melanoma, lung tumors, breast carcinoma, hepatocellular carcinoma, ovarian carcinoma
  (c) retroperitoneal lymphangioma / hemangioma

Microcystic Lesion of Pancreas

= pancreatic lesion with >6 cysts each <2 cm in size

1.	Pancreatic adenocarcinoma	50%
2.	Microcystic adenoma	19%
3.	Pancreatitis	11%
4.	Metastases	6%
5.	Mucinous cystadenocarcinoma	5%
6.	Islet cell carcinoma	3%
7.	Lymphoma	3%
8.	Sarcoma	3%

Hyperamylasemia

A. PANCREATIC
  1. Acute / chronic pancreatitis
  2. Pancreatic trauma
  3. Pancreatic carcinoma

B. GASTROINTESTINAL
  1. Perforated peptic ulcer
  2. Intestinal obstruction
  3. Peritonitis
  4. Acute appendicitis
  5. Afferent loop syndrome
  6. Mesenteric ischemia / infarction
  7. Portal vein thrombosis

C. TRAUMA
  1. Burns
  2. Cerebral trauma
  3. Postoperative

D. OBSTETRICAL
  1. Pregnancy
  2. Ruptured ectopic pregnancy

E. RENAL
  1. Transplantation
  2. Renal insufficiency

F. METABOLIC
  1. Diabetic ketoacidosis
  2. Drugs

G. PNEUMONIA

H. SALIVARY GLAND LESION
  1. Facial trauma
  2. Mumps

SPLEEN

Nonvisualization of Spleen

1. Asplenia syndrome
2. Polysplenia syndrome
3. Traumatic fragmentation of spleen
4. Wandering spleen

Small Spleen

1. Infarction
2. Celiac disease
3. Congenital / hereditary hypoplasia
   ◊ associated with recurrent bacterial infections
4. Fanconi anemia
5. Irradiation
6. Partial splenectomy
7. Polysplenia syndrome
8. Atrophy

Splenomegaly

√ inferior tip of spleen extends below tip of right lobe of liver
√ AP diameter of spleen >2/3 of abdominal diameter

A. CONGESTIVE SPLENOMEGALY
   heart failure, portal hypertension, cirrhosis, cystic fibrosis, portal / splenic vein thrombosis, acute splenic sequestration crisis of sickle cell anemia

B. NEOPLASM
   leukemia, lymphoma, lymphoproliferative disease, Langerhans cell histiocytosis, metastases, primary neoplasm

C. STORAGE DISEASE
   Gaucher disease, Niemann-Pick disease, mucopolysaccharidoses, gargoylism, amyloidosis, diabetes mellitus, hemochromatosis

D. INFECTION
  (a) bacterial: TB, subacute bacterial endocarditis, typhoid fever, syphilis, brucellosis
  (b) viral: hepatitis, infectious mononucleosis
  (c) protozoal: echinococcosis, malaria, kala azar, American leishmaniosis
  (d) fungal: histoplasmosis

E. HEMOLYTIC ANEMIA
   hemoglobinopathy, hereditary spherocytosis, primary neutropenia, thrombotic thrombocytopenic purpura, extracorporeal membrane oxygenation (due to RBC damage)

F. EXTRAMEDULLARY HEMATOPOIESIS
   osteopetrosis, myelofibrosis

G. COLLAGEN VASCULAR DISEASE
systemic lupus erythematosus, rheumatoid arthritis, Felty syndrome
H. SPLENIC TRAUMA
I. OTHERS
1. Sarcoidosis
√ splenomegaly in up to 60%
√ inhomogeneous enhancement after bolus injection (multiple 2–3-cm hypodense nodular lesions)
√ necrotic mass with focal calcifications
2. Hemodialysis
3. Autoimmune lymphoproliferative syndrome

Solitary Splenic Lesion

mnemonic: "L'CHAIM"
Lymphoma
Cyst
Hematoma, **H**emangioma, **H**amartoma
Abscess
Infarct
Metastasis

Solid Splenic Lesion

A. MALIGNANT TUMOR
1. Lymphoma (Hodgkin disease, non-Hodgkin lymphoma, primary splenic lymphoma)
◊ Splenomegaly in non-Hodgkin lymphoma indicates involvement in most patients
◊ 30% of patients with splenomegaly have no involvement from non-Hodgkin lymphoma
◊ 30% of patients with lymphoma of any kind have splenic involvement without splenomegaly
√ homogeneous splenomegaly (from diffuse infiltration)
√ miliary nodules
√ large 2–10-cm nodules (10–25%)
√ nodes in splenic hilum (50%) in NHL; uncommon in Hodgkin disease
2. Metastasis (7%)
melanoma (6–34%), breast carcinoma (12–21%), bronchogenic carcinoma (9–18%), colon carcinoma (4%), renal cell carcinoma (3%), ovary (8%), prostate (6%), stomach (7%), pancreas, endometrial cancer
3. Angiosarcoma
4. Malignant fibrous histiocytoma, leiomyosarcoma, fibrosarcoma
5. Langerhans cell histiocytosis
√ splenomegaly
√ multiple hypoechoic nodules (less often)

B. BENIGN TUMOR
1. Hamartoma = splenoma
2. Hemangioma
3. Hematopoietic
4. Sarcoidosis
√ nodular lesions in liver and spleen in 5–15% (= coalescent granulomata) occurring within 5 years of diagnosis
√ hepatosplenomegaly
√ abdominal adenopathy (mean size of 2.6 cm)
5. Gaucher disease (islands of RES cells laden with glucosylceramide)
6. Inflammatory pseudotumor
7. Lymphangioma

C. SPLENIC INFARCTION

Cystic Splenic Lesion

A. CONGENITAL
1. Epidermoid cyst = true cyst = congenital cyst

B. VASCULAR
1. Splenic laceration / fracture
2. Hematoma
3. **False cyst** = posttraumatic cyst = nonpancreatic pseudocyst of the spleen
◊ 80% of all splenic cysts are pseudocysts (= secondary cysts)
Cause: cystic end stage of trauma, infection, infarction
√ internal echoes from debris
√ calcifications within cyst wall may resemble eggshell
√ smaller size than true cyst
4. Cystic degeneration of infarct
(a) occlusion of splenic a. / branches (hemolytic anemia, endocarditis, SLE, arteritides, pancreatic cancer)
(b) venous thrombosis of splenic sinusoids (massive splenomegaly)
5. Peliosis

C. INFECTION / INFLAMMATION
1. Pyogenic abscess
Prevalence: 0.1–0.7%
Cause: hematogenous spread in sepsis (75%), penetrating trauma (15%), infarction (10%)
Predisposed: endocarditis, drug abuse, penetrating trauma, neoplasm, sickle cell disease
• fever, chills, LUQ pain (in <50%)
√ irregular borders without capsule
√ gas bubbles within abscess
√ rim enhancement
Rx: 76% success rate for percutaneous drain
2. Microabscesses
Organism: fungus (especially Candida, Aspergillus, Cryptococcus)
Prevalence: 26% of splenic abscesses
Predisposed: immunocompromised patient
√ hepatosplenomegaly
√ multiple round hypoechoic / hypoattenuating "target" lesions of 5–10 mm often associated with hepatic + renal involvement
√ "wheel-in-wheel" appearance when central hyperechoic portion becomes necrotic + hypoechoic

3. Granulomatous infection
   (a) Mycobacterium tuberculosis: miliary TB
      √ mild splenomegaly uncommon
   (b) M. avium-intracellulare
      √ marked splenomegaly in 20%
4. Pneumocystis carinii infection
   √ splenomegaly + multiple hypoattenuating foci
5. Parasitic cyst (Echinococcus)
   Prevalence: in <2% of patients with hydatid disease
   Cause: systemic dissemination, intraperitoneal spread of ruptured liver cyst
   √ solitary cyst ± subjacent daughter cysts
   √ hydatid sand ± infolded membranes
   √ ± linear calcification
6. Intrasplenic pancreatic pseudocyst
   Prevalence: in 1–5% of patients with pancreatitis

D. CYSTIC NEOPLASM
1. Cavernous hemangioma
   ◊ Most common primary neoplasm of the spleen!
2. Lymphangioma / lymphangiomatosis
   √ septate subcapsular cystic lesions
3. Lymphoma (most common malignant neoplasm!)
4. Necrotic metastasis:
   ◊ In 7% of patients with widespread metastasis!
   malignant melanoma (in 50%); breast, lung, ovarian, pancreatic, endometrial, colonic, prostatic, carcinoma; chondrosarcoma

E. TRUE CYST (with epithelial lining)
1. Congenital cyst = epidermoid cyst
2. Parasitic cyst

F. FALSE CYST = PSEUDOCYST (lacking epithelial lining)
1. Traumatic cyst
2. Postinfarct cyst

Increased Splenic Density

1. Sickle cell anemia (in 5% of sicklers)
2. Hemochromatosis
3. Thorotrast exposure
4. Lymphangiography

Splenic Calcification

A. DISSEMINATED
1. Phlebolith: visceral angiomatosis
2. Granuloma (most common): histoplasmosis, TB, brucellosis

B. CAPSULAR & PARENCHYMAL
1. Pyogenic / tuberculous abscess
2. Pneumocystis carinii infection
2. Infarction (multiple)
3. Hematoma

C. VASCULAR
1. Splenic artery calcification
2. Splenic artery aneurysm
3. Splenic infarct

D. CALCIFIED CYST WALL
1. Congenital cyst
2. Posttraumatic cyst
3. Echinococcal cyst
4. Cystic dermoid
5. Epidermoid

mnemonic: "HITCH"
Histoplasmosis (most common)
Infarct (sickle cell disease)
Tuberculosis
Cyst (Echinococcus)
Hematoma

Iron Accumulation in Spleen

A. DIFFUSE
1. Multiple blood transfusions
2. Sickle cell anemia

B. FOCAL
1. Gamna Gandy bodies
2. Angiosarcoma

Hyperechoic Splenic Spots

1. Granulomas: miliary tuberculosis, histoplasmosis
2. Phleboliths
3. Lymphoma / leukemia
4. Myelofibrosis
5. Gamna-Gandy nodules (in portal hypertension)

Spontaneous Splenic Rupture

1. Posttraumatic delayed rupture
2. Splenomegaly
3. Hemangioma
4. Epidermoid cyst
5. Peliosis
6. Previous splenic infarction

ANATOMY OF LIVER, BILE DUCTS, AND PANCREAS

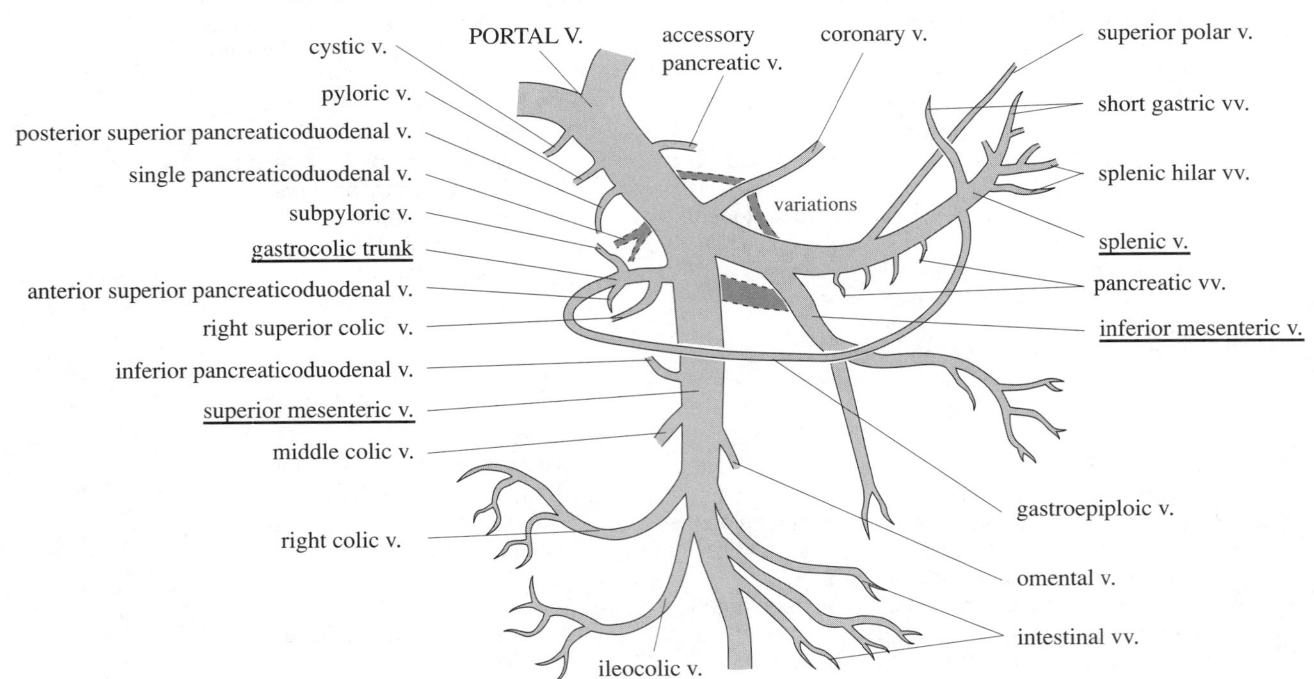

Extrahepatic Portal Vein Tributaries

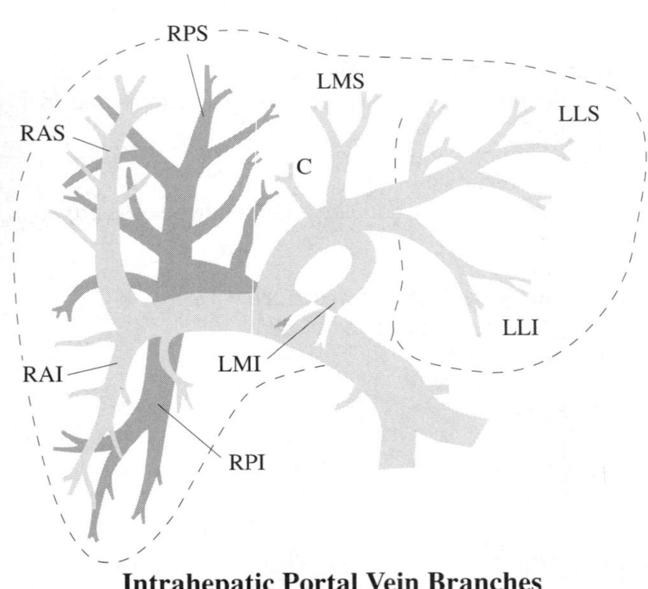

Intrahepatic Portal Vein Branches

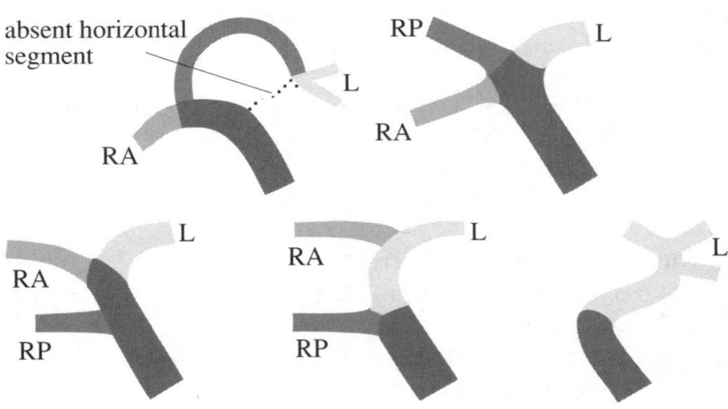

Variations of Intrahepatic Portal Venous System
(20%)

A. LEFT PORTAL VEIN
   1. Absence of horizontal segment (0.2%)
B. RIGHT PORTAL VEIN
   1. Trifurcation of main portal vein (11%)
   2. Origin of RP segment from main portal vein (5%)
   3. Origin of RA segment from left portal vein (4%)
   4. Absence of main right, RA, and RP portal segments

RA = right anterior segment
RAI = right anterior inferior
RAS = right anterior superior
RP = right posterior segment
RPI = right posterior inferior
RPS = right posterior superior
C = caudate lobe
L = left portal vein
LMI = left median inferior
LMS = left median superior
LLI = left lateral inferior
LLS = left lateral superior

LIVER

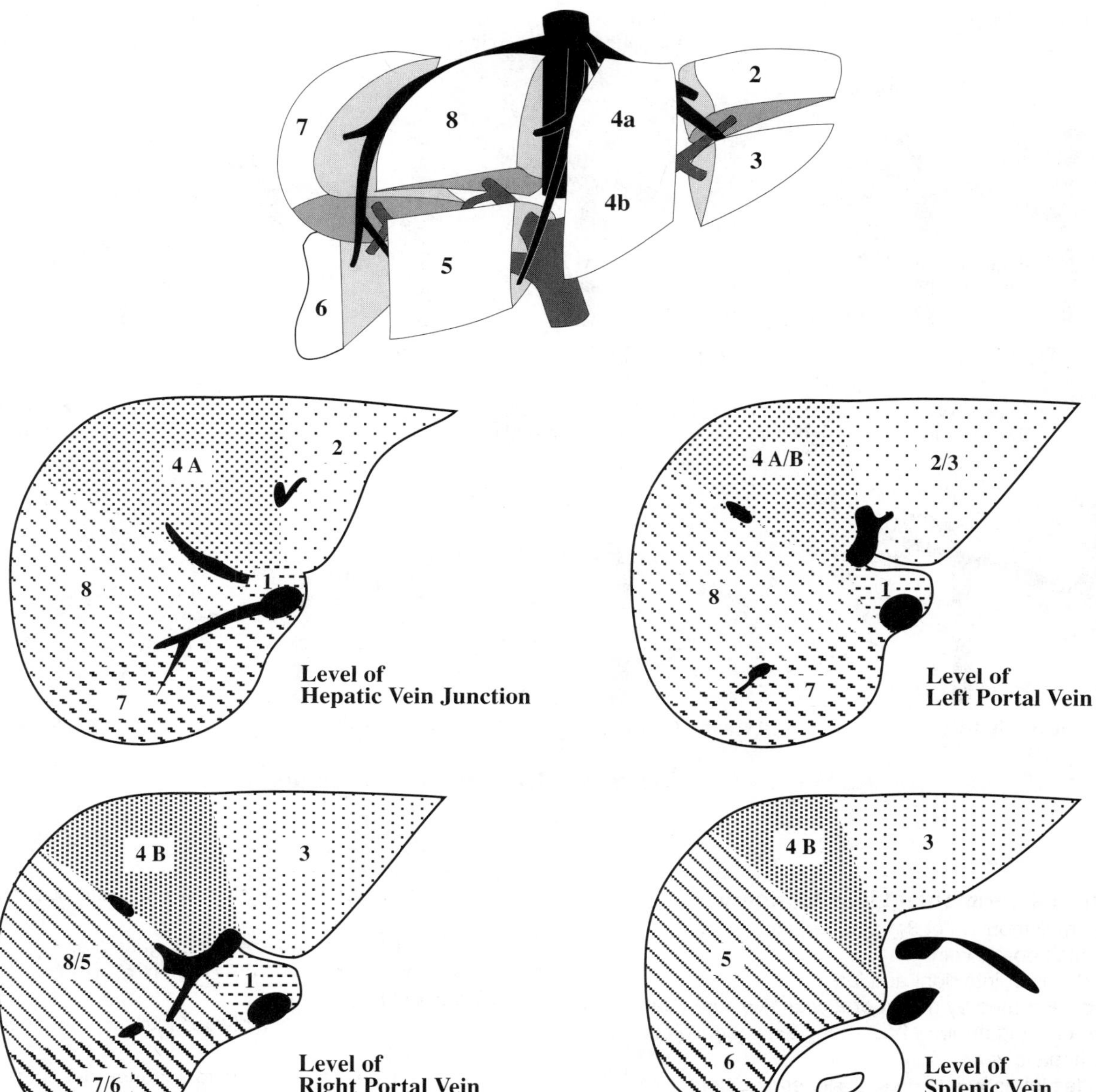

Functional Segmental Liver Anatomy			
Goldsmith & Woodburne		*Couinaud & Bismuth*	
CAUDATE LOBE		Caudate lobe	1
LEFT LOBE	Left lateral segment	Left lateral superior subsegment	2
		Left lateral inferior subsegment	3
	Left medial segment	Left medial superior subsegment	4 a
		Left medial inferior subsegment	4 b
RIGHT LOBE	Right anterior segment	Right anterior inferior subsegment	5
		Right anterior superior subsegment	8
	Right posterior segment	Right posterior inferior subsegment	6
		Right posterior superior subsegment	7

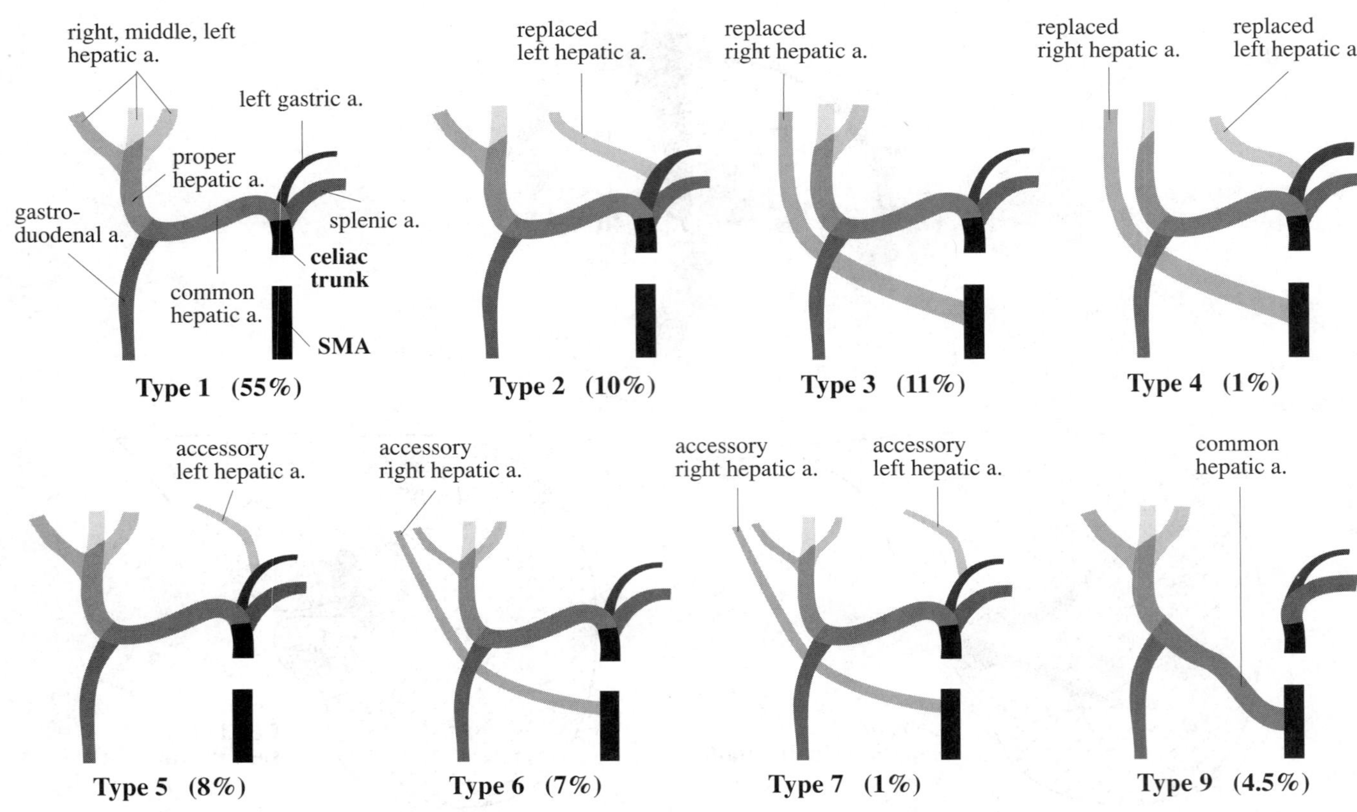

Michels Classification of Hepatic Arterial Anatomy

LIVER

Functional Segmental Liver Anatomy

based on distribution of 3 major hepatic veins:

(a) middle hepatic vein
divides liver into right and left lobe
also separated by main portal vein scissura (Cantlie line) passing through IVC + long axis of gallbladder)

(b) left hepatic vein
divides left lobe into medial + lateral sectors

(c) right hepatic vein
divides right lobe into anterior + posterior sectors

Each of the four sections is further divided:
by an imaginary transverse line drawn through the right + left portal vein into anterior + posterior segments; the segments are numbered counterclockwise from IVC

Hepatic Arterial Anatomy (Michels classification)

Type 1 (55%):
- celiac trunk trifurcates into LT gastric a. + splenic a. + common hep. a.
- common hep. a. divides into gastroduodenal a. + proper hep. a.
- RT hep. a. + LT hep. a. arise from proper hep. a.
- middle hep. a. (supplying caudate lobe) arises from
  (a) LT / RT hep. a.
  (b) proper hep. a. (in 10%)

Type 2 (10%):
- common hep. a. divides into gastroduodenal + RT hep. a.
- LT hep. a. replaced to LT gastric a.
- middle hep. a. from RT hep. a.

Type 3 (11%):
- common hep. a. divides into gastroduodenal + LT hep. a.
- RT hep. a. replaced to superior mesenteric a.
- middle hep. a. from LT hep. a.

Type 4 (1%):
- common hep. a. divides into middle hep. a. + gastroduodenal a.
- RT hep. a. + LT hep. a. are both replaced

Type 5 (8%):
- accessory LT hep. a. arises from LT gastric a.

Type 6 (7%):
- accessory RT hep. a. arises from superior mesenteric a.

Type 7 (1%):
- accessory RT + LT hepatic a.

Type 8 (2%):
- combinations of accessory + replaced hepatic aa.

Type 9 (4.5%):
- hepatic trunk replaced to superior mesenteric a.

Type 10 (0.5%):
- hepatic trunk replaced to LT gastric a.

Aberrant Hepatic Artery

= hepatic artery coursing between IVC + portal vein

1. Replaced right hepatic artery (50%)
2. Right hepatic artery with early bifurcation of common hepatic artery into right + left hepatic arteries (20%)
3. Accessory right hepatic artery (15%)
4. Replacement of entire hepatic trunk to SMA (15%)

Third Inflow to Liver

= aberrant veins supplying small areas of liver tissue + communicating with intrahepatic portal vein branches

Effect: focal decrease of portal vein perfusion resulting in areas of fat-sparing / fat accumulation

1. Cholecystic veins
   - directly entering liver segments 4 + 5
   - veins joining the parabiliary veins via triangle of Calot
2. Parabiliary venous system
   = venous network within hepatoduodenal ligament anterior to main portal vein
   Tributaries:
   - cholecystic vein through triangle of Calot
   - pancreaticoduodenal vein
   - right gastric / pyloric vein

   √ pseudolesion at dorsal aspect of segment 4
3. Epigastric-paraumbilical venous system
   = small veins around falciform ligament draining anterior part of abdominal wall directly into liver
   Subgroups:
   (a) superior vein of Sappey
   - drains upper portion of falciform ligament + medial part of diaphragm
   - enters peripheral left portal vein branches
   - communicates with superior epigastric + internal thoracic veins

   (b) inferior vein of Sappey
   - drains lower portion of falciform ligament
   - enters peripheral left portal vein branches
   - communicates with branches of inferior epigastric vein around the umbilicus

   (c) vein of Burow
   - terminates in middle portion of collapsed umbilical vein
   - communicates with branches of inferior epigastric vein around the umbilicus

   (d) intercalary veins
   - interconnect vein of Burow + inferior vein of Sappey

Hepatic Fissures

1. Fissure for **ligamentum teres** = umbilical fissure
   = invagination of ligamentum teres = embryologic remnant of obliterated umbilical vein connecting placental venous blood with left portal vein
   — located at dorsal free margin of **falciform ligament**
   — runs into liver with visceral peritoneum
   — divides left hepatic lobe into medial + lateral segments (divides subsegment 3 from 4)

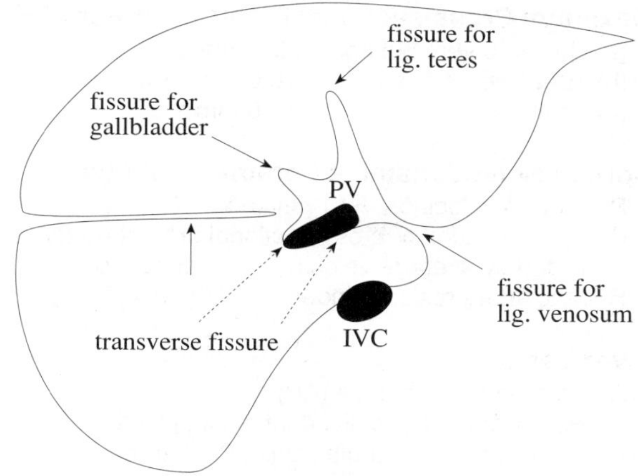

Hepatic Fissures

2. Fissure for **ligamentum venosum**
   = invagination of obliterated ductus venosus
   = embryologic connection of left portal vein with left hepatic vein
   — separates caudate lobe from left lobe of liver
   — lesser omentum within fissure separates the greater sac anteriorly from lesser sac posteriorly
3. Fissure for gallbladder (GB)
   = shallow peritoneal invagination containing the GB
   — divides right from left lobe of liver
4. Transverse fissure
   = invagination of hepatic pedicle into liver
   — contains horizontal portion of left + right portal veins
5. Accessory fissures
   (a) Right inferior accessory fissure
   = from gallbladder fossa / just inferior to it to lateroinferior margin of liver

   (b) Others (rare)

Size of Liver

A. YOUNG INFANT
   right hepatic lobe should not extend >1 cm below right costal margin

B. CHILD
   right hepatic lobe should not extend below right costal margin

C. ADULT
   (a) midclavicular line (vertical / craniocaudad axis):
   <13 cm = normal
   13.0–15.5 cm = indeterminate (in 25%)
   >15.5 cm = hepatomegaly (87% accuracy)

   (b) preaortic line <10 cm
   (c) prerenal line <14 cm

Liver Echogenicity & Attenuation

US: pancreatic > hepatic > renal echogenicity
CT: 40–70 HU (precontrast)
CECT: early arterial phase (20 sec), late arterial phase (30–40 sec), portal venous phase (60–70 sec); maximal enhancement at 45–60 sec

LIVER

Maximum Cross-sectional Diameter of Portal Vein

(a) child <10 years of age: 8.5 mm
(b) 10–20 years of age: 10.0 mm
(c) adult: 13.0 mm

Normal Hemodynamics Parameter of Liver

Portal vein velocity: >11 cm/sec
Congestion index (= cross-sectional area of portal vein divided by average velocity): 0.070 ± 0.09
Hepatic artery resistive index: 0.60–0.64 ± 0.06

Liver Tests

A. Alkaline phosphatase (AP)
Formation: bone, liver, intestine, placenta
High increase: cholestasis with extrahepatic biliary obstruction (confirmed by rise in γGT), drugs, granulomatous disease (sarcoidosis), primary biliary cirrhosis, primary + secondary malignancy of liver
Mild increase: all forms of liver disease, heart failure

B. Gamma-glutamyl transpeptidase (γGT)
very sensitive in almost all forms of liver disease
Utility: confirms hepatic source of elevated AP, may indicate significant alcohol use

C. Transaminases
high increase: viral / toxin-induced acute hepatitis
(a) aspartate aminotransferase (AST; formerly serum glutamic oxaloacetic transaminase [SGOT])
Formation: liver, muscle, kidney, pancreas, RBCs
(b) alanine aminotransferase (ALT; formerly serum glutamic pyruvic transaminase [SGPT])
Formation: primarily in liver
• rather specific elevation in liver disease

D. Bilirubin
helps differentiate between various causes of jaundice
(a) unconjugated / indirect bilirubin = insoluble in water
Formation: breakdown of senescent RBCs
Metabolism: tightly bound to albumin in vessels, actively taken up by liver, cannot be excreted by kidneys
(b) conjugated / direct bilirubin = water-soluble
Formation: conjugation in liver cells
Metabolism: excretion into bile; not reabsorbed by intestinal mucosa + excreted in feces

Elevation:
– overproduction: hemolytic anemia, resorption of hematoma, multiple transfusions
– decreased hepatic uptake: drugs, sepsis
– decreased conjugation: Gilbert syndrome, neonatal jaundice, hepatitis, cirrhosis, sepsis
– decreased excretion into bile: hepatitis, cirrhosis, drug-induced cholestasis, sepsis, extrahepatic biliary obstruction

E. Lactic dehydrogenase (LDH)
nonspecific and therefore not helpful
high increase: primary or metastatic liver involvement

F. Alpha fetoprotein (AFP)
>400 ng/mL strongly suggests that focal mass represents a hepatocellular carcinoma

BILE DUCTS

Normal Size of Bile Ducts

@ CBD at point of maximum diameter = free edge of gastrohepatic ligament (point of least constraint):
(a) adolescents & adults
≤5 mm = normal; 6–7 mm = equivocal; ≥8 mm = dilated
◊ In patient >60 years of age add 1 mm/decade
◊ Following cholecystectomy up to 8 mm
(b) neonates: <1 mm
(c) infants up to 1 year of age: <2 mm
(d) older children: <4 mm

@ CHD at porta hepatis + CBD in head of pancreas: 5 mm

@ right intrahepatic bile duct just proximal to CHD: 2–3 mm / <40% of diameter of accompanying portal vein

@ Cystic duct diameter: 1.8 mm
average length of 1–2 cm
distal cystic duct posterior to CBD (in 95%), anterior to CBD (in 5%)

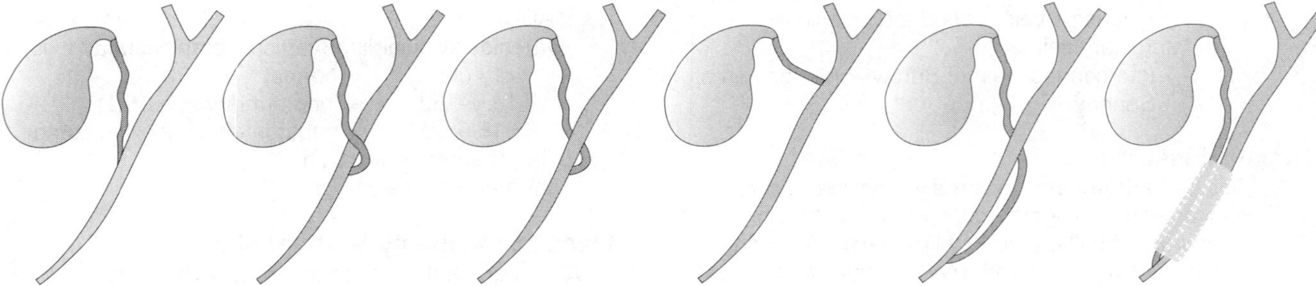

Anatomic Variants of Cystic Duct Insertion

LIVER

Bile Duct Variants

Prevalence: 2.4% of autopsies; 13–18.5% of operative cholangiograms
Significance: aberrant ducts near cystic duct / gallbladder have the greatest risk of iatrogenic injury at cholecystectomy
Cx: (1) postoperative bile leak if severed
(2) segmental biliary obstruction if ligated

A. ABERRANT INTRAHEPATIC DUCT
may join CHD, CBD, cystic duct, right hepatic duct, gallbladder
— major right segmental bile duct joins extrahepatic bile duct at / near cystic duct insertion (4–5%)
— cysticohepatic duct (1–2%) = anomalous right hepatic duct inserts into cystic duct
— anomalous left hepatic ducts: not susceptible to injury + therefore of no clinical significance
B. CYSTIC DUCT ENTERING RIGHT HEPATIC DUCT
C. DUCTS OF LUSCHKA
= small ducts from hepatic bed draining directly into gallbladder
D. DUPLICATION OF CYSTIC DUCT / CBD
± duplication of gallbladder
E. CONGENITAL TRACHEOBILIARY FISTULA
= fistulous communication between carina and left hepatic duct
• infants with respiratory distress
• productive cough with bilious sputum
√ pneumobilia

Variants of Cystic Duct Insertion

Prevalence: variations occur in 18–23%
(a) Craniocaudad direction:
– proximal third = common hepatic duct high in porta hepatis
– middle third of extrahepatic bile duct in 75%
– distal third of extrahepatic bile duct in 10%
√ cystic duct parallels extrahepatic bile duct (implies common fibrous sheath)
Cx: during cholecystectomy
(1) common hepatic duct stricture
(2) inadvertent ligation / transection of extrahepatic bile duct
(3) long cystic duct remnant

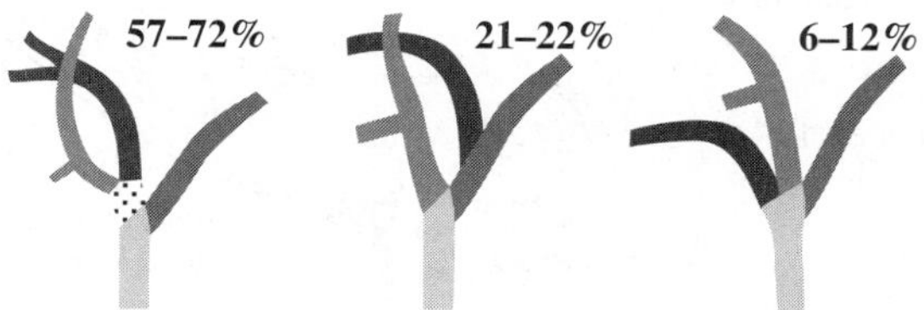

Bile Duct Variants
right posterior segmental duct
right anterior segmental duct
common hepatic duct
right hepatic duct
left hepatic duct

(b) Mediolateral direction:
– right lateral
– anterior spiral
– posterior spiral
– low lateral (with common sheath)
– low medial (at / near ampulla of Vater)
(c) Insertion into intrahepatic bile duct
– right hepatic duct (0.3%)
– left hepatic duct (rare)
(d) absence of cystic duct
√ gallbladder drains directly into common bile duct

GALLBLADDER

Size & Capacity & Wall Thickness

Length:
(a) infant < 1 year old: 1.5–3 cm in length
(b) older child: 3–7 cm in length
(c) adult: 7–10 cm in length; 2–3.5 cm in width
Capacity: 30–50 mL
Wall thickness: 2–3 mm
Bile volume: 250–1,000 mL/day secreted by hepatocytes
GB function: concentration of bile through absorption of 90% of water

Congenital Gallbladder Anomalies

Agenesis of Gallbladder

Incidence: 0.04–0.07 % (autopsy)
Associated with:
common: rectovaginal fistula, imperforate anus, hypoplasia of scapula + radius, intracardiac shunt
rare: absence of corpus callosum, microcephaly, atresia of external auditory canal, tricuspid atresia, TE fistula, dextroposition of pancreas + esophagus, absent spleen, high position of cecum, polycystic kidney

Hypoplastic Gallbladder

(a) congenital
(b) associated with cystic fibrosis

Septations of Gallbladder

A. LONGITUDINAL SEPTA
1. Duplication of gallbladder
= two separate lumens + two cystic ducts
Incidence: 1:3,000–1:12,000
2. Bifid gallbladder = double gallbladder
= two separate lumens with one cystic duct
3. Triple gallbladder (extremely rare)
B. TRANSVERSE SEPTA
1. Isolated transverse septum
2. PHRYGIAN CAP (2–6% of population)
= kinking / folding of fundus ± septum
3. Multiseptated gallbladder (rare)
= multiple cystlike compartments connected by small pores
Cx: stasis + stone formation
C. GALLBLADDER DIVERTICULUM
= persistence of cystohepatic duct

LIVER

Gallbladder Ectopia

Most frequent locations:
(1) beneath the left lobe of the liver > (2) intrahepatic > (3) retrohepatic

Rare locations:
(4) within falciform ligament, (5) within interlobar fissure, (6) suprahepatic (lodged between superior surface of right hepatic lobe + anterior chest wall), (7) within anterior abdominal wall, (8) transverse mesocolon, (9) retrorenal, (10) near posterior spine + IVC, (11) intrathoracic GB (inversion of liver)
Associated with: eventration of diaphragm

"Floating GB"
= gallbladder with loose peritoneal reflections, may herniate through foramen of Winslow into lesser sac

"Torqued GB"
= results in hydrops

PANCREAS

Size

- pancreatic head: 1.0–2.2 cm
- pancreatic body: 0.4–1.0 cm
- pancreatic tail: 0.8–1.8 cm

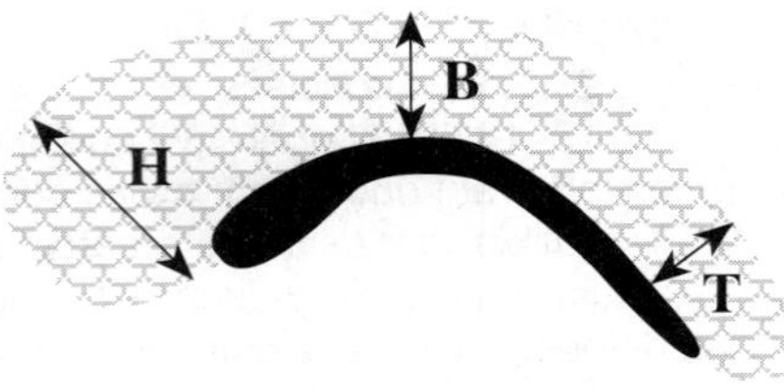

Pancreatic Diameters (on TRV image)

H	=	head	=	1.0–2.0 cm
B	=	body	=	0.4–1.0 cm
T	=	tail	=	0.8–2.2 cm

Pancreatic Development & Anatomy

during the 4th week of gestation 2 endodermal diverticula form in the foregut near its junction with the yolk sac
— dorsal diverticulum forms dorsal pancreas
— ventral diverticulum forms liver, gallbladder, bile ducts, ventral pancreas

A. DORSAL ANLAGE (in mesoduodenum)
Origin: arises from dorsal wall of duodenum + is later displaced to the left
◊ Forms cranial portion of head + isthmus + body + tail of pancreas
– prone to atrophy (poor in polypeptides)
√ drains to the minor papilla through accessory duct of Santorini

B. VENTRAL ANLAGE (below primordial liver bud)
Origin: ventral bud arises from ventral wall of duodenum and is composed of right + left lobes (the left ventral bud regresses completely), rotates dorsally and inferiorly + then to the left of the duodenum + fuses with dorsal anlage during 6–7th week GA
◊ Forms caudal portion of the pancreatic head + uncinate process + CBD
– not prone to atrophy (rich in polypeptides)
√ ventral duct drains with CBD through ampulla of Vater + becomes the major drainage pathway for the entire pancreas after fusion with dorsal duct

C. MAIN PANCREATIC DUCT OF WIRSUNG
distal portion of dorsal duct connects with ventral duct; proximal portion of dorsal duct may disappear
√ measures 1–2–3 mm in diameter
√ receives 20–35 tributaries / side branches that enter at right angles
√ usually drains through major papilla
◊ Major drainage route in 91% of individuals

D. ACCESSORY PANCREATIC DUCT OF SANTORINI
= proximal portion of dorsal duct, which has not atrophied
◊ Present in 44% of individuals

E. AMPULLA OF VATER
= space within medial wall of second portion of duodenum below surface of papilla of Vater

F. MAJOR DUODENAL PAPILLA = papilla of Vater
◊ Drainage of common bile duct in 100%
◊ Drainage of main pancreatic duct of Wirsung in 90%

G. MINOR DUODENAL PAPILLA (present in 60%)
◊ Drainage of accessory pancreatic duct of Santorini
◊ Drainage of main pancreatic duct in 10%
√ located a few cm orad to papilla of Vater

Pancreaticobiliary Junction Variants

A. Angle between CBD + pancreatic duct:
(a) usually acute at 5°–30°
(b) occasionally abnormal at up to 90°

B. Sphincter of Oddi = sphincter of hepaticopancreatic ampulla
= muscle fibers encircling the CBD + pancreatic duct at choledochoduodenal junction

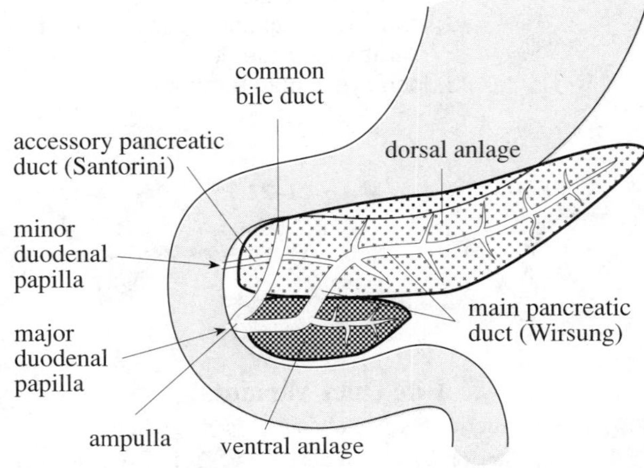

Embryologic Development of Pancreas

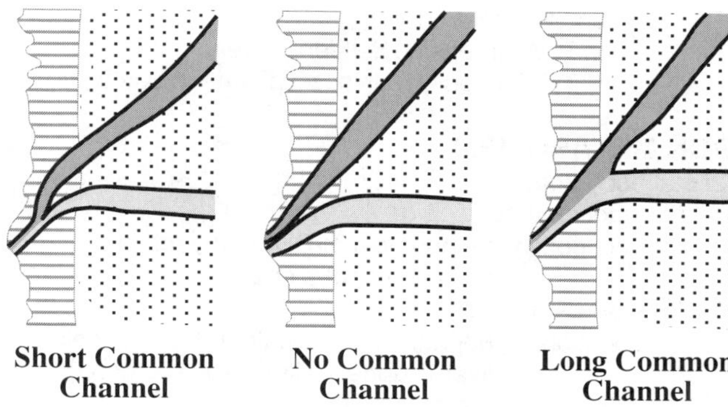

Normal Union between CBD & Pancreatic Duct

(a) choledochal sphincter (Boyden) = encircles distal CBD
(b) pancreatic duct sphincter (in 33% separate)
(c) ampullary sphincter

C. Types of union between CBD + pancreatic duct:
   1. Normal junction = union inside duodenal wall
      (a) 2–10 (mean 5) mm short common channel (55–85%) with a diameter of 3–5 mm
      (b) separate entrances into duodenum (42%)
      (c) 8–15 mm long common channel
   2. Anomalous junction = union outside duodenal wall beyond the influence of the sphincter of Boyden (1.5–3.2%)
      (a) pancreatic duct inserting into CBD >15 mm from entrance into duodenum
      (b) CBD inserting into pancreatic duct

SPLEEN

Size of Spleen

in adults: 12 cm length, 7–8 cm anteroposterior diameter, 3–4 cm thick; splenic index (L x W x H) of <480
in children: logarithmic increase in length with increasing age; formula for length = 5.7 + 0.31 x age (in years)
in infants (0–3 months of age): <6.0 cm in length

Weight of Spleen

at birth: 15 g
in adults: 150 (100–265) g
estimated weight = splenic index x 0.55

Embryology of Spleen

– spleen arises from mesenchymal cells between layers of dorsal mesogastrium during 5th week GA
– splenic primordium differentiates to form capsule, connective tissue framework, splenic parenchyma
– major site of hematopoiesis until 28 weeks GA; retains capacity for extramedullary hematopoiesis well into adult life
√ spleen recognizable by 12th week GA (as fusion of mesenchymal aggregates occurs)
√ splenic clefts / notches / lobules may persist
√ accessory spleen (in up to 30% by autopsy)

Histology of Spleen

(a) RED PULP = numerous vascular sinuses
(b) WHITE PULP = lymphoid follicles + cells of RES

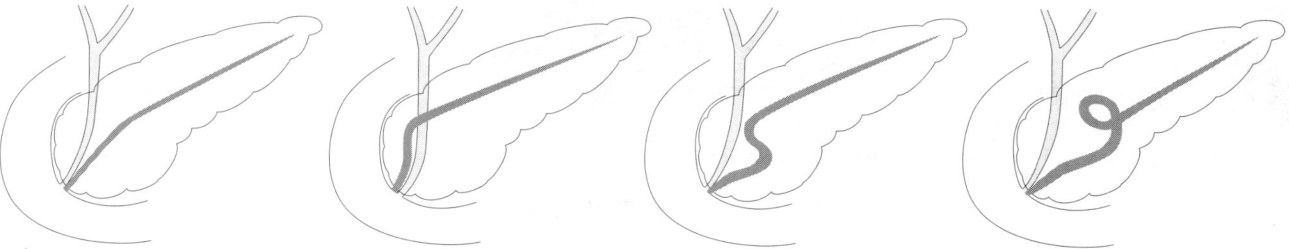

Descending Pancreatic Duct 50% | **Vertical Pancreatic Duct** | **Sigmoid Pancreatic Duct** | **Looped Pancreatic Duct**

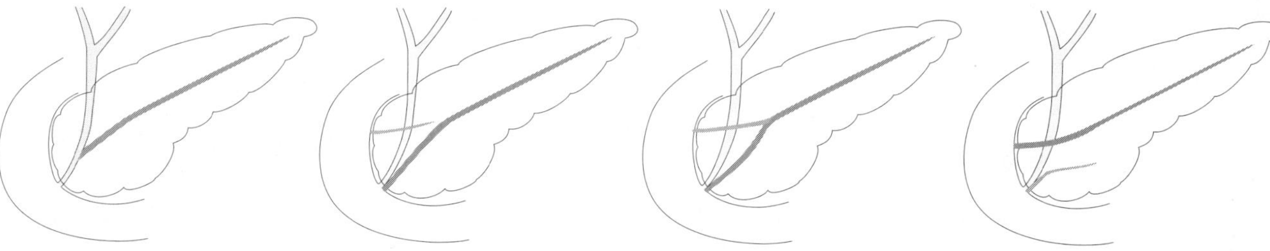

Anomalous Union of Pancreatic Duct and Bile Duct | **Persistent Duct of Santorini** duct of Wirsung as major drainage route in 91% | **Persistent Duct of Santorini (44%)** duct of Santorini as major drainage route in 9% | **Pancreas Divisum (7%)**

Variations in Pancreatic Duct Anatomy

Development: ratio of white to red pulp increases with age + progressive antigenic stimulation

Imaging Characteristics of Spleen

A. CT ATTENUATION
   (a) without enhancement:
      40–60 HU; 5–10 HU less than liver
   (b) with enhancement:
      normal heterogeneous enhancement during first minute after bolus injection (due to different blood flow rates through the cords of the red + white pulp)
      √ arciform (alternating bands of high + low attenuation) / focal / diffuse heterogeneity
      √ heterogeneity resolved in portal venous phase

B. MR SIGNAL INTENSITY
   directly related to ratio of white to red pulp
   (a) neonate <8 months of age:
      √ T1WI- and T2WI-intensity: spleen < liver (due to predominance of red pulp)
      DDx: hemochromatosis
   (b) adult + older child:
      √ T2WI-intensity: spleen > liver
      √ T1WI-intensity: liver > spleen > muscle

IRON METABOLISM

Total body iron: 5 g
   (a) functional iron: 4 g
      Location: hemoglobin of RBCs, myoglobin of muscle, various enzymes
   (b) stored iron: 1 g
      Location: hepatocytes, reticuloendothelial cells of liver (Kupffer cells) + spleen + bone marrow

Absorption: 1–2 mg/day through gut
Transport: bound to transferrin intravascularly
Deposition:
   (a) transferrin-transfer to:
      hepatocytes, RBC precursors in erythron, parenchymal tissues (eg, muscle)
   (b) phagocytosis by:
      reticuloendothelial cells phagocytize senescent erythrocytes (= extravascular hemolysis); RBC iron stored as ferritin / released and bound to transferrin

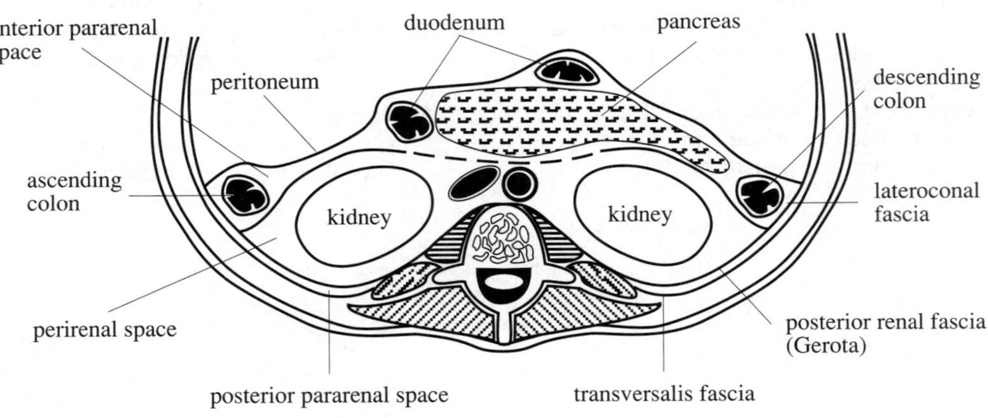

Extraperitoneal Spaces

LIVER

DISORDERS OF LIVER, BILIARY TRACT, PANCREAS, AND SPLEEN

ACCESSORY SPLEEN

= failure of coalescence of several small mesodermal buds in the dorsal mesogastrium that comprise the spleen

Incidence: 10–30% of population; multiple (up to 6) in 10%

◊ Undergoes hypertrophy after splenectomy and is responsible for recurrence of hematologic disorders (idiopathic thrombocytopenic purpura, hereditary spherocytosis, acquired autoimmune hemolytic anemia, hypersplenism)

Location:
- (a) near splenic hilum along the course of splenic vessels (most common)
- (b) within layers of omentum (gastrosplenic ligament, other suspensory ligaments of spleen)
- (c) anywhere in abdomen (eg, pancreas, pelvis)
- (d) attached to left ovary / testis =**splenogonadal fusion** (due to close relationship between developing spleen + mesonephros + left gonadal anlage)

NUC (Tc-99m sulfur colloid scan / spleen-specific Tc-99m denatured RBCs):
- √ usually <1 cm in diameter
- √ <10% identified when normal spleen present

Cx: disease recurrence due to hypertrophy of accessory spleen after splenectomy for hypersplenism

AMPULLARY TUMOR

= benign / malignant tumors arising from glandular epithelium of ampulla of Vater

Age: 6th + 7th decade; M:F = 2:1

Path: average diameter of <3 cm

Histo:
- (a) dysplastic epithelium in glandular / villous structures of tubular / villous adenoma
- (b) carcinoma in situ
- (c) invasive carcinoma often with desmoplastic reaction

Associated with: familial adenomatous polyposis syndromes (eg, familial polyposis coli, Gardner syndrome) [100–200-fold risk], colon carcinoma

- • malaise, epigastric pain, weight loss
- • intestinal bleeding (tumor ulceration)
- • intermittent jaundice (ductal obstruction)
- • gray "aluminum / silver-colored" stools (3%)
- • chills, fever, RUQ pain (ascending cholangitis) in up to 20%
- • endoscopy: tumor extending through orifice (63%), prominent papilla / submucosal mass (25%), not visualized (9%)

TNM staging:
- T1 : tumor confined to ampulla
- T2 : tumor extending into duodenal wall
- T3 : invasion of pancreas <2 cm deep
- T4 : invasion of pancreas >2 cm deep

International Union Against Cancer Staging:
- I = tumor confined to ampulla
- II = tumor extension into duodenal wall / pancreas
- III = regional lymph node involvement (Lnn stations around head + body of pancreas, anterior + posterior pancreaticoduodenal, pyloric, common bile duct, proximal mesenteric)
- IV = invasion of pancreas >2 cm deep

√ tumor often inapparent due to small size

UGI:
- √ indentation of duodenal lumen at papilla of Vater with filling defect >1.5 cm
- √ surface irregularity + deep barium-filled crevices in villous tumor

Biliary imaging:
- √ dilatation of most distal segment of common bile duct
- √ stenosis (circumferential tumor growth around ampulla / desmoplastic reaction)
- √ irregular predominantly polypoid filling defect
- √ ± pancreatic dilatation = double-duct sign (may be absent if tumor small / accessory pancreatic duct decompresses pancreatic system / main pancreatic duct drains into minor papilla)

Endoscopic US (most sensitive technique): 87% staging accuracy

Rx: Whipple procedure (= pancreaticoduodenectomy)

Prognosis: 28–70% 5-year survival for ampullary carcinomas (depending on stage)

DDx:
1. Periampullary duodenal adenoma / adenocarcinoma (usually larger lesion with significant intraduodenal extension)
2. Choledochocele (cystic lesion filling with biliary contrast)
3. Brunner gland tumor, pancreatic rest ("myoepithelial hamartoma"), leiomyoma, carcinoid (often produce somatostatin)
4. Duodenitis, pancreatitis
5. Stone impaction in ampulla

ANNULAR PANCREAS

= second most common congenital anomaly wherein a ring of normal pancreatic tissue encircles the duodenum secondary to abnormal migration of ventral pancreas (head + uncinate)

Incidence: 1:20,000 autopsies

Age at discovery: childhood (52%); adulthood (48%)

Associated with: other congenital anomalies (in 75%): esophageal atresia, TE fistula, duodenal atresia / stenosis, duodenal diaphragm, imperforate anus, malrotation, Down syndrome

Location: 2nd portion of duodenum (85%); 1st / 3rd portion of duodenum (15%)

- • mostly asymptomatic with incidental discovery
- • neonate : persistent vomiting (duodenal obstruction)

• adult : nausea, vomiting (60%), abdominal pain (70%), hematemesis (10%), jaundice (50%)
√ polyhydramnios (in utero)
√ "double bubble" = dilated duodenal bulb + stomach
√ proximal duodenal dilatation
√ enlargement of pancreatic head
UGI:
√ eccentric narrowing with lateral notching + medial retraction of 2nd part of duodenum
√ concentric narrowing of mid-descending duodenum
√ reverse peristalsis, pyloric incompetency
CT:
√ pancreatic tissue surrounding descending duodenum
ERCP (most specific) / MR pancreatography:
√ normally located main duct in pancreatic body + tail
√ small duct originating on anterior left + passing posteriorly around duodenum communicates with main duct (in 85%)
Cx: increased incidence of
(1) periampullary peptic ulcers
(2) pancreatitis (15–20%) usually confined to pancreatic head and annulus
Rx: gastrojejunostomy / duodenojejunostomy

ASCARIASIS

Most frequent helminthic infection in humans
Organism: Ascaris lumbricoides, 25–35 cm long as adult worm; life span of 1 year
Country: 644 million humans harbor the roundworm; 70– 90% in America; in United States endemic in: Appalachian range, southern + Gulf coast states
Prevalence: 25% of world population infected
(a) in United States: 12% in blacks, 1% in whites
(b) in parts of Africa, Asia, South America: 90%
Cycle:
ingestion of contaminated water / soil / vegetable; larvae penetrate intestinal wall; migrate into mesenteric lymphatics + veins into liver; reach lung via right heart + pulmonary artery; mature in pulmonary capillary bed to 2–3 mm length; burrow into alveoli; ascend in respiratory tract; are swallowed and again reach small intestine, where they become adult worms whose eggs leave the body by the fecal route
• abnormal liver function tests + biliary colic
• hypereosinophilia only present during acute stage of larval migration
√ barium study
√ cholangiography (49%)
US:
√ tubular echogenic filling defect with 2–4-mm wide central sonolucent line (= worm with digestive tract) within dilated common bile duct
Cx: (1) Intestinal obstruction
(2) Intermittent biliary obstruction with acute cholangitis, cholecystitis, pancreatitis
(3) Liver abscess (rare)
(4) Granulomatous stricture of extrahepatic bile ducts (rare)
Rx: Mebendazole

BANTI SYNDROME

= NONCIRRHOTIC IDIOPATHIC PORTAL HYPERTENSION = NONCIRRHOTIC PORTAL FIBROSIS = HEPATOPORTAL SCLEROSIS
= syndrome characterized by
(1) splenomegaly
(2) hypersplenism
(3) portal hypertension
Etiology: increased portal vascular resistance possibly due to portal fibrosis + obliterative venopathy of intrahepatic portal branches
Histo: slight portal fibrosis, dilatation of sinusoids, intimal thickening with eccentric sclerosis of peripheral portal vein walls
Age: middle-aged women; rare in America + Europe but common in India + Japan
• elevated portal vein pressure (without cirrhosis, parasites, venous occlusion)
• normal liver function tests
• cytopenia (due to hypersplenism)
• normal / slightly elevated hepatic venous wedge pressure
√ esophageal varices
√ patent hepatic veins
√ patent extrahepatic portal vein + multiple collaterals
Prognosis: 90% 5-year survival; 55% 30-year survival

BILIARY CYSTADENOCARCINOMA

= BILE DUCT CYSTADENOCARCINOMA
= rare malignant multilocular cystic tumor originating from biliary cystadenoma
Histo: (a) with ovarian stroma (good prognosis), in females only
(b) without ovarian stroma (bad prognosis)
• hemorrhagic internal fluid
√ nodularity with septations are suggestive of malignancy
√ coarse calcifications
DDx: no image differentiation from biliary cystadenoma

BILIARY CYSTADENOMA

= BILE DUCT CYSTADENOMA
= rare benign premalignant multilocular cystic tumor originating in bile ducts; probably deriving from ectopic nests of primitive biliary tissue
Incidence: 4.6% of all intrahepatic cysts of bile duct origin
Age: >30 years (82%), peak incidence in 5th decade; M:F = 1:4; predominantly Caucasian
Path: multilocular cystic tumor containing proteinaceous fluid with well-defined thick capsule
Histo: single layer of cuboidal / tall columnar biliary-type epithelium with papillary projections, subepithelial stroma resembling that of the ovary
◊ Similar to mucinous cystic tumors of pancreas + ovary
Location: intrahepatic:extrahepatic bile ducts = 85:15; right lobe (48%); left lobe (20–35%); both lobes (15–30%); gallbladder (rare)
• chronic abdominal pain
• dyspepsia, anorexia, nausea + vomiting
• jaundice

• abdominal swelling with palpable mass (90%)
√ mass of 1.5–35 cm in size
√ up to 11 liters of clear / cloudy, serous / mucinous / gelatinous, purulent / hemorrhagic / bilious fluid containing hemosiderin / cholesterol / necrosis
√ papillary excrescences + mural nodules
√ septations between cysts

US:
√ ovoid multiloculated anechoic mass with highly echogenic septations / papillary growths
√ may contain fluid-fluid levels

CT:
√ multiloculated mass of near water density
√ contrast enhancement in wall + internal septa

MR:
√ locules with variable signal intensity on T1WI + T2WI depending on their protein content

Angio:
√ avascular mass with small clusters of peripheral abnormal vessels
√ stretching + displacement of vessels
√ thin subtle blush of neovascularity in septa + wall

Cx: (1) malignant transformation into cystadenocarcinoma (indicated by invasion of capsule)
(2) rupture into peritoneum / retroperitoneum

Rx: surgical resection (recurrence common)

DDx: liver abscess, echinococcal cyst, cystic mesenchymal hamartoma (children + young adults), undifferentiated sarcoma (children + young adults), necrotic hepatic metastasis, cystic primary hepatocellular carcinoma

BILIARY-ENTERIC FISTULA

Incidence: 5% at cholecystectomy; 0.5% at autopsy

Etiology: cholelithiasis (90%), acute / chronic cholecystitis, biliary tract carcinoma, regional invasive neoplasm, diverticulitis, inflammatory bowel disease, peptic ulcer disease, echinococcal cyst, trauma, congenital communication

Communication with:
duodenum (70%), colon (26%), stomach (4%), jejunum, ileum, hepatic artery, portal vein (caused death of Ignatius Loyola), bronchial tree, pericardium, renal pelvis, ureter, urinary bladder, vagina, ovary

A. CHOLECYSTODUODENAL FISTULA (51–80%)
   1. Perforated gallstone (90%): associated with gallstone ileus in 20%
   2. Perforated duodenal ulcer (10%)
   3. Surgical anastomosis
   4. Gallbladder carcinoma
B. CHOLECYSTOCOLIC FISTULA (13–21%)
C. CHOLEDOCHODUODENAL FISTULA (13–19%) due to perforated duodenal ulcer disease
D. MULTIPLE FISTULAE (7%)

√ pneumobilia = branching tubular radiolucencies, more prominent centrally within the liver
√ barium filling of biliary tree
√ shrunken gallbladder mimicking pseudodiverticulum of duodenal bulb
√ multiple hyperechoic foci with dirty shadowing

DDx: patulous sphincter of Oddi, ascending cholangitis, surgery (choledochoduodenostomy, cholecystojejunostomy, sphincterotomy)

BUDD-CHIARI SYNDROME

= syndrome of global / segmental hepatic venous outflow obstruction

Cause:
A. IDIOPATHIC (66%)
B. THROMBOSIS
   (a) hypercoagulable state: polycythemia rubra vera (1/3), oral contraceptives, pregnancy + postpartum state, paroxysmal nocturnal hemoglobulinuria (12%), sickle cell disease
   mnemonic: "5 P's"
   Paroxysmal nocturnal hemoglobulinuria
   Platelets (thrombocytosis)
   Pill (birth control pills)
   Pregnancy
   Polycythemia rubra vera
   (b) injury to vessel wall: phlebitis, trauma, hepatic radiation injury, chemotherapeutic + immunosuppressive drugs in patients with bone marrow transplants, venoocclusive disease from pyrrolizidine alkaloids (senecio) found in medicinal bush teas in Jamaica
C. NONTHROMBOTIC OBSTRUCTION
   (a) Tumor growth into IVC / hepatic veins (renal cell carcinoma, hepatoma, adrenal carcinoma, metastasis, primary leiomyosarcoma of IVC)
   (b) Membranous obstruction of suprahepatic IVC = IVC diaphragm (believed to be a congenital web or an acquired lesion from long-standing IVC thrombosis); common in Oriental + Indian population (South Africa, India, Japan, Korea); very rare in Western countries
   (c) Right atrial tumor
   (d) Constrictive pericarditis
   (e) Right heart failure

Pathophysiology: hepatic venous thrombosis leads to elevation of sinusoidal pressure, which causes delayed / reversed portal venous inflow, ascites, alteration in hepatic morphology

Age: all ages; M < F

• right upper quadrant pain
• shortness of breath (due to decreased cardiac return)
• nonspecific elevated transaminases, jaundice
• lower-extremity edema

Location:
Type I : occlusion of IVC ± hepatic veins
Type II : occlusion of major hepatic veins ± IVC
Type III : occlusion of small centrilobar veins

√ hepatosplenomegaly (early sign)
√ caudate lobe hypertrophy (88%) [DDx: cirrhosis]
√ ascites
√ gallbladder wall thickening >6 mm
√ nonvisualization of hepatic veins (75%) / vein diameter <3 mm (measured 2 cm from IVC)

LIVER

√ communications between right / middle hepatic vein and inferior right hepatic vein
√ enlarged inferior right hepatic vein (18%)
√ portal vein diameter >12 mm (in adults), >8 mm (in children)
√ visualization of collateral pathways:
(a) portosystemic: paraumbilical vein
(b) bypassing IVC: azygos, hemiazygos
√ ± narrowing / obstruction of intrahepatic IVC

NECT:
√ global liver enlargement + diffuse hypoattenuation

CT:
√ "flip-flop" enhancement pattern:
√ prominent enhancement of central liver + weak enhancement of peripheral liver on early images
√ enhancement of liver periphery + wash-out of contrast from central liver on delayed images
√ normal enhancement of enlarged caudate lobe (due to separate venous drainage directly into IVC)
√ mottled liver enhancement pattern (due to hepatic congestion):
√ patchy liver enhancement (85%) with normal portal blood flow
√ hypodensity in atrophic areas / periphery (82%) with inversion of portal blood flow (= reversed portal venous blood flow due to increased postsinusoidal pressure produced by hepatic venous obstruction / rarely infarcts)
√ failure to identify hepatic veins
√ hepatic vein thrombi (18–53%)

MRI:
√ reduction in caliber / complete absence of hepatic veins
√ "comma sign" = multiple comma-shaped intrahepatic flow voids (due to intrahepatic collaterals)

Doppler US (85–100% sensitive, 85% specific):
√ one / more major hepatic veins reduced in size to <3 mm / filled with thrombus / not visualized
√ communicating intrahepatic venous collaterals
√ decreased / absent / reversed blood flow in hepatic veins
√ flat flow / loss of cardiac modulation in hepatic veins
√ demodulated portal venous flow = disappearance of portal vein velocity variations with breathing
√ slow flow (<11 cm/sec) / hepatofugal flow in portal vein
√ portal vein congestion index >0.1
√ portal vein thrombosis (20%)
√ compression of IVC by enlarged liver / caudate lobe
√ sluggish / reversed / absent blood flow within IVC
√ hepatic artery resistive index >0.75

NUC (Tc-99m sulfur colloid):
√ central region of normal activity (hot caudate lobe) surrounded by greatly diminished activity (venous drainage of hypertrophied caudate lobe into IVC by separate vein)
√ colloid shift to spleen + bone marrow
√ wedge-shaped focal peripheral defects

Angio (inferior venocavography, hepatic venography):
√ absence of main hepatic veins
√ spider web pattern of collateral + recanalized veins
√ high-pressure gradient between infra- and suprahepatic portion of IVC (due to enlarged liver)
√ stretching + draping of intrahepatic arteries with hepatomegaly
√ inhomogeneous prolonged intense hepatogram with fine mottling
√ large lakes of sinusoidal contrast accumulation

Portography:
√ central hepatic enhancement (normal hepatopetal flow)
√ reversed portal flow in liver periphery (supplied only by hepatic artery)
√ bidirectional / hepatofugal main portal vein flow

Acute Budd-Chiari Syndrome (1/3)

◊ Caudate lobe has not had time to hypertrophy!
• rapid onset of abdominal pain (liver congestion)
• insidious onset of intractable ascites
√ hepatomegaly without derangement of liver function
√ ascites (97%)

CT:
√ diffuse hypodensity on NECT
√ early enhancement of caudate lobe + central portion around IVC with decreased enhancement peripherally
√ hypodense lumina of hepatic veins on CECT
√ decreased attenuation of enhancing areas with patchy inhomogeneous enhancement in liver periphery on delayed scans

MR:
√ peripheral liver parenchyma of moderately low signal intensity on T1WI + moderately high signal intensity on T2WI compared with central portion
√ diminished + mottled peripheral enhancement

Chronic Budd-Chiari Syndrome (2/3)

• insidious onset of jaundice, intractable ascites
• portal hypertension, variceal bleeding
√ enlargement of central region (= caudate lobe + adjacent central part of right lobe + medial segment of left lobe
√ nonsegmental / lobar atrophy of affected liver (due to extensive fibrosis) with diminished attenuation before + after contrast administration
√ progressive patchy enhancement radiating outward from major portal vessels (on dynamic bolus CT)
√ "reticulated mosaic" enhancement = diffuse patchy lobular enhancement separated by irregular linear areas of low density in central area
√ delayed homogeneous enhancement of entire liver after several minutes
√ ascites

Color Doppler:
√ "bicolored" hepatic veins (due to intrahepatic collateral pathways) are PATHOGNOMONIC

MR:
√ absence of flow within hepatic veins
√ minimal differences in signal intensity between central and peripheral portions of liver
√ intrahepatic collateral vessels

Dx: liver biopsy
Rx: control of ascites with diuretics + sodium restriction; anticoagulation, thrombolytic therapy, surgery / balloon dilatation (depending on etiology); transjugular portosystemic shunt; orthotopic liver transplantation (for advanced cases)

CANDIDIASIS OF LIVER

= almost exclusively seen in immunocompromised patients (acute leukemia, chronic granulomatous disease of childhood, renal transplant, chemotherapy for myeloproliferative disorders)

Prevalence: at time of autopsy in 50–70% of acute leukemia, in 50% of lymphoma patients
◊ Most common systemic fungal infection in immunocompromised patients!

• abdominal pain
• persistent fever in neutropenic patient whose leukocyte count is returning to normal
• elevated alkaline phosphatase
√ hepatomegaly
√ "target" / "bull's-eye" sign = multiple small hypoechoic / hypoattenuating masses with centers of increased echogenicity / attenuation distributed throughout liver
◊ Bull's-eye lesion becomes visible only when neutropenia resolves!
√ hyperintense lesions on T2WI

NUC:
√ uniform uptake / focal photopenic areas
√ diminished Ga-67 uptake

Dx: biopsy evidence of yeast / pseudohyphae in central necrotic portion of lesion
DDx: metastases, lymphoma, leukemia, sarcoidosis, septic emboli, other infections (MAI, CMV), Kaposi sarcoma

CAROLI DISEASE

= COMMUNICATING CAVERNOUS ECTASIA OF INTRAHEPATIC DUCTS
= rare congenital probably autosomal recessive disorder characterized by segmental saccular cystic dilatation of major intrahepatic bile ducts

Etiology: (a) ? perinatal hepatic artery occlusion
(b) ? hypoplasia / aplasia of fibromuscular wall components

Age: childhood + 2nd–3rd decade, occasionally in infancy; M:F = 1:1

Associated with:
benign renal tubular ectasia, medullary sponge kidney (in 80%), infantile polycystic kidney disease, choledochal cyst (rare), congenital hepatic fibrosis

• recurrent cramplike upper abdominal pain
• fever, transient jaundice
• cirrhosis / portal hypertension (very rare)
√ multiple cystic structures converging toward porta hepatis as either localized / diffusely scattered cysts communicating with bile ducts (DDx: polycystic liver disease)
√ portal radicles completely surrounded by dilated bile ducts = central dot sign on CT
√ sludge / calculi in dilated ducts

Cholangiography (diagnostic):
√ segmental saccular / beaded appearance of intrahepatic bile ducts extending to periphery of liver
√ bridge formation across dilated lumina
√ intraluminal bulbar protrusions
√ frequent ectasia of extrahepatic ducts + CBD

Cx: (1) Bile stasis with recurrent cholangitis
(2) Biliary calculi
(3) Liver abscess
(4) Septicemia
(5) Increased risk for cholangiocarcinoma

CHOLANGIOCARCINOMA

Incidence: 0.5–1% of all cancers, 30% of hepatic primary malignancies

◊ Cholangiocarcinomas occur in 10–15% of patients with primary sclerosing cholangitis!

Location:
A. INTRAHEPATIC
1. PERIPHERAL distal to 2nd-order branches
2. HILAR / CENTRAL at bifurcation / in 1st-order branches = Klatskin tumor
confluence of hepatic ducts in 10–26%
left / right hepatic duct in 8–13%

B. EXTRAHEPATIC
common hepatic duct in 14–37%
proximal CBD in 15–30%
distal CBD in 30–50%
cystic duct in 6%

Path:
(a) **exophytic** (= mass-forming / nodular) type: commonly in peripheral cholangiocarcinoma
√ large irregular hypoattenuating mass
√ stippled / punctate hyperattenuating foci
√ thin rimlike / thick bandlike enhancement around the tumor (early)
√ progressive concentric filling in of contrast (late) due to slow diffusion into interstitial tumor spaces
(b) diffuse = **infiltrative** (periductal) type: commonly in hilar + extrahepatic cholangiocarcinoma
√ mural thickening / encircling mass of bile duct wall
√ focal or diffuse stricture / complete obstruction of bile ducts
(c) **polypoid** = papillary (intraductal) type: infrequent
√ intraluminal polypoid mass
(d) combination

Histo: well / moderately / poorly differentiated ductal (most common), papillary, mucinous, signet-ring cell, mucoepidermoid, adenosquamous, cystadenocarcinoma

Unusual manifestation:
1. Mucin-hypersecreting cholangiocarcinoma
√ severe diffuse dilatation of intra- and extrahepatic bile ducts proximal + distal to tumor
2. Squamous cell carcinoma
= metaplastic transformation of adenocarcinoma cells

LIVER

Predisposed:
(1) Inflammatory bowel disease (10 x increased risk); incidence of 0.4–1.4% in ulcerative colitis; latent period of 15 years; tumors usually multicentric + predominantly in extrahepatic sites; GB involved in 15% (simultaneous presence of gallstones is rare)
(2) Biliary lithiasis: cholecystolithiasis (20–50%), intrahepatic lithiasis (5–10%)
(3) Primary sclerosing cholangitis (10%)
(4) Clonorchis sinensis infestation (Far East); most common cause worldwide
(5) Choledochal cyst / congenital hepatic cyst / congenital biliary atresia
(6) Ductal plate malformation:
- Biliary hamartoma
- Autosomal dominant polycystic disease
- Congenital hepatic fibrosis
- Caroli disease (due to chronic biliary stasis)

(7) Papillomatosis of bile ducts
(8) Recurrent pyogenic cholangitis
(9) Choledochoenteric anastomosis
(10) History of other malignancy (10%)
(11) Thorotrast exposure
(12) Alpha-1 antitrypsin deficiency

Prognosis: median survival of 7 months, 0–10% 5-year survival

Intrahepatic Cholangiocarcinoma

= CHOLANGIOCELLULAR CARCINOMA

Incidence: 1/3 of all malignancies originating in the liver; 8–13% of all cholangiocarcinomas; 2nd most common primary hepatic tumor after hepatoma

Histo: adenocarcinoma arising from the epithelium of a small intrahepatic bile duct with prominent desmoplastic reaction (fibrosis); ± mucin and calcifications

Average age: 50–60 years; M > F

- abdominal pain (47%)
- palpable mass (18%)
- weight loss (18%)
- painless jaundice (12%)

Spread: (a) local extension along duct
(b) local infiltration of liver substance
(c) metastatic spread to regional lymph nodes (in 15%)

√ mass of 5–20 cm in diameter
√ satellite nodules in 65%
√ punctate / chunky calcifications in 18%
√ calculi in biliary tree

NUC:
√ cold lesion on sulfur colloid / IDA scans
√ segmental biliary obstruction
√ may show uptake on gallium scan

US:
√ dilated biliary tree
√ predominantly homo- / heterogeneous mass
√ hyper- (75%) / iso- / hypoechoic (14%) mass
√ mural thickening

CT:
√ single predominantly homogeneous round / oval hypodense mass with irregular borders
√ "peripheral washout sign" = early minimal / moderate rim enhancement with progressive concentric filling and clearing of contrast material in rim of lesion on delayed images
√ marked homogeneous delayed enhancement (74%)

MR:
√ large central heterogeneous hypointense mass on T1WI
√ hyperintense periphery (viable tumor) + large central hypointensity (fibrosis) on T2WI
√ gadolinium enhancement of lesion

Angiography:
√ avascular / hypo- / hypervascular mass
√ stretched / encased arteries (frequent)
√ neovascularity in 50%
√ lack of venous invasion

Prognosis: <20% resectable; 30% 5-year survival

Klatskin Tumor

= INTRAHEPATIC CENTRAL CHOLANGIOCARCINOMA
= tumor at confluence of hepatic ducts (up to 70% of cholangiocarcinomas)

√ direct signs of Klatskin tumor:
√ iso- to hyperechoic central porta hepatis mass / focal irregularity of ducts (for infiltrating cholangiocarcinoma = more common subtype)
√ polypoid / smooth nodular intraluminal mass (for papillary + nodular types of cholangiocarcinoma) with associated mural thickening

√ indirect signs of Klatskin tumor:
√ segmental dilatation with nonunion of right and left ducts at porta hepatis + normal caliber of extrahepatic ducts
√ pressure effect / encasement / invasion / obliteration of portal vein and hepatic artery
√ lobar atrophy (14%) = dilated crowded ducts extending to liver surface ± geographic fatty change in one lobe

Intrahepatic Peripheral Cholangiocarcinoma

- no jaundice

Location: right lobe predilection

√ solitary mass (nodular form) without hypoechoic halo
√ diffusely abnormal liver texture (infiltrative form):
√ tumor more hypoechoic if <3 cm
√ tumor more hyperechoic if >3 cm
√ well-marginated cystic mass (papillary mucin-producing tumor) ± diffuse hyperechoic flecks of tumor calcification
√ dilatation of bile ducts peripheral to tumor (31%)

DDx: metastatic adenocarcinoma / leiomyosarcoma; sclerosing hepatocellular carcinoma

Extrahepatic Cholangiocarcinoma

= BILE DUCT CARCINOMA

Age peak: 6th–7th decade, M:F = 3:2

Incidence: <0.5% of autopsies; 90% of all cholangiocarcinomas; more frequent in Far East

Histo: well-differentiated sclerosing adenocarcinoma (2/3), anaplastic carcinoma (11%), cystadenocarcinoma, adenoacanthoma, malignant adenoma, squamous cell = epidermoid carcinoma, leiomyosarcoma

- gradual onset of fluctuating painless jaundice
- cholangitis (10%)
- weight loss, fatigability
- intermittent epigastric pain
- elevated bilirubin + alkaline phosphatase
- enlarged tender liver

Growth pattern:

(1) Obstructive type (70–85%)
  √ U- / V-shaped obstruction with nipple, rattail, smooth / irregular termination
(2) Stenotic type (10–25%)
  √ strictured rigid lumen with irregular margins + prestenotic dilatation
(3) Polypoid / papillary type (5–6%)
  √ intraluminal filling defect with irregular margins

Spread:
(a) lymphatic spread: cystic + CBD nodes (>32%), celiac nodes (>16%), peripancreatic nodes, superior mesenteric nodes
(b) infiltration of liver (23%)
(c) peritoneal seeding (9%)
(d) hematogenous (extremely rare): liver, peritoneum, lung

UGI:
√ infiltration / indentation of stomach / duodenum

Cholangiography (PTC or ERC best modality to depict bile duct neoplasm):
√ exophytic intraductal tumor mass (46%), 2–5 mm in diameter
√ frequently long / rarely short concentric focal stricture in infiltrating sclerosing cholangitic type with wall irregularities
√ prestenotic diffuse / focal biliary dilatation (100%)
√ progression of ductal strictures (100%)

US / CT:
√ dilatation of intrahepatic ducts without extrahepatic duct dilatation
√ failure to demonstrate the confluence of L + R hepatic ducts
√ mass within / surrounding the ducts at point of obstruction (21% visible on US, 40% visible on CT)
√ infiltrating tumor visible as highly attenuating lesion in 22% on CT, in 13% on US
√ exophytic tumor visible in 100% on CT as low-attenuation mass, in 29% on US
√ polypoid intraluminal tumor visible as isoechoic mass within surrounding bile in 100% on US, in 25% on CT

CECT:
√ hyperattenuating lesion at delayed imaging (due to delayed accumulation + washout of fibrous center)

Angiography:
√ hypervascular tumor with neovascularity (50%)
√ arterioarterial collaterals along the course of bile ducts associated with arterial obstruction
√ poor / absent tumor stain
√ displacement / encasement / occlusion of hepatic artery + portal vein

Cx:
(1) Obstruction leading to biliary cirrhosis
(2) Hepatomegaly
(3) Intrahepatic abscess (subdiaphragmatic, perihepatic, septicemia)
(4) Biliary peritonitis
(5) Portal vein invasion

Dx: endoscopic brush biopsy (30–85% sensitive)

Prognosis: median survival of 5 months; 1.6% 5-year survival; 39% 5-year survival for carcinoma of papilla of Vater

DDx: sclerosing cholangitis, AIDS cholangitis, benign stricture, chronic pancreatitis, edematous papilla, idiopathic inflammation of CBD

CHOLANGITIS

Acute Obstructive / Ascending Cholangitis

= biliary duct obstruction associated with biliary infection

Cause:
(a) benign disease:
(1) stricture from prior surgery (36%) after bile duct exploration / bilioenteric anastomosis, (2) calculi (30%), (3) sclerosing cholangitis, (4) obstructed drainage catheter, (5) parasitic infestation
(b) malignant disease: ampullary carcinoma

Types:

A. ACUTE NONSUPPURATIVE ASCENDING CHOLANGITIS
- bile remains clear
- patient nontoxic

B. ACUTE SUPPURATIVE ASCENDING CHOLANGITIS (14%)
Associated with: obstructing biliary stone or malignancy
- septicemia, CNS depression, lethargy, mental confusion, shock (50%)

√ purulent material fills biliary ducts
Prognosis: 100% mortality if not decompressed; 40–60% mortality with treatment; 13–16% overall mortality rate

Organism: gram-negative enteric bacteria = E. coli > Klebsiella > Pseudomonas > Enterococci

- recurrent episodes of sepsis + RUQ pain
- Charcot triad (70%): fever + chills + jaundice
- bile cultures in 90% positive for infection

√ may have gas in biliary tree

CECT:
√ transient hepatic parenchymal enhancement in periportal location on hepatic arterial phase (= hyperemic changes around bile ducts)

Cx: miliary hepatic abscess formation; secondary sclerosing cholangitis

LIVER

AIDS-related Cholangitis

= AIDS CHOLANGIOPATHY
= infectious cholangitis characterized by opportunistic organisms

Organism: Cryptosporidium (protozoan parasite typically infecting GI tract epithelium), CMV

Histo: marked periductal inflammatory response with interstitial edema + interstitial inflammatory cell infiltrates + necrotic biliary epithelium

• RUQ pain, fever, nausea, jaundice
• elevated WBC count
• abnormal LFT (esp. serum alkaline phosphatase)
• opportunistic organism isolated from bile (in 50%)

√ irregular mild dilatation of intra- and extrahepatic bile ducts resembling sclerosing cholangitis

US:
√ stricture of distal CBD / papillary stenosis (due to papillitis)
√ echogenic nodule at the distal end of the CBD
√ mural thickening of gallbladder + bile ducts
√ periductal echogenicity
√ ± pericholecystic fluid

CT:
√ "pseudogallstone" appearance = marked circumferential edema of gallbladder wall + mucosal enhancement
√ periportal edema

Cholangiography:
√ strictures + beading of central intrahepatic bile ducts
√ pruning of peripheral bile ducts

DDx: acalculous cholecystitis, papillary stenosis, sclerosing cholangitis

LIVER

Chemotherapy-induced Cholangitis

= inflammatory fibrosing process about the portal triads simulating primary sclerosing cholangitis

Predisposed: patients with liver metastases from colon cancer

Cause: direct effect of hepatic arterial infusion with chemotherapeutic agents (eg, floxuridine) / ischemia secondary to thrombosis of intrahepatic arterial branches

√ bile duct strictures as early as 2 months after therapy (in up to 15%)
√ stricture of common hepatic duct + sparing of distal CBD

Primary Sclerosing Cholangitis

= insidious progressive obliterative fibrosing inflammation of the biliary tree causing multifocal strictures, bile duct obliteration, cholestasis, and biliary cirrhosis

Etiology: idiopathic, ? autoimmune process (speculative); altered bile acid metabolism with increase in lithocholic acid by bacterial overgrowth

Prevalence: 1% as common as alcoholic liver disease

Age: <45 years (2/3); mean 39 (range 21–67) years; M:F = 7:3

Histo:
Stage 1: degeneration of epithelial bile duct cells + infiltration with lymphocytes ± neutrophils; inflammation + scarring + enlargement of periportal triads (pericholangitis)
Stage 2: fibrosis + inflammation infiltrating periportal parenchyma with piecemeal necrosis of hepatocytes; enlargement of portal triads; bile ductopenia
Stage 3: portal-to-portal fibrous septa; severe degenerative changes + disappearance of bile ducts; cholestasis in periportal + paraseptal hepatocytes
Stage 4: frank cirrhosis

Associated with:
(1) Inflammatory bowel disease (ulcerative colitis in 50–74%, Crohn disease in 13%)
  ◊ 1–4% of patients with inflammatory bowel disease develop secondary sclerosing cholangitis!
(2) Cirrhosis, chronic active hepatitis, pericholangitis, fatty degeneration
(3) Pancreatitis
(4) Retroperitoneal / mediastinal fibrosis
(5) Peyronie disease
(6) Riedel thyroiditis, hypothyroidism
(7) Retroorbital pseudotumor
(8) Sjögren syndrome

• abnormal liver function tests: serum bilirubin, serum alkaline phosphatase, γ-glutamyltransferase
• progressive chronic / intermittent obstructive jaundice (75%)
• history of previous biliary surgery (53%) + chronic / recurrent pancreatitis (14%)
• fever, night sweats, chills, RUQ pain, pruritus (10–15%)

Location:
1. CBD almost always involved
2. Intra- and extrahepatic ducts (68–89%)
3. Cystic duct involved in 15–18%
4. Intrahepatic ducts only (1–11–25%)
5. Extrahepatic ducts only (2–3%)

√ intrahepatic bile duct calculi (8–30%): soft black crushable stones / sandlike grit

US:
√ brightly echogenic portal triads
√ echogenic biliary casts / punctate coarse calcifications along portal vein branches
√ ± gallbladder wall thickening

CT:
√ dilatation, stenosis, pruning (decreased arborization), beading of tortuous intrahepatic bile ducts = "tree-in-winter" appearance (80%)
√ wall nodularity, duct wall thickening, mural contrast enhancement of extrahepatic bile ducts (100%)
√ hepatic metastases + lymph nodes in porta hepatis
√ subtle foci of high attenuation in intrahepatic bile ducts
√ lobar atrophy in preferentially affected portions

Cholangiography:
- √ multifocal strictures with predilection for bifurcations + skip lesions (uninvolved duct segments of normal caliber) involving intra- and extrahepatic bile ducts:
  - √ CLASSIC "string-of-beads" appearance (= alternating segments of dilatation and focal annular stenoses)
  - √ "pruned tree" appearance (= opacification of central ducts + nonvisualization of peripheral smaller radicles due to diffuse obstruction)
  - √ "cobblestone" appearance (= coarse nodular mural irregularities) in 50%
  - √ new strictures + lengthening of strictures between 6 months and 6 years (<20%)
  - √ minimal duct dilatation due to periductal inflammation + fibrosis
  - √ marked ductal dilatation (24%)
    DDx: ascending cholangitis, cholangiocarcinoma
- √ small eccentric saccular outpouchings (diverticula / pseudodiverticula) [up to 27%] = PATHOGNOMONIC
- √ webs = focal 1–2-mm-thick areas of incomplete circumferential narrowing
- √ angles formed between central and peripheral ducts change from acute to obtuse
- √ polypoid mass (7%)
- √ gallbladder irregularities uncommon

MR:
- √ periportal intermediate intensity on T1WI + hyperintense on T2WI (due to inflammation)

NUC (Tc-99m-IDA scan):
- √ multiple persistent focal areas of retention in distribution of intrahepatic biliary tree
- √ marked prolongation of hepatic clearance
- √ gallbladder visualized only in 70%

Cx: (1) Biliary cirrhosis (up to 49%)
(2) Portal hypertension
(3) Cholangiocarcinoma (clinically in 4–19%; in 7–36% at autopsy / liver transplantation)
(4) Secondary cholangitis

Rx: (1) Palliative: ursodeoxycholic acid, dilatation of dominant strictures
(2) Curative: liver transplantation (4th leading indication)

DDx:
(1) Sclerosing cholangiocarcinoma (progressive cholangiographic changes within 0.5–1.5 years of initial diagnosis, marked ductal dilatation upstream from a dominant stricture, intraductal mass >1 cm in diameter)
(2) Acute ascending cholangitis (history)
(3) Primary biliary cirrhosis (disease limited to intrahepatic ducts, strictures less pronounced, pruning + crowding of bile ducts, normal AMA titer)
(4) AIDS cholangiopathy (same on cholangiography)

Recurrent Pyogenic Cholangitis

= PRIMARY CHOLANGITIS = RECURRENT PYOGENIC HEPATITIS / CHOLANGITIS = ORIENTAL CHOLANGIO-HEPATITIS = ORIENTAL CHOLANGITIS = HONG KONG DISEASE = INTRAHEPATIC PIGMENT STONE DISEASE

= chronic recurrent parasitic cholangitis resulting in progressive destructive cholangiopathy + liver failure

Etiology: ? Clonorchis sinensis infestation, coliform infection of bile, portal bacteremia, malnutrition

Incidence: 3rd most common cause of an acute abdomen in Hong Kong after appendicitis and perforated ulcer; uncommon in United States

Epidemiology: endemic to Southeast Asia (South China, Indochina, Taiwan, Japan, Korea); Asian immigrants in United States

Associated intrabiliary infestation:
Clonorchis sinensis, Ascaris lumbricoides, E. coli

Path: pericholangitis, periductal abscesses, fibrosis of bile duct walls, heavy infiltration of portal tracts by PMNs, intraductal bile pigment calculi

Age: 20–50 years; M:F = 1:1

• recurrent attacks of fever, chills, abdominal pain, jaundice

Location: particularly in lateral segment of L lobe + posterior segment of R lobe

- √ marked dilatation of proximal intrahepatic ducts (3–4 mm) in 100%
- √ decreased arborization of intrahepatic radicles
- √ intra- and extrahepatic bile ducts filled with nonshadowing soft mudlike pigment (= calcium bilirubinate) stones (74%)
- √ dilatation of CBD (68%) + choledocholithiasis (30%)
- √ multifocal bile duct strictures (22%)
- √ pneumobilia (3–52%)
- √ biloma
- √ segmental hepatic atrophy (36%)
- √ hepatic abscesses

CT:
- √ high-attenuation biliary calculi
- √ enhancement of bile duct wall

Associated findings:
- √ gallstones
- √ splenomegaly
- √ varices

ERCP:
- ◊ Worsening of cholangitis / sepsis if patients do not receive antibiotics!
- √ acute tapering + straightening + rigidity of bile ducts
- √ decreased arborization + increased branching angle of bile ducts

Cx: liver abscess (18%), splenomegaly (14%), biloma (4%), pancreatitis (4%), cholangiocarcinoma (2.5–6%)

Rx: endoscopic sphincterotomy, choledochoduodenostomy

DDx: (1) Caroli disease (saccular dilatation of intrahepatic bile ducts)
(2) Primary sclerosing cholangitis (focal discontinuous bile duct dilatation)
(3) Clonorchiasis (biliary ductal dilatation limited to intrahepatic bile ducts)

Secondary Sclerosing Cholangitis

Cause:
(1) chronic bacterial cholangitis from bile duct stricture / choledocholithiasis
(2) ischemic bile duct damage from treatment with floxuridine
(3) infectious cholangiopathy in AIDS
(4) previous biliary tract surgery
(5) congenital biliary tree anomalies
(6) bile duct neoplasm

CHOLECYSTITIS

Acute Calculous Cholecystitis

Etiology: (a) in 80–95% cystic duct obstruction by impacted calculus; 85% disimpact spontaneously if stone <3 mm
(b) in 10% acalculous cholecystitis

Pathogenesis: chemical irritation from concentrated bile, bacterial infection, reflux of pancreatic secretions

Age peak: 5th–6th decade; M:F = 1:3

Associated with: choledocholithiasis (15–25%)

- persisting (>6 hours) RUQ pain radiating to right shoulder / scapula / interscapular area (DDx: biliary colic usually <6 hours)
- nausea, vomiting, chills, fever
- RUQ tenderness + guarding
- ± leukocytosis, elevated levels of alkaline phosphatase and transaminase and amylase
- mild hyperbilirubinemia (20%)
- Murphy sign = inspiratory arrest upon palpation of GB area (falsely positive in 6% of patients with cholelithiasis)

Oral cholecystography:
√ nonvisualization / poor visualization of gallbladder

US (81–100% sensitivity, 60–100% specificity, 92% PPV, 95% NPV):
√ ± GB wall thickening >3 mm (45–72% sensitive, 76–88% specific):
√ hazy delineation of GB wall
√ "halo sign" = GB wall lucency (in 8%) = 3-layered configuration with sonolucent middle layer (edema)
√ striated wall thickening (62%) = several alternating irregular discontinuous lucent + echogenic bands within GB wall (100% PPV)
√ GB hydrops = distension with AP diameter >5 cm or enlargement of greater than 4 x 10 cm
√ positive sonographic Murphy sign (in 85–88%) = maximum tenderness during compression with transducer directly over gallbladder (63–94% sensitive, 85–93% specific, 72% NPV)
False-negative sonographic Murphy sign:
lack of patient responsiveness, pain medication, inability to press directly on GB (position deep to liver / protected by ribs), GB wall necrosis
√ crescent-shaped / loculated pericholecystic fluid (in 20%) = inflammatory intraperitoneal exudate / abscess
√ gallstones (83–98% sensitive, 52–77% specific):
√ impacted gallstone in GB neck / cystic duct
√ echogenic shadowing fat within hepatoduodenal ligament ± conspicuous color Doppler flow (due to inflammation)
DDx: bowel gas
√ sludge

Color Doppler US:
√ visualization of cystic artery >50% of the length of the gallbladder (30% sensitive, 98% specific)

CECT:
√ distended gallbladder
√ gallbladder wall thickness >3 mm
√ increased gallbladder wall attenuation
√ transient focal increased attenuation around gallbladder fossa on hepatic arterial phase (due to hepatic arterial hyperemia + early venous drainage)
√ haziness of pericholecystic fat
√ pericholecystic fluid
√ increased attenuation of bile

NUC (86–97% sensitivity, 73–100% specificity , 95–98% accuracy):
= functional information about gallbladder + cystic duct patency
◊ Tracer uptake hinges on adequate hepatic function + fasting status
√ nonvisualization of GB during 1st hour (in 83%) = evidence of cystic duct obstruction
√ nonvisualization of GB by 4 hours (99% specific)
√ nonvisualization of GB + CBD (in 13%)
√ pericholecystic rim sign (34% sensitive) on initial images = increased hepatic activity adjacent to empty GB fossa (= local hepatocyte inflammation + hyperemia in transmural process); 57% PPV for gangrenous GB + 94% PPV for acute cholecystitis
√ increased perfusion to GB fossa during "arterial phase" (in up to 80%)

Endpoint of imaging
— when tracer fills GB
— 4 hours of delayed imaging after tracer injection
— 45 minutes after morphine injection

False-positive scans (10–12%) = nonvisualization of GB without acute cholecystitis:
prolonged fasting, total parenteral nutrition, hyperalimentation, recent feeding <4–6 hours prior to study, severe intercurrent illness, CBD obstruction, congenital absence of GB, post-cholecystectomy, carcinoma of GB, chronic cholecystitis, acute pancreatitis, alcoholic liver disease, hepatocellular disease
Reduction to 2% false-positive scans through:
(1) delayed images up to 4 hours
(2) cholecystokinin (Sincalide®) injection 15 minutes prior to study
(3) morphine IV (0.04 mg/kg) at 40 minutes + reimaging after 20 minutes (contraction of sphincter of Oddi + rise in intrabiliary pressure)

False-negative scans (4.8%) = visualization of GB despite acute cholecystitis:
rare calculous / acalculous cholecystitis without cystic duct obstruction

Cholangiography:
√ sharply defined filling defect in contrast-material filled lumen of cystic duct

MR cholangiopancreatogram (high sensitivity):
√ low-signal–intensity defect surrounded by high-signal–intensity bile on T2WI

Cx:
mnemonic: "GAME BEG"
Gangrene
Abscess (pericholecystic)
Mirizzi syndrome
Emphysematous cholecystitis
Bouveret syndrome (= gallstone erodes into duodenum leading to duodenal obstruction)
Empyema
Gallstone ileus

(1) Gangrene of gallbladder
• positive Murphy sign (33%)
√ shaggy, irregular, asymmetric wall (mucosal ulcers, intraluminal hemorrhage, necrosis)
√ hyperechoic foci within GB wall (microabscesses in Rokitansky-Aschoff sinuses)
√ intraluminal pseudomembranes (gangrene)
√ coarse nonshadowing nondependent echodensities (= sloughed necrotic mucosa / sludge / pus / clotted blood within gallbladder)

(2) Perforation of gallbladder (in 2–20%)
(a) acute free perforation with peritonitis causing pericholecystic abscess in 33%
(b) subacute localized perforation causing pericholecystic abscess in 48%
(c) chronic perforation resulting in internal biliary fistula causing pericholecystic abscess in 18%
Location: most commonly at fundus
√ gallstone lying free in peritoneal cavity
√ sonolucent / complex collection surrounding GB
√ collection in liver adjacent to gallbladder

(3) Empyema of gallbladder
√ multiple medium / coarse highly reflective intraluminal echoes without shadowing / layering / gravity dependence (purulent exudate / debris)

Acute Acalculous Cholecystitis

Frequency: 5–15% of all acute cholecystitis cases
Associated with: recent surgery in 50%
Etiology: probably caused by decreased blood flow within cystic artery
(1) depressed motility / starvation in trauma, burns, surgery, total parenteral nutrition, anesthesia, positive pressure ventilation, narcotics, shock, vasoactive amines, congestive heart failure, arteriosclerosis, polyarteritis nodosa, SLE, diabetes mellitus
(2) obstruction of cystic duct by extrinsic inflammation, lymphadenopathy, metastases
(3) infection (only in 50%) from Salmonella, cholera, Kawasaki syndrome

√ thickened gallbladder wall >4–5 mm
√ echogenic bile / sludge
√ gallbladder distension
√ pericholecystic fluid in absence of ascites
√ subserosal edema
√ sloughed mucosal membrane
√ Murphy sign = pain + tenderness with transducer pressure over the gallbladder
√ intramural gas
√ decreased response to cholecystokinin

NUC: same criteria as for calculous cholecystitis
Cx: gallbladder perforation, gangrene
Prognosis: 6.5% mortality rate

Chronic Cholecystitis

◊ Most common form of gallbladder inflammation
√ gallstones
√ smooth / irregular GB wall thickening (mean of 5 mm)
√ mean volume of 42 mL

NUC:
√ normal GB visualization in majority of patients
√ delayed GB visualization (1–4 hours)
√ visualization of bowel prior to GB (sensitivity 45%, specificity 90%)
√ noncontractility / decreased response after CCK injection (decreased GB ejection fraction)

Emphysematous Cholecystitis

= ischemia of gallbladder wall + infection with gas-producing organisms
Etiology: small-vessel disease with cystic artery occlusion, complication of acute cholecystitis
Organism: Clostridium perfringens, Clostridium welchii, E. coli, staphylococcus, streptococcus
Age: >50 years; M:F = 5:1
Predisposed: diabetics (20–50%), debilitating diseases; calculous (70–80%) / acalculous cystic duct obstruction
• WBC count may be normal (1/3)
• point tenderness rare (diabetic neuropathy)

Plain film:
√ gas appears 24–48 hours after onset of symptoms
√ air-fluid level in GB lumen, air in GB wall within 24–48 hours after acute episode
√ pneumobilia (rare)

US:
√ arclike high-level echoes outlining GB wall
√ cholecystolithiasis (50%)

Cx: gangrene (75%); gallbladder perforation (20%)
Mortality: 15%
DDx: (1) Enteric fistula
(2) Incompetent sphincter of Oddi
(3) Air-containing periduodenal abscess
(4) Periappendiceal abscess in malpositioned appendix
(5) Lipomatosis of gallbladder

Xanthogranulomatous Cholecystitis

= FIBROXANTHOGRANULOMATOUS INFLAMMATION
= CEROID GRANULOMAS OF THE GALLBLADDER
= uncommon inflammatory disease of gallbladder characterized by presence of multiple intramural nodules

Etiology:
rupture of occluded Rokitansky-Aschoff sinuses with subsequent intramural extravasation of inspissated bile + mucin attracting histiocytes to phagocytose the insoluble cholesterol

Incidence: 1–2%
Age: 7th + 8th decade
Histo: mixture of ceroid (waxlike) xanthogranuloma with foamy histiocytes + multinucleated foreign body giant cells + lymphocytes + fibroblasts containing areas of necrosis (in newer lesions)
May be associated with: gallbladder carcinoma (11%)

√ preservation of 2–3-mm thick mucosal lining (in 82%)
√ thickened gallbladder wall: 91% diffuse, 9% focal
√ infiltration of pericholecystic fat: in 45% focal, in 54% diffuse
√ hepatic extension (45%)
√ biliary obstruction (36%)
√ lymphadenopathy (36%)

US:
√ intramural hypoechoic nodules

CT:
√ 5–20-mm small intramural hypoattenuating nodules
√ poor / heterogeneous contrast enhancement

DDx: gallbladder carcinoma (in 59% focal, in 41% diffuse thickening of gallbladder wall, multiple masses within liver)

CHOLEDOCHAL CYST

= CYSTIC DILATATION OF EXTRAHEPATIC BILE DUCT
= segmental aneurysmal dilatation of common bile duct without involvement of gallbladder / cystic duct; most common congenital lesion of bile ducts

Etiology: anomalous junction of pancreatic duct and CBD proximal to duodenal papilla; higher pressure in pancreatic duct and absent ductal sphincter allows free reflux of enzymes into CBD resulting in weakening of CBD wall

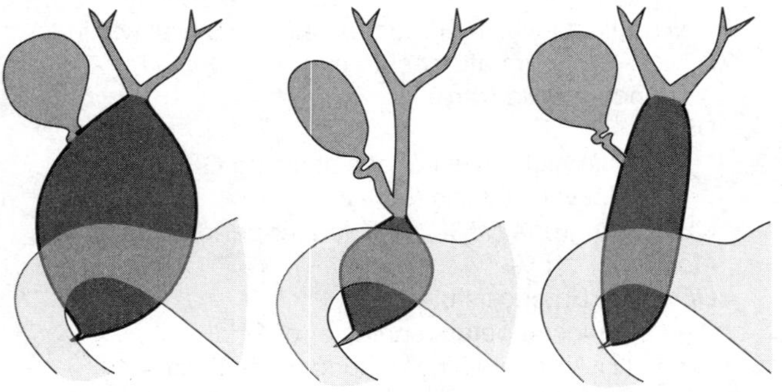

Choledochal Cysts

Classification:
malunion of pancreaticobiliary duct
Kimura type I = pancreatic duct enters the proximal / mid CBD (10–58%) at right angle
Kimura type II = CBD drains into pancreatic duct

Prevalence: 1:13,000 admissions; high prevalence in Japanese / Asian infants
Age: <10 years (60%) + young adulthood; 80% diagnosed in childhood; 7% during pregnancy; occasionally detected up to 8th decade; M:F = 1:4
Histo: fibrous cyst wall without epithelial lining
Associated with:
(1) dilatation, stenosis or atresia of other portions of the biliary tree (2%)
(2) gallbladder anomaly (aplasia, double GB)
(3) failure of union of left + right hepatic ducts
(4) pancreatic duct + accessory hepatic bile ducts may drain into cyst
(5) polycystic liver disease

• Classic triad (20–30% of adult patients):
  (1) intermittent obstructive jaundice (33–50%)
    ◊ Uncommon cause of obstructive jaundice!
  (2) recurrent RUQ colicky pain (>75–90%), back pain
  (3) intermittent palpable RUQ abdominal mass (<25%)
• recurrent fever, chills, weight loss, pruritus

Types:
(a) marked cystic dilatation of CBD + CHD
(b) focal segmental dilatation of CBD distally
(c) cylindric dilatation of CBD + CHD

√ size: diameter of 2 cm up to 15 cm
(the largest choledochal cyst contained 13 liters)
√ NO / mild peripheral intrahepatic bile duct dilatation
√ may contain stones / sludge

UGI:
√ soft-tissue mass in RUQ
√ anterior displacement of 2nd portion of duodenum + distal portion of stomach (on LAT view)
√ widening of C-loop with inferior displacement of duodenum (on AP view)

US:
√ ballooned / fusiform cyst beneath porta hepatis separate from gallbladder
  ◊ Communication with common hepatic / intrahepatic ducts needs to be demonstrated!
√ abrupt change of caliber at junction of dilated segment to normal ducts
√ intrahepatic bile duct dilatation (16%) secondary to stenosis

OB-US (earliest diagnosis at 25 weeks MA):
√ right-sided cyst in fetal abdomen + adjacent dilated hepatic ducts
  DDx: duodenal atresia; cyst of ovary, mesentery, omentum, pancreas, liver

NUC with HIDA:
◊ At times the choledochal cyst does not fill with radionuclide!
√ photopenic area within liver that fills within 60 minutes + stasis of tracer within cyst
√ lack of tracer passage into small intestine
√ prominent hepatic ductal activity (dilatation of ducts)

DDx: often excludes hepatic cyst, pancreatic pseudocyst, enteric duplication, spontaneous loculated biloma

Cholangiography / MR cholangiography (confirms diagnosis):

√ anomalous junction of panreaticobiliary ductal system
√ dilated intrahepatic bile ducts
√ intraductal calculi

Cx:
(1) Stones in gallbladder, in CBD, within cyst, in intrahepatic biliary tree, in pancreatic duct (8–50%)
(2) Malignant transformation into bile duct carcinoma + gallbladder carcinoma (increasing with age, <1% in 1st decade, 7–14% > age 20)
(3) Recurrent pancreatitis (33%)
(4) Cholangitis / cholecystitis (20%)
(5) Cyst rupture with bile peritonitis (1.8%)
(6) Bleeding
(7) Biliary cirrhosis + portal hypertension
(8) Portal vein thrombosis
(9) Hepatic abscess

Rx: excision of cyst + Roux-en-Y hepaticojejunostomy

DDx: mesenteric, omental, ovarian, renal, adrenal, hepatic, enteric duplication cyst, pancreatic pseudocyst, hydronephrotic kidney, hepatic artery aneurysm, biloma (from spontaneous perforation of CBD)

CHOLEDOCHOCELE

= DUODENAL DUPLICATION CYST = ENTEROGENOUS CYST OF AMPULLA OF VATER / DUODENUM = INTRADUODENAL CHOLEDOCHAL CYST = DIVERTICULUM OF COMMON BILE DUCT

= cystic dilatation of the distal / intramural duodenal portion of the CBD with herniation of CBD into duodenum (similar to ureterocele)

Etiology:
(1) congenital:
(a) originates from tiny bud / diverticulum of distal CBD (found in 5.7% of normal population)
(b) stenosis of ductal orifice / weakness of ductal wall
(2) acquired:
stone passage followed by stenosis + inflammation

Age: 33 years (manifestation usually in adulthood)

Types:
(a) CBD terminates in cyst, cyst drains into duodenum (common)
(b) cyst drains into adjacent intramural portion of CBD (less common)

• biliary colic, episodic jaundice, nausea, vomiting

Associated with: stones / sludge (frequent)

UGI:

√ smooth well-defined intraluminal duodenal filling defect in region of papilla
√ change in shape with compression / peristalsis

Cholangiography (diagnostic):

√ opacified smooth clublike / saclike dilatation of intramural segment of CBD prolapsed into duodenum

Cx: pancreatitis, duodenal obstruction

Rx: sphincterotomy / sphincteroplasty

DDx: choledochal cyst (involves more than only terminal portion of CBD)

CHOLELITHIASIS

Prevalence:
25 million adults in United States ; 10% of population + 2% of children;
increasing with age (40% of women in 9th decade);
in 3rd decade M:F = 2%:4%
in 7th decade M:F = 10%:25%

Predisposing factors: "female, forty, fair, fat, fertile, flatulent"

Pathogenesis:
supersaturation of bile constituents, most notably cholesterol, related to defects in biliary lipid metabolism; biliary dysmotility; prolonged intestinal transit; aggravated by sedentary lifestyle + diet

(a) Hemolytic disease
sickle cell disease (7–37%), hereditary spherocytosis (43–85%), thalassemia, pernicious anemia (16–20%), prosthetic cardiac valves + mitral stenosis (hemolysis), cirrhosis (hemolysis secondary to hypersplenism), Rhesus / ABO blood group incompatibility (perinatal period)

(b) Metabolic disorder = disruption of biliary lithogenic index
diabetes mellitus, obesity, pancreatic disease, cystic fibrosis, hypercholesterolemia, type 4 hyperlipidemia, hemosiderosis (20%), hyperparathyroidism, hypothyroidism, prolonged use of estrogens / progesterone, pregnancy

(c) Cholestasis
— hepatic dysfunction: hepatitis, neonatal sepsis
— biliary tree malformation: Caroli disease
— biliary obstruction: parasitic infection, benign / malignant strictures, foreign bodies (sutures, ascariasis)
— prolonged fasting (total parenteral nutrition)
— methadone intake

(d) Intestinal malabsorption
has a 10 x increased risk of stone formation
— Inflammatory bowel disease: Crohn disease (28–34%)
— ileal resection
— bypass surgery

(e) Genetic predisposition = familial
Navaho, Pima, Chippewa Indians

(f) Others
muscular dystrophy

GALLSTONES IN NEONATE

◊ Rare without predisposing factors

Associated with: obstructive congenital biliary anomaly, total parenteral nutrition, furosemide, GI dysfunction (short-gut syndrome), prolonged fasting, phototherapy, dehydration, infection, hemolytic anemia

GALLSTONES IN OLDER CHILDREN

Associated with: sickle cell disease, cystic fibrosis, malabsorption, total parenteral nutrition, Crohn disease, intestinal resection, hemolytic anemia, choledochal cyst

Composition:

A. CHOLESTEROL STONE (70%)
 = main component of most calculi
 √ lucent (93%), calcified (7%)
 √ slightly hypodense compared with bile
 (a) pure cholesterol stones (10%): yellowish, soft
  √ buoyancy in contrast-enhanced bile
  √ density of <100 HU
 (b) mixture of cholesterol + calcium carbonate / bilirubinate (70%)
  √ laminated appearance
  √ radiopaque on plain film (15–20%)

B. PIGMENT STONE (30%)
 • brown (common) = granular precipitate of calcium bilirubinate containing <25% cholesterol (by definition)
 Cause: inflammation / infection of gallbladder, status post cholecystectomy
 • black (less common) = compact "lacquer" of bilirubin derivatives with a high affinity for calcium carbonate
 √ multiple tiny faceted / spiculated homogeneously radiopaque stones
 CT:
  √ usually denser than bile

Radiopacity:
 √ lucent stones (84%):
 cholesterol (85%), pigment (15%)
 √ calcified stones (15–20% on plain film, 60% on CT):
 cholesterol (33%), pigment (67%)
 Location of calcium:
  √ calcium phosphate deposited centrally within cholesterol stones
  √ calcium carbonate deposited radially within aging cholesterol / peripherally around cholesterol + pigmented stones

FLOATING GALLSTONES (20–25%)
 (a) relatively pure cholesterol stones
 (b) gas-containing stones
 (c) rise in specific gravity of bile (1.03) from oral cholecystopaques (specific gravity of 1.06) causing stones (specific gravity of 1.05) to float

GAS-CONTAINING GALLSTONES

Mechanism: dehydration of older stones leads to internal shrinkage + dendritic cracks + subsequent nitrogen gas–filling from negative internal pressure

√ "crow-foot" = "Mercedes-Benz" sign = radiating streaklike lucencies within stone, also responsible for buoyancy

SLUDGE
 = calcium-bilirubinate granules + cholesterol crystals associated with biliary stasis
 Cause: prolonged fasting, parenteral nutrition, hyperalimentation, hemolysis, extrahepatic bile duct obstruction, cystic duct obstruction, acute + chronic cholecystitis
 √ nonshadowing homogeneously echogenic material:
  √ fluid-sludge level
 √ "sludge ball" = tumefactive sludge:
  √ slowly shifting with repositioning of patient
  DDx: gallbladder cancer
 Prognosis: may cause acute cholecystitis
 DDx: hemobilia with blood clot, parasitic infestation, mucus

Cholecystolithiasis

• asymptomatic (60–65%); become symptomatic at a rate of 2% per year
• **biliary colic** (misnomer) due to transient obstruction of cystic duct / common bile duct develops in 33% (18% overall risk in 20 years):
 = acute RUQ / epigastric / LUQ / precordial / lower abdominal pain increasing over seconds / minutes + remaining fairly steady for 1–3(–6) hours associated with nausea + vomiting
 • no tenderness upon palpation

Abdominal plain film (10–16% sensitive):
 √ calcified gallstones

OCG (65–90% sensitive):
 √ filling defect in contrasted gallbladder lumen:
  √ allows determination of size + number of gallstones
  √ demonstrates cystic duct patency
  √ shows contractility after a fatty meal
 √ nonvisualization of gallbladder (25%) = inconclusive

CT (80% sensitive):
 √ hyperdense calcified gallstones in 60%
 √ hypodense cholesterol stones ≤140 HU = pure cholesterol stone (= ≥80% cholesterol content):
  ◊ Inverse relationship between CT attenuation number + cholesterol content
 √ gallstones isointense to bile in 21–24% and thus undetectable by CT (<30 HU)

US (91–98% sensitive; in 5% falsely negative):
 √ bright (= highly reflective) echo from anterior surface of gallstone within gallbladder:
  √ marked posterior acoustic shadowing
  √ mobile upon repositioning of patient (may infrequently be adherent to wall)
  √ reverberation artifact
  ◊ Small calcifications <2 mm may not shadow
 √ nonvisualization of GB + collection of echogenic echoes with acoustic shadowing (15–25%):
  √ "wall-echo-shadow" = "double-arc shadow" sign = 2 echogenic curvilinear parallel lines separated by sonolucent line (ie, anterior GB wall + bile + stone with acoustic shadowing)

√ focal nonshadowing opacities <5 mm in diameter (in 70% gallstones)
False-negative US (5%):
contracted GB, GB in anomalous / unusual location, small gallstone, gallstone impacted in GB neck / cystic duct, immobile patient, obese patient, extensive RUQ bowel gas
Prognosis: stones <3 mm may pass through cystic duct
Cx: acute cholecystitis (in 30%), choledocholithiasis, cholangitis, pancreatitis, duodenitis, biliary fistula, gallstone ileus, Mirizzi syndrome; cancer of GB + bile ducts (2–3 x more frequent)

Cholangiolithiasis

A. CHOLEDOCHOLITHIASIS
◊ Most common cause of bile duct obstruction!
Etiology: (a) passed stones originating in GB
(b) primary development in intra- / extrahepatic ducts
Incidence: in 12–15% of cholecystectomy patients; in 3–4% of postcholecystectomy patients; in 75% of patients with chronic bile duct obstruction
Risk indicators for CBD stone:
(1) recent history of jaundice
(2) recent history of pancreatitis
(3) elevated serum bilirubin >17 μmol/L
(4) elevated serum amylase >120 IU/L
(5) dilated CBD >6 mm (16%)
(6) obscured bile duct
• recurrent episodes of right upper quadrant pain, jaundice, chills, fever (25–50%)
• elevated transaminase (75%)
• spontaneous passage with stones <6 mm size
Cholangiography (most specific technique):
√ stone visualization in 92%
Peroperative cholangiography:
prolongs operation by 30 minutes;
4% false-negatives; 4–10% false-positives
√ dependent round filling defects
DDx: air bubbles
US (22–82% sensitive):
√ stone visualization in 13–75% (more readily with CBD dilatation + good visibility of pancreatic head)
√ dilated ducts in 64–77% / duct <8 mm in diameter in 24–36%
√ increased dilatation of CBD with administration of fatty meal / cholecystokinin
√ no stone in gallbladder (1.2–11%)
CT (88% sensitive, 97% specific, 94% accurate):
√ stone visualization in 75–88% (isoattenuating to bile in 12–25%)
√ target sign = intraluminal mass with crescentic ring (= stone of soft-tissue density) in 85%
√ subtle alternating low- and high-attenuation rings (= mixed cholesterol-calcium stones)
MRCP (81–100% sensitive, 85–100% specific):
√ dark filling defect within hyperintense fluid (stone must be >2 mm in diameter)
NUC:
√ delayed bowel activity beyond 2 hours
√ persistent hepatic + common bile duct activity to 24 hours
√ prominent ductal activity beyond 90 minutes with visualization of secondary ducts
DDx: air bubbles, neoplasm, concentrated bile
B. STONE IN CYSTIC DUCT REMNANT:
retained in 0.4% after surgery for choledocholithiasis

CHRONIC GRANULOMATOUS DISEASE OF CHILDHOOD

= recessive X-linked (60%) / autosomal (40%) immunodeficiency disorder resulting in purulent infections + granuloma formation primarily involving lymph nodes, skin, lungs
Etiology: polymorphonuclear leukocyte dysfunction characterized by inability to generate hydrogen peroxide causing prolonged intracellular survival of phagocytized catalase-positive bacteria with dissemination in reticuloendothelial system
Organism: most commonly staphylococcus, Serratia marcescens, Nocardia species, mycobacteria, fungi
Path: chronic infection with granuloma formation / caseation / suppuration
Age: onset in childhood; M > F (more severe in boys)
• recurrent chronic infections
• nitroblue tetrazolium test: low percentage of WBCs that reduce the dye after stimulation by phagocytosis / contact with endotoxin (normally >90%)
@ Bone
√ osteomyelitis (commonly of spine, ribs, metatarsals)
@ Chest
√ chronic pneumonia
√ hilar lymphadenopathy
√ pleural + pericardial effusions
@ Liver
√ hepatosplenomegaly
√ hepatic abscess (most common abdominal process)
√ liver calcifications
@ GI tract
• chronic diarrhea with malabsorption
• vomiting, anorexia, heartburn, weight loss
√ esophageal dysmotility, esophagitis, stricture
√ gastric antral narrowing ± gastric outlet obstruction
√ perianal fistula + abscess
@ GU tract
• dysuria
√ cystitis
√ obstruction of urethra + ureters
@ Lymph nodes
√ suppurative lymphadenitis
@ Skin
• pyoderma
Rx: prophylactic long-term trimethoprim-sulfamethoxazole + interferon gamma therapy

CIRRHOSIS

= chronic liver disease characterized by diffuse parenchymal necrosis, regeneration and scarring with abnormal reconstruction of preexisting lobular architecture

Etiology:

A. TOXIC
  (1) Alcoholic liver disease in 75%
  (2) Drug-induced (prolonged methotrexate, oxyphenisatin, alpha- methyldopa, nitrofurantoin, isoniazid)
  (3) Iron overload (hemochromatosis, hemosiderosis)

B. INFLAMMATION
  (1) Viral hepatitis
  (2) Schistosomiasis

C. BILIARY OBSTRUCTION
  (1) Cystic fibrosis
  (2) Inflammatory bowel disease
  (3) Primary biliary cirrhosis
  (4) Obstructive infantile cholangiopathy

D. VASCULAR
  (1) Prolonged CHF = cardiac cirrhosis
  (2) Hepatic venoocclusive disease (Budd-Chiari syndrome)

E. NUTRITIONAL
  (1) Intestinal bypass
  (2) Severe steatosis
  (3) Abetalipoproteinemia

F. HEREDITARY
  (1) Wilson disease
  (2) Alpha-1 antitrypsin deficiency
  (3) Juvenile polycystic kidney disease
  (4) Galactosemia
  (5) Type IV glycogen storage disease
  (6) Hereditary fructose intolerance
  (7) Tyrosinemia
  (8) Hereditary tetany
  (9) Osler-Weber-Rendu syndrome
  (10) Familial cirrhosis

G. IDIOPATHIC / CRYPTOGENIC

Cirrhosis in children: chronic hepatitis, congenital hepatic fibrosis, cystic fibrosis, biliary atresia, alpha-1 antitrypsin deficiency, tyrosinemia, galactosemia, hemochromatosis, Wilson disease, schistosomiasis, total parenteral nutrition

Morphology:

(a) micronodular cirrhosis (<3 mm): usually due to alcoholism, biliary obstruction, hemochromatosis, venous outflow obstruction, previous small-bowel bypass surgery, Indian childhood fibrosis
(b) macronodular cirrhosis (3–15 mm, up to several cm): usually due to chronic viral hepatitis, Wilson disease, alpha-1 antitrypsin deficiency
(c) mixed cirrhosis

Nodular lesions:

(a) **regenerative nodules** = localized proliferation of hepatocytes + supporting stroma
(b) cirrhotic nodule = regenerative nodule largely / completely surrounded by fibrous septa
(c) dysplastic nodule [adenomatous hyperplasia] = cluster of hepatocytes >1 mm in diameter with evidence of dysplasia; common in hepatitis B and C, alpha-1 antitrypsin deficiency, tyrosinemia
(d) hepatocellular carcinoma

Associated with: anemia, coagulopathy, hypoalbuminemia, cholelithiasis, pancreatitis, peptic ulcer disease, diarrhea, hypogonadism

• anorexia, weakness, fatigue, weight loss
• jaundice, continuous low-grade fever
• ascites, bleeding from esophageal varices, hepatic encephalopathy

√ enlarged (early stage) / normal / shrunken liver
√ shrinkage of right lobe (segments 5–8) and medial segment of left lobe (segments 4a + 4b) with concomitant hypertrophy of lateral segment of left lobe (segments 2 + 3) and caudate lobe (segment 1):
  √ ratio of caudate to right lobe >0.65 on transverse images [sensitivity 43–84%, least sensitive in alcoholic cirrhosis, most sensitive in cirrhosis caused by hepatitis B; specificity 100%; 26% sensitivity; 84–96% accuracy] (DDx: Budd-Chiari syndrome)
  √ diameter of quadrate lobe (segment 4) <30 mm (= distance between left wall of gallbladder and ascending portion of left portal vein) due to selective atrophy (95% specific)
√ widened porta hepatis + interlobar fissure
√ surface nodularity + indentations (regenerating nodules)
√ signs of portal hypertension
√ splenomegaly
√ ascites (failure of albumin synthesis, overproduction of lymph due to increased hydrostatic pressure in sinusoids / decreased splanchnic output due to portal hypertension)
√ associated with fatty infiltration (in early cirrhosis)

US (sensitivity 65–80%; DDx: chronic hepatitis, fatty infiltration):

  Hepatic signs:
    √ hepatomegaly (63%)
    √ hypertrophy of caudate lobe (26%):
      √ ratio of width of caudate lobe to width of right hepatic lobe >0.65 (43–84% sensitive, 100% specific)
    √ surface nodularity (88% sensitive, 82–95% specific)
    √ increased hepatic parenchymal echogenicity in 66% (as a sign of superimposed fatty infiltration):
      √ increased sound attenuation (9%)
      √ decreased / normal definition of walls of portal venules (sign of associated fatty infiltration NOT of fibrosis)
    √ heterogeneous coarse (usually) / fine echotexture (7%)
    √ occasional depiction of isoechoic regenerative nodules
    √ dilatation of hepatic arteries (increased arterial flow) with demonstration of intrahepatic arterial branches (DDx: dilated biliary radicals)

√ increase in hepatic artery resistance after meal ingestion
√ "portalization" of hepatic vein waveform = dampened oscillations of hepatic veins resembling portal vein flow

Extrahepatic signs:
√ splenomegaly
√ ascites
√ signs of portal hypertension

CT:
√ native + enhanced parenchymal inhomogeneity
√ decreased attenuation (steatosis) in early cirrhosis
√ isodense / hyperdense (siderotic) regenerative nodules
√ nodular / lobulated liver contour
√ predominantly portal venous supply to dysplastic nodules
√ hypodense area adjacent to portal vein (= peribiliary cysts from obstructed extramural peribiliary glands)
√ rapid tapering of intrahepatic portal + hepatic venous branches

CECT:
√ enlarged tortuous hepatic artery (compensatory increase in arterial blood flow)
√ arterioportal shunts (through trans-sinusoidal shunts in liver periphery + transplexal shunts with hypertrophy of peribiliary plexus) in hepatic arterial phase:
√ poorly demarcated transient peripheral wedge-shaped hepatic parenchymal enhancement
DDx: hepatocellular carcinoma (defect on portal venous phase)
√ early retrograde enhancement of portal vein branches
√ hepatofugal flow
Cause: with occlusion of small hepatic venules the portal vein turns from a supplying vein into a draining vein

MR (problem-solving tool):
√ no alteration of liver parenchyma
√ regenerating nodules = hypointense lesions (due to iron deposits within nodules) with hyperintense septa (due to vascularity) on T2WI
√ dysplastic nodule = iso- / hyperintense on T1WI + iso- / hypointense on T2WI
√ HCC nodule = hypo- / iso- / hyperintense on T1WI + usually hyperintense on T2WI with marked enhancement during arterial phase

Angio:
√ stretched hepatic artery branches (early finding)
√ enlarged tortuous hepatic arteries = "corkscrewing" (increase in hepatic arterial flow)
√ shunting between hepatic artery and portal vein
√ mottled parenchymal phase
√ delayed emptying into venous phase
√ pruning of hepatic vein branches (normally depiction of 5th order branches) = postsinusoidal compression by developing nodules

NUC (Tc-99m–labeled sulfur colloid):
√ high blood pool activity secondary to slow clearance
√ colloid shift to bone marrow + spleen + lung
√ shrunken liver with little or no activity + splenomegaly
√ mottled hepatic uptake (pseudotumors) on colloid scan (normal activity on IDA scans!)
√ displacement of liver + spleen from abdominal wall by ascites

Cx: (1) Ascites: cause / contributor to death in 50%
(2) Portal hypertension
(3) Hepatocellular carcinoma (in 7–12%)
(4) Cholangiocarcinoma

Fatality from:
esophageal variceal bleeding (in 25%), hepatorenal syndrome (10%), spontaneous bacterial peritonitis (5–10%), complications from treatment of ascites (10%)

Primary Biliary Cirrhosis

= CHRONIC NONSUPPURATIVE DESTRUCTIVE CHOLANGITIS

Histo: idiopathic progressive destructive cholangitis of interlobar and septal bile ducts, portal fibrosis, nodular regeneration, shrinkage of hepatic parenchyma

Age: 35–55 years; M:F = 1:9

Associated autoimmune disorders:
rheumatoid arthritis, Hashimoto thyroiditis, Sjögren syndrome, scleroderma, sarcoidosis
◊ 66–100% of patients with primary biliary cirrhosis have sicca-complex signs of the Sjögren syndrome

- fatigue, pruritus
- xanthelasma / xanthoma (25%)
- hyperpigmentation (50%)
- insidious onset of pruritus (60%)
- IgM increased (95%)
- positive antimitochondrial antibodies (AMA) in 85–100%

√ normal extrahepatic ducts
√ cholelithiasis in 35–39%

CT:
√ scattered dilated intrahepatic ducts with no apparent connection to main bile ducts
√ caudate lobe hypertrophy (in 98%):
√ hypertrophied hyperattenuating caudate lobe surrounded by hypoattenuating rindlike right lobe (pseudotumor)
√ atrophy of lateral segment of left hepatic lobe
√ intrahepatic biliary calculi (20%)

NUC:
√ marked prolongation of hepatic Tc-99m IDA clearance
√ uniform hepatic isotope retention
√ normal visualization of GB and major bile ducts in 100%

DDx: (1) Sclerosing cholangitis (young men)
(2) CBD obstruction

Prognosis: mean survival 6 (range 3–11) years after onset of cholestatic symptoms

Complications of End-Stage Liver Disease

Hepatopulmonary Syndrome

Dx: (1) chronic liver disease
(2) increased alveolar-arterial gradient
(3) intrapulmonary vascular dilatation

• hypoxemia (in 1/3 of decompensated cirrhotic patients)

Pathomechanism:
elevation of unknown vasoactive substances in cirrhotic patient cause pulmonary vascular dilatation (from 8–15 μm to 15–500 μm) + result in diffusion-perfusion mismatch

√ basilar nodular / reticulonodular areas of increased opacity (in 46–100%)
√ dilated arterioles with an increased number of terminal branches extending to pleura
√ intrapulmonary arteriovenous shunt (demonstrated with Tc-99m macroaggregated albumin imaging, microbubble echocardiography)

Hepatic Hydrothorax

= large pleural effusion in cirrhotic patient without primary pulmonary / cardiac disease

Prevalence: 10%
Mechanism: pressure gradient favors fluid movement from peritoneal to pleural cavity through small diaphragmatic defects

√ pleural fluid: right in 67%, left in 17%, bilateral in 17%

Pulmonary Hypertension

Prevalence: 0.73% in patients with liver cirrhosis (versus 0.13% in all patients)

Cause:
(a) thromboembolic: portal venous thrombus reaches lung through spontaneous / surgically created portosystemic shunts
(b) plexogenic: vasoactive substances (serotonin, thromboxane, neuropeptide Y, elastase) bypass the liver through portosystemic shunts

Prognosis: mean survival of 15 months

CLONORCHIASIS

Rarely of clinical significance

Country: endemic to Southeast Asia: Japan, Korea, Central + South China, Taiwan, Indochina
Organism: Chinese liver fluke = Clonorchis sinensis
Cycle: parasite cysts digested by gastric juice, larvae migrate up the bile ducts, remain in small intrahepatic ducts until maturity (10–30 mm in length), travel to larger ducts to deposit eggs
Infection: snail + freshwater fish serve as intermediate hosts; infection occurs by eating raw fish; hog, dog, cat, man are definite hosts
Path: (a) desquamation of epithelial bile duct lining with adenomatous proliferation of ducts + thickening of duct walls (inflammation, necrosis, fibrosis)
(b) bacterial superinfection with formation of liver abscess

• remittent incomplete obstruction + bacterial superinfection

√ multiple crescent- / stiletto-shaped filling defects within bile ducts:
 √ echogenic focus / cast on US
√ diffusely thickened bile ducts

Cx: (1) Bile duct obstruction (conglomerate of worms / adenomatous proliferation)
(2) Calculus formation (stasis / dead worms / epithelial debris)
(3) Jaundice in 8% (stone / stricture / tumor)
(4) Generalized dilatation of bile ducts (2%)

CONGENITAL BILIARY ATRESIA

Etiology: ? variation of same infectious process as in neonatal hepatitis with additional component of sclerosing cholangitis or vascular injury
Prevalence: <10 in 100,000 live births
Age: neonate; M:F = 2:1
Histo: periportal fibrosis, proliferation of small intrahepatic bile ducts, mixed inflammatory infiltrates
In 15% associated with: polysplenia, trisomy 18

Types:
I Focal = intrauterine vascular insult (extremely rare)
II Intrahepatic biliary atresia = paucity of intrahepatic bile ducts (uncommon)
III Extrahepatic biliary atresia = atresia of CBD + patent intrahepatic bile ducts

<u>Subtype 1</u> = perinatal type (66%)
• jaundice develops after regression of physiologic jaundice
√ bile duct remnant in porta hepatis

<u>Subtype 2</u> = embryonic / fetal type (34%)
• normal decline in bilirubin does not occur
√ NO bile duct remnant in porta hepatis

Associated with: polysplenia (10–12%), intestinal malrotation, azygos continuation of IVC, symmetric bilobed liver, situs inversus, preduodenal portal vein, anomalous hepatic arteries, bilobed right lung, complex CHD

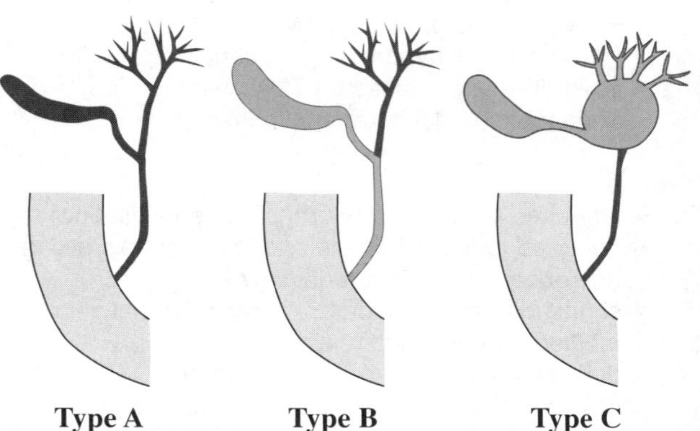

Biliary Atresia

US:
- √ normal / increased size of liver
- √ normal / increased liver echogenicity
- √ decreased visualization of peripheral portal veins (due to fibrosis)
- √ "triangular cord" / tubular echogenic structure in porta hepatis (due to fibrous tissue) = PATHOGNOMONIC
- √ gallbladder findings:
  - √ nonvisualization of gallbladder
  - √ small gallbladder <1.5 cm in length + varying degrees of luminal compromise (DDx: hepatitis)
  - √ normal gallbladder >1.5 cm in length (19%) when atresia of CBD distal to insertion of cystic duct
- √ bile duct findings:
  - √ no dilatation of intrahepatic bile ducts (due to panductal sclerosis)
  - √ ± visualization of bile duct remnant in porta hepatis (depending on type of biliary atresia)
  - √ small focal cystic dilatation of extrahepatic bile duct (= choledochal cyst) = patent segment of CBD with other parts being occluded due to fibrosis ± communication with gallbladder / intrahepatic bile ducts

NUC [phenobarbital-augmented cholescintigraphy] (90–97% sensitive, 60–94% specific, 75–90% accurate):
- » preparation of patient with 5 ng/kg/d phenobarbital twice a day for 3–7 days to stimulate biliary secretion (via induction of hepatic enzymes + increase in conjugation + excretion of bilirubin)
- √ good hepatic activity within 5 min (infants of <3 months of age have a normal hepatic extraction fraction)
- √ NO biliary excretion:
  - √ NO visualization of bowel on delayed images at 6 and 24 hours
- √ delayed clearance from cardiac blood pool
- √ increased renal excretion + bladder activity

DDx: severe hepatocellular dysfunction (DDx from neonatal hepatitis impossible in the absence of small bowel activity) requires liver biopsy

MR cholangiography:
- √ nonvisualization of extrahepatic bile ducts
- √ atrophic gallbladder
- √ periportal thickening

Cholangiography (percutaneous / endoscopic / intraoperative)

Liver Bx (60–97% accurate)

Rx: (1) Roux-en-Y choledochojejunostomy (20%);
(2) Kasai procedure = portoenterostomy (80%)
- (a) child <60 days of age: 91% success rate
- (b) child between 60 and 90 days of age: 50% success rate (due to developing cirrhosis)
- (c) child >90 days of age: 17% success rate

(3) Liver transplant

DDx:
(1) Neonatal hepatitis
(2) Sclerosing cholangitis
(3) **Alagille syndrome** = arteriohepatic dysplasia (abnormal facies, butterfly vertebra, pulmonic stenosis, complex CHD)

CONGENITAL HEPATIC FIBROSIS

= congenital cirrhosis with rapid + fatal progression

Histo: fibrous tissue within hepatic parenchyma with excess numbers of distorted terminal interlobular bile ducts + cysts that rarely communicate with bile ducts

Age: usually present in childhood resulting in early death

Associated with:
autosomal recessive polycystic kidney disease (invariably), Meckel-Gruber syndrome, vaginal atresia, tuberous sclerosis, nephronophthisis, medullary sponge kidney (80%), autosomal dominant polycystic kidney disease (rare)

- • hepatosplenomegaly, portal hypertension
- • predisposed to cholangitis + calculi
- √ "lollipop-tree" = ectasia of peripheral biliary radicles
- √ hepatosplenomegaly
- √ periportal fibrosis + portosystemic collaterals

Cx: portal hypertension, hepatocellular carcinoma, cholangiocellular carcinoma

ECHINOCOCCAL DISEASE OF LIVER

Echinococcus Granulosus

= HYDATID DISEASE = unilocular form

= E. cysticus (more common); man is accidental host
- (a) pastoral (European) form: dog is definite host; intermediate hosts are cattle, sheep, horses, hogs; endemic in sheep-raising countries: Australia, New Zealand, North + East Africa, USSR, Mediterranean countries, Near + Middle East, Japan, Argentina, Chile, Uruguay
- (b) sylvatic (northern) form: wolf is definite host; intermediate hosts are deer, moose; endemic in northwestern Canada, Alaska

Cycle: ingestion of contaminated material (eggs passed in feces of dog / other carnivore); eggs hatch in duodenum; larvae penetrate intestinal wall + mesenteric venules; larvae carried into portal circulation; larvae are filtered in capillaries of liver (first line of defense) > lung > other organs

Histo:
A. CYST FLUID = antigenic clear / pale yellow fluid with neutral pH containing sodium chloride, proteins, glucose, ions, lipids, polysaccharides

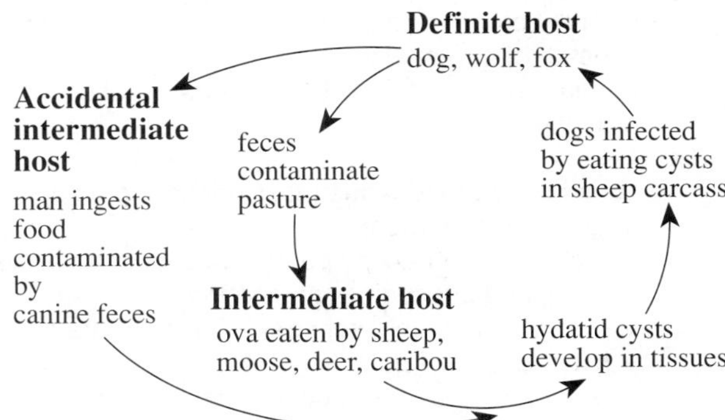

Parasitic Cycle of Echinococcus Granulosus

LIVER

B. ENDOCYST (parasitic component of capsule) = inner GERMINATIVE LAYER (resembling wet tissue paper) giving rise to brood capsules (daughter vesicles), which may
   (a) remain attached to cyst wall harboring up to 400,000 scolices
   (b) detach + form sediment in cyst fluid = "hydatid sand"
   (c) break up into numerous self-contained daughter cysts
C. ECTOCYST = CYST MEMBRANE = acellular laminated chitinlike substance secreted by parasite, allowing passage of nutrients
D. PERICYST = dense fibrous protective zone of host granulation tissue replacing tissue necrosis (from compression by the expanding cyst); marginal vascular rim of 0.5–4 mm

- pain / asymptomatic
- recurrent jaundice + biliary colic (transient obstruction by membrane fragments + daughter cysts expelled into biliary tree)
- blood eosinophilia (20–50%)
- urticaria + anaphylaxis (following rupture)
- Tests:
  1. Casoni intradermal test (60% sensitivity; may be falsely positive)
  2. Complement fixation double diffusion (65% sensitivity)
  3. Immunoelectrophoresis (most specific)
  4. Indirect hemagglutination (85% sensitivity)

Time to diagnosis: 11–81 (mean 51) years

Affected organs:
liver (73%); lung (14%); peritoneum (12%); kidney (3–6%); spleen (0.9–8%); CNS (1%); orbit (1%); bone (0.5–4%); bladder; thyroid; prostate; heart

Location: right lobe > left lobe of liver; multiple cysts in 20%

Size: up to 50 cm (average size of 5 cm), up to 16 liters of fluid; grows 2–3 cm annually

Stages of cyst growth:
(1) Unilocular cyst
(2) Cyst with daughter vesicles / daughter cysts
(3) Partially / completely calcified

Plain film:
√ peripheral crescentic / curvilinear / polycyclic calcifications (10–20–33%), located in pericyst:
  ◊ Only complete calcification of all layers implies death of parasite!
√ pneumohydrocyst (infection / communication with bronchial tree)

US:
√ complex heterogeneous mass mimicking a solid mass (most common):
  ◊ Look for membranes / peripheral daughter vesicles
√ well-defined anechoic cyst (common):
  √ cyst wall of double echogenic lines separated by hypoechoic layer
  √ "snowstorm sign" = multiple internal echogenic foci settling to most dependent portion of cyst (= hydatid sand)
√ multivesicular cyst of "racemose" / honeycomb appearance = multiple septa between daughter cysts inside mother cyst, CHARACTERISTIC but rare:
  √ "wheel spoke" pattern = daughter cysts separated by echogenic material of hydatid matrix composed of broken daughter vesicles + scolices + hydatid sand
  √ HIGHLY SPECIFIC serpentine linear structures within hydatid matrix
√ partial / complete detachment of endocyst from pericyst (due to decreasing intracystic pressure as a sign of degeneration / trauma / host response / response to therapy):
  √ localized split in wall with floating undulating membrane, CHARACTERISTIC but rare
  √ "water lily sign" = complete detachment of membrane
  ◊ Floating membrane does not indicate death of parasite!
√ eggshell calcification in cyst wall (least common)

CT:
√ well-demarcated round low-density mass of fluid attenuation (3–30 HU):
  √ cyst wall of high attenuation on NECT
  √ linear areas of increased attenuation = detached laminated membrane
  √ round peripheral fluid collection of lower attenuation (= daughter cysts)
√ enhancement of cyst wall + septations
√ calcification of cyst wall / internal septa

MR:
√ cyst with hypointense rim (= collagenous pericyst) on T1WI + T2WI
√ peripheral cysts within cyst hypointense on T1WI + hyperintense on T2WI (= daughter cysts)
√ twisted linear structures within cyst = collapsed parasitic membrane

Angio:
√ avascular area with splaying of arteries
√ halo of increased density around cyst (inflammation / compressed liver)

Cholangiography:
√ cyst may communicate with bile ducts: right hepatic duct (55%), left hepatic duct (29%), CHD (9%), gallbladder (6%), CBD (1%)

Percutaneous aspiration:
- fluid analysis positive for hydatid disease in 70% (fragments of laminated membrane in 54%; scolices in 15%; hooklets in 15%)
◊ Risk of anaphylactic shock (0.5%), asthma (3%), implantation of spilled protoscoleces

Local Cx:
(1) Rupture (50–90%)
   (a) contained = rupture of laminated membrane of endocyst, pericyst remains intact
      √ floating membranes
   (b) communicating = cyst contents escapes through biliary (5–15%) / bronchial tree

(c) direct = tear of endocyst + ectocyst + pericyst with cyst contents spilling into pleural / peritoneal cavity (anaphylaxis, metastatic hydatidosis)
(2) Infection (5–8%) following rupture
(3) Transdiaphragmatic growth (0.6–16%) through bare area of liver
(a) rupture into pleural cavity
(b) seeding in pulmonary parenchyma
(c) chronic bronchial fistula
(4) Perforation into hollow viscus (0.5%)
(5) Peritoneal seeding (13%) = encysted peritoneal hydatidosis
(6) Compression of vital structures (bile ducts, portal vein)

Rx: (1) Surgery (in 10% recurrence)
(2) Anthelmintics (albendazole, medendazole)
(3) Injection of scolecidal agents (silver nitrate, 20 / 30% hypertonic saline solution, 0.5% cetrimide solution, 95% ethanol)

Echinococcus Multilocularis

= E. alveolaris = less common but more aggressive form of echinococcal disease
Primary host: fox, wolf
Secondary host: rodents (moles, lemmings, wild mice); domestic cat; dog
Endemic to: eastern France, southern Germany, western Austria, much of Soviet Union, Japan, Alaska, Canada, some areas in Turkey
Infection: eating wild fruits contaminated with fox / wolf feces; direct contact with fox / wolf; contact with dogs / cats that have ingested infested rodents
Path: larvae proliferate by exogenous extension + penetration of surrounding tissue (= diffuse + infiltrative process resembling malignancy); chronic granulomatous reaction with central necrosis, cavitation, calcification
Histo: daughter cysts with thick lamellar wall arising on outer surface of original cyst, rarely containing scolices
Location: liver (access via portal vein); widespread hematogenous dissemination not uncommon

• clinical manifestation 5–20 years after ingestion
• abdominal discomfort, jaundice, hepatomegaly
• eosinophilia

√ aggressive growth pattern:
√ geographic infiltrating lesion with ill-defined margins
√ invasion of IVC, diaphragm
√ metastases to lung, heart, brain (in 10%)
√ faint / dense amorphous coalescent nodular / flame-shaped calcifications (dystrophic central calcifications scattered throughout necrotic + granulomatous tissue)

US:
√ echogenic geographic ill-defined single / multiple solid masses
√ ± irregular cystic areas
√ propensity of spread to liver hilum

CT:
√ heterogeneous hypodense poorly marginated infiltrating masses
√ pseudocystic necrotic regions of near water density surrounded by hyperdense solid component
√ little / no enhancement

Angio:
√ intrahepatic arterial tapering + obstruction

Cx: Budd-Chiari syndrome, IVC thrombosis, portal hypertension
Prognosis: fatal within 10–15 years (if left untreated)
DDx: hepatocellular carcinoma (biopsy!), large hemangioma (characteristic enhancement pattern), metastasis, epithelial hemangioendothelioma

EMBRYONAL RHABDOMYOSARCOMA OF BILIARY TREE

= rare tumor most commonly arising from CBD
Median age: 3 years; M > F
Path: intraluminal biliary mass / cluster of grapelike masses (similar to rhabdomyosarcoma of bladder)
Histo: same as sarcoma botryoides

• malaise, fever, jaundice
• elevation of conjugated bilirubin

Metastases (in up to 30%) to:
retroperitoneal +mesenteric lymph nodes, lung
Location: common bile duct (most frequently)
√ 8–20-cm bulky heterogeneous mass in porta hepatis
√ intrahepatic bile duct dilatation
√ displacement of duodenum, stomach, pancreas

Cholangiography:
√ large bulky intraluminal mass / grapelike cluster of intraluminal masses focally distending common bile duct + obstructing proximal bile ducts

EPIDERMOID CYST OF SPLEEN

= EPITHELIAL CYST = PRIMARY CYST OF SPLEEN
Incidence: 10% of all benign nonparasitic cysts
Cause: infolding of peritoneal mesothelium / collection of peritoneal mesothelial cells trapped within splenic sulci
Histo: (1) mesothelial lining
(2) squamous epithelial lining = epidermoid cyst = squamous metaplasia from embryonic inclusions within preexisting mesothelial surface epithelium
Age: 2nd–3rd decade (average age of 18 years)
May be associated with: polycystic kidney disease
(a) unilocular + solitary (80%)
(b) multiple + multilocular (20%)
√ well-defined thin-walled anechoic lesion of water density
√ average size of 10 cm
√ peripheral septations / cyst wall trabeculations (in 86%)
√ curvilinear calcification in wall (9–25%)
√ may contain cholesterol crystals, fat, blood
Cx: trauma, rupture, infection

EPITHELIOID HEMANGIOENDOTHELIOMA

= rare primary malignant vascular tumor of liver (soft tissue, bone, lung)

Age: average age of 45 years; M:F = 1:2

Possibly associated with: oral contraceptives, exposure to vinyl chloride

Path: multifocal nodules varying in size from a few mm to several cm involve both lobes of the liver (due to rapid perivascular extension); nodules may coalesce in liver periphery

Histo: dendritic spindle-shaped cells + epithelioid round cells in a matrix of myxoid + fibrous stroma; neoplastic endothelial cells invade sinusoids + terminal hepatic + portal veins cutting off the tumor's blood supply

• in 80%: abdominal pain, weakness, anorexia, jaundice

Metastases to: spleen, mesentery, lymph nodes, lung, bone

√ multiple nodules (nodular form)
√ peripheral subcapsular growth (diffuse form) without deforming liver contour
√ increased tumor vascularity
√ hypertrophy of uninvolved liver

Plain film:
- √ hepatic calcifications within myxoid stroma (15%)

US:
- √ typically hypoechoic lesions (due to central core of myxoid stroma)

CT:
- √ low-attenuation masses on NECT, may become isoattenuating with rest of liver on CECT (due to vasoformative growth + compensatory hepatic arterial flow with portal vein occlusion)

Angio:
- √ hyper- and hypovascularity (dependent upon degree of sclerosis + hyalinization)
- √ invasion ± occlusion of portal + hepatic veins

NUC:
- √ decreased perfusion to central myxoid tumor portion + increased perfusion to cellular areas on sulfur colloid scan
- √ photopenic defect on static sulfur colloid scan
- √ NOT gallium avid

Prognosis: 20% die within 2 years, 20% survive for 5–28 years ± treatment

DDx of multiple nodules: metastatic disease

DDx of diffuse form: sclerosing carcinoma, vaso-occlusive disease

FATTY LIVER

= FATTY INFILTRATION OF THE LIVER = HEPATIC STEATOSIS

Cause:

A. METABOLIC DERANGEMENT
poorly controlled diabetes mellitus (50%), obesity, hyperlipidemia, acute fatty liver of pregnancy, protein malnutrition, total parenteral hyperalimentation (TPN), malabsorption (jejunoileal bypass), glycogen storage disease, glycogen synthetase deficiency, cystic fibrosis, Reye syndrome, corticosteroids, severe hepatitis, trauma, chronic illness (TB, CHF)

B. HEPATOTOXINS
alcohol (>50%), carbon chlorides, phosphorus, amiodarone, chemotherapy

Histo: hepatocytes with large cytoplasmic fat vacuoles containing triglycerides; >5% fat of total liver weight

• NO abnormal liver function tests

√ rapid change with time (few days to >10 months) depending on clinical improvement (abstinence from alcohol, improved nutrition) + degree of severity

Diffuse Fatty Infiltration

√ hepatomegaly (75–80%) / normal sized liver

Plain film:
- √ radiolucent liver sign = enlarged radiolucent liver

US (sensitivity >90%, accuracy 85–97%):
- √ increased sound attenuation (scattering of sound beam) = poor definition of posterior aspect of liver
- √ fine (more typical) / coarsened hyperechogenicity (compared with kidney)
- √ impaired visualization of borders of hepatic vessels
- √ attenuation of sound beam (feature of fat, NOT fibrosis)

CT:
- √ areas of lower attenuation than normal portal vein / IVC density
- √ reversal of liver-spleen density relationship (liver density is normally 6–12 HU greater than spleen)
- √ hyperdense intrahepatic vessels

NUC:
- Tc-99m sulfur colloid scan:
  - √ diffuse heterogeneous uptake (68%)
  - √ reversal of liver-spleen uptake (41%)
  - √ increased bone marrow uptake (41%)
- Xe-133 ventilation scan:
  - √ increased activity during washout phase (38%)

MR:
- √ slightly increased signal on T1WI + T2WI; relatively insensitive (10% fat by weight will alter SE signal intensities only by 5–15%)
- √ fat turns black with Dixon technique

FAT-SPARED AREA in diffuse fatty infiltration

Cause: direct drainage of systemic blood into liver

Location:
(a) posterior edge of segment 4 = anterior to portal vein bifurcation (drainage of aberrant gastric vein)
(b) next to gallbladder bed (drainage of cystic vein)
(c) subcapsular skip areas

√ hypoechoic ovoid / spherical / sheetlike mass
√ NO mass effect (undisplaced course of vessels)

DDx: tumor mass

Focal Fatty Infiltration

Etiology: ? vascular origin, focal tissue hypoxia

LIVER

Distribution: (a) lobar / segmental uniform lesions
(b) lobar / segmental nodular lesions
(c) perihilar lesions
(d) diffuse nodular lesions
(e) diffuse patchy lesions
predominantly in centrilobar + periportal regions, subcapsular distribution may be due to variants of blood supply (due to "third inflow" from connection between peripheral portal radicles + perforating capsular / accessory cystic veins)

Location: right lobe, caudate lobe, perihilar region

√ fan-shaped lobar / segmental distribution with angulated / interdigitating geographic margins
√ lesions extend to periphery of liver
√ NO mass effect (undisplaced course of vessels, no bulging of liver contour)

US:
√ hyperechoic area with poorly defined / sharp margins
√ multiple / rarely single echogenic nodules simulating metastases (rare)

CT:
√ patchy areas of decreased attenuation ranging from –40 to +10 HU (DDx: liver tumor)
√ NO contrast enhancement

MR (not sensitive for fat):
√ high signal on T1WI + low / isointense signal on T2WI

NUC with colloid:
√ no significant changes on sulfur colloid images (SPECT imaging may detect focal fatty infiltration)

DDx: primary / secondary hepatic tumor

FOCAL NODULAR HYPERPLASIA

= FNH = rare benign congenital hamartomatous malformation or reparative process in areas of focal injury; SPECIFIC DIAGNOSIS RARELY POSSIBLE

Incidence: 2nd most common benign tumor of liver after hemangioma; 4% of all primary hepatic tumors in pediatric population, 3–8% in adult population; twice as common as hepatocellular adenoma; only 357 cases reported

Cause: (?) congenital arteriovenous malformation triggers focal hepatocellular hyperplasia owing to a regional increase in blood flow
◊ Oral contraceptives DO NOT cause FNH, but exert a trophic effect on its growth!

Path: localized, well-delineated, usually solitary (80–95%), subcapsular mass of numerous small lobules within an otherwise normal liver; no true capsule; frequently central fibrous scar in area of interconnection of fibrous bands (HALLMARK) containing centrally an arteriovenous malformation with spiderlike branches supplying the component nodules

Histo: composed of multiple spherical aggregates of <u>hepatocytes</u> often containing increased amounts of fat + triglycerides + glycogen; <u>Kupffer cells</u>; <u>bile duct</u> proliferation within fibrous septa <u>without connection to biliary tree</u>; thick-walled arteries within fibrous septa radiating from the center toward the periphery; absent portal triads + central veins; difficult differentiation from regenerative nodules of cirrhosis + hepatocellular adenoma

Age peak: 3rd–4th decade (range: 7 months to 75 years); M:F = 1:2–4

Associated with: hepatic hemangioma (in 23%), meningioma, astrocytoma, arterial dysplasia of other organs in case of multiple FNH

- initially often asymptomatic (in 50–90% incidental discovery)
- vague abdominal pain (10–15%) due to mass effect
- normal liver function
- hepatomegaly / abdominal mass

Location: right lobe:left lobe = 2:1

Size: <5 cm (in 85%)

√ well-circumscribed <u>nonencapsulated</u> nodular cirrhotic-like mass in an otherwise normal liver:
  √ often near liver surface
  √ pedunculated mass (in 5–20%)
  √ multiple masses (in 20%)
√ central scar containing arteriovenous malformation
√ highly vascular tumor
  √ hemorrhage is unlikely
√ calcifications are EXTREMELY rare

NECT:
√ iso- / slightly hypoattenuating homogeneous mass

CECT:
√ transient intense hyperdensity (after 30–60 sec) on bolus injection followed rapidly by isodensity:
  √ hypodense mass during peak portal venous phase
  √ isodense mass during equilibrium phase
  ◊ Lesion may be missed without precontrast study!
√ hypodense central stellate scar = central fibrous core with radiating fibrous septa (15–33%) (DDx: fibrolamellar HCC):
  √ ± early enhancement of vessels traversing central scar
  √ hyperdense central scar on delayed images (delayed washout of contrast from myxomatous scar tissue)

US:
√ iso- / hypo- / hyperechoic (33%) homogeneous mass
√ hyperechoic central scar in 18%
√ displacement of hepatic vessels

Doppler:
√ enlarged afferent blood vessel with central arterial hypervascularity + centrifugal filling to the periphery in "spoke-wheel" pattern
√ large draining veins at tumor margins
√ may show high-velocity Doppler signals with arterial pulsatility from arteriovenous shunts

NUC:
Sulfur colloid scan:
√ normal uptake (50–70%), hot spot (7–10%)
◊ Only FNH contains sufficient Kupffer cells to cause normal / increased uptake (almost PATHOGNOMONIC)!

√ cold spot (30–50%)
(DDx: hepatic adenoma, hemangioma, hepatoblastoma, liver herniation, hepatocellular carcinoma)

Tc-HIDA:
√ normal / increased uptake (40–70%), cold spot (60%)

Tc-99m–tagged RBCs:
√ increased uptake during early phase
√ defect relative to liver on delayed images

MR:
√ usually homogeneous signal intensity of lesion
√ T1WI:
√ iso- to hypointense (94–100%)
√ atypically hyperintense lesion in 6%
√ T2WI: slightly hyper- to isointense (94–100%)
√ central scar
√ hypointense on T1WI
√ hyperintense on T2WI in 75% (due to vascular channels + edema)
√ hypointense on T2WI in 25% (absent or minimal edema)

CEMR:
√ dense enhancement in arterial phase:
√ isointense during portal venous phase
√ hyperintense on delayed images
√ occasionally prolonged enhancement (due to entrapment of Gd-DTPA by functioning hepatocytes inside tumor followed by 1% excretion into biliary tree)
√ late + prolonged enhancement of central scar
√ less uptake of IV superparamagnetic iron oxide than surrounding liver (uptake mechanism similar to that of sulfur colloid)

Angio:
√ discretely marginated hypervascular mass (90%) with intense capillary blush / hypovascular (10%)
√ enlargement of main feeding artery with central blood supply (= "spoke-wheel" pattern in 33%)
√ homogeneous parenchymal stain
√ decreased vascularity in central stellate fibrous scar

Rx: (1) Discontinuation of oral contraceptives
(2) Resection of pedunculated mass
(3) Diagnostic excisional biopsy for extensive tumor (FNH seldom requires surgery)

Cx: rarely rupture with hemoperitoneum (increased incidence in patients on oral contraceptives — 14%)

DDx:
(1) Fibrolamellar carcinoma (scar calcified, metastases, retroperitoneal adenopathy, tumor hemorrhage + necrosis causing pain, hypointense scar on T2WI)
(2) Hepatic adenoma (10 cm large tumor, symptomatic due to propensity for hemorrhage in 50%, central scar atypical)
(3) Well-differentiated hepatocellular carcinoma (internal necrosis + hemorrhage, vascular invasion, metastases, rim-enhancement of pseudocapsule)
(4) Giant cavernous hemangioma (larger tumor, may calcify, globular peripheral enhancement followed by centripetal filling, retention of contrast on delayed images, CSF-like behavior on MRI)
(5) Hypervascular metastasis (hypovascular during portal venous phase, older patient)
(6) Intrahepatic cholangiocarcinoma (less vascular, dominant large central scar, metastases)

GALLBLADDER CARCINOMA

Incidence: 0.4–4.6% of biliary tract operations; most common biliary cancer (9 x more common than extrahepatic bile duct cancer); 6th most common gastrointestinal malignancy (after colon, pancreas, stomach, liver, esophagus); 3% of all intestinal neoplasms; 6,500 deaths/ year in United States

Demographics: most common in Israel, Bolivia, Chile, northern Japan, New Mexico

Ethnicity: Native Americans + Hispanic Americans (associated with increased prevalence of gallstones)

Median age: 73 years; M:F = 1:3–1:4
◊ 85% occur in 6th decade or later!

Risk factors: increased body mass, female gender, postmenopausal status, cigarette smoking, chronic Salmonella typhi infection, exposure to chemicals (rubber, automobile, wood finishing, metal fabricating industries)

Associated with:
(1) Disorder of gallbladder:
(a) Cholelithiasis in 74–92%
◊ Gallbladder carcinoma occurs in only 1% of all patients with gallstones!
(b) Porcelain gallbladder (in 4–60%): prevalence of gallbladder carcinoma in 10–25% of autopsies
(c) Chronic cholecystitis
(d) Gallbladder polyp: a polyp >2 cm is likely malignant!
(2) Disorder of bile ducts:
(a) Primary sclerosing cholangitis
(b) Congenital biliary anomalies: cystic dilatation of biliary tree, choledochal cyst, anomalous junction of pancreaticobiliary ducts, low insertion of cystic duct
(3) Inflammatory bowel disease (predominantly ulcerative colitis, less common in Crohn disease)
(4) Familial polyposis coli

Path: diffusely infiltrating lesion (68%), intraluminal polypoid growth (32%)

Histo: (a) adenocarcinoma (76%):
– papillary (6% with tendency to fill gallbladder lumen)
– intestinal type (variant of well-differentiated adenocarcinoma with intestinal glands)
– mucinous (5%, with >50% extracellular mucin)
– signet-ring cell (abundant intracytoplasmic mucin)
– clear cell (well-defined cytoplasmic borders)

LIVER

(b) rare epithelial cell types:
- adenosquamous carcinoma (3%)
- squamous cell carcinoma (1%)
- small (oat) cell carcinoma (0.5%, highly aggressive, ± paraneoplastic Cushing syndrome)
- undifferentiated carcinoma

(c) nonepithelial cell types (2%): carcinoid, carcinosarcoma, basal cell carcinoma, lymphoma

Modified Nevin Stage:
- I mucosa only (in situ carcinoma)
- II mucosal + muscular invasion
- III mucosa + muscularis + serosa
- IV gallbladder wall + lymph nodes
- V hepatic / distant metastases

• Early diagnosis usually unsuspected due to lack of specific signs + symptoms:
  • history of past GB disease (50%)
  • malaise, vomiting, weight loss
  • chronic RUQ pain (54–76%)
  • obstructive jaundice (35–74%)
  • abnormal liver function tests (20–75%)
  • ± elevated α-fetoprotein and CEA

Location: fundus (60%), body (30%), neck (10%)

Growth types:
- √ mass replacing the gallbladder (40–65%)
- √ thickening of GB wall (20–30%) due to submucosal spread:
  - √ focal (59%) / diffuse (41%) wall thickening
  - *DDx:* acute / chronic inflammation (usually <10 mm)
- √ intraluminal polypoid / fungating "cauliflower-like" mass with wide base (15–25%)

√ replacement of gallbladder by mass (37–70%)
√ pericholecystic infiltration: in 76% focal, in 24% diffuse
√ dilatation of biliary tree (38–70%):
- √ infiltrative tumor growth along cystic duct
- √ lymph node enlargement causing biliary obstruction
- √ intraductal tumor spread

√ fine granular / punctate flecks of calcification (mucinous adenocarcinoma)
√ lymph node enlargement in porta hepatis

N.B.: misdiagnosis by US / CT in 50%, especially in the presence of gallstones

Abdominal radiograph:
- √ calcified gallstones
- √ porcelain gallbladder
- √ RUQ gas collection (after invasion of adjacent bowel)

Cholangiography:
- √ malignant stricture / obstruction of extrahepatic bile ducts / right and left bile duct confluence, intrahepatic duct of right lobe
- √ intraluminal GB filling defect (= tumor / stones)
- √ mass displacing / invading gallbladder
- √ intraductal filling defects (= tumor / stones)

US:
- √ gallbladder replaced by mass with irregular margins + heterogenous echotexture (= tumor necrosis)
- √ immobile intraluminal well-defined round / oval mass
  - *DDx:* tumefactive sludge
- √ echogenic foci = coexisting gallstones / wall calcifications / tumoral calcification
- √ tumor inseparable from liver

CT:
- √ hypo- / isoattenuating mass in gallbladder fossa:
  - √ low-attenuation areas of necrosis
  - √ areas of enhancement (= viable tumor)
- √ subtle extension beyond wall of GB
- √ invasion of liver with protrusion of anterior surface of medial segment of left lobe

MR:
- √ hypointense mass on T1WI + ill-defined early contrast enhancement

Metastases: in 75–77% at time of diagnosis

(a) direct extension (most common mode): invasion of liver (34–65–89%), duodenum (12–15%), colon (9–15%), pancreas (6%), stomach, bile duct, right kidney, abdominal wall

Cause: thin GB wall with only a single muscle layer + no substantial lamina propria + perimuscular connective tissue continuous with interlobular connective tissue of liver

(b) lymphatic spread (26–41–75%): cystic, pericholedochal, celiac, superior mesenteric, foramen of Winslow, paraaortic nodes, superior + posterior pancreaticoduodenal

(c) intraperitoneal seeding (common)

(d) hematogenous spread (less common): liver, lung, bones, heart, pancreas, kidney, adrenal, brain

(e) neural spread (frequent): associated with more aggressive tumors

(f) intraductal spread (least common): particularly in papillary adenocarcinoma

Cx: perforation of gallbladder + abscess formation
- √ gallstones located within abscess

Prognosis: 75% unresectable at presentation; average survival is 6 months; 5% 1-year survival rate; 6% 5-year survival rate

DDx:
(1) Xanthogranulomatous cholecystitis (lobulated mass filling gallbladder + stones)
(2) Acute / chronic cholecystitis (generalized gallbladder wall thickening <10 mm)
(3) Liver tumor invading gallbladder fossa
(4) Tumors from adjacent organs (pancreas, duodenum)
(5) Metastases (melanoma, leukemia, lymphoma)
(6) Polyps: cholesterol polyp, hyperplastic polyp, granulation polyp
(7) Adenomyomatosis

GLYCOGEN STORAGE DISEASE

= autosomal recessive diseases with varying severity and clinical syndromes

A. VON GIERKE DISEASE (TYPE I)

Etiology: defect in glucose-6-phosphatase with excess deposition of glycogen in liver, kidney, intestines

Dx: failure of rise in blood glucose after glucagon administration

Age at presentation: infancy
√ hepatomegaly
US:
√ increased echogenicity (glycogen / fat)
CT:
√ increased (glycogen) / normal / decreased (fat) parenchymal attenuation
Prognosis: death in infancy, may survive into adulthood with early therapy
Cx: (1) Hepatic adenoma
(2) Hepatocellular carcinoma

B. POMPE DISEASE (TYPE II)
= abnormal metabolism with enlargement of myocardial cells due to glycogen deposition; similar to endocardial fibroelastosis
Etiology: defect in lysosomal glucosidase
√ massive cardiomegaly with CHF
√ hepatomegaly
Prognosis: sudden death in 1st year of life (due to conduction abnormalities); survival rarely beyond infancy

C. CORI DISEASE (TYPE III)
D. ANDERSEN DISEASE (TYPE IV)
E. McARDLE DISEASE (TYPE V)
F. HERS DISEASE (TYPE VI)

HEMOCHROMATOSIS

= excess iron deposition in various parenchymal organs (liver, pancreas, spleen, kidneys, heart) leading to cirrhosis with portal hypertension
Cause: excess iron deposition from
(a) increased GI absorption:
1. Genetic hemochromatosis
2. Erythropoietic hemochromatosis
3. Bantu siderosis
(b) IV blood transfusion
(c) intravascular (extrasplenic) hemolysis

CT (60% sensitivity for iron):
√ diffuse / rarely focal increase in liver density (up to 75–130 HU)
√ depiction of portal + hepatic veins against background of hyperattenuating liver on NECT
√ dual energy CT (at 80 + 120 kVp) can quantitate amount of iron deposition

Genetic Hemochromatosis

= IDIOPATHIC / PRIMARY HEMOCHROMATOSIS
= excessive absorption + parenchymal retention of dietary iron that favors accumulation within non-RES organs (liver, pancreas, heart, pituitary gland)
Cause: autosomal recessive disorder (human-leukocyte antigen [HLA]-linked abnormal gene located on short arm of chromosome 6) with mucosal defect in intestinal wall / increased absorption of intestinal iron
Prevalence: 1:220 whites of northern European ancestry; homozygote frequency up to 0.25–0.50%; heterozygote carriers >10%
Pathophysiology:
absorbed iron is selectively bound to transferrin; increased transferrin saturation in portal circulation favors selective iron uptake by periportal hepatocytes as initial site of iron accumulation; RES cells are incapable of storing excess iron
Path: excess iron stored as crystalline iron oxide (ferric oxyhydroxide) within cytoplasmic ferritin + lysosomal hemosiderin; iron overload affects parenchymal cells (liver, pancreas, heart) NOT Kupffer cells / RE cells of bone marrow + spleen (abnormal function of RES)

- asymptomatic during 1st decade of disease
- hyperpigmentation (90%)
- hepatomegaly (90%)
- arthralgias (50%)
- diabetes mellitus (30%) secondary to insulin resistance by hepatocytes + pancreatic β-cell damage from iron deposition
- CHF + arrhythmia (15%)
- loss of libido, impotence, amenorrhea, testicular atrophy, loss of body hair
- liver iron index > 2 (= liver iron concentration [micromoles per gram of dry weight] per patient's age)

MR:
(skeletal muscle = good signal intensity reference)
√ significant signal loss in liver on T2WI with signal intensity equal to background noise (paramagnetic susceptibility of ferritin + ferric ions leads to profound shortening of T1 + T2 relaxation times of adjacent protons)
√ normal pancreatic signal intensity in noncirrhotics
√ pancreatic signal intensity equal to / less than muscle (in 90% of cirrhotic patients)
√ normal signal intensity of spleen (in 86%) due to abnormal RES function

Dx: liver biopsy
Cx: (1) Periportal fibrosis resulting in cirrhosis (if iron concentration >22,000 μg/g of liver tissue)
(2) Hepatocellular carcinoma (14–30%)
(3) Insulin-dependent diabetes mellitus (30–60%)
(4) Congestive cardiomyopathy (15%)
Rx: phlebotomies in precirrhotic stage
Prognosis: normal life expectancy with early diagnosis and treatment

Secondary Hemochromatosis

[= HEMOSIDEROSIS = increased iron deposition without organ damage]
Cause:
(1) Erythrogenic hemochromatosis = increased absorption of iron secondary to erythroid hyperplasia in ineffective erythropoiesis (eg, thalassemia, NOT in sickle cell anemia)
Path: no excess Kupffer cell iron
(2) Bantu siderosis = excessive dietary iron from food preparation in iron containers (Kaffir beer)
(3) Transfusional iron overload = patients receiving >40 units of blood (iron storage capacity of RES = 10 g of iron)

Path: iron deposition initially in RES (phagocytosis of intact RBC) with sparing of parenchymal cells of pancreas; after saturation of RES storage capacity parenchymal cells of other organs accumulate iron (liver, pancreas, myocardium)

Age: 4th–5th decade; M:F = 10:1

• little clinical significance

MR:

√ signal loss in liver on T2WI with signal intensity greater than background noise (iron in Kupffer cells with sparing of parenchymal liver cells)
√ splenic signal intensity less than muscle
√ low signal intensity of bone marrow

HEPATIC ABSCESS

= localized collection of pus in the liver resulting from any infectious process with destruction of the hepatic parenchyma + stroma

Types: pyogenic (85%), fungal (9%), amebic (6%)

Location: multiple in 50%

◊ A pyogenic abscess tends to be centrally located, an amebic abscess peripherally!

√ hepatomegaly
√ elevation of right hemidiaphragm
√ pleural effusion
√ right lower lobe atelectasis / infiltration
√ gas within abscess (esp. Klebsiella)

MR:

√ hypointense on T1WI + hyperintense on T2WI (72%)
√ perilesional edema (35%)
√ "double target sign" on T2WI = hyperintense center (fluid) + hypointense sharply marginated inner ring (abscess wall) + hyperintense poorly marginated ring (perilesional edema)
√ rim enhancement (86%)

Amebic Abscess

Organism: Entamoeba histolytica

Etiology: spread of viable amebae from colon to liver via portal system

Incidence: in 1–25% of intestinal amebiasis

Age: 3rd–5th decade; M:F = 4:1

• amebic dysentery
• amebic hepatitis (15%)

Location: liver abscess (right lobe) in 2–25%; systemic dissemination by invasion of lymphatics / portal system (rare); liver:lung:brain = 100:10:1

Size: 2–12 cm; multiple liver abscesses in 25%

√ nonspecific variable appearance
√ nodularity of abscess wall (60%)
√ internal septations (30%)
√ not gas-containing (unless hepatobronchial / hepatoenteric fistula present)
√ ± disruption of diaphragm

CT:

√ nonspecific hypoattenuating area
√ enhancing wall

US:

√ homogeneous hypoechoic area
√ posterior acoustic enhancement
√ well-defined smooth thin wall

NUC:

√ sensitivity of sulfur colloid scan is 98%
√ photon-deficient area surrounded by rim of uptake on Ga-67 scan

Aspiration:

typically opaque reddish / dirty brown / pink material ("anchovy paste" / "chocolate sauce"), usually sterile, parasite confined to margin of abscess

Cx: (1) Diaphragmatic disruption (rare) is strongly suggestive of amebic abscess
(2) Fistulization into colon, right adrenal gland, bile ducts, pericardium

Rx: conservative treatment with chloroquine / metronidazole (Flagyl®); percutaneous drainage for left hepatic abscess (spontaneous rupture into pericardium + tamponade possible)

Prognosis: resolution under therapy may take from 1 month to 2 years; permanent cysts may remain behind

Pyogenic Liver Abscess

◊ Most common type of liver abscess

Organisms: E. coli, aerobic streptococci, St. aureus, anaerobic bacteria (45%)

Incidence: 0.016%

Etiology: (1) Ascending cholangitis from obstructive biliary tract disease (malignant / benign)
(2) Portal phlebitis (suppurative appendicitis, colitis, diverticular disease)
(3) Infarction from sickle cell / embolism / postembolization / septicemia
(4) Indwelling arterial catheters
(5) Direct spread from contiguous infection (cholecystitis, peptic ulcer, subphrenic sepsis)
(6) Trauma (rupture, penetrating wounds, biopsy, surgery)
(7) Cryptogenic in 45% (invasion of cysts / dead tissue by pyogenic intestinal flora)

Age: 6th–7th decade; M > F

• pyrexia (79%)
• abdominal pain (68%)
• nocturnal sweating (43%)
• vomiting / malaise (39%)
• jaundice (0–20%)
• positive blood culture (50%)

Location: solitary abscess in right lobe (40–75%), in left lobe (2–10%); multiple abscesses in 10–34–73% (more often of biliary than hematogenous origin)

US:

√ hypoechoic round lesion with well-defined mildly echogenic rim
√ posterior acoustic enhancement
√ coarse clumpy debris / low-level echoes / fluid-debris level

√ intensely echogenic reflections with reverberations (from gas) in 20–30%

CT:
√ inhomogeneous hypoattenuating (0–45 HU) single / multiloculated cavity
√ "double target sign" = wall-enhancement + surrounding hypodense zone (6–30%)
√ "cluster sign" = several abnormal foci within the same anatomic area; suggestive of biliary origin
√ air density

MR:
√ decreased T1 signal + increased T2 signal
√ enhancement of peripheral rim

NUC:
√ photon-deficient area on sulfur colloid + IDA scan
√ Ga-67 citrate uptake in 80%
√ In-111 tagged WBC uptake is highly specific (since WBCs normally go to liver, may need sulfur colloid test for correlation)

Cx: (1) Septicemia
(2) Rupture into right subphrenic space
(3) Rupture into abdominal cavity
(4) Rupture into pericardium
(5) Empyema
(6) Common hepatic duct obstruction

Mortality: 20–80%; 100% if unrecognized / untreated

HEPATIC ADENOMA

= HEPATOCELLULAR ADENOMA = LIVER CELL ADENOMA

◊ The most frequent hepatic tumor in young women after use of contraceptive steroids!

Prevalence: half as common as FNH

Path: pseudocapsule due to compression of liver tissue containing multiple large vessels; high incidence of hemorrhage + necrosis + fatty change; no scar

Histo: solitary spherical benign growth of hepatocytes; sheets of hepatocytes without portal veins or central veins; scattered thin-walled vascular channels + bile canaliculi; decrease in number of abnormally functioning Kupffer cells; hepatocytes contain increased amounts of glycogen ± fat

Age: young women in childbearing age; not seen in males unless on anabolic steroids; rare in children

Associated with: oral contraceptives (2.5 x risk after 5-year use, 7.5 x risk after 9-year use, 25 x risk >9-year use), steroids, pregnancy, diabetes mellitus, type Ia glycogen storage disease (von Gierke) in 60%, Fanconi anemia

◊ Pregnancy may increase tumor growth rate + lead to tumor rupture!

◊ Tumor regression may occur with dietary therapy leading to normal insulin, glucagon, and serum glucose levels

- asymptomatic (20%)
- RUQ pain as sign of mass effect (40%) / intratumoral or intraperitoneal hemorrhage (40%)
- hepatomegaly

Location: right lobe of liver in subcapsular location (75%)

Size: between 6 and 30 cm in size (average size of 8–10 cm)

√ round well-circumscribed pseudo-encapsulated mass
√ intraparenchymal / pedunculated (in 10%)
√ unusual "nodule-in-nodule" appearance in large tumors (DDx: hepatocellular carcinoma)
√ occasional eccentric dystrophic calcifications

CT:
√ round mass of decreased density; areas of necrosis (30–40%)
√ hyperdense areas of fresh intratumoral hemorrhage (22–50%)

CECT:
√ transient enhancement on arterial-phase images (due to supply by hepatic artery)
√ iso- / hypoattenuating on delayed-phase images

US:
√ usually small well-demarcated solid heterogeneous mass of variable echogenicity (echogenic / complex hyper- and hypoechoic):
√ hyperechoic lesion with well-defined hypoechoic rim
√ anechoic cystic areas if large

MR:
√ inhomogeneous on all pulse sequences (indistinguishable from HCC)
√ often hyperintense areas on T1WI (due to presence of fat-laden hepatocytes / hemorrhage)
√ isointense (sheets of hepatocytes) and hyperintense areas (necrosis, hemorrhage) on T2WI

NUC:
√ focal photopenic lesion on sulfur colloid scan (because lesion composed of hepatocytes + nonfunctioning Kupffer cells) surrounded by rim of increased uptake (due to compression of adjacent normal liver containing Kupffer cells); may show uptake equal to / slightly less than liver (23%)
√ usually increased activity on HIDA scan
√ NO gallium uptake

Angio:
√ usually hypervascular mass
√ homogeneous but not intense stain in capillary phase
√ enlarged hepatic artery with feeders at tumor periphery (50%)
√ hypo- / avascular regions (secondary to hemorrhage / necrosis)
√ neovascularity

CAVE: percutaneous biopsy carries high risk of bleeding!

Cx: (1) Spontaneous hemorrhage with subcapsular hematoma / hemoperitoneum (41%)
(2) Malignant transformation (? contiguous development of hepatocellular carcinoma)
(3) Recurrence after resection

Rx: surgical resection (to prevent rupture)

DDx: FNH, hemangioma, hepatocellular carcinoma

HEPATIC ANGIOMYOLIPOMA

= rare benign mesenchymal tumor

Associated with: tuberous sclerosis

Histo: smooth muscle cells, fat, proliferating blood vessels

• asymptomatic
√ intratumoral fat is DIAGNOSTIC
√ soft-tissue component may enhance
Cx: intratumoral hemorrhage

HEPATIC ANGIOSARCOMA

= HEMANGIOENDOTHELIAL SARCOMA = KUPFFER CELL SARCOMA = HEMANGIOSARCOMA

Prevalence: 0.14–0.25 per million; <2% of all primary liver neoplasms; most common sarcoma of liver (followed by fibrosarcoma > malignant fibrohistiocytoma > leiomyosarcoma)

Etiology: (a) thorotrast = thorium dioxide (7–10%) with latent period of 15–24 years
(b) arsenic
(c) polyvinyl chloride (latent period of 4–28 years)

Associated with: hemochromatosis, von Recklinghausen disease

Path: (a) multifocal / multinodular lesions (71%) of up to >5 cm in size
(b) large solitary mass with hemorrhage + necrosis

Histo:
(a) vessels lined with malignant endothelial cells (eg, sinusoids) causing atrophy of surrounding liver
(b) vasoformative = forming poorly organized vessels
(c) forming solid nodules of malignant spindle cells

Age: 6th–7th decade; M:F = 4:1

• abdominal pain, weakness, fatigue, weight loss
• spontaneous hemoperitoneum (27%)
• jaundice
• NO elevation of α-fetoprotein

Early metastases to:
lung, spleen (16%), porta hepatis nodes, portal vein, thyroid, peritoneal cavity, bone marrow (rapid metastatic spread)

√ portal vein invasion
√ hemorrhagic ascites

Plain film:
√ circumferential displacement of residual thorotrast

NUC:
√ single / multiple photopenic areas on sulfur colloid scan
√ increased gallium uptake
√ perfusion blood pool mismatch (initial decrease followed by slow increase in RBC concentration) as in hemangioma on 3-phase red blood cell scan

US:
√ solid / mixed mass with anechoic areas (hemorrhage / necrosis)
√ multiple nodules

CT:
√ hypodense masses with high-density regions (hemorrhage) / low-attenuation regions (old hemorrhage / necrosis)
√ striking peripheral enhancement on dynamic CT as in large hemangioma

MR:
√ hypointense on T1WI + hyperintense on T2WI
√ peripheral Gd-pentetate enhancement on T1WI

Angio:
√ hypervascular stain around tumor periphery in late arterial phase with puddling; NO arterial encasement

CAVE: Biopsy may lead to massive bleeding in 16%! Opt for open rather than percutaneous biopsy!

Prognosis: rapid deterioration with median survival of 6 months (13 months under chemotherapy)

DDx for multiple lesions: metastases
DDx for single lesion: cavernous hemangioma

HEPATIC CYST

◊ Second most common benign hepatic lesion after hemangioma

Prevalence: 2–7%; increasing with age; M < F

A. ACQUIRED HEPATIC CYST
secondary to trauma, inflammation, parasitic infestation, neoplasia

B. CONGENITAL HEPATIC CYST
= defective development of aberrant intrahepatic bile ducts; derived from bile duct hamartoma
Incidence: liver cysts detected at autopsy in 50%; in 22% detected during life
Age of detection: 5th–8th decade
Histo: cysts surrounded by fibrous capsule + lined by columnar epithelium, related to bile ducts within portal triads; no communication with bile ducts
Associated with:
(1) Tuberous sclerosis
(2) Polycystic kidney disease (25–33% have liver cysts)
(3) Polycystic liver disease: autosomal dominant; M:F = 1:2; (50% have polycystic kidney disease)

• hepatomegaly (40%); pain (33%); jaundice (9%)

Size of cyst: range from microscopic to huge (average 1.2 cm; in 25% largest cyst <1 cm; in 40% largest cyst >4 cm; maximal size of 20 cm); multiple cysts spread throughout liver (in 60%) / solitary cyst

√ unilocular simple cyst:
√ imperceptible wall
√ may show fluid-fluid interface
√ water attenuation (0–10 HU)
√ "cold spot" on IDA, Ga-68, Tc-99m sulfur colloid scans

Rx: sclerosing therapy with minocycline hydrochloride (Dose: 1 mg per 1-mL cyst content up to 500 mg in 10 mL of 0.9% saline + 10 mL 1% lidocaine) following contrast opacification of cyst to confirm absence of communication with biliary tree / leakage into peritoneal cavity

HEPATIC HEMANGIOMA

Cavernous Hemangioma of Liver

= most common benign liver tumor (78%); second most common liver tumor after metastases

Incidence: 1–4%; autopsy incidence 0.4–7.3%; increased with multiparity

LIVER

Cause: ? enlarging hamartoma present since birth, ? true vascular neoplasm
Age: rarely seen in young children; M:F = 1:5
Path: large vascular channels filled with slowly circulating blood; lined by single layer of mature flattened endothelial cells separated by thin fibrous septa; no bile ducts; thrombosis of vascular channels common resulting in fibrosis + hemorrhage + myxomatous degeneration + calcifications

Pathophysiology: large blood volume with low blood flow
Associated with: (1) Hemangiomas in other organs
(2) Focal nodular hyperplasia
(3) Rendu-Osler-Weber disease

- asymptomatic if tumor small (50–70%)
- may present with spontaneous life-threatening hemorrhage if large (5%)
- hepatomegaly
- may enlarge during pregnancy
- abdominal discomfort + pain (from thrombosis in large hemangioma)
- Kasabach-Merritt syndrome (= hemangioma + thrombocytopenia) rare

Location: frequently peripheral / subcapsular in posterior right lobe of liver; 20% are pedunculated; multiple in 10–20%
Size: <4 cm (90%);
>4–6–12 cm = **giant cavernous hemangioma**

√ blood supply from hepatic artery
√ may have central area of fibrosis = areas of nonenhancement / nonfilling / cystic space (occurrence increases with age)
√ central septal calcifications within areas of fibrosis / phleboliths (5–20%)

US:
√ uniformly hyperechoic (60–70%) mass due to multiple interfaces created by blood-filled spaces separated by fibrous septa
√ inhomogeneous hypoechoic mass (up to 40%) in larger hemangiomas with well-defined thick / thin echogenic lobulated border due to hemorrhagic necrosis, scarring, myxomatous change centrally
√ homogenous (58–73%) / heterogeneous (fibrosis, thrombosis, hemorrhagic necrosis)
√ hypoechoic center possible
√ may show acoustic enhancement (37–77%)
√ unchanged in size / appearance (82%) on 1–6-year follow-up
√ no Doppler signals / signals with peak velocity of <50 cm/sec

CT (combination of precontrast images, good bolus, dynamic scanning):
√ well-circumscribed spherical / ovoid low-density mass:
√ may have areas of higher / lower density within mass
√ typical pattern of low density on NECT + peripheral enhancement + complete fill-in on delayed images 3–30 minutes post IV bolus (55–89%):
√ peripheral (72%) / central (in 8%) / diffuse dense (in 8%) enhancement
√ complete (75%) / partial (24%) / no (2%) fill-in to isodensity in delayed phase
√ rapid contrast filling (16%), more often in small lesions (in 42% of hemangiomas <1 cm)
DDx: hypervascular tumor (do not remain hyperattenuating on delayed-phase images)
√ central scar may not enhance at any time

MR (90–95% accuracy):
√ spheroid / ovoid (87%) mass with smooth well-defined lobulated margins (87%); no capsule
√ homogeneous internal architecture if <4 cm, hypointense internal inhomogeneities if >4 cm (due to fibrosis)
√ T1WI: hypo- / isointense
√ T2WI: hyperintense "light bulb" appearance (due to slow flowing blood) increasing with echo time
(*DDx:* hepatic cyst, hyper-vascular tumor, necrotic tumor, cystic neoplasm)
√ same enhancement pattern as CT:
√ uniform enhancement at 1 second in 40% of small hemangiomas <1.5 cm after gadolinium-DTPA
√ peripheral nodular enhancement progressing centripetally with centrally uniform enhancement (50%) / persistent hypointensity (30%)
√ mildly hyperintense on T2WI for hyalinized hemangioma + lack of enhancement in early phase + slight peripheral enhancement in late phase (DDx: malignant hepatic tumor)

Angio (historical gold standard):
√ dense opacification of well-circumscribed, dilated, irregular, punctate vascular lakes / puddles in late arterial + capillary phase starting at periphery in ring- / C-shaped configuration
√ normal-sized feeders; AV shunting (very rare)
√ contrast persistence late into venous phase

NUC (95% accuracy with SPECT):
Indication: lesions >2 cm (detectable in 70–90%)
√ initially cold lesion on Tc-99m labeled RBC scans (dose of 15–20 mCi) with increased activity on delayed images at 1–2 hours
√ cold defect on sulfur colloid scans

Bx: may be biopsied safely provided normal liver is present between tumor + liver capsule
√ nonpulsatile blood (73%)
√ endothelial cells without malignancy (27%)

Prognosis: no growth when <4 cm in diameter; giant cavernous hemangiomas may enlarge
Cx (rare): (1) Spontaneous rupture (4.5%)
(2) Abscess formation
(3) Kasabach-Merritt syndrome (platelet sequestration)
DDx: hypervascular malignant neoplasm / metastasis (quick homogeneous filling during arterial phase of small hemangiomas)

Giant Hepatic Cavernous Hemangioma

= at least one dimension exceeding 8 cm (in literature no agreement on size)

Associated with: coexistent smaller <5 cm hemangioma in 13%

Histo: hemorrhage, thrombosis, extensive hyalinization, liquefaction, fibrosis; central cleft due to cystic degeneration / liquefaction

• RUQ pain / fullness; abdominal mass

US:
- √ heterogeneous mass

NECT:
- √ heterogeneous hypoattenuating mass with marked central areas of low attenuation

CECT:
- √ early peripheral globular enhancement
- √ incomplete filling of central portions

MR:
- √ sharply marginated hypointense mass with cleftlike area of lower intensity on T1WI
- √ markedly hyperintense cleftlike area with some hypointense internal septa inside a hyperintense mass on T2WI
- √ cleftlike area remains hypointense during enhancement

DDx: metastasis, hepatocellular carcinoma, cholangiocarcinoma, hepatic adenoma, FNH, focal fatty infiltration

Infantile Hemangioendothelioma of Liver

= INFANTILE HEPATIC HEMANGIOMA = CAPILLARY / CAVERNOUS HEMANGIOMA

◊ Most common benign hepatic tumor during first 6 months of life!

Histo: multiple anastomosing thick-walled vascular spaces similar to cavernous hemangioma lined by plump immature endothelial cells in single or (less often) multiple cell layers; areas of extramedullary hematopoiesis / thrombi; scattered bile ducts; involutional changes (infarction, hemorrhage, necrosis, scarring)

Classification:

(a) Hemangioendothelioma type 1 (more common): orderly proliferation of small blood vessels

(b) Hemangioendothelioma type 2: more aggressive histologic pattern
DDx: angiosarcoma

(c) Cavernous hemangioma: dilated vascular spaces lined by flat endothelial cells
◊ Relationship to adult cavernous hemangioma unknown!

Age at presentation: <6 months in 85%, during 1st month in 33%, >1 year in 5%; M:F = 1:1.4–1:2

• abdominal mass secondary to hepatomegaly

• cutaneous hemangiomas (9–45–87%) occur with multinodular form

• may present with high-output CHF secondary to AV shunts within tumor (8 –15–25%)

• **Kasabach-Merritt syndrome** (in 11%)
= hemorrhagic diathesis due to platelet sequestration by tumor / disseminated intravascular coagulation; characterized by an association of hemangioma, or hemangioendothelioma, or angiosarcoma with thrombocytopenia and purpura (secondary to increased systemic fibrinolysis)
Prognosis: fatal outcome in 20–30%

• hemolytic anemia

Size: several mm up to 20 cm (average size of 3 cm)

- √ diffuse involvement of entire liver, rarely focal
- √ single mass (50%) / multiple masses (50%)
- √ enlargement of celiac + hepatic arteries + proximal aorta
- √ rapid decrease in aortic caliber below celiac trunk
- √ enlarged hepatic veins (increased venous flow)

Plain film:
- √ fine speckled / fibrillary calcifications in 16–25% (DDx: hepatoblastoma, hamartoma, metastatic neuroblastoma)

US:
- √ heterogeneous predominantly hypoechoic / complex / hyperechoic lesion
- √ multiple sonolucent areas (= enlarging vascular channels secondary to initial rapid growth) (DDx: mesenchymal hamartoma):
  - √ vascular components demonstrated by color Duplex
- √ calcifications (in up to 50%)

OB-US:
- √ polyhydramnios + fetal hydrops

NECT:
- √ large well-defined hypoattenuating mass
- √ hemorrhage (not uncommon)
- √ calcifications (in up to 16%)

CECT (similar to cavernous hemangioma):
- √ early peripheral enhancement (72%)
- √ variable delayed central enhancement

MR:
- √ heterogeneous hypointense multinodular lesion on T1WI ± hyperintense areas of hemorrhage
- √ varying degrees of hyperintensity on T2WI (resembling adult hemangioma)
- √ decreasing signal intensity with fibrotic replacement on T2WI

NUC (sulfur colloid, tagged RBC):
- √ increased flow in viable portions of lesion during angiographic phase
- √ increased activity mixed with central photopenic areas (hemorrhage, necrosis, fibrosis) on delayed tagged RBC images
- √ photopenic defect on delayed sulfur colloid images

Angio:
- √ enlarged, tortuous feeding arteries and stretched intrahepatic vessels
- √ hypervascular tumor with inhomogeneous stain; clusters of small abnormal vessels
- √ pooling of contrast material in sinusoidal lakes with rapid clearing through early draining veins (AV shunting)

Prognosis: rapid growth in first 6 months followed by tendency to involute within 6–8 months; 32–75% survival rate in complicated cases

Cx: (1) Congestive heart failure
(2) Hemorrhagic diathesis
(3) Obstructive jaundice
(4) Hemoperitoneum (rupture of tumor)
(5) Malignant transformation into angiosarcoma (rare)

Rx: (1) No treatment if asymptomatic
(2) Reduction in size with steroids / radiotherapy / chemotherapy
(3) Embolization
(4) Surgical resection / liver transplantation

DDx: (1) Hepatoblastoma (>1 year of age, elevated α-fetoprotein, more heterogeneous)
(2) Mesenchymal hamartoma (usually multilocular cystic mass)
(3) Metastatic neuroblastoma (elevated catecholamines in urine, adrenal mass, nonenhancing multiple liver masses)

HEPATIC VENOOCCLUSIVE DISEASE

= occlusion of small centrilobular veins without involvement of major hepatic veins

Etiology: radiation and chemotherapy in bone-marrow transplant patients; bush tea (alkaloid) consumption in Jamaica

√ main hepatic veins + IVC normal
√ bidirectional / reversed portal venous flow
√ gallbladder wall thickening

HEPATITIS

Cause: alcohol, medication, viral infection, NASH (nonalcoholic steatohepatitis)

Acute Hepatitis

• markedly elevated AST + ALT
• increase in serum-conjugated bilirubin
√ hepatomegaly / normal size of liver
√ gallbladder wall thickening
√ lymphadenopathy

CT:
√ periportal low attenuation (lymph edema)

US:
√ diffuse decrease in liver echogenicity
√ increased brightness of portal triads ("starry sky" pattern) = centrilobular pattern due to edema in hepatocytes (DDx: leukemic infiltrate, diffuse lymphomatous involvement, toxic shock syndrome)
√ edema of gallbladder fossa + gallbladder wall thickening
√ thickening + increase in echogenicity of fat within falciform ligament, ligamentum venosum, porta hepatis, periportal connective tissue

Chronic Hepatitis

= process present for at least 6 months

Viral Markers of Hepatitis

Virus	*Tests*	*Interpretation*
HAV	Anti-HAV IgM	acute hepatitis (can remain positive for >1 year)
	Anti-HAV IgG	past hepatitis, lifelong immunity
HBV	HBsAg	acute / chronic disease
	Anti-HBc IgM	acute infection (if titer high); chronic infection (if titer low)
	Anti-HBc IgG	past / recent HBV contact (may be only serum indicator of past infection)
	HBe	active viral replication
	Anti-HBe	low / absent replicative state (typically present in long-standing HBV carriers)
	Anti-HBs	imunity after vaccination
	HBV-DNA	active viral replication
HCV	Anti-HCV	past / current infection
	RIBA	test for various viral components
	HCV-RNA	active viral replication
HDV	Anti-HDV IgM	acute / chronic infection
	Anti-HDV IgG	chronic infection (if titer high + IgM positive); past infection if titer low + IgM negative)
	HDV-RNA	active viral replication
HEV	Anti-HEV IgM	acute hepatitis
	Anti-HEV IgG	past hepatitis
	HEV-RNA	viral replication

Diseases: autoimmune hepatitis; hepatitis B, C, D; cryptic hepatitis; chronic drug hepatitis; primary biliary cirrhosis; primary sclerosing cholangitis; Wilson disease; alpha-1 antitrypsin deficiency

US:
√ increased liver echogenicity
√ coarsening of hepatic echotexture
√ silhouetting / loss of definition of portal venules = decreased visualization of the walls of the peripheral portal veins
√ NO sound attenuation

Cx: cirrhosis (10% for hepatitis B; 20–50% for hepatitis C)

Neonatal Hepatitis

Cause:
A. INFECTION: virus, protozoa, spirochete, toxoplasmosis, rubella, CMV, herpes, hepatitis A/ B, syphilis
B. METABOLIC: alpha-1 antitrypsin deficiency, familial recurrent cholestasis, errors of metabolism (nesidioblastosis = idiopathic hyperinsulin hypoglycemia of infancy)
C. IDIOPATHIC

Age: 1–4 weeks of age; M > F

Histo: multinucleated giant cells with hepatic parenchymal disruption, relatively little bile within bile duct canaliculi

US:
√ normal-sized / enlarged liver
√ increase in parenchymal echogenicity
√ decreased visualization of peripheral portal veins
√ normal bile duct system
√ gallbladder of normal size / small (with decrease in bile volume in severe hepatocellular dysfunction)
√ decrease in gallbladder size after milk feeding (DDx: congenital biliary atresia)

NUC:
Technique: often performed after pretreatment with phenobarbital (5 mg/kg x 5 days) to maximize hepatic function
√ normal / decreased hepatic tracer accumulation
√ prolonged clearance of tracer from blood pool
√ bowel activity faint / delayed usually by 24 hours (best seen on lateral view; covering liver activity with lead shielding is helpful)
√ gallbladder may not be visualized

Prognosis: spontaneous remission
DDx: biliary atresia (NO small bowel activity)

Radiation Hepatitis

Acute Radiation-induced Hepatitis

Time of onset: 2–6 weeks after completion of radiation therapy with dose >3,500 rad (35 Gy)
• abnormal liver function tests
• right upper quadrant discomfort
√ hepatomegaly
√ ascites

Prognosis: complete recovery in majority

Chronic Radiation-induced Hepatitis

√ increased attenuation in irradiated parenchyma (no fatty infiltration)
√ geographic areas of hypointensity on T1WI + hyperintensity on T2WI (due to increased water content)

HEPATOBLASTOMA

Incidence: 3rd most common abdominal tumor in children; most frequent malignant hepatic tumor in infants + children <3 years of age
Incidence increased with: hemihypertrophy, Beckwith syndrome
Histo: (a) epithelial type = small cells resembling embryonal / fetal liver
(b) mixed type = epithelial cells + mesenchymal cells (osteoid, cartilaginous, fibrous tissue)
Age: <3 years; <18 months (in 50%); peak age between 18 and 24 months; range from newborn to 15 years; M:F = 2:1
• upper abdominal mass, weight loss, nausea, vomiting
• jaundice, pain
• precocious puberty (production of endocrine substances)
• persistently + markedly elevated α-fetoprotein (66%)

Metastases to: lung (frequent)
Location: right lobe of the liver
√ usually solitary mass with an average size of 10–12 cm
√ multifocal (20%)
√ coarse calcifications / osseous matrix (12–30%)

US:
√ large heterogeneous echogenic mass, often with calcifications, occasionally cystic areas (necrosis / extramedullary hematopoiesis)

CT:
√ hypointense tumor with peripheral rim enhancement

MR:
√ inhomogeneously hypointense on T1WI with hyperintense foci (hemorrhage)
√ inhomogeneously hyperintense with hypointense bands (fibrous septa) on T2WI

NUC:
√ photopenic defect

Angio:
√ hypervascular mass with dense stain
√ marked neovascularity; NO AV-shunting
√ vascular lakes may be present
√ avascular areas (secondary to tumor necrosis)
√ may show caval involvement (= unresectable)

Prognosis: 60% resectable; 75% mortality; better prognosis than hepatoma; better prognosis for epithelial type than mixed type
DDx: hemangioendothelioma (fine granular calcifications), metastatic neuroblastoma, mesenchymal hamartoma, hepatocellular carcinoma (>5 years of age, no calcifications)

HEPATOCELLULAR CARCINOMA

= HEPATOMA
= most frequent primary visceral malignancy in the world; 80–90% of all primary liver malignancies; 2nd most frequent malignant hepatic tumor in children (39%) after hepatoblastoma

Incidence: (a) in industrialized world: 0.2–0.8%
(b) in sub-Saharan Africa, Southeast Asia, Japan, Greece, Italy: 5.5–20%
Peak age: (a) industrialized world: 6th–7th decade; M:F = 2.5:1; fibrolamellar subtype (in 3–10%) below age 40 years
(b) high incidence areas: 30–40 years; M:F = 5:1
(c) in children: >5 years of age (peak at 12–14 years); M:F = 4:3

Etiology:
1. Cirrhosis (60–90%)
Latent period: 8 months to 14 years from onset of cirrhosis
Incidence of HCC:
— 44% in macronodular (= postnecrotic) cirrhosis due to hepatitis B virus, alcoholism, hemochromatosis
— 6% in micronodular cirrhosis due to alcoholism
◊ 5% of alcoholic cirrhotics develop HCC!
(a) alcohol (c) cardiac
(b) hemochromatosis (d) biliary atresia

LIVER

2. Chronic hepatitis B / C: 12% develop HCC
3. Carcinogens
   (a) aflatoxin
   (b) siderosis
   (c) thorotrast
   (d) oral contraceptives / anabolic androgens
4. Inborn errors of metabolism
   (a) alpha-1 antitrypsin deficiency
   (b) galactosemia
   (c) type I glycogen storage disease (von Gierke)
   (d) Wilson disease
   (e) tyrosinosis

mnemonic: "WHAT causes HCC?"
Wilson disease
Hemochromatosis
Alpha-1-antitrypsin deficiency
Tyrosinosis
Hepatitis
Cirrhosis (alcoholic, biliary, cardiac)
Carcinogens (aflatoxin, sex hormones, thorotrast)

Path: soft tumor due to lack of stroma, often hemorrhagic + necrotic

Histo: HCC cells resemble hepatocytes in appearance + structural pattern (trabecular, pseudoglandular = acinar, compact, scirrhous);
(a) expansive encapsulated HCC: collapsed portal vein branches at capsule
(b) infiltrative nonencapsulated HCC: portal venules communicate with tumoral sinusoids = often invasion of portal ± hepatic veins

GROWTH PATTERN:
(a) solitary massive (27–50–59%):
bulk in one (most often right) lobe with satellite nodules
(b) multicentric small nodular (15–25%):
small foci of usually <2 cm (up to 5 cm) in both hepatic lobes
(c) diffuse microscopic (10–15–26%):
tiny indistinct nodules closely resembling cirrhosis

Vascular supply: hepatic artery, portal vein in 6%

- α-fetoprotein elevated in 75–90% (DDx: negative α-fetoprotein in cholangiocarcinoma)
- elevated liver function tests
- persistent RUQ pain, hepatomegaly, ascites
- fever, weight loss, malaise
- Paraneoplastic syndromes:
  (a) sexual precocity / gynecomastia
  (b) hypercholesterolemia
  (c) erythrocytosis (tumor produces erythropoietin)
  (d) hypoglycemia
  (e) hypercalcemia
  (f) carcinoid syndrome

Metastases to: lung (most common = 8%), adrenal, lymph nodes, bone

√ portal vein invasion (25–33–48%)
√ arterioportal shunting (4–63%)
√ invasion of hepatic vein (16%) / IVC (= Budd-Chiari syndrome)
√ occasionally invasion of bile ducts
√ calcifications in ordinary HCC (2–9–25%); however, common in fibrolamellar (30–40%) and sclerosing HCC
√ hepatomegaly and ascites
√ tumor fatty metamorphosis (2–17%)

CT (sensitivity of 63% in cirrhosis, 80% without cirrhosis):
√ hypodense mass / rarely isodense / hyperdense in fatty liver:
  √ dominant mass with satellite nodules
  √ mosaic pattern = multiple nodular areas with differing attenuation on CECT (up to 63%)
  √ diffusely infiltrating neoplasm
√ encapsulated HCC = circular zone of radiolucency surrounding the mass (12–32–67%)

False-positive: confluent fibrosis, regenerative nodule

Biphasic CECT:
√ enhancement during hepatic arterial phase (80%)
√ decreased attenuation during portal venous phase with inhomogeneous areas of contrast accumulation
√ isodensity on delayed scans (10%)
√ thin contrast-enhancing capsule (50%) due to rapid washout
√ wedge-shaped areas of decreased attenuation (segmental / lobar perfusion defects due portal vein occlusion by tumor thrombus)

CT with intraarterial ethiodol injection:
√ hyperdense mass detectable as small as 0.5 cm US (86–99% sensitivity, 90–93% specificity, 50–94% accuracy):
√ hyperechoic HCC (13%) due to fatty metamorphosis or marked dilatation of sinusoids
√ hypoechoic HCC (26%) due to solid tumor
√ HCC of mixed echogenicity (61%) due to nonliquefactive tumor necrosis
√ Doppler peak velocity signals >250 cm/sec

US:
√ variable echogenicity
√ calcifications (rare)

MR:
√ hypointense (50%) / iso- to hyperintense (with fatty metamorphosis) on T1WI
√ ring sign = well-defined hypointense capsule on T1WI (24–44%), double layer of inner hypointensity (fibrous tissue) + outer hyperintensity (compressed blood vessels + bile ducts) on T2WI in expansive type of HCC
√ mildly hyperintense on T2WI
√ Gd-DTPA enhancement peripherally (21%) / centrally (7%) / mixed (10%) / no enhancement (21%)
√ improved lesion detectability after intravenous administration of superparamagnetic iron oxide

NUC:
√ Sulfur colloid scan: single cold spot (70%), multiple defects (15–20%), heterogeneous distribution (10%)
√ Tc-HIDA scan: cold spot / atypical uptake in 4% (delayed images)
√ Gallium-scan: avid accumulation in 70–90% (in 63% greater, in 25% equal, in 12% less uptake than liver)

Angio:
√ "thread and streaks" = linear parallel vascular channels coursing along portal venous radicles seen with portal venous involvement
√ in differentiated HCC: enlarged arterial feeders, coarse neovascularity, vascular lakes, dense tumor stain, arterioportal shunts
√ in anaplastic HCC: vascular encasement, fine neovascularity, displacement of vessels + corkscrew-like vessels of cirrhosis

Prognosis: >90% overall mortality; 17% resectability rate; 6 months average survival time; 30% 5-year survival time

Cx: spontaneous rupture (in 8%)

Rx: (1) Resection
(2) I-131 antiferritin IgG (remission rate >40% up to 3 years)

DDx: hepatocarcinoma, cholangiocarcinoma, focal nodular hyperplasia, hemangioma, hepatic adenoma

Fibrolamellar Carcinoma of Liver

= uncommon variant of hepatocellular carcinoma

Prevalence: 1–9% of all HCCs; up to 35% of HCCs in patients <50 years of age

Age: 5–69 (mean 23) years; mostly 2nd–3rd decade; M:F = 1:1

Path: large well-circumscribed lobulated nonencapsulated strikingly desmoplastic tumor with calcifications + fibrous central scar

Histo: large hepatocyte-like cells with granular eosinophilic cytoplasm growing in sheets / cords / trabeculae separated by broad bands of fibrous stroma arranged in parallel lamellae resulting in compartmentalized appearance

Risk factors: NONE known; underlying cirrhosis or hepatitis in <5%

Demographics: less common in Europe; rare in Japan + China

- pain, cachexia; palpable RUQ mass, hepatomegaly
- gynecomastia (rare) from conversion of androgens to estrogens by tumor-elaborated enzyme aromatase
- jaundice (5%) from biliary compression
- α-fetoprotein usually negative / mildly elevated to <200 ng/μL (in up to 10%)
- transaminase levels <100 IU/L

√ partially / completely encapsulated solitary mass (in 80–90%):
  √ intrahepatic (80%) / pedunculated (20%)
  √ 5–20 (mean 13) cm in diameter
  √ prominent central fibrous scar (45–60%)
  √ capsular retraction (10%)
  √ punctate / nodular / stellate calcifications located within scar (33–55%)
  √ intratumoral hemorrhage + necrosis (10%)
  √ vascular invasion (<5%)
√ mass + small peripheral satellite lesions (10–15%)
√ diffuse multifocal masses (<1%)
√ regional adenopathy (50–70%): porta hepatis
√ distant metastases (20%): lung, peritoneal implants

US:
√ mixed echogenicity (60%)
√ central hyperechoic scar (33–60%)

CT:
√ mass of low attenuation
√ enhancement of non-scar portion:
  √ prominent heterogeneous enhancement in arterial + portal venous phase
  √ less pronounced enhancement during equilibrium phase
√ delayed enhancement of scar (25%)
+ pseudocapsule of compressed liver tissue (15%)

MRI:
√ large lobulated mass
  √ T1WI:
    √ hypointense (86%) / isointense (14%)
    √ homogeneous (80%) / heterogeneous (20%)
  √ T2WI:
    √ hyperintense / heterogeneous (85%)
    √ isointense / homogeneous (15%)
√ hypointense central scar on T1WI + T2WI

Angio:
√ dense tumor stain
√ enlarged feeding arteries
√ NO arteriovenous / arterioportal shunting
√ avascular central scar

NUC:
√ photopenic defect on sulfur colloid scan
√ increased activity during arterial phase + photopenic during delayed imaging on labeled RBC scan

Prognosis: 48% resectability rate; 32 months average survival time; 67% 5-year survival time

DDx: focal nodular hyperplasia (young + middle-aged women, <5 cm in size, calcifications uncommon, isointense to liver on all CT + MR images with pronounced homogeneous enhancement during arterial phase, hyperintense central scar on T2WI, uptake of sulfur colloid / super paramagnetic iron oxide)

HYPERPLASTIC CHOLECYSTOSIS

= variety of degenerative + proliferative changes of gallbladder wall characterized by hyperconcentration, hyperexcitability, and hyperexcretion

Incidence: 30–50% of all cholecystectomy specimens; M:F = 1:6

Adenomyomatosis of Gallbladder

= increase in number + height of mucosal folds

Histo: hyperplasia of epithelial + muscular elements with mucosal outpouching of epithelium-lined cystic spaces into (46%) or all the way through (30%) a thickened muscular layer as tubules / crypts / saccules (= intramural diverticula = Rokitansky-Aschoff sinus); develop with increasing age

Incidence: 5% of all cholecystectomies

Age: >35 years; M:F = 1:3

Associated with: (1) Gallstones in 25–75%
(2) Cholesterolosis in 33%

(a) generalized form = ADENOMYOMATOSIS
√ "pearl necklace gallbladder" = tiny extraluminal extensions of contrast on OCG (enhanced after contraction)
√ "comet-tail" = sound reverberation artifact between cholesterol crystals in Rokitansky-Aschoff sinuses (PATHOGNOMONIC)
(b) segmental form
compartmentalization most often in neck / distal 1/3
(c) localized form in fundus = ADENOMYOMA
√ smooth sessile mass in GB fundus
= solitary adenomyoma + extraluminal diverticula-like formation
(d) annular form
√ "hourglass" configuration of GB with transverse congenital septum

Cholesterolosis

= abnormal deposits of cholesterol esters in macrophages within lamina propria (foam cells) + in mucosal epithelium

1. STRAWBERRY GALLBLADDER
= LIPID CHOLECYSTITIS = CHOLESTEROSIS
= planar form = seedlike patchy / diffuse thickening of the villous surface pattern (disseminated micronodules)
Associated with: cholesterol stones in 50–70%
• not related to serum cholesterol level
√ radiologically not demonstrable
2. CHOLESTEROL POLYP (90%)
= polypoid form
= abnormal deposit of cholesterol ester producing a villouslike structure covered with a single layer of epithelium and attached via a delicate stalk
Prevalence: 4%; most common fixed filling defect of gallbladder
Location: commonly in middle 1/3 of gallbladder
√ multiple small filling defects <10 mm in diameter
DDx: papilloma, adenopapilloma, inflammatory granuloma

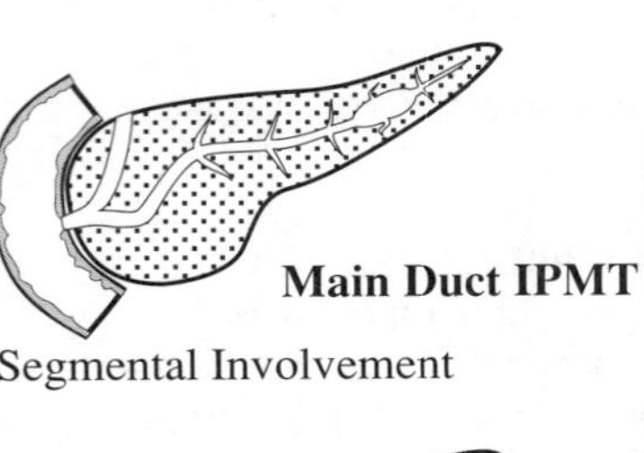
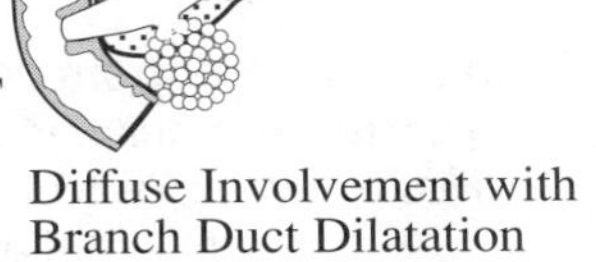

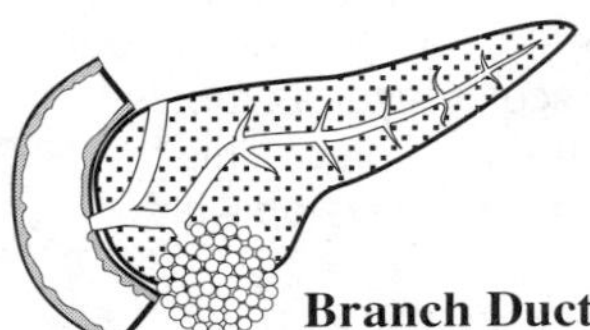
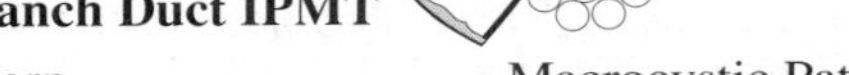

Intraductal Papillary Mucinous Tumor (IPMT)

INSPISSATED BILE SYNDROME

= uncommon cause of jaundice in neonate
Associated with: massive hemolysis (Rh incompatibility), hemorrhage (intraabdominal, intracranial, retroperitoneal), increased enterohepatic circulation (Hirschsprung disease, intestinal atresia, stenosis)

US:
√ sludge in gallbladder
√ sludge within bile ducts + partial / complete obstruction (affected ducts may blend with surrounding hepatic parenchyma)

INTRADUCTAL PAPILLARY MUCINOUS TUMOR OF PANCREAS

= IPMT = MUCINOUS DUCTAL ECTASIA = DUCTECTATIC MUCINOUS CYSTIC TUMOR OF PANCREAS
= INTRADUCTAL MUCIN-HYPERSECRETING NEOPLASM
= MUCIN-PRODUCING PANCREATIC TUMOR = MUCINOUS VILLOUS ADENOMATOSIS
= rare intraductal tumor originating from epithelial lining typified by voluminous mucin secretions

Path: conglomeration of communicating cysts covered by a rim of normal pancreatic parenchyma + thin fibrous capsule
Histo: cysts represent a dilated duct lined with innumerable papillae coated with hyperplastic / atypical / malignant epithelium (adenoma-carcinoma sequence)

• recurrent episodes of dull pain / acute pancreatitis (due to impaired outflow of pancreatic secretions)
• viscosity of fluid greater than normal serum (89% sensitive, 100% specific)

Prognosis: low-grade malignancy with better prognosis than pancreatic adenocarcinoma
Rx: Whipple operation (main duct IPMT / partial pancreatectomy (branch duct IPMT)
DDx: chronic obstructive pancreatitis, serous / mucinous cystic tumors, pseudocyst

Main Duct IPMT

Age: 57 (range, 34–75) years; M:F = 1:1
√ hyperechoic, hyperdense, T2-hypointense filling defect within dilated duct (= enhancing papillary mural nodule / gravity-dependent mucin glob)
√ dilatation of main pancreatic duct:
(a) dilatation of entire main pancreatic duct
√ homogeneous hypoechoic, hypodense, T1-hypointense and T2-hyperintense main duct
√ pancreatic parenchymal atrophy
√ dilatation of branch ducts (usually in pancreatic tail + uncinate process)
√ dilatation of major ± minor papilla bulging into duodenal lumen
√ ± obstruction of CBD (due to tumor / impacted mucin)
Cx: pancreato-biliary / -duodenal fistula, pseudomyxoma peritonei
DDx: chronic obstructive pancreatitis

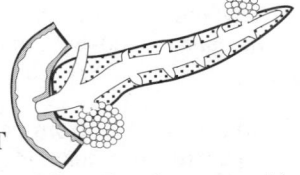

LIVER

(b) segmental dilatation of main pancreatic duct
√ cyst in pancreatic body / tail + normal remaining pancreatic parenchyma
√ cyst in pancreatic head + upstream dilatation of main pancreatic duct
DDx: peripheral mucinous cystic tumor (main duct almost always normal)

ERCP:
• thick jellylike mucus protruding from a bulging patulous duodenal papilla
√ plugging of the papilla of Vater
√ amorphous intraluminal filling defects in main pancreatic duct
√ usually small mural polypoid / flat tumor
√ dilated main + branch pancreatic ducts without obstructive ductal stricture
N.B.: reflux of contrast material due to excess of mucin / patent papillary orifice hinders filling of ductal tree

Branch Duct IPMT

Age: 63 (range, 37–76) years; M:F=1:1
• usually incidental finding when tumor small
• symptoms mimicking acute / chronic pancreatitis
Location: mainly in uncinate process >> pancreatic tail > pancreatic body
Path: macrocystic / microcystic pattern; malignancy suggested by irregular thick wall + septa and solid nodules
√ round / ovoid small lobulated intraductal mass (frequently not visualized):
√ dilated main pancreatic duct
√ normal main pancreatic duct (almost always normal in small tumor)
◊ Secretin administration distends ducts and enhances detection of communication with main pancreatic duct!
√ uni- / multilocular cyst 10-20 mm large with sparse septa
DDx: mucinous cystadenoma (no communication with main pancreatic duct); pseudocyst (no intraluminal filling defects)
√ multiple thin septa separating fluid-filled lacunae
DDx: serous cystadenoma (no communication with main pancreatic duct)
√ ± severe pancreatic atrophy
√ protrusion of papilla into duodenum

ERCP:
√ contrast spills from main duct into cystically dilated branch ducts
√ elongated band- / threadlike or nodular filling defects in dilated ducts (= depiction of mucin)
Cx: seeding to main pancreatic duct resulting in main duct IPMT

LIPOMA OF LIVER

Extremely rare
• asymptomatic
May be associated with: tuberous sclerosis
Size: few mm – 13 cm

US:
√ echogenic mass
√ striking acoustic refraction (sound velocity in soft tissue 1,540 m/sec, in fat 1,450 m/sec)
Prognosis: no malignant potential

LIVER TRANSPLANT

Indication:
– chronic viral hepatitis: chronic active hepatitis (4% in childhood)
– metabolic disease: alpha-1 antitrypsin deficiency (9% in childhood), hemochromatosis, Wilson disease
– cholestatic liver disease: primary biliary cirrhosis, primary sclerosing cholangitis, biliary atresia (52% in childhood)
– autoimmune hepatitis
– cryptogenic cirrhosis (6% in childhood)
– alcoholic liver disease
– acute fulminant hepatic failure (11% in childhood): viral hepatitis, drug-induced hepatitis (eg, by acetaminophen, isoniazid), hepatotoxins (eg, mushrooms)

Contraindications: AIDS, extrahepatic malignant tumors, active IVDA / alcohol abuse

NORMAL POSTTRANSPLANT FINDINGS
(1) Periportal edema (21%)
Cause: lymphedema in early posttransplantation period (= dilatation of lymphatic channels due to lack of normal lymphatic drainage)
√ "periportal collar" of low attenuation on CT + hyperechogenicity on US
√ resolution within weeks to months
(2) Fluid collection around falciform ligament (11%), at vascular anastomoses (liver hilum, IVC), biliary anastomosis, lesser sac
(3) Small right pleural effusion
(4) Peri- / subhepatic hematoma / free intraabdominal fluid

Vascular Complications in Liver Transplant (9%)

◊ Most frequent cause of graft loss
• liver failure, bile leak, abdominal bleeding, septicemia
1. Anastomotic narrowing of IVC / portal vein
◊ Discrepancies in caliber between donor + recipient vessel have no pathologic significance!
• venous hypertension of lower part of body
• portal hypertension
√ narrowing of portal vein + poststenotic dilatation
√ 3–4-fold velocity increase compared with prestenotic segment
2. Thrombosis / stenosis of portal vein (1–3%)
Cause: faulty surgical technique, vessel misalignment, differences in vessel caliber creating turbulent flow, hypercoagulable state, prior portal vein surgery, prior thrombosis in recipient portal vein

LIVER

- portal hypertension, liver failure, massive ascites, edema

√ filling defect / focal narrowing at anastamosis

Rx: percutaneous transluminal angioplasty ± stent placement, surgical thrombectomy, venous jump graft, creation of portosystemic shunt, retransplantation

3. Thrombosis / stenosis of IVC (<1%)
   - pleural effusions, hepatomegaly, ascites, extremity edema

   √ compression of IVC (due to swelling of graft)
   √ size discrepancy between donor + recipient IVC
4. Hepatic artery stenosis (5–13%)
   Location: at / near anastomotic site
   Time of onset: within 3 months
   √ marked focal increase in velocity >200–300 cm/sec + poststenotic turbulence (in >50% stenosis)
   √ intrahepatic tardus et parvus waveform = slowed systolic acceleration time (SAT >0.08 sec) distal to stenosis (73% sensitive)
   √ diminished pulsatility (RI <0.5) due to ischemia
   DDx: normal in early post-transplantation period
   √ biliary dilatation (due to stricture), infarction, biloma
   Rx: revascularization surgery, balloon angioplasty
5. Hepatic artery thrombosis (3–9–16% in adults, 9–19–42% in children)
   Risk factors: significant caliber difference between donor + recipient artery, preexisting celiac artery stenosis, prolonged cold ischemia of donor liver, ABO blood type incompatibility, rejection
   Time of onset: usually within first 2 months
   - Three types of clinical presentation:
     (1) fulminant hepatic necrosis + rapid deterioration
     (2) bile leak, bile peritonitis, bacteremia, sepsis
     (3) relapsing bacteremia

   √ absence of hepatic artery flow
   False-positive Doppler (10%):
   low flow state, small vessel size, severe liver edema (in first 72 hours after transplantation, viral hepatitis, rejection)
   False-negative Doppler: arterial collaterals
   √ multiple hypoechoic lesions in liver periphery (= infarcts)
   Mortality: 27–58%
6. Hepatic artery pseudoaneurysm (uncommon)
   Location: at vascular anastomosis
   Cx: massive intraperitoneal hemorrhage, portal vein fistula, biliary fistula
   Rx: surgical resection, embolization, exclusion by stent placement

Parenchymal Complications in Liver Transplant

1. Rejection
   ◊ Can ONLY be diagnosed with liver biopsy!
2. Infarction (10%)
   √ may calcify
   √ may liquefy developing into intrahepatic biloma
3. Graft infection

Biliary Complications in Liver Transplant (6–34%)

◊ Second most common cause of liver dysfunction after rejection

Time of onset: within first 3 months

1. Biliary obstruction
   (a) anastomotic stricture (extrahepatic)
   Cause: iatrogenic trauma resulting in ischemia + scar formation
   (b) nonanastomotic (intrahepatic) stricture
   Cause: hepatic arterial thrombosis / stenosis (in 50%), prolonged preservation time, bacterial / viral cholangitis, rejection, recurrent primary sclerosing cholangitis, cholangiocarcinoma, kinking of redundant CBD, sphincter of Oddi dysfunction
   (c) tension mucocele of allograft cystic duct remnant
   Cause: ligation of cystic duct proximally + distally
   √ extrinsic mass compressing CHD
   √ fluid collection adjacent to CHD
   Cx: ascending cholangitis
2. Bile leak
   (a) T-tube exit site: 50% within 10 days
   (b) anastomotic site of choledochocholedochostomy: 70% within 1st month
   (c) bile duct necrosis (hepatic artery occlusion)
   ◊ The intrahepatic biliary epithelium is perfused solely by the hepatic artery!
   (d) after liver biopsy
   (e) common hepatic duct leak
   Incidence: 4.3–23%
3. Stone / sludge formation
   Cause: alteration in bile composition

LYMPHOMA OF LIVER

A. PRIMARY LYMPHOMA (rare)
   √ solid solitary mass
B. SECONDARY LYMPHOMA (common)
   autoptic incidence of liver involvement:
   60% in Hodgkin disease
   50% in non-Hodgkin lymphoma

Pattern:
(a) infiltrative diffuse (most common): no alteration in hepatic architecture
(b) focal nodular: detectable by cross-sectional imaging
(c) combination of diffuse + nodular (3%)

Detection rate (for CT, MRI): <10%

MACROCYSTIC ADENOMA OF PANCREAS

= MUCINOUS CYSTIC NEOPLASM = MUCINOUS CYSTADENOMA / CYSTADENOCARCINOMA

= thick-walled uni- / multilocular low-grade malignant tumor composed of large mucin-containing cystic spaces

Frequency: 10% of pancreatic cysts; 1% of pancreatic neoplasms

Mean age: 50 years (range of 20–95 years); in 50% between 40–60 years;
M:F = 1:19

Path: large smooth round / lobulated multiloculated cystic mass encapsulated by a layer of fibrous connective tissue

Histo: similar to biliary and ovarian mucinous tumors; cysts lined by tall columnar, mucin-producing cells subtended by a densely cellular mesenchymal stroma (reminiscent of ovarian stroma), often in papillary arrangement, lack of cellular glycogen

(a) mucinous cystadenoma

(b) mucinous cystadenocarcinoma = stratified papillary epithelium

◊ All mucinous cystic neoplasms should be considered as malignant neoplasms of low-grade malignant potential

Location: often in pancreatic tail (90%) / body, infrequently in head

- asymptomatic
- abdominal pain, anorexia

√ well-demarcated thick-walled mass of 2–36 (mean 10–12) cm in diameter

√ multi- / unilocular large cysts >2 cm with thin septa <2 mm:

◊ A tumor with <6 cysts of >2 cm in diameter is in 93–95% a mucinous cystic neoplasm!

√ solid papillary excrescences protrude into the interior of tumor (sign of malignancy)

√ amorphous discontinuous peripheral mural calcifications (10–15%)

√ hypovascular mass with sparse neovascularity

√ vascular encasement and splenic vein occlusion may be present

√ great propensity for invasion of adjacent organs

US:

√ cysts may contain low-level echoes

CT:

√ internal septations may not be visualized without contrast enhancement

√ cysts with attenuation values of water; may have different levels of attenuation within different cystic cavities

√ enhancement of cyst walls

Angio:

√ predominantly avascular mass

√ cyst wall + solid components may demonstrate small areas of vascular blush + neovascularity

√ displacement of surrounding arteries + veins by cysts

Metastases:

√ round thick-walled cystic lesions in liver

Prognosis: invariable transformation into cystadenocarcinoma

Rx: complete surgical excision (5-year survival rate of 74–90%)

DDx:

(1) Pseudocyst: inflammatory changes in peripancreatic fat, pancreatic calcifications, temporal evolution, history of alcoholism, elevated levels of amylase

(2) Lymphangioma / hemangioma

(3) Variants of ductal adenocarcinoma:

(a) mucinous colloid adenocarcinoma / ductectatic mucinous tumor of pancreas = mucin-hypersecreting carcinoma

(b) papillary intraductal adenocarcinoma

(c) adenosquamous carcinoma: squamous component predisposes to necrosis + cystic degeneration

(d) anaplastic adenocarcinoma: lymphadenopathy + metastases at time of presentation

(4) Solid and cystic papillary epithelioid neoplasm: hemorrhagic cystic changes in 20%

(5) Cystic islet cell tumor: hypervascular component

(6) Cystic metastases: history of malignant disease

(7) Atypical serous cystadenoma: smaller tumor with greater number of smaller cysts

(8) Sarcoma

(9) Infection: amebiasis, Echinococcus multilocularis

MESENCHYMAL HAMARTOMA OF LIVER

= rare developmental cystic liver tumor

Histo: disordered arrangement of primitive fluid-filled mesenchyme, bile ducts, hepatic parenchyma; stromal / cystic predominance with cysts of a few mm up to 14 cm in size; no capsule

Age peak: 15–24 months (range from newborn to 19 years); M:F = 2:1

- slow progressive abdominal enlargement
- ± respiratory distress and lower extremity edema

Location: right lobe:left lobe = 6:1; 20% pedunculated

Size: 5–29 (mean 16) cm

√ grossly discernible cysts in 80%

US:

√ multiple rounded cystic areas on an echogenic background

√ may appear solid in younger infant (when cysts are still small)

CT:

√ multiple lucencies of variable size + attenuation (depending on composition of stromal versus cystic elements)

√ hemorrhage (rare)

√ enhancement of stromal component

MR:

√ varying signal intensity (varying concentrations of protein in cystic predominance type) / hypointense on T1WI (mesenchymal predominance type)

√ marked hyperintensity of cystic locules / hypointense fibrosis on T2WI

NUC:

√ one / more areas of diminished uptake on sulfur colloid scan

Angio:

√ hypovascular mass

√ may show patchy areas of neovascularity

√ enlarged irregular tortuous feeding vessels

METASTASES TO GALLBLADDER

Organ of origin:
melanoma, renal cell carcinoma (late in course of disease), lymphoma (in AIDS), malignant fibrous histiocytoma
– in children: embryonal cell sarcoma, rhabdomyosarcoma

METASTASES TO LIVER

◊ Most common malignant lesion of the liver

Incidence: the liver is the most common metastatic site after regional lymph nodes; incidence of metastatic carcinoma is 20 x greater than primary carcinoma; metastases represent 22% of all liver tumors in patients with known malignancy

Organ of origin: colon (42%), stomach (23%), pancreas (21%), breast (14%), lung (13%)

√ involvement of liver + spleen typical in leukemia/ lymphoma + melanoma

IN CHILDREN: neuroblastoma, Wilms tumor

- hepatomegaly (70%)
- abnormal liver enzymes (50–75%)

Location: both lobes (77%), right lobe (20%), left lobe (3%)
Number: multiple (50–98%), solitary (2%)
Size: >33% smaller than 2 cm

Enhancement characteristics compared with normal liver:

√ lesion enhancement during arterial phase (metastases are supplied by hepatic artery)
√ less enhancement during portal venous phase (metastases have a negligible portal venous supply)
√ extracellular space agents accumulate more in tumor tissue (metastases have a larger interstitial space)

NUC: 80–95% sensitivity in lesions >1.5 cm; lesions <1.5 cm are frequently missed; sensitivity increases with metastatic deposit size, peripheral location, and use of SPECT

NECT: important for hypervascular tumors (eg, renal cell carcinoma, carcinoid, islet cell tumors), which may be obscured by CECT

CECT:

Technique:
optimal is bolus technique with dynamic incremental scanning; sensitivity is decreased relative to NCCT if scans are obtained during equilibrium phase of contrast administration

√ circumferential bead- or bandlike enhancement during arterial phase + peripheral washout on delayed images
√ no (35%), peripheral (37%), mixed (20%), central (8%) enhancement
√ complete isodense fill-in on delayed scans in 5% (DDx: hemangioma)

◊ CT-sensitivity 88–90%; specificity 99%; lesions of approx. 1 cm can usually be detected!

CT-Angiography (most sensitive imaging modality):

Indication: patients with potentially resectable isolated liver metastases / preoperative to partial hepatectomy for detection of additional metastases (additional lesions detected in 40–55%)

(1) CT arteriography = angiography catheter in hepatic artery, detects lesions by virtue of increased enhancement
(2) CT arterial portography = angiography catheter in SMA, detects hypodense lesions on a background of increased enhancement of normal surroundings in portal venous phase

CT-delayed iodine scanning:
= CT performed 4–6 hours following administration of 60 mg iodine results in detection of additional lesions in 27%

Rx: Exclusion criteria for metastasectomy:
(1) advanced stage of primary tumor
(2) >4 metastases
(3) extrahepatic disease
(4) <30% normal liver tissue / function available after resection

Calcified Liver Metastases

Incidence: 2–3%

1. Mucinous carcinoma of GI tract (colon, rectum, stomach)
2. Endocrine pancreatic carcinoma
3. Leiomyosarcoma, osteosarcoma
4. Malignant melanoma
5. Papillary serous ovarian cystadenocarcinoma
6. Lymphoma
7. Pleural mesothelioma
8. Neuroblastoma
9. Breast cancer
10. Medullary carcinoma of the thyroid
11. Renal cell carcinoma
12. Lung carcinoma
13. Testicular carcinoma

mnemonic for mucinous adenocarcinoma: "COBS"
Colon carcinoma
Ovarian carcinoma
Breast carcinoma
Stomach carcinoma

Hypervascular Liver Metastases

1. Renal cell carcinoma
2. Carcinoid tumor
3. Pancreatic islet cell tumor
4. Melanoma
5. Thyroid cancer
6. Choriocarcinoma
7. Ovarian cystadenocarcinoma
8. Sarcomas
9. Pheochromocytoma

mnemonic: "CHIMP"
Carcinoid
Hypernephroma
Islet cell carcinoma
Melanoma
Pheochromocytoma

Hypovascular Liver Metastases

1. Stomach
2. Colon
3. Pancreas
4. Lung
5. Breast

Hemorrhagic Liver Metastases

mnemonic: "CT BeComes MR"

Colon carcinoma
Thyroid carcinoma
Breast carcinoma
Choriocarcinoma
Melanoma
Renal cell carcinoma

Echogenic Liver Metastases

Incidence: 25%

1. Colonic carcinoma (mucinous adenocarcinoma) 54%
2. Hepatoma 25%
3. Treated breast carcinoma 21%

Liver Metastases of Mixed Echogenicity

Incidence: 37.5%

1. Breast cancer 31%
2. Rectal cancer 20%
3. Lung cancer 17%
4. Stomach cancer 14%
5. Anaplastic cancer 11%
6. Cervical cancer 5%
7. Carcinoid 1%

Cystic Liver Metastases

1. Mucinous ovarian carcinoma
2. Colonic carcinoma
3. Sarcoma
4. Melanoma
5. Lung carcinoma
6. Carcinoid tumor

mnemonic: "LC GOES"

Leiomyosarcoma (and other sarcomas)
Choriocarcinoma
Gastric carcinoma
Ovarian carcinoma
Endometrial carcinoma
Small cell carcinoma

Echopenic Liver Metastases

Incidence: 37.5%

1. Lymphoma 44%
2. Pancreas 36%
3. Cervical cancer 20%
4. Lung (adenocarcinoma)
5. Nasopharyngeal cancer

METASTASES TO PANCREAS

Frequency: 3–10% (autopsy)

Organ of origin: renal cell carcinoma (30%), bronchogenic carcinoma (23%), breast carcinoma (12%), soft-tissue sarcoma (8%), colonic carcinoma (6%), melanoma (6%)

√ solitary (78%) / multiple (17%) ovoid masses with discrete smooth margins
√ diffuse pancreatic enlargement (5%)

CECT:
- √ heterogeneously (60%) / homogeneously (17%) hyperattenuating relative to pancreas
- √ hypoattenuating relative to pancreas (20%)
- √ isoattenuating relative to pancreas (5%)

Concomitant intraabdominal metastases to:
liver (36%), lymph nodes (30%), adrenal glands (30%)

DDx: ductal pancreatic adenocarcinoma (uniformly nonenhancing mass, encasement of vessels)

MICROCYSTIC ADENOMA OF PANCREAS

= SEROUS CYSTADENOMA = GLYCOGEN-RICH CYSTADENOMA
= benign lobulated neoplasm composed of innumerable small cysts (1–20 mm) containing proteinaceous fluid separated by thin connective tissue septa

Incidence: approximately 50% of all cystic pancreatic neoplasms

Histo: cyst walls lined by cuboidal / flat glycogen-rich epithelial cells derived from centroacinar cells of pancreas (DDx: lymphangioma), thin fibrous pseudocapsule

Age: 34–88 years; mean age 65 years; 82% over 60 years of age; M:F = 1:4

Associated with: von Hippel-Lindau syndrome

- pain, weight loss, jaundice
- palpable mass

Location: any part of pancreas affected, slight predominance for head

√ well-demarcated lobulated mass 1–25 (mean 5) cm in diameter with smooth / nodular contour
√ innumerable small <2 cm cysts; uncommonly few large cysts (in <5%) / cyst up to 8 cm in diameter
√ prominent central stellate scar (CHARACTERISTIC)
√ amorphous central calcifications (in 33% on plain film) in dystrophic area of stellate central scar ("sunburst")
√ pancreatic duct + CBD may be displaced, encased, or obstructed

US:
- √ solid predominantly echogenic mass with mixed hypoechoic + echogenic areas

CT:
- √ attenuation values close to water
- √ contrast enhancement

Angio:
- √ hypervascular mass with dilated feeding arteries, dense tumor blush, prominent draining veins, neovascularity, occasional AV shunting, NO vascular encasement

MR:
√ delayed enhancement of scar on contrast-enhanced FLASH images
Prognosis: no malignant potential
Rx: surgical excision / follow-up examinations

MILK OF CALCIUM BILE

= LIMY BILE = CALCIUM SOAP
= precipitation of particulate material with high concentration of calcium carbonate, calcium phosphate, calcium bilirubinate
Associated with: chronic cholecystitis + gallstone obstruction of cystic duct
√ diffuse opacification of GB lumen with dependent layering
√ usually functionless GB on oral cholecystogram
US:
√ intermediate features between sludge + gallstones

MIRIZZI SYNDROME

= extrinsic right-sided compression of common hepatic duct by large gallstone impacted in cystic duct / gallbladder neck / cystic duct remnant; accompanied by chronic inflammatory reaction
Frequently associated with: formation of fistula between gallbladder and common hepatic duct
• jaundice
√ cystic duct course usually parallel to CHD
√ normal CBD below level of impacted stone
√ TRIAD:
(1) gallstone impacted in GB neck
(2) dilatation of bile ducts above level of cystic duct
(3) smooth curved segmental stenosis of CHD
Cholangiography:
√ partial obstruction of CHD due to external compression on lateral side of duct / eroding stone
DDx: lymphadenopathy, neoplasm of GB / CHD

MULTIPLE BILE DUCT HAMARTOMA

= VON MEYENBURG COMPLEX
Incidence: 0.15–2.8% of autopsies
Etiology: failure of involution of embryonic bile ducts

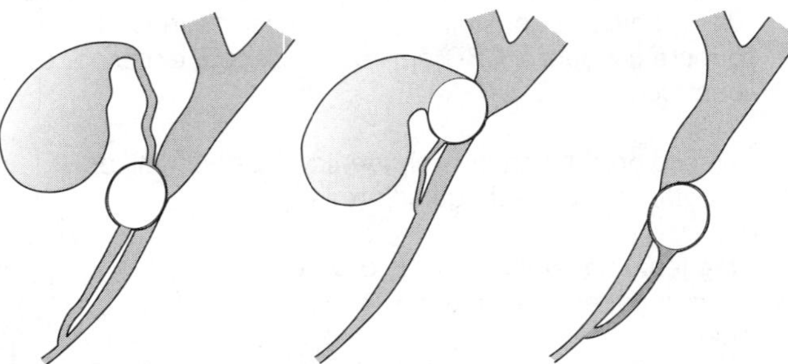

Mirizzi Syndrome

Histo: cluster of proliferated bile ducts lined by single layer of cuboidal cells embedded in fibrocollagenous tissue with single ramified lumen, communication with biliary system usually obliterated
Associated with: polycystic liver disease
Size: 0.1–10 mm
• asymptomatic
√ nonspecific imaging appearance
CT:
√ multiple irregular hypodense lesions of up to 10 mm
√ little / no enhancement
US:
√ multiple small cysts / echogenic areas (if size not resolved) up to 10 mm ± comet-tail artifact
MR:
√ hypointense on T1WI
√ iso- / slightly hyperintense on T2WI
√ hypointense after gadopentetate dimeglumine
Angio:
√ multiple areas of abnormal vascularity in form of small grapelike clusters persisting into venous phase
DDx: metastatic liver disease, hepatic abscesses

MULTIPLE ENDOCRINE NEOPLASIA

= MEN = MULTIPLE ENDOCRINE ADENOMAS (MEA)
= familial autosomal dominant adenomatous hyperplasia characterized by neoplasia of more than one endocrine organ

Theory: cells of involved principal organs originate from neural crest and produce polypeptide hormones in cytoplasmic granules, which allow **a**mine **p**recursor **u**ptake and **d**ecarboxylation = APUD cells

		reminder:
Type I	= Wermer syndrome	PPP
Type II	= Sipple syndrome (type IIA)	PMP
Type III	= Mucosal neuroma syndrome (type IIB)	MPM

MEA	*Type I*	*Type II*	*Type III*
Pituitary adenoma	+		
Parathyroid adenoma	+	+	
Medullary thyroid carcinoma		+	+
Pancreatic island cell tumor	+		
Pheochromocytoma		+	+
Ganglioneuromatosis			+

MEN I Syndrome

= WERMER SYNDROME
= autosomal dominant trait with high penetrance; M:F = 1:1
Cause: genetic defect in chromosome 11
Organ involvement:
1. Parathyroid hyperplasia (97%): multiglandular
2. Pancreatic islet cell tumor (30–80%):
◊ Likely multiple + behaving malignant!
◊ Primary cause of morbidity + mortality!

LIVER

(a) gastrinoma = Zollinger-Ellison syndrome (most common type, in 50%), usually multicentric
(b) insulinoma
(c) VIPoma = WDHH-syndrome (watery diarrhea, hypokalemia, hypochlorhydria)
3. Anterior pituitary gland tumor (15–50%):
(a) nonfunctioning
(b) prolactin, growth hormone, corticotropin, TSH
4. Combination of parathyroid + pancreas + pituitary involvement (40%)
5. Adrenocortical hyperplasia (up to 33–40%)
6. Carcinoid
7. Lipoma

• usually asymptomatic

May be associated with:
thyroid tumor (20%), thymoma, buccal mucosal tumor, colonic polyposis, Ménétrier disease

MEN II Syndrome

= SIPPLE DISEASE = MEN Type IIA

Organ involvement:
1. Medullary carcinoma of thyroid
2. Pheochromocytoma: bilateral in 50%; malignant in 3%
diagnosed before (in 10%) / after detection (in 17%) of medullary thyroid carcinoma
3. Parathyroid neoplasia
• ± hyperparathyroidism

May be associated with: carcinoid tumors, Cushing disease

MEN III Syndrome

= MUCOSAL NEUROMA SYNDROME = MEN Type IIB

Organ involvement:
1. Medullary carcinoma of thyroid
2. Pheochromocytoma
3. Oral + intestinal neuroganglioneuromatosis
◊ Usually precedes the appearance of thyroid carcinoma + pheochromocytoma!

• long slender extremities (Marfanoid appearance)
• thickened lips (due to submucosal nodules)
• nodular deformity of tongue (mucosal neuromas of tongue often initially diagnosed by dentists)
• prognathism
• corneal limbus thickening
• constipation alternating with diarrhea

@ GI tract
√ thickened / plaquelike colonic wall
√ dilated colon with abnormal haustral markings
√ alternating areas of colonic spasm + dilatation
√ multiple submucosal neuromas throughout small bowel, may act as lead point for intussusception

PANCREAS DIVISUM

= most common anatomic variant of pancreas due to failure of fusion of the ventral and dorsal anlage at 8th week of fetal life with main dorsal pancreatic duct (Santorini) draining through minor (accessory) papilla + ventral pancreatic duct (Wirsung) with CBD draining through major papilla

Prevalence: 4–9–14% in autopsy series;
2–8% in ERCP series;
3–7% in normal population;
12–26% in patients with idiopathic recurrent pancreatitis

Hypothesis: relative / actual functional stenosis of minor papilla predisposes to nonalcoholic recurrent pancreatitis in dorsal segment

Age: young / middle-aged adult

• chronic relapsing pancreatitis (clinical relevance continues to be debated)

Pancreatography:
◊ The ONLY reliable means for diagnosis
√ contrast injection into major papilla demonstrates CBD + only short ventral pancreatic duct with early arborization
√ contrast injection into minor papilla fills dorsal pancreatic duct
√ no communication between ventral + dorsal ducts

CT:
√ oblique fat cleft between ventral + dorsal pancreas (25%)
√ failure to see union of dorsal + ventral pancreatic ducts (rare)

PANCREATIC ACINAR CELL CARCINOMA

= rare neoplasm of exocrine origin

Age: 40–81 (mean 62) years; M:F = 86:14; 87% Caucasian

• increased serum lipase ± amylase
• syndrome of elevated lipase:
  • disseminated subcutaneous + intraosseous fat necrosis (usually distal to knees / elbows)
  • polyarthropathy
  • skin lesions resembling erythema nodosum
• biliary obstruction distinctly uncommon

√ lobulated well-defined mass of 2–15 cm in diameter
√ thin enhancing capsule
√ tumor necrosis usually present
√ moderately vascular tumor + neovascularity + arterial and venous encasement

Prognosis: median survival of 7–9 months

DDx: (1) pancreatic adenocarcinoma (small, irregular, locally invasive, without capsule, biliary obstruction if located in head of pancreas)
(2) Nonfunctioning islet-cell tumor
(3) Microcystic cystadenoma
(4) Solid and papillary epithelial neoplasm
(5) Oncocytic tumor of pancreas

PANCREATIC DUCTAL ADENOCARCINOMA

= DUCT CELL ADENOCARCINOMA

◊ duct cells comprise only 4% of pancreatic tissue

Incidence: 80–95% of nonendocrine pancreatic neoplasms; 5th leading cause of cancer death in the United States (27,000 per year)

Etiology: alcohol abuse (4%), diabetes (2 x more frequent than in general population, particularly in females), hereditary pancreatitis (in 40%); cigarette smoking (risk factor 2 x)

LIVER

Path: scirrhous infiltrative adenocarcinoma with a dense cellularity + sparse vascularity

Mean age at onset: 55 years; peak age in 7th decade; M:F = 2:1

STAGE I = confined to pancreas
II = + regional lymph node metastases
III = + distant spread

◊ At presentation
- 65% of patients have advanced local disease / distant metastases
- 21% of patients have localized disease with spread to regional lymph nodes
- 14% of patients have tumor confined to pancreas

Extension:
(a) local extension beyond margins of organ (68%): posteriorly (96%), anteriorly (30%), into porta hepatis (15%), into splenic hilum (13%)
(b) invasion of adjacent organs (42%): duodenum > stomach > left adrenal gland > spleen > root of small bowel mesentery

Metastases: liver (30–36%), regional lymph nodes >2 cm (15–28%), ascites from peritoneal carcinomatosis (7–10%), lungs (pulmonary nodules / lymphangitic), pleura, bone

- weight loss, anorexia, fatigue
- pain in hypochondrium radiating to back
- obstructive jaundice (75%): most frequent cause of malignant biliary obstruction
- new onset diabetes (25–50%), steatorrhea
- thrombophlebitis

Location: pancreatic head (56–62%); body (26%); tail (12%)

Size: 2–10 cm (in 60% between 4–6 cm)

UGI:
√ "antral padding" = extrinsic indentation of the posteroinferior margin of antrum
√ "Frostberg inverted-3" sign = inverted 3 contour to the medial portion of the duodenal sweep
√ spiculated duodenal wall + traction + fixation (neoplastic infiltration of duodenal mucosa / desmoplastic response)
√ irregular / smooth nodular mass with ampullary carcinoma

BE:
√ localized haustral padding / flattening / narrowing with serrated contour at inferior aspect of transverse colon / splenic flexure
√ diffuse tethering throughout peritoneal cavity (from intraperitoneal seeding)

CT (99% detection rate for dynamic CT scan; 89% in predicting nonresectability):
√ pancreatic mass (95%) / diffuse enlargement (4%) / normal scan (1%)
√ mass with central zone of diminished attenuation (75– 83%)
√ pancreatic + bile duct obstruction without detectable mass (4%)
√ duct dilatation (58%): 3/4 biductal, 1/10 isolated to one duct; dilated pancreatic duct (67%); dilated bile ducts (38%)
√ atrophy of pancreatic body + tail (20%)
√ calcifications (2%)
√ postobstructive pseudocyst (11%)
√ obliteration of retropancreatic fat (50%)
√ thickening of celiac axis / SMA (invasion of perivascular lymphatics) in 60%
√ dilated collateral veins (12%)
√ thickening of Gerota fascia (5%)
√ local tumor extension posteriorly, into splenic hilum, into porta hepatis (68%)
√ contiguous organ invasion (duodenum, stomach, mesenteric root) in 42%

US:
√ hypoechoic pancreatic mass
√ focal / diffuse (10%) enlargement of pancreas
√ contour deformity of gland; rounding of uncinate process
√ dilatation of pancreatic ± biliary duct

MR (no diagnostic improvement over CT):
√ hypointense lesion on fat-suppressed T1WI
√ diminished enhancement on dynamic contrast images

Angiography (70% accuracy):
√ hypovascular tumor / neovascularity (50%)
√ arterial encasement: SMA (33%), splenic artery (14%), celiac trunk (11%), hepatic artery (11%), gastroduodenal artery (3%), left renal artery (0.6%)
√ venous obstruction: splenic vein (34%), SMV (10%)
√ venous encasement: SMV (23%), splenic vein (15%), portal vein (4%)

Cholangiography:
√ "rat tail / nipplelike" occlusion of CBD
√ nodular mass / meniscuslike occlusion in ampullary tumors

Pancreatography (abnormal in 97%):
√ irregular, nodular, rat-tailed, eccentric obstruction
√ localized encasement with prestenotic dilatation
√ acinar defect

Prognosis:
10% 1-year survival, 2% 3-year survival, <1% 5-year survival; 14 months medial survival after curative resection, 8 months after palliative resection, 5 months without treatment; tumors resectable in only 8–15% at presentation, 5% 5-year survival rate after surgery

DDx: focal pancreatitis, islet cell carcinoma, metastasis, lymphoma, normal variant

PANCREATIC ISLET CELL TUMORS

Origin: embryonic neuroectoderm, derivatives of APUD (amine precursor uptake and decarboxylation) cell line arising from islet of Langerhans (APUDoma)

Prevalence: 1:1,000,000 population/year; isolated or part of MEN I syndrome (= Wermer syndrome)

Path: (a) small tumor: solid well-demarcated
(b) large tumor: cystic changes + necrosis + calcifications

Histo: sheets of small round cells + numerous stromal vessels

Average time from onset of symptoms to diagnosis is 2.7 years

Classification: (a) functional (85%)
(b) nonfunctional (below threshold of detectability) / hypofunctional

Metastases: in 60–90% to liver ± regional lymph nodes

◊ Hyperechoic liver metastasis is suggestive of islet cell tumor rather than pancreatic adenocarcinoma!

√ calcifications highly suggestive of malignancy

NUC:

√ somatostatin receptor imaging with octreotide

DDx:

(1) Pancreatic ductal adenocarcinoma (hypovascular, smaller, encasement of SMA + celiac trunk)
(2) Microcystic adenoma (benign tumor, small cysts, older women)
(3) Metastatic tumor: renal cell carcinoma (clinical Hx)
(4) Solid and papillary epithelial neoplasm (young female, hemorrhagic areas)
(5) Paraganglioma
(6) Sarcoma (rare)

ACTH-producing Tumor

rare cause of Cushing syndrome

- increased level of serum cortisol
- impaired glucose tolerance > central obesity > hypertension, oligomenorrhea > osteoporosis > purpura > striae > muscle atrophy

Prognosis: almost all malignant with metastases at time of diagnosis

Gastrinoma

2nd most common islet cell tumor; in α cells / δ cells

Age: 8% in patients <20 years; M > F

Path: (a) islet cell hyperplasia (10%)
(b) benign adenoma (30%): in 50% solitary, in 50% multiple (especially in MEN I)
(c) malignant (50–60%) with metastases to liver, spleen, lymph nodes, bone

Associated with: MEN Type I (in 10–40%)

- Zollinger-Ellison syndrome: severe recurrent peptic ulcer disease (>90%), malabsorption, hypokalemia, gastric hypersecretion, hyperacidity / occasionally hypoacidity, diarrhea (from gastric hypersecretion)
  ◊ Only 1:1,000 patients with peptic ulcer disease has a gastrinoma!
- GI bleeding
- elevated serum levels of gastrin

Location:

(a) 87% in pancreas (50% solitary in head / tail)
(b) ectopic (7–33%):
— duodenal wall (13% in medial wall of duodenum = gastrinoma triangle)
— peripancreatic nodes / spleen
— stomach, jejunum
— omentum, retroperitoneum
— ovary

frequently in “gastrinoma triangle” (= triangle defined by porta hepatis as apex of triangle + 2nd and 3rd parts of duodenum as the base)

√ average tumor size 3.4 cm (up to 15 cm)
√ occasionally calcifications
√ homogeneous hypoechoic mass

Angio:

√ hypervascular lesion (70%)
√ hepatic venous sampling after intraarterial stimulation with secretin

CT:

√ transiently hyperdense on dynamic CT (majority)
√ thickening of gastric rugal folds

MR:

√ low-intensity mass on fat-suppressed T1WI
√ diminished central + peripheral ring enhancement
√ high-intensity mass on fat-suppressed T2WI

Sensitivity of preoperative localization:
25% for US, 35% for CT, 20% for MRI, 42–63% for transhepatic portal venous sampling for gastrin, 68–70% for selective angiography, 77% for arteriography combined with intra-arterial injection of secretin

Rx: surgery curative in 30%

Glucagonoma

Uncommon tumor; derived from α cells; M < F

Associated with: MEN

- necrolytic erythema migrans (erythematous macules / papules on lower extremity, groin, buttocks, face) in >70% of patients
- diarrhea, diabetes, painful glossitis, weight loss, anemia
- plasma glucagon level > 1,000 ng/L

Location: predominantly in pancreatic body / tail

√ tumor size 2.5–25 cm (mean 6.4 cm) with solid + necrotic components
√ hypervascular in 90%; successful angiographic localization in 15%

Cx: deep vein thrombosis + pulmonary embolism

Prognosis: in 60–80% malignant transformation (liver metastases at time of diagnosis in 50%); 55% 5-year survival rate

Insulinoma

Most common functioning islet cell tumor

Age: 4th–6th decade; M:F = 2:3

Associated with: MEN type I

Path: (a) single benign adenoma (80–90%)
(b) multiple adenomas / microadenomatosis (5–10%)
(c) islet cell hyperplasia (5–10%)
(d) malignant adenoma (5–10%)

- Whipple triad: starvation attack + hypoglycemia (fasting glucose <50 mg/dL) + relief by IV dextrose
- neuroglycopenic symptoms: headaches, confusion, coma
- hypoglycemia exacerbated by fasting results in frequent meals to avoid symptoms

- sweating, palpitations, tremor (secondary to catecholamine release in response to hypoglycemia)
- obesity
- firm rubbery palpable mass at surgery (in >90%)

Location: no predilection for any part of pancreas, 2–5% in ectopic location; 10% multiple (especially in MEN I)

√ average tumor size 1–2 cm; <1.5 cm in 70%

US (20–75% preoperative and 75–100% endoscopic + intraoperative sensitivity):
√ round / oval smoothly marginated solid homogeneously hypoechoic mass

Angio:
√ hypervascular tumor (66%): accurate angiographic localization in 50–90%
√ transhepatic portal venous sampling (correct localization in 95%)
√ hepatic venous sampling after intraarterial stimulation with calcium gluconate

CECT (30–75% sensitivity):
√ hypo- / iso- / hyperattenuating lesion

MR:
√ low signal intensity on fat-suppressed T1WI
√ hyperintense on T2WI + dynamic contrast-enhanced + suppressed inversion recovery images

Prognosis: malignant transformation in 5–10%

Rx: surgery curative

Nonfunctioning Islet Cell Tumor

Incidence: 3rd most common islet cell tumor after insulinoma + gastrinoma; 15–25% of all islet cell tumors

derived from either α or β cells

Age: 24–74 (mean 57) years

- mostly asymptomatic (hormonally quiescent)
- abdominal pain, jaundice, gastric variceal bleeding
- palpable mass, gastric outlet obstruction

Location: predominantly in pancreatic head

√ tumor size 6–20 cm (>5 cm in 72%) with solid + necrotic components
√ coarse nodular calcifications (20–25%)
√ CT contrast enhancement in 83%
√ hypoechoic mass
√ late dense capillary stain
√ large irregular pathologic vessels with early venous filling

Prognosis: in 80–100% malignant transformation with metastases to liver + regional nodes; 60% 3-year survival; 44% 5-year survival

Rx: may respond to systemic chemotherapy

Somatostatinoma

Origin: derived from δ cells

- inhibitory syndrome = inhibitory action of somatostatin on other pancreatic + bowel peptides (growth hormone, TSH, insulin, glucagon, gastric acid, pepsin, secretin)
- diabetes, cholelithiasis, steatorrhea
- elevated level of somatostatin

Location: predominantly in pancreatic head

√ tumor size 0.6–20 cm (average >4 cm)
√ hypervascular

Prognosis: 50–90% malignant transformation; metastatic disease in 70% at time of initial diagnosis

VIPoma

= solitary tumor liberating **V**asoactive **I**ntestinal **P**eptides acting directly on cyclic adenosine monophosphate (AMP) within epithelial cells of bowel relaxing vascular smooth muscle; sporadic occurrence

Histo: adenoma / hyperplasia

M:F = 1:2

- **WDHA syndrome** = **w**atery **d**iarrhea + **h**ypokalemia + **a**chlorhydria (more recently + more accurately described as) **WDHH syndrome** = **w**atery **d**iarrhea + **h**ypokalemia + **h**ypochlorhydria = "pancreatic cholera" = **Verner-Morrison syndrome**
- dehydration due to massive diarrhea (>1 L/day)

Location:
(1) pancreas: from δ cells predominantly in pancreatic body / tail
(2) extrapancreatic: retroperitoneal ganglioblastoma, pheochromocytoma, lung, neuroblastoma (in children)

√ average size 5–10 cm with solid + necrotic tissue
√ mostly hypervascular tumor
√ dilatation of gallbladder

Prognosis: in 50–80% malignant transformation

DDx: small cell carcinoma of lung / neuroblastoma may also cause WDHH syndrome

PANCREATIC LIPOMATOSIS

= FATTY REPLACEMENT = FATTY INFILTRATION
= deposition of fat cells in pancreatic parenchyma

Predisposing factors:
1. Atherosclerosis of elderly
2. Obesity
3. Steroid therapy
4. Diabetes mellitus
5. Cushing syndrome
6. Chronic pancreatitis
7. Main pancreatic duct obstruction
8. Cystic fibrosis (most common cause in childhood)
9. Malnutrition / dietary deficiency
10. Hepatic disease
11. Hemochromatosis
12. Viral infection
13. Schwachman-Diamond syndrome
14. Johanson-Blizzard syndrome

√ fatty replacement often uneven:
√ increase in AP diameter of pancreatic head with focal fatty replacement = lipomatous pseudohypertrophy
√ prominently lobulated external contour

US:
√ increased pancreatic echogenicity

CT:
√ "marbling" of pancreatic parenchyma / total fatty replacement / lipomatous pseudohypertrophy

Pancreatic Fatty Sparing

= sparing of fatty change in pancreatic head + uncinate process (ventral pancreatic anlage) as initial stage in pancreatic lipomatosis

Histo: ventral pancreatic anlage has smaller + more densely packed acini with scanty / absent interacinar fat

US:
- √ rounded / triangular hypoechoic area within pancreatic head / uncinate process + diffusely increased echogenicity in remainder of gland

CT:
- √ higher-density region of pancreatic head + uncinate process with diffusely decreased attenuation of pancreatic body + tail

PANCREATIC PSEUDOCYST

= collection of pancreatic fluid encapsulated by fibrous tissue

Etiology:
(1) Acute pancreatitis ; requires >4 weeks to form; pseudocysts mature in 6–8 weeks
(2) Chronic pancreatitis
(3) Posttraumatic
(4) Pancreatic cancer

Incidence: 2–4% in acute pancreatitis; 10–15% in chronic pancreatitis

Location: 2/3 within pancreas

Atypical location (may dissect along tissue planes in 1/3):
(a) intraperitoneal: mesentery of small bowel / transverse colon / sigmoid colon
(b) retroperitoneal: along psoas muscle; may present as groin mass / in scrotum
(c) intraparenchymal: liver, spleen, kidney
(d) mediastinal (through esophageal hiatus > aortic hiatus > foramen of Morgagni > erosion through diaphragm): may present as neck mass

May communicate with: duodenum, stomach, spleen

Plain film / contrast radiograph:
- √ smooth extrinsic indentation of posterior wall of stomach / inner duodenal sweep (80%)
- √ indentation / displacement of splenic flexure / transverse colon (40%)
- √ downward displacement of duodenojejunal junction
- √ gastric outlet obstruction
- √ splaying of renal collecting system / ureteral obstruction

US (pseudocyst detectable in 50–92%; 92–96% accuracy):
- √ usually single + unilocular cyst
- √ multilocular in 6%
- √ fluid-debris level / internal echoes (may contain sequester, blood clot, cellular debris from autolysis)
- √ septations (rare; sign of infection / hemorrhage)
- √ may increase in size (secondary to hypertonicity of fluid, communication with pancreatic duct, hemorrhage, erosion of vessel)
- √ obstruction of pancreatic duct / CBD

CT:
- √ fluid in pseudocyst (0–30 HU)
- √ cyst wall calcification (extremely rare)

Pancreatography:
- √ communication with pancreatic duct in up to 50–70%

Indications for pseudocyst drainage:
pain, suspected infection, persistence of pseudocyst >5 cm, increasing size, biliary / gastrointestinal obstruction

Cx (in 40%):
1. Rupture into abdominal cavity, stomach, colon, duodenum
2. Hemorrhage / formation of pseudoaneurysm
3. Infection = **pancreatic abscess**
   - usually occurs >4 weeks after acute pancreatitis
   - symptomatology of infection
   - √ gas bubbles (DDx: fistulous communication to GI tract)
   - √ increase in attenuation of fluid contents

   Dx: transcutaneous needle aspiration
4. Intestinal obstruction

Prognosis: spontaneous resolution (in 20–50%) secondary to rupture into GI tract / pancreatic / bile duct

DDx: pancreatic cystadenoma, cystadenocarcinoma, necrotic pancreatic carcinoma, fluid-filled bowel loop, fluid-filled stomach, duodenal diverticulum, aneurysm

PANCREATIC TRANSPLANTATION

Complications: sepsis, rejection, pancreatitis, pseudocyst, pancreatic abscess (22%), anastomotic leak

Prognosis: 40% survival rate >1 year

Graft-vessel Thrombosis in Pancreatic Transplant (2–19%)

A. Early thrombosis (<1 month after transplantation)
   Cause: technical error in fashioning anastomosis, microvascular damage due to preservation injury
B. Late thrombosis (>1 month after transplantation)
   Cause: alloimmune arteritis with gradual occlusion of small blood vessels

Acute Rejection of Pancreatic Transplant

- focal tenderness over transplant
- measurement of urinary + serum amylase, blood glucose (nonspecific for diagnosis of rejection)

US:
- √ poor margination of transplant
- √ acoustic inhomogeneity
- √ dilated pancreatic duct

PANCREATITIS

Cause:
A. IDIOPATHIC (20%)
B. ALCOHOLISM (<50%): acute pancreatitis (15%); chronic pancreatitis (70%)
C. CHOLELITHIASIS (<50%): acute pancreatitis (75%); chronic pancreatitis (20%)

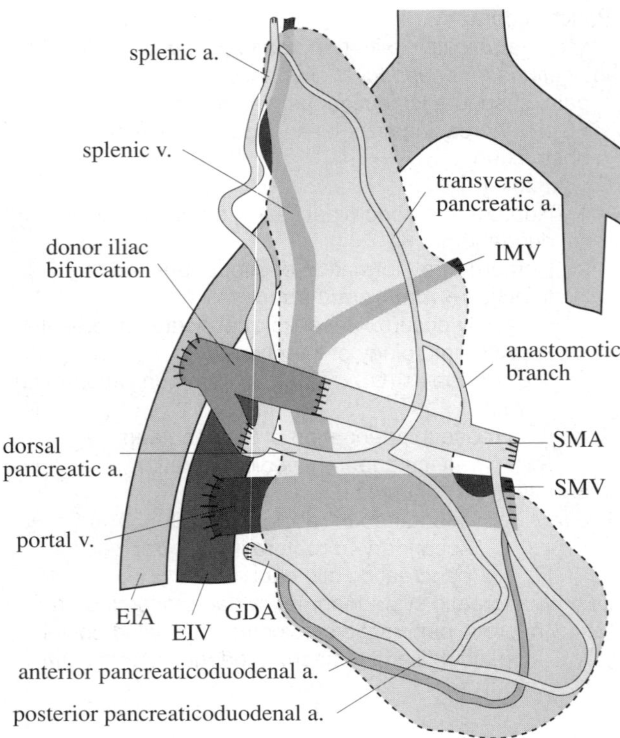

Pancreatic Transplantation
EIA = external iliac artery, EIV = external iliac vein,
GDA = gastroduodenal artery, IMV = inferior mesenteric vein,
SMA = superior mesenteric artery, SMV = superior mesenteric vein

D. METABOLIC DISORDERS
1. Hypercalcemia in hyperparathyroidism (10%), multiple myeloma, amyloidosis, sarcoidosis
2. **Hereditary pancreatitis**: autosomal dominant, only Caucasians affected, most common cause of large spherical pancreatic calcifications in childhood (in 50%), recurrent episodes of pancreatitis, development into pancreatic carcinoma in 20–40%; pronounced dilatation of pancreatic duct; pseudocyst formation (50%); associated with type I hypercholesterolemia
3. Hyperlipidemia types I and V
4. Cystic fibrosis

E. INFECTION / INFESTATION
1. Viral infection (mumps, hepatitis, Coxsackie virus, mononucleosis)
2. Parasites (ascariasis, clonorchis)

F. TRAUMA
◊ One of the most common causes of pancreatitis in childhood!
1. Penetrating ulcer
2. Blunt / penetrating trauma; nonaccidental trauma
3. Surgery (in 0.8% of Billroth-II resections, 0.8% of splenectomies, 0.7% of choledochal surgery, 0.4% of aortic graft surgery)

G. STRUCTURAL ABNORMALITIES
1. Pancreas divisum
◊ In 12–50% of cases with no other underlying abnormalities
2. Choledochocele

H. DRUGS
Azathioprine, thiazide, furosemide, ethacrynic acid, sulfonamides, tetracycline, phenformin, steroids (eg, renal transplant), l-asparaginase, acetaminophen, procainamide

I. MALIGNANCY
Pancreatic carcinoma (in 1%), metastases, lymphoma

J. MULTISYSTEM CONDITIONS
1. Sepsis and shock
2. Hemolytic-uremic syndrome
3. Reye syndrome
4. Systemic lupus erythematosus

Theories of pathogenesis:
Reflux of bile / pancreatic enzymes / duodenal succus
(a) terminal duct segment shared by common bile duct + pancreatic duct
(b) obstruction at papilla of Vater from inflammatory stenosis, edema / spasm of sphincter of Oddi, tumor, periduodenal diverticulum
(c) incompetent sphincter of Oddi

Acute Pancreatitis

= inflammatory disease of pancreas producing temporary changes with potential for restoration of normal anatomy + function following resolution

Path:
1. INTERSTITIAL EDEMATOUS PANCREATITIS (75–95%): edema, congestion, leukocytic infiltrates; mortality rate of 4%
2. NECROTIZING PANCREATITIS (5–25%): proteolytic destruction of pancreatic parenchyma; mortality rate of 80–90%
   (a) HEMORRHAGIC PANCREATITIS:
   + fat necrosis and hemorrhage (due to erosion of small vessels)
   • falling hematocrit
   (b) SUPPURATIVE PANCREATITIS:
   + bacterial infection

A. Diffuse pancreatitis (52%)
B. Focal pancreatitis (48%): location of head:tail = 3:2

Mild Acute Pancreatitis (75%)

• minimal organ dysfunction
Path: interstitial edema
Prognosis: improvement within 48–72 hours following conservative therapy with gradual decrease of elevated enzymes
Mortality: 1–5%

Severe Acute Pancreatitis

◊ Develops shortly after onset of untreated mild acute pancreatitis

• increased abdominal tenderness, rebound distension, hypoactive bowel sounds
Associated with: organ failure / local complications
Path: pancreatic cell breakdown + necrosis
Cx: acute fluid collection, pancreatic necrosis, pseudocyst, abscess

ACUTE FLUID COLLECTIONS (30–50%)
= early form of acute pseudocyst / pancreatic abscess
Path: lack of a defined wall of fibrous / granulation tissue; **pancreatic phlegmon** [misnomer, no infection] = solid boggy inflammatory mass characterized by edema, infiltration of inflammatory cells + necrosis of retroperitoneal fat
Location: extension into lesser sac, anterior pararenal space, transverse mesocolon, small bowel mesentery, retroperitoneum, pelvis
√ near 0 HU on CT
Prognosis: spontaneous regression (in 40–50%)

PANCREATIC NECROSIS
= focal / diffuse area of nonviable pancreatic parenchyma
Path: clumps of devitalized pancreatic parenchyma + hemorrhage in pancreatic and peripancreatic tissues
Histo: extensive interstitial fat necrosis with vessel damage + necrosis of acinar cells, islet cells, ductal system
Associated with: peripancreatic fat necrosis
√ focal / diffuse well-marginated zones of unenhanced pancreatic parenchyma > 3 cm / involving >30% of the pancreatic gland

ACUTE PSEUDOCYST
= collection of pancreatic fluid enclosed by a wall of fibrous granulation tissue
Cause: acute pancreatitis, pancreatic trauma, chronic pancreatitis
Time of onset: >4 weeks after acute pancreatitis
• amylase-rich fluid
Prognosis: spontaneous resolution in 44%

PANCREATIC ABSCESS
= well-demarcated fluid collection of pus usually close to the pancreas
Time of onset: 2–4 weeks after severe acute pancreatitis
Organism: most commonly due to E. coli
• liquefied tissue with little / no necrosis
√ may contain gas within pancreatic bed in 30–50% (DDx of gas: cutaneous / enteric fistula, ruptured duodenum, iatrogenic gas collection)
DDx: infected necrosis

Clinical stages:
I = EDEMATOUS PANCREATITIS (75%)
• rapid improvement following conservative therapy
• gradual decrease of elevated enzymes
Mortality: 1–5%
II = PARTIALLY NECROTIZING PANCREATITIS
• delayed / no response to conservative therapy
• delayed / no normalization of enzymes:
  • hyperglycemia of <200 mg/100 mL
  • hypocalcemia of >4 mval/L
  • base deficit of <4 mval/L
• leukocytosis of <16,000
Mortality: 30–75%
III = TOTALLY NECROTIZING PANCREATITIS
• deterioration under conservative therapy:
  • hyperglycemia of >200 mg/100 mL
  • hypocalcemia of <4 mval/L
  • base deficit of >4 mval/L
  • leukocytosis of >16,000
Mortality: 100% (40% by 2nd day, 75% by 5th day, 100% by 10th day)

• acute abdominal pain (peaking after a few hours, resolving in 2–3 days), nausea, vomiting
• raised pancreatic amylase + lipase in blood + urine
• increased amylase-creatinine clearance ratio
• signs of hemorrhagic pancreatitis:
  • Cullen sign = periumbilical ecchymosis
  • Grey-Turner sign = flank ecchymosis
  • Fox sign = infrainguinal ecchymosis
• subcutaneous nodules + fat necrosis + polyarthritis

√ NO findings on US / CT in 29%
Abdominal film:
√ "colon cutoff" sign (2–52%) = dilated transverse colon with abrupt change to a gasless descending colon (inflammation via phrenicocolic ligament causes spasm + obstruction at the splenic flexure impinging on a paralytic transverse colon)
√ "sentinel loop" (10–55%) = localized segment of gas-containing bowel in duodenum (in 20–45%) / terminal ileum / cecum
√ "renal halo" sign = water-density of inflammation in anterior pararenal space contrasts with perirenal fat; more common on left side
√ mottled appearance of peripancreatic area (secondary to fat necrosis in pancreatic bed, mesentery, omentum)
√ intrapancreatic gas bubbles (from acute gangrene / suppurative pancreatitis)
√ "gasless abdomen" = fluid-filled bowel associated with vomiting
√ ascites
CXR (findings in 14–71%):
√ pleural effusion (in 5%), usually left-sided, with elevated amylase levels (in 85%)
√ left-sided diaphragmatic elevation
√ left-sided subsegmental atelectasis (20%)
√ parenchymal infiltrates, pulmonary infarction

√ pulmonary edema, ARDS
√ pleural empyema, pericardial effusion
√ mediastinal abscess, mediastinal pseudocyst
√ pancreatico-bronchial / -pleural / -pulmonary fistula

UGI:
√ esophagogastric varices (from splenic vein obstruction)
√ enlarged tortuous edematous rugal folds along antrum + greater curvature (20%)
√ widening of retrogastric space (from pancreatic enlargement / inflammation in lesser sac)
√ diminished duodenal peristalsis + edematous folds
√ widening of duodenal sweep + downward displacement of ligament of Treitz
√ Poppel sign = edematous swelling of papilla
√ Frostberg inverted-3 sign = segmental narrowing with fold thickening of duodenum
√ jejunal + ileal fold thickening (proteolytic spread along mesentery)

BE:
√ narrowing, nodularity, fold distortion along inferior haustral row of transverse colon ± descending colon

Cholangiography:
√ long gently tapered narrowing of CBD
√ prestenotic biliary dilatation
√ smooth / irregular mucosal surface

Bone films (findings in 6%):
Cause: metastatic intramedullary lipolysis + fat necrosis + trabecular bone destruction
Time of onset: usually 3–6 weeks after peak of clinical pancreatitis
√ punched out / permeative mottled destruction of cancellous bone + endosteal erosion
√ aseptic necrosis of femoral / humeral heads
√ metaphyseal infarcts, predominantly in distal femur + proximal tibia

US (pancreatic visualization in 62–78%):
√ hypoechoic diffuse / focal enlargement of pancreas
√ dilatation of pancreatic duct (if head focally involved)
√ perivascular cloaking = spread of inflammatory exudate along perivascular spaces
√ extrapancreatic hypoechoic mass with good acoustic transmission (= phlegmonous pancreatitis)
√ fluid collection: lesser sac (60%), L > R anterior pararenal space (54%), posterior pararenal space (18%), around left lobe of liver (16%), in spleen (9%), mediastinum (3%), iliac fossa, along transverse mesocolon / mesenteric leaves of small intestine
Fate of fluid collection:
(a) complete resolution
(b) pseudocyst formation
(c) bacterial infection = abscess
√ pseudocyst formation (52%): extension into lesser sac, transverse mesocolon, around kidney, mediastinum, lower quadrants of abdomen

CT (pancreatic visualization in 98%):
√ no detectable change in size / appearance (29%)
√ enlargement of pancreas with convex margins + indistinctness of gland + parenchymal heterogeneity:
  √ hypodense (5–20 HU) mass in phlegmonous pancreatitis; may persist long after complete recovery
  √ hyperdense areas (50–70 HU) in hemorrhagic pancreatitis for 24–48 hours
√ thickening of anterior pararenal fascia
√ "halo sign" = sparing of perirenal space
√ non–contrast-enhancing parenchyrna during bolus injection (= pancreatic necrosis)
√ fluid collection

Angiography:
√ may be normal
√ hypovascular areas (15–56%)
√ hypervascularity + increased parenchymal stain (12– 45%)
√ venous compression secondary to edema
√ formation of pseudoaneurysms (in 10% with chronic pancreatitis): splenic artery (50%), pancreatic arcades, gastroduodenal artery

Cx:
1. Phlegmon (18%)
2. Pseudocyst formation (10%)
3. Hemorrhagic pancreatitis (2–5%)
4. Abscess (2–10%)
5. Pancreatic ascites
6. Biliary duct obstruction
7. Thrombosis of splenic vein / SMV
8. Pseudoaneurysm
   (a) rupture into preexisting pseudocyst
   (b) digestion of arterial wall by enzymes
   Incidence: in up to 10% of severe pancreatitis
   Location: splenic artery (most common), gastroduodenal, pancreatico-duodenal, hepatic, left gastric artery
   Mortality: 37% for rupture, 16–50% for surgery
9. Thoracopancreatic fistula
   (a) pancreaticopleural fistula
   (b) pancreaticopericardial fistula
   (c) pancreaticoesophageal fistula
   (d) pancreaticobronchial fistula
   (e) mediastinal pseudocyst

Rx:
1. Conservative (NPO, gastric tube, atropine, analgesics, sedation, prophylactic antibiotics) for stage I
2. Early surgery in stages II and III

Chronic Pancreatitis

= continued inflammatory disease of pancreas characterized by irreversible permanent damage to anatomy + function

LIVER

Etiology:
A. CHRONIC CALCIFYING PANCREATITIS
1. **Juvenile tropical pancreatitis** = Kwashiorkor: in equatorial third-world countries, associated with pure protein malnutrition, patients present with diabetes + chronic abdominal pain
2. Hereditary pancreatitis
3. Inborn errors of metabolism
4. Hyperlipidemia
5. Hypercalcemia

√ protein plugs / calculi within ductal system

B. CHRONIC OBSTRUCTIVE PANCREATITIS:
1. Congenital / acquired lesions of pancreatic duct
2. Trauma / surgical duct ligation
3. Sphincter of Oddi dysfunction, ampullary stenosis
4. Sclerosing cholangitis
5. Idiopathic fibrosing pancreatitis
6. Renal failure
7. Slow growing ampullary tumor

√ dilatation of pancreatic duct
√ normal sized / focally or diffusely enlarged / small atrophic gland
√ calcifications uncommon

- acute exacerbation of epigastric pain (93%): decreasing with time due to progressive destruction of gland, usually painless after 7 years
- jaundice (42%) from common bile duct obstruction
- steatorrhea (80%)
- diabetes mellitus (58%)
- secretin test with decreased amylase + bicarbonate in duodenal fluid

Plain film:
√ numerous irregular calcifications (in 20–50% of alcoholic pancreatitis) PATHOGNOMONIC

UGI:
√ displacement of stomach / duodenum by pseudocyst
√ shrinkage / fold induration of stomach (DDx: linitis plastica)
√ stricture of duodenum

Cholangiopancreatography (most sensitive imaging modality):
√ side-branch ectasia = slight ductal ectasia / clubbing of side branches (minimal disease)
√ "nipping" = narrowing of the origins of side branches
√ dilatation >2 mm, tortuosity, wall rigidity, main ductal stenosis (moderate disease)
√ "beading, chain of lakes, string of pearls" = multifocal dilatation, stenosis, obstruction of main pancreatic duct + side branches (severe disease)
√ intraductal filling defects due to mucinous protein plugs / calculi / debris
√ prolonged emptying of contrast material
√ may have stenosis / obstruction + prestenotic dilatation of CBD
√ filling of pseudocysts (<50%)

US / CT:
√ irregular (73%) / smooth (15%) / beaded (12%) pancreatic ductal dilatation (in 41–68%)
√ small atrophic gland (in 10–54%)
√ pancreatic mostly intraductal calcifications (4–68%)
√ inhomogeneous gland with increased echogenicity (62%)
√ irregular pancreatic contour (45–60%)
√ focal (12–32%) / diffuse (27–45%) pancreatic enlargement during flare up (DDx: pancreatic carcinoma)
√ mostly mild biliary ductal dilatation (29%)
√ intra- / peripancreatic pseudocysts (20–34%)
√ segmental portal hypertension (= splenic vein thrombosis + splenomegaly) in 11%
√ arterial pseudoaneurysm formation
√ peripancreatic fascial thickening + blurring of organ margins (16%)
√ ascites / pleural effusion (9%)

MR:
√ loss of signal intensity on fat-suppressed T1WI (from loss of aqueous protein in pancreatic acini secondary to fibrosis)
√ diminished contrast enhancement (from loss of normal capillary network replaced by fibrous tissue)

Angiography:
√ increased tortuosity + angulation of pancreatic arcades + intrahepatic arteries (88%)
√ luminal irregularities / focal fibrotic arterial stenoses (25–75%) / smooth beaded appearance
√ irregular parenchymal stain
√ venous compression / occlusion (20–50%)
√ portoportal shunting + gastric varices without esophageal varices

Cx: pancreatic carcinoma (2–4%), jaundice, pseudocyst formation, pancreatic ascites, thrombosis of splenic / mesenteric / portal vein
Rx: surgery for infected pseudocyst, GI bleeding from portal hypertension, common bile duct obstruction, gastrointestinal obstruction
DDx: pancreatic carcinoma (extrapancreatic spread)

PANCREATOBLASTOMA

= rare childhood tumor often misdiagnosed as neuroblastoma / hepatoblastoma
Age: <7 years
- palpable mass, anorexia, vomiting

√ up to 10 cm large well-defined lobulated solid / multiloculated mass in region of lesser sac

PAPILLARY ADENOMA OF BILE DUCTS

= very rare benign tumor of biliary tract
Path: usually solitary tumor / papillomatosis with papillary fronds extending into lumen
Histo: columnar epithelium supported by connective tissue from lamina propria
- biliary obstruction

Location: common bile duct > right / left hepatic duct

√ usually small intraductal mass
√ visualized at cross-sectional imaging only if large enough
Prognosis: high rate of recurrence after surgical resection
Cx: malignant transformation (rare)

PASSIVE HEPATIC CONGESTION

Cause: CHF, constrictive pericarditis
Pathophysiology: chronic central venous hypertension transmitted to hepatic sinusoids results in centrilobular congestion + eventually hepatic atrophy, necrosis, fibrosis
• abnormal liver function tests
CT:
√ globally delayed enhancement (36%)
√ enhancement of portal veins + hepatic arteries + immediately adjacent parenchyma (56%)
√ "reticulated mosaic" pattern = lobular patchy areas of enhancement separated by coarse linear regions of diminished attenuation (100%)
√ diminished periportal attenuation (24%)
√ diminished attenuation around intrahepatic IVC (8%)
√ prominent IVC + hepatic vein enhancement (due to contrast reflux from right atrium into dilated IVC)
DDx: Budd-Chiari syndrome (regional / lobular distribution of reticulated mosaic pattern, caudate lobe hypertrophy)

PELIOSIS

[*pelios* , Greek = purple]
= rare benign disorder characterized by multiple blood-filled cavities within organs of the RES
Cause: (a) ? acquired: chronic infection (disseminated TB), hepatotoxic drugs (androgen-anabolic steroids, corticosteroids, tamoxifen citrate, chemotherapeutic agents, azathioprine, oral contraceptives, thorium dioxide injection), diabetes mellitus, chronic renal failure, advanced malignancy (Hodgkin disease, myeloma, disseminated cancer)
(b) bacillary peliosis hepatis in AIDS (lesions contain bacilli of Rochalimaea species) responsive to antibiotics
(c) ? congenital: angiomatous malformation
Histo: (1) **Phlebectatic** peliosis hepatis (early stage)
= endothelial-lined cysts (= ? dilatation of central veins) communicating with dilated hepatic sinusoids + compression of surrounding liver
(2) **Parenchymal** peliosis hepatis (late stage)
= irregularly shaped cysts without lining communicating with dilated hepatic sinusoids + areas of liver cell necrosis
Associated with: hormonally induced benign / malignant tumors
Location: liver (most common), spleen, bone marrow, lymph nodes, lungs)
Age: fetal life (rare) to adult life
• incidental discovery
√ hepatomegaly, splenomegaly
US:
√ multiple indistinct areas of hypo- / hyperechogenicity
CECT:
√ initially hypoattenuating, with passage of time isoattenuating / enhancing round lesions
MR:
√ mixed signal intensity due to repeated hemorrhage (deoxyhemoglobin + methemoglobin + siderotic nodules)
Angio:
√ multiple small (several mm to 1.5 cm) round collections of contrast medium scattered throughout liver in late arterial phase of hepatic arteriogram
√ ± simultaneous opacification of hepatic veins
Prognosis: reversible after drug withdrawal / progression to hepatic failure / intraperitoneal hemorrhage leading to death

PERICHOLECYSTIC ABSCESS

Cause: subacute perforation of gallbladder wall subsequent to gangrene + infarction due to acute cholecystitis
Prevalence: 2–20%
Location: (a) gallbladder bed (most common)
√ area of low-level echoes in liver adjacent to gallbladder
(b) intramural
√ small area of low-level echoes within thickened gallbladder wall
(c) intraperitoneal
√ area of low-level echoes within peritoneal cavity adjacent to gallbladder
Rx: (1) Emergency operation
(2) Antibiotic treatment + elective operation
(3) Percutaneous abscess drainage

PORCELAIN GALLBLADDER

= calcium carbonate incrustation of gallbladder wall
Incidence: 0.6–0.8% of cholecystectomy patients; M:F = 1:5
Histo: (a) flakes of dystrophic calcium within chronically inflamed + fibrotic muscular wall
(b) microliths scattered diffusely throughout mucosa, submucosa, glandular spaces, Rokitansky-Aschoff sinuses
Associated with: gallstones in 90%
• minimal symptoms
√ curvilinear (muscularis) / granular (mucosal) calcifications in segment of wall / entire wall
√ nonfunctioning GB on oral cholecystogram
√ highly echogenic shadowing curvilinear structure in GB fossa (DDx: stone-filled contracted GB)
√ echogenic GB wall with little acoustic shadowing (DDx: emphysematous cholecystitis)
√ scattered irregular clumps of echoes with posterior acoustic shadowing
Cx: 10–20% develop carcinoma of gallbladder

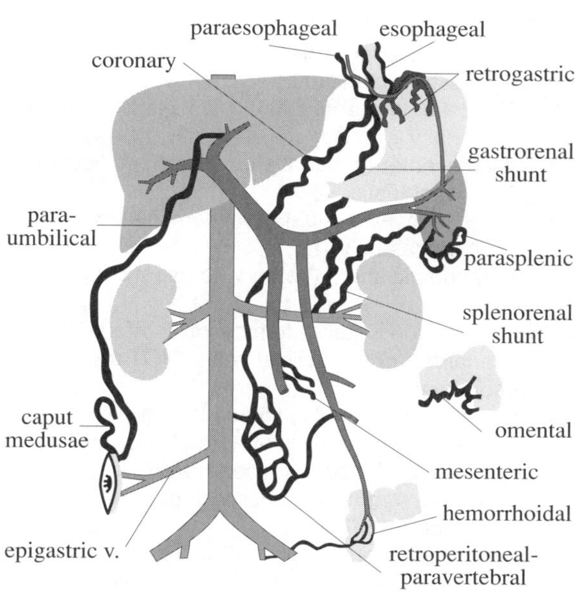

Portosystemic Collateral Vessels in Portal Hypertension

PORTAL HYPERTENSION

= portal venous pressure >10 mm Hg

- normal hepatic blood flow of 550–900 mL/min (= 25% of cardiac output) passes through portal system (2/3) + through hepatic artery (1/3)

Classification:

A. DYNAMIC / HYPERKINETIC PORTAL HYPERTENSION
   congenital / traumatic / neoplastic arterioportal fistula
B. INCREASED PORTAL RESISTANCE
   @ Prehepatic
   — portal vein thrombosis (portal phlebitis, oral contraceptives, coagulopathy, neoplastic invasion, pancreatitis, neonatal omphalitis)
   — portal vein compression (tumor, trauma, lymphadenopathy, portal phlebosclerosis, pancreatic pseudocyst)
   @ Intrahepatic (= obstruction of portal venules)
   — presinusoidal
   1. Congenital hepatic fibrosis
   2. Idiopathic noncirrhotic fibrosis
   3. Primary biliary cirrhosis
   4. alpha-1 antitrypsin deficiency
   5. Wilson disease
   6. Sarcoid liver disease
   7. Toxic fibrosis (arsenic, copper, PVC)
   8. Reticuloendotheliosis
   9. Myelofibrosis
   10. Felty syndrome
   11. Schistosomiasis
   12. Cystic fibrosis
   13. Chronic malaria
   — sinusoidal
   1. Hepatitis
   2. Sickle cell disease
   — postsinusoidal
   1. Cirrhosis (most frequent): Laennec cirrhosis, postnecrotic cirrhosis from hepatitis
   2. Venoocclusive disease of liver
   @ Posthepatic
   1. Budd-Chiari syndrome
   2. Constrictive pericarditis
   3. CHF (tricuspid incompetence)

Pathophysiology:

continued elevated pressure despite formation of portal venous collateral vessels may be explained by
(a) backward flow theory = hypodynamic flow theory
   = increase in sinusoidal pressure due to deposition of collagen in the spaces of Disse + hepatocyte swelling
   • low / stagnant portal venous flow rates
(b) forward flow theory = hyperdynamic flow theory
   = splanchnic flow increases secondary to mesenteric vasodilators + increase in cardiac output to preserve hepatic perfusion + intrahepatic endogenous vasoconstrictors
   • increased portal venous flow rates >15 mL/min/kg

Flow direction:

(a) hepatopetal (*petere* , Latin = to seek)
(b) hepatofugal (*fugere* , Latin = to flee) = flow reversal
   Cause: intrahepatic arterioportal communications (inside portal triads vasa vasorum of portal veins + hepatic arteries connect via bile duct capillaries to portal vein)

- elevated hepatic wedge pressure (HWP) = portal venous pressure; normal values seen in presinusoidal portal hypertension
- **caput medusae** = drainage from paraumbilical + omental veins through superficial veins of chest (lateral thoracic vein to axillary vein; superficial epigastric vein to internal mammary vein and subclavian vein) + abdominal wall (circumflex iliac vein and superficial epigastric vein to femoral vein; inferior epigastric vein to external iliac vein)
- hemorrhaging esophageal varices (50%)

@ Splanchnic system:
   √ portal vein >13 mm (57% sensitivity, 100% specificity)
   √ SMV + splenic vein >10 mm; coronary vein >4 mm; recanalized umbilical vein >3 mm (size of vessels not related to degree of portal hypertension or presence of collaterals)
   √ loss of respiratory increase of splanchnic vein diameters of <20% (81% sensitive, 100% specific)
   √ portal vein aneurysm
   √ portal vein thrombosis
   √ cavernous transformation of portal vein
   √ increased echogenicity + thickening of portal vein walls

LIVER

Doppler US:
- √ continuous monophasic portal venous flow pattern without respiratory fluctuations
- √ reduction of mean portal vein velocities to 7–12 cm/sec (normally 12–30 cm/sec)
- √ loss of flow increase in portal venous system during expiration
- √ congestive index >0.13 cm/sec (= ratio of area of portal vein divided by flow velocity; 67% sensitive)
- √ may have bidirectional / hepatofugal (<10%) flow within spontaneous splenorenal shunts (indicates high incidence of hepatic encephalopathy)
- √ dilated hepatic artery may demonstrate elevated resistive index >0.78

@ Spontaneous portosystemic shunts:
- • high frequency of hepatic encephalopathy
- √ varices = serpentine tubular rounded structures
- √ coronary (left gastric) vein >5–6 mm (in 26%)
- √ gallbladder wall varices in thickened gallbladder wall (in 80% associated with portal vein thrombosis)

Type of Varices	*Frequency (%)*
Coronary venous	80–86
Esophageal	45–65
Paraumbilical	10–43
Abdominal wall	30
Perisplenic	30
Retrogastric / gastric	2–27
Paraesophageal	22
Omental	20
Retroperitoneal-paravertebral	18
Mesenteric	10
Splenorenal	10
Gastrorenal	7

(a) connection to SVC
1. Esophageal varices (= subepithelial + submucosal veins) supplied by anterior branch of left gastric vein
2. Paraesophageal varices (endoscopically not visible) supplied by posterior branch of coronary (= left gastric) vein draining into azygos + hemiazygos vv. + vertebral plexus
   ◊ NOT connected to esophageal varices!
   √ mediastinal / lung mass on CXR in 5–8%

(b) connection to pulmonary circulation
1. Gastropulmonary shunt (between gastric / esophageal vv. and left pericardiophrenic / inferior pulmonary vv.)
   √ nodularity along left cardiac border on CXR

(c) retrograde mesenteric flow
1. Veins of Retzius (= anastomoses between portal vein and IVC)
   — ileocolic veins – right gonadal vein – IVC
   — pancreaticoduodenal vein – IVC
   — proximal small left branches of SMV – left gonadal vein – left renal vein
   — ileocolic veins – directly into IVC

(d) retroperitoneal collaterals
1. Splenorenal / splenoadrenorenal shunt
2. Gastrorenal shunt
3. Mesenterorenal shunt (between SMV + right renal v.)
4. Mesenterogonadal shunt (between ileocolic v. + right testicular v.)
5. Splenocaval shunt (between splenic v. + left hypogastric v.)

(e) intrahepatic shunt (portal v. to hepatic v.)

@ Cruveilhier-von Baumgarten syndrome (20–35%)
= recanalized paraumbilical veins (NOT recanalized umbilical veins)
- √ hypoechoic channel in ligamentum teres
  - (a) size <2 mm (in 97% of normal subjects; in 14% of patients with portal hypertension)
  - (b) size ≥2 mm (86% sensitivity for portal hypertension)
- √ arterial signal on Doppler US in 38%
- √ hepatofugal venous flow (82% sensitivity, 100% specificity for portal hypertension)

@ Spleen
- √ splenomegaly (absence does not rule out portal hypertension)
- √ siderotic Gamna-Gandy nodules in 13% (= small foci of perifollicular + trabecular hemorrhage):
  - √ multiple 3–8-mm low-intensity spots on FLASH / GRASS images
  - √ multiple hyperechoic spots on US
- √ multiple faint calcifications on CT

√ ascites

Cx: Acute gastrointestinal bleeding (mortality of 30–50% during 1st bleeding)

Segmental Portal Hypertension

= splenic vein occlusion / superior mesenteric vein occlusion

Portosystemic Surgical Connections

A. NONSELECTIVE SHUNT
= decompression of the entire portal system with increased risk of hepatic encephalopathy
1. Portacaval shunt
   = portal vein to IVC end-to-side / side-to-side
2. Mesocaval shunt
   = synthetic graft between SMV and IVC
   (a) short "H-graft" to posterior wall of SMV
   (b) long "C-graft" to anterior wall of SMV
   (c) direct mesocaval shunt dividing IVC (rare)
3. Mesorenal shunt
4. Mesoatrial shunt
   = polytetrafluoroethylene (PTFE) graft between anterior wall of SMV superior to pancreas and right atrium coursing through abdomen + diaphragm into right thoracic cavity

B. SELECTIVE SHUNT
= decompression of parts of the portal system with preservation of blood flow to the liver

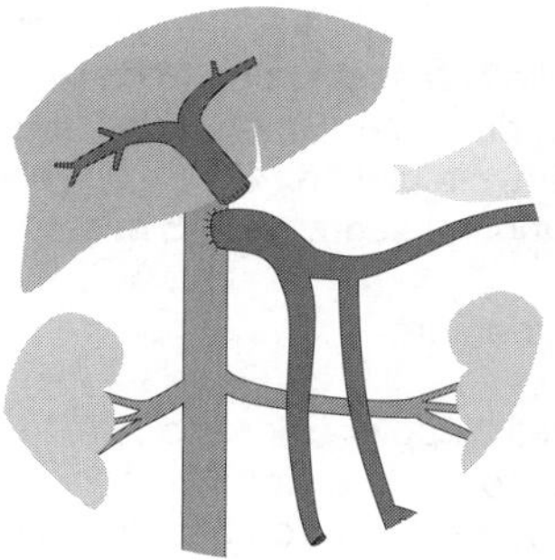
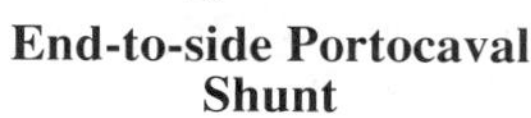
End-to-side Portocaval Shunt

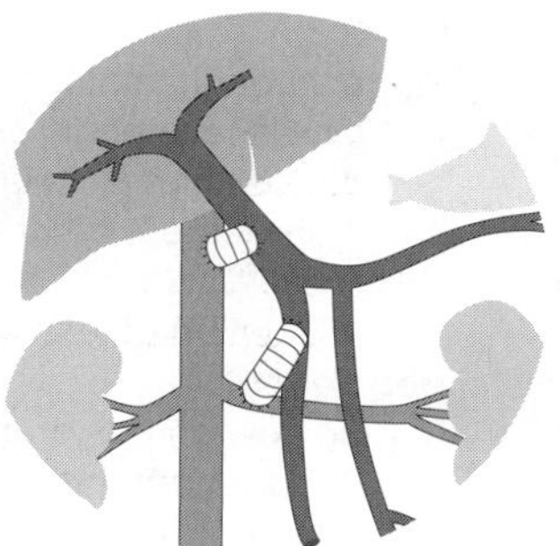
Side-to-side Portocaval and Mesorenal Shunt

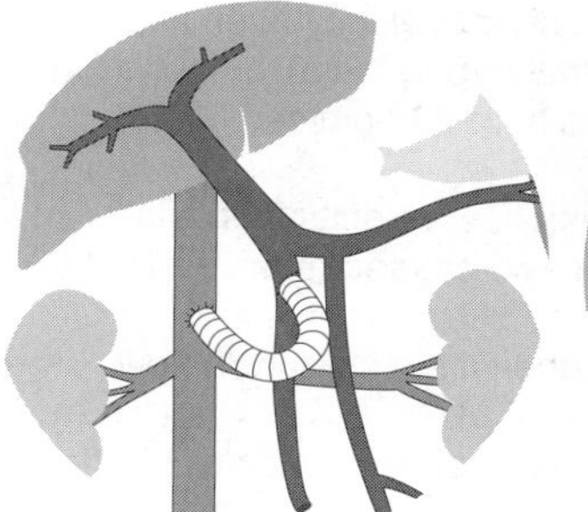
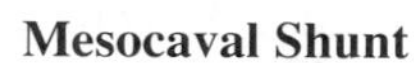
Mesocaval Shunt

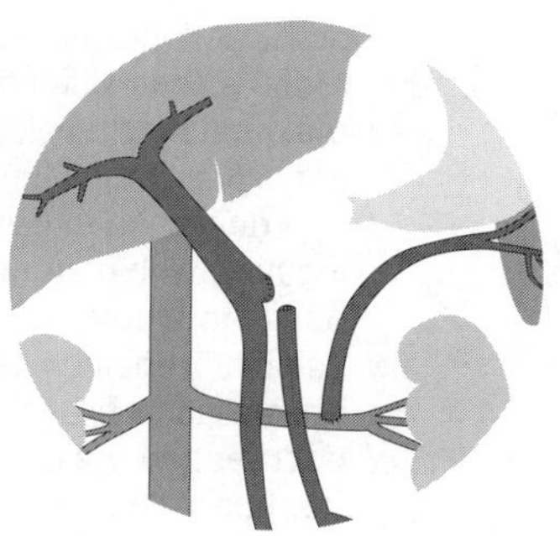
Splenorenal (Warren) Shunt

Surgical Portosystemic Shunts

◊ Contraindicated in patients with ascites

1. Distal splenorenal shunt = Warren shunt (popular) = splenic vein to left renal vein

Doppler criteria for shunt patency:

√ increased local velocities
√ turbulence + severe spectral broadening
√ dilatation of recipient vein at shunt site
√ phasic flow pattern in portal tributaries
√ hepatofugal flow in intrahepatic portal vein branches
√ reduction in size + number of portosystemic collaterals
√ reduction / absence of ascites or splenomegaly

Transjugular Intrahepatic Portosystemic Shunt (TIPS)

= portal decompression through percutaneously established shunt with expandable metallic stent between hepatic + portal veins within the liver

Indication: patients with esophageal + gastric variceal hemorrhage / refractory ascites due to advanced liver disease with portal hypertension, hepatorenal syndrome

Type of stent: 10-mm Wall stent (curved), Palmaz stent (straight), Strecker stent, spiral Z stent

Shunt surveillance: at regular 3–6-month intervals for

A. MORPHOLOGY
   1. Ascites
   2. Portosystemic collaterals
   3. Size of spleen
   4. Diameter of stent (usually 8–10 mm)
   5. Configuration of stent: areas of narrowing
   6. Extension of stent into portal + hepatic veins

B. HEMODYNAMICS
   1. Direction of flow in: extrahepatic portal vein, RT + LT portal vein, SMV, splenic vein, all 3 hepatic veins, intrahepatic IVC, paraumbilical vein, coronary vein
   2. Peak blood flow velocity within main portal vein
   3. Peak blood flow velocity within proximal + mid + distal aspects of stent
   4. Hepatic artery: PSV, EDV, RI

Pre- and post-TIPS baseline study under stable fasting conditions:

	Pre-TIPS	*Post-TIPS*
Portal vein velocity (cm/s)	10–30	40–60
Mean portal vein velocity (cm/s)	18 ± 6	55 ± 7
Portal pressure (mm Hg)	37 ± 8	22 ± 6
Shunt peak velocity (cm/s)		95 ± 58

√ high-velocity turbulent flow (50–270 cm/s) at least double that of pre-TIPS values
√ superimposed cardiac + respiratory variations
√ increase in hepatic artery velocities from 77 cm/s (pre-TIPS) to 119 cm/s (post-TIPS)
√ reversed flow direction within portal vein branches

Cx:
(1) Shunt obstruction (38%)
(2) Hepatic vein stenosis
(3) Vascular injury: hepatic artery pseudoaneurysm, arterioportal fistula
(4) Intrahepatic / subcapsular hematoma
(5) Hemoperitoneum (due to penetration of liver capsule)
(6) Transient bile duct dilatation (due to hemobilia)
(7) Bile collection
(8) Stent dislodgment with embolization to right atrium, pulmonary artery, internal jugular vein

Mortality: <2% (intraperitoneal hemorrhage)

TIPS failure

Cause: acute thrombosis, improper stent placement, intimal hyperplasia, hepatic vein stenosis, change in stent configuration, bulging of liver parenchyma into shunt

Prevalence: 31% at 1 year, 42% at 2 years

• recurrent bleeding = shunt abnormality in 100%

A. >50% stenosis (in 30–80% within 12 months)
   √ irregular filling defects along wall of shunt on color Doppler
   ◊ Pseudointimal hyperplasia is isoechoic to blood!

LIVER

√ gradual decrease in shunt velocity over 1–6 months (due to intimal hyperplasia)
√ maximal shunt velocity of <60 cm/sec (>95% sensitive + specific)
√ in- / decrease in peak flow velocity in similar location within stent >50 cm/sec relative to initial baseline study
√ velocity transition zone within stent with flow acceleration by a factor of 2
√ decrease in maximal portal vein velocity >33% from baseline
√ reversal of portal venous flow direction (100% sensitive, 92% specific, 71% PPV, 100% NPV)
√ loss of pulsatility of portal / shunt flow
√ change in flow direction in collateral veins from baseline
√ retrograde flow in RHV (developing stenosis of right hepatic venous outflow tract)
√ developing / worsening ascites/splenomegaly

B. Occlusion
√ absent flow within shunt
√ echogenic material within stent
– acute cause: prolonged procedural catheterization, leakage of bile into / around stent
– delayed cause: pseudointimal hyperplasia, stent shortening with delayed stent expansion

PORTAL VEIN THROMBOSIS

Etiology:
A. IDIOPATHIC (mostly): ? neonatal sepsis
B. SECONDARY:
(1) Cirrhosis + portal hypertension (5%)
(2) Malignancy: tumor invasion by HCC, cholangiocarcinoma, pancreatic carcinoma, gastric carcinoma, metastasis / extrinsic compression by tumor
(3) Trauma: umbilical venous catheterization; surgery; Cx of splenectomy (7%, higher in patients with myeloproliferative disorders)
(4) Hypercoagulable state: blood dyscrasia; clotting disorder; estrogen therapy; severe dehydration
(5) Intraperitoneal inflammatory process (portal vein phlebitis): perinatal omphalitis; pancreatitis; appendicitis; ascending cholangitis

Age: predominantly children, young persons
• abdominal pain
• portal systemic encephalopathy
• hematemesis (esophageal varices)

Acute Portal Vein Thrombosis

Plain film:
√ hepatosplenomegaly
√ enlarged azygos vein
√ paraspinal varices

UGI:
√ esophageal varices
√ thickening of bowel wall

US:
√ echogenic material within vessel lumen (67%)
√ increase in portal vein diameter (57%)
√ portosystemic collateral circulation (48%)
√ enlargement of thrombosed segment >15 mm (38%)
√ thickening of lesser omentum

Doppler-US:
√ no flow on postprandial Doppler color scans:
◊ Malignant thrombus tends to distend vein + exhibit pulsatile flow, a bland thrombus does not!
√ decrease in hepatic artery resistive index:
√ RI <0.50 (in acute occlusive portal vein thrombosis)
√ minimal decrease / normal RI (in chronic portal vein thrombosis / nonocclusive thrombosis)

NECT:
√ decreased attenuation of affected hepatic parenchyma (due to edema, depletion of hepatocytes, fibrosis)

CECT:
√ transient high attenuation during hepatic arterial phase (due to increased arterial flow)
√ low-density center of portal vein thrombus surrounded by peripheral enhancement:
√ portal vein density 20–30 HU less than aortic density

MR:
√ absent flow void in portal area + abnormal signal intensity in main portal vein
√ hyperintense thrombus on T1WI + T2WI (if <5 weeks old)
√ filling defect on MRA

Angio:
√ "thread and streaks" sign of tumor thrombus (streaky contrast opacification of tumor vessels)

Cx: (1) Cavernous transformation (19%)
(2) Hepatic infarction
(3) Bowel infarction

Chronic Portal Vein Thrombosis

Pathophysiology:
central part (caudate lobe + lateral segment) is well supplied by collateral venous vessels; the peripheral zone (mainly right lobe) receives less portal venous blood resulting in increased arterial flow
√ nonvisualization of extrahepatic portal vein (= fibrotic portal vein)
√ calcification within clot / wall of portal vein
√ cavernous transformation (= **cavernoma**) of portal vein:
√ presence of a racemose conglomerate of collateral veins with portal venous flow linking pancreas + duodenum + gallbladder fossa
√ splenomegaly
√ ascites

CECT:
√ peripheral scattered areas of high attenuation in liver during hepatic arterial phase

LIVER

US:
√ echogenic / nonvisualized portal vein
MR:
√ hypointense portal vein on T1WI + hyperintense on T2WI (2–18 months old)
√ numerous abnormal flow voids in porta hepatis

POSTCHOLECYSTECTOMY SYNDROME

= symptoms recurring / persisting after cholecystectomy
Incidence:
mild recurrent symptoms in 9–25%; severe symptoms in 2.6–32% (result of 1,930 cholecystectomies):
— completely cured (61%)
— satisfactory improvement with
(a) persistent mild dyspepsia (11%)
(b) mild attacks of pain (24%)
— failure with
(a) occasional attacks of severe pain (3%)
(b) continuous severe distress (1.7%)
(c) recurrent cholangitis (0.7%)
Cause:
A. BILIARY CAUSES
(a) Incomplete surgery
1. Gallbladder / cystic duct remnant
2. Retained stone in cystic duct remnant (1%)
3. Overlooked CBD stone (5%)
(b) Operative trauma
1. Bile duct stricture
2. Bile peritonitis
3. Suture granuloma of cystic duct remnant
(c) Bile duct pathology
1. Fibrosis of sphincter of Oddi
2. Biliary dyskinesia
3. Biliary fistula
4. Cystic duct mucocele
(d) Residual disease in neighboring structures
1. Pancreatitis
2. Hepatitis
3. Cholangitis
(e) Overlooked bile duct neoplasia
B. EXTRABILIARY CAUSES (erroneous preoperative diagnosis)
(a) Other GI tract disease:
1. Inadequate dentition
2. Hiatus hernia
3. Peptic ulcer
4. Spastic colon
(b) Anxiety state, air swallowing
(c) Abdominal angina
(d) Carcinoma outside gallbladder
(e) Coronary artery disease

RICHTER SYNDROME

= development of large cell / diffuse histiocytic lymphoma in patients with CLL
Etiology: transformation / dedifferentiation of CLL lymphocytes
Incidence in CLL patients: 3–10%
Median age: 59 years
Medium time interval after diagnosis of CLL: 24 months
• fever (65%) without evidence of infection
• increasing lymphadenopathy + hepatosplenomegaly (46%)
• weight loss (26%), abdominal pain (26%)
Location: bone marrow, lymph nodes, liver, spleen, bowel, lung, pleura, kidney, dura
Prognosis: median survival time: 4 months from diagnosis of lymphoma; 14% rate of remission rate

SCHISTOSOMIASIS

◊ Major cause of portal hypertension worldwide: 200 million people affected
Types:
A. SCHISTOSOMA MANSONI
occurs in >70 million inhabitants of parts of Africa, Caribbean, Arabic peninsula, West Indies, northern part of South America
B. SCHISTOSOMA JAPONICUM
coastal areas of China, Japan, Formosa, Philippines, Celebes
C. SCHISTOSOMA HAEMATOBIUM
in Africa, Mediterranean, Southwest Asia
→ typically affects urinary tract
Cycle:
cercariae enter lymphatics + blood system via thoracic duct; larvae are transported into mesenteric capillaries; mature in portal system + liver into worms; worms live in pairs in copula within portal vein + tributaries for 10–15 years; female swims against blood flow to reach venules of urinary bladder (S. haematobium) or intestine + rectum (S. mansoni, S. japonicum); deposits eggs in wall of urinary bladder or intestines, eggs pass with urine + feces; hatch within water to release miracidia which infect snail hosts; cercariae emerge after maturation from snails
Infection: cercariae penetrate human skin / buccal mucosa from contaminated water (slow-moving streams, irrigation canals, paddy fields, lakes)
Histo: granulomatous reaction + fibrosis along portal vein branches
• clinically mild infection with chronic course
@ Liver & spleen (10%)
√ hepatosplenomegaly
√ portal vein dilatation in 73% (= presinusoidal portal hypertension)
√ marked diffuse thickening of echogenic walls of portal venules = periportal fibrosis
◊ Schistosoma infection is the most frequent cause of liver fibrosis worldwide!
√ normal parenchymal echogenicity + small peripheral hyperechoic foci in 50%
√ hyperechoic gallbladder bed
√ thickened gallbladder wall
√ peripheral septal + capsular "turtle back" calcifications (Schistosomiasis japonicum)
@ GI tract
√ gastric + esophageal varices
√ polypoid bowel wall masses (esp. in sigmoid)

√ granulomatous colitis
√ strictures with extensive pericolic inflammation
Cx: ileus

SCHWACHMAN-DIAMOND SYNDROME

= rare probably autosomal recessive condition characterized by congenital absence of pancreatic exocrine tissue
◊ 2nd most frequent cause of exocrine pancreatic insufficiency in childhood after cystic fibrosis!
• pancreatic insufficiency, steatorrhea
• recurrent respiratory and skin infections (secondary to bone marrow hypoplasia)
• normal electrolytes in sweat
• failure to thrive
• tends to improve with time
√ total fatty replacement of pancreas
√ metaphyseal chondrodysplasia resulting in dwarfism
DDx: cystic fibrosis (pancreatic calcifications, cyst formation, abnormal sweat test)

SOLID AND PAPILLARY NEOPLASM OF PANCREAS

= SOLID AND CYSTIC TUMOR = PAPILLARY-CYSTIC NEOPLASM = SOLID AND PAPILLARY EPITHELIAL NEOPLASM = HAMOUDI TUMOR
= rare, low-grade malignant tumor; often misclassified as nonfunctioning islet cell tumor, cystadenoma, cystadenocarcinoma of pancreas
Prevalence: 0.17–2.7% of all nonendocrine pancreatic tumors
Mean age: 25 (range 10–74) years ; M:F = 1:9; especially in black and East Asian patients
Path: large well-encapsulated mass with considerable hemorrhagic necrosis + cystic degeneration
Histo: sheets + cords of cells arranged around a fibrovascular stroma
• vague upper abdominal discomfort and pain
• gradually enlarging abdominal mass
Location: tail of pancreas (most frequently)
√ well-encapsulated inhomogeneous round / lobulated pancreatic mass with solid + cystic portions
√ may be completely cystic (when complicated by extensive necrosis + internal hemorrhage)
√ fluid-debris level (20%)
√ mean diameter of 9 cm (range 3–15 cm)
√ ± stippled / punctate / amorphous dystrophic calcification (33%)
√ hypovascular with no contrast enhancement / enhancement of solid tissue projecting toward center of mass
US:
√ echogenic mass with necrotic center
MR:
√ high signal intensity on T1WI (consistent with hemorrhagic necrosis)
Prognosis: (1) excellent after excision
(2) metastases (in 4%): omentum, lymph nodes, liver

DDx: (1) Microcystic adenoma (innumerable tiny cysts, older age group)
(2) Mucinous cystic neoplasm (large uni- / multilocular cysts, older age group)
(3) Nonfunctioning islet cell tumor (hypervascular)
(4) Pleomorphic carcinoma of pancreas (smaller tumor in older patient)
(5) Pancreatoblastoma (childhood tumor)
(6) Calcified hemorrhagic pseudocyst

SPLENIC ANGIOSARCOMA

Incidence: rare, <100 cases in literature
Cause: usually not due to thorotrast or toxic exposure to vinyl chloride / arsenic as in liver angiosarcoma
Age: 50–60 years
• splenomegaly, abdominal pain
√ multiple nodules of varying size usually enlarging the spleen
√ solitary complex mass with variable contrast enhancement
√ metastasizes to liver (70%)
√ spontaneous rupture (33%)
MR:
√ focal / diffuse hypointense foci on T1WI + T2WI (iron deposition from hemorrhage)
Prognosis: 20% survival rate after 6 months

SPLENIC HAMARTOMA

= SPLENOMA
= rare typically single nonneoplastic lesion composed of a mixture of normal splenic elements
Etiology: congenital
May be associated with: hamartomas elsewhere as in tuberous sclerosis
Histo: (a) mixture of white + red pulp (most common)
(b) white pulp subtype = aberrant lymphoid tissue
(c) red pulp subtype = aberrant complex of sinusoids
• asymptomatic
CT:
√ attenuation equal to / hypodense to splenic tissue
√ prolonged heterogenous enhancement
MR:
√ heterogeneously hyperintense on T2WI
√ diffuse heterogeneous enhancement, more homogeneous on delayed images

SPLENIC HEMANGIOMA

Cause: congenital, arising from sinusoidal epithelium
Prevalence: 0.03–14% (autopsy); M > F
◊ Most common primary splenic tumor!
Age: 20–50 years
Histo: proliferation of vascular channels lined by single layer of endothelium; mostly of cavernous type; may contain areas of infarction, hemorrhage, thrombosis, fibrosis
Associated with: generalized angiomatosis Klippel-Trénaunay-Weber syndrome, Beckwith-Wiedemann syndrome, Turner syndrome

• asymptomatic / pain + fullness in LUQ
√ usually small single lesion <4 cm, up to 17 cm in size
√ foci of speckled / snowflakelike calcifications
US:
√ well-marginated predominantly hyperechoic lesion
CT:
√ predominantly cystic lesion is avascular
√ solid areas hypo- / isodense to normal spleen and enhancing
MR:
√ hypo- / isointense on T1WI + hyperintense on T2WI
√ hypointense areas due to hemosiderin deposits
√ progressive centripetal enhancement with persistent uniform enhancement on delayed images
NUC:
√ no uptake of Tc-99m sulfur colloid
Prognosis: slow growth, thus becoming symptomatic in adulthood
Cx: (1) Spontaneous splenic rupture (in up to 25%)
(2) Kasabach-Merritt syndrome (= anemia, thrombocytopenia, coagulopathy) with large hemangioma
(3) Portal hypertension
(4) Malignant degeneration

SPLENIC INFARCTION

◊ Most common cause of focal defects!
Cause:
1. Embolic: bacterial endocarditis (responsible in 50%), atherosclerosis with plaque emboli, cardiac thrombus (atrial fibrillation, left ventricular thrombus), metastatic carcinoma
2. Local thrombosis: sickle cell disease (leading to functional asplenia), myelo- / lymphoproliferative disorders (CML most common), polycythemia vera, myelofibrosis with myeloid metaplasia + splenomegaly, Gaucher disease, collagen vascular disease, portal hypertension
3. Vasculitis: periarteritis nodosa
4. Vascular compromise of splenic artery: focal inflammatory process (eg, pancreatitis), thrombus from splenic artery aneurysm, splenic torsion
5. Therapeutic complication: transcatheter hepatic arterial embolization

mnemonic: "PSALMS"
Pancreatic carcinoma, **P**ancreatitis
Sickle cell disease / trait
Adenocarcinoma of stomach
Leukemia
Mitral stenosis with emboli
Subacute bacterial endocarditis

Anatomy: branches of the splenic artery are noncommunicating end arteries
• LUQ pain, fever
• elevated erythrocyte sedimentation rate, leukocytosis
• abnormal lactate dehydrogenase levels
√ single / multiple focal wedge-shaped peripheral defects
√ global infarction
US:
√ initially ill-defined hypoechoic lesion (due to inflammation, edema, necrosis)
√ later increasingly well-defined echogenic lesion (due to organization of infarct with fibrosis)
CT phases:
(a) hyperacute phase (day 1)
√ mottled area of increased attenuation on NECT (hemorrhage)
√ large focal hyperattenuating lesion on CECT
√ mottled pattern of contrast enhancement
(b) acute (days 2–4) + subacute phase (days 4–8)
√ focal progressively more well-demarcated areas of decreased attenuation without enhancement
(c) chronic phase (2–4 weeks)
√ size decreases + attenuation returns to normal
√ complete resolution / residual contour defect
√ areas of calcification
Cx: acute febrile illness, abscess formation, pseudocyst formation, splenic rupture, hemorrhage

SPLENOSIS

= posttraumatic autotransplantation of splenic tissue to other sites
Age: young men with history of trauma / splenectomy
Time of detection: mean of 10 years (range of 6 months to 32 years) after trauma
Location: diaphragmatic surface, liver, omentum, mesentery, peritoneum, pleura (attaches to peritoneal / pleural surface)
√ multiple small encapsulated sessile implants (few mm to 3 cm)
√ demonstrated by Tc-99m sulfur colloid; In-111 labeled platelets; Tc-99m heat-damaged RBC (best detection rate)
Significance:
(1) protects against infection in pediatric patients
(2) may be confused with metastases / lymphoma
(3) responsible for disease recurrence after splenectomy (eg, idiopathic thrombocytopenic purpura)
DDx: accessory spleen

SPONTANEOUS PERFORATION OF COMMON BILE DUCT

Pathogenesis: unknown (? CBD obstruction, localized mural malformation, ischemia, trauma)
Age: 5 weeks to 3 years of age
• vague abdominal distension
• mild persistent hyperbilirubinemia
• varying acholic stools
US:
√ biliary ascites / loculated subhepatic fluid
√ localized pseudocholedochal cyst in porta hepatis
Hepatobiliary scintigraphy:
√ radioisotope diffusely throughout peritoneal cavity

THOROTRASTOSIS

Thorotrast = 25% colloidal suspension of thorium dioxide; used as contrast agent between late 1920s and mid 1950s, in particular for cerebral angiography and liver spleen imaging; chemically inert with high atomic number of 90; >100,000 people injected

Thorium dioxide = consists of 11 radioactive isotopes (thorium-232 is major isotope); decay by means of alpha, beta, and gamma emission; biologic half-life of 1.34 x 10^{10} years; hepatic dose of 1,000–3,000 rads in 20 years

Distribution: phagocytosed by RES + deposited in liver (70%), spleen (30%), bone marrow, abdominal lymph nodes (20%)

√ linear network of metallic density contrast material in spleen, lymph nodes, liver
√ spleen may be shrunken / nonfunctional

Cx: hepatic fibrosis, angiosarcoma (50%), cholangiocarcinoma, hepatocellular carcinoma (latency period of 3–40 years; mean 26 years)

TYROSINEMIA

= rare autosomal recessive metabolic disorder

Country: increased prevalence in Canadian province of Quebec and parts of Scandinavia

Biochemistry: deficiency of enzyme fumarylacetoacetase (last step in catabolic pathway of tyrosine, serum methionine, urinary succinylacetone); elevated levels of serum tyrosine as a precursor of dopamine, norepinephrine, epinephrine, melanin, thyroxin

A. ACUTE FORM
  • fulminant liver failure, often by 1 year of age

B. CHRONIC FORM
  = Fanconi syndrome with renal tubular dysfunction
  • vitamin D-resistant rickets
  • intermittent porphyria-like symptoms

• progressive liver failure in early childhood
• anemia, abnormal liver function tests
• elevated levels of α-fetoprotein
√ hepatosplenomegaly
√ micro- and macronodular cirrhosis (early childhood):
  √ regenerating nodules of 2–20 mm: hyper- (mostly) / iso- / hypoattenuating; hypo- / occasionally hyperechoic
  √ portal hypertension
  √ increased echogenicity (fibrosis + fatty infiltration)
√ nephromegaly with uniformly thickened renal cortices
√ nephrocalcinosis

Prenatal Dx: enzyme deficiency demonstrable in hepatocytes, skin fibroblasts, lymphocytes, amniocytes

Cx: hepatocellular carcinoma (in 37% beyond 2 years of age)

Rx: (1) Diet restricted in phenylalanine + tyrosine (alleviates kidney damage but does not prevent fatal outcome)
(2) 2-2-nitro-4-trifluoro-methylbenzoyl-1,3-cyclohexanedione (NTBC) inhibits 4-hydroxyphenylpyruvate dioxygenase + prevents formation of maleylacetoacetate and fumarylacetoacetate
(3) Liver transplantation (before HCC develops)

UNDIFFERENTIATED SARCOMA OF LIVER

= EMBRYONAL SARCOMA

Incidence: 4th / 5th most common liver tumor in pediatric population

Age: <2 months (in 5%); 6–10 years (in 52%); by 15 years (in 90%); up to 49 years; M:F = 1:1

Histo: primitive undifferentiated stellate / spindle-shaped sarcomatous cells closely packed in whorls + sheets / scattered loosely in a myxoid ground substance with foci of hematopoiesis (50%)

• painful RUQ mass and fever
• mild anemia + leukocytosis (50%)
• elevated liver enzymes (33%)
• fever (5%)

Location: right lobe (75%); left lobe (10%); both lobes (15%)

√ 7–14–21 cm in size
√ well-defined margins (fibrous pseudocapsule)

NUC:
  √ photodefect on sulfur colloid scan

US / CT:
  √ large intrahepatic mass with cystic areas up to 4 cm in diameter (myxoid stroma + necrosis + hemorrhage)
  √ discordant finding between US (solid) + CT (cystlike)

Angio:
  √ hypo- / hypervascular with stretching of vessels
  √ scattered foci of neovascularity

Prognosis: mostly results in death within 12 months

DDx: mesenchymal hamartoma
(a) solid lesion + cystic degeneration:
hepatocellular carcinoma, fibrolamellar carcinoma, intrahepatic cholangiocarcinoma, angiosarcoma, epithelioid hemangio-endothelioma, other sarcomas, lymphoma, metastatic disease, hepatocellular adenoma
(b) solitary cystic lesion:
biliary cystadenoma / biliary carcinoma, cystic degeneration of hepatocellular carcinoma, bacterial / parasitic abscess, metastatic disease, posttraumatic resolving hematoma

WANDERING SPLEEN

= ABERRANT / FLOATING / PTOTIC / DRIFTING / DYSTOPIC / DISPLACED / PROLAPSED SPLEEN

= excessively mobile spleen on an elongated pedicle displaced from its usual position in LUQ

Cause: embryologically absent / malformed gastrosplenic + splenorenal ligaments; deficient / lax abdominal musculature (prune-belly syndrome, pregnancy)

Age: any (higher frequency in women of childbearing age)
- asymptomatic mobile abdominal / pelvic mass
- chronic vague lower abdominal / back pain
- nausea, vomiting, eructation, flatulence
- acute abdomen (with splenic infarction from torsion)

√ empty splenic fossa + associated soft-tissue mass in center of abdomen / pelvis
√ inverted malpositioned stomach
√ splenic hilum often located anteriorly
√ displaced large spleen (congestion during torsion)

Cx:
1. Torsion with prolonged venous occlusion: perisplenitis, localized peritonitis, adhesions, venous thrombosis, hypersplenism
   √ no flow within spleen on Doppler US
   √ elevated resistive index in proximal splenic artery
   √ low attenuation with heterogeneous enhancement on CT
   √ whorled appearance of twisted splenic pedicle
2. Torsion with arterial occlusion: hemorrhagic infarction, subcapsular / intrasplenic hemorrhage, gangrene, degenerative cysts, functional asplenism
3. GI complications:
   @ Stomach: compression, distension, volvulus, traction diverticulum, varices
   @ Small bowel: dilatation, obstruction
   @ Colon: compression, volvulus, laxity, ptosis

Rx:
1. Splenectomy (4% postsplenectomy sepsis)
2. Splenopexy
3. Conservative treatment (if asymptomatic)

DIFFERENTIAL DIAGNOSIS OF GASTROINTESTINAL DISORDERS

ACUTE ABDOMEN IN CHILD
1. Intussusception
2. Appendicitis
3. Obstruction (previous surgery, hernia)
4. Acute gastroenteritis
5. Basilar pneumonia

GASTROINTESTINAL HEMORRHAGE
Mortality: approx. 10%

◊ Barium examination should be avoided in acute bleeders!

Source:

A. UPPER GASTROINTESTINAL HEMORRHAGE
= bleeding site proximal to ligament of Treitz
@ Esophagogastric junction
1. Esophageal varices (17%): 50% mortality
2. Mallory-Weiss syndrome (7–14%): very low mortality

@ Stomach
1. Acute hemorrhagic gastritis (17–27%)
2. Gastric ulcer (10%)
3. Pyloroduodenal ulcer (17–25%)

Mortality: <10% if under age 60; >35% if over age 60

@ Other causes (14%): visceral artery aneurysm, vascular malformation, neoplasm, vascular-enteric fistula
Average mortality: 8–10%

Rx:
(1) Transcatheter embolization (method of choice) abundant collaterals except for postoperative stomach
(2) Intraarterial vasopressin infusion (0.2–0.4 U/min)
Prognosis: controls 73% of gastric mucosal bleeding; high recurrence rate

B. LOWER GASTROINTESTINAL HEMORRHAGE
= bleeding site distal to ligament of Treitz
@ Small intestine
tumor (eg, leiomyoma, hemangioma, metastases), ulcers, diverticula (eg, Meckel diverticulum), inflammatory bowel disease (eg, Crohn disease), vascular malformation, visceral artery aneurysm, aortoenteric fistula

@ Colorectal (70%)
– massive bleeding
1. Diverticula (most common): hemorrhage in 25% of patients with diverticulosis; spontaneous cessation of bleeding in 80%; recurrent bleeding in 25%
2. Colonic angiodysplasia = dilated submucosal arteries + veins overlying mucosal thinning (? secondary to mucosal ischemia)
3. Biopsy

– low-rate bleeding
1. Inflammatory bowel disease
2. Benign / malignant tumor
3. Mesenteric varices

Rx:
(1) Intraarterial vasopressin infusion
Prognosis: 90% initial control rate; in 30% recurrent bleeding
(2) Transcatheter embolization
Requires superselective catheterization using microcatheters + microembolic agents
Cx: 25% risk of bowel infarction + stricture

Gastrointestinal Bleeding in Infant
(1) Peptic ulcer
(2) Varices
(3) Ulcerated Meckel diverticulum

Gastrointestinal Bleeding in Child
(1) Meckel diverticulum
(2) Juvenile polyp
(3) Inflammatory bowel disease

Intramural Hemorrhage
A. VASCULITIS
1. Henoch-Schönlein purpura

B. TRAUMA

C. COAGULATION DEFECT
1. Anticoagulant therapy
2. Thrombocytopenia
3. Disseminated intravascular coagulation

D. DISEASES WITH COAGULATION DEFECT
1. Hemophilia
2. Leukemia, lymphoma
3. Multiple myeloma
4. Metastatic carcinoma
5. Idiopathic thrombocytopenic purpura

E. ISCHEMIA (often fatal)

• abdominal pain
• melena

Site: submucosal / intramural / mesenteric

√ “stacked coin” / “picket fence” appearance of mucosal folds (due to symmetric infiltration of submucosal blood)
√ “thumbprinting” = rounded polypoid filling defect (due to focal accumulation of hematoma in bowel wall)
√ separation + uncoiling of bowel loops
√ narrowing of lumen + localized filling defects (asymmetric hematoma)
√ no spasm / irritability
√ mechanical obstruction + proximal distension of loops

Prognosis: resolution within 2–6 weeks

GI ABNORMALITIES IN CHRONIC RENAL FAILURE AND RENAL TRANSPLANTATION

@ Esophagus
1. Esophagitis: candida, CMV, herpes

@ Stomach & duodenum
1. Gastritis
   √ thickened gastric folds (38%)
   √ edema + erosions
   Cause:
   (a) imbalance of gastrin levels + gastric acid secretion due to
      (1) reduced removal of gastrin from kidney with loss of cortical mass
      (2) impaired acid feedback mechanism
      (3) hypochlorhydria
   (b) opportunistic infection (eg, CMV)
2. Gastric ulcer (3.5%)
3. Duodenal ulcer (2.4%)
4. Duodenitis (47%)

@ Colon
More severely + frequently affected after renal transplantation
1. Progressive distention + pseudoobstruction
   Contributing factors: dehydration, alteration of diet, inactivity, nonabsorbable antacids, high-dose steroids
2. Ischemic colitis
   (a) primary disease responsible for end-stage renal disease (eg, diabetes, vasculitis)
   (b) trauma of renal transplantation
3. Diverticulitis
   Contributing factors: chronic obstipation, steroids, autonomic nervous dysfunction
4. Pseudomembranous colitis
5. Uremic colitis = nonspecific colitis
6. Spontaneous colonic perforation
   Cause: nonocclusive ischemia, diverticula, duodenal + gastric ulcers

@ Pancreas
1. Pancreatitis
   Cause: hypercalcemia, steroids, infection, immunosuppressive agents, trauma

@ General
1. GI hemorrhage
   Cause: gastritis, ulcers, colonic diverticula, ischemic bowel, infectious colitis, pseudomembranous colitis, nonspecific cecal ulceration
2. Bowel perforation (in 1–4% of transplant recipients)
3. Opportunistic infection
   Organism: Candida, herpes, CMV, strongyloides
4. Malignancy
   (a) skin tumors
   (b) lymphoma

ENTEROPATHY

Protein-losing Enteropathy

A. DISEASE WITH MUCOSAL ULCERATION
   1. Carcinoma
   2. Lymphoma
   3. Inflammatory bowel disease
   4. Peptic ulcer disease
B. HYPERTROPHIED GASTRIC RUGAE
   1. Ménétrier disease
C. NONULCERATIVE MUCOSAL DISEASE
   1. Celiac disease
   2. Tropical sprue
   3. Whipple disease
   4. Allergic gastroenteropathy
   5. Gastrocolic fistula
   6. Villous adenoma of colon
D. LYMPHATIC OBSTRUCTION
   1. Intestinal lymphangiectasia
E. HEART DISEASE
   1. Constrictive pericarditis
   2. Tricuspid insufficiency

Malabsorption

= deficient absorption of any essential food materials within small bowel

A. PRIMARY MALABSORPTION
   = the digestive abnormality is the only abnormality present
   1. Celiac disease = nontropical sprue
   2. Tropical sprue
   3. Disaccharidase deficiencies

B. SECONDARY MALABSORPTION
   = occurring during course of gastrointestinal disease
   (a) enteric
      1. Whipple disease
      2. Parasites: hookworm, Giardia, fish tapeworm
      3. Mechanical defects: fistulas, blind loops, adhesions, volvulus, short circuits
      4. Neurologic: diabetes, functional diarrhea
      5. Inflammatory: enteritis (viral, bacterial, fungal, nonspecific)
      6. Endocrine: Zollinger-Ellison syndrome
      7. Drugs: neomycin, phenindione, cathartics
      8. Collagen disease: scleroderma, lupus, polyarteritis
      9. Lymphoma
      10. Benign + malignant small bowel tumors
      11. Vascular disease
      12. CHF, agammaglobulinemia, amyloid, abetalipoproteinemia, intestinal lymphangiectasia
   (b) gastric
      vagotomy, gastrectomy, pyloroplasty, gastric fistula (to jejunum, ileum, colon)
   (c) pancreatic
      pancreatitis, pancreatectomy, pancreatic cancer, cystic fibrosis
   (d) hepatobiliary
      intra- and extrahepatic biliary obstruction, acute + chronic liver disease

Roentgenographic Signs in Malabsorption

√ SMALL BOWEL WITH NORMAL FOLDS + FLUID
1. Maldigestion (deficiency of bile salt / pancreatic enzymes)
2. Gastric surgery
3. Alactasia

√ SMALL BOWEL WITH NORMAL FOLDS + WET
1. Sprue
2. Dermatitis herpetiformis

√ DILATED DRY SMALL BOWEL
1. Scleroderma
2. Dermatomyositis
3. Pseudoobstruction: no peristaltic activity

√ DILATED WET SMALL BOWEL
1. Sprue
2. Obstruction
3. Blind loop

√ THICKENED STRAIGHT FOLDS + DRY SMALL BOWEL
1. Amyloidosis (malabsorption is unusual)
2. Radiation
3. Ischemia
4. Lymphoma (rare)
5. Macroglobulinemia (rare)

√ THICKENED STRAIGHT FOLDS + WET SMALL BOWEL
1. Zollinger-Ellison syndrome
2. Abetalipoproteinemia: rare inherited disease characterized by CNS damage, retinal abnormalities, steatorrhea, acanthocytosis

√ THICKENED NODULAR IRREGULAR FOLDS + DRY SMALL BOWEL
1. Lymphoid hyperplasia
2. Lymphoma
3. Crohn disease
4. Whipple disease
5. Mastocytosis

√ THICKENED NODULAR IRREGULAR FOLDS + WET SMALL BOWEL
1. Lymphangiectasia
2. Giardiasis
3. Whipple disease (rare)

Small Bowel Nodularity with Malabsorption

mnemonic: "**W**hat **I**s **H**is **M**ain **A**im? **L**ay **E**ggs, **B**y **G**od"

Whipple disease
Intestinal lymphangiectasia
Histiocytosis
Mastocytosis
Amyloidosis
Lymphoma, **L**ymph node hyperplasia
Edema
Blood
Giardiasis

ABDOMINAL MASS

Abdominal Mass in Neonate

A. RENAL (55%)
1. Hydronephrosis (25%)
2. Multicystic dysplastic kidney (15%)
3. Polycystic kidney
4. Mesoblastic nephroma
5. Renal vein thrombosis

B. GENITAL (15%)
1. Ovarian cyst
2. Hydrometrocolpos

C. GASTROINTESTINAL (15%)
1. Duplication
2. Volvulus
3. Cystic meconium peritonitis
4. Mesenteric cyst

D. NONRENAL RETROPERITONEAL (10%)
1. Adrenal hemorrhage
2. Neuroblastoma
3. Teratoma

E. HEPATOBILIARY (5%)
1. Hemangioendothelioma
2. Choledochal cyst
3. Hydrops of gallbladder

Abdominal Mass in Infant & Child

A. RENAL (55%)
1. Wilms tumor (22%)
2. Hydronephrosis (20%)
3. Cystic renal mass
4. Congenital anomaly

B. NONRENAL RETROPERITONEAL (23%)
1. Neuroblastoma (21%)
2. Teratoma

C. GASTROINTESTINAL (18%)
1. Appendiceal abscess (10%)
2. Hepatobiliary (6%)

D. GENITAL (4%)
1. Ovarian cyst / teratoma
2. Hydrometrocolpos

ABNORMAL INTRAABDOMINAL AIR

Abnormal Air Collection

1. Abnormally located bowel
   Chilaiditi syndrome (= colon interposed between liver and chest wall), inguinal hernia
2. Pneumoperitoneum
3. Retropneumoperitoneum
   perforation of duodenum / rectum / ascending + descending colon, diverticulitis, ulcerative disease, endoscopic procedure
4. Gas in bowel wall
   gastric pneumatosis, phlegmonous gastritis, endoscopy, rupture of lung bulla

5. Gas within abscess
located in subphrenic, renal, perirenal, hepatic, pancreatic space, lesser sac
6. Gas in biliary system = pneumobilia
7. Gas in portal venous system

Pneumoperitoneum

Etiology:

A. DISRUPTION OF WALL OF HOLLOW VISCUS
  (a) blunt / penetrating trauma
    1. Perforating foreign body (eg, thermometer injury to rectum, vaginal stimulator in rectum)
    2. Compressor air directed toward anus
  (b) iatrogenic perforation
    1. Laparoscopy / laparotomy (58%): absorbed in 1–24 days dependent on initial amount of air introduced and body habitus (80% in asthenic, 25% in obese patients)
       ◊ After 3 days free air should be followed with suspicion!
    2. Leaking surgical anastomosis
    3. Endoscopic perforation
    4. Enema tip injury
    5. Diagnostic pneumoperitoneum
  (c) diseases of GI tract
    1. Perforated gastric / duodenal ulcer
    2. Perforated appendix
    3. Ingested foreign-body perforation
    4. Diverticulitis (ruptured Meckel diverticulum / sigmoid diverticulum, jejunal diverticulosis)
    5. Necrotizing enterocolitis with perforation
    6. Inflammatory bowel disease (eg, toxic megacolon)
    7. Obstruction† (gas traversing intact mucosa): neoplasm, imperforate anus, Hirschsprung disease, meconium ileus
    8. Ruptured pneumatosis cystoides intestinalis† with "balanced pneumoperitoneum" (= free intraperitoneal air acts as tamponade of pneumatosis cysts thus maintaining a balance between intracystic air + pneumoperitoneum)
    9. Idiopathic gastric perforation = spontaneous perforation in premature infants (congenital gastric muscular wall defect)

B. THROUGH PERITONEAL SURFACE
  (a) transperitoneal manipulation
    1. Abdominal needle biopsy / catheter placement
    2. Mistaken thoracentesis / chest tube placement
    3. Endoscopic biopsy
  (b) extension from chest†
    1. Dissection from pneumomediastinum (positive pressure breathing, rupture of bulla / bleb, chest surgery)
    2. Bronchopleural fistula
  (c) rupture of urinary bladder
  (d) penetrating abdominal injury

C. THROUGH FEMALE GENITAL TRACT†
  (a) iatrogenic
    1. Perforation of uterus / vagina
    2. Culdocentesis
    3. Rubin test = tubal patency test
    4. Pelvic examination
  (b) spontaneous
    1. Intercourse, orogenital insufflation
    2. Douching
    3. Knee-chest exercise, water skiing, horseback riding

D. INTRAPERITONEAL
    1. Gas-forming peritonitis
    2. Rupture of abscess

Note † = asymptomatic spontaneous pneumoperitoneum without peritonitis

√ air in lesser peritoneal sac
√ gas in scrotum (through open processus vaginalis)

<u>Large collection of gas</u>:
√ abdominal distension, no gastric air-fluid level
√ "football sign" = large pneumoperitoneum outlining entire abdominal cavity
√ "double wall sign" = "Rigler sign" = "bas-relief sign" = air on both sides of bowel as intraluminal gas + free air outside (usually requires >1,000 mL of free intraperitoneal gas + intraperitoneal fluid)
√ "telltale triangle sign" = triangular air pocket between 3 loops of bowel
√ depiction of diaphragmatic muscle slips = two or three 6–13-cm long and 8–10-mm wide arcuate soft-tissue bands directed vertically inferiorly + arching parallel to diaphragmatic dome superiorly
√ outline of ligaments of anterior inferior abdominal wall:
√ "inverted V sign" = outline of both lateral umbilical ligaments (containing inferior epigastric vessels)
√ outline of medial umbilical ligaments (obliterated umbilical arteries)
√ "urachus sign" = outline of middle umbilical ligament

<u>RUQ gas</u> (best place to look for small collections):
√ single large area of hyperlucency over the liver
√ oblique linear area of hyperlucency outlining the posteroinferior margin of liver
√ doge's cap sign = triangular collection of gas in Morison pouch (posterior hepatorenal space)
√ outline of falciform ligament = long vertical line to the right of midline extending from ligamentum teres notch to umbilicus; most common structure outlined
√ ligamentum teres sign = air outlining fissure of ligamentum teres hepatis (= posterior free edge of falciform ligament) seen as vertically oriented sharply defined slitlike / oval area of hyperlucency between 10th and 12th rib within 2.5–4.0 cm of right vertebral border 2–7 mm wide and 6–20 mm long

√ ligamentum teres notch = inverted V-shaped area of hyperlucency along undersurface of liver
√ "saddlebag / mustache / cupola sign" = gas trapped below central tendon of diaphragm
√ parahepatic air = gas bubble lateral to right edge of liver

Pseudopneumoperitoneum

= process mimicking free air

A. ABDOMINAL GAS
  (a) gastrointestinal gas
    1. Pseudo-wall sign = apposition of gas-distended bowel loops
    2. Chilaiditi syndrome
    3. Diaphragmatic hernia
    4. Diverticulum of esophagus / stomach / duodenum
  (b) extraintestinal gas
    1. Retroperitoneal air
    2. Subdiaphragmatic abscess
B. CHEST
  1. Pneumothorax
  2. Empyema
  3. Irregularity of diaphragm
C. FAT
  1. Subdiaphragmatic intraperitoneal fat
  2. Interposition of omental fat between liver + diaphragm

Pneumoretroperitoneum

Cause: (1) Traumatic rupture (usually duodenum)
(2) Perforation of duodenal ulcer
(3) Gas abscess of pancreas (usually extends into lesser sac)
(4) Urinary tract gas (trauma, infection)
(5) Dissected mediastinal air

√ kidney outlined by gas
√ outline of psoas margin ± gas streaks in muscle bundles

Pneumatosis Intestinalis

= PNEUMATOSIS CYSTOIDES INTESTINALIS = BULLOUS EMPHYSEMA OF THE INTESTINE = INTESTINAL GAS CYSTS = PERITONEAL LYMPHOPNEUMATOSIS

◊ Attributed to at least 58 causative factors!

A. BOWEL NECROSIS / GANGRENE
  ◊ Most common + life-threatening cause!
  Pathogenesis: damage + disruption of mucosa with entry of gas-forming bacteria into bowel wall (cysts contain 50% hydrogen = evidence of bacterial origin)
  necrotizing enterocolitis, ischemia + infarction (mesenteric thrombosis), neutropenic colitis, sepsis, volvulus, emphysematous gastritis, caustic ingestion
B. MUCOSAL DISRUPTION
  Pathogenesis: increased intestinal gas pressure leads to overdistension and dissection of gas into bowel wall
  (a) intestinal obstruction:
  pyloric stenosis, annular pancreas, imperforate anus, Hirschsprung disease, meconium plug syndrome, obstructing neoplasm
  (b) intestinal trauma:
  endoscopy ± biopsy, biliary stent perforation, sclerotherapy, bowel surgery, postoperative bowel anastomosis, penetrating / blunt abdominal trauma, trauma of child abuse, intracatheter jejunal feeding tube, barium enema
  (c) infection / inflammation:
  peptic ulcer disease, intestinal parasites, tuberculosis, peritonitis, inflammatory bowel disease (Crohn disease, ulcerative colitis, pseudomembranous colitis), ruptured jejunal diverticula, Whipple disease, systemic amyloidosis
C. INCREASED MUCOSAL PERMEABILITY
  Pathogenesis: defects in lymphoid tissue of bowel wall allows bacterial gas to enter bowel wall
  (a) immunotherapy:
  graft-versus-host disease, organ transplantation, bone marrow transplantation
  (b) others:
  AIDS enterocolitides, steroid therapy, chemotherapy, radiation therapy, collagen vascular disease (scleroderma, systemic lupus erythematosus, periarteritis dermatomyositis), intestinal bypass enteropathy, diabetes mellitus
D. PULMONARY DISEASE
  Pathogenesis: alveolar rupture with air dissecting interstitially along bronchovascular bundles to mediastinum + retroperitoneally along vascular supply of viscera
  Chronic obstructive pulmonary disease (chronic bronchitis, emphysema, bullous disease of lung), asthma, cystic fibrosis, chest trauma (barotrauma from artificial ventilation, chest tube), increased intrathoracic pressure associated with retching + vomiting

Path: (a) microvesicular type = 10–100-mm cysts / bubbles within lamina propria
(b) linear / curvilinear type = streaks of gas oriented parallel to bowel wall

Location: any part of GI tract; may be discontinuous with spread to distant sites along mesentery

Site: subserosa > submucosa > muscularis > mesentery; mesenteric side >> antimesenteric side

√ radiolucent clusters of cysts along contour of bowel wall (best demonstrated on CT)
√ segmental mucosal nodularity (DDx: polyposis)
√ ± pneumoperitoneum / pneumoretroperitoneum (asymptomatic large pneumoperitoneum may persist for months / years)
√ ± gas in mesenteric + portal vein

Prognosis:
wide spectrum from innocuous to fatal; clinical outcome impossible to predict based on x-ray findings

GI

◊ Linear gas collections probably have a more severe connotation
◊ Pneumatosis of the colon is likely clinically insignificant
◊ Extent of pneumatosis is inversely related to severity of disease

Soap-bubble Appearance in Abdomen of Neonate

1. Feces in infant fed by mouth
2. Meconium ileus:
gas mixed with meconium, usually RLQ
3. Meconium plug:
gas in and around plug, in distribution of colon
4. Necrotizing enterocolitis: submucosal pneumatosis
5. Atresia / severe stenosis: pneumatosis
6. Hirschsprung disease:
impacted stool, sometimes pneumatosis

ABDOMINAL CALCIFICATIONS & OPACITIES

Opaque Material in Bowel

mnemonic: "CHIPS"
Chloral hydrate
Heavy metals (lead)
Iron
Phenothiazines
Salicylates

Diffuse Abdominal Calcifications

1. Cystadenoma of ovary
√ granular, sandlike psammomatous calcifications
2. Pseudomyxoma peritonei
(a) pseudomucinous adenoma of ovary
(b) mucocele of appendix
3. Undifferentiated abdominal malignancy
4. Tuberculous peritonitis
√ mottled calcifications simulating residual barium
5. Meconium peritonitis
6. Oil granuloma
√ annular / plaquelike calcifications

Focal Alimentary Tract Calcifications

A. ENTEROLITHS
1. Appendicolith: in 10–15% of acute appendicitis
2. Stone in Meckel diverticulum
3. Diverticular stone
4. Rectal stone
5. Proximal to partial obstruction (eg, tuberculosis, Crohn disease)

B. MESENTERIC CALCIFICATIONS
1. Dystrophic calcification of omental fat deposits + appendices epiploicae (secondary to infarction / pancreatitis / TB)
2. Cysts: mesenteric cyst, hydatid cyst
3. Calcified mesenteric lipoma

C. INGESTED FOREIGN BODIES
trapped in appendix, diverticula, proximal to stricture
1. Calcified seeds + pits (bezoar)
2. Birdshot
Location of intraluminal lodgement:
esophagus (68%), stomach (11.6%), small bowel (3.3%), colon (11.6%)

D. TUMOR
1. Mucocele of appendix
√ crescent-shaped / circular calcification
2. Mucinous adenocarcinoma of stomach / colon
= COLLOID CARCINOMA
√ small mottled / punctate calcifications in primary site ± in regional lymph node metastases, adjacent omentum, metastatic liver foci
3. Gastric / esophageal leiomyoma: calcifies in 4%
4. Lipoma

Abdominal Wall Calcifications

A. IN SOFT TISSUES
1. Hypercalcemic states
2. Idiopathic calcinosis

B. IN MUSCLE
(a) parasites:
1. Cysticercosis = Taenia solium
√ round / slightly elongated calcifications
2. Guinea worm = dracunculiasis
√ stringlike calcifications up to 12 cm long
(b) injection sites
from quinine, bismuth, calcium gluconate, calcium penicillin
(c) myositis ossificans

C. IN SKIN
1. Soft-tissue nodules: papilloma, neurofibroma, melanoma, nevi
2. Scar:
√ linear density
3. Colostomy / ileostomy
4. Tattoo markings

Abdominal Vascular Calcifications

A. ARTERIES
1. Atheromatous plaques
2. Arterial calcifications in diabetes mellitus

B. VEINS
phleboliths = calcified thrombus, generally seen below interspinous line
1. Normal / varicose veins
2. Hemangioma

C. LYMPH NODES
1. Histoplasmosis / tuberculosis
2. Chronic granulomatous disease
3. Residual lymphographic contrast
4. Silicosis

ABNORMAL INTRAABDOMINAL FLUID

Ascites

A. TRANSUDATE
(1) Cirrhosis (75%): poor prognostic sign
(2) Hypoproteinemia
(3) CHF
(4) Constrictive pericarditis
(5) Chronic renal failure

(6) Budd-Chiari syndrome

B. EXUDATE
(1) Carcinomatosis
(2) Polyserositis
(3) TB peritonitis
(4) Pancreatitis
(5) Meigs syndrome

C. HEMORRHAGIC / CHYLOUS FLUID

Early signs (accumulation in pelvis):
- √ round central density in pelvis + ill-defined bladder top
- √ thickening of peritoneal flank stripe
- √ space between properitoneal fat and gut >3 mm

Late signs:
- √ Hellmer sign = medial displacement of lateral liver margins
- √ medial displacement of ascending + descending colon
- √ obliteration of hepatic + splenic angles
- √ bulging flanks
- √ gray abdomen
- √ floating centralized loops
- √ separation of loops

High-density Ascites

1. Tuberculosis: 20–45 HU; may be lower
2. Ovarian tumor
3. Appendiceal tumor

Neonatal Ascites

A. GASTROINTESTINAL
(a) perforation of hollow viscus
1. Meconium peritonitis
(b) inflammatory lesions
1. Meckel diverticulum
2. Appendicitis
(c) cyst rupture
1. Mesenteric cyst
2. Omental cyst
3. Choledochal cyst
(d) bile leakage
1. Biliary obstruction
2. Biliary perforation

B. PORTOHEPATIC
(a) extrahepatic portal vein obstruction
1. Atresia of veins
2. Compression by mass
(b) intrahepatic portal vein obstruction
1. Portal cirrhosis (neonatal hepatitis)
2. Biliary cirrhosis (biliary atresia)

C. URINARY TRACT
◊ Urine ascites (most common cause) from lower urinary tract obstruction + upper urinary tract rupture: posterior / anterior urethral valves, ureterovesical / ureteropelvic junction obstruction, renal / bladder rupture, anterior urethral diverticulum, bladder diverticula, neurogenic bladder, extrinsic bladder mass

D. GENITAL
1. Ruptured ovarian cyst
2. Hydrometrocolpos

E. HYDROPS FETALIS
1. Immune hydrops
2. Nonimmune hydrops (usually cardiac causes)

F. MISCELLANEOUS
1. Chylous ascites
2. Lymphangiectasia
3. Congenital syphilis, trauma
4. Idiopathic

Chylous Ascites

IN ADULTS:	1. Inflammatory process	(35%)
	2. Tumor	(30%)
	3. Idiopathic	(23%)
	4. Trauma	(11%)
	5. Congenital	(1%)
IN CHILDREN:	1. Congenital	(39%)
	2. Inflammatory process	(15%)
	3. Trauma	(12%)
	4. Tumor	(3%)
	5. Idiopathic	(33%)

Fluid Collections

mnemonic: "BLUSCHINGS"

Biloma
Lymphocele, **L**ymphangioma, **L**ymphoma (almost anechoic by US)
Urinoma
Seroma
Cyst (pseudocyst, peritoneal inclusion cyst)
Hematoma (aneurysm, AVM)
Infection, **I**nfestation (empyema, abscess, Echinococcus)
Neoplasm (necrotic)
GI tract (dilated loops, ileus, duplication)
Serosa (ascites, pleural fluid, pericardial effusion)

Intraabdominal Cyst in Childhood

1. Omental cyst (greater omentum / lesser sac, multilocular)
2. Mesenteric cyst (between leaves of small bowel mesentery)
3. Choledochal cyst
4. Intestinal duplication
5. Ovarian cyst
6. Pancreatic pseudocyst
7. Cystic renal tumor
8. Abscess
9. Meckel diverticulum (communicates with GI tract)
10. Lymphangioma
11. Mesenteric lymphoma
12. Intramural tumor

MECHANICAL INTESTINAL OBSTRUCTION

= occlusion / constriction of bowel lumen

Prevalence: 20% of acute abdominal admissions
- 80% small bowel obstruction
- 20% large bowel obstruction

GI

Air Progression in Neonates

stomach	within minutes after birth
entire small bowel	within 3 hours
sigmoid colon	after 8–9 hours

Cause of Absent Gas in Neonate

1. GI obstruction
2. Mechanical ventilation in severe respiratory distress
3. Continuous gastric suction

Cause of Delayed Passage of Gas in Neonate

1. Traumatic delivery
2. Septicemia
3. Hypoglycemia
4. Brain damage

Passage of Meconium

A. NORMAL
   - in 94% within 24 hours
   - in 99% within 48 hours

   exceptions: prematurity, severely asphyxiated term infants

B. DELAYED PASSAGE
   1. Hirschsprung disease
   2. Ileal / jejunal atresia
   3. Meconium ileus
   4. Meconium plug syndrome
   5. Colon atresia
   6. Imperforate anus

Common Causes of Obstruction in Children

Nursery	Intestinal atresia, midgut volvulus, meconium ileus, Hirschsprung disease, small bowel atresia with meconium ileus, meconium plug syndrome, small left colon syndrome, imperforate anus, obstruction from duplication cyst
First 3 months	Hypertrophic pyloric stenosis, inguinal hernia, Hirschsprung disease, midgut volvulus
6—24 months	Ileocolic intussusception
Childhood	Appendicitis

Terminology:

High obstruction = proximal to midileum
- ◊ Rarely needs further radiologic evaluation
- • bilious vomiting (after first feeding)
- • abdominal distention
- √ few dilated bowel loops

Low obstruction = distal ileum / colon
- ◊ More difficult to accurately localize
- ◊ Requires contrast enema examination to diagnose microcolon, position of cecum, level of obstruction
- • abdominal distention + vomiting
- • failure to pass meconium
- √ many dilated intestinal loops

Intestinal Obstruction in Neonate

- • abdominal distension
- • vomiting
- • failure to pass meconium

1. Duodenal atresia (50%), stenosis (40%), web (10%)
2. Midgut volvulus
3. Jejunal / ileal atresia
4. Meconium ileus
5. Meconium plug syndrome
6. Hirschsprung disease
7. Necrotizing enterocolitis

Neonatal Obstruction with Microcolon

1. Ileal atresia
2. Distal jejunal atresia
3. Meconium ileus

Neonatal Obstruction with Normal Colon

1. Meconium plug
2. Hirschsprung disease

Intestinal Obstruction in Infant & Child

1. Hypertrophic pyloric stenosis
2. Appendicitis
3. Intussusception

Gastric Outlet Obstruction

A. CONGENITAL LESION
   1. Antral mucosal diaphragm = antral web
   2. Gastric duplication: usually along greater curvature, abdominal mass in infancy
   3. Hypertrophic pyloric stenosis

B. INFLAMMATORY NARROWING
   1. Peptic ulcer disease: cause in adults in 60–65%
   2. Corrosive gastritis
   3. Crohn disease, sarcoidosis, syphilis, tuberculosis

C. MALIGNANT NARROWING
   1. Antral carcinoma: cause in adults in 30–35%
   2. Scirrhous carcinoma of pyloric channel

D. OTHERS
   1. Prolapsed antral polyp / mucosa
   2. Bezoar
   3. Gastric volvulus
   4. Postoperative stomal edema

Abdominal plain film:
- √ large smoothly marginated homogeneous mass displacing transverse colon + small bowel inferiorly
- √ one / two air-fluid levels

Duodenal Obstruction

A. CONGENITAL
   1. Annular pancreas
   2. Peritoneal bands = Ladd bands
   3. Aberrant vessel

B. INFLAMMATORY NARROWING
   1. Chronic duodenal ulcer scar
   2. Acute pancreatitis: phlegmon, abscess, pseudocyst
   3. Acute cholecystitis: perforated gallstone

GI

C. INTRAMURAL HEMATOMA
   1. Blunt trauma (accident, child abuse)
   2. Anticoagulant therapy
   3. Blood dyscrasia
D. TUMORAL NARROWING
   1. Primary duodenal tumors
   2. Tumor invasion from pancreas, right kidney, lymph node enlargement
E. EXTRINSIC COMPRESSION
   1. Aortic aneurysm
   2. Pseudoaneurysm
F. OTHERS
   1. Superior mesenteric artery syndrome from extensive burns, body cast, rapid weight loss, prolonged bed rest
   2. Bezoar (in gastrectomized patient)

mnemonic: "VA BADD TU BADD"

child	adult
Volvulus	**T**umor
Atresia	**U**lcer
Bands	**B**ands
Annular pancreas	**A**nnular pancreas
Duplication	**D**uplication
Diverticulum	**D**iverticulum

Abdominal plain film:
√ double-bubble sign = air-fluid levels in stomach + duodenum
√ frequently normal due to absence of gas from vomiting

Jejunal and Ileal Obstruction

= SMALL BOWEL OBSTRUCTION (SBO)

Mortality: 5.5% (*dictum:* "Never let the sun rise or set on small-bowel obstruction")

A. CONGENITAL
   1. Jejunal atresia
   2. Ileal atresia / stenosis
   3. Enteric duplication: located on antimesenteric side, mostly in ileum
   4. Midgut volvulus from arrest in rotation + fixation of small bowel during fetal life
   5. Mesenteric cyst from meconium peritonitis: located on mesenteric side
   6. Meckel diverticulum
B. EXTRINSIC BOWEL LESION
   1. Fibrous adhesions (50–75%) from previous surgery (80%), peritonitis (15%), congenital / uncertain cause (5%)
   2. Hernia (10%)
   3. Volvulus
   4. Masses: extrinsic neoplasm (most commonly advanced peritoneal carcinomatosis), abscess, aneurysm, hematoma, endometriosis
C. LUMINAL OCCLUSION
   (a) swallowed:
      1. Foreign body: in children; mentally disturbed / disabled patients
      2. Bezoar
      3. Gallstone
      4. Inspissated milk
      5. Bolus of Ascaris lumbricoides
   (b) after birth:
      1. Meconium ileus:
         √ microcolon in cystic fibrosis
      2. Meconium ileus equivalent
   (c) other:
      1. Intussusception
      2. Tumor (rare): eg, lipoma
D. INTRINSIC BOWEL WALL LESION
   (a) neoplasm
      1. Adenocarcinoma
      2. Carcinoid tumor
      3. Lymphoma
      4. Gastrointestinal stromal tumor
   (b) inflammatory lesion
      1. Crohn disease
      2. Tuberculous enteritis
      3. Eosinophilic gastroenteritis
      4. Parasitic disease
   (c) vascular insufficiency
      1. Ischemia (arterial / venous occlusion)
      2. Radiation enteropathy
   (d) intramural hemorrhage
      1. Blunt trauma
      2. Henoch-Schönlein purpura
      3. Anticoagulants
   (e) strictures
      1. Surgical anastomosis
      2. Irradiation
      3. Potassium chloride tablets
      4. Massive deposition of amyloid

Plain abdominal radiograph (50–66% sensitive):
√ "candy cane" appearance in erect position = >3 distended small bowel loops >3 cm with gas-fluid levels (>3–5 hours after onset of obstruction)
√ disparity in size between obstructed loops and contiguous small bowel loops of normal caliber beyond site of obstruction
√ small bowel positioned in center of abdomen
√ little / no gas + stool in colon with complete mechanical obstruction after 12–24 hours
√ "stretch sign" = erectile valvulae conniventes completely encircle bowel lumen
√ "stepladder appearance" in low obstruction (the greater the number of dilated bowel loops, the more distal the site of obstruction)
√ "string-of-beads" indicate peristaltic hyperactivity to overcome mechanical obstruction
√ hyperactive peristalsis / aperistalsis = fatigued small bowel

CAVE: little / no gas in small bowel from fluid-distended loops may lead one to overlook obstruction

Location of obstruction:
   (a) valvulae conniventes high + frequent = jejunum
   (b) valvulae conniventes sparse / absent = ileum

Plain abdominal radiographic categories:
1. Normal
   = absence of small intestinal gas / gas within 3–4 variably shaped loops <2.5 cm in diameter
2. Mild small bowel stasis
   = single / multiple loops of 2.5–3 cm in diameter with ≥3 air-fluid levels
3. Probable SBO pattern
   = dilated multiple gas- / fluid-filled loops with air-fluid levels + moderate amount of colonic gas
4. Definite SBO pattern
   = clearly disproportionate gaseous / fluid distension of small bowel relative to colonUGI:

√ "snake head" appearance = active peristalsis forms bulbous head of barium column in an attempt to overcome obstruction
√ barium appears in colon >12 hours

Enteroclysis for adhesive obstruction:
√ abrupt change in caliber of bowel with normal caliber / collapsed bowel distal to obstruction
√ stretched folds of normal pattern
√ angulated + fixed bowel segment

Enteroclysis categories of SBO (Shrake):
(a) low-grade partial SBO
   = sufficient flow of contrast material through point of obstruction so that fold pattern beyond obstruction is readily defined
(b) high-grade partial SBO
   = stasis + delay in arrival of contrast so that contrast material is diluted in distended prestenotic loop with minimal contrast in postobstructive loop leading to difficulty in defining fold pattern after transition point
(c) complete SBO
   = no passage of contrast material 3–24 hours after start of examination

CT (66% accurate, 78% specific, 63% sensitive, [81% sensitive for high-grade obstruction, 48% sensitive for low-grade partial obstruction])
√ small bowel dilatation >2.5 cm (not reliable to distinguish from adynamic ileus):
  √ "small bowel feces" sign = gas bubbles mixed with particulate matter proximal to obstruction
√ discrepant caliber at transition zone from dilated to nondilated bowel:
  √ level of obstruction best determined by relative lengths of dilated versus collapsed bowel
  √ passage of contrast material through transition zone indicates incomplete obstruction

DDx: adynamic ileus (distension of entire small bowel)

US:
√ small bowel loops dilated >3 cm
√ length of dilated segment >10 cm
√ increased peristalsis of dilated segment (may become paralytic in prolonged obstruction)
√ colon collapsed

Closed-loop Obstruction
= obstruction at two points along the course of the bowel at a single site usually with involvement of mesentery

◊ Most common cause of strangulation!

Cause: adhesion (75%), incarcerated hernia

√ fixation of bowel loop = no change in position:
  √ "coffee bean sign" = gas-filled loop
  √ "pseudotumor" = fluid-filled loop
  √ U- or C-shaped dilated bowel loop on CT
√ increasing intraluminal fluid
√ "beak sign" = point of obstruction on CT / UGI
√ "whirl sign" = twisting of bowel + mesentery on CT:
  √ stretched mesenteric vessels converging toward site of obstruction / torsion

Cx: volvulus

Strangulated Obstruction
= impaired circulation of obstructed segment

Prevalence: 5–10–42% of patients with SBO

At risk: patients with acute complete / high-grade SBO; risk increases over time

TRIAD:
(1) closed-loop obstruction of the involved segment (majority of cases)
(2) mechanical obstruction proximal to the involved segment
(3) venous congestion of the involved loop

CT (63–100% detection rate):
√ slight circumferential thickening of bowel wall:
  √ increased wall attenuation
  √ target / halo sign
√ serrated beaklike narrowing at site of obstruction (32–100% specific) = closed loop with regional mesenteric vascular engorgement + bowel wall thickening at the obstructed segment
√ unusual course of mesenteric vasculature
√ vascular compromise of affected bowel:
  √ poor / no enhancement of bowel wall (100% SPECIFIC)
  √ delayed prolonged enhancement of bowel wall
  √ mesenteric haziness due to edema (95% specific)
  √ diffuse engorgement of mesenteric vasculature
  √ localized mesenteric fluid / hemorrhage
√ large amount of ascites
√ pneumatosis intestinalis
√ gas in portal vein

Prognosis:
20–37% mortality rate (compared with 5–8% for a recently reduced simple obstruction) due to delay in diagnosis: 8% for surgery performed in <36 hours, 25% mortality for surgery performed in >36 hours

Acquired Small Bowel Obstruction in Childhood
mnemonic: "AAIIMM"
Adhesions
Appendicitis
Intussusception
Incarcerated hernia

Malrotation
Meckel diverticulum

Small Bowel Obstruction in Adulthood

mnemonic: "SHAVIT"
Stone (gallstone ileus)
Hernia (21%)
Adhesion (49%)
Volvulus
Intussusception
Tumor (16%)

Colonic Obstruction

Incidence: 25% of all intestinal obstructions

A. NEONATAL COLONIC OBSTRUCTION
1. Meconium plug syndrome
2. Colonic atresia
3. Anorectal malformation: rectal atresia, imperforate anus
4. Hirschsprung disease
5. **Functional colonic immaturity** (especially in premies + infants of mothers treated with magnesium or high doses of sedatives / opiates, children with septicemia, hypothyroidism, hypoglycemia, diabetic mothers)
— small left colon syndrome
— meconium plug syndrome

B. LUMINAL OBTURATION
1. Fecal impaction
√ bubbly pattern of large mass of stool
2. Fecaloma
3. Gallstone (in sigmoid narrowed by diverticulitis)
4. Intussusception

C. BOWEL WALL LESION
(a) malignant (60–70% of obstructions): predominantly in sigmoid
(b) inflammatory
1. Crohn disease
2. Ulcerative colitis
3. Mesenteric ischemia
4. Sigmoid diverticulitis (15%)
√ stenotic segment >6 cm
5. Acute pancreatitis
(c) infectious:
– infectious granulomatous process
1. Actinomycosis
2. Tuberculosis
3. Lymphogranuloma venereum
– parasitic disease
1. Amebiasis
2. Schistosomiasis
(d) wall hematoma:
blunt trauma, coagulopathy

D. EXTRINSIC
(a) mass impression
1. Endometriosis
2. Large tumor mass: prostate, bladder, uterus, tubes, ovaries
3. Pelvic abscess
4. Hugely distended bladder
5. Mesenteritis
6. Poorly formed colostomy
(b) severe constriction
1. Volvulus (3rd most common cause): sigmoid colon, cecum, transverse colon, compound volvulus (= ileosigmoid knot)
2. Hernia: transverse colon in diaphragmatic hernia, sigmoid colon in left inguinal hernia
3. Adhesion

Abdominal plain-film patterns:
(a) dilated colon only = competent ileocecal valve
(b) dilated small bowel (25%) = incompetent ileocecal valve
(c) dilated colon + dilated small bowel = ileocecal valve obstruction secondary to cecal overdistension

√ gas-fluid levels distal to hepatic flexure (fluid is normal in cecum + ascending colon); sign not valid with diarrhea / saline catharsis / enema
√ cecum most dilated portion (in 75% of cases); critical at 10 cm diameter (high probability for impending perforation)
◊ The lower the obstruction, the more proximal the distension!

BE: Emergency barium enema of unprepared colon in suspected obstruction!
Contraindicated in toxic megacolon, pneumatosis intestinalis, portal vein gas, extraluminal gas

ILEUS

[ileus = stasis / inability to push fluid along (term does not distinguish between mechanical and nonmechanical causes)]
= ADYNAMIC / PARALYTIC / NONOBSTRUCTIVE ILEUS
= derangement impairing proper distal propulsion of intestinal contents

Cause:
— in neonate:
1. Hyperbilirubinemia
2. Intracranial hemorrhage
3. Aspiration pneumonia
4. Necrotizing enterocolitis
5. Aganglionosis

— in child / adult:
1. Postoperative ileus
• usually resolves by 4th postoperative day
2. Visceral pain: obstructing ureteral stone, common bile duct stone, twisted ovarian cyst, blunt abdominal / chest trauma
3. Intraabdominal inflammation / infection: peritonitis, appendicitis, cholecystitis, pancreatitis, salpingitis, abdominal abscess, hemolytic-uremic syndrome, gastroenteritis
4. Ischemic bowel disease
5. Anticholinergic drugs: atropine, propantheline, morphine + derivatives, tricyclic antidepressants, dilantin, phenothiazines, hexamethonium bromide

6. Neuromuscular disorder: diabetes, hypothyroidism, porphyria, lead poisoning, uremia, hypokalemia, amyloidosis, urticaria, sprue, scleroderma, Chagas disease, vagotomy, myotonic dystrophy, CNS trauma, paraplegia, quadriplegia
7. Systemic disease: septic / hypovolemic shock, urticaria
8. Chest disease: lower lobe pneumonia, pleuritis, myocardial infarction, acute pericarditis, congestive heart failure
9. Retroperitoneal disease: hemorrhage (spine trauma), abscess

mnemonic: "Remember the P's"
Pancreatitis
Pendicitis
Peptic ulcer
Perforation
Peritonitis
Pneumonia
Porphyria
Postoperative
Potassium deficiency
Pregnancy
Pyelonephritis

• intestinal sounds decreased / absent
• abdominal distension
√ large + small bowel ± gastric distension
√ decreased small bowel distension on serial films
√ delayed but free passage of contrast material
Rx: not amenable to surgical correction

Localized Ileus
= isolated distended loop of small / large bowel
= SENTINEL LOOP
Often associated with: adjacent acute inflammatory process
Etiology:
1. Acute pancreatitis: duodenum, jejunum, transverse colon
2. Acute cholecystitis: hepatic flexure of colon
3. Acute appendicitis: terminal ileum, cecum
4. Acute diverticulitis: descending colon
5. Acute ureteral colic: GI tract along course of ureter

GI

Intestinal Pseudoobstruction
A. TRANSIENT PSEUDOOBSTRUCTION
1. Electrolyte imbalance
2. Renal failure
3. Congestive heart failure

B. CHRONIC PSEUDOOBSTRUCTION
1. Scleroderma
2. Amyloidosis

C. IDIOPATHIC PSEUDOOBSTRUCTION
1. Chronic intestinal pseudoobstruction syndrome
   • persistently decreased peristalsis + clinical obstruction

   Age: neonatal period / delayed for months + years
2. Megacystis-microcolon-intestinal-hypoperistalsis syndrome

ESOPHAGUS
Esophageal Contractions
◊ Esophageal motor activity needs to be evaluated in recumbent position without influence of gravity!
PERISTALTIC EVENT = coordinated contractions of esophagus
PERISTALTIC SEQUENCE = aboral stripping wave clearing esophagus

A. PRIMARY PERISTALSIS
= orderly peristaltic sequence with progressive aboral stripping traversing entire esophagus with complete clearance of barium; centrally mediated (medulla) swallow reflex via glossopharyngeal + vagal nerve; initiated by swallowing
√ rapid wave of inhibition followed by slower wave of contraction
◊ Normal peristaltic sequence will be interrupted by repetitive swallowing before peristaltic sequence is complete!

B. SECONDARY PERISTALSIS
= local peristaltic wave identical to primary peristalsis but elicited through esophageal distension = sensorimotor stretch reflex
◊ Esophageal motility can be evaluated with barium injection through nasoesophageal tube despite patient's inability to swallow!

C. TERTIARY CONTRACTIONS
= nonpropulsive esophageal motor event characterized by disordered up-and-down movement of bolus without clearing of esophagus
Cause:
1. Presbyesophagus
2. Diffuse esophageal spasm
3. Hyperactive achalasia
4. Neuromuscular disease:
   diabetes mellitus, parkinsonism, amyotrophic lateral sclerosis, multiple sclerosis, thyrotoxic myopathy, myotonic dystrophy
5. Obstruction of cardia:
   neoplasm, distal esophageal stricture, benign lesion, S/P repair of hiatal hernia

◊ Tertiary activity does not necessarily imply a significant motility disturbance!
Age: in 5–10% of normal adults during 4th–6th decade
(a) nonsegmental = partial luminal indentation
Location: in lower 2/3 of esophagus
√ spontaneous repetitive nonpropulsive contraction
√ "yo-yo" motion of barium
√ "corkscrew" appearance = scalloped configuration of barium column
√ "rosary bead" / "shish kebab" configuration = compartmentalization of barium column
√ no lumen-obliterating contractions

(b) segmental = luminal obliteration (rare)
  √ "curling" = erratic segmental contractions
  √ "rosary-bead" appearance

Abnormal Esophageal Peristalsis

A. PRIMARY MOTILITY DISORDERS
1. Achalasia
2. **Diffuse esophageal spasm**
   - severe intermittent pain while swallowing
   - √ compartmentalization of esophagus by numerous tertiary contractions

   Dx: extremely high pressures on manometry
3. Presbyesophagus
4. Chalasia
5. Congenital TE fistula
6. Intestinal pseudoobstruction

B. SECONDARY MOTILITY DISORDERS
(a) connective tissue disease
1. Scleroderma
2. SLE
3. Rheumatoid arthritis
4. Polymyositis
5. Dermatomyositis
6. Muscular dystrophy

(b) chemical / physical injury
1. Reflux / peptic esophagitis
2. S/P vagotomy
3. Caustic esophagitis
4. Radiotherapy

(c) infection
- — fungal: candidiasis
- — parasitic: Chagas disease
- — bacterial: TB, diphtheria
- — viral: herpes simplex

(d) metabolic disease
1. Diabetes mellitus
2. Amyloidosis
3. Alcoholism
4. Electrolyte disturbances

(e) endocrine disease
1. Myxedema
2. Thyrotoxicosis

(f) neoplasm

(g) drug-related
atropine, propantheline, curare

(h) muscle disease
1. Myotonic dystrophy
2. Muscular dystrophy
3. Oculopharyngeal dystrophy
4. Myasthenia gravis (disturbed motility only in striated muscle of upper 1/3 of esophagus)
   √ persistent collection of barium in upper third of esophagus
   √ findings reversed by cholinesterase inhibitor edrophonium (Tensilon®)

(i) neurologic disease
1. Parkinsonism
2. Multiple sclerosis
3. CNS neoplasm
4. Amyotrophic lateral sclerosis
5. Bulbar poliomyelitis
6. Cerebrovascular disease
7. Huntington chorea
8. Ganglioneuromatosis
9. Wilson disease
10. Friedreich ataxia
11. Familial dysautonomia (Riley-Day)
12. Stiff-man syndrome

Diffuse Esophageal Dilatation

= ACHALASIA PATTERN = MEGAESOPHAGUS

A. ESOPHAGEAL MOTILITY DISORDER
1. Idiopathic achalasia
2. Chagas disease: patients commonly from South America; often associated with megacolon + cardiomegaly
3. Postvagotomy syndrome
4. Scleroderma
5. Systemic lupus erythematosus
6. Presbyesophagus
7. Ehlers-Danlos syndrome
8. Diabetic / alcoholic neuropathy
9. Anticholinergic drugs
10. Idiopathic intestinal pseudoobstruction = degeneration of innervation
11. Amyloidosis: associated with macroglossia, thickened small bowel folds
12. Esophagitis

B. DISTAL OBSTRUCTION
1. Infiltrating lesion of distal esophagus / gastric cardia (eg, carcinoma) = pseudoachalasia
2. Benign stricture
3. Extrinsic compression

mnemonic: "MA'S TACO in a SHell"
Muscular disorder (eg, myasthenia gravis)
Achalasia
Scleroderma
Trypanosomiasis (Chagas disease)
Amyloidosis
Carcinoma
Obstruction
Stricture (lye, potassium, tetracycline)
Hiatal hernia

Air Esophagogram

1. Normal variant
2. Scleroderma
3. Distal obstruction: tumor, stricture, achalasia
4. Thoracic surgery
5. Mediastinal inflammatory disease
6. S/P total laryngectomy (esophageal speech)
7. Endotracheal intubation + PEEP

Abnormal Esophageal Folds

A. TRANSVERSE FOLDS
1. **Feline esophagus**
   frequently seen with gastroesophageal reflux; normally found in cats
   √ transient contraction of longitudinally oriented muscularis mucosae

2. Fixed transverse folds
   due to scarring from reflux esophagitis
   √ stepladder appearance in distal esophagus

B. LONGITUDINAL FOLDS
   normal: 1–2 mm wide, best seen in collapsed esophagus
   √ >3 mm with submucosal edema / inflammation
   1. Gastroesophageal reflux
   2. Opportunistic infection
   3. Caustic ingestion
   4. Irradiation

DDx: (1) Varices
   √ tortuous / serpentine folds that can be effaced by esophageal distension
   (2) Varicoid carcinoma
   √ fixed rigid folds with abrupt demarcation due to submucosal spread

Esophageal Inflammation

A. CONTACT INJURY
   (a) reflux related
   1. Peptic ulcer disease
   2. Barrett esophagus
   3. Scleroderma (patulous LES)
   4. Nasogastric intubation
   (b) caustic
   1. Foreign body
   2. Corrosives
   (c) thermic
   Habitual ingestion of excessively hot meals / liquids

B. RADIATION INJURY

C. INFECTION
   1. Candidiasis
   2. Herpes simplex virus / CMV
   3. Diphtheria

D. SYSTEMIC DISEASE
   (a) dermatologic disorders
   • blistering of skin + mucous membranes in response to minor trauma
   1. Epidermolysis bullosa dystrophica
      Histo: intraepidermal bullae
   2. Benign mucous membrane pemphigoid
      = rare disease of unknown cause
      Histo: subepidermal bullae without acantholysis
      Age: 4th decade; M < F
      √ esophageal lesions (in 2–13%) most frequent at sites of relative stasis (aortic knob, carina, GE junction):
      √ thin smooth webs arising from anterior aspect
      √ stenoses of variable length
   3. Pemphigus vulgaris
   (b) others:
   1. Crohn disease
   2. Graft-versus-host disease
   3. Behçet disease
   4. Eosinophilic gastroenteritis

Esophageal Ulcer

A. PEPTIC
   1. Reflux esophagitis: scleroderma
   2. Barrett esophagus
   3. Crohn disease
   4. Dermatologic disorders: benign mucous membrane pemphigoid, epidermolysis bullosa dystrophica, Behçet disease

B. INFECTIOUS
   1. Herpes
   2. Cytomegalovirus

C. CONTACT INJURY / EXTERNAL INJURY
   1. Corrosives: alkali, strictures in 50%
   2. Alcohol-induced esophagitis
   3. Drug-induced esophagitis
   4. Radiotherapy: smooth stricture >4,500 rads
      √ shallow / deep ulcers conforming to radiation portal
   5. Nasogastric tube
      √ elongated stricture in middle + distal 1/3
   6. Endoscopic sclerotherapy

D. MALIGNANT
   1. Esophageal carcinoma

Location:
   @ Upper esophagus
   1. Barrett ulcer in islets of gastric mucosa
   @ Midesophagus
   1. Herpes esophagitis
   2. CMV esophagitis
   3. Drug-induced esophagitis
   @ Distal esophagus
   1. Reflux esophagitis
   2. CMV esophagitis

DDx:
   (1) Sacculation
   = outpouching in distal esophagus due to asymmetric scarring in reflux esophagitis
   (2) Esophageal intramural pseudodiverticula
   (3) Artifact
   (a) tiny precipitates of barium
   (b) transient mucosal crinkling in inadequate distension
   (c) irregular Z-line

Small Esophageal Ulcer (<1 cm)

1. Herpes simplex virus type I
2. Drug-induced
3. Reflux esophagitis
4. Behçet syndrome
5. Benign mucous membrane pmephigoid
6. Acute radiation change

Large Esophageal Ulcer (>1 cm)

1. Cytomegalovirus
2. Human immunodeficiency virus
3. Carcinoma
4. Drug-induced
5. Barrett esophagus
6. Sclerotherapy for varices

Double-barrel Esophagus

1. Dissecting intramural hematoma from emetogenic injury
2. Mallory-Weiss tear
   trauma, esophagoscopy (in 0.25%), bougienage (in 0.5%), ingestion of foreign bodies, spontaneous (bleeding diathesis)
3. Intramural abscess
4. Intraluminal diverticulum
5. Esophageal duplication (if communication with esophageal lumen present)

Esophageal Diverticulum

1. Zenker diverticulum (pharyngoesophageal)
2. Interbronchial diverticulum
   = traction diverticulum
   response to pull from fibrous adhesions following lymph node infection (TB), contains all 3 esophageal layers
   Location: usually on right anterolateral wall of interbronchial segment
   √ calcified mediastinal nodes
3. Interaorticobronchial diverticulum
   = thoracic pulsion diverticulum
   Location: on left anterolateral wall between inferior border of aortic arch + upper margin of left main bronchus
4. Epiphrenic diverticulum (rare)
   Location: usually on lateral esophageal wall, right > left, in distal 10 cm
   √ often associated with hiatus hernia
5. Intramural esophageal pseudodiverticulosis
   √ outpouching from mucosal glands

Tracheobronchoesophageal Fistula

A. CONGENITAL
   1. Congenital tracheoesophageal fistula
B. MALIGNANCY (in 60%)
   1. Lung cancer
   2. Metastases to mediastinal lymph nodes
   3. Esophageal cancer
      ◊ In 5–10% of patients with advanced esophageal cancer
   4. Radiation treatment of mediastinal malignancy
C. TRAUMATIC
   1. Instrumentation (esophagoscopy, bougienage, pneumatic dilatation)
   2. Blunt ("crush injury") / penetrating chest trauma
   3. Surgery
   4. Foreign-body perforation
   5. Corrosives
   6. Postemetic rupture = Boerhaave syndrome
D. INFECTIOUS / INFLAMMATORY
   1. TB, syphilis, histoplasmosis, actinomycosis, Crohn disease
   2. Perforated diverticulum
   3. Pulmonary sequestration / cyst

Long Smooth Esophageal Narrowing

1. Congenital esophageal stenosis
   √ at junction between middle + distal third
   √ weblike / tubular stenosis of 1 cm in length
2. Surgical repair of esophageal atresia
   √ interruption of primary peristaltic wave at anastomosis
   √ secondary contractions may produce retrograde flow with aspiration
   √ impaction of food
3. Caustic burns = alkaline burns
4. Alendronate (= inhibitor of osteoclastic activity)
5. Gastric acid: reflux, hyperemesis gravidarum
6. Intubation: reflux + compromise of circulation
7. Radiotherapy for esophageal carcinoma; tumor of lung, breast, or thymus; lymphoma; metastases to mediastinal lymph nodes
   Onset of stricture: usually 4–8 months post Rx
   Dose: 3,000–5,000 rad
8. Postinfectious: moniliasis (rare)

Lower Esophageal Narrowing

mnemonic: "SPADE"

Scleroderma
Presbyesophagus
Achalasia; **A**nticholinergics
Diffuse esophageal spasm
Esophagitis

Focal Esophageal Narrowing

1. **Esophageal web**
   = 1–2-mm thick (vertical length) area of complete / incomplete circumferential narrowing
2. **Ring**
   = 5–10-mm thick (vertical length) area of complete / incomplete circumferential narrowing
3. **Stricture**
   = >10 mm in vertical length

mnemonic: "LETTERS MC"

Lye ingestion
Esophagitis
Tumor
Tube (prolonged nasogastric intubation)
Epidermolysis bullosa
Radiation
Surgery, **S**cleroderma
Moniliasis
Congenital

Midesophageal Stricture

1. Barrett esophagus
2. Radiation injury
3. Caustic esophagitis
4. Primary carcinoma: squamous cell carcinoma
5. Metastatic cancer (from subcarinal nodes / left mainstem bronchus)
6. Drug-induced stricture (esp. potassium chloride)
7. Esophageal intramural pseudodiverticulosis

8. Dermatologic disorder: benign mucous membrane pemphigoid, epidermolysis bullosa
9. Graft-versus-host disease

Long Distal Esophageal Stricture

A. SEVERE ACID EXPOSURE
   1. Nasogastric intubation
   2. Zollinger-Ellison syndrome
   3. Alkaline reflux esophagitis
B. INFLAMMATION
   1. Crohn disease

Short Distal Esophageal Stricture

1. Reflux esophagitis
2. Carcinoma (adenocarcinoma)
3. Crohn disease
4. Schatzki ring

Esophageal Filling Defect

A. BENIGN TUMORS
   <1% of all esophageal tumors
   (a) Submucosal tumor (75%)
      = nonepithelial, intramural
      1. Leiomyoma (50% of all benign tumors)
         ◊ Most common submucosal mass in esophagus
      2. Granular cell myoblastoma
      3. Lipoma, fibroma, lipoma, fibrolipoma, myxofibroma, hamartoma, hemangioma, lymphangioma, neurofibroma, schwannoma,
         √ primary wave stops at level of tumor
         √ proximal esophageal dilatation + hypotonicity
         √ rigid esophageal wall at site of tumoral implant
         √ disorganized / altered / effaced mucosal folds around defect
         √ tumor shadow on tangential view extending beyond esophageal margin
   (b) Mucosal tumor (25%) = epithelial, intraluminal
      1. **Squamous papilloma**
         = most common benign mucosal tumor; rarely multiple (esophageal papillomatosis)
         √ small sessile slightly lobulated polyp
      3. **Fibrovascular polyp**
         Path: fibrovascular + adipose tissue
         Location: cervical esophagus near cricopharyngeus
         √ giant sausage-shaped intraluminal mass
         Cx: regurgitation into larynx causes sudden death
      2. **Inflammatory esophagogastric polyp**
         = sentinel polyp = bulbous tip of thickened gastric fold
         Cause: sequelae of chronic reflux esophagitis
         Prognosis: no malignant potential
      3. **Adenoma**
         = originates in Barrett mucosa
         √ sessile / pedunculated polyp
         Cx: malignant degeneration
      4. Glycogen acanthosis
B. MALIGNANT TUMORS
   1. Esophageal cancer
      (a) squamous / varicoid squamous cell carcinoma
      (b) adenocarcinoma
      (c) spindle cell carcinoma: leiomyosarcoma, carcinosarcoma, pseudosarcoma
   3. Carcinoma of cardia (gastric cancer)
   4. Metastases: malignant melanoma, lymphoma (<1% of gastrointestinal lymphomas), stomach, lung, breast
C. VASCULAR
   1. Varices
D. INFECTION / INFLAMMATION
   1. Candida / herpes esophagitis
   2. Drug-induced inflammatory reaction
E. CONGENITAL / NORMAL VARIANT
   1. Prolapsed gastric folds
   2. Esophageal duplication cyst (0.5–2.5% of all esophageal tumors)
F. FOREIGN BODIES
   1. Retained food particles (chicken bone, fish bone, pins, coins, small toys, meat)
   2. Undissolved effervescent crystals
   3. Air bubbles

Esophageal Mucosal Nodules / Plaques

plaque = discrete irregular / ovoid elevation barely protruding above mucosal surface
nodule = small more rounded elevation

1. Candida esophagitis
2. Reflux esophagitis (early stage)
3. Barrett esophagus
4. Glycogen acanthosis
5. Superficial spreading carcinoma
6. Artifacts (undissolved effervescent agent, air bubbles, debris)

Extrinsic Esophageal Impression

Cervical Causes of Esophageal Impression

A. OSSEOUS LESIONS
   1. Anterior marginal osteophyte / DISH
   2. Anterior disk herniation
   3. Cervical trauma + hematoma
   4. Osteomyelitis
   5. Bone neoplasm
B. ESOPHAGEAL WALL LESIONS
   (a) muscle
      1. Cricopharyngeus
      2. Esophageal web
   (b) vessel
      1. Pharyngeal venous plexus
      2. Lymph node enlargement

C. ENDOCRINE ORGANS
  1. Thyroid / parathyroid enlargement (benign / malignant)
  2. Fibrotic traction after thyroidectomy
D. Retropharyngeal / mediastinal abscess

Thoracic Causes of Esophageal Impression

A. NORMAL INDENTATIONS
aortic arch, left mainstem bronchus, left inferior pulmonary vein, diaphragmatic hiatus
B. ABNORMAL VASCULATURE
right-sided aortic arch, cervical aortic arch, aortic unfolding, aortic tortuosity, aortic aneurysm, double aortic arch ("reverse S"), coarctation of aorta ("reverse figure 3"), aberrant right subclavian artery
= arteria lusoria (semilunar / bayonet-shaped imprint upon posterior wall of esophagus), aberrant left pulmonary artery (between trachea + esophagus), anomalous pulmonary venous return (anterior), persistent truncus arteriosus (posterior)
C. CARDIAC CAUSES
  (a) enlargement of chambers
  left atrial / left ventricular enlargement: mitral disease (esophageal displacement backward + to the right)
  (b) pericardial masses
  pericardial tumor / cyst / effusion
D. MEDIASTINAL CAUSES
mediastinal tumor, lymphadenopathy (metastatic, tuberculous), inflammation, cyst
E. PULMONARY CAUSES
pulmonary tumor, bronchogenic cyst, atypical pulmonary fibrosis (retraction)
F. ESOPHAGEAL ABNORMALITIES
  1. Esophageal diverticulum
  2. Paraesophageal hernia
  3. Esophageal duplication

STOMACH

Gastric Tumor

Classification based on Biologic Behavior

A. MALIGNANT (10–15%)
  1. Adenocarcinoma (>95%)
  2. Lymphoma, mucosa-associated lymphoid tissue (MALT)
  3. Sarcoma: leiomyosarcoma, Kaposi sarcoma
  4. Carcinoid tumor
  5. Metastasis
    (a) hematogenous: malignant melanoma, breast cancer
      √ one / more submucosal masses
      √ target / bull's-eye lesion if centrally ulcerated
      √ giant cavitated lesion
      √ linitis plastica (usually in breast cancer)
    (b) direct invasion
      – Barrett cancer: gastric fundus
      – Pancreatic cancer: stomach / duodenal sweep
      – Colonic cancer: greater gastric curvature
      – Omental cake: greater gastric curvature
B. BENIGN (85–90%)
  (a) epithelial / mucosal tumor (50%)
    1. Hyperplastic polyp
    2. Adenomatous polyp
    3. Brunner gland hyperplasia
  (b) mesenchymal tumor (50%)
    1. Leiomyoma
    2. Ectopic pancreatic rest

Mesenchymal Tumors of GI Tract

A. SOMATIC SOFT TISSUE TUMOR
  (a) smooth muscle tumor
    1. True leiomyoma
    2. True leiomyosarcoma
  (b) neural tumor
    ◊ 4% of all benign gastric tumors
    1. Schwannoma
    2. Neurofibroma
    3. Plexosarcoma
  (c) lipocytic tumor
    1. Lipoma (2–3% of all benign gastric tumors)
    2. Liposarcoma
  (d) vascular / perivascular tissue
    ◊ 2% of all benign gastric tumors
    1. Glomus tumor (most common)
    2. Hemangioma
    3. Lymphangioma
B. GASTROINTESTINAL STROMAL TUMOR
= SPINDLE CELL / EPITHELIOID TUMOR
Origin: interstitial cell of Cajal
◊ Largest category of primary nonepithelial neoplasms

Calcified Gastric Tumor

1. Mucinous adenocarcinoma: miliary / punctate
2. Stromal tumors: amorphous calcifications
3. Hemangioma: clusters of phleboliths

Congenital Gastric Obstruction

A. COMPLETE OBSTRUCTION
  1. **Gastric atresia**
  Frequency: <1% of all GI obstructions
  May be associated with: epidermolysis bullosa
  Site: antrum + pylorus
  • regurgitation of bile-free vomitus within first few hours after birth
  √ "single bubble" appearance of air in stomach
  √ membranous mucosal diaphragm
  2. Congenital peritoneal bands
  3. Annular pancreatic tissue
B. PARTIAL GASTRIC OUTLET OBSTRUCTION
  • cyclic transient postprandial vomiting
  1. Incomplete prepyloric diaphragm
  2. Antral stenosis
  3. Aberrant pancreatic tissue in gastric antrum
  4. Antral duplication cyst

Widened Retrogastric Space

A. PANCREATIC MASSES (most common cause)
1. Acute + chronic pancreatitis
2. Pancreatic pseudocyst
3. Pancreatic cystadenoma + carcinoma

B. OTHER RETROPERITONEAL MASSES
1. Sarcoma
2. Renal tumor, adrenal tumor
3. Lymph node enlargement
4. Abscess, hematoma

C. GASTRIC MASSES
1. Leiomyoma, leiomyosarcoma

D. OTHERS
1. Aortic aneurysm
2. Choledochal cyst
3. Obesity
4. Postsurgical disruptions + adhesions
5. Ascites
6. Gross hepatomegaly + enlarged caudate lobe
7. Hernia involving omentum

Gas within Stomach Wall

A. NONINFECTIOUS
1. **Interstitial gastric emphysema**
   = gas accumulation in submucosa / subserosa / or both
   Cause: air from an extrinsic source
   (a) obstructive (due to raised intragastric pressure): gastric outlet obstruction, volvulus, overinflation during gastroscopy, profuse severe vomiting
   (b) pulmonary (due to rupture + dissection of subpleural blebs in bullous emphysema along esophageal wall / mediastinum): pulmonary emphysema
   (c) traumatic (due to mucosal trauma): instrumentation of stomach, recent gastroduodenal surgery, endoscopy (1.6%)
   • benign clinical course with spontaneous resolution
   √ linear lucency conforming to contour of a thin-walled distended stomach
2. **Cystic pneumatosis**
   = PNEUMATOSIS CYSTOIDES INTESTINALIS
   Cause: similar to interstitial gastric emphysema
   • little / no gastrointestinal symptoms
   √ multiple 1–2-mm gas-filled cysts in wall of stomach and intestines

B. INFECTIOUS
1. Emphysematous gastritis
   predisposing: corrosive gastritis, acid ingestion, severe necrotizing gastroenteritis, gastric ulcer disease with intramural perforation, gastric carcinoma, volvulus, gastric infarction

Gastric Atony

= gastric retention in the absence of mechanical obstruction

Pathophysiology: reflex paralysis
• abdominal distension
• vascular collapse (decreased venous return)
• vomiting
√ large stomach filled with air + fluid (up to 7,500 mL)
√ retention of barium
√ absent / diminished peristaltic activity
√ patulous pylorus
√ frequently dilated duodenum

DDx: gastric volvulus, pyloric stenosis

A. ACUTE GASTRIC ATONY
(may develop within 24–48 hours)
1. Acute gastric dilatation: secondary to decreased arterial perfusion (ischemia, congestive heart failure) in old patients, usually fatal
2. Postsurgical atony, ureteral catheterization
3. Immobilization: body cast, paraplegia, postoperative state
4. Abdominal trauma: especially back injury
5. Severe pain: renal / biliary colic, migraine headaches, severe burns
6. Infection: peritonitis, pancreatitis, appendicitis, subphrenic abscess, septicemia

B. CHRONIC GASTRIC ATONY
1. Neurologic abnormalities: brain tumor, bulbar poliomyelitis, vagotomy, tabes
2. Muscular abnormalities: scleroderma, muscular dystrophy
3. Drug-induced atony: atropine, morphine, heroin, ganglionic blocking agents
4. Electrolyte imbalance: diabetic ketoacidosis, hypercalcemia, hypocalcemia, hypokalemia, hepatic coma, uremia, myxedema
5. Diabetes mellitus = gastroparesis diabeticorum (0.08% incidence)
6. Emotional distress
7. Lead poisoning
8. Porphyria

Narrowing of Stomach

= **linitis plastica** type of stenosis

A. MALIGNANCY
1. Scirrhous gastric carcinoma (involving portion / all of stomach)
2. Hodgkin lymphoma, NHL
3. Metastatic involvement (carcinoma of breast, pancreatic carcinoma, colonic carcinoma)

B. INFLAMMATION
1. Chronic gastric ulcer disease with intense spasm
2. Pseudo-Billroth-I pattern of Crohn disease
3. Sarcoidosis
   √ polypoid appearance, pyloric hypertrophy
   √ gastric ulcers, duodenal deformity
4. Eosinophilic gastritis
5. Polyarteritis nodosa
6. Stenosing antral gastritis / hypertrophic pyloric stenosis

C. INFECTION
1. Tertiary stage of syphilis
   √ absent mucosal folds + peristalsis

√ no change over years
2. Tuberculosis (rare)
   √ hyperplastic nodules / ulcerative lesion / annular lesion
   √ pyloric obstruction, may cross into duodenum
3. Histoplasmosis
4. Actinomycosis
5. Strongyloidiasis
6. Phlegmonous gastritis
7. Toxoplasmosis

D. TRAUMA
1. Corrosive gastritis
2. Radiation injury
3. Gastric freezing
4. Hepatic arterial chemotherapy infusion

E. OTHERS
1. Perigastric adhesions (normal mucosa, no interval change, normal peristalsis)
2. Amyloidosis
3. Pseudolymphoma
4. Exogastric mass (hepatomegaly, pancreatic pseudocyst)

mnemonic: "SLIMRAGE"
Scirrhous carcinoma of stomach
Lymphoma
Infiltration from adjacent neoplasm
Metastasis (breast carcinoma)
Radiation therapy
Acids (corrosive ingestion)
Granulomatous disease (TB, sarcoidosis, Crohn)
Eosinophilic gastroenteritis

Antral Narrowing

mnemonic: "SPICER"
Sarcoidosis, **S**yphilis
Peptic ulcer disease
Infection (tuberculosis, chronic granulomatous disease of childhood)
Cancer (linitis plastica), **C**rohn disease, **C**austic ingestion
Eosinophilic gastritis
Radiation

Intramural-extramucosal Lesions of Stomach

√ sharply delineated marginal / contour defect
√ stretched folds over intact mucosa
√ acute angle at margins
√ may ulcerate centrally
√ may become pedunculated and acquire polypoid appearance over years

A. NEOPLASTIC
1. Leiomyoma (48%)
2. Neurogenic tumors (14%)
3. Heterotopic pancreas (12%)
4. Fibrous tumor (11%)
5. Lipoma (7%)
6. Hemangioma (7%)
7. Glomus tumor (rare)
8. Carcinoid
9. Metastatic tumor

B. INFLAMMATION / INFECTION
1. Granuloma
   (1) Foreign-body granuloma
   (2) Sarcoidosis
   (3) Crohn disease
   (4) Tuberculosis
   (5) Histoplasmosis
2. Eosinophilic gastritis
3. Tertiary syphilis: infiltrative / ulcerative / tumorous type
4. Echinococcal cyst

C. PANCREATIC ABNORMALITIES
1. Ectopic pancreas
2. Annular pancreas
3. Pancreatic pseudocyst

D. DEPOSITS
1. Amyloid
2. Endometriosis
3. Localized hematoma

E. OTHERS
1. Varices (ie, fundal)
2. Duplications (4% of all GI tract duplications)

Gastric Filling Defects

A. INTRINSIC WALL LESIONS
(a) benign (most common)
   1. Polyps: hyperplastic, adenomatous, villous, hamartomatous (Peutz-Jeghers syndrome, Cowden disease)
   2. Leiomyoma
   3. Granulomatous lesions
      (1) Eosinophilic granuloma
      (2) Crohn disease
      (3) Tuberculosis
      (4) Sarcoidosis
   4. Pseudolymphoma = benign reactive proliferation of lymphoid tissue
   5. Extramedullary hematopoiesis
   6. Ectopic pancreas
   7. Gastric duplication cyst
   8. Intramural hematoma
   9. Esophagogastric herniation
(b) malignant
   1. Gastric carcinoma, lymphoma
   2. Gastric sarcoma: leiomyosarcoma, liposarcoma, leiomyoblastoma
   3. Gastric metastases: melanoma, breast, pancreas, colon

B. EXTRINSIC IMPRESSIONS ON STOMACH
in 70% nonneoplastic (extrinsic pseudotumors in 20%)
(a) normal organs: organomegaly, tortuous aorta, heart, cardiac aneurysm
(b) benign masses:
   cysts of pancreas, liver, spleen, adrenal, kidney; gastric duplication, postoperative deformity (eg, Nissen fundoplication)
(c) malignant masses: enlarged celiac nodes

GI

(d) inflammatory lesion:
left subphrenic abscess / hematoma
— lateral displacement: enlarged liver, aortic aneurysm, enlarged celiac nodes
— medial displacement: splenomegaly, mass in colonic splenic flexure, cardiomegaly, subphrenic abscess

C. INTRALUMINAL GASTRIC MASSES
1. Bezoar
2. Foreign bodies: food, pills, blood clot, gallstone

D. TUMORS OF ADJACENT ORGANS
1. Pancreatic carcinoma + cystadenoma
2. Liver carcinoma
3. Carcinoma of gallbladder
4. Colonic carcinoma
5. Renal carcinoma
6. Adrenal carcinoma
7. Lymph node involvement

E. THICKENED GASTRIC FOLDS

Filling Defect of Gastric Remnant

A. IATROGENIC
surgical deformity / plication defect, suture granuloma

B. INFLAMMATORY
bile reflux gastritis, hyperplastic polyps

C. INTUSSUSCEPTION
1. **Jejunogastric intussusception**
(efferent loop in 75%, afferent loop in 25%)
(a) acute form: high intestinal obstruction, left hypochondriac mass, hematemesis
(b) chronic / intermittent form: may be self-reducing
√ "coiled spring" appearance of gastric filling defect
2. Gastrojejunal / gastroduodenal mucosal prolapse
• often asymptomatic
• bleeding partial obstruction

D. NEOPLASTIC
1. Gastric stump carcinoma: >5 years after resection for benign disease; 15% within 10 years; 20% after 20 years
2. Recurrent carcinoma (10%) secondary to incomplete removal of gastric cancer
3. Malignancy at anastomosis (incomplete resection)

E. INTRALUMINAL MATTER: bezoar

mnemonic: "PUBLICS"
Polyp (hyperplastic polyp due to bile reflux)
Ulcer (anastomotic)
Bezoar, **B**lind loop syndrome
Loop (afferent loop syndrome)
Intussusception at gastrojejunostomy
Cancer (recurrent, residual, de novo)
Surgical deformity, **S**uture granuloma

Thickened Gastric Folds

A. INFLAMMATION / INFECTION
1. Inflammatory gastritis:
alcoholic, hypertrophic, antral, corrosive, postirradiation, gastric cooling
2. Crohn disease
3. Sarcoidosis
4. Infectious gastritis:
bacterial invasion, bacterial toxins from botulism, diphtheria, dysentery, typhoid fever, anisakiasis, TB, syphilis
5. Pseudolymphoma

B. MALIGNANCY
1. Lymphoma
2. Gastric carcinoma

C. INFILTRATIVE PROCESS
1. Eosinophilic gastritis
2. Amyloidosis

D. PANCREATIC DISEASE
1. Pancreatitis
2. Direct extension from pancreatic carcinoma

E. OTHERS
1. Zollinger-Ellison syndrome
2. Ménétrier disease
3. Gastric varices

mnemonic: "ZEAL VOLUMES C^3P^3"
Zollinger-**E**llison syndrome
Amyloidosis
Lymphoid hyperplasia
Varices
Operative defect
Lymphoma
Ulcer disease (peptic)
Ménétrier disease
Eosinophilic gastroenteritis
Syphilis
Crohn disease, **C**arcinoma, **C**orrosive gastritis
Pancreatitis, **P**ancreatic carcinoma, **P**ostradiation gastritis

Bull's-eye Lesions

A. PRIMARY NEOPLASMS
1. Leiomyoma, leiomyosarcoma
2. Lymphoma
3. Carcinoid
4. Primary carcinoma

B. HEMATOGENOUS METASTASES
1. Malignant melanoma
√ usually spares large bowel
2. Breast cancer (15%)
√ scirrhous appearance in stomach
3. Cancer of lung
4. Renal cell carcinoma
5. Kaposi sarcoma
6. Bladder carcinoma

C. ECTOPIC PANCREAS
in duodenum / stomach

D. EOSINOPHILIC GRANULOMA
most frequently in stomach

Complications of Postoperative Stomach

1. Filling defect of gastric remnant
2. Retained gastric antrum
3. Dumping syndrome
4. Afferent loop syndrome

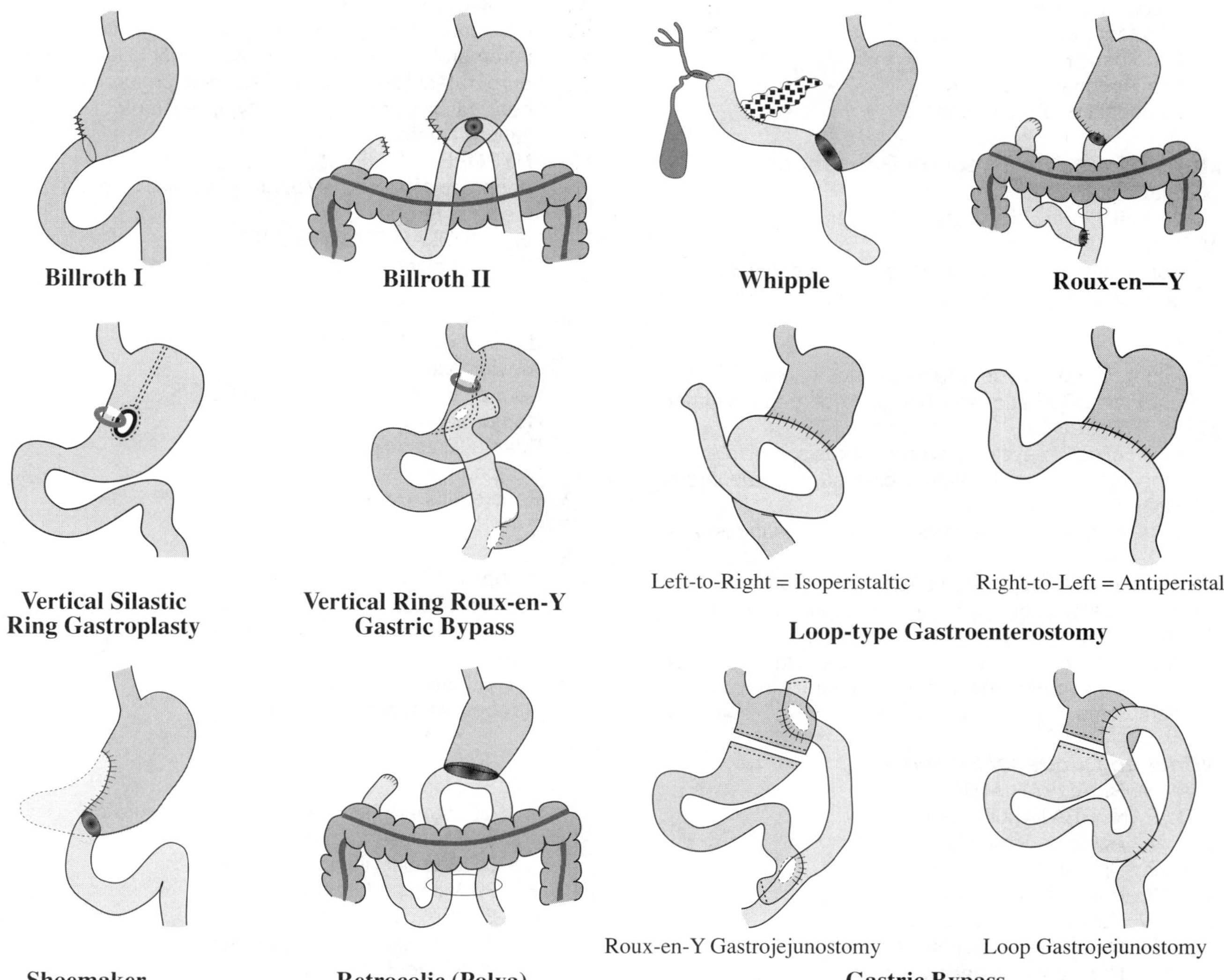

Gastric Surgical Procedures

5. Stomal obstruction
   (a) temporary reversible: edema of suture line, abscess / hematoma, potassium deficiency, inadequate electrolyte replacement, hypoproteinemia, hypoacidity
   (b) late mechanical: stomal ulcer (75%)

mnemonic: "LOBULATING"

Leaks (early)
Obstruction (early)
Bezoar
Ulcer (especially marginal)
Loop (afferent loop syndrome)
Anemia (macrocytic secondary to decreased intrinsic factor)
Tumor (? increased incidence)
Intussusception
Not feeling well after meals (dumping syndrome)
Gastritis (bile reflux)

Lesions Involving Stomach and Duodenum = Transpyloric Involvement

1. Lymphoma: in up to 40% of patients with lymphoma
2. Gastric carcinoma: in 5–25%, but 50 x more common than lymphoma
3. Peptic ulcer disease
4. Tuberculosis: in 10% of gastric TB
5. Crohn disease: pseudo-Billroth-I pattern
6. Strongyloidiasis
7. Eosinophilic gastroenteritis

DUODENUM

Congenital Duodenal Obstruction

- bile-stained vomiting delayed until after first feeding and increasing progressively

√ "double bubble" sign

1. Duodenal atresia / severe stenosis
2. Annular pancreas

GI

3. Midgut volvulus
4. Duodenal web
5. Ladd bands
6. Preduodenal portal vein
7. Duodenal duplication cyst

Extrinsic Pressure Effect on Duodenum

A. BILE DUCTS
normal impression, dilated CBD, choledochal cyst
B. GALLBLADDER
normal impression, gallbladder hydrops, Courvoisier phenomenon, gallbladder carcinoma, pericholecystic abscess
C. LIVER
hepatomegaly, hypertrophied caudate lobe, anomalous hepatic lobe, hepatic cyst, hepatic tumor
D. RIGHT KIDNEY
bifid collecting system, hydronephrosis, multiple renal cysts, polycystic kidney disease, hypernephroma
E. RIGHT ADRENAL
adrenal carcinoma, enlargement in Addison disease
F. COLON
duodenocolic apposition due to anomalous peritoneal fixation, carcinoma of hepatic flexure
G. VESSELS
lymphadenopathy, duodenal varices, dilated arterial collaterals, aortic aneurysm, intramural / mesenteric hematoma

Widened Duodenal Sweep

A. NORMAL VARIANT
B. PANCREATIC LESION
 1. Acute pancreatitis
 2. Chronic pancreatitis
 3. Pancreatic pseudocyst
 4. Pancreatic carcinoma
 5. Metastasis to pancreas
 6. Pancreatic cystadenoma
C. VASCULAR LESION
 1. Lymph node enlargement: lymphoma, metastasis, inflammation
 2. Cystic lymphangioma of the mesentery
D. RETROPERITONEAL MASS
 1. Aortic aneurysm
 2. Choledochal cyst

Thickened Duodenal Folds

A. INFLAMMATION
 (a) within bowel wall:
 peptic ulcer disease, Zollinger-Ellison syndrome, regional enteritis, lymphoid hyperplasia, uremia
 (b) surrounding bowel wall:
 pancreatitis, cholecystitis
B. INFECTION
giardiasis, TB, strongyloidiasis, celiac disease
C. NEOPLASIA
lymphoma, metastases to peripancreatic nodes
D. DIFFUSE INFILTRATIVE DISORDER
Whipple disease, amyloidosis, mastocytosis, eosinophilic enteritis, intestinal lymphangiectasia
E. VASCULAR DISORDER
duodenal varices, mesenteric arterial collaterals, intramural hemorrhage (trauma, Schönlein-Henoch purpura), chronic duodenal congestion (congestive heart failure, portal venous hypertension); lymphangiectasia
F. HYPOPROTEINEMIA
nephrotic syndrome, Ménétrier disease, protein-losing enteropathy
G. GLANDULAR ENLARGEMENT
Brunner gland hyperplasia, cystic fibrosis

mnemonic: "BAD HELP"
Brunner gland hyperplasia
Amyloidosis
Duodenitis (Z-E syndrome, peptic)
Hemorrhage
Edema, **E**ctopic pancreas
Lymphoma
Pancreatitis, **P**arasites

Duodenal Filling Defect

A. EXTRINSIC
gallbladder impression, CBD impression, gas-filled diverticulum
B. INTRINSIC TO WALL
 (a) benign neoplastic mass
 1. Adenoma
 2. Leiomyoma
 3. Lipoma
 4. Hamartoma (Peutz-Jeghers syndrome)
 5. Prolapsed antral polyp
 6. Brunner gland adenoma
 7. Villous adenoma
 8. Islet cell tumor
 9. Gangliocytic paraganglioma
 (b) malignant neoplastic mass
 1. Carcinoid tumor
 2. Adenocarcinoma
 3. Ampullary carcinoma
 4. Lymphoma
 5. Sarcoma
 6. Metastasis (stomach, pancreas, gallbladder, colon, kidney, melanoma)
 7. Retroperitoneal lymph node involvement
 (c) nonneoplastic mass
 1. Papilla of Vater
 2. Choledochocele
 3. Duplication cyst
 4. Pancreatic pseudocyst
 5. Duodenal varix
 6. Mesenteric artery collaterals
 7. Intramural hematoma
 8. Adjacent abscess, stitch abscess
 9. Ectopic pancreas, heterotopic gastric mucosa
 10. Prolapsed antral mucosa
 11. Brunner gland hyperplasia
 12. Benign lymphoid hyperplasia

GI

C. INTRALUMINAL
   1. Blood clot
   2. Foreign body: fruit pit, gallstone, feeding tube

Duodenal Tumor

Benign Duodenal Tumors

1. Leiomyoma (27%)
2. Adenomatous polyp (21%)
3. Lipoma (21%)
4. Brunner gland adenoma (17%)
5. Angiomatous tumor (6%)
6. Ectopic pancreas (2%)
7. Duodenal cyst (2%)
8. Neurofibroma (2%)
9. Hamartoma (2%)

Malignant Duodenal Tumors

1. Adenocarcinoma (73%)
   Location: 40% in duodenum, most often in 2nd + 3rd portion = periampullary neoplasm
   (a) suprapapillary: apt to cause obstruction + bleeding
   (b) peripapillary: extrahepatic jaundice
   (c) intrapapillary: GI bleeding
   Predisposed: Gardner syndrome, celiac disease
   May be associated with: Peutz-Jeghers syndrome
   √ annular / polypoid / ulcerative
   Metastases: regional lymph nodes (2/3)
   DDx: (1) Primary bile duct carcinoma
   (2) Ampullary carcinoma
2. Leiomyosarcoma (14%)
   most often beyond 1st portion of duodenum
   √ up to 20 cm in size
   √ frequently ulcerated exophytic mass
3. Carcinoid (11%)
4. Lymphoma (2%)
   √ marked wall thickening
   √ bulky periduodenal lymphadenopathy

Enlargement of Papilla of Vater

A. Normal variant
   identified in 60% of UGI series; atypical location in 3rd portion of duodenum in 8%; 1.5 cm in diameter in 1% of normals
B. Papillary edema
   1. Impacted stone
   2. Pancreatitis (Poppel sign)
   3. Acute duodenal ulcer disease
   4. Papillitis
C. Perivaterian neoplasms
   = tumor mass + lymphatic obstruction
   1. Adenocarcinoma
   2. Adenomatous polyp (premalignant lesion)
   √ irregular surface + erosions
D. Lesions simulating enlarged papilla
   1. Benign spindle cell tumor
   2. Ectopic pancreatic tissue

Duodenal Narrowing

A. DEVELOPMENTAL ANOMALIES
   1. Duodenal atresia
   2. Congenital web / duodenal diaphragm
   3. Intraluminal diverticulum
   4. Duodenal duplication cyst
   5. Annular pancreas
   6. Midgut volvulus, peritoneal bands (Ladd bands)
B. INTRINSIC DISORDERS
   (a) inflammation / infection
   1. Postbulbar ulcer
   2. Crohn disease
   3. Sprue
   4. Tuberculosis
   5. Strongyloidiasis
   (b) tumor
   duodenal / ampullary malignancy
C. DISEASE IN ADJACENT STRUCTURES
   1. Pancreatitis, pseudocyst, pancreatic carcinoma
   2. Cholecystitis
   3. Contiguous abscess
   4. Metastases to pancreaticoduodenal nodes (lymphoma, lung cancer, breast cancer)
D. TRAUMA
   1. Duodenal rupture
   2. Intramural hematoma
E. VASCULAR
   1. Superior mesenteric artery syndrome
   2. Aorticoduodenal fistula
   3. Preduodenal portal vein (anterior to descending duodenum)

Dilated Duodenum

Megaduodenum = marked dilatation of entire C-loop
Megabulbus = dilatation of duodenal bulb only

A. VASCULAR COMPRESSION
   superior mesenteric artery syndrome, abdominal aortic aneurysm, aorticoduodenal fistula
B. PRIMARY DUODENAL ATONY
   (a) scleroderma, dermatomyositis, SLE
   (b) Chagas disease, aganglionosis, neuropathy, surgical / chemical vagotomy
   (c) focal ileus: pancreatitis, cholecystitis, peptic ulcer disease, trauma
   (d) altered emotional status, chronic idiopathic intestinal pseudoobstruction
C. INFLAMMATORY / NEOPLASTIC INDURATION OF MESENTERIC ROOT
   Crohn disease, tuberculous enteritis, pancreatitis, peptic ulcer disease, strongyloidiasis, metastatic disease
D. FLUID DISTENSION
   celiac disease, Zollinger-Ellison syndrome

Postbulbar Ulceration

1. Benign postbulbar peptic ulcer
   √ medial aspect of upper 2nd portion
   √ incisura pointing to ulcer
   √ occasionally barium reflux into common bile duct
   √ ring stricture

√ stress- and drug-induced ulcers heal without deformity
2. Zollinger-Ellison syndrome
   √ multiple ulcers distal to duodenal bulb
   √ thickening of folds + hypersecretion
3. Leiomyoma
4. Malignant tumors:
   (a) primaries
   adenocarcinoma, lymphoma, sarcoma
   (b) contiguous spread
   pancreas, colon, kidney, gallbladder
   (c) hematogenous spread
   melanoma, Kaposi sarcoma
   (d) lymphogenic spread
   metastases to periduodenal lymph nodes
5. Granulomatous disease: Crohn disease, TB
6. Aorticoduodenal fistula
7. Mimickers: ectopic pancreas, diverticulum

SMALL BOWEL

Anatomic Predilection for Intestinal Involvement

@ proximal jejunum	diverticulosis, giardiasis, adenocarcinoma, Whipple disease, ZE syndrome, celiac disease
@ distal ileum	Crohn disease, TB, infectious enteritis, lymphoma, carcinoid, metastases
@ mesenteric border	diverticulosis, Crohn disease, mesenteric hematoma, intraperitoneal spread of tumor
@ antimesenteric border	Meckel diverticulum, sacculations in scleroderma, hematogenous metastases

Increased Fluid within Small Bowel

1. Ingestion
2. Resection / removal of stomach
3. Small-bowel obstruction
4. Enteritis
5. Malabsorption: celiac disease, Whipple disease
6. Peritoneal carcinomatosis

Small Bowel Diverticula

A. TRUE DIVERTICULA
   (a) Duodenal diverticula
      1. Racemose diverticula: bizarre, lobulated
      2. Giant diverticula
      3. Intraluminal diverticula: result of congenital web / diaphragm
   (b) Jejunal diverticulosis
   (c) Meckel diverticulum
B. PSEUDODIVERTICULA
   1. Scleroderma
   2. Crohn disease
   3. Lymphoma
   4. Mesenteric ischemia
   5. Communicating ileal duplication

6. Giant duodenal ulcer

Small Bowel Ulcer

Aphthous Ulcers of Small Bowel

A. INFECTION
   1. Yersinia enterocolitis (25%)
   2. Salmonellosis
   3. Tuberculosis
   4. Rickettsiosis
B. INFLAMMATION
   1. Crohn disease (22%)
   2. Behçet syndrome
   3. Reiter syndrome
   4. Ankylosing spondylitis

Large Nonstenotic Ulcers of Small Bowel

1. Primary nonspecific ulcer	47% incidence
2. Yersiniosis	33%
3. Crohn disease	30%
4. Tuberculosis	18%
5. Salmonellosis / shigellosis	7%
6. Meckel diverticulum	5%

Multiple Small Bowel Ulcers

A. DRUGS
   1. Potassium tablets
   2. Steroids
   3. Nonsteroidal antiinflammatory drugs
B. INFECTION / INFLAMMATION
   1. Bacillary dysentery
   2. Ischemic enteritis
   3. Ulcerative jejunoileitis as complication of celiac disease
C. TUMOR
   1. Neoplasms
   2. Intestinal lymphoma

Cavitary Small Bowel Lesion

A. PRIMARY TUMOR
   1. Lymphoma (exoenteric form)
   2. Leiomyosarcoma (exoenteric form)
   3. Primary adenocarcinoma
B. METASTASIS
   1. Malignant melanoma
   2. Lung cancer
C. INFLAMMATION
   1. Diverticulitis with abscess (Meckel, jejunal)
   2. Communicating duplication cyst

Separation of Bowel Loops

A. INFILTRATION OF BOWEL WALL / MESENTERY
   (a) inflammation / infection
      1. Crohn disease
      2. TB
      3. Radiation injury
      4. Retractile mesenteritis
      5. Intraperitoneal abscess
   (b) deposits
      1. Intestinal hemorrhage / mesenteric vascular

occlusion
2. Whipple disease
3. Amyloidosis

(c) tumor
1. Carcinoid tumor: local release of serotonin responsible for muscular thickening + fibroplastic proliferation = desmoplastic reaction
2. Primary carcinoma of small bowel (unusual presentation)
3. Lymphoma
4. Neurofibromatosis

B. ASCITES / INTRAPERITONEAL BLEEDING
hepatic cirrhosis (75%), peritonitis, peritoneal carcinomatosis, congestive heart failure, constrictive pericarditis, primary / metastatic lymphatic disease

C. EXTRINSIC MASS
1. Intraperitoneal spread of tumor: peritoneal mesothelioma, mesenteric tumors (fibroma, lipoma, fibrosarcoma, leiomyosarcoma, malignant mesenteric lymphoid tumor, metastases)
2. Interloop abscesses / loculated fluid collection
3. Endometriosis
4. Retractile mesenteritis (fibrosis, fatty infiltration, panniculitis)
5. Mesenteric fat deposits
6. Fibrofatty proliferation: Crohn disease, mesenteric panniculitis

Normal Small Bowel Folds & Diarrhea

1. Pancreatic insufficiency
2. Lactase deficiency
3. Lymphoma / pseudolymphoma

Dilated Small Bowel & Normal Folds

mnemonic: "SOS"

Sprue
Obstruction
Scleroderma

A. EXCESSIVE FLUID

(a) mechanical obstruction
due to adhesion, hernia, neoplasm
√ "string-of-beads sign" = air bubbles between mucosal folds in a fluid-filled small bowel
√ "pseudotumor sign" = closed-loop obstruction

(b) malabsorption syndromes
1. Celiac disease, tropical + nontropical sprue
2. Lactase deficiency

B. BOWEL WALL PARALYSIS
= functional ileus = adynamic ileus
1. Surgical vagotomy
2. Chemical vagotomy from drug effects: atropine-like substances, morphine, L-dopa, glucagon
3. Chagas disease
4. Metabolic: hypokalemia, diabetes
5. Intrinsic + extrinsic intraabdominal inflammation
6. Chronic idiopathic pseudoobstruction

C. VASCULAR COMPROMISE
1. Mesenteric ischemia (atherosclerosis)
2. Acute radiation enteritis
3. Amyloidosis
4. SLE

D. BOWEL WALL DESTRUCTION
1. Lymphoma
2. Scleroderma (smooth muscle atrophy)
3. Dermatomyositis

Abnormal Small Bowel Folds

Abnormal Folds + Increased Intraluminal Fluid

1. Malabsorption syndrome
2. Crohn disease, infectious enteritis
3. Parasitic infestation / giardiasis
4. Ischemia proximal to an obstruction
5. Zollinger-Ellison syndrome
6. Lymphangiectasia, mesenteric lymphadenopathy

Thickened Folds of Stomach & Small Bowel

1. Lymphoma
2. Crohn disease
3. Eosinophilic gastroenteritis
4. Zollinger-Ellison syndrome
5. Ménétrier disease
6. Cirrhosis = gastric varices + hypoproteinemia
7. Amyloidosis
8. Whipple disease
9. Systemic sclerosis

Thickened Smooth Folds ± Dilatation

A. EDEMA

(a) hypoproteinemia
1. Cirrhosis
2. Nephrotic syndrome
3. Protein-losing enteropathy (celiac disease, Whipple disease)

(b) increased capillary permeability
1. Angioneurotic edema
2. Gastroenteritis

(c) increased hydrostatic pressure
1. Portal venous hypertension

(d) Zollinger-Ellison syndrome

B. HEMORRHAGE

(a) vessel injury
1. Ischemia
2. Infarction
3. Trauma

(b) vasculitis
1. Connective tissue disease
2. Henoch-Schönlein purpura
3. Thrombangitis obliterans, irradiation

(c) hypocoagulability
1. Hemophilia
2. Anticoagulant therapy
3. Hypofibrinogemia
4. Circulating anticoagulants
5. Fibrinolytic system activation
6. Idiopathic thrombocytopenic purpura

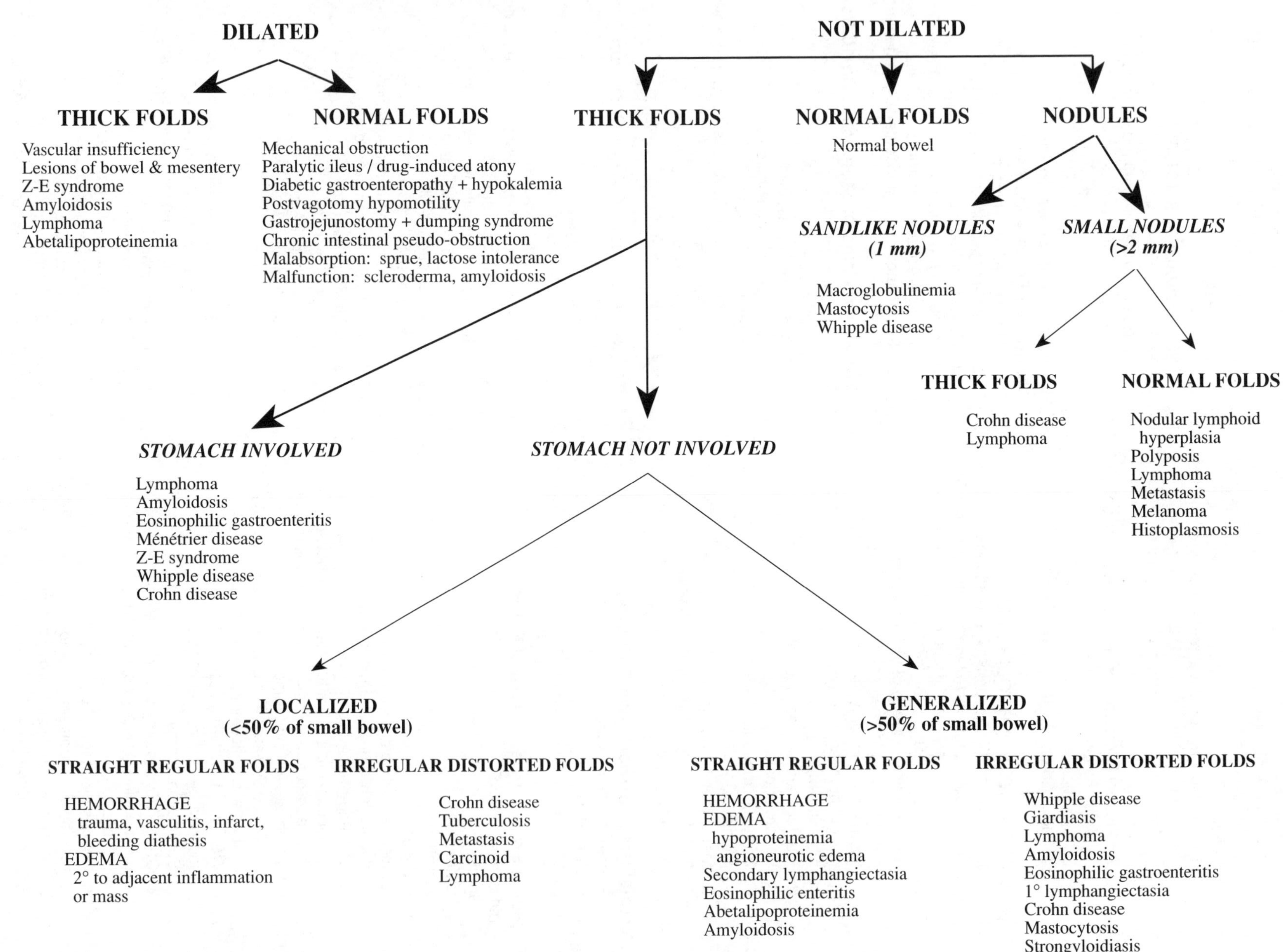
ABNORMAL SMALL BOWEL CALIBER & CONTOUR
DILATED
THICK FOLDS
Vascular insufficiency
Lesions of bowel & mesentery
Z-E syndrome
Amyloidosis
Lymphoma
Abetalipoproteinemia
NORMAL FOLDS
Mechanical obstruction
Paralytic ileus / drug-induced atony
Diabetic gastroenteropathy + hypokalemia
Postvagotomy hypomotility
Gastrojejunostomy + dumping syndrome
Chronic intestinal pseudo-obstruction
Malabsorption: sprue, lactose intolerance
Malfunction: scleroderma, amyloidosis
NOT DILATED
THICK FOLDS
STOMACH INVOLVED
Lymphoma
Amyloidosis
Eosinophilic gastroenteritis
Ménétrier disease
Z-E syndrome
Whipple disease
Crohn disease
STOMACH NOT INVOLVED
LOCALIZED
(<50% of small bowel)
STRAIGHT REGULAR FOLDS
HEMORRHAGE
trauma, vasculitis, infarct,
bleeding diathesis
EDEMA
2° to adjacent inflammation
or mass
IRREGULAR DISTORTED FOLDS
Crohn disease
Tuberculosis
Metastasis
Carcinoid
Lymphoma
GENERALIZED
(>50% of small bowel)
STRAIGHT REGULAR FOLDS
HEMORRHAGE
EDEMA
hypoproteinemia
angioneurotic edema
Secondary lymphangiectasia
Eosinophilic enteritis
Abetalipoproteinemia
Amyloidosis
IRREGULAR DISTORTED FOLDS
Whipple disease
Giardiasis
Lymphoma
Amyloidosis
Eosinophilic gastroenteritis
1° lymphangiectasia
Crohn disease
Mastocytosis
Strongyloidiasis
NORMAL FOLDS
Normal bowel
NODULES
SANDLIKE NODULES
(1 mm)
Macroglobulinemia
Mastocytosis
Whipple disease
SMALL NODULES
(>2 mm)
THICK FOLDS
Crohn disease
Lymphoma
NORMAL FOLDS
Nodular lymphoid
hyperplasia
Polyposis
Lymphoma
Metastasis
Melanoma
Histoplasmosis

7. Coagulation defects (leukemia, lymphoma, multiple myeloma, metastatic carcinoma)
8. Hypoprothrombinemia

C. LYMPHATIC BLOCKAGE
1. Tumor infiltration: lymphoma, pseudolymphoma
2. Irradiation
3. Mesenteric fibrosis
4. Intestinal lymphangiectasia
5. Whipple disease

D. DEPOSITS
1. Eosinophilic enteritis
2. Pneumatosis intestinalis
3. Amyloidosis
4. Abetalipoproteinemia
5. Crohn disease
6. Graft-versus-host disease
7. Immunologic deficiency: hypo- / dysgammaglobulinemia

Thickened Irregular Folds ± Dilatation

A. INFLAMMATION
1. Crohn disease

B. NEOPLASTIC
1. Lymphoma, pseudolymphoma

C. INFECTION
(a) protozoan
giardiasis, strongyloidiasis, hookworm
(b) bacterial
Yersinia enterocolitica, typhoid fever, tuberculosis
(c) fungal: histoplasmosis
(d) AIDS-related infection

D. IDIOPATHIC
(a) lymphatic dilatation
1. Lymphangiectasia
2. Inflammatory process, tumor growth, irradiation fibrosis
3. Whipple disease

(b) cellular infiltration
1. Eosinophilic enteritis
2. Mastocytosis

(c) deposits
1. Zollinger-Ellison syndrome
2. Amyloidosis
3. Alpha chain disease: defective secretory IgA system
4. A-β-lipoproteinemia: recessive, retinitis pigmentosa, neurologic disease
5. A-α-lipoproteinemia
6. Fibrocystic disease of the pancreas
7. Polyposis syndrome

mnemonic: "G. WILLIAMS"
Giardiasis
Whipple disease, **W**aldenström macroglobulinemia
Ischemia
Lymphangiectasia
Lymphoma
Inflammation
Amyloidosis, **A**gammaglobulinemia
Mastocytosis, **M**alabsorption
Soft-tissue neoplasm (carcinoid, lipoma)

Tethered Folds

= indicative of desmoplastic reaction
√ kinking, angulation, tethering, separation of bowel loops

1. Carcinoid
2. Postoperative in Gardner syndrome
3. Retractile mesenteritis
4. Hodgkin disease
5. Peritoneal implants
6. Endometriosis
7. Tuberculous peritonitis
8. Mesothelioma
9. Postoperative adhesions

Atrophy of Small Bowel Folds

1. Chronic malabsorption: celiac disease
2. Chronic ischemic changes: radiation injury, amyloidosis
3. Crohn disease in burned-out stage
4. Parasitic infestation: strongyloidiasis
5. Graft-versus-host disease

Ribbonlike Small Bowel

= featureless / tubular nature of small bowel with effacement of folds

1. Graft-versus-host disease
2. Celiac disease
3. Small bowel infection (eg, viral enteritis)
4. Injury from radiation / corrosive medication
5. Allergy (eg, soybeans)
6. Ischemia
7. Amyloid, mastocytosis
8. Lymphoma, pseudolymphoma
9. Crohn disease

Delayed Small Bowel Transit

= transit time >6 hours
mnemonic: "SPATS DID"
Scleroderma
Potassium (hypokalemia)
Anxiety
Thyroid (hypothyroidism)
Sprue
Diabetes (poorly controlled)
Idiopathic
Drugs (opiates, atropine, phenothiazine)

Constricting Lesion of Small Bowel

1. Primary adenocarcinoma (proximal jejunum)
2. Carcinoid (distal ileum)
3. Lymphoma, metastasis
4. Endometriosis
5. Adhesion, mucosal diaphragm
6. Strictures: Crohn disease, radiation enteritis, ischemia, potassium chloride tablets

Multiple Stenotic Lesions of Small Bowel
1. Crohn disease
2. End-stage radiation enteritis
3. Metastatic carcinoma
4. Endometriosis
5. Eosinophilic gastroenteritis
6. Tuberculosis
7. Drug-induced (eg, potassium chloride tablets, NSAIDs)

Small Bowel Filling Defects
Solitary Filling Defect of Small Bowel
A. INTRINSIC TO BOWEL WALL
   (a) benign neoplasm: leiomyoma (97%), adenoma, lipoma, hemangioma, neurofibroma
   (b) malignant primary: adenocarcinoma, lymphoma (desmoplastic response), sarcoma, carcinoid
   (c) metastases: from melanoma, lung, kidney, breast
   (d) inflammation: inflammatory pseudotumor
   (e) infection: parasites
B. EXTRINSIC TO BOWEL WALL
   1. Duplication cyst
   2. Endometrioma
C. INTRALUMINAL
   1. Gallstone ileus
   2. Parasites (ascariasis, strongyloidiasis)
   3. Inverted Meckel diverticulum
   4. Blood clot
   5. Foreign body, bezoar, pills, seeds

Multiple Filling Defects of Small Bowel
A. POLYPOSIS SYNDROMES
   1. Peutz-Jeghers syndrome
   2. Gardner syndrome
   3. Disseminated gastrointestinal polyposis
   4. Generalized gastrointestinal juvenile polyposis
   5. Cronkhite-Canada syndrome
B. BENIGN TUMORS
   1. Multiple simple adenomatous polyps
   2. Hemangioma, blue rubber bleb nevus syndrome
   3. Leiomyoma, neurofibroma, lipoma
   4. Nodular lymphoid hyperplasia
      = normal terminal ileum in children + adolescents; may be associated with dysgammaglobulinemia
      √ symmetric fairly sharply demarcated filling defects
   5. Varices (= multiple phlebectasia in jejunum, oral mucosa, tongue, scrotum)
C. MALIGNANT TUMORS
   1. Carcinoid tumor
   2. Lymphoma
      (a) primary lymphoma (rarely multiple)
      (b) secondary lymphoma: gastrointestinal involvement in 63% of disseminated disease; 19% in small intestine
   3. Kaposi sarcoma
   4. Submucosal metastases: melanoma > lung > breast > choriocarcinoma > kidney > stomach, uterus, ovary, pancreas
D. INTRALUMINAL
   1. Gallstones
   2. Foreign bodies, food particles, seeds, pills
   3. Parasites: ascariasis, strongyloidiasis, hookworm, tapeworm

Sandlike Lucencies of Small Bowel
1. Waldenström macroglobulinemia
2. Mastocytosis
3. Histoplasmosis
4. Nodular lymphoid hyperplasia
5. Intestinal lymphangiectasia
6. Eosinophilic gastroenteritis
7. Lymphoma
8. Crohn disease
9. Whipple disease
10. Yersinia enterocolitis
11. Cronkhite-Canada syndrome
12. Cystic fibrosis
13. Food particles / gas bubbles
14. Strongyloides stercoralis

Small Bowel Tumors
Incidence: 1:100,000; 1.5–6% of all GI neoplasms
Malignant:benign = 1:1
Symptomatic malignant:symptomatic benign = 3:1
Location of small bowel primaries:
ileum (41%), jejunum (36%), duodenum (18%)

ROENTGENOGRAPHIC APPEARANCE:
(1) pedunculated intraluminal tumor, usually originating from mucosa
   √ smooth / irregular surface without visible mucosal pattern
   √ moves within intestinal lumen twice the length of the stalk
(2) sessile intraluminal tumor without stalk, usually from tissues outside mucosa
   √ smooth / irregular surface without visible mucosal pattern
(3) intra- / extramural tumor
   √ base of tumor greater than any part projecting into the lumen
   √ mucosal pattern visible, may be stretched
(4) serosal tumor
   √ displacement of adjacent loops
   √ small bowel obstruction (rare)
   √ coil-spring pattern of intussusceptum

CT: small bowel wall >1.5 cm thick

Cx: small-bowel obstruction (in up to 10%)

Benign Small Bowel Tumors
• asymptomatic (80%)
• melena, intermittent abdominal pain, weakness
• palpable abdominal mass (20%)

GI

Types:
1. Leiomyoma (36–49%)
   Location: any segment
2. Adenoma (15–20%)
3. Lipoma (14–16%)
   Location: duodenum (32%), jejunum (17%), ileum (51%)
   √ fat-density on CT
4. Hemangioma (13–16%)
5. Lymphangioma (5%)
   Location: duodenum > jejunum > ileum
6. Neurogenic tumor (1%)

Malignant Small Bowel Tumors

At risk: Crohn disease, celiac disease, polyposis syndromes, history of small-bowel diverting surgery

- asymptomatic (10–30%)
- pain due to intermittent obstruction (80%)
- weight loss (66%)
- gastrointestinal blood loss (50%)
- palpable abdominal mass (50%)

PRIMARY MALIGNANT SMALL BOWEL TUMOR

1. Carcinoid (25–41%)
   ◊ Most common primary small bowel tumor!
   Location: predominantly distal ileum
   √ calcified mesenteric mass on CT
2. Adenocarcinoma (25–26%)
   Location: duodenum (48%), jejunum (44%), ileum (8%)
3. Lymphoma (16–17%)
   √ aneurysmal dilatation
4. Gastrointestinal stromal tumor (GIST) = leiomyosarcoma (9–10%)
   Location: ileum (50%)
5 Vascular malignancy (1%)
6. Fibrosarcoma (0.3%)

SECONDARY MALIGNANT SMALL BOWEL TUMOR

◊ Most common neoplasm of small intestines!

CECUM

Ileocecal Valve Abnormalities

A. Lipomatosis: >40 years of age, female
   √ stellate / rosette pattern
B. NEOPLASM
   1. Lipoma, adenomatous polyp, villous adenoma
   2. Carcinoid tumor
   3. Adenocarcinoma: 2% of all colonic cancers
   4. Lymphoma: often involving terminal ileum
C. INFLAMMATION
   1. Crohn disease
   2. Ulcerative colitis
      √ patulous valve, fixed in open position
   3. Tuberculosis
   4. Amebiasis
      √ terminal ileum not involved (in USA)
   5. Typhoid fever, anisakiasis, schistosomiasis, actinomycosis
   6. Cathartic abuse
D. PROLAPSE
   (a) antegrade: indistinguishable from lipomatosis / prolapsing mucosa / neoplasm
   (b) retrograde
E. INTUSSUSCEPTION
F. LYMPHOID HYPERPLASIA

Coned Cecum

A. INFLAMMATION
   1. Crohn disease
      √ involvement of ascending colon + terminal ileum
   2. Ulcerative colitis
      √ backwash ileitis (in 10%)
      √ gaping ileocecal valve
   3. Appendicitis
   4. Typhlitis
   5. Perforated cecal diverticulum
B. INFECTION
   1. Tuberculosis
      √ colonic involvement more prominent than that of terminal ileum
   2. Amebiasis
      √ involvement of cecum in 90% of amebiasis
      √ thickened ileocecal valve fixed in open position
      √ reflux into normal terminal ileum
      √ skip lesions in colon
   3. Actinomycosis
      - palpable abdominal mass
      - indolent sinus tracts in abdominal wall
   4. Blastomycosis
   5. Anisakiasis
   6. Typhoid, Yersinia
C. TUMOR
   1. Carcinoma of the cecum
   2. Metastasis to cecum

Cecal Filling Defect

A. ABNORMALITIES OF THE APPENDIX
   1. Acute appendicitis / appendiceal abscess
   2. Crohn disease
   3. Inverted appendiceal stump / appendiceal intussusception
   4. Mucocele
   5. Myxoglobulosis
   6. Appendiceal neoplasm: carcinoid tumor (90%), leiomyoma, neuroma, lipoma, adenocarcinoma, metastasis
B. COLONIC LESION
   1. Ameboma
   2. Primary cecal neoplasm
   3. Ileocolic intussusception
   4. Lipomatosis of ileocecal valve
C. UNUSUAL ABNORMALITIES
   1. Ileocecal diverticulitis (in 50% < age 30 years)
   2. Solitary benign ulcer of the cecum
   3. Adherent fecolith (eg, in cystic fibrosis)
   4. Endometriosis
   5. Burkitt lymphoma

mnemonic: "CECUM TIPSALE"
Carcinoma
Enteritis
Carcinoid
Ulcerative colitis
Mucocele of appendix
Tuberculosis
Intussusception
Periappendiceal abscess
Stump of the appendix
Ameboma
Lymphoma
Endometriosis

Appendiceal Intussusception

1. Mucocele
2. Endometrioma
3. Fecolith
4. Foreign body
5. Polyp (juvenile, inflammatory)
6. Papilloma
7. Adenoma / adenocarcinoma
8. Carcinoid tumor
9. Postappendectomy stump

Pericecal Fat-Stranding on CT

1. Appendicitis
2. Crohn disease
3. Tuboovarian abscess
4. Cecal diverticulitis
5. Perforated cecal carcinoma

COLON

Colon Cutoff Sign

= abrupt termination of colonic gas column at splenic flexure with decompression of the distal colon due to spasm + obstruction at the splenic flexure impinging on a paralytic transverse colon

A. IMPINGEMENT VIA PHRENICOCOLIC LIGAMENT
   1. Acute pancreatitis / postpancreatitic stricture
   2. Pancreatic / gastric carcinoma
   3. Hemorrhage from rupture of splenic artery / abdominal aortic aneurysm

B. COLONIC DISEASE
   1. Colon cancer
   2. Mesenteric thrombosis
   3. Ischemic colitis
   4. Perforated appendicitis (in 20%)
      N.B.: amputation of gas at the hepatic flexure due to spastic ascending colon

Colonic Thumbprinting

= sharply defined fingerlike marginal indentations at contours of wall

1. ISCHEMIA = Ischemic colitis
   occlusive vascular disease, hypercoagulability state, hemorrhage into bowel wall (bleeding diathesis, anticoagulants), traumatic intramural hematoma
2. INFLAMMATION
   ulcerative colitis, Crohn colitis
3. INFECTION
   acute amebiasis, schistosomiasis, strongyloidiasis, cytomegalovirus (in renal transplant recipients), pseudomembranous colitis
4. MALIGNANT LESIONS
   localized primary lymphoma, hematogenous metastases
5. MISCELLANEOUS
   endometriosis, amyloidosis, pneumatosis intestinalis, diverticulosis, diverticulitis, hereditary angioneurotic edema

mnemonic: "PSALM II"
Pseudomembranous colitis
Schistosomiasis
Amebic colitis
Lymphoma
Metastases (to colon)
Ischemic colitis
Inflammatory bowel disease

Colonic Urticaria Pattern

A. OBSTRUCTION
   1. Obstructing carcinoma
   2. Cecal volvulus
   3. Colonic ileus
B. ISCHEMIA
C. INFECTION / INFLAMMATION
   1. Yersinia enterocolitis
   2. Herpes
   3. Crohn disease
D. URTICARIA

Colonic Ulcers

A. IDIOPATHIC
   1. Ulcerative colitis
   2. Crohn colitis
B. ISCHEMIC
   1. Ischemic colitis
C. TRAUMATIC
   1. Radiation injury
   2. Caustic colitis
D. NEOPLASTIC
   1. Primary colonic carcinoma
   2. Metastases (prostate, stomach, lymphoma, leukemia)
E. INFLAMMATORY
   1. Pseudomembranous colitis
   2. Pancreatitis
   3. Diverticulitis
   4. Behçet syndrome
   5. Solitary rectal ulcer syndrome
   6. Nonspecific benign ulceration
F. INFECTION
   (a) protozoan
      1. Amebiasis
      2. Schistosomiasis
      3. Strongyloidiasis
   (b) bacterial
      1. Shigellosis, salmonellosis
      2. Staphylococcal colitis

GI

3. Tuberculosis
4. Gonorrheal proctitis
5. Yersinia colitis
6. Campylobacter fetus colitis

(c) fungal
histoplasmosis, mucormycosis, actinomycosis, candidiasis

(d) viral
1. Lymphogranuloma venereum
2. Herpes proctocolitis
3. Cytomegalovirus (transplants)

Aphthous Ulcers of Colon

1. Crohn disease
2. Amebic colitis
3. **Yersinia enterocolitis**
   Organism: Gram-negative
   • fever, diarrhea, RLQ pain
   Location: terminal ileum
   √ thickened folds + ulceration
   √ lymphoid nodular hyperplasia
4. Salmonella, shigella infection
5. Herpes virus infection
6. Behçet syndrome
7. Lymphoma
8. Ischemia

Multiple Bull's-eye Lesions of Colonic Wall

mnemonic: "MaCK CLaN"
Melanoma and
Carcinoma
Kaposi sarcoma
Carcinoid
Lymphoma and
Neurofibromatosis

Double-tracking of Colon

= longitudinal extraluminal tracks paralleling the colon
1. Diverticulitis: generally 3–6 cm in length
2. Crohn disease: generally >10 cm
3. Ulcerative colitis
4. Primary carcinoma: wider + more irregular

Colonic Narrowing

A. CHRONIC STAGE OF ANY ULCERATING COLITIS
(a) inflammatory:
1. Ulcerative colitis
2. Crohn colitis
3. Solitary rectal ulcer syndrome
4. Nonspecific benign ulcer

(b) infectious:
1. Amebiasis
2. Schistosomiasis
3. Bacillary dysentery
4. Tuberculosis
5. Fungal disease
6. Lymphogranuloma venereum
7. Herpes zoster
8. Cytomegalovirus
9. Strongyloides

(c) ischemic
1. Ischemic colitis

(d) traumatic
1. Radiation injury
2. Cathartic colon
3. Caustic colitis

B. MALIGNANT LESION
(a) primary
1. Colonic carcinoma (annular / scirrhous)
2. Complication of ulcerative colitis + Crohn colitis

(b) metastatic:
from prostate, cervix, uterus, kidney, stomach, pancreas, primary intraperitoneal sarcoma
— hematogenous (eg, breast)
— lymphangitic spread
— peritoneal seeding

C. EXTRINSIC PROCESS
(a) inflammation
1. Retractile mesenteritis
2. Diverticulitis
3. Pancreatitis

(b) deposits
1. Amyloidosis
2. Endometriosis
3. Pelvic lipomatosis

D. POSTSURGICAL
1. Adhesive bands
2. Surgical anastomosis

E. NORMAL
1. Cannon point

Localized Colonic Narrowing

mnemonic: "SCARED CELL-MATE"
Schistosomiasis
Carcinoid
Actinomycosis
Radiation
Endometriosis
Diverticulitis
Colitis
Extrinsic lesion
Lymphoma
Lymphogranuloma venereum
Metastasis
Adenocarcinoma
Tuberculosis
Entamoeba histolytica

Microcolon

mnemonic: "MI MCA"
Meconium ileus, **M**econium peritonitis (cystic fibrosis)
Ileal / jejunal atresia
Megacystis-microcolon-hypoperistalsis syndrome
Colonic atresia (distal to atretic segment)
Aganglionosis (Hirschsprung disease)

GI

Colonic Filling Defects

Submucosal Tumor of Colon

1. Lipoma
2. Carcinoid
3. Leiomyoma
4. Lymphangioma, hemangioma

Single Colonic Filling Defect

A. BENIGN TUMOR
   1. Polyp
      (hyperplastic, adenomatous, villous adenoma, villoglandular); most common benign tumor
   2. Lipoma
      Most common intramural tumor; 2nd most common benign tumor; M < F
      Location: ascending colon + cecum > left side of colon
   3. Carcinoid: 10% metastasize
   4. Spindle cell tumor
      (leiomyoma, fibroma, neurofibroma); 4th most common benign tumor; rectum > cecum
   5. Lymphangioma, hemangioma

B. MALIGNANT TUMOR
   (a) primary tumor:
      carcinoma, sarcoma
   (b) secondary tumor:
      metastases (breast, stomach, lung, pancreas, kidney, female genital tract), lymphoma, invasion by adjacent tumors

C. INFECTION
   1. Ameboma
   2. Polypoid granuloma: schistosomiasis, TB

D. INFLAMMATION
   1. Inflammatory pseudopolyp: ulcerative colitis, Crohn disease
   2. Periappendiceal abscess
   3. Diverticulitis
   4. Foreign-body perforation

E. NONSESSILE INTRALUMINAL BODY
   1. Fecal impaction
   2. Foreign body
   3. Gallstone
   4. Bolus of Ascaris worms

F. MISCELLANEOUS
   1. Endometriosis
      3rd most common benign tumor
      Location: sigmoid colon, rectosigmoid junction (at level of cul-de-sac)
      - may cause bleeding (after invasion of mucosa)
   2. Localized amyloid deposition
   3. Suture granuloma
   4. Intussusception
   5. Pseudotumor (adhesions, fibrous bands)
   6. Colitis cystica profunda

Multiple Colonic Filling Defects

A. NEOPLASMS
   (a) polyposis syndrome:
      familial polyposis, Gardner syndrome, Peutz-Jeghers syndrome, Turcot syndrome, juvenile polyposis syndrome, disseminated gastrointestinal polyps, multiple adenomatous polyps
   (b) hematogenous metastases:
      from breast, lung, stomach, ovary, pancreas, uterus
   (c) multiple tumors
      – benign:
        neurofibromatosis, colonic lipomatosis, multiple hamartoma syndrome (Cowden disease)

Differential Diagnosis of Colonic Polyps

	Single Polyp	*Multiple Polyps*
Neoplastic (10 %)		
— epithelial (adenomatous)	1. Tubular adenoma 2. Tubulovillous adenoma 3. Villous adenoma	1. Familial multiple polyposis 2. Adenomatosis of GI tract 3. Gardner syndrome 4. Turcot syndrome
— nonepithelial	1. Carcinoid 2. Leiomyoma 3. Lipoma 4. Hemangioma, lymphangioma 5. Fibroma, neurofibroma	
Nonneoplastic (90%)		
— unclassified	1. Hyperplastic polyp	1. Hyperplastic polyposis
— hamartomatous	1. Juvenile polyps	1. Juvenile polyposis 2. Peutz-Jeghers syndrome 3. Cronkhite-Canada syndrome
— inflammatory	1. Benign lymphoid polyp 2. Fibroid granulation polyp	1. Ulcerative colitis

GI

– malignant:
lymphoma, leukemia, adenocarcinoma

B. INFLAMMATORY PSEUDOPOLYPS
ulcerative colitis, Crohn colitis, ischemic colitis, amebiasis, schistosomiasis, strongyloidiasis, trichuriasis

C. ARTIFACTS
feces, air bubbles, oil bubbles, mucous strands, ingested foreign body (eg, corn kernels)

D. MISCELLANEOUS
nodular lymphoid hyperplasia, lymphoid follicular pattern, hemorrhoids, diverticula, pneumatosis intestinalis, colitis cystica profunda, colonic urticaria, submucosal colonic edema secondary to obstruction, cystic fibrosis, amyloidosis, ulcerative pseudopolyps, proximal to obstruction

mnemonic: "MILL P³"
Metastases (to colon)
Ischemia (thumbprinting)
Lymphoma
Lymphoid hyperplasia
Polyposis
Pseudopolyposis (with inflammatory bowel disease); **P**neumatosis cystoides

Carpet Lesions of Colon

= flat lobulated lesions with alteration of surface texture + little / no protrusion into lumen

Location: rectum > cecum > ascending colon

Cause:

A. NEOPLASMS
1. Tubular / tubulovillous / villous adenoma
2. Familial polyposis
3. Adenocarcinoma
4. Submucosal tumor spread (from adjacent carcinoma)

B. MISCELLANEOUS
1. Nonspecific follicular proctitis
2. Biopsy site
3. Endometriosis
4. Rectal varices
5. Colonic urticaria

Colonic Polyp

Terminology:

1. **Polyp**
= mass projecting into the lumen of a hollow viscus above the level of the mucosa; usually arises from mucosa, may derive from submucosa / muscularis propria
(a) neoplastic: adenoma / carcinoma
(b) nonneoplastic: hamartoma / inflammatory polyp

2. **Pseudopolyp**
= scattered island of inflamed edematous mucosa on a background of denuded mucosa
(a) pseudopolyposis of ulcerative colitis
(b) "cobblestoning" of Crohn disease

3. **Postinflammatory (filiform) polyp**
= fingerlike projection of submucosa covered by mucosa on all sides following healing + regeneration of inflammatory (most common in ulcerative colitis) / ischemic / infectious bowel disease

Histologic classification:

A. ADENOMATOUS POLYPS
= **Familial adenomatous polyposis syndrome**
Cause: abnormality on chromosome 5
Cx: adenomatous polyps are premalignant eventually leading to colorectal carcinoma
1. Familial (multiple) polyposis
2. Gardner syndrome
3. Turcot syndrome

B. HAMARTOMATOUS POLYPS
= **Hamartomatous polyposis syndromes**
1. Peutz-Jeghers syndrome (most in small bowel)*
2. Cowden disease*
3. Juvenile polyposis*
4. Cronkhite-Canada syndrome
5. Bannayan-Riley-Ruvalcaba syndrome

* = increased prevalence of coexisting adenomas and adenoma-carcinoma sequence

C. POLYPOSIS LOOK-ALIKES
1. Inflammatory polyposis
2. Lymphoid hyperplasia
3. Lymphoma
4. Metastases
5. Pneumatosis coli

Polyposis Syndromes

= more than 100 polyps in number

Mode of transmission:

A. HEREDITARY
(a) autosomal dominant
1. Familial (multiple) polyposis
2. Gardner syndrome
3. Peutz-Jeghers syndrome
4. Juvenile polyposis coli
(b) autosomal recessive
1. Turcot syndrome

B. NONHEREDITARY
1. Cronkhite-Canada syndrome
2. Juvenile polyposis

GI

MURAL STRATIFICATION OF INTESTINAL TRACT

= abnormal separation of bowel layers on cross-sectional imaging

CECT:
√ "doubel halo / target" sign during arterial phase:
√ contrast enhancement of inner layer:
(1) mucosa + (2) muscularis propria
√ interposed edema (water) / hemorrhage (blood) / inflammatory cell infiltrate (pus, cells) / fatty proliferation:
(3) submucosa
√ contrast enhancement of outer layer:
(4) muscularis propria + (5) serosa

Cause:
◊ Tumor has not been reported to cause stratification!
A. EDEMA
√ low-density / water-density separation
1. Ulcerative colitis (50%): rectum
2. Proximal to obstructing tumor / intussusception
B. INFLAMMATORY CELL INFILTRATE
1. Crohn disease (in up to 50%)
2. Mycobacterium tuberculosis
3. Eosinophilic enteritis
4. Cytomegalovirus
5. Clostridium difficile
6. Entamoeba histolytica
7. Vibrio cholera
8. Shigella
9. Escherichia coli
C. ISCHEMIA / INFARCTION
1. Arterial obstruction: thromboembolism, plaque thrombus
2. Peripheral vasculopathy
3. Venous obstruction: thrombosis, bowel torsion, closed-loop obstruction
4. Hypoperfusion: proximal arterial stenosis potentiated by myocardial infarction, bradycardia, dehydration

N.B.: closed-loop obstruction with signs of bowel infarction is a surgical condition!
√ signs of bowel infarction:
√ free peritoneal fluid
√ asymmetric bowel wall enhancement
√ persistent enhancement of bowel wall / segmental arteries
√ arterial / venous filling defects
√ increased density of mesentery
√ bowel obstruction

D. INTESTINAL WALL HEMORRHAGE
1. Anticoagulation
2. Blood dyscrasia: thrombocytopenic purpura
3. Blunt trauma
√ "snow-cone" appearance of duodenum
7. Intramural hemorrhage

Pseudomembranous Colitis
1. Clostridium difficile
2. Ischemic colitis: acute / subacute
3. Staphylococcus
4. Shigella
5. Pseudomonas aeruginosa
6. Drugs: chlorpropamide, mercuric compounds, gold, NSAIDs

Accordion Sign
= gross irregular polypoid thickening of colonic wall with wide separation of inner + outer walls
1. Radiation-induced colitis
2. Ischemic colitis
3. Infectious colitis: Clostridium difficile, tuberculosis
4. Typhlitis, neutropenic colitis
5. Inflammation: Crohn disease, ulcerative colitis
◊ The only 2 conditions with wall thickening >10 mm
6. Lymphangiectasia

RECTUM & ANUS

Rectal Narrowing
1. Pelvic lipomatosis + fibrolipomatosis
2. Lymphogranuloma venereum
3. Radiation injury of rectum
4. Chronic ulcerative colitis

Enlarged Presacral Space
Normal width <5 mm in 95%; abnormal width >10 mm
A. RECTAL INFLAMMATION / INFECTION
ulcerative colitis, Crohn colitis, idiopathic proctosigmoiditis, radiation therapy
B. RECTAL INFECTION
1. Proctitis (TB, amebiasis, lymphogranuloma venereum, radiation, ischemia)
2. Diverticulitis
C. BENIGN RECTAL TUMOR
1. Developmental cyst (dermoid, enteric cyst, tailgut cyst)
2. Lipoma, neurofibroma, hemangioendothelioma
3. Epidermal cyst
4. Rectal duplication
D. MALIGNANT RECTAL TUMOR
1. Adenocarcinoma, cloacogenic carcinoma
2. Lymphoma, sarcoma, lymph node metastases
3. Prostatic carcinoma, bladder tumors, cervical cancer, ovarian cancer
E. BODY FLUIDS / DEPOSITS
1. Hematoma: surgery, sacral fracture
2. Pus: perforated appendix, presacral abscess
3. Serum: edema, venous thrombosis
4. Deposit of fat: pelvic lipomatosis, Cushing disease
5. Deposit of amyloid: amyloidosis
F. SACRAL TUMOR
1. Sacrococcygeal teratoma, anterior sacral meningocele
2. Chordoma, metastasis to sacrum
G. MISCELLANEOUS
1. Inguinal hernia containing segment of colon
2. Colitis cystica profunda
3. Pelvic lipomatosis

Lesions of Ischiorectal Fossa
A. Congenital and developmental anomalies
1. Gartner duct cyst
2. Klippel-Trenaunay syndrome
3. Tailgut cyst
B. Inflammatory and hemorrhagic lesions
1. Fistula in ano
2. Ischiorectal / perirectal abscess
3. Extraperitoneal pelvic hematoma
4. Rectal perforation
C. Secondary neoplasm
per direct extension / hematogenous spread: anorectal / prostatic / pelvic / sacral tumor; lung cancer; melanoma; lymphoma

D. Primary neoplasm
   1. Aggressive angiomyxoma
   2. Lipoma
   3. Plexiform neurofibroma
   4. Anal adenocarcinoma
   5. Squamous cell carcinoma

PERITONEUM

Peritoneal Mass

A. SOLID MASS
   1. Peritoneal mesothelioma
   2. Peritoneal carcinomatosis

B. INFILTRATIVE PATTERN
   1. Peritoneal mesothelioma

C. CYSTIC MASS
   1. Cystic mesothelioma
   2. Pseudomyxoma peritonei
   3. Bacterial / mycobacterial infection

MESENTERY & OMENTUM

Short mesentery

= shortened line of fixation

1. Malrotation + midgut volvulus
2. Omphalocele
3. Gastroschisis
4. Congenital diaphragmatic hernia
5. Asplenia + polysplenia

"Apple peel" Small Bowel

= distal small intestines spirals around its vascular supply resembling an apple peel resulting in a very short intestine

1. Proximal jejunal atresia
2. Absence of distal superior mesenteric artery
3. Shortening of small bowel distal to atresia
4. Absence of dorsal mesentery

Cx: propensity toward necrotizing enterocolitis
Prognosis: high mortality

Omental Mass

◊ 33% of primary omental tumors are malignant!
◊ Secondary neoplasms are more frequent than primary!

A. SOLID MASS
   (a) benign
      1, Leiomyoma
      2. Lipoma
      3. Neurofibroma
   (b) malignant
      1. Leiomyosarcoma
      2. Liposarcoma
      3. Fibrosarcoma
      4. Lymphoma
      5. Peritoneal mesothelioma
      6. Hemangiopericytoma
      7. Metastases
   (c) Infection: tuberculosis

B. CYSTIC MASS
   1. Hematoma

Mesenteric Mass

A. ROUND SOLID MASSES
   ◊ Benign primary tumors are more common than malignant primary tumors!
   ◊ Secondary neoplasms more frequent than primary
   ◊ Cystic tumors more common than solid tumors!
   ◊ Malignant solid tumors have a tendency to be located near root of mesentery, benign solid tumors in periphery near bowel!
   1. Metastases especially from colon, ovary (most frequent neoplasm of mesentery)
   2. Lymphoma
   3. Leiomyosarcoma (more frequent than leiomyoma)
   4. Neural tumor (neurofibroma, ganglioneuroma)
   5. Lipoma (uncommon), lipomatosis, liposarcoma
   6. Fibrous histiocytoma
   7. Hemangioma
   8. Desmoid tumor (most common primary)
   9. Desmoplastic small round cell tumor of peritoneum

B. ILL-DEFINED MASSES
   1. Metastases (ovary)
   2. Lymphoma
   3. Fibromatosis, fibrosing mesenteritis (associated with Gardner syndrome)
   4. Lipodystrophy
   5. Mesenteric panniculitis

C. STELLATE MASSES
   1. Peritoneal mesothelioma
   2. Retractile mesenteritis
   3. Fibrotic reaction of carcinoid
   4. Radiation therapy
   5. Desmoid tumor
   6. Hodgkin disease
   7. Tuberculous peritonitis
   8. Ovarian metastases
   9. Diverticulitis
   10. Pancreatitis
   ◊ A calcified mesenteric mass suggests carcinoid tumor!

D. LOCULATED CYSTIC MASSES (2/3)
   1. Cystic lymphangioma (most common)
   2. Pseudomyxoma peritonei
   3. Cystic mesothelioma
   4. Mesenteric cyst
   5. Mesenteric hematoma
   6. Benign cystic teratoma
   7. Cystic spindle cell tumor (= centrally necrotic leiomyoma / leiomyosarcoma)

Mesenteric / Omental Cysts

= "BUBBLES OF THE BELLY"

◊ The first step is to determine the organ of origin!

1. Lymphangioma
2. Nonpancreatic pseudocyst
   = sequelae of mesenteric / omental hematoma / abscess
   Path: thick-walled, usually septated cystic mass with hemorrhagic / purulent contents
3. Duplication cyst

GI

4. Mesothelial cyst
5. Enteric cyst

Mesenteric Edema / Congestion

√ increase of mesenteric fat attenuation to –40 to –60 HU
√ loss of sharp interfaces between mesenteric vessels + fat

A. SYSTEMIC FLUID OVERLOAD
   1. Hypoalbuminemia
   2. Liver cirrhosis
   3. Nephrosis
   4. Heart failure
B. LOCAL VESSEL DISEASE
   1. Portal vein thrombosis
   2. Mesenteric vein / artery thrombosis
   3. Vasculitis
   4. SMA dissection
C. CELL INFILTRATE
   1. Malignant neoplasm
   2. Inflammation
   3. Trauma (small hemorrhage)

Umbilical Tumor

A. PRIMARY (38%)
   benign / malignant neoplasm, skin tumor
B. METASTASES (30%)
   = "Sister Joseph nodule"
   • firm painful nodule
   • ± ulceration with serosanguinous / purulent discharge

   Cause: gastrointestinal cancer (50%), undetermined (25%), ovarian cancer, pancreatic cancer, small cell carcinoma of lung (very rare)

   Spread:
   (a) direct extension from anterior peritoneal surface
   (b) extension along embryonic remnants: falciform, median umbilical, omphalomesenteric ligaments
   (c) hematogenous
   (d) retrograde lymphatic flow from inguinal, axillary, paraaortic nodes
   (e) iatrogenic: laparoscopic tract, tract of percutaneous needle biopsy
C. NONNEOPLASTIC
   1. Endometriosis (32%)
   2. Granuloma
   3. Incarcerated hernia

ABDOMINAL LYMPHADENOPATHY

Regional Patterns of Lymphadenopathy

@ Retrocrural nodes
   Abnormal size: >6 mm
   Common cause: lung carcinoma, mesothelioma, lymphoma

@ Gastrohepatic ligament nodes
   = superior portion of lesser omentum suspending stomach from liver
   Abnormal size: >8 mm
   Common cause: carcinoma of lesser curvature of stomach, distal esophagus, lymphoma, pancreatic cancer, melanoma, colon + breast cancer
   DDx: coronary varices

@ Porta hepatis nodes
   = in porta hepatis extending down hepatoduodenal ligament, anterior + posterior to portal vein
   Abnormal size: >6 mm
   Common cause: carcinoma of gallbladder + biliary tree, liver, stomach, pancreas, colon, lung, breast
   Cx: high extrahepatic biliary obstruction

@ Pancreaticoduodenal nodes
   = between duodenal sweep + pancreatic head anterior to IVC
   Abnormal size: >10 mm
   Common cause: lymphoma, pancreatic head, colon, stomach, lung, breast cancer

@ Perisplenic nodes
   = in splenic hilum
   Abnormal size: >10 mm
   Common cause: NHL, leukemia, small bowel neoplasm, ovarian cancer, carcinoma of right / transverse colon

@ Retroperitoneal nodes
   = periaortic, pericaval, interaortocaval
   Abnormal size: >10 mm
   Common cause: lymphoma, renal cell, testicular, cervical, prostatic carcinomas

@ Celiac and superior mesenteric artery nodes
   = preaortic nodes
   Abnormal size: >10 mm
   Common cause: any intraabdominal neoplasm

@ Pelvic nodes
   = along common, external + internal iliac vessels
   Abnormal size: >15 mm
   Common cause: carcinoma of bladder, prostate, cervix, uterus, rectum

Enlarged Lymph Node with Low-density Center

1. Tuberculosis, Mycobacterium avium-intracellulare
2. Pyogenic infection
3. Whipple disease
4. Lymphoma
5. Metastatic disease after radiation + chemotherapy
6. Lymphangioleiomyomatosis
7. Neurofibromatosis type I

ANATOMY AND FUNCTION OF GASTROINTESTINAL TRACT

GASTROINTESTINAL HORMONES

Cholecystokinin

= CCK = 33 amino acid residues (former name: Pancreozymin); the 5 C-terminal amino acids are identical to those of gastrin, causing similar effects as gastrin

Produced in: duodenal + upper intestinal mucosa

Released by: fatty acids, some amino acids (phenylalanine, methionine), hydrogen ions

Effects:

@ Stomach
- (1) weakly stimulates HCl secretion
- (2) given alone: inhibits gastrin, which leads to decrease in HCl production
- (3) stimulates pepsin secretion
- (4) stimulates gastric motility

@ Pancreas
- (1) stimulates secretion of pancreatic enzymes (= Pancreozymin)
- (2) stimulates bicarbonate secretion (weakly by direct effect; strongly through potentiating effect on secretin)
- (3) stimulates insulin release

@ Liver
- (1) stimulates water + bicarbonate secretion

@ Intestine
- (1) stimulates secretion of Brunner glands
- (2) increases motility

@ Biliary tract
- (1) strong stimulator of gallbladder contraction
- (2) relaxation of sphincter of Oddi

Medication:

sincalide (Kinevac®) = cholecystokinin-C-terminal octapeptide

Use: may be used to empty gallbladder about 30 minutes (to 4 hours) before tracer injection in patients on prolonged fasting (gallbladder atony + retained bile and sludge secondary to absence of endogenously produced CCK)

Dose for radiologic imaging:

slow IV injection of 0.02 µg/kg Kinevac® over >3 minutes

Useful in:
- (a) patient fasting >24 hours / on total parenteral nutrition
- (b) acalculous cholecystitis
- (c) chronic GB dysfunction

Side effect: increase in biliary-to-bowel transit time, nausea, abdominal cramps

Gastrin

= 17 amino acid peptide amide;

PENTAGASTRIN

= acyl derivative of the biologic active C-terminal tetrapeptide amide

Produced in: antral cells + G cells of pancreas

Released by:
- (a) vagal stimulation, gastric distension
- (b) short-chain alcohol (ethanol, propanol)
- (c) amino acids (glycine, ß-alanine)
- (d) caffeine
- (e) hypercalcemia

mediated by neuroendocrine cholinergic reflexes

Inhibited by: drop in pH of antral mucosa to <3.5

Effects:

@ Stomach:
- (1) stimulation of gastric HCl secretion from parietal cells, which in turn:
- (2) increases pepsinogen production by chief cells through local reflex
- (3) increase in antral motility
- (4) trophic effect on gastric mucosa (parietal cell hyperplasia)

@ Pancreas
- (1) strong increase in enzyme output
- (2) weakly stimulates fluid + bicarbonate output
- (3) stimulates insulin release

@ Liver
- (1) water + bicarbonate secretion

@ Intestine
- (1) stimulates secretion of Brunner glands
- (2) increases motility

@ Gallbladder
- (1) stimulates contraction

@ Esophagus
- (1) increases resting pressure of LES

Glucagon

Produced in: α cells (and β cells) of pancreas

Released by: low blood glucose levels

Effects:

@ Intestines
- (1) lowers pressure of GE sphincter
- (2) hypotonic effect on duodenum > jejunum > stomach > colon

@ Hormones
- (1) releases catecholamines from the adrenal gland that paralyze intestinal smooth muscle
- (2) increases serum insulin + glucose levels (mobilization of hepatic glycogen)

@ Biliary tract
- (1) increases bile flow
- (2) relaxes gallbladder + sphincter of Oddi

Dose for radiologic imaging: 1 mg maximum

◊ IV administration causes a quick response + rapid dissipation of action!

◊ IM administration prolongs onset + increases length of action!

Half-life: 3–6 minutes

Side effects: nausea + vomiting, weakness, dizziness (delayed onset of 1.5–4 hours after IM administration)

Contraindication:
- (1) hypersensitivity / allergy to glucagon: urticaria, periorbital edema, respiratory distress, hypotension, coronary artery spasm (?), circulatory arrest
- (2) known hypertensive response to glucagon
- (3) pheochromocytoma: glucagon stimulates release of catecholamines
- (4) insulinoma: insulin-releasing effect may result in hypoglycemia
- (5) glucagonoma
- (6) poorly controlled diabetes mellitus

Secretin

Produced in: duodenal mucosa
Released by: hydrogen ions providing a pH <4.5
Effects:
@ Stomach
- (1) inhibits gastrin activity, which leads to decrease in HCl secretion
- (2) stimulates pepsinogen secretion by chief cells (potent pepsigogue)
- (3) decreases gastric and duodenal motility + contraction of pyloric sphincter

@ Pancreas
- (1) increases alkaline pancreatic secretions ($NaHCO_3$)
- (2) weakly stimulates enzyme secretion
- (3) stimulates insulin release

@ Liver
- (1) stimulates water + bicarbonate secretion (most potent choleretic)

@ Intestine
- (1) stimulates secretion of Brunner glands
- (2) inhibits motility

@ Esophagus
- (1) opens LES

EMBRYOLOGY OF ALIMENTARY TRACT

Origin: as a pouchlike extension of the yolk sac

Development of GI tube:
continuous tubular structure by 6 weeks GA;
divided into:
- (a) foregut (supplied by celiac artery)
- (b) midgut (supplied by superior mesenteric artery)
- (c) hindgut (supplied by inferior mesenteric artery)

Rotation about omphalomesenteric vessels by 270°:

<u><6 weeks GA</u>
90° counterclockwise rotation of duodenojejunal segment toward the right of SMA
90° counterclockwise rotation of ileocolic segment toward the left of SMA

<u>during 6th week GA</u>
additional 90° counterclockwise rotation of duodenum posterior to SMA
remainder of midgut within umbilical cord

<u>10–12 weeks GA</u>
intestines slides back into peritoneal cavity
final 90° counterclockwise rotation of duodenum
final 180° counterclockwise rotation of cecum

Peritoneal fixation of small bowel
broad-based mesentery extending from ligament of Treitz to ileocecal valve

ESOPHAGUS

Lower Esophageal Anatomy

A. **Esophageal Vestibule**
= saccular termination of lower esophagus with upper boundary at tubulovestibular junction + lower boundary at esophagogastric junction
√ collapsed during resting state
√ assumes bulbous configuration with swallowing

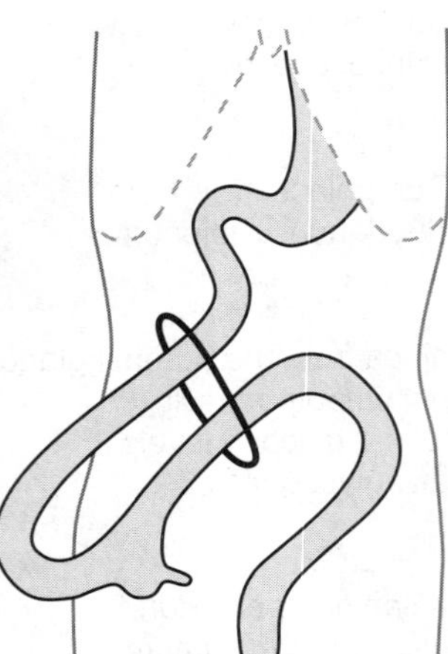
Rotation of duodenum + distal large bowel by 90° counterclockwise

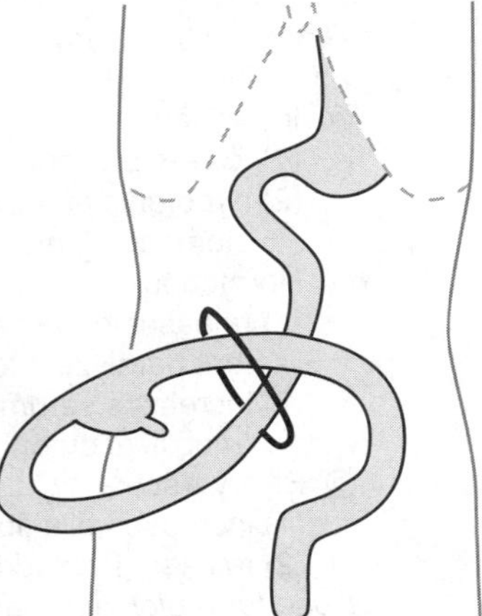
Rotation of duodenum by an additional 90° counterclockwise

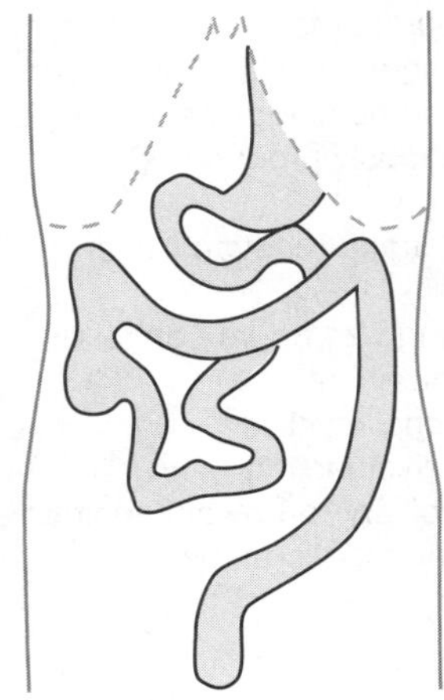
Final 90° counterclockwise rotation of duodenum

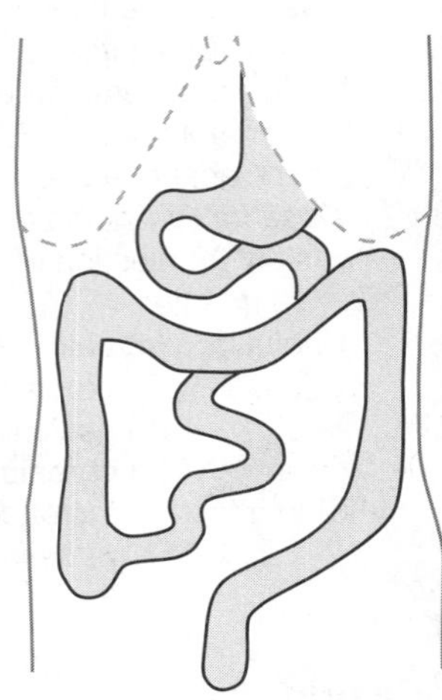
Final position of normal bowel rotation

Stages of Intestinal Rotation

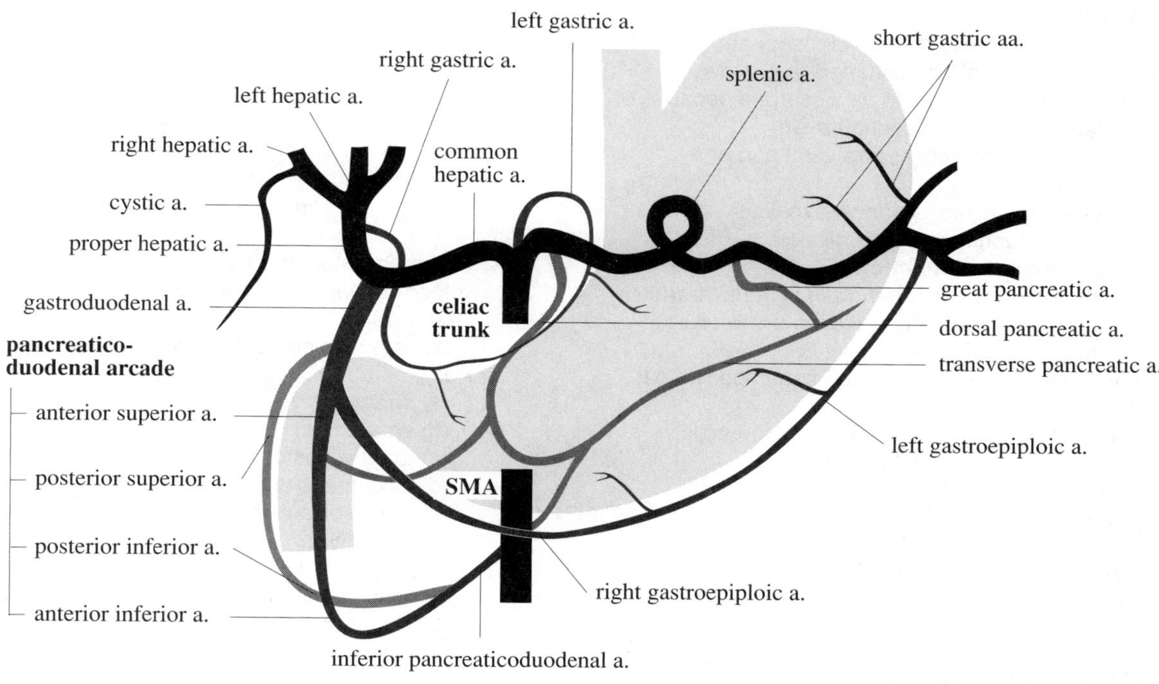

Blood Supply of Stomach, Duodenum, and Pancreas

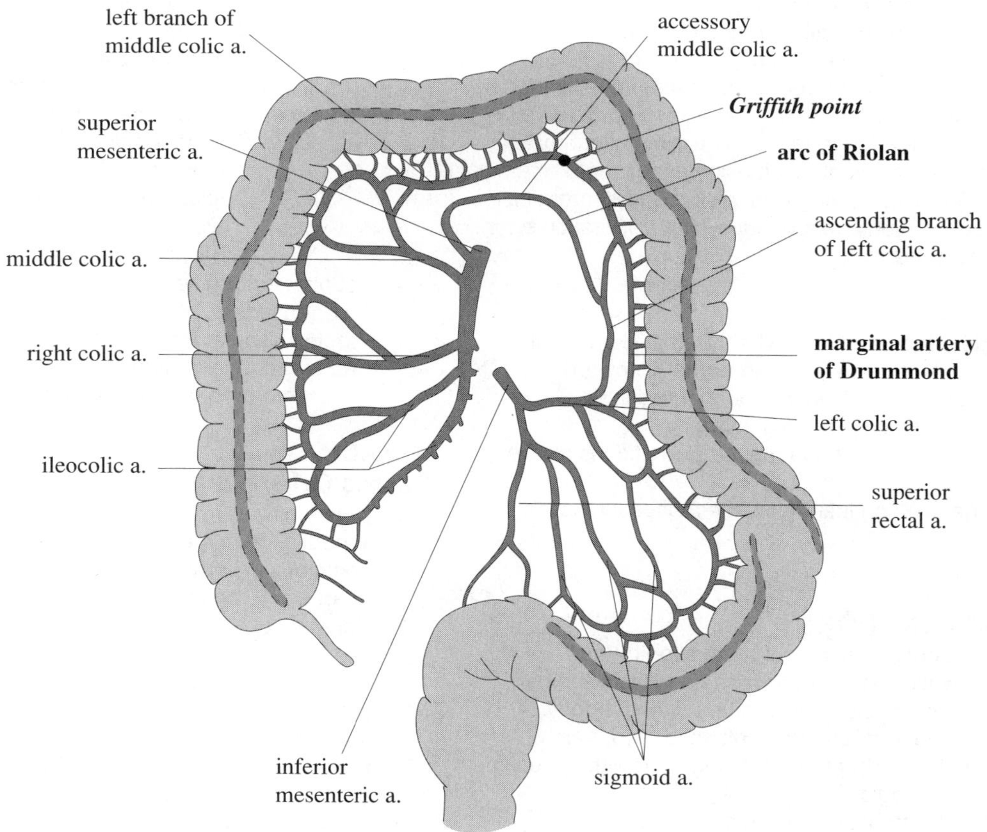

Blood Supply of Large Intestine

GI

(a) tubulovestibular junction = A level = junction between tubular and saccular esophagus
(b) phrenic ampulla = bell-shaped part above diaphragm (term should be discarded because of dynamic changes of configuration)
(c) submerged segment = infrahiatal part of esophagus
√ widening / disappearance is indicative of gastroesophageal reflux disease (GERD)

B. **Gastroesophageal Junction**
Site: at upper level of gastric sling fibers, straddles cardiac incisura demarcating the left lateral margin of GE junction

C. **Z line** = B level = zigzag-shaped squamocolumnar junction line
not acceptable criterion for locating GE junction
Site: 1–2 cm above gastric sling fibers

D. **Lower Esophageal Sphincter**
= physiologic 2–4-cm high pressure zone corresponding to esophageal vestibule
√ tightly closed during resting state
√ assumes bulbous configuration with swallowing

Muscular Rings of Esophagus

A Ring

= contracted / hypertrophied muscles in response to incompetent GE sphincter
• rarely symptomatic / dysphagia
Location: at tubulovestibular junction = superior aspect of vestibule
√ usually 2 cm proximal to GE junction at upper end of vestibule
√ varies in caliber during the same examination, may disappear on maximum distension
√ broad smooth narrowing with thick rounded margins
√ visible only if tubular esophagus above + vestibule below are distended

B Ring

= sling fibers representing a U-shaped thickening of inner muscle layers with open arm of U toward lesser curvature = inferior aspect of vestibule
Location: < 2 cm from hiatal margins
√ only visible when esophagogastric junction is above hiatus
√ thin ledge-like ring just below the mucosal junction (Z line)

SWALLOWING FUNCTION

Technique: videofluoroscopy of a modified barium swallow study to assess handling of bolus (with consistency of nectar liquid, honey liquid, pureed food, soft solid food, hard solid food); preferrably together with speech pathologist

Document patient behavior + reaction:
episode of refusal, cough, silent aspiration, apnea, bradycardia

CNS involved: cranial nerves V, VII, IX, X, XII; 5 cervical nerves; cortical + subcortical pathways; midbrain; brainstem
Muscles involved: 32 groups of muscles
Developmental: swallowing as early as 11 weeks GA; suckling at 18–24 weeks GA; nonnutritive sucking at 27–28 weeks GA; single breath sucking at 35–36 weeks GA

Phases:

1. Oral preparatory phase
√ food chewed + mixed with saliva
2. Oral phase
√ bolus propelled posteriorly to tongue
Path:
(a) spillage from mouth
(b) small bolus formation
(c) tongue tremor
(d) incomplete tongue elevation
(e) early spillage into valleculae prior to initiation of swallow
3. Pharyngeal phase
√ elevation of soft palate + valleculae (to seal nasopharynx)
√ elevation of larynx (to close vestibule)
√ relaxation of cricopharyngeal muscle
√ contraction of lateral pharyngeal wall
Path:
(a) nasopharyngeal reflux
(b) laryngeal penetration (= contrast material enters laryngeal vestibule
Cause: delayed elevation of larynx
(c) tracheal aspiration (= contrast material enters airway below vocal cord level)
Cause: delayed elevation of larynx, delayed pharyngeal transit time, decreased clearance of bolus with residual in vallecula + pyriform sinus spilling into larynx + trachea
4. Esophageal phase
√ contraction of cricopharyngeal muscle
√ bolus transfer into esophagus
Path: cricopharyngeal achalasia (with reflux of bolus into oropharynx / pooling in pyriform sinus)

STOMACH

Gastric Cells

1. Chief cells
= peptic / zymogenic cells
Location: body + fundus
produce: pepsinogen
2. Parietal cells
= oxyntic cells
Location: body + fundus
produce: H^+, Cl^-, intrinsic factor, prostaglandins
3. Mucous neck cells
produce: mucoprotein, mucopolysaccharide, aminopolysaccharide sulfate
4. Argentaffine cells
= enteroendocrine cells
Location: body + fundus

GI

produce: glucagon-like substance (A-cells), somatostatin (D-cells), vasoactive intestinal polypeptide (D_1-cells), 5-hydroxytryptamine (EC-cells)

5. G-cells
   Location: pylorus
   produce: gastrin

Effect of Bilateral Vagotomy

= cholinergic denervation

(1) decreased MOTILITY of stomach + intestines
(2) decreased GASTRIC SECRETION
(3) decreased TONE OF GALLBLADDER + bile ducts
(4) increased TONE OF SPHINCTERS (Oddi + lower esophageal sphincter)

Pylorus

= fan-shaped specialized circular muscle fibers with:

(a) distal sphincteric loop = right canalis loop
   √ corresponds to radiologic pyloric sphincter
(b) proximal sphincteric loop = left canalis loop
   √ 2 cm proximal to distal sphincteric loop on greater curvature (seen during complete relaxation)
(c) torus
   = fibers of both sphincters converge on the lesser curvature side to form a muscular prominence; prolapse of mucosa between sphincteric loops produces a niche simulating ulcer

√ pyloric channel 5–10 mm long, wall thickness of 4–8 mm
√ concentric indentation of the base of the duodenal bulb

SMALL BOWEL

◊ Longest tubular organ in body measuring 550–600 cm (18–22 feet) in length

Segments:
- duodenum of 25–30 cm in length
- jejunum of 10–12 feet in length (= proximal 60%)
- ileum of 6–8 feet in length (= distal 40%)

Mesentery: 15 cm long between ligament of Treitz + ileocecal junction

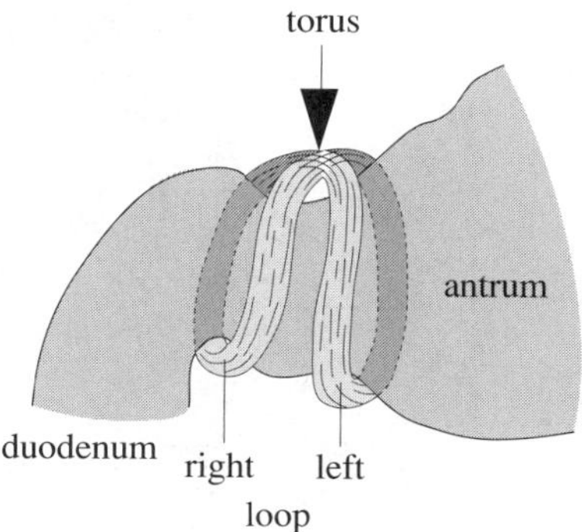

Pyloric Muscular Anatomy

Duodenal Segments

(1) duodenal bulb + short postbulbar segment:
   intraperitoneal + freely movable
(2) descending duodenum:
   retroperitoneal attached to head of pancreas
(3) horizontal = transverse segment:
   retroperitoneal crossing the spine
(4) ascending portion
   retroperitoneal ascending to level of duodenojejunal junction

VARIATIONS:
(1) "mobile duodenum" / "water-trap duodenum"
   = long postbulbar segment with undulation / redundancy
(2) duodenum inversum / duodenum reflexum
   = distal duodenum ascends to the right of spine to the level of duodenal bulb + then crosses spine horizontally + fixated in normal location

Small Bowel Folds

◊ Circular small bowel folds = folds of Kerckring
   = valvulae conniventes = two mucosal layers around a core of submucosa

A. NORMAL FOLD THICKNESS

@ jejunum	1.7–2.0 mm	>2.5 mm pathologic
@ ileum	1.4–1.7 mm	>2.0 mm pathologic

B. NORMAL NUMBER OF FOLDS

@ jejunum	4–7 / inch
@ ileum	2–4 / inch

C. NORMAL FOLD HEIGHT

@ jejunum	3.5–7.0 mm
@ ileum	2.0–3.5 mm

D. NORMAL LUMEN DIAMETER

@ upper jejunum	3.0–4.0 cm	>4.5 cm pathologic
@ lower jejunum	2.5–3.5 cm	>4.0 cm pathologic
@ ileum	2.0–2.8 cm	>3.0 cm pathologic

RULE OF 3's:
◊ Wall thickness <3 mm
◊ Valvulae conniventes <3 mm
◊ Diameter <3 cm
◊ Air-fluid levels <3

Normal Bowel Caliber

mnemonic: "3-6-9-12"

3 cm	maximal size of small bowel
6 cm	maximal size of transverse colon
9 cm	maximal size of cecum
12 cm	maximal caliber of cecum before it may burst

Small Bowel Peristalsis

A. INCREASED
   1. Vagal stimulation
   2. Acetylcholine
   3. Anticholinesterase (eg, neostigmine)
   4. Cholecystokinin
B. DECREASED
   1. Atropine (eg, Pro-Banthine®)
   2. Bilateral vagotomy

INTESTINAL FUNCTION

Intestinal Gas

A. INFLUX
1. Aerophagia .... 2 L
2. Liberation from intestinal tract
   (a) neutralization of bicarbonate in secretions (CO_2) .... 8 L
   (b) bacterial fermentation (CO_2, H_2, CH_4, H_2S) .... 15 L
3. Diffusion from blood (N_2, O_2, CO_2)

B. EFFLUX
1. Diffusion from intestines into blood and expulsion from lung .... 50 L
2. Expulsion from anus .... 2 L

Intestinal Fluid

A. INFLUX
1. Oral ingestion .... 2.5 L
2. Intestinal secretions .... 8.2 L
   saliva .... 1.5 L
   bile .... 0.5 L
   gastric secretions .... 2.5 L
   pancreatic secretions .... 0.7 L
   intestinal secretions .... 3.0 L

B. EFFLUX
1. Peranal .... 0.1 L
2. Intestinal resorption (primarily in ileum + ascending colon) .... 10.6 L

Defecography / Evacuation Proctography

evacuation time = 15 (range 5–40) seconds

anorectal angle = angle formed between central axis of anal canal + line parallel to posterior wall of rectum
√ 90° at rest and during voluntary contraction (squeeze maneuver)
√ more obtuse during defecation straining (void)

anorectal junction = point of taper of distal rectal ampulla as it merges with the anal canal; position of anorectal junction referenced to plane of ischial tuberosities = 0–3.5 cm; elevation during squeeze of 0–4.5 cm; elevation during void of –3.0–0 cm

rectovaginal space = space between vagina and rectum

perineum = area between external genital organs and anal verge

rectocele = measurement of anteroposterior depth of convex wall protrusion extending beyond expected margin of normal rectal wall
small <2 cm;
moderate = 2–4 cm;
large >4 cm

peritoneocele = extension of rectouterine excavation to below upper third of vagina; containing liquid / bowel / omentum

enterocele = bowel present in peritoneocele

rectal prolapse = descent of entire thickness of rectal wall through anal verge

rectal intussusception
= descent of the entire thickness of the rectal wall possibly extending into anal canal; starting 6–11 cm above anus; accompanied by formation of a circular indentation forming a ring pocket
√ infolding of <3 mm in width / > 3 mm in width / intraluminal narrowing / descent into anal canal / external prolapse

PERITONEUM

Peritoneal Spaces

Definitions:

Ligament = formed by two folds of peritoneum supporting a structure within the peritoneal cavity

Omentum = specialized structure connecting stomach to an additional structure

Mesentery = two peritoneal folds connecting a portion of bowel to the retroperitoneum

Embryology:

above transverse mesocolon:

A. RIGHT PERITONEAL SPACE
forms perihepatic space + lesser sac:
1. Right subphrenic space:
   — located between right hepatic lobe + diaphragm
   — limited posteriorly by right superior reflection of coronary lig. + right triangular ligament
2. Right subhepatic space:
   — divided into
     • anterior right subhepatic space: located just posterior to porta hepatis, communicating with lesser sac via epiploic foramen (= foramen of Winslow)

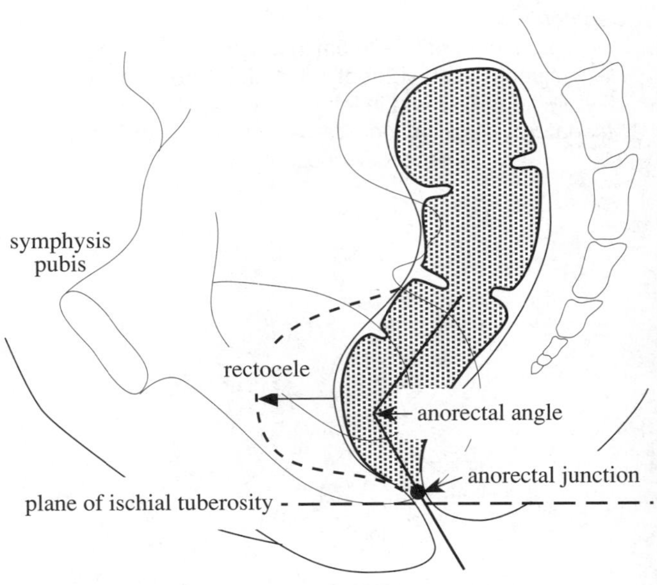

Defecographic Measurements

GI

- posterior right subhepatic space
  = Morison pouch = hepatorenal fossa
  ◊ Most dependent portion of the abdomen in supine patient!
3. Bare area of liver
   — situated between reflections of right + left coronary ligaments
   — continuous with right anterior pararenal space
4. Lesser sac:
   - superior recess:
     — surrounds medial aspect of caudate lobe
     — separated from splenic recess by gastropancreatic fold
   - splenic recess:
     — extends across midline to splenic hilum
   - inferior recess:
     — separates stomach from pancreas + transverse mesocolon
     — anteriorly covered by lesser omentum
5. Lesser omentum = combination of gastrohepatic ligament + hepatoduodenal ligament
6. Right triangular ligament:
   — forms from coalescence of superior and inferior reflections of right coronary ligament
   — divides posterior aspect of right perihepatic space into right subphrenic space + posterior right subhepatic space

B. LEFT PERITONEAL SPACE
forms left subphrenic space
1. Left subphrenic space:
   — artificially divided into
   - immediate subphrenic space: between diaphragm + gastric fundus
   - perisplenic space: bounded inferiorly by phrenicocolic lig.
   - subhepatic space = gastrohepatic recess: located between lateral segment of left hepatic lobe + stomach
   — separated from right subphrenic space by falciform ligament
2. Left triangular ligament:
   — forms from coalescence of superior and inferior reflections of left coronary ligament
   — located along superior aspect of left hepatic lobe

C. DORSAL MESENTERY gives rise to:
1. Gastrophrenic ligament
   — courses through immediate subphrenic space
   — suspends stomach from dome of diaphragm
2. Gastropancreatic ligament
   — formed by proximal left gastric artery
   — attaches posterior aspect of gastric fundus to retroperitoneum
   – partially separates superior recess of lesser sac from splenic recess
3. Phrenicocolic ligament
   — major suspensory ligament of spleen
   — attaches proximal descending colon to left hemidiaphragm
   — separates left subphrenic space from left paracolic gutter
4. Gastrosplenic ligament
   — remnant of dorsal mesentery
   — connects greater curvature of stomach with splenic hilum
   — contains short gastric vessels

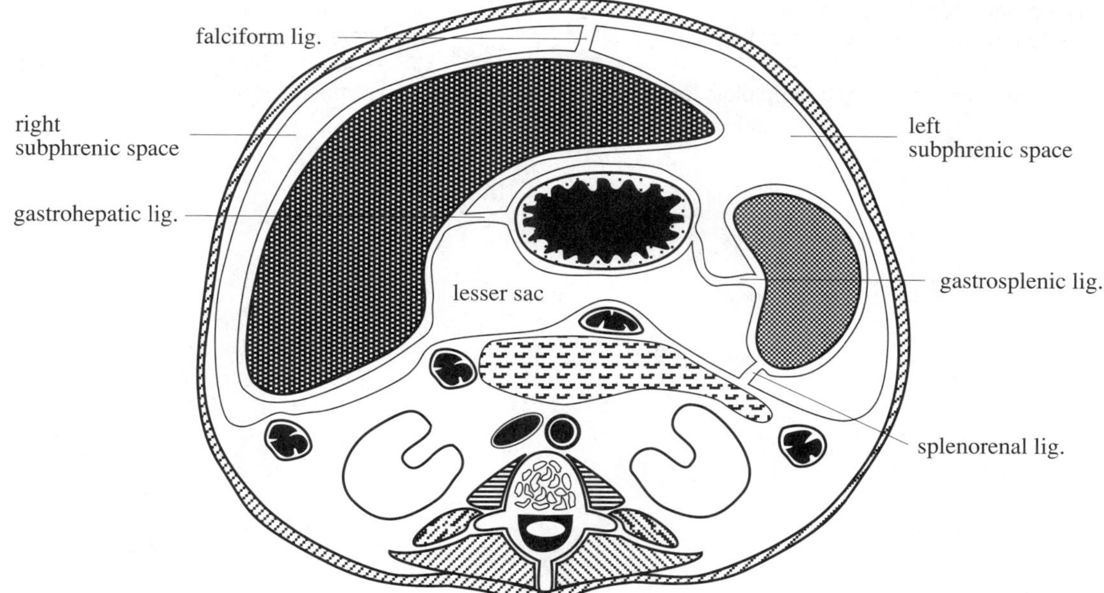

Ligaments and Peritoneal Spaces in Upper Abdomen

GI

5. Splenorenal ligament
   — connects posterior aspect of spleen to anterior pararenal space
   — contributes to left lateral + posterior border of lesser sac
   — encloses tail of pancreas + distal splenic artery + proximal splenic vein
6. Gastrocolic ligament
   — forms portion of anterior border of lesser sac
   — forms superior aspect of greater omentum
   — connects greater curvature of stomach with superior aspect of transverse colon
   — contains gastroepiploic vessels

D. VENTRAL MESENTERY gives rise to:
1. Falciform ligament
   = sickle-shaped fold composed of two layers of peritoneum
   — attaches ventral surface of liver to anterior abdominal wall
   — its right layer continues into the superior layer of the coronary ligament, its left layer continues into the anterior layer of the left triangular ligament
   — contains ligamentum teres (= obliterated umbilical vein) in its free inferoposterior margin
   — continuous with fissure for ligamentum venosum
2. Gastrohepatic ligament:
   — arises in fissure of ligamentum venosum
   — connects medial aspect of liver to lesser curvature of stomach as part of lesser omentum
   — contains left gastric artery, coronary vein, lymph nodes
3. Hepatoduodenal ligament:
   — forms inferior edge of gastrohepatic ligament
   — forms anterior margin of epiploic foramen
   — extends from proximal duodenum to porta hepatis
   — contains common hepatic duct, common bile duct, hepatic artery, portal vein

<u>below transverse mesocolon</u>:

A. VENTRAL MESENTERY regresses

B. DORSAL MESENTERY forms:
1. Transverse mesocolon:
   — suspends transverse colon from retroperitoneum along anteroinferior edge of pancreas
   — forms posteroinferior border of lesser sac
   — contains middle colic vessels
2. Small bowel mesentery:
   — suspends small bowel from retroperitoneum
   — extends from ligament of Treitz to ileocecal valve
   — contains superior mesenteric vessels + lymph nodes
3. Sigmoid mesocolon:
   — attaches sigmoid colon to posterior pelvic wall
   — contains sigmoid + hemorrhoidal vessels
4. Greater omentum:
   — inferior continuation of gastrocolic ligament
   — formed by double reflection of dorsal mesogastrium thus composed of 4 layers of peritoneum
5. Superior + inferior ileocecal recesses:
   — located above + below terminal ileum
6. Retrocecal space:
   — present only if peritoneum reflects posterior to cecum
7. Right + left paracolic gutters:
   — located lateral to ascending + descending colon
8. Intersigmoid recess:
   — located along undersurface of sigmoid mesocolon

GASTROINTESTINAL DISORDERS

ACHALASIA

= failure of organized peristalsis + relaxation at level of lower esophageal sphincter

Etiology: (a) idiopathic: abnormality of Auerbach plexus / medullary dorsal nucleus; ? neurotropic virus, ? gastrin hypersensitivity
(b) Chagas disease

√ megaesophagus = dilatation of esophagus beginning in upper 1/3, ultimately entire length
√ absence of primary peristalsis below level of cricopharyngeus
√ nonperistaltic contractions
√ "bird-beak" / "rat tail" deformity = V-shaped conical + symmetric tapering of stenotic segment with most marked narrowing at GE junction
√ Hurst phenomenon = temporary transit through cardia when hydrostatic pressure of barium column is above tonic LES pressure
√ sudden esophageal emptying after ingestion of carbonated beverage (eg, Coke)
√ "vigorous achalasia" = numerous tertiary contractions in nondilated distal esophagus of early achalasia
√ prompt relaxation of LES upon amyl nitrate inhalation (smooth-muscle relaxant)

CXR:
√ right convex opacity behind right heart border; occasionally left convex opacity if thoracic aorta tortuous
√ right convex opacity may be tethered by azygos arch allowing for greater dilatation above + below
√ air-fluid level (stasis in thoracic esophagus filled with retained secretions + alimentary residue)
√ small / absent gastric air bubble
√ anterior displacement + bowing of trachea (LAT view)
√ patchy bilateral alveolar opacities resembling acute / chronic aspiration pneumonia (M. fortuitum-chelonei infection)

Cx: esophageal carcinoma in 2–7% (usually midesophagus)
Rx: pneumatic dilatation / surgical myotomy

DDx: (1) Neoplasm (separation of gastric fundus from diaphragm; normal peristalsis; asymmetric tapering)
(2) Peptic stricture of esophagus

Secondary Achalasia

= carcinoma of cardia / gastric fundus invading esophagus

Age: >50 years
• duration of symptoms for <6 months
√ irregular / asymmetric narrowing
√ abrupt transition
√ associated fundal lesion

ADENOMA OF SMALL BOWEL

Location: duodenum (21%), jejunum (36%), ileum (43%) esp. ileocecal valve

Histo: (1) Hamartomatous polyp (77%), multiple in 47%, 1/3 of multiple lesions associated with Peutz-Jeghers syndrome
(2) adenomatous polyp (13%), may have malignant potential
(3) polypoid gastric heterotopic tumor (10%)

ADENOMATOUS COLONIC POLYP

= EPITHELIAL POLYP

Most common benign colonic tumor (68–79%)

Predisposed: previously detected polyp / cancer; family history of polyps / cancer; idiopathic inflammatory bowel disease; Peutz-Jeghers syndrome; Gardner syndrome; familial polyposis

Prevalence: 3% in 3rd decade; 10% in 7th decade; 26% in 9th decade

Location: rectum (21–34%); sigmoid (26–38%); descending colon (6–18%); transverse colon (12–13%); ascending colon (9–12%); multiple in 35–50% (usually <5–10 in number)

Histo:

1. Tubular adenoma (75%)
   = cylindrical glandular formation lined by stratified columnar epithelium + containing nests of epithelium within lamina propria
   √ usually <10 mm in diameter
   √ often pedunculated if >10 mm
   malignant potential: <10 mm in 1%; 10–20 mm in 10%; >20 mm in 35%
2. Tubulovillous adenoma (15%)
   = mixture between tubular + villous adenoma
   malignant potential: <10 mm in 4%; 10–20 mm in 7%; >20 mm in 46%
3. Villous adenoma (10%)
   = thin frondlike surface projections ("villous fronds")
   • potassium depletion
   √ often >20 mm in diameter with papillary surface
   √ often broad-based sessile lesion
   malignant potential: <10 mm in 10%; 10–20 mm in 10%; >20 mm in 53%

Adenoma size & incidence of malignancy:
<5 mm in 0.5%; 5–9 mm in 1%; 10–20 mm in 5–10%; >20 mm in 10–50% malignant

◊ Invasive carcinoma (= penetration of muscularis mucosa):
(a) rare in a pedunculated adenoma of <15 mm
(b) in 30% of villous adenomas of >50 mm

◊ All polyps >10 mm should be removed!

◊ Time for adenoma-carcinoma sequence probably averages 10–15 years!

Probability of coexistent colonic growth:
— synchronous adenoma in 50%
— metachronous adenoma in 30–40%
— synchronous adenocarcinoma in 1.5–5%
— metachronous adenocarcinoma in 5–10%
• asymptomatic (75%)
• diarrhea, abdominal pain
• peranal hemorrhage (67%)
Colonoscopy (incomplete in 16–43%)
BE:
Sensitivity of DCBE in detecting polyps:
<10 mm 80–83%; >10 mm 96–97%; all 84–88%; rate of detection of polyps <10 mm higher with DCBE than SCBE
√ sessile flat / round polyp
√ pedunculated polyp: stalk >2 cm in length almost always indicative of a benign polyp
√ suggestive of malignancy: irregular lobulated surface, broad base = width of the base greater than height, retraction of colonic wall = dimpling / indentation / puckering at base of tumor, interval growth
√ lacelike / reticular surface pattern CHARACTERISTIC for villous adenoma (occasionally in tubular adenoma)

DDx: (1) Nonneoplastic: hyperplastic polyp, inflammatory pseudopolyp, lymphoid tissue, ameboma, tuberculoma, foreign-body granuloma, malacoplakia, heterotopia, hamartoma
(2) Neoplastic subepithelial: lipoma, leiomyoma, neurofibroma, hemangioma, lymphangioma, endothelioma, myeloblastoma, sarcoma, lymphoma, enteric cyst, duplication, varix, pneumatosis, hematoma, endometriosis

ADENOCARCINOMA OF SMALL BOWEL

Frequency: about 50 x less common than colonic carcinoma
Risk factors: Crohn disease, sprue, Peutz-Jeghers syndrome, Lynch syndrome II, congenital bowel duplication, ileostomy, duodenal / jejunal bypass surgery
Histo: mostly moderately to well differentiated; may arise in villous tumors / de novo; no correlation between size and invasiveness
Location: duodenum (~50%, especially near ampulla), jejunum > ileum
√ annular stricture with "overhanging edges" (60%)
√ lobulated / ovoid polypoid sessile mass (41%)
◊ Duodenal tumors tend to be papillary / polypoid!
√ ulcerated mass (27%)
CT:
√ soft-tissue mass with heterogeneous attenuation
√ moderate contrast enhancement
Cx: intussusception
DDx: lymphoma (lymphadenopathy more bulky)

AFFERENT LOOP SYNDROME

= PROXIMAL LOOP / BLIND LOOP SYNDROME
= partial intermittent obstruction of afferent loop leading to overdistension of loop by gastric juices after Billroth-II gastrojejunostomy

Cause: gastrojejunostomy with left-to-right anastomosis (= proximal jejunal loop attached to greater curvature instead of lesser curvature), mechanical factors (intussusception, adhesion, kinking), inflammatory disease, neoplastic infiltration of local mesentery or anastomosis, idiopathic motor dysfunction
• postprandial epigastric fullness relieved by bilious vomiting
• vitamin B_{12} deficiency with megaloblastic anemia
• afferent loop with abnormal bacterial flora (Gram negative, resembling colon in quality + quantity)
Abdominal plain film:
√ normal in 85% (no air in lumen of afferent loop)
UGI:
√ preferential emptying of stomach into proximal loop
√ proximal loop stasis
√ regurgitation
CT:
√ rounded water-density masses adjacent to head + tail of pancreas forming a U-shaped loop
√ oral contrast material may not enter loop
√ may result in biliary obstruction (increased pressure at ampulla)
Rx: antibiotic therapy

AIDS

◊ Gastrointestinal involvement due to opportunistic infections + AIDS-associated neoplasms!
◊ Pathologic abnormalities at multiple sites with single / several opportunistic organisms are frequent!

A. VIRAL PATHOGENS
1. **Cytomegalovirus infection**
◊ Most common cause of life-threatening opportunistic viral infection in AIDS patients!
Organism: double-stranded DNA virus of the herpes family
Infection: ubiquitous among humans occurring at an early age in populations with poor sanitation + crowded living conditions
◊ Result of reactivation of latent virus in previously infected host!
Prevalence: 13% of all gastrointestinal diseases in AIDS patients
Path: infection of endothelial cells leads to small vessel vasculitis resulting in hemorrhage, ischemic necrosis, ulceration
Histo: large mononuclear epithelial / endothelial cells that contain intranuclear / cytoplasmatic inclusions with surrounding inflammation
Location: colon > small bowel (terminal ileum) > esophagus > stomach
@ Esophagus
√ single / multiple large superficial ulcers
@ Small bowel
√ luminal narrowing secondary to marked bowel wall thickening

√ thickened irregular folds (vasculitis leading to thrombosis + ischemia)
√ penetrating ulcer ± perforation
√ CMV pseudotumor (uncommon)

@ Colon (CMV colitis)
• hematochezia, crampy abdominal pain, fever
√ findings of toxic megacolon
√ discrete small well-defined nodules (similar to lymphoid nodular hyperplasia) throughout entire colon
√ aphthous ulcers on background of normal mucosa
√ marked bowel wall thickening
√ double-ring / target sign on CT (due to increased submucosal edema)
√ ascites
√ inflammation of pericolonic fat + fascia

Rx: ganciclovir (effective in 75%)

2. **Herpes simplex virus infection**
◊ Result of reactivation of latent virus in previously infected host
Organism: neurotropic DNA virus of herpes family
Prevalence: 70% for type 1, 16% for type 2 (endemic in United States); type 2 much more common in AIDS
Infection: direct inoculation through mucous membrane contact; from dormant state in root ganglia reactivated + transported via efferent nerves to mucocutaneous surface
Location: oral cavity, esophagus, rectum, anus
√ multiple small discrete ulcers

3. **HIV infection**
◊ Not an AIDS-defining illness!
Infection: acute HIV-infection with transient immunosuppression / during AIDS
√ >2-cm large solitary ulcer in the mid- or distal esophagus (HIV-infected cells cause alterations in cytokines resulting in infiltration of inflammatory cells into submucosa + destruction of mucosa)
Rx: corticosteroids

B. FUNGAL PATHOGENS

1. **Candidiasis**
◊ The absence of thrush does not exclude the diagnosis of candida esophagitis!
Organism: commensal fungus Candida albicans
Prevalence: 10–20% (in United States); up to 80% in developing countries
Location: oral cavity, esophagus
√ discrete linear / irregular longitudinally oriented filling defects in esophagus
Cx: disseminated systemic candidiasis (rare + indicative of granulocytopenia from chemotherapy / direct inoculation via catheter)

2. **Histoplasmosis**
Organism: dimorphic opportunistic fungus
Prevalence: 10% GI involvement with disseminated histoplasmosis in AIDS patients
Location: colon > terminal ileum
√ segmental inflammation / apple core lesion / bowel stricture
√ hepatosplenomegaly
√ mesenteric lymphadenopathy
√ diffuse hypoattenuation of spleen

C. PROTOZOAN PATHOGENS

1. **Cryptosporidiosis**
◊ One of the most common causes of enteric + biliary disease in AIDS patients!
Organism: intracellular parasite Cryptosporidium
Prevalence: isolated in 6% of all patients with AIDS; in 16% (in United States) + in up to 48% (in developing countries) in patients with diarrhea
• severe choleralike debilitating diarrhea with fluid loss of 10–17 L/day
Location: jejunum > other small bowel > stomach > colon
√ Cryptosporidium antritis (= area of focal gastric thickening + ulceration)
√ small bowel dilatation (increased secretions)
√ regular fold thickening + effacement (atrophy, blunting, fusion, loss of villi)
√ "toothpaste" appearance of small bowel (mimicking sprue)
√ dilution of barium (hypersecretion)
√ marked antral narrowing (extensive inflammation)
√ AIDS-related cholangitis
Dx: microscopic identification in stool / biopsy

2. **Pneumocystosis**
◊ Likely to occur in patients treated with aerosolized pentamidine!
Organism: eukaryotic microbe Pneumocystis carinii
Prevalence: pulmonary infection in 75% of AIDS patients; in <1% dissemination
Location: liver, spleen, lymph nodes
√ hepatic + splenic + nodal punctate calcifications
√ multiple tiny echogenic foci in spleen
√ multiple low-attenuation lesions of varying size in spleen (foamy eosinophilic material) with subsequently progressive rimlike / punctate calcifications

D. BACTERIAL PATHOGENS

1. **Tuberculosis**
◊ Most common cause of serious HIV-related infection worldwide with tendency to occur earlier than other AIDS-defining opportunistic infections!
Prevalence: 4% (in United States) + 43% (in developing countries) of HIV-infected persons

Infection: swallowing of infected sputum; hematogenous spread from pulmonary focus; direct extension from lymph node
Location: lymph nodes, liver, spleen, peritoneum, GI tract (especially ileum, colon, ileocecal valve)
√ low-attenuation mesenteric lymphadenopathy (suggestive of necrosis)
√ segmental ulceration
√ inflammatory stricture
√ hypertrophic lesion resembling polyp or mass

2. **Mycobacterium avium complex infection**
= PSEUDO-WHIPPLE DISEASE in AIDS
◊ Most common opportunistic infection of bacterial origin in AIDS patients!
◊ Most common nontuberculous mycobacterial infection in AIDS patients!
Organism: facultative intracellular acid-fast bacillus M. avium / M. intracellulare
Infection: invasion of Peyer patches + adjacent mesenteric lymph nodes
Histo: true granulomas with Langhans giant cells and caseous necrosis are rare because infection occurs in patients with advanced disease and a CD4 cell count of <100/μL
• diarrhea, malabsorption (similar clinical picture as in Whipple disease caused by Mycobacterium avium-intracellulare)
Location: jejunum (most common)
√ mild dilatation of middle + distal small bowel
√ wall thickening of small bowel loops
√ diffuse irregular mucosal fold thickening and nodularity without ulceration
√ mesenteric + retroperitoneal lymphadenopathy (1.0–1.5 cm in size) with homogeneous soft-tissue attenuation causing segmental separation of small bowel loops
√ hepatosplenomegaly
√ multiple tiny echogenic foci in liver + spleen (occasionally large hypoechoic / low-attenuation lesions)
Dx: (1) Visualization of large numbers of intracellular acid-fast bacilli in foamy histiocytes of tissue specimens
(2) Tissue culture
DDx: Whipple disease (positive with periodic acid-Schiff stain just like M. avium, but not with acid-fast stain, responsive to tetracyclines)

E. OTHER INFECTIONS
1. **Bacillary angiomatosis**
Organism: Rickettsiales Bartonella henselae
Histo: characteristic pattern of vascular proliferation with bacilli
Location: cutis (mimicking Kaposi sarcoma), liver, spleen, lymph nodes
√ peliosis (blood-filled cystic spaces) of liver / spleen
√ abdominal lymphadenopathy with contrast enhancement

2. **Isospora belli**
◊ Infection resembles cryptosporidiosis
Organism: protozoan pathogen
Histo: oval oocysts within bowel lumen / epithelial cells; localized inflammation; fold atrophy
Location: small intestine
• severe watery diarrhea
√ fold thickening

F. AIDS-ASSOCIATED NEOPLASMS
1. Kaposi sarcoma

2. **Non-Hodgkin lymphoma**
◊ 2nd most common AIDS-associated neoplasm
Prevalence: in 4–10% of AIDS patients (60 times higher risk compared with general population); occurs in all AIDS risk groups
Histo: multiclonal B-cell lymphoma of high or intermediate grade
• at initial presentation widely disseminated disease often with extranodal involvement
Location: CNS, bone marrow, GI tract (stomach, small bowel)
@ Stomach
√ circumferential / focal wall thickening
√ mural mass ± ulceration
@ Small bowel
√ diffuse / focal wall thickening
√ excavated mass
√ solitary / multiple liver lesions

Differential diagnostic considerations:
1. Splenomegaly (31–45%)
Cause: nonspecific (most), lymphoma, infection (M. avium-intracellulare, P. carinii)
2. Lymphadenopathy (21–60%)
Cause: reactive hyperplasia (most), Kaposi sarcoma, lymphoma, infections
Size: <3 cm in diameter (in 95%)
3. Hepatomegaly (20%)
Cause: nonspecific, hepatitis, fatty infiltration, lymphoma, Kaposi sarcoma
4. AIDS-related cholangiopathy:
Organism: CMV, Cryptosporidium
√ papillary stenosis of CBD
√ dilatation of extra- and intrahepatic bile ducts
√ periductal fibrosis
√ strictures + irregularities of bile ducts resembling primary sclerosing cholangitis
√ intraluminal polypoid filling defects
5. AIDS-related esophagitis:
Organism: Candida, herpes simplex, CMV
√ giant esophageal ulcer: HIV (76%), CMV (14%)
√ esophageal fistula / perforation: tuberculosis, actinomycosis

6. Gastritis
   Organism: CMV (GE junction + prepyloric antrum), Cryptosporidium (antrum)
7. AIDS enteritis
   Organism: Cryptosporidium, M. avium complex
8. AIDS colitis
   — ischemic bowel
   — acute appendicitis
   — neutropenic colitis
   — pseudomembranous colitis
   — infectious colitis / ileitis
9. Bowel obstruction
   (a) infection
   (b) intussusception: Kaposi sarcoma, lymphoma

AMEBIASIS

= primary infection of the colon by protozoan Entamoeba histolytica

Countries: worldwide distribution, most common in warm climates; South Africa, Egypt, India, Asia, Central + South America (20%); United States (5%)

Route: contaminated food / water (human cyst carriers); cyst dissolves in small bowel; trophozoites settle in colon; proteolytic enzymes + hyaluronidase lyse intestinal epithelium; may embolize into portal venous + systemic blood system

Histo: amebic invasion of mucosa + submucosa causing tiny ulcers, which spread beneath mucosa + merge into larger areas of necrosis; mucosal sloughing; secondary bacterial infection

- asymptomatic for months / years
- acute attacks of diarrhea (loose mucoid bloodstained stools)
- fever, headache, nausea

Location: (areas of relative stasis) right colon + cecum (90%) > hepatic + splenic flexures > rectosigmoid

√ loss of normal haustral pattern with granular appearance (edema, punctate ulcers)
√ "collarbutton" ulcers
√ cone-shaped cecum
√ several cm long stenosis of bowel lumen in transverse colon, sigmoid colon, flexures (result of healing + fibrosis); in multiple segments
√ ameboma = hyperplastic granuloma with bacterial invasion of amebic abscess; usually annular + constricting / intramural mass / cavity continuous with bowel lumen; shrinkage under therapy in 3–4 weeks
√ ileocecal valve thickened + fixed in open position with reflux
√ involvement of distal ileum (10%)

Dx: stool examination / rectal biopsy

Cx: (1) Toxic megacolon with perforation
(2) Amebic abscess in liver (2%), brain, lung (transdiaphragmatic spread of infection), pericolic, ischiorectal, subphrenic space
(3) Intussusception in children (due to ameboma)
(4) Fistula formation (colovesical, rectovesical, rectovaginal, enterocolic)

AMYLOIDOSIS

= group of heterogeneous disorders caused by interstitial deposits of a protein-polysaccharide in various organs leading to hypoxia, mucosal edema, hemorrhage, ulceration, mucosal atrophy, muscle atrophy

Cause: (a) prolonged antigenic stimulation of RES by chronic infection
(b) disorder of immunoincompetence
(c) aging
(d) idiopathic

Histo: amorphous eosinophilic hyaline material deposited around terminal blood vessels, stains with Congo red + crystal violet; green birefringence under polarizing light; amyloid fibrils have β-pleated sheet structure (= β fibrilloses)

Biochemical classification (1979):

1. AL amyloidosis
   (A = amyloidosis, L = light chain immunoglobulin)
   - monoclonal protein in serum + urine
   - occurs in primary amyloidosis + myeloma-associated amyloidosis

   Histo: massive deposits in muscularis mucosae + submucosa

   √ thickening of folds with polyps / large nodules
2. SAA amyloidosis (S = serum, AA = amyloid A)
   - occurs in secondary = reactive amyloidosis

   Histo: expansion of lamina propria

   √ coarse mucosal pattern + innumerable fine granular elevations
3. AF amyloidosis (A = amyloid, F = familial)
   - AF prealbumin as precursor of fibrils
   - occurs in familial amyloidosis
4. AS amyloidosis (A = amyloid, S = senile)
   - AS prealbumin as precursor of fibrils
   - occurs in senile amyloidosis

   √ massive amyloid deposition
5. AH amyloidosis (A = amyloid, H = hemodialysis)
   - β_2 microglobulin as precursor of fibrils
6. AE amyloidosis (A = amyloid, E = endocrine)
   - calcitonin produced by medullary thyroid carcinoma is precursor of fibrils

GI

Reimann classification (1935):

1. Primary = idiopathic amyloidosis
   = probably autosomal dominant inheritance with immunologically determined dysfunction of plasma cells
   - absence of discernible preceding / concurrent disease

   Location: (predominant involvement of connective tissues + mesenchymal organs) heart (90%), lung (30–70%), liver (35%), spleen (40%), kidneys (35%), adrenals, tongue (40%), GI tract (70%), skin + subcutis (25%)

   √ tendency to nodular deposition

2. Secondary amyloidosis (most common form)
   - following / coexistent with prolonged infectious / inflammatory processes

   Cause: rheumatoid arthritis (in 20%), Still disease, tuberculosis, osteomyelitis, leprosy, chronic pyelonephritis, bronchiectasis, ulcerative colitis, Waldenström macroglobulinemia, familial Mediterranean fever, lymphoreticular malignancy, paraplegia

   Location: spleen, liver, kidneys (>80%), breast, tongue, GI tract, connective tissue

   √ small amyloid deposits
3. Amyloidosis associated with multiple myeloma
   - may precede development of multiple myeloma

   Incidence: 10–15%

   √ primary amyloidosis with osteolytic lesions in myelomatous disease
4. Tumor-forming / organ-limited amyloidosis
   - related to primary type

   (a) hereditary = familial amyloidosis

   (b) senile amyloidosis (limited to heart / brain / pancreas / spleen)

   √ large localized masses

◊ GI involvement in primary more common than in secondary amyloidosis!

- malabsorption (diarrhea, protein loss)
- occult GI bleeding
- obstruction
- macroglossia

@ Esophagus (11%)
√ loss of peristalsis
√ megaesophagus

@ Stomach (37%)
- postprandial epigastric pain + heartburn
- acute erosive hemorrhagic gastritis

(a) diffuse infiltrative form
√ small-sized stomach with rigidity + loss of distensibility simulating linitis plastica (from thickening of gastric wall)
√ effaced rugal pattern
√ diminished / absent peristalsis
√ marked retention of food

(b) localized infiltration (often located in antrum)
√ irregularly narrowed + rigid antrum
√ thickened rugae
√ superficial erosions / ulcerations

(c) amyloidoma = well-defined submucosal mass

@ Small bowel (74%)

(a) diffuse form (more common)
√ diffuse uniform thickening of valvulae conniventes in entire small bowel
√ broadened flat undulated mucosal folds (mucosal atrophy)
√ "jejunalization" of ileum
√ impaired intestinal motility
√ small bowel dilatation

(b) localized form (less common)
√ multiple pea- / marble-sized deposits
√ pseudoobstruction = physical + plain-film findings suggesting mechanical obstruction with patent large + small bowel on barium examination (involvement of myenteric plexus)

Cx: small bowel infarction

@ Colon (27%):
√ pseudopolyps in colon

@ Bone:
√ bone cysts

@ Liver:

Path: extracellular deposition of amyloid in the spaces of Disse (= narrow gaps between endothelial linings of sinusoids and hepatocytes of hepatic lamina) with progressive encroachment on hepatic parenchymal cells + sinusoids

- hepatic function usually preserved

CT:
√ hepatomegaly
√ regions of low attenuation with decreased contrast enhancement

@ Spleen:

Histo: (a) nodular form involving lymph follicles
(b) diffuse form infiltrating red pulp

√ discrete masses
√ splenomegaly (4–13%)

MR:
√ T2 values significantly lower than normal

Cx: spontaneous splenic rupture (from vascular fragility + acquired coagulopathy)

Dx: by rectal / gingival biopsy

DDx: Whipple disease, intestinal lymphangiectasia, lymphosarcoma

ANGIODYSPLASIA OF COLON

= VASCULAR ECTASIA = ARTERIOVENOUS MALFORMATION

Cause: ?; acquired lesion

Associated with: aortic stenosis (20%)

Incidence at autopsy: 2%

Age: majority >55 years

Location: (a) cecum + ascending colon (majority)
(b) descending + sigmoid colon (25%)

Site: usually at antimesenteric border

- chronic intermittent low-grade bleeding
- occasionally massive bleeding

√ "arterial tuft" = cluster of vessels during arterial phase along antimesenteric border
√ early opacification of draining ileocolic vein
√ densely opacified dilated tortuous ileocolic vein into late venous phase
√ contrast extravasation (unusual)

ANISAKIASIS

= parasitic disease of GI tract

Cause: ingestion of Anisakis larvae present in raw / undercooked fish (mackerel, cod, pollack, herring, whiting, bonito, squid) consumed as sashimi, sushi, ceviche, lomi-lomi

Organism: worm with straight / serpentine / circular threadlike appearance

◊ Site of penetration by larvae determines clinical form!

GI

@ Gastric anisakiasis
- acute gastric pain, nausea, vomiting a few hours after ingestion (DDx: acute gastritis, peptic ulcer, food poisoning, neoplasia)
- eosinophilia

√ mucosal edema
√ about 3-cm-long threadlike filling defects (= larvae)

@ Intestinal anisakiasis
- diffuse abdominal tenderness / colicky abdominal pain, nausea, vomiting (DDx: acute appendicitis, regional enteritis, intussusception, ileus, diverticulitis, neoplasia)
- leukocytosis without eosinophilia (frequent)

Histo: marked edema, eosinophilic infiltrates, granuloma formation
√ thickened folds
√ disappearance of Kerckring folds
√ thumbprinting / saw-tooth appearance
√ irregular luminal narrowing
√ eosinophilic ascites (DDx: eosinophilic gastroenteritis, hypereosinophilic syndrome)
Cx: ileus

@ Colonic anisakiasis (rare)
DDx: colonic tumor

ANORECTAL MALFORMATION

(1) Rectal atresia
= open anus + atretic rectal segment superior to anus + no fistula

(2) Ectopic anus
= fistulous opening of bowel due to failure of terminal bowel to descend normally
Site of arrest: high / low colon arrest = above / below puborectal sling
- most common anomaly of anorectal segment
- anal dimple + external sphincter in normal position

Location of fistula: perineum, vestibule, vagina, urethra, bladder, cloaca
√ low small bowel / colonic obstruction
√ "M" line accurately represents level of puborectal muscle = line drawn horizontally through junction of lower 1/3 + upper 2/3 of ischium on lateral radiograph

(3) Imperforate anus
= blind ending of terminal bowel + no fistula

(4) Cloacal malformation

(5) Cloacal exstrophy

Embryology:
during weeks 3 and 4 the dorsal part of the yolk sac folds are incorporated into embryo forming the *primitive hindgut* consisting of distal part of transverse + descending + sigmoid colon, rectum, superior portion of anal canal, epithelium of urinary bladder, and most of the urethra; at 4 weeks the transverse *rectovesical septum* descends caudally between allantois and hindgut dividing the *cloaca* into *urogenital sinus* ventrally + *anorectal canal* dorsally; by 7th week the rectovaginal septum fuses with cloacal membrane creating a *urogenital membrane* ventrally + anal membrane dorsally; perineum is formed by fusion of rectovesical septum + cloacal membrane; *anal membrane* ruptures by 9th week

In 48% associated with: (part of VACTERL syndrome)
(1) GU anomalies (20%):
renal agenesis / ectopia, vesicoureteral reflux, obstruction, hypospadia (3.1%); M > F
(2) Lumbosacral segmentation anomalies (30%):
dysplasia, agenesis, hemivertebrae
(3) GI anomalies (11%):
esophageal atresia ± tracheoesophageal fistula (4%), duodenal atresia / stenosis
(4) Cardiovascular anomalies (8%)
(5) Abdominal wall (2%)
(6) Cleft lip–cleft palate (1.6%)
(7) Down syndrome (1.5%)
(8) Meningomyelocele (0.5%) + occult myelodysplasia
(9) Others (8%)

ANTRAL MUCOSAL DIAPHRAGM

= ANTRAL WEB
Age range: 3 months to 80 years
Associated with: gastric ulcer (30–50%)
- symptomatic if opening <1 cm

Location: usually 1.5 cm from pylorus (range 0–7 cm)
√ constant symmetric band of 2–3 mm thickness traversing the antrum perpendicular to long axis of stomach
√ "double bulb" appearance (in profile)
√ concentric / eccentric orifice
√ normal peristaltic activity

APPENDICITIS

Prevalence: 1–4% in children with acute abdominal pain
Lifetime risk: 7–9% in Western world population
Etiology: obstruction of appendiceal lumen by lymphoid hyperplasia (60%), fecolith (33%), foreign bodies (4%), stricture, tumor, parasite; Crohn disease (in 25%)
Cause: luminal obstruction from
(a) fecolith (11–52%) = hard crushable concretions from inspissation of fecal material + inorganic salts
(b) appendiceal calculus = hard noncrushable calcified stone (7–15%)
(c) lymphoid hyperplasia
(d) foreign body
(e) parasite
(f) primary tumor: carcinoid, adenocarcinoma, Kaposi sarcoma, lymphoma
(g) metastatic tumor: colon cancer, breast cancer

Pathogenesis:
continued secretion of mucus in appendiceal obstruction elevates intraluminal pressure + distends lumen; venous engorgement + arterial compromise + tissue ischemia ensues after intraluminal pressure exceeds capillary perfusion pressure

Peak age: 2nd decade; thereafter declining incidence; M:F = 3:2 (in teens / young adults, thereafter 1:1)
◊ Rare under the age of 2 years!

- 80% clinical accuracy (78–92% in males, 58–85% in females):
  Diagnostic dilemma (20–35%):
  in elderly, ovulating women, infants / young children
  ◊ 32–45% rate of misdiagnosis in women between ages 20–40!
  ◊ 5–25% false-negative appendectomy rate for pediatric population!
  - pain
    - mild poorly localized visceral pain of 4–6 hours duration referred to epigastrium + periumbilical region
    - crampy pain migrates into RLQ pain over appendix = McBurney sign (72%) and becomes continuous + more severe (somatic pain)
  - anorexia, nausea, vomiting (40%)
  - afebrile / low-grade fever (56%)
    ◊ Suspect perforation with temperature >38.3°C
  - leukocytosis with left shift (88%)

Clinical scoring system: "MANTRELS" score of 10

Migration of pain to RLQ 1
Anorexia 1
Nausea and vomiting 1
Tenderness in RLQ 2
Rebound pain 1
Elevated temperature 1
Leukocytosis 2
Shift of WBC count to left 1

Location:
(a) base of appendix: posteromedial wall of cecum 3 cm below ileocecal valve
(b) tip of appendix: retrocecal, subcecal, retroileal, preileal, within pelvis (30%), extraperitoneal (5%)

Abdominal plain film (abnormalities seen in <50%):
◊ Plain-film findings become more distinctive after perforation, while clinical findings subside / simulate other diseases!
√ usually laminated calcified appendicolith in RLQ (in 7–15%):
  ◊ Appendicolith + abdominal pain = 90% probability of acute appendicitis!
  ◊ Appendicolith in acute appendicitis means a high probability for gangrene / perforation!
√ cecal changes:
  √ thickening of cecal wall
  √ water-density mass + paucity / absence of intestinal gas in RLQ (in 24% of perforations)
  √ "cecal ileus" = gas-fluid level in cecum in gangrene (= local paralysis)
  √ colon cutoff sign = amputation of gas at the hepatic flexure (in 20% of perforations) due to spastic ascending colon
√ small bowel obstruction pattern = small bowel dilatation with air-fluid levels (in 43% of perforations)
√ extraluminal gas (in 33% of perforations):
  √ gas loculation
  √ mottled bacteriogenic gas
  √ pneumoperitoneum (rare)
√ loss of fat planes:
  √ focal increase in thickness of lateral abdominal wall in 32% (= edema between properitoneal fat line + cecum)
  √ loss of properitoneal fat line
  √ loss of pelvic fat planes around the bladder / right obturator (= fluid / pus in cul-de-sac)
  √ loss of definition of right inferior hepatic outline (= free peritoneal fluid)
  √ distortion of psoas margin + flank stripes
√ scoliosis (due to muscle irritation)

BE / UGI (accuracy 50–84%):
√ failure to fill appendix with barium (normal finding in up to 35%)
√ indentation along medial wall of cecum (= edema at base of appendix / matted omentum / periappendiceal abscess)

Graded-compression US (85% sensitive, 92% specific, 78–96% accurate, 91–94% PPV, 89–97% NPV):
◊ Nondiagnostic study in 4% due to inadequate compression of RLQ
◊ Useful in ovulating women (false-negative appendectomy rate in males 15%, in females 35%) + infants / children
√ visualization of noncompressible appendix as a blind-ending tubular aperistaltic structure (seen only in 2% of normal adults, but in 50% of normal children)
√ laminated wall with target appearance of ≥6 mm in total diameter on cross section (81% SPECIFIC) / mural wall thickness ≥2 mm
√ lumen may be distended with anechoic / hyperechoic material
√ pericecal / periappendiceal fluid
√ increased periappendiceal echogenicity (= infiltration of mesoappendix / pericecal fat)
√ enlarged mesenteric lymph nodes
√ loss of wall layers = gangrenous appendix
√ perforated appendix (23–73%):
  √ loss of echogenic submucosal layer
  √ appendix no longer visualized (40–60%)
  √ loculated periappendiceal / pelvic fluid collection ± gas bubbles (= abscess)
  √ prominent hyperechoic mesoappendix / pericecal fat
  √ visualization of appendicolith (6%) = bright echogenic focus with clean distal acoustic shadowing
  √ gas bubbles localized to perforation site
√ hypoechoic zones with poor margination within inflamed fat (= phlegmonous appendicitis)
√ sympathetic thickening of adjacent terminal ileum + ascending colon

False-negative US:
(a) failure to visualize appendix
  — inability of adequate compression
  — aberrant location of appendix (eg, retrocecal)
  — appendiceal perforation
(b) early inflammation limited to appendiceal tip

False-positive US:
(a) normal appendix mistaken for appendicitis

GI

(b) alternate diagnosis: Crohn disease, pelvic inflammatory disease, inflamed Meckel diverticulum
(c) spontaneous resolution of acute appendicitis

Color Doppler US:
√ increased conspicuity (= increase in size + number) of circumferential vessels in and around the wall of the appendix (= hyperemia)
√ decreased resistance of arterial waveforms
√ continuous / pulsatile venous flow
√ decreased / no perfusion = gangrenous appendicitis

CT (87–100% sensitive, 89–98% specific, 93–98% accurate, 92–98% PPV, 95–100% NPV):
√ normal appendix visualized in 67–100%:
 √ 1–2 cm below ileocecal junction from posteromedial aspect of cecum with a diameter of up to 10 mm
√ abnormal appendix:
 √ distended lumen (appendix >7 mm in diameter)
 √ circumferential wall thickening
 √ homogeneously enhancing wall ± mural stratification ("target sign")
 √ appendicolith = homogeneous / ringlike calcification (25%)
 √ distal appendicitis = abnormal tip of appendix + normal proximal appendix and normal cecal apex
√ periappendicular inflammation (98%):
 √ linear streaky densities in periappendicular / pericecal / mesenteric / pelvic fat
 √ subtle clouding of mesentery
 √ local fascial thickening
 √ free peritoneal fluid
 √ mesenteric lymphadenopathy
√ circumferential / focal cecal apical thickening (80%):
 √ "arrowhead sign" = funnel of contrast medium in cecum symmetrically centering about occluded orifice of appendix
√ perforation of appendix:
 √ nonvisualization of appendix (due to fragmentation)
 √ pericecal phlegmon = pericecal soft-tissue mass (DDx: ileocolitis with secondary inflammation of appendix)
 √ pericecal / mesenteric / pelvic abscess = poorly encapsulated single / multiple fluid collection with air / extravasated contrast material
 √ appendicolith
 √ extraluminal air
 √ marked ileocecal thickening
 √ localized lymphadenopathy
 √ peritonitis
 √ small-bowel obstruction

False-negative CT:
(a) overlapping range in maximal appendiceal diameter between inflamed + uninflamed appendix
(b) appendix mistaken for unopacified bowel
(c) inflammation limited to appendiceal tip

Prognosis:
(1) mild acute appendicitis may resolve spontaneously (after relief of inciting obstruction)
(2) recurrent appendicitis (10%) = repeated similar episodic attacks of RLQ pain leading to appendectomy + showing acute inflammation
(3) chronic appendicitis (1%) = RLQ pain of >3 weeks + no alternative diagnosis + chronic active inflammation on histology + relief of symptoms after appendectomy
(4) Mortality rate of 1% (associated with perforation)

Cx: perforation (13–30–73%), abscess formation, peritonitis, wound infection, sepsis, infertility, adhesions, bowel obstruction, death

Rx: finding of appendicolith is sufficient evidence to perform prophylactic appendectomy in asymptomatic patients (50% have perforation / abscess formation at surgery)

DDx: colitis, diverticulitis, epiploic appendagitis, small bowel obstruction, infectious enteritis, duodenal ulcer, pancreatitis, intussusception, Crohn disease, mesenteric lymphadenitis, ovarian torsion, pelvic inflammatory disease
 ◊ Only 22–38% of children referred for suspected appendicitis actually have appendicitis

ASCARIASIS

= most common parasitic infection in world; cosmopolitan occurrence; endemic along Gulf Coast, Ozark Mountains, Nigeria, Southeast Asia

Organism: Ascaris lumbricoides = roundworm parasite, 15–35 cm in length; production of 200,000 eggs daily

Cycle: infection by contaminated soil, eggs hatch in duodenum, larvae penetrate into venules / lymphatics, carried to lungs, migrate to alveoli and up the bronchial tree, swallowed, maturation in jejunum within 2.5 months

Age: children age 1–10 years
• colic
• eosinophilia
• appendicitis
• hematemesis / pneumonitis
• jaundice (if bile ducts infested)

Location: jejunum > ileum (99%), duodenum, stomach, CBD, pancreatic duct
√ 15–35-cm-long tubular filling defects
√ barium-filled enteric canal outlined within Ascaris
√ whirled appearance, occasionally in coiled clusters ("bolus of worms")

Cx: (1) Perforation of bowel
(2) Mechanical obstruction

BANNAYAN-RILEY-RUVALCABA SYNDROME

= RUVALCABA-MYHRE-SMITH SYNDROME

Cause: autosomal dominant transmission
• pigmented genital lesions
√ hamartomatous intestinal polyps (in 45%): usually in distal ileum + colon
√ macrocephaly
√ subcutaneous and visceral lipomas + hemangiomas

GI

BARRETT ESOPHAGUS

= BARRETT SYNDROME

= replacement of stratified squamous epithelium by metaplastic columnar epithelium (Barrett epithelium) containing goblet cells but no parietal cells

Cause: chronic gastroesophageal reflux with epithelial injury from esophagitis

Contributing factors:

genetic influence, reduced LES pressure, transient LES relaxation, hiatal hernia, delayed acid clearance, reduced acid sensitivity, duodenogastroesophageal reflux, alcohol, tobacco, chemotherapy, scleroderma (37%), S/P repair of esophageal atresia / esophagogastric resection / Heller esophagomyotomy

Histo: (1) specialized columnar epithelium (proximal)
(2) junctional-type epithelium (distal to above)
(3) fundic-type epithelium (most distally)

Prevalence: in general 0.3–4%; 7–10% of patients with advanced chronic reflux esophagitis

Associated with: moderate + severe esophagitis (94%), no / mild esophagitis (6%)

Age: 0–15 years and 40–88 years (mean of 55 years); M > F; mainly among Whites

- dysphagia (due to esophageal stricture)
- signs of reflux esophagitis: heartburn, substernal chest pain, regurgitation
- low-grade upper intestinal bleeding
- asymptomatic

Location: middle to lower esophagus

N.B.: the squamocolumnar junction does not coincide with the GE junction, is irregular and lies >2–3 cm orad from the gastroesophageal junction

Distribution: circumferential / focal

√ several-cm-long stricture (71%) in midesophagus (40%) or lower esophagus (60%) [DDx: peptic stricture without Barrett esophagus]

√ large deep wide-mouthed peptic ulcer (= Barrett ulcer) at upwardly displaced squamocolumnar junction / within columnar epithelium

√ fine reticular mucosal pattern (3–30%) resembling areae gastricae of the stomach = netlike web of barium-filled grooves surrounding small tufts of mucosa; located distally from stricture (DDx: gastroesophageal reflux, monilial + viral esophagitis, superficial spreading carcinoma)

√ thickened irregular mucosal folds (28–86%)

√ fine granular mucosal pattern (DDx: reflux esophagitis, acanthosis, leukoplakia, superficial spreading carcinoma, moniliasis / herpes simplex / CMV esophagitis)

√ gastroesophageal reflux (45–63%)

√ distal esophageal widening (34–66%; due to abnormal motility)

√ hiatal hernia (75–94%)

√ uptake of Tc-99m pertechnetate by columnar epithelium

Dx: velvety pinkish red appearance of gastric-type mucosa extending from gastric mucosa into distal esophagus (endoscopy with biopsy)

Cx: (1) Ulceration ± penetration into mediastinum
(2) Stricture
3. Adenocarcinoma (0–10–46%;) 40-fold higher risk than general population
√ plaquelike / focal irregularity / nodularity / sessile polyps

Rx: (1) stop smoking, avoid bedtime snacks + foods that lower LES pressure, lose excess weight
(2) suppress gastric acidity: antacids, H_2-receptor antagonists (cimetidine, ranitidine, famotidine), H^+K^+-adenosintriphosphatase inhibitor (omeprazole)
(3) improve LES pressure: metoclopramide, bethanechol
(4) esophageal resection in high-grade dysplasia

BEHÇET SYNDROME

= uncommon chronic multisystem inflammatory disorder of unknown etiology with relapsing course characterized by mucocutaneous-ocular symptoms as a triad of aphthous stomatitis, genital ulcers, ocular inflammation

Countries: worldwide, most common in eastern Mediterranean countries, eastern rim of Asia

Histo: nonspecific necrotizing vasculitis with deposition of immune complexes in walls of small blood vessels

Age at onset: 3rd decade; M:F = 2:1

Major criteria: buccal + genital ulceration, ocular inflammation, skin lesions

Minor criteria: thrombophlebitis, GI + CNS lesions, arthritis, family history

- abdominal pain + diarrhea (50%)

@ Mucocutaneous: aphthous stomatitis, papules, pustules, vesicles, folliculitis, erythema nodosum-like lesions

@ Genital: ulcers on penis + scrotum / vulva + vagina

@ Ocular: relapsing iridocyclitis, hypopyon, choroiditis, papillitis, retinal vasculitis

@ Articular: mild nondestructive arthritis

@ Vascular: migratory thrombophlebitis

@ CNS: chronic meningoencephalitis

DDx: Reiter syndrome, Stevens-Johnson syndrome, SLE, ulcerative colitis, ankylosing spondylitis

Intestinal Behçet Disease

= large deeply penetrating intestinal ulcers (HALLMARK)

Incidence: 10–40%

Location: terminal ileum, cecum, ascending colon, transverse colon

√ deep round ulcers similar in appearance to peptic ulcers of stomach / duodenum

√ multiple shallow / longitudinal / aphthoid ulcers

CT:

√ polypoid lesion / thickened bowel wall (mural edema associated with deep ulcer penetration)

√ contrast enhancement (71%)

√ minimal lymphadenopathy, mostly <10 mm

Cx (56%): panperitonitis with high mortality due to tendency for perforation at multiple sites; fistula; hemorrhage

Prognosis: recurrence in 40–45% adjacent to surgical anastomosis

GI

DDx: ulcerative colitis, Crohn disease

BEZOAR

[*padzahr*, Persian = antidote, counterpoison]
= persistent concretions of foreign matter composed of accumulated ingested material in intestines
Incidence: 0.4% (large endoscopic series)
Etiology: material unable to exit stomach because of large size, indigestibility, gastric outlet obstruction, poor gastric motility (diabetes, mixed connective tissue disease, myotonic dystrophy, hypothyroidism)
Predisposition:
previous gastric surgery (vagotomy, pyloroplasty, antrectomy, partial gastrectomy), inadequate chewing, missing teeth, dentures, massive overindulgence of food with high fiber contents
• anorexia, bloating, early satiety / may be asymptomatic

Phytobezoar

Incidence: 55% of all bezoars
= poorly digested fibers, skin + seeds of fruits and vegetables usually forming in stomach, may become impacted in small bowel
• history of recent ingestion of pulpy foods
Food: oranges, persimmons (most common, unripe persimmons contain the tannin shibuol that forms a gluelike coagulum after contact with dilute acid)
Site of impaction: stomach, jejunum, ileum
√ intraluminal filling defect without constant site of attachment to bowel wall
√ interstices filled with barium
√ coiled-spring appearance (rare)
√ partial / complete obstruction
Cx: decubitus ulceration + pressure necrosis of bowel wall, perforation, peritonitis
DDx: lobulated / villous adenoma, leiomyosarcoma, metastatic melanoma, intussusception

Trichobezoar

[*trikho-*, *thrix*, Greek = hair]
80% are < age 30, almost exclusively in females;
Associated with: gastric ulcer in 24–70%

BLUE RUBBER BLEB NEVUS SYNDROME

= rare disorder characterized by vascular hamartomas of skin + visceral hemangiomas predominantly afflicting the GI tract (but also liver, spleen, heart, skeletal muscle, lung, kidney, thyroid, eyes, CNS)
Etiology: sporadic / autosomal dominant
Path: thin layer of connective tissue + single layer of endothelial cells surrounding blood-filled ectatic vessels
• red to deep blue soft painless cutaneous lesions evacuating under pressure + slow refilling (commonly present at birth ± increase in size and number with age)
• iron deficiency anemia (due to spontaneous hemorrhage)
√ nodular filling defects throughout small bowel

MR:
√ hyperintense lesions on T2WI (due to slow flow / thrombosis)
Cx: intussusception, volvulus; pressure erosion of bone, osseous + soft-tissue hypertrophy (secondary to hypervascularity)
DDx:
(1) Mafucci syndrome (dyschondroplasia + osteochondromas + vascular malformations)
(2) Klippel-Trenaunay-Weber syndrome (port wine stain, vascular malformations, limb hypertrophy)
(3) Kasabach-Merritt syndrome (large vascular malformations + consumptive coagulopathy)
(4) Kaposi sarcoma
(5) Peutz-Jeghers syndrome (congenital polyposis + melanotic cutaneous lesions)
(6) Gardner syndrome (soft-tissue tumors + sebaceous cysts)

BLUNT ABDOMINAL TRAUMA

CT is imaging method of choice for evaluation of stable patients
US imaging in the detection of intraabdominal injury: 86% sensitive, 99% specific, 98% accurate

Hemoperitoneum

Frequency: 29–34% of patients with abdominal visceral injury have no hemoperitoneum
Location: paracolic gutters, pelvis
CT (negative predictive value of 99.6%):
Attenuation values of blood:
during IV contrast administration and assuming an initially normal hematocrit without significant dilution from intraperitoneal fluid (ascites, urine, succus, lavage fluid)
— serum (after hematocrit effect) 0–20 HU
— fresh unclotted blood 30–45 HU
— clotted blood 60–100 HU
— active arterial extravasation >180 HU
√ "sentinel clot" sign = the highest attenuation value of blood clot marks the anatomic site of visceral injury
√ high-density active arterial extravasation always surrounded by lower-density hematoma (DDx: extravasated oral contrast is not surrounded by lower-density material)
US:
√ usually anechoic fluid accumulation in subhepatic space (= Morison pouch) > pouch of Douglas / paravesical space > between bowel loops
DDx: bowel contents, urine, bile, ascites
√ hemoperitoneum score = depth of largest fluid collection in cm + 1 point for each additional site with fluid (score of ≤2 managed conservatively)
√ hyperechoic / occasionally isoechoic masses (= intraperitoneal clot)
Prognosis: 17% of patients without hemoperitoneum require surgical / angiographic intervention
◊ Peritoneal lavage cannot quantify amount of hemoperitoneum + results in a 19–39% rate of nontherapeutic surgeries

Hypovolemia = Hypoperfusion complex

√ "collapsed cava" sign = persistent flattening of IVC (due to decreased venous return)
N.B.: abort CT examination as shock is imminent!
√ small hypodense spleen (decreased enhancement)
√ small aorta + mesenteric arteries (due to intense vasoconstriction)
√ shock nephrogram = lack of renal contrast excretion
√ "shock bowel" = dilatation of fluid-filled intestines + generalized thickening of small bowel folds + increased enhancement (due to vasoconstriction of mesenteric vessels)
√ marked enhancement of adrenal gland
√ intense pancreatic enhancement

Blunt Trauma To Spleen

◊ Most frequently injured intraperitoneal organ in blunt abdominal trauma

Associated with: other solid visceral / bowel injuries (29%); lower rib fractures in 44%, injury to left kidney in 10%, injury to left diaphragm in 2%

◊ 20% of left rib fractures have splenic injury!
◊ 25% of left renal injury have splenic injury!

Technique: scanning delay of 60–70 seconds to avoid heterogeneous splenic enhancement

Categories of Splenic Injury

Grade	*Injury*	*Description*
I	hematoma	subcapsular <25% surface area
	laceration	capsular tear <1 cm parenchymal depth
II	hematoma	subcapsular 25–50% surface area; intraparenchymal <5 cm in diameter
	laceration	1–3 cm deep without involvement of trabecular vessel
III	hematoma	subcapsular >50% surface area; ruptured subcapsular / parenchymal; intraparenchymal >10 cm / expanding
	laceration	>3 cm parenchymal depth / involvement of trabecular vessels
IV	laceration	involving segmental / hilar vessels with devascularization of >25%
V	laceration	completely shattered spleen
	vascular	total splenic devascularization

CECT (95% accurate):
◊ CT not reliable to determine need for surgical intervention!
√ hemoperitoneum (indicates disruption of splenic capsule)
√ "sentinel clot" (= area of >60 HU adjacent to spleen) sensitive predictor of splenic injury = **perisplenic hematoma**
√ high-attenuation area (80–370 HU) = **active extravasation** / pseudoaneurysm:
N.B.: active extravasation of contrast material usually requires surgery
√ mottled parenchymal enhancement = **contusion**
√ hypoattenuating line connecting opposing visceral surfaces = linear parenchymal defect = **splenic laceration**:
  √ almost always associated with hemoperitoneum
√ crescentic region of low attenuation along splenic margin flattening / indenting / compressing the normal parenchyma = **subcapsular hematoma**
√ round hypodense inhomogeneous region ± hyperdense clot = **intrasplenic hematoma**
√ hypoattenuating hematoma with complete separation of splenic fragments = laceration traversing two capsular surfaces = **splenic fracture**
√ multiple lacerations = **"shattered spleen"**

US:
√ hyperechoic intraparenchymal region (= acute hematoma / laceration)
√ anechoic intralesional collection (= brisk hemorrhage)
√ diffusely heterogeneous parenchymal pattern containing hyper- and hypoechoic areas (= extensive splenic injury)
√ loss of normal organ contour (= perisplenic clot)

Sequelae:
(1) scar / fibrosis
(2) splenic pseudocyst (20–30 HU)
(3) pseudoaneurysm formation
(4) delayed splenic rupture
  = hemorrhage >48 hours after trauma
  Cause: subcapsular hematoma
  Prevalence: 0.3–20% of blunt splenic injuries
  Time of onset: in 70% within 2 weeks of injury, in 90% within 4 weeks of injury

Prognosis: 52% surgery (splenectomy [8%], splenorrhaphy), 48% nonsurgical management

Rx: up to 91% of stable patients can be treated conservatively with observation; transcatheter embolization

DDx:
(1) Normal lobulation / splenic cleft (smoothly contoured, medially located)
(2) Adjacent unopacified jejunum simulating splenic tissue
(3) Early differential enhancement of red and white pulp (scan obtained within 20–50 seconds)
(4) Perisplenic fluid from ascites / urine / succus / bile / lavage

Blunt Trauma To Liver (20%)

◊ Second most frequently injured intraabdominal viscus

Associated with: splenic injury in 45%

• clinical manifestation often delayed by days / weeks

Location: R > L lobe

Site: perivascular, paralleling right + middle hepatic arteries + posterior branches of right portal vein, avulsion of right hepatic vein from IVC (13%)
◊ Left lobe injury more often associated with damage to duodenum, pancreas, transverse colon

GI

Categories of Liver Injury		
Grade	*Injury*	*Description*
I	hematoma	subcapsular <10% surface area
	laceration	capsular tear <1 cm parenchymal depth
II	hematoma	subcapsular 10–50% surface area; intraparenchymal <10 cm in diameter
	laceration	1–3 cm deep and <10 cm long
III	hematoma	subcapsular >50% surface area; ruptured subcapsular / parenchymal; intraparenchymal >10 cm / expanding
	laceration	>3 cm parenchymal depth
IV	laceration	parenchymal disruption 25–75% of lobe; 1–3 Couinaud segments in single lobe
V	laceration	disruption >75% of single lobe; >3 Couinaud segments in single lobe
	vascular	juxtahepatic venous injury (HV, IVC)
VI	vascular	hepatic avulsion

CECT:
- √ hypoattenuating hematoma:
  - √ lenticular configuration (= subcapsular hematoma) usually resolving within 6–8 weeks
  - √ irregular linear branching / round regions of low attenuation = laceration
  - √ focal / diffuse periportal tracking (in up to 22%) due to dissecting hemorrhage / bile / dilated periportal lymphatics (secondary to elevated central venous pressure / injury to lymphatics)
  - √ alteration in distribution of vessels + ducts
- √ hypodense wedge extending to liver surface = focal hepatic devascularization
- √ focal hyperdense (80–350 HU) area = active hemorrhage / pseudoaneurysm
- √ hemoperitoneum (inability of liver veins to contract)
- √ intrahepatic / subcapsular gas (usually due to necrosis)

US:
- √ localized area of increased intraparenchymal echogenicity (= acute hematoma / laceration)

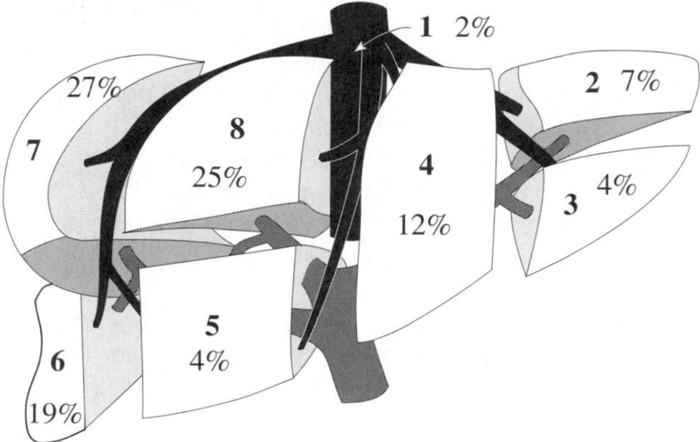

Distribution of Traumatic Hepatic Lesions

- √ widespread heterogeneous liver echogenicity + absence of normal vascular pattern (= global parenchymal injury)

Cx: in up to 20%
(1) delayed rupture (rare)
(2) hemobilia
(3) arteriovenous fistula / pseudoaneurysm
(4) biloma ± infection
(5) superinfection of hematoma / devascularized hepatic parenchyma

Rx: conservative treatment in up to 80% in adults + 97% in children; transcatheter embolization

Healing: 1–6–15 months

DDx: (1) beam-hardening artifact from adjacent ribs / from air-contrast level in stomach
(2) Focal fatty infiltration

Blunt Trauma to Gallbladder (2%)

Associated with: injury to liver, duodenum
- √ pericholecystic fluid (extraperitoneal location of GB)
- √ free intraperitoneal fluid

CECT:
- √ blurred contour of GB
- √ focal thickening / discontinuity of GB wall
- √ intraluminal enhancing mucosal flap
- √ hyperattenuating blood within GB lumen
- √ mass effect on adjacent duodenum
- √ collapsed GB = GB rupture
- √ focal periportal tracking = GB rupture

US:
- √ focal hypoechoic thickening
- √ echogenic mass within GB lumen

Blunt Trauma to GI Tract (5%)

Cause in children: MVA (lap belts), bicycle handle bar, child abuse

May be associated with: Chance fracture; traumatic hernia (disruption of the rectus abdominis muscle)

Location: jejunum distal to ligament of Treitz > duodenum > ascending colon at ileocecal valve > descending colon

- • abdominal tenderness (100% sensitive)
- • increased temperature + heart rate
- • decreased urine output over 24 hours
- • lap belt ecchymosis

NECT:
- √ pneumoperitoneum (15–32%):
- √ small gas bubbles anteriorly near liver / trapped within leaves of mesentery (with small bowel perforation)
- √ retroperitoneal air (with disruption of duodenum / colon)
- √ hypodense free fluid (58–85%), particularly in interloop location due to perforation
  DDx: parenchymal organ injury / osseous injury / large vessel injury / bladder perforation
- √ sentinel clot sign adjacent to bowel

CECT (88–92% sensitive):
- √ focal discontinuity of bowel wall = direct evidence

GI

√ focal bowel wall thickening > 3 mm (= intramural hematoma (75%) / vascular compromise and inflammation due to spilling of bowel contents):
  √ ± intestinal obstruction
√ hyperdense contrast enhancement of injured bowel wall = delayed venous transit time (20%)
√ stranding of mesentery = streaky hyperattenuating infiltration / fluid at mesenteric root (due to hemorrhage + inflammatory response)
√ mesenteric hematoma (39%)
√ extravasation of oral contrast material (uncommon), most dense near perforation
  DDx: hyperattenuating blood, extravasating vascular contrast material, leak of contrast material from urinary tract
√ mesenteric pseudoaneurysm

US:
√ nonspecific free fluid (98% sensitive)

N.B.: clinical signs + symptoms may be delayed for 24 hours (increasing mortality to 65%)

Blunt Trauma to Pancreas (3%)

Mechanism: compression against vertebral column with shear across pancreatic neck
Incidence: <10% of childhood trauma
Cause: motor vehicle accident, fall onto handle bars of a bicycle, child abuse
Associated with: injury to liver, duodenum
Classification:
I minor contusion / hematoma, capsule + major duct intact
II parenchymal injury without major duct injury
III major ductal injury
IV severe crush injury

Location: junction of body + tail
√ posttraumatic pancreatitis:
  √ edema / fluid in peripancreatic fat
  √ focal / diffuse pancreatic enlargement
  √ irregularity of pancreatic contour
√ area of low-attenuation = contusion / laceration (actual site of laceration difficult to visualize)
√ fluid around superior mesenteric artery
√ fluid in transverse mesocolon / lesser sac
√ fluid between pancreas and splenic vein
√ thickening of anterior pararenal fascia

N.B.: 24–48-hour delayed scans uncover findings not present earlier
Rx: I + II conservative management;
III + IV need surgery within 24 hours
Cx: recurrent pancreatitis, pseudocyst, pseudoaneurysm, fistula, abscess (attendant mortality of 20%)

BOERHAAVE SYNDROME

= complete transmural disruption of esophageal wall with extrusion of gastric content into mediastinum / pleural space secondary to food bolus impaction
• forceful vomiting with sudden onset of pain (substernal, left chest, in neck, pleuritic, abdominal)
• dyspnea
• NO hematemesis (blood escapes outside esophageal lumen)
√ rent of 2–5 cm in length, 2–3 cm above GE junction, predominantly on left posterolateral wall
√ pleural effusion on left >> right side / hydropneumothorax
√ pneumomediastinum (single most important plain-film finding), pneumopericardium, subcutaneous air
√ "V sign of Naclerio" = localized mediastinal emphysema with air between lower thoracic aorta + diaphragm
√ mediastinal widening
√ air-fluid level within mediastinum
√ extravasation of contrast medium into mediastinum / pleura

BRUNNER GLAND HYPERPLASIA

= BRUNNER GLAND HAMARTOMA
Incidence: 1.2% of all gastric polyps
Etiology: response to increased acid secretion
Histo: diffusely enlarged hyperplastic glands with Swiss cheese appearance
Physiology: secrete a clear viscous alkaline mucus into crypts of Lieberkühn

MORPHOLOGIC TYPES:
1. Diffuse nodular hyperplasia
2. Circumscribed nodular hyperplasia: in suprapapillary portion
3. Single adenomatous hyperplastic polyp: in duodenal bulb

Location: duodenum, prepyloric region (duodenal glands begin in vicinity of pylorus extending distally within proximal 2/3 of duodenum)
√ multiple nodular filling defects (usually limited to 1st portion of duodenum) with "cobblestone appearance" (most common finding)
  DDx: polyposis syndromes, lymphoid hyperplasia, heterotopic gastric mucosa, nodular duodenitis
√ occasionally single mass up to 5 cm ± central ulceration
  DDx: adenomatous polyp, various submucosal tumors
Cx: GI bleeding, obstruction, intussusception

BURKITT LYMPHOMA

= most common type of pediatric non-Hodgkin lymphoma; initially described in a 7-year old Ugandan child in 1958 by Dennis Burkitt, a British surgeon
Etiology: tumor from undifferentiated small noncleaved B-cell–derived lymphocytes
Path: resemblance to Hodgkin disease
Histo: characteristic "starry sky" pattern
• fastest growing tumor in humans with a potential doubling time of 24 hours
• paraplegia
• NO peripheral leukemia
√ conspicuous absence of lymph node disease
√ tendency to permeate / destroy bone

MR:
√ isointense to muscle on T1WI + T2WI
√ intense homogeneous enhancement

A. ENDEMIC FORM OF BURKITT LYMPHOMA
Endemic in areas with malaria:
sub-Saharan Africa, New Guinea (exposure to Plasmodium falciparum has a synergistic effect causing a marked decrease in T-cell surveillance)
Incidence in central Africa:
50–80% of all childhood neoplasms
Associated with: Epstein-Barr virus infection in 95% (implicated as a B-cell mitogen in the oncogenesis)
Age: 3–10 years
@ Mandible (first) / maxilla / facial bones
- jaw mass
- exophthalmos (orbital extension)

√ grossly destructive lesion, spicules of bone growing at right angles
√ large soft-tissue mass

@ Other skeleton (multifocal in 10%)
√ reminiscent of Ewing tumor / reticulum cell sarcoma
√ lamellated periosteal reaction around major long bones

B. NONENDEMIC / SPORADIC FORM OF BURKITT LYMPHOMA
Incidence in Europe + North America:
35–45% of all pediatric NHL; 3% of all childhood tumors
Age: 6–15 years
- Epstein-Barr virus genome found in only a minority

@ Abdomen (69%)
tumors of small bowel (Peyer patches of terminal ileum), mesentery
- abdominal mass
- intestinal obstruction

√ usually intraabdominal extranodal involvement with sparing of spleen
√ well-defined sharply marginated homogeneous tumors (75%)
√ ascites (13%)

@ Genitourinary tract (20%)
ovary, uterus, kidneys, retroperitoneum
√ renal masses / diffuse enlargement (5%)
√ hydronephrosis (28%)

@ Chest
√ pleural effusion (most common chest abnormality)

@ CNS
√ meningeal infiltration (most commonly)
√ cavernous sinus invasion
√ supra- and parasellar tumor
√ epidural spinal mass ± spinal cord compression

@ Others
salivary glands, thyroid, bone marrow

Rx: dramatic response to chemotherapy
Prognosis: long-term survival in 50%

CARCINOID

= most common primary tumor of small bowel + appendix (>95% of all carcinoids); belongs to APUDomas (like pheochromocytoma, medullary carcinoma of thyroid, islet cell tumors of pancreas); M:F = 2:1

Path: firm yellow submucosal nodule arising from argentophil Kulchitsky cells in the crypts of Lieberkühn (= argentaffinoma due to affinity for silver stain); invasion into mesentery incites an intense fibrotic reaction
Histo: low-grade malignancy = resemble adenocarcinomas but do not have their aggressive behavior; malignant through invasion of muscularis
Biochemistry:
tumor elaborates (1) ACTH, (2) histamine, (3) bradykinin (4) kallikrein, (5) serotonin = 5-hydroxytryptamine (from tryptophan over 5-hydroxytryptophan), which is metabolized in liver by monamine oxidase into 5-hydroxyindole acetic acid (5-HIAA) and excreted in urine; 5-hydroxytryptophan is destroyed in pulmonary circulation
Associated with: other synchronous / metachronous malignancies (36% at necropsy)

- asymptomatic (66%)
- abdominal pain / obstruction (19%)
- nausea, weight loss (16%)
- palpable mass (14%)
- GI bleeding
- **Carcinoid syndrome** (in 7% of small bowel carcinoids):
  = constellation of clinical findings related to hormone secretion by tumor
  Cause: excess serotonin levels when the metabolic pathway to 5-HIAA (in liver) is bypassed
  (a) with liver metastases
  (b) with primary pulmonary / ovarian carcinoids
  - recurrent diarrhea (70%)
  - right-sided endocardial fibroelastosis (35%) resulting in tricuspid regurgitation + pulmonary valve stenosis + right heart failure
  - attacks precipitated by ingestion of food / alcohol
  - asthmatic wheezing from bronchospasm (15%)
  - desquamative skin lesions (5%)
  - pellagra (7%) from niacin deficiency as a result of preferential conversion of dietary tryptophan to serotonin rather than niacin
  - multiple telangiectasias (25%)
  - nausea & vomiting, fever
  - hypotension (vasomotor instability)
  - cutaneous flushing (rare)
  - excess 5-HIAA in urine

  Prognosis: carcinoid syndrome has a higher morbidity & mortality than does the tumor itself!

RULE OF 1/3:
◊ 1/3 occur in small bowel
◊ 1/3 have metastases
◊ 1/3 are multiple
◊ 1/3 have a second malignancy

Metastases:
to lymph nodes, liver (in 90% of patients with carcinoid syndrome), lung, bone (osteoblastic)
(a) incidence versus tumor size

tumor of	<1 cm	(in 75%)	metastasizes in	2%
tumor of	1–2 cm	(in 20%)	metastasizes in	50%
tumor of	>2 cm	(in 5%)	metastasizes in	85%

GI

(b) incidence versus location

tumor in ileum	(in 28%)	metastasizes in 35%
tumor in appendix	(in 46%)	metastasizes in 3%
tumor in rectum	(in 17%)	metastasizes in 1%

Liver metastases seen: best / (only) on:
(a) NECT 35% (3%)
(b) CECT in HAP 35% (14%)
(c) CECT in PVP 30% (3%)
HAP = hepatic arterial-dominant phase of triple phase CT
PVP = portal venous-dominant phase of triple phase CT

Location: between gastric cardia and anus
@ Appendix (30–45%)
Commonly benign: slow growth, rarely metastasizing
Incidence at surgery: 0.03–0.7%
Site: tip (70%), middle (20%), base (10%) of appendix
• symptoms of appendicitis
√ invasion of mesoappendix (11%)
@ Small bowel (25–35%)
Incidence: 25% of all small bowel tumors
Location: ileum (91%); jejunum (7%), duodenum (2%); multiple in 15–35%
◊ 75% of patients with symptomatic spread have midgut carcinoids
◊ Duodenal carcinoids are associated with multiple endocrine neoplasia
@ Rectum (10–15%): metastasize in 10%
@ Colon (5%): ascending colon, often malignant
@ Stomach (<3%): lesser curvature of distal antrum
√ one / more 1–4-cm submucosal masses:
√ bull's eye appearance when ulcerated
√ one / more sessile / pedunculated polyps
@ Other organs (5%): bronchus, thyroid, pancreas, biliary tract, teratomas (ovarian, sacrococcygeal, testicular)
@ may be multicentric

UGI:
√ small smooth submucosal mass (usually <2 cm) impinging eccentrically on lumen
√ desmoplastic response of mesentery from locally high levels of serotonin causes:
√ angulation + kinking of loops leading to obstruction (DIAGNOSTIC)
√ spiculated / tethered appearance of mucosal folds
√ matting of multiple loops
√ separation of loops due to large mesenteric metastases
CT:
√ focal calcified mesenteric mass surrounded by thickened mesentery
√ stellate radiating pattern + beading of mesenteric neurovascular bundles (desmoplastic reaction)
√ retraction + shortening of mesentery√ displacement + kinking + separation of adjacent bowel loops
√ segmental thickening of adjacent bowel loops (encasement of mesenteric vessels leads to chronic ischemia)
√ low-density lymphadenopathy (due to necrosis)
√ hypoattenuating liver metastases:
√ may appear hyperdense in arterial phase
√ may become isodense after slow contrast infusion
Angio:
√ "sunburst" appearance:
√ kinking of small- and medium-sized vessels with a stellate configuration
√ simulated hypervascularity with thickening + foreshortening of mesenteric vessels secondary to fibrotic retraction
√ mesenteric ischemia:
√ arterial branch stenoses from encasement of medium-sized vessels (due to elastic vascular sclerosis with locally elevated serotonin levels)
√ venous occlusion / mesenteric varices
√ tumor may be identified as hypervascular mass
NUC (I-123 MIBG imaging):
√ uptake in 44–63% (higher frequency of radiotracer uptake in midgut carcinoids + with elevated serotonin levels)
US:
√ persistent fluid-distended appendix without typical signs of appendicitis
Prognosis: slow progression with average survival time of 3.2 years after diagnosis of liver metastases
Rx: Somatostatin / SMS 201-995; chemoembolization of hepatic arteries
DDx: oat-cell carcinoma, pancreatic carcinoma, medullary thyroid carcinoma, retractile mesenteritis, desmoplastic carcinoma / lymphoma

CATHARTIC COLON

= prolonged use of stimulant-irritant cathartics (>15 years) resulting in neuromuscular incoordination from chronically increased muscular activity + tonus
Agents: castor oil, senna, phenolphthalein, cascara, podophyllum, aloin
Location: involvement of colon proximal to splenic flexure
√ effaced mucosa with flattened smooth surface
√ diminished / absent haustrations
√ "pseudostrictures" = smoothly tapered areas of narrowing are typical (sustained tonus of circular muscles)
√ poor evacuation of barium
√ flattened + gaping ileocecal valve
√ shortened but distensible ascending colon
DDx: "burned-out" ulcerative colitis with right-sided predominance (very similar)

CHAGAS DISEASE

= damage of ganglion cells by neurotoxin liberated from protozoa Trypanosoma cruzi resulting in aperistalsis of GI tract + dilatation
Endemic to Central + South America (esp. eastern Brazil)
Histo: decreased number of cells in medullary dorsal motor nucleus + Wallerian degeneration of vagus + decrease / loss of argyrophilic cells in myenteric plexus of Auerbach
Peak age: 30–50 years; M:F = 1:1

GI

- intermittent / persistent dysphagia
- odynophagia (= fear of swallowing)
- foul breath, regurgitation, aspiration
- Mecholyl test: abnormal response indicative of deficient innervation; 2.5–10 mg methacholine subcutaneously followed by severe tetanic nonperistaltic contraction 2–5 minutes after injection, commonly in distal half of esophagus, accompanied by severe pain

@ Dilatative cardiomyopathy (myocarditis)
@ Megacolon (bowels move at intervals of 8 days to 5 months)
Cx: impacted feces, sigmoid volvulus
@ Esophagus: changes as in achalasia

CHALASIA

= continuously relaxed sphincter with free reflux in the absence of a sliding hernia
Etiology: elevated submerged segment
Causes: (1) Delayed development of esophagogastric region in newborns
(2) Scleroderma, Raynaud disease
(3) S/P forceful dilatation / myotomy for achalasia
√ free / easily induced reflux

CHRONIC IDIOPATHIC INTESTINAL PSEUDOOBSTRUCTION

= nonpropulsive intestine characterized by impaired response to intestinal dilatation without definable cause; ? autosomal dominant
Age: all ages, M:F = 1:1
- recurrent attacks of abdominal distension, periumbilical pain, nausea, vomiting, constipation

√ mild to marked gaseous distension of duodenum + proximal small bowel
√ esophageal dilation + hypoperistalsis (lower third)
√ excessive duodenal dilation (DDx: megaduodenum, superior mesenteric artery syndrome)
√ ligament of Treitz may be placed lower than usual
√ delayed transit of barium through affected segments
√ disordered motor activity (fluoroscopy)

COLITIS CYSTICA PROFUNDA

= rare benign condition characterized by submucosal mucus-containing cysts lined by normal colonic epithelium
Etiology: probably related to chronic inflammation
Associated with: solitary rectal ulcer syndrome (in localized form)
Age: primarily disease of young adults
- brief periods of bright red rectal bleeding
- mucous / bloody discharge
- intermittent diarrhea

Location: (a) localized to rectum (most commonly) / sigmoid
(b) generalized colonic process (less common)
√ nodular polypoid / cauliflower-like lesions <2 cm in size, containing no gas
√ spiculations mimicking ulcers (barium-filled clefts between nodules)
DDx: pneumatosis (rarely affects rectum)

COLONIC ATRESIA

Incidence: less common than ileal atresia
Plain radiograph:
√ massive dilatation of colon proximal to obstruction
√ mottled pattern of gas + feces proximal to point of atresia
DDx: often indistinguishable from obstruction of distal ileum
BE:
√ functional microcolon
√ obstruction to retrograde flow of barium
US:
√ dilated hyperechoic distal small bowel + proximal colon (from retained meconium)

COLORECTAL CARCINOMA

Most common cancer of GI tract; 3rd most commonly diagnosed malignancy in developed countries in men (after lung + prostate cancer) and women (after lung + breast cancer); 2nd leading cause of cancer deaths
Incidence: 11% of all newly diagnosed cancers; 13% of all cancer deaths; 150,000 new cases/year with 57,000 deaths in United States (1999); 6% lifetime probability of any White person to develop colorectal cancer; 3:100,000 in 30–34-year-olds; 532:100,000 for >85-year-olds
Lifetime probability: 4%
Risk factors:
1. Personal history of colonic adenoma / carcinoma
— malignancy in 5% of tubular adenomas
— malignancy in 30–40% of villous adenomas
Proof of adenoma-carcinoma sequence:
(a) frequent coexistence of adenoma + carcinoma
(b) similar distribution within colon
(c) consistent proportional prevalence in population having varied magnitudes of colon cancer risk
(d) increased frequency of carcinoma in patients with adenomas
(e) reduction of cancer incidence following endoscopic removal of polyps
(f) all patients with familial adenomatous polyposis syndrome develop colon carcinoma if colon not removed
(g) similarity of DNA + chromosomal constitution
◊ 93% of colorectal carcinomas arise from adenomatous polyp!
◊ A patient with one adenoma has a 9% chance of having a colorectal carcinoma in next 15 years!
◊ It takes about 7 years for a 1-cm adenoma to become an invasive cancer!
◊ 5% of adenomas 5 mm in size develop into invasive cancers (5 mm is considered critical mass of intraepithelial neoplasia)!

2. Family history of benign / malignant colorectal tumors in first-degree relatives (3–5 x risk)
3. Personal history of ovarian / endometrial / breast cancer
4. Dysplasia of colon within flat mucosa
5. Inflammatory bowel disease:
   (a) Ulcerative colitis (3–5% incidence; cumulative incidence of 26% after 25 years of colitic symptoms)
   (b) Crohn disease affecting the colon + rectum (particularly in bypassed loops / in vicinity of chronic fistula)

   Time delay: >8–10 years of colitis
   Underlying lesion: dysplasia within flat mucosa
6. Prominent lymphoid follicular pattern
7. Pelvic irradiation
8. Ureterosigmoidostomy

Environmental risk factors:
   (a) low fiber diet: prevents rapid transit time thus increasing contact time between potential toxins and colonic mucosa
   (b) increased ingestion of fat + animal protein
   (c) obesity
   (d) asbestos worker

Genetic risk factors (6% of colorectal carcinomas):
   (a) familial adenomatous polyposis syndrome: familial polyposis, Gardner syndrome, Turcot syndrome
   Age: approximately at 40 years
   (b) certain hamartomatous polyposis syndromes: Peutz-Jeghers syndrome, juvenile polyposis, Cowden disease
   (c) hereditary nonpolyposis colon cancer syndrome = Lynch syndrome *(see below)*

Screening recommendations (American Cancer Society): as / more effective than mammographic screening
   (a) for persons >50 years of age: annual fecal occult-blood test + sigmoidoscopy / BE every 3–5 years
   (b) for first-degree relatives of patients with colon cancer screening should start at age 40

Age: median age of 71 years for colon cancer; median age of 69 years for rectal cancer; M:F = 3:2

Histo: (1) Adenocarcinoma with varied degrees of differentiation
   (2) Mucinous carcinoma (uncommon)
   (3) Squamous cell carcinoma + adenoacanthoma (rare)

Staging (modified Dukes = Astler-Coller classification):

Stage		*Findings*
A		limited to mucosa
B		involvement of muscularis propria
	B_1	extension into muscularis propria
	B_2	extension through muscularis propria into serosa / mesenteric fat (35%)
C		lymph node metastases (50%)
	C_1	+ growth limited to bowel wall
	C_2	+ growth extending into adipose tissue
D		distant metastases

Staging (UICC-AJCC Colorectal Cancer Staging System):

Stage	*Grouping*			*5-year Survival*
0	Tis	N0	M0	>95%
I	T1	N0	M0	75–100%
	T2	N0	M0	
II	T3	N0	M0	50–75%
	T4	N0	M0	
III	any T	N1	M0	30–50%
	any T	N2,3	M0	
IV	any T	any N	M1	<10%

Legend:

Tis	carcinoma in situ
T1	invasion of submucosa
T2	invasion of muscularis propria
T3	invasion of subserosa / pericolic tissue
T4	invasion of visceral peritoneum / other organs
N1	1–3 pericolic Lnn
N2	>4 pericolic Lnn
N3	any Lnn along course of a vascular trunk

Metastases (lymphatic / hematogenous venous):
1. Liver (75%; 15–20% at time of surgery) due to portal venous drainage route
2. Mesentery + mesenteric nodes (10–15%)
3. Adrenal (10–14%)
4. Lung (5–50%)
5. Ovary (3–8%) = Krukenberg tumor
6. Psoas muscle tumor deposit
7. Peritoneal metastases:
   (a) malignant ascites: usually associated with poorly differentiated colonic carcinoma
   (b) pseudomyxoma peritonei (<5%): low-grade colonic adenocarcinoma
8. Bone (5%)
9. Brain (5%)

◊ Because of absence of lymphatics in lamina propria colon cancer will not metastasize until it penetrates the muscularis mucosa!

- rectal bleeding, iron deficiency anemia
- change in bowel habits / caliber of stools
- obstruction (poor prognostic indicator)
- hydronephrosis (13%)
- positive fecal occult blood testing (2–6% positive-result rate ; 5–10% positive predictive value; fails to detect 30–50% of colorectal carcinomas + up to 75% of adenomas): Hemoccult (hematein), Hemoquant (porphyrins), Haemselect (hemoglobin)
- progressive elevation of carcinoembryonic antigen (CEA) >10 μg/L indicative of recurrent / metastatic disease
- watery diarrhea + potassium depletion / excessive secretion of mucus + hypoalbuminemia (in large mucin-secreting villous tumor)

Location: "aging gut" = number of right-sided lesions increasing with age ("changing distribution")
   (a) left colon (52–61%):
   rectum (15–33 –41%), sigmoid (20–37%), descending colon (10–11%)
   √ commonly annular strictures with obstruction

GI

(b) right colon:
transverse colon (12%), ascending colon (8–16%), cecum (8–10%)
√ commonly polypoid lesions with chronic bleeding + intussusception

Colonoscopy: cecum not visualized in 10–36%; fails to detect 12% of colonic polyps (10% in areas never reached by colonoscope)
Cx: perforation in 0.2% (0.02% for BE); death in 1:5,000 (1:50,000 for BE)

BE (sensitivities in detection of polyps >1 cm: SCBE 77–94%, DCBE 82–97%; for polyps <1 cm: SCBE 18–72%, DCBE 61–83%):
√ fungating polypoid carcinoma:
• chronic bleeding, intussusception
√ annular ulcerating carcinoma = "apple core lesion"
= annular constriction is a result of tumor growing along the lymphatic channels, which parallel the circular muscle fibers of the inner layer of the muscularis propria; longitudinal growth is limited with abrupt transition to normal mucosa
• colonic obstruction
√ "saddle lesion" = growth characteristics between polypoid mass + annular constricting lesion
√ scirrhous carcinoma (signet-ring type)
= long-segment stricture without significant mucosal abnormality similar to linitis plastica due to diffuse circumferential + longitudinal tumor infiltration within the loose submucosal tissue between muscularis mucosa + muscularis propria
• often seen in ulcerative colitis
√ curvilinear / mottled calcifications (rare) are CHARACTERISTIC of mucinous adenocarcinoma

CT (48–90% staging accuracy, 25–73% for lymph node metastases):
CT staging (poor accuracy compared with Astler-Coller classification):
Stage 1 intramural polypoid mass
Stage 2 thickening of bowel wall
Stage 3 slight invasion of surrounding tissues
Stage 4 massive invasion of surrounding tissue + adjacent organs / distant metastases
√ low-density mass + low-density lymph nodes in mucinous adenocarcinoma (= >50% of tumor composed of extracellular mucin)
√ psammomatous calcifications in mucinous adenocarcinoma
√ signs of Lnn involvement: single lymph node >1 cm in diameter / cluster of ≥3 nodes <1 cm / node of any size within mesentery
MR (staging accuracy of 73%, 40% sensitivity for lymph node metastases)

Prognosis:
Survival rate of 40–50% overall in 5 years (unchanged over past 40 years); 80–90% with Duke A; 70% with Duke B; 33% with Duke C; 5% with Duke D
Recurrence in 1/3 of patients:
(a) local recurrence at line of anastomosis (60%) within 1 year after resection in 50%, within 2 years after resection in 70–80%
(b) distant metastases (26%)
(c) local recurrence + metastases (14%)
Risk after detection of colon cancer:
5% for synchronous colon cancer
14% for synchronous cancer with "sentinel polyp"
35% for additional adenomatous polyp
3% for metachronous colon cancer
4% for extracolonic malignancy
Cx: (1) Obstruction (frequently in descending + sigmoid colon)
(2) Perforation
(3) Intussusception
(4) Abscess formation
(5) Fistula formation
(6) Pneumatosis cystoides intestinalis
(7) Pseudomyxoma peritonei (from low-grade adenocarcinoma of colon)
Rx: (1) Local surgical excision / polypectomy for stage I disease
(2) Right / left hemicolectomy with eventual anastomosis of proximal + distal excision sites
(3) Low anterior resection: >2 cm of rectum must remain to anastomose the colon
(4) Abdominoperineal resection with colostomy for low rectal carcinoma
(5) Adjuvant chemotherapy for stage II disease (fluorouracil / levamisole)
DDx: (1) Prolapsing ileocecal valve (change on palpation)
(2) Spasm (intact mucosa, released by propantheline bromide)
(3) Diverticulitis

Lynch Syndrome
= HEREDITARY NONPOLYPOSIS COLORECTAL CANCER SYNDROME
= families with high incidence of colorectal cancers + increased incidence of synchronous and metachronous colorectal cancers
Amsterdam criteria:
(a) ≥3 family members of whom 2 are 1st degree relatives of the third
(b) family members in ≥2 generations
(c) one family member diagnosed <50 years of age
A. Lynch I = no associated extracolonic cancer
B. Lynch II = associated with extracolonic malignancy: transitional cell carcinoma of ureter + renal pelvis; adenocarcinoma of endometrium, stomach, small bowel, pancreas, biliary tract, brain; hematologic malignancy; carcinoma of skin + larynx
Etiology: autosomal dominant abnormality of chromosome 2 with defect in DNA replication-repair process
(a) accelerated adenoma-carcinoma sequence
(b) dysplasia in flat mucosa of colon

GI

Prevalence: 5–10% of patients with colon cancer; 5 x more common than familial adenomatous polyposis syndrome
Mean age: 45 years
Location: 70% proximal to splenic flexure
Prognosis: better stage for stage than in other cancers (5-year survival rate of 65% versus 44% in sporadic cases)
Surveillance: colonoscopy every 1–2 years from ages 22–35 years

Rectal Cancer

Incidence: 45,000 rectal cancers/year in United States
Pathologic staging of rectal cancer:

Astler-Coller/TNM		*Description*	*5-year Survival*
A	T1,N0,M0	limited to submucosa	80%
B1	T2,N0,M0	limited to muscularis propria	70%
B2	T3,N0,M0	transmural extension	60–65%
C1	T2,N1,M0	nodes (+), into muscularis	35–45%
C2	T3,N1,M0	nodes (+), transmural	25%
	T4	invasion of adjacent organs	
D	M1	distant metastasis	<25%

Hematogenous metastasis:
dual venous drainage into portal + systemic veins
√ may have lung without liver metastases
Risk of recurrence:
5% for T1
10% for T2 33% for T1,N1 + T2N1
25% for T3 66% for T3N1
50% for T4
Staging accuracy:
(1) Digital rectal examination: 68–75–83%; limited to lesions within 10 cm of anal verge
(2) CT: 48–72–92%, better for more extensive regional spread; 25–73% for lymph node involvement
(3) MR: 74–84–93% with tendency for overstaging
(4) Transrectal ultrasound: 64–77–94% with tendency for overstaging; limited to lesions <14 cm from anal verge + nonstenotic lesions; 50–83% sensitivity for lymph node involvement

Transrectal US (81% accuracy):
Normal layers:
(a) hyperechoic interface of balloon + mucosa
(b) hypoechoic mucosa + muscularis mucosa
(c) hyperechoic submucosa
(d) hypoechoic muscularis propria
(e) hyperechoic serosa

√ hypoechoic mass disrupting rectal wall:
√ no interruption of hyperechoic submucosa = tumor confined to mucosa + submucosa
√ no interruption of hyperechoic serosa = tumor confined to rectal wall
√ break in outermost hyperechoic layer = tumor penetrates into perirectal fat
√ irregular serrated outer border of muscularis propria (pseudopodia through serosa)
√ hypoechoic perirectal lymph nodes (= tumor involvement)

COLONIC VOLVULUS

= most common form of volvulus
Incidence: 10% of large-bowel obstruction

Cecal Volvulus

= VOLVULUS OF CECUM
Incidence: 40% of colonic volvulus
Cause: sudden distension by trauma, pressure, constipation, distal colonic obstruction
Associated with: malrotation + long mesentery resulting in poor fixation of right colon (10–25% of population)
Pathophysiology of vascular compromise:
(1) Acute mesenteric torsion + strangulation causes arterial + venous obstruction
(2) Gradual distension + increase in intraluminal pressure interferes with blood supply; perforation in 65%

Age peak: 20–40 years; M > F
√ cecal gaseous distension:
√ cecum rotates anterior to ascending colon = **cecal bascule** [French = seesaw] (type I cecal volvulus)
√ "kidney-shaped" distended cecum rotates into left upper quadrant (type II cecal volvulus)
√ tapered end of barium column points toward torsion
Cx: (1) cecal distension >10–12 cm means risk of bowel perforation / infarction
(2) **Abdominal compartment syndrome** = increase in abdominal pressure diminishes respiratory function + cardiac output

Sigmoid Volvulus

= VOLVULUS OF SIGMOID
Cause: sigmoid twists on mesenteric axis
Age: usually in elderly / psychiatrically disturbed
Degree of torsion: 360° (50%), 180° (35%), 540° (10%)
√ greatly distended paralyzed loop with fluid-fluid levels, mainly on left side, extending toward diaphragm (erect film)
√ "coffee-bean sign" = distinct midline crease corresponding to mesenteric root in largely gas-distended loop (supine)
√ "bird-of-prey sign" = tapered hooklike end of barium column
CT:
√ "whirl sign" = tightly torsioned mesentery formed by twisted afferent + efferent loop

CONGENITAL ESOPHAGESOPHAGEAL ATRESIA & TRACHEOESOPHAGEAL FISTULA

= complex of congenital anomalies characterized by failed / incomplete formation of the tubular esophagus or an abnormal communication between esophagus + trachea
Cause: developmental disorder in formation and separation of primitive foregut into trachea + esophagus / vascular compromise

GI

Embryology:
primitive foregut tube develops lateral wall folds that may incompletely connect at any point leaving a fistulous communication; occurs at 3rd–5th week of intrauterine life

Incidence: 1:2,000–4,000 livebirths; most common sporadic congenital anomaly diagnosed in childhood

Risk of recurrence in sibling: 1%

Associated anomalies (17–56–70%):

1. Gastrointestinal (20–25%): imperforate anus, pyloric stenosis, duodenal atresia, annular pancreas
2. Cardiac (15–39%): patent ductus arteriosus, ASD, VSD, right-sided aortic arch (5%)
3. Musculoskeletal (24%): radial ray hypoplasia, vertebral anomalies
4. Genitourinary (12%): unilateral renal agenesis
5. Chromosomal (3–19%): trisomy 18, 21, 13
   ◊ Trisomy 18 is present in 75–100% of fetuses + in 3–4% of neonates with esophageal atresia!

mnemonic: "ARTICLES"
Anal atresia
Renal anomalies
TE fistula
Intestinal atresia / malrotation
Cardiac anomaly (PDA, VSD)
Limb anomalies (radial ray hypoplasia, polydactyly)
Esophageal atresia
Spinal anomalies

mnemonic: "VACTERL"
Vertebral anomalies
Anorectal anomaly
Cardiovascular anomalies
Tracheo-
Esophageal fistula
Renal anomalies
Limb anomalies

- drooling from excessive accumulation of pharyngeal secretions (esophageal atresia = EA)
- obligatory regurgitation of ingested fluids (EA)
- aspiration with coughing + choking during feeding (TEF)
- recurrent pneumonia + progressive respiratory distress of variable severity (tracheoesophageal fistula = TEF) in neonate

Location: between upper 1/3 + lower 1/3 of esophagus just above carina

@ Mediastinum
√ "coiled tube" = inability to pass feeding tube into stomach (esophageal atresia)
√ retrotracheal air-distended pouch of proximal esophagus causing compression / displacement of trachea
√ non- / hypoperistaltic esophageal segment (6–15 cm) in midesophagus
√ food impaction

@ Abdomen
√ gasless abdomen (esophageal atresia ± proximal TE fistula = types A + B)
√ abdomen distended by bowel gas in 90% (distal TE fistula / H-type fistula = types C + D)

@ Chest
√ bronchopneumonia with patchy airspace opacity, esp. in dependent upper lobes (in 50%)

OB-US (anomalies not identified before 24 weeks GA):
√ polyhydramnios in 33–60%:
  ◊ TE-fistula with esophageal atresia is cause of polyhydramnios in only 3%!
√ absence of fluid-distended stomach (in 10–41%; in remaining cases TE-fistula / gastric secretions allow some gastric distension)
√ reduced intraluminal fluid in fetal gut
√ small abdomen (birth weight <10th percentile in 40%)
√ distended proximal pouch of atretic esophagus

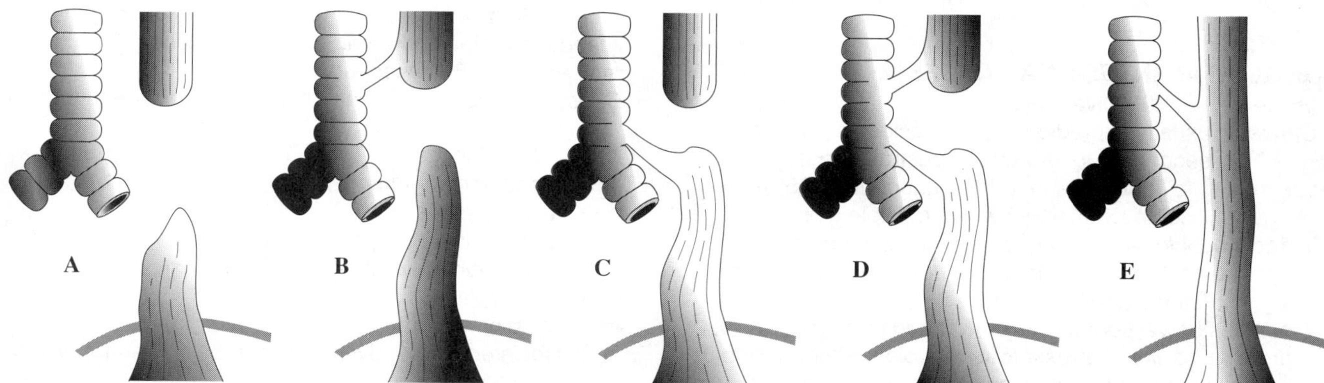

Esophageal Atresia	Esophageal Atresia + Proximal TE Fistula	Esophageal Atresia + Distal TE Fistula	Esophageal Atresia + Proximal and Distal TE Fistula	TE Fistula without Esophageal Atresia
10%	1%	77%	2%	10%

Esophageal Atresia with Tracheo-esophageal Fistula

Cx after repair:
(1) Anastomotic leak
(2) Recurrent TE fistula
(3) Aspiration pneumonia secondary to
(a) esophageal stricture
(b) disordered esophageal motility distal to TE fistula
(c) gastroesophageal reflux

DDx: pharyngeal pseudodiverticulum (traumatic perforation of posterior pharynx from finger insertion into oropharynx during delivery / tube insertion)

Esophageal Atresia without Fistula = Type A

Frequency: 8–10%
Associated anomalies in 17% (mostly Down syndrome + other atresias of GI tract)

Esophageal Atresia with Fistula

Associated anomalies in 30% (mostly cardiovascular)
Type B = esophageal atresia + proximal TE fistula
Frequency: 0.9–1%
Type C = esophageal atresia + distal TE fistula
Frequency: 53–86%
Type D = esophageal atresia + proximal and distal TE fistula
Frequency: 1–2.1%

Tracheoesophageal Fistula without Atresia

= H-shaped fistula **= Type E**
Frequency: 6–10%
Associated anomalies in 23% (mostly cardiovascular)
- feeding difficulties with choking
- diagnosis may not be made for several years

√ fistula courses forward and upward from esophagus

mnemonic:

type A = esophageal atresia	– **NO fistula**	=	**10%**
type B = esophageal atresia	– **PROX** fistula	=	**1%**
type C = esophageal atresia	– **DIST** fistula	=	**80%**
type D = esophageal atresia	– **PROX + DIST**	=	**1%**
type E = H-type fistula	– **NO atresia**	=	**10%**

CONGENITAL INTESTINAL ATRESIA

Incidence: 1:300 livebirths
Cause: usually sporadic vascular accidents (primary / secondary to volvulus or gastroschisis)
Location: jejunum + ileum (70%), duodenum (25%), colon (5%); may involve multiple sites

√ "triple bubble sign" = intraluminal gas in stomach + duodenal bulb + proximal jejunum as pathognomonic sign for jejunal atresia
√ bulbous bowel segment sign = dilated loop of bowel just proximal to site of atresia (due to prolonged impaction of intestinal contents) with curvilinear termination
√ gasless lower abdomen (gut usually air-filled by 4 hours after birth)
√ meconium peritonitis (6%)
√ polyhydramnios (in 50% with duodenal / proximal jejunal atresia; rarely in ileal / colonic atresia)

Prognosis: 88% survival for isolated atresia

CRICOPHARYNGEAL ACHALASIA

= hypertrophy of cricopharyngeus muscle (= upper esophageal sphincter) with failure of complete relaxation

Etiology:
1. Normal variant without symptoms: seen in 5–10% of adults
2. Compensatory mechanism to gastroesophageal reflux
3. Neuromuscular dysfunction of deglutition
   (a) primary neural disorders:
   brainstem disorder (bulbar poliomyelitis, syringomyelia, multiple sclerosis, amyotrophic lateral sclerosis); central / peripheral nerve palsy; cerebrovascular occlusive disease; Huntington chorea
   (b) primary muscle disorder:
   myotonic dystrophy; polymyositis; dermatomyositis; sarcoidosis; myopathies secondary to steroids / thyroid dysfunction; oculopharyngeal myopathy
   (c) myoneural junction disorder:
   myasthenia gravis; diphtheria; tetanus

- mostly asymptomatic
- dysphagia

◊ Cineradiography / videotape recording required for demonstration!
√ distension of proximal esophagus + pharynx
√ smoothly outlined shelf- / liplike projection posteriorly at level of cricoid (= pharyngoesophageal junction) = level of C5/6
√ barium may overflow into larynx + trachea

Cx: Zenker diverticula
Rx: cricopharyngeal myotomy

COWDEN DISEASE

= MULTIPLE HAMARTOMA SYNDROME
= autosomal dominant disease with high penetrance characterized by multiple hamartomas + neoplasms of endodermal, ectodermal, mesodermal origin

Incidence: 160 cases reported
Cause: susceptibility gene on long arm of chromosome 10 (10q23)
Age: 2nd decade

@ Mucocutaneous tumors
- facial papules
- oral papillomas (lips, gingiva, tongue)
- palmoplantar keratosis, acral keratosis

@ CNS neoplasia
meningioma; glioma
Associated with: dysplastic cerebellar gangliocytoma
- macrocephaly

@ Breast lesions (in 50%):
√ fibrocystic disease + fibroadenomas
√ breast cancer (20–30%): often bilateral + ductal

@ GI tract
√ multiple hamartomatous polyps (in 30–60%, commonly in rectosigmoid)

GI

@ Thyroid abnormalities (in 60–70%):
√ adenomas + goiter
√ follicular thyroid adenocarcinoma (3–4%)
@ Genitourinary lesions
@ Skeletal abnormalities

CROHN DISEASE

= REGIONAL ENTERITIS
= disease of unknown etiology with prolonged + unpredictable course characterized by discontinuous + asymmetric involvement of entire GI tract

Prevalence: 2–3:100,000 white adults
Path: transmural inflammation (noncaseating granuloma with Langhans giant cells and epithelioid cells, edema, fibrosis); obstructive lymphedema + enlargement of submucosal lymphoid follicles; ulceration of mucosa overlying lymphoid follicles
Age: onset between 15 and 30 years; M:F = 1:1

- recurrent episodes of diarrhea
- colicky / steady abdominal pain
- low-grade fever
- weight loss, anorexia
- occult blood + anemia
- perianal abscess / fistula (40%)
- malabsorption (30%)

Associated with: erythema nodosum, pyoderma gangrenosum

INTESTINAL MANIFESTATIONS
@ Esophagus (3%)
√ "aphthous" ulcers (early)
√ esophagitis, stricture, fistula (late)
@ Stomach (1–2%) = granulomatous gastritis
√ aphthous ulcers (= pinpoint erosions)
√ pseudo–post Billroth-I appearance
√ "ram's horn sign" = poorly distensible smooth tubular narrowed antrum + widened pylorus + narrow duodenal bulb
√ cobblestone appearance of mucosa
√ antral-duodenal fistula
@ Duodenum (4–10%)
almost always associated with gastric involvement
Location: duodenal bulb + proximal half of duodenum
√ superficial erosions / aphthoid ulcers (early lesion)
√ thickened duodenal folds
@ Small bowel (80%) = REGIONAL ENTERITIS
terminal ileum (alone / in combination in 95%); jejunum / ileum (15–55%)
√ thickening + slight nodularity of circular folds
√ aphthous ulcers
√ cobblestone mucosa / ulceration
√ commonly associated with medial cecal defect
@ Colon (22–55%) = GRANULOMATOUS COLITIS
Location: particularly on right side with rectum + sigmoid frequently spared
√ tiny 1–2-mm nodular filling defects (lymphoid follicular pattern)
√ aphthous ulcers with "target / bull's-eye" appearance
√ "transverse stripe sign" = 1-cm-long straight stripes representing contrast medium within deep grooves of coarse mucosal folds
√ long fistulous tracts parallel to bowel lumen
@ Appendicitis (20%)
@ Rectum (14–50%)
√ deep / collarbutton ulcers
√ rectal sinus tracts

Phases:
(a) Earliest changes
√ nodular enlargement of lymphoid follicles
√ blunting / flattening / distortion / straightening / thickening of valvulae conniventes (obstructive lymphedema, usually first seen in terminal ileum)
√ aphthous ulcers = nodules with shallow central barium collection up to 5 mm in diameter
Location: duodenal bulb, second portion of duodenum, terminal ileum
(b) Advanced nonstenotic phase
√ skip lesions (90%) = discontinuous involvement with intervening normal areas
√ cobblestone appearance = serpiginous longitudinal + transverse ulcers separated by areas of edema
√ thick + blunted small bowel folds (inflammatory infiltration of lamina propria + submucosa)
√ straightening + rigidity of small bowel loops with luminal narrowing (spasm + submucosal edema)
√ separation + displacement of small bowel loops (from lymphedematous wall thickening / increase in mesenteric fat / enlarged mesenteric lymph nodes / perforation with abscess formation)
√ pseudopolyps = islands of hyperplastic mucosa between denuded mucosa
√ inflammatory polypoid masses
√ sessile / pedunculated / filiform postinflammatory polyps
√ diffuse mucosal granularity due to 0.5–1-mm round lucencies (= blunted + fused villi seen en face)
√ pseudodiverticula = pseudosacculations = bulging area of normal wall opposite affected scarred wall on antimesenteric side
(c) Stenotic phase
√ "string sign" = strictures (in 21%, most frequently in terminal ileum) / marked narrowing of rigid loops
√ normal proximal loops may be dilated with stasis ulcers + fecoliths

CT:
√ homogeneous density of thickened bowel wall (DDx: ulcerative colitis with heterogeneous attenuation):
√ "double halo configuration" (50%) = intestinal lumen surrounded by inner ring of low attenuation (= edematous mucosa) + outer ring of soft-tissue density (= thickened fibrotic muscularis + serosa) (DDx: radiation enteritis, ischemia, mesenteric venous thrombosis, acute pancreatitis)

√ skip areas of asymmetric bowel wall thickening of 11 (range 10–20) mm in 82% (DDx: ulcerative colitis with a mean thickness of 8 mm)
√ "creeping fat" = massive proliferation of mesenteric fat (40%) with mass effect separating small bowel loops
√ "Comb" sign = vascular dilatation + tortuosity indicative of active disease
√ luminal narrowing + proximal dilatation
√ fistula / sinus tract (15–40%)
√ mesenteric adenopathy (18%)
√ mesenteric abscess in 15–20% (DDx: postoperative blind loop)

US:
√ "pseudokidney" / target sign = thickening of bowel wall (22–65–89%) of 5–20 mm (DDx: ulcerative colitis)
√ circumferential diffusely hypoechoic bowel wall with loss of normal layering (due to transmural edema, inflammation, fibrosis)
√ rigid + noncompressible bowel segment with reduction / loss of peristalsis
√ hyperemia of gut wall + adjacent fat on color Doppler
√ inflammatory mass = phlegmon (14%), abscess (4%)
√ distended fluid-filled loops (12%)
√ hypoechoic fistulous tract

Prognosis: recurrence rate of up to 39% after resection (commonly at the site of the new terminal ileum, most frequently during first 2 years after resection); mortality rate of 7% at 5 years, 12% at 10 years after 1st resection

Cx: (1) Fistula (33%):
(a) enterocolic: most frequently between ileum and cecum
(b) enterocutaneous (8–21%): rectum-to-skin; rectum-to-vagina
(c) perineal fistula + sinus tracts
◊ Crohn disease is 3rd most common cause of fistula / sinus tracts (*DDx:* iatrogenic [most common cause], diverticula [2nd most common cause])!
(2) Intramural sinus tracts
(3) Abscess (DDx: acute appendicitis)
(4) Free perforation (1–2%)
(5) Toxic megacolon
(6) Small bowel obstruction (15%)
(7) Hydronephrosis (from ureteric compression, generally on right side)
(8) Adenocarcinoma in ileum / colon (particularly in bypassed loops / in vicinity of chronic fistula)
◊ 4–20 x increased risk of colonic adenocarcinoma compared with general population with a latency period of 25–30 years!
(9) Lymphoma in large + small bowel

DDx: (1) Yersinia (in terminal ileum, resolution within 3–4 months)
(2) Tuberculosis (more severe involvement of cecum, pulmonary TB)
(3) Actinomycosis, histoplasmosis, blastomycosis, anisakiasis
(4) Segmental infarction (acute onset, elderly patient)
(5) Radiation ileitis (appropriate history)
(6) Lymphoma (no spasm, luminal narrowing is uncommon, tumor nodules)
(7) Carcinoid tumor (tumor nodules)
(8) Eosinophilic gastroenteritis
(9) Potassium stricture

EXTRAINTESTINAL MANIFESTATIONS

@ Hepatobiliary
1. Fatty infiltration of liver (steroid therapy, hyperalimentation)
2. Hepatic abscess
3. Gallstones (15–34%): predominantly cholesterol;
Risk: 3–5 x higher risk than expected; risk correlates with length of diseased ileum / resected ileum / duration of disease
Cause: interrupted enterohepatic circulation with malabsorption of bile salts in terminal ileum
4. Acute cholecystitis
5. Sclerosing cholangitis (10%) + hepatoma
6. Bile duct + gallbladder carcinoma

@ Genitourinary
1. Urolithiasis (5–10%): oxalate (steatorrhea leads to excess colonic absorption of oxalate) / urate stones
2. Hydronephrosis
3. Renal amyloidosis
4. Focal cystitis
5. Ileoureteral / ileovesical fistula (5–20%)

@ Musculoskeletal
- digital clubbing (11–40%)
- mild self-limiting seronegative peripheral migratory arthritis (15–22%): may precede bowel disease in 10%; severity + course correlates well with severity of intestinal disease; resection of diseased bowel leads to regression of symptoms

1. Hypertrophic osteoarthropathy
2. Ankylosing spondylitis (in 3–16%)
◊ Axial skeletal involvement usually precedes onset of GI symptoms!
• unrelated in severity / course to activity level of bowel disease
√ symmetric bilateral sacroiliitis
√ spondylitis with syndesmophytes
3. Peripheral erosive arthritis
√ small marginal erosions
√ periostitis
√ propensity for osseous ankylosis
4. Avascular necrosis of femoral head (steroid Rx)
5. Pelvic osteomyelitis (contiguous involvement)
6. Septic arthritis
7. Muscle abscess
8. Retarded skeletal growth + maturation

@ Erythema nodosum, uveitis

CRONKHITE-CANADA SYNDROME

= nonneoplastic nonhereditary polyps (as in juvenile polyposis) associated with ectodermal abnormalities; no familial predisposition

Incidence: >100 cases described
Histo: hamartomatous polyps resembling juvenile / retention polyps = multiple cystic spaces filled with mucin secondary to degenerative changes; expansion + inflammation of lamina propria
Age: 62 years (range 42–75 years); M < F
- exudative protein-losing enteropathy
- diarrhea (disaccharidase deficiency, bacterial overgrowth in small intestine)
- severe weight loss, anorexia
- abdominal pain
- nail atrophy
- brownish macules of hand + feet
- alopecia

√ multiple polyps
√ thickened gastric rugae
Location: stomach (100%); small bowel (>50%); colon (100%)
Prognosis: rapidly fatal in women within 6–18 months (cachexia); tendency toward remission in men

DESMOPLASTIC SMALL ROUND CELL TUMOR

= INTRAABDOMINAL DESMOPLASTIC SMALL ROUND CELL TUMOR OF PERITONEUM
= highly malignant tumor belonging to a generic group of small round blue cell tumors (Ewing sarcoma, neuroblastoma, Wilms tumor, rhabdomyosarcoma, primitive neuroendocrine tumor)
Incidence: <50 cases in literature
Median age: 21 years; affects children + young adults; up to 6th decade; M:F = 4:1
Origin: mesothelial / submesothelial / subserosal mesenchyme of the abdominal cavity
Histo: islands of small blue cells surrounded by fibrous stroma; immunohistochemically positive for epithelial, neural, muscular markers (cytoplasmic keratin + desmin); abnormal chromosome 11
- gastrointestinal / genitourinary discomfort / pain
- abdominal distension
- palpable abdominal mass

Location: mesentery (spread to omentum), retroperitoneum, paratesticular, posterior mediastinum, pleura, meninges
√ multiple scattered necrotic tumor masses in abdomen + pelvis with no definite visceral organ of origin:
 √ nodular peritoneal thickening
 √ serosal hepatic metastases
 √ punctate peritoneal calcifications
√ enlarged lymph nodes
√ scant ascites
Cx: hydronephrosis, bowel obstruction
Prognosis: mean survival time of 17 months
DDx:
 (a) in infants / adolescents: rhabdomyosarcoma; neuroblastoma; mesenteric carcinoid; Burkitt lymphoma
 (b) in adults: diffuse omental / peritoneal carcinomatosis (carcinoma of stomach, colon, ovary, pancreas); melanoma; leiomyosarcoma; lymphoma; desmoid tumor; mesothelioma; tumefactive tuberculosis; actinomycosis; Castleman disease

DIAPHRAGM DISEASE

= small bowel webs due to NSAIDs
Effect of NSAID: gastric irritation, ulceration of small intestines
Frequency: in 10% of patients receiving long-term NSAID therapy
Path: foci of submucosal fibrosis with interruption of adjacent muscularis mucosae
- blood + protein loss
- intermittent intestinal obstruction

Location: ileum > jejunum
Enteroclysis:
 √ multiple concentric diaphragm-like strictures
DDx: Crohn disease

DISACCHARIDASE DEFICIENCY

= enzyme deficiencies for any of the disaccharides (maltose, lactose, etc.)
A. PRIMARY
B. SECONDARY to other diseases (eg, Crohn disease)
Pathophysiology:
 (a) unabsorbed disaccharides produce osmotic diarrhea
 (b) bacterial fermentation produces short-chain volatile fatty acids causing further osmotic + irritant diarrhea
√ normal small bowel series without added lactose
√ abnormal small bowel series done with lactose (50 g added to 600 cm^3 of barium suspension)
√ small + large bowel distension
√ dilution of barium
√ shortening of transit time

DISTAL INTESTINAL OBSTRUCTION SYNDROME

= MECONIUM ILEUS EQUIVALENT
= impaction of inspissated stool in distal part of ileum + proximal part of colon
Prevalence: 7–15–41% of children / adolescents with cystic fibrosis; 2% in patients <5 years of age
Cause: tenacious intestinal mucus, steatorrhea due to pancreatic insufficiency, undigested food residue, disordered intestinal motility with increase in intestinal transit time, fecal stasis, dehydration
Age: 2nd–3rd decade of life
- recurrent bouts of colicky abdominal pain (from fecal impaction / constipation) in RLQ
- palpable cecal mass

√ bubbly granular ileocecal soft-tissue mass in RLQ
√ partial / complete small bowel obstruction (due to puttylike fecal material in terminal ileum / right colon)
√ thickening of mucosal folds
√ cystic fibrosis of lung
CT:
 Location: cecum > ascending colon > transverse colon > descending colon (contiguous involvement)
 √ diffuse colonic thickening

√ mural striation (50%)
√ mesenteric soft-tissue infiltration (100%)
√ increased pericolonic fat (60%)

Cx: intussusception, volvulus

Rx: stool softeners, oral polyethylene glycol-electrolyte solution (Golytely®), increasing dose of pancreatic enzyme supplements, mucolytic agents (N-acetylcysteine) orally / with Gastrografin® enema

DDx: appendicitis, partial intestinal obstruction (adhesion / stricture from previous bowel surgery)

DIVERTICULAR DISEASE OF COLON

= overactivity of smooth muscle causing herniation of mucosa + submucosa through muscle layers

Incidence: 5–10% in 5th decade; 33–48% over age 50; 50–65% past 7th decade; M:F = 1:1; most common affliction of colon in developed countries

Cause: decreased fecal bulk (diet high in refined fiber + low in roughage)

Location: in 80% in sigmoid (= narrowest colonic segment with highest pressure); in 17% distributed over entire colon; in 4–12% isolated to cecum / ascending colon

Prediverticular Disease of Colon

= longitudinal + circular smooth muscle thickening with redundancy of folds secondary to myostatic contracture

√ "saw-tooth sign" = crowding + thickening of haustral folds (shortening of colonic segment)
√ plump marginal indentations
√ superimposed muscle spasm (relieved by antispasmodics)

DDx: hemorrhage; ischemia; radiation changes; pseudomembranous colitis

Colonic Diverticulosis

= acquired herniations of mucosa + muscularis mucosae through the muscularis propria with wall components of mucosa, submucosa, serosa = false diverticula of pulsion type

Location: predominantly left-sided colon

Site:
(a) lateral diverticula arise between mesenteric + antimesenteric teniae on opposite sides
(b) antimesenteric intertaenial diverticula opposite of mesenteric side

Intramural type vasa recta (= nutrient arteries) pass through the circular muscle (weakness in muscular wall) and are carried over the fundus of the diverticula as it enlarges

√ size: initially tiny (3–10-mm) V-shaped protrusions increasing up to several cm in diameter
√ bubbly appearance of air-containing diverticula
√ residual barium within diverticula from previous study
√ spiky irregular outline (antimesenteric intertaenial ridge is typical site for intramural diverticula)
√ smooth dome-shaped appendages with a short neck
√ may be pointed, attenuated, irregular with variable filling
√ circular line with sharp outer edge + fuzzy blurred inner edge (en face view in double contrast BE)
√ **Giant sigmoid diverticulum** = large gas-containing cyst (air entrapment secondary to ball-valve mechanism) arising in left iliac fossa

CT:
√ rounded outpouchings containing air ± contrast material (= diverticula)
√ circumferential sawtooth-like thickening of colonic haustra + distorted luminal contour (= muscular hypertrophy)

Cx: bleeding (usually right colon), diverticulitis (usually sigmoid colon)

Colonic Diverticulitis

= perforation of diverticulum with intramural / localized pericolic inflammatory mass

Incidence: 5% of population; in 10–35% of diverticular disease; increasing frequency with age (in 5–10% >45 years of age, in 80% >85 years of age)

Pathogenesis: mucosal abrasion from inspissated fecal material leads to perforation of thin wall

• pain + local tenderness + mass in LLQ
• fever (25%), leukocytosis (36%)
• clinical misdiagnosis rate of 34–67%

Location: sigmoid colon (95%), cecum (4%)

√ localized ileus
√ ± pattern of small bowel obstruction (kinking / edema if small bowel adheres to abscess)
√ extraluminal gas in abscess / fistula
√ pneumoperitoneum (rare)

BE (77–86% sensitive):
√ focal area of eccentric luminal narrowing caused by pericolic / intramural inflammatory mass:
√ annular lesion mimicking carcinoma

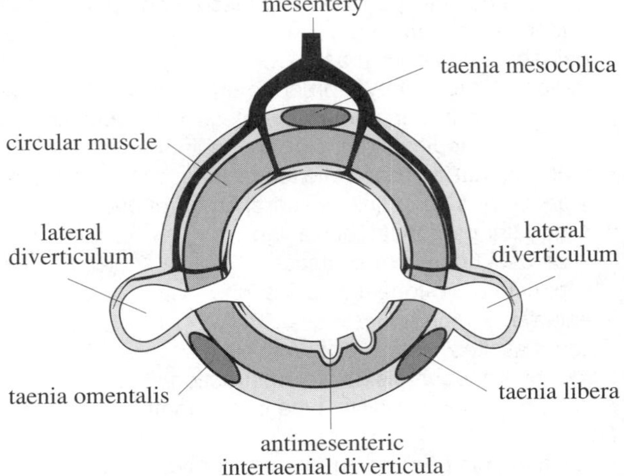

Cross Section through Colon

GI

√ marked thickening + distortion of mucosal folds
√ tethered spiculated mucosal folds
√ centrally amputated diverticulum
√ extraluminal contrast = **peridiverticulitis**:
√ "double-tracking" = pericolonic longitudinal sinus tract
√ pericolonic collection = peridiverticular abscess
√ fistula to bladder / small bowel / vagina

CT (79–93% sensitive, 77% specific):
√ inflamed diverticulum:
√ pericolic fat stranding = poorly marginated hazy area of increased attenuation ± fine linear strands within pericolic fat (98%)
√ diverticula (84%) = flask-shaped structures projecting through colonic wall + filled with air / barium / fecal material
√ "centipede" sign = hyperemic engorged vasa recta
√ bowel wall thickening:
√ circumferential bowel wall thickening of >4 mm (70%)
√ focally thickened + inflamed colonic wall
√ "arrowhead sign" = funnel of intraluminal contrast medium / air in focally thickened colonic wall centering about occluded orifice of inflamed diverticulum (27%)
√ fluid collection:
√ frank abscess (47%) = central liquid / gas
√ fluid ± air of peritonitis (16%)
√ fluid at root of sigmoid mesentery
√ tract formation:
√ fistula formation (14%): most commonly colovesical, also colovaginal, coloenteric, colocutaneous
√ intramural sinus tracts (9%)
√ fecolith
√ colonic obstruction (12%)
√ ureteral obstruction (7%)

US (85–98% sensitive, 80–97% specific):
√ thickening of bowel wall = >4 mm distance between echogenic lumen interface and serosa
√ diverticula = round / oval hypo- / hyperechoic foci protruding from colonic wall with focal disruption of normal layer continuity ± internal acoustic shadowing
√ inflammatory pericolic fat = regionally increased echogenicity adjacent to colonic wall ± ill-defined hypoechoic zones
√ pericolic abscess

Prognosis: (a) self-limiting (usually)
(b) transmural perforation
(c) superficial ulceration
(d) chronic abscess

Cx: (1) Colonic obstruction
(2) Fistula to bladder / vagina / small bowel
(3) Free perforation (rare)

DDx: (1) Colonic neoplasm (shorter segment, heaped-up margins, ulcerated mucosa)
(2) Crohn colitis (double-tracking longer than 10 cm)

Rx: antibiotics, surgery (in 25%), percutaneous abscess drainage

Colonic Diverticular Hemorrhage

Not related to diverticulitis
Incidence: in 3–47% of diverticulosis
Location: 75% located in ascending colon (larger neck + dome of diverticula)
• massive rectal hemorrhage without pain
√ extravasation of radionuclide tracers
√ angiographic contrast pooling in bowel lumen
Rx: (1) transcatheter infusion of vasoconstrictive agents (Pitressin®)
(2) embolization with Gelfoam®

Right Colonic Diverticulitis

= congenital true diverticulum
Frequency: 1:34–1:300 appendectomies
Age: any; peak prevalence at 35–45 years of age
• protracted mild pain; palpable mass in 33%
√ solitary diverticulum containing a 12-mm fecolith surrounded by inflamed fat
√ marked circumferential colonic wall thickening
Cx: pericolonic abscess
Prognosis: spontaneous evacuation into colonic lumen
Rx: conservative
DDx: appendicitis

DUMPING SYNDROME

= early postprandial vascular symptomatology of sweating, flushing, palpitation, feeling of weakness and dizziness
Pathophysiology: rapid entering of hypertonic solution into jejunum resulting in fluid shift from blood compartment into small bowel
Incidence: 1–5%; M:F = 2:1
◊ Roentgenologic findings not diagnostic!
√ rapid emptying of barium into small bowel (= loss of gastric reservoir function)
Rx: lying down, diet
DDx: late postprandial hypoglycemia (90–120 minutes after eating)

DUODENAL ATRESIA

= most common cause of congenital duodenal obstruction; second most common site of gastrointestinal atresias after ileum
Incidence: 1:10,000; M:F = 1:1
Etiology: defective vacuolization of duodenum between 6th and 11th weeks of fetal life; rarely from vascular insult (extent of obstruction usually involves larger regions with vascular insult)
Age at presentation: first few days of life
• persistent bilious vomiting a few hours after birth / following 1st feeding (75%)
• rapid deterioration secondary to loss of fluids + electrolytes

Isolated sporadic anomaly (30–52%)
Associated anomalies (in 50–60%):
(1) Down syndrome (20–33%);
◊ 25% of fetuses with duodenal atresia have Down syndrome!
◊ <5% of fetuses with Down syndrome have duodenal atresia!

(2) CHD (8–30–50%): endocardial cushion defect, VSD
(3) Gastrointestinal anomalies (26%):
esophageal atresia, biliary atresia, duodenal duplication, imperforate anus, small bowel atresia, malrotation, Ladd bands, Meckel diverticulum, transposed liver, annular pancreas (20%), preduodenal portal vein
(4) Urinary tract anomalies (8%)
(5) Vertebral + rib anomalies (37%)

Location: (a) usually distal to ampulla of Vater (80%)
(b) proximal duodenum (20%)

√ "double bubble sign" = gas-fluid levels in duodenal bulb + gastric fundus
√ total absence of intestinal gas in small / large bowel
√ colon of normal caliber

OB-US (usually not identified prior to 24 weeks GA):
- ± elevated AFP
√ "double bubble sign" = simultaneous distension of stomach + 1st portion of duodenum, continuity of fluid between stomach + duodenum must be demonstrated
√ increased gastric peristalsis
√ polyhydramnios in 3rd trimester (100%)

Prognosis: 36% mortality in neonates

DDx: (1) Prominent incisura angularis causing bidissection of stomach
(2) Choledochal cyst
(3) Annular pancreas
(4) Peritoneal bands
(5) Intestinal duplication

Cx: prematurity (40%) secondary to preterm labor related to polyhydramnios

DUODENAL DIVERTICULUM

Incidence: 1–5% of GI studies; 22% of autopsies

A. PRIMARY DIVERTICULUM
= mucosal prolapse through muscularis propria posteriorly (8%), lateral wall (4%)

B. SECONDARY DIVERTICULUM
= all layers of duodenal wall = true diverticulum as complication of duodenal / periduodenal inflammation
Location: almost invariably in 1st portion of duodenum

- mostly asymptomatic

Cx: (1) Perforation + peritonitis
(2) Bowel obstruction
(3) Biliary obstruction
(4) Bleeding
(5) Diverticulitis

DUODENAL ULCER

Incidence: 200,000 cases/year; 2–3 x more frequent than gastric ulcers; M:F = 3:1

Pathophysiology: too much acid in duodenum from
(a) abnormally high gastric secretion
(b) inadequate neutralization

Predisposed: cortisone therapy, severe cerebral injury, after surgery, chronic obstructive pulmonary disease

Location: (a) bulbar (95%):
anterior wall (50%), posterior wall (23%), inferior wall (22%), superior wall (5%)
√ bulbar deformity in 85%
(b) postbulbar (3–5%): M:F = 7:1;
majority on medial wall above papilla;
- hemorrhage in 66%
√ edema + spasm may obscure ulcer
√ smooth rounded indentation of lateral wall

√ frequently <1 cm round / ovoid (5% linear) ulcer niche
√ "kissing ulcers" = ulcers opposite from each other on anterior + posterior wall
√ giant duodenal ulcer >2 cm (rare) with higher morbidity + mortality; may be overlooked by simulating a normal / deformed scarred duodenal bulb
√ "cloverleaf deformity, hourglass stenosis" (healed stage) with prestenotic dilatation of recesses

Cx: (1) Obstruction (5%)
(2) Perforation (<10%): anterior > posterior wall; fistula to gallbladder
(3) Penetration (<5%) = sealed perforation
(4) Hemorrhage (15%): melena > hematemesis

Rx: antral resection (Billroth I) + vagotomy

DUODENAL VARICES

= dilated collateral veins secondary to portal hypertension (posterior superior pancreaticoduodenal vein)

√ lobulated filling defects (best demonstrated in prone position, maximal luminal distension will obliterate them)
√ commonly associated with fundal + esophageal varices

DUPLICATION CYST

= uncommon congenital anomaly found anywhere along alimentary tract from tongue to anus

Incidence: 15% of pediatric abdominal masses are gastrointestinal duplication cysts

Theories of formation:
(1) Abortive twinning
(2) Persistent embryologic diverticula
(3) Split notochord

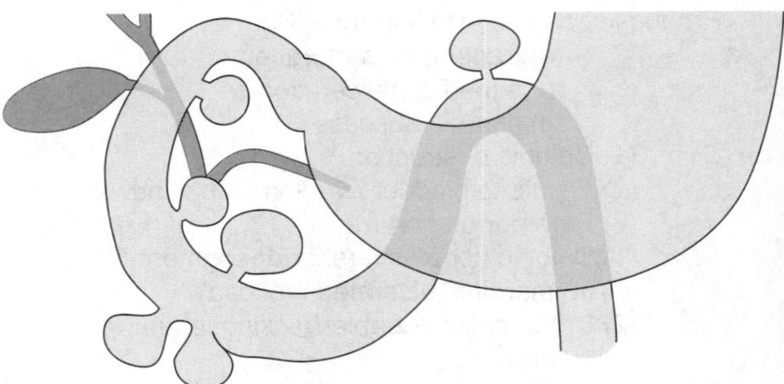

Duodenal Diverticula

(4) Aberrant luminal recanalization (Bremer): foregut epithelium grows and obliterates lumen (solid stage for esophagus, small bowel, colon); later produces secretions that form vacuoles in the intercellular space; vacuoles line up longitudinally and coalesce to form new lumen; failure of an aberrant vacuole to coalesce creates a wall cyst
(5) Intrauterine vascular accident (Favara)
associated with alimentary tract atresia in 9%

Age: presentation often in infancy / early childhood
Path: spherical cyst / tubular structure located in / immediately adjacent to gastrointestinal tract; shares a common muscle wall + blood supply; has a separate mucosal lining; cyst contents are usually serous
Histo: smooth muscle wall + lined with alimentary tract mucosa; ectopic mucosa; squamous, transitional, ciliated mucosa; lymphoid aggregates; ganglion cells
◊ Gastric mucosa + pancreatic tissue are the only ectopic tissues of clinical importance!

• respiratory distress (with esophageal duplication)
• palpable abdominal mass
• nausea, emesis (due to partial / complete obstruction)

Location: ileum (30–33%), esophagus (17–20%), colon (13–30%), jejunum (10–13%), stomach (7%), pylorus (4%), duodenum (4–5%), ileocecal junction (4%), rectum (4%);
◊ In 7–15% concomitant duplications elsewhere in the alimentary tract!

Site: on mesenteric aspect of alimentary canal
Morphology:
(a) large spherical / saccular cyst (82%)
(b) small intramural cyst
(c) tubular sausage-shaped cyst (18%): commonly along small + large bowel; frequently communicates with lumen of adjacent gut

BE:
√ mass extrinsic to bowel lumen

US:
√ elongated tubular / spherical cystic mass:
√ sonolucent mass with good through transmission (due to clear fluid content)
√ echogenic mass (due to hemorrhage + inspissated material)
√ muscular rim sign (= echogenic inner mucosal lining + hypoechoic outer rim) in 47%
√ cyst paralleling normal bowel lumen

CT:
√ smoothly rounded fluid-filled cyst / tubular structure
√ thin slightly enhancing wall

MR:
√ heterogeneous signal intensity of intracystic fluid on T1WI + homogeneous high signal intensity on T2WI

Cx: bowel obstruction, intussusception (due to cyst at ileocecal junction), small bowel volvulus (due to weight of duplication), bleeding (due to presence of gastric mucosa / pressure necrosis of adjacent mucosa by cyst expansion / from intussusception)

DDx:
(1) Omental cyst (greater omentum / lesser sac, multilocular)
(2) Mesenteric cyst (between leaves of small bowel mesentery)
(3) Choledochal cyst
(4) Ovarian cyst
(5) Pancreatic pseudocyst
(6) Cystic renal tumor
(7) Abscess
(8) Meckel diverticulum (communicates with GI tract)
(9) Lymphangioma
(10) Mesenteric lymphoma
(11) Intramural tumor

Colonic Duplication Cyst

Incidence: 13% of all alimentary tract duplications

A. CYSTIC COLONIC DUPLICATION (7%)
Path: closed spherical cyst; contains gastric mucosa in 2% + ectopic pancreatic tissue in 5%
• abdominal mass, bowel obstruction / constipation
• GI hemorrhage
Location: cecum (40%) ± intussusception
√ air / intestinal matter can enter cyst (20%)

B. COLORECTAL TUBULAR DUPLICATION (6%)
= DUPLICATION OF THE HINDGUT
= double-barreled duplication involving part / all of large bowel with "twin" segment on mesenteric / antimesenteric side
Symptomatic age: neonatal period / infancy; M:F = 1:2
May be associated with:
rectogenital / rectourinary fistula, duplication of internal / external genitalia, vertebral anomalies, multisystem congenital anomaly complex
• bowel obstruction / constipation
• passage of feces through vagina
√ simultaneous opacification of true + twin colon
√ duplication may terminate at
(a) 2nd functional anus
(b) imperforate perineal orifice
(c) fistulous communication with GU tract

C. DOUBLE APPENDIX

Duodenal Duplication Cyst

Incidence: 5% of all alimentary tract duplications
Path: noncommunicating spherical cyst; may contain ectopic gastric mucosa in 21%, small bowel mucosa, pancreatic tissue

• obstructive symptoms, palpable abdominal mass
• hemorrhage (due to peptic ulceration)
• jaundice (due to biliary obstruction)
• pancreatitis (due to ectopic pancreatic tissue)

Site: on mesenteric side of anterior wall of 1st + 2nd portion of duodenum
√ mass in concavity of duodenal C-loop
√ compression + displacement of 1st / 2nd portion of duodenum superiorly + anteriorly

Cholangiography:
√ may communicate with pancreatic ductal system through the aberrant duct of an accessory lobe
Cx: pancreatitis from perforation of duplication cyst
DDx: pancreatic cyst, pancreatic pseudocyst, choledochal cyst, choledochocele, duodenal intramural tumor, pancreatic tumor

Esophageal Duplication Cyst

arises from foregut
Incidence: 10–20% of all alimentary tract duplications; 0.5–2.5% of all esophageal masses; M:F = 2:1
Path: contains ectopic gastric mucosa in 43%
Histo: contains no cartilage, lined by alimentary tract mucosa
Associated with: vertebral anomalies (spina bifida, hemivertebra, fusion defects), esophageal atresia, small bowel duplication (18%)
Location: adjacent to esophagus / within esophageal musculature at any level, paraspinal position; R:L = 2:1; in right pleural space detached from esophagus (rare)

A. CERVICAL ESOPHAGUS (23%)
- asymptomatic enlarging lateral neck mass
- upper airway obstruction in newborn

DDx: thyroglossal duct cyst, branchial cleft cyst, cystic hygroma, cervical tumor, cervical lymphadenopathy

B. MIDESOPHAGUS (17%)
- severe upper airway obstruction in early infancy

DDx: bronchogenic cyst, neurenteric cyst, intramural esophageal tumor

C. DISTAL ESOPHAGUS (60%)
- frequently asymptomatic

Location: paraspinal
DDx: bronchogenic cyst, neurenteric cyst, intramural esophageal tumor

√ thick-walled closed spherical cyst, almost never communicating
CXR:
√ posterior mediastinal mass ± air-fluid level
√ lobar consolidation + central cavitation (from autodigestion of lung tissue by gastric secretions)
√ thoracic vertebral anomalies
UGI:
√ displacement of esophagus by paraesophageal mass
√ intramural extramucosal mass
US:
√ hypoechoic fluid-filled cyst + inner mucosal lining
CT:
√ sharply marginated homogeneous near-water density mass without enhancement
Cx: (1) Peptic ulceration (secondary to gastric mucosa)
(2) Perforation (secondary to penetrating ulcer)
(3) Hematemesis (from erosion into esophagus)
(4) Hemoptysis + autodigestion of pulmonary tissue (from erosion into tracheobronchial tree)

Gastric Duplication Cyst

= intramural gastric cyst lined with secretory epithelium
Incidence: 7% of all alimentary tract duplications
Path: noncommunicating spherical cyst (majority); may communicate with aberrant pancreatic duct; ectopic pancreatic tissue found in 37%
Symptomatic age: infancy; in 75% detected before age 12; M:F = 1:2
- pain (from overdistension of cyst, rupture with peritonitis, peptic ulcer formation, internal pancreatitis)
- vomiting, anemia, fever
- symptoms mimicking congenital hypertrophic pyloric stenosis (if duplication in antrum / pylorus)

Most common site: greater curvature (65%)
√ paragastric cystic mass up to 12 cm in size, indenting greater curvature
√ seldom communicates with main gastric lumen at one or both ends
√ may enlarge + ulcerate
√ Tc-99m uptake
US:
√ cyst with two wall layers: inner echogenic layer of mucosa + outer hypoechoic layer of muscle
√ clear / debris-containing fluid
Cx: (1) Partial / complete small bowel obstruction
(2) Relapsing pancreatitis (with ductal communication)
(3) Ulceration, perforation, fistula formation
DDx: pancreatic cyst, pancreatic pseudocyst, mesenteric cyst, leiomyoma, adenomatous polyp, hamartoma, lipoma, neurofibroma, teratoma

Rectal Duplication Cyst

Incidence: 4% of all alimentary tract duplications
Path: spherical fluid-filled cyst; may contain duodenal / gastric mucosa + pancreatic tissue
Site: posterior to rectum / anus
√ communication with rectum / perianal fistula (in 20%)
Symptomatic age: childhood
- constipation + fecal soiling
- palpable retrorectal / retroanal mass
- intractable excoriation of perianal skin (with chronic perianal fistula)

√ cystic mass; may be echogenic (due to solid material ± gas from communication with rectum)
DDx: anterior meningocele, sacrococcygeal teratoma, retrorectal abscess, pilonidal cyst, sacral bone tumor

Small Bowel Duplication Cyst

Incidence: most common of all alimentary tract duplications
Symptomatic age: neonatal period (1/3); <2 years of age (in 72%)

Path: contains ectopic gastric mucosa in 24%; ectopic pancreatic tissue in jejunum (8%)
May be associated with: small bowel atresia
• neonatal bowel obstruction
• intussusception, palpable mass
• acute abdominal pain, hemorrhage
Location: ileum (33%), jejunum (10%), ileocecal (4%)
√ low small bowel obstruction ± soft-tissue mass
√ cyst may serve as lead point for intussusception
DDx: mesenteric cyst, pancreatic pseudocyst, omental cyst, exophytic hepatic cyst, ovarian cyst

Thoracoabdominal Duplication

= FOREGUT DUPLICATION
= long tubular cyst closed at its cranial end, passing through diaphragm through its own hiatus, in 60% communicating with normal duodenum / jejunum / ileum
Incidence: 2% of all alimentary tract duplications
Associated with: thoracic vertebral anomalies
Histo: gastric mucosa in 29%
Symptomatic age: 50% during neonatal period; 80% within 1st year of life
• severe respiratory distress
• chest pain, GI bleeding, anemia
√ tubular right posterior mediastinal mass ± air
√ thoracic vertebral anomaly
√ contrast material may enter through distal connection

ECTOPIC PANCREAS

= PANCREATIC REST = MYOEPITHELIAL HAMARTOMA
Incidence: 2–10% of autopsies; M:F = 2:1
• asymptomatic
Location: lesions may be multiple
(a) greater curvature of antrum 1–6 cm from pylorus, pylorus, duodenal bulb, proximal jejunum (in 80%)
(b) ileum, Meckel diverticulum
√ smooth cone- / nipple-shaped submucosal nodule 1–5 cm in size
√ central umbilication representing orifice of filiform duct

ENTERIC CYST

= cyst lined by gastrointestinal mucosa without bowel wall
Etiology: migration of small bowel / colonic diverticulum into mesentery / mesocolon
Path: unilocular thin smooth-walled cyst with serous contents lined by enteric epithelium + thin fibrous wall
US:
√ hypoechoic cystic mass, occasionally with septations
DDx: duplication cyst (reduplication of bowel wall)

EOSINOPHILIC GASTROENTERITIS

= uncommon self-limited form of gastroenteritis with remissions + exacerbations characterized by infiltration of eosinophilic leukocytes into stomach / small bowel wall + usually marked peripheral eosinophilia
Cause: unknown
Histo: fibrous tissue + eosinophilic infiltrate of gastrointestinal mucosa
Age: in children + young adults with allergy + eosinophilia
A. EOSINOPHILIC GRANULOMA
= FIBROUS POLYPOID LESION
= INFLAMMATORY PSEUDOTUMOR
= localized form / circumscribed type
Location: almost exclusively in stomach (most common in antrum + pylorus)
√ submucosal polypoid mass / pedunculated polyp
B. EOSINOPHILIC GASTROENTERITIS
= diffuse type
= eosinophilic infiltration of mucosa, submucosa, and muscular layers of small intestine ± stomach by mature eosinophils (? gastric pendant to Löffler syndrome)
• recurrent episodes of abdominal pain, diarrhea, vomiting
• weight loss
• hematemesis (from ulceration)
• peripheral eosinophilia, anemia
• history of systemic allergy / food allergy
Location: entire small bowel (particularly jejunum), distal stomach, omentum, mesentery
Site: (a) mucosal
(b) muscular
(c) serosal (rare)
@ Stomach (almost always limited to antrum)
√ "wet stomach"
√ ulcers are rare
(a) mucosal type
√ enlarged gastric rugae / cobblestone nodules / polyps
(b) muscular type
√ thickened + rigid wall with narrowed gastric antrum / pylorus
√ bulky intraluminal mass up to 9 cm in size
Cx: pyloric obstruction
DDx: hypertrophic gastritis, lymphoma, carcinoma
@ Small bowel (involved in 50%)
√ separation of small bowel loops
(a) mucosal type
• malabsorption + hypoproteinemia
√ thickening + distortion of folds predominantly in jejunum
(b) submucosal / muscular type
√ motility disturbance
√ small-bowel obstruction
√ effacement of mucosal pattern + narrowing of lumen
(c) serosal type
√ ascites
Prognosis: tendency toward spontaneous remission
Rx: steroids / removal of sensitizing agent

EPIPLOIC APPENDAGITIS

= rare inflammation of one of the 100 epiploic appendages
Cause: (a) primary: torsion (exercise), venous thrombosis
(b) secondary: inflammation of adjacent organ (eg, diverticulitis, appendicitis)

Histo: acute infarction with fat necrosis, inflammation, thrombosed vessels with hemorrhagic suffusion
• abrupt onset of localized abdominal pain (RLQ in 50%), gradually resolving over 3–7 days
• palpable mass (10–30%)
• ± peritoneal signs
• normal / mildly increased WBCs
◊ Almost never suspected preoperatively!
Location: anterolaterally / (occasionally) anteromedially to ascending / descending / sigmoid colon
US:
√ solid hyperechoic noncompressible ovoid mass
√ hypoechoic margin (93%)
CT:
√ pericolic oval-shaped pedunculated mass, 1–4 cm in diameter, with fat attenuation (approx. –60 HU):
√ hyperattenuating peripheral rim
√ internal fat stranding
√ periappendigeal fat infiltration
√ thickening of adjacent visceral peritoneal lining (93%)
Prognosis: spontaneous resolution
Rx: conservative management
DDx: torsion / infarction of greater omentum, diverticulitis, appendicitis

ESOPHAGEAL CANCER

Incidence: <1% of all cancers; 4–10% of all GI malignancies; 11,000 cases/year (USA in 1994); M:F = 4:1; Blacks:Whites = 2:1
High-risk regions: Iran, parts of Africa, Italy, China
Predisposing factors:
achalasia (risk factor of 1,000 x), asbestosis, Barrett esophagus, celiac disease, radiation exposure, caustic stricture (risk factor of 1,000 x), Plummer-Vinson syndrome, tannins, alcohol, tobacco, history of oral / pharyngeal cancer, tylosis palmaris et plantaris

mnemonic: "BELCH SPAT"
Barrett esophagus
EtOH abuse
Lye stricture
Celiac disease
Head and neck tumor
Smoking
Plummer-Vinson syndrome
Achalasia, **A**sbestosis
Tylosis

Cancer Staging:
TNM system:
T1 tumor invades lamina propria / submucosa
T2 tumor invades muscularis propria
T3 tumor invades adventitia
T4 tumor invades adjacent structures

Stage I = T1,N0,M0
Stage IIA = T2/3,N0,M0
Stage IIB = T1/2,N1,M0
Stage III = T3,N1,M0 or T4,N0/1,M0
Stage IV = T1-4,N0/1,M1

CT staging (Moss):
Stage 1 intraluminal tumor / localized wall thickening of 3–5 mm
Stage 2 localized / circumferential wall thickening >5 mm
Stage 3 contiguous spread into adjacent mediastinum (trachea, bronchi, aorta, pericardium)
√ loss of fat planes (nonspecific due to cachexia, often still resectable)
√ mass in contact with aorta >90° arc (in 20–70% still resectable)
√ displacement / compression of airway (90–100% accuracy for invasion)
√ esophagotracheal / -bronchial fistula (unresectable)
Stage 4 distant metastases
√ enlarged abdominal lymph nodes >10 mm (12–85% accuracy)
√ hepatic, pulmonary, adrenal metastases
√ direct erosion of vertebral body
√ tumor >3 cm wide = high frequency of extraesophageal spread
Histo:
(1) Squamous cell carcinoma (50–70%)
(2) Adenocarcinoma (30–50%) arising from mucosal / submucosal glands or heterotopic gastric mucosa or columnar-lined epithelium (Barrett)
(a) in 70% from Barrett esophagus
(b) gastric adenocarcinoma involving GE junction
(c) in submucosal / deep esophageal glands
(d) ectopic gastric mucosa in esophagus
◊ 2,500 new cases each year; M:F = 7:1
√ tendency to invade gastric cardia + fundus
(3) Spindle-cell squamous carcinoma = carcinosarcoma = pseudosarcoma
Histo: squamous + sarcomatous elements
Age: in men >45 years
Location: usually middle third of esophagus
√ large bulky polypoid smooth, lobulated, scalloped intraluminal mass; may be pedunculated
DDx: lymphoma, other sarcomas
(4) Mucoepidermoid carcinoma, adenoid cystic carcinoma
(5) Leiomyosarcoma, rhabdomyosarcoma, fibrosarcoma, malignant lymphoma
(6) Secondary tumor involvement from: thyroid, larynx
(7) Metastasis from: breast, melanoma, GI tract

• dysphagia (87–95%) of <6 months' duration
• weight loss (71%)
• retrosternal pain (46%)
• regurgitation (29%)
Location: upper 1/3 (15–20%); middle 1/3 (37–44%); lower 1/3 (38–43%)

Radiologic types:
(1) Polypoid / fungating form (most common)
√ sessile / pedunculated tumor with lobulated surface

√ protruding, irregular, polycyclic, overhanging, steplike "apple core" lesion
(2) Ulcerating form
√ large ulcer niche within bulging mass
(3) Infiltrating form
√ gradual narrowing with smooth transition (DDx: benign stricture)
(4) Varicoid form = superficial spreading carcinoma
Histo: longitudinal extension confined to mucosa / submucosa
√ focal area of confluent mucosal nodules / plaques
DDx: Candida esophagitis

Metastases:
(a) lymphogenic: anterior jugular chain + supraclavicular nodes (primary in upper 1/3); paraesophageal + subdiaphragmatic nodes (primary in middle 1/3); mediastinal + paracardial + celiac trunk nodes (primary in lower 1/3)
(b) hematogenous: lung, liver, adrenal gland

CXR:
√ widened azygoesophageal recess with convexity toward right lung (in 30% of distal + midesophageal cancers)
√ thickening of posterior tracheal stripe + right paratracheal stripe >4 mm (if tumor located in upper third of esophagus)
√ widened mediastinum
√ tracheal deviation
√ posterior tracheal indentation / mass
√ retrocardiac mass
√ esophageal air-fluid level
√ lobulated mass extending into gastric air bubble
√ repeated aspiration pneumonia (with tracheoesophageal fistula)

Cx: fistula formation to trachea (5–10%) / bronchi / mediastinum
Prognosis: 3–5–20% 5-year survival rate; 0% 5-year survival rate for cancer of cervical esophagus
Mean survival time:
90 days with subdiaphragmatic lymphadenopathy
180 days with local invasion + abdominal metastases
480 days without evidence of invasion / metastases

Rx: (1) chemotherapy (fluorouracil, cisplatin, bleomycin sulfate, mitomycin) + surgery
(2) chemotherapy + irradiation (~4,000 cGy)
(3) chemotherapy + irradiation + surgery
Operative mortality: 3–8%

ESOPHAGEAL INTRAMURAL PSEUDODIVERTICULOSIS

= dilated excretory ducts of deep mucous glands
Etiology: uncertain
Incidence: about 100 cases in world literature
Site: diffuse / segmental involvement
In 90% associated with:
diabetes, alcoholism, any severe esophagitis (most often reflux / Candida), esophageal stricture

√ multiple tiny rounded / flask-shaped barium collections in longitudinal rows parallel to long axis of esophagus:
√ appear to "float" outside esophagus without apparent communication with lumen
√ esophageal stricture:
√ short stricture in distal esophagus (common)
√ long stricture in cervical / upper thoracic esophagus (classic)

ESOPHAGEAL PERFORATION

= ESOPHAGEAL RUPTURE
Cause:
(1) Iatrogenic injury (most common cause, 55%): complication of endoscopy, dilatation of stricture, bougie, disruption of suture line following surgical anastomosis, attempted intubation
(2) Spontaneous rupture = Boerhaave syndrome (15%): emetogenic injury of the esophagus from sudden increase in intraabdominal pressure + relaxation of distal esophageal sphincter in the presence of a moderate to large amount of gastric contents
(3) Closed chest trauma (10%)
Incidence: 1% of all blunt chest trauma
Location:
(a) cervical / upper thoracic esophagus (82%)
(b) just above gastroesophageal junction along posterolateral wall on the left side
(4) Esophageal carcinoma
(5) Retained foreign body (14%): coin, aluminum pop-tops, metallic button, safety pin, invisible plastic toy) leading to perforation (in pediatric age group)
(6) Barrett ulcer

• pain, dysphagia, odynophagia
• rapid onset of overwhelming sepsis: fever, tachycardia, hypotension, shock

Plain film (normal in 9–12%):
√ extensive pneumomediastinum
√ V sign of Naclerio = extrapleural air within lower mediastinum between parietal pleura + diaphragm (usually on left)
√ subcutaneous emphysema of the neck
√ delayed widening of the mediastinum (secondary to mediastinitis)
√ hydrothorax (after rupture into pleural cavity), usually unilateral on left side
√ hydropneumothorax (often not initially seen)
√ left lower lobe atelectasis
√ confirmation with contrast study (90% of contrast esophagograms are positive)

CT:
√ focal extraluminal air collection at site of tear (92%; most useful sign)
√ periesophageal / mediastinal hematoma / fluid (92%)
√ pleural effusion (75%)
√ esophageal wall thickening
√ extravasation of oral contrast material

Esophagography with:
(1) water-soluble contrast material (10% false-negative results)

(2) barium (if result with water-soluble material negative)

A. UPPER / MID-ESOPHAGEAL PERFORATION
Location: at level of cricopharyngeus muscle (most frequent)
√ widening of upper mediastinum
√ right-sided hydrothorax

B. DISTAL ESOPHAGEAL PERFORATION (more common, but not in blunt chest trauma)
Cause: biopsy, dilatation of stricture, Boerhaave syndrome
√ left-sided hydrothorax
√ little mediastinal changes

Cx: (1) Acute mediastinitis
(2) Obstruction of SVC
(3) Mediastinal abscess

Prognosis: 20–60% mortality

ESOPHAGEAL VARICES

= plexuses formed by dilated subepithelial veins + submucosal veins + dilated venae commitantes of the vagus nerves outside the tunica muscularis

Anatomy:
(a) anterior branch connected to left gastric vein
(b) posterior branch connected to azygos + hemiazygos system

A. UPHILL VARICES
= collateral blood flow from portal vein via azygos vein into SVC (usually lower esophagus drains via left gastric vein into portal vein)
Cause:
(a) intrahepatic obstruction from cirrhosis
◊ In <5% of patients with portal hypertension
(b) splenic vein thrombosis (usually gastric varices)
(c) obstruction of hepatic veins
(d) IVC obstruction below hepatic veins
(e) IVC obstruction above hepatic vein entrance / CHF
(f) marked splenomegaly / splenic hemangiomatosis (rare)
√ varices in lower half of esophagus

B. DOWNHILL VARICES
= collateral blood flow from SVC via azygos vein into IVC / portal venous system (upper esophagus usually drains via azygos vein into SVC)
Cause: obstruction of superior vena cava distal to entry of azygos vein (= superior vena cava syndrome) most commonly due to lung cancer, lymphoma, retrosternal goiter, thymoma, mediastinal fibrosis
√ varices in upper 1/3 of esophagus

EXAMINATION TECHNIQUE
(a) small amount of barium (not to obscure varices)
(b) relaxation of esophagus (not to compress varices): refrain from swallowing because succeeding swallow initiates a primary peristaltic wave that lasts for 10–30 seconds; sustained Valsalva maneuver precludes from swallowing
(c) in LAO projection with patient recumbent / in Trendelenburg position ± Valsalva maneuver / deep inspiration

Plain film:
√ lobulated masses in posterior mediastinum (visible in 5–8% of patients with varices)
√ silhouetting of descending aorta
√ abnormal convex contour of azygoesophageal recess at level of gastroesophageal junction

UGI:
√ thickened sinuous interrupted mucosal folds (earliest sign)
√ tortuous radiolucencies of variable size + location
√ "worm-eaten" smooth lobulated filling defects
√ findings may be accentuated after sclerotherapy

CT:
√ thickened esophageal wall + lobulated outer contour
√ scalloped esophageal luminal masses
√ right- / left-sided soft-tissue masses (= paraesophageal varices)
√ marked enhancement following dynamic CT

Cx: bleeding in 28% within 3 years; exsanguination in 10–15%

DDx: varicoid carcinoma of esophagus

ESOPHAGEAL WEB

= complete / incomplete circumferential narrowing caused by 1–2-mm thick (vertical length) mucosal membrane projecting into esophageal lumen; covered by squamous epithelium on superior + inferior surfaces

Age: middle-aged females

? Association with:
Plummer-Vinson syndrome = Paterson-Kelly syndrome (iron deficiency anemia, stomatitis, glossitis, dysphagia, thyroid disorder, spoon-shaped nails)

Cause: *mnemonic:* "BIEP"
B-ring (Schatzki ring)
Idiopathic (= transverse mucosal fold)
Epidermolysis bullosa
Plummer-Vinson disease

Path: hyperkeratosis + chronic inflammation of submucosa

• mostly asymptomatic (unless severely stenosing)

Location: in cervical esophagus near cricopharyngeus (most common) > thoracic esophagus; occasionally multiple

√ visualized during maximal distension (in one-tenth of a second)
√ arises at right angles from anterior esophageal wall
√ thin delicate membrane of uniform thickness of <3 mm

Cx: high risk of upper esophageal + hypopharyngeal carcinoma

Rx: (1) balloon dilatation
(2) bougienage during esophagoscopy

DDx: stricture (circumferential + thicker = 1–2-mm thick [vertical length] area of complete / incomplete circumferential narrowing

GI

ESOPHAGITIS

Acute Esophagitis

mnemonic for cause: "CRIER"

Corrosives, **C**rohn disease
Reflux
Infection, **I**ntubation
Epidermolysis bullosa
Radiation therapy

√ thickened >3-mm-wide folds with irregular lobulated contour
√ mucosal nodularity (= multiple ulcerations + intervening edema)
√ erosions
√ vertically oriented ulcers usually 3–10 mm in length
√ inflammatory esophagogastric polyp = proximal gastric fold extending across esophagogastric junction (rare)
√ abnormal motility

Candida Esophagitis

= MONILIASIS = CANDIDIASIS

◊ Most common cause of infectious esophagitis!

Organism: C. albicans, C. tropicalis; endogenous (majority) / transmitted by another human / animal; often discovered in diseased skin, GI tract, sputum, female genital tract, urine with an indwelling Foley catheter

Predisposed:
(a) individuals with depressed immunity: hematologic disease, renal transplant, leukemia, chronic debilitating disease, diabetes mellitus, steroids, chemotherapy, radiotherapy, AIDS
◊ Most common type of fungi found with opportunistic infections!
(b) delayed esophageal emptying: scleroderma, strictures, achalasia, S/P fundoplication
(c) antibiotics

Path: patchy, creamy-white plaques covering a friable erythematous mucosa

Histo: mucosal plaques = necrotic epithelial debris + fungal colonies

• dysphagia (= difficulty swallowing)
• severe odynophagia (= painful swallowing from segmental spasm)
• intense retro- / substernal pain
• associated with thrush (= oropharyngeal moniliasis) in 20–50–80%

Location: predilection for upper 1/2 of esophagus

√ involvement of long esophageal segments:
√ "cobblestone" appearance = mucosal nodularity in early stage (from growth of colonies on surface)
√ longitudinal plaques = grouping of tiny 1–2-mm nodular filling defects with linear orientation (= heaped-up areas of mucosal plaques)
√ shaggy / fuzzy / serrated contour (from coalescent plaques, pseudomembranes, erosions, ulcerations, intramural hemorrhage) in fulminant candidiasis of AIDS

√ narrowed lumen (from spasm, pseudomembranes, marked edema)
√ "intramural diverticulosis" = multiple tiny indentations + protrusions
√ sluggish / absent primary peristalsis
√ strictures (rare)
√ mycetoma resembling large intraluminal tumor (rare)

Diagnostic sensitivity: endoscopy (97%), double contrast (88%), single contrast (55%)

Cx: (1) Systemic candidiasis ("microabscesses" in liver, spleen, kidney)
(2) Gastric bezoar due to large fungus ball (after long-standing esophageal candidiasis)

Rx: ketoconazole / fluconazole

DDx: glycogen acanthosis, reflux esophagitis, superficial spreading carcinoma, artifacts (undissolved effervescent crystals, air bubbles, retained food particles), herpes esophagitis, acute caustic ingestion, intramural pseudodiverticulosis, squamous papillomatosis, Barrett esophagus, epidermolysis bullosa, varices

Caustic Esophagitis

= CORROSIVE ESOPHAGITIS

Corrosive agents:
lye (sodium hydroxide), washing soda (sodium carbonate), household cleaners, iodine, silver nitrate, household bleaches, Clinitest® tablets (tend to be neutralized by gastric acid)

◊ Severity of injury dependent on contact time + concentration of corrosive material!

Associated with: injury to pharynx + stomach (7–8%): antral burns more common with acid (buffering effect of gastric acid on alkali)

Location: middle + lower thirds of esophagus

Stage I : acute necrosis from protein coagulation
√ mucosal blurring (edema)
√ diffusely atonic + dilated esophagus
√ tertiary contractions / spasm

Stage II : frank ulceration in 3–5 days
√ ulceration + pseudomembranes

Stage III : scarring + stricture from fibroblastic activity
√ long segmental stricture after 10 days when acute edema subsides (7–30%)

Cx: (1) Esophageal / gastric perforation during ulcerative stage
(2) Squamous cell carcinoma in injured segment

Rx: dilatation procedure / esophageal replacement surgery

Chronic Esophagitis

√ luminal narrowing with tapered transition to normal + proximal dilatation
√ circumferential / eccentric stricture
√ sacculations = pseudodiverticula

GI

Drug-induced Esophagitis

= contact esophagitis due to oral medications = "pill esophagitis"

Agents: antibiotics (tetracycline, doxycycline), quinidine, potassium chloride, nonsteroidal antiinflammatory agents (aspirin), ascorbic acid, alprenolol chloride, emepronium bromide, alendronate (= inhibitor of osteoclastic activity)

- severe odynophagia
- history of taking medication with little / no water immediately before going to bed
- rapid clinical improvement after withdrawal of offending agent

Location: midesophagus at site of normal extrinsic impressions by aortic arch / left mainstem bronchus / left atrium

√ localized cluster of tiny ulcers distributed circumferentially (most commonly)

√ superficial solitary / several discrete ulcers

Prognosis: ulcers heal within 7–10 days after cessation of offending medication

DDx: herpes esophagitis (immunosuppressed patient, less localized); reflux esophagitis (heartburn, distal esophagus near esophagogastric junction)

Reflux Esophagitis

= esophageal inflammation secondary to reflux of acid-peptic contents of the stomach; reflux occurs if resting pressure of LES <5 mm Hg (may be normal event if followed by rapid clearing)

Prevalence: in 20% of gastroesophageal reflux

Histo: basal cell hyperplasia with wall thickening + thinning of epithelium, mucosal edema + erosions, inflammatory infiltrate

Determinants: (1) Frequency of reflux
(2) Adequacy of clearing mechanism
(3) Volume of refluxed material
(4) Potency of refluxed material
(5) Tissue resistance

Reflux preventing features:
(1) Lower esophageal sphincter
(2) Phrenoesophageal membrane
(3) Length of subdiaphragmatic esophagus
(4) Gastroesophageal angle of His (70–110°)

May be associated with: sliding hiatal hernia (in most patients), scleroderma, nasogastric intubation

- heartburn, epigastric discomfort
- choking, globus hystericus
- retrosternal pain
- thoracic / cervical dysphagia

Site: usually lower 1/3 / lower 1/2 with continuous disease extending proximally from GE junction

√ segmental esophageal narrowing (edema / spasm / stricture)

√ poorly defined tiny mucosal elevations ("mucosal granularity") on thickened / nodular longitudinal folds (mucosal edema + inflammation) in early stages

√ single marginal ulcer / erosion at or adjacent to gastroesophageal junction

√ multiple areas of superficial ulceration in distal esophagus

√ prominent mucosal fold ending in polypoid protuberance within hiatal hernia / cardia

√ interruption of primary peristalsis at inflamed segment

√ nonperistaltic waves in distal esophagus following deglutition (85%)

√ incomplete relaxation of LES (75%), incompetent sphincter (33%)

√ acid test = abnormal motility elicited by acid barium (pH 1.7)

√ "felinization" = transverse ridges of esophagus secondary to contraction of muscularis mucosae (similar to cat esophagus)

NUC (pertechnetate):
√ esophageal activity (Barrett esophagus similar to ectopic gastric mucosa)

Reflux tests:

1. Reflux of barium in RPO position, may be elicited by coughing / deep respiratory movements / swallowing of saliva + water / anteflexion in erect position: only in 50% accurate
2. Water-siphon test: in 5% false negative; large number of false positives
3. Tuttle test = measurement of esophageal pH: 96% accurate
4. Radionuclide gastroesophageal reflux test (typically combined with gastric emptying test):
   Technique: ROI drawn over distal esophagus + compared with time-activity curve over stomach, scaled to 4%
   √ esophageal activity >4% stomach activity

Cx of reflux:
(a) from acid + pepsin acting on esophageal mucosa:
1. Motility disturbance
2. Stricture
3. Schatzki ring
4. Barrett esophagus
5. Iron-deficiency anemia
6. Reflux / peptic esophagitis

(b) from aspiration of gastric contents
1. Acute aspiration pneumonia
2. Mendelson syndrome
3. Pulmonary fibrosis

Viral Esophagitis

Predisposed: immunocompromised, eg, underlying malignancy, debilitating illness, radiation treatment, steroids, chemotherapy, AIDS

Cytomegalovirus Esophagitis

Organism: member of herpesvirus group

Associated with: AIDS

- severe odynophagia

√ diffusely normal mucosal background

√ one / more giant ovoid flat ulcers (up to several cm in size) near gastroesophageal junction

√ discrete small superficial ulcers indistinguishable from herpes esophagitis (uncommon)
Rx: ganciclovir (relatively toxic)
Dx: endoscopic brushings, biopsy specimen, cultures

Herpes Esophagitis

◊ 2nd most common cause of opportunistic infection!
Organism: Herpes simplex virus type I (DNA core virus) secreted in saliva of 2% of healthy population
Age: 15–30 years; usually males
Predisposed: immunosuppressed patient
- history of recent exposure to sexual partners with herpetic lesions on lips / buccal mucosa
- flulike prodrome of 3–10 days (headaches, fever, sore throat, upper respiratory symptoms, myalgia)
- severe acute dysphagia / odynophagia

May be associated with: oropharyngeal herpetic lesions / oropharyngeal candidiasis
Location: midesophagus (level of left main bronchus)
√ initially vesicles / blisters that subsequently rupture
√ multiple small discrete superficial punctate / round / linear / serpentine / stellate (often "diamond-shaped") ulcers surrounded by radiolucent halos of edematous mucosa (in >50%)
√ intervening mucosa normal (without plaques)
√ multiple plaquelike lesions (only with severe infection)
Dx: rising serum titer for HSV type I, viral culture, biopsy (immunofluorescent staining for HSV antigen, demonstration of intranuclear inclusions)
Rx: oral / intravenous acyclovir
Prognosis: resolution of symptoms in 3–14 days
DDx: drug-induced esophagitis, Crohn disease, esophageal intramural pseudodiverticulosis

Human Immunodeficiency Virus Esophagitis

- maculopapular rash + ulcers of soft palate (occasionally)
- recent seroconversion / known AIDS

√ one / more giant (>1 cm) flat ovoid / diamond-shaped ulcers (at time of seroconversion) indistinguishable from CMV esophagitis
Dx: per exclusion (brushings, biopsies, cultures negative for CMV)
Rx: oral steroids
DDx: CMV esophagitis, mycobacterial esophagitis, actinomycosis, potassium chloride, quinidine, caustic ingestion, nasogastric intubation, radiation therapy, endoscopic sclerotherapy

FAMILIAL ADENOMATOUS POLYPOSIS

= FAMILIAL MULTIPLE POLYPOSIS
= autosomal dominant disease with 80% penetrance (gene for familial polyposis localized on chromosome 5); sporadic occurrence in 1/3

Incidence: 1:7,000 to 1:24,000 live births
Histo: tubular / villotubular adenomatous polyps; usually about 1,000 adenomas
Age: polyps appear around puberty
- family history of colonic polyps (66%)
  ◊ Screening of family members after puberty!
- clinical symptoms begin during 3rd–4th decade (range 5–55 years)
- vague abdominal pain, weight loss
- diarrhea, bloody stools
- protein-losing enteropathy (occasionally)

Associated with: (1) Hamartomas of stomach in 49%
(2) Adenomas of duodenum in 25%
(3) Periampullary carcinoma
√ "carpet of polyps" = myriad of 2–3 mm (up to 2 cm) polypoid lesions
@ Colon (100%): more numerous in distal colon; always affecting rectum
√ normal haustral pattern
@ Stomach (5%)
@ Small bowel (<5%)
Cx: malignant transformation: colon > stomach > small bowel (in 12% by 5 years; in 30% by 10 years; in 100% by 20 years after diagnosis; age at carcinomatous development usually 20–40 years; multiple carcinomas in 48%)
◊ Periampullary carcinoma is the most common cause of death after prophylactic colectomy!
Rx: prophylactic total colectomy in late teens / early twenties before symptoms develop +
(1) Permanent ileostomy
(2) Continent endorectal pull-through pouch
(3) Kock pouch (= distal ileum formed into a one-way valve by invaginating the bowel at skin site)
DDx: other polyposes, lymphoid hyperplasia, lymphosarcoma, ulcerative colitis with inflammatory pseudopolyps

GALLSTONE ILEUS

Incidence: 0.4–5% of all intestinal obstructions (20% of obstruction in patients >65 years; 24% of obstructions in patients >70 years); develops in <1% of patients with cholelithiasis; in 1 of 6 perforations; risk increases with age
Etiology: biliary disease (90%), peptic ulcer disease, cancer, trauma
Age: average 65–75 years; M:F = 1:4 –1:7
- previous history of gallbladder disease
- intermittent episodes of acute colicky abdominal pain (20–30%)
- nausea, vomiting, fever, distension, obstipation

√ **Rigler triad** on plain film (in 10%):
1. Partial / complete intestinal obstruction (usually small bowel), "string of rosary beads" = multiple small amounts of air trapped between dilated + stretched valvulae conniventes (in 86%)
2. Gas in biliary tree (in 69%)
3. Ectopic calcified gallstone (in 25%): stones are commonly >2.5 cm in diameter

√ change in position of previously identified gallstone

UGI / BE:
- √ well-contained localized barium collection lateral to first portion of duodenum (barium-filled collapsed GB + possibly biliary ducts)
  Fistulous communication:
  Cholecystoduodenal (60%), choledochoduodenal, cholecystocolic, choledochocolic, cholecystogastric
- √ identification of site of obstruction: terminal ileum (60–70%), proximal ileum (25%), distal ileum (10%), pylorus, sigmoid, duodenum (Bouveret syndrome)

Cx: recurrent gallstone ileus in 5–10% (additional silent calculi more proximally)

Prognosis: high mortality

GANGLIOCYTIC PARAGANGLIOMA

= rare benign tumor of the GI tract

Frequency: <100 cases reported

Origin: pancreatic endocrine rest that remained when the ventral primordium rotated around the duodenum

Age: 50–60 years of age; M:F = 2:1

Location: almost exclusively in 2nd portion of duodenum near the ampulla of Vater on the medial / lateral wall of duodenum

- GI hemorrhage, abdominal pain
- √ polypoid smooth-surfaced intraluminal mass
- √ homogeneously enhancing mural / extrinsic solid mass of soft-tissue attenuation
- √ well-circumscribed hypoechoic mass contiguous with bowel
- √ no biliary duct dilatation

DDx: adenocarcinoma (biliary duct dilatation, hypovascular), leiomyosarcoma (cystic internal hemorrhage / necrosis), hemangioma, duplication cyst, choledochal cyst, lipoma, hamartoma, inflammatory fibroid polyp (distal small bowel), lymphoma (isolated in stomach and ileum)

GARDNER SYNDROME

= autosomal dominant disease (? variant of familial polyposis) characterized by a triad of
(1) colonic polyposis
(2) osteomas
(3) soft-tissue tumors

Cause: adenomatous polyposis gene on chromosome 5-q21; in 20% new mutations
◊ Familial polyposis + Gardner syndrome may occur in the same family!

Histo: adenomatous polyps

Age: 15–30 years (2 months – 70 years)

Associated with: ? MEA complex
(1) periampullary / duodenal carcinoma (12%)
(2) papillary thyroid carcinoma (often multicentric)
(3) adrenal adenoma / carcinoma
(4) parathyroid adenoma
(5) pituitary chromophobe adenoma
(6) carcinoid, adenoma of small bowel
(7) retroperitoneal leiomyoma

◊ Extraintestinal manifestations occur usually earlier than in intestinal polyposis!
- skin pigmentation
- cramping abdominal pain
- weight loss, diarrhea

@ Polyposis
Location: colon (100%), stomach (5–68%), duodenum (90%), small bowel (<5%)
- √ multiple colonic polyps appearing during puberty, increasing in number during 3rd–4th decade
- √ lymphoid hyperplasia of terminal ileum
- √ hamartomas of stomach
- √ intussusception

Cx: small bowel / colonic obstruction

@ Soft-tissue tumors
(a) sebaceous / epidermoid inclusion cysts (scalp, back, face, extremities)
(b) fibroma, lipoma, leiomyoma, neurofibroma
(c) desmoid tumors (3–29%); peritoneal adhesions (desmoplastic tendency); mesenteric fibrosis, retroperitoneal fibrosis
- urinary tract obstruction
(d) mammary fibromatosis
(e) marked keloid formation, hypertrophied scars (anterior abdominal wall) arise 1–3 years after surgery

@ Osteomatosis of membranous bone (50%)
Location: calvarium, mandible (81%), maxilla, ribs, long bones

@ Long bones
- √ localized wavy cortical thickening / exostoses
- √ slight shortening + bowing

@ Teeth
- √ odontoma, unerupted / supernumerary teeth, hypercementosis
- √ tendency toward numerous caries (dental prosthesis at early age)

Cx: malignant transformation of colonic polyps in 100% (average age at death is 41 years if untreated)

Prophylaxis: gastrointestinal surveillance, thyroid screening, ophthalmologic evaluation for retinal pigmentation anomalies; screening of family members starting at age 15

Rx: prophylactic total colectomy at about 20 years of age

GASTRIC CARCINOMA

◊ 3rd most common GI malignancy after colorectal + pancreatic cancer, 6th leading cause of cancer deaths

Prevalence: declining; 24,000 cases/year in USA

Risk factors: smoking, nitrites, nitrates, pickled vegetables

Predisposing factors:
H. pylori gastritis, chronic atrophic gastritis, adenomatous + villous polyp (7–27% are malignant), gastrojejunostomy, partial gastrectomy (Billroth II > Billroth I), pernicious anemia (risk factor of 2), Ménétrier disease (?)

Histo: adenocarcinoma (95%); rarely squamous cell carcinoma / adenoacanthoma

Staging:

- T1 tumor limited to mucosa / submucosa
- T2 tumor involves muscle / serosa
- T3 tumor penetrates through serosa
- T4a invasion of adjacent contiguous tissues
- T4b invasion of adjacent organs, diaphragm, abdominal wall
- N1 involvement of perigastric nodes within 3 cm of primary along greater / lesser curvature
- N2 involvement of regional nodes >3 cm from primary along branches of celiac axis
- N3 paraaortic, hepatoduodenal, retropancreatic, mesenteric nodes
- M1 distant metastases

Location: mostly distal third of stomach + cardia; 60% on lesser curvature, 10% on greater curvature; esophagogastric junction in 30%; transpyloric spread in 5–25% (for lymphoma 40%)

Probability of malignancy of an ulcer: at lesser curvature 10–15%, at greater curvature 70%, in fundus 90%

Morphology:

1. Polypoid / fungating carcinoma
2. Ulcerating / penetrating carcinoma (70%)
3. Infiltrating / scirrhous carcinoma (5–15%)
   = linitis plastica
   Histo: frequently signet ring cell type + increase in fibrous tissue
   Location: antrum, fundus + body (38%)
   √ firmness, rigidity, reduced capacity of stomach, aperistalsis in involved area
   √ granular / polypoid folds with encircling growth
4. Superficial spreading carcinoma
   = confined to mucosa / submucosa; 5-year survival of 90%
   √ patch of nodularity
   √ little loss of elasticity
5. Advanced bulky carcinoma

• GI bleeding, abdominal pain, weight loss

UGI:
- √ rigidity
- √ filling defect
- √ amputation of folds ± ulceration ± stenosis
- √ miliary / punctate calcifications (mucinous adenocarcinoma)

CT:
- √ irregular nodular luminal surface
- √ asymmetric thickening of folds
- √ mass of uniform density / varying attenuation
- √ wall thickness >6 mm with gas distension + 13 mm with positive contrast material distension:
  - √ diffuse low attenuation in mucinous carcinoma
- √ increased density in perigastric fat
- √ enhancement exclusively in linitis plastica type
- √ nodules of serosal surface (= dilated surface lymphatics)
- √ diameter of esophagus at gastroesophageal junction larger than adjacent aorta (DDx: hiatal hernia)
- √ lymphadenopathy below level of renal pedicle (3%)

Prognostic Parameters of Gastric Carcinoma

Tumor Size	*Metastases*	*Limited to Submucosa*	*5-Year Survival Rate*
1 cm	11%		87%
2 cm	25%	70%	67%
3 cm	45%		35%
4 cm	59%	60%	33%
>4 cm	72%	33%	

Metastases:

1. along peritoneal ligaments
   (a) gastrocolic lig.: transverse colon, pancreas
   (b) gastrohepatic + hepatoduodenal lig.: liver
2. local lymph nodes
3. hematogenous: liver (most common), adrenals, ovaries, bone (1.8%), lymphangitic carcinomatosis of lung (rare)
4. peritoneal seeding:
   on rectal wall = Blumer shelf
   on ovaries = Krukenberg tumor
5. left supraclavicular lymph node = Virchow node

Prognosis:

overall 5-year survival rate of 5–18%, mean survival time of 7–8 months;
- — 85% 5-year survival in stage T1
- — 52% 5-year survival in stage T2
- — 47% 5-year survival in stage T3
- — 17% 5-year survival in stage N1-2
- — 5% 5-year survival in stage N3

Early Gastric Cancer (20%)

= invasion limited to mucosa + submucosa (T1 lesion) regardless of lymph node involvement

Classification of Japan Research Society for Gastric Cancer:

- Type I protruded type = >5 mm in height with protrusion into gastric lumen (10–20%)
- Type II superficial type = <5 mm in height
  - IIa slightly elevated surface (10–20%)
  - IIb flat / almost unrecognizable (2%)
  - IIc slightly depressed surface (50–60%)
- Type III excavated / ulcerated type (5–10%)

Advanced Gastric Cancer (T2 lesion and higher)

Bormann classification:

- Type 1 broad-based elevated polypoid lesion
- Type 2 elevated lesion + ulceration + well-demarcated margin
- Type 3 elevated lesion + ulceration + ill-defined margin
- Type 4 ill-defined flat lesion
- Type 5 unclassified, no apparent elevation

GASTRIC DIVERTICULUM

stomach is least common site of diverticula

Incidence: 1:600–2,400 of UGI studies

Etiology: (a) traction secondary to scarring / periantral inflammation = true diverticulum
(b) pulsion (less common) = false diverticulum
Age: beyond 40 years
Often associated with: aberrant pancreas in antral location
Location: juxtacardiac on posterior wall (75%), prepyloric (15–22%), greater curve (3%)
√ pliability + varying degrees of distension
√ NO mass, edema or rigidity of adjacent folds
DDx: small ulcer in intramural-extramucosal mass

GASTRIC POLYP

Incidence: 1.5–5%, most common benign gastric tumor
Associated with: hyperacidity + ulcers, chronic atrophic gastritis, gastric carcinoma

A. NONNEOPLASTIC
1. **Inflammatory polyp of stomach** (75–90%)
= HYPERPLASTIC POLYP = REGENERATIVE POLYP
Histo: cystically dilated glands lined by gastric epithelium + acute and chronic inflammatory infiltrates in lamina propria
Associated with: chronic atrophic gastritis, pernicious anemia
Location: predominantly in fundus + body; usually multiple
√ sharply delineated polyp with smooth circular border
√ "Mexican hat sign" = stalk seen en face overlying the head of polyp
√ sessile / pedunculated
√ usually <2 cm in diameter without progression
√ no contour defect of stomach
Prognosis: no malignant potential
2. **Hamartomatous polyp of stomach** (rare)
Histo: densely packed gastric glands + bundles of smooth muscle
Associated with: Peutz-Jeghers syndrome
√ sessile / pedunculated
√ usually <2 cm in diameter
3. **Retention polyp of stomach** (rare)
Histo: dilated cystic glands + stroma
Associated with: Cronkhite-Canada syndrome

B. NEOPLASTIC
1. **Adenomatous polyp of stomach** (10–20%)
= true neoplasm with malignant potential (10–80%, increasing with size)
Age: increasing incidence with age; M:F = 2:1
Histo: intestinal metaplasia (common) + marked cellular atypism
Associated with: Gardner syndrome; coexistent with gastric carcinoma in 35%
Location: more commonly in antrum (antrum spared in Gardner syndrome)
√ broad-based elliptical / mushroom-shaped polyp ± pedicle; usually solitary
√ usually >2 cm in diameter (in 80%)
√ smooth / irregular lobulated contour
2. **Villous polyp of stomach** (rare)
√ trabeculated / lobulated slightly irregular contour
Cx: malignant transformation

DDx: (1) Ménétrier disease (antrum spared)
(2) Eosinophilic polyp (peripheral eosinophilia, linitis plastica appearance, small bowel changes)
(3) Lymphoma
(4) Carcinoma

GASTRIC ULCER

Benign Gastric Ulcer

95% of all gastric ulcers
Cause:
A. HORMONAL
1. Zollinger-Ellison syndrome
2. Hyperparathyroidism (in 1.3–24%)
duodenum:stomach = 4:1; M:F = 3:1
◊ Duodenal ulcers predominate in females!
◊ Gastric ulcers predominate in males!
• absence of gastric hypersecretion
3. Steroid-induced ulcer
gastric > duodenal location;
frequently multiple + deep ulcers;
commonly associated with erosions
• bleeding (in 1/3)
4. Stress, severe prolonged illness
5. Cerebral disease = Cushing ulcer
6. Curling ulcer (burns) (in 0.09–2.6%)
7. Retained gastric antrum
8. Uremia

B. INFLAMMATION
1. Peptic ulcer disease
2. Gastritis
3. Radiation-induced ulcer
4. Intubation
5. Stasis ulcer proximal to pyloric / duodenal obstruction

C. BENIGN MASS
1. Leiomyoma
2. Granulomatous disease
3. Pseudolymphoma (lymphoid hyperplasia)

D. DRUGS
ASA: greater curvature

Pathophysiology:
disrupted mucosal barrier (Helicobacter pylori) with vulnerability to acid + secretion of large volume of gastric juice containing little acid
Incidence: 5:10,000; 100,000/year (United States)
Age peak: 55–65 years; M:F = 1:1
Multiplicity:
(a) multiple in 2–8% (17–24% at autopsy), especially in patients on aspirin

Gastric Ulcer

Sign	*Benign*	*Malignant*
Crater	round, ovoid	irregular
Radiating folds	symmetric	nodular, clubbed, fused
Areae gastricae	preserved	destroyed
Projection	outside lumen	inside lumen
Ulcer mound	smooth	rolled edge

GI

(b) coexistent duodenal ulcer in 5–64%;
gastric:duodenal = 1:3 (adults) = 1:7 (children)
• abdominal pain: in 30% at night, in 25% precipitated by food
Location: lesser curvature at junction of corpus + antrum within 7 cm from pylorus; proximal half of stomach in older patients (geriatric ulcer); adjacent to GE junction within hiatal hernia
√ ulcer size usually <2 cm (range 1–250 mm); in 4% >40 mm
√ round / ovoid / linear shape
√ Haudek niche = conical / collar button-shaped barium collection projecting outside gastric contour (profile view)
√ Hampton line = 1-mm thin straight lucent line traversing the orifice of the ulcer niche (seen on profile view + with little gastric distension) = ledge of touching overhanging gastric mucosa of undermined benign ulcer
√ ulcer collar = smooth thick lucent band interposed between the niche and gastric lumen (thickened rim of edematous gastric wall) in well-distended stomach
√ ulcer mound = smooth, sharply delineated, gently sloping extensive tissue mass surrounding a benign ulcer (edema + lack of wall distensibility) in well-distended stomach
√ ulcer crater = round / oval barium collection with smooth border on dependent side (en face view)
√ halo defect = wide lucent band symmetrically surrounding ulcer resembling extensive ulcer mound (viewed en face)
√ ring shadow: ulcer on nondependent side (en face view)
√ radiating thick folds extending directly to crater edge fusing with the effaced marginal fold of the ulcer collar / halo of ulcer mound
√ incisura defect = smooth, deep, narrow, sharp indentation on greater curvature opposite a niche on lesser curvature at / slightly below the level of the ulcer (spastic contraction of circular muscle fibers)
Prognosis: healing in 50% by 3 weeks, in 100% by 6–8 weeks; slower healing in older patients; only complete healing proves benignancy
Cx: bleeding, perforation, fistula
◊ Most common cause of gastrocolic fistula!

Malignant Gastric Ulcer

Incidence: 5% of ulcers are malignant
Cause:
1. Gastric carcinoma
2. Lymphoma (2% of all gastric neoplasms)
   √ multiple ulcers with aneurysmal appearance
3. Leiomyosarcoma, neurogenic sarcoma, fibrosarcoma, liposarcoma
4. Metastases
   (a) hematogenic: malignant melanoma, breast cancer, lung cancer
   (b) per continuum: pancreas, colon, kidney

Prognosis: partial healing may occur
Location: anywhere within stomach; fundal ulcers above level of cardia are usually malignant
√ ulcer location within gastric lumen, ie, not projecting beyond expected margin of stomach (profile view)
√ eccentrically located ulcer within the tumor
√ irregularly shaped ulcer
√ shallow ulcer with width greater than depth
√ nodular ulcer floor
√ abrupt transition between normal mucosa + abnormal tissue at some distance (usually 2–4 cm) from ulcer edge
√ rolled / rounded / shouldered edges surrounding ulcer
√ nodular irregular folds approaching ulcer with fused / clubbed / amputated tips
√ rigidity / lack of distensibility
√ associated large irregular mass
√ **Carman meniscus sign** = curvilinear lens-shaped intraluminal form of crater with convexity of crescent toward gastric wall and concavity toward gastric lumen (profile view, usually under compression) found in specific type of ulcerating carcinoma, seen only infrequently; wall aspect can also be concave / flat
√ **Kirklin meniscus complex** = Carman sign (appearance of crater) + radiolucent slightly elevated rolled border

GASTRIC VARICES

Cause: portal hypertension (varices seen in 2–78%); splenic vein obstruction (from pancreatitis, pancreatic carcinoma, pseudocyst)
Location: (a) esophagogastric junction (most common)
(b) along lesser curvature (in 11–75% of patients with portal hypertension / cirrhosis)
Feeding vessels:
1. Left gastric vein (between splenic vein + stomach)
2. Short gastric veins (between spleen + fundus)
3. Retrogastric vein (between splenic vein + esophagogastric junction)

• increased prevalence of portosystemic encephalopathy
√ barium study: 65–89% rate of detection:
  √ lobulated folds / polypoid masses in fundus
√ endoscopy: most practical method
√ splenic portography
√ hepatofugal blood flow along SMV into left gastric + splenic vein
Cx: variceal bleeding in 3–10–36%
◊ Gastric varices bleed less frequently but more severely than esophageal varices!

GASTRIC VOLVULUS

= abnormal degree of rotation of one part of stomach around another part, usually requires >180° twisting to produce complete obstruction
Etiology: (a) abnormality of suspensory ligaments (hepatic, splenic, colic, phrenic)
(b) unusually long gastrohepatic + gastrocolic mesenteries

GI

Usually associated with: diaphragmatic abnormality:
1. Paraesophageal hiatus hernia in 33%
2. Eventration

Types:
- A. ORGANOAXIAL VOLVULUS
  rotation around a line extending from cardia to pylorus
- B. MESENTEROAXIAL VOLVULUS
  rotation around an axis extending from lesser to greater curvature

- severe epigastric pain
- vigorous attempts to vomit without results
- inability to pass tube into stomach

√ massively distended stomach in LUQ extending into chest
√ incomplete / absent entrance of barium into stomach
√ barium demonstrates area of twist

Cx: intramural emphysema, perforation
DDx: gastric atony, acute gastric dilatation, pyloric obstruction

GASTRITIS

Corrosive Gastritis

Agents:
(a) acid, formaldehyde
- clinically usually silent

Location: esophagus usually unharmed, severe gastric damage, duodenum may be involved (newer potent materials cause atypical distribution)

(b) alkaline
Location: pylorus + antrum most frequently involved

A. ACUTE CHANGES (edema + mucosal sloughing)
√ marked enlargement of gastric rugae + erosions / ulceration
√ complete cessation of motor activity
√ gas in portal venous system
Cx: perforation

B. CHRONIC CHANGES
√ firm thick nonpliable wall
√ stenotic / incontinent pylorus (if involved)
√ gastric outlet obstruction (cicatrization) after 3–10 weeks

Emphysematous Gastritis

= rare but severe form of widespread phlegmonous gastritis subsequent to mucosal disruption characterized by gas in wall of stomach

Cause of mucosal disruption:
ingestion of toxic / corrosive substances (37%), alcohol abuse (22%), gastroenteritis (15%), recent abdominal surgery (15%), gastric infarction, necrotizing enterocolitis, ulcer, acute pancreatitis, adenocarcinoma of stomach, phytobezoar, leukemia, diabetes mellitus, disseminated strongyloidiasis, gastric muormycosis, after ingestion of large amounts of carbonated beverages

Histo: bacterial invasion of submucosa + subserosa
Organism: hemolytic streptococcus, Clostridium welchii, Clostridium perfringens, E. coli, S. aureus, enterobacter, Pseudomonas aeruginosa

- explosive onset of severe abdominal pain
- nausea, diarrhea, chills, fever, leukocytosis
- bloody foul-smelling emesis ± PATHOGNOMONIC vomiting of a necrotic cast of stomach (due to dissection along plane of muscularis mucosae)

CT:
√ gastric wall thickening (DDx: emphysematous gastritis)

Plain radiographs:
√ innumerable small gas bubbles silhouetting the stomach in a mottled fashion without positional change
√ thickening of rugal folds
√ ± portal venous gas

GI:
√ cobblestone appearance of mucosa on upper GI
√ intramural penetration of contrast material

Cx: cicatricial stenosis (21%), sinus tract formation
Prognosis: 60–80% mortality
Rx: broad-spectrum antibiotics + intravenous fluids; emergent surgery for acute perforation

Erosive Gastritis

= HEMORRHAGIC GASTRITIS
Incidence: 0.5–10% of GI studies
Etiology (in 50% without causative factors):
(1) Peptic disease: emotional stress, alcohol, acid, corrosives, severe burns, anti-inflammatory agents (aspirin, steroids, phenylbutazone, indomethacin)
(2) Infection: herpes simplex virus, CMV, Candida
(3) Crohn disease: aphthoid ulcers identical in appearance to varioliform erosions

Histo: epithelial defect not penetrating beyond muscularis mucosae

- 10–20% of all GI hemorrhages (usually without significant blood loss)
- vague dyspepsia, ulcerlike symptoms

Location: antrum, rarely extending into fundus; aligned on surface of gastric rugal folds

√ varioliform complete erosion (95%) = tiny fleck of barium surrounded by radiolucent halo ("target lesion") <5 mm, usually multiple
√ incomplete erosion (5%) = linear streaks / dots of barium without surrounding mound of edema / inflammation
√ nodularity / scalloping of prominent antral folds
√ contiguous duodenal disease may be present
√ limited distensibility, poor peristalsis / atony, delayed gastric emptying

Phlegmonous Gastritis

Etiology: septicemia, local abscess, postoperative stomach, complication of gastric ulcer / cancer
Organism: Streptococcus

Path: multiple gastric wall abscesses, which may communicate with lumen

• severe fulminating illness
• patient may vomit pus

Location: usually limited to stomach not extending beyond pylorus; submucosa is the most severely affected gastric layer

√ barium dissection into submucosa + serosa

GIARDIASIS

= overgrowth of commensal parasite Giardia lamblia

Organism:
Giardia lamblia (flagellated protozoan); often harmless contaminant of duodenum + jejunum in motile form (= trophozoite) attached to mucosa by suction disk, nonmotile form (= cyst) shed in feces; capable of pathogenic behavior with invasion of gut wall

Incidence: 1.5–2% of population in United States, infests 4–16% of inhabitants of tropical countries, found in 3–20% of children in parts of southern United States

Predisposed: altered immune mechanism (dysgammaglobulinemia, nodular lymphoid hyperplasia of ileum)

Histo: blunted villi (may be misdiagnosed as celiac disease especially in children), cellular infiltrate of acute + chronic inflammation in lamina propria

• abdominal pain, weight loss, failure to thrive (especially in children)
• spectrum from asymptomatic to severe debilitating diarrhea, steatorrhea (related to number of organisms)
• reduced fat absorption (simulating celiac disease)

Location: most pronounced in duodenum + jejunum

√ thickened distorted mucosal folds in duodenum + jejunum (mucosal edema) with normal ileum
√ marked spasm + irritability with rapid change in direction + configuration of folds
√ hypersecretion with blurring + indistinctness of folds
√ hyperperistalsis with rapid transit time
√ segmentation of barium (from motility disturbance + excess intraluminal fluid)
√ ± lymphoid hyperplasia (associated with immunoglobulin deficiency state)

Dx: (1) Detection of Giardia lamblia cysts in formed feces or trophozoites in diarrheal stools
(2) Trophozoites in duodenal aspirate / jejunal biopsy

DDx: Strongyloides / hookworm infection

Rx: quinacrine (Atabrine®)

GLOMUS TUMOR OF STOMACH

◊ Most common benign vascular gastric tumor

Histo: dilated irregularly shaped thin-walled vessels (= modified capillaries) covered by nests / strands / sheets of glomus cells

• asymptomatic / upper GI bleeding

Location: gastric antrum

√ single smooth submucosal mass ± ulceration
√ tiny flecks of calcification (occasionally)
√ strong enhancement in early arterial phase

GLYCOGEN ACANTHOSIS

= benign degenerative condition with accumulation of cellular glycogen within squamous epithelial lining of esophagus

Incidence: in up to 15% of endoscoped patients

Etiology: unknown

Age: middle-aged / elderly individuals

Histo: hyperplasia + hypertrophy of squamous mucosal cells secondary to increased glycogen; no malignant potential

• asymptomatic
• white oval mucosal plaques of 2–15 mm in diameter on otherwise normal appearing mucosa

Location: middle (common) / upper esophagus, in random distribution

√ multiple 1–3-mm rounded nodules / plaques

Dx: biopsy

DDx: candida esophagitis (lesions disappear under treatment in contrast to glycogen acanthosis), reflux esophagitis

GRAFT-VERSUS-HOST DISEASE

= T lymphocytes from donor bone marrow cause selected epithelial damage of recipient target organs

Bone marrow transplantation for treatment of:
leukemia, lymphoma, aplastic anemia, immunologic deficit, metabolic disorders of hematopoietic system, some metastatic disease

Incidence: 30–70% of patients with allogeneic (= donor genetically different from host) transplant

Target organs: GI tract (small bowel), skin, liver

@ Skin
• maculopapular rash on face, trunk, extremities

@ Liver
• elevation of hepatic enzymes ± liver failure

@ GI tract
• profuse secretory diarrhea
• abdominal cramping, fever, nausea, vomiting

Path: severe mucosal atrophy / destruction

√ shaggy fold thickening
√ "ribbon bowel" = small bowel fold effacement with tubular appearance (DDx: viral enteritis, ischemia, celiac disease, radiation, soybean allergy)
√ loss of haustration, spasm, edema, ulceration, granular mucosal pattern of colon (simulating ulcerative colitis)
√ small bowel "cast" = prolonged coating of abnormal bowel for hours to days
√ circular collections of contrast material on cross section + parallel tracks on longitudinal section
√ severely decreased transit time

CT:
√ abnormally enhancing thin layer of mucosa diffusely involving small + large bowel
√ fluid-filled distended poorly opacified bowel (oral contrast material not given!)
√ barium (from previous contrast enema) may become incorporated into bowel wall

GI

Cx: infection with opportunistic organisms, eg, Candida albicans, herpes virus, invasive fungal organisms, CMV, varicella-zoster virus, Epstein-Barr virus, hepatitis viruses, rotavirus, adenovirus, Coxsackie virus A and B, P. carinii, pneumococcus
Prognosis: fatal in up to 15% (due to opportunistic infections)
Rx: steroids + cyclosporine
DDx: superinfection with enteroviruses

HELICOBACTER PYLORI INFECTION

Organism: worldwide Gram-negative spiral-shaped bacillus [formerly Campylobacter pylori]
Prevalence: increasing with age; >50% of Americans >60 years of age
Path: surface epithelial damage + inflammation with mucosal infiltration by neutrophils, plasma cells, and lymphoid nodules
Location: gastric antrum > proximal half of stomach
Site: beneath mucus layer on surface epithelial cells
• asymptomatic (vast majority)
• dyspepsia, epigastric pain
√ gastritis (75% prevalence of H. pylori):
  √ thickened gastric folds
  √ polypoid gastritis mimicking malignant tumor
  √ enlarged areae gastricae
√ gastric ulcer (60–80% prevalence of H. pylori)
√ duodenal ulcer (90–100% prevalence of H. pylori)
Dx: (1) Endoscopic brushings + biopsy
(2) Breath test measuring urease activity after ingestion of carbon-14–labeled urea
(3) Serologic test for IgG antibodies
Rx: triple therapy (= bismuth + metronidazole + tetracycline / amoxicillin) results in 95% cure rate after 2 weeks of therapy

HEMANGIOMA OF SMALL BOWEL

Incidence: 7–10% of all benign small bowel tumors
Increased incidence in: Turner syndrome, tuberous sclerosis, Osler-Weber-Rendu disease
• symptomatic (80%):
  • acute intermittent severe bleeding (melena)
  • acute / chronic life-threatening anemia
  • intestinal obstruction, intussusception, perforation
Path: submucosal soft infiltrative polypoid mass
Location: jejunum (55%), ileum (42%), duodenum (2%)
√ multiple sessile compressible intraluminal filling defects
√ nodular segmental mucosal abnormality
√ ± phleboliths in intestinal wall
CT:
  √ well-circumscribed lobulated mass of mixed attenuation supplied by large artery

HENOCH-SCHÖNLEIN PURPURA

= most common systemic allergic hypersensitivity-related acute small-vessel vasculitis in children
Precipitated by: bacterial / viral infection, allergies, insect sting, drugs (eg, penicillin, sulfonamides, aspirin), certain foods
Cause: deposition of IgA-dominant immune complexes in venules, capillaries, and arterioles
Age: children (peak age of 5, range 3–10 years) + adults >20 years (in up to 30%)
• most frequent manifestations:
  • purpuric skin rash on legs + extensor surfaces on arms
  • colicky abdominal pain + GI bleeding
  • microscopic hematuria + proteinuria in 50% (from proliferative glomerulonephritis with IgA deposits demonstrated by immunofluorescence)
• often begins as an upper respiratory tract infection
• arthralgias of large joints
√ multifocal bowel wall thickening (due to intramural hemorrhage + edema)
Cx: (1) Bowel infarct / perforation / irreducible intussusception (3–5%)
(2) Renal insufficiency (10–20%), end-stage renal disease (5%)
Rx: high doses of corticosteroids + azathioprine

HERNIA

Prevalence: 10% of SBO; 2nd most common cause of small bowel obstruction!
Nomenclature: indicates anatomic site of its orifice

External Hernia

= bowel extending outside the abdominal cavity
Incidence: 95% of all hernias
Location:
@ Ventral
1. Postoperative hernia
2. Trocar site hernia
   Incidence: 1–3.6%
   √ often Richter type hernia
2. Umbilical hernia
3. Epigastric hernia
4. **Spigelian hernia**
   Frequency: 2% of anterior abdominal hernias
   = acquired ventrolateral hernia through defect in aponeurosis between transverse and rectus muscle of abdomen at junction of semilunar + arcuate lines below umbilicus
   √ hernia sac dissects laterally to rectus abdominis muscle through a fibrous groove (= semicircular / spigelian line)
   √ hernia sac lies beneath an intact external oblique aponeurosis
@ Diaphragm
1. Bochdalek hernia
2. Morgagni hernia
@ Lumbar
1. Grynfelt (upper)
2. Petit lumbar triangle (lower)
@ Pelvic floor
1. Obturator foramen
   √ hernia between pectineus + external obturator muscles

GI

2. Sciatic notch
3. Perineal hernia (rare)
   (a) anterior perineal hernia = defect of urogenital diaphragm anterior to superficial transverse perineal m. + lateral to bulbocavernosus m. + medial to ischiocavernosus m. (only in females)
   (b) posterior perineal hernia = defect in levator ani m. / between levator ani m. and coccygeus m. posterior to superficial transverse perineal m.
   √ defecating proctography

@ Groin
1. Inguinal hernia
   (a) direct inguinal hernia
      = defect in Hesselbach triangle (bounded by inguinal ligament inferiorly, inferior epigastric artery superolaterally, fused aponeuroses of internal oblique + transverse abdominal muscles medially)
      √ medial to inferior epigastric vessels
      √ hernia contains bowel, mesenteric fat, vessels
   (b) indirect inguinal hernia
      √ lateral to inferior epigastric vessels originating at deep inguinal ring
2. Femoral hernia
   √ medial to femoral vein within femoral canal
   Cx: high probability of incarceration
3. **Richter hernia** = entrapment of antimesenteric border of bowel in hernia orifice, usually seen in older women with femoral hernias
   • no palpable mass = difficult to diagnose
   √ partial obstruction with patent bowel lumen

Internal Hernia

= herniation of bowel through a developmental / surgically created defect of the peritoneum, omentum, mesentery or through an adhesive band

Incidence: 5% of all hernias, responsible for <1% of mechanical small bowel obstruction

Classification of internal hernias:

(a) retroperitoneal: usually congenital containing a hernial sac
   1. paraduodenal (ligament of Treitz)
   2. foramen of Winslow
   3. intersigmoid
   4. pericecal / ileocolic
   5. supravesical

(b) anteperitoneal:
   small group of hernias without a peritoneal sac
   1. transmesenteric (transverse / sigmoid mesocolon)
   2. transomental
   3. pelvic (including broad ligament)

• intermittent nausea, abdominal pain, distension (made worse by eating + standing and relieved by fasting + assuming a recumbent position)

√ signs of bowel obstruction (only during symptomatic period)

√ mass effect with displacement of other abdominal organs

Cx: volvulus

Paraduodenal Hernia (53%)

= congenital defect in descending mesocolon

• frequently asymptomatic

(a) LEFT through fossa of Landzert (75%)
   Location:
      to the left of 4th portion of duodenum at duodenujejunal junction (paraduodenal fossa = confluent zone of descending mesocolon + transverse mesocolon + small bowel mesentery
   √ cluster of dilated small-bowel loops between pancreas + stomach
   √ displacement of gastric wall anteriorly
   √ displacement of duodenojejunal flexure + transverse colon inferiorly
   √ engorged crowded vessels at entrance of hernia sac
   CT:
      √ encapsulated bowel loop displacing the <u>inferior mesenteric vein</u> (= landmark of the right margin of the descending mesocolon) anterolaterally

(b) RIGHT through mesentericoparietal fossa of Waldeyer (25%)
   Predisposed: nonrotation of small bowel
   Location: behind the root of small bowel mesentery caudal to SMA and inferior to 3rd portion of duodenum on right side
   CT:
      √ encapsulated bowel loop displacing the <u>right colic vein</u> (= landmark of left margin of the ascending mesocolon) anteriorly
      √ looping of small intestine behind SMA + SMV below transverse portion of duodenum
      √ SMV located ventral + to left of SMA
      √ absence of normal horizontal duodenum

Cx: partial / complete obstruction of small intestine (in 50%)

Lesser Sac Hernia (<10%)

through foramen of Winslow in retrogastric location

Invaginated gut:
   ileum > jejunum, cecum, appendix, ascending colon, Meckel diverticulum, gallbladder, greater omentum

√ gas-containing bowel loops in center of upper abdomen

√ distended small bowel loops occupying space between stomach + liver

Iatrogenic Hernia

Transmesenteric Hernia

Cause: fenestration of transverse mesocolon in construction of Roux-en-Y loop

√ cluster of small-bowel loops (70%)

GI

√ clustered small bowel outside colon compressed against abdominal wall without overlying omental fat (85%)
√ central displacement of colon (92%)
√ displacement of mesenteric trunk (85%)
√ engorged mesenteric vessels (85%)

HERNIA THROUGH BROAD LIGAMENT (very rare)
after laceration / fenestration during surgery or during pregnancy

Hiatal Hernia

Associated with: diverticulosis (25%), reflux esophagitis (25%), duodenal ulcer (20%), gallstones (18%)

Sliding Hiatal Hernia (99%)

= AXIAL HERNIA = CONCENTRIC HERNIA
= esophagogastric junction remains in chest with portion of peritoneal sac forming part of wall of hernia
Etiology: rupture of phrenicoesophageal membrane due to repetitive stretching with swallowing
Incidence: increasing with age
√ reducible in erect position
√ epiphrenic bulge = entire vestibule + sleeve of stomach are intrathoracic
√ distance between B ring (if visible) and hiatal margin >2 cm
√ peristalsis ceases above hiatus (end of peristaltic wave delineates esophagogastric junction)
√ tortuous esophagus having an eccentric junction with hernia
√ numerous coarse thick gastric folds within suprahiatal pouch (>6 longitudinal folds)
√ ± gastroesophageal reflux
CT:
√ dehiscence of diaphragmatic crura >15 mm
√ pseudomass within / above esophageal hiatus
√ increase in fat surrounding distal esophagus (= herniation of omentum through phrenicoesophageal ligament)
DDx: normal temporary cephalad motion of esophagogastric junction by 1–2 cm into chest due to contraction of longitudinal muscle during esophageal peristalsis

Paraesophageal Hernia (1%)

= ROLLING HIATAL HERNIA = PARAHIATAL HERNIA
= portion of stomach superiorly displaced into thorax with esophagogastric junction remaining in subdiaphragmatic position
√ cardia in normal position
√ herniation of portion of stomach anterior to esophagus
√ frequently nonreducible
√ may be associated with gastric ulcer of lesser curvature at level of diaphragmatic hiatus

Totally Intrathoracic Stomach

= defect in central tendon of diaphragm in combination with slight volvulus in transverse axis of stomach behind heart
√ cardia may be intrathoracic (usually) / subdiaphragmatic
√ great gastric curvature either on right / left side

Congenitally Short Esophagus

(not true hernia, very rare)
= gastric ectopy by lack of lengthening of esophagus
√ nonreducible intrathoracic gastric segment (in erect / supine position)
√ cylindrical / round intrathoracic segment with large sinuous folds
√ short straight esophagus
√ circular narrowing at gastroesophageal junction, frequently with ulcer
√ gastroesophageal reflux

Umbilical Hernia

= protrusion of abdominal contents / fat into anterior abdominal wall via umbilical ring
Prevalence: 4% of all hernias; M < F
Cause: failed closure of umbilical ring, obesity, multiple pregnancies, intraabdominal masses, liver failure, increased intraabdominal pressure, weak abdominal wall
√ may contain fat / small bowel / colon
√ herniation of antimesenteric border of intestine (Richter hernia)
√ Meckel diverticulum in hernial sac (Littre hernia)
Cx: strangulation, incarceration
DDx: paraumbilical, spigelian, epigastric, incisional hernia

HIRSCHSPRUNG DISEASE

= AGANGLIONOSIS OF THE COLON = AGANGLIONIC MEGACOLON
= absence of parasympathetic ganglia in muscle (Meissner plexus) + submucosal layers (Auerbach plexus) secondary to an arrest of craniocaudal migration of neuroblasts along vagal trunks before 12th week leading to relaxation failure of the aganglionic segment
Incidence: 1:5,000–8,000 live births; 15–20% of all neonatal bowel obstructions; usually sporadic; familial in 4%
Age: during first 6 weeks of life of a full-term infant (70–80%); M:F = 4–9:1; extremely rare in premature infants
Associated with: trisomy 21 (in 2%)
Location: at varying distances proximal to anus, usually rectosigmoid (in 80%)
(a) ultrashort segment (= internal sphincter) .. (very rare)
(b) short segment disease .... (80%)
(c) long segment disease .... (15%)
(d) total colonic aganglionosis .... (5%)
(e) skip aganglionosis = sparing of rectum .... (very rare)

GI

- failure to pass meconium within first 48 hours of life
- intermittent constipation + paradoxical diarrhea (25%)
- bilious vomiting, abdominal distention
- rectal manometry with absence of spike activity

√ generalized gaseous distention of bowel loops

BE:
- √ short patent colon usually of normal caliber
- √ inverted cone shape at transition between abnormal + normal bowel (MOST CHARACTERISTIC):
  - √ "transition zone" = aganglionic segment appearing normal in size (seen in 50% during 1st week of life)
  - √ dilatation of large + small bowel aborally from transition zone
- √ normal-appearing rectum in 33%
- √ marked retention of barium on delayed postevacuation films after 12–24 hours
- √ 10–15-cm segment of persistent corrugated / convoluted rectum (= abnormal uncoordinated contractions of the aganglionic portion of colon) in 31% (DDx: colitis, milk allergy, normal intermittent spasm of rectum)

N.B.: avoid digital exam / cleansing enema prior to radiographic studies!

OB-US:
- √ dilated small bowel / dilated colon

Cx: (1) Necrotizing enterocolitis
(2) Cecal perforation (secondary to stasis, distension, ischemia)
(3) Obstructive uropathy

Dx: suction mucosal biopsy of rectum (increased acetylcholinesterase activity)

Rx: (1) Swenson pull-through procedure
(2) Duhamel operation
(3) Soave procedure

HYPERPLASTIC POLYP OF COLON

= intestinal metaplasia consisting of mucous glands lined by a single layer of columnar epithelium; NO malignant potential

Path: infolding of epithelium into the glandular lumen

Location: rectosigmoid

√ smooth rounded sessile elevation
√ usually <5 mm in diameter

HYPERTROPHIC PYLORIC STENOSIS

= idiopathic hypertrophy and hyperplasia of circular muscle fibers of pylorus with proximal extension into gastric antrum

Incidence: 3:1,000; M:F = 4–5:1

Etiology: inherited as a dominant polygenic trait; increased incidence in firstborn boys; acquired rather than congenital condition

Infantile Form of Hypertrophic Pyloric Stenosis

Age: manifestation between 2–8 weeks of life

- nonbilious projectile vomiting (sour formula / clear gastric contents) with progression over a period of several weeks after birth (15–20%)
- positive family history
- palpable olive-shaped mass (80% sensitive in experienced hands, up to 14% false positive)
- nasogastric aspirate >10 mL (92% sensitive, 86% specific)

UGI (95% sensitivity):

Precautions: (1) empty stomach via nasogastric tube before study
(2) remove contrast at end of study

- √ elongation + narrowing of pyloric canal (2–4 cm in length):
  - √ "double / triple track sign" = crowding of mucosal folds in pyloric channel
  - √ "string sign" = passing of small barium streak through pyloric channel
  - √ Twining recess = "diamond sign" = transient triangular tentlike cleft / niche in midportion of pyloric canal with apex pointing inferiorly secondary to mucosal bulging between two separated hypertrophied muscle bundles on the greater curvature side within pyloric channel
- √ abnormal configuration of antrum:
  - √ "pyloric teat" = outpouching along lesser curvature due to disruption of antral peristalsis
  - √ "antral beaking" = mass impression upon antrum with streak of barium pointing toward pyloric channel
  - √ Kirklin sign = "mushroom sign" = indentation of base of bulb (in 50%)
- √ gastric distension with fluid
- √ active gastric hyperperistalsis:
  - √ "caterpillar sign" = gastric hyperperistaltic waves

US:
- √ "target sign" = hypoechoic ring of hypertrophied pyloric muscle around echogenic mucosa centrally on cross-section
- √ elongated pylorus with thickened muscle:
  - √ pyloric muscle wall thickness ≥3 mm
  - √ pyloric volume >1.4 cm^3 (= 1/4 π x [maximum pyloric diameter]^2 x pyloric length); most criteria independent of contracted or relaxed state (33% false negative)
  - √ pyloric length (mm) + 3.64 x muscle thickness (mm) > 25

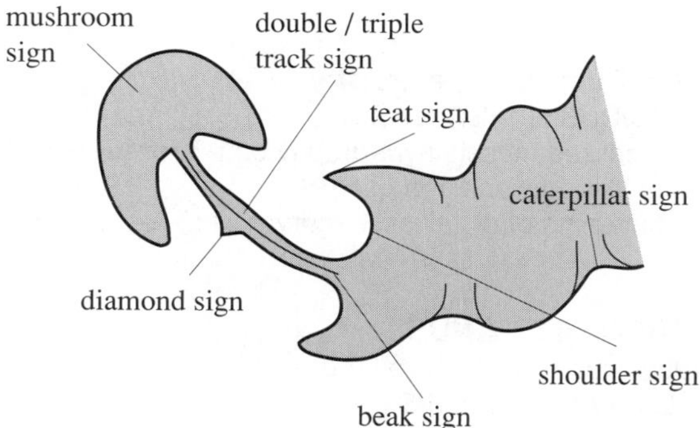

Hypertrophic Pyloric Stenosis

√ pyloric transverse diameter ≥13 mm with pyloric channel closed
√ elongated pyloric canal ≥17 mm in length
√ "cervix sign" = indentation of muscle mass on fluid-filled antrum on longitudinal section
√ "antral nipple sign" = redundant pyloric channel mucosa protruding into gastric antrum
√ exaggerated peristaltic waves
√ delayed gastric emptying of fluid into duodenum

Cx: hypochloremic metabolic alkalosis
DDx:
1. **Infantile pylorospasm**
   √ muscle thickness between 1.5 and 2 mm
   √ variable caliber of antral narrowing
   √ antral peristalsis
   √ delayed gastric emptying
   √ elongation of pylorus
   Prognosis: resolves in several days / ? early stage of evolving pyloric stenosis
   Rx: effective with metachlopromide / bentyl
2. Gastritis / milk allergy
   √ circumferential / eccentric thickening of antral mucosa >2–3 mm
3. Duodenal obstruction from midgut volvulus
   √ distended descending duodenum
   √ reversal of SMA and SMV relationship
   √ whirlpool sign = twisting of small bowel mesentery
4. Gastric diaphragm

Adult Form of Hypertrophic Pyloric Stenosis
Cause: secondary to mild infantile form
- acute obstructive symptoms uncommon
- nausea, intermittent vomiting
- postprandial distress, heartburn

Associated with:
(1) peptic ulcer disease (in 50–74%) (prolonged gastrin production secondary to stasis of food)
(2) chronic gastritis (54%)

√ persistent elongation (2–4 cm) + concentric narrowing of pyloric channel
√ parallel + preserved mucosal folds
√ antispasmodics show no effect on narrowing
√ proximal benign ulcer (74%), usually near incisura

GI

Focal Pyloric Hypertrophy
= TORUS HYPERPLASIA
= localized muscle hypertrophy on the lesser curvature
= milder atypical form of HPS
√ flattening of distal lesser curvature

IMPERFORATE ANUS
Prevalence: 1:5,000 live births

A. LOW ANOMALY (55%)
   = bowel has passed through levator sling
   - fistula to perineum / vulva

   Rx: readily reparable
B. INTERMEDIATE DEFECT (least common)
   = bowel ends within levator muscle as a result of abnormality in posterior migration of rectum
   - fistula opening low in vagina / vestibule

   Rx: 2- / 3-stage operation
C. HIGH ANOMALY
   = bowel ends above levator sling; M > F
   - fistulous connection to perineum / vagina / posterior urethra (air in bladder in males; air in vagina in females)

   Cx: associated malformations more common + more severe
   Rx: multiple surgical procedures

√ distance between rectal air and skin will not accurately outline the extent of atretic rectum and anus (varying length during crying with increase in abdominal pressure + contraction of levator ani muscle)

US:
√ ≤15 mm distance between anal dimple + distal rectal pouch on transperineal images indicates low lesion

OB-US (earliest detection by 20–29 weeks GA):
- absent / low disaccharidase level in amniotic fluid

√ dilated colon in lower pelvis with U- / S-shaped configuration ± intraluminal calcifications
√ normal amniotic fluid (unless also TE fistula)
√ absence of anal characteristics (= hypoechoic circular rim with central echogenic stripe)

INFECTIOUS COLITIS
Cause:
(1) bacterium: Shigella, Salmonella, Yersinia, Campylobacter, Staphylococcus, Chlamydia trachomatis, amebiasis, tuberculosis
(2) fungus: histoplasmosis, mucormycosis, actinomycosis
(3) virus: herpesvirus, CMV, rotavirus

Location:
- diffuse involvement = CMV, E. coli
- limited to right colon = Shigella, Salmonella
- descending + sigmoid colon = schistosomiasis
- rectosigmoid = gonorrhea, herpesvirus, C. trachomatis (lymphogranuloma venereum)

CT:
√ wall thickening + low attenuation
√ homogeneous wall enhancement
√ multiple air-fluid levels
√ inflammation of pericolic fat
√ ascites

Dx: clinical

INTESTINAL LYMPHANGIECTASIA
A. CONGENITAL LYMPHANGIECTASIA
   = PRIMARY PROTEIN-LOSING ENTEROPATHY
   = generalized congenital malformation of lymphatic system with atresia of the thoracic duct + gross dilatation of small bowel lymphatics; usually sporadic; may be inherited

   Age: presentation before 30 years
   - asymmetric generalized lymphedema (due to protein-losing enteropathy with hypoproteinemia)

- chylous pleural effusions (45%)
- diarrhea (60%), steatorrhea (20%)
- vomiting (15%)
- abdominal pain (15%) + distension
- decreased albumin + globulin
- lymphocytopenia (90%)
- decreased serum fibrinogen, transferrin, ceruloplasmin

B. ACQUIRED LYMPHANGIECTASIA

Causes leading to dilatation of intestinal lymphatics:

1. Mesenteric adenitis
2. Retroperitoneal fibrosis
3. Diffuse small bowel lymphoma
4. Pancreatitis
5. Pericardial effusion with obstruction of thoracic duct

- peripheral edema / anasarca (KEY SYMPTOM)
- chylous + serous effusion
- diarrhea, vomiting, abdominal pain, malabsorption, steatorrhea
- hypoproteinemia secondary to protein loss into intestinal lumen

Path: dilatation of lymph vessels in mucosa + submucosa + abundance of foamy fat-staining macrophages (negative for PAS)

√ diffuse symmetric marked enlargement of folds in jejunum + ileum (due to dilated intestinal lymphatics + hypoproteinemic edema)
√ slight separation + rigidity of folds
√ dilution of barium column (considerable increase in intestinal secretions from malabsorption)
√ no / mild dilatation of bowel

Lymphangiogram (not always diagnostic):
- √ hypoplasia of lower extremity lymphatics
- √ occlusion of thoracic duct / large tortuous thoracic duct
- √ obstruction of cisterna chyli with backflow into mesenteric + intestinal lymphatics
- √ hypoplastic lymph nodes

Dx: small bowel biopsy (dilated lymphatics in lamina propria + vascular core)

Rx: low-fat diet with medium-chain triglycerides (direct absorption into portal venous system)

DDx: (1) Whipple disease (more segmentation + fragmentation, wild folds)
(2) Amyloidosis (edema + secretions usually absent)
(3) Hypoalbuminemia (less pronounced symmetric thickening of folds, less prominent secretions)

INTRALUMINAL DUODENAL DIVERTICULUM

= congenital lesion secondary to elongation of an incomplete duodenal diaphragm

Age at presentation: in young adult

- easy satiety
- vomiting
- upper abdominal cramping pain

Location: 2nd–3rd portion of duodenum

√ barium-filled sac within duodenal lumen (pathognomonic picture) = "windsock, comma, teardrop" appearance
√ anchored to the lateral wall of the duodenum
√ "halo" sign = duodenal mucosa covers outer + inner wall of diverticulum

INTRAMURAL ESOPHAGEAL RUPTURE

= DISSECTING INTRAMURAL HEMATOMA
= mucosal tear with dissecting hemorrhage into submucosa and involvement of venous plexus

- hematemesis

√ intramural hematoma simulates retained solid material within lumen
√ "mucosal stripe sign" = dissected mucosa floating within lumen

INTUSSUSCEPTION

= telescope-like invagination or prolapse of a segment of intestinal tract (= intussusceptum = donor loop) into the lumen of the adjacent intestine (= intussuscipiens = receiving loop)

◊ The intussuscipiens contains the folded intussusceptum with entering limb + returning limb + their mesentery

A. IN CHILDREN (94%)

Incidence: 2–4:1,000 live births; most common abdominal emergency of early childhood

◊ Leading cause of acquired bowel obstruction in childhood!

Etiology:

(1) idiopathic (over 95%): mucosal edema + lymphoid hyperplasia following viral gastroenteritis; predominantly at ileocecal valve
(2) lead point (5%):
(a) infants <3 months: Meckel diverticulum (most common), duplication cyst
(b) children >3 years of age: Burkitt lymphoma, polyp in Peutz-Jeghers syndrome, polypoid hemangioma, enterogenous cyst, ectopic pancreas, suture granuloma, periappendicitis, Henoch-Schönlein purpura, coagulopathy, inspissated meconium

mnemonic: "H DIMPL"

Henoch-Schönlein purpura
Duplication
Idiopathic
Meckel diverticulum
Polyp
Lymphosarcoma

Age: peak incidence between 6 months and 2 years; 3–9 months (40%); <1 year (50%); <2 years (75%); >3 years (<10%); M:F = 2:1

- abrupt onset of violent crampy pain (94%)
- vomiting (91%)
- red "currant jelly" stools / hematochezia (66%) usually only after >48 hours duration
- palpable abdominal mass (59%)
- diarrhea
- restlessness, pallor, fever

Types: ileocolic (75–95%) > ileoileocolic (9%) > ileoileal (4%) > colocolic

Location: transverse colon + hepatic flexure + ascending colon (90%)

Cx: vascular compromise secondary to incorporation of mesentery (hemorrhage, infarction, acute inflammation)

B. IN ADULTS (6%)
◊ Accounts for <16% of all bowel obstructions!
Etiology:
(a) specific cause (80%):
1. Tumor: benign (1/3), malignant (1/5)
2. Postsurgical changes (1/3): adhesions adjacent to sutures / submucosal bowel edema / discoordinated motility
3. Invaginated (= inverted) Meckel diverticulum
4. Prolapsed gastric mucosa
5. Aberrant pancreas
6. Foreign body, feeding tube
7. Chronic ulcer (TB, typhoid)
8. Prior gastroenteritis
9. Gastroenterostomy, trauma

spontaneous without anatomic lead point: celiac disease, scleroderma, Whipple disease, fasting, anxiety, agonal state

(b) idiopathic (20%)

- recurrent episodes of colicky pain, nausea, vomiting
- abdominal tenderness, distention
- change in bowel habits
- palpable mass (in up to 50%)
- bloody stool (in majority)

Location: ileoileal (40%) > ileocolic (15%)
small bowel (55%): benign neoplasm (40%), malignant neoplasm (17%), nonneoplastic (43%)
colon (45%): malignant neoplasm (48%), benign neoplasm (21%), nonneoplastic (31%)

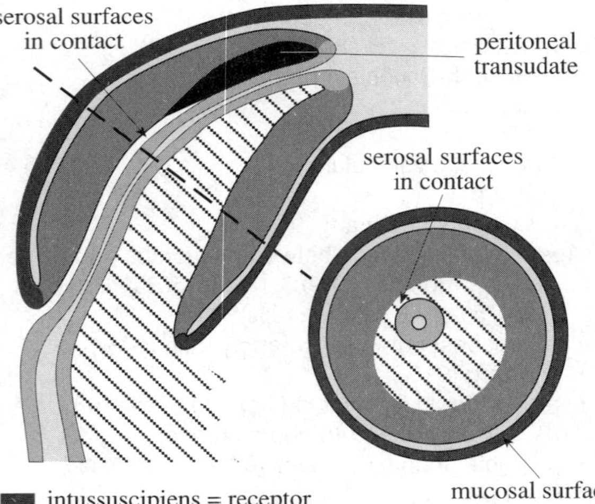

Anatomy of Intussusception

Plain film (40–90% accuracy):
√ no abnormality in 25%
√ abdominal soft-tissue mass (50–60%), usually in RUQ:
√ target sign = soft-tissue mass with concentric circular areas of lucency (due to mesenteric fat of intussusceptum)
√ meniscus sign = crescent of gas within colonic lumen that outlines the apex of the intussusceptum
√ loss of inferior hepatic margin
√ little air in small intestine / gasless abdomen
√ air in displaced appendix
√ small bowel obstruction (25%)

Antegrade barium study:
√ "coiled spring" appearance
√ beaklike abrupt narrowing of barium column demonstrating a central channel

Diagnostic Enema:
Indication: unusual age of child (<2 months, >4 years), high fever, peritoneal signs
Contraindication: free air
√ meniscus sign = convex intracolic mass = rounded apex of intussusceptum protrudes into contrast column
√ "coiled spring" sign = edematous mucosal folds of returning limb of intussusceptum outlined by contrast material within lumen of colon

US (98–100% sensitive, 88–100% specific):
√ readily detectable mass over 5.0 x 2.5 cm
√ "crescent-in-doughnut / target / bull's eye sign" (on transverse scan) = concentric rings of alternating hypoechoic + hyperechoic layers (= intussuscipiens) with central hyperechoic portion (= mesentery of intussusceptum)
√ "pseudokidney / sandwich / hay fork sign" (on longitudinal scan) = hypoechoic layers on each side of echogenic center of mesenteric fat
√ peritoneal fluid trapped inside intussusception in <15% (associated with irreducibility + ischemia)
√ echogenic mesentery contains lymph nodes + ceco-appendiceal complex close to base of intussusception
√ color Doppler demonstrates mesenteric vessels dragged between entering + returning wall of intussusceptum
◊ Absence of blood flow within the intussusceptum suggests bowel necrosis (47%)!
◊ Presence of blood flow within the intussusceptum is a good predictor of reducibility!

CT:
√ "multiple concentric rings" = 3 concentric cylinders (central cylinder = canal + wall of intussusceptum; middle cylinder = crescent of mesenteric fat; outer cylinder = returning intussusceptum + intussuscipiens)
√ proximal obstruction

HYDROSTATIC / PNEUMATIC REDUCTION
◊ <1% mortality if reduction occurs <24 hours after onset!
Overall success rate: 70–85%
Contraindications: pneumoperitoneum, peritonitis, hypovolemic shock
◊ Obtain abdominal radiograph to document absence of perforation before reduction!

Technique:
(1) Sedation (debated) with morphine sulfate (0.2 mg/kg IM) / fentanyl citrate IV (straining increases intraluminal pressure of distended colon)
(2) Anal seal with 24-F Foley catheter + balloon inflation to size equal to interpediculate distance of L5; balloon pulled down to levator sling; taped to buttocks; both buttocks firmly taped together
(3) 60% wt/vol barium sulfate with container between 24–36 inches above level of anus
(4) Maximally 3 attempts for 3 minutes each
(5) Manual manipulation increases colonic pressure
(6) Reduction should be accomplished within 10 minutes
(7) Extensive reflux into small bowel desirable to exclude residual ileoileal intussusception

"Rule of 3s":
(1) 3.5 feet (105 cm) above table (= 120 mm Hg)
(2) 3 attempts
(3) 3 minutes between attempts (delay allows venous congestion + edema to subside)

Alternative medium:
(1) 1:4 Gastrografin®-water solution raised to a height of 5 feet (150 cm)
(2) air: delivers higher intracolonic pressures, faster, less fluoroscopic time, smaller tears, less contamination of peritoneal cavity
(3) Ultrasound-guided saline enema: no limit to procedure time, low perforation rate

Cx: perforation (0.4–3%; colonic bursting pressure ~200 mm Hg); reduction of nonviable bowel; incomplete reduction; missed lead point
Prognosis: 3.5–10% rate of recurrence

ISCHEMIC COLITIS

= nonocclusive ischemic disease (major mesenteric vessels usually patent) characterized by acute onset + rapid clinical and radiographic evolutionary changes

Etiology: decrease in blood flow to 20% of normal flow associated with small vessel disease (hypoxia) + reperfusion injury when blood flow is reestablished; injury more severe if terminal vascular branches obstructed rather than proximal mesenteric arcades

Path: (a) mucosal congestion, patchy necrosis, ulcerations + submucosal edema and hemorrhage (mucosa + submucosa most sensitive to ischemia)
◊ Early mucosal injury is reversible
(b) injury of muscularis propria (after severe + prolonged ischemia) can lead to transmural necrosis
◊ Fibrotic stricture, perforation, severe sepsis

Precipitating factors:
(a) bowel obstruction: volvulus, carcinoma (proximal dilatation with increased intraluminal pressure and reduced blood flow)
(b) thrombosis: cardiovascular disease, myocardial infarction, digitalis treatment, arrhythmia, oral contraceptives, hypotensive episode, collagen vascular disease, sickle cell disease, hemolytic-uremic syndrome
(c) trauma: aortoiliac reconstruction (2%) with ligation of IMA, cardiac surgery
(d) idiopathic / spontaneous: mainly in elderly

mnemonic: "VINTS"
Vasculitis
Incarceration (hernia, volvulus)
Nonocclusive ischemia (shock, CHF)
Thrombosis (atherosclerosis, emboli, polycythemia vera, hyperviscosity)
Spontaneous

Age: usually >50 years; M = F
• abrupt onset of lower abdominal pain + rectal bleeding
• abdominal tenderness, diarrhea
• lack of sepsis
• negative stool cultures

Location: segmental involvement of any part of colon; entire colon (11%); right colon (30%); transverse colon (9%); left colon (46–90%); sigmoid colon (4%); rectum spared;
most commonly affected segments:
(a) **Griffith point** (80%) = junction between distribution of superior + inferior mesenteric arteries at the splenic flexure
(b) **point of Sudeck** = anastomotic plexus between inferior mesenteric artery + hypogastric vascular supply at rectosigmoid junction

Mean length of segmental involvement: 19 cm

Plain film (usually normal):
√ segmental thumbprinting = marginal indentations on mesenteric side (rare finding on plain film)

BE (in 90% abnormal):
◊ Single contrast may efface thumbprinting, but double contrast overall is more sensitive!
√ thumbprinting (75%) due to submucosal hemorrhage + edema
√ transverse ridging = markedly enlarged mucosal folds (spasm), some wall pliability is preserved
√ serrated mucosa = inflammatory edema + superficial longitudinal / circumferential ulceration
√ deep penetrating ulcers (late)

CT (detection rate of 26–39%):
√ symmetric / lobulated segmental thickening of colonic wall between 2 and 20 (mean 8) mm:
√ shaggy configuration + alternate layers of high and low attenuation (double halo sign) + marked pericolic streakiness of edema (wet appearance in 61%)
√ sharply defined homogeneously enhancing wall + mild mural thickening (dry appearance in 33%)
√ loss of haustral markings
√ irregular narrowed atonic lumen (= thumbprinting)
√ curvilinear collection of intramural gas (6%) suggests bowel infarction
√ portal + mesenteric venous air
√ blood clot in SMA / SMV

GI

US:
- √ absence / barely visible color flow
- √ absence of arterial signals
- √ nonstratified (= indistinct layers) thickened bowel wall >3 mm

Angio (findings similar to inflammatory disease):
- √ normal / slightly attenuated arterial supply
- √ mild acceleration of arteriovenous transit time
- √ small tortuous ectatic draining veins

Prognosis:
(1) Transient ischemia = complete resolution within 1–3 months (76%)
(2) Stricturing ischemia = incomplete delayed healing
  √ narrowed foldless segment of several cm in length with smooth tapering margins
(3) Gangrene with necrosis + perforation (extremely uncommon)
(4) Mortality rate of 11–36%

DDx: (a) dry appearance: ulcerative / granulomatous colitis
(b) wet appearance: pseudomembranous colitis, CMV colitis

JEJUNAL ATRESIA

◊ Air may be injected through nasogastric tube
◊ BE to exclude 2nd and 3rd areas of atresia

Cause: intrauterine ischemic injury to developing gut
Age: majority presenting during 1st day of life
In 25% associated with: malrotation, volvulus, gastroschisis, omphalocele

- bilious vomiting, abdominal distension, failure to pass meconium

Plain film:
N.B.: difficult to tell colon from small bowel in neonate
- √ 2–3 dilated bowel loops
- √ absence of gas in lower portion of abdomen

BE:
Purpose: to exclude large-bowel causes of obstruction, show anatomical size of colon, demonstrate meconium ileus
- √ microcolon / small colon / colon of normal caliber (due to sufficient intestinal secretions in remaining small bowel)

Cx: meconium peritonitis (5%)

JEJUNOILEAL DIVERTICULAR DISEASE

= JEJUNAL DIVERTICULOSIS
= rarest form of gastrointestinal diverticular disease

Cause: disordered contractions of smooth muscle results in increased intraluminal pressure and mucosal herniation (= pulsion diverticula = false diverticula)
Incidence: 0.5–1.1–2.3% on UGI; 0.3–4.5% of autopsy series; M > F
Age: 6th–7th decades
Location: 80% in jejunum, 15% in ileum (usually solitary), 5% in jejunum + ileum
Site: on mesenteric border near entrance of vasa recti

- intermittent upper abdominal pain, flatulence, episodes of diarrhea (30%)

Size: a few milimeters to >10 cm
Plain film:
- √ air-fluid levels in multiple diverticula
- √ slight dilatation of intestinal loops in area of diverticula

BE:
- √ may not fill (narrow neck / stagnant secretions)
- √ trapped barium on delayed film after 24 hours

Cx:
(1) Blind loop syndrome with bacterial overgrowth
  - steatorrhea, diarrhea, malabsorption, weight loss
  - megaloblastic anemia (overgrowth of coliform bacteria leads to deconjugation of bile acids + intraluminal metabolism of vitamin B12)
(2) Free perforation = leading cause of pneumoperitoneum without peritonitis (21–40% mortality)
(3) Hemorrhage (few cases)
(4) Diverticulitis
(5) Intestinal obstruction (enterolith ileus)

JUVENILE POLYPOSIS

= rare autosomal dominant disease with variable penetrance characterized by development of multiple (>5) juvenile polyps in GI tract
◊ Most common familial / nonfamilial colonic polyp in children (75%)!

Categories:
A. Juvenile polyposis of infancy
  Age: 4–6 years (range 1–10 years); M:F = 3:2
  - protein-losing enteropathy, diarrhea, hemorrhage
  - rectal prolapse
  - √ intussusception
B. Colonic & generalized juvenile polyposis
  Age: in 85% manifested by 20 years of age
  - prolapse of polyp / rectum
  - rectal bleeding, anemia

Path: hamartomatous polyps; adenomas may coexist
Histo: little / no smooth muscle; hyperplasia of mucous glands; retention cysts develop with obstruction of gland orifices (multiple mucin-filled spaces); edematous inflamed expanded lamina propria
DDx: familial adenomatous polyposis, Peutz-Jeghers syndrome

- rectal bleeding (95%) most commonly as intermittent bright red hematochezia
- anemia, pain
- diarrhea, constipation
- abdominal pain (from intussusception)
- rectal prolapse (rare)

Location: rectosigmoid (80%); rare in small bowel + stomach; not in esophagus
- √ solitary polyp (75%); multiple polyps (1/3) of smooth round contour
- √ lesion of pinpoint size / up to several cm in diameter
- √ invariably on stalk of variable length

Dx: (1) Any number of polyps with family history
(2) Polyps throughout the GI tract
(3) >5–10 polyps in colon

Cx: colorectal cancer by 35 years of age (in 15%)
DDx: solitary juvenile polyps (<5 polyps, 1% prevalence in children)

GI

KAPOSI SARCOMA

= multicentric malignant neoplasm originating from endothelial cells of lymphatic / blood vessels

Cause: HIV regulatory protein (trans-activator target [TAT]) important for viral replication is thought to cause proliferation of Kaposi sarcoma cells

Incidence: most common AIDS-related neoplasm (10–20–34%); in 51% of homosexual / bisexual men with AIDS; rare in hemophiliacs; M:F = 50:1

Histo: proliferation of spindle cells with numerous extravasated RBCs located in clefts between stromal cells

Types:

1. Classic Kaposi sarcoma
   affecting men of Mediterranean origin in 7th decade
2. Central African Kaposi sarcoma
3. AIDS-related Kaposi sarcoma

@ Skin (most frequent site)
- multiple bluish red slightly elevated skin lesions

@ Lymph nodes (2nd most frequent site):
√ abdominal + pelvic lymphadenopathy with high contrast-enhancement (secondary to vascularity)
Associated with high frequency of GI tract involvement

@ GI tract (40–50%, 3rd most frequent site):
- usually clinically silent
- concurrent with / after cutaneous disease

◊ GI tract is the only site of involvement in <5%!
Location: anywhere within GI tract; often multifocal
√ thickened nodular folds
√ multiple submucosal nodules ± central umbilication
√ polypoidal mass
√ infiltrating linitis plastica lesion (rare)

@ Liver (34% at autopsy)
infrequently contributes to morbidity + mortality
√ multiple 5–12-mm nodules hyperechoic on US, hypoattenuating on NECT/CECT indistinguishable from multiple hemangiomas
DDx: metastatic disease, fungal microabscesses, multiple areas of bacillary angiomatosis (= swollen venous lakes in liver)

@ Lung (18–47% of patients with cutaneous sarcoma):
= late complication of AIDS
Site: peribronchial + perivascular axial interstitium (91%); middle / lower lung zones (92%)
√ coarsening of bronchovascular bundles:
  √ tram track opacities
  √ peribronchial cuffing
  √ septal lines (38–71%)
√ central perihilar coalescent consolidation ± air bronchograms in 45% (= confluent tumor)
√ small (50%) / large (28%) pulmonary nodules (= tumor proliferation extending into parenchyma)
√ pleural effusion (33–67%), chylothorax (rare)
√ moderate lymphadenopathy (16%)

@ Lower extremities
√ lytic cortical lesion
√ subcutaneous nodules

Dx: visualization + biopsy of mass with red-purple color

LADD BANDS

= congenital peritoneal bands extending from cecum / hepatic flexure over anterior surface of 2nd / 3rd portion of duodenum causing duodenal obstruction at its 2nd portion (even without volvulus)

Associated with: malrotation

√ oblique termination of duodenal contrast column

LEIOMYOMA

Location: 2/3 occur in stomach

Path: arising from muscularis propria / submucosa / muscularis mucosae / smooth muscle of blood vessels within wall of viscus

Histo: intersecting bands of muscle + fibrous tissue in a well-defined capsule

√ difficult to differentiate from leiomyosarcoma

DDx: fibroma, neurofibroma, hemangioma

Esophageal Leiomyomatosis

Age: 6–18 (mean of 11) years; M > F

Cause: (1) sporadic (50%)
(2) familial disease (20%): leiomyomas of uterus, vulva, tracheobronchial tree, small bowel, rectum
(3) Alport syndrome (30%) = nephritis, high-frequency sensorineural hearing loss, congenital cataract

Site: distal third / half of esophagus ± extension into proximal stomach
- slowly progressive dysphagia over years

√ smooth tapered narrowing of distal esophagus over an average length of 6 cm
√ decreased / absent esophageal peristalsis
√ smooth relatively symmetric defect at cardia (from thickened muscle bulging into gastric fundus)

CT:
√ marked circumferential wall thickening of up to 4 cm from mass with relatively low soft-tissue attenuation

DDx: (1) Primary achalasia (shorter narrowed segment)
(2) Secondary achalasia (older individual, recent onset of dysphagia)
(3) Stricture from reflux esophagitis
(4) Idiopathic muscular hypertrophy of the esophagus (in late adulthood, corkscrew appearance of esophagus with nonperistaltic contractions, cardia rarely involved)

Leiomyoma of Esophagus

◊ Most common benign submucosal tumor of esophagus

Incidence: 1:1,119 (autopsy study); 50% of all benign esophageal tumors

Age: young adults; 3% in children; M > F
- usually asymptomatic (due to slow growth)
- dysphagia, odynophagia, dyspepsia
- hematemesis if large (rare)

Site: frequently lower + mid 1/3 of esophagus; intramural; multiple leiomyomas in 3–4%

√ 2–15-cm large smooth well-defined intramural mass causing eccentric thickening of wall + deformity of lumen

√ may have coarse calcifications:
◊ Leiomyoma is the only calcifying esophageal tumor!
√ ulceration extremely uncommon
CT:
√ uniform soft-tissue density
√ diffuse contrast enhancement
CAVE: high percentage misdiagnosed as extrinsic lesion!

Leiomyoma of Small Bowel

Most common benign tumor of small bowel
Location: duodenum (21%), jejunum (48%), ileum (31%); single in 97%
Site: mainly serosal (50%), mainly intraluminal (20%), intramural (10%)
Size: <5 cm (50%), 5–10 cm (25%), >10 cm (25%)
√ small ulcer + large barium-filled cavity (central necrosis + communication with lumen)
√ hypervascular

Leiomyoma of Stomach

◊ 2nd most common benign gastric tumor (after gastric polyp), most common of calcified benign tumors
Location: pars media (39%), antrum (26%), pylorus (12%), fundus (12%), cardia (10%)
Site: intraluminal submucosal (60%), exophytic subserosal (35%), combined intramural-extramural dumbbell type mass (5%)
◊ 90% of all submucosal tumors!
√ average size of 4.5 cm
√ ovoid mass with smooth margin + smooth surface (most frequently)
√ forms right angle with gastric wall
√ ulcerated in 50%
√ pedunculated intraluminal tumor in submucosal growth (rare)
√ "iceberg phenomenon" = large extraluminal component in subserosal growth
√ calcifies in 4%
Cx: (1) Hemorrhage (acute / chronic)
(2) Obstruction (tumor bulk / intussusception)
(3) Infection
(4) Fistulization / perforation
(5) Malignant degeneration (benign:malignant = 3:1)

GI

LEIOMYOSARCOMA

Leiomyosarcoma of Small Bowel

Location: duodenum (26%), jejunum (34%), ileum (40%)
√ usually >6 cm in size
√ nodular mass: intraluminal (10%), intraluminal pedunculated (5%), intramural (15%), chiefly extrinsic (66%)
√ mucosa may be stretched + ulcerated (50%)
√ may show central ulcer pit / fistula communicating with a large necrotic center
√ intussusception

Leiomyosarcoma of Stomach

Incidence: 0.1–3% of all gastric malignancies
Age: 10–73 years; M > F
Histo: pleomorphism, hypercellularity, mitotic figures, cystic degeneration, necrosis
• GI bleeding (from ulceration)
• obstruction
Metastases:
(a) hematogenous to liver, lung, peritoneum; rarely to bone + soft tissue
(b) direct extension into omentum, retroperitoneum
(c) lymph nodes (rare)
Location: 90% in fundus / body of stomach
Site: anterior / posterior wall; endo- / exogastric
√ average size of 12 cm
√ intramural mass
√ may be pedunculated
√ large masses tend to be exogastric
√ very frequently ulcerated
CT:
√ lobulated irregular outline
√ heterogenous exogastric mass with central zones of low density (necrosis with liquefaction)
√ air / positive contrast within tumor (= ulceration)
√ dystrophic calcifications

Carney Syndrome

Triad of (1) Gastric epithelioid leiomyosarcoma
(2) Functioning extraadrenal paraganglioma
(3) Pulmonary chondromas
Incidence: 24 patients reported; M:F = 1:11

LIPOMA

= benign submucosal tumor composed of mature adipose tissue
◊ Most common submucosal tumor in colon
Incidence: in colon in 0.25% (autopsy); 2–3% of benign gastric tumors
Location: colon (particularly cecum + ascending colon) > duodenum > ileum > stomach (gastric antrum) > jejunum > esophagus
• asymptomatic
• crampy pain, hemorrhage (rare)
√ smooth, sharply outlined, round / ovoid globular mass of 1–3 cm in diameter
√ short thick pedicle in 1/3 caused by repeated peristaltic activity (prone to intussuscept)
√ marked radiolucency
√ change in shape + size on compression due to softness:
√ "squeeze sign" = sausage-shaped mass on postevacuation radiographs
CT:
√ well-circumscribed submucosal mass of uniform fat density
Cx: (1) Intussusception (rare)
(2) Ulceration (from pressure necrosis of overlying mucosa by large lipoma; rare)
Prognosis: NO liposarcomatous degeneration

LYMPHANGIOMA

= congenital malformation of lymphatic vessels

Path: usually multiloculated large thin-walled cystic mass with chylous / serous / hemorrhagic fluid contents

Location: mesentery; rarely affecting GI tract

√ proximal bowel dilatation (in partial bowel obstruction)

US:
- √ multiseptated cystic mass with lobules
- √ fluid anechoic / with internal echoes / sedimentation

CT:
- √ cystic mass with contents of water- to fat-density

MR:
- √ serous contents: hypointense on T1WI + hyperintense on T2WI
- √ hemorrhage / fat: hyperintense on T1WI + T2WI

Rx: surgery (difficult due to intimate attachment to bowel wall)

LYMPHOGRANULOMA VENEREUM

= LGV = sexually transmitted disease caused by virus Chlamydia trachomatis producing a nonspecific granulomatous inflammatory response in infected mucosa (mononuclear cells + macrophages), perirectal lymphatic invasion

Location: rectum, may extend to sigmoid + descending colon

M:F = 3.4:1

√ narrowing + shortening + straightening of rectosigmoid
√ widening of retrorectal space
√ irregularity of mucosa + ulcerations
√ paracolic abscess
√ fistula to pericolic area, rectum, vagina (common)

Rx: tetracyclines effective in acute phase before scarring has occurred

LYMPHOID HYPERPLASIA

Incidence: normal variant in 13% of BE examinations

Histo: hyperplastic lymph follicles in lamina propria (Peyer patches), probably compensatory attempt for immunoglobulin deficiency

Etiology:
- (1) Normal in child / young adult
- (2) Self-limiting local / systemic inflammation / infection / allergy
- (3) May be related to immunodeficiency / dysgammaglobulinemia with small bowel involvement

Age: (a) generally in children <2 years
(b) in adults invariably associated with late onset immunoglobulin deficiency (IgA, IgM)

Associated with: splenomegaly, large tonsils, eczematous dermatitis, achlorhydria, pernicious anemia, acute pancreatitis, colonic carcinoma

At risk for:
- (1) **Good syndrome** (10%)
  = gastric carcinoma + benign thymoma + lymphoid hyperplasia
- (2) Respiratory infections
- (3) Giardia lamblia infection (90%)
- (4) Functional thyroid abnormalities

Location: primarily jejunum, may involve entire small bowel, ascending colon + hepatic flexure, seldom in sigmoid / rectum

- • malabsorption (diarrhea + steatorrhea)
- • low serum concentrations of IgA, IgG, IgM

√ mucosa studded with innumerable 1–3-mm small uniform polypoid lesions
√ lesions may be umbilicated (uncommon)

LYMPHOMA OF GASTROINTESTINAL TRACT

Classification:

A. PRIMARY LYMPHOMA OF BOWEL
(a) localized (b) diffuse
Predisposed: Arabs + Middle Eastern Jews
Associated with: celiac disease

B. SECONDARY INTESTINAL LYMPHOMA
as part of generalized systemic process

Incidence: 4–20% of all NHL; 10% of patients with abdominal lymphoma have bowel involvement

At risk: long-standing celiac disease, AIDS, systemic lupus erythematosus, Crohn disease, history of chemotherapy

Median age: 60 years

Histo:
- (1) T-cell malignant lymphoma (in celiac disease)
- (2) B-cell lymphoma
- (3) Immunoproliferative small intestinal disease (= Mediterranean lymphoma)
- (4) Low-grade B-cell lymphoma (= low-grade mucosa-associated lymphoid tissue = MALT lymphoma) 50–72% of all primary gastric lymphomas;
  Associated with: Helicobacter pylori gastritis in 90% (may regress completely after antibiotic therapy)
- (5) Follicular lymphoma
- (6) Burkitt lymphoma (in children)
- (7) Mantle cell lymphoma
- (8) Hodgkin disease (<15%)

May be associated with: enlargement of extraabdominal lymph nodes, malabsorption

Radiographic types:
1. Polypoid / nodular (47%)
   √ enlarged nodular folds
2. Ulcerative (42%)
   √ ulcerative lesions, may be complicated by perforation
   √ aneurysmal configuration
3. Diffusely infiltrating (11%)
   √ diffuse hoselike thickening of bowel wall
   √ decreased / absent peristalsis

CT staging:

Stage I	tumor confined to bowel wall
Stage II	limited to local nodes
Stage III	widespread nodal disease
Stage IV	disseminated to bone marrow, liver, other organs

GI

Location: 10–25% of NHL are extranodal; stomach (50%) > small bowel > colon > esophagus; multicentric in 10–50%

√ enlargement of spleen
√ bulky enlargement of regional lymph nodes

@ Esophagus
least common site of GI involvement (in <1%)

@ Stomach
1–5% of all gastric malignancies; most common site of extranodal lymphoma (25%); most frequent site of involvement by NHL (50%); isolated primary gastric malignancy in 10%
Location: no predilection for any particular region of stomach
Site: arises in lymphoid tissue of lamina propria that forms secondary to chronic Helicobacter pylori gastritis (normally gastric mucosa has no lymphoid tissue!)
Direct extension into: pancreas, spleen, transverse colon, liver
√ pliant gastric wall
√ duodenum often affected when antrum involved
√ circumscribed mass with endogastric / exogastric (25%) growth
√ broad tortuous mucosal folds over large portions of stomach (diffuse form):
  √ polypoid / nodular
√ large irregular ulcer
√ rarely luminal narrowing
CT:
  √ diffuse involvement of entire stomach (50%), typically more than half of gastric circumference
  √ segmental involvement (15%)
  √ ulcerated mass (8%)
  √ average wall thickness of 4–5 cm
  √ luminal irregularity (66%)
  √ hyperrugosity (58%)
Prognosis: 55% 5-year survival rate after resection
DDx: gastric adenocarcinoma (wall thickening less pronounced, perigastric fat plane not likely preserved, luminal narrowing, rigid wall, smaller lymph nodes above the level of renal veins)

@ Small bowel
1/5 of all small bowel malignancies; most common malignant small bowel tumor; multiple sites of involvement in 1/5; most common cause of intussusception in children >6 years
Location: ileum (51%), jejunum (47%), duodenum (2%),
Site: arising from lymphoid patches of Peyer
Types:
1. Infiltrating lymphoma with plaquelike involvement of wall >5 cm in length (80%) / >10 cm in length (20%) (DDx: Crohn disease)
   √ ± ulceration (considerable excavation)
   √ desmoplastic response
   √ thickened valvulae with corrugated appearance
   √ aneurysmal dilatation (secondary to destruction of autonomic nerve plexus + muscle / tumor necrosis)
2. Single / multiple polypoid mucosal / submucosal masses
   √ cobblestone defects due to lymphomatous polyps
   √ nodules may ulcerate
   √ may cause intussusception
   √ sprue pattern
3. Endoexoenteric mass
   √ large mass with only small intramural component
   √ ± ulcer + fistulas + aneurysmatic dilatation
4. Mesenteric / retroperitoneal adenopathy
   √ single / multiple extraluminal masses displacing bowel
   √ ill-defined confluent mass engulfing + encasing multiple loops of adjacent bowel
   √ "sandwich configuration" = mass surrounding mesenteric vessels that are separated by perivascular fat
   √ conglomerate mantle of retroperitoneal + mesenteric mass

@ Colon
Less commonly involved than stomach / small bowel; 1.5% of all abdominal lymphomas
Location: cecum most commonly involved (85%)
√ single mass > diffuse infiltration > polypoid lesion
√ paradoxical dilatation
√ gross mural circumferential / focal soft-tissue thickening (average size of 5 cm)
√ slight enhancement
√ massive regional + distant mesenteric + retroperitoneal adenopathy
DDx: frequently resembles inflammatory disease / polyposis

Prognosis: (a) 71–82% 2-year survival rate in isolated bowel lymphoma
(b) 0% 2-year survival rate in stage IV disease with bowel involvement

Cx during chemotherapy: perforation (9–40%), hemorrhage

MALIGNANT MELANOMA

= develops from melanocytes derived from neural crest cells, arising in preexisting benign nevi (in 20%)
Incidence: 1% of all cancers; increasing at 3.9% per year
Peak prevalence: 40–60 years of age
Risk factors: dysplastic mole, atypical melanocytic hyperplasia, xeroderma pigmentosum, melanoma in first-degree relative, sun-sensitive phenotype, excessive sun exposure
Primary sites: skin, mucous membranes, leptomeninges, eye

- areas of red / white / blue in addition to brown and black colors of benign nevi
- irregular borders with notching + striking protrusions

@ Skin primary
Clark staging:
Level I all tumor cells above basement membrane (in situ lesion)
Level II tumor extends to papillary dermis
Level III tumor extends to interface between papillary + reticular dermis
Level IV tumor extends between bundles of collagen of reticular dermis
Level V tumor invasion of subcutaneous tissue (in 87% metastatic)
Breslow staging:
thin <0.75 mm depth of invasion
intermediate 0.76–3.99 mm depth of invasion
thick >4 mm depth of invasion
METASTASES:
latent period of 2–20 years after initial diagnosis (most commonly 2–5 years)
Primary site: head + neck (79%), eye (77%), GU system (67%), GI tract (in up to 60%)
@ Lymphadenopathy
— in 23% with level II + IV
— in 75% with level V
• sentinel node biopsy:
√ intraoperative intradermal injection of dye
√ preoperative lymphoscintigraphy
@ Bone (7–17%)
Prevalence: 30–40% at autopsy
• often initial manifestation of recurrence
• poor prognosis
√ predominantly osteolytic
Location: axial skeleton (80%), ribs (38%)
@ Lung (70% at autopsy)
most common site of relapse;
respiratory failure most common cause of death
@ Liver (17–23%; 58–66% at autopsy)
√ single / multiple lesions 0.5–15 cm in size
√ larger lesion often necrotic
√ may be partially calcified
@ Spleen (1–5%; 33% at autopsy)
√ single / multiple lesions of variable size
√ solid / cystic
@ GI tract + mesentery (4–8%)
• abdominal pain, GI bleeding
Location: small intestine (35–50%), colon (14–20%), stomach (7–20%)
√ multiple submucosal nodules ± "bull's-eye / target" appearance = central ulceration
√ irregular amorphous cavity (exoenteric growth)
√ intussusception (10–20%)
@ Kidney (up to 35% at autopsy)
@ Adrenal (11%, up to 50% at autopsy)
@ Subcutis

MR of melanotic melanoma:
√ hypo- / isointense on T1WI + T2WI + STIR images (most commonly)
√ hyperintense on T1WI + hypointense on T2WI (due to T1-shortening effect of the paramagnetic metals iron + copper bound to melanin)
DDx: melanotic / amelanotic hemorrhagic tumor (hyperintense on T1WI + iso- / hyperintense on T2WI)
Prognosis: 30–40% eventually die from this tumor

MALLORY-WEISS SYNDROME

= mucosal + submucosal tear with involvement of venous plexus
Pathophysiology: violent projection of gastric contents against lower esophagus
Age: 30–60 years; M > F
Predisposed: alcoholics
• history of repeated vomiting prior to hematemesis
• massive painless hematemesis
Location: at / above / below (76%) esophagogastric junction
√ longitudinal single tear in 77%, in 23% multiple tears
√ extravasation of barium
Angio:
√ bleeding site at gastric cardia
DDx: peptic ulcer / ulcerative gastritis

MALROTATION

= abnormal position of gut secondary to a narrow mesenteric attachment as a result of arrest in the embryologic development of gut rotation + fixation
Embryology:
duodenojejunal + ileocolic segments of primitive digestive tube rotate by 270° in a counterclockwise direction about the omphalomesenteric vessels to cross beneath the vessels (future SMA + SMV); normally LUQ fixation at ligament of Treitz (an extension of the right crus of diaphragm) + fibrous tissue around celiac artery, located to left of L2) + RLQ fixation of cecum
Abnormal fixation of mesentery: shorter than usual, its upper point below the normal position of ligament of Treitz, its lower point superior + medial to normal cecal position

Definition:
Nonrotation
= midgut loop returns to peritoneal cavity without rotation resulting in weak peritoneal fixation
Frequency: common
• generally asymptomatic: often incidental finding in older children + adults
√ SMA to right of SMV
√ large intestine on left + small intestine on right
Cx: volvulus (as a result of local clockwise rotation) with "whirl sign" around SMA

Incomplete rotation
= failure of midgut loop to complete final 90° of rotation
• prearterial segment of midgut reenters abdomen first toward left side
√ cecum just inferior to pylorus
Cx: duodenal obstruction (peritoneal bands pass over duodenum)

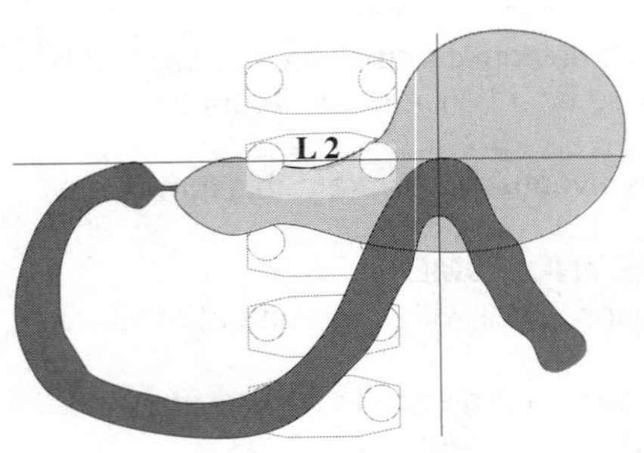

Normal Duodenal Position

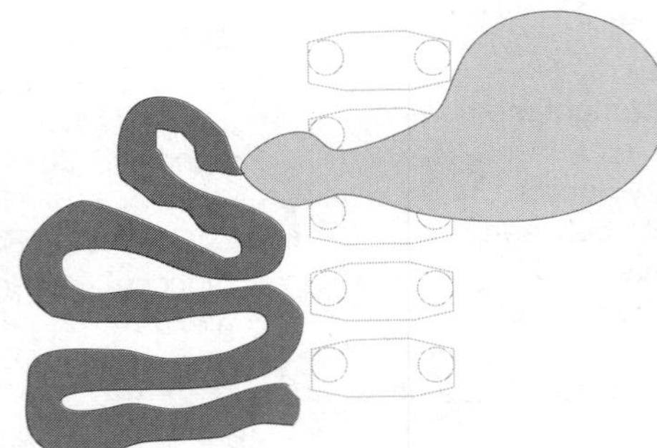
Nonrotation of Duodenum

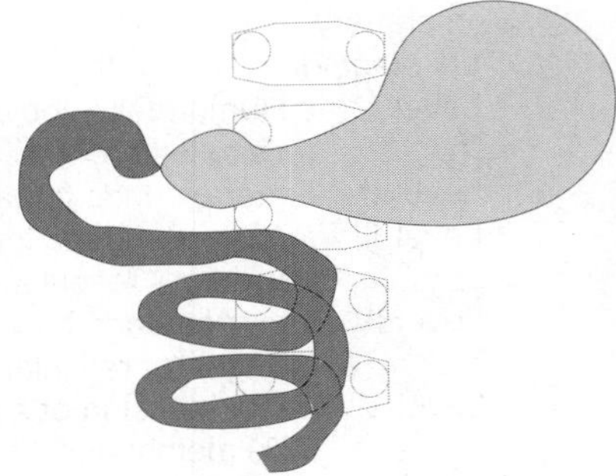
Corkscrew Duodenum + Jejunum

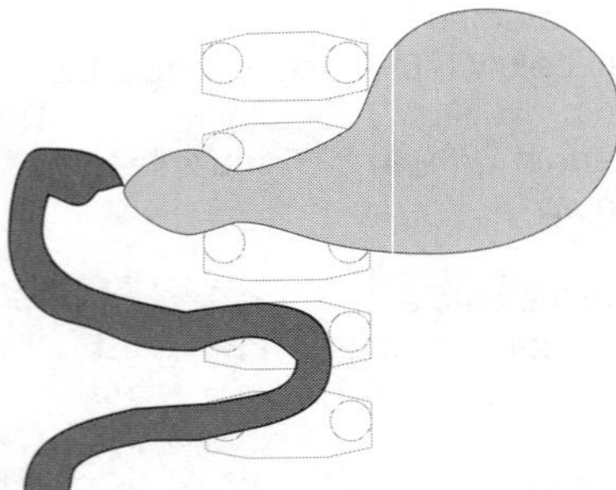
Partial Duodenal Rotation with Jejunum in Right Upper Quadrant

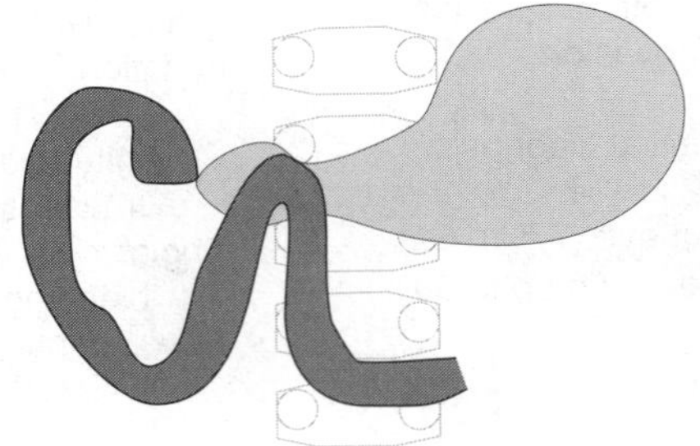
Partial Duodenal Rotation with Duodenojejunal Junction over Right Pedicle

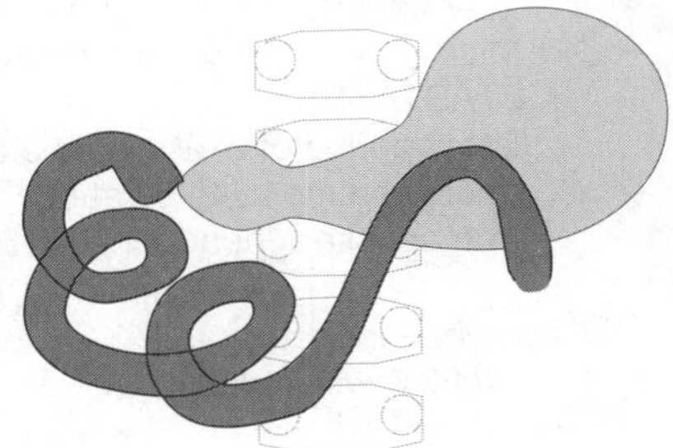
Redundant-Duodenum Malrotation to Right of Spine

Malrotation

Reversed rotation

Frequency: rare

- postarterial segment of midgut reenters abdomen first

= cecum migrates first passing behind SMA toward right thus unwinding the normal counterclockwise rotation of the first stage with additional final 90° clockwise rotation

√ duodenum anterior to SMA

√ transverse colon behind duodenum + SMA

Cx: obstruction of transverse colon by pressure from SMA

Associated with: urinary pseudoobstruction, prune-belly syndrome, cloacal exstrophy

- symptoms of partial / complete proximal bowel obstruction:
  - vomiting (77% of neonates; in 39% within 1st week of life)
  - recurrent attacks of vomiting + distension (in older children)

Barium meal & barium enema:

Purpose: guess the location of abnormal peritoneal fixation from position of bowel!

√ clearly abnormal position of duodenum (81%):
  √ duodenum + jejunum to the right of spine (30%)
  √ corkscrew duodenum + jejunum (29%)
  √ duodenojejunal junction low + in midline (22%)
√ unusual abnormal position of duodenum (16%):
  √ duodenojejunal junction over right pedicle
  √ duodenojejunal junction to left of spine but low
  √ duodenal redundancy to right of spine
  √ Z-shape configuration of duodenum + jejunum
√ small bowel on right + colon on left side of abdomen (in 0.2% incidental finding in adults)
√ abnormal position of duodenum + cecum (84%)
√ normal position of duodenum (3%)
√ normal position of cecum (in 5–20%)

DDx: mobile cecum (15%)

CT:

√ SMV positioned to left of SMA (80%)
√ aplastic / hypoplastic uncinate process of pancreas

Cx: midintestinal / midgut volvulus, duodenal obstruction, Ladd bands, internal herniation

MASTOCYTOSIS

= URTICARIA PIGMENTOSA

= systemic disease with mast cell proliferation in skin and RES (lamina propria of small bowel; bone; lymph nodes; liver; spleen) associated with eosinophils + lymphocytes

Age: <6 months old (in 50%)

Associated with: myeloproliferative disorders, acute nonlymphatic leukemia, malignant lymphoma, mast cell leukemia

Categories:

I indolent mastocytosis (most frequent)

II mastocytosis associated with myeloproliferative / myelodysplastic hematologic disorder

III aggressive / lymphadenopathic mastocytosis with eosinophilia

IV mast cell leukemia (rare)
- diarrhea, malabsorption, steatorrhea, anorexia
- urticaria pigmentosa = cutaneous form (in 80–90%):
  - hyperpigmented skin lesions exhibiting "wheal and flare" phenomenon when disturbed
- abdominal pain, nausea, vomiting
- tachycardia, asthma, flushing, gastrointestinal upset, headache, pruritus (due to liberation of histamine / prostaglandin D_2)

  caused by: physical exertion, heat, certain foods, alcohol, nonsteroidal antiinflammatory drugs
- pancytopenia (chronic neutropenia)

@ Skeletal involvement (70%)
- bone and joint pain

√ osteoporosis (due to release of heparin + prostaglandin by mast cells activating osteoclasts)
√ scattered well-defined sclerotic foci with focal / diffuse involvement (due to release of histamine by mast cells promoting osteoblastic activity); often alternating with areas of bone rarefaction

Predilected sites: skull, spine, ribs, pelvis, humerus, femur

@ Reticuloendothelial system
√ hepatomegaly
√ splenomegaly (43–61%)
√ lymphadenopathy: retroperitoneal, periportal, mesenteric
√ Budd-Chiari hepatic venoocclusive disease
√ reversed portal venous flow
√ cavernous transformation of portal vein

@ Abdomen
- nausea, vomiting, diarrhea

√ thickening of omentum, + mesentery
√ ascites: (a) transudative secondary to liver disease
(b) exudative from mast cell proliferation of peritoneum

@ Small bowel
√ generalized irregular distorted nodular thickened folds ± wall thickening (due to infiltration by mast cells, lymphocytes, plasma cells)
√ diffuse pattern of 2–3-mm sandlike mucosal nodules
√ urticaria-like lesions of gastric + intestinal mucosa

Dx: skin / bone marrow biopsy; jejunal biopsy demonstrates an excess of mast cells

Cx: (1) Peptic ulcer disease (release of histamine increases gastric acid secretion)
(2) Leukemia

Rx: antihistamines, histamine decarboxylase inhibitors, sodium chromoglycase; steroids; splenectomy (for symptomatic splenomegaly / hypersplenism)

DDx: carcinoid, pheochromocytoma

MECKEL DIVERTICULUM

= persistence of the omphalomesenteric duct (= vitelline duct), which usually obliterates by 5th embryonic week

◊ Most common congenital abnormality of the GI tract!

Incidence: 0.3–2–3% of population (at autopsy)

Age: majority in children <10 years of age; M:F = 3:1

Histo: contains ectopic mucosa in 50%: gastric / pancreatic / colonic mucosa
◊ Frequency of ectopic gastric mucosa: 15–34% overall; 60% in symptomatic children; in >95% with GI hemorrhage

Location: within terminal 6 feet of ileum (= 30–90 cm from ileocecal valve); in 94% on antimesenteric border
- asymptomatic (20–40%)

RULE OF 2s: (1) in 2% of population
(2) symptomatic usually before age 2
(3) located within 2 feet of ileocecal valve
(4) length of 2 inches

NUC (>85% sensitive, >95% specific, >83–88% accurate):
◊ Tc-99m pertechnetate is excreted by mucoid cells of gastric mucosa, excretion is not dependent on presence of parietal cells

N.B.: sensitivity drops after adolescence, because patients asymptomatic throughout childhood are less likely to have ectopic gastric mucosa

Preparation:
(1) No irritative measures for 48 hours (contrast studies, endoscopy, cathartics, enemas, drugs irritating GI tract)
(2) Fasting for 3–6 hours (results in decreased gastric secretion + diminished bowel peristalsis)
(3) Evacuation of bowel + bladder prior to study

Dose: 5–10–20 mCi (100 µCi/kg) Tc-99m pertechnetate (adult dose!)

Radiation dose: 0.54 rad/2 mCi for thyroid;
0.3 rad/2 mCi for large intestine;
0.2 rad/2 mCi for stomach

Imaging: immediate continuous anterior imaging for 30–45 minutes / serial images in 5–10-minute intervals for up to 1 hour

√ small focal collection of tracer in RLQ appearing at the same time / shortly after gastric activity
√ tracer activity increases in intensity with time parallel to that of stomach
√ improved visualization through
(a) pentagastrin = stimulates uptake (6 µg/kg SC 20 minutes prior to pertechnetate)
(b) cimetidine = inhibits secretion (maximum 300 mg/dose IV 1 hour prior)
(c) glucagon = decreases peristalsis (50 µg/kg IM 5–10 minutes prior)
√ poor visualization with use of perchlorate + atropine (= depressed uptake)

False-positive results:
(1) Ectopic gastric mucosa in gastrogenic cyst, enteric duplication, normal small bowel, Barrett esophagus
(2) Increased blood pool in AVM, hemangioma, hypervascular tumor, aneurysm
(3) Duodenal ulcer, ulcerative colitis, Crohn disease, appendicitis, laxative abuse
(4) Intussusception, intestinal obstruction, volvulus
(5) Urinary tract obstruction, caliceal diverticulum
(6) Anterior meningomyelocele
(7) Poor technique

mnemonic: "HA GUIDI"
Hemangioma
Appendicitis
Gastric ectopia
Urinary obstruction
Intussusception
Duplication of bowel
Inflammatory bowel disease

False-negative results:
(1) Insufficient mass of ectopic gastric mucosa
(2) Dilution of intraluminal activity (hemorrhage / hypersecretion)
mnemonic: "MIS"
Malrotation of ileum
Irritable bowel in RLQ (rapid transit)
Small amount of ectopic gastric mucosa

Enteroclysis:
√ elongated, smoothly marginated, clublike, intraluminal mass parallel to long axis of distal ileum = inverted Meckel diverticulum (20%)
√ 0.5–20-cm-long blind pouch on the antimesenteric border of ileum with junctional fold pattern

Angio (59% accuracy):
√ presence of vitelline artery (= anomalous end branch of superior mesenteric artery) is PATHOGNOMONIC

Cx (in 20%):
(1) GI bleeding secondary to ulceration (in 95% due to ectopic gastric mucosa)
(2) Acute diverticulitis
(3) Intestinal obstruction secondary to intussusception (diverticulum acts as lead point) / volvulus (when omphalomesenteric diverticulum attached to umbilicus by fibrous band)
(4) Malignant tumor (rare): carcinoma, sarcoma, carcinoid
(5) Chronic abdominal pain

MECONIUM ILEUS

= small bowel obstruction secondary to desiccated meconium pellets impacted in distal ileum

Age: may develop in utero (in 15%)

Associated with:
cystic fibrosis with tenacious + sticky meconium due to deficiency of pancreatic secretions (in almost 100%)
◊ Earliest clinical manifestation of cystic fibrosis!
◊ Virtually all infants with meconium ileus prove to have cystic fibrosis
◊ 10–15% of infants with cystic fibrosis present with meconium ileus!

• abdominal distension, bilious emesis
• failure to pass meconium within 48 hours

√ numerous dilated small bowel loops without air-fluid levels (fluid not present)
√ "bubbly" / "frothy" appearance of intestinal contents
√ "soap-bubble" / "applesauce" appearance in RLQ (in 50–66%) due to admixture of gas with meconium
√ multiple round / oval filling defects in distal ileum + colon
√ functional microcolon (unused colon in antenatal obstruction)

OB-US:
√ unusual echogenic intraluminal areas in small bowel (DDx: normal transient inspissated meconium)
√ usually polyhydramnios
√ fluid-filled dilated small bowel

Cx (in 40–50%): volvulus, ischemia, necrosis, stenosis, atresia, perforation, meconium peritonitis, pseudocyst

Rx:
(1) Nonionic contrast media enema (because of risk of bowel perforation)
(2) 17% Hypaque / Conray enema mixed with acetylcysteine (Mucomyst®)
(3) Gastrografin® enema with Tween 80 (attention to fluid + electrolyte balance)

DDx: Hirschsprung disease, small bowel atresia with meconium ileus, meconium plug syndrome, small left colon syndrome, imperforate anus, obstruction from duplication cyst

MECONIUM PERITONITIS

= sterile chemical peritonitis secondary to perforation of bowel proximal to high-grade / complete obstruction that seals in utero due to inflammatory response

Incidence: 1:35,000 livebirths

Age: antenatal perforation after 3rd month of gestation

Cause:
(1) Atresia (secondary to ischemic event) (50%)
(a) of small bowel (usually ileum or jejunum)
(b) of colon (uncommon)
(2) Bowel obstruction (46%)
(a) meconium ileus
(b) volvulus, internal hernia
(c) intussusception, congenital bands, Meckel diverticulum
(3) Hydrometrocolpos
◊ Meconium peritonitis due to cystic fibrosis diagnosed in utero in 8% + at birth in 15–40%!
◊ Intraperitoneal meconium may calcify within 24 hours!

Types:
(a) fibroadhesive type (most common):
= intense chemical reaction of peritoneum, which seals off the perforation
• no evidence for active leak at birth
√ dense mass with calcium deposits
√ calcific plaques scattered throughout peritoneal cavity
(b) cystic type:
= cystic cavity formed by fixation of bowel loops surrounding the perforation site, which continues to leak meconium
√ cyst outlined by calcific rim
(c) generalized type:
• perforation occurs immediately antenatally
• active leakage of bowel contents
√ complicated ascites

GI

√ intraabdominal calcifications (conspicuously absent in cystic fibrosis):
√ peripherally calcified pseudocysts
√ small flecks of calcifications scattered throughout abdomen
√ larger aggregates of calcifications along inferior surface of liver / flank / processus vaginalis / scrotum
√ obstructive roentgen signs following birth
√ separation of bowel loops by fluid
√ microcolon = "unused colon"
√ meconium hydrocele producing labial mass

US:
√ highly echogenic linear / clumped foci with posterior acoustic shadowing in scrotum
√ "snowstorm appearance" = highly echogenic material throughout abdomen in between bowel loops
√ ill- / well-defined homo- / heterogeneous encysted collections of meconium

OB-US:
√ polyhydramnios (64–71%)
√ fetal ascites (54–57%)
√ bowel dilatation (27–29%)
√ intraabdominal bright echogenic mass
√ multiple linear / clumped foci of calcifications (84%); may develop within 12 hours after perforation
√ meconium pseudocyst = well-defined hypoechoic mass surrounded by an echogenic calcified wall (= contained perforation)

DDx: (1) Intraabdominal teratoma
(2) Fetal gallstones
(3) Isolated liver calcifications

Mortality: up to 62%
Prognosis: generally good; surgery may not be required when perforation site is completely healed

MECONIUM PLUG SYNDROME

= local inspissation of meconium leading to low colonic obstruction; probably related to small left colon syndrome as part of same spectrum of functional immaturity

Age: newborn infant (symptomatic within first 24 hours of life)
Cause: cystic fibrosis (25%), Hirschsprung disease, prematurity, maternal magnesium sulfate treatment

• abdominal distension
• vomiting
• failure to pass meconium

√ distended transverse + ascending colon + dilated small bowel (proximal to obstruction)
√ small left colon with change in caliber at splenic flexure
√ occasionally bubbly appearance in colon (DDx: submucosal air in necrotizing enterocolitis)
√ presacral pseudotumor (no gas in rectum)

BE:
√ double-contrast effect = barium between meconium plug + colonic wall

Rx: water-soluble enema
DDx: Hirschsprung disease

MELANOSIS COLI

= benign brown-black discoloration of colonic mucosa

Incidence: 10% of autopsies
Cause: ? chronic anthracene cathartic usage

• asymptomatic

Prognosis: no malignant potential

MÉNÉTRIER DISEASE

= GIANT HYPERTROPHIC GASTRITIS = HYPERPLASTIC GASTROPATHY
= characterized by excessive mucus production and TRIAD of (1) Giant mucosal hypertrophy
(2) Hypoproteinemia
(3) Hypochlorhydria

Path: mucosal thickness up to 6 mm (normal range: 0.6–1.0 mm)
Histo: hyperplasia of glandular tissue + microcyst formation
Age: 20–70 years; M:F = 2:1
Associated with: benign gastric ulcer (13–72%)

• epigastric pain, vomiting, weight loss
• gastrointestinal bleeding
• protein-losing enteropathy with hypoproteinemia + peripheral edema
• absent / decreased acid secretion (>50%)

Location: throughout fundus + body, particularly prominent along greater curvature, antrum usually spared (DDx to lymphoma: usually in antrum)

√ markedly enlarged + tortuous gastric rugae in spite of adequate gastric distension:
√ relatively abrupt demarcation between normal antrum + abnormal fundus + body
√ marked hypersecretion (mucus)
√ preserved pliability of stomach

CT:
√ wall thickening of proximal stomach
√ nodular symmetric folds

Cx: development of gastric cancer reported
DDx: lymphoma, polypoid variety of gastric carcinoma, acute gastritis, chronic gastritis, gastric varices

MESENTERIC LYMPHADENITIS

= clinical entity whose symptoms relate to benign inflammation of lymph nodes in the bowel mesentery

Cause: Yersinia enterocolitica, Y. pseudotuberculosis, viral infection
Age: children, young adults

• nausea, vomiting, diarrhea, fever
• diffuse / RLQ pain + tenderness

Location: usually RLQ (immediately anterior to right psoas muscle in 78%, small bowel mesentery in 56%)

√ enlarged mesenteric lymph nodes
√ isolated ileal wall thickening (33%)
√ colonic wall thickening (18%)

N.B.: visualization of entire normal appendix is necessary to differentiate from acute appendicitis!

DDx: appendicitis (enlarged nodes immediately anterior to right psoas muscle in 40–82%, nodes less numerous + smaller), Crohn disease

MESENTERIC ISCHEMIA

= BOWEL ISCHEMIA

Etiology:

(a) arterial occlusion: atheromatous disease, embolic disease, dissecting aortic aneurysm, fibromuscular hyperplasia, arteritis, endotoxin shock, hypoperfusion (shock, hypovolemia), disseminated intravascular coagulation, direct trauma, radiation, antiphospholipid antibody syndrome

— **occlusive mesenteric infarction** (90% mortality)

1. Embolus (40–50%) just distal to middle colic a.
2. SMA thrombosis (20–40%) at origin + site of atherosclerotic narrowing (ostium stenosis)

— **nonocclusive mesenteric ischemia** (10% mortality)

1. Preexisting atherosclerosis with systemic low-flow state (hypovolemia, cardiac failure, intraoperative hypotension)
2. Bowel vasoconstriction = spasm (reflex hypotension, digitalis, ergot preparation, vasopressin, amphetamine, cocaine)
3. **Shock bowel** = diffuse small bowel ischemia in hypovolemia (due to increased bowel permeability to macromolecules + albumin)
   √ diffuse bowel wall thickening
   √ increased enhancement on CT (due to slowed perfusion + interstitial leakage of contrast material)
   √ accumulation of intraluminal fluid (due to failed resorption capacity)

(b) venous (<10%): young patient, often following abdominal surgery
Location: superior mesenteric vein > inferior mesenteric vein > portal vein

(c) bowel obstruction: strangulation by adhesions + bands, incarceration of hernia, volvulus, intussusception, ischemic colitis in colonic carcinoma (1–7%)

(d) vasculitis: polyarteritis nodosa (50–70%)
√ relatively long segment of bowel involved
√ multiple skip areas in nonsegmental distribution
√ involvement of duodenum is indicative

(e) abdominal inflammation: pancreatitis, appendicitis, diverticulitis, diffuse peritonitis, parasitic infestation

(f) cytotoxic drugs: long-term immunosuppressive drugs for rejection, chemotherapy for leukemia / lymphoma

(g) radiation: >4,500 cGy

Prevalence: 5% for SMA; 4% for celiac artery; 11% for inferior mesenteric artery

Pathophysiology: mucosa is most sensitive area to anoxia from arterial / venous occlusion with early ulcerations leading to formation of strictures

Acute Mesenteric Ischemia

Cause:

(a) acute occlusive SMA embolus (in >50%): usually lodges at bifurcation of middle colic artery + SMA
(b) SMA thrombosis (4–18%; nonocclusive in 25%): frequently involves the proximal SMA
(c) SMA dissection (due to cystic medial necrosis, fibromuscular dysplasia)
(d) venous occlusion in 5–10–15% (due to hypercoagulability, trauma, portal hypertension, infection, carcinoma, oral contraceptives)

- first crampy, then continuous abdominal pain with acute event
- cardiac disease predisposing to embolization
- gut emptying (vomiting / diarrhea)
- WBC >12,000/μl with left shift (80%)
- gross rectal bleeding

Location: (a) any segment of small bowel
(b) distal transverse colon, splenic flexure, cecum (most common)

Consequences:
dependent on magnitude of insult, duration of process, adequacy of collaterals

(a) reversible ischemia
1. Complete restitution of bowel wall secondary to abundant collaterals
2. Healing with fibrosis + stricture formation

(b) irreversible ischemia
1. Transmural infarction with bowel perforation

Plain film:
√ gasless abdomen (= fluid-filled loops from exudation) (21%)
√ bowel distension to splenic flexure (= perfusion territory of SMA) in 43%
√ "thumbprinting" (36%) = thickening of bowel wall + valvulae (edema)
√ small bowel pseudoobstruction (most frequently in thrombosis)
√ pneumatosis = dissection of luminal gas into bowel wall (28%)
√ mesenteric + portal vein gas (14%)
√ ascites (14%)

Barium:
√ "scalloping / thumbprinting" = thickening of wall + valvulae
√ "picket fencing"
√ separation + uncoiling of loops
√ narrowed lumen
√ circumferential ulcer

CT (26–73–82% sensitive):
√ circumferential bowel wall thickening (52%):
  √ target sign (20%) = alternating layers of high and low attenuation (from submucosal edema + hemorrhage of ischemic segment)
  √ thinning of bowel wall if it becomes gangrenous
√ focal / diffuse bowel dilatation (10–56–71%) with gas (43%) / fluid (29%) due to interruption of peristaltic activity
√ variable enhancement pattern:
  √ decreased enhancement of bowel wall (due to compromised blood flow)

GI

√ engorgement of mesenteric vessels = venous congestion secondary to stasis
√ increased wall enhancement (due to hyperemia)
√ delayed + persistent enhancement (due to delayed venous return and arteriospasm)
√ increased attenuation of mesenteric fat (edema)
√ pneumatosis intestinalis (22–30%) = dissection of luminal gas into bowel wall across compromised mucosa signaling irreveresible disease
√ portal venous gas (5–13–36%) / mesenteric vein gas (28%) = propagation of intramural gas into mesenteric venous system
√ pneumoperitoneum (7%) = perforation of infarcted bowel segment
√ ascites (43%)
√ mesenteric edema
(a) arterial occlusion:
√ hyperattenuating SMA on NECT
√ filling defect with ring enhancement on CECT
√ thumbprinting (26%) = thickening of bowel wall
√ lack of bowel wall enhancement with arterial occlusion
√ concurrent embolic infarction of kidney / spleen
(b) venous thrombosis (15%):
√ enlarged diameter + increased attenuation of SMV on NECT
√ filling defect in SMV / portal vein thrombosis on CECT
√ thickened intestinal wall (64%) due to edema
√ "waterlogging" with marked contrast enhancement of mesentery + bowel wall
Cx: bowel necrosis (with occlusion of small vasa recta disallowing collateral flow)

Angio (AP and LAT views):
√ occlusion / vasoconstriction / vascular beading
√ embolus lodged at major branching points distal to first 3 cm of SMA
Rx for nonocclusive mesenteric ischemia:
via SMA catheter 60 mg papaverin slowly injected followed by papaverin infusion of 1 mg/min
NUC:
(a) IV / IA Tc-99m sulfur colloid / labeled leukocytes, Ga-citrate, Tc-99m pyrophosphate:
√ tracer accumulation 5 hours after onset of ischemia (more intense uptake with transmural infarcts)
(b) intraperitoneal injection of Xe-133 in saline is absorbed by intestine:
√ decreased washout with abnormal perfusion of strangulated bowel

Prognosis:
(1) Massive infarction of small + large bowel if mesenteric embolization occurs proximal to middle colic artery (= limited collateral flow)
(2) Focal segments of intestinal ischemia if mesenteric embolization occurs distal to middle colic artery (= good collateral flow)
Mortality: 70–80–92% for intestinal infarction

Chronic Mesenteric Ischemia

= ABDOMINAL ANGINA
= intermittent mesenteric ischemia in severe arterial stenosis with inadequate collateralization provoked by food ingestion
• postprandial abdominal pain 15–20 minutes after food intake (due to "gastric steal" diverting blood flow away from intestine)
• fear of eating large meals
• weight loss, malabsorption
• reflex emptying of bowel after eating
Barium:
(a) Subacute:
√ flattening of one border
√ pseudosacculation / pseudodiverticula on antimesenteric border
(b) Chronic:
√ 7–10-cm-long smooth pliable strictures
√ dilatation of gut between strictures
√ thinned + atrophic valvulae
Cx: obstruction
Duplex US:
√ celiac trunk occlusion + retrograde perfusion of hepatic artery through SMA
√ PSV >300 cm/sec and EDV >45 cm/sec in SMA
√ peak systolic velocity >160 cm/sec in celiac trunk for >50% stenosis (57% sensitivity, 100% specificity) during fasting state

Mesenteric Venous Thrombosis

Cause:
(1) Infection: sepsis, diverticulitis, appendicitis, Crohn disease, peritonitis, abdominal abscess
(2) Hypercoagulable state: antithrombin III / protein C or S deficiency, oral contraceptives
(3) Trauma
(4) Mechanical: volvulus, bowel obstruction, postoperative state
Location: SMV > IMV (6%)
• subacute symptomatology over 1–4 weeks
• severe abdominal pain with rebound / guarding
• nausea, vomiting, diarrhea
• hematemesis, hematochezia (after bowel necrosis)
√ ileus
√ ascites
√ bowel wall thickening with "thumbprinting"
√ dilated vein with echogenic thrombus

MESOTHELIAL CYST

= MESENTERIC / OMENTAL CYST
Etiology: failure of mesothelial peritoneal surfaces to coalesce
Path: unilocular thin-walled cyst usually with serous, occasionally chylous / hemorrhagic fluid contents
Histo: lined by mesothelial cells + surrounded by thin layer of fibrous tissue
Location: small bowel, mesentery (78%), mesocolon
• asymptomatic
√ single cyst up to several cm in size
√ omental cysts may be pedunculated

CT:
√ near-water density / soft-tissue density
√ ± fluid levels related to fat + water components
Cx: torsion, hemorrhage, intestinal obstruction
DDx: lymphangioma (septations)

METASTASES TO COLON

Spread:
(1) Hematogenous
√ submucosal masses / bull's-eye lesions
√ diffusely infiltrating lesions mimicking inflammatory bowel disease
(2) Direct invasion by contiguous tumor
– ovary — inferior border of sigmoid
– left kidney — splenic flexure
– pancreatic tail — splenic flexure
– pelvis (uterus, bladder) — anterior border of rectum
– prostate — rectosigmoid
(3) Direct invasion along mesenteric reflections
– stomach — transverse colon superior margin
– pancreas — transverse colon inferior margin
– omental cake — transverse colon superior margin
(4) Intraperitoneal seeding
Origin: ovarian, gastric, colonic, pancreatic cancers (most commonly)
Classic sites of seeding:
– pouch of Douglas (50%): anterior border of rectosigmoid
– lower small bowel mesentery (40%): medial border of cecum
– sigmoid mesocolon (20%): superior border of sigmoid colon
– right paracolic gutter (10%): lateral border of ascending colon

METASTASES TO SMALL BOWEL

Origin: colon > stomach > breast > ovary > uterine cervix > melanoma > lung > pancreas
Spread:
(1) Intraperitoneal seeding: primary mucinous tumor of ovary, appendix, colon; breast cancer
(2) Hematogenous dissemination with submucosal deposits: malignant melanoma, breast carcinoma, lung carcinoma, Kaposi sarcoma
(3) Direct extension from adjacent neoplasm: ovary, uterus, prostate, pancreas, colon, kidney
√ fixation + tenting + transverse stretching (= across long axis) of folds secondary to mesenteric + peritoneal infiltration (most common form)
UGI:
√ single mass protruding into lumen resembling annular carcinoma
√ "bull's-eye" lesions = multiple polypoid masses with sizable ulcer craters
√ obstruction from kinking / annular constriction / large intraluminal mass
√ compression by direct extension of primary tumor / involved nodes

CT:
√ soft-tissue density nodules / masses
√ sheets of tissue causing thickening of bowel wall + mesenteric leaves
√ fixation + angulation of bowel loops (in tumors with desmoplastic response)
√ ascites

METASTASES TO STOMACH

Organ of origin: malignant melanoma, breast, lung, colon, prostate, leukemia, secondary lymphoma
- GI bleeding + anemia (40%)
- epigastric pain

√ solitary mass (50%)
√ multiple nodules (30%)
√ linitis plastica (20%): especially breast
√ multiple umbilicated nodules: melanoma

MIDGUT VOLVULUS

= torsion of entire gut around SMA due to a short mesenteric attachment of small intestine in malrotation
Age: neonate / young infant (= acute intestinal obstruction); occasionally older child / adult (= chronic intestinal obstruction)
In 20% associated with: (1) Duodenal atresia
(2) Duodenal diaphragm
(3) Duodenal stenosis
(4) Annular pancreas
Pathophysiology:
degree of twisting can change due to natural movement of bowel + determines symptomatology; severe volvulus (= twist of 3 and a half turns) causes bowel necrosis
- acute symptoms within first 3 weeks of life in 75% (MEDICAL EMERGENCY): bilious vomiting (postprandial, intermittent, projectile) is HALLMARK; abdominal distension; shock
- intermittent obstructive symptoms in older child: recurring attacks of nausea, vomiting, and abdominal pain
- failure to thrive (hypoproteinemic gastroenteropathy as a result of lymphatic + venous obstruction)
- "currant jelly" stools / melena (implying vascular compromise)

Plain film:
√ dilated air-filled duodenal bulb + paucity of gas distally
√ "double bubble sign" = air-fluid levels in stomach + duodenum
√ isolated collection of gas-containing bowel loops distal to obstructed duodenum = gas-filled volvulus = closed-loop obstruction (from nonresorption of intestinal gas secondary to obstruction of mesenteric veins)
UGI:
N.B.: exclude perforation on plain films!
√ dilated proximal duodenum terminating in a distinctive conical shape
√ duodenal-fold thickening + thumbprinting (mucosal edema + hemorrhage)

√ duodenojejunal junction (ligament of Treitz) located lower than duodenal bulb + to the right of expected position
√ spiral course of midgut loops beyond point of obstruction = "apple-peel / twisted ribbon / corkscrew" appearance (in 81%)
√ abnormally high position of cecum (on barium enema)

CT:
√ whirl-like pattern of small bowel loops + adjacent mesenteric fat converging to the point of torsion (during volvulus)
√ transposition of SMA/SMV = SMV to the left of SMA (NO volvulus)
√ chylous mesenteric cyst (from interference with lymphatic drainage)

US:
√ clockwise whirlpool sign = color Doppler depiction of superior mesenteric vein wrapping clockwise around superior mesenteric artery
√ distended proximal duodenum with arrowhead-type compression over spine
√ superior mesenteric vein to the left of SMA
√ thick-walled bowel loops below duodenum + to the right of spine associated with free intraperitoneal fluid

Angio:
√ "barber pole sign" = spiraling of SMA
√ tapering / abrupt termination of mesenteric vessels
√ marked vasoconstriction + prolonged contrast transit time
√ absent venous opacification / dilated tortuous superior mesenteric vein

Cx: intestinal ischemia + necrosis in distribution of SMA with occlusion of lymphatics, SMV + SMA (bloody diarrhea, ileus, abdominal distension)

DDx: pyloric stenosis (same age group, no bilious vomiting)

MUCOCELE OF APPENDIX

Mucocele

= distension of appendix with sterile mucus

Etiology:
(a) (perhaps) cystic dilatation of lumen secondary to obstruction by fecolith, foreign body, carcinoid, endometriosis, adhesions, volvulus
(b) mucosal hyperplasia (25%)
(c) mucinous cystadenoma due to hyperplasia with epithelial atypia (63%)
(d) mucinous cystadenocarcinoma with stromal invasion (12%)
(e) accumulation of thick mucus in cystic fibrosis

Incidence: 0.07–0.3% of appendectomy specimens
Mean age: 55 years; M:F = 1:4
Associated with: colonic adenocarcinoma (6-fold risk), mucin-secreting tumor of ovary

- asymptomatic (25%)
- palpable mass (in up to 50%)
- acute / chronic right lower quadrant pain

√ globular, smooth-walled, broad-based mass invaginating into cecum
√ nonfilling of the appendix on BE
√ peripheral punctate / rimlike calcifications frequent

CT:
√ round sharply defined paracecal mass with homogeneous content of near-water / soft-tissue attenuation (depending on amount of mucin)

US:
√ purely cystic / cystic with fine internal echoes / complex cystic mass with high-level echoes
√ gravity-dependent echoes = layering of protein macroaggregates / inspissated mucoid material
√ acoustic shadowing if calcifications present

NUC:
√ intense early gallium uptake (affinity to acid mucopolysaccharides of mucus)

Cx: (1) Rupture with pseudomyxoma peritonei
(2) Torsion with gangrene + hemorrhage
(3) Herniation into cecum with bowel obstruction
(4) Intussusception

Myxoglobulosis

= rare variant of mucocele of the appendix characterized by clusters of pearly white mucous balls intermixed with mucus

- usually asymptomatic
- may appear as acute appendicitis

√ multiple 1–10-mm small rounded annular, nonlaminated calcified spherules (PATHOGNOMONIC)

DDx: inverted appendiceal stump, acute appendicitis, carcinoma of the cecum

NECROTIZING ENTEROCOLITIS

= NEC = ischemic bowel disease secondary to hypoxia, perinatal stress, infection (endotoxin), congenital heart disease

Incidence: most common GI emergency in premature infants
Age: develops 2–3 days after birth; in 90% within first 10 days of life
Path: acute inflammation + mucosal ulceration + widespread transmural necrosis
Organism: not yet isolated; often occurs in miniepidemics within nursery
Predisposed: premature infant (50–80%), Hirschsprung disease, bowel obstruction (small bowel atresia, pyloric stenosis, meconium ileus, meconium plug syndrome)

- abdominal distension, bilious emesis
- blood-streaked stools (in 50%); explosive diarrhea
- mild respiratory distress
- generalized sepsis

Location: usually in terminal ileum (most commonly involved), cecum, right colon; rarely in stomach, upper bowel

√ distension of small bowel and colon (loops wider than vertebral body L1) ± air-fluid levels, commonly in RLQ (1st sign)
√ disarrayed bowel gas pattern (no longer normal array of polygons)

√ tubular loops of bowel
√ bowel wall thickening + "thumbprinting"
√ "fixed" bowel = persistent abnormal loop of bowel without change on supine vs. prone films / for >24 hours
√ pneumatosis intestinalis (80%):
— in curvilinear shape (= subserosal) or
— bubbly / cystic (= submucosal gas collection from gas-forming organisms / dissection of intraluminal gas)
√ "bubbly" appearance of bowel due to gas in wall / intraluminal gas / fecal matter (intraluminal contents are composed of blood, sloughed colonic mucosa, intraluminal gas, some fecal material)
√ gas in portal venous system (frequently transient, does not imply hopeless outcome)
√ ascites
√ pneumoperitoneum (immediate surgery required)

N.B.: barium enema is contraindicated! May be used judiciously in selected cases with radiologic + clinical doubt!

Cx: (1) Inflammatory stricture after healing in 10–30%, in 30% multiple, in 80% in left colon (BE follow-up in survivors)
(2) Bowel perforation in 12–32%

PELVIC LIPOMATOSIS + FIBROLIPOMATOSIS

= nonmalignant overgrowth of adipose tissue with minimal fibrotic + inflammatory components compressing soft-tissue structures within pelvis

Age: 9–80 years (peak 25–60 years); M:F = 10:1; NO racial predominance for Blacks; obesity NOT contributing factor

• often incidental finding
• urinary frequency, flank pain, suprapubic tenderness
• recurrent urinary tract infections
• low back pain, fever

√ elongation + narrowing of rectum
√ elevation of rectosigmoid + sigmoid colon out of pelvis
√ increase in sacrorectal space >10 mm
√ stretching of sigmoid colon
√ elongation + elevation of urinary bladder with symmetric inverted pear shape
√ elongation of posterior urethra
√ pelvic lucency; CT confirmatory
√ medial / lateral displacement of ureters

Cx of fibrolipomatosis:
(1) Ureteral obstruction (40% within 5 years)
(2) IVC obstruction

GI

PERITONEAL MESOTHELIOMA

= only primary tumor of peritoneum arising from mesothelial cells lining peritoneal cavity

Age: 55–66 years; M >> F
Associated with: asbestos exposure
Spread: intraperitoneal along serosal surfaces; direct invasion of liver, pancreas, bladder, bowel
Location: pleura (67%), peritoneum (30–40%), pericardium (2.5%), processus vaginalis (0.5%)

√ thickening of mesentery, omentum, peritoneum, bowel wall
√ nodular masses in anterior parietal peritoneum becoming confluent and cakelike
√ disproportionately small amount of ascites
√ areas of calcification (rare)

CT:
√ nodular irregular thickening of peritoneal surfaces
√ localized masses
√ infiltrating sheets of tissue
√ foci of calcifications
√ ascites of near-water density
√ stellate configuration of neurovascular bundles
√ pleated thickening of mesenteric leaves

NUC:
√ diffuse uptake of gallium-67

Prognosis: extremely poor due to advanced disease at presentation (most patients die within 1 year)

Cystic Mesothelioma

= rare benign neoplasm without metastatic potential but tendency for local recurrence (in 27–50%)

Path: multiple thin-walled cysts lined by mesothelial cells + filled with watery fluid; intermediate form between benign adenomatoid tumor + malignant peritoneal mesothelioma

◊ Not associated with asbestos exposure!

Median age: 37 years; M << F
Location: any peritoneal / omental surface, most frequently in pelvis

• contains watery fluid

√ uni- / multilocular cystic tumor (cysts of 1 mm to 6 cm) without calcifications

DDx: lymphangioma, ovarian carcinoma

PERITONEAL METASTASES

= PERITONEAL CARCINOMATOSIS
= intraabdominal spread of malignant tumors

Origin: (a) common: ovary, stomach, colon
(b) less common: pancreas, uterus, bladder

√ massive ascites
√ desmoplastic reaction at (a) anterior border of rectum (Blumer shelf), (b) mesenteric side of terminal ileum

CT:
√ increased density of linear network in mesenteric fat
√ loculated fluid collections in peritoneal cavity
√ apparent thickening of mesenteric vessels (= fluid within leaves of mesentery)
√ adnexal mass of cystic / soft-tissue density (= Krukenberg tumor)
√ small nodular densities on peritoneal surface
√ "omental cake" = thickening of greater omentum
√ lobulated mass in pouch of Douglas
√ calcified peritoneal implants in serous cystadenocarcinoma of ovary (in up to 40% with stage III / IV disease)

PEUTZ-JEGHERS SYNDROME

= rare autosomal dominant disease with incomplete penetrance characterized by intestinal polyposis + mucocutaneous pigmentation (= hamartomatosis); often spontaneous mutation

Incidence: 1:7,000 live births; in 50% familial, in 50% sporadic; most frequent of polyposis syndromes to involve small intestines
Age: 25 years at presentation (range 10–30 years); M:F = 1:1
Path: multiple small sessile / large pedunculated polyps
Histo: benign hamartomatous polyp with smooth muscle core arising from muscularis mucosae + extending treelike into lamina propria of polyp; misplaced epithelium in submucosa, muscularis propria, subserosa frequently surrounding mucin-filled spaces

- mucocutaneous pigmentation (similar to freckles):
  = 1–5-mm small elongated melanin spots on mucous membranes (lower lips, gums, palate) + facial skin (nose, cheeks, around eyes) + volar aspects of toes and fingers (100%), becoming noticeable in first few years of life
- cramping abdominal pain (small bowel intussusception in 47%)
- rectal bleeding, melena (30%)
- prolapse of polyp through anus
- chronic hypochromic microcytic anemia

Location: small bowel (jejunum + ileum > duodenum) > colon > stomach; mouth + esophagus spared
@ Small bowel (>95%)
  √ multiple usually broad-based polyps separated by wide areas of intervening flat mucosa
  √ multilobulated surface of larger polyps
  √ myriad of 1–2-mm nodules of up to several cm = carpet of polyps
  √ intussusception usually confined to small bowel
@ Colon + rectum (30%)
  √ multiple scattered 1–30-mm polyps; NO carpeting
@ Stomach + duodenum (25%)
  √ diffuse involvement with multiple polyps
@ Respiratory + urinary tract
  √ adenoma of bronchus + bladder

Cx:
(1) Transient intussusception (pedunculated polyp)
(2) Carcinoma of GI tract (2–3%)
(3) Carcinoma of pancreas (13%)
(4) Carcinoma of breast (commonly bilateral + ductal)
(5) Ovarian tumor (5%), commonly bilateral: sex cord-stromal tumor of ovary (almost in 100% of patients), mucinous cystic tumor, cystadenoma, granulosa cell tumor
(6) Endometrial cancer: adenoma malignum of cervix (= minimal deviation adenocarcinoma = low-grade mucinous tumor of cervix)
(7) Testicular tumor: feminizing Sertoli cell tumor

Rx: (1) Endoscopic removal of all polyps >5 mm
(2) Surgery is reserved for obstruction, severe bleeding, malignancy
Prognosis: decreased life expectancy (risk of cancer approaching 40% by 40 years of age)

DDx: familial adenomatous polyposis, juvenile polyposis (similar age), Cowden syndrome, Cronkhite-Canada syndrome

POSTCRICOID DEFECT

= variable defect seen commonly in the fully distended cervical esophagus; no pathologic value
Etiology: redundancy of mucosa over rich postcricoid submucosal venous plexus
Incidence: in 80% of normal adults
Location: anterior aspect of esophagus at level of cricoid cartilage
√ tumor- / weblike lesion with variable configuration during swallowing
DDx: submucosal tumor, esophageal web (persistent configuration)

POSTINFLAMMATORY POLYPOSIS

= PSEUDOPOLYPOSIS
= reepithelialized inflammatory polyps as sequelae of mucosal ulceration
Etiology: ulcerative colitis (10–20%); granulomatous colitis (less frequent); schistosomiasis (endemic); amebic colitis (occasionally); toxic megacolon
Location: most common in left hemicolon, may occur in stomach / small intestine
√ sessile + frondlike appearance (often)
√ filiform polyposis = multiple wormlike projections only attached at their bases (CHARACTERISTIC)
Pathogenesis: ulcerative undermining of strips of mucosa with reepithelialization of denuded surfaces of tags + bowel wall
Prognosis: NO malignant potential
DDx: familial polyposis (polyps terminate in bulbous heads)

PRESBYESOPHAGUS

= defect in primary peristalsis + LES relaxation associated with aging
Incidence: 15% in 7th decade; 50% in 8th decade; 85% in 9th decade
Associated with: hiatus hernia, reflux
- usually asymptomatic

√ impaired / no primary peristalsis
√ often repetitive nonperistaltic tertiary contractions in distal esophagus
√ mild / moderate esophageal dilatation
√ poor LES relaxation
DDx: diabetes, diffuse esophageal spasm, scleroderma, esophagitis, achalasia, benign stricture, carcinoma

PROGRESSIVE SYSTEMIC SCLEROSIS

= PSS = multisystem connective tissue disorder (collagen-vascular disease) of unknown etiology characterized by widespread disorder of the microvasculature and overproduction of collagen causing exuberant interstitial fibrosis with atrophy + sclerosis of many organ systems

= SCLERODERMA = variety of skin disorders associated with hardening of skin;
by extent of cutaneous involvement divided into:
(a) DIFFUSE SCLERODERMA
tends to involve older women;
interstitial pulmonary fibrosis more severe;
organ failure more likely
(b) SYSTEMIC SCLEROSIS WITH LIMITED SCLERODERMA (formerly CREST syndrome)
CREST features more common; pulmonary arterial hypertension more common + more severe)

May be associated with:
other connective tissue diseases (especially SLE and polymyositis/dermatomyositis)

Cause: autoimmune condition with genetic predisposition, may be initiated by environmental antigen (eg, toxic oil syndrome in Spain through ingestion of adulterated rape seed oil / ingestion of L-tryptophan)

Peak age: 30–50 years; M:F = 1:3

Histo: vasculitis + submucosal fibrosis extending into muscularis, smooth muscle atrophy (initially hypertrophy and finally atrophy of collagen fibers)

• CREST: **C**alcinosis of skin
Raynaud phenomenon
Esophageal dysmotility
Sclerodactyly
Telangiectasia
• antinuclear antibodies (30–80%):
  • centromere antibody (ACA) specific for limited disease
  • anti–topoisomerase-1 (= antiScl-70) identifies patients with diffuse cutaneous disease
• antibodies to extracellular matrix proteins and type I + IV collagen
• rheumatoid factor (35%)
• LE cells (5%)
• weakness, generalized debility

Prognosis: 50–67% 5-year survival rate

Gastrointestinal Scleroderma (in 40–45%)

◊ Third most common manifestation of scleroderma (after skin changes + Raynaud phenomenon)
◊ May precede other manifestations!
• abdominal pain, diarrhea
• multiple episodes of pseudoobstruction
√ hepatomegaly

@ Esophagus (in 42–95%)
◊ First GI tract location to be involved!
• dysphagia (50%)
• heartburn (30%)
√ normal peristalsis above aortic arch (striated muscle in proximal 1/3 of esophagus)
√ hypotonia / atony + hypokinesia / aperistalsis in lower 2/3 of esophagus (>50%)
√ deficient emptying in recumbent position
√ thin / vanished longitudinal folds
√ mild to moderate dilatation of esophagus
√ chalasia (= patulous lower esophageal sphincter)
√ gastroesophageal reflux (70%)
√ erosions + superficial ulcers (from asymptomatic reflux esophagitis: NO protective esophageal contraction)
√ fusiform stricture usually 4–5 cm above gastroesophageal junction (from reflux esophagitis)
√ esophageal shortening + sliding hiatal hernia
Cx: peptic stricture, aspiration, Barrett esophagus, adenocarcinoma

@ Stomach (less frequent involvement)
√ gastric dilatation
√ decreased motor activity + delayed emptying

@ Small bowel (in up to 45%)
◊ PSS is rapidly progressing once small intestine is involved!
• malabsorption (delayed intestinal transit time + bacterial overgrowth)
√ marked dilatation of small bowel (in particular duodenum = megaduodenum, jejunum) simulating small bowel obstruction
CAVE: misdiagnosis of obstruction may lead to exploratory surgery!
√ abrupt cutoff at SMA level (atrophy of neural cells with hypoperistalsis)
√ prolonged transit time with barium retention in duodenum up to 24 hours
√ "hidebound / accordion" pattern (60%) = sharply defined folds of normal thickness with decreased intervalvular distance (tightly packed folds) within dilated segment (due to predominant involvement of circular muscle)
√ pseudodiverticula (10–40%) = asymmetric sacculations with squared tops + broad bases on mesenteric side (due to eccentric smooth muscle atrophy)
√ pneumatosis cystoides intestinalis + pneumoperitoneum (occasionally)
√ excess fluid with bacterial overgrowth (= "pseudo–blind loop syndrome")
√ normal mucosal fold pattern
Cx: intussusception without anatomic lead point

@ Colon (up to 40–50%)
• constipation (common), may alternate with diarrhea
√ pseudosacculations + wide-mouthed "diverticula" on antimesenteric side (formed by repetitive bulging through atrophic areas) in transverse + descending colon
√ eventually complete loss of haustrations (simulating cathartic colon)
√ marked dilatation (may simulate Hirschsprung disease)
√ stercoral ulceration (from retained fecal material)

Cx: life-threatening barium impaction

DDx: (1) Dermatomyositis (similar radiographic findings)
(2) Sprue (increased secretions, segmentation, fragmentation, dilatation most significant in midjejunum, normal motility)

(3) Obstruction (no esophageal changes, no pseudodiverticula)
(4) Idiopathic intestinal pseudoobstruction (usually in young people)

Pulmonary Scleroderma (in 10–66%)

Path: almost 100% involvement in autopsy series
Histo: thickening of basement membrane of alveoli + small arteries and veins; pattern of usual interstitial pneumonia / nonspecific interstitial pneumonitis

- slightly productive, mostly dry cough
- exertional progressive dyspnea
- hematemesis
- pulmonary function abnormalities in the absence of frank roentgenographic changes (typical dissociation of clinical, functional, and radiologic evidence)
- pericarditis

Location: peripherally, most prominent at both lung bases (where blood flow greatest)

√ bibasilar pulmonary fibrosis:
Prevalence: 20–65% on CXR, up to 90% on HRCT
√ fine / coarse reticulations / diffuse interstitial infiltrates
√ subpleural fibrocystic spaces (honeycombing)
√ low lung volumes from progressive volume loss
√ alveolar changes (secondary to aspiration of refluxed gastric contents with disturbed esophageal motility / mineral oil taken to combat constipation)
√ dilated esophagus with air esophagogram (DDx: achalasia, mediastinitis) with increased frequency of aspiration pneumonia
√ pleural reaction / effusion distinctly uncommon

HRCT:
√ areas of ground-glass attenuation
√ poorly defined subpleural nodules
√ reticular pattern of attenuation
√ traction bronchiectasis
√ honeycombing

Cx: (1) Pulmonary arterial hypertension (6–60%)
(2) Aspiration pneumonia
(3) Increased incidence of lung cancer

@ Heart: sclerosis of cardiac muscle ± cor pulmonale

Renal Scleroderma (25%)

Onset: common within 3 years
Histo: fibrinoid necrosis of afferent arterioles (also seen in malignant hypertension)

√ renal cortical necrosis
√ spotty inhomogeneous nephrogram (constriction + occlusion of arteries)
√ concomitant arterial ectasia

Cx: renal failure (from nephrosclerosis)

Musculoskeletal Scleroderma

- edema of distal portion of extremities
- thickened inelastic waxy skin most prominent about face + extremities
- symmetrical polyarthralgias (50–80%)
- Raynaud phenomenon (may precede other symptoms by months / years)
- atrophy + thickening of skin and musculature (78%)

@ Fingers
- "sausage digit" = edema of digits associated with loss of transverse skin folds + lack of definition of subcutaneous fat

√ "tapered fingers" = sclerodactyly = atrophy + resorption of soft tissues of fingertips + soft-tissue calcifications
√ acroosteolysis = "penciling" / "autoamputation" = resorption of distal phalanges of hand (63%) beginning at volar aspect of terminal tufts with proximal progression
√ calcinosis (25%) = punctate soft-tissue calcifications of fingertips, axilla, ischial tuberosity, forearm, elbow (over pressure area), lower leg, face
√ calcifications around tendons. bursae, within joints

@ Arthritis
- stiffness in small joints, occasionally in knee, shoulder, wrist
- lack of motility, eventually contractures

√ arthritis of interphalangeal joints of hands (25%)
Location: 1st CMC, MCP, DIP, PIP
√ central / marginal erosions (50%):
√ resorption of palmar aspect of terminal phalanges (most frequent sign)
√ bony erosions of carpal bones (trapezium), distal radius + ulna, mandible, ribs, lateral aspect of clavicle, humerus, acromion, mandible, cervical spine
√ joint-space narrowing (late)
DDx: rheumatoid, psoriatic, erosive arthritis
√ soft-tissue swelling ± periarticular osteoporosis
√ NO significant osteoporosis
√ ± flexion contractures of fingers (from tendon sheath inflammation + fibrosis)

@ Ribs
√ erosion of superior aspect of ribs

@ Teeth
√ widening of periodontal membrane

PROLAPSED ANTRAL MUCOSA

= prolapse of hypertrophic + inflammatory mucosa of gastric antrum into duodenum resulting in pyloric obstruction

√ mushroom- / umbrella- / cauliflower-shaped filling defect at duodenal base
√ filling defect varies in size + shape
√ redundant gastric rugae can be traced from pyloric antrum through pyloric channel
√ gastric hyperperistalsis

PSEUDOMEMBRANOUS COLITIS

= CLOSTRIDIUM DIFFICILE DISEASE
= nosocomial epidemic / endemic acute infectious colitis due to Clostridium difficile toxins

Cause: unopposed proliferation of Gram-positive Clostridium difficile in response to a decrease in normal intestinal flora

Etiologic agent: toxin A (enterotoxin) + toxin B (cytotoxin) produced by C. difficile

Predisposed:
- (a) complication of antibiotic therapy with tetracycline, penicillin, ampicillin, clindamycin, lincomycin, amoxicillin, chloramphenicol, cephalosporins
- (b) complication of some chemotherapeutic agents: methotrexate, fluorouracil
- (c) following abdominal surgery / renal transplantation / irradiation
- (d) prolonged hypotension / hypoperfusion of bowel
- (e) shock, uremia
- (f) proximal to colonic obstruction
- (g) debilitating diseases: lymphosarcoma, leukemia, advanced HIV infection
- (h) immunosuppressive therapy with actinomycin D

Histo: pseudomembranes (exudate composed of leukocytes, fibrin, mucin, sloughed necrotic epithelium held in columns by strands of mucus) on a partially denuded colonic edematous mucosa (mucosa generally intact); reactive edema in lamina propria, submucosa, and eventually subserosa

Clinical manifestations of C. difficile infection:
- (a) absence of symptoms (majority)
- (b) antibiotic-associated colitis without pseudomembrane formation
- (c) pseudomembranous colitis
- (d) fulminant colitis

- • profuse watery diarrhea, abdominal cramps, tenderness
- • fever, fecal blood, leukocytosis
- • less common: chronic diarrhea, dehydration, toxic megacolon, hyperpyrexia, leukemoid reaction, hypoalbuminemia with anasarca

Location: rectum (95%); confined to right + transverse colon (5–27–40%)

◊ Radiographic abnormalities in 32% with a positive stool toxin assay!

Plain film:
- √ adynamic ileus pattern = moderate gaseous distension of small bowel + colon:
  - √ small bowel ileus (20%)
  - √ colonic ileus (32%)
- √ nodular haustral thickening (18%):
  - √ "thumbprinting" = "transverse banding" = marked thickening + distortion of haustral folds most prominent in transverse colon
  - √ diffusely shaggy + irregular surface (confluent pseudomembranes)
- √ ascites (7%)

BE (CONTRAINDICATED in severe cases):
- √ pseudoulcerations = barium filling clefts between pseudomembranes
- √ irregular ragged polypoid contour of colonic wall
- √ discrete multiple plaquelike lesions of 2–4 mm in size (DDx: polyposis, nodular form of lymphoma)

N.B.: risk of colonic perforation in toxic megacolon!

CT (85% sensitive, 48% specific):
- √ NO colonic abnormality (12–39%)
- √ colonic wall thickening of 3–32 (mean of 14.7) mm in 61–88%:
  - √ circumferential / eccentric
  - √ smooth (44%) / irregular / polypoid (17%)
  - √ "target sign" = submucosal edema + mucosal hyperemia (best seen during arterial enhancement)

  DDx: wall thickening is greater than in any other colitis except Crohn disease!
- √ "accordion sign" (51–70%) = orally administered intraluminal contrast material trapped between distorted thickened closely spaced transverse edematous folds of low attenuation (simulating intramural tracts), TYPICAL but only in severe cases
- √ colonic dilatation frequent due to transmural inflammation
- √ homogeneous enhancement due to hyperemia
- √ usually disproportionately mild pericolonic stranding (42%) relative to marked wall thickening
- √ ascites in severe cases (15–35%)
- √ pneumatosis coli ± portal vein gas in severe cases

Dx:
- (1) Stool assay for Clostridium difficile cytotoxin (detects toxin B): cumbersome to perform
- (2) Enzyme immunoassay test (up to 33% false-negative results): detects toxin A + B
- (3) Stool culture (95% sensitive): not available for 2 days
- (4) Pseudomembranes of adherent yellow plaques 2–10 mm in diameter on proctosigmoidoscopy

Cx: peritonitis, toxic megacolon, perforation

Prognosis: 1.1–3.5% overall mortality; most patients recover within 2 weeks

Rx:
- (1) Discontinuation of suspected antibiotic
- (2) Administration of vancomycin / metronidazole (response within 3–4 days)
- (3) Attention to fluid and electrolyte balance
- (4) Life-saving partial colectomy required in <1%

DDx: acute stage of ulcerative / granulomatous colitis, inflammatory colitis, ischemic colitis, colonic wall hemorrhage, colonic lymphangiectasia, leukemic infiltration, diverticulitis

PSEUDOMYXOMA PERITONEI

= "jelly belly" = "gelatinous ascites"

= slow insidious accumulation of large amounts of intraperitoneal gelatinous material

Etiology: spillage of mucin from ruptured mucocele with foreign body peritonitis; spread of cystadenocarcinoma of appendix (male) / ovary (female)

Rarely associated with: malignancy of colon (<5%), stomach, uterus, pancreas, common bile duct, urachal duct, omphalomesenteric duct

- • slowly progressive massive abdominal distension
- • recurrent abdominal pain
- √ thickening of peritoneal + omental surfaces
- √ omental cake
- √ posterior fixation of bowel loops + mesentery
- √ voluminous septated / loculated pseudoascites

√ several thin-walled cystic masses of different size throughout abdominal cavity
√ scalloped contour of liver + splenic margins
√ annular / semicircular calcifications (rare but highly suggestive)
CT:
√ intraperitoneal collection of very low attenuation (common) / soft-tissue density (rare)
√ may contain enhancing septa ± calcifications
√ discrete hypoattenuating masses (infrequent)
US:
√ hypoechoic collection (common) / more solid appearance (rare)
Prognosis: bowel obstruction with need for multiple surgical debulkings
DDx: peritoneal metastases, pancreatitis with pseudocysts, pyogenic peritonitis, widespread echinococcal disease, ascites
Prognosis: 50% 5-year survival rate
Rx: often requires repeated laparotomies for drainage

RADIATION INJURY

= obliterative endarteritis with irradiation in excess of 4,000–4,500 rads
Incidence: 5%; increased risk after pelvic surgery
√ radiographic changes within field of radiation only

Radiation Gastritis

◊ Permanent radiographic findings of radiation injury appear 1 month to 2 years after therapy
√ gastric ulceration + deformity (pylorus)
√ enlargement + effacement of gastric folds
√ antral narrowing + rigidity (similar to linitis plastica)

Radiation Enteritis

◊ Permanent radiographic findings of radiation injury appear >1–2 years following irradiation
Predisposed: women (cancer of cervix, endometrium, ovary), patients with bladder cancer
• crampy abdominal pain (from intermittent obstruction)
• persistent diarrhea
• occult intestinal hemorrhage
Location: ileum; concomitant radiation damage to colon / rectum
√ irregular nodular thickening of folds with straight transverse course ± ulcerations
√ serrated bowel margin
√ thickened bowel wall with luminal narrowing
√ multiple strictures + partial mechanical obstruction
√ separation of adjacent bowel loops by >2 mm
√ shortening of small bowel
√ fixation + immobilization of bowel loops with similar radiographic appearance between examinations (from dense desmoplastic response to irradiation)
CT: √ increased attenuation of mesentery
DDx: Crohn disease, lymphoma, ischemia, hemorrhage

Radiation Injury of Rectum

◊ Manifestation of radiation colitis can occur up to 15 years following irradiation
Predisposed: 90% in women (carcinoma of cervix)
• tenesmus, diarrhea, bleeding, constipation
√ ridgelike appearance of mucosa (submucosal fibrosis)
√ irregularly outlined ulcerations (rare)
CT:
√ narrowed partially distensible rectum
√ thick homogeneous rectal wall
√ "target sign" = submucosal circumferential lucency
√ proliferation of perirectal fat >10 mm
√ thickening of perirectal fascia
√ "halo sign" = increase in pararectal fibrosis
Cx: (1) Obstruction
(2) Colovaginal / coloenteric fistula formation

RETAINED GASTRIC ANTRUM

Cause: retention of endocrinologically active gastric antrum in continuity with pylorus + duodenum
Pathophysiology: bathing of antrum in alkaline duodenal juice stimulates secretion of gastrin
Associated with: gastric ulcers in 30–50%
√ duodenogastric reflux of barium through pylorus (diagnostic)
√ giant marginal ulcer / several marginal ulcers usually on jejunal side of anastomosis (large false-negative + false-positive rates; correct-positive rate of 28–60%)
√ large amount of secretions
√ edematous mucosa of jejunal anastomotic segment
√ lacy / cobweblike small bowel pattern (hypersecretion)
Cx: gastrojejunocolic fistula

RETRACTILE MESENTERITIS

= CHRONIC FIBROSING MESENTERITIS = CHRONIC SUBPERITONEAL SCLEROSIS = MESENTERIC PANNICULITIS = LIPOSCLEROTIC MESENTERITIS = LIPOGRANULOMA OF THE MESENTERY = MESENTERIC LIPODYSTROPHY = ISOLATED LIPODYSTROPHY = RETROPERITONEAL XANTHOGRANULOMA = MESENTERIC WEBER-CHRISTIAN DISEASE
= rare benign disorder of unknown etiology characterized by fibrofatty thickening of small bowel mesentery
Etiology: ? trauma, previous surgery, ischemia
Age: most common in 6th decade; M:F = 2–3:1
Associated with:
(1) Gardner syndrome, familial polyposis
(2) Fibrosing mediastinitis, retroperitoneal fibrosis
(3) Lymphoma, lymphosarcoma (in 15%)
(4) Carcinoid tumor
(5) Metastatic gastric / colonic carcinoma
(6) Whipple lipodystrophy
(7) Weber-Christian disease
Location: root of mesentery extending toward mesenteric border of bowel
Site: small bowel mesentery; occasionally mesocolon, sigmoid mesentery, omentum, retroperitoneum
Plain film:
√ soft-tissue mass with calcifications
√ ± thumbprinting (from vascular congestion)
UGI:
√ compression / distortion of duodenum near ligament of Treitz

√ separation of small bowel loops with fixation, kinking, and angulation

CT:

√ mass of fat density interspersed with soft-tissue density (fibrous tissue) + calcifications
√ mesenteric thickening with fine stellate pattern extending to bowel border
√ retraction of small bowel loops
√ single mesenteric soft-tissue mass (fibroma)
√ multiple nodules throughout mesentery (fibromatosis)

Dx: supported by absence of pancreatitis / inflammatory bowel disease

Prognosis: usually benign course with spontaneous resolution

Rx: steroids

DDx: pseudomyxoma peritonei (from metastatic gastric / colonic adenocarcinoma); carcinoid / desmoid tumor; mesenteric lymphoma, lymphosarcoma; liposarcoma of mesentery; pyogenic peritonitis

Mesenteric Lipodystrophy (1st stage)

= degeneration of mesenteric fat

Path: diffuse mesenteric thickening (42%); solitary (32%) / multiple (26%) discrete mesenteric masses

Histo: sheets of foamy macrophages with scattered lymphocytic infiltration replacing mesenteric fat

• asymptomatic

√ ± chylous ascites

Prognosis: spontaneous recovery

Mesenteric Panniculitis (2nd stage)

= inflammatory changes in mesenteric adipose tissue

Path: diffuse mesenteric thickening with puckering of mesenteric surface due to desmoplastic reaction; adherent mass(es) in root of mesentery; fat necrosis

Histo: infiltrate of plasma cells, foreign body giant cells, foamy macrophages

• crampy abdominal pain; bowel disturbances
• nausea + vomiting; malaise; mild weight loss
• poorly defined mass (50%) / abdominal fullness
• low-grade fever

Retractile Mesenteritis (3rd stage)

= fibrosis of adipose tissue

Histo: collagen deposition, fibrosis, inflammation; calcifications

√ intestinal obstruction

SCHATZKI RING

= LOWER ESOPHAGEAL MUCOSAL RING

= constant lower esophageal ring (mucosal thickening) presumed to result from reflux esophagitis = thin annular peptic stricture

Incidence: 6–14% of population; old age > young age; M > F

Histo: usually squamous epithelium on upper surface + columnar epithelium on undersurface; may be covered totally by squamous epithelium or columnar epithelium

• asymptomatic (if ring >20 mm)
• dysphagia (if ring <12 mm)

Location: near the squamocolumnar junction; in region of B ring at inferior margin of lower esophageal sphincter

√ permanently present nondistensible transverse ring with constant shape + size (range of 3–18 mm)
√ 2–4-mm-thick shelflike projection into lumen with smooth symmetric margins
√ visible only with adequate distension of esophagogastric region and when located above the esophageal hiatus of the diaphragm
√ best demonstrated in prone position during arrested deep inspiration with Valsalva maneuver while solid barium column passes through esophagogastric region
√ short esophagus + intrahiatal / intrathoracic gastric segment = sliding hiatal hernia if Schatzki ring located 1–2 cm above diaphragmatic hiatus

Prognosis: decrease in caliber over 5 years (in 25–33%)

Cx: impaction of food bolus (associated with severe chest pain)

Rx:
(1) Proper mastication of food
(2) Endoscopic rupture
(3) Esophageal dilatation (radiographically often lack of caliber change after successful dilatation)

DDx: annular peptic stricture (usually thicker, asymmetric, irregular surface, associated with thickened esophageal folds, serration of esophageal margins)

SCHWANNOMA

= rare neurogenic tumor

Incidence: 4% of all benign gastric tumors are neurogenic tumors

Location: stomach

√ discrete submucosal mass

Cx:
(1) Ulceration (pressure necrosis of overlying mucosa)
(2) Central necrosis (after outgrowing its blood supply)

SMALL LEFT COLON SYNDROME

Cause: transient functional colonic obstruction due to immaturity of mesenteric plexus

Age: newborn infant

Associated with: maternal diabetes mellitus (most common), maternal substance abuse; NOT related to cystic fibrosis

√ colonic caliber becomes abruptly diminutive distal to splenic flexure
√ bowel dilatation proximal to splenic flexure
√ ± meconium plug (as a result and not the cause of obstruction)

Prognosis: gradual resolution of functional immaturity over days to weeks

SOLITARY RECTAL ULCER SYNDROME

= MUCOSAL PROLAPSE SYNDROME

Related disorders with common pathogenesis:
hamartomatous inverted polyp, colitis cystica profunda

Cause: prolapse of anterior rectal wall resulting in mucosal ischemia due to traumatization of rectal mucosa by anal sphincter during defecation (rectal straining / prolapse)

Age: young patients (especially women)

Path: small / large, single / multiple shallow ulcers; 25% broad-based, 18% patchy granular / velvety hyperemic mucosa; rectal stenosis through confluent circumferential lesion

Histo: obliteration of lamina propria mucosae by fibromuscular proliferation of muscularis mucosae, streaming of fibroblasts + muscle fibers between crypts, misplaced mucosal glands deep to muscularis mucosae; diffuse increase in mucosal collagen

- chronic rectal bleeding
- passage of mucus
- disordered defecation
- tenesmus

BE:
- √ ulcer (ulcerative type) on anterior rectal wall
- √ polypoid lesion / nodules (polypoid type)
- √ flat granular mucosa (flat type)
- √ thickened valves of Houston without ulcer
- √ stricture

Evacuation proctography:
- √ failure of anorectal angle to open while straining
- √ excessive perineal descent

Prognosis:
(1) Little change over time
(2) Considerable change in appearance of lesion
(3) Transfusions necessitated by massive blood loss

Dx: rectal biopsy

DDx: invasive rectal carcinoma, Crohn disease

SPRUE

= classic disease of malabsorption

Path: villous atrophy (truncation) + elongation of crypts of Lieberkühn (crypt hyperplasia) + round cell infiltration of lamina propria and epithelium (plasma cells, mast cells, lymphocytes, eosinophils)

- severe diarrhea, steatorrhea (CLASSIC but found only in minority of patients); flatulence
- crampy abdominal pain (from intussusception)
- lassitude, fatigue, weight loss
- stomatitis, neuropathy, depression
- bleeding diathesis
- infertility
- osteomalacia with bone pain
- dermatitis herpetiformis
- anemia from iron / folate / vitamin B_{12} deficiency
- low serum levels of cholesterol, calcium, albumin
- elevated alkaline phosphatase + liver enzymes
- prolonged prothrombin time

Location: patchy involvement of duodenum + jejunum > remainder of small bowel

Small bowel follow-through:
- √ small bowel dilatation is HALLMARK in untreated celiac disease (70–95%), best seen in mid + distal jejunum (due to intestinal hypomotility); degree of dilatation related to severity of disease
- √ hypersecretion-related artifacts:
  - √ air-fluid levels in small bowel (rare)
  - √ segmentation = breakup of normal continual column of barium creating large masses of barium in dilated segments separated by stringlike strands from adjacent clumps due to excessive fluid; best seen on delayed films
  - √ flocculation = coarse granular appearance of small clumps of disintegrated barium due to excess fluid best seen at periphery of intestinal segment; occurs especially with steatorrhea
  - √ fragmentation = scattering = faint irregular stippling of residual barium resembling snowflakes associated with segmentation due to excessive fluid
- √ "moulage sign" (50%) = smooth contour with effaced featureless folds resembling tubular wax mold (due to atrophy of the folds of Kerckring); CHARACTERISTIC of sprue if seen in duodenum + jejunum
- √ long / normal / short transit time
- √ nonpropulsive peristalsis (flaccid + poorly contracting loops)
- √ normal / thickened / effaced mucosal folds (depending on degree of hypoproteinemia)
- √ colonlike haustrations in well-filled jejunum (secondary to spasm + cicatrization from transverse ulcers)
- √ "jejunization" of ileal loops (= adaptive response to decreased jejunal mucosal surface) = SPECIFIC
- √ transient nonobstructive intussusception (20%) without anatomic lead point
- √ "bubbly bulb" = peptic duodenitis = mucosal inflammation, gastric metaplasia, Brunner gland hyperplasia

Enteroclysis:
- √ decreased number of folds in proximal jejunum (≤3 folds per inch)
- √ increased number of folds in distal ileum (>5 folds per inch)
- √ tubular featureless lumen
- √ mosaic pattern = 1–2-mm polygonal islands of mucosa surrounded by barium-filled distinct grooves (10%)

CT:
- √ small bowel dilatation + increased fluid content ± mucosal fold thickening
- √ mild to moderate lymphadenopathy in mesentery / retroperitoneum (up to 12%)

US:
- √ moderately dilated fluid-filled small intestine
- √ thickening of small bowel wall
- √ hyperperistalsis (82%)
- √ dilated superior mesenteric artery + portal vein
- √ liver steatosis (metabolic derangement from malabsorption)
- √ mesenteric + retroperitoneal lymphadenopathy (12%)
- √ slight ascites (76%)

Dx: (1) Jejunal / duodenal biopsy
(2) Improvement of small bowel abnormalities after a few months of a gluten-free diet

Cause for relapse: hidden dietary gluten, diabetes, bacterial overgrowth, intestinal ulceration, development of lymphoma

Cx:
(1) Ulcerative jejunoileitis
= multiple chronic benign ulcers (sausage appearance of small bowel) with hemorrhage, perforation + obstruction
Age: 5th–6th decade
Location: jejunum > ileum > colon
• response to gluten-free diet ceases
Prognosis: frequently fatal
Rx: small bowel resection
(2) Hyposplenism (30–50%)
√ small atrophic spleen
(3) Cavitary mesenteric lymph node syndrome characterized by:
(a) mesenteric lymph node cavitation
(b) splenic atrophy
(c) villous atrophy of small intestinal mucosa
√ enlarged lymph nodes of low attenuation ± fat-fluid levels (filled with lipid-rich hyaline material) within jejunoileal mesentery
Prognosis: usually fatal disorder
(4) Malignant tumors
(a) lymphoma (in 8%): commonly diffuse + nodular and of C-cell type
Peak prevalence: 7th decade
√ enlarged nodular folds, ulcers, extrinsic mass effect
(b) adenocarcinoma of small bowel (6%), rectum, stomach
(c) squamous cell carcinoma of pharynx / esophagus (in 6%) during 6th–7th decade
(5) Generalized lymphadenopathy with lymphocytosis (mimicking lymphoma)
(6) Sigmoid volvulus (rare)

DDx:
(1) Esophageal hypoperistalsis: scleroderma, idiopathic pseudoobstruction
(2) Gastric abnormalities: Zollinger-Ellison syndrome, chronic granulomatous disease, eosinophilic enteritis, amyloidosis, malignancy
(3) Tiny nodular defects on thickened folds: Whipple disease, intestinal lymphangiectasia, Waldenström macroglobulinemia
(4) Small 1–3-mm nodules: lymphoid hyperplasia associated with giardiasis and immunoglobulin deficiency disease, diffuse lymphoma
(5) Small nodules of varying sizes: systemic mastocytosis, amyloidosis, eosinophilic enteritis, Cronkhite-Canada syndrome
(6) Bowel wall narrowing, kinking, scarring, ulceration: regional enteritis, bacterial / parasitic infection, carcinoid, vasculitis, ischemia, irradiation

Celiac Disease

= NONTROPICAL SPRUE = GLUTEN-SENSITIVE ENTEROPATHY
= characterized by malabsorption resulting from atrophy of small intestinal villi

Irritating agent: gliadin polypeptides in wheat, rye, barley, oats
May be hereditary: detected in 15% of 1st-degree relatives
Countries: North America, Europe, Australia, India, Pakistan, Middle East, Cuba
Prevalence: 1:1,000 to 1:2,000; western Ireland 1:300
Age: childhood by age 2 years; 30–40 years with M < F; 40–60 years with M > F
Rx: gluten-free diet: corn, rice, tapioca, soya, millet, vitamin supplements

Tropical Sprue

Etiology: infectious agent cured with antibiotics; geographic distribution (India, Far East, Puerto Rico)
Age: any age group
• glossitis
• hepatosplenomegaly
• macrocytic anemia + leukopenia
Prognosis: spontaneous resolution after months / years
Rx: responds well to folic acid + broad-spectrum antibiotics

STRONGYLOIDIASIS

Organism: helminthic parasite Strongyloides stercoralis (2.2 mm long, 50 μm in diameter); capable of reproducing within human host
Prevalence: 100 million cases globally; 0.4–4% in USA
Country: tropical + subtropical regions, parts of Europe, southeastern USA (eastern Kentucky, rural Tennessee), Puerto Rico
Primary host: humans
Infection: filiform larva enters body through skin / mucous membranes (from contaminated soil)
Cycle: filariform larva penetrates skin and passes from subcutaneous / submucosal sites via lymphatic + venous circulation to lung; larva breaks into alveolar spaces and ascends bronchi + trachea; larva swallowed; settles in duodenum + upper jejunum (lives in tunnels between enterocytes); larva matures into parasitic adult female worm; worm deposits eggs into the intestinal lumen; ova hatch immediately into nonmigratory rhabditiform larvae, which are excreted in feces
Autoinfection (endogenous reinfection): rhabditiform larva may remain in intestines long enough to metamorphose into infective filariform larva, which penetrates intestinal mucosa / perianal skin and reenters venous system repeating life cycle in same host
Path: edema + inflammation of intestinal wall secondary to invasion by larvae; flattening of villi; ova in mucosal crypts

Histo: intact larvae with Gomori methenamine silver stain
- asymptomatic for many years (in majority)
- midepigastric pain mimicking peptic ulcer disease
- weight loss
- severe malnutrition (malabsorption, steatorrhea)
- larva currens = recurrent allergic pruritic cutaneous skin reaction at site of larval penetration within 24 hours in area of buttocks + upper thighs in patients with autoinfection
- worms, larvae, eggs in stool
- blood eosinophilia (extremely common)
- elevated levels of immunoglobulin E

√ paralytic ileus (due to massive intestinal infestation):
  √ mild to moderate dilatation of proximal 2/3 of duodenum + jejunum
  √ edematous irregular mucosal folds
√ ulcerations
√ stricture of 3rd + 4th part of duodenum
  √ rigid pipestem appearance + irregular narrowing of duodenum (in advanced cases)

Rx: thiabendazole (90% efficacy rate)
Prognosis: high mortality in undernourished patients

Strongyloides Hyperinfection Syndrome

= widespread dissemination + extensive tissue invasion in immunocompromised host with malignancy, autoimmune disease, malnutrition

- Gram-negative bacteremia, septicemia (due to spillage of gut organisms into bloodstream at time of larval penetration of intestinal wall)
- crampy abdominal pain, nausea, diarrhea
- persistent vomiting, hematemesis

√ thickened colonic wall (due to florid transmural granulomatous inflammatory colitis caused by invasive larvae)

@ Heart, skeletal muscle, lymph nodes, liver
  - endocarditis, peritonitis

@ CNS
  (a) meningitis due to larvae in pia arachnoid
  (b) global ischemia, atrophy, microinfarcts (from capillary obstruction)

@ Lung
  Histo: foreign body reaction resulting in inflammatory pneumonitis + pulmonary hemorrhage
  - ± dyspnea, cough, sputum production, wheezing
  - hemoptysis
  √ fine miliary nodules
  √ diffuse reticulonodular interstitial opacities
  √ fleeting bilateral patchy alveolar / segmental / lobar opacities (with heavy infestation)
  √ adult ARDS may develop

Dx: filariform larvae in stool (single stool sample in 70% negative), sputum samples / bronchial washings / bronchial / lung biopsy specimens, CNS samples

SUPERIOR MESENTERIC ARTERY SYNDROME

= VASCULAR COMPRESSION OF DUODENUM = WILKIE SYNDROME = CHRONIC DUODENAL ILEUS = BODY CAST SYNDROME
= vascular compression of 3rd portion of duodenum within aortomesenteric compartment; probably representing a functional reflex dilatation

Etiology: narrowing of angle between SMA + aorta to 10–22° (normal 45–65°)
  Cause: congenital, weight loss, visceroptosis due to loss of abdominal muscle tone (as in pregnancy), asthenic build, exaggerated lumbar lordosis, prolonged bed rest in supine position (body cast, whole-body burns, surgery)

- repetitive vomiting
- abdominal cramping

√ megaduodenum = pronounced dilatation of 1st + 2nd portion of duodenum + frequently stomach, best seen in supine position
√ vertical linear compression defect in transverse portion of duodenum overlying spine
√ abrupt change in caliber distal to compression defect
√ relief of compression by postural change into prone knee-elbow position

TAILGUT CYST

= RETRORECTAL CYSTIC HAMARTOMA

Cause: incomplete regression of embryonic tailgut (= the portion distal to future anus)
Average age: 35 years; M < F
Histo: several types of epithelia + elements of intestinal epithelium, smooth muscle within cyst wall

- asymptomatic / perirectal pain, rectal bleeding, urinary frequency

Location: retrorectal / presacral space ± extension into ischiorectal fossa

√ thin-walled multicystic / unilocular cyst adhering to sacrum / rectum
√ clear fluid / mucoid fluid with internal echoes

Cx: (1) Repeated perirectal abscesses, recurring anorectal fistula
(2) Degeneration into mucinous adenocarcinoma

TOXIC MEGACOLON

= acute transmural fulminant colitis with neurogenic loss of motor tone + rapid development of extensive colonic dilatation >5.5 cm in transverse colon (damage to entire colonic wall + neuromuscular degeneration)

Etiology:
1. Ulcerative colitis (most common)
2. Crohn disease
3. Amebiasis, salmonellosis
4. Pseudomembranous colitis
5. Ischemic colitis

Histo: widespread sloughing of mucosa + thinning of frequently necrotic muscle layers

GI

• systemic toxicity
• profuse bloody diarrhea
√ colonic ileus with marked dilatation of transverse colon
√ few air-fluid levels
√ increasing caliber of colon on serial radiographs without redundancy
√ loss of normal colonic haustra + interhaustral folds
√ coarsely irregular mucosal surface
√ pseudopolyposis = mucosal islands in denuded ulcerated colonic wall
√ pneumatosis coli ± pneumoperitoneum

CT:
√ distended colon filled with large amounts of fluid + air
√ distorted haustral pattern
√ irregular nodular contour of thin wall
√ intramural air / small collections

BE: CONTRAINDICATED due to risk of perforation

Prognosis: 20% mortality

TUBERCULOSIS

Rarely encountered in Western Hemisphere, increased incidence in AIDS; usually associated with pulmonary tuberculosis (in 6–38%)

Etiology:
(1) Ingestion of tuberculous sputum
(2) Hematogenous spread from tuberculous focus in lung to submucosal lymph nodes
◊ Radiographic evidence of pulmonary TB in <50%
(3) Primary infection by cow milk (Mycobacterium bovis)

Path:
(a) ulcerative form (most frequent): ulcers with their long axis perpendicular to axis of intestine, undermining + pseudopolyps
(b) hypertrophic form: thickening of bowel wall (transmural granulomatous process)

Organism: M. tuberculosis, M. bovis, M. avium-intracellulare

Age: 20–40 years

• weight loss, abdominal pain (80–90%)
• nausea, vomiting
• tuberculin skin test negative in most patients with primary intestinal TB

Location: ileocecal area > ascending colon > jejunum > appendix > duodenum > stomach > sigmoid > rectum

@ Tuberculous peritonitis (in 1/3)
◊ Most common presentation associated with widespread abdominal disease!
Cause: hematogenous spread / rupture of mesenteric node
Types:
(a) wet type (most common) = exudative ascites with high protein contents + leukocytes
• large amount of freely distributed / loculated viscous fluid
√ high-density ascites of 20–45 HU (due to high protein + cellular content)
(b) dry / plastic type = caseous adenopathy + adhesions
√ caseous nodules, fibrous peritoneal reaction, dense adhesions
(c) fibrotic-fixed type = omental cakelike mass with separation + fixation of bowel loops
√ irregular masses of soft-tissue density in omentum + mesentery (common)
√ matted loops of bowel and mesentery
√ loculated ascites (occasionally)

CT:
√ enlarged lymph nodes (90%) with low-density centers in 40% (due to caseous necrosis)
Location: peripancreatic, mesenteric, omental, retroperitoneal Lnn
√ infiltration of mesentery

Cx: small bowel obstruction (adhesions from serosal tubercles)

@ Ileocecal area (80–90%)
◊ Most commonly affected bowel segment!
Cause: relative stagnation of intestinal contents + abundance of lymphoid tissue (Peyer patches)
√ Stierlin sign = rapid emptying (hypermotility) of narrowed terminal ileum (spasm) into shortened rigid obliterated cecum on BE
√ thickened ileocecal valve (mass effect)
√ Fleischner sign = "inverted umbrella" defect = wide gaping patulous ileocecal valve associated with narrowing of the immediately adjacent terminal ileum
√ deep fissures + large shallow linear / stellate ulcers with CHARACTERISTIC elevated margins following the orientation of lymphoid follicles (ie, longitudinal in terminal ileum and transverse in colon)
√ sinus tracts (rare) / enterocutaneous fistulas / perforation
√ symmetric annular "napkin ring" stenoses

CT:
√ circumferential wall thickening of cecum + terminal ileum
√ asymmetric thickening of ileocecal valve + medial wall of cecum
√ exophytic extension engulfing terminal ileum
√ adjacent massive mesenteric lymphadenopathy with central areas of low attenuation

DDx: Crohn disease, amebiasis, cecal carcinoma

@ Colon
Site: segmental colonic involvement, esp. on right side
√ rigid contracted cone-shaped cecum (spasm / transmural fibrosis)
√ spiculations + wall thickening
√ diffuse ulcerating colitis + pseudopolyps
√ short hourglass strictures
√ shortened "amputated" cecum secondary to retraction of cecum out of the iliac fossa (due to fibrosis of mesocolon)

DDx: ulcerative colitis, Crohn disease, amebiasis (spares terminal ileum), colitis of bacillary dysentery, ischemic colitis, pseudomembranous colitis

@ Gastroduodenal
Site: simultaneous involvement of pylorus + duodenum
√ stenotic pylorus with gastric outlet obstruction
√ narrowed antrum (linitis plastica appearance)
√ antral fistula
√ multiple large and deep ulcerations on lesser curvature
√ thickened duodenal folds with irregular contour / dilatation
DDx: carcinoma, lymphoma, syphilis

@ Esophagus
◊ Least common GI tract manifestation
Cause: secondary involvement from adjacent tuberculous lymphadenitis / primary TB
√ deep ulceration
√ stricture
√ mass
√ intramural dissection / fistula formation
= sinus tract formation

TURCOT SYNDROME

= autosomal recessive disease with
(a) colonic polyposis
(b) CNS tumors (especially supratentorial glioblastoma, occasionally medulloblastoma)
Age: symptomatic during 2nd decade
Histo: adenomatous polyps
- diarrhea
- seizures

√ multiple 1–30-mm polyps in colon + rectum
Cx: malignant transformation of colonic polyps in 100%
Prognosis: death from brain tumor in 2nd + 3rd decade

TYPHLITIS

= ILEOCECAL SYNDROME = NEUTROPENIC COLITIS
= acute inflammation of cecum, appendix, and occasionally terminal ileum; initially described in children with leukemia + severe neutropenia;
[*typhlos* , Greek = blind sac = cecum]
Cause: leukemic / lymphomatous infiltrate, ischemia, focal pseudomembranous colitis, infection (CMV)
Histo: edema + ulceration of entire bowel wall; transmural necrosis with perforation possible
Organism: CMV, Pseudomonas, Candida, Klebsiella, E. coli, B. fragilis, Enterobacter
Predisposed: common in childhood leukemia, aplastic anemia, lymphoma, immunosuppressive therapy (eg, renal transplant), cyclic neutropenia, myelodysplastic syndrome, clinical AIDS
- abdominal pain, may be localized to RLQ
- watery / bloody diarrhea
- fullness / palpable mass in RLQ
- fever, neutropenia
- hematochezia / occult blood

Location: cecum + ascending colon, appendix + distal ileum may become secondarily involved
√ fluid-filled masslike density in RLQ
√ distension of nearby small bowel loops
√ thumbprinting of ascending colon
√ circumferential thickening of cecal wall >4 mm
√ occasionally pneumatosis
CT (preferable examination due to risk of perforation):
√ circumferential wall thickening (>1–3 mm) of cecum ± terminal ileum
√ decreased bowel wall attenuation (edema)
√ increased attenuation of adjacent fat + thickening of fascial planes (pericolonic inflammation)
√ ± pericolonic fluid + intramural pneumatosis
Cx: (1) Perforation (BE is a risky procedure)
(2) Abscess formation
Rx: (1) Early aggressive medical support (high doses of antibiotics + IV fluids), bowel rest, total parenteral nutrition, electrolyte replacement prior to development of transmural necrosis
(2) Surgery with uncontrollable GI bleeding, obstruction, abscess, transmural necrosis, free perforation, uncontrollable sepsis
DDx: (1) Leukemic / lymphomatous deposits (more eccentric thickening)
(2) Appendicitis with periappendicular abscess (normal cecal wall thickness)
(3) Diverticulitis
(4) Inflammatory bowel disease

ULCERATIVE COLITIS

= common idiopathic inflammatory bowel disease with continuous concentric + symmetric colonic involvement
Etiology: ? hypersensitivity / autoimmune disease
Prevalence: 50–80:100,000 In high incidence areas of North America, Northern Europe, Australia
Path: predominantly mucosal + submucosal disease with exudate + edema + crypt abscesses (HALLMARK) resulting in shallow ulceration
Age peak: 20–40 years + 60–70 years; M:F = 1:1
- alternating periods of remission + exacerbation
- bloody diarrhea
- electrolyte depletion, fever, systemic toxicity
- abdominal cramps

Extracolonic manifestations:
- iritis, erythema nodosum, pyoderma gangrenosum
- pericholangitis, chronic active hepatitis, primary sclerosing cholangitis, fatty liver
- spondylitis, peripheral arthritis, coincidental rheumatoid arthritis (10–20%)
- thrombotic complications

Location: begins in rectum with proximal progression (rectum spared in 4%); relatively uniform symmetric involvement of bowel
(a) rectosigmoid in 95% (diagnosed by rectal biopsy); continuous circumferential involvement often limited to left side of colon

(b) colitis extending proximally to splenic flexure = universal colitis
(c) terminal ileum in 10–25% ("backwash ileitis")

Plain film:
√ hyperplastic mucosa, polypoid mucosa, deep ulcers
√ diffuse dilatation with loss of haustral markings
√ toxic megacolon√ free intraperitoneal gas
√ complete absence of fecal residue (due to inflammation)

BE:
(a) acute stage
√ narrowing + incomplete filling (spasm + irritability)
√ fine mucosal granularity = stippling of barium coat (from diffuse mucosal edema + hyperemia + superficial erosions)
√ spicules + serrated bowel margins (tiny superficial ulcers)
√ "collar button" ulcers (= undermining of ulcers)
√ "double-tracking" = longitudinal submucosal ulceration over several cm
√ hazy / fuzzy quality of bowel contour (excessive secretions)
√ "thumbprinting" = symmetric thickening of colonic folds
√ pseudopolyps = scattered islands of edematous mucosa + reepithelialized granulation tissue within areas of denuded mucosa
√ widening of presacral space
√ obliterated rectal folds = valves of Houston (43%)
(b) subacute stage
√ distorted irregular haustra
√ inflammatory polyps = sessile frondlike / rarely pedunculated lesions (= localized mucosal inflammation resulting in polypoid protuberance)
√ coarse granular mucosa (= mucosal replacement by granulation tissue)
(c) chronic stage
√ shortening of colon (= reversible spasm of longitudinal muscle) with depression of flexures
√ "leadpipe" colon = rigidity + symmetric narrowing of lumen
√ widening of haustral clefts / complete loss of haustrations (DDx: cathartic colon)
√ "burnt-out colon" = fairly distensible colon without haustral markings + without mucosal pattern
√ hazy / fuzzy quality of bowel contour (excessive secretions)
√ postinflammatory polyps (12–19%) = small sessile nodules / long wormlike branching + bridging outgrowths (= filiform polyposis)
√ "backwash ileitis" (5–30%) involving 4–25 cm of terminal ileum with patulous ileocecal valve + absent peristalsis + granularity

CT:
√ wall thickening <10 mm

Cx:
(1) Toxic megacolon ± perforation in 5–10% (DDx: granulomatous / ischemic / amebic colitis)
◊ Most common cause of death in ulcerative colitis!
(2) Colonic adenocarcinoma (3–5%):
risk starts after 8–10 years of onset of disease; risk progresses at 0.5%/ year for 10–20 years + at 0.9%/ year thereafter; higher risk with pancolitis + onset of disease in <15 years of age
Usually associated with: total colitis
Location: rectosigmoid > descending colon, distal transverse colon
√ narrowed segment of 2–6 cm in length with eccentric lumen + irregular contour + flattened rigid tapered margins = scirrhous carcinoma
√ annular / polypoid carcinoma
Prognosis: synchronous lesions in 35%
(3) Colonic strictures (10%)
smooth contour with fusiform pliable tapering margins, usually short + single stricture; commonly in sigmoid / rectum / transverse colon; usually after minimum of 5 years of disease; rarely cause for obstruction (DDx: colonic carcinoma)
(4) Perforation

DDx: (1) Familial polyposis (no inflammatory changes)
(2) Cathartic colon (more extensive in right colon)

DDx between Crohn Disease and Ulcerative Colitis

	Crohn Disease	*Ulcerative Colitis*
mnemonic: "LUCIFER M"		
Location	right side	left side
Ulcers	deep	shallow
Contraction	no	yes
Ileocecal valve	thickened	gaping
Fistulae	yes	no
Eccentricity	yes	no
Rate of carcinoma	slight increase	marked increase
Megacolon	unusual	yes

VILLOUS ADENOMA

Villous Adenoma of Colon

Incidence: 7% of all colonic tumors
Age: presentation late in life; M = F
Location: rectum + sigmoid (75%), cecum, ileocecal valve; 2% of all tumors in rectum + colon
Associated with: other GI tumors (25%)
• sensation of incomplete evacuation
• rectal bleeding
• excretion of copious amounts of thick mucus
• fatigability, weakness
• diarrhea + electrolyte depletion syndrome in 4% (dehydration, hypokalemia, hyponatremia)
√ may completely encircle the colon
√ broad-based sessile bulky tumor often >20 mm in diameter:
√ innumerable papillary mucosal projections ("villous fronds") with reticular / granular surface pattern (if villous elements constitute >75% of tumor, diagnosis can be made on BE):
√ spongelike corrugated appearance (barium within interstices)

GI

√ striated "brushlike" surface
√ soft pliable tumor with change in shape:
√ apparent decrease in size on postevacuation films
CT:
√ heterogeneous low attenuation on CT (due to capacious mucin becoming trapped within papillary projections + crevices)
Prognosis: higher malignant potential than tubular adenoma
Cx: malignant transformation / invasion (in 36%) related to size of tumor <5 cm (9%); >5 cm (55%); >10 cm (100%)

Villous Adenoma of Duodenum

More common in colon + rectum; fewer than 50 cases in world literature
√ sessile, soft nonobstructive mass
√ "lace" / "soap bubble" pattern
√ preservation of peristaltic activity + bowel distensibility

WALDENSTRÖM MACROGLOBULINEMIA

= low-grade lymphoid malignancy composed of mature plasmacytoid lymphocytes with production of abnormal monoclonal IgM protein
Incidence: 0.53 / 100,000 annually; frequency 10–15% that of multiple myeloma
Histo: macroglobulin proteinaceous hyaline material fills lacteals in lamina propria of small bowel villi with secondary lymphatic distension + edema
Mean age: 63 years; M > F
• fatigue, weight loss
• diarrhea, steatorrhea, malabsorption
• anemia, bleeding diathesis
• IgM elevation
• hyperviscosity syndrome (20%) = bleeding, visual changes, neurologic abnormalities
@ Small bowel (rarely involved)
√ small bowel dilatation
√ uniform diffuse thickening of valvulae conniventes with spikelike configuration (jejunum + proximal ileum)
√ granular surface of punctate filling defects (distended villi)
@ Bone marrow involvement (91–98%)
(a) diffuse replacement of bone marrow (56%)
(b) variegated replacement of bone marrow (35%)
√ compression fractures of spine (48%)
√ diffuse demineralization of spine
√ lytic lesions on bone surveys (in up to 20%)
MR (pre- and postcontrast T1WI preferred):
√ marrow iso- / hypointense to muscle on T1WI
√ enhancement of abnormal marrow on T1WI
@ Lymph nodes
√ lymphadenopathy (43%)
@ Liver & spleen
√ hepatosplenomegaly
Dx: (1) characteristic M-spike in serum / urine electrophoresis
(2) abnormal lymphplasmacytoid cells in bone marrow / lymph nodes
DDx: multiple myeloma (lymphadenopathy rare, lytic lesions in 31%)

WHIPPLE DISEASE

= INTESTINAL LIPODYSTROPHY
= sporadically occurring chronic multisystem disease
Etiology: thought to be caused by infection with an as yet unidentified Gram-positive bacterium (Tropheryma whippelii) closely related to actinobacteria
Histo: PAS-positive material (periodic acid Schiff) = glycoprotein (from bacterial cell wall) within foamy macrophages in the submucosa of the jejunum + fat deposits within intestinal submucosa and lymph nodes causing lymphatic obstruction + dilatation
Age: 4th–6th decade (mean age of onset, 50 years); M:F = 8:1; Caucasians
• recurrent and migratory arthralgias / nondeforming arthritis (65–95%); arthritis may precede Whipple disease in 10% up to 10 years
• malabsorption, steatorrhea, abdominal pain
• weight loss, low-grade fever
• polyserositis
• generalized peripheral lymphadenopathy (50%)
• hyperpigmentation of skin similar to Addison disease
• pale shaggy yellow plaques / erosions in postbulbar duodenum on endoscopy
Organ involvement: liver, intestines, joints, heart, lung, CNS, eyes, skin (virtually every organ system)
√ moderate thickening of jejunal + duodenal folds (from mucosal + submucosal infiltration by PAS-positive macrophages combined with lymphatic obstruction)
√ micronodularity (= swollen villi) and wild mucosal pattern
√ hypersecretion, segmentation, fragmentation (occasionally if accompanied by hyperproteinemia)
√ NO / minimal dilatation of small bowel
√ NO rigidity of folds, NO ulcerations
√ normal transit time (approximately 3 hours)
√ hepatosplenomegaly
CT:
√ bulky 3–4-cm large low-density lymph nodes in mesenteric root + retroperitoneum (due to extracellular neutral fat + fatty acids)
√ thickening of bowel wall
√ splenomegaly
√ ascites
√ pleuropericarditis
√ sacroiliitis

Dx: endoscopically guided biopsy of small bowel mucosa, abdominal / peripheral lymph node biopsy
Rx: long-term broad-spectrum antibiotics (tetracycline)
DDx: (1) Sprue (marked dilatation, no fold thickening, pronounced segmentation + fragmentation)
(2) Intestinal lymphangiectasia (thickened folds throughout small bowel)
(3) Amyloidosis
(4) Lymphoma

ZENKER DIVERTICULUM

= PHARYNGOESOPHAGEAL DIVERTICULUM
= outpouching of posterior hypopharyngeal wall = pulsion diverticulum with herniation of mucosa + submucosa through oblique + transverse muscle bundles (pseudodiverticulum) of the cricopharyngeal muscle

Prevalence: 0.01–0.11% (overall); higher in elderly women (50% occur in 7th–8th decade)

Etiology: cricopharyngeal dysfunction (cricopharyngeal achalasia / premature closure) results in increased intraluminal pressure

Associated with: hiatal hernia, gastroduodenal ulcer, midesophageal diverticulum, esophageal spasm, achalasia

- compressible neck mass
- upper esophageal dysphagia (98%)
- regurgitation + aspiration of undigested food
- noisy deglutition
- halitosis (= foul breath)

Location: at pharyngoesophageal junction in midline of Killian dehiscence / triangle of Laimer, at level of C5/6

√ posterior barium extension in upper half of semilunar depression on the posterior wall of esophagus (cricopharyngeal muscle)
√ barium-filled sac extending caudally behind + usually to left of esophagus
√ partial / complete obstruction of esophagus from external pressure of sac contents
√ partial barium reflux from diverticulum into hypopharynx
√ continual growth with successive enlargement

CXR:
√ air-fluid level in superior mediastinum

Cx: aspiration pneumonia (30%); esophageal perforation; carcinoma (0.48%)

Rx: surgical excision

ZOLLINGER-ELLISON SYNDROME

= peptic ulcer diathesis associated with marked hypersecretion of gastric acid + gastrin-producing non-β islet cell tumor of pancreas

Cause:

A. GASTRINOMA (90%)
   = non-β islet cell tumor with continuous gastrin production
B. PSEUDO Z-E SYNDROME = COWLEY SYNDROME
   = antral G-cell hyperplasia (10%) = increase in number of G-cells in gastric antrum
   - lack of gastrin elevation after secretin injection
   - exaggerated gastrin elevation after protein meal

Age: middle age; M > F

- Clinical tetrad:
  (1) Gastric hypersecretion: refractory response to histamine stimulation test concerning HCl concentration; increased basal secretion (>60% of augmented secretion is diagnostic)
  (2) Hypergastrinemia >1000 ng/L (during fasting)
  (3) Hyperacidity with basal acid output >15 mEq/h
  (4) Diarrhea (30%), steatorrhea (40%): may be sole complaint in 10%, frequently nocturnal; secondary to inactivation of pancreatic enzymes by large volumes of HCl
- severe intractable pain (90%)
- ulcer perforation (30%)
- positive secretin test = increase in serum gastrin level by >200 ng/L after administration of 2 IU/kg of secretin

√ ulcers (atypical location + course should suggest diagnosis):
  Location: duodenal bulb (65%) + stomach (20%), near ligament of Treitz (25%), duodenal C-loop (5%), distal esophagus (5%)
  Multiplicity: solitary ulcer (90%), multiple ulcers (10%)
  √ recurrent / intractable ulcers
  √ marginal ulcers in postgastrectomy patient
    (a) on gastric side of anastomosis
    (b) on mesenteric border of efferent loop
√ prominence of area gastricae (hyperplasia of parietal cell mass)
√ enlargement of rugal folds
√ sluggish gastric peristalsis (? hypokalemia)
√ "wet stomach" = dilution of barium by excess secretions in nondilated nonobstructed stomach
√ gastroesophageal reflux (common) + esophagitis
√ dilatation of duodenum + upper small bowel (fluid overload)
√ thickened folds in duodenum + jejunum (edema)
√ rapid small-bowel transit time

mnemonic: "FUSED"
Folds (thickened, gastric folds)
Ulcers (often multiple, postbulbar)
Secretions increased (refractory to histamine)
Edema (of proximal small bowel)
Diarrhea

Cx: (1) Malignant islet cell tumor (in 60%)
(2) Liver metastases will continue to stimulate gastric secretion

Rx:
(1) Control of gastric hypersecretion:
  (a) H2-receptor antagonist: cimetidine, ranitidine, famotidine
  (b) Hydrogen-potassium adenosine triphosphatase inhibitor (omeprazole)
(2) Resection of gastrinoma if found (because of malignant potential)
(3) Total gastrectomy

DIFFERENTIAL DIAGNOSIS OF UROGENITAL DISORDERS

RENAL FAILURE
= reduction in renal function
- rise in serum creatinine >2.5 mg/dL

Acute Renal Failure
= clinical condition associated with rapid steadily increasing azotemia ± oliguria (<500 mL urine per day) over days / weeks

Etiology:

A. PRERENAL
   = renal hypoperfusion secondary to systemic illness
   1. Fluid + electrolyte depletion
   2. Hemorrhage
   3. Hepatic failure + hepatorenal syndrome
      √ abnormally elevated resistive index
   4. Cardiac failure
   5. Sepsis
      √ resistive index <0.75 in 80% of kidneys

B. RENAL (most common)
   1. Acute tubular necrosis:
      ischemia, nephrotoxins, radiographic contrast, hemoglobulinuria, myoglobulinuria, myocardial infarction, burns
      √ resistive index ≥0.75 in 91% of kidneys
   2. Acute glomerulonephritis + small vessel disease:
      acute poststrep glomerulonephritis, rapidly progressive glomerulonephritis, lupus, polyarteritis nodosa, Schönlein-Henoch purpura, subacute bacterial endocarditis, serum sickness, Goodpasture syndrome, malignant hypertension, hemolytic uremic syndrome, drug-related vasculitis, abruptio placentae
      √ normal resistive index <0.70
   3. Acute tubulointerstitial nephritis:
      drug reaction, pyelonephritis, papillary necrosis
      √ abnormal resistive index
   4. Intrarenal precipitation (hypercalcemia, urate, myeloma protein)
   5. Arterial / venous obstruction
   6. Acute cortical necrosis

C. POSTRENAL (5%)
   = result of outflow obstruction (rare)
   1. Prostatism
   2. Tumors of bladder, retroperitoneum, pelvis
   3. Calculus
   √ hydronephrosis

D. CONGENITAL
   bilateral renal agenesis / dysplasia / infantile polycystic kidney disease, congenital nephrotic syndrome, congenital nephritis, perinatal hypoxia

Incidence: ATN + prerenal disease account for 75% of acute renal failure

Chronic Renal Failure
= decrease in renal function over months / years

Incidence:
end-stage renal disease in 0.01% of U.S. population; 85,000 patients/year undergo hemodialysis; 8,000 renal transplantations/year

Etiology:

A. INFLAMMATION / INFECTION
   1. Glomerulonephritis
   2. Chronic pyelonephritis
   3. Tuberculosis
   4. Sarcoidosis

B. VASCULAR
   1. Renal vascular disease
   2. Bilateral renal vein thrombosis

C. DYSPROTEINEMIA
   1. Myeloma
   2. Amyloid
   3. Cryoglobulinemia
   4. Waldenström macroglobulinemia

D. METABOLIC
   1. Diabetes
   2. Gout
   3. Hypercalcemia
   4. Hyperoxaluria
   5. Cystinosis
   6. Fabry disease

E. CONGENITAL
   1. Polycystic kidney disease
   2. Multicystic dysplastic kidney
   3. Medullary cystic disease
   4. Alport syndrome
   5. Infantile nephrotic syndrome

F. MISCELLANEOUS
   1. Hepatorenal syndrome
   2. Radiation

Musculoskeletal Manifestations of CRF
1. Renal osteodystrophy = combination of 2° HPT, osteoporosis, osteosclerosis, osteomalacia, soft-tissue and vascular calcifications
2. Aluminum toxicity (1–30%)
   Cause: ingestion of aluminum salts phosphate-binding antacids (to control hyperphosphatemia)
   - aluminum serum level >100 ng/mL
   √ signs of osteomalacia (>3 insufficiency fractures with predominant involvement of ribs)
   √ avascular necrosis
   √ lack of osteosclerosis
   √ less evidence of subperiosteal resorption
3. Amyloid deposition
   Path: amyloid consists of β_2-microglobulin

Organs: bone, tenosynovium (carpal tunnel syndrome), vertebral disk, articular cartilage + capsule, ligament, muscle

4. Destructive spondyloarthropathy (15%)
   √ diskovertebral junction erosion + sclerosis
   √ vertebral body compression
   √ disk space narrowing
   √ Schmorl node formation
   √ lack of osteophytosis
   √ facet involvement with subluxation
5. Tendon rupture
6. Crystal deposition disease
   Type: calcium hydroxyapatite, CPPD, calcium oxalate, monosodium urate
7. Osteomyelitis + septic arthritis
8. Avascular necrosis (in up to 40%)

DIABETES INSIPIDUS

= characterized by daily production of very large volume of dilute urine (specific gravity <1.005, <200 mOsm/L)

Pituitary Diabetes Insipidus

= HYPOTHALAMIC DIABETES INSIPIDUS
= VASOPRESSIN-SENSITIVE DIABETES INSIPIDUS
= vasopressin (ADH) production is reduced to <10%

Cause:
(a) idiopathic (27%)
   septooptic dysplasia / rare familial (autosomal dominant X-linked) / sporadic disorder
   Histo: atrophic supraoptic nucleus
   • never associated with anterior pituitary dysfunction
(b) pituitary destruction by tumor / infiltrative disorder (32%):
   in childhood: hypothalamic glioma, tuber cinereum hamartoma, craniopharyngioma, Langerhans histiocytosis, germinoma, leukemia, complication of meningitis
   in adulthood: sarcoidosis, TB, metastasis
   • in 60% associated with anterior pituitary dysfunction
(c) pituitary destruction by surgery (20%)
   • always associated with anterior pituitary dysfunction
(d) head injury (17%)
   • in 20% associated with anterior pituitary dysfunction

◊ A lesion in the posterior pituitary will NOT produce diabetes insipidus, because it is simply the storage space for vasopressin!

Psychogenic Water Intoxication

= compulsive intake of large amounts of fluid, which leads to inhibition of normal vasopressin production
• water deprivation test

Nephrogenic Diabetes Insipidus

= poor reabsorption of water in collecting ducts due to end-organ resistance to vasopressin

Cause:
(a) congenital
   1. Rare X-linked recessive genetic disorder with unresponsiveness of tubules + collecting system to vasopressin (in infants + young males) with variable expression
   2. Autosomal dominant form (rare)
(b) acquired = nephrogenic DI syndrome
   = disorders affecting the medulla / distal nephrons: medullary + polycystic disease, sickle cell nephropathy, postobstructive uropathy, reflux nephropathy, chronic uremic nephropathy, unilateral renal artery stenosis, acute tubular necrosis, drug toxicity, analgesic nephropathy, hypokalemic + hypercalcemic nephropathy, amyloidosis, sarcoidosis

• symptoms in infancy:
  • vomiting secondary to hypernatremic dehydration
  • mental retardation
  • caloric growth failure (water favored over formula)
• symptoms after infancy:
  • increased fluid intake
  • avoiding urination

√ bilateral hydroureteronephrosis

Rx: thiazide diuretics, low-salt diet, encouragement of frequent micturition, indomethacin

HYPERCALCEMIA

mnemonic: "SHAMPOO DIRT"
Sarcoidosis
Hyperparathyroidism, **H**yperthyroidism
Alkali-milk syndrome
Metastases, **M**yeloma
Paget disease
Osteogenesis imperfecta
Osteopetrosis
D vitamin intoxication
Immobility
Renal tubular acidosis
Thiazides

POLYCYTHEMIA

Cause: increased level of erythropoietin (acting on erythroid stem cells) secondary to a decrease in pO_2; erythropoietin precursor is produced in juxtaglomerular epithelioid cells of kidney + converted in blood

A. RENAL
   (a) intrarenal
      1. Vascular impairment
      2. Renal cell carcinoma (5%)
      3. Wilms tumor
      4. Benign fibroma
      5. Simple cyst (14%)
      6. Polycystic kidney disease
   (b) postrenal
      1. Obstructive uropathy (14%)

GU

B. EXTRARENAL
   (a) liver disease
      1. Hepatoma
      2. Regenerating hepatic cells
   (b) adrenal disease
      1. Pheochromocytoma
      2. Aldosteronoma
      3. Cushing disease
C. CNS DISEASE
   1. Cerebellar hemangioblastoma
D. Large uterine myomas

NOT in: renal vein thrombosis, multicystic dysplastic kidney, medullary sponge kidney

ARTERIAL HYPERTENSION

A. PRIMARY / ESSENTIAL HYPERTENSION (85–90%)
B. SECONDARY HYPERTENSION
   (a) Renal parenchymal disease (5–10%)
   (b) Potentially curable secondary hypertension (1–2%)
      — vascular
         1. Renovascular disease 0.18–4.4%
         2. Coarctation 0.6%
      — hormonal
         1. Pheochromocytoma 0.04–0.2%
         2. Cushing syndrome 0.3%
         3. Primary aldosteronism 0.01–0.4%
         4. Hyperthyroidism
         5. Myxedema
      — renal
         1. Unilateral renal disease

Renovascular Hypertension

= normalization of blood pressure following nephrectomy / reestablishment of normal renal blood flow (Dx made in retrospect)

Incidence: 1–5% of general population; 2nd most common cause of potentially curable hypertension

Pathophysiology:
usually >50% stenosis at any level in renovascular bed leads to mildly reduced pressure in glomerular afferent arteriole (pressure falls precipitously in >80% stenosis); reduced pressure stimulates release of renin followed by angiotensin-II, and aldosterone causing
(a) constriction of efferent glomerular arterioles
(b) increase in systemic hypertension
(c) sodium retention

Cause:
1. Atherosclerosis (60–90%) in individuals >50 years of age
2. Fibromuscular dysplasia (10–35%) in women <40 years of age
3. Neurofibromatosis
4. Pheochromocytoma
5. Fibrous bands (congenital stenosis, retroperitoneal fibrosis, postradiation artery stenosis)
6. Arteritis (Buerger disease, polyarteritis nodosa, Takayasu disease, thrombangitis obliterans, syphilitic arteritis)
7. Arteriovenous malformation / fistula
   • renin-mediated hypertension (due to renal ischemia distal to fistula)
8. Thromboembolic disease (eg, atrial fibrillation, prosthetic valve thrombi, cardiac myxoma, paradoxical emboli, atheromatous emboli)
9. Renal artery aneurysm
10. Extrinsic compression (eg, renal cyst, neoplasm, chronic subcapsular hematoma) = Page kidney
11. Middle aortic syndrome, aortic dissection, dissecting aortic aneurysm
12. Posttraumatic renovascular hypertension
   (a) occlusion of main renal artery
   (b) significant stenosis by intimal flap
   (c) severe renal contusion
   (d) segmental renal artery branch injury

◊ Renal artery stenosis is present in 77% of hypertensive patients!
◊ Renal artery stenosis is present in 32–49% of normotensive patients!
◊ 15–20% of patients remain hypertensive after restoration of normal renal blood flow!

Clinical findings that suggest renovascular disease:
1. Onset of HTN <30 years and >50 years of age
2. Hypertension refractory to therapy
3. Accelerated / malignant hypertension
4. Unexplained large increases in blood pressure above previously controlled / baseline values
5. Symptomatic hypertension

Rx: (1) Relieving renal artery stenosis
(2) Angiotensin-converting enzyme inhibitor

Hypertension in Children

Prevalence: 1–3%
1. Coarse renal cortex scarring (36%)
2. Glomerulonephritis (23%)
3. Coarctation of aorta (10%)
4. Renovascular disease (10%)
5. Polycystic renal disease (6%)
6. Hemolytic-uremic syndrome (4%)
7. Catecholamine excess [pheochromocytoma, neuroblastoma] (3%)
8. Renal tumor (2%)
9. Essential hypertension (3%)

ARTERIAL HYPOTENSION

Cause: intrarenal hypovolemia, primary vasoconstriction, reduced glomerular filtration, depletion of intratubular urine volume

◊ May occur as a contrast reaction!
◊ Urogram reverts to normal after reversion of hypotension!
√ bilateral small smooth kidneys (compared with size on preliminary films)
√ increasingly dense nephrogram

√ usually NO opacification of collecting system
√ initially opacification of collecting system if hypotension occurs during contrast injection

URINARY TRACT INFECTION

= pure growths of >100,000 organisms/mL urine

Prevalence: 3% of girls + 1% of boys during first 10 years of life

Underlying radiologic abnormality:
1. Vesicoureteral reflux = VUR (30–40%)
2. Obstructive uropathy (8%)
3. Reflux nephropathy / scar formation (6%)
   ◊ The prevalence of an underlying radiologic abnormality depends on age, sex, and frequency of previous infections!

Imaging objective:
1. Identify patients at risk for reflux nephropathy
2. Detect reflux nephropathy / scars
3. Detect obstructive uropathy
4. Minimize radiation, morbidity, and cost

VCUG:
for children <5 years of age with infection; normal results in 60–70%

Renal cortical scintigraphy (DMSA / glucoheptonate):
to detect acute pyelonephritis (risk for scarring) / scar; with VUR there is twice the risk of cortical defects than without VUR

GAS IN URINARY TRACT

A. Renal emphysema = renal / perirenal gas
   1. Emphysematous pyelonephritis
   2. Emphysematous pyelitis
   3. Gas-forming perinephric abscess
   4. Perinephric emphysema

B. Bladder
   1. Emphysematous cystitis

C. Trauma
   1. Penetrating trauma
   2. Ureterosigmoidostomy, ileal conduit, catheterization with vesicoureteral reflux, percutaneous procedure
      CAVE: anomalous posterior position of colon
   3. Infarction of renal carcinoma (therapeutic / spontaneous)

D. Fistula to urinary tract
   Connection: bronchus / cutis / GI tract (colon > duodenum > stomach > small bowel > appendix
   1. Inflammation: chronic purulent renal infection, diverticulitis, Crohn disease
   2. Neoplastic: colonic carcinoma

ADRENAL GLAND

Adrenal Medullary Disease
1. Neuroblastoma
2. Ganglioneuroblastoma
3. Ganglioneuroma
4. Pheochromocytoma

Adrenal Cortical Disease
1. Adrenal hyperplasia
2. Adrenocortical adenoma
3. Adrenocortical carcinoma
4. Cushing syndrome
5. Conn syndrome
6. Adrenogenital syndrome

Adrenocortical Hyperfunction
1. Adrenogenital syndrome
2. Conn syndrome = hyperaldosteronism
   √ solitary unilateral adrenal adenoma + normal contralateral gland on CT may be due to:
   (a) aldosterone-producing adrenocortical adenoma
   (b) renin-responsive aldosterone-producing adenoma
   (c) idiopathic hyperaldosteronism with dominant hyperplastic / nonfunctional adenoma
3. Cushing syndrome = hypercortisolism
   DDx of Cushing syndrome
   A. FOCAL UNILATERAL ADRENAL MASS
      √ 2–4-cm focal mass in one adrenal gland + atrophy of contralateral gland = adrenal adenoma
      √ >4-cm large focal mass with central necrosis in one adrenal gland + atrophy of contralateral gland = adrenal adenocarcinoma
   B. BILATERAL ADRENAL ENLARGEMENT
      √ diffuse uniform thickening = Cushing disease
   C. MULTIPLE BILATERAL ADRENAL NODULES
      √ macronodules = multinodular hyperplasia of long-standing Cushing disease
      √ large nodules (autonomous ACTH-independent) = massive macronodular hyperplasia
      √ small nodules = primary pigmented nodular adrenal disease

Bilateral Large Adrenals
mnemonic: "4 H PM"
Hodgkin disease
Hyperplasia
Hemorrhage
Histoplasmosis / TB
Pheochromocytoma
Metastasis

Unilateral Adrenal Mass
Criteria to differentiate benign from malignant:

A. NECT attenuation
   <10 HU = benign lipid-rich adenoma / cyst
   >10 HU = indeterminate
   Reason: 60–70% of benign adrenocortical tumors contain intracytoplasmic fat

B. CECT (15-minute delay):
<35 HU = lipid-poor adenoma
>35 HU = indeterminate lesion
Cause: rapid contrast washout from benign lesions
N.B.: an initial dynamic CECT is not useful for lesion characterization!

C. CECT relative enhancement washout (15-minute HU / initial peak HU x 100%):
washout >50% = lipid-poor adenoma
washout <50% = indeterminate mass
Cause: nonadenomas have a disturbed capillary permeability with prolonged retention of contrast material

D. Chemical shift MRI:
Reason: fat protons precess faster than water
√ fat + water summate to intermediate signal intensity on in-phase images
√ fat + water signals cancel each other out to low signal intensity on out-of-phase images = adenoma

E. A lesion without change in size over 6 months is likely benign!

F. Large size, irregularity, inhomogeneity are suggestive of malignancy

mnemonic: "PLAN My HAM"
Pheochromocytoma
Lymphoma
Adenoma
Neuroblastoma
Myelolipoma
Hemorrhage
Adenocarcinoma
Metastasis

Small Unilateral Adrenal Tumor

◊ Incidental discovery of adrenal mass in 1% of all CT!
(a) mass <3 cm in diameter is likely (in 87%) benign
(b) mass >5 cm in diameter is likely malignant

1. Cortical adenoma (in 1–9% of autopsies)
   √ <10 HU imply (in 96%) an adenoma
2. Metastasis
3. Pheochromocytoma
4. Asymmetric hyperplasia
5. Granulomatous disease (TB, histoplasmosis)
   √ diffuse enlargement / discrete mass
   √ ± central cystic changes ± calcification
6. Myelolipoma

Large Solid Adrenal Mass

1. Cortical carcinoma
2. Pheochromocytoma
3. Neuroblastoma / ganglioneuroma
4. Myelolipoma
5. Metastasis
6. Hemorrhage
7. Inflammation
8. Abscess (eg, histoplasmosis, tuberculosis)
9. Hemangioma

Cystic Adrenal Mass

1. Pseudocyst: old hemorrhage / infarction
2. Vascular cystic space (endothelial lining): lymphangioma, hemangioma
3. True cyst (epithelial lining): glandular cyst, embryonal cyst, mesothelial inclusion cyst
4. Parasitic cyst: hydatid cyst
5. Hemorrhagic complication / degeneration of a tumor: cystic adenoma, cystic pheochromocytoma, cystic adenomatoid tumor, cystic adrenocortical carcinoma, schwannoma
6. Neuroblastoma (rare)
7. Cortical adenoma with low density

Adrenal Calcification

A. TUMOR
   1. Neuroblastoma
   2. Pheochromocytoma
   3. Adrenal adenoma
   4. Adrenal carcinoma
   5. Dermoid

B. VASCULAR
   1. Hemorrhage (neonatal, sepsis)

C. INFECTION
   1. Tuberculosis
   2. Histoplasmosis
   3. Waterhouse-Friderichsen syndrome

D. ENDOCRINE
   1. Addison disease (TB)

E. OTHERS
   1. Wolman disease

KIDNEY

Developmental Renal Anomalies

Numerary Renal Anomaly

1. Supernumerary kidney
2. Complete / partial renal duplication
3. Abortive calyx
4. Unicaliceal (unipapillary) kidney

Renal Underdevelopment

1. Congenital renal hypoplasia
2. Renal agenesis
3. Renal dysgenesis

Renal Ectopia

Normal location of kidneys: 1st–3rd lumbar vertebra
Incidence: 0.2% (autopsy series)
Cause: failure of kidney to ascend by 8 weeks GA
At risk of: hydronephrosis due to UPJ obstruction, infection, calculi
√ unusual developmental "funny-looking calices" often misinterpreted as obstructive

LONGITUDINAL RENAL ECTOPIA

Location: pelvic, sacral, lower lumbar level, intrathoracic; L > R

√ must demonstrate aberrant arteries

DDx: displacement through diaphragmatic hernia (nonaberrant); hypermobile kidney

Pelvic kidney

= ectopic kidney due to failure of renal ascent

Incidence: 1:725 births

May be associated with:

(1) vesicoureteral reflux
(2) hydronephrosis due to abnormally high insertion of ureter into renal pelvis
(3) hypospadia (common)
(4) contralateral renal agenesis

√ blood supply via iliac vessels / aorta

√ nonrotation = anteriorly positioned renal pelvis (common)

CROSSED RENAL ECTOPIA

= kidney located on opposite side of midline from its ureteral orifice; usually L > R and crossed kidney inferior to normal kidney

Cause: ? faulty development of ureteral bud, vascular obstruction of renal ascent

Associated with: obstruction urolithiasis, infection, reflux, megaureter, hypospadia, cryptorchidism, urethral valves, multicystic dysplasia

(a) fused (common)
(b) separate (rare)

√ invariably aberrant renal arteries

√ distal ureter inserts into trigone on the side of origin

RENAL FUSION

= "lump, cake, disk, horseshoe"

Cx: aberrant arteries may cross and obstruct ureter

Horseshoe kidney

Discoid / pancake kidney

= bilateral fused pelvic kidneys

Associated with:

abnormal testicular descent, tetralogy of Fallot, vaginal agenesis, sacral agenesis, caudal regression, anal anomalies

RENAL MALROTATION

√ collecting structures may be positioned ventrally (most common), lateral (rare), dorsal (rarer), transverse (along AP axis)

√ "funny-looking calices" = developmental usually nonobstructive ectasia

Absent Renal Outline on Plain Film

A. ABSENT KIDNEY
   1. Congenital absence
   2. S/P nephrectomy
B. SMALL KIDNEY
   1. Renal hypoplasia
   2. Renal atrophy
C. RENAL ECTOPIA
   1. Pelvic kidney
   2. Crossed fused ectopia
   3. Intrathoracic kidney
D. OBLITERATION OF PERIRENAL FAT
   1. Perirenal abscess
   2. Perirenal hematoma
   3. Renal tumors

Nonvisualized Kidney on Excretory Urography

A. ABSENCE OF KIDNEY
   1. Agenesis
   2. Surgical absence
   3. Renal ectopia
B. LOSS OF PERFUSION
   1. Chronic infarction
   2. Unilateral renal vein thrombosis
C. TRAUMA
   1. Thrombosis of main renal artery
   2. Severe contusion (with renal vascular spasm)
   3. Avulsion of renal pedicle
D. HIGH-GRADE URINARY OBSTRUCTION
   1. Hydronephrosis
   2. Ureteropelvic junction obstruction
E. REPLACED NORMAL RENAL PARENCHYMA
   1. Multicystic dysplastic kidney
   2. Unilateral polycystic kidney disease
   3. Renal tumor (RCC, TCC, Wilms tumor)
   4. Xanthogranulomatous pyelonephritis

Unilateral Large Smooth Kidney

A. PRERENAL
   (a) arterial: acute arterial infarction
   (b) venous: acute renal vein thrombosis
B. INTRARENAL
   (a) congenital: duplicated pelvicaliceal system, crossed fused ectopia, multicystic dysplastic kidney, adult polycystic kidney (in 8% unilateral)
   (b) infectious: acute bacterial nephritis
   (c) adaptation: compensatory hypertrophy
C. POSTRENAL
   (a) collecting system: obstructive uropathy

mnemonic: "AROMA"

Acute pyelonephritis
Renal vein thrombosis
Obstructive uropathy
Miscellaneous (compensatory hypertrophy, duplication)
Arterial obstruction (infarction)

Bilateral Large Kidneys

Average renal length by x-ray: M = 13 cm; F = 12.5 cm

1. PROTEIN DEPOSITION
   amyloidosis, multiple myeloma
2. INTERSTITIAL FLUID ACCUMULATION
   acute tubular necrosis, acute cortical necrosis, acute arterial infarction, renal vein thrombosis
3. CELLULAR INFILTRATION
   (a) Inflammatory cells: acute interstitial nephritis, acute bacterial nephritis
   (b) Malignant cells: leukemia / lymphoma, bilateral Wilms tumor, nephroblastomatosis
4. PROLIFERATIVE / NECROTIZING DISORDERS
   (a) Glomerulonephritis (GN)
   acute (poststreptococcal) GN, rapidly progressive GN, idiopathic membranous GN, lobular GN, membranoproliferative GN, IgA nephropathy, glomerulosclerosis, glomerulosclerosis related to heroin abuse
   (b) Multisystem disease
   polyarteritis nodosa, systemic lupus erythematosus, Wegener granulomatosis, allergic angitis, diabetic glomerulosclerosis, Goodpasture syndrome (lung hemorrhage + glomerulonephritis), Schönlein-Henoch syndrome (anaphylactoid purpura), thrombotic thrombocytopenic purpura, focal glomerulonephritis associated with subacute bacterial endocarditis
5. URINE OUTFLOW OBSTRUCTION
   bilateral hydronephrosis: congenital / acquired
6. HORMONAL STIMULUS
   acromegaly, compensatory hypertrophy, nephromegaly associated with cirrhosis / hyperalimentation / diabetes mellitus
7. DEVELOPMENTAL
   bilateral renal duplication, horseshoe kidney, polycystic kidney disease
8. MISCELLANEOUS
   acute urate nephropathy, glycogen storage disease, hemophilia, sickle cell disease, Fabry disease, physiologic response to contrast material and diuretics

mnemonic: "FOG P"

Fluid:	= edema of kidney (ATN, acute cortical necrosis)
Other:	leukemia, acromegaly, sickle cell anemia, bilateral duplication, acute urate nephropathy
Glomerular disease:	acute GN, lupus, polyarteritis nodosa, diabetes mellitus
Protein deposition:	multiple myeloma, amyloidosis

Bilateral Small Kidneys

A. PRERENAL = VASCULAR
   1. Arterial hypotension (acute)
   2. Generalized arteriosclerosis
   3. Atheroembolic disease
   4. Benign & malignant nephrosclerosis

B. INTRARENAL
   1. Hereditary nephropathies:
      medullary cystic disease, hereditary chronic nephritis (Alport syndrome)
   2. Chronic glomerulonephritis
   3. Amyloidosis (late)

C. POSTRENAL
   1. Papillary necrosis

D. CAUSES OF UNILATERAL SMALL KIDNEY occurring bilaterally

mnemonic: "CAPE HANA"
Chronic glomerulonephritis
Arteriosclerosis
Papillary necrosis
Embolic disease (secondary to atherosclerosis)
Hypotension
Alport syndrome
Nephrosclerosis
Amyloidosis (late)

Unilateral Small Kidney

A. PRERENAL = VASCULAR
   1. Lobar infarction
   2. Chronic infarction
   3. Renal artery stenosis
   4. Radiation nephritis

B. INTRARENAL = PARENCHYMAL
   1. Congenital hypoplasia
   2. Multicystic dysplastic kidney (in adult)
   3. Postinflammatory atrophy

C. POSTRENAL = COLLECTING SYSTEM
   1. Reflux nephropathy = chronic atrophic pyelonephritis
   2. Postobstructive atrophy

mnemonic: "RIP R HIP"
Reflux atrophy
Ischemia (renal artery stenosis)
Postobstructive atrophy
Radiation therapy
Hypoplasia (congenital)
Infarction
Postinflammatory atrophy

Increased Echogenicity of Renal Cortex

= RENAL MEDICAL DISEASE
= diffuse increase in cortical echogenicity with preservation of corticomedullary junction

Path: deposition of collagen / calcium in interstitial, glomerular, tubular, vascular disease

√ echointensity of cortex greater than liver / spleen ± equal to renal sinus
√ renal size may be normal; enlarged kidneys suggest active stage of renal disease; small kidneys suggest chronic + often end-stage renal disease

GU

1. Acute / chronic glomerulonephritis
2. Renal transplant rejection
3. Lupus nephritis
4. Hypertensive nephrosclerosis
5. Renal cortical necrosis
6. Methemoglobulinuric renal failure
7. Alport syndrome
8. Amyloidosis
9. Diabetic nephrosclerosis
10. Nephrotoxin-induced acute tubular necrosis
11. End-stage renal disease

Hyperechoic Renal Pyramids in Children

A. NEPHROCALCINOSIS
   (a) iatrogenic (most common cause): furosemide (Rx for BPD), vitamin D (Rx for hypophosphatemic rickets)
   (b) noniatrogenic:
      1. Idiopathic hypercalcemia
      2. Williams syndrome
      3. Absorptive hypercalcemia
      4. Hyperparathyroidism
      5. Milk-alkali syndrome
      6. Kenny-Caffey syndrome
      7. Distal renal tubular acidosis
      8. Malignant tumors
      9. Chronic glomerulonephritis
      10. Sjögren syndrome (distal RTA)
      11. Sarcoidosis

B. METABOLIC DISEASE
   1. Gout
   2. Lesch-Nyhan syndrome (urate)
   3. Fanconi syndrome
   4. Glycogen storage disease (distal RTA)
   5. Wilson disease (distal RTA)
   6. Alpha-1 antitrypsin deficiency
   7. Tyrosinemia
   8. Cystinosis
   9. Oxalosis
   10. Crohn disease

C. HYPOKALEMIA
   1. Primary aldosteronism
   2. Pseudo-Bartter syndrome

D. PROTEIN DEPOSITS
   1. Infant dehydration with presumed Tamm-Horsfall proteinuria
   2. Toxic shock syndrome

E. VASCULAR CONGESTION
   1. Sickle cell anemia

F. INFECTION
   1. Candida / CMV nephritis
   2. AIDS-associated Mycobacterium avium-intracellulare

G. FIBROSIS OF RENAL PYRAMIDS

H. CYSTIC MEDULLARY DISEASE
   1. Medullary sponge kidney
   2. Congenital hepatic fibrosis with tubular ectasia

I. INTRARENAL REFLUX
   1. Chronic pyelonephritis

Iron Accumulation in Kidney

A. RENAL CORTEX
   1. Paroxysmal nocturnal hemoglobulinuria (= intravascular extrasplenic hemolysis)
   2. Sickle cell anemia

B. RENAL MEDULLA
   1. Hemorrhagic fever with renal syndrome (uncommon viral illness caused by Hanta virus)
      Triad: (1) renal medullary hemorrhage
      (2) right atrial hemorrhage
      (3) necrosis of anterior pituitary

Depression of Renal Margins

1. Fetal lobation
   √ notching between normal calices
2. Splenic impression
   √ flattened upper outer margin of left kidney
3. Chronic atrophic pyelonephritis
   √ indentation over clubbed calices
4. Renal infarct
   √ normal calices
5. Chronic renal ischemia
   √ normal calices

Enlargement of Iliopsoas Compartment

A. INFECTION
   (a) from retroperitoneal organs
      1. Renal infection
      2. Complicated pancreatitis
      3. Postoperative aortic graft infection
   (b) from spine
      1. Osteomyelitis / postoperative complication of bone surgery
      2. Diskitis / postoperative complication from disk surgery
   (c) from GI tract
      1. Crohn disease
      2. Appendicitis
   (d) others
      1. Pelvic inflammatory disease / postpartum infection
      2. Sepsis

B. HEMORRHAGE
   1. Coagulopathy and anticoagulant therapy
   2. Ruptured aortic aneurysm
   3. Postoperative aneurysm repair / other surgery / trauma

C. NEOPLASTIC DISEASE
   (a) extrinsic
      1. Lymphoma
      2. Metastatic lymphadenopathy
      3. Bone metastases with soft-tissue involvement
      4. Retroperitoneal sarcoma
   (b) intrinsic
      1. Muscle tumors
      2. Nervous system tumors
      3. Lipoma / liposarcoma

D. MISCELLANEOUS
1. Pseudoenlargement of psoas muscle compared with de facto atrophy of contralateral side in neuromuscular disease
2. Fluid collections
urinoma, lymphocele, pancreatic pseudocyst, enlargement of iliopsoas bursa
3. Pelvic venous thrombosis
√ diffuse swelling of all muscles (edema)

RENAL MASS

Bilateral Renal Masses

A. MALIGNANT TUMOR
1. Malignant lymphoma / Hodgkin disease
2. Metastases
3. Renal cell carcinoma
4. Wilms tumor

B. BENIGN TUMOR
1. Angiomyolipoma
2. Nephroblastomatosis

C. CYSTS
1. Adult polycystic kidney disease
2. Acquired cystic kidney disease

Renal Mass in Neonate

A. UNILATERAL
1. Multicystic kidney (15%)
2. Hydronephrosis (25%)
(a) UPJ obstruction
(b) upper moiety of duplication
3. Renal vein thrombosis
4. Mesoblastic nephroma
5. Rare: Wilms tumor, teratoma

B. BILATERAL
1. Hydronephrosis
2. Polycystic kidney disease
3. Multicystic kidney + contralateral hydronephrosis
4. Nephroblastomatosis
5. Bilateral multicystic kidney

Renal Mass in Older Child

A. SINGLE MASS
(a) single solid mass
1. Wilms tumor (87%)
2. Clear cell sarcoma of kidney (6%)
3. Mesoblastic nephroma (2%)
4. Rhabdoid tumor (2%)
5. Renal cell carcinoma (<0.5%)
6. Teratoma
7. Intrarenal neuroblastoma

(b) single cystic mass
1. Focal hydronephrosis
2. Multilocular cystic nephroma
3. Traumatic cyst, abscess

B. MULTIPLE MASSES
1. Nephroblastomatosis
2. Multiple Wilms tumors
3. Angiomyolipoma
4. Lymphoma (<0.5%)
5. Leukemia
6. Adult polycystic kidney disease
7. Abscesses

Growth Pattern of Renal Lesions

Renal Lesion with Expansile Growth Pattern

1. Renal cell carcinoma
2. Oncocytoma
3. Angiomyolipoma
4. Juxtaglomerular tumor
5. Metastatic tumor (eg, lymphoma)
6. Mesenchymal tumor

Renal Lesions with Infiltrative Growth Pattern

Imaging hallmarks:
√ growth initially respects renal contour
√ invasion of normal structures
√ poorly defined interface between normal renal parenchyma and lesion
√ enlarged kidney with preservation of reniform shape

IVP:
√ decreased / absent nephrogram

Angio:
√ vascular encasement, pruning, amputation
√ no vascular displacement

CT:
√ poorly marginated area of diminished enhancement
√ encasement of collecting system without displacement
√ replacement of renal sinus fat

US:
√ poorly circumscribed hypo-/hyperechoic regions

A. NEOPLASM
(a) lymphoproliferative
1. Lymphoma / leukemia
2. Extramedullary plasmacytoma

(b) epithelial tumor of renal parenchyma
1. Renal cell carcinoma (unusual)
2. High-grade and sarcomatoid carcinoma

(c) epithelial tumors of the renal pelvis
1. Invasive transitional cell carcinoma
2. Squamous cell carcinoma

(d) medullary tumor of uncertain cell origin
1. Collecting duct carcinoma
2. Renal medullary carcinoma

(e) metastases
(f) renal sarcomas
(g) pediatric tumor
1. Mesoblastic nephroma
2. Rhabdoid tumor of the kidney
3. Nephroblastomatosis
4. Primitive neuroectodermal tumor
5. Wilms tumor (unusual)

B. INFLAMMATION
1. Bacterial pyelonephritis
2. Xanthogranulomatous pyelonephritis
3. Renal parenchymal malacoplakia

Local Bulge in Renal Contour

A. CYST
   1. Simple renal cyst
B. TUMOR
   1. Adenocarcinoma
   2. Angiomyolipoma
   3. Pseudotumor
C. INFECTION
   1. Subcapsular abscess
   2. XGP
D. TRAUMA
   1. Subcapsular hematoma
E. DILATED COLLECTING SYSTEM

Unilateral Renal Mass

Solid Renal Mass

A. TUMORS
   (a) primary malignant:
   - epithelial tumor of renal parenchyma: adenocarcinoma (83%), papillary neoplasm (14%), chromophobe carcinoma (4%), renal neuroendocrine tumors (carcinoid, small cell carcinoma), Wilms tumor (6%),
   - epithelial tumor of renal pelvis: TCC (8%), squamous cell carcinoma
   - medullary tumor: renal medullary carcinoma, renal collecting duct carcinoma = Bellini duct carcinoma (1%)
   - renal sarcoma (2%)

   in horseshoe kidney: adenocarcinoma (45%), Wilms tumor (28%), transitional cell carcinoma (20%)

   (b) secondary malignant: malignant lymphoma / Hodgkin disease, metastases, invasive transitional cell carcinoma

   (c) benign: adenoma, oncocytoma, hamartoma (mesoblastic nephroma, angiomyolipoma, myolipoma, lipoma, leiomyoma, fibroma), hemangioma

B. INFLAMMATORY MASSES
   acute focal pyelonephritis, renal abscess, xanthogranulomatous pyelonephritis, malacoplakia, tuberculoma

Fluid-filled Mass

A. CYSTS
   1. Simple renal cyst
   2. Inherited cystic disease: multicystic dysplastic kidney disease (Potter type II), multilocular cystic nephroma
   3. Focal hydronephrosis
B. VASCULAR
   1. Arteriovenous malformation
   2. Arteriovenous fistula
      = single dilated artery + vein
      √ tortuous varices over time
      √ enlargement of renal vein
      Cx: hydronephrosis

◊ Lesions <1 cm often cannot be clearly characterized
◊ Lesions 1–1.5 cm can often be ignored, particularly in elderly / patients with significant other disease

Calcified Renal Mass

◊ A calcified renal mass is malignant in 75% of cases!
◊ Lesions with
   (a) nonperipheral calcifications are malignant in 87%!
   (b) peripheral calcifications are malignant in 20%!

A. TUMOR
   1. Renal cell carcinoma (calcifies in 8–20%)
      √ calcifications generally nonperipheral, sometimes along fibrous capsule
   2. Wilms tumor
   3. Transitional cell carcinoma (rare)
   4. Osteosarcoma of renal capsule
   5. Metastasis

B. INFECTION
   1. Abscess
      ◊ Tuberculous abscess frequently calcifies!
      ◊ Pyogenic abscess rarely calcifies!
   2. Echinococcal cyst
      Renal involvement in 3% of hydatid disease; 50% of echinococcal cysts calcify
   3. Xanthogranulomatous pyelonephritis
      √ large obstructive calculus in >70%

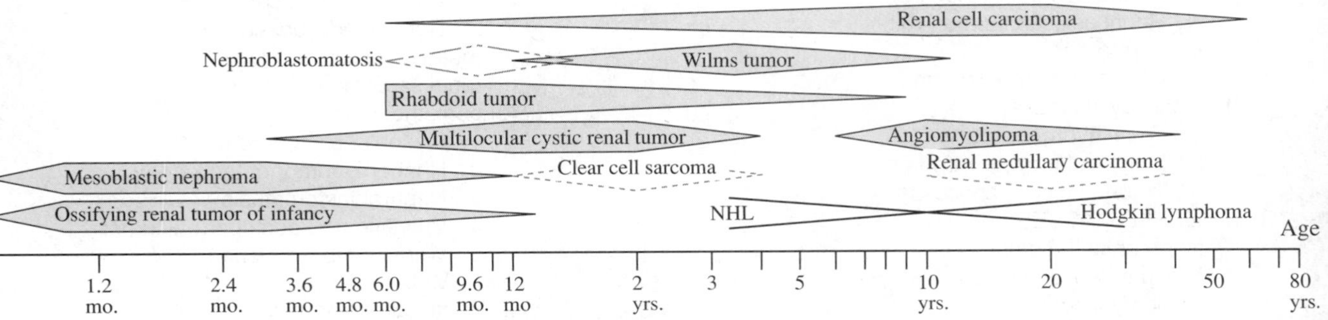

Most Common Age at Presentation for Solid Renal Malignancies

C. CYSTS
◊ Calcification is related to prior hemorrhage or infection!
1. Simple renal cyst (calcifies in 1–3%)
√ thin peripheral "eggshell"-like calcification
2. Multicystic dysplastic kidney (in adult)
3. Autosomal dominant polycystic kidney disease
4. Milk of calcium (cyst, caliceal diverticulum, obstructed hydrocalyx)
DDx: residual pantopaque used in cyst puncture

D. VASCULAR
1. Subcapsular / perirenal hematoma
2. Renal artery aneurysm
√ circular cracked eggshell appearance
3. Congenital / posttraumatic arteriovenous malformation
4. Arteriosclerosis in severe atherosclerotic disease, diabetes mellitus, hyperparathyroidism
5. Sloughed papilla in papillary necrosis

Avascular Mass in Kidney

mnemonic: "CHEAT"
Cyst
Hematoma
Edema
Abscess
Tumor

Hyperechoic Renal Nodule

A. MALIGNANT TUMOR
1. Renal cell carcinoma
2. Angiosarcoma
3. Liposarcoma
4. Undifferentiated sarcoma
5. Lymphoma

B. BENIGN TUMOR
1. Angiomyolipoma
2. Lipoma
3. Oncocytoma
4. Cavernous hemangioma

C. INFARCT

D. HEMATOMA

Hyperattenuating Renal Mass on NECT

A. BENIGN
1. Complicated benign cyst: hemorrhagic, protein-rich, gelatinous
2. Leiomyoma
3. Angiomyolipoma (rare)
4. Thrombosed renal vein

B. MALIGNANT
1. Metastasis from thyroid carcinoma
2. Renal cell carcinoma

Primary Malignant Tumor of Retroperitoneum

1. Liposarcoma
2. Malignant fibrous histiocytoma
√ dystrophic calcifications in 25%
3. Leiomyosarcoma

Low-density Retroperitoneal Mass

1. Lipoma
√ sharply marginated, homogeneously fatty mass
2. Lymphangioma
√ similar to lipoma if enough fat content
3. Renal angiomyolipoma
√ intrarenal component
√ hypervascular with large feeding arteries, multiple aneurysms, laking without shunting, tortuous circumferential vessels, whorled parenchymal + venous phase
4. Adrenal myelolipoma
√ density between fat + water
√ usually nonhomogeneous, occasionally with hemorrhage ± calcifications
5. Xanthogranulomatous pyelonephritis
√ nonfunctioning kidney replaced by low-density material + central staghorn calculus
6. Metastatic retroperitoneal tumors
7. Renal cell carcinoma
8. Fibrosarcoma, fibrous histiocytoma, mesenchymal sarcoma, malignant teratoma
√ density close to muscle
9. Liposarcoma

Focal Area of Increased Renal Echogenicity

A. NONNEOPLASTIC
1. Chronic renal infarction
2. Acute focal bacterial nephritis

B. BENIGN TUMOR
1. Angiomyolipoma
2. Cavernous renal hemangioma
3. Oncocytoma

C. MALIGNANCY
1. Renal cell carcinoma
2. Angiosarcoma
3. Undifferentiated sarcoma
4. Metastasis

Fat-containing Renal Mass

1. Angiomyolipoma
2. Lipoma, liposarcoma
3. Teratoma
4. Wilms tumor
5. Xanthogranulomatous pyelonephritis
6. Oncocytoma engulfing renal sinus fat
7. Renal cell carcinoma
(a) invasion of perirenal fat
(b) intratumoral metaplasia into fatty marrow (in 32% if RCCs <3 cm)

Renal Sinus Mass

A. TUMORS
1. Transitional cell carcinoma
2. Lymphoma
3. Metastasis to sinus lymph nodes
4. Mesenchymal tumor: lipoma, fibroma, myoma, hemangioma
5. Plasmacytoma
6. Myeloid metaplasia

B. MISCELLANEOUS
1. Sinus lipomatosis
2. Parapelvic cyst
3. Saccular aneurysm
4. Urinoma

Hypoechoic Renal Sinus

A. SOLID
1. Fibrolipomatosis
2. Column of Bertin
3. Duplex kidney
4. TCC / RCC

B. CYSTIC
1. Renal sinus cysts
2. Caliectasis
3. Dilated veins, varix
4. Aneurysm, arteriovenous malformation

Renal Pseudotumor

= anomalies of lobar anatomy that may simulate a tumor

A. PRIMARY
1. **Large column of Bertin**
= large septum / cloison of Bertin = large cloison = focal cortical hyperplasia = benign cortical rest = focal renal hypertrophy
= persistence of normal septal cortex / excessive infolding of cortex usually in the presence of partial or complete duplication
Location: between upper and interpolar portion
√ mass <3 cm in largest diameter
√ lateral indentation of renal sinus
√ "deformation" of adjacent calices + infundibula
√ mass continuous with renal cortex
√ enhancement pattern like renal cortex
√ echogenicity similar to cortex
2. **Dromedary hump**
= subcapsular nodule = splenic bump
= secondary to prolonged pressure by spleen during fetal development
Location: in mid portion of lateral border of left kidney
√ triangular contour + elongation of middle calyx
√ enhancement pattern like renal cortex
3. **Hilar lip**
= supra- / infrahilar bulge = medial part of kidney above / below sinus
Location: most frequently medial to left kidney just above renal pelvis (on transaxial scan)
√ enhancement pattern like cortex with medulla
4. **Fetal lobation**
= persistent cortical lobation = ren lobatus
14 individual lobes with centrilobar cortex located around calices
5. **Lobar dysmorphism**
complete diminutive lobe situated deep within renal substance with its own diminutive calyx in its central portion = calyx of nonresorbed normal junctional parenchyma between upper + lower subkidneys

B. ACQUIRED
1. **Nodular compensatory hypertrophy**
areas of unaffected tissue in the presence of focal renal scarring from chronic atrophic pyelonephritis (= reflux nephropathy), surgery, trauma, infarction;
√ hypertrophy usually evident within 2 months; less likely to occur > age 50
DDx: accessory spleen, medial lobule of spleen, splenosis, normal / abnormal bowel, pancreatic disease, gallbladder, adrenal abnormalities
Dx: static radionuclide imaging / renal arteriography / CT

Pseudokidney Sign

= sonographic mass of reniform appearance with a central hyperechoic region surrounded by a hyperechoic region
1. Intussusception
2. Necrotizing enterocolitis
3. Midgut volvulus
4. Sigmoid volvulus
5. Crohn disease

False-positive:
feces in colon, perforated Meckel diverticulum with malrotation + Ladd bands, psoas muscle, hematoma

RENAL CYSTIC DISEASE

Potter Classification

= POTTER SYNDROME
= any renal condition associated with severe oligohydramnios
• peculiar facies with wide-set eyes, parrot-beak nose, pliable low-set ears, receding chin

Type I : infantile PCKD
Type II : multicystic dysplastic kidney disease, multilocular cystic nephroma
IIa : kidneys of normal / increased size
IIb : kidneys reduced in size
Type III : adult PCKD, tuberous sclerosis, medullary sponge kidney
Type IV : small cortical cysts / cystic dysplasia secondary to ureteropelvic junction obstruction

Renal Cystic Disease

A. GENETIC CYSTIC DISEASE
1. Autosomal dominant polycystic kidney disease
2. Autosomal recessive polycystic kidney disease
3. Medullary sponge kidney
4. Medullary cystic disease
5. Glomerulocystic kidney disease
= congenital disease with extremely variable presentation + prognosis
Path: cysts within Bowman capsule ± tubular cysts
√ multiple macroscopic cortical cysts

GU

B. OBSTRUCTIVE CYSTIC DISEASE
1. Multicystic dysplastic kidney
2. Segmental / focal renal dysplasia
3. Familial renal dysplasia

C. ACQUIRED CYSTIC DISEASE
1. Simple cyst
2. Parapelvic cyst
3. Acquired cystic disease of uremia
4. Infectious cysts (TB, Echinococcus, abscess)
5. Medullary necrosis
6. Pyelogenic cyst

D. CYSTS ASSOCIATED WITH SYSTEMIC DISEASE
1. Tuberous sclerosis
2. von Hippel-Lindau disease

E. CYSTIC TUMORS
1. Multilocular cystic nephroma
2. Cystic Wilms tumor
3. Cystic renal cell carcinoma

Syndromes with Multiple Cortical Renal Cysts

1. Von Hippel-Lindau syndrome
2. Tuberous sclerosis
3. Meckel-Gruber syndrome
4. Jeune syndrome
5. Zellweger syndrome = cerebrohepatorenal syndrome
6. Conradi syndrome = chondrodysplasia punctata
7. Oro-facial-digital syndrome
8. Trisomy 13
9. Turner syndrome
10. Dandy-Walker malformation

Multiloculated Renal Mass

A. NEOPLASTIC DISEASE
1. Cystic renal cell carcinoma
2. Multilocular cystic renal tumor
   (a) cystic nephroma
   (b) cystic partially differentiated nephroblastoma
3. Cystic Wilms tumor
4. Necrotic tumor
   (a) mesoblastic nephroma
   (b) clear cell sarcoma

B. RENAL CYSTIC DISEASE
1. Localized renal cystic disease
2. Septated cyst
3. Multicystic dysplastic kidney
3. Segmental multicystic dysplasia
4. Complicated cyst

C. INFLAMMATORY DISEASE
1. Echinococcus
2. Segmental XGP
3. Abscess
4. Malacoplakia

D. VASCULAR LESIONS
1. AV fistula
2. Organizing hematoma

ABNORMAL NEPHROGRAM

Absence of Nephrogram

Global Absence of Nephrogram

Pathophysiology: complete renal ischemia secondary to occlusion of main renal artery

1. Injury to vascular pedicle during blunt abdominal trauma
2. Thromboembolic disease
3. Renal artery dissection: spontaneous, traumatic, iatrogenic

Segmental Absence of Nephrogram

A. SPACE-OCCUPYING PROCESS
1. Neoplasm
2. Cyst
3. Abscess

B. FOCAL RENAL INFARCTION
1. Arterial embolus / thrombosis
2. Vasculitis, collagen-vascular disease
3. Sickle cell anemia
4. Septic shock
5. Renal vein thrombosis

Rim Nephrogram

= rim of cortex receiving collateral blood flow from capsular, peripelvic, and periureteric vessels

◊ Most specific indicator of renovascular compromise!

√ 2–4-mm peripheral band of cortical opacification

Cause:
1. Acute total main renal artery occlusion: seen in 50% of cases with renal infarction
2. Renal vein thrombosis
3. Acute tubular necrosis
4. Severe chronic urinary obstruction

DDx: severe hydronephrosis (rim/shell nephrogram surrounding dilated calices)

Unilateral Delayed Nephrogram

A. OBSTRUCTIVE UROPATHY

B. REDUCTION IN RENAL BLOODFLOW
1. Renal artery stenosis
2. Renal vein thrombosis

Striated Nephrogram

= streaky linear bands of alternating hyper- and hypoattenuation parallel to axis of tubules + collecting ducts *during excretory phase*

Cause: stasis of contrast material in dilated collecting ducts on background of edematous renal parenchyma (diminished concentration of contrast material in tubules from ischemia + tubular obstruction by inflammatory cells + debris)

A. UNILATERAL
1. Acute ureteric obstruction
2. Acute bacterial nephritis / pyelonephritis
3. Renal contusion
4. Renal vein thrombosis

B. BILATERAL
   1. Acute pyelonephritis
   2. Intratubular obstruction: Tamm-Horsfall proteinuria, rhabdomyolysis with myoglobinuria
   3. Systemic hypotension
   4. Autosomal recessive PCKD
   5. Medullary sponge kidney
   6. Medullary cystic disease

mnemonic: "CHOIR BOY"
- **C**ontusion
- **H**ypotension (systemic)
- **O**bstruction (ureteral)
- **I**ntratubular obstruction
- **R**enal vein thrombosis
- **B**acterial nephritis (acute)
- **O**bstruction (ureteral) — it is so common!
- **Y**es, also cystic diseases: infantile PCKD, medullary cystic disease, medullary sponge kidney

Persistent Nephrogram

A. BILATERAL GLOBAL
   1. Systemic hypotension
   2. Intratubular obstruction from protein: Tamm-Horsfall, Bence Jones, myoglobin
   3. Tubular damage by contrast material

B. UNILATERAL GLOBAL
   1. Renal artery stenosis
   2. Renal vein thrombosis
   3. Urinary tract obstruction

C. SEGMENTAL
   1. Obstructed moiety of duplicated collecting system
   2. Obstructing renal calculus
   3. Obstructing neoplasm
   4. Focal stricture
   5. Focal parenchymal disease: tubulointerstitial infection

Abnormal Nephrogram due to Impaired Perfusion

A. SYSTEMIC HYPOTENSIVE REACTION
   as reaction to contrast material / cardiac failure / dehydration / shock
   Pathophysiology:
   drop in perfusion pressure after contrast reaches kidney leads to increased salt + water reabsorption and slowed tubular transit
   √ prolonged bilateral dense nephrograms = persistent increasing nephrogram
   √ decrease in renal size
   √ loss of pyelogram after initial opacification
   NUC (use of glomerular filtration agent [eg, Tc-99m DTPA] preferred)
   √ prolonged cortical transit + reduced excretion

B. RENAL ARTERY STENOSIS
   √ decreased nephrographic opacity + rim nephrogram
   √ hyperconcentration in collecting system
   √ ureteral notching
   NUC (glomerular filtration agent [eg, Tc-99m DTPA] preferred):
   √ decreased perfusion with prolonged excretory phase

C. IMPAIRED PERFUSION OF SMALL ARTERIES
   Trueta shunting = transient rerouting of blood flow from cortex to medulla
   Cause:
   (a) reflex spasm during arterial angiography secondary to catheter trauma / pressure injection of highly concentrated contrast medium
   (b) chronic renal disorders (collagen vascular disease, malignant nephrosclerosis, chronic glomerulonephritis)
   (c) necrotizing vasculitis (polyarteritis nodosa, scleroderma, hypertensive nephrosclerosis)
   CT, Angio:
   √ inhomogeneous opacification of cortex
   IVP:
   √ irregular cortical nephrogram = spotted nephrogram

D. ACUTE VENOUS OUTFLOW OBSTRUCTION
   in renal vein thrombosis
   √ obstructive nephrogram
   √ progressive increase in opacity of entire kidney

Abnormal Nephrogram due to Impaired Tubular Transit

Cause:

A. EXTRARENAL: ureteric obstruction (eg, stone)
   √ obstructive nephrogram
   NUC:
   before decrease in renal function use of glomerular filtration agent (eg, Tc-99m DTPA); with decrease in renal function use of plasma flow agents (eg, Tc-99m MAG3 / I-123 Hippuran) preferred
   √ continuous increase in renal activity
   √ dilatation of collecting system

B. INTRARENAL
   (a) segmental: limb of duplication system, caliceal obstruction, interstitial edema
   √ segmental nephrogram
   (b) protein precipitation: **Tamm-Horsfall protein** (a normal mucoprotein product of proximal nephrons), **Bence-Jones protein** (multiple myeloma), uric acid precipitation (acute urate nephropathy), myoglobulinuria, hyperproteinuric state
   √ striated nephrogram
   NUC:
   before decrease in renal function use of glomerular filtration agent (eg, Tc-99m DTPA); with decrease in renal function use of plasma flow agents (eg, Tc-99m MAG3 / I-123 Hippuran) preferred
   √ prolonged cortical transit time + prolonged excretory phase

GU

Abnormal Nephrogram due to Abnormal Tubular Function

Pathophysiology:

A. PROXIMAL TUBULE
reabsorbs almost all of glucose, amino acids, phosphate, bicarbonate
- glycosuria (Toni-Fanconi syndrome)
- aminoaciduria (cystinuria)
- phosphaturia (phosphate diabetes, thiazides)
- HCO_3^- wasting (proximal renal tubular acidosis)

B. DISTAL TUBULE
absorbs most of water
- diabetes insipidus, secretes H^+
- distal renal tubular acidosis

1. Acute tubular necrosis
   √ immediate persistent nephrogram (common)
   √ progressive increasing opacity (rare)
2. Contrast-induced renal failure

Striated Angiographic Nephrogram

= random patchy densities reflecting redistribution of blood flow from the cortical vasculature to the vasa recta of the medulla

1. Obliterative diseases of the renal microvasculature: polyarteritis nodosa, scleroderma, necrotizing angitis, catheter-induced vasospasm
2. Acute bacterial nephritis
3. Renal vein thrombosis

Increasingly Dense Nephrogram

= initially faint nephrogram becoming increasingly dense over hours to days

Mechanism:

(a) diminished plasma clearance of contrast material
(b) leakage of contrast material into renal interstitial spaces
(c) increase in tubular transit time

Cause:

A. VASCULAR = diminished perfusion
   1. Systemic arterial hypotension (bilateral)
   2. Severe main renal artery stenosis (unilateral)
   3. Acute tubular necrosis (in 33%): due to contrast material nephrotoxicity
   4. Acute renal vein thrombosis

B. INTRARENAL
   1. Acute glomerular disease

C. COLLECTING SYSTEM
   1. Intratubular obstruction
      (a) Uric acid crystals (acute urate nephropathy)
      (b) Precipitation of Bence Jones protein (myeloma nephropathy)
      (c) Tamm-Horsfall protein (severely dehydrated infants / children)
   2. Acute extrarenal obstruction: ureteral calculus

Vicarious Contrast Material Excretion during IVP

= biliary contrast material detected radiographically following intravenous administration of contrast material

Normal contrast excretion:
<2% of urographic dose of diatrizoates + iothalamates are handled by hepatobiliary excretion

Pathophysiology:
increase in protein binding due to prolonged intravascular contact + acidosis

Cause:

1. Uremia (reduction in glomerular filtration + uremia-associated acidosis)
2. Acute unilateral obstruction (increase in circulation time + transient intracellular acidosis)
3. Spontaneous urinary extravasation (prolonged vascular contact of contrast material)

COLLECTING SYSTEM

Spontaneous Urinary Contrast Extravasation

= SPONTANEOUS PYELORENAL BACKFLOW

Etiology: physiologic "safety valve" for obstructed urinary tract with pressures of 80–100 mm Hg in collecting system due to ipsilateral ureteral obstruction from distal stone impaction; pressure is proportional to degree + duration of acute obstruction + dose of contrast material

Incidence: 0.1–18%; M > F (male ureter less compliant)

Criteria:

(a) absence of recent ureteral instrumentation
(b) absence of previous renal / ureteral surgery
(c) absence of destructive urinary tract lesion
(d) absence of external trauma
(e) absence of external compression
(f) absence of pressure necrosis due to stone

Types:

1. Pyelotubular backflow
   = opacification of terminal portions of collecting ducts (= papillary ducts = ducts of Bellini) as a physiologic phenomenon (in 13% with low osmolality + in 0.4% with high osmolality contrast media), wrongly termed "backflow"
   √ wedge-shaped brushlike lines from calyx toward periphery
2. Pyelosinus backflow
   = contrast extravasation from ruptured fornices along infundibula, renal pelvis, proximal ureter; most common form
   Cx: urinoma, retroperitoneal fibrosis
3. Pyelointerstitial backflow
   = contrast flow from pyramids into subcapsular tubules
4. Pyelolymphatic backflow
   = contrast extravasation into periforniceal + peripelvic lymphatics
   √ visualization of small lymphatics draining medially

5. Pyelovenous backflow
   = forniceal rupture into interlobar / arcuate veins; very rare

Widened Collecting System & Ureter

Fetal pyelectasis:

AP diameter of renal pelvis	<5 mm	<20 weeks MA
	<8 mm	20–30 weeks MA
	<10 mm	>30 weeks MA

A. OBSTRUCTIVE UROPATHY
B. NONOBSTRUCTIVE WIDENING
   (a) congenital
      1. Megacalicosis
         underdevelopment of papillae, usually unilateral
      2. Congenital primary megaureter
         = widened ureter with normally tapered distal end
      3. Megacystis-megaureter syndrome
      4. Prune-belly syndrome
      5. Bardet-Biedl syndrome
      6. Beckwith-Wiedemann syndrome
      7. Megalourethra
   (b) increased urine volume
      1. High-flow states: diabetes insipidus, osmotic diuresis, dehydrated patient undergoing rehydration, unilateral kidney
      2. Vesicoureteral reflux
   (c) atony of renal collecting system
      1. Infection: ie, acute pyelonephritis
      2. Pregnancy
      3. Retroperitoneal fibrosis
   (d) overdistended urinary bladder
   (e) previous long-standing significant obstruction: dilatation remains in spite of relief of obstruction

Caliceal Abnormalities

A. OPACIFICATION OF COLLECTING TUBULES
   1. Pyelorenal backflow
   2. Medullary sponge kidney
B. PAPILLARY CAVITY
   1. Papillary necrosis
   2. Caliceal diverticulum
   3. Tuberculosis / brucellosis
C. LOCALIZED CALIECTASIS
   1. Reflux nephropathy = chronic atrophic pyelonephritis
   2. Compound calyx
   3. Hydrocalyx
   4. Congenital megacalyx
   5. Localized postobstructive caliectasis
   6. Localized tuberculosis / papillary necrosis
D. GENERALIZED CALIECTASIS
   1. Postobstructive atrophy
   2. Congenital megacalices
   3. Obstructive uropathy (hydronephrosis)
   4. Nonobstructive hydronephrosis
   5. Diabetes insipidus

Filling Defect in Collecting System

mnemonic: "6 C's & 2 P's"
- **C**lot
- **C**ancer
- **C**yst
- **C**alculus
- **C**andida + other fungi
- **C**ystitis cystica
- **P**olyp
- **P**apilla (sloughed)

Nonopaque Intraluminal Mass in Collecting System

A. NONOPAQUE CALCULUS
   uric acid, xanthine, matrix
   √ smooth, rounded, not attached
B. TISSUE SLOUGH
   1. Papillary necrosis
   2. Cholesteatoma
   3. Fungus ball = conglomeration of fibrillar hyphae
   4. Inspissated debris ("mucopus")
C. VASCULAR
   1. Blood clot: history of hematuria
   √ change in appearance over time
D. FOREIGN MATERIAL
   1. Air
      from bladder via reverse peristalsis, direct trauma, renoalimentary fistula
   2. Foreign matter

Mucosal Mass in Collecting System

A. NEOPLASTIC
   (a) benign tumor
      1. Aberrant papilla = papilla without calyx protruding into major infundibulum
      2. Endometriosis
      3. **Fibroepithelial polyp** = fibrous polyp
         = FIBROEPITHELIOMA = VASCULAR FIBROUS POLYP = POLYPOID FIBROMA
         = mesodermal tumor with fibrovascular stroma + normal transitional cell epithelium
         Age: 20–40 years
         • intermittent abdominal / flank pain
         • gross hematuria (rare)
         √ elongated cylindrical filling defect with smooth margins
         √ mobile on thin pedicle
   (b) malignant tumor
      — Uroepithelial tumors
         1. Transitional cell carcinoma (85–91%)
         2. Squamous cell carcinoma (10–15%)
            Predisposing factors:
               calculi (50–60%), chronic infection, leukoplakia, phenacetin abuse
               √ infiltrating / superficially spreading
         3. Mucinous adenocarcinoma
            = metaplastic transformation
         4. Sarcoma (extremely rare)

— Metastases: breast (most common), melanoma, stomach, lung, cervix, colon, prostate

B. INFLAMMATION / INFECTION
1. Tuberculosis
2. Candidiasis
3. Schistosomiasis
4. Pyeloureteritis cystica
5. Leukoplakia
6. Malacoplakia
7. Xanthogranulomatous pyelonephritis

C. VASCULAR
(a) submucosal hemorrhage
1. Trauma
2. Anticoagulant therapy
3. Acquired circulating anticoagulants
4. Complication of crystalluria / microlithiasis

√ thumbprinting with progressive improvement

(b) vascular notching
1. Ureteropelvic varices
2. Renal vein occlusion
3. IVC occlusion
4. Vascular malformation
5. Retroaortic left renal vein
6. "Nutcracker" effect on left renal vein between aorta and SMA
7. Polyarteritis nodosa

D. PROMINENT MUCOSAL FOLDS
1. Redundant longitudinal mucosal folds of intermittent hydronephrosis (UPJ obstruction, vesicoureteral reflux) or after relief of obstruction
2. Chemical / mechanical irritation
3. Urticaria (Stevens-Johnson syndrome = erythema multiforme bullosa)
4. Leukoplakia (= squamous metaplasia)
5. Ureteral diverticulosis
= rupture of the roofs of cysts in ureteritis cystica

Effaced Collecting System

A. EXTRINSIC COMPRESSION
(a) Unilateral / bilateral global enlargement of renal parenchyma
(b) Renal sinus masses
1. Hemorrhage
2. Parapelvic cyst
3. Sinus lipomatosis

B. SPASM / INFLAMMATION
(a) infection
1. Acute pyelonephritis
2. Acute bacterial nephritis
3. Acute tuberculosis

(b) Hematuria

C. INFILTRATION
1. Malignant uroepithelial tumors

D. OLIGURIA
1. Antidiuretic state
2. Renal ischemia
3. Oliguric renal failure

RENAL CALCIFICATION

Retroperitoneal Calcification

A. NEOPLASM
1. Wilms tumor (in 10%)
2. Neuroblastoma (in 50%): fine granular / stippled / amorphous
3. Teratoma: cartilage / bone / teeth, pseudodigits, pseudolimbs
4. Cavernous hemangioma: phleboliths

B. INFECTION
1. Tuberculous psoas abscess
2. Hydatid cyst

C. TRAUMA
1. Old hematoma

Nephrocalcinosis

= NEPHROLITHIASIS
= deposition of calcium salts in renal parenchyma

Incidence: 0.1–6%; M > F

mnemonic: "MARCH"

Medullary sponge kidney
Alkali excess
Renal medullary / cortical necrosis, **R**TA
Chronic glomerulonephritis
Hyperoxaluria, **H**ypercalcemia, **H**ypercalciuria

Medullary Nephrocalcinosis

= calcifications involving the distal convoluted tubules in the loops of Henle

Incidence: 95% of all nephrocalcinoses

Cause:

A. HYPERCALCIURIA
(a) endocrine
1. Hyperparathyroidism in 5% (primary >> secondary)
2. Paraneoplastic syndrome of lung + kidney primary (ectopic parathormone production)
3. Cushing syndrome
4. Diabetes insipidus
5. Hyperthyroidism / hypothyroidism

(b) alimentary
1. Milk-alkali syndrome (excess calcium + alkali = milk + antacids)
2. Hypervitaminosis D
3. Beryllium poisoning

(c) osseous
1. Osseous metastases, multiple myeloma
2. Prolonged immobilization
3. Progressive senile osteoporosis

(d) renal
1. Medullary sponge kidney
2. Renal tubular acidosis (in 73% of primary RTA)
3. **Bartter syndrome**
tubular disorder with potassium + sodium wasting, hyperplasia of juxtaglomerular apparatus, hyperaldosteronism, hypokalemic alkalosis, and normal blood pressure

(e) drug therapy
  1. Furosemide (in infants)
  2. Prolonged ACTH therapy
  3. Vitamin E (orally)
  4. Vitamin D excess
  5. Calcium (orally)
  6. Nephrotoxic drugs: outdated tetracycline, amphotericin B

(f) miscellaneous
  1. Sarcoidosis
  2. Idiopathic hypercalciuria
  3. Idiopathic hypercalcemia

B. HYPEROXALURIA = OXALOSIS
  1. **Primary hyperoxaluria**
     = Hereditary hyperoxaluria (more common)
     = rare autosomal recessive inherited enzyme deficiency of carboligase with diffuse oxalate deposition in kidneys, heart, blood vessels, lung, spleen, bone marrow

     Type I = α-ketoglutarate-glyoxylate carboxylase deficiency
       • glycolic aciduria

     Type II = D-glycerate dehydrogenase deficiency
       • 1-glyceric aciduria

     Age: usually <5 years
     Prognosis: early death in childhood
  2. **Secondary hyperoxaluria**
     = enteric hyperoxaluria (rare)
     Cause: disturbance of bile acid metabolism after jejunoileal bypass, ileal resection, blind loop syndrome, Crohn disease, increased ingestion (green leafy vegetables), pyridoxine deficiency, ethylene glycol poisoning, methoxyflurane anesthesia

C. HYPERURICOSURIA
  1. Gouty kidney
  2. Lesch-Nyhan syndrome

D. URINARY STASIS
  1. Milk-of-calcium in pyelocaliceal diverticulum
  2. Medullary sponge kidney

E. DYSTROPHIC CALCIFICATION
  1. Renal papillary necrosis (especially analgesic nephropathy)
  2. Chronic pyelonephritis
  3. Sickle cell disease
  4. Renal tuberculosis

mnemonic: "HAM HOP"
Hyperparathyroidism
Acidosis (renal tubular)
Medullary sponge kidney
Hypercalcemia / hypercalciuria (sarcoidosis, milk-alkali syndrome, hypervitaminosis D)
Oxalosis
Papillary necrosis

GU

√ normal-sized / occasionally enlarged kidneys (medullary sponge kidney)
√ small poorly defined / large coarse granular calcifications in renal pyramids:
  √ uniform deposition: hyperparathyroidism / distal renal tubular acidosis (type 1)
  √ asymmetric deposition in dilated collecting ducts within papillary tips: medullary sponge kidney

US:
  √ absence of hypoechoic papillary structures (earliest sign)
  √ hyperechoic rim at corticomedullary junction + around tip and sides of pyramids
  √ solitary focus of hyperechogenicity at tip of pyramid near fornix
  √ increased echogenicity of renal pyramids ± shadowing (no acoustic shadowing with small + light calcifications)

DDx of hyperechoic medulla in newborns:
  oliguria with transient tubular blockage by Tamm-Horsfall proteinuria

Cx: often followed by urolithiasis

Cortical Nephrocalcinosis

= calcium deposition in renal cortex
Incidence: 5% of all nephrocalcinoses
Cause:
  1. Acute cortical necrosis
  2. Chronic glomerulonephritis
  3. Alport syndrome = hereditary nephritis + deafness
  4. Congenital oxalosis, primary hyperoxaluria
  5. Chronic paraneoplastic hypercalcemia
  6. Toxic: ethylene glycol, methoxyflurane
  7. Sickle cell disease
  8. Rejected renal transplant

mnemonic: "COAG"
Cortical necrosis (acute)
Oxalosis
Alport syndrome
Glomerulonephritis (chronic)

√ thin rim of calcification with a "tramline" appearance
√ spotty appearance (= preferential deposition in necrotic glomeruli)

US:
  √ homogeneously increased echogenicity of renal parenchyma > liver echogenicity

RENOVASCULAR DISEASE

Renal Artery Aneurysm

Prevalence: 0.01–0.1%; 22% of visceral aneurysms
Types:
  (a) saccular: near first bifurcation of main renal artery; associated with medial fibroplasia + atherosclerosis
  (b) fusiform: in medial fibroplasia; not calcified

(c) dissecting: traumatic, spontaneous (atherosclerosis, intimal fibroplasia, perimedial fibroplasia), iatrogenic

Cx: (1) Hypertension (unusual)
(2) Perinephric / retroperitoneal hemorrhage [rare]
(3) Formation of AV fistula
(4) Peripheral renal embolization [from mural thrombus] (5) Thrombosis

Extrarenal Aneurysm (2/3)

(a) True aneurysm
1. Atherosclerotic (most common)
2. Fibromuscular dysplasia
3. Pregnancy
4. Mesenchymal disease: neurofibromatosis, Ehlers-Danlos syndrome

(b) False aneurysm
1. Trauma; renal artery angioplasty
2. Behçet disease
3. Mycotic aneurysm
2.5% of all aneurysms
Cause: bacteremia, SBE, perivascular extension of inflammation
Organism: Streptococcus, Staphylococcus, Pneumococcus, Salmonella

√ incomplete / complete ring of calcification
√ variable enhancement (depending on amount of thrombus)

Rx: (1) conservative in asymptomatic patient for well-calcified aneurysm <2 cm in diameter
(2) surgery for (a) interval growth, (b) emboli to kidney, (c) in woman of childbearing age, (d) diminished renal function / ischemia / hypertension / dissection

Intrarenal Aneurysm (1/3)

in interlobar and more peripheral branches

A. CONGENITAL
1. Congenital renal aneurysm
Age at Dx: 30 years; M:F = 1:1
• hypertension in 25% (from segmental renal ischemia)
√ aneurysm close to vascular bifurcations, may calcify

B. ARTERITIS
1. Polyarteritis nodosa
2. SLE
3. Allergic vasculitis
4. Wegener granulomatosis
5. Transplant rejection
6. Drug-abuse vasculitis
Kidney most commonly affected organ
Cause:
(a) immunologic injury from circulating hepatitis antigen-antibody complexes producing a necrotizing angitis
(b) bacterial endocarditis
(c) drug-related
(d) impurity-related
Drugs: methamphetamine, heroin, LSD
√ multiple small aneurysms in interlobar branches near corticomedullary junction
√ inhomogeneous spotty nephrogram

C. DEGENERATIVE: Atherosclerosis (may calcify)

D. TUMOR
1. Neoplasm (RCC in 14%; adult Wilms tumor)
2. Hamartoma (angiomyolipoma in 50%)
3. Metastatic arterial myxoma
4. Vascular malformation

E. MESENCHYMAL DISEASE:
1. Neurofibromatosis
2. Fibroplasia

F. TRAUMA

G. INFECTION: syphilis, tuberculosis

Spontaneous Retroperitoneal Hemorrhage

A. RENAL TUMOR (57–63%)
(a) malignant tumor (30–33%)
1. RCC (33%)
2. TCC of renal pelvis
3. Wilms tumor
4. Lipo-, fibro-, angiosarcoma
(b) benign tumor (24–33%):
1. Angiomyolipoma (16–24%)
2. Lipoma
3. Adenoma
4. Fibromyoma
5. Ruptured hemorrhagic cyst

B. VASCULAR DISEASE (18–26%)
1. Ruptured renal artery aneurysm
2. Vasculitis (eg, polyarteritis nodosa in 13%)
3. Arteriovenous malformation
4. Segmental renal infarction

C. INFLAMMATION / INFECTION (7–10%)
1. Abscess (in 50% of infections)
2. Acute / chronic nephritis

D. COAGULOPATHY
1. Anticoagulant therapy (in 4.3–6.6% of IV heparin, in 01.–0.6% of oral anticoagulants)
Source: idiopathic (42%), tumor (21%), stone disease (17%), hemorrhagic cystitis
2. Bleeding diathesis
3. Long-term hemodialysis

E. PRIMARY ADRENAL CYST / TUMOR
1. Pheochromocytoma
◊ Massive bleed due to an undiagnosed pheochromocytoma has been lethal in 50%!
2. Pseudocyst
3. Myelolipoma
4. Hemangioma
5. Adrenocortical adenoma / carcinoma
6. Metastasis

• flank pain of sudden onset
◊ Follow-up CT may be indicated at 3 and 6 months if the source of blood remains indeterminate!
◊ Surgical exploration must be considered to uncover a small renal tumor if the cause of hemorrhage is not determined radiologically!

Subcapsular Hematoma

√ subcapsular mass with flattening of renal parenchyma
√ total resorption / formation of pseudocapsule with calcification
Angio:
√ avascular mass
Cx: Page kidney (ischemia, release of renin, hypertension)

Renal Doppler

A. NORMAL RENAL DOPPLER
√ resistive index (RI) of 0.70 = upper limit of normal
Elevation of RI:
— significant systemic hypotension
— markedly decreased heart rate
— perinephric / subcapsular fluid collection
— in neonates + infants

B. RENAL MEDICAL DISEASE
Elevation of RI more likely with vascular / tubulointerstitial process, less likely with glomerular disease
May be useful in predicting clinical outcome in:
— hemolytic-uremic syndrome
— acute renal failure
— nonazotemic patients with severe liver disease

C. RENAL ARTERIAL STENOSIS

D. RENAL VEIN THROMBOSIS

URETER

Ureteral Deviation

A. LUMBAR URETER
(a) lateral deviation (common)
1. Hypertrophy of psoas muscle
2. Enlargement of paracaval / paraaortic lymph nodes
3. Aneurysmal dilatation of aorta
4. Neurogenic tumors
5. Fluid collections (abscess, urinoma, lymphocele, hematoma)
(b) medial deviation
1. Retrocaval ureter (on right side only)
2. Retroperitoneal fibrosis

B. PELVIC URETER
(a) medial deviation
1. Hypertrophy of iliopsoas muscle
2. Enlargement of iliac lymph nodes
3. Aneurysmal dilatation of iliac vessels
4. Bladder diverticulum at UVJ (Hutch)
5. Following abdominoperineal surgery + retroperitoneal lymph node dissection
6. Pelvic lipomatosis
(b) lateral deviation with extrinsic compression
1. Pelvic mass (eg, fibroids, ovarian tumor)

Megaureter

A. VESICOURETERAL REFLUX
(a) primary vesicoureteral reflux
1. Primary reflux megaureter
abnormal ureteral tunnel at UVJ
2. Prune belly syndrome
(b) secondary vesicoureteral reflux
1. Hypertonic neurogenic bladder
2. Bladder outlet obstruction
3. Posterior urethral valves

B. OBSTRUCTION
(a) primary obstruction
1. Intrinsic ureteral obstruction (stone, stricture, tumor)
2. Ectopic ureter
3. Ureterocele
4. Ureteral duplication: tortuous dilated ureter of upper moiety
(b) secondary obstruction
1. Retroperitoneal obstruction: tumor, fibrosis, aortic aneurysm
2. Bladder wall mass
3. Bladder outlet obstruction:
eg, prostatic enlargement

C. NONREFLUX-NONOBSTRUCTED MEGAURETER
1. Congenital primary megaureter = megaloureter
2. Polyuria: eg, diabetes insipidus, acute diuresis
3. Infection
4. Ureter remaining wide after relief of obstruction

mnemonic: "DiaPOUR"
Diabetes insipidus
Primary megaureter
Obstruction (recent / old)
UVJ obstruction
Reflux

Ureteral Stricture

A. INTRINSIC CAUSE
(a) mucosal
1. Primary ureteral tumors
(b) mural
1. **Endometriosis**
common disorder in menstruating women (15%); ureteral involvement is rare and indicates widespread pelvic disease
√ abrupt smooth stricture of 0.5–2.5 cm length
√ rectosigmoid involvement on BE
2. Tuberculosis, schistosomiasis
3. Traumatic
ureterolithotomy, endoscopic stone extraction, hysterectomy
4. Amyloidosis
√ distal stricture with submucosal calcification
5. Nonspecific (rare)

B. EXTRINSIC CAUSE
1. Endometriosis
extrinsic form:intrinsic form = 4:1
2. Abscess
tuboovarian, appendiceal, perisigmoidal
3. Inflammatory bowel disease
(eg, Crohn disease, diverticulitis)
4. Radiation fibrosis

5. Metastases
   cervix, endometrium, ovary, rectum, prostate, breast, lymphoma
6. Iliac artery aneurysm (with perianeurysmal fibrosis)

mnemonic: "MISTER"
Metastasis (extrinsic / intrinsic)
Inflammation from calculus
Schistosomiasis
Tuberculosis, **T**ransitional cell carcinoma, **T**rauma
Endometriosis + other periureteral inflammatory process
Radiation therapy, **R**etroperitoneal fibrosis

Ureteral Filling Defect
A. FIXED
   (a) neoplasm
      1. Urothelial neoplasm
      2. Metastasis
      3. Fibroepithelial polyp
   (b) inflammation
      1. Ureteritis cystica
      2. Tuberculosis
      3. Endometriosis
B. MOBILE
   1. Calculus
   2. Sloughed papilla
   3. Blood clot

Ureteral Calcification
A. URETERAL LUMEN
   1. Stone migrated from kidney
   2. Stone in ureteral diverticulum / ureterocele
   3. "Steinstrasse" (stone street) = collection of stone fragments in distal ureter following lithotripsy
B. URETERAL WALL
   1. Schistosomiasis
   2. Tuberculosis
   3. Amyloid infiltration
   4. Ureteral tumor

DDx: (1) Phlebolith in gonadal vein (multiple, not along course of ureter, centrally radiolucent)
(2) Silastic fallopian tube band

URINARY BLADDER
Bilateral Narrowing of Urinary Bladder
A. WITH ELEVATION OF BLADDER FLOOR
   1. Pelvic lipomatosis
   2. Pelvic hematoma
      Cause: trauma, anticoagulant therapy, spontaneous rupture of blood vessels, blood dyscrasia (rare), bleeding neoplasm (rare)
   3. Chronic cystitis
B. WITH SUPERIOR COMPRESSION OF BLADDER
   1. Thrombosis of IVC
      Cause: trauma, hypercoagulability state (oral contraceptives), extension of thrombi from lower extremity, abdominal sepsis, Budd-Chiari syndrome, compression of IVC by neoplasm
      √ collaterals through gonadal veins, ascending lumbar veins, vertebral plexus, retroperitoneal veins, portal vein (via hemorrhoidal veins)
      √ notching of distal ureter by ureteral veins
   2. Pelvic lymphadenopathy
      Cause: lymphoma (most often)
      √ polycyclic asymmetric compression of bladder
      √ medial displacement of pelvic segment of ureters
      √ lateral displacement of upper ureters
   3. Hypertrophy of iliopsoas muscles
   4. Bilateral pelvic masses
      (a) bilateral lymphocysts (following radical pelvic surgery)
      (b) bilateral urinomas
      (c) bilateral pelvic abscesses

Pear-shaped Urinary Bladder
mnemonic: "HALL"
Hematoma
Aneurysm (bilateral common / external iliac artery)
Lipomatosis
Lymphadenopathy (pelvic)

Small Bladder Capacity
Cause:
A. Thickened / fibrotic bladder wall
   1. Interstitial cystitis
   2. Tuberculous cystitis
   3. Cystitis cystica
   4. Schistosomiasis
   5. Trauma: surgical resection, radiation therapy
B. Disuse of bladder

• urinary frequency
• progressive rise in bladder pressure during filling
√ reduced bladder compliance
√ thickened bladder wall + decreased bladder volume
√ vesicoureteral reflux

Bladder Wall Thickening
Normal bladder wall thickness (regardless of age + gender):
<5 mm in nondistended bladders
<3 mm in well-distended bladders

A. TUMOR
   1. Neurofibromatosis
B. INFECTION / INFLAMMATION
   1. Cystitis
C. MUSCULAR HYPERTROPHY
   1. Neurogenic bladder
   2. Bladder outlet obstruction (eg, posterior urethral valves)
D. UNDERDISTENDED BLADDER

Urinary Bladder Wall Masses

A. CONGENITAL
  1. Congenital septum
  2. Simple ureterocele
  3. Ectopic ureterocele

B. BLADDER TUMORS

C. INFLAMMATION / INFECTION
  1. Cystitis: hemorrhagic cystitis, abacterial cystitis, bullous cystitis, edematous cystitis, interstitial cystitis, eosinophilic cystitis, granulomatous cystitis, emphysematous cystitis, cystitis cystica, cyclophosphamide cystitis, cystitis glandularis (premalignant lesion with villous lesions in bladder dome from proliferation of "intestinelike" glands in submucosa)
  2. Tuberculosis
  3. Schistosomiasis
  4. Malacoplakia
  5. Extravesical inflammation:
     (a) Diverticulitis
     (b) Crohn disease
     (c) endometriosis

D. HEMATOMA
after instrumentation, surgery, trauma

Bladder Tumor

A. EPITHELIAL TUMORS (95%)
  1. Transitional cell carcinoma (90%)
     multicentric, aniline dyes
  2. Squamous cell carcinoma (4%)
     worst prognosis; secondary to chronic disorders (infection, stricture, calculi), bladder diverticula, schistosomiasis
  3. Adenocarcinoma (1%)
     most common in bladder exstrophy, less common in cystitis glandularis + urachal carcinoma (at dome of bladder in urachal remnant)

B. NONEPITHELIAL TUMORS
  (a) primary benign tumors
    1. Leiomyoma (most common)
       • hematuria secondary to ulceration
       Site: submucosal / intramural / subserosal
    2. Rhabdomyoma (rare)
    3. Hemangioma
    4. Neurofibroma / neurofibromatosis
       generalized neurofibromatosis in 60%
    5. Nephrogenic adenoma
       Associated with: cystitis cystica / cystitis glandularis
    6. Endometriosis
       Location: on posterior wall
       • urinary symptoms in 80%
    7. Pheochromocytoma (0.5%)
       Origin: from paraganglia of bladder wall
       • adrenergic attack at micturition / bladder filling (headaches, weakness)
       • intermittent hypertension
       • elevated catecholamine levels
       Prognosis: 7% are malignant
  (b) primary malignant tumors
    1. Primary lymphoma
       ◊ 2nd most common nonepithelial tumor of urinary bladder
       Age: 40 years; M:F = 1:3
       Location: submucosal; at bladder base + trigone
    2. Rhabdomyosarcoma
       Age: 1st and 2nd decades of life
    3. Leiomyosarcoma
       Age: mainly >40 years of age
       Location: rarely at trigone
  (c) secondary tumors
    1. Metastases
       1.5% of all bladder malignancies
       Origin: melanoma > stomach > breast > kidney > lung
       √ solitary / multiple nodules
    2. Lymphoma
       bladder involved at autopsy: in 15% of NHL, in 5% of Hodgkin disease
    3. Leukemia
       microscopic involvement in 22% at autopsy
    4. Direct extension (common)
       from prostate, rectum, sigmoid, cervix, ovary

Bladder Calcification

Bladder Calculi

1. Stasis calculi (70%)
   in bladder outflow obstruction, bladder diverticula, cystocele, neuropathic bladder dysfunction
   Associated with: Gram-negative lower urinary tract infection (in 30%), in particular Proteus
2. Migrant calculi
   = renal calculi spontaneously passing into bladder
3. Foreign body nidus calculi
   from self-introduced objects, urinary stent, chronic catheterization, bladder wall-penetrating bone fragments, prostatic chips, nonabsorbable suture material, fragments of Foley balloon catheter, pubic hair, presence of intestinal mucosa (in bladder augmentation, ileal conduit, repaired bladder exstrophy)
4. Idiopathic/ primary/ endemic calculi
   Countries: in North Africa, India, Indonesia
   Age: in young boys of low socioeconomic class (nutritional deficiency?)
   √ single stone in 86%

Incidence: India (13:100,000); less common in western hemisphere
Number of stones: solitary; multiple (in up to 25%)
Composition: magnesium ammonium phosphate (50%), calcium salts (31%), uric acid origin (5%)
• hematuria, recurrent UTIs, pelvic pain, irritative / obstructive voiding symptoms
Rx: surgical extraction, lithotripsy, alkalinization of urine
Rate of recurrence: 41%

Bladder Wall Calcification

A. INFLAMMATION
  1. Schistosomiasis (50%)
     √ relatively normal distensibility of bladder
     √ thin arcuate pattern of calcification
  2. Tuberculosis
     √ bladder markedly contracted
  3. Cystitis:
     postirradiation cystitis, alkaline incrusted cystitis, cytotoxin cystitis
  4. Bacillary UTI (extremely uncommon)
  5. Encrusted foreign material

B. NEOPLASM
  1. Primary neoplasm of bladder: TCC, squamous cell carcinoma, leiomyosarcoma, hemangioma, neuroblastoma, osteogenic sarcoma
  2. Urachal carcinoma

mnemonic: "SCRITT"
Schistosomiasis
Cytoxan
Radiation
Interstitial cystitis
Tuberculosis
Transitional cell carcinoma

Masses Extrinsic to Urinary Bladder

A. NORMAL / ENLARGED ORGANS
  1. Uterus, leiomyomatous uterus, pregnant uterus
  2. Distended rectosigmoid
  3. Ectopic pelvic kidney
  4. Prostate cancer / BPH

B. SOLID PELVIC TUMORS
  1. Lymphadenopathy
  2. Bone tumor from sacrum / coccyx
  3. Rectosigmoid mass
  4. Hip arthroplasty
  5. Neurogenic neoplasm, meningomyelocele
  6. Pelvic lipomatosis / liposarcoma

C. CYSTIC PELVIC LESIONS
  (a) congenital / developmental
    1. Urachal cyst
    2. Müllerian duct cyst
    3. Gartner duct cyst
    4. Anterior meningocele
    5. Hydrometrocolpos
  (b) related to trauma
    1. Hematoma (eg, rectus sheath hematoma)
    2. Urinoma
    3. Lymphocele
    4. Abscess
    5. Aneurysm
    6. Mesenteric cyst
  (c) cyst of genitalia
    1. Prostatic cyst
    2. Cyst of seminal vesicle
    3. Cyst of vas deferens
    4. Ovarian cyst
    5. Hydrosalpinx
    6. Vaginal cyst
  (d) cyst of urinary bladder
    1. Bladder diverticulum
  (e) cyst of GI tract
    1. Peritoneal inclusion cyst
    2. Fluid-filled bowel

VOIDING DYSFUNCTION

A. FAILURE TO STORE URINE
  • urinary frequency, urgency, incontinence
  (a) bladder causes
    1. involuntary detrusor contractions
       – detrusor instability (idiopathic / neurogenic)
       – detrusor hyperreflexia (upper cord lesion)
    2. poor bladder compliance
       – detrusor hyperreflexia
       – bladder wall fibrosis
    3. sensory urgency
       – infection, inflammation, irritation
       – neoplasia
    4. vesicovaginal fistula
    5. psychogenic condition
  (b) sphincter causes
    1. Stress incontinence
    2. Sphincteric incontinence
  (c) extravesical ectopic insertion of ureter in females

B. FAILURE TO EMPTY BLADDER
  • poor flow, straining, hesitancy
  • inability to completely empty bladder
  (a) bladder causes
    1. Detrusor areflexia (sacral arc lesion)
    2. Impaired detrusor contractility (myogenic)
    3. Psychogenic condition
  (b) bladder outlet obstruction:
    1. Bladder neck contracture
    2. Prostatic enlargement
    3. Detrusor-external sphincter dyssynergia
    4. Scarring from surgery / radiation therapy
    5. Ectopic ureterocele
    6. Urethral stenosis
    7. Urethral kinking (eg, due to cystocele)

Incontinence

1. Stress incontinence
2. Vesicovaginal / ureterovaginal fistula
3. Urge incontinence
4. Psychogenic incontinence
5. Overflow incontinence
   secondary to lesions of sacral spinal cord / sacral reflex arc or severe outlet obstruction
6. Reflex voiding
   (a) hyperreflexive lesion (lesion of upper spinal cord)
   (b) uninhibited / unstable bladder
7. Continual dribbling
   (extravesical ectopic termination of ureter)

Stress Incontinence

= SPHINCTER WEAKNESS INCONTINENCE

Cause:
  A. Male: S/P prostatectomy with damage to distal sphincter

B. Female: congenital bladder neck weakness, pregnancy, childbirth, aging (secondary to changes in anatomic relationship of urethra + bladder base)
• frequency, urgency (involuntary filling of bladder neck)
√ opening of bladder neck during coughing
√ impairment of milk-back mechanism (= retrograde emptying of urethra during interruption of voiding phase does not occur)
√ urethrovesical descent (in types I + II)
Chain cystography:
√ posterior urethrovesical angle (= angle between posterior urethra + bladder base) increased >100°
√ upper urethral axis (= angle between upper urethra + vertical line) increased >35°

Detrusor Instability

= MOTOR URGE INCONTINENCE = UNSTABLE BLADDER
◊ Condition resembles that of immature bladder before toilet training
Patient groups:
(1) symptoms of nocturnal enuresis + frequency / incontinence dating back to childhood
(2) idiopathic instability occurring in middle age
(3) outflow obstruction commonly in men
(4) degenerative instability secondary to cardiovascular + neurologic disease later in life
• frequency, urgency, urge incontinence, occasionally nocturia
• hesitancy + difficulty in voiding may occur in men without significant prostatic hypertrophy
√ involuntary bladder contractions with no relationship to bladder distension
√ progressively vigorous contractions during bladder filling
√ postural instability limited to upright position
√ impaired milk-back mechanism due to high bladder pressure
√ strong after contractions following bladder emptying
Cx: thickening of bladder wall, bladder diverticula
Rx: treatment of obstruction, anticholinergic drug (oxybutynin), operative increase in bladder capacity

Sensitive Bladder (Sensory Urgency)

Cause:
cystitis (reduced compliance), some cases of stress incontinence (filling of bladder neck induces urgency)
• frequency, urgency, sometimes nocturia
√ patient uncomfortable with low bladder filling
√ no abnormal rise in bladder pressure
√ normal voiding function

Detrusor-sphincter Dyssynergia

= overactivity of bladder neck muscle with failure to relax at beginning of voiding
Cause: spinal cord lesion / trauma above level of sacral outflow
• difficulty in voiding ± frequency
• lifelong history of poor stream
√ collarlike indentation of bladder neck during voiding (= persistent / intermittent narrowing of membranous urethra)
√ may have high voiding pressure + reduced flow
√ trapping of contrast in urethra during interruption of flow
√ massive reflux into prostatic ducts during voiding (due to high pressure within prostatic urethra)
√ severely trabeculated **"Christmas-tree" bladder** + bilateral hydroureteronephrosis
Rx: bladder neck incision

Hinman Syndrome

= NONNEUROGENIC NEUROGENIC BLADDER [NNNB]
= DETRUSOR-SPHINCTER DYSSYNERGIA
Cause: no neurologic / anatomic obstructive disease; distinctly abnormal family dynamics (in 50%)
Age: some time after toilet training with onset during early / late childhood / puberty
• clinical criteria:
(1) intact perineal sensation + anal tone
(2) normal anatomy + function of lower extremities
(3) absence of skin lesions overlying sacrum
(4) normal lumbosacral spine at plain radiography
(5) normal spinal cord at MR imaging
√ high-pressure uninhibited detrusor contractions
√ lack of coordination between detrusor contraction + periurethral striated sphincter relaxation
√ inability to suppress bladder contractions
√ normal response of detrusor muscle to reflex stimulation
√ increased bladder capacity + pressure
√ sphincter activity may increase paradoxically during detrusor contraction
US:
√ trabeculated bladder
√ dilatation of upper urinary tracts
√ renal damage
VCUG:
√ urethra normal during early voiding
√ urethral distension after contraction of external sphincter as voiding progresses
√ ureterovesical obstruction / reflux
Rx: suggestion therapy + hypnosis, bladder retraining, biofeedback, anticholinergic drugs

Wetting

1. **Enuresis**
= manifestation of neuromuscular vesicourethral immaturity; M:F = 3:2
• intermittent wetting, usually at night during sleep
• often positive history of enuresis from one parent
• normal physical examination
√ no structural abnormality; urography NOT indicated

GU

2. Epispadia
3. Sacral agenesis
   = segmental defect (below S2) with deficiency of nerves that innervate bladder, urethra, rectum, feet
   ◊ Children of diabetic mothers are affected in 17%!
4. **Extravesical infrasphincteric ectopic ureter**
   only affects girls as boys do NOT have infrasphincteric ureteral orifices
   (a) ureter draining upper pole of duplex system exits below urethral sphincter (90%)
   (b) ureter draining single system with ectopic extravesical orifice (10%)
5. **Synechia vulvae**
   = adhesive fusion of minor labia directs urine primarily into vagina from where it dribbles out post micturition
6. **Vaginal reflux**
   in obese older girls with fat thighs and fat labia
7. Miscellaneous
   posterior urethral valves, urethral stricture, urethral diverticula

Prostatic Obstruction

= urethral compression by hypertrophic prostatic tissue
• difficulty in voiding
• reduction in flow rate
√ high-pressure bladder
√ slow + prolonged flow
√ increase in bladder capacity with reduced contractility (late)

SCROTUM

Acutely Symptomatic Scrotum

= acute unilateral scrotal swelling ± pain
Cause:
   epididymitis:torsion = 3:2 <20 years of age
   epididymitis:torsion = 9:1 >20 years of age

A. TORSION
   1. Torsion of testis (20%)
      = most common acute process in prepubertal age
   2. Torsion of testicular appendages
      accounts for 5% of scrotal pathology; both appendages located near upper pole of testes
      Frequency:
         appendix testis:appendix epididymis = 9:1
      √ 8–9-mm complex mass in superior aspect of scrotum without color Doppler flow signals
      √ mildly enlarged epididymis (75%)
      √ blood flow increased in epididymis (60%), scrotal wall (53%), testis (13%) simulating acute epididymoorchitis
B. INFECTION / INFLAMMATION (75–80%)
   1. Acute epididymitis
      = most common acute process in postpubertal age
   2. Orchitis
   3. Intrascrotal abscess
   4. Schönlein-Henoch purpura
   5. Kawasaki syndrome
   6. Insect bite
   7. Acute hydrocele
C. HEMORRHAGE
   1. Testicular trauma
      Location: hematoma in scrotal wall, between layers of tunica vaginalis (= hematocele), in epididymis, in testis
      √ rapid change in echo character over time
      √ disruption of tunica albuginea (= testicular rupture)
   2. Hemorrhage into testicular tumor
D. HERNIA
   1. Scrotal fat necrosis
   2. Strangulated hernia

Scrotal Wall Thickening

1. Acute idiopathic scrotal edema
   Incidence: 20–30% of all acute scrotal disorders
   Age: 5–11 years (range 18 months to 14 years)
   • subcutaneous scrotal edema, erythema
   • minimal pain, afebrile, peripheral eosinophilia
2. Epididymoorchitis
3. Testicular torsion
4. Torsion of testicular / epididymal appendage
5. Trauma
6. Henoch-Schönlein purpura
7. Cx of ventriculoperitoneal shunt
8. Cx of peritoneal dialysis (? leakage of fluid into the anterior abdominal wall + dissection into scrotum)

Testicular Blood Flow

Increased Testicular Blood Flow

1. Orchitis
2. Torsion-detorsion sequence
3. Torsion of appendix testis / epididymis
4. Abscess
5. Tumor

Decreased Testicular Blood Flow

1. Torsion
2. Infarct

Scrotal Gas

1. Fournier gangrene
2. Scrotal abscess
3. Scrotal hernia with gas-containing bowel
4. Scrotal emphysema from bowel perforation
5. Extension of subcutaneous emphysema
6. Air leakage + dissection due to faulty chest tube positioning

Groin Mass

A. CONGENITAL
   1. Encysted hydrocele
      = peritoneal fluid remnant of processus vaginalis
      (a) of spermatic cord (male)
      (b) of canal of Nuck (female equivalent)
   2. Retractile testis

B. HERNIA
  1. Inguinal hernia
  2. Femoral hernia
C. VASCULAR
  1. Hematoma
  2. Pseudoaneurysm
  3. Varicocele
  4. Varices of greater saphenous vein
D. INFECTIOUS / INFLAMMATORY
  1. Inflammation of ileopectineal bursa
  2. Synovial osteochondromatosis of hip joint
  3. Groin abscess
E. NEOPLASM
  1. Lipoma (most common benign tumor)
  2. Inguinal lymph node metastases (from cancer of lower vagina, vulva, penis, lower rectum, anus, lower extremity)

Scrotal Mass

Most frequent conditions:

1.	Inflammation	(48%)
2.	Hydrocele	(24%)
3.	Torsion	(9%)
4.	Varicocele	(7%)
5.	Spermatocele	(4%)
6.	Cysts	(4%)
7.	Malignant tumor	(2%)
8.	Benign tumor	(0.7%)

◊ Sonographic differentiation of intra- from extratesticular mass is 80–95% accurate!

Intratesticular Mass

◊ 90–95% of testicular tumors are malignant!
1. Testicular cancer
2. Inflammation: focal orchitis
3. Abscess
4. Testicular infarction
   • soft to palpation
   √ hypoechoic wedge-shaped peripheral defect
5. Hematoma
6. Benign gonadal tumor
7. Granulomatous orchitis:
   (a) TB, syphilis, fungi, parasites
      √ tendency to involve epididymis first
   (b) sarcoidosis (genital tract affected in 5%)
      √ multiple hypo- / hyperechoic masses within testis / epididymis
8. Testicular cyst / tunica albuginea cyst
9. Postbiopsy defect
10. **Adrenal rest**
   Prevalence: in 7–15% of newborns; in 1.6% of adults
   Associated with: congenital adrenal hyperplasia, Cushing syndrome
   • increase in cortisol levels (testicular vein sampling is diagnostic)
     ◊ Adrenal rests only form masses after exposure to elevated levels of adrenocorticotropic hormone
   √ bilateral eccentric nodular masses <5 mm:
     √ predominantly hypoechoic
     √ occasionally heterogeneously hyperechoic ± acoustic shadowing

Multiple Intratesticular Masses

1. Lymphoma / leukemia
2. Primary testicular tumor
3. Chronic infections
4. Metastases: prostate, kidney, melanoma
5. Granulomatous disease: sarcoidosis

◊ The prevalence of synchronous / metachronous bilateral testicular neoplasms is 1–3%!

Prepubertal Testicular Mass

◊ Only 0.5–5% of all intratesticular tumors occur in patients <15 years of age

A. PRIMARY TUMOR
  (a) Germ cell tumors (70–90%):
    1. Yolk sac tumor (≤2 years)
    2. Teratoma (≤5 years)
  (b) Sex cord-stromal tumors (10–30%):
    1. Leydig cell tumor (3–9 years)
    2. Sertoli cell tumor (commonly <1 year)
    3. Gonadoblastoma (after puberty)
    4. Fibroma, lipoma, hemangioma, sarcoma, adrenal rest
B. SECONDARY TUMOR
  1. Lymphoproliferative tumor: leukemia, lymphoma
  2. Solid tumor: Wilms, neuroblastoma, rhabdomyosarcoma, retinoblastoma
  3. Others: sinus histiocytosis, Langerhans cell histiocytosis, tuberculous orchitis

Paratesticular Mass

◊ Only 4% of all scrotal tumors!

A. INFLAMMATORY MASS
  1. Sarcoidosis of epididymis
  2. Inflammatory nodule of epididymitis
  3. Sperm granuloma
     Cause: sperm extravasation with granuloma formation
  4. Scrotal calculi = "scrotal pearls"
     Cause: fibrinous debris in long-standing hydrocele / following torsion of appendix testis or epididymis
B. PARATESTICULAR TUMOR
  ◊ The majority of paratesticular tumors are derived from the spermatic cord!
  ◊ Sarcomas are the most common spermatic cord tumors after lipomas!
  — Benign paratesticular tumor (70%)
    1. Cord lipoma (vast majority)
    2. **Adenomatoid tumor** (30%)
       = benign slow-growing mesothelial neoplasm
       Age: 2nd–4th decade

GU

Histo: epithelial-like cells + fibrous stroma
Location: epididymis (particularly in globus minor), tunica albuginea, spermatic cord (rare)
√ well-marginated solid mass with echogenicity equal to / greater than testis
√ 0.4–5.0 cm in size
3. Epidermoid inclusion cyst
4. Polyorchidism
5. Others: herniated omentum, adrenal rest, carcinoid, papillary cystadenoma of epididymis, cord leiomyoma, cord fibroma (= reactive nodular proliferation of paratesticular tissues), adrenal rest, cholesteatoma

— Malignant paratesticular tumor (3–16%)
1. Sarcomas:
   (a) primarily in adults: undifferentiated sarcoma (30%), leiomyo-, lipo-, fibro-, myxochondro-sarcoma
   (b) children: rhabdomyosarcoma (20%), embryonal sarcoma
   ◊ Rhabdomyosarcoma is the most common extratesticular neoplasm in children!
2. Mesothelioma of tunica (in 15% malignant)
3. Metastases

Extratesticular Fluid Collection

1. Hydrocele, pyocele, hematocele (surgery, trauma, neoplasm)
2. Varicocele
3. **Spermatocele** (after puberty)
   = single / multiple retention cysts filled with fluid + spermatozoa + cellular debris
   • frequently following vasectomy
   Location: commonly in head of epididymis
   √ up to a few cm in size ± septations
4. **Epididymal cyst**
   = cyst without spermatozoa (less common than spermatoceles)
   • status post vasectomy
   Location: anywhere within epididymis
   √ wide range of sizes
5. Lymphangioma, hemangioma
6. Lymphocele
7. Abscess
8. Scrotal hernia = bowel in inguinal hernia
   √ hypoechoic bowel musculature + peristalsis

Cystic Lesions of Testis

Incidence: 4–10% (increasing with age)
• asymptomatic

A. NONNEOPLASTIC
1. **Intratesticular cyst**
   Prevalence: 8–10%
   Cause: ? trauma, prior inflammation, surgery
   Age: >40 years
   • nonpalpable
   Often associated with: spermatocele, dilated rete testis
   Location: related to rete testis (in 92%)
   √ usually solitary 2–20-mm simple cyst
   DDx: cystic neoplasm
2. **Tunica albuginea cyst**
   = mesothelial rests
   Cause: fluid within mesothelial rests; fluid from blind-ending efferent ductules
   Mean age: 40 years
   • palpable firm nodule
   Location: upper anterior / lateral aspect of testis
   √ solitary uni- / multilocular 2–5-mm marginally located cyst
3. **Intratesticular tubular ectasia**
   = DILATATION OF RETE TESTIS = CYSTIC TRANSFORMATION OF THE RETE TESTIS
   Cause: partial / complete obliteration of efferent ductules
   Age: >55 years
   Often associated with: spermatocele
   • nonpalpable
   Location: mediastinum testis, frequently asymmetrically bilateral
   √ elliptical hypoechoic branching tubular structures ± cysts
   √ ± epididymal cysts / spermatoceles
   MR:
   √ hypointense on T1WI
   √ iso- to hyperintense on T2WI
   DDx: teratoma
4. Intratesticular spermatocele
   = cyst containing mature spermatozoa
   Location: attached to mediastinum testis
5. Intratesticular varicocele
   • ± pain (related to passive congestion)
   √ multiple anechoic serpiginous tubules
   √ characteristic venous flow pattern increasing with Valsalva on Doppler
   Infrequently associated with: extratesticular varicocele
6. Intratesticular abscess
   Cause: epididymoorchitis, trauma, testicular infarction, mumps
   √ collection with low-level echoes, shaggy irregular wall, occasionally hypervascular margin
7. Intratesticular infarction
   √ avascular hypoechoic mass
8. Congenital cystic dysplasia of testis (extremely rare)

B. BENIGN TUMOR
1. Epidermoid cyst / keratin cyst of testis

C. MALIGNANCY
◊ 24% of all testicular tumors have cystic component!
• palpable
√ in combination with solid elements

DDx: hematoma, inflammation, seminoma, Leydig cell tumor

Epididymal Enlargement with Hypoechoic Foci

1. Epididymitis
2. Sperm granulomas
3. Tuberculosis
4. Lymphogranuloma venereum
5. Granuloma inguinale
6. Filarial granuloma
7. Fungal disease
8. Lymphoproliferative disease
9. Metastases

Cystic Lesions of Epididymis

1. Epididymal cyst
   Incidence: in up to 40%
   May be associated with: intratesticular tubular ectasia
   √ single / multiple / bilateral
   DDx: loculated hydrocele
2. Spermatocele
   √ may contain low-level echoes
3. Cystic degeneration of epididymis

PROSTATE

Large Utricle

1. Prune belly syndrome
2. Imperforate anus of high type
3. Down syndrome
4. Hypospadia
5. Posterior urethral valves

Prostatic Cysts

1. **Müllerian duct cyst**
   from remnants of paramesonephric (= müllerian) duct which has regressed by 3rd fetal month
   Prevalence: 4–5% of male newborns; in 1% of men
   Age: discovered in 3rd–4th decade
   • obstructive / irritative urinary tract symptoms
   • suprapubic / rectal pain
   • hematuria
   • infertility (most common cause of ejaculatory duct obstruction)
   Location: arise from region of verumontanum slightly lateral to midline
   ◊ No communication with genital tract / urethra
   √ large intraprostatic cyst usually with extension superolaterally above prostate
   √ aspirate contains serous / mucous clear brown / green fluid (hemorrhage + debris), NOT spermatozoa
   √ rarely contains calculi
   Cx: infection, hemorrhage, carcinomatous transformation
2. **Utricle cyst**
   Secondary to dilatation of prostatic utricle (sometimes believed to be a remnant of the müllerian duct)
   Age: 1st–2nd decade
   • postvoid dribbling
   • obstructive / irritative urinary tract symptoms
   • suprapubic / rectal pain
   • hematuria
   Often associated with:
   hypospadia, intersex disorders, incomplete testicular descent, ipsilateral renal agenesis
   Location: arise in midline from verumontanum
   ◊ Free communication with urethra
   √ usually 8–10-mm-long cyst
   √ NO extension above prostate
   Dx: endoscopic catheterization with aspiration of white / brown fluid occasionally containing spermatozoa
   Cx: infection, hemorrhage, carcinomatous metaplasia
3. **Ejaculatory duct cyst**
   Cause: congenital / acquired obstruction of ejaculatory duct
   • perineal pain, dysuria, ejaculatory pain
   • hematospermia
   Location: along expected course of ejaculatory duct
   √ intraprostatic cyst within central zone
   √ aspirate contains spermatozoa with normal testicular function
   √ cyst commonly contains calculi
   √ cystic dilatation of ipsilateral seminal vesicle
   √ contrast injection into cyst outlines seminal vesicle
4. **Cystic degeneration of BPH**
   Most common cystic lesion of prostate
   Location: transition zone
   √ usually small cyst within nodules of benign prostatic hyperplasia
5. **Retention cyst**
   = dilatation of glandular acini
   Cause: acquired obstruction of glandular ductule
   Age: 5th–6th decade
   Location: transition / central / peripheral zone
   √ 1–2-cm smooth-walled unilocular cyst
6. **Cavitary / diverticular prostatitis**
   Cause: fibrosis of chronic prostatitis constricts ducts leading to stagnation of exudate + breakdown of intraacinar septa with cavity formation
   • history of long-standing inflammatory condition
   √ "Swiss cheese" prostate
7. **Prostatic abscess**
   Age: 5th–6th decade
   • fever, chills
   • urinary frequency, urgency, dysuria, hematuria
   • perineal / lower back pain
   • focally enlarged tender prostate
   √ hypo- / anechoic mass with irregular wall + septations
8. Parasitic cyst (Echinococcus, bilharziasis)
9. Cystic carcinoma
   • hemorrhagic aspirate
   √ solid tissue invaginating into cyst

Hypoechoic Lesion of Prostate

1. Adenocarcinoma (35%)
2. Benign prostatic hyperplasia (18%)
   √ rarely may originate in the peripheral zone
3. "Normal" prostatic tissue (18%)
   (a) cluster of prostate retention cysts
   (b) prominent ejaculatory ducts
4. Acute / chronic prostatitis (14%)
5. Granulomatous prostatitis (0.8%): most frequently due to intravesical Calmette-Guérin bacillus (BCG) therapy in treatment of bladder cancer
6. Atrophy (10%)
   • occurs in 70% of young healthy men
   ◊ May be confused with carcinoma histologically!
7. Prostatic dysplasia (6%)

URETHRA

Congenital Urethral Anomalies

A. Anomaly of number
   1. Duplication of urethra
B. Anomalies of form
   1. Posterior urethral valves
   2. Congenital stricture
   3. Congenital polyp
   4. Congenital diverticulum
C. Malformation of urethral groove
   1. **Epispadia**
      = absent roof of urethra with opening anywhere between base of bladder and glans penis
      Associated with: bladder exstrophy
      • urinary incontinence from incompetent bladder neck / urethral sphincter
      √ abnormally wide symphysis pubis (>1 cm)
   2. **Hypospadia**
      = congenital defect of anterior urethra with opening anywhere along ventral aspect of penile shaft

Cowper (Bulbourethral) Gland Lesions

Analogous to Bartholin glands in females
Prevalence: 2.3% (autopsy)
Location: within urogenital diaphragm
1. Retention cyst
   Cx: prenatal death from urinary obstruction
2. Infectious / traumatic cyst
   • asymptomatic (most)
   • hematuria, bloody urethral discharge
   • postvoid dribbling

Urethral Tumors

Benign Urethral Tumor

1. **Fibroepithelial polyp**
   Age: in child / young adult
   Histo: transitional cell epithelium
   √ solitary, pedunculated fingerlike filling defect attached near verumontanum
   Cx: bladder outlet obstruction
2. **Transitional cell papilloma**
   Age: older patient
   Location: in prostatic / bulbomembranous urethra
   ◊ Frequently associated with concomitant bladder papillomas
3. **Adenomatous polyp**
   Age: young men
   Histo: columnar epithelium from aberrant prostatic epithelium
   Location: adjacent to verumontanum
   • hematuria
4. **Penile squamous papilloma / condyloma acuminata**
   ◊ In 5% of patients with cutaneous disease (glans penis)
   √ verrucous lesion in distal urethra, rarely extension into bladder
5. Others: caruncle, urethral mucosal prolapse, inflammatory tags (in female)

Malignant Urethral Neoplasm

Incidence: 6th–7th decade, M:F = 1:5
A. FEMALE
   • urethral bleeding
   • obstructive symptoms
   • dysuria
   • mass at introitus
   1. Squamous cell carcinoma (70%): distal 2/3 of urethra
   2. Transitional cell carcinoma (8–24%): posterior 1/3 of urethra
   3. Adenocarcinoma (18–28%): from periurethral glands of Skene
B. MALE
   • palpable urethral mass
   • periurethral abscess
   • obstructive symptoms
   • cutaneous fistula
   • bloody discharge
   Site: bulbomembranous urethra (60%); penile urethra (30%); prostatic urethra (10%)
   1. Squamous cell carcinoma (70%)
      secondary to chronic urethritis from venereal disease (44%) + urethral strictures (88%)
   2. Transitional cell carcinoma (16%)
      part of multifocal urothelial neoplasia, in 10% after cystectomy for bladder tumor
   3. Adenocarcinoma (6%)
      in bulbous urethra originating in glands of Cowper / Littre
   4. Melanoma, rhabdomyosarcoma, fibrosarcoma (rare)
   5. Metastases from bladder / prostatic carcinoma (rare)

CALCIFICATIONS OF MALE GENITAL TRACT

A. VAS DEFERENS
   1. Diabetes mellitus: in muscular outer layer
   2. Degenerative changes
   3. TB, syphilis, nonspecific UTI: intraluminal

B. SEMINAL VESICLES
gonorrhea, TB, schistosomiasis, bilharziasis
C. PROSTATE
calcified corpora amylacea, TB

AMBIGUOUS GENITALIA

= external genitalia that are not clearly of either sex
Prevalence: 1:1,000 live births
• cryptorchidism • labial fusion
• epi- / hypospadia • clitoromegaly
Cause:
A. Abnormal hormone levels
1. Congenital adrenal hyperplasia
2. Transplacental passage of hormones
3. True hermaphroditism
B. Anomalies of external genitalia not hormonally mediated (eg, micropenis)
Terminology:
SEX = what a person is biologically; sex assignment based on
(1) karyotype
(2) gonadal biopsy
(3) genital anatomy
GENDER = what a person becomes socially

Female Pseudohermaphroditism

= FEMALE INTERSEX
Cause: exposure to excessive androgens in 1st trimester due to
(a) congenital adrenogenital syndrome
(b) maternal drug ingestion (progestational agents, androgens)
(c) masculinizing ovarian tumor
Karyotype: 46,XX
• masculinized external genitalia:
  • penislike clitoris (due to prominent corpora cavernosa + corpus spongiosum)
  • rugose labioscrotum
• uterus + vagina may be filled with urine through urogenital sinus
√ normal ovaries, fallopian tubes, uterus, vagina
√ enlarged adrenal glands (adrenal hyperplasia)
√ no testicular tissue / internal wolffian duct derivatives

Male Pseudohermaphroditism

Cause: within fetal testis
(a) decreased testosterone synthesis
(b) decreased dihydrotestosterone production (= substance responsible for masculinization of external genitalia) due to 5α-reductase deficiency
(b) no testosterone production due to early destruction / dysgenesis of testes
(c) complete / incomplete androgen insensitivity due to androgen receptor defect (= testicular feminization)
Karyotype: 46,XY
• incompletely masculinized / ambiguous external genitalia
[• apparent hypergonadotropic primary amenorrhea]
√ commonly undescended normal / mildly defective bilateral testes
√ prostatic tissue
√ no müllerian duct derivatives (production of müllerian regression factor by testes not affected)
√ occasionally blind-ending vaginal pouch emptying into perineum (= pseudovagina) / through urethra (= urogenital sinus)

Gonadal Dysgenesis

characterized by abnormal gonadal organization and function with gonads often partially / completely replaced by fibrous stroma
(1) Mixed gonadal dysgenesis
= testis on one side + gonadal streak on other side
Karyotype: 45,XO/46,XY karyotype or other mosaics with a Y chromosome
• ambiguous external genitalia
√ small / rudimentary uterus + vagina
√ fallopian tube present on side of streak gonad
√ urogenital sinus commonly empties at base of phallus
√ dysgenetic gonads (with inability to secrete müllerian regression factor)
Cx: gonadal neoplasia
(2) Pure XY gonadal dysgenesis
Karyotype: 46, XY
√ bilateral streak gonads / dysgenetic testes
√ müllerian + wolffian duct derivatives both absent / partially developed
(3) XY gonadal agenesis
= vanishing testes syndrome = testicular resorption in early fetal life of unknown cause
Karyotype: 46,XY
• ambiguous external genitalia / female phenotype
√ absent testes
√ müllerian + wolffian duct derivatives both absent / partially developed

True Hermaphroditism

= TRUE INTERSEX
= condition characterized by presence of ovarian + testicular tissue either separate or in same gonad (= ovotestis in 64%)
Gonads: (a) ovary on one + testis on other side (30%)
(b) ovary / testis on one + ovotestis on other side (50%)
(c) bilateral ovotestes (20%)
Location: in pelvis (predominantly ovarian tissue); in scrotum / inguinal region (predominantly testicular tissue)
Incidence: rare (500 cases in world literature); <10% of all intersex conditions
Age: diagnosed within first 2 decades (75%)
Karyotype: 46,XX (80%) / 46,XY (10%) / mosaicism (10%)
Classification:
Class I : normal female genitalia (80%)

Class II : enlarged clitoris
Class III : partially fused labioscrotal folds
Class IV: fused labioscrotal folds
Class V : hypoplastic scrotum + penoscrotal hypospadia
Class VI: normal male genitalia

- ambiguous external genitalia
- inguinal hernia
- lower abdominal pain (due to endometriosis)
- lower abdominal tumor (dysgerminoma, myomatous uterus)

Reared as boy:

- cryptorchidism
- short penis
- slight degree of hypospadia
- urogenital sinus at base of penis
- penile urethra (extremely rare)
- effective spermatogenesis (rare)

Reared as girl:

- development of breasts
- hematuria (= menstruation via urogenital sinus opening) in 50%
- internal female organs + female fertility
- amenorrhea
- separate urethral + vaginal openings (uncommon)

√ hypoplastic uterus (in virtually 100%)
√ ovotestis with heterogeneous appearance due to combination of testicular tissue + ovarian follicles
√ internal gonadal duct fits the gonad:
 √ deferent duct on side of testis
 √ fallopian tube on side of ovary
 √ ipsilateral fallopian tube absent (suppression of development by fetal testis)
√ testis / testicular portion of ovotestis usually dysgenetic

MALE INFERTILITY

A. CONGENITAL
 (a) Wolffian duct anomalies
  1. Renal agenesis / atrophy
  2. Vas deferens agenesis / cyst
  3. Seminal vesicle agenesis / cyst
  4. Ejaculatory duct cyst
 (b) Müllerian duct anomalies
  1. Müllerian duct cyst
  2. Utricle cyst

B. ACQUIRED
 1. Cowper duct cyst
 2. Prostatic cyst in peripheral zone

C. INFECTIOUS
 1. Prostatitis

D. HORMONAL
 - semen low in volume, acid pH, without fructose
 1. Seminal vesicle atrophy
  = seminal vesicles <7 mm in width
 2. Seminal vesicle hypoplasia
  = seminal vesicles <11 mm + >7 mm in width

GU

ANATOMY AND FUNCTION OF UROGENITAL TRACT

UROGENITAL EMBRYOLOGY

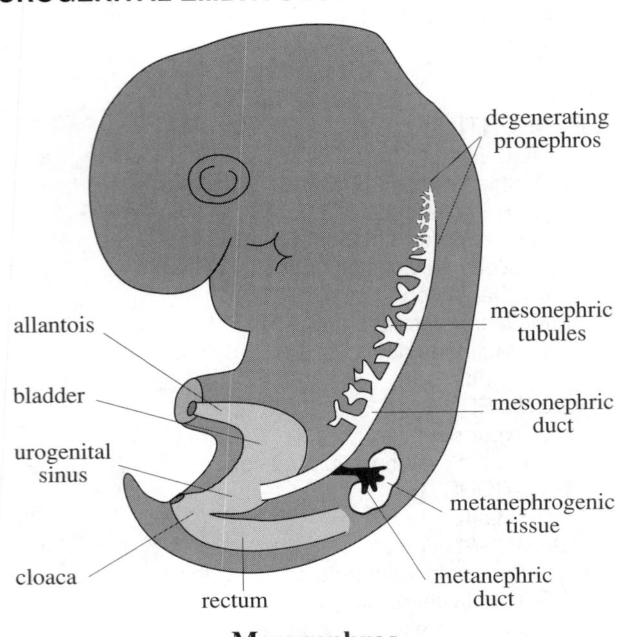

Mesonephros
(embryo at 6th week)

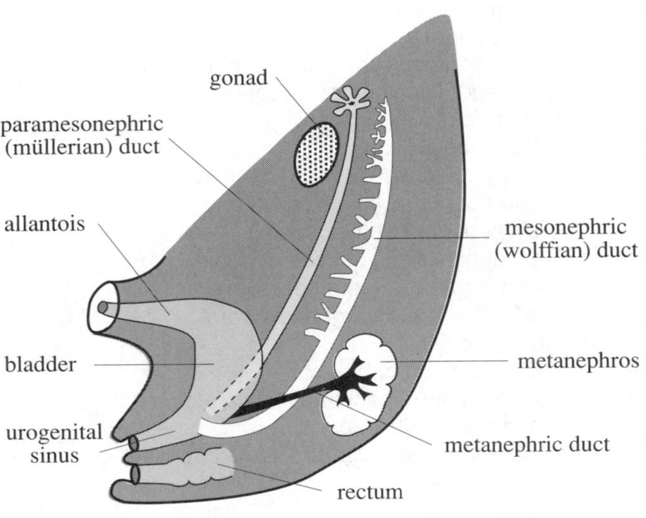

Metanephros
(embryo at 7th week)

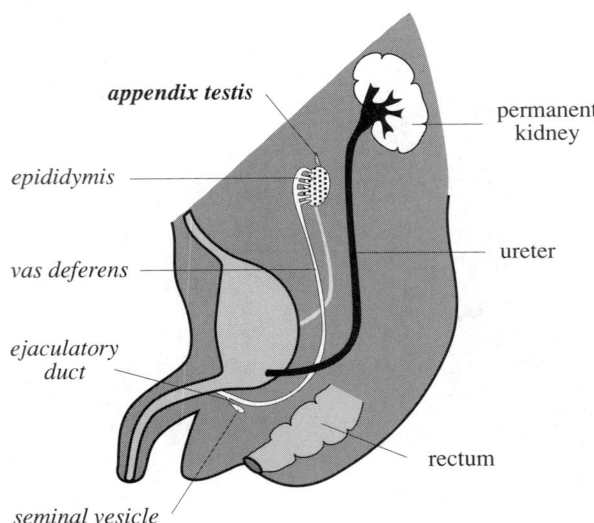

Male Metanephros Differentiation

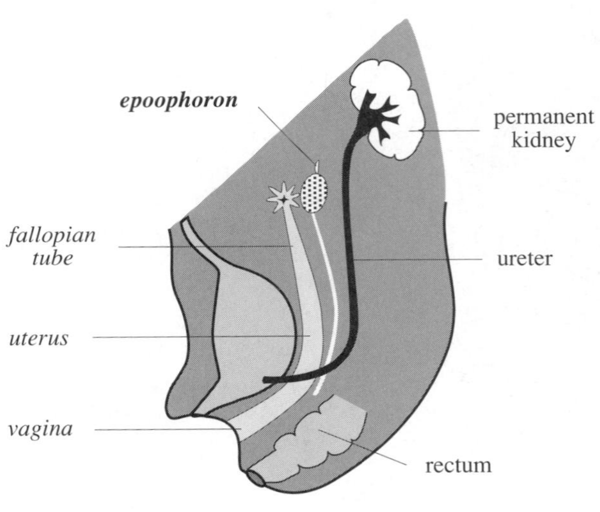

Female Metanephros Differentiation

GU

Pronephros = forekidney
develops from mesoderm during 3rd week of gestation; involutes during 4th week of gestation;
→ vestigial remnant / completely absent

Mesonephros = midkidney
develops during 4th week of gestation immediately caudal to pronephros, functions as interim kidney; degenerates around 8 weeks of gestation

(a) mesonephric tubules
→ paradidymis, epididymis, efferent ductules (M); epinephron (F)

(b) mesonephric (wolffian) duct
→ appendix epididymis, vas deferens, ejaculatory duct, seminal vesicles (M); vanishes (F)

Paramesonephric (Müllerian) Duct

(grows along mesonephric duct)

Male: degenerates due to production of müllerian inhibiting factor (MIF) by Sertoli cells of testis at about 6 weeks GA
→ prostatic utricle + appendix testis

Female: induced by wolffian duct at 5 weeks GA; grows caudally + joins in midline + fuses with outgrowth of urogenital sinus
→ uterus, fallopian tubes

Metanephros = hindkidney = permanent kidney

(1) metanephric diverticulum (**ureteric bud**) buds from mesonephric duct near its entry into the cloaca at 4th week; it lengthens + grows toward nephrogenic cord which becomes the metanephric blastema + divides and forms
→ ureter (mesonephric duct)
→ renal pelvis (first 4 dividing generations of duct)
→ calices (second 4 dividing generations of duct)
→ collecting tubules (10–12 generations of duct)

(2) **metanephric blastema** (= nephrogenic mesoderm) forms nephrons under the influence of ureteral bud, ie, the end of collecting tubules induce clusters of metanephric blastema cells located at the periphery and along the sides of the medullary ray (= pyramid) except around the papilla

(3) **metanephric vesicles** form within clusters of metanephric blastema cells + elongate into S-shaped tubules which, by 12th week of gestation, result in
→ glomerulus
→ proximal convoluted tubule
→ loop of Henle
→ distal convoluted tubule
→ connective tissue
◊ Polycystic kidney disease is believed to be a failure of linkage!

Urogenital Sinus

forms from cloaca
→ develops into bladder + urethra (+ prostate)

Sex Development

Indifferent Stage of Sex

Period: until 7th week of GA

Composition of Undifferentiated Gonad:

(1) Mesenchyme
condensation of mesenchyme forms genital ridges on both sides of midline between 6th thoracic and 2nd sacral segments; differentiates into interstitial (Leydig) cells within seminiferous tubules

(2) Mesothelium
genital ridges are covered by proliferating mesothelium (coelomic epithelium); differentiates into Sertoli / supporting cells of the seminiferous tubules; forms tunica albuginea

(3) Germ cells
form in wall of yolk sac and migrate along hindgut into genital ridge; differentiate into spermatogonia within seminiferous tubules

Formation of Testis

Period: around 8 weeks GA

- testis-determining factor localized on short arm of Y chromosome forms seminiferous tubules
- Leydig cells secrete testosterone supporting the mesonephric (wolffian) duct development
- Sertoli cells secrete müllerian-inhibiting factor leading to regression of paramesonephric (müllerian) duct

Testicular Migration

testes remain near deep inguinal canal until 7th month and then descend through inguinal canal into twin scrotal sacs

RENAL ANATOMY

Adult Kidney

— forms by fusion of superior + inferior subkidneys (= metanephric lobes); the line of fusion runs obliquely forward and upward
√ separation of upper + lower groups of calices
√ indentation of cortical contour + echogenic line (= interrenicular septum = **junctional parenchymal defect**) delineates junctional parenchyma (often referred to as hypertrophic column of Bertin)

— consists of 20,000 lobules within 14 lobes (reniculi)

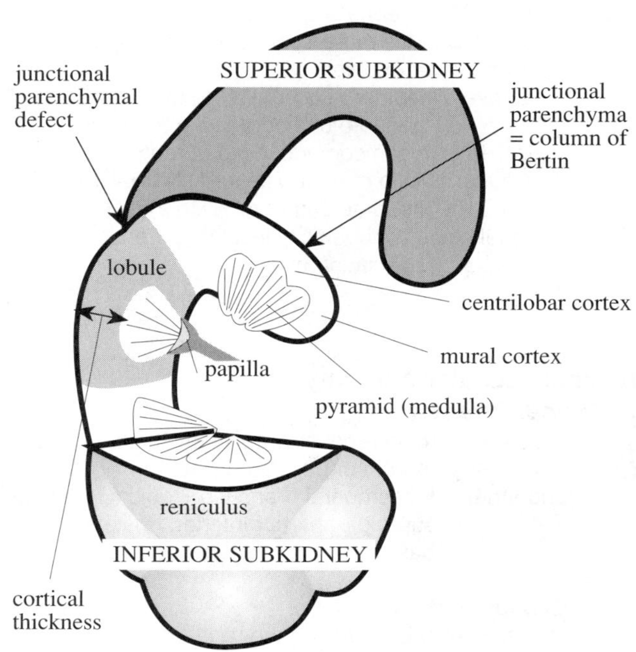

Renal Anatomy

GU

— initially located in pelvic region ventral to sacrum, ascending cranially at 9 weeks of gestation secondary to body growth caudal to kidneys + straightening of body curvature
— renal hilum at first ventrally located, eventually rotating medially by 90 degrees with renal ascent

Reniculus = *renal lobe*
= central core of medullary tissue enveloped by
(a) centrilobar cortex (= cortical arch) that covers the base of the pyramid subsequently forming the renal cortex with loss of grooves
(b) mural cortex that wraps around sides of pyramid and fuses with the mural cortex of adjacent lobe to form renal septum (= column of Bertin)
• renal lobes completed by 28 weeks GA
√ ren lobatus (= interlobar surface grooves) present in fetus + infant, rare in adulthood
√ assimilation of independent lobes >28 weeks GA makes renal surface smoother
• nephrogenesis completed by 36 weeks GA

Renal Size (in cm)
— <1 year of age: 4.98 + 0.155 x age (months)
— >1 year of age: 6.79 + 0.22 x age (years)
— adulthood: R kidney 10.74 ± 1.35 (SD); L kidney 11.10 ± 1.15 (SD);
— ratio of renal length (RL) to distance between first 4 lumbar transverse processes (4TP) = 1.04 ± 0.22

Renal Echogenicity
A. ADULTHOOD
liver ≥ spleen ≥ renal cortex > renal medulla
B. INFANCY (in neonate up to 6 months of age)
√ cortex may be more echogenic than adjacent normal liver / spleen
Cause: glomeruli occupy 18% of cortex in neonate compared with 9% in adult
√ increase in corticomedullary differentiation
Cause: ratio of cortex to medulla 1.64:1 in neonate compared with 2.59:1 in adult
√ renal sinus echogenicity less prominent
Cause: paucity of fat

Renal Vascular Anatomy

Renal Arteries

1st order: main renal arteries at level of L1 / upper margin of L2
2nd order: 5 segmental branches = apical, anterior superior, anterior inferior, posterior, basilar

Capsular artery
= tiny vessels perfusing the renal capsule
Origin: main renal a., branch renal a., other retroperitoneal aa. (lumbar a.)

ANATOMIC RENAL ARTERY VARIANTS

Multiple renal arteries (25–30%)
unilaterally (32%); bilaterally (12%)

Polar artery
Entry: without going through renal hilum directly into renal parenchyma
(a) superior polar artery
Origin: main renal artery (12%), aorta (7%)
(b) inferior polar artery
Origin: aorta (5.5%), main renal artery (1.4%)

Supplementary artery
Entry: renal hilum
Origin: aorta, iliac a., internal spermatic a., SMA, IMA, celiac trunk, middle colic a., lumbar a., middle sacral a., contralateral renal a.
Supply: lower pole (72%) > upper pole

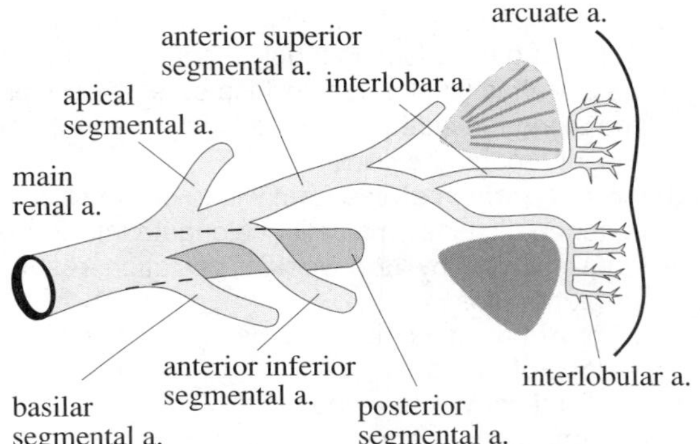

Anatomy of Renal Arteries

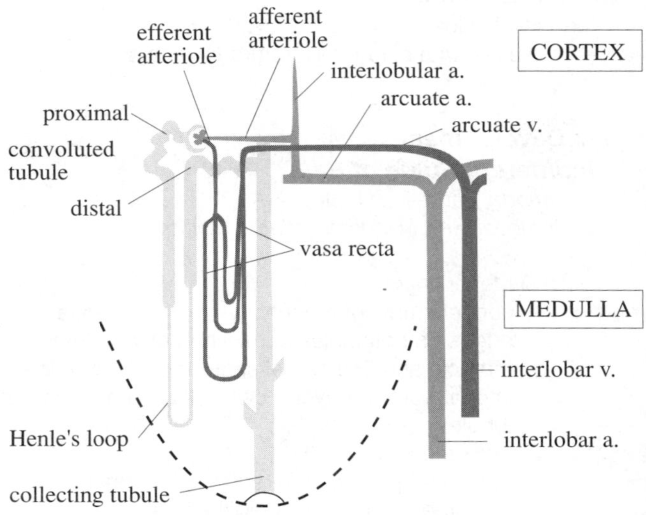

Renal Parenchymal Blood Supply

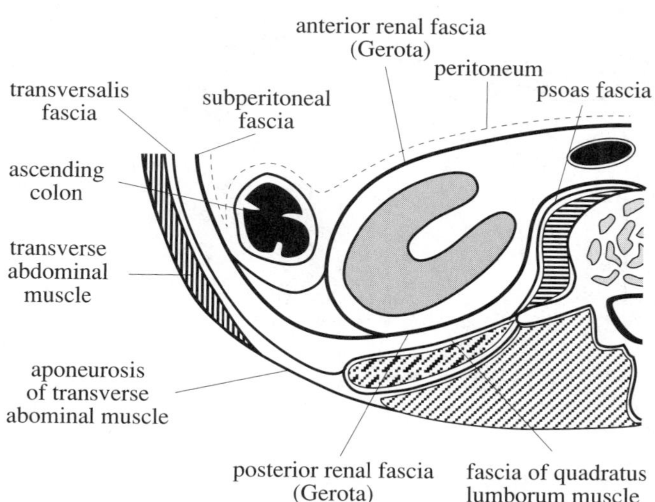

Gerota's Fascia

anterior pararenal space
anterior renal fascia = Gerota fascia = fascia of Toldt
peritoneum
lateroconal fascia
transverse fascia
posterior pararenal space
posterior renal fascia = Zuckerkandl fascia
perirenal space

Pararenal Spaces

Extrahilar branching
= branching of main renal artery prior to reaching hilum
Entry: renal hilum / direct as polar arteries
— early branching: within 1.5 cm from aorta

Accessory renal artery
= segmental artery originating from aorta / iliac a.

Aberrant renal artery
= segmental artery arising from superior mesenteric artery / internal spermatic artery

Resistive index: <0.70
1 SD of several measurements = 0.04

Renal Veins
Single right renal vein (85%) without major extrarenal tributaries
Single preaortic left renal vein (86%) with several major extrarenal tributaries
(a) left adrenal vein
(b) left gonadal vein
(c) lumbar, ascending lumbar, hemiazygos vv.

Anatomic Renal Vein Variants
Multiple right renal veins (28–30%)
(a) single right renal vein divides just before union with IVC (4%)
(b) right gonadal vein joins the renal vein (6%)
(c) accessory branch of adrenal vein enters right renal vein (31%)
(d) lumbar / azygos vv. enter right renal vein (3%)

Circumaortic left renal vein (5–17%)
Single retroaortic left renal vein (2–3%)
Lumbar veins joining left renal vein (75%)

RETROPERITONEUM
= space between transversalis fascia + parietal peritoneum extending from diaphragm to pelvic brim

Perirenal Compartments

A. Anterior border: anterior renal fascia
B. Anterior pararenal space
  → superiorly joins with posterior renal fascia and attaches to crux of diaphragm
  → in the middle blends with connective tissues of central prevertebral space around great vessels
  → inferiorly joins with posterior renal fascia and attaches to great vessels
  contains: pancreas, duodenum, ascending + descending colon
C. Perirenal space
  subdivided into multiple compartments by incomplete bridging septa that attach to anterior + posterior renal fascia
  → forms inverted cone around adrenal gland + perirenal fat + upper half of kidney
  → forms cone around perirenal fat + lower pole of kidney
  → medially open communicating with central prevertebral space
  contains: kidneys, adrenals
D. Posterior pararenal space
  contains: fat, no organs
E. Posterior border: posterior renal fascia (attaches to psoas muscle)

RENAL HORMONES
Antidiuretic Hormone (ADH)
Production site: supraoptic nuclei of hypothalamus, transported to neurohypophysis
Stimulus: fluid loss with increase in osmolality

GU

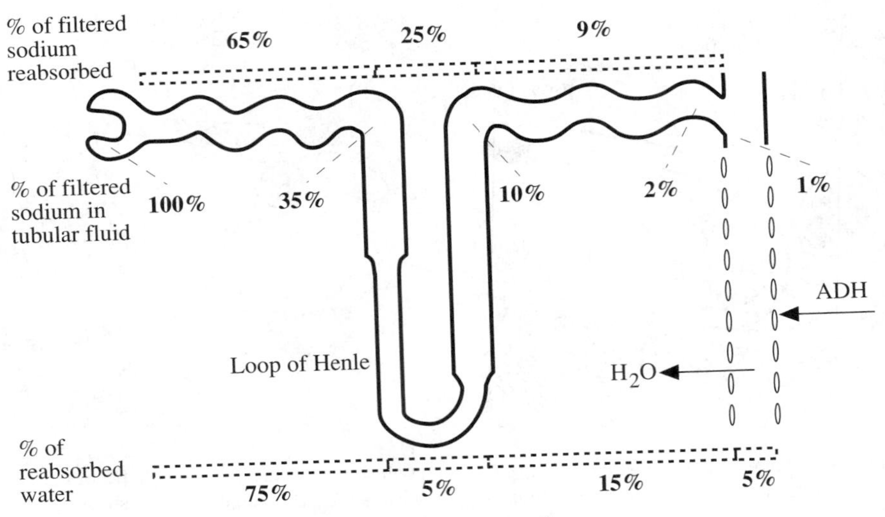

Sodium Reabsorption

hypertonicity is maintained within the medullary interstitium by the countercurrent multiplier system of the loop of Henle and the vasa recta; ADH increases permeability of collecting ducts for water

Effects:
(1) 10 x increase in permeability of collecting ducts (= concentrated urine)
(2) decreased blood flow through vasa recta leads to increased hypertonicity of interstitium (= countercurrent multiplier mechanism)

Renin-aldosterone Mechanism

receptors in juxtaglomerular apparatus register the intraglomerular capillary hydraulic pressure, which is one of the main determinants of the glomerular filtration rate (GFR);

the receptors regulate the release of **renin** as an autoregulatory feedback mechanism to maintain the intraglomerular hydraulic pressure;

renin mediates conversion of angiotensin to angiotensin-I, which is then cleaved by a converting enzyme into angiotensin-II

Angiotensin-II effect:
(a) constriction of efferent postglomerular arterioles, which increases intraglomerular capillary hydraulic pressure + GFR
(b) systemic arteriolar constriction (= most potent vasoconstrictor of biologic systems), which causes systemic hypertension
(c) release of **aldosterone**, which increases sodium retention by renal tubules
— leads to an increase in blood volume + pressure if both kidneys are affected
— leads to compensatory natriuresis if only one kidney is affected

◊ ACE inhibitors (eg, captopril) produce a dramatic decrease in blood pressure!

RENAL PHYSIOLOGY

Perfusion: 1.2–1.3 L of blood per minute (= 20–25% of total cardiac output)
Urine output: 1 L/d
Filtration: substances of up to 4 nm (excluding substances >8 nm), threshold at molecular weight of approximately 40,000

Glomerular Filtration Rate (GFR)

$[P] \times GFR = [U] \times U_{vol}$

GFR $= \{[U] \times U_{vol}\} / [P]$ = 125 mL/min = 20% of RPF

Substrate: inulin; Tc-99m DTPA

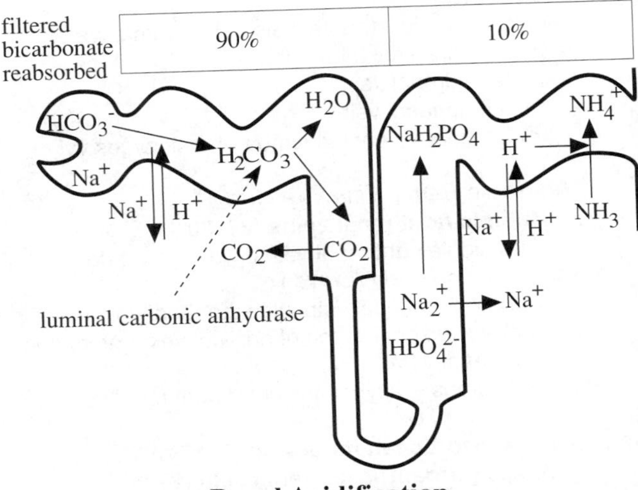

Renal Acidification

GU

Tubular Secretion (Tm)

$[U] \times U_{vol} = [P] \times GFR + Tm$

$\mathbf{Tm = \{[U] \times U_{vol}\} - \{[P] \times GFR\}}$

Substrate: p-aminohippurate (PAH); I-131 Hippuran

Renal Plasma Flow (RPF)

$[P] \times RPF = [U] \times U_{vol}$

$\mathbf{RPF = \{[U] \times U_{vol}\} / [P]}$

Substrate: p-aminohippurate

[P] = concentration in plasma
GFR = glomerular filtration rate
[U] = concentration in urine
U_{vol} = urine volume
Tm = transport maximum (across tubular cells)
RPF = renal plasma flow

Renal Acidification Mechanism

Proximal tubule:
reabsorption of 90% of filtered bicarbonate by luminal Na^+/H^+ exchange and Na^+/HCO_3^- cotransport at basolateral membrane
regulated by: luminal carbonic anhydrase
influenced by: luminal HCO_3^- concentration, extracellular fluid volume, parathormone, K^+, aldosterone

Distal nephron:
active secretion of H^+ against a steep urine-to-blood gradient across luminal cell membrane by H^+-ATPase pump facilitated by Na^+ reabsorption resulting in reabsorption of 10% of filtered bicarbonate, formation of ammonium (NH_4^+) and titratable acidity

Ammonium excretion:
Ammonia (NH_3) is formed in proximal tubule as a product of catabolism of glutamine + other amino acids; combination with secreted H^+ to NH_4^+ takes place in distal nephron

Titratable acidity:
divalent basic phosphate is converted into monovalent acid form in distal tubule

Renal Imaging in Newborn Infant

◊ Low glomerular filtration rate (GFR):
- — on first day of life: 21% of adult values
- — by 2 weeks of age: 44% of adult values
- — at end of 1st year: close to adult values

◊ Limited capacity to concentrate urine

IVP:
√ occasional failure of renal visualization

NUC:
√ improved visualization on radionuclide studies

Normal Nephrographic Phases / Progression

1. Vascular phase (= cortical arteriogram)
   = contrast material visible in interlobular arteries + glomeruli
   Timing after IV injection: 10–15–25 seconds (arm-to-kidney circulation time)
   Duration: transient vascular phase of <0.5 seconds
2. Cortical phase (= cortical nephrogram)
   = contrast medium within cortical capillaries + peritubular spaces + cortical tubular lumina
   Timing after IV injection: 25–45–70 seconds
   Timing after intraarterial injection: 2–3 seconds
   CT:
   √ exclusive renal cortical enhancement with minimally enhancing renal medulla (= corticomedullary differentiation)
3. Parenchymal phase (= generalized / diffuse / tubular nephrogram)
   = contrast material within loops of Henle + collecting tubules
   Timing after IV injection: 60–85–120 seconds (maximum)
   √ enhancement of both cortex and medulla
   N.B.: most valuable phase for detecting renal masses
4. Excretory phase
   = contrast material within collecting system
   Timing after IV injection: beginning at 2–3–5 minutes

Contrast Excretion

UROGRAPHIC DENSITY depends on

$$[U] = \{[P] \times GFR\} / U_{vol}$$

1. Concentration of contrast material in plasma [P] is a function of
   (a) total iodine dose
   (b) contrast injection rate
   (c) volume distribution
   Rapid decline of concentration of contrast material in vessels is due to:
   (1) rapid mixing within vascular compartment
   (2) diffusion into extravascular extracellular fluid space (capillary permeation)
   (3) renal excretion
2. Glomerular filtration rate (GFR): 99% filtered
3. Urine volume (U_{vol}), ie, activity of ADH:
   (a) in dehydrated state with increased ADH activity concentrations of contrast material are higher
   ◊ Dehydration is considered a risk-potentiating factor for nephrotoxicity!
   (b) in volume-expanded state with decreased ADH activity concentrations of contrast material are lower
   ◊ Patients with CHF require higher doses of contrast material!

A. MEGLUMINE
no metabolization, excreted by glomerular filtration alone

Meglumine effect of osmotic diuresis:
(a) lower concentration of urinary iodine per mL urine
(b) greater distension of collecting system
N.B.: Avoid meglumine in "at risk" patients (higher incidence of contrast reactions than sodium!)

B. SODIUM
extensive reabsorption by tubules with delayed excretion
Sodium effect of reabsorption:
(a) increased concentration of urinary iodine (improved visualization)
(b) less distension of collecting system (ureteral compression necessary)

ADRENAL ANATOMY

from periphery to centrum:
(a) renin-angiotensin–dependent outer adrenal cortex:
zona glomerulosa = mineralocorticoid (aldosterone)
(b) corticotropin-dependent inner adrenal cortex:
zona fasciculata = cortisol
zona reticularis = sex hormones (androgen, estrogen)
(c) medulla = norepinephrine, epinephrine
mnemonic: "**G**lomerular **F**iltration **R**ate **M**ay **G**ive **A**nswers"
Glomerulosa
Fasciculata
Reticulosa
Mineralocorticoids
Glucocorticoids
Androgens

Normal size : 3–5 (L) x 3 (W) x 1 cm (thick)
◊ Each limb of the adrenal gland should not be thicker than the crus of the diaphragm
Normal weight : 3–5 g (5–10 g at birth)
Visualization by CT : left side 100%, right side 99%
by US : left side 45%, right side 80%

@ IN NEONATAL PERIOD
Normal weight : 5–10 g at birth
◊ Rapid regression of fetal cortex during first 6 weeks of life!

Adrenal Vascular Anatomy

Adrenal Arteries

50–60 small adrenal branches from 3 main adrenal arteries form a subcapsular plexus that drains into medullary sinusoids
Supply: inferior phrenic artery, renal artery, directly from aorta
(a) all 3 sources in 34%
(b) two sources in 61%
(c) single source in 5% (renal a. only in 2%)
forming superior, middle, inferior adrenal arteries
◊ The renal artery contributes in 71%!
◊ Gonadal artery contributes in 60% in fetal circulation!

Adrenal Veins

"Vascular dam" = gland is drained by an intrinsically vulnerable network of relatively few venules
Single right adrenal v. drains into IVC (69%)
Accessory right adrenal v. drains into renal v. (31%)
Left adrenal v. almost always enters left renal v.

BLADDER

Bladder capacity [mL] = (age in years + 2) x 30

SCROTAL ANATOMY

Scrotal wall thickness: 2–8 mm (3–6 mm in 89%)
Tunica vaginalis
= inferior extension of processus vaginalis of the peritoneum
Hydrocele: small to moderate in 14% of normals

Testis

Average size of testis: 3.8 x 3.0 x 2.5 cm (decreasing with age)
Length of testis: 3–5.5 cm (mature); 1–1.5 cm (newborn)
Testicular cysts: in 8% of normals (average size 2–3 mm), numbers increasing with age
Anatomy: 200–300 lobules each containing 400–600 seminiferous tubules; each tubule is 30–80 cm long with a total length of 300–980 m
Histo: (1) spermatogonia (adjacent to basement membrane) → spermatocytes → spermatids → spermatozoa
(2) nondividing Sertoli cells provide the support structure; their tight cell junctions are responsible for the blood-testis barrier
(3) interstitium (= space between seminiferous tubules) contains connective tissue, lymphatics, blood vessels, mast cells, Leydig cells (= principal source of testosterone production)

Appendix Testis

= small stalked appendage at upper pole of testis
= remnant of paramesonephric duct

Tunica Albuginea

= fibrous covering of testis, invaginating into testicular parenchyma at mediastinum testis; externally covered by visceral layer of tunica vaginalis (= flattened layer of mesothelium); internally applied to tunica vasculosa carrying the capsular artery

Mediastinum Testis

= converging point of ~400 cone-shaped lobules separated by fibrous septa + seminiferous tubules forming larger tubuli recti and draining into the rete testis (= 15–20 efferent ductules)
= entry and exit point for ducts, nerves, vessels (hilum of testis)

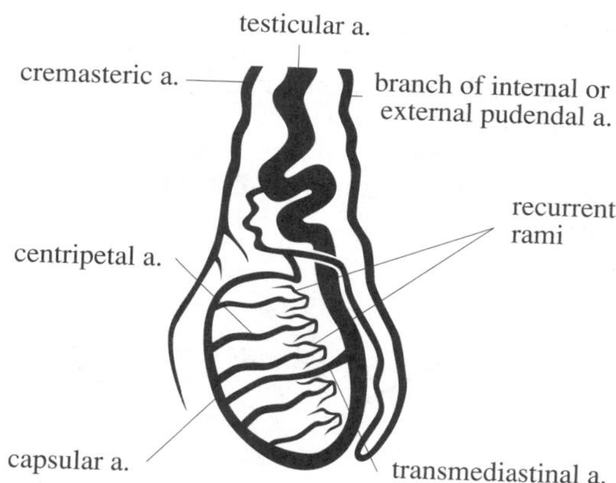

Arterial Supply of Scrotum

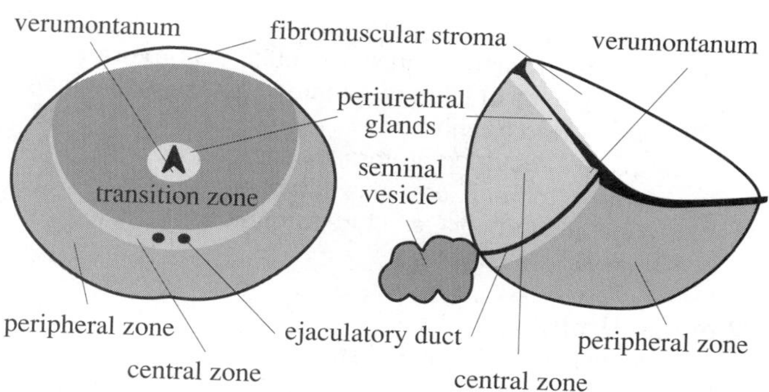

Transverse Section through Prostate with BPH

Midsagittal Section through Normal Prostate

√ posteriorly located linear echogenic region extending longitudinally 5–8 mm from the edge

Blood Flow To Testis

PSV: 4–10–19 cm/s
EDV: 2–5–8 cm/s
RI: 0.44–0.60–0.75

Epididymis

= tortuous tightly folded canal forming the efferent route from testis; consists of head (= globus major), body, tail (= globus minor)

Length: 7 cm
Size of globus major: 11 x 7 x 6 mm (decreasing with age)
Epididymal cysts: occur in 30% of normals (average size of 4 mm)
Epididymal calcification: in 3%
Appendix epididymis = small stalked appendage of globus major (in 33%); occasionally duplicated

Spermatic Cord

= testicular + deferential + cremasteric aa., pampiniform plexus of veins, vas deferens, nerves, lymphatics

Gonadal Vascular Anatomy

Gonadal Artery

Origin: ventral surface of aorta a few cm below the origin of renal arteries (83%);
from renal artery / arteries (17%):
(a) RT from renal a. + LT from aorta (6%)
(b) RT from aorta + LT from renal a. (4%)
(c) RT + LT from both renal arteries (4%)

Course: LT anterior to left renal v. (20%);
RT behind IVC + anterior to right renal v.

Gonadal Vein

RT: drains into IVC (93%) / right renal v. (7%)
LT: left renal v.
Multiple gonadal veins (15%)

ZONAL ANATOMY OF PROSTATE

Normal weight: 20 ± 6 g
Normal size: 2.8 cm (craniocaudad), 2.8 cm (anteroposterior), 4.8 cm (width)

A. OUTER GLAND
1. Central zone: surrounds ejaculatory ducts from their entrance at prostatic base to verumontanum; 25% of glandular tissue
2. Peripheral zone: extends from base of prostate to apex along rectal surface; 70% of glandular tissue

B. INNER GLAND
1. Transition zone: on each side of internal sphincter; 4% of glandular tissue; enlarges with BPH
2. Periurethral zone: surrounding urethra; 1% of glandular tissue

ANATOMY OF URETHRA

Male Urethra

extends through corpus spongiosum (composed of large venous sinuses)

A. POSTERIOR URETHRA
1. Prostatic urethra
   = from vesical neck to triangular ligament
   – orifices of ducts from prostatic acini at floor
   – verumontanum = colliculus seminalis
     = prostatic utricle (fused end of müllerian ducts)
   – orifice of the two ejaculatory ducts
2. Membranous urethra
   = portion traversing urogenital diaphragm
   – pea-sized bulbourethral glands of Cowper lie laterally + posteriorly between fasciae and sphincter urethrae within urogenital diaphragm

B. ANTERIOR = CAVERNOUS URETHRA
1. Bulbous urethra

GU

2. Penile (= pendulous) urethra
   - many small branched tubular periurethral glands of Littre terminate in recesses (lacunae of Morgagni)

   Cx: recurring urethral discharge following chronic urethritis, latent gonorrheal urethritis, stricture formation
3. Fossa navicularis

Female Urethra

3–5 cm in length, 6 mm in diameter
urethral crest = posteriorly located prominent fold
Two sets of glands:

(a) urethral glands
   - terminate separately along entire length of urethra

(b) paraurethral glands = glands of Skene (= homologues of prostatic ducts)
   - formed by an interdependent conducting system
   - exit on either side of midline just posterior to urethral meatus draining into vaginal vestibule

   Cx: chronic gonorrheal urethritis

1. Intrapelvic urethra
   = upper 2/3 of urethra that lies behind symphysis pubis
2. Membranous urethra
   surrounded by sphincter membranacea urethrae (weaker less important structure than in male)
3. Perineal urethra
   lower 1/3 extending from superior fascia of urogenital diaphragm to meatus between labia minora

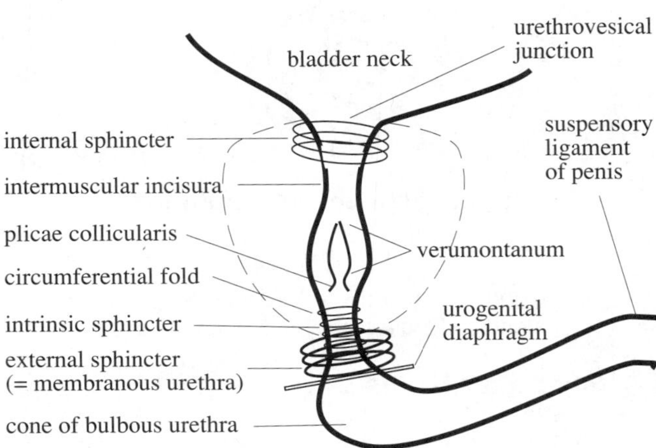

Urethrogram: Normal Urethral Folds in LPO

RENAL, ADRENAL, URETERAL, VESICAL, AND SCROTAL DISORDERS

ABORTIVE CALYX

= developmental anomaly with short blind-ending outpouching of pyramid without papillary invagination

Location: (a) renal pelvis
(b) infundibulum (mostly upper pole)

ACQUIRED CYSTIC KIDNEY DISEASE

= ACQUIRED CYSTIC DISEASE OF UREMIA
= development of numerous fluid-filled renal cysts in patients with chronic renal failure undergoing hemodialysis

◊ Successful transplant probably stops development of additional cysts, but does not affect malignant potential!

Prevalence: in 10–20% after 1–3 years,
in 40–60% after 3–5 years,
in 90% after 5–10 years of hemodialysis;
in 25% of renal allograft recipients

Proposed etiologies:
(a) altered compliance of tubular basement membrane
(b) intra- and extratubal obstruction due to focal proliferation of tubular epithelium
(c) obstruction of ducts by interstitial fibrosis / oxalate crystals
(d) toxicity from circulating metabolites (endogenous / exogenous toxins, mutagens, mitogens, growth factors)
(e) vascular insufficiency

At increased risk: older men

Histo: cysts lined by flattened cuboidal / papillary epithelium

Associated with:
(a) small papillary / tubular / solid clear-cell adenomas (in 13–20%): approximately 1 cm in diameter
(b) renal cell carcinoma (in 3–6%): 7-year interval between transplantation + detection of RCC

√ small end-stage kidneys (<280 g)
√ multiple 0.5–3-cm cysts bilaterally (early = small, late = large)
√ occasionally progressive renal enlargement due to cysts

Dx: >3 cysts + NO history of hereditary cystic disease

Cx: spontaneous hemorrhage into cyst (macrohematuria / retroperitoneal hemorrhage from cyst rupture)

AIDS

• azotemia, proteinuria, hematuria, pyuria (in 38–68% sometime during illness)
• progressive renal failure (10%)

1. **HIV nephropathy** (40%)
   = characterized by nephrotic-range proteinuria + rapidly progressive renal failure, primarily occurring in Black patients
   Histo: focal + segmental glomerulosclerosis, sparse interstitial infiltrates, severe tubular degenerative changes, interstitial tubular microcystic ectasia containing protein casts
   • mild hypertension
   • early + rapidly progressive renal failure with 100% mortality within 6 months
   √ global enlargement of both kidneys
   US (best screening test):
   √ increased cortical echogenicity (33–68%)
   CT:
   √ medullary hyperattenuation (14%)
   √ striated nephrogram on CECT
   MRI:
   √ loss of corticomedullary differentiation
   Prognosis: death within 6 months
2. Renal infection with Pneumocystis carinii (8%)
   ◊ More frequent since introduction of prophylactic aerosolized pentamidine therapy encouraging extrapulmonic spread (<1%) due to inadequate systemic distribution of drug!
   √ punctate renal calcifications confined to cortex (DDx: CMV, Mycobacterium avium-intracellulare)
   √ associated calcifications in spleen, liver, lymph nodes, adrenal glands
3. Renal lymphoma (3–12%)
   AIDS-related lymphoma:
   highly aggressive B-cell lymphomas (centroblastic, lymphoblastic, immunoblastic); NHL > Burkitt lymphoma, Hodgkin disease
   √ bilateral multiple renal masses
   √ direct extension of retroperitoneal lymphadenopathy engulfing kidney, renal sinus, ureter
4. Cystitis (22%)
   Organism: routine Gram-negative species, Candida, beta-hemolytic streptococci, Salmonella, CMV
   √ bladder wall thickening

ACUTE CORTICAL NECROSIS

= rare form of acute renal failure

Etiology:
(a) ischemia due to vasospasm of small vessels
(b) toxic damage to glomerular capillary endothelium
(c) primary intravascular thrombosis

At risk:
(a) Obstetric patient (most often): abruptio placentae
= premature separation of placenta with concealed hemorrhage (50%), septic abortion, placenta previa
(b) Children: severe dehydration + fever, infection, hemolytic uremic syndrome, transfusion reaction
(c) Adults: sepsis, severe dehydration, acute prolonged shock, myocardial failure, burns, venomous snakebite, abdominal aortic surgery, hyperacute renal transplant rejection

Histo: patchy / universal necrosis of renal cortex + proximal convoluted structures (secondary to distension of glomerular capillaries with dehemoglobulinized RBCs); medulla and 1–2 mm of peripheral cortex are spared

• protracted + severe oliguria / anuria
Distribution: diffuse / multifocal; mostly bilateral

A. EARLY SIGNS
√ diffusely enlarged smooth kidneys
√ absent / faint nephrogram
CT:
√ enhancing interlobar and arcuate arteries adjacent to nonenhancing cortex (arterial phase)
√ enhancement of medulla + nonenhancement of cortex (parenchymal phase)
√ rim of subcapsular cortical enhancement (due to collateral blood flow from cortical vessels)
√ enhancement of juxtamedullary zone of cortex
US:
√ loss of normal corticomedullary region with hypoechoic outer rim of cortex
NUC:
√ severely impaired renal perfusion
B. LATE SIGNS
√ small kidney (after a few months)
√ "tramline" / punctate calcifications along margins of viable and necrotic tissue (as early as 1–2 months)
US:
√ hyperechoic cortex with acoustic shadowing
Prognosis: poor chance of recovery

ACUTE DIFFUSE BACTERIAL NEPHRITIS

= ACUTE SUPPURATIVE PYELONEPHRITIS
= more severe and extensive form of acute pyelonephritis, which may lead to diffuse necrosis (phlegmon)
Organism: Proteus, Klebsiella > E. coli
Predisposed: diabetics (60%)

ACUTE INTERSTITIAL NEPHRITIS

= infiltration of interstitium by lymphocytes, plasma cells, eosinophils, few PMNs + edema
Cause: allergic / idiosyncratic reaction to drug exposure (methicillin, sulfonamides, ampicillin, cephalothin, penicillin, anticoagulants, phenindione, diphenylhydantoin)
• eosinophilia (develops 5 days to 5 weeks after exposure)
√ large smooth kidneys with thick parenchyma
√ normal / diminished contrast density
US:
√ normal / increased echogenicity

ACUTE TUBULAR NECROSIS

= temporary reversible marked reduction in tubular flow rate
Etiology:
(a) DRUGS: bichloride of mercury, ethylene glycol (antifreeze), carbon tetrachloride, bismuth, arsenic, uranium, urographic contrast material (especially when associated with glomerulosclerosis in diabetes mellitus), aminoglycosides (gentamicin, kanamycin)
(b) ISCHEMIA: major trauma, massive hemorrhage, postpartum hemorrhage, crush injury, myoglobulinuria, compartmental syndrome, septic shock, cardiogenic shock, burns, transfusion reaction, severe dehydration, pancreatitis, gastroenteritis, renal transplantation, cardiac surgery, biliary surgery, aortic resection
Pathophysiology: profound reduction in renal blood flow due to elevated arteriolar resistance
√ smooth large kidneys, especially increase in AP diameter >4.63 cm (due to interstitial edema)
√ diminished / absent opacification of collecting system
√ immediate persistent dense nephrogram (75%)
√ increasingly dense persistent nephrogram (25%)
√ diffuse calcifications (rare)
US:
√ normal to diminished echogenicity of medulla
√ sharp delineation of swollen pyramids
√ normal (89%) / increased (11%) echogenicity of cortex
√ elevated resistive index ≥0.75 (in 91% excluding patients with hepatorenal syndrome); unusual in prerenal azotemia
Angio:
√ normal arterial tree with delayed emptying of intrarenal vessels
√ slightly delayed / normal venous opacification
NUC:
√ poor concentration of Tc-99m glucoheptonate / Tc-99m DTPA
√ well-maintained renal perfusion
√ better renal visualization on immediate postinjection images than on delayed images
√ progressive parenchymal accumulation of I-131 Hippuran / Tc-99m MAG3
√ no excretion

ADDISON DISEASE

= PRIMARY ADRENAL INSUFFICIENCY
◊ 90% of adrenal cortex must be destroyed!
Course: acute (adrenal apoplexy), subacute (disease present for <2 years), chronic

Acute Primary Adrenal Insufficiency

= ADDISONIAN CRISIS = ADRENAL APOPLEXY
Cause: bilateral adrenal hemorrhage most commonly due to stress from surgery / sepsis / hypotension with shock / hemorrhagic diathesis, anticoagulation therapy
• abdominal / back pain
• fever (70%), hyperpyrexia, lethargy, nausea, vomiting
√ bilateral adrenal enlargement with areas of increased attenuation
Cx: catastrophic hypotension + shock

Chronic Primary Adrenal Insufficiency

Cause:
1. Idiopathic adrenal atrophy (60–70%): likely autoimmune disorder
2. Fungal infection: histoplasmosis, blastomycosis, coccidioidomycosis

3. Granulomatous disease: tuberculosis, sarcoidosis
4. Bilateral metastatic disease (rare)

• hyponatremia, hyperkalemia, azotemia, hypercalcemia
√ diminutive glands (in idiopathic atrophy + chronic inflammation)
√ calcifications (in 25% of chronic course)

ADRENAL CYST

Prevalence: 0.064–0.180%
Age: 3rd–6th decades (most commonly); M:F = 1:3
Path:
(a) endothelial lining (45–48%):
1. Lymphangioma (93%)
2. Hemangioma

(b) pseudocyst (39–42%):
1. Previous hemorrhage / infarction
2. Hemorrhagic complication of benign vascular neoplasm / malformation
3. Cystic degeneration / hemorrhage of primary adrenal mass

(c) epithelial lining = true cyst (9–10%):
1. Glandular / retention cyst
2. Embryonal cyst
3. Cystic adenoma
4. Mesothelial inclusion cyst

(d) parasitic cyst (7%): usually echinococcal

Location: mostly solitary; R:L = 1:1; bilateral in 8–10%
√ well-defined uni- / multilocular
√ wall thickness of up to 3 mm
√ <5 cm in diameter in 50% (up to 20 cm)
√ usually homogeneous with near-water density; higher attenuation with hemorrhage / intracystic debris / crystals
√ lack of central enhancement ± wall enhancement
√ calcifications:
(a) peripheral / mural: rimlike / nodular (51–69%)
(b) central: in intracystic septation (19%) / punctate within intracystic hemorrhage (5%)

Cx: hypertension; hemorrhage; infection; rupture with retroperitoneal hemorrhage
DDx:
1. Cystic pheochromocytoma
2. Cystic adenomatoid tumor
3. Schwannoma
4. Cystic adrenocortical carcinoma (thick-walled lesion >7 cm in size; extremely rare)
5. Adrenal adenoma (contrast enhancement, no wall, no peripheral calcification)

ADRENAL HEMORRHAGE

Traumatic Adrenal Hemorrhage

Cause: blunt abdominal trauma, adrenal venous sampling
Prevalence: 2% (in 28% of autopsies)
Location: R:L = 9:1, bilateral in 20%
√ round / oval hematoma (in 83%) located in medulla + stretching cortex around hematoma
√ obliteration of gland by diffuse irregular hemorrhage (in 9%)
√ uniform adrenal enlargement (in 9%)
√ periadrenal hemorrhage causes ill-defined adrenal margin + stranding + asymmetric thickening of diaphragmatic crus

Nontraumatic Adrenal Hemorrhage

◊ Most common neonatal lesion of adrenal gland
Cause:
A. NEONATAL STRESS
1. Difficult labor / delivery: forceps / breech delivery
2. Asphyxia / hypoxia due to prematurity
3. Septicemia
4. Hemorrhagic disorders: DIC, hypoprothrombinemia
5. Extracorporeal membrane oxygenation (in 4%)
6. Thrombus extending from renal vein thrombosis

Predisposed: infants large for gestational age, infants of diabetic mothers
Age: 1st week of life
Site: R:L = 7:3; bilateral in 10%

B. STRESS
Pathophysiology:
stress increases endogenous secretion of adrenocorticotropic hormone severalfold causing an increase in adrenal vascularity; venoconstriction + venous thrombosis (due to catecholamines, thrombin , fibrin, endotoxin) during shock lead to intraglandular hemorrhage
1. Surgery: orthotopic liver transplantation
2. Sepsis: **Waterhouse-Friderichsen syndrome** (= fulminant meningococcemia); Pseudomonas infection; other Gram-negative organisms
3. Burns
4. Hypotension
5. Pregnancy
6. Cardiovascular disease
7. Exogenous adrenocorticotropic hormone
8. Exogenous steroids

C. HEMORRHAGIC DIATHESIS & COAGULOPATHY
1. Anticoagulant therapy (heparin, coumadin): during initial 3 weeks
2. Disseminated intravascular coagulopathy
3. Antiphospholipid syndrome ± systemic lupus erythematosus (hypercoagulable state causes adrenal vein thrombosis + venous infarction)

D. UNDERLYING ADRENAL TUMOR
1. Pseudocyst
2. Myelolipoma
3. Hemangioma
4. Pheochromocytoma
5. Adrenocortical adenoma / carcinoma
6. Metastasis: bronchogenic carcinoma, angiosarcoma, melanoma

• sudden / gradual onset of lower chest / upper abdominal / flank / back pain
• signs of massive blood loss
• acute primary adrenal insufficiency (rare but life-threatening)

√ mass displacing kidney inferiorly + IVC anteriorly
√ gradual decrease in size over weeks (follow-up for 2–3 months)
√ developing rimlike curvilinear / eggshell calcification

US (modality of choice for neonate):
√ complex solid echogenic mass during early stage
√ mixed echogenicity with centrally hypoechoic region (as liquefaction occurs)
√ completely anechoic / cystlike in chronic stage
√ peripheral calcifications in 1–2 weeks
√ avascular on color Doppler / power Doppler

CT:
√ round / oval mass (similar to traumatic causes)
√ periadrenal fat stranding
√ mass + hypoattenuating center ± calcifications in chronic stage = **adrenal pseudocyst**
√ calcification >1 year

NECT:
√ high-attenuation mass (50–90 HU) in acute / subacute stage

MR:
@ acute stage (<7 days):
= high concentration of intracellular deoxyhemoglobin with preferential T2 proton relaxation enhancement
√ isointense / slightly hypointense on T1WI
√ markedly hypointense on T2WI

@ subacute stage (7 days – 7 weeks):
= T1 shortening due to paramagnetic effect of free methemoglobin (Fe^{3+}) produced by oxidation of hemoglobin (Fe^{2+})
√ hyperintense on T1WI + T2WI appearing at periphery filling in over several weeks
√ hematoma may be multilocular, each locule with its own different signal intensity

@ chronic stage (>7 weeks):
= T2 proton relaxation enhancement due to hemosiderin deposition + presence of a fibrous capsule
√ hypointense rim on T1WI + T2WI
√ "blooming effect" (= magnetic susceptibility) of hemosiderin in gradient-echo imaging

Cx: acute primary adrenal insufficiency (rare) is life-threatening

DDx: neuroblastoma (stippled calcifications, increase in vanillylmandelic acid, no decrease on follow-up)

ADRENOCORTICAL ADENOMA

Histo: clear cells arranged in cords with abundant intracytoplasmic lipid

A. NONHYPERFUNCTIONING
characterized by
(a) normal lab values of adrenal hormones
(b) NO pituitary shutdown of the contralateral gland
(c) activity on NP-59 radionuclide scans

Incidence: incidental finding in 0.6–1.5% of CT examinations, in 3–9% at autopsy
√ surveillance CT to confirm lack of growth

Rx: surgical removal for masses 3–5 cm as indeterminate potentially malignant neoplasms

DDx: metastasis

B. HYPERFUNCTIONING
1. Primary hyperaldosteronism = Conn syndrome (80%)
Pathophysiology: secretion of aldosterone by an adenoma is pulsatile
√ ACTH infusion incites a dramatic increase in levels of cortisol + aldosterone for venous sampling
2. Cushing syndrome (10%)
3. Virilization
(a) hirsutism + clitoromegaly in girls
(b) pseudopuberty in boys
most common type of hormone elevation in children
• elevated testosterone levels >0.55 ng/mL
4. Feminization (estrogen production)
√ contralateral atrophic gland (secondary to ACTH suppression with autonomous adenoma)
√ unilateral focus of I-131 NP-59 radioactivity + contralateral absence of iodocholesterol accumulation (DDx: hyperplasia [bilateral activity])

√ well-defined sharply marginated mass <5 cm in size (average size 2.0–2.5 cm)
√ mild homogeneous enhancement
√ adenoma may calcify

CT:
√ soft-tissue density / cystic density (mimicked by high cholesterol content) with poor correlation between functional status and HU number
√ <0 HU on NECT (47% sensitive, 100% specific)
√ <10 HU on NECT (73% sensitive, 96% specific)
√ <18 HU on NECT (85% sensitive, 100% specific)
√ <37 HU on delayed CECT (>5–15 minutes after contrast injection) is DIAGNOSTIC of adenoma
√ small adenomas <1 cm often go undetected
√ contralateral gland often normal / atrophic

Angio:
√ tumor blush + neovascularity; occasionally hypovascular
√ pooling of contrast material
√ enlarged central vein with high flow
√ arcuate displacement of intraadrenal veins
√ bilateral adrenal venous sampling in up to 40% unsuccessful in localizing

MR:
√ mass iso- / hypointense (rarely hyperintense) to spleen on T2WI
√ marked hypointensity compared with liver / spleen on out-of-phase GRE images (95% of adenomas)
√ India ink effect = characteristic black lines outlining interface between organ + adjacent fat (chemical shift artifact)
√ mild enhancement + quick washout on Gd-dimeglumine–enhanced study
(DDx: metastases tend to have higher signal intensities [however 20–30% overlap])

ADRENOCORTICAL CARCINOMA

Prevalence: 1:1,000,000 people; 0.3–0.4% of all pediatric neoplasms (3 times more likely than adrenal adenoma)
Age: 4th–7th decade
May be associated with: hemihypertrophy, Beckwith-Wiedemann syndrome, astrocytomas
Path: large lobulated tumor, often with cystic / necrotic / hemorrhagic center
Histo: differentiation of benign from malignant solely on the basis of histologic features may be difficult

- abdominal pain, palpable abdominal mass
- 20% nonfunctioning
- 50% hyperfunctioning (in 10–15% Cushing syndrome)

Size: usually >5 cm (median size 12 cm; in 16% <6 cm)
√ frequently heterogeneous mass with irregular margins
√ occasionally calcified (in 30%)
√ invasion of IVC, liver, kidney, diaphragm
√ metastases to regional lymph nodes, lung, bone, brain
◊ Metastases are the only reliable sign of malignancy!
◊ Large size + calcifications suggest malignancy!
CT:
√ central areas of low attenuation (tumor necrosis)
√ heterogeneous enhancement (foci of hemorrhage + central necrosis)
CECT:
√ peripheral nodular enhancement (in 88%)
US:
√ complex echo pattern (due to hemorrhage + necrosis)
MR:
√ heterogeneously hyperintense to liver on T1WI + T2WI (due to frequent presence of internal hemorrhage + necrosis)
√ nodular enhancement + central hypoperfusion + delayed washout
Angio:
√ enlarged adrenal arteries
√ neovascularity, occasionally with parasitization
√ AV shunting; multiple draining veins
NUC:
√ usually bilateral nonvisualization with I-131 NP-59 (carcinomatous side does not visualize because amount of uptake is small for size of lesion; contralateral side does not visualize because carcinoma is releasing sufficient hormone to cause pituitary feedback shutdown of contralateral gland)
Biopsy: may appear histologically benign in well-differentiated adenocarcinoma
◊ Sampling error with fine-needle aspiration possible; use core biopsy instead
Prognosis: 0% 5-year survival rate
DDx: metastasis (similar signal intensities on MR)

Adrenocortical Neoplasm in Children

Incidence: 3:1,000,000 annually; less common than neuroblastomas but more common than pheochromocytoma
Age: 6 months to 19 years (mean age of 8 years); 2/3 younger than 5 years of age; M:F = 2.2:1.0
Path: adenoma = solitary spherical well-demarcated unencapsulated tumor of <50 g;
carcinoma = multinodular tumor with areas of hemorrhage + necrosis of >100–500 g
Histo: no reliable features to distinguish between adenoma and carcinoma
Associated with:
(1) Congenital hemihypertrophy (3%)
(2) **Li-Fraumeni syndrome** = SBLA (sarcoma, breast and brain tumors, laryngeal carcinoma, adrenocortical carcinoma)
- alteration of p53 tumor suppressor gene located on short arm of chromosome 17, band 13

- palpable abdominal mass (57%)
- gonadotropin-independent production of endogenous androgens + cortisol (92%):
  - virilization in female
    = herculean habitus (increased muscle mass), clitoromegaly, facial hair, advanced pubic + axillary hair development, advanced bone age
  - isosexual precocious puberty in male
    = early development of acne, pubic hair, penile enlargement
  - mixed endocrine syndrome with cushingoid features (less frequent)
- other endocrine abnormalities (unusual):
  - pure Cushing syndrome
  - feminization in boys (caused by secretion of estrogen)
  - Conn syndrome (primary hyperaldosteronism)
- increase in 24-hour urinary ketosteroid excretion
- increased levels of serum cortisol, testosterone, androstenedione, estradiol

Metastases: lung > liver > tumor invasion of IVC (35%) > peritoneum (29%) > pleura + diaphragm (24%) > abdominal lymph nodes (24%) > kidney (18%)
US:
√ 3–22-cm round / ovoid well-circumscribed mass
√ lobulated border (common)
√ thin echogenic capsule-like rim (27%)
√ homogeneous mass hypo- / isoechoic to kidney
√ heterogeneous mass with centrally hypoechoic regions (= tumor necrosis) if large
√ tumor calcification (19%)
CECT:
√ well-circumscribed mass with thin rim
√ heterogeneous enhancement if lesion large
√ calcification (24%)
MR:
√ isointense to liver on T1WI
√ hyperintense to liver on T2WI
√ secondary findings due to excess serum cortisol:
√ hyperattenuating / hyperechoic renal pyramids (due to hypercalcemia of Cushing syndrome)
√ increase in retroperitoneal fatty tissue (obesity due to Cushing syndrome)
Rx: surgery

GU

Prognosis of adrenocortical carcinoma:
survival rate of 70% for children <5 years of age and 13% for children >5 years of age;
death within 1–2 years after diagnosis

DDx: (1) Neuroblastoma (encasing vascular structures, punctate calcifications, extradural extension, ill child, often already metastatic, increase in catecholamines)
(2) Pheochromocytoma (older child, headaches)
(3) Adrenal hemorrhage (neonate, temporal evolution)
(4) Metastasis (extremely rare)

ADRENOCORTICAL HYPERPLASIA

◊ Responsible for 8% of Cushing syndrome and 10–20% of hyperaldosteronism!

Cause:
1. Corticotropin-dependent (85%): pituitary causes, ectopic corticotropin production, production of corticotropin-releasing factor
2. Primary pigmented nodular adrenocortical hyperplasia
   Associated with: Carney complex
3. Primary aldosteronism (rare)

Incidence: 4 x increased in patients with malignancy
Age: 70–80% in adults; 19% in children
Types:
(1) Smooth hyperplasia (common)
√ bilateral normal-sized glands
√ thickened + elongated glands
(2) Cortical nodular hyperplasia (less common)
√ normal glands ± appreciable micronodular configuration
√ thickened gland with macronodular configuration (nodules up to 2.5 cm)

Angio:
√ minimally increased hypervascularity
√ focal accumulation of contrast medium
√ normal venogram / may show enlarged gland

NUC:
√ asymmetric bilateral NP-59 uptake (related to urinary cortisol excretion) without dexamethasone suppression in Cushing syndrome
√ bilateral foci of NP-59 uptake with dexamethasone suppression (nondiagnostic ≥5 days)

ADRENOGENITAL SYNDROMES

A. CONGENITAL TYPE
= impaired cortisol + aldosterone synthesis secondary to enzyme defect (21-hydroxylase) with increased ACTH stimulation by pituitary gland (negative feedback mechanism)
M < F
- excess of androgenic steroids
- ± salt wasting due to diminished mineralocorticoids
- virilization of female fetus
- precocious puberty in male
- pseudohermaphroditism (clitoral hypertrophy, ambiguous external genitalia, urogenital sinus)

√ symmetrically enlarged + thickened adrenal glands
Rx: cortisone ± mineralocorticoids

B. ACQUIRED TYPE
M < F
(a) adrenal hyperplasia / adenoma / carcinoma
(b) ovarian / testicular tumor
(c) gonadotropin-producing tumor: pineal, hypothalamic, choriocarcinoma
- virilization
- Cushing syndrome

AMYLOIDOSIS

= accumulation of extracellular eosinophilic protein substances

@ Renal involvement
Incidence: 1° amyloidosis (35%), 2° amyloidosis (in >80%)
√ smooth normal to large kidneys with increase in parenchymal thickness (early stage)
√ small kidneys = renal atrophy (late stage)
√ occasionally attenuated collecting system
√ increase in cortical echogenicity (deposition of amyloid in glomeruli and interstitium) + prominence of corticomedullary junction + obscuration of arcuate aa.
√ nephrographic density normal to diminished
US:
√ normal to increased echogenicity
Cx: renal vein thrombosis

ANALGESIC NEPHROPATHY

= renal damage from ingestion of salicylates in combination with phenacetin / acetaminophen in a cumulative dose of 1 kg

Incidence: United States (2–10%), Australia (20%)
Age: middle-aged; M:F = 1:4
- gross hematuria
- hypertension
- renal colic (passage of renal tissue)
- renal insufficiency (2–10% of all end-stage renal failures)
- **Analgesic syndrome**: history of psychiatric therapy, abuse of alcohol + laxatives, headaches, pain in cervical + lumbar spine, peptic ulcer, anemia, splenomegaly, arteriosclerosis, premature aging

√ papillary necrosis
√ scarring of renal parenchyma ("wavy outline"); bilateral in 66%, unilateral in 5%
√ renal atrophy
√ papillary urothelial tumors in calyces / pelvis (mostly TCC / squamous cell carcinoma), in 5% bilateral

ANGIOMYOLIPOMA

= AML = RENAL CHORISTOMA (benign tumor composed of tissues not normally occurring within the organ of origin)
= RENAL HAMARTOMA (improper name since fat and smooth muscle do not normally occur within renal parenchyma)
= benign mesenchymal tumor of kidney

Prevalence: 0.3–3%

Path: no true capsule, 88% extending through renal capsule, hemorrhage (characteristic lack of complete elastic layer of vessels predisposes to aneurysm formation); tumor continues to grow during childhood + early adulthood
Histo: tumor composed of fat, smooth muscle, aggregates of thick-walled blood vessels
Types:
(1) Isolated AML (80%) = sporadic AML
√ solitary + unilateral (in 80% on R side) AML, NO stigmata of tuberous sclerosis
Age: 27–72 (mean 43) years of age; M:F = 1:4
(2) AML associated with tuberous sclerosis (20%)
◊ In 80% of patients with tuberous sclerosis
◊ May be the only evidence of tuberous sclerosis
√ commonly large + bilateral + multifocal AMLs
Mean age: 17 years; usually present by 10 years; M:F = 1:1
(3) AML associated with neurofibromatosis + von Hippel-Lindau syndrome
- small lesions are asymptomatic (60%)
◊ Angiomyolipomas >4 cm are symptomatic in 82–94%!
- acute flank / abdominal pain in 87%
- **Wunderlich syndrome** = hemorrhagic shock due to massive bleeding into angiomyolipoma or into retroperitoneum
◊ AMLs >4 cm bleed spontaneously in 50–60%!
Rx: (1) annual follow-up of lesions <4 cm
(2) semiannual follow-up of lesions ≥4 cm
(3) emergency laparotomy (in 25%): nephrectomy, tumor resection
(4) selective arterial embolization
DDx: renal / perirenal lipoma or liposarcoma; Wilms tumor / renal cell carcinoma (occasionally contains fat)

ARTERIOVENOUS CONNECTION

√ early enhancement of draining vein + renal vein + IVC
√ intraparenchymal / subcapsular / perirenal hematoma (as a result of bleeding)
Rx: transcatheter intraarterial occlusion, surgery

Arteriovenous Malformation (20–30%)

(1) Congenital AVM
- asymptomatic; M < F
(2) Acquired AVM: trauma, spontaneous rupture of aneurysm, very vascular malignant neoplasm
Histo:
(a) cirsoid AVM = multiple coiled vascular channels grouped in cluster
(b) cavernous AVM = single well-defined artery feeding into a single vein (rare)
- gross hematuria
Location: adjacent to collecting system
√ supplied by multiple segmental / interlobar arteries of normal caliber
√ draining into one / more veins
√ large unifocal mass
√ focally attenuated and displaced collecting system
√ homogeneously enhancing mass
√ curvilinear calcification

US:
√ tubular anechoic structure (DDx: hydronephrosis, hydrocalyx)
Cx: subcapsular / perinephric hematoma (rare)

Arteriovenous Fistula (70–80%)

M > F
Cause: trauma (stab wound, percutaneous needle biopsy, percutaneous nephrostomy, nephrolithotripsy), surgery, tumor, inflammation, erosion of aneurysm into vein
Path: single feeding artery + single draining vein
- asymptomatic with abnormal bruit
- persistent / delayed hematuria (common)
√ diminished nephrogram ± cortical atrophy distal to fistula (due to reduced flow to renal segment)
Cx: cardiomegaly + CHF (50%), renin-mediated hypertension
Prognosis: spontaneous closure within a few months

BENIGN PROSTATIC HYPERTROPHY

= BENIGN PROSTATIC HYPERPLASIA
Prevalence: 50% between ages 51 + 60 years; 75–80% of all men >80 years of age
Histo: fibromyoadenomatous nodule (most common), muscular + fibromuscular + fibroadenomatous + stromal nodules
Age: initial growth onset <30 years of age; onset of clinical symptoms at 60 ± 9 years
- sensation of full bladder, nocturia
- trouble initiating micturition
- decreased urine caliber + force
- dribbling at termination of micturition
Location: transition + periurethral zone proximal to verumontanum forming "lateral lobes" (82%), "median lobe" (12%)
√ oval (61%) / round (22%) / pear-shaped (17%) enlargement of central gland
√ posterior + lateral displacement of outer gland (= prostate proper) creating cleavage plane of fibrous tissue between hyperplastic tissue + compressed prostatic tissue (= surgical capsule) often demarcated by displaced intraductal calcifications
Cx: bladder outflow obstruction
Rx:
(1) Surgery: open prostatectomy (glands >80 g), transurethral resection of prostate = TURP (glands <80 g)
◊ Only 4–5% of patients need surgical treatment!
(2) Drugs: α-blockers (for stromal hyperplasia); androgen deprivation (suppression of LHRH / inhibition of Leydig cell synthesis of testosterone / competition for androgen receptor binding sites) + α-blockers (for glandular hyperplasia)

BLADDER DIVERTICULUM

= cavity formed by herniation of bladder mucosa through muscular wall, joined to the bladder cavity by a constricted neck

Prevalence: 1.7% in children
Etiology:
A. PRIMARY / CONGENITAL / IDIOPATHIC DIVERTIVULA (40%)
√ in 3% single diverticulum
(a) with vesicoureteral reflux
1. Hutch diverticulum in paraureteral region
(b) without vesicoureteral reflux
B. SECONDARY DIVERTICULA (60%)
√ in 50% multiple diverticula
(a) postoperative state
(b) associated with bladder outlet obstruction
1. Posterior urethral valves
2. Urethral stricture
3. Large ureterocele
4. Neurogenic dysfunction
5. Enlarged prostate
6. Bladder neck stenosis
(c) associated with syndromes
1. Prune belly syndrome
2. Menkes kinky-hair syndrome
3. Williams syndrome
4. Ehlers-Danlos type 9 syndrome
5. Diamond-Blackfan syndrome
C. MULTIPLE DIVERTICULA IN CHILDREN
1. Neurogenic dysfunction
2. Posterior urethral valves
3. Prune belly syndrome

Average age: 57 years; M:F = 9:1
Site: areas of congenital weakness of muscular wall at
(a) ureteral meatus
(b) posterolateral wall (Hutch diverticulum = paraureteral)
Cx: (1) Vesical carcinoma in 0.8–7% secondary to chronic inflammation (average age 66 years)
(2) Ureteral obstruction
(3) Ureteral reflux

BLADDER EXSTROPHY

= EPISPADIA-EXSTROPHY COMPLEX
Prevalence: 1:33,000 to 1:40,000 live births
Etiology: incomplete retraction of cloacal membrane prevents normal midline migration of mesoderm resulting in incomplete midline closure of infraumbilical abdominal wall; size of persistent cloacal membrane at time of rupture accounts for different degrees of severity

- urinary bladder exposed + open anteriorly
- mucosa everted through abdominal wall defect
- bladder margins continuous with margins of abdominal wall
- epispadia (male); bifid clitoris (female)

May be associated with:
wide linea alba, omphalocele, limb defects (eg, club feet), renal malformation (horseshoe kidney, renal agenesis), incomplete testicular descent, GI obstruction, bilateral inguinal hernias, imperforate anus, cardiac anomalies, hydrocephalus, meningomyelocele

√ ventral defect of infraumbilical abdominal wall
√ low position of umbilicus
√ pubic diastasis = widening of pubic symphysis
Cx: urinary incontinence, infertility, pyelonephritis, bladder carcinoma (4%)
Rx: primary closure, bladder excision with urinary diversion

Closed Exstrophy = Pseudoexstrophy

= persistent large cloacal membrane without rupture
- anterior wall of bladder covered by thin bilaminar epithelial membrane

√ infraumbilical musculoskeletal defect
√ subcutaneous position of bladder

CHOLESTEATOMA

= keratin ball = keratinized squamous epithelium shed into lumen
Pathogenesis: long-standing urinary infection may result in squamous metaplasia of transitional epithelium

- history of UTIs
- repeated episodes of renal colic with passage of "white tissue flakes"

Location: renal pelvis > upper ureter
√ mottled / stringy "onion-skin" filling defect in calices / renal pelvis
√ dilatation of pelvicaliceal system (with obstruction)
√ calcification of keratinized material possible
◊ Not a premalignant condition!

CHROMOPHOBE CARCINOMA OF KIDNEY

Prevalence: 4% of renal cell neoplasms
Age: median in 6th decade (31–75 years)
Histo: cells with abundant cytoplasm containing numerous microvesicles
√ average size of 8 cm (range 1.3–20 cm)
Prognosis: probably better than RCC

CHRONIC GLOMERULONEPHRITIS

Cause: after acute poststreptococcal glomerulonephritis

- late presentation without prior clinically apparent acute phase
- hypertension
- renal failure

√ small smooth kidneys with wasted parenchyma
√ normal papillae + calyces
√ patchy nephrogram with diminished density of contrast material
√ cortical calcification (uncommon)
US:
√ increased echogenicity
√ small kidneys with vicarious sinus lipomatosis
Angio:
√ marked reduction in renal blood flow + reflux of contrast material into aorta
√ severely pruned + tortuous interlobar and arcuate arteries
√ nonvisualization of interlobular arteries
√ delayed contrast clearance from interlobar arteries

GU

CLEAR CELL SARCOMA OF KIDNEY

= BONE-METASTASIZING RENAL TUMOR OF CHILDHOOD
= rare highly malignant renal tumor of childhood with predilection for bone metastasis

Incidence: 4–5% of renal tumors in childhood
Age: peak age at 2 years (range, 1–6 years); M > F
Path: soft well-circumscribed tumor
Histo: composed of well-defined polygonal to stellate cells with vacuolization, ovoid to rounded nuclei, prominent capillary pattern + tendency toward cyst formation separated by slightly thickened septa

• increasing abdominal girth + palpable abdominal mass
• lethargy, weight loss
• hematuria

√ expansile well-demarcated mass (8–16 cm) with dominant soft-tissue component
√ cystic component of varying size (few mm to 5 cm) + multiplicity (58%)
√ amorphous / linear calcifications (25%)
√ renal mass crossing midline (58%)
√ WITHOUT intravascular extension

Metastases to: bone, lymph nodes, brain, liver, lung

US:
√ inhomogeneous renal mass of soft-tissue density
√ well-defined hypoechoic central area (= necrosis)
√ mass of fluid-filled cystic spaces

CT:
√ inhomogeneous enhancement less than that of normal renal parenchyma
√ low-attenuation areas (= necrosis)
√ water-density areas (= cysts)

Prognosis: 60–70% long-term survival rate; aggressive behavior (worse than Wilms tumor) with higher rate of relapse + mortality
DDx: cystic form of Wilms tumor (vascular invasion), multilocular cystic nephroma, cystic dysplasia

CONGENITAL RENAL HYPOPLASIA

= miniaturization with reduction in number of renal lobes, number of calyces and papillae, amount of nephrons (+ smallness of cells)

VARIANT: **Ask-Upmark kidney** = aglomerular focal hypoplasia

√ unilateral small kidney
√ decreased number of papillae + calyces (5 or less)
√ hypertrophied contralateral kidney
√ absent renal artery
√ hypoplastic disorganized renal veins

CONN SYNDROME

= PRIMARY HYPERALDOSTERONISM = PRIMARY ALDOSTERONISM
= autonomous excess secretion of the mineralocorticoid aldosterone with hypertension + spontaneous hypokalemia

Incidence: 0.05–2% of hypertensive population
Age: 3rd–5th decade; M:F = 1:2

• hypertension (secondary to hypernatremia)
• hypokalemia (80–90%, induced by administering large amounts of sodium chloride for 3–5 days):
  • muscle weakness, cardiac arrhythmia
  • carbohydrate intolerance
  • nephrogenic diabetes insipidus
• depletion of magnesium
• metabolic alkalosis
• increased urinary excretion of aldosterone + metabolites
• nonsuppressible elevation in plasma aldosterone concentration
• suppressed plasma renin levels

Path:
(a) adenoma (65–89%): solitary aldosteronoma (65–70%); multiple (13%); microadenomatosis (6%)
(b) bilateral adrenal hyperplasia (11–25–30%):
= idiopathic hyperaldosteronism = focal / diffuse hyperplasia of glomerular zone accompanied by micro- / macroscopic nodules
(c) adrenocortical carcinoma (<1%)

√ small aldosteronoma of 1.7 cm average size (range 0.5–3.5 cm); L > R, bilateral in 6%:
  √ soft-tissue density / low attenuation
    ◊ Among hyperfunctioning adrenal adenomas aldosteronomas have the lowest attenuation!
  √ usually hypervascular, rarely hypovascular
√ normal / nodular / multinodular adrenal gland(s) (with hyperplasia)

Adrenal venography : 76% accuracy
Adrenal venous blood sampling : 95% accuracy, 75% sensitivity
CT : 60–80% sensitivity

NUC:
√ I-131 NP-59 uptake following dexamethasone suppression:
  √ bilateral early visualization (<5 days) implies adrenal hyperplasia
  √ unilateral early visualization implies adenoma
  √ late bilateral visualization (>5 days) may be normal

Dx: elevated plasma aldosterone concentration + suppressed plasma renin activity
Diagnostic endocrine tests:
postural stimulation test, short saline infusion test, 18-hydroxycorticosterone concentration

Rx: adrenalectomy for neoplasms (75% long-term cure rate for hypertension); medical treatment for hyperplasia

CONTRAST NEPHROPATHY

= CONTRAST-INDUCED RENAL FAILURE
= increase in serum creatinine of ≥1 mg/dL ± 25–50% of the baseline creatinine level after intravascular contrast administration

Patients at risk:
1. Preexisting renal insufficiency
2. Insulin-dependent diabetes mellitus
3. Large volume of contrast media
4. Concomitant administration of other nephrotoxic drugs: aminoglycosides, nonsteroidal anti-inflammatory agents

5. American Heart Association class IV congestive heart failure
6. Hyperuricemia

◊ A serum creatinine level of >4.5 mg/dL causes acute renal failure in 60% of nondiabetics + 100% of diabetics!

Previously considered but no longer accepted risk factors: dehydration, hypertension, proteinuria, peripheral vascular disease, age >65 years, multiple myeloma

Mechanism:
increase in renal perfusion by vasodilatation (via prostaglandin I2 ± E2) followed by vasoconstriction (via angiotensin II, norepinephrine, vasopressin)

Time course:
(a) rise in serum creatinine within 1–2 days
(b) peak at 4–7 days
(c) return to normal by 10–14 days

√ persistent nephrogram on plain film
√ cortical attenuation >140 HU on CT with 24-hour delay

Recommendation:
◊ Employ nonionic contrast media (LOCM appears safe in patients without renal dysfunction / underlying risk factors in doses as large as 800 mL [300 mg iodine per mL])
◊ Do not exceed maximum allowed dose (Cigarroa formula for HOCM):

$$\text{Contrast limit (mL) 60\% by weight} = \frac{5 \text{ mL} \times \text{body weight (kg)}}{\text{serum creatinine (mg/100 mL)}}$$

CUSHING SYNDROME

= HYPERCORTISOLISM
= excessive glucocorticoid secretion from either exogenous / endogenous sources

Etiology:

A. ACTH-INDEPENDENT
  1. Exogenous cortisol
  2. Primary adrenal abnormality (20%):
    (a) primary pigmented nodular adrenocortical hyperplasia (children, young adults)
    (b) adrenocortical adenoma (10–20% of cases; 10% in adults, 15% in children)
    (c) adrenocortical carcinoma (5–10% of cases; 10% in adults, 66% in children)

B. ACTH-DEPENDENT
  = overproduction of corticotropin with adrenal hyperplasia (in up to 85%)
  1. Exogenous ACTH
  2. Paraneoplastic ectopic ACTH production (20%): oat cell carcinoma of lung (8%), liver cancer, prostate cancer, ovarian cancer, breast cancer, bronchial / thymic carcinoid, bronchial adenoma, pancreatic islet cell tumor (10%), medullary carcinoma of thyroid, thymoma, pheochromocytoma
    ◊ Bronchial + thymic carcinoids are often <1 cm at the time they produce Cushing syndrome!
    ◊ Islet cell tumors are large + often metastatic by the time they produce Cushing syndrome!
  3. **Cushing disease** (70% of endogenous causes)
    = adrenal hyperplasia due to overproduction of pituitary ACTH
    Cause: (1) basophilic / chromophobe adenoma
    (2) overactive pituitary
    (3) ACTH-producing primary elsewhere
  4. Hypothalamic dysfunction
  5. Production of corticotropin-releasing factor (rare)

Incidence: 1:1,000 autopsies; M:F = 1:4
Age: 30–40 years (highest incidence); more often following pregnancy

• central / truncal obesity, buffalo hump, moon face, facial plethora
• purple abdominal striae, acne, hirsutism
• fatigue, proximal muscle weakness, amenorrhea
• impaired glucose tolerance = glycosuria / diabetes
• hypertension, atherosclerosis, edema
• elevated plasma cortisol levels
• excessive excretion of urinary 17-hydroxy-corticosteroids
• dexamethasone suppression test / metyrapone test

√ retarded bone maturation
√ most often axial osteoporosis
√ stippled calvarium
√ demineralized dorsum sellae
√ excess callus formation

Cx: (1) Pathologic fractures of vertebrae + ribs with excessive callus formation
(2) Aseptic necrosis of hips
(3) Bone infarcts
(4) Delayed skeletal maturation in children

CYSTITIS

= bacterial infection; M < F
• frequency, dysuria, hematuria
• reduced bladder capacity
√ cystogram insensitive

US:
√ focal / multifocal / circumferential isoechoic bladder wall thickening
√ decrease in bladder wall thickening during bladder distension (eg, instillation of sterile saline via a urethral catheter)
√ bullous lesions
√ intact mucosa

DDx: bladder neoplasm, ureterocele, pseudoureterocele, neurofibromatosis, pseudosarcomatous myofibroblastic proliferations

Cystitis Cystica

= CYSTITIS FOLLICULARIS = CYSTITIS GLANDULARIS = BULLOUS CYSTITIS
= nonspecific inflammatory process of bladder wall
√ multiple small round cystlike mucosal elevations

Prognosis: potentially malignant in adults

Emphysematous Cystitis

= uncommon complication of urinary tract infection by gas-forming organism almost PATHOGNOMONIC of poorly controlled diabetes (= bacterial fermentation of glucose)

Age: >50 years; M:F = 1:2
Predisposed: diabetes mellitus, neurogenic bladder, bladder outlet obstruction, chronic UTI
Organism: E. coli, E. aerogenes, P. mirabilis, S. aureus, streptococci, Clostridium perfringens, Nocardia, Candida
May be associated with: emphysematous pyelitis / pyelonephritis
• pneumaturia (rare)
Plain film:
√ translucent streaky irregular area / ring of air bubbles in bladder wall
√ intraluminal air-fluid level
US:
√ shadowing echogenic foci within area of bladder wall thickening
CT (most specific modality)
DDx: (a) Gas within bladder:
trauma, urinary tract instrumentation, enterovesical fistula
(b) Gas external to bladder:
rectal gas, emphysematous vaginitis, pneumatosis cystoides intestinalis, gas gangrene of uterus

Granulomatous Cystitis = Tuberculous Cystitis
√ irritable hypertonic bladder with decreased capacity
√ disease process usually starts at trigone spreading upward and laterally
√ calcification of bladder wall (rare)

Hemorrhagic Cystitis
Cause: unclear
(a) nonspecific: negative culture
(b) bacterial: E. coli (in 17%)
(c) viral (adenovirus in 19%): negative culture, viral exanthem
(d) cytotoxic: cyclophosphamide (Cytoxan®), in 15% of patients within 1st year of treatment
√ echogenic mobile clumps of solid material (= intraluminal blood clots)

Interstitial Cystitis
Age: postmenopausal female
• pink pseudoulceration of bladder mucosa characteristically at vertex of bladder (= Hunner ulcer)

Bullous Edema of Bladder Wall
Cause: continuous internal contact with Foley catheter, involvement of bladder wall by external contact in pelvic inflammatory conditions (eg, Crohn disease, appendicitis, diverticulitis)
√ smoothly thickened / polypoid redundant hypoechoic mucosa

DIABETES MELLITUS
= multisystem disorder
Prevalence: 14 million patients in United States
Path: macro- and microvascular disease; neuropathy; increased susceptibility to infection
A. CHRONIC EFFECTS
1. Papillary necrosis
2. Renal artery stenosis
3. Vas deferens calcification
B. URINARY TRACT INFECTIONS
1. Renal and perirenal abscess
2. Emphysematous pyelonephritis
3. Emphysematous cystitis
4. Fungal infection: Candida, Aspergillus
5. Xanthogranulomatous pyelonephritis
C. GENITAL INFECTION
1. Fournier gangrene
2. Postmenopausal tuboovarian abscess

Diabetic Nephropathy
= defined as persistent proteinuria (>500 mg of albumin/ 24 hours) + retinopathy + elevated blood pressure
◊ Most common cause of end-stage renal disease!
Incidence: 35–45% of IDDM; <20% of NIDDM; M > F
Histo: diffuse intercapillary glomerulosclerosis
Mortality: 90% after 40 years
Early:
√ renal enlargement (renal hypertrophy with glomerular expansion)
Late:
√ progressive decrease in size
√ diffuse cortical hyperechogenicity with gradual loss of corticomedullary differentiation
√ resistive index >0.7 (very late)
IVP:
√ contrast material may induce renal failure (= rise in serum creatinine level 1–5 days after exposure)
◊ Keep patient well hydrated with 0.45% saline!

Diabetic Cystopathy
Cause: autonomous peripheral neuropathy
Histo: vacuolation of ganglion cells in bladder wall, giant sympathetic neurons, hypochromatic ganglion cells, demyelination
• insidious impairment of bladder sensation
• decreased reflex detrusor activity
√ enlarged postvoid residual urine volume
Cx: vesicoureteral reflux, recurrent pyelonephritis, pyohydronephrosis, overflow incontinence

EPIDIDYMITIS
Acute Epididymitis
= ACUTE EPIDIDYMOORCHITIS
◊ Most common acute pathologic process in postpubertal age
Cause: ascending urinary tract infection; instrumentation + prostatitis (in older men)
Incidence: 634,000 cases/year
Age: adolescence to middle age; <10 years in 0%; 20–30 years in 72%

Organism: E. coli + S. aureus (85%), Gonococcus (12%), TB (2%); nonspecific epididymitis in 20%
(a) >35 years of age: Escherichia coli + Proteus mirabilis, CMV with AIDS
(b) <35 years of age: Chlamydia trachomatis, Neisseria gonorrheae

- fever
- increasing pain over 1–2 days
- hemiscrotal swelling + tenderness + erythema
- pyuria (95%)
- positive urine culture
- leukocytosis (50%)
- dysuria + frequency (25%)
- prostatic tenderness (infrequent)

Location: may have focal involvement as in focal epididymitis (25%) often in epididymal tail
◊ Subsequent spread to testis is common: global orchitis (frequent), focal orchitis (10%)

US:
√ enlarged epididymis with decreased echogenicity:
√ enlarged head suggests hematogenous spread
√ enlarged tail suggest retrograde reflux from prostate / urine
√ reactive hydrocele ± thickening of scrotal wall
√ enlarged spermatic cord containing hyperechoic fat
√ thickening of tunica albuginea (in severe infection)

Color Duplex (91% sensitive, 100% specific):
√ increased number + concentration of identifiable vessels in affected region (= hyperemia)
√ peak systolic velocity (PSV) >15 cm/s with PSV ratio >1.9 compared with normal side
√ detection of venous flow
√ diastolic flow reversal in testicular artery (due to epididymal edema with obstruction of venous outflow)

NUC (true positive rate of 99%):
√ symmetric perfusion of iliac + femoral vessels
√ markedly increased perfusion through spermatic cord vessels (testicular + deferential arteries)
√ curvilinear increased activity laterally in hemiscrotum on static images (also centrally if testis involved)
√ increased activity of scrotal contents on static images (hyperemia + increased capillary permeability)

Rx: antimicrobial therapy, scrotal elevation, bed rest, analgesics, ice packs

Cx:
(1) Focal / diffuse orchitis (20–40%)
(2) Epididymal abscess (6%)
(3) Testicular abscess (6%)
(4) Testicular infarction (3%) from extrinsic compression of testicular blood flow
(5) Late testicular atrophy (21%)
(6) Hydropyocele
(7) Fournier gangrene

DDx:
(1) Testicular abscess (increased perfusion with centrally decreased uptake)
(2) Hydrocele (normal perfusion, no uptake)
(3) Testicular tumor (slightly increased perfusion; in- / decreased uptake; no associated epididymal hyperemia on CFI; positive tumor markers: hCG, AFP)

Chronic Epididymitis

US:
√ enlarged hyperechoic epididymis

ERECTILE DYSFUNCTION

= IMPOTENCE (term replaced due to negative connotation)
= inability to have / maintain a penile erection sufficient for vaginal penetration in 50% or more attempts during intercourse

Incidence: 10 million Americans

Physiology:
(a) psychogenic phase:
- stimuli from thalamic nuclei, rhinencephalon, limbic system converge in medial preoptic anterior hypothalamic area

(b) neurologic phase:
- sacral nerve roots (S2–S4) contribute fibers to pelvic sympathetic plexus
- stimulation of cavernous n. (parasympathetic nerve) causes changes in blood flow resulting in full erection
- stimulation of pudendal n. (motor nerve) causes contraction of bulbocavernosus + ischiocavernosus muscle resulting in occlusion of veins + rigid erection

Risk factors: hypertension, diabetes, smoking, CAD, peripheral vascular disease, pelvic trauma / surgery, blood lipid abnormalities,

Cause:
A. ORGANIC (majority)
1. Endocrine disorder reducing serum testosterone / increasing serum prolactin
2. Vascular disease (10–20%): increasing with age
(a) failure to fill (arteriogenic)
(b) failure to store (venogenic)
3. Neurogenic disease (10%) = failure to initiate:
(a) neurologic disorder: multiple sclerosis, spinal cord injury, cervical spondylosis, spinal arachnoiditis, pelvic trauma, temporal lobe / idiopathic epilepsy, Alzheimer disease, Parkinson disease, tabes dorsalis, amyloidosis, primary autonomic insufficiency, cerebrovascular accidents, primary / metastatic tumor
(b) surgical injury to nerves: damage to pelvic sympathetic nerves / cavernous n. during radical prostatectomy / cystectomy
4. Chronic disease: diabetes mellitus (2 million); drugs (antihypertensives, anticonvulsants, alcohol, narcotics, psychotropic agents)
5. Endorgan disease: priapism

B. PSYCHOGENIC

Penile-brachial index (normal >1.0)
= highest penile artery pressure over mean brachial pressure
√ <0.70 suggests large vessel disease
Rx: (1) Surgery:
(a) vascular reconstructive surgery
(b) penile prosthesis placement
— nonhydraulic: semirigid, malleable, positionable
— hydraulic
(2) Oral / intracavernosal injection of vasoactive agents
(3) Nonsurgical external devices: vacuum erection devices
(4) Sex therapy

FOURNIER GANGRENE

= FULMINANT FASCIITIS
= uncommon potentially lethal necrotizing fasciitis of the scrotum
Incidence: 500 cases in literature
Organism: (a) aerobes: S. aureus, E. coli, Proteus species, enterococci
(b) anaerobes: Bacteroides fragilis, anaerobic streptococci, clostridia
Path: cellulitis, myositis, fasciitis with soft-tissue necrosis
Histo: thrombosis of subcutaneous vessels with gangrene of overlying skin
Age: newborn to elderly
Predisposed: diabetes mellitus (present in 40–60%)
• pain, fever, leukocytosis
• scrotal tenderness, erythema, swelling, crepitation
◊ In 95% primary focus of infection is recognizable (urethra, soft tissue of anorectal area, genital skin)!
√ gas in scrotal wall + perineum
√ scrotal skin thickening + normal testes
Mortality: 7–75%
Rx: antibiotic therapy + surgery + hyperbaric oxygen
DDx: epididymoorchitis, gas-containing scrotal abscess, scrotal hernia with gas-containing bowel, scrotal emphysema from bowel perforation, extension of subcutaneous emphysema, air leakage + dissection due to faulty chest tube positioning

GANGLIONEUROBLASTOMA

= tumor of sympathetic nervous system that is intermediate in cellular maturity between neuroblastoma and ganglioneuroma; metastatic potential
Incidence: less common than neuroblastoma / ganglioneuroma
Age: early childhood; M:F = 1:1
Location: posterior mediastinum, abdomen
√ extension through neural foramen into epidural space
√ nerve root / spinal cord compression

GANGLIONEUROMA

= benign neoplastic growth of autonomic ganglia
= may represent end-stage of maturation of a neuroblastoma induced by chemotherapy / occurring spontaneously
Histo: mixture of mature ganglion + Schwann cells
Age: 42–60% <20 years, 39% aged 20–39 years, 19% aged 40–80 years; M:F = 1:1
Location: posterior mediastinum (25–43%); abdomen (52%), adrenal gland (20%); pelvis and neck (9%); oral + intestinal ganglioneuromatosis associated with MEN IIb
• respiratory symptoms, local pressure (40%)
• rarely hormone-active: diarrhea, sweating, hypertension, virilization, myasthenia gravis
√ spherical / elliptical large well-defined encapsulated slow-growing mass
√ tendency to surround blood vessels without compromising the lumen
√ dumbbell-shaped large mass extending from paraspinous region through neural foramen into epidural space
√ calcifications (8–27%)
CT:
√ homogeneous attenuation less than that of muscle
MR:
√ homogeneous + isointense with muscle on T1WI
√ heterogeneous + hyperintense to muscle on T2WI
DDx: neurofibroma (no calcification), schwannoma (no calcification), neuroblastoma (calcified)

HEMANGIOMA OF ADRENAL GLAND

= rare benign stromal tumor of adrenal gland
√ often large mass (usually >10 cm in diameter, up to 22 cm)
√ multiple peripheral nodular areas of marked enhancement after contrast bolus injection
√ NO complete fill in of contrast material
√ calcifications (28–87%) from previous hemorrhage
CT:
√ central low attenuation (necrosis / fibrosis)
MR:
√ mass hypointense relative to liver on T1WI + central hyperintensity (due to hemorrhage)
√ markedly hyperintense on T2WI, especially in central portion
√ variable appearance after hemorrhage, thrombosis, necrosis, fibrosis
Cx: hemorrhage

HEMANGIOMA OF URINARY BLADDER

Incidence: 0.6% of primary bladder neoplasms; 0.3% of all bladder tumors
Age: <20 years (in >50%), M:F = 1:1
May be associated with:
(a) additional hemangiomas in 30%
(b) Klippel-Trenaunay syndrome
(c) Sturge-Weber syndrome
Histo: capillary / venous / cavernous / hemangiolymphomatous form
• recurrent gross painless hematuria
• cutaneous hemangiomas over abdomen, perineum, thighs in 25–30%
Location: dome, posterolateral wall

Site: limited to submucosa (33%), muscular wall, perivesical tissue
√ compressible solitary (2/3) / multiple (1/3) masses:
 √ rounded well-marginated intraluminal mass
 √ diffuse bladder wall thickening + punctate calcifications (phleboliths)
IVP:
 √ rounded / lobulated filling defect
US:
 √ solid predominantly hyperechoic mass
 √ hypoechoic spaces within thickened bladder wall
CAVE: high risk of intractable hemorrhage at biopsy!

HEMOLYTIC-UREMIC SYNDROME

◊ Most common cause of acute renal failure in children requiring dialysis!
= characterized by thrombotic microangiopathy with typical features of DIC

Cause:
 (1) Infection: enterotoxic E. coli, Shigella dysenteriae I, Streptococcus pneumoniae, Salmonella typhi, Coxsackie virus, echovirus, adenovirus
 (2) Associated medical condition: pregnancy, SLE + other collagen vascular disease, malignancy, malignant hypertension
 (3) Drugs: oral contraceptives, cyclosporine, mitomycin, 5-fluorouracil

Pathogenesis: capillary and endothelial injury to kidney leads to mechanical damage of RBCs + formation of hyaline microthrombi within renal vasculature + focal infarction
Age: usually children <2 years
Histo: microangiopathy including endothelial swelling + thrombus formation in glomerulus + renal arterioles

CLASSIC TRIAD:
 (1) microangiopathic hemolytic anemia
 (2) thrombocytopenia
 (3) acute oliguric / anuric renal failure leading to uremia
• recent bout of gastroenteritis (commonly with E. coli)
• sudden pallor, irritability
• bloody diarrhea
• dyspnea (due to fluid retention, heart failure, pleural effusion)
• convulsions
• rapid rise in blood urea nitrogen level out of proportion to plasma creatinine level (= result of cell lysis)

@ Kidney (sometimes only organ involved):
 √ kidneys of normal / slightly increased size
 √ hyperechoic cortex
 Doppler-US:
  √ diastolic flow absent / reversed / reduced (= increase in resistance to flow)
  √ return to normal waveforms predates return of urine output
 Scintigraphy:
  √ lack of renal perfusion
@ Liver: hepatomegaly, hepatitis
@ Pancreas: diabetes mellitus
@ Heart: myocarditis
@ Muscle: rhabdomyolysis
@ Intestines: perforation, intussusception, pseudomembranous colitis
@ Brain (20–50%): drowsiness, personality changes, coma, hemiparesis, seizures (up to 40%)

Prognosis: complete spontaneous recovery (in 85%)

HEREDITARY CHRONIC NEPHRITIS

= ALPORT SYNDROME
= probably autosomal dominant trait with presence of fat-filled macrophages ("foam cells") in the corticomedullary junction and medulla
(a) males: progressive renal insufficiency, death usually < age 50
(b) females: nonprogressive
• polyuria
• anemia
• salt wasting
• hyposthenuria
• nerve deafness
• ocular abnormalities (congenital cataracts, nystagmus, myopia, spherophakia)
• NO hypertension
√ small smooth kidneys
√ diminished density of contrast material
√ cortical calcifications

HORSESHOE KIDNEY

= two kidneys joined at poles by parenchymal / fibrous isthmus

Incidence: 1–4:1,000 births; 0.2–1% (autopsy series); M:F = 2–3:1
 ◊ Most common fusion anomaly

Associated with:
cardiovascular anomaly, skeletal anomaly, CNS anomaly, anorectal malformation, genitourinary anomaly (hypospadia, undescended testis, bicornuate uterus, ureteral duplication), trisomy 18, Turner syndrome (60%)

In 50% associated with:
 (1) Caudal ectopia
 (2) Vesicoureteral reflux
 (3) Hydronephrosis 2° to UPJ obstruction
√ fusion of R + L kidney at lower (90%) / upper (10%) pole
√ renal long axis medially oriented
√ isthmus at L4/5 between aorta + inferior mesenteric a.
√ renal pelves and ureters situated anteriorly
√ multiple renal arteries including isthmus artery

Cx: infection, renal calculi

HYDROCELE

= collection of fluid between parietal and visceral layers of tunica vaginalis
◊ Most common cause of testicular swelling
◊ Most common type of fluid collection in scrotum
US:
 √ anechoic, good back wall, through transmission
 √ COMPLICATED HYDROCELE = hydrocele with low-level echoes ± septations: hematocele / pyocele / cholesterol crystals

Primary = Idiopathic Hydrocele

without predisposing lesion as congenital defect of lymphatic drainage

Secondary Hydrocele

(a) inflammation (epididymitis, epididymoorchitis)
(b) testicular tumor (in 10–40% of malignancies)
(c) trauma / postsurgical
◊ 50% of acquired hydroceles are due to trauma!
(d) torsion, infarction

Congenital Hydrocele

= ascites trapped in scrotum through communication with peritoneal cavity (= open processus vaginalis); may be associated with inguinal hernia

- should resolve within 2 years

Infantile Hydrocele

= hydrocele with fingerlike extension into funicular process but without communication with peritoneal cavity

HYDRONEPHROSIS

A. OBSTRUCTIVE UROPATHY = HYDRONEPHROSIS
= dilatation of collecting structures without functional deficit
B. OBSTRUCTIVE NEPHROPATHY = dilatation of collecting system with renal functional impairment

US:

Grading system of hydronephrosis:

Grade 0 = homogeneous central renal sinus complex without separation
Grade 1 = separation of central sinus echoes of ovoid configuration; continuous echogenic sinus periphery; 52% predictive value for obstruction
Grade 2 = separation of central sinus echoes of rounded configuration; dilated calyces connecting with renal pelvis; continuity of echogenic sinus periphery
Grade 3 = replacement of major portions of renal sinus; discontinuity of echogenic sinus periphery

Amount of collecting system dilatation depends on:
(a) duration of obstruction
(b) renal output
(c) presence of spontaneous decompression
◊ Amount of residual renal cortex is of prognostic significance!

Acute Hydronephrosis

Cause:
(1) Passage of calculus
(2) Passage of blood clot (from carcinoma, AV malformation, trauma, anticoagulant therapy), sloughed necrotic papilla
(3) Suture on ureter
(4) Ureteral edema following instrumentation
(5) Sulfonamide crystallization in nonalkalinized urine
(6) Normal pregnancy

- pain (50%)
- urinary tract infection (36%)
- nausea + vomiting (33%)

√ normal-sized kidney with normal parenchymal thickness
√ increasingly dense nephrogram
√ delayed opacification of collecting system (decreased glomerular filtration)
√ increasingly dense nephrogram over time ("obstructed nephrogram")
√ dilated collecting system + ureter
√ widening of forniceal angles
√ delayed images demonstrate site of obstruction at the end of a persistent column of contrast material in a dilated urinary collecting system
√ vicarious contrast excretion through gallbladder (uncommon)

US:
√ separation of renal sinus echoes
False-negatives: staghorn calculus filling entire collecting system, hyperacute renal obstruction (system not yet dilated), spontaneous decompression of obstruction, fluid-depleted patient with partial obstruction, dehydrated neonate
False-positives: full bladder, increased urine flow (overhydration, medications, following urography, diabetes insipidus, diuresis in nonoliguric azotemia), acute pyelonephritis, postobstructive / postsurgical dilatation, vesicoureteral reflux
Imposters: parapelvic cysts, sinus vessels, prominent extrarenal pelvis
√ ureteral jet not detectable / trickling flow
CAVE: in 25% ureteral jets not detectable (insufficient differences in specific gravity between ureteral urine and urine in the bladder)
√ ureteral jet absent in 13% of pregnant patients without ureteral obstruction
N.B.: turning pregnant patient into contralateral decubitus position will make jet visible

Duplex US:
√ mean RI of 0.77 ± 0.05 (0.63 ± 0.06 in nonobstructed kidney)
Caution: RI often normal in chronic obstruction; nonobstructive renal disease may elevate RIs
√ ≥0.08 difference in RI in right-to-left comparison with unilateral obstruction

Cx: spontaneous urinary extravasation (10–18%) from forniceal / pelvic tear (= pyelosinus reflux)

Chronic Hydronephrosis

= most frequent cause of abdominal mass in first 6 months of life (25% of all neonatal abdominal masses)

Cause:
(a) acquired: benign + malignant tumors of the ureter; ureteral strictures; retroperitoneal tumor / fibrosis; neurogenic bladder; benign prostatic hyperplasia; cervical / prostatic carcinoma; pelvic mass (lymphoma, abscess, ovarian); urethral polyps; urethral neoplasm; acquired urethral strictures
(b) congenital: ureteropelvic junction obstruction (most common), posterior urethral valves, ectopic ureterocele, congenital ureterovesical obstruction, prune-belly syndrome, primary megaureter

• insidious course
√ large kidney with wasted parenchyma
√ diminished nephrographic density (decreased clearance)
√ early "rim" sign (= thin band of radiodensity surrounding calyces)
√ delayed opacification of collecting system
√ moderate to marked widening of collecting system
√ tortuous dilated ureter

NUC:
√ photopenic area during vascular phase
√ accumulation of radionuclide tracer within hydronephrotic collecting system on delayed images

Cx: superimposed infection (= pyonephrosis)

Congenital Hydronephrosis

Mostly isolated malformation
Incidence: 1:100–300 births
Risk of recurrence: 2–3% for siblings
Age at presentation: 25% by age 1 year, 55% by age 5 years
Cause:
1. UPJ obstruction (22–40–67%)
2. Posterior urethral valves (18%)
3. Ectopic ureterocele (14%)
4. Prune belly syndrome (12%)
5. Ureteral + UVJ obstruction (8%)
6. Others: severe vesicoureteral reflux, bladder neck obstruction, hypertrophy of verumontanum, urethral diverticulum, congenital urethral strictures, anterior urethral valves, meatal stenosis

May be associated with: Down syndrome (17–25%)
• palpable abdominal mass
• intermittent flank + periumbilical pain
• failure to thrive
• vomiting
• hematuria, infection

Location: 70% unilateral

OB-US:
√ AP diameter of renal pelvis ≥5 mm between 15–20 weeks, ≥8 mm at 20–30 weeks, ≥10 mm after 30 weeks MA
√ ratio of AP diameter of renal pelvis to kidney >50%
√ caliceal distension communicating with renal pelvis
◊ Postnatal evaluation after 4–7 days of age (because of decreased GFR + relative dehydration in first days of life)!

Prognosis: parenchymal atrophy + renal impairment (dependent on severity + duration)

Focal Hydronephrosis

= HYDROCALICOSIS = HYDROCALYX
= obstructed drainage of one portion of kidney
Cause:
(1) Congenital: partial / complete duplication
(2) Infectious stricture: eg, TB
(3) Infundibular calculus
(4) Tumor
(5) Trauma

√ unifocal mass, commonly in upper pole
√ absent polar group of calyces (early)
√ dilated polar group (late) with displacement of adjacent calyces
√ delayed opacification in obstructed group
√ focally replaced nephrogram

US:
√ anechoic cystic lesion with smooth margins

CT:
√ focal area of water density with smooth margin and thick wall

Hydronephrosis in Pregnancy

1. Physiologic dilatation
   Incidence: 80%; in up to 90% by 3rd trimester
   Cause: hormonal (relaxation of ureteric smooth muscle in response to progesterone), mechanical (gravid uterus compresses ureter at pelvic brim near crossing of iliac vessels with right ureter taking a more acute angle)
   • asymptomatic
   √ as early as 6–10 weeks of gestation
   √ right side (85–90%), left side (15–67%)
   √ ureter widened only to pelvic brim
   Prognosis: resolution within a few weeks to 6 months after delivery
2. "Overdistension syndrome"
   Cause: obstruction by gravid uterus
   • pain mimicking renal colic
3. Acute hydronephrosis
   Cause: change in position of fetus, diuresis, passage of stone into ureter
   • constant pain ± nausea and vomiting

JUXTAGLOMERULAR TUMOR

= RENINOMA
= very rare benign tumor arising from renin-producing juxtaglomerular cells
Incidence: <30 cases reported
Age: mean age of 24 (range, 7–58) years; 50% <21 years; M:F = 1:2
Origin: arising from afferent arterioles of glomeruli
Path: small foci of hemorrhage + pseudocapsule
Histo: tumor resembles hemangiopericytoma

GU

- typical features of primary reninism:
  - marked + sustained hypertension, often accelerated and poorly controlled
  - secondary hyperaldosteronism with hypokalemia
  - hyperreninemia
- moderate to severe headaches
- hypertensive retinopathy
- polydipsia, polyuria, enuresis

Location: just beneath renal capsule
√ renal mass of usually 2–3 (range, 0.8–6.5) cm in size
US:
√ echogenic mass ± areas of necrosis / hemorrhage
CT (thin overlapping cuts):
√ isodense tumor on NECT, hypodense on CECT
MR:
√ early peripheral enhancement on T1WI
√ washout of contrast material from periphery + filling in of central tumor portion on delayed T1WI
Angio:
√ (easily overlooked) hypo- / avascular tumor (in 43%)
√ renal vein sampling yields high renin level on affected side
Dx: combination of elevated renin without renal arterial lesion + hypovascular solid renal mass
Rx: surgical excision
DDx of renin elevation:
Wilms tumor, hypernephroma, lung cancer, paraovarian tumor, fallopian tube adenocarcinoma, epithelial liver hamartoma, orbital hemangiopericytoma, pancreatic cancer, angiolymphoid hyperplasia

LEUKEMIA

= clonal proliferation of lymphoblasts (acute leukemia) or small lymphocytes (chronic leukemia)
◊ Most common malignant cause of bilateral global renal enlargement!
Incidence: renal involvement in 50% of children + in 65% of adults at autopsy

A. DIFFUSE INVOLVEMENT (most common)
leukemic cells infiltrate the interstitial tissue + renal sinus; tubules are replaced (more common in lymphocytic than in granulocytic forms); no relationship to peripheral white blood cell count
- renal impairment (from leukemic infiltrate, hyperuricemia, septicemia, hemorrhage)
- hypertension

√ moderate to massive nephromegaly bilaterally with smooth contours
√ normal or diminished density on nephrogram
√ occasionally attenuated collecting system (DDx: renal sinus lipomatosis)
√ nonopaque filling defects on IVP (clot, uric acid)
√ renal / subcapsular / perinephric hemorrhage frequent
√ retroperitoneal lymphadenopathy
US:
√ loss of definition + distortion of central sinus complex
√ normal to increased coarse echoes throughout renal cortex + preservation of renal medullae
√ single / multiple focal anechoic masses

B. FOCAL ACCUMULATION OF LEUKEMIC CELLS (rare)
chloroma (= granulocytic sarcoma) of acute myeloblastic leukemia, myeloblastoma, myeloblastic sarcoma
- may antedate other manifestations of leukemia

√ unifocal mass in renal cortex / renal sinus
DDx: Hodgkin disease, malignant lymphoma, multiple myeloma

LEUKOPLAKIA

= KERATINIZING SQUAMOUS METAPLASIA / DYSPLASIA
= DYSKERATOSIS
Cause: chronic infection (80%) / stones (40%)
Histo: large confluent areas / scattered patches of squamous metaplasia of transitional cell epithelium with keratinization + cellular atypia in deeper layers
Peak age: 4th–5th decade;
M:F = 1:1 (with involvement of renal pelvis)
M:F = 4:1 (with involvement of bladder)
- hematuria (30%)
- recurrent UTIs
- pathognomonic passage of gritty flakes, soft-tissue stones, white chunks of tissue (desquamated keratinized epithelial layers) leading to colic, fever, chills

Location: bladder > renal pelvis > ureter; bilateral in 10%
√ corrugated / striated irregularities of pelvicaliceal walls, localized / generalized
√ plaquelike intraluminal mass with "onion skin" pattern of contrast material in interstices
√ caliectasis + pyelectasis common (with obstruction)
√ ridging / filling defects of ureter
√ associated with calculi in 25–50%
Cx: premalignant condition for epidermoid carcinoma in 12% (controversial!)

LOCALIZED CYSTIC DISEASE

= multiple simple cysts involving only one portion of the kidney
- no family history

Histo: dilated ducts and tubules varying in size from mm to several cm
Prognosis: not progressive

LYMPHOMA OF KIDNEY

Incidence: in 3–8% (by CT), 30–60% (by autopsy)
◊ The kidneys are one of the most common extranodal sites of lymphoma!
Types:
A. NON-HODGKIN LYMPHOMA (more common)
(a) SECONDARY due to systemic disease
renal involvement detected in 3–8% of abdominal CT, in 33–65% of autopsies; occurs usually late in disease
At risk: immunocompromised patients with HIV infection / organ transplantation (esp. after cyclosporine therapy), ataxia-telangiectasia
(b) PRIMARY renal lymphoma (rare)
arising in renal hilar nodes / renal parenchyma

GU

B. HODGKIN DISEASE (rare)
renal involvement in 13% of autopsies

Patterns of involvement:
(a) hematogenous dissemination (bilateral in 75%):
— single / multiple foci (most common)
√ resembling primary renal neoplasm
— diffuse infiltration (less common)
√ preservation of renal parenchyma + contour
(b) contiguous extension from adjacent pararenal lymphomatous disease, usually extranodal

- clinically silent (50%)
- flank pain, weight loss
- palpable mass, hematuria
- compromised renal function (urinary tract obstruction, renal vein compression, diffuse infiltration of kidney, superimposed infarct, amyloidosis, hypercalcemia)

Associated with: splenomegaly, lymphadenopathy
◊ Look for other sites of multisystemic involvement in bone marrow, liver, GI tract, lung, heart, CNS!

√ unilateral:bilateral = 1:3
√ multiple nodular masses (29–61%), 1–3 cm in size
√ spread from retroperitoneal disease (25–30%) with involvement by transcapsular / hilar invasion
√ solitary tumor (10–20%): bulky up to 15 cm in size (7%) / small (7–48%)
√ perinephric lymphoma:
(a) direct extension from retroperitoneal disease
(b) transcapsular growth of renal parenchymal disease
◊ A tumor surrounding kidney without parenchymal compression or compromise in function is virtually PATHOGNOMONIC of lymphoma
√ renal sinus infiltration
√ small curvilinear areas of high attenuation
√ thickening of fascia of Gerota
√ perirenal nodules / masses of soft-tissue density
√ mass contiguous with retroperitoneal disease
√ nephromegaly due to diffuse infiltration of interstitium (6–19%) with sparing of glomeruli and tubules:
√ preservation of renal contour
√ almost always bilateral
√ encasement / deformation of pelvocaliceal system
• clinically silent poor renal function
√ patency of renal vessels despite tumor encasement is CHARACTERISTIC

CT (nephrographic phase most sensitive for detection):
√ usually homogeneous poorly marginated masses less dense than renal parenchyma + decreased enhancement compared with renal parenchyma

US:
√ single / multiple anechoic / hypoechoic masses:
√ may show increased through transmission
√ renal enlargement + decreased parenchymal echoes
√ loss of renal sinus echoes

Angio:
√ neovascularity, encasement, vascular displacement (occasionally palisade-like configuration)

DDx of nodular mass:
(1) RCC (more heterogeneous, vascular invasion)
(2) Metastases from lung, breast, synchronous renal cell cancer

DDx of infiltrative tumor:
TCC, acute / xanthogranulomatous pyelonephritis

MALACOPLAKIA

= MALAKOPLAKIA [*malacoplakia*, Greek = soft plaque]
= uncommon chronic inflammatory response to Gram-negative infection

Frequency: <200 cases reported
Organism: E. coli (in 94%)
Predisposed: diabetes mellitus, immunocompromise
Pathogenesis: altered host response to infection at the macrophage level = engulfed organisms remain viable + become a source for recurring infection
Histo: submucosal histiocytic granulomas containing large foamy mononuclear cells (**Hansemann macrophages**) with intracytoplasmic basophilic PAS-positive inclusion bodies (**Michaelis-Gutmann bodies** = calculospherules) consisting of incompletely destroyed E. coli bacterium surrounded by lipoprotein membranes
Peak age: 5th–7th decade; M:F = 1:4

- history of recurrent urinary tract infections
- hematuria
- raised yellow lesion <3 cm in diameter

Location:
1. bladder > lower 2/3 of ureter > upper ureter > renal pelvis; multifocal in 75%; bilateral in 50%
2. outside urinary tract

@ Bladder / ureter
√ multiple nodular dome-shaped smooth mural filling defects of collecting system
√ scalloped appearance if lesions confluent
√ generalized pelviureteral dilatation (if obstructive)
DDx: pyeloureteritis cystica

@ Kidney
√ diffuse enlargement of kidney (bilateral involvement unusual)
√ displacement of pelvicaliceal system + distortion of central sinus complex
√ multifocal parenchymal masses may cause diminished / absent nephrogram
√ urinary tract calcification rare
US:
√ lesions of variable echogenicity
CT:
√ ill-defined low-attenuation lesions
√ ± perinephric extension
DDx: infiltrative neoplasm; XGP (unilateral, urinary tract calcification)

MALPOSITIONED TESTIS

= MALDESCENDED TESTIS

Testicles are normally within scrotum by 28–32 weeks MA

Prevalence: early 3rd trimester in 10%; at birth in 3.7–6% (in babies >2,500 g in 3.4%; in premature babies in 30%); beyond 3 months of age in 1%

Test sensitivity:
- MR : modality of choice
- US : 20–88%; very sensitive in inguinal canal
- CT : 95% (testis <1 cm cannot be detected)
  √ no spermatic cord in inguinal canal
- Venography : 50–90%
- Laparoscopy: most reliable method

Cx: (1) Sterility
(2) Malignancy: most commonly seminoma, 30–50 x risk increase = 1:1,000 men/year; 4–11% of all testicular tumors found in cryptorchidism; risk remains increased even after orchidopexy
◊ Annual screening until at least age 35!
(3) Torsion: 10 x risk in cryptorchidism

Rx: surgery / orchidopexy at 9–12 months of age

DDx: (1) Rudimentary testis
(2) Pars intravaginalis gubernaculum = nonatrophied bulbous termination
(3) Congenital absence = monorchia / anorchia (in 3–5%)
◊ Nonpalpable testes are agenetic in 15–63% of term infants!

Cryptorchidism (20–29%)
= arrested descent of testis along its normal course
Pathophysiologic theory:
generalized defect in embryogenesis results in bilateral dysgenetic gonads
Theory supported by:
- cancer risk extends to contralateral testis
- orchiopexy does not decrease cancer risk
- cancer risk increases with degree of ectopy

Associated with:
prune belly syndrome (bilateral cryptorchidism), Prader-Willi syndrome, Beckwith-Wiedemann syndrome, Noonan syndrome, Laurence-Moon-Biedl syndrome, trisomies 13, 18, 21
- nonpalpable testis

Location: high scrotal position (50%); canalicular = between internal + external inguinal ring (20%); abdominal (10%); bilateral in 10%
◊ The most craniad possible point of an undescended testis is the lower pole of the ipsilateral kidney!
√ failure to visualize testis within scrotum
√ small atrophic testis with generalized decreased echogenicity:
√ identification of mediastinum testis is necessary
DDx: lymph node

Ectopia Testis (1%)
= deviation from the usual pathway
Location: interstitial = groin (on external oblique muscle), pubopenile = root of penis, perineal, femoral triangle, on opposite side

Pseudocryptorchidism (70%)
= RETRACTILE TESTIS
= unusually spastic cremasteric muscle

Undescended Testis
= retractile testis + cryptorchidism

MECKEL-GRUBER SYNDROME
= autosomal recessive disease characterized by occipital encephalocele, polycystic kidneys, polydactyly
Incidence: 1:12,000–50,000; more common among Yemenite Jews
Risk of recurrence: 25%; carrier frequency of 1:56
- history of affected siblings

OB-US:
√ large polycystic kidneys containing 2–10-mm cysts
√ occipital encephalocele
√ postaxial polydactyly
√ microcephaly
√ cleft lip and palate
√ moderate-to-severe oligohydramnios (onset midtrimester)
√ inability to visualize urine within fetal bladder

OB management:
1. Chromosomal analysis to exclude trisomy 13 (if no prior family history)
2. Option of pregnancy termination <24 weeks GA
3. Nonintervention for fetal distress >24 weeks GA

Prognosis: invariably fatal at birth due to pulmonary hypoplasia + renal failure
DDx: trisomy 13

MEDULLARY CYSTIC DISEASE
= NEPHRONOPHTHISIS
= salt-wasting nephropathy causing chronic renal failure in adolescents / young adults
Histo: variable number of medullary cysts (100 μm to 2 cm) + progressive periglomerular and interstitial fibrosis + tubular atrophy with dilatation of some proximal tubules
Types:
(1) **Medullary Cystic Disease** = ADULT ONSET
autosomal dominant, in young adults, rapidly progressive course with uremia + death in 2 years
(2) **Juvenile Nephronophthisis** = JUVENILE ONSET
= UREMIC MEDULLARY CYSTIC DISEASE
autosomal recessive, in children 3–5 years, average duration of 10 years before uremia and death occurs
- salt-wasting, polyuria, hyposthenuria, polydipsia
- failure to thrive, growth retardation (in early teens)
- uremia, severe anemia, normal sediment, hypertension (only in late phase)

√ bilateral normal / small kidneys with smooth contour
√ thin cortex
IVP:
√ poor opacification of renal collecting system
√ "medullary nephrogram" = medullary striations persistent for up to 2 hours; occasionally replaced by sharply defined multiple thin-walled lucencies
Retrograde pyelogram:
√ communication between collecting system + cysts

US / CT:
- √ increased parenchymal echogenicity + loss of corticomedullary junction
- √ multiple small corticomedullary / medullary cysts

MEDULLARY RENAL TUMOR

Incidence: 1–2% of all renal cancers

Collecting Duct Carcinoma

= BELLINI DUCT CARCINOMA

Frequency: ~100 cases reported in literature

Age: mean age of 55 years (range of 13–80 years)

Histo: mostly high-grade tumor

- • abdominal pain, flank mass, hematuria
- ◊ In 40% metastasized at presentation

Prognosis: aggressive clinical course with 33% surviving >2 years

- √ infiltrative neoplasm centered in medulla:
  - √ renal sinus invasion
  - √ extension into cortex is frequent
  - √ ± coexisting expansile component
- √ large tumor at presentation

US: √ hyperechoic mass

Angio: √ hypovascular mass

MR: √ hypointense mass on T2WI

Renal Medullary Carcinoma

= highly aggressive malignant tumor of epithelial origin occurring almost exclusively in adolescent / young adult blacks with sickle cell trait / hemoglobin SC disease (termed "seventh sickle cell nephropathy") but NOT with hemoglobin SS (sickle cell) disease

Origin: distal collecting duct / epithelium of papilla; ? aggressive form of collecting duct carcinoma

Mean age: 20 (range, 11–39) years; M:F = 3:1 (if <24 years of age) and 1:1 (if >24 years of age)

Histo: poorly differentiated tumor cells within a desmoplastic stroma + mixed with reticular, yolk saclike, adenoid cystic components

- • abdominal / flank pain, gross hematuria
- • palpable mass, weight loss, fever
- • metastases at presentation common: regional lymph nodes, liver, lung, bone
- √ large ill-defined mass centered in renal medulla:
  - √ heterogenous due to varying amounts of hemorrhage and necrosis
  - √ extension into renal sinus and cortex
  - √ ± peripheral caliectasis
  - √ heterogeneous enhancement
- √ reniform enlargement with shape of kidney preserved
- √ small peripheral satellite nodules

Prognosis: mean survival rate of 15 weeks from diagnosis

DDx: transitional cell carcinoma, rhabdoid tumor

MEDULLARY SPONGE KIDNEY

= dysplastic cystic dilatation of papillary + medullary portions of collecting ducts (first few generations of metanephric duct branchings)

Incidence: 0.5%

Age: young to middle-aged adults; sporadic

May be associated with: Ehlers-Danlos syndrome, parathyroid adenoma, Caroli disease

- • often asymptomatic
- √ medullary nephrocalcinosis (40–80%) with one / more calculi of up to 5 mm clustered in papillary region
- √ "bunch of flowers" = thick dense streaks of contrast material radiating from pyramids peripherally representing papillary cysts / ectatic ducts (DDx: dense papillary blush in normals)
- √ may be unilateral in 25%
- √ may involve <u>only one</u> pyramid / all pyramids (25%)

US:
- √ echogenic medulla (in absence of stones)

Cx: urolithiasis, hematuria, infection

Dx: (1) opacification of stone-free papillary cysts
(2) accumulation of contrast material around calculi within ectatic tubules / cysts

DDx:
1. (1) Normal variant ("papillary blush" without distinct streaks / nephrocalcinosis / pyramidal enlargement)
2. (2) Renal tuberculosis (larger more irregular calcifications + cavitations + strictures + ulcerations)
3. (3) Papillary necrosis (sloughed papilla + caliceal ring sign)
4. (4) Medullary nephrocalcinosis (no ectatic ducts / cysts, calcifications beyond pyramids)
5. (5) Juvenile polycystic kidney disease (bilateral renal enlargement + hepatic periportal fibrosis)
6. (6) Caliceal diverticulum (small, solitary, located between pyramid)

MEGACALICOSIS

= CONGENITAL MEGACALICES

= nonprogressive caliceal dilatation caused by hypoplastic medullary pyramids

Age: any age; M >> F

May be associated with: primary megaureter

- • normal glomerular filtration rate

Site: entire kidney / part of kidney; unilateral >> bilateral

- √ kidney usually enlarged with prominent fetal lobation
- √ reduced parenchymal thickness (medulla affected, NOT cortex):
  - √ normal DMSA scintigram
- √ mosaic-like arrangement of dilated calyces (polygonal + faceted appearance, NOT globular as in obstruction)
- √ increased number of calyces (>15)
- √ ABSENT caliceal cupping (semilunar instead of pyramidal configuration of papillae)
- √ NO dilatation of pelvis / ureters, NORMAL contrast excretion

Cx: (1) Hematuria
(2) Stone formation

MEGACYSTIS-MICROCOLON SYNDROME

= MEGALOCYSTIS-MICROCOLON-INTESTINAL HYPOPERISTALSIS SYNDROME (MMIH)

= functional obstruction of bladder + colon characterized by
(1) enlarged urinary bladder

GU

(2) small colon
(3) strikingly short small intestine suspended on a primitive dorsal mesentery
(4) markedly enlarged hydronephrotic kidneys with little remaining parenchyma

Incidence: 26 cases reported; M:F = 1:7

May be associated with: diaphragmatic hernia, PDA, teeth at birth

- distended abdomen (large bladder + dilated small bowel loops)
- overflow incontinence
- intestinal pseudoobstruction (poor emptying of stomach, NO peristaltic activity of small bowel)

OB-US:
√ normal amount of amniotic fluid / polyhydramnios (in spite of dilated bladder = "nonobstructive obstruction")
√ massive + progressive bladder distension with poor emptying
√ bilateral megaloureters
√ ± hydronephrosis
√ female sex

BE:
√ microcolon (transient feature of "unused colon") with narrow rectum + sigmoid
√ malrotation / malfixation or foreshortening of small bowel

VCUG
√ distended unobstructed bladder with poor / absent muscular function

Prognosis: lethal in most cases (a few months of age)

MEGALOURETER

= CONGENITAL PRIMARY MEGAURETER = TERMINAL URETERECTASIS = ACHALASIA OF URETER = URETEROVESICAL JUNCTION OBSTRUCTION
= intrinsic congenital dilatation of lower juxtavesical orthotopic ureter

Cause: aperistaltic juxtavesical (1.5 cm long) segment secondary to faulty development of muscle layers of ureter with too much collagen / too much muscle (functional, NOT mechanical obstruction)

Incidence: all ages; second most common cause of hydronephrosis in fetus and newborn; M:F = 2–5:1

Associated disorders (in 40%):
(a) contralateral: UPJ obstruction, reflux, ureterocele, ureteral duplication, renal ectopia, renal agenesis
(b) ipsilateral: caliceal diverticulum, megacalicosis, papillary necrosis

- asymptomatic (mostly)
- pain
- abdominal mass
- hematuria
- infection

Location: L:R = 3:1, bilateral in 15–40%

√ prominent localized dilatation of pelvic ureter (up to 5 cm in diameter) usually not progressive, but may involve entire ureter + collecting system
√ vigorous nonpropulsive to-and-fro motion in dilated segment
√ functional smoothly tapered narrowing of intravesical ureter
√ NO reflux, NO stenosis

MESOBLASTIC NEPHROMA

= FETAL RENAL HAMARTOMA = LEIOMYOMATOUS HAMARTOMA = BENIGN CONGENITAL WILMS TUMOR = BENIGN FETAL HAMARTOMA = FETAL MESENCHYMAL TUMOR = FIBROMYXOMA = BOLANDE TUMOR = CONGENITAL FIBROSARCOMA
= nonfamilial benign fibromyomatoid mass arising from renal connective tissue

Incidence: most common solid renal neoplasm in neonate; 3% of all renal neoplasms in children

Age: peak age 1–3 months; 90% within 1st year of life; rare after the age of 6 months; may occasionally go undetected until adulthood; M > F

Path: solid unencapsulated mass infiltrating renal parenchyma (derived from early nephrogenic mesenchyme)

Histo: monomorphic tumor composed of smooth muscle cells + immature fibroblasts resembling leiomyoma containing trapped islands of embryonic glomeruli, tubules, vessels, hematopoietic cells, cartilage

In 14% associated with: prematurity, polyhydramnios, GI + GU tract malformations, neuroblastoma

- large palpable flank mass (most common)
- hematuria (20%) / hypertension (4%), anemia

√ large usually solid intrarenal mass:
  √ usually replaces 60–90% of renal parenchyma
  √ typically involves renal sinus
  √ may produce multiple cystic spaces (hemorrhage, necrosis)
√ infiltrative growth:
  √ NO sharp cleavage plane toward normal parenchyma
  √ may extend beyond capsule (common)
√ calcifications (rare)
√ NO venous extension (DDx from Wilms tumor)
√ NO invasion of collecting system

IVP:
√ large noncalcified renal mass with distortion of collecting system
√ usually NO herniation into renal pelvis (DDx from MLCN)

CECT:
√ uniform enhancement of less than normal renal parenchyma
√ areas of low attenuation in large lesions (hemorrhage / necrosis)

US:
√ evenly echogenic tumor resembling uterine fibroids
√ concentric rings of alternating echogenicity
√ homogeneously hypoechoic tumor
√ complex heterogeneous mass with hemorrhage + cyst formation + necrosis

OB-US:
- premature delivery, increased renin levels
- √ polyhydramnios, hydrops

Angio:
- √ hypervascular mass with neovascularity + displacement of adjacent vessels

Cx: (1) Transformation to metastasizing spindle cell sarcoma (rare)
(2) Metastases to lung, brain, bone (rare)

Rx: nephrectomy with wide surgical margin

Prognosis: excellent (imaging follow-up for 1 year)

METANEPHRIC ADENOMA

= NEPHROGENIC ADENOFIBROMA = EMBRYONAL ADENOMA

Age: any (range, 15 months – 83 years); M < F

Histo: proliferation of spindle-shaped mesenchymal cells encasing nodules of embryonal epithelium; numerous psammoma bodies

- pain, hypertension, hematoma, flank mass, hypercalcemia, polycythemia

US:
- √ well-defined solid hypovascular mass
- √ hypo- / hyperechoic / cystic with mural nodule

CT:
- √ iso- / hypoattenuating mass + little enhancement
- √ ± small calcifications

Rx: local resection with sparing of kidney

METASTASES TO ADRENAL GLAND

Frequency: 4th most common site of metastatic disease in the body
◊ 50% of adrenal masses in oncologic patients represent benign nonhyperfunctioning adenomas!
◊ An adrenal mass in a patient with malignancy is a metastasis in 30–40%!

Origin: lung (40%), breast 920%), thyroid, colon, melanoma, renal cell carcinoma, lymphoma

√ large heterogeneously attenuating mass with irregular contour

Dx: biopsy

DDx: adenoma (intracytoplasmic lipid causing chemical shift artifact + significant decrease in signal intensity on out-of-phase GRE)

GU

METASTASES TO KIDNEY

◊ Most common malignant tumor of the kidney (2–3 times as frequent as primaries in autopsy studies)!
◊ 5th most common site of metastases (after lung, liver, bone, adrenals)!
◊ Renal metastases means typically advanced disease!

Frequency: 7–13% in large autopsy series

most common primaries: bronchus, breast, GI tract, opposite kidney, non-Hodgkin lymphoma, colon, neuroblastoma (in children)

less common primaries: stomach, cervix, ovary, pancreas, prostate, chloroma, myeloblastoma, myeloblastic sarcoma, melanoma (45% incidence), osteogenic sarcoma, choriocarcinoma (10–50% incidence), Hodgkin lymphoma, rhabdomyosarcoma

- usually asymptomatic
- √ bilateral multiple small masses (due to brief survival of patient)
- √ solitary exophytic mass (in colon cancer)
- √ perinephric tumor (in melanoma)
- √ infiltrative growth pattern

DDx on CT: lymphoma, bilateral RCC, multiple renal infarcts, acute focal bacterial nephritis, infiltrating TCC

MULTICYSTIC DYSPLASTIC KIDNEY

= MULTICYSTIC DYSGENETIC KIDNEY (MCDK)
= MULTICYSTIC KIDNEY (MCK) = Potter Type II

◊ Second most common cause of an abdominal mass in neonate (after hydronephrosis)!
◊ Most common form of cystic disease in infants!

Incidence: 1:4,300 (for unilateral MCDK), 1:10,000 (for bilateral MCDK) live births; M:F = 2:1 (for unilateral MCDK); more common among infants of diabetic mothers

Risk of recurrence: 2–3%

Etiology: sporadic NOT familial; obstruction / atresia of ureter during metanephric stage before 8–10 weeks' GA

Pathophysiology: ureteral obstruction / atresia interferes with ureteral bud division + inhibits induction and maturation of nephrons; collecting tubules enlarge into cysts

Histo: immature glomeruli + tubules reduced in number + whirling mesenchymal tissue, cartilage (33%), cysts

- abdominal mass
- asymptomatic if unilateral (may go undetected until adulthood)
- recurrent urinary tract infections, intermittent abdominal pain, nausea + vomiting, hematuria, failure to thrive
- fatal due to pulmonary hypoplasia if bilateral
  Fatal form: bilateral MCDK (4.5–21%), contralateral renal agenesis (0–11%)

Location:
1. UNILATERAL multicystic dysplastic kidney
   most common form (80–90%); L:R = 2:1
   secondary to pelvoinfundibular atresia
   In 20–33–50% associated with anomalies of contralateral kidney:
   (1) Vesicoureteral reflux (15–43%)
   (2) Ureteropelvic junction obstruction (7–27%)
   (3) Horseshoe kidney (5–9%)
   (4) Ureteral anomalies (5%)
   (5) Renal hypoplasia (4%)
   (6) Megaloureter
   (7) Malrotation
   (8) Renal agenesis

Associated with anomalies of ipsilateral kidney:
(1) Vesicoureteral reflux (25%)
(2) Ectopic ureter

2. SEGMENTAL / focal renal dysplasia
= "multilocular cyst" secondary to
(a) high-grade obstruction of upper pole moiety in duplex kidney from ectopic ureterocele
(b) single obstructed infundibulum
3. BILATERAL cystic dysplasia
in the presence of severe obstruction in utero from posterior urethral valves / urethral atresia with oligohydramnios + pulmonary hypoplasia
Prognosis: lethal

Potter types:
(1) Multicystic kidney (Potter IIa)
√ large kidney with multiple large cysts + little visible renal parenchyma
(2) Hypoplastic / diminutive form (Potter IIb)
√ echogenic small kidney

APPEARANCE RELATED TO SITE OF OBSTRUCTION
@ ureteropelvic junction
√ single / several large / multiple medium-sized cysts in large kidney
@ distal ureter / urethra
√ small / no cysts in small kidney

APPEARANCE RELATED TO TIME OF INSULT
(a) early onset between 8th and 11th week
√ small / atretic renal pelvis + calyces
√ 10–20 cysts + loss of reniform appearance
(b) late onset = HYDRONEPHROTIC FORM
√ large central cyst (= dilated pelvis) often communicating with cysts
√ some renal function may be demonstrated

√ large kidney with lobulated contour in infancy
√ often incidental finding of small kidney in adults (as little as 1 g secondary to arrested growth)
√ ipsilateral atretic ureter associated with hemitrigone
√ contralateral renal hypertrophy
√ calcification: curvilinear / ringlike in wall of cysts in 30% of adults, rarely in children

NUC (99m-Tc MAG 3):
◊ NUC preferred over IVP in first month of life as concentrating ability of even normal neonatal kidneys is suboptimal!
√ no function
DDx: severe hydronephrosis (peripheral activity), UPJ obstruction (minimal uptake)

US:
√ normal renal architecture replaced by:
√ random cysts of varying shape + size ("cluster of grapes") with largest cyst in peripheral nonmedial location (100% accurate)
√ cysts separated by septa (100% accurate)
√ no communication between multiple cysts (93% accurate)
√ cysts begin to disappear in infancy
√ central sinus complex absent (100% accurate)
√ no identification of parenchymal rim or corticomedullary differentiation (74% accurate)
√ oligohydramnios in bilateral MCDK / unilateral MCDK + contralateral urinary obstruction

Angio:
√ absent / hypoplastic renal artery; angiography unnecessary since a DDx to long-standing functionless kidney is not possible

OB management:
(1) Routine antenatal care + evaluation by pediatric urologist following delivery if unilateral
(2) Option of pregnancy termination if ≤24 weeks GA
(3) Nonintervention for fetal distress if >24 weeks GA

Cx: (1) Renin-dependent hypertension (rare)
(2) Malignancy in <1:330

Rx: (1) Follow-up in 3–4-month intervals in first year (isolated reports of developing malignancy)
(2) Nephrectomy (in hypertension / massive renal enlargement)

DDx: (1) Hydronephrosis
(2) Renal dysplasia with cysts (associated with partial obstruction)

MULTILOCULAR CYSTIC RENAL TUMOR

= BENIGN MULTILOCULAR CYSTIC NEPHROMA (MLCN) = POLYCYSTIC NEPHROBLASTOMA = WELL-DIFFERENTIATED POLYCYSTIC WILMS TUMOR = BENIGN CYSTIC DIFFERENTIATED NEPHROBLASTOMA = CYSTIC PARTIALLY DIFFERENTIATED NEPHROBLASTOMA = MULTILOCULAR CYSTIC NEPHROMA = PERLMANN TUMOR = MULTILOCULAR RENAL CYST = CYSTIC ADENOMA / HAMARTOMA / LYMPHANGIOMA = PARTIALLY POLYCYSTIC KIDNEY

= rare nonhereditary benign renal neoplasm originating from metanephric blastema possibly representing the benign end of a spectrum with solid Wilms tumor at the malignant end

Age: biphasic age + sex distribution: <4 years in 73% male, >4 years in 89% female
(a) 3 months to 2 years of age (65%), 5–30 years (5%); M:F = 2:1
(b) >30 years (30%); M:F = 1:8
◊ 90% of tumors in males occur in first 2 years of life (peak 3–24 months)!
◊ Most of the lesions in females occur between ages 4 and 20 or 40 and 60!

Path: solitary large well-circumscribed multiseptated mass of noncommunicating fluid-filled loculi, surrounded by thick fibrous capsule + compressed renal parenchyma; cyst size between mm up to 4 cm

Histo: (gross anatomic + radiologic features are identical)
1. **Cystic nephroma**
fibrous tissue septa of undifferentiated mesenchymal and primitive glomerulotubular elements surround cysts lined by flattened cuboidal epithelium;
NO blastemal / other embryonal elements
• typically seen in adult women

GU

2. **Cystic partially differentiated nephroblastoma**
   = CPDN
   predominantly cystic lesion with septa containing primitive metanephric blastema
   • primarily in young boys
   ◊ No association with Wilms tumor!

• commonly asymptomatic painless abdominal mass
• ± sudden and rapid enlargement
• pain, hematuria, urinary tract infection

Location: unilateral, often replacing an entire renal pole (usually lower pole)
Size: average size of 10 cm (few cm to 33 cm)
√ sharply well-circumscribed (characteristic) multiseptated cystic renal mass
√ tumor surrounded by thick fibrous capsule
√ cluster of noncommunicating "honeycombed" cysts of various sizes (several mm to 4 cm) separated by thick septa
√ smaller closely spaced cysts appear as solid nodules
√ contrast enhancement of septations (secondary to tortuous fine vessels coursing through septa)
√ curvilinear to flocculent calcification of septa / capsule
IVP:
√ distortion of calyces / hydronephrosis secondary to nonfunctional mass
√ tendency for <u>herniation of tumor cysts into renal pelvis</u> (nonspecific, also seen with Wilms tumor + RCC)
US:
√ cluster of cysts separated by thick septa (SUGGESTIVE PATTERN)
√ occasionally solid echogenic character (due to very small cysts / jellylike contents)
CT:
√ cysts with attenuation equal to / higher than water (gelatinous fluid)
MR:
√ multicystic masses of low signal intensity on T1WI + hyperintense on T2WI
Cx: local recurrence / coexistent Wilms tumor (extremely rare)
Rx: nephrectomy with excellent prognosis
DDx: (1) Cystic Wilms tumor (overlapping age, expansile solid masses of nephroblastomatous tissue)
(2) Clear cell sarcoma (poor prognosis)
(3) Cystic mesoblastic nephroma (most common renal tumor of infancy)
(4) Cystic RCC (mean age of 10 years)
(5) Segmental form of multicystic dysplastic kidney

GU

MULTIPLE MYELOMA

◊ It is essential that dehydration be avoided!

Impairment of renal function:
(1) Precipitation of abnormal proteins (Bence Jones ± Tamm-Horsfall protein casts) into tubule lumen (30–50%)
(2) Toxicity of Bence Jones proteins on tubules
(3) Impaired renal blood flow secondary to increased blood viscosity
(4) Amyloidosis
(5) Nephrocalcinosis from hypercalcemia
◊ Contrast-induced renal failure in multiple myeloma is not seen with greatly increased frequency!

• Tamm-Horsfall proteinuria (tubular cell secretion)
√ smooth normal to large kidneys (initially), become small with time
√ occasionally attenuated pelvo-infundibulo-caliceal system
√ normal to diminished contrast material density; increasingly dense in acute oliguric failure
US:
√ normal to increased echogenicity
NUC in bone scintigraphy:
√ nonspecific increased parenchymal activity

MYCETOMA

= FUNGUS BALL

Organism: typically Candida, Aspergillus, Mucor, Cryptococcus, Phycomycetes, Actinomycetes mostly mycelial (M-form) or occasionally yeast cells (Y-form)
Predisposed: diabetics, debilitating illness, prolonged antibiotic therapy, leukemia, lymphoma, thymoma, immunosuppression

• flank pain, passing of tissue, hematuria (extremely rare)
• renal candidiasis associated with candidemia
• Candida cystitis preceded by vaginal candidiasis

√ unilateral nonvisualization of kidney (most frequent)
√ large irregular filling defect extending into dilated calyces (retrograde contrast study)
√ necrotizing papillitis from Candida nephritis (common)
√ lacelike pattern (on antegrade contrast study)

MYELOLIPOMA

= rare benign tumor composed of hematopoietic cells + fat similar to bone marrow

Prevalence: 0.08–0.2% (autopsy series)
Cause: ? metaplasia of adrenal cortical cells precipitated by chronic stress / degeneration
Path: mature fat interspersed with hematopoietic cells resembling bone marrow + pseudocapsule
Histo: variable mixture of myeloid cells, erythroid cells, megakaryocytes, lymphocytes
Associated with: endocrine disorders in 7% (Cushing syndrome, 21-hydroxylase deficiency), nonhyperfunctioning adenoma (15%)

• pain (from spontaneous hemorrhage if large)

Location: (a) adrenal gland (85%)
(b) extraadrenal (15%): retroperitoneal (12%), intrathoracic (3%)
Site: unilateral:bilateral = 10:1
Size: mean diameter of 10.4 cm
X-ray:
√ lucent mass with rim of residual normal adrenal cortex
√ calcifications (in up to 22% from previous hemorrhage)
US:
√ heterogeneous predominantly hyperechoic (= fatty + myeloid tissue) mass with interspersed hypoechoic (= pure fat) regions

CT:
- √ fatty tissue mass of –30 to –115 HU
- √ large amounts of fat with interspersed "smoky" areas of higher attenuation of 20–30 HU (= admixture of fat + marrowlike elements)

MR:
- √ hyperintense areas on T1WI (= predominantly fatty areas)
- √ intermediate intensity on T2WI similar to spleen
- √ focal reduction in signal intensity on fat-suppressed images (in fatty areas)

Cx: acute retroperitoneal hemorrhage with increase in size (12%)
Dx: percutaneous needle biopsy
Rx: surgical excision not necessary
DDx: liposarcoma, fat-containing adrenocortical carcinoma

NEPHROBLASTOMATOSIS

= multiple / diffuse NEPHROGENIC RESTS
= dysontogenetic process with persistence of embryonic renal parenchyma (= metanephric blastema) within the renal cortex >36 weeks GA

Incidence: 1% of infant kidneys; in 41% with unilateral Wilms tumor, in 94% with metachronous contralateral Wilms tumor, in 99% with bilateral Wilms tumor
◊ Usually absent in infants >4 months of age

Pathogenesis: metanephric blastema (= persistent embryonal tissue) normally present up to 36 weeks of gestational age; embryonal renal tissue in mature kidney after birth retains potential to form nephroblastoma / Wilms tumor

A. PERILOBAR NEPHROGENIC REST (0.87%)
Path: multiple rests forming a well-circumscribed smooth band at periphery of lobe
Histo: predominant tissue is blastema
Associated with:
(1) Beckwith-Wiedemann syndrome (gigantism, macroglossia, omphalocele, genitourinary anomalies)
(2) Hemihypertrophy
◊ 3% develop Wilms tumor
(3) Perlman syndrome (visceromegaly, gigantism, cryptorchidism, polyhydramnios, characteristic facies)
(4) Trisomy 18 syndrome
- Abnormal chromosome band 11p15 (Wilms tumor gene 2) in up to 77% of patients with perilobar rests
- Mean age presenting with neoplasia: 36 months

B. INTRALOBAR NEPHROGENIC REST (0.10%)
Path: single / few rests with irregular indistinct margins randomly anywhere within lobe
Histo: predominant tissue is stroma + epithelium
Associated with:
(1) Drash syndrome (ambiguous genitalia in genotypic males, progressive renal failure): 78% with intralobar rests + 11% with perilobar rests
(2) Sporadic aniridia: 100% with intralobar rests + 20% with perilobar rests
◊ 33% likelihood of Wilms tumor
(3) WAGR syndrome (Wilms tumor, aniridia, genital abnormalities, mental retardation)
- Abnormal chromosome band 11p13 (Wilms tumor gene 1)
- Mean age presenting with neoplasia: 16 months

Age: <2 years of age; neonatal period, infancy, childhood
- clinically occult in vast majority / renal enlargement

Histologic subtypes:
(a) dormant (nascent): nephrogenic rests the size of a glomerulus primarily composed of blastemal + epithelial elements; no malignant potential
(b) sclerosing (regressing / obsolescent): microscopic rests primarily composed of stromal elements
(c) hyperplastic: spherical / irregular / oval proliferation of most or all cell elements
(d) neoplastic: expansile mass due to proliferation of a single cell line

1. **Multifocal (juvenile) nephroblastomatosis**
most common form
= isolated macroscopic nephrogenic rests
√ may escape detection with imaging
√ ± nodular mass effect on pelvicaliceal structures
√ kidneys may be enlarged
√ lobulated contour of kidney
US:
√ hypoechoic / isoechoic / hyperechoic nodules
CECT (preferred study):
√ nodules with less enhancement than renal parenchyma

2. **Superficial diffuse (late infantile) nephroblastomatosis**
= superficial continuous rind of rests around medulla (= perilobar type)
Age: <2 years
√ nephromegaly
US:
√ loss of corticomedullary differentiation
√ kidneys diffusely echogenic / of normal echogenicity
√ cysts of variable size
CECT:
√ thick rind at periphery of kidney with poor / striated enhancement
DDx: autosomal recessive polycystic kidney disease, leukemia, lymphoma
◊ Strong association with Wilms tumor!

3. **Universal / panlobar (infantile) nephroblastomatosis**
rare form
= entire renal parenchyma diffusely involved
- may develop renal failure
√ bilateral renal enlargement (infiltrative growth)

MR (43% sensitivity, 58% sensitivity with enhancement):
√ homogeneously hypointense lesions on T1WI
√ homogeneously hypointense lesions on T2WI for sclerosing / involuting type of nephroblastomatosis

GU

√ isointense lesions on T2WI for hyperplastic / neoplastic type of nephroblastomatosis
√ hypointense lesions on enhanced T1WI

Cx: malignant transformation (enlargement of rest / development of mass) into cystic partially differentiated nephroblastoma / Wilms tumor
◊ 1% of patients with nephrogenic rests undergo neoplastic transformation!

Screening: for children with associated syndromes baseline CT at diagnosis / 6 months of age + follow-up sonograms every 3 months until age 7 years

Rx: radiologic follow-up / chemotherapy (for biopsy-proved hyperplastic nephrogenic rests similar to stage I Wilms tumor)

NEPHROGENIC ADENOMA

= uncommon benign metaplastic response to urothelial injury / prolonged irritation

Cause: (a) trauma: pelvic trauma, surgery in lower urinary tract, endoscopic procedure, renal transplantation (after a mean of 50 months)
(b) irritation: calculi, chronic bacterial infection, irradiation, intravesical chemotherapy, immunosuppressive therapy

Age: 3 weeks to 83 years; M:F = 3:1 (more common in females if <20 years of age)

Path: discrete raised papillary / polypoid / cystic areas projecting from epithelial surface

Histo: variable number of small tubules (resembling loops of Henle and collecting ducts) + cysts + papillae lined with a single layer of cuboidal / low columnar cells

- hematuria, dysuria, bladder instability
- asymptomatic

Location: bladder (72%), renal pelvis, ureter, urethra; strong correlation between location + site of insult to urothelium

Size: usually 1 mm, up to 7 cm in diameter

√ papillary / polypoid filling defect

Prognosis: high likelihood of recurrence; rarely malignant transformation

Rx: resection / fulguration

DDx: inflammatory / malignant urothelial lesions

GU

NEUROBLASTOMA

Most common solid abdominal mass of infancy (12.3% of all perinatal neoplasms), 3rd most common malignant tumor in infancy (after leukemia + CNS tumors); 2nd most common tumor in childhood (Wilms tumor more common in older children), 8–10% of all childhood cancers; 15% of cancer deaths in children

Incidence: 1:7,100 to 1:10,000 live births; 500 cases per year in USA; 20% hereditary

Origin: neural crest

Path: round irregular lobulated mass of 50–150 g with areas of hemorrhage + necrosis

Histo: small round cells slightly larger than lymphocytes with scant cytoplasm; Horner-Wright rosettes = one / two layers of primitive neuroblasts surrounding a central zone of tangled neurofibrillary processes

Age: peak age at 2 years; 25% during 1st year; 50% <2 years; 79% in <4 years; 97% in <10 years; occasionally present at birth; M:F = 1:1

Median age: 22 months

May be associated with: aganglionosis of bowel, CHD

- pain + fever (30%)
- palpable abdominal mass (45–54%)
- bone pain, limp, inability to walk (20%)
- cerebellar ataxia:
  - myoclonus of trunk + extremities
  - opsoclonus (20%) = spontaneous conjugate + chaotic eye movements (sign of cerebellar disease)
- orbital ecchymosis / proptosis (12%)
- increased catecholamine production (75–90%):
  - in 95% excreted in urine as vanillylmandelic acid (VMA) / homovanillic acid (HVA)
  - hypertension (up to 30%)
  - intractable diarrhea (9%) due to increase in vasoactive intestinal polypeptides (VIP)
  - acute cerebellar encephalopathy
  - paroxysmal episodes of flushing, tachycardia, headaches, sweating
  - rise in body temperature
  - hyperglycemia

Stage:

I	limited to organ of origin
II	regional spread not crossing midline
III	extension across midline
IV	metastatic to distant lymph nodes, liver, bone, brain, lung
IVs	stages I + II with disease confined to liver, skin, bone marrow WITHOUT radiographic evidence of skeletal metastases

Metastases:

bone (60%), regional lymph nodes (42%), orbit (20%), liver (15%), intracranial (14%), lung (10%)

◊ Metastases are first manifestation in up to 60%!

Hutchinson syndrome
(1) primary adrenal neuroblastoma
(2) extensive skeletal metastases, particularly skull
(3) proptosis
(4) bone pain

Pepper syndrome
(1) primary adrenal neuroblastoma
(2) massive hepatomegaly from metastases

Blueberry muffin syndrome
(1) primary adrenal neuroblastoma
(2) multiple metastatic skin lesions

◊ Bone marrow aspirate positive in 50–70% at time of initial diagnosis!

◊ 2/3 of patients >2 years have disseminated disease!

@ Skeletal metastases:
- paraplegia / extremity weakness from spinal canal extension

√ periosteal reaction
√ osteolytic focus / multicentric lytic lesions
√ lucent horizontal metaphyseal line
√ vertical linear radiolucent streaks in metadiaphysis of long bones
√ pathologic fracture
√ vertebral collapse
√ widened cranial sutures (subjacent dural metastases)
√ sclerotic lesions with healing
DDx: Ewing sarcoma, rhabdomyosarcoma, leukemia, lymphoma

@ Intracranial + maxillofacial metastases:
Site: dura, brain substance

@ Pulmonary metastases:
√ nodular infiltrates
√ rib erosion
√ mediastinal + retrocrural lymphadenopathy (common)

Location: anywhere within sympathetic neural chain

@ Abdomen
(a) adrenal (36%): almost always unilateral
(b) both adrenals (7–10%)
(c) extraadrenal in sympathetic chain (18%)

@ Thorax + posterior mediastinum (14%): aortic bodies
@ Neck (5%): carotid ganglia
@ Pelvis (5%): organ of Zuckerkandl
@ Skull / esthesioneuroblastoma of olfactory bulb, cerebellum, cerebrum (2%)
@ Other sites (10%): eg, intrarenal (very rare)
@ Unknown (10%)

√ large suprarenal mass with irregular shape + margins (82%):
√ displacement of kidney
√ inseparable from kidney ± invasion of kidney (10–32%) along the vascular pathways
√ propensity for extension into spinal canal through neural foramen with erosion of pedicles (15%)
√ extension across midline (55%) (DDx: Wilms tumor)
√ stippled / coarse calcifications frequent

√ retroperitoneal adenopathy / contiguous extension (73%)
√ retrocrural adenopathy (27%)
√ encasement of IVC + aorta, celiac axis, SMA (32%):
N.B.: caval involvement = indicator of unresectability
√ liver metastases (18–66%); invasion of liver (5%)

IVP:
√ "drooping lily" sign = displacement of kidney inferolaterally without distortion of collecting system
√ hydronephrosis (24%)
√ calcifications in 36–50% on KUB

CT:
√ heterogeneous texture with low-density areas from hemorrhage + necrosis (55%)
√ calcifications in up to 85%

MR:
√ hyperintense heterogenous mass on T2WI

Angio:
√ hypo- / hypervascular mass

US:
√ hyperechoic poorly defined mass with acoustic shadowing (calcifications):
√ hypoechoic areas (representing necrosis + hemorrhage)

NUC:
√ focal uptake of I-131 / I-123 MIBG radioactivity (82% sensitivity; 88% specificity)
√ tracer uptake on bone scan (60%)

OB-US:
• maternal symptoms of catecholamine excess
√ mixed cystic + solid mass in adrenal region
√ may exhibit acoustic shadowing (calcifications)
√ hydrops fetalis (severe anemia secondary to metastases to bone marrow, mechanical compression of IVC, hypersecretion of aldosterone)
√ polyhydramnios

2-year survival rate versus age at presentation:
60% if patient's age <1 year
20% if patient's age 1–2 years
10% if patient's age >2 years
◊ May revert to benign ganglioneuroma in 0.2%!

Survival rate versus stage:
80% for stage I
60% for stage II
30% for stage III
7% for stage IV
75–87% for stage IVs

DDx: exophytic Wilms tumor, mesoblastic nephroma, multicystic kidney, retroperitoneal teratoma, adrenal hemorrhage, hepatic hamartoma / hemangioma, infradiaphragmatic sequestration

NEUROGENIC BLADDER

Neuroanatomy: bladder innervation of detrusor muscle by parasympathetic nerves S2–S4

Etiology: congenital (myelomeningocele); trauma; neoplasm (spinal, CNS); infection (herpes, polio); inflammation (multiple sclerosis, syrinx); systemic disorder (diabetes, pernicious anemia)

A. SPASTIC BLADDER
"upper motor neuron" lesion above conus

B. ATONIC BLADDER
"lower motor neuron lesion" below conus

ONCOCYTOMA

= PROXIMAL TUBULAR ADENOMA = BENIGN OXYPHILIC ADENOMA

Prevalence: 1–2–13% of renal tumors

Age: median age around 65 (range of 26–94) years; M:F = 1.6:1 to 2.5:1

Path: well-encapsulated tan-colored tumor of well-differentiated proximal tubular cells (benign adenoma) + oncocytes

Histo: oncocytes = large epithelial cells with granular oxyphilic / eosinophilic cytoplasm (due to large number of mitochondria); no clear cytoplasm; similar oncocytic tumors seen in thyroid, parathyroid, salivary glands, adrenals

• majority asymptomatic, occasionally hypertension
√ renal mass of 6–7.5 cm average size (0.1–26 cm)
√ tumor of homogeneous low attenuation / hypoechogenicity (>50%)
√ well-demarcated with pseudocapsule
√ central stellate scar in 30% (in lesions >3 cm in diameter due to organization of central infarction + hemorrhage after tumor growth has outstripped blood supply)
√ invasion of renal capsule / renal vein in large tumors

Angio:
  √ spoke-wheel configuration (80%), homogeneously dense parenchymal phase (71%)
  √ NO contrast puddling / arteriovenous shunting / renal vein invasion

NUC:
  √ photopenic area (tubular cells do not function normally) on Tc-99m DMSA

Dx: percutaneous needle biopsy unreliable
◊ Pathologic diagnosis requires entire tumor because well-differentiated renal cell carcinoma may have oncocytic features!

Rx: local resection / heminephrectomy

Prognosis: death from malignancy following surgery (3%)

ORCHITIS

• unusual without epididymitis

Etiology:
(a) bacterial infection
(b) viral infection
  — complication of mumps in 20%: in adolescents + young adults; usually developing 4–5 days later; unilateral involvement in >90%; parotitis precedes orchitis in 84%, simultaneous in 3%, later in 4%; without parotitis in 10%
  — Coxsackie virus

√ increased testicular blood flow
√ ± enlargement of testis
√ ± hydrocele + thickening of scrotal wall

DDx: neoplasm (mimicked by focal orchitis)

OSSIFYING RENAL TUMOR OF INFANCY

= rare benign renal mass originating from urothelium

Incidence: only 11 cases in literature
Age: 6 days – 14 months; M > F
Histo: osteoid core, osteoblasts, spindle cells

• hematuria

Location: L > R kidney
Site: upper pole

√ 2–3-cm polypoid mass:
  √ calcified (in 80%)
  √ filling defect of collecting system
  √ partial obstruction of collecting system
√ echogenic mass + shadowing
√ poor enhancement on CT

DDx: staghorn calculus

PAGE KIDNEY

= renin-angiotensin–mediated hypertension caused by reduction of blood flow to kidney secondary to renal compression in a perinephric / subcapsular location

Etiology:
(1) Spontaneous hematoma (most common)
(2) Blunt trauma with chronic contained subcapsular hematoma / perirenal scarring
(3) Cyst
(4) Tumor

√ stretching + splaying of intrarenal vessels
√ slow arterial washout
√ distortion of renal contour + thinning of renal parenchyma
√ enlarged + displaced capsular artery

PAPILLARY NECROSIS

= NECROTIZING PAPILLITIS
= ischemic necrobiosis of medulla (loops of Henle + vasa recta) secondary to interstitial nephritis (interstitial edema) or intrinsic vascular obstruction

Cause:
mnemonic: "POSTCARD"
Pyelonephritis
Obstructive uropathy
Sickle cell disease
Tuberculosis, **T**rauma
Cirrhosis = alcoholism, **C**oagulopathy
Analgesic nephropathy
Renal vein thrombosis
Diabetes mellitus (50%)
also: dehydration, severe infantile diarrhea, hemophilia, Christmas disease, acute tubular necrosis, transplant rejection, postpartum state, high-dose urography, intravesical instillation of formalin, thyroid cancer

Types:
1. Necrosis in situ = necrotic papilla detaches but remains unextruded within its bed
2. Medullary type (partial papillary slough) = single irregular cavity located concentric / eccentric in papilla with long axis paralleling the long axis of the papilla + communicating with calyx
3. Papillary type (total papillary slough)

Phases:
(1) Enlargement of papilla (papillary swelling)
(2) Fine projections of contrast material alongside papilla (tract formation)
(3) Medullary cavitation / complete slough of papilla

• flank pain, dysuria, fever, chills
• ureteral colic
• acute oliguric renal failure
• hypertension
• proteinuria, pyuria, hematuria, leukocytosis

Location: (a) localized / diffuse
(b) bilateral distribution (systemic cause)
(c) unilateral (obstruction, renal vein thrombosis, acute bacterial nephritis)

√ normal or small kidney (analgesic nephropathy) / large kidney (acute fulminant)
√ smooth / wavy renal contour (analgesic nephropathy)
√ calcification of necrotic papilla: papillary / curvilinear / ringlike

IVP:
- √ subtle streak of contrast material extending from fornix parallel to long axis of papilla
- √ centric / eccentric, thin and short / bulbous cavitation of papilla
- √ widened fornix (necrotic shrinkage of papilla)
- √ ring shadow of papilla (outlining detached papilla within contrast material-filled cavity)
- √ club-shaped / saccular calyx (sloughed papilla)
- √ intraluminal nonopaque filling defect (sloughed papilla) in calyx / pelvis / ureter
- √ diminished density of contrast material in nephrogram; rarely increasingly dense
- √ wasted parenchymal thickness
- √ displaced collecting system (enlarged septal cortex from edema)

US:
- √ multiple round / triangular cystic spaces in medulla with echo reflections of arcuate arteries at periphery of cystic spaces

Cx: higher incidence of transitional cell carcinoma in analgesic abusers (8 x); higher incidence of squamous cell carcinoma

DDx:
(1) Postobstructive renal atrophy
(2) Congenital megacalices (normal renal function)
(3) Hydronephrosis (dilated infundibula)

PAROXYSMAL NOCTURNAL HEMOGLOBINURIA

= rare acquired disorder of nonmalignant hematopoietic stem cells

Cause: infection, transfusion, radiographic contrast material, exercise, drugs, immunization, surgery

Pathophysiology:
destruction of abnormally sensitive RBCs + granulocytes + platelets by activated complement; complement activation of abnormal platelets + release of thrombogenic material from lysed RBCs

- increased susceptibility to infections
- intravascular hemolysis:
  - hemoglobinuria
  - pancytopenia / aplasia
  - chronic iron deficiency anemia
- venous thrombosis in uncommon sites:
  - cerebral vein thrombosis
  - acute (tubulointerstitial nephritis) / chronic renal failure (small vessel thrombosis)
  - mesenteric + splenic vein thrombosis
  - hepatic vein thrombosis (= Budd-Chiari syndrome) involving tertiary + secondary venous radicles
  - portal vein thrombosis

MR:
- √ low signal intensity of renal cortex on T1WI + T2WI due to hemosiderin deposition in proximal convoluted tubules (secondary to intravascular hemolysis)
- √ usually decreased iron concentration in liver + spleen unless transfusions were given (DDx to other hemolytic anemias)

Prognosis: venous thrombosis is a major cause of death

PHEOCHROMOCYTOMA

= ADRENAL PARAGANGLIOMA

= rare catecholamine-secreting tumor of chromaffin tissue; responsible for 0.1% of hypertensions

Incidence: 0.13% in autopsy series; sporadic occurrence in 94%

Origin: neuroectodermal tissue

Histo: chromaffin tumor cells contain chromagranin within secretory granules, tumor tends to form "Zellballen" (cell balls)

Age: 5% in childhood

- symptomatology secondary to excess catecholamine production (norepinephrine / epinephrine):
  - asymptomatic (9%)
  - headaches, sweating, flushing, palpitations, tachycardia, anxiety, tremor
  - nausea, vomiting, abdominal pain, chest pain
  - paroxysmal (47%) / sustained (37%) hypertension
    (a) elevated catecholamine
    (b) functional renal vasoconstriction
    (c) renal artery stenosis (fibrosis, intimal proliferation, tumor encasement)
  - hypoglycemia during hypertensive crisis
  - elevated urine vanillylmandelic acid (VMA) in 54%; in up to 22% false-negative result because VMA not excreted

◊ Most common cause of spontaneous retroperitoneal hemorrhage from a primary adrenal tumor!

Associated with heritable conditions (10%):
√ usually with bilateral pheochromocytomas

(1) Multiple endocrine neoplasia (MEN) in 6%:
- pheochromocytoma asymptomatic in 50%

(a) Sipple syndrome = MEN type II (= type 2A)
= medullary carcinoma of thyroid + parathyroid adenoma + pheochromocytoma
(b) Mucosal neuroma syndrome = MEN type III (= type IIB)
= medullary carcinoma of thyroid + intestinal ganglioneuromatosis + pheochromocytoma

(2) Neuroectodermal disorder
(a) tuberous sclerosis
(b) von Hippel-Lindau disease
(c) neurofibromatosis

(3) Familial pheochromocytosis
(4) Carney syndrome

mnemonic: "VEIN"
Von Hippel-Lindau
Endocrine neoplasia (MEA 2)
Inherited (congenital pheochromocytoma)
Neurofibromatosis

Location: anywhere in sympathetic nervous system from neck to sacrum; subdiaphragmatic in 98%
(a) adrenal medulla (85–90%) = **pheochromocytoma**
(b) extraadrenal (10–15% in adults, 31% in children) = **paraganglioma**:
paraaortic sympathetic chain (8%), organ of Zuckerkandl at origin of inferior mesenteric artery (2–5%), gonads, urinary bladder (1%)

GU

Multiplicity: 10% in nonfamilial adult cases
32% in nonfamilial childhood cases
65% in familial syndromes

RULE OF TENS ("ten-percent tumor"):
10% bilateral / multiple **10%** extraadrenal
10% malignant **10%** familial

√ discrete round / oval mass with a mean size of 5 cm (range 3–12 cm)
√ calcifications in 10%

CT (93–100% sensitive):
Localization accurate in 91% with tumor >2 cm in size; up to 40% in extraadrenal location are missed by CT
√ solid / cystic / complex mass with low-density areas secondary to hemorrhage / necrosis
√ marked contrast enhancement
◊ IV injection of iodinated contrast material may precipitate hypertensive crisis in patients not on alpha-adrenergic blockers!

NUC: I-131 / I-123 MIBG (metaiodobenzylguanidine) scan (80–90% sensitive; 98% specific):
Useful:
(a) with clear clinical / laboratory evidence of tumor but no adrenal abnormality on CT / MRI
(b) in detecting extraadrenal pheochromocytomas by whole-body scintigraphy

US:
√ well-marginated purely solid (68%) / complex (16%) / cystic tumor (16%)
√ homo- (46%) / heterogeneously (54%) solid tumor: isoechoic + hypoechoic (77%) / hyperechoic (23%) to renal parenchyma

MRI:
√ iso- / slightly hypointense to liver on T1WI
√ extremely hyperintense on T2WI (60%) due to intratumoral cystic regions
√ contains areas of decreased signal intensity in 35%
√ rapid marked homo- / inhomogeneous enhancement

Angio:
N.B.: intraarterial injection CONTRAINDICATED (induces hypertensive crisis)
√ localization by aortography in >91%
√ usually hypervascular lesion with intense tumor blush
√ slow washout of contrast material
√ enlarged feeding arteries + neovascularity ("spoke-wheel" pattern)
√ parasitization from intrarenal perforating branches
√ venous blood sampling (at different levels in IVC)

Cx: (1) malignancy in 2–14% with metastases (may be hormonally active) to bone, lymph nodes, liver, lung
(2) Spontaneous retroperitoneal hemorrhage (was lethal in 50% if tumor previously undiagnosed)

Rx: (1) Surgical removal curative
(2) Alpha-adrenergic blocker (phenoxybenzamine / phentolamine)
(3) Beta-adrenergic blocker (propranolol)
(4) I-131 MIBG used to treat metastases

DDx: nonfunctioning adrenal adenoma, adrenocortical carcinoma, adrenal cyst

PLASMACYTOMA OF KIDNEY

= group of malignant disorders involving differentiated B lymphocytes or plasma cells

Classification:
(a) solitary = plasmacytoma (5%)
(b) multiple = multiple myeloma (95%): involvement of kidney in 17% at autopsy

Distribution of primary extramedullary plasmacytoma:
(a) skeleton (95%)
(b) nonskeletal sites (5%): upper respiratory tract

• monoclonal immunoglobulin / Bence Jones proteinuria
√ well-circumscribed mass / infiltrative lesion

DDx: indistinguishable from other renal primaries

POLYCYSTIC KIDNEY DISEASE

Autosomal Dominant Polycystic Kidney Disease

= ADULT POLYCYSTIC KIDNEY DISEASE = ADPKD
= Potter type III
= slowly progressive disease with nearly 100% penetrance and great variation in expressivity

Cause: gene located on short arm of chromosome 16 (in 90%); spontaneous mutation in 10%

Incidence: 1:1,000 people carry the mutant gene; 3rd most prevalent cause of chronic renal failure

Risk of recurrence: 50%

Histo: abnormal rate of tubule divisions (Potter type III) with hypoplasia of portions of tubules left behind as the ureteral bud advances; cystic dilatation of Bowman capsule, loop of Henle, proximal convoluted tubule, coexisting with normal tissue

Mean age at diagnosis:
43 years (neonatal / infantile onset has been reported); M:F = 1:1
Onset of cyst formation:
— 54% in 1st decade
— 72% in 2nd decade
— 86% in 3rd decade
morphologic evidence in all patients by age 80

Associated with:
(1) Cysts in: liver (25–50–80%), pancreas (9%); rare in lung, spleen, thyroid, ovaries, uterus, testis, seminal vesicles, epididymis, bladder
(2) Aneurysm: saccular "berry" aneurysm of cerebral arteries (3–13%), aortic aneurysm
(3) Mitral valve prolapse
(4) Colonic diverticulosis
◊ Consider ADPKD a systemic disease due to a generalized collagen defect!

• symptomatic at mean age of 35 years (cysts are growing with age)
• hypertension (50–70%)
• azotemia
• hematuria, proteinuria
• lumbar / abdominal pain

√ bilaterally large kidneys with multifocal round lesions; unilateral enlargement may be the first manifestation of the disease

√ cysts may calcify in curvilinear rim- / ringlike irregular amorphous fashion
√ elongated + distorted + attenuated collecting system
√ nodular puddling of contrast material on delayed images
√ "Swiss cheese" nephrogram = multiple lesions of varying size with smooth margins
√ polycystic kidneys shrink after beginning of renal failure, after renal transplantation, or on chronic hemodialysis

NUC: poor renal function on Tc-99m DTPA scan
√ multiple areas of diminished activity, cortical activity only in areas of functioning cortex

US:
√ multiple cysts in cortical region (usually seen in 50% by 10 years of age)
√ diffusely echogenic when cysts small (children)
√ renal contour poorly demarcated

OB-US:
√ large echogenic kidneys similar to infantile PCKD (usually in 3rd trimester, earliest sonographic diagnosis at 14 weeks), can be unilateral
√ macroscopic cysts (rare)
√ normal amount of amniotic fluid / oligohydramnios (renal function usually not impaired)

Atypical rare presentation:
(a) unilateral adult PCKD
(b) segmental adult PCKD
(c) adult PCKD in utero / neonatal period

Cx:
(1) Death from uremia (59%) / cerebral hemorrhage (secondary to hypertension or ruptured aneurysm [13%]) / cardiac complications (mean age 50 years)
(2) Renal calculi (20%): mostly urate
(3) Urinary tract infection
(4) Cyst rupture
(5) Cyst hemorrhage (66%):
• common cause of acute flank pain
√ hyperattenuated cyst content on CT
√ calcifications frequent, which may take years
(6) Renal cell carcinoma (increased risk if in renal failure)

DDx:
(1) Multiple simple cysts (less diffuse, no family history)
(2) von Hippel-Lindau disease (cerebellar hemangioblastoma, retinal hemangiomas, occasionally pheochromocytomas)
(3) Acquired uremic cystic disease (kidneys small, no renal function, transplant)
(4) Infantile PCKD (usually microscopic cysts)

Autosomal Recessive Polycystic Kidney Disease

= INFANTILE POLYCYSTIC KIDNEY DISEASE = POLYCYSTIC DISEASE OF CHILDHOOD = Potter Type I

Frequency: 1: 6,000 to 1:55,000 live births; F > M; carrier frequency of 1:70

Cause: chromosomal abnormality on 6p21 (gene not yet identified) resulting in abnormal epithelium

Pathogenesis:
symmetric circumferential epithelial proliferation results in tubular lengthening + fusiform dilatation of collecting ducts; abnormal epithelium becomes secretory instead of resorptive; secreted fluid is rich in epithelial growth factors stimulating further epithelial proliferation

Path:
@ Kidney: numerous dilated + elongated collecting tubules with radial orientation extending from medulla into cortex; associated renal interstitial edema + fibrosis; increased separation of a normal number of glomeruli
• spongelike texture of renal parenchyma
• azotemia
• diminished concentrating ability of kidneys
@ Liver: **congenital hepatic fibrosis** = irregularly formed dilated nonobstructive intrahepatic bile ducts increased in number with atypical branching pattern + fibrosed portal tracts
@ Pancreas: pancreatic fibrosis

◊ The greater the percentage of abnormal collecting tubules, the more severe the renal compromise and the earlier the clinical presentation!
◊ The less severe the renal findings, the more severe the hepatic findings!

Blythe & Ockenden classification:

A. PERINATAL FORM (most common)
90% of tubules show cystic changes
• onset of renal failure in utero
• Potter sequence
√ both kidneys enlarged
√ oligohydramnios and dystocia (large abdominal mass)
Prognosis: death from renal failure / respiratory insufficiency (pulmonary hypoplasia) within 24 hours in 75%, within 1 year in 93%; uniformly fatal

B. NEONATAL FORM
60% of tubules show ectasia + minimal hepatic fibrosis + bile duct proliferation
• onset of renal failure within 1st month of life
Prognosis: death from renal failure / hypertension / left ventricular failure within 1st year of life

C. INFANTILE FORM
25% of renal tubules involved + mild / moderate periportal fibrosis
• disease appears by 3–6 months of age
Prognosis: death from chronic renal failure / systemic arterial hypertension / portal hypertension

D. JUVENILE FORM
10% of tubules involved + gross hepatic fibrosis + bile duct proliferation
• disease appears at 6 months to 5 years of age
Prognosis: death from portal hypertension

@ Abdominal radiograph
√ abdominal distension
√ gas-filled bowel loops deviated centrally
@ Lung
√ severe pulmonary hypoplasia
√ pneumothorax / pneumomediastinum
@ Liver
• portal venous hypertension (between 5 and 13 years of age)
√ tubular cystic dilatation of small intrahepatic bile ducts
√ patchy / diffuse increase in liver echogenicity
√ increased echogenicity of portal tracts
√ hepatosplenomegaly
√ enlarged splenic and portal veins
@ Kidneys
√ bilateral gross smooth renal enlargement
√ faint nephrogram + blotchy opacification on initial images
√ increasingly dense nephrogram
√ poor visualization of collecting system
√ "sunburst nephrogram" = striated nephrogram with persistent radiating opaque streaks (collecting ducts) on delayed images
√ prominent fetal lobation
√ poor opacification + contrast excretion with impaired renal function
CT:
√ kidneys low in attenuation
√ prolonged corticomedullary phase
√ striated pattern of contrast media excretion (due to contrast material in dilated tubules)
MR:
√ hyperintense renal parenchyma on T2WI
US:
√ hyperechoic enlarged kidneys (unresolved 1–2-mm cystic / ectatic dilatation of renal tubules increases the number of acoustic interfaces)
√ increased renal through-transmission (due to fluid content of cysts)
√ loss of corticomedullary differentiation, poor visualization of renal sinus + renal borders
√ thin rim of hypoechoic cortex
√ occasionally discrete macroscopic cysts <1 cm with tendency to become larger + more numerous over time (in older children resembling adult medullary sponge kidney)
√ compressed / minimally dilated collecting system
√ small bladder
OB-US (diagnostic as early as 17 weeks GA):
• decreased fetal urine output
• Potter facies: low-set + flattened ears, short + snubbed nose, deep eye creases, micrognathia
√ progressive massive renal enlargement (10–20 x larger than normal):
√ renal:abdominal circumference ratio >0.30
√ hyperechoic renal parenchyma
√ nonvisualization of urine in fetal bladder (in severe cases)
√ oligohydramnios (33%)
√ small fetal thorax with pulmonary hypoplasia
√ club foot
OB management:
(1) Chromosome studies to determine if other malformations present (eg, trisomy 13 / 18)
(2) Option of pregnancy termination <24 weeks
(3) Nonintervention for fetal distress >24 weeks if severe oligohydramnios present
Risk of recurrence: 25%
DDx: Meckel-Gruber syndrome, adult polycystic kidney disease

POSTERIOR URETHRAL VALVES

= congenital thick folds of mucous membrane located in posterior urethra (prostatic + membranous portion) distal to verumontanum
Type I: (most common) mucosal folds (vestiges of wolffian duct) extend anteroinferiorly from the caudal aspect of the verumontanum, often fusing anteriorly at a lower level
Type II: (rare) mucosal folds extend anterosuperiorly from the verumontanum toward the bladder neck (nonobstructive normal variant, probably a consequence of bladder outlet obstruction)
Type III: diaphragm-like membrane located below the verumontanum (= abnormal canalization of urogenital membrane)
Incidence: 1:5,000–8,000 boys; most common cause of urinary tract obstruction + leading cause of end-stage renal disease among boys
Time of discovery: prenatal (8%), neonatal (34%), 1st year (32%), 2nd–16th year (23%), adult (3%)
• urinary tract infection (fever, vomiting) in 36%
• obstructive symptoms in 32% (hesitancy, straining, dribbling [20%], enuresis [20%])
• palpable kidneys / bladder in neonate (21%)
• failure to thrive (13%)
• hematuria (5%)
VCUG:
√ vesicoureteral reflux, mainly on left side (in 33%)
√ fusiform distension + elongation of proximal posterior urethra persisting throughout voiding
√ transverse / curvilinear filling defect in posterior urethra
√ diminution of urethral caliber distal to severe obstruction
√ hypertrophy of bladder neck√trabeculation + sacculation of bladder wall
√ large postvoid bladder residual
US:
√ male gender
√ oligohydramnios (related to severity + duration of obstruction)
√ hypoplastic / multicystic dysplastic kidney (if early occurrence)

GU

√ bilateral hydroureteronephrosis (+ pulmonary hypoplasia)
√ dilated renal pelvis may be absent in renal dysplasia / rupture of bladder / pelviureteral atresia
√ overdistended urinary bladder (megacystis) in 30%
√ thick-walled urinary bladder + trabeculations (best seen after decompression)
√ urine leak: urinoma, urine ascites, urothorax
√ "pear / keyhole" bladder = posterior urethral dilatation (on perineal scan)
√ dilated utricle (perineal scan)

OB management:
(1) Induction of labor as soon as fetal lung maturity established if diagnosed during last 10 weeks of pregnancy
(2) Vesicoamniotic shunting may be contemplated if diagnosed remote from term (68% survivors) with good prognostic parameters of fetal urinary sodium <100 mEq/dL + chloride <90 mEq/dL + osmolality <210 mOsm/dL

Cx: (1) Neonatal urine leak (ascites, urothorax, urinoma) in 13%
(2) Neonatal pneumothorax / pneumomediastinum in 9%
(3) Prune belly syndrome
(4) Renal dysplasia (if obstruction occurs early during gestation)

Prognosis: depends upon duration of obstruction prior to corrective surgery; poor prognosis if associated with vesicoureteral reflux; nephrectomy for irreversible damage (13%)

DDx: (1) UPJ obstruction
(2) UVJ obstruction
(3) Primary megaureter
(4) Massive vesicoureteral reflux
(5) Megacystis-microcolon-intestinal hypoperistalsis syndrome

POSTINFLAMMATORY RENAL ATROPHY

= acute bacterial nephritis with irreversible ischemia as an unusual form of severe Gram-negative bacterial infection in patients with altered host resistance in spite of proper antibiotic treatment

Histo: occlusion of interlobar arteries / vasospasm
√ small smooth kidney
√ papillary necrosis in acute phase

POSTOBSTRUCTIVE RENAL ATROPHY

= generalized papillary atrophy usually following successful surgical correction of urinary tract obstruction and progressing in spite of relief of obstruction
√ small smooth kidney, usually unilateral
√ dilated calyces with effaced papillae
√ thinned cortex

PRIAPISM

= prolonged penile erection not associated with sexual arousal

Types:
(1) Low-flow form = venoocclusive form (common) characterized by ischemia, venous stasis, pooling of blood within corpora cavernosa
Cause: sickle cell disease, hematopoietic malignancy, hypercoagulable state
• painful erection
√ sluggish intracavernosal flow
√ decreased venous outflow
√ decreased arterial inflow
√ intracavernosal thrombosis
Rx: cavernosal aspiration + irrigation, anticoagulation, shunt procedure
Cx: impotence (in 50% in spite of Rx)
(2) High-flow form (rare)
characterized by unregulated arterial inflow of blood into corpora cavernosa usually due to arterial injury
Cause: perineal / penile trauma
• subsequent persistent painless erection
Color Doppler US:
√ focal blush of abnormal intracavernosal flow adjacent to cavernosal artery from arterial-sinusoidal fistula
Rx: percutaneous transcatheter embolization; arterial ligation

PROSTATE CANCER

Incidence:
8.7% in White males, 9.4% in Black males, increasing with age; less common in Asian population; 200,000 new cases in USA (1994); 2nd most common malignancy in males (after lung cancer); in 35% of men >45 years of age (autopsies)
◊ One out of 11 males will develop prostate cancer!

Risk factors: advancing age, presence of testes, cadmium exposure, animal fat intake

Histo:
nuclear anaplasia + large nucleoli in secretory cells, disturbed architecture, invasive growth
Premalignant change:
(1) Prostatic intraepithelial neoplasia (PIN)
= premalignant lesion frequently associated with invasive carcinoma next to it / elsewhere in the gland
(2) Atypical adenomatous hyperplasia = proliferation of newly formed small acini

Grading (Gleason score 2–10):
1,2,3 glands surrounded by 1 row of epithelial cells
4 absence of complete gland formation
5 sheets of malignant cells

low numbers refer to well-differentiated, high numbers to anaplastic tumors; primary predominant grade (1–5) is added to secondary less representative area with highest degree of dedifferentiation (1–5)
◊ Gleason grading is in only 80% reproducible!

• Clinical categories:
1. Latent carcinoma = usually discovered at autopsy of a patient without signs or symptoms referable to the prostate (26–73%)

2. Incidental carcinoma = discovered in 6–20% of specimens obtained during transurethral resection for clinically benign prostatic hyperplasia
3. Occult carcinoma = found at biopsy of metastatically involved bone lesion / lymph node in a patient without symptoms of prostatic disease
4. Clinical carcinoma = cancer detected by digital rectal examination based on induration / irregularity / nodule
   - digital rectal exam is 30–60% accurate for differentiating stage B from stage C disease

- **Prostate-specific antigen** (PSA = glycoprotein produced by prostatic epithelium) may be elevated
  (a) monoclonal radioimmunoassay (Hybritech®); most commonly used: normal value of 0.1–4 ng/mL
    ◊ Cancers of <1 mL usually do not elevate PSA!
    ◊ 16% of normal men have PSA >4 ng/mL
    ◊ 19% of prostate cancers have normal PSA!
    ◊ Benign conditions with PSA elevation: benign prostatic hypertrophy, prostatitis, prostatic intraepithelial neoplasia
    Confined disease (stage B and less) & PSA level:
      75% of patients with PSA of <4 ng/mL
      53% of patients with PSA of 4–10 ng/mL
      2% of patients with PSA of >30 ng/mL
  (b) polyclonal radioimmunoassay (Proscheck®, Abbott PSA®)
  (c) enzyme-linked immunosorbent assay

  PSA density = volume corrected PSA level [= prostate volume (height x width x length x 0.523) / Hybritech® PSA value]:
    >0.12 (90% sensitive, 51% specific for cancer)
    ◊ Each gram of malignant prostate tissue results in about 10 x as much PSA in the serum as its benign counterpart!

  PSA "velocity" = serial PSA evaluation
    ◊ If annual rate of PSA increase is >20% / >0.75 ng/ mL, the chances of cancer increase sharply!

Staging (American Urological Association System, modified Jewitt-Whitmore staging system):

- A No palpable lesion
  - A_1 focal well-differentiated tumor <1.5 cm
  - A_2 diffuse poorly differentiated tumor; >5% of chips from transurethral resection contain cancer
- B Palpable tumor confined to prostate
  - B_1 lesion <1.5 cm in diameter confined to one lobe
  - B_2 tumor ≥1.5 cm / involving more than one lobe
- C Localized tumor with capsular involvement
  - C_1 capsular invasion
  - C_2 capsular penetration
  - C_3 seminal vesicle involvement
- D Distant metastasis
  - D_1 involvement of pelvic lymph nodes
  - D_2 distant nodes involved
  - D_3 metastases to bone / soft tissues / organs

◊ At initial presentation >75% have stage C + D!
◊ Escape routes through prostatic capsule are: (1) apex, (2) capsular margin at neurovascular bundle posterolaterally, (3) seminal vesicles!

Staging (American Joint Committee on Cancer):

- T0 No evidence of primary tumor
- T1 Clinically inapparent nonpalpable nonvisible tumor
  - T1a <3 microscopic foci of cancer / <5% of resected tissue
  - T1b >3 microscopic foci of cancer / <5% of resected tissue
  - T1c tumor identified by needle biopsy
- T2 Tumor clinically present + confined to prostate
  - T2a tumor ≤1.5 cm, normal tissue on 3 sides
  - T2b tumor >1.5 cm / in one lobe (unilateral)
  - T2c tumor involves both lobes (bilateral)
- T3 Extension through prostatic capsule
  - T3a unilateral extracapsular extension
  - T3b bilateral extracapsular extension
  - T3c invasion of seminal vesicles
- T4 Tumor fixed / invading adjacent structures other than seminal vesicles
  - T4a invasion of bladder neck, external sphincter, rectum
  - T4b invasion of levator anus muscle and/or fixed to pelvic wall
- N Involvement of regional lymph nodes
  - N1 metastasis in a single node ≤2 cm
  - N2 metastasis in a single node >2 and <5 cm / multiple lymph nodes affected
  - N3 metastasis in a lymph node ≥5 cm
- M Distant metastasis
  - M1a nonregional lymph nodes
  - M1b bone
  - M1c other site

Staging accuracy for local / advanced disease:
  46 / 66% for US, 57 / 77% for MR
◊ Extracapsular disease is common at a tumor volume of >3.8 cm³!

Metastases to lymph nodes:
  0% in stage A_1, 3–7% in stage A_2 5% in stage B_1, 10–12% in stage B_2, 54–57% in stage C; 10% with Gleason grade ≤5, 70–93% with Gleason grade 9 / 10

Location: peripheral zone (70%), transition zone (20%), central zone (10%)

US (21% positive predictive value):
- √ hypoechoic (61%) / mixed (2%) / hyperechoic (2%) lesion; not detectable isoechoic lesion (35%)
- √ asymmetric enlargement of gland
- √ deformed contour of prostate = irregular bulge sign (75% PPV)
- √ heterogeneous texture

Size versus rate of detection:
  ≤5 mm (36%), 6–10 mm (65%), 11–15 mm (53%), 16–20 mm (84%), 21–25 mm (92%), ≥26 mm (75%)

DDx of hypoechoic lesion: external sphincter, veins, neurovascular bundle, seminal vesicle, dilated duct, small prostatic cyst, acute prostatitis, benign prostatic hyperplasia, dysplasia, sonographic artifact

MR:
- √ low-signal abnormality within the normally high-signal glandular tissue on T2WI
- √ extracapsular extension (90% specific, 15% sensitive):
  - √ obliteration of rectoprostatic angle
  - √ asymmetry of neurovascular bundle
  - √ low-signal lesion on T2WI within seminal vesicles that are normally of high-signal intensity

DDx: post-biopsy hemorrhage (low signal on T2WI + high signal on T1WI)

Prognosis: increase in tumor volume increases probability of capsular penetration, metastasis, histologic dedifferentiation

Mortality: 2.6% for White males, 4.5% for Black males; 34,000 deaths/1992

Screening recommendation (American Urological Association, American Cancer Society):
PSA level measurements + digital rectal exam annually

Rx:
(1) Watchful waiting
(2) Radical prostatectomy for disease confined to capsule + life expectancy >15 years
(3) Radiation therapy for
(a) disease confined to capsule, life expectancy <15 years
(b) disease outside capsule, no spread
(4) Hormonal therapy (orchiectomy, diethylstilbestrol, leuprolide acetate) for widely metastatic disease
(5) Cryosurgery
(6) Chemotherapy

PRUNE BELLY SYNDROME

= EAGLE-BARRETT SYNDROME
= congenital nonhereditary multisystem disorder; almost exclusively in males

TRIAD:
1. Abdominal wall muscle deficiency ("prune belly")
2. Nonobstructed markedly distended redundant ureters ± hydronephrosis and variable degree of renal dysplasia
3. Bilateral undescended testes (cryptorchidism)

Etiology:
(1) primary mesodermal arrest at 6–10 weeks GA: abundance of fibrous tissue with sparsely placed smooth muscle throughout urinary tract
(2) massive abdominal distension with pressure effects on abdominal wall musculature:
secondary to bladder outlet obstruction (10–20%) / urine ascites / intestinal perforation with ascites / cystic abdominal masses / megacystis-microcolon-intestinal hypoperistalsis syndrome causing pressure atrophy of abdominal wall muscles; bladder distension interferes with descent of testes
(3) dysgenesis of yolk sac

Incidence: 1:29,000 to 1:50,000 live births; M:F = 19:1; increased prevalence in Nigeria + Saskatchewan, Canada

Groups:
(1) Severe urethral obstruction (urethral atresia [most commonly] / valves)
Associated with:
malrotation (most common anomaly), intestinal atresia, imperforate anus, skeletal abnormalities (meningomyelocele, scoliosis, pectus carinatum / excavatum, arthrogryposis, clubfoot, dislocation of hip, lower limb hemimelia, sacral agenesis, polydactyly), CHD (VSD, pulmonary artery stenosis), Hirschsprung disease, congenital cystic adenomatoid malformation of lung
- √ bladder wall hypertrophy
- √ bilateral cystic renal dysplasia

Prognosis: in 20% death within 1 month; in 50% death within 2 years (due to renal failure ± pulmonary insufficiency)

(2) Functional abnormality of bladder emptying (more common) with no associated abnormalities
- √ large floppy urinary bladder
- √ large urachal remnant
- √ dilated posterior urethra (without obstruction)
- √ utricle
- √ vesicoureteral reflux
- √ dilated tortuous ureters + focal areas of narrowing
- √ lobulated kidneys with dilated collecting system of bizarre shape

Prognosis: chronic urinary tract problems

- • wrinkled flaccid appearance of hypotonic abdominal wall with bulging flanks (agenesis / hypoplasia of muscles in lower parts of abdominal wall ventrally + laterally):
transverse m. > rectus abdominis m. below umbilicus > internal + external oblique m. > rectus abdominis m. above umbilicus
- • bilateral cryptorchidism (ESSENTIAL COMPONENT) with increased risk for malignant degeneration
- • ± impaired renal function

@ Bladder
- √ thickened bladder wall without trabeculations (due to presence of fibrocytes + collagen)
- √ large distended urinary bladder with a capacity of 600–800 mL
- √ intramural bladder calcifications
- √ persistence of patent urachus ± calcification
- √ widely patent bladder neck
- √ laterally placed ureteric orifices

@ Urethra
- √ elongated + dilated prostatic urethra with tapering of the membranous urethra
- √ small / absent verumontanum
- √ absent / hypoplastic prostate (cause of infertility)
- √ enlarged prostatic utricle (= small epithelium-lined diverticulum representing the remnant of the fused caudal ends of the müllerian ducts)
- √ urethral obstruction (stenosis / atresia / dorsal chordae / posterior urethral valves) in 20%
- √ megalourethra (70%)
  (a) complete / fusiform megalourethra (rare)
  = complete absence / marked deficiency of corpora cavernosa + corpus spongiosum

(b) incomplete / scaphoid megalourethra (common)
= congenital absence / deficiency of corpus spongiosum with a normal glans + navicular fossa

@ Ureters
Histo: diffuse increase in connective tissue with replacement of smooth muscle
√ massively dilated tortuous elongated ureters affecting the lower third more profoundly (HALLMARK)
√ poor ureteral peristalsis (due to decrease in number of nerves + degeneration of nonmyelinated Schwann fibers)
√ alternating narrowed + dilated ureteral segments
√ vesicoureteral reflux (>70%)

@ Kidneys
√ asymmetry of renal size + lobulated contours
√ no / mild hydronephrosis
√ caliceal dilatation ± diverticula
√ renal calcifications
√ renal dysplasia with cystic dysplastic changes oligohydramnios, pulmonary hypoplasia (in severe cases due to a combination defect of ureteric bud + metanephron)

@ Lung (55%)
√ pulmonary hypoplasia
√ cystic adenomatoid malformation
Cx: respiratory infections (ineffective cough)

@ Musculoskeletal (50%)
scoliosis, pectus deformity, arthrogryposis, clubfoot, valgus foot, hemimelia, dislocation of hip, sacral agenesis, polydactyly

@ Gastrointestinal anomalies (30%)
malrotation, atresia, stenosis, volvulus, imperforate anus, Hirschsprung disease, gastroschisis

@ Cardiovascular (10%)
VSD, PDA, tetralogy of Fallot

Cx: death from chronic renal failure / urosepsis / respiratory failure
Rx: internal urethrotomy, cutaneous vesicostomy, reduction cystoplasty, ureteral reimplantation, orchidopexy at 1–2 years of age, renal transplantation after bilateral nephroureterectomy, abdominoplasty

GU

PYELOCALICEAL DIVERTICULUM

= PYELOGENIC CYST = PERICALICEAL CYST = CALICEAL DIVERTICULUM
= uroepithelium-lined pouch extending from a peripheral point of the collecting system into adjacent renal parenchyma

TYPE I (calyx):
more common; connected to caliceal cup, usually at fornix; bulbous shape; narrow connecting infundibulum of varying length; few millimeters in diameter; in polar region especially upper pole

TYPE II (pelvis):
interpolar region; communicates directly with pelvis; usually larger and rounder; neck short and not easily identified

Cause:
(1) Developmental origin from ureteral bud remnant (obstruction of peripheral aberrant "minicalyx")
(2) Acquired: reflux, infection, rupture of simple cyst / abscess, infundibular achalasia / spasm, hydrocalyx secondary to inflammatory fibrosis of an infundibulum

√ formation of single / multiple stones (50%) or milk of calcium (fluid-calcium level)
√ opacification may be delayed and remain so for prolonged period
√ mass effect on adjacent pelvicaliceal system if large enough

Cx: recurrent infection
DDx: ruptured simple nephrogenic cyst, evacuated abscess / hematoma, renal papillary necrosis, medullary sponge kidney, hydrocalyx due to infundibular narrowing from TB / crossing vessel / stone / infiltrating carcinoma

PYELONEPHRITIS

= upper urinary tract infection with pelvic + caliceal + parenchymal inflammation

◊ Society of Uroradiology recommends eliminating the terms (acute focal) bacterial nephritis, lobar nephritis, lobar nephronia, preabscess, renal cellulitis, renal phlegmon, renal carbuncle!

Acute Pyelonephritis

= episodic bacterial infection of kidney with acute inflammation, usually involving pyelocaliceal lining + renal parenchyma centrifugally along medullary rays

Risk factors:
1. Vesicoureteral reflux in children
2. Obstruction, stasis, stone in adults (5%)

Pathway of infection:
(a) ascending bacterial infection usually due to P-fimbriated E. coli (fimbriae facilitate adherence to mucosal surface): initial colonization of ureter in areas of turbulent flow leads to paralysis of ureteral smooth muscle function with dilatation + functional obstruction of collecting system
(b) vesicoureteral reflux + pyelotubular backflow: P-fimbriated E. coli not necessary for infection
(c) hematogenous spread (12–20%) with Gram-positive cocci

Path: thickened urothelium with multifocally / globally edematous kidney; radiating yellow-white stripes / wedges extending from papillary tip to cortical surface in a patchy distribution + sharply demarcated from adjacent spared parenchyma by 48–72 hours
Histo: tubulointerstitial nephritis = leukocytic migration from interstitium into lumen of tubules with destruction of tubule cells by released enzymes, bacterial invasion of interstitium by 48–72 hours

Organism: E. coli > Proteus > Klebsiella, Enterobacter, Pseudomonas
Age: most commonly 15–30 years; M << F
Prevalence: 1–2% of all pregnant women
• fever, chills, flank pain + tenderness
• leukocytosis
• pyuria, bacteriuria, positive urine culture
• ± microscopic hematuria / bacteremia
Indication for imaging in adults:
(1) diabetes
(2) analgesic abuse
(3) neuropathic bladder
(4) history of urinary tract stones
(5) atypical organism
(6) poor response to antibiotics
(7) frequent recurrences
(8) immunocompromised
(9) atypical organism (eg, proteus)

IVP (abnormal in 25%):
√ smooth normal / enlarged kidney(s), focal >> diffuse involvement of kidney
√ diminished nephrographic density (global / wedge-shaped / patchy)
√ immediate persistent dense nephrogram, rarely striated
√ nonvisualization of kidney (in severe pyelonephritis, rare)
√ "tree-barking" = mucosal striations (rare)
√ compression of collecting system (edema)
√ delayed opacification of collecting system
√ nonobstructive ureteral dilatation (rare, effect of endotoxins)

CT:
√ thickening of Gerota fascia + thickened bridging septa / stranding (= perinephric inflammation)
√ generalized renal enlargement / focal swelling
√ obliteration of renal sinus
√ thickening of walls of renal pelvis + calices
√ mild dilatation of renal pelvis + ureter
√ area of high attenuation on unenhanced scan (= hemorrhagic bacterial nephritis)

CECT (abnormal in 65–90%):
√ hypoattenuating (80–90 HU) wedge-shaped area of cortex extending from papilla to renal capsule *during nephrographic phase* (= lobar segments of hypoperfusion + edema)
√ striated nephrogram
√ poor corticomedullary differentiation
√ dense parenchymal staining on scan delayed 3–6 hours in area of earlier diminished enhancement (= functioning renal parenchyma)
√ soft-tissue filling defect in collecting system (= papillary necrosis, inflammatory debris, blood clot)
√ caliceal effacement

US (abnormal in <50%):
◊ Pyelonephritis is difficult to detect sonographically
√ swollen kidney of decreased echogenicity
√ loss of central sinus complex
√ wedge-shaped hypo- / isoechoic zones, rarely hyperechoic (due to hemorrhage)
√ thickened sonolucent corticomedullary bands
√ blurred corticomedullary junctions
√ localized increase in size + echogenicity of perinephric fat ± fat within renal sinus
√ localized perinephric exudate
√ thickening of wall of renal pelvis
√ focally decreased blood flow on power Doppler

MR:
√ wedge-shaped foci of persistent increased signal intensity on contrast-enhanced fast inversion recovery / T2WI

Renal cortical scintigraphy (Tc-99m DMSA):
√ focal areas of diminished uptake (in 90%)

Prognosis:
(1) Quick response to antibiotic treatment will leave no scars
(2) Delayed treatment of acute pyelonephritis during first 3 years of life can severely affect renal function later in life: decreased renal function, hypertension (33%), end-stage renal disease (10%)

Cx: (1) Renal abscess (near-water density lesion without enhancement)
(2) Scarring of affected renal lobes often in children + in up to 43% in adults
(3) Maternal septic shock (3%)
(4) Premature labor (17%)

Acute Focal Pyelonephritis

= LOBAR NEPHRONIA = ACUTE FOCAL BACTERIAL NEPHRITIS = CARBUNCLE = RENAL CELLULITIS = RENAL PHLEGMON
= focal variant of acute pyelonephritis with single / multiple areas of suppuration + necrosis
Organism: E. coli > Proteus > Klebsiella
Predisposed: patients with altered host resistance (diabetes [60%], immunosuppression), chronic catheterization, mechanical / functional obstruction, trauma
• fever, flank pain, pyuria
Site: usually involves entire renal lobe
√ Ga-67 uptake
√ vesicoureteral reflux often present

IVP:
√ focal area of absent nephrogram / distorted pyelogram

US:
√ hypoechoic mass with ill-defined margins and disruption of corticomedullary border
√ NOT a fluid collection

CT:
√ hypoattenuating zone with poorly defined transition to surrounding parenchyma
√ less than normal parenchymal enhancement

Angio:
√ renal arteries displaced, renal veins compressed

DDx: abscess (no enhancement on CT)
Cx: scarring, abscess

GU

Emphysematous Pyelitis

= gas confined to renal pelvis + calyces

Organism: E. coli

Predisposed: diabetes mellitus (50%); M:F = 1:3

May be associated with: emphysematous cystitis (rare)

• pyuria

√ gas pyelogram outlining pelvicaliceal system

√ dilated renal collecting system (frequent)

√ ± gas in ureters

DDx: reflux of gas / air from bladder or urinary diversion

Emphysematous Pyelonephritis

= life-threatening acute fulminant necrotizing infection of kidney and perirenal tissues associated with gas formation

Organism: E. coli (68%), Klebsiella pneumoniae (9%), Proteus mirabilis, Pseudomonas, Enterobacter, Candida, Clostridia (exceptionally rare)

Path: acute and chronic necrotizing pyelonephritis with multiple cortical abscesses

Mechanism: pyelonephritis leads to ischemia + low O_2 tension with anaerobic metabolism; facultative anaerobe organisms form CO_2 with fermentation of necrotic tissue / tissue glucose

Predisposed: immunocompromised patients, esp. diabetics (in 87–97% of cases); ureteral obstruction (in 20–40%)

Average age: 54 years; M:F = 1:2

May be associated with: XGP

• features of acute severe pyelonephritis (chills, fever, flank pain, lethargy, confusion) not responding to Rx

• positive blood + urine cultures (in majority)

• urosepsis, shock

• fever of unknown origin + NO localizing signs in 18%

• multiple associated medical problems: uncontrolled hyperglycemia, acidosis, dehydration, electrolyte imbalance

Location: in 5–7% bilateral

Type I (33%):

√ streaky / mottled gas in interstitium of renal parenchyma radiating from medulla to cortex

√ crescent of subcapsular / perinephric gas

√ NO fluid collection (= no effective immune response)

Prognosis: 69% mortality

Type II (66%):

√ bubbly / loculated intrarenal gas (infers presence of abscess)

√ renal / perirenal fluid collection

√ gas within collecting system (85%)

Prognosis: 18% mortality

√ parenchymal destruction

√ absent / decreased contrast excretion (due to compromised renal function)

US:

√ high-amplitude echoes within renal sinus / renal parenchyma associated with "dirty" shadowing / "comet tail" reverberations

CAVE: (1) kidney may be completely obscured by large amount of gas in perinephric space (DDx: surrounding bowel gas)

(2) gas may be confused with renal calculi

CT (most reliable + sensitive modality):

√ mottled areas of low attenuation extending radially along the pyramids

√ extensive involvement of kidney + perinephric space

√ air extending through Gerota's fascia into retroperitoneal space

√ occasionally gas in renal veins

MR:

√ signal void on T1WI + T2WI (DDx: renal calculi, rapidly flowing blood)

Mortality: 60–75% under antibiotic Rx; 21–29% after antibiotic Rx + nephrectomy; 80% with extension into perirenal space

Rx: antibiotic therapy + nephrectomy; drainage procedure with coexisting obstruction

DDx: emphysematous pyelitis (gas in collecting system but not in parenchyma, diabetes in 50%, less grave prognosis)

Fungal Pyelonephritis

Organism: Candida, Aspergillus, Mucor, Coccidioides, Cryptococcus, Actinomyces, Nocardia, Torulopsis

At risk: diabetes, drug addiction, leukemia, immunosuppression, debilitation

√ pyelonephritis, papillary necrosis, renal abscess

√ fungus ball

Xanthogranulomatous Pyelonephritis

= chronic suppurative granulomatous infection in chronic renal obstruction (calculus, stricture, carcinoma) arising from an abnormal host response to bacterial infection

Incidence: 681,000 surgically proven cases of chronic pyelonephritis

Organism: Proteus mirabilis, E. coli, S. aureus

Path: replacement of corticomedullary junction with soft yellow nodules; calyces filled with pus and debris

Histo: diffuse infiltration by plasma cells + histiocytes + lipid-laden macrophages (xanthoma cells)

Pathophysiology: infection of renal pelvis, which the host is unable to eradicate; macrophages become enlarged with undigested bacteria gradually replacing the renal parenchyma + perinephric space

Peak age: 45–65 years; all ages affected, may occur in infants; M:F = 1:3–1:4

• pyuria (95%)

• flank pain (80%)

• fever (70%)

• palpable mass (50%)

• weight loss (50%)

• microscopic hematuria (50%)

- elevated ESR
- reversible elevated liver function tests (50%) caused by inflammation in portal triads

◊ Symptomatic for 6 months prior to diagnosis in 40%!

A. DIFFUSE XGP (83–90%)
B. SEGMENTAL / FOCAL XGP (10–17%)
 = tumefactive form due to obstructed single infundibulum / one moiety of duplex system
 DDx: renal cell carcinoma

√ kidney globally enlarged (smooth contour uncommon) / focal renal mass (less frequent)
√ contracted pelvis with dilated calyces
√ totally absent / focally absent nephrogram (80%)
√ centrally obstructing calculus:
 √ staghorn calculus in 75%
√ extension of inflammation into perirenal space, pararenal space, ipsilateral psoas muscle, colon, spleen, diaphragm, posterior abdominal wall, skin

Retrograde:
 √ complete obstruction at ureteropelvic junction / infundibulum / proximal ureter
 √ contracted renal pelvis, dilated deformed calyces + nodular filling defects
 √ irregular parenchymal masses with cavitation

CT:
 √ low-attenuation fatty masses replacing renal parenchyma (= replacement fibrolipomatosis with attenuation values of less than water)

US:
 √ hypoechoic dilated calyces with echogenic rim
 √ hypoechoic masses frequently with low-level internal echoes replacing renal parenchyma
 √ loss of corticomedullary junction
 √ parenchymal calcifications are uncommon

Angio:
 √ stretching of segmental / interlobar arteries around large avascular masses
 √ hypervascularity / blush around periphery of masses in late arterial phase (= granulation tissue)
 √ venous encasement + occlusion

DDx: hydronephrosis, avascular tumor
Rx: nephrectomy

PYELOURETERITIS CYSTICA

= hyperplastic transitional epithelial cell collections projecting into ureteral lumen

◊ Indicative of past / present urinary tract infection!

Cause: chronic urinary tract irritant (stone / infection)
Histo: numerous small submucosal epithelial-lined cysts representing cystic degeneration of epithelial cell nests within lamina propria (cell nests of von Brunn) formed by downward proliferation of buds of surface epithelium that have become detached from the mucosa
Organism: E. coli > M. tuberculosis, Enterococcus, Proteus, schistosomiasis
Predisposed: diabetics
Age: 6th decade; more prevalent in women

- no specific symptoms; ± hematuria

Location: bladder >> proximal 1/3 of ureter > ureteropelvic junction; unilateral >> bilateral

√ multiple small round smooth lucent filling defects of 1–3 mm in size; scattered discrete / clustered
√ persist unchanged for years in spite of antibiotic therapy

Cx: increased incidence of transitional cell carcinoma
DDx:
(1) Spreading / multifocal TCC
(2) Vascular ureteral notching
(3) Multiple blood clots
(4) Multiple polyps
(5) Allergic urticaria of mucosa
(6) Submucosal hemorrhage (eg, anticoagulation)

PYONEPHROSIS

= presence of pus in dilated collecting system (= infected hydronephrosis)

Path: purulent exudate composed of sloughed urothelium + inflammatory cells from early formation of microabscesses + necrotizing papillitis
Organism: most commonly E. coli

US:
 √ dispersed / dependent internal echoes within dilated pelvicaliceal system
 √ shifting urine-debris level
 √ dense peripheral echoes in nondependent location + shadowing (gas from infection)

Cx:
(1) Renal microabscesses + necrotizing papillitis
(2) XGP
(3) Renal / perinephric abscess
(4) Fistula to duodenum, colon, pleura

RADIATION NEPHRITIS

Histo: interstitial fibrosis, tubule atrophy, glomerular sclerosis, sclerosis of arteries of all sizes, hyalinization of afferent arterioles, thickening of renal capsule

Threshold dose: 2,300 rads over 5 weeks

- clinically resembling chronic glomerulonephritis

√ normal / small smooth kidney consistent with radiation field
√ parenchymal thickness diminished (globally / focally; related to radiation field)
√ diminished nephrographic density

REFLUX ATROPHY

Cause: increased hydrostatic pressure of pelvicaliceal urine with atrophy of nephrons secondary to long-standing vesicoureteral reflux

√ small smooth kidney with loss of parenchymal thickness
√ widened collecting system with effaced papillae
√ longitudinal striations from redundant mucosa when collecting system is collapsed

◊ Do NOT confuse with reflux nephropathy!

REFLUX NEPHROPATHY

= CHRONIC ATROPHIC PYELONEPHRITIS
= ascending bacterial urinary tract infection secondary to reflux of infected urine from lower tract + tubulointerstitial inflammation in childhood (hardly ever endangers adult kidney); most common cause of small scarred kidney

Etiology: 3 essential elements:
(1) Infected urine
(2) Vesicoureteral reflux
(3) Intrarenal reflux

Age: usually young adults (subclinical diagnosis starting in childhood); M < F

- fever, flank pain, frequency, dysuria
- hypertension, renal failure
- may have no history of significant symptoms

Site: predominantly affecting poles of kidneys secondary to presence of compound calyces having distorted papillary ducts of Bellini (= papillae with gaping openings instead of slitlike openings of interpolar papillae)

√ normal / small kidney; uni- / bilateral; uni- / multifocal
√ focal parenchymal thinning with contour depression in upper / lower pole (more compound papillae in upper pole), scar formation only up to age 4
√ retracted papilla with clubbed calyx subjacent to scar
√ contralateral / focal compensatory hypertrophy (= renal pseudotumor)
√ dilated ureters (secondary to reflux) sometimes with linear striations (redundant / edematous mucosa)

US:
√ focally increased echogenicity within cortex (scar)

Angio:
√ small tortuous intrarenal arteries, pruning of intrarenal vessels
√ vascular stenoses, occlusion, aneurysms
√ inhomogeneous nephrographic phase

NUC (Tc-99m glucoheptonate / DMSA with SPECT most sensitive method):
√ focal / multifocal photon-deficient areas

Cx: (1) Hypertension
(2) Obstetric complications
(3) Renal failure

RENAL / PERIRENAL ABSCESS

= usually complication of renal inflammation with liquefactive necrosis; 2% of all renal masses

Pathway of infection:
(a) ascending (80%): associated with obstruction (UPJ, ureter, calculus)
Organism: E. coli, Proteus
(b) hematogenous (20%): infection from skin, teeth, lung, tonsils, endocarditis, intravenous drug abuse
Organism: staphylococcus aureus

Predisposed: diabetics (twice as frequent compared with nondiabetics)

- positive urine culture in 33%
- positive blood culture in 50%
- pyuria, hematuria (absent if abscess isolated within parenchyma)

Renal Abscess

- may have negative urine analysis / culture (in up to 20%)

IVP:
√ focal mass displacing collecting system

CT:
√ hypoattenuating irregular / sharply defined focal renal mass:
√ thick enhancing wall / pseudocapsule
√ no enhancement of center of abscess
√ ± presence of gas
√ thickened septa + Gerota fascia
√ perinephric fat obliteration

US:
√ slightly hypoechoic (early), hypo- to anechoic (late) mass with irregular margins + increased through-transmission ± septations ± microbubbles of gas

NUC (Ga-67 citrate / In-111 leukocytes):
√ hot spot

DDx: cystic renal cell carcinoma

Carbuncle

= multiple coalescent intrarenal abscesses
◊ Term should not be used in radiology reports!

Perinephric Abscess

Cause:
(1) acute pyelonephritis with extension of renal abscess through capsule
(2) from adjacent retroperitoneal infection (eg, perforation of colon cancer, psoas abscess)
(3) deep penetration from SQ abscess
(4) hematogenous spread

Predisposed: diabetics (in 30%), urolithiasis, septic emboli

Organism: in up to 30% different from abscess

◊ 14–75% of patients with perinephric abscess have diabetes mellitus!

√ loss of psoas margin / obscuration of renal contour
√ renal displacement
√ focal renal mass
√ scoliosis concave to involved side
√ respiratory immobility of kidney = renal fixation
√ occasionally gas in renal fossa
√ unilateral impaired excretion
√ pleural effusion

RENAL ADENOMA

◊ Small adenoma <3 cm should be considered a renal cell carcinoma of low metastatic potential = borderline renal cell carcinoma!

Incidence: in 7–15–23% of adults (autopsies); most common cortical lesion; increasing with age (in 10% of patients >80 years of age); increased frequency in tobacco users + patients on long-term dialysis

Age: usually >30 years; M:F = 3:1

Types:
(1) Papillary / cystadenoma (38%)
(2) Tubular adenoma (38%)

(3) Mixed type adenoma (21%)
(4) Alveolar adenoma (3%) = precursor of RCC
√ solitary in 75%, multiple in 25%
√ usually <3 cm in size; subcapsular cortical location
√ impossible to differentiate from renal cell carcinoma
Cx: premalignant / potentially malignant
Prognosis: average growth rate of 0.4 (range, 0.2–3.5) cm/year; tumors growing <0.25 cm/year rarely metastasize; tumors growing >0.6 cm/year frequently metastasize

RENAL AGENESIS

Mechanism:
(a) formation failure
= failure of ureteral bud to form
• hemitrigone = absence of ipsilateral trigone + ureteral orifice
(b) induction failure
= failure of growing ureteral bud to induce metanephric tissue
• blind-ending ureter

Unilateral Renal Agenesis

Incidence: 1:600–1,000 pregnancies; M:F = 1.8:1
Risk of recurrence: 4.5%
Often coexisting with other anomalies:
1. Genital abnormalities:
(a) in male (10–15%): hypoplasia or agenesis of testis / vas deferens, seminal vesicle cyst (Zinner syndrome)
(b) in female (25–50%): unicornuate / bicornuate / hypoplastic / absent uterus, absent / aplastic vagina
◊ 90% of women with renal agenesis have uterine anomalies
◊ 30–40% of women with uterine anomalies have renal agenesis
2. Turner syndrome, trisomy, Fanconi anemia, Laurence-Moon-Biedl syndrome

Location: L > R
√ visualization of single kidney (DDx: additional kidney in ectopic location)
√ absent adrenal gland (11%)
√ absent / rudimentary renal vessels
√ colon occupies renal fossa
√ compensatory contralateral renal hypertrophy (50%)

Bilateral Renal Agenesis

= Potter syndrome
Incidence: 1:3,000 to 1:10,000 pregnancies; M:F = 2.5:1
Risk of recurrence: <1%
• Potter's facies = low-set ears, redundant skin, parrot-beaked nose, receding chin
◊ US sensitivity is ONLY 69–73% due to decreased visualization from oligohydramnios + discoid-shaped adrenal glands simulating kidneys!
√ severe oligohydramnios (after 14 weeks MA)
√ bilateral absence of kidneys (after 12 weeks), ureters, renal arteries
√ inability to visualize renal arteries by color duplex
√ inability to visualize urine in fetal bladder (after 13 weeks) = bladder agenesis / hypoplasia; negative furosemide test (20–60 mg IV) not diagnostic (fetuses with severe IUGR may not be capable of diuresis)
√ flattened discoid shape of adrenals (due to absence of pressure by kidney)
√ bell-shaped thorax (pulmonary hypoplasia) in mid to late 3rd trimester
√ compression deformities of extremities = clubfoot, flexion contractures, joint dislocations (eg, hip)
Prognosis: stillbirths (24–38%); invariably fatal in the first days of life (pulmonary hypoplasia)
DDx: functional cause of in utero renal failure (eg, severe IUGR)

Potter Sequence

= hypoplasia of lungs, bowing of legs, broad hands, loose skin, growth retardation associated with long-standing severe oligohydramnios
Cause: renal agenesis, urethral obstruction, prolonged rupture of membranes, severe IUGR

RENAL ARTERY STENOSIS

Prevalence: 1–2–4% of hypertensive individuals; 4.3 % of autopsies; 10% of hypertensive individuals with coronary artery disease; 25% of patients with hypertension that is difficult to control; in 45% of patients with malignant hypertension; in 45% of patients with peripheral vascular disease
Cause:
1. Atherosclerosis (60–90%) mostly in proximal 2 cm of main renal artery
◊ Any of multiple renal arteries (occurring in 14–28% of the population) may be affected!
2. Fibromuscular dysplasia (10–30%)
3. Others (<10%): thromboembolic disease, arterial dissection, infrarenal aortic aneurysm, arteriovenous fistula, vasculitis (Buerger disease, Takayasu disease, polyarteritis nodosa, postradiation), neurofibromatosis, retroperitoneal fibrosis

Pathophysiology:
decreased perfusion pressure of glomeruli stimulates production of renin in juxtaglomerular apparatus + angiotensin II in kidney; renin converts circulating angiotensinogen (α_2-globulin) into angiotensin I, subsequently converted by angiotensin-converting enzyme (ACE present in vascular endothelium) into angiotensin II, which releases aldosterone; aldosterone increases salt + water retention; angiotensin II + aldosterone vasoconstrict vessels (especially intraglomerular efferent arteriole to maintain filtration pressure)
◊ ACE inhibition may impair overall renal function due to disruption of autoregulatory mechanism of GFR (with renal artery stenosis in both kidneys / solitary kidney)

Renin production stimuli:
(a) baroreceptors in the afferent glomerular arteriole sense a decreased stretching of arteriolar wall with diminished blood flow
(b) chemoreceptors of the macula densa located in first part of the distal tubule sense a decreased amount of sodium and chloride (which have been largely reabsorbed due to a low GFR)

Histo: tubular atrophy and shrinkage of glomeruli
- abdominal / flank pain
- hematuria
- oliguria, anuria
- hypertension (= renin-mediated hypertension in response to ischemia)
- low urine sodium concentration

Hemodynamic significance determined by:
(a) elevated renin levels in ipsilateral renal vein ≥1.5:1
(b) presence of collateral vessels
(c) greater than 70% stenosis with poststenotic dilatation
(d) transstenotic pressure gradient ≥40 mm Hg
(e) decrease in renal size
◊ 15–20% of patients remain hypertensive after restoration of normal renal blood flow (= renal artery stenosis without renovascular hypertension)!

Patient selection criteria for screening test:
Prevalence of renovascular hypertension: 20–30%
1. Hypertension + epigastric / flank bruit
2. Accelerated / malignant hypertension
3. Unilateral small kidney
4. Severe hypertension in patients <25 years of age or >50 years of age
5. Recent-onset / worsening of hypertension with diastolic pressure ≥105 mm Hg
6. Hypertension + unexplained impairment of renal function
7. Sudden worsening of long-standing well-controlled hypertension
8. Hypertension refractory to an appropriate 3-drug regimen
9. Impairment of renal function after treatment with ACE inhibitor
10. Generalized vascular disease + hypertension

√ normal / decreased renal size (R 2 cm < L; L 1.5 cm < R) with smooth contour
√ vascular calcifications (aneurysm / atherosclerosis)

IVP (60% true-positive rate, 22% false-negative rate):
√ delayed appearance of contrast material (decreased glomerular filtration)
√ increased density of contrast material (increased water reabsorption)
√ delayed washout of contrast material (prolonged urine transit time)
√ lack of distension of collecting system
√ global attenuation of contrast density; urogram may be normal with adequate collateral circulation
√ notching of proximal ureter (enlargement of collateral vessels)

CT:
√ prolongation of cortical nephrographic phase + persistent corticomedullary differentiation
√ CT angiography (2–3-mm collimation, pitch ≤1.5–2.0): specificity of real-time interactive volume rendering > maximum-intensity projection > shaded-surface display

MRA (>95% sensitive, >90% specific):
√ tendency to overestimate stenosis
Limitations:
— evaluation of branch vessels
— presence of metallic stent
— detection of accessory arteries
— evaluation of small renal arteries

Angiography:
(a) conventional angiography = "gold standard" test
(b) intravenous digital subtraction angiography: does not address hemodynamic significance

NUC: ACE inhibitor scintigraphy (51–96% sensitive, 80–93% specific)

Duplex US:
(1) direct signs = visualization of renal artery stenosis
√ peak systolic velocity >150 cm/sec for angles <60° or 180 cm/sec for angles >70° (with many false positives due to suboptimal Doppler angles)
√ ratio of peak renal artery velocity to peak aortic center stream velocity >3.5 (for >60% stenosis; 0–91% sensitive, 37–97% specific)
√ poststenotic spectral broadening ± flow reversal

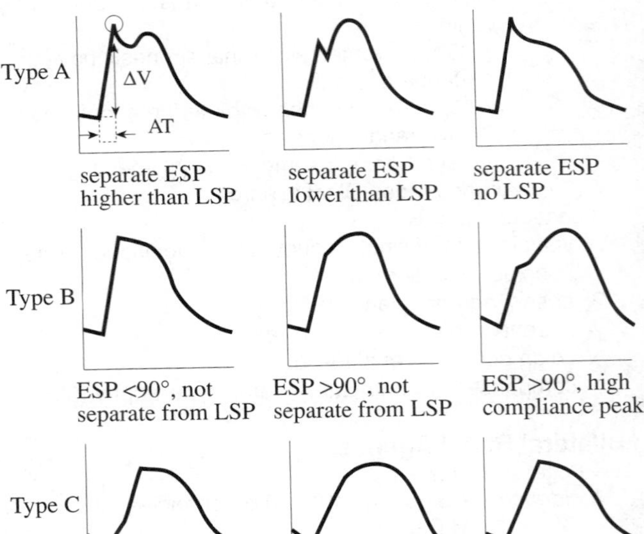

Renal Artery Doppler Waveform Patterns

Type A: early systolic peak (ESP) at the end of the early rise
Type B: no peak but rise remains straight
Type C: abnormal spectra with slowed early rise
AT = acceleration time; ΔV = velocity difference between ESP velocity and late diastolic velocity; ESP = early systolic peak; LSP = late systolic peak; acceleration index (AI) = ΔV/AT

√ absence of blood flow during diastole (for >50% stenosis)
√ no detectable Doppler signal with good visualization of renal artery (= arterial occlusion)
Problems:
(a) technically inadequate examination (gas, corpulence, respiratory motion) in 6–49%; usually limited to children + thin adults
(b) multiple renal arteries in 16–28%
(c) "false" tracings from large collateral vessels / reconstituted segments of main renal artery
(d) need to visualize entire length of renal artery
(e) transmitted cardiac / aortic pulsations obscure renal artery waveform recordings

(2) indirect signs = analysis of intrarenal arterial Doppler waveforms
(a) pattern recognition
√ dampened appearance = tardus-parvus pulse (tardus = late arrival, parvus = attenuated peak)
√ loss of early systolic peak (not necessarily abnormal!)
√ segmental arterial flow detectable with renal artery occlusion (due to collateral circulation)
(b) quantitative criteria
√ acceleration index of <370–470 cm/s^2 = $\Delta V/\Delta T$ = tangential inclination of Doppler waveform in early systole (single most sensitive screening parameter)
√ delay in acceleration / pulse rise time of >0.05–0.08 seconds = gradual slope of Doppler waveform during early systole
√ ΔRI >5% between both kidneys (82% sensitive + 92% specific for stenosis >50%, 100% sensitive + 94% specific for stenosis ≥60%)
√ RI <0.56
√ attenuated (= parvus) Doppler waveform amplitude = decrease in peak systolic velocity to <20–30 cm/s
Problems: technically inadequate examination in 0–2%

False-negative US: stenosis in accessory renal artery
False-positive US: coarctation

Results for >60% renal artery stenosis:

	Sensitivity	*Specificity*	*Accuracy*
AT ≥ 0.07 s	81%	95%	91%
AI < 300 cm/s^2	89%	86%	87%
Absent ESP	92%	96%	95%

Arteriosclerotic Renal Artery Disease

Incidence: in up to 6% of hypertensive patients; most common cause of secondary hypertension
Age: >50 years; M > F
Path: lesion primarily involving intima
• worsening of preexistent hypertension
• abrupt onset of severe hypertension >180/110 mm Hg
• vascular bruit in 40–50% (present in 20% of hypertensive patients without renal artery stenosis)

Associated with: severe arteriosclerosis of aorta, cerebral, coronary, peripheral arteries
Location: main renal artery (93%) + additional stenosis of renal artery branch (7%); bilateral in 31%
√ eccentric stenosis in proximal 2 cm of renal artery, frequently involving orifice
√ decrease in renal length over time (= high-grade renal artery stenosis with risk for occlusion)
Prognosis: progression of atherosclerotic lesion (40–45%) to renal atrophy, arterial occlusion, ischemic renal failure
Cx: azotemia with
(a) bilateral renal artery stenoses
(b) unilateral renal artery stenosis + poorly functioning contralateral kidney
◊ Reversible azotemia may be induced by treatment with angiotensin-converting enzyme inhibitors / sodium nitroprusside!
Rx: (1) Three-step antihypertensive therapy (control of hypertension difficult)
(2) Angiotensin-converting enzyme inhibitors (eg, captopril PO, enalaprilat IV)
(3) Renal artery angioplasty (80% success for nonostial lesion, 25–30% for ostial lesion)
(4) Surgical revascularization (80–90% success for any lesion location)
– hypertension improved in 66%
– improvement / stabilization of renal function in 27–80%

Fibromuscular Dysplasia of Renal Artery

Incidence: 35% of renal artery stenoses; 1,100 patients reported (by 1982) with involvement of renal artery in 60% + extracranial carotid artery in 30%; 25% of all cases of renovascular hypertension
Age: most common cause of renovascular hypertension in children + young adults <30–40 years; M:F = 1:3
Associated with: fibromuscular dysplasia of other aortic branches in 1–2%: celiac a., hepatic a., splenic a., mesenteric a., iliac a., internal carotid a.
• hypertension
• progressive renal insufficiency
Sites: mid and distal main renal artery (79%), renal artery branches (4%), combination (17%); proximal third of main renal artery spared in 98%; bilateral in 2/3; R:L = 4:1
Types:
1. Intimal fibroplasia = intimal hyperplasia
√ narrow annular radiolucent band in main renal artery + major segmental branches; often bilateral
√ poststenotic fusiform dilatation
2. Medial fibroplasia with microaneurysm
√ "string-of-beads" sign = alternating areas of stenoses + aneurysms in mid + distal renal artery + branches; usually bilateral

3. Medial / fibromuscular hyperplasia
   √ long smooth tubular narrowing of main renal artery and branches
4. Perimedial fibroplasia
   √ beading without aneurysm formation of distal (mostly right) main renal artery
5. Medial dissection
   √ false channel in main renal artery + branches
6. Adventitial fibroplasia
   √ long segmental stenosis of main renal artery + large branches

Prognosis: progression of lesions in 20% causing decline in renal function

Cx: (1) Giant aneurysm
(2) AV fistula between renal artery + vein (in medial fibroplasia)

Rx: (1) Resection of diseased segment with end-to-end anastomosis
(2) Replacement by autogenous vein graft, excision + repair by patch angioplasty
(3) Transluminal balloon angioplasty (90% success rate with very low restenosis rate)

Neurofibromatosis

Hypertension in neurofibromatosis due to:
(1) Pheochromocytoma
(2) Renal artery stenosis

◊ Renal artery involvement mainly seen in children!

Types:
(a) mesodermal dysplasia of arterial wall with fibrous transformation (common)
(b) narrowing of main renal artery by periarterial neurofibroma (rare)

√ saccular funnel-shaped aneurysm involving aorta / main renal artery
√ smooth / nodular stenosis (mural / adventitial neurofibroma) in proximal renal artery
√ intrarenal aneurysm (rare)

DDx: fibromuscular dysplasia; congenital renal artery stenosis

RENAL CELL CARCINOMA

= RCC = RENAL ADENOCARCINOMA = HYPERNEPHROMA

Incidence: 80–90% of all renal malignant primaries in adults; 2% of all visceral cancers (frequency approximates ovarian cancer, gastric cancer, pancreatic cancer, leukemia); 31,200 new RCCs in the USA diagnosed in 2000

Age: 6th–7th decade (generally >40 years); median age of 55 years; 2% occur in children in first 2 decades of life; M:F = 1.6:1; frequency increasing with age

Path: arises from proximal tubular cells; 30% found incidentally with imaging;
Tumor growth pattern:
papillary (5–15%, best prognosis); trabecular / tubular / cystic / solid (poorer prognosis)

Histo subtypes:
(a) clear cell (70–80%) = rich in cytoplasmic glycogen + lipid content, which wash away during histologic preparation
(b) papillary (10–15%)
(c) chromophobe (5%)
(d) sarcomatoid (1.5%)

Predisposed:
(1) von Hippel-Lindau syndrome (10–25%): multiple often small intracystic tumors (hemangioblastoma, retinal angioma, renal cysts) manifesting at a young age
(2) Hemodialysis (in 1.4–2.6%)
(3) Acquired cystic disease of uremia (3.3–6.1%; 7 x increased risk)
(4) Tobacco; phenacetin abuse

Staging classification:

Robson Stage	*TNM Class*	
I		tumor confined within renal capsule √ sharply defined convex interface with perirenal fat
	T1	tumor <7 cm
	T2	tumor ≥7 cm
II	T3	extension into perinephric fat but confined to Gerota fascia √ irregular interface between tumor + fat
III A		extension into renal vein or IVC
	T3b	renal vein only
	T3c	infradiaphragmatic IVC
	T4b	supradiaphragmatic IVC
III B	N	regional lymph nodes metastases
III C		extension into renal vein + lymph nodes
IV A	T4a	invasion of adjacent organs (other than ipsilateral adrenal)
IV B	M	distant metastases

Staging accuracy: 84–91% for CT
82–96% for MR
poor for US

Regional extension: into lymph nodes (9–23%); into main renal vein (21–35%); into IVC (4–10%)

Multiple RCC: commonly in von Hippel-Lindau syndrome; hereditary RCC; sporadic in 4–15%; bilateral in 1–3%

METASTASES

• bone pain, cough, hemoptysis (as initial symptoms of metastatic disease present in 9%)

◊ 28% of patients have clinically apparent multiple distant metastases at presentation!

√ tumor metastases tend to be hypervascular

Spread to:
lung (55%); lymph nodes (34%); liver (33%); bone (32%); adrenals (4.3–19%); contralateral kidney (11%); brain (6%); heart (5%); spleen (5%); bowel (4%); skin (3%); ureter (rare)

Incidence of metastatic disease:
(a) tumors <3 cm : 2.6%
(b) tumors 3–5 cm : 15.4%
(c) tumors >5 cm : 78.6%

• hematuria (56%), flank pain (36%), weight loss (27%), fever (11–15%)
• classic triad of flank pain + gross hematuria + palpable renal mass (4–9%)
• varicocele (2%)
• normochromic normocytic anemia (28–40%)
• Stauffer syndrome (15%) = nephrogenic hepatopathy = hepatosplenomegaly + abnormal liver function in absence of hepatic metastases (? tumor hepatotoxin)
• Paraneoplastic syndromes: erythrocytosis (2%); hypercalcemia (parathormone, prostaglandin, vitamin D metabolites)

√ well-marginated often lobulated solitary mass:
  √ focal bulge in renal contour
  √ enlargement of affected part of kidney
√ calcification (15–20%): usually central + amorphous or peripheral + curvilinear in cystic RCC
√ extrinsic compression / displacement / invasion of renal pelvis + calyces
√ cysts:
  (a) cystic necrotic tumor (40%)
  (b) cystadenocarcinoma (2–5%)
  (c) renal cell carcinoma in wall of cyst (3%)
√ tumor growth into renal vein / IVC (in up to 16%) conveys poor prognosis
√ infiltrative growth pattern (6%) with ill-defined margin

IVP:
  √ diminished function (parenchymal replacement, hydronephrosis)
  √ absence of contrast excretion (renal vein occlusion)
  √ pyelotumoral backflow = necrotic part of tumor fills with contrast material

NECT:
  √ homogeneous (if ≤3 cm) solid lesion of >20 HU
  √ heterogenous mass (if >3 cm) due to hemorrhage / necrosis
  √ calcifications in up to 30%
  √ perinephric fat stranding (50%) due to edema, vascular engorgement, previous inflammation, tumor invasion

CECT:
  √ mostly heterogeneous enhancement (due to cystic areas or necrosis):
    √ enhancement of >12 HU compared with NECT
  √ enhancing nodule in perinephric space (46% sensitive for perinephric spread)
  √ renal vein thrombus (92% PPV, 97% NPV):
    √ low-attenuation filling defect in corticomedullary phase (most specific sign)
    √ abrupt change in caliber of vein
    √ presence of collateral veins
    √ heterogenous enhancement of malignant thrombus
  √ ± subcapsular / perinephric hemorrhage
  √ nodal enlargement of >1 cm (4% FN) (DDx: benign inflammation as reactive immune response in >50%)

  False negatives in corticomedullary phase:
    (1) in a small tumor may enhance to the same degree as renal parenchyma
    (2) centrally located tumor mistaken for medulla

US:
  √ hyperechoic (50–61%), mostly in small tumors <3 cm (78%), occasionally in large tumors (32%):
    √ markedly hyperechoic, ie, isoechoic to renal sinus fat in 4–12% of small tumors (DDx: angiomyolipoma)
    √ anechoic rim (in 84% of small hyperechoic RCCs), probably due to pseudocapsule of compressed renal tissue (NOT seen in angiomyolipoma)
  √ isoechoic (30–86%) / hypoechoic (10–12%), mostly in larger tumors
  √ cystic lesion with increase in acoustic transmission (2–13%) due to extensive liquefaction necrosis (DDx: complicated cyst)
  √ inhomogeneity due to hemorrhage, necrosis, cystic degeneration

MRI (best modality to assess stage III + IV disease):
  √ hyper- / iso- / hypointense relative to renal parenchyma:
    √ often low to medium signal intensity on T1WI
    √ hyperintense areas usually due to hemorrhage
  √ heterogeneous signal intensity on T2WI

Angio:
  √ typically hypervascular (95%) with puddling of contrast + occasional AV shunting
  √ enlarged tortuous poorly tapering feeding vessels
  √ coarse neovascularity + formation of small aneurysms
  √ parasitization of lumbar, adrenal, subcostal, mesenteric artery branches
  √ poorly defined tumor margins

Prognosis:
  ◊ Tumor stage + histologic grade are the most important prognosticators!
  — 5-year survival rates for stages I, II, III, IV are 85–100%, 45–65%, 20–40%, 0–10%;
  — 10-year survival rates for stages I, II, III, IV are 56%, 28%, 20%, 3%
  — 4.4% 3-year survival rate if untreated
  — papillary carcinomas have a better prognosis than nonpapillary carcinomas!
  — clear cell + granular cell cancers have a better prognosis than spindle cell + anaplastic cancers

Recurrence: in 11% after 10 years

Rx:
  (1) Radical nephrectomy (2–5% operative mortality)
  (2) Nephron-sparing surgery (partial nephrectomy) with solitary functioning kidney, compromised renal function, multiple bilateral tumors, small RCC (<4 cm in diameter, polar, cortical, far from renal hilum / collecting system)

Cystic Renal Cell Carcinoma

A. UNILOCULAR CYSTIC RCC (50%)
  = extensive necrosis of a previously solid RCC / intrinsic cystic growth of a cystadenocarcinoma
  √ fluid-filled mass without criteria of a renal cyst
B. MULTILOCULAR RCC (30%)
  = intrinsic multilocular growth
  √ impossible to distinguish from multilocular cystic nephroma

C. MURAL NODULE IN CYSTIC RCC (20%)
   (a) asymmetric cystic tumor necrosis
   (b) tumor arising in wall of preexisting cyst
   (c) tubular dilatation with secondary cyst formation from tumor obstruction

Papillary Renal Cell Carcinoma

Incidence: 5–15% of all RCC
Age: 40–50 years
Path: cystic necrosis + degeneration frequent; familial form associated with trisomy 17
Histo: cells surrounding fronds of fibrovascular stroma; macrophages infiltrating the papillary stalks
√ slow growing well-encapsulated tumor
√ peripheral calcification frequent
√ usually hypovascular
√ little / no contrast enhancement
√ frequently hypoechoic mass
Prognosis: favorable (metastasize late)

Renal Cell Carcinoma in Childhood

Incidence: 7% of all primary renal tumors during first 2 decades of life;
in childhood: Wilms tumor:RCC = 30:1
in 2nd decade: Wilms tumor:RCC = 1:1
Mean age: 9 years
- palpable abdominal mass (60%)
- abdominal pain (50%)
- hematuria (30–60%)
- hypertension due to renin production
- polycythemia due to erythropoietin production
- bone resorption due to parathyroid hormone production

Increased risk of renal cell carcinoma:
von Hippel-Lindau disease in 10–25% (cerebellar hemangioblastoma, retinal angioma, pancreatic cysts + tumors, pheochromocytoma, renal cysts + tumors)
Metastases (20%): lung, bone, liver, brain

Cx: intravascular extension (25%)
Prognosis: 64% overall survival rate
DDx: Wilms tumor (younger age, larger at presentation, calcifications less frequent [9% versus 25%], less dense / homogeneous)

RENAL CYST

Simple Cortical Renal Cyst

= acquired lesion possibly secondary to tubular obstruction; accounts for 62% of all renal masses
Incidence: in 1–2% of all urograms; in 3–5% of all autopsies
Age: peak incidence after age 30 years; increasing frequency with age (in 0.22% in pediatric age group, in 50% over age 50)
Path: low cuboidal / flattened epithelium surrounded by 1–2-mm-thick fibrous wall containing clear / slightly yellow serous fluid
May be associated with: tuberous sclerosis, von Hippel-Lindau disease, Caroli disease, neurofibromatosis

√ large and unifocal when peripheral
√ focal attenuation + displacement of collecting system
√ focally replaced nephrogram with smooth margin
√ "beak / claw sign" = effaced wedge of renal parenchyma
√ delicate filamentous often undulating septa (10–15%)
√ curvilinear calcification (1%) in wall / septa

US (90–100% accuracy of US & CT):
√ spherical / ovoid in shape
√ anechoic without internal echoes
√ smooth clearly demarcated walls
√ acoustic enhancement beyond cyst

CT:
√ near-water–density lesion (<20–25 HU), thin wall, smooth interface with renal parenchyma, no enhancement

Cystography:
√ smooth wall, clear aspirate with low lactic dehydrogenase, no fat content

Cx: (1) Hemorrhage in 1–11.5%
(2) Infection in 2.5%
(3) Tumor within cyst in <1%

Atypical / Complicated Renal Cyst

A. HEMORRHAGIC CYST
Cause: trauma, varices, bleeding diathesis
- rust-colored puttylike material

√ uni- / multilocular cyst separated by thick septa
√ thick fibrous ± calcified wall
√ fibrin ball inside cyst (rare)

CT:
√ increased density secondary to acute hemorrhage / high protein contents (= hyperattenuating cyst with approximately 50–90 HU)
√ no contrast enhancement

MR:
√ usually iso- to hyperintense on T1WI (owing to methemoglobin) + hyperintense on T2WI (due to lysis of RBCs)
√ variable signal intensities (dependent on amount + acuity of hemorrhage, hemoglobin degradation product, degree of RBC lysis, protein content)
√ hematocrit effect (= RBCs settle to cyst bottom)

B. INFECTED CYST
Cause: hematogenous dissemination of bacteria, ascending urinary tract infection
Mean age: 61 years; in 94% females
- history of no response to antibiotic Rx for acute pyelonephritis
- leukocyturia

US:
√ thickened irregular cyst wall (22%)
√ internal septations (11%)
√ wall calcification (occasionally)
√ minute debris either diffusely / fluid-fluid level in dependent portion of cyst
√ amorphous solid conglomerates
√ round sharply marginated lesion

GU

Dx: cyst puncture
DDx: renal abscess, hematoma, renal artery aneurysm, cystic tumor
Rx: surgery, aspiration, serial follow-up

High-density Renal Cyst

= cyst content ≥20 HU
1. Proteinaceous content
2. Hemorrhage
3. Infection
4. Calcification
5. Communication with calyx
6. Streak artifact

◊ Considered a Bosniak Class II lesion if: ≤3 cm in size, partially exophytic, round, sharply marginated, homogeneous, nonenhancing

Renal Sinus Cyst

= PERIPELVIC / PARAPELVIC CYST = PARAPELVIC LYMPHANGIECTASIA = PARAPELVIC LYMPHATIC CYST
= spherical fluid-filled masses intimately attached to renal pelvis without connection to pelvicaliceal system arising either from renal sinus or parenchyma

Incidence: 1.5% (autopsies); 4–6% of all renal cysts
Etiology:
probably ectatic lymphatic channels from lymphatic obstruction; ? posttraumatic extravasation of urine / blood; ? protrusion of parenchymal cysts into sinus; ? mesonephric remnant; ? remnant of wolffian body; ? outpouchings of renal pelvis; ? duplication anomaly
Age: mostly during 5th–6th decade

- almost always asymptomatic
- pain (from obstructive caliectasis)
- renal vascular hypertension (compression of renal aa.)
- clear straw-colored serous fluid

√ soft-tissue density in renal sinus
√ focal displacement + smooth effacement of collecting system
√ stretching of collecting system when generalized (indistinguishable from sinus lipomatosis)

CT Features of Cystic Renal Lesions (Bosniak Classification)

I	simple cyst	well-defined round homogeneous lucent mass + thin imperceptible wall, no enhancement
II	minimally complicated cystic lesion	cluster of cysts, septated cysts, minimal curvilinear calcifications, minimally irregular wall, high-density content
III	complicated (surgical) cystic lesion	irregular thickened septa ± enhancement, coarse irregular calcification, irregular margin, multiloculated lesion, uniform wall thickening, nonenhancing nodular mass
IV	clearly malignant cystic lesion	large cystic / necrotic component, irregular wall thickening, solid enhancing elements

Differentiation of Renal Lesions

CT Feature	*Cyst*	*Neoplasm*
Shape	round, oval	irregular
Margin	smooth	lobulated
Wall	thin, not measurable	thick
Interface	sharp, distinct	indistinct
Density	0–20 HU	>30 HU
Enhancement	<10–20 HU	>10–20 HU
Vascular invasion	no	yes

√ rarely curvilinear calcification of cyst wall (4%)
US:
√ anechoic mass(es) with acoustic enhancement, irregular shape

Cx: obstructive caliectasis (rarely hydronephrosis)
Rx: cyst ablation with 95% ethanol if symptomatic
DDx: hydronephrosis

RENAL DYSGENESIS

= undifferentiated tissue of renal anlage
◊ Pathologic NOT radiologic diagnosis
√ renal vessels usually absent; occasionally small vascular channels

RENAL INFARCTION

Causes:
1. TRAUMA: blunt abdominal trauma with traumatic avulsion / occlusion of renal artery, penetrating vascular injury, surgery
2. EMBOLISM:
   (a) Cardiac: rheumatic heart disease with arrhythmia (atrial fibrillation), myocardial infarction, prosthetic valve, myocardial trauma, left atrial / mural thrombus, myocardial tumor, subacute bacterial endocarditis (septic emboli)
   (b) Catheters: angiographic catheter manipulation, transcatheter embolization, umbilical artery catheter above level of renal arteries
3. ARTERIAL THROMBOSIS:
   arteriosclerosis, aneurysm or dissection of aorta / renal artery, thrombangitis obliterans, polyarteritis nodosa, syphilitic cardiovascular disease, sickle cell disease, paraneoplastic syndrome (Trousseau syndrome), hypercoagulable state
4. VASCULITIS
   polyarteritis nodosa, SLE, drug-induced vasculitis
5. Sudden complete renal vein thrombosis

Acute Renal Infarction

- sudden onset of flank / back pain
- ± hematuria, proteinuria, fever, leukocytosis

√ normal / large kidney with smooth contour
√ normal / expanded parenchymal thickness
√ normal / attenuated collecting system, often only opacified by retrograde pyelography
√ absent / diminished nephrogram with cortical rim enhancement, rarely striations

CT:
- √ wedge-shaped area of absent enhancement
- √ edematous enlargement of kidney (with large infarct)
- √ cortical rim sign within several days after global infarction

US:
- √ diminished echogenicity (within <24 hours)
- √ normal echogenicity (echoes appear within 7 days)

NUC (SPECT imaging with Tc-99m DMSA):
- √ photon-deficient area

Rx: thrombolytic therapy, , supportive hemodialysis, transcatheter thrombembolectomy, surgery

Lobar Renal Infarction

EARLY SIGNS:
- √ focal attenuation of collecting system (tissue swelling)
- √ focally absent nephrogram (triangular with base at cortex)

LATE SIGNS:
- √ normal / small kidney(s)
- √ focally wasted parenchyma with NORMAL interpapillary line (portion of lobe / whole lobe / several adjacent lobes)

CT:
- √ nonperfused area corresponding to vascular division, cortical rim sign

US:
- √ focally increased echogenicity

Chronic Renal Infarction

Path: all elements of kidney atrophied with replacement by interstitial fibrosis
- √ normal / small kidney with smooth contour
- √ globally wasted parenchyma
- √ diminished / absent contrast material density

US:
- √ increased echogenicity (by 17 days)

Angio:
- √ normal intrarenal venous architecture
- √ late visualization of renal arteries on abdominal aortogram

Atheroembolic Renal Disease

= dislodgment of multiple atheromatous emboli from the aorta into renal circulation (below level of arcuate arteries)
- √ normal / small kidneys with smooth contour or shallow depressions
- √ wasted parenchymal thickness
- √ diminished density of contrast material

CT:
- √ patchy nephrographic distribution

Angio:
- √ embolic occlusion

Arteriosclerotic Renal Disease

= disseminated process involving most of the interlobar + arcuate arteries causing uniform shrinkage of kidney

Age: generally over 60 years

Accelerated development in: scleroderma, polyarteritis nodosa, chronic tophaceous gout

- • often associated with hypertension (**nephrosclerosis**)
- √ normal / small kidneys
- √ smooth contour with random shallow contour depressions (infarctions)
- √ uniform loss of cortical thickness
- √ normal / effaced collecting system (fat proliferation)
- √ increased pelvic radiolucency (vicarious sinus fat proliferation)
- √ calcification of medium-sized intrarenal arteries

US:
- √ increased echogenicity possible
- √ increased size of renal sinus echoes (fatty replacement)

Nephrosclerosis

Histo: thickening + hyalinization of afferent arterioles, proliferative endarteritis, necrotizing arteriolitis, necrotizing glomerulitis

- • arterial hypertension

(a) BENIGN NEPHROSCLEROSIS
(b) MALIGNANT NEPHROSCLEROSIS (rapid deterioration of renal function)

- √ radiographic appearance similar to arteriosclerotic kidney

RENAL LEIOMYOMA

= CAPSULOMA

Prevalence: 5% at autopsy (average size of 5 mm)

Median age: 42 years; M < F

Path: well-encapsulated solid mass with mean size of 12 cm containing hemorrhage (17%) / cystic degeneration (27%)

Histo: smooth muscle cells in a whorled arrangement

Location: 53% subcapsular, 37% capsular, 10% attached to renal pelvis

Associated with: tuberous sclerosis

- • palpable mass (50%), hematuria (20%)
- √ well-circumscribed exophytic solid lesion ± cleavage plane between tumor and cortex
- √ dense calcifications

Angio:
- √ hypo- to hypervascular nonspecific mass

DDx: renal leiomyosarcoma, adenocarcinoma

RENAL SARCOMA

Frequency: 1% of malignant renal parenchymal tumors

Subtypes: leiomyosarcoma (>50%), angiosarcoma, hemangiopericytoma, rhabdomyosarcoma, fibrosarcoma, osteosarcoma

- √ considerable variation in growth pattern:
  - √ expansile mass (most commonly)
  - √ infiltrative growth (rhabomyosarcoma, angiosarcoma)

Dx: by exclusion of sarcomatoid renal carcinoma + primary retroperitoneal sarcoma with direct extension into kidney

GU

RENAL TRANSPLANT

Frequency: 11,000 transplants per year in USA (1994)
Complications in 10%:
◊ Problematic period between 4 days and 3 weeks after surgery!
• hypertension in 50% (from rejection / arterial stenosis)
Prognosis: organ survival at 1 year in 80–95%; 13–24 years half-life for transplant from living related donor

Acute Tubular Necrosis in Renal Transplant

= primary nonfunction within 72 hours of transplantation followed by improvement within a few days to 1 month
◊ Most common cause of "delayed" graft function"
Cause: prolonged ischemia (cold ischemia time >24–30 hours), reperfusion injury
— ATN more frequent in cadaveric than living-related donor transplant (donor hypotension)
— ATN greater in transplants with more than one renal artery
— ATN related to length of ischemic interval (prolonged organ storage)
• no constitutional symptoms
• elevated urine sodium
• oliguria may begin immediately after transplantation / may be delayed for several days
US:
√ transient enlargement of transplant
√ transient increase in resistive index
Scintigram:
√ normal / slightly decreased transplant perfusion:
√ delayed time from T_{max} to one-half maximal activity
√ decreased + delayed radiopharmaceutical uptake:
√ delayed transit time + delayed T_{max}
√ delayed / decreased / absent excretion of Tc-99m with parenchymal retention:
√ high 20-minute to 3-minute ratio
DDx: acute rejection (serial renal studies help to differentiate)

Rejection of Renal Transplant

◊ Most common cause of parenchymal failure!
◊ Rejection occurs in all transplants to some degree!

1. **Hyperacute rejection** (rare)
= humeral rejection with preformed circulating antibodies present in recipient at time of transplantation, usually following retransplantation
Path: thrombosed arterioles + cortical necrosis
Time of onset: within minutes after transplantation
√ complete absence of renal perfusion + renal function on Tc-99m DTPA scan (DDx: complete arterial / venous occlusion)
Rx: requires immediate reoperation
2. **Accelerated acute rejection**
= combination of antibody + cell-mediated rejection
Time of onset: 2–5 days after transplantation
3. **Acute rejection**
= cellular rejection predominantly dependent on cellular immunity
Time of onset: any time, typically within 5 days to 6 months; peak incidence at 2nd–5th week
Prevalence: in 50% at least 1 episode in 1st year
Path:
(a) acute interstitial rejection
= edema of interstitium with lymphocytic infiltration of capillaries + lymphatics
(b) acute vascular rejection (rare)
= proliferative endovasculitis + vessel thrombosis
• malaise, fever, weight gain
• tenderness of transplant
• low urine sodium, increase in serum creatinine
• hypertension, oliguria
US (30–50% negative predictive value):
√ increase in renal volume from edema:
√ decreased renal sinus fat + increased cortical thickness (most predictive)
√ conspicuous pyramids + decreased cortical echogenicity
√ thickening of pelvoinfundibular wall
√ diminished echogenicity of renal sinus fat
Doppler US (higher accuracy than morphologic parameters):
√ initially <u>decrease</u> in resistive index (? autoregulatory mechanism)
√ increase in resistive index > 0.80 (with increasing severity of rejection)
(a) ≤0.70 without any form of rejection (57% negative predictive value)
(b) >0.90 (100% positive predictive value, 26% sensitivity)
√ reversal of diastolic flow
NUC:
√ may show decreased renal perfusion + renal function
√ initially perfusion may be normal with only function decreased (DDx to ATN may not be possible on single study)
√ subsequent exams (1–3-day intervals) demonstrate decreasing renal perfusion
√ prolonged excretory phase
√ poor and inhomogeneous nephrogram
Angio:
√ rapid tapering + pruning of interlobar arteries
√ multiple stenoses + occlusions
√ nonvisualization of interlobular arteries
√ prolonged arterial opacification (normally <2 s)
DDx: acute tubular necrosis (develops within first few days)
4. **Chronic rejection**
= slow relentless progressive process resulting in interstitial scarring
◊ Most common cause of late graft loss
Histo: endothelial proliferation in small arteries + arterioles; interstitial cellular infiltration + fibrosis; tubular atrophy; glomerular lesions (? recurrence of patient's original glomerulonephritis)

GU

Time of onset: months to years after transplantation
- progressive decline of renal function
- √ small kidney with thin cortex
- √ diminished number of intrarenal vessels
- √ vascular pruning / stenoses / occlusions
- √ mild hydronephrosis

NUC:
- √ diminished uptake of radiopharmaceuticals
- √ normal parenchymal transit
- √ abnormal cortical retention

Drug Nephrotoxicity

Nephrotoxic potential:
cyclosporine (vasoconstrictive effect on afferent glomerular arterioles) > OKT3 > FK506
◊ Effects are dose-dependent and accentuated by dehydration + decreased renal perfusion

Action: impedes rejection process with narrow therapeutic window

Histo: (a) acutely: damage to tubules, microthrombosis of kidney (secondary to activation of coagulation cascade)
(b) chronically: hyaline deposition within arterial walls

- √ no change in renal size
- √ no change (?) / elevation of resistive index

NUC:
- √ depressed effective renal plasma flow
- √ no parenchymal retention

Urologic Problems with Renal Transplant

1. **Ureteral obstruction** (1–5–10%)
   (a) acute: secondary to technical problems
   (b) late: secondary to ischemia or previous extravasation
   Causes: stricture (most commonly at ureterovesical junction), ureteral kinking, (transient) edema at ureteroneocystostomy, ureteropelvic fibrosis, crossing vessels, blood clot, hematoma, lymphocele, fungus ball, calculus
   - rising creatinine level
   - √ pyelocaliectasis
   - √ normal resistive index strongly argues against obstruction unless ureteral leak is present

   DDx: diminished ureteral tone due to denervation

Causes of Renal Allograft Dysfunction	
Immediate to 1st 48 hours	*Day 2 to day 7*
1. Hyperacute rejection 2. Renal vein thrombosis 3. Discordant size	1. ATN 2. RVT
>1 Week post-op	*Delayed*
1. Acute rejection 2. ATN	1. Chronic rejection 2. Drug toxicity 3. Obstruction 4. Infection 5. Extrinsic compression

2. **Urine extravasation** (3–10%)
   Cause:
   (1) Distal ureteral necrosis secondary to interruption of blood supply (early) / vascular insufficiency due to rejection (late)
   (2) Leakage from ureteroneocystostomy site (related to surgical technique / distal ureteral necrosis)
   (3) Leakage from anterior cystostomy closure site
   (4) Segmental renal infarction
   - high creatinine level in fluid collection

   Prognosis: high morbidity + mortality (death from transplant infection + septicemia)
3. **Pararenal fluid collection**
   Incidence: in up to 50% of transplantations
   Dx: percutaneous fluid aspiration
   Cx: Page kidney
   (1) Lymphocele (in up to 15%)
   Onset: within 4–8 weeks after transplantation
   - mostly asymptomatic
   - creatinine + urea nitrogen + protein + electrolyte components similar to serum
   - predominantly lymphocytes, few leukocytes
   - √ mean diameter of 11 cm
   - √ thick septa (50%) + internal debris
   - √ photopenic region with displacement / impression on renal transplant / urinary bladder

   Cx: hydronephrosis; edema of leg / abdominal wall / scrotum / labia
   Rx: sclerotherapy with povidone-iodine / ethanol; long-term catheter drainage / surgical marsupialization
   (2) Urinoma (rare)
   - pain, swelling, discharge from wound (in early postoperative period)
   - √ rarely septated + smaller than lymphoceles
   - √ progressive radiotracer activity within collection

   (3) Hematoma, seroma, abscess
   - √ small crescentic peritransplant fluid collection (as normal sequelae of surgery)
   - √ photopenic region with displacement / impression on renal transplant / urinary bladder

   Prognosis: small hematomas typically resolve spontaneously within a few weeks

   mnemonic: "HAUL"
   Hematoma
   Abscess
   Urinoma
   Lymphocele

Vascular Problems with Renal Transplant (10%)

A. PRERENAL
1. **Renal artery stenosis** (1–12%)
   ◊ Transient elevation of velocities in immediate postoperative period is due to vessel wall edema / arterial spasm!
   Time of onset: within 3 years; cadaver kidney > young donor kidney > living-related donor kidney

Location:
- (a) short-segment stenosis at anastomosis: technical (75%), use of clamp / cannula, trauma, ischemia of donor vessel
- (b) long-segment stenosis of proximal artery (close to anastomosis) > distal artery: trauma during allograft harvesting, faulty operative technique, chronic rejection, atherosclerosis, kinking, scar formation

• recent onset of hypertension / severe hypertension refractory to medical therapy
◊ 65% of transplant recipients have nonrenovascular hypertension
• unexplained graft dysfunction
• audible bruit over graft site (occasionally)
√ increase in peak systolic velocity >200–210 cm/sec
√ 2:1 ratio between peak stenotic and poststenotic velocities
√ main renal artery/external iliac artery ratio >3.5
√ marked poststenotic turbulence (supportive evidence)
√ dampened signals distal to stenosis (= tardus-parvus waveform)
√ increase in acceleration time (= pulse rise time) of intrarenal arteries

Angio:
√ standard test for detection of arterial stenosis ± intravascular treatment

Cx (0.5–2.3%): hemorrhage, intimal flap, arteriovenous fistula

2. **Renal artery thrombosis** (1–5%)

Cause: rejection, faulty surgical technique
Time of onset: within 1st week
Predisposed: allografts with disparate vessel size, multiple anastomoses, intramural vessel injury due to faulty handling, rejection

• early sudden onset of anuria
• graft tenderness + swelling

(a) global
√ absence of perfusion, uptake, excretion
√ failure to demonstrate intrarenal arterial / venous flow
Prognosis: graft loss

(b) segmental
√ segmental infarction due to occlusion of polar artery
√ hypo- / hyperechoic area ± cortical thickening
√ no flow in affected area

3. **Pseudoaneurysm** (in up to 17%)

Cause: percutaneous biopsy with vascular injury, faulty surgical technique, perivascular infection

Location:
- (a) extrarenal at anastomotic site: due to suture rupture, anastomotic leakage, vessel wall ischemia
- (b) intrarenal, mostly of arcuate arteries: following needle biopsy, mycotic infection

√ mimics renal cyst
√ disorganized flow / to-and-fro waveform
Prognosis: spontaneous regression frequent
Cx: spontaneous rupture

4. **Arteriovenous fistula** (in 2%)

Cause: percutaneous biopsy with vascular injury, faulty surgical technique, perivascular infection

• hypertension, hematuria, high-output cardiac failure
√ high-velocity low-resistance flow in feeding artery
√ pulsatile "arterialized" waveform in draining vein
√ turbulence + high-frequency velocity shift
√ exaggerated focal color around lesion (= bruit = perivascular soft-tissue vibration)
Cx: renal ischemia (with large lesion)

5. **Renal allograft necrosis**

= total lack of perfusion in an area of renal cortex associated with variable degrees of medullary necrosis

Cause: rejection, surgical ligature, preexistent arterial lesion, severe ATN, prolonged time of warm ischemia

Pattern:
1. Small focal necrosis
2. Large isolated area of infarction (segmental arterial occlusion)
3. Outer cortical necrosis
4. Cortical necrosis with large patches
5. Diffuse cortical necrosis
6. Cortical + medullary necrosis
7. Necrosis of whole kidney (occlusion of main renal artery)

Renal Transplant Scintigram

	Early study (<24 hours post transplantation)		Late study (>5 days post transplantation)	
	Flow	Excretion	Flow	Excretion
Acute tubular necrosis	nl / mildly decreased	decreased	nl / mildly decreased	mildly decreased
Hyperacute rejection	absent	absent		
Acute rejection	decreased	decreased	worsening	worsening
Chronic rejection	decreased	decreased	decreased	decreased

GU

MR:
√ slightly hyperintense (ischemic necrosis) / hypointense (hemorrhagic necrosis) / isointense area on T2WI
√ hypointense areas on Gd-DTPA images

US:
√ hypoechoic (ischemic necrosis) / iso- or hyperechoic (hemorrhagic necrosis) areas
√ swollen area (probably cortical edema)
√ absence of arterial perfusion by color duplex (not sensitive for small infarcts / superficial cortical necrosis)
√ elevated resistive indexes + no / reversed diastolic flow

B. POSTRENAL
1. **Renal / iliac vein thrombosis** (4.2–5%)
Cause:
(a) immediately: injury to epithelium at site of renal vein anastomosis, extrinsic compression by fluid collection
(b) after 1st week: acute rejection, reduced intrarenal arterial flow, hypovolemia
• abrupt onset of oliguria
• graft tenderness
• hematuria, proteinuria
√ enlarged hypoechoic transplant
√ prolonged arterial transit time without arterial occlusions + arterial spasms
√ diminished cortical perfusion
√ absent venous flow
√ "U-shaped" / plateau-like reversal of diastolic arterial flow
√ decreased systolic rise time
2. **Renal vein stenosis**
Cause: perivascular fibrosis, compression from adjacent perinephric fluid collection
√ color aliasing
√ 3–4-fold increase in velocity

HIGH VASCULAR IMPEDANCE OF RENAL TRANSPLANT
= pulsatility index (A – B / mean) greater than 1.8 or resistive index (A – B / B) of Doppler signals of 0.75–0.80 indicate a reduction in diastolic flow velocity
Causes:
(a) intrinsic vascular obstruction
1. Acute vascular rejection (later stage)
2. Renal vein obstruction
(b) increased intraparenchymal pressure
1. Severe ATN
2. Severe pyelonephritis: CMV, herpes, E. coli, C. albicans
3. Extrarenal compression: large collection, hematoma, discordant size
4. Urinary obstruction (doubted!)
5. Excessive pressure by transducer

Gastrointestinal Problems with Renal Transplant
Incidence: 40%
1. Gastrointestinal hemorrhage
(a) Upper GI tract bleeding
gastric erosions, gastric / duodenal ulcers
Mortality rate: 2–3 x of normal
(b) Lower GI tract bleeding
hemorrhoids, pseudomembranous colitis, cecal ulcers, colonic polyps
2. GI tract perforation (3%)
Causes: spontaneous, antacid impaction, perinephric abscess, diverticular disease
Location: colon > small bowel > gastroduodenal
Mortality rate: approaches 75% (because of delayed diagnosis)

Hypertension with Renal Transplant
◊ Leading cause of death in renal transplant recipient!
Prevalence: up to 60% 1 year after transplantation
Cause:
A. TRANSPLANT RELATED
1. Acute transplant rejection
2. Chronic rejection
3. Cyclosporine toxicity
4. Ureteral obstruction
5. Renal artery stenosis
(a) Accelerated atherosclerosis
(b) Postsurgical fibrosis at anastomosis
B. NOT TRANSPLANT RELATED
1. Renin production of native kidney
2. Original renal disease involving transplant
3. Development of essential hypertension

Aseptic Necrosis with Renal Transplant
Most common long-term disabling complication; femoral head most common site, bilateral in 59–80%
Frequency: 6–15–29% within 3 years after surgery
Time of onset: symptoms develop 5–126 (mean 9–19) months after transplantation
Risk factors:
dose + method of glucocorticoid administration, duration + quality of dialysis before transplantation, secondary hyperparathyroidism, allograft dysfunction, liver disease, previous transplantation, iron overload, increased protein catabolism during dialysis
Pathophysiology of corticosteroid therapy:
(1) Fat embolism (fat globules occlude subchondral end arteries)
(2) Increase in fat cell volume in closed marrow space (increase in intramedullary pressure leads to diminished perfusion)
(3) Osteopenia (increased bone fragility)
(4) Reduced sensibility to pain (loss of protection against excessive stress)
Histo: fragmentation, compression, resorption of dead bone, proliferation of granulation tissue, revascularization, production of new bone
• 40% asymptomatic
• joint pain

• restriction of movement
Sites: femoral head, femoral condyles (lateral > medial condyle), humeral head
√ subchondral bone resorption
√ patchy osteosclerosis
√ collapse / fragmentation of bone
MR with abbreviated T1WI protocol = test of choice!
see AVASCULAR NECROSIS

Posttransplant Lymphoproliferative Disease

= abnormal proliferation of B-cell lymphocytes strongly associated with Epstein-Barr virus infection (in 80%); up to 11% may arise from T-cell lymphocytes

Incidence:
0.6% after bone marrow transplantation,
1–6% after kidney transplantation (in 20% NHL, especially affecting CNS)
1.8–20% after cardiac transplantation
◊ Prevalence of NHL is 35 x greater than in general population!

Cause: sequelae of chronic immunosuppression with limited ability to suppress neoplastic activity

Types:
1. Polyclonal B-cell hyperplasia (nearly identical to infectious mononucleosis)
2. Monoclonal non-Hodgkin lymphoma

Time of onset: as early as 1 month after transplantation depending on immunosuppressive regimen

Location:
@ Lymph nodes: tonsils, cervical neck nodes
@ Gastrointestinal tract
Cx: visceral perforation (frequent)
@ Thorax
√ multiple / solitary well-circumscribed pulmonary nodules ± mediastinal lymphadenopathy (DDx: cryptococcosis, fungus, Kaposi sarcoma)
√ patchy airspace consolidation (DDx: edema, infection, rejection)

DDx: lymphoid hyperplasia (spontaneous resolution)
Rx: (1) Antiviral agents (controversial)
(2) Reduction / cessation of immunosuppressive agents
(3) Surgical resection of tumor mass (complete resolution in 63%)

RENAL TUBULAR ACIDOSIS

= clinical syndrome characterized by tubular insufficiency to resorb bicarbonate, excrete hydrogen ion, or both (= nonanion gap metabolic acidosis)
• failure to thrive

Proximal Renal Tubular Acidosis

= TYPE 2 RTA
= impaired capacity to absorb HCO_3^- in proximal tubule leads to presence of bicarbonate in urine at lower plasma levels than normal

Pathogenesis:
? defect in Na^+/HCO_3^- cotransport at basolateral membrane; deficit of carbonic anhydrase; parathyroid hormone activates cyclic AMP, which inhibits carbonic anhydrase (hypocalcemia of hyperparathyroidism + various types of Fanconi syndrome)
• self-limited acidosis (bicarbonate loss stops once bicarbonate threshold of about 15 mEq/L is reached)
• unimpaired ability to lower urine pH (pH 4.5–7.8 depending on level of plasma bicarbonate) by normal excretion of hydrogen ions
• hypokalemia (due to hyperaldosteronism secondary to decreased proximal resorption of NaCl)
√ rickets / osteomalacia

N.B.: NEVER nephrocalcinosis / nephrolithiasis (due to normal urinary citrate excretion, low urine pH, self-limited less severe acidosis with less calcium release from bone

Dx: bicarbonate titration test, large requirement of alkali to sustain plasma bicarbonate level at 22 mmol/L

Rx: administration of alkali ± potassium ± hydrochlorothiazide

1. INFANTILE TYPE OF PRIMARY PROXIMAL RTA
Age: diagnosed within first 18 months of life; usually male patients
• excessive vomiting in early infancy
• growth retardation (<3rd percentile)
• metabolic hyperchloremic acidosis
• normal quantities of net acid excretion
Prognosis: transient type with spontaneous remission
2. SECONDARY PROXIMAL RTA
= tubular defect of bicarbonate resorption associated with other tubular dysfunction / generalized disease
Cause:
— Fanconi syndrome, cystinosis, Lowe syndrome, hereditary fructose intolerance, glycogen storage disease, galactosemia, tyrosinemia, Wilson disease, Leigh syndrome
— 1° + 2° hyperparathyroidism, vitamin D deficiency, mineralocorticoid deficiency, osteopetrosis
— medullary cystic disease, renal transplantation, vascular accident to kidney in newborn period, multiple myeloma, amyloidosis, nephrotic syndrome, cyanotic CHD, Sjögren syndrome
— intoxication with cadmium, outdated tetracycline, methylchromone, 6-mercaptopurine

GU

Distal Renal Tubular Acidosis

= TYPE 1 RTA (first type discovered)
= impaired ability to secrete H^+ in distal tubule despite low levels of plasma bicarbonate (urine cannot be acidified with pH invariably high at >5.5–6.0)

Pathophysiology:
primary defect of nonacidification of urine followed by
(a) hyperchloremia
small constant loss of serum sodium bicarbonate ($NaHCO_3$) without concomitant loss of chloride (NaCl retention) leads to shrinkage of ECF volume
(b) chronic severe + progressive acidosis (due to inability to excrete the usual endogenously produced nonvolatile acid) leads to
— mobilization of calcium + phosphate from bone (osteomalacia)
— growth retardation
— hypercalciuria (+ 2° hyperparathyroidism)
— loss of phosphate (osteomalacia / rickets)
(c) nephrocalcinosis + nephrolithiasis (due to combination of hypercalciuria + elevated urine pH + marked reduction in urinary citrate)
(d) potassium wastage with hyperkaliuria + hypokalemia (due to constant small loss of sodium bicarbonate in urine, reduction of ECF space, 2° hyperaldosteronism, increase in sodium-potassium exchange in distal tubule)

Path: calcium deposits accompanied by chronic interstitial nephritis with cellular infiltration, tubular atrophy, glomerular sclerosis

- muscle weakness, hyporeflexia, paralysis (due to hypokalemia)
- bone pain (due to osteomalacia)
- polyuria (from defect in urinary concentrating ability as a result of nephrocalcinosis + potassium deficiency)
- low plasma bicarbonate
- hyperchloremic acidosis (from impaired ability to excrete the usual endogenous load of nonvolatile acid)
- alkaline urine (pH >5.0–5.5)
- hypokalemia, loss of sodium
- hypercalciuria (continued mobilization of calcium phosphate from bone due to metabolic acidosis)
- hypocitraturia (increased proximal tubular reabsorption of citrate)

Dx: acid load test with ammonium chloride (NH_4Cl)
Rx: administration of mixture of sodium + potassium bicarbonate
Cx: interstitial nephritis, chronic renal failure (damage from nephrocalcinosis + secondary pyelonephritis), bone lesions, nephrocalcinosis, nephrolithiasis

1. PERMANENT DISTAL RTA
= ADULT TYPE OF PRIMARY DISTAL RTA = BUTLER-ALBRIGHT SYNDROME
Genetics: mostly sporadic, may be autosomal dominant
Age: children + adults (usually not diagnosed before age 2); F > M
- vomiting, constipation, polyuria, dehydration
- failure to thrive, growth retardation, anorexia
- polyuria (due to renal concentrating defect)
- potassium loss resulting in flaccid paralysis
- bone pain + pathologic fractures in adolescents + adults (from osteomalacia)
- low serum pH, low bicarbonate concentration
- elevation of chloride
- urinary pH of 6.0–6.5

√ rickets / osteomalacia
√ moderately retarded bone age
√ medullary nephrocalcinosis / nephrolithiasis (as early as 1 month of age)

2. SECONDARY DISTAL RTA
(a) systemic conditions:
— starvation, malnutrition, sickle cell disease
— primary hyperthyroidism + nephrocalcinosis, 1° hyperparathyroidism + nephrocalcinosis, vitamin D intoxication, idiopathic hypercalcemia, idiopathic hypercalciuria + nephrocalcinosis
— amphotericin B nephropathy, toxicity to lithium, toluene sniffing
— hepatic cirrhosis, fructose intolerance with nephrocalcinosis, Ehlers-Danlos syndrome, Marfan syndrome, elliptocytosis
(b) renal conditions:
renal tubular necrosis, renal transplantation, medullary sponge kidney, obstructive uropathy
(c) hypergammaglobulinemic states (? autoimmune process):
idiopathic hypergammaglobulinemia, chronic active hepatitis, hyperglobulinemic purpura, Sjögren syndrome, cryoglobulinemia, systemic lupus erythematosus, lupoid hepatitis, fibrosing alveolitis

TRANSIENT DISTAL RENAL TUBULAR ACIDOSIS
= INFANTILE TYPE OF PRIMARY DISTAL RTA
= LIGHTWOOD SYNDROME = SALT-LOSING NEPHRITIS
= transient self-limited form of infancy (only observed within 1st year of life) with unclear pathophysiology, probably due to vitamin D intoxication]
- NO nephrocalcinosis

RENAL VEIN THROMBOSIS

Prevalence: 0.5% (autopsy)
Causes:
A. Intrinsic
= thrombotic process begins intrarenally within small intrarenal veins due to acidosis, hemoconcentration, disseminated intravascular coagulation, intrarenal arteriolar constriction reducing venous flow
(a) antenatally: abruptio placentae
(b) neonates (most common): advanced maternal age, glycosuria in infants of diabetic mothers, dehydration from vomiting, diarrhea, enterocolitis, sepsis, polycythemia, birth trauma, left adrenal hemorrhage, prematurity
(c) adults: pyelonephritis, amyloidosis, polyarteritis nodosa, sickle cell anemia, thrombosis of IVC, low flow states (CHF, constrictive pericarditis), diabetic nephropathy, sarcoidosis
– hypercoagulable state

GU

-- nephrotic syndrome:
membranous + membranoproliferative glomerulonephritis (most common), lupoid nephrosis
-- SLE
-- inherited hypercoagulable state:
antithrombin III deficiency, protein C deficiency, protein S deficiency
– mechanical process
-- trauma
-- neoplasm: renal neoplasia (50%: RCC, TCC, Wilms tumor), left adrenal carcinoma
-- abscess
-- aneurysm
– left ovarian vein thrombosis

B. Extrinsic
umbilical vein catheterization, thrombosis of IVC with extension into renal vein, malpositioned IVC filter, carcinoma of pancreatic tail invading renal vein (in 75%), pancreatitis, lymphoma, retroperitoneal sarcoma, retroperitoneal fibrosis, metastases to retroperitoneum (bronchogenic carcinoma)

mnemonic: "TEST MAN"
Thrombophlebitis
Enterocolitis (dehydration)
Sickle cell disease, **S**ystemic lupus erythematosus
Trauma
Membranous glomerulonephritis
Amyloidosis
Neoplasm

Radiographic appearance varies with:
(1) rapidity of venous occlusion
(2) extent of occlusion
(3) availability of collateral circulation
(4) site of occlusion in relation to collateral pathways

Pathophysiology: formation of collateral channels develops at 24 hours + peaks at 2 weeks after onset of occlusion

Collaterals: ureteral v. to vesicular vv., pericapsular vv. to lumbar vv., azygos v., portal v.
on left: in addition gonadal v., adrenal v., inferior phrenic vv.

Acute Renal Vein Thrombosis

Path: hemorrhagic renal infarction from ruptured venules + capillaries without time for effective development of collaterals
• gross hematuria, proteinuria
• asymptomatic / painful flank mass
• consumptive thrombocytopenia
• anuria, hypertension, azotemia

Location: more common on left (longer left renal vein)
√ focal hemorrhagic infarction + capsular rupture
√ smooth enlargement of kidney (edema + blood)

IVP:
√ initially faint + delayed dense nephrogram
√ completely normal to pyelocaliceal nonvisualization

US:
√ focal / generalized areas of increased echogenicity (from hemorrhage / edema)
√ loss of corticomedullary differentiation
√ thrombus within distended renal vein / IVC

Doppler-US:
√ venous flow present in segmental veins + collateral veins overlying renal hilum mimicking patency of main renal vein
√ steady / less pulsatile venous flow compared with contralateral main renal vein
√ main renal vein not traceable into IVC on color Doppler
√ elevated resistive index >0.70 ± reversed end-diastolic renal arterial flow in native kidney

CT:
√ prolonged cortical nephrographic phase with coarse striations + persistent corticomedullary differentiation
√ edema in renal sinus + perinephric space
√ thickened renal fascia + perirenal stranding
√ development of collateral venous vessels
√ retroperitoneal hemorrhage

MR:
√ high signal intensity on T1WI + T2WI

Angio:
√ poorly filling cortical arteries
√ absent inflow from renal vein into IVC
√ thrombus extending into IVC

NUC:
√ no characteristic pattern on sequential functional study

Cx: (1) Pulmonary emboli (50%)
(2) Severe renal atrophy (may show complete recovery)

Subacute Renal Vein Thrombosis

= good collateral drainage; impaired function with steady state or recanalization
√ enlarged edematous boggy kidney
√ slightly diminished / normal nephrographic density (may increase over time)
√ compression of collecting system ("spidery calyces")
√ hypoechoic large kidney
√ collateral veins allow venous efflux normalizing arterial waveform
√ main renal vein appears small due to recanalization

Chronic Renal Vein Thrombosis

= indolent stage
• 80–90% asymptomatic
• nephrotic syndrome (proteinuria, hypercholesterolemia, anasarca)
√ normal excretory urogram in 25% (with good collateral circulation especially if left side affected)
√ notching of collecting system + proximal ureter
√ retroperitoneal dilated collaterals
√ lacelike intrarenal pattern of calcifications

US:
- √ branching linear calcifications (calcified thrombus)
- √ small atrophic echogenic kidney

CT:
- √ attenuated renal vein (due to retraction of blood clot) + IVC thrombus (24%)
- √ collaterals along proximal + middle ureter + perirenal
- √ prolonged corticomedullary differentiation
- √ delayed / absent pyelocaliceal opacification + attenuated collecting system
- √ thickening of Gerota fascia

Arteriography:
- √ enlarged venous collaterals on delayed images

RETROCAVAL URETER

= CIRCUMCAVAL URETER

Etiology: abnormality in embryogenesis of IVC with persistence of right posterior cardinal vein ventral to ureter + failure of right supracardinal system to develop

Incidence: 0.07%; M:F = 3:1

- • symptoms of right ureteral obstruction
- √ proximal right ureter swings medially over pedicle of L3/4, passes behind IVC, and emerges to right of aorta, returns to its normal position anterior to iliac vessels
- √ varying degrees of hydronephrosis + proximal hydroureteronephrosis

Cx: recurrent urinary tract infections

RETROPERITONEAL FIBROSIS

= ORMOND DISEASE = CHRONIC PERIAORTITIS

Path: dense hard fibrous tissue enveloping the retroperitoneum with effects on ureter, lymphatics, great vessels

Causes:

A. PRIMARY RETROPERITONEAL FIBROSIS (2/3)
Probably autoimmune disease with antibodies to ceroid (by-product of aortic plaque, which has penetrated into media) leading to systemic vasculitis;
Associated with fibrosis in other organ systems (in 8–15%):
mediastinal fibrosis, Riedel fibrosing thyroiditis, sclerosing cholangitis, fibrotic orbital pseudotumor
Age: 31–60 years (in 70%); M:F = 2:1
Rx: responsive to corticoids

B. SECONDARY RETROPERITONEAL FIBROSIS (1/3)
(1) Drugs (12%): methysergide, beta-blocker, phenacetin, hydralazine, ergotamine, methyldopa, amphetamines, LSD
(2) Desmoplastic response to malignancy (8%): lymphoma, Hodgkin disease, carcinoid, retroperitoneal metastases (breast, lung, thyroid, GI tract, GU organs)
(3) Retroperitoneal fluid collection: from trauma, surgery, infection
(4) Aneurysm of aorta / iliac arteries (desmoplastic response)
(5) Connective tissue disease: eg, polyarteritis nodosa
(6) Radiation therapy

Peak age: 40–60 years; M:F = 2:1

- • weight loss, nausea, malaise
- • dull pain in flank, back, abdomen (90%)
- • renal insufficiency (50–60%)
- • hypertension
- • leg edema, fever, hydrocele (10%)
- • claudication (occasionally)

Location:
plaque typically begins around aortic bifurcation extending cephalad to renal hilum / surrounding kidney; rarely extends below pelvic rim, but may extend caudad to bladder + rectosigmoid

IVP
Classic TRIAD:
(1) ureterectasis above L4/5 (interference with peristalsis)
(2) medial deviation of ureters in middle third, typically bilateral
(3) gradual tapering of ureter (extrinsic compression)
- √ usually mild pyelocaliectasis

US:
- √ hypoechoic homogeneous mass in paraaortic region / perinephric space

CT:
- √ periaortic mass of attenuation similar to muscle
- √ may show contrast enhancement (active inflammation)

MR:
- √ low to medium homogeneous signal intensity on T1WI
- √ heterogeneous high signal intensity on T2WI (with malignancy / associated inflammatory edema)
- √ low signal intensity on T2WI (in dense fibrotic plaque)

NUC:
- √ gallium uptake during active inflammation

DDx: lymphoma, retroperitoneal adenopathy

Rx: (1) Withdrawal of possible causative agent
(2) Interventional relief of obstruction
(3) Corticosteroids

RETROPERITONEAL LEIOMYOSARCOMA

Incidence: 2nd most common primary retroperitoneal malignancy (after liposarcoma)

Origin:
(a) retroperitoneal space without attachment to organs
(b) wall of inferior vena cava

Age: 5th–6th decade; M:F = 1:6

- • abdominal mass, pain, weight loss, nausea, vomiting
- • abdominal distension, change in defecation habits, leg edema, back / radicular pain, frequency of urination
- • hemoperitoneum, GI bleeding, dystocia, paraplegia

Metastases:
frequently hematogenous, less commonly lymphatic dissemination
(a) common sites: liver, lung, brain, peritoneum
(b) rare sites: skin, soft tissue, bone, kidney, omentum
◊ Distant metastases present at time of diagnosis in 40%

DDx: (1) Liposarcoma (fat content)
(2) Malignant fibrous histiocytoma (not as necrotic)

GU

(3) Lymphoma (nonnecrotic, tends to envelop IVC + aorta)
(4) Primary adrenal tumor
(5) IVC thrombus (no luminal enlargement, no neovascularity)

Rx: (1) Complete excision (resectable in 10–75%)
(2) Partial resection (reduction in tumor size)
(3) Adjuvant chemotherapy / radiotherapy

Prognosis: local recurrence in 40–70%; death within 5 years in 80–87% with extraluminal tumors

Extravascular Leiomyosarcoma (62%)

Path: extraluminal (= completely extravascular) large tumor with extensive necrosis

IVP:
- √ large soft-tissue mass with
  (a) displacement of kidney + ureter
  (b) gas-containing ascending / descending colon
- √ well-defined fat plane between mass and kidney
- √ obstruction of kidney (ureteral involvement)
- √ usually not calcified

US:
- √ solid mass isoechoic to liver / rarely hyperechoic
- √ complex mass with cystic spaces + irregular walls

CT:
- √ lobulated mass often >10 cm in size
- √ large cystic areas of tumor necrosis in center of mass
- √ areas of high attenuation with recent hemorrhage

MR:
- √ intermediate intensity on T1WI with low-intensity areas of necrosis
- √ inhomogeneous intermediate to high signal intensity on T2WI (due to high water content of cystic areas)

Angio:
- √ hypervascular tumor with blood supply from lumbar, celiac, mesenteric, renal arteries
- √ avascular center surrounded by thick hypervascular rind

Intravascular Leiomyosarcoma (5%)

Path: intraluminal (= completely intravascular) polypoid mass firmly attached to vessel wall

Location: between diaphragm + renal veins, may extend along entire length of IVC + into heart
- √ small solid mass within IVC
- √ gradually dilatation / obstruction of IVC
- √ intratumoral vascularity confirmed by Doppler
- √ irregular enhancement (CT bolus injection)

Cx:
(1) Budd-Chiari syndrome (extension into hepatic veins)
(2) Nephrotic syndrome (extension into renal veins)
(3) Edema of lower extremities (extension into lower IVC without adequate collateralization)
(4) Tumor embolus to lung

Extra- & Intravascular Leiomyosarcoma (33%)
- √ solid / necrotic extraluminal mass not originating from a retroperitoneal organ with contiguous intravascular enhancing component (PATHOGNOMONIC)

Intramural Leiomyosarcoma (extremely rare)

RETROPERITONEAL LIPOSARCOMA

= slow-growing tumor that displaces rather than infiltrates surrounding tissue and rarely metastasizes

Incidence: most common primary malignant retroperitoneal tumor, 95% of all fatty retroperitoneal tumors

Histo:
(a) lipogenic type:
  √ radiodensity of fat
(b) myxoid type (most common):
  √ radiodensity between water + muscle
(c) pleomorphic type (least common):
  √ radiodensity of muscle

Age: most commonly 40–60 years; M > F
- • abdominal pain, weight loss, anemia, palpable mass

Site: anterior to spine + psoas muscle > paraspinal + posterior pararenal space

CT:
- √ solid pattern: inhomogeneous poorly marginated infiltrating mass with contrast enhancement
- √ mixed pattern: focal fatty areas (–40 to –20 HU) + areas of higher density (+20 HU)
- √ pseudocystic pattern: water-density mass (averaging of fatty + solid connective-tissue elements)
- √ calcifications in up to 12%

Angio:
- √ hypovascular without vessel dilatation / capillary staining / laking

Prognosis: most radiosensitive of soft-tissue sarcomas; 32% overall 5-year survival

DDx: malignant fibrous histiocytoma, leiomyosarcoma, desmoid tumor

RHABDOID TUMOR OF KIDNEY

◊ Most aggressive renal neoplasm of childhood!

Frequency: 2% of pediatric renal tumors

Mean age: 11–17 months; 6–12 months of age (25%), <1 year of age (60%), <2 years of age (80%); M:F = 1.5:1

Origin: renal sinus

Histo: monomorphic noncohesive large cells with prominent nucleoli + abundant eosinophilic cytoplasm (superficial resemblance to skeletal muscle, hence name); filamentous intracytoplasmic inclusions (CHARACTERISTIC)

Associated with: syn- / metachronous primary brain tumor of neuroectodermal origin (medulloblastoma, ependymoma, cerebellar / brainstem astrocytoma, PNET)

Metastatic to: lung, liver, brain
- • paraneoplastic hypercalcemia (occasionally)

√ centrally located heterogeneous renal mass:
  √ indistinct borders with infiltration of medulla + sinus
  √ PROMINENT peripheral crescent-shaped subcapsular fluid collection in 70% (subcapsular hematoma in 47% / necrotic cavity in 53%)
  √ linear calcifications outlining tumor lobules
√ midline posterior fossa mass
√ metastases (in 80%) to lung, liver, abdomen, brain, lymph nodes, bone

Prognosis: 20% 18-month survival rate

DDx: Wilms tumor, mesoblastic nephroma

RHABDOMYOSARCOMA, GENITOURINARY

Frequency:
4–8% of all malignant solid tumors in children <15 years of age (ranking 4th after CNS neoplasm, neuroblastoma, Wilms tumor); 10–25% of all sarcomas; annual incidence of 4.5:1,000,000 white + 1.3:1,000,000 black children

Age: mean age of 7 years; white:black = 3:1; M:F = 6:4

Origin: mesenchyme of the urogenital ridge

Path: firm fleshy lobulated mass with infiltrative margin / well-defined pseudocapsule; composed of smooth grapelike clusters if intraluminal (= sarcoma botryoides)

Histo (Horn & Enterline):
(a) embryonal (56%)
(b) botryoid = "grapelike" (5%) = subtype of embryonal rhabdomyosarcoma
(c) alveolar (20%): worst prognosis
(d) pleomorphic (1%): mostly in adults

DDx: primitive neuroectodermal tumor, extraosseous Ewing sarcoma, synovial cell sarcoma, fibrosarcoma, alveolar soft part sarcoma, hemangiopericytoma, undifferentiated sarcoma, neuroblastoma

Metastases: lung, cortical bone, lymph nodes > bone marrow, liver
◊ Metastases in 10–20% at time of diagnosis!

√ nonspecific imaging features:
  √ homogeneous echogenicity similar to muscle ± hypoechoic areas (hemorrhage / necrosis)
  √ hyperemia with high diastolic flow component
  √ bulky pelvic mass of heterogeneous attenuation
  √ hypointense on T1WI + hyperintense on T2WI with heterogeneous enhancement
  √ diffuse tumor vascularity on angio

Prognosis:
(a) 14–35% 5-year survival with radical surgery
(b) 60–90% 3-year survival with chemotherapy added
◊ Local recurrence is common!

Bladder-prostate Rhabdomyosarcoma

Age: in first 3 years of life

Location: trigone of urinary bladder / prostate (tumor infiltrating both)

- abdominal pain + distension (from bladder outlet obstruction)
- urinary frequency + dysuria (from urinary tract infection) + retention
- palpable bladder
- hematuria (unusual late manifestation)
- strangury (= painful urge to void without success)

√ polypoid intraluminal tumor mass
√ elevation of bladder floor with obstruction of bladder neck + large postvoid residual
√ ± invasion of periurethral / perivesical tissues
√ retroperitoneal lymph node enlargement

DDx: polyp, hemangioma, ectopic ureterocele, hemorrhagic cystitis

Rhabdomyosarcoma of Female Genital Tract

Location: vulva / vagina (infancy), cervix (reproductive years), uterine corpus (postmenopausal)

- vulvar / perineal / vaginal mass
- vaginal bleeding / discharge / protruding grapelike mass

DDx: polyp, urethral prolapse, hydrometrocolpos, neoplasm

Prognosis: 91% 5-year survival rate for nonmetastatic rhabdomyosarcoma of genital tract

Vaginal Rhabdomyosarcoma

Age: very young children (almost exclusively)

Histo: commonly botryoid

US:
√ large solid heterogenous hypoechoic mass posterior to urinary bladder

Paratesticular Rhabdomyosarcoma

Age: childhood, 2nd age peak in adolescence

Location: spermatic cord, testis, penis, epididymis

- painless scrotal swelling
- palpable nontransilluminating intrascrotal tumor
- bulky abdominal (lymphadenopathy)

√ displacement / compression / infiltration of adjacent testis

Prognosis: 73–89% 3-year survival rate

DDx: hydrocele, epididymitis, testicular neoplasm

SCHISTOSOMIASIS

= BILHARZIASIS

Organism: trematodes of species:
S. haematobium (GU tract) >95%;
S. mansoni, S. japonicum (GI tract) <5%

Life cycle:
female parasite discharges eggs into vesicular venules; eggs erode bladder mucosa, are excreted with urine + feces, and hatch in fresh water into larval miracidia; larvae invade snail (= intermediate host) of genus Bulinus, Biomphalaria, Oncomelania; resulting daughter sporocytes develop into cercariae and pass into surrounding body of water; penetrate human skin (usually foot) + pass into lymphatics; schistosoma settles in portal veins + migrates into pelvic venous plexus

Incidence: 8% of world's population; 25% in Africa (endemic in South Africa, Egypt, Nigeria, Tanzania, Zimbabwe); endemic in Puerto Rico

@ Urinary tract
- frequency, urgency, dysuria
- hematuria, albuminuria (most common)
- dull flank pain (from hydronephrosis)
- index of infectious severity = urine egg count

Location: lower ureters + bladder
√ bladder wall calcifications (in 4–56%): linear / coarse / floccular, beginning at base, parallel to upper aspect of pubic bone, involving all wall layers
√ vesical calculi (in 39%), distal ureteral calcification (in 34%), honeycombed calcification of seminal vesicles
√ striation of renal pelvis + proximal ureter in 21% (DDx: normal in 3%, other urinary tract infection, vesicoureteric reflux
√ ureterectasis (focal egg deposition leads to peristaltic disorganization)
√ ureteral strictures in distal third (in 8%, L > R), most commonly in intravesical portion with cobra-head configuration = pseudoureterocele); Makar stricture = focal stricture at L3
√ multiple inflammatory pseudopolyps in ureter secondary to granulomas (= bilharziomas)
√ ureteritis cystica
√ ureterolithiasis / ureteritis calcinosa (= punctate / linear calcifications)
√ vesicoureteral reflux
√ polypoid filling defects + mucosal irregularities in urinary bladder (pseudotubercles, papillomas)
√ thick-walled fibrotic "flat-topped" bladder with high insertion of ureters
√ reduced bladder capacity with significant postvoid residual (fibrotic stage)
√ urethral stricture with perineal fistulas

Cx: Squamous cell carcinoma of bladder
Age: 30–50 years (exposed early in childhood with 20–30-year latency period)
Location: posterior bladder wall, rarely trigone
√ irregular filling defect
√ discontinuous calcifications

@ GI tract
√ portal hypertension (ova migrating into portal venous system incite fibrosing granulomatous reaction within presinusoidal portal veins)
√ esophageal varices (from portal hypertension)
√ polypoid calcifying bowel lesions (from eggs of S. mansoni trapped in bowel wall + inciting granulomatous reaction)

@ Chest
√ enlargement of RV + pulmonary artery + azygos vein (from portal hypertension)
√ diffuse granulomatous lung lesions

Rx: praziquantel

SCROTAL ABSCESS

Etiology:
(1) Complication of epididymoorchitis (often in diabetics), missed testicular torsion, gangrenous tumor, infected hematoma, primary pyogenic orchitis
(2) Systemic infection: mumps, smallpox, scarlet fever, influenza, typhoid, syphilis, TB
(3) Septic dissemination from: sinusitis, osteomyelitis, cholecystitis, appendicitis

Predisposed: diabetics

NUC:
√ marked increase in perfusion, hot hemiscrotum with photon-deficient area representing the abscess on Tc-99m pertechnetate scan (DDx: chronic torsion)
√ increased scrotal uptake with leukocyte imaging

US:
√ hypoechoic / complex fluid collection with low-level echoes (differentiation of intra- from extratesticular abscess location possible)
√ skin thickening
√ hydrocele

Cx: (1) Pyocele
(2) Fistulous tract to skin

SEMINAL VESICLE CYST

A. ACQUIRED SEMINAL VESICLE CYST
1. Autosomal dominant polycystic kidney disease
   √ bilateral seminal vesicle cysts
2. Invasive bladder tumor
3. Infection
4. Benign prostatic hypertrophy
5. Ejaculatory duct obstruction

B. CONGENITAL SEMINAL VESICLE CYST
Associated with: anomalies of ipsilateral mesonephric duct:
(1) Ectopic insertion of ipsilateral ureter (92%) into bladder neck / posterior prostatic urethra / ejaculatory duct / seminal vesicle
(2) Ipsilateral renal dysgenesis (80%)
(3) Duplication of collecting system (8%)
(4) Vas deferens agenesis

Symptomatic age: 21–41 years
- abdominal / flank / pelvic / perineal pain exacerbated by ejaculation
- dysuria, frequent urination
- epididymitis in prepubertal boy
- recurrent urinary tract infection

√ cystic mass posterior to urinary bladder (DDx: müllerian duct cyst)
√ dilated ejaculatory duct

SINUS LIPOMATOSIS

= PERIPELVIC LIPOMATOSIS = PELVIC FIBROLIPOMATOSIS = PERIPELVIC FAT PROLIFERATION

Etiology:
(1) Normal increase with aging and obesity
(2) Vicarious proliferation of sinus fat with destruction / atrophy of kidney (= replacement lipomatosis)
(3) Extravasation of urine leading to proliferation of fatty granulation tissue
(4) Normal variant

Age: 6th–7th decade
√ kidney may be enlarged
√ elongated "spiderlike / trumpetlike" pelvicaliceal system

√ infundibula arranged in "spoke-wheel" pattern
√ parenchymal thickness diminished with underlying disease
√ occasionally focal fat deposit with localized deformity of collecting system

Plain film:
√ diminished sinus density

CT:
√ unequivocal fat values

US:
√ echodense / patchy hypoechoic sinus complex

Replacement Lipomatosis

= REPLACEMENT FIBROLIPOMATOSIS
= extreme form of renal sinus lipomatosis

Associated with: infection, long-term hydronephrosis, calculi (70%)

Path: marked proliferation of hyperplastic sinus fat with extremely atrophied cortex + varying degrees of hydro- / pyonephrosis, acute / chronic pyelonephritis

√ kidney enlarged by a fatty sinus mass and outlined by an extremely thin cortex:
  √ fat characteristically distributed within renal sinus + perinephric space
√ staghorn calculus inside an enlarged renal outline
√ poorly functioning / nonfunctioning kidney

DDx: xanthogranulomatous pyelonephritis, lipoma, angiomyolipoma, liposarcoma

SQUAMOUS CELL CARCINOMA OF KIDNEY

Incidence: 5–10% of all urothelial tumors; 1% of renal neoplasms; 2nd most common malignancy of pelvic urothelium after TCC

Age: 60–70 years; M:F = 2:1

Path: flat ulcerating mass + extensive induration

Associated with: chronic irritation of urothelium by renal infection + calculi (25–60%)

• painless hematuria
• flank pain (with ureteropelvic junction obstruction)

√ infiltrating renal process
√ nonfunctional kidney:
  √ ureteropelvic junction obstruction (common)
√ presence of faceted calculi (40–80%)

IVP:
√ stricture that may simulate extrinsic cause

Angio:
√ arterial encasement + occlusion + neovascularity
√ enlarged pelvic + ureteric arteries
√ occlusion of renal vein / branches (41%)

CT:
√ thickening of pelvicaliceal wall (with superficial spread over large areas)
√ enlarged kidney maintaining reniform shape:
  √ infiltrating growth into sinus + parenchyma
  √ tumor mass infrequent
√ no contrast excretion (due to obstruction)

Prognosis: worse than TCC due to early metastases; 33% 1-year survival rate

DDx: xanthogranulomatous pyelonephritis (radiologically indistinguishable)

SUPERNUMERARY KIDNEY

= aberrant division of nephrogenic cord into two metanephric tails (rare)

Associated with: horseshoe kidney, vaginal atresia, duplicated female urethra, duplicated penis

Location: most commonly on left side of abdomen caudal to normal kidney

√ supernumerary ureter may insert into ipsilateral kidney / directly into bladder / ectopic site

Cx: hydronephrosis, pyonephrosis, pyelonephritis, cysts, calculi, carcinoma, papillary cystadenoma, Wilms tumor

TESTICULAR INFARCTION

Etiology: torsion, trauma, leukemia, embolus (eg, bacterial endocarditis), vasculitis (eg, polyarteritis nodosa, Henoch-Schönlein purpura)

√ diffusely hypoechoic small testis / focal mass
√ hyperechoic regions (hemorrhage / fibrosis)
√ decrease in size over time
√ low signal intensity on T1WI + T2WI

DDx: malignancy (difficult differentiation)

TESTICULAR MICROLITHIASIS

Etiology: defect in phagocytotic activity of Sertoli cells leaving degenerated intratubular debris behind

Prevalence: 0.6%

May be associated with:
Klinefelter syndrome, cryptorchidism, testicular infarcts, granulomas, subfertility, infertility, testicular germ cell tumor (40%), male pseudohermaphroditism, Down syndrome, alveolar microlithiasis

Histo: laminated concretions within lumen of seminiferous tubules

• asymptomatic, uncommon incidental finding

√ 1–2-mm hyperechoic nonshadowing foci (>5) scattered throughout the parenchyma of both testes (PATHOGNOMONIC):
  √ may be asymmetrically distributed, unilateral, clustered in periphery

Cx: concurrent germ cell tumor in up to 40% (21.6 x risk)

Recommendation: follow up in 6-month intervals to screen for testicular tumors (contested)

DDx: postinflammatory changes, scars, granulomatous changes, benign adenomatoid tumor, hemorrhage with infarction, large-cell calcifying Sertoli cell tumor

TESTICULAR RUPTURE

◊ Testicular rupture is indication for immediate surgical intervention!

Cause: scrotal trauma

Salvageability:
80–90% if surgical repair occurs <72 hours after trauma;
30–55% if surgical repair occurs >72 hours after trauma

GU

√ areas of decreased / increased echogenicity (hemorrhage ± necrosis)
√ loss of testicular outline
√ thickened scrotal wall (= hematoma)
√ visualization of fracture plane
√ hematocele, may show thickening + calcification of tunica vaginalis if chronic
√ uriniferous hydrocele from perforated bulbous urethra
√ avascular region on color duplex

Cx: torsion (due to stimulation of a forceful cremasteric contraction)

DDx: laceration, contusion, hemorrhage

TESTICULAR TORSION

= SPERMATIC CORD TORSION

Most common scrotal disorder in children, 20% of acute scrotal pathology

Incidence: 1:160, 10-fold risk in undescended testis compared with normal annual incidence of 1:4,000 males

Etiology:

(1) "Bell and clapper" deformity = high insertion of tunica vaginalis on spermatic cord
(2) Abnormally loose mesorchium between testis + epididymis
(3) Extravaginal torsion involving testis + tunica vaginalis due to loose attachment of testicular tunics to scrotum during in utero + perinatal period

Peak age: newborn period + puberty (13–16 years); <20 years in 74–85%; >21 years in 26%; >30 years in 9%

• sudden severe pain in 100% (frequently at night)
• negative urine analysis (98%)
• history of similar episode in same / contralateral testis (42%)
• nausea + vomiting (50%)
• scrotal swelling + tenderness (42%)
• leukocytosis (32%)
• low-grade fever (20%)
• history of trauma / extreme exertion (13%)

Location: in 5% bilateral (anomalous suspension of contralateral testis found in 50–80%)

Salvage rate:

versus time interval between onset of pain and surgery

80–100%	<6 hours
76%	6–12 hours
20%	12–24 hours
near 0%	>24 hours

spontaneous detorsion in 7%

◊ Irreversible ischemic damage in only 3–6 hours!

Cx: testicular atrophy (in 33–45%)

Acute Testicular Torsion

= symptoms present for <24 hours

• 70% of patients present within first 6 hours from onset of pain

US (80–90% sensitivity):

√ normal grey-scale appearance (within 6 hours)
√ diffusely hypoechoic echotexture (>6 hours)
√ testicular + epididymal enlargement with decreased echogenicity (within 8–24 hours)
√ visualization of twisted enlarged spermatic cord
√ scrotal skin thickening
√ hydrocele (occasionally)

Color duplex (86% sensitive, 100% specific, 97% accurate):

√ loss of spermatic cord Doppler signal (sensitivity 44%, specificity 67%)
√ absence of testicular + epididymal flow (DDx: global testicular infarction)

False-negative: torsion-detorsion sequence, incomplete torsion <360 degrees

Degree of torsion and blood flow:

• testis usually turns medially up to 1,080°
√ diminished blood flow in <180°-torsion at 1 hour
√ absent blood flow in any degree of torsion >4 hours
√ hyperemia after spontaneous detorsion

NUC (98% accuracy):

Dose: 5–15 mCi Tc-99m pertechnetate

Imaging: at 2- to 5-second intervals for 1 minute (vascular phase); at 5-minute intervals for 20 minutes (tissue phase)

√ decreased perfusion / occasionally normal
√ nubbin sign = bump of activity extending medially from iliac artery denoting reactive increased blood flow in spermatic cord with abrupt termination
√ rounded cold area replacing testis (requires knowledge of side + location of painful testis)

Subacute Testicular Torsion

= MISSED TESTICULAR TORSION

= symptoms present for >24 hours + less than 10 days

US:

√ enlarged / normal-sized testis with heterogeneous punctate / diffusely increased echotexture
√ increased peritesticular flow without parenchymal blood flow

NUC:

√ normal NUC angiogram / nubbin sign
√ "doughnut" sign = decreased testicular activity with rim hyperemia of dartos perfusion

MRI:

√ enlarged spermatic cord without increase in vascularity
√ whirlpool pattern (twisting of spermatic cord)
√ torsion knot = low-signal-intensity focus at point of twist (displacement of free protons from epicenter of twist)

Chronic Testicular Torsion

√ small atrophied homogeneously hypoechoic testis
√ enlarged echogenic epididymis

TESTICULAR TUMOR

Most common neoplasm in males between ages 15 and 34 years; 1–2% of all cancers in males; 4–6% of all male genitourinary tumors; 1.5% of all childhood malignancies; 4th most common cause of death from malignancy between ages 15–34 years (12%)

Incidence per year: 3–5:100,000; 7,200 new cases in 2001 (100% increase since 1936)

Peak age: 25–35 years and 71–90 years and infants up to 10 years: yolk sac tumor + teratoma

Risk factors:
(1) Prior testicular cancer (20 x risk = 2–5%)
(2) Family history of testicular cancer (6 x risk for 1st-degree relative)
more prevalent in Caucasian race, Jewish religion
(3) Cryptorchidism (10 x risk):
5% for abdominal site, 1.25% for inguinal site
(4) Infertility (0.4–1.1% prevalence of intratubular germ cell neoplasia)
(5) Intersex syndrome: gonadal dysgenesis, true hermaphroditism, pseudohermaphroditism

- painless enlarging testis / mass (most common)
- "heaviness / fullness" in lower abdomen / scrotum
- acute scrotal pain (10%, from intratumoral hemorrhage)
- gynecomastia, virilization

Location: mostly unilateral; contralateral tumor develops eventually in 8%

Metastases: at presentation in 4–14%
(a) lymphatic dissemination
along testicular lymphatic drainage to
- interaortocaval chain at 2nd lumbar vertebra (for right testicular tumor)
- left paraaortic nodes between renal vein, aorta, ureter and inferior mesenteric artery
- along thoracic duct
- left supraclavicular nodes
- lungs

(b) hematogenous dissemination (usually late) to lung, liver, brain, bone
◊ Choriocarcinoma has a proclivity for early hematogenous spread (especially to brain)!

Histo: may be different from that of primary tumor indicating totipotential nature of germ cells

Staging:

Stage I		limited to testis + spermatic cord
Stage II		metastases to lymph nodes below diaphragm
	II A	nonpalpable
	II B	bulky mass
Stage III		metastases to lymph nodes above diaphragm
	III A	confined to lymphatic system
	III B	extranodal metastases

Staging (American Joint Committee on Cancer):

pTX	primary tumor not available (no orchiectomy)
pT0	no primary tumor found
pTis	intratubular germ cell tumor (carcinoma in situ)
pT1	limited to testis + epididymis
pT2	as pT1 + vascular / lymphatic invasion or involvement of tunica vaginalis
pT3	invasion of spermatic cord
pT4	invasion of scrotum

pN0	negative lymph nodes
pN1	node ≤20 mm; or ≤5 nodes involved all <20 mm
pN2	node between 20 and 50 mm; or >5 nodes none >50 mm
pN3	node mass >50 mm

M0	no distant metastasis
M1	distant metastasis

S0	all markers normal
S1	LDH <1.5 x ULM + hCG <5,000mmIU/mL + AFP <1,000 ng/mL
S2	LDH <1.5–10 x ULM ± hCG 5,000–50,000 mIU/mL ± AFP 1,000–10,000 ng/mL
S3	LDH >10 x ULM ± hCG >50,000 mIU/mL ± AFP >10,000 ng/mL

ULM = upper limits of normal

Tumor markers (elevated in 80% at time of diagnosis):

α-fetoprotein:	yolk sac tumors, mixed germ cell tumors with yolk sac elements
β-hCG:	seminoma, choriocarcinoma (tumors containing syncytiotrophoblasts)
LDH:	correlates with bulk of disease (nonspecific as it is produced by multiple organs throughout the body)

Color duplex:
√ tumor <1.5 cm is hypovascular in 86%, >1.6 cm hypervascular in 95% (DDx: orchitis associated with epididymal hyperemia)
√ distortion of vessels

MRI:
√ tumors isointense to testicular parenchyma on T1WI + T2WI

Prognosis: >93% 5-year survival rate for stage I; 85–90% 5-year survival rate for stage II; complete remission under chemotherapy in 65–75%; relapse in 10–20% within 18 months

Rx: inguinal orchiectomy (first-line treatment)

Germ Cell Tumors (95%)

Origin: spermatogenic cells
(a) one histologic type in 65%
- from unipotential gonadal line:
  1. Seminoma
- along a totipotential line forming nonseminatous tumors:
  1. Embryonal carcinoma (largely undifferentiated)
  2. Teratoma (embryonic differentiation)
  3. Yolk sac tumor (extraembryonic differentiation)
  4. Choriocarcinoma (extraembryonic differentiation)

(b) mixed lesion in 35–40%
- from totipotential cells developing along several pathways (embryonal carcinoma being the most common component of mixed lesions)
  1. Teratocarcinoma (= teratoma + embryonal cell carcinoma)

GU

◊ 2nd most common after seminoma, may occasionally undergo spontaneous regression
2. Embryonal cell carcinoma + seminoma
3. Seminoma + teratoma

Growing Teratoma Syndrome
= evolution of mixed germ cell tumor into mature teratoma after chemotherapy (in 40%) followed by interval growth despite maintaining a benign histologic type

mnemonic: "YES CT"
Yolk sac tumor
Embryonal cell carcinoma
Seminoma
Choriocarcinoma
Teratoma

Seminoma *(35–50%)*
◊ Most common tumor in undescended testis!
◊ Most common pure germ cell tumor!
Average age: 40.5 years
Histo: uniform cellular morphology resembles primitive germ cells
Presentation: in 75% limited to testis; in 20% retroperitoneal lymphadenopathy; in 5% extranodal metastases
• serum α-fetoprotein usually normal
• β-hCG elevation in 10–15%
√ usually uniformly hypoechoic + confined within tunica albuginea:
√ lobulated / multiple confluent nodules
√ may be multifocal
√ bilateral in 1–3%, almost always asynchronous
MR:
√ homogeneously hypointense on T2WI
Rx: very sensitive to radiation ± chemotherapy
Prognosis: 10-year survival rate of 75–85%; 19% develop pulmonary metastases

Nonseminomatous Tumor
Age: 20–30 years

EMBRYONAL CELL CARCINOMA (20–25%)
◊ Second most common testicular tumor!
◊ Most common component of mixed germ cell tumors (embryonal cells present in 87%); often associated with teratoma
Histo: primitive anaplastic epithelial cells resembling early embryonic cells
Age: 25–35 years and <2 years

Age Group of Testicular Tumors	
Endodermal sinus tumor / teratoma	1st decade
Choriocarcinoma	2nd + 3rd decade
Embryonal cell carcinoma	3rd decade
Seminoma	4th decade

Spread: most aggressive testicular tumor, visceral metastases
• ± α-fetoprotein elevation
√ hypoechoic mass with heterogeneous areas:
√ ill-defined borders
√ areas of increased echogenicity (hemorrhage)
√ cystic areas (necrosis)
√ may show invasion of tunica albuginea
Rx: less sensitive to radiation
Prognosis: 30–35% 5-year survival rate

TERATOMA (4–10%)
◊ 2nd most common testicular tumor in young boys ≤5 years (75%)
Prevalence: 1:1,000,000
Histo: consists of elements from more than one germ cell layer (keratin, muscle, bone, cartilage, hair, mucous glands, neural tissue)
(a) mature
(b) immature
(c) malignant areas
Age: within first 4 years of life; benign in children; may transform into malignancy in adulthood
• serum α-fetoprotein usually normal
√ well-circumscribed heterogeneous complex mass:
√ anechoic / complex cysts with variable echogenicity (serous, mucoid, keratinous fluid)
√ markedly echogenic components (cartilage, calcification, fibrosis, scar formation)
Prognosis:
variable biologic behavior: benign in prepubertal testes BUT may metastasize in postpubertal testes with nonteratomatous germ cell elements; metastases to lymph nodes, bone, liver in 30% within 5 years

EPIDERMOID CYST / KERATIN CYST OF TESTIS (1%)
= "monodermal dermoid"
= benign teratoma with only ectodermal components / squamous metaplasia of surface mesothelium
Age: 20–40 years; primarily in Whites
Histo: cyst contains keratin debris, wall composed of fibrous tissue + lined by keratinizing stratified squamous epithelium
• painless testicular nodule
• negative tumor marker status
√ sharply circumscribed encapsulated round lesion of 1–3 (range 0.5–10.5) cm in diameter:
√ "onion-skin" / ringed appearance of alternating hypo- and hyperechogenicity (= alternating layers of compacted keratin + loosely arranged desquamated squamous cells):
√ hyperechoic fibrous cyst wall ± shadowing from calcifications / ossification
√ hypoechoic cyst contents (= laminated keratin debris)
√ "target / bull's eye" appearance due to an echogenic center (secondary to compacted keratin / calcification)
√ confined by tunica albuginea

√ diffuse testicular enlargement (10%)
√ no blood flow on Doppler (avascular lesion)
MR:
√ target appearance:
√ fibrous capsule of low signal intensity on T1WI + T2WI
√ cyst content (water and lipid) of high signal intensity on T1WI + T2WI
√ central calcification with center of low signal intensity

Prognosis: no malignant potential
Rx: enucleation + frozen section (to avoid orchiectomy)

CHORIOCARCINOMA (1–3%)

Prevalence: <1% in pure form; 8% in mixed germ cell tumors
Peak age: 20–30 years
Histo: admixture of cytotrophoblastic + syncytiotrophoblastic cells
Spread: may rapidly metastasize (lung, liver, GI tract, brain) without evidence of choriocarcinoma in primary lesion, pulmonary metastases develop in 81%

• symptoms of metastatic disease while primary not yet palpable
• serum β-hCG always elevated (gynecomastia in 10%)

N.B.: Choriocarcinoma has a proclivity for hemorrhage in primary site and metastases!

√ often small tumor of mixed echotexture (hemorrhage, necrosis, calcifications)
√ indistinct margins of pulmonary metastases (due to hemorrhage)

Prognosis: death usually within 1 year of diagnosis; nearly 0–48% 5-year survival rate

YOLK SAC TUMOR = ENDODERMAL SINUS TUMOR

Equivalent to endodermal sinus tumor of ovary
◊ 80% of childhood testicular tumors!
◊ Present in 44% of mixed germ cell tumors of adults

Age: ≤2 years (80%)

• serum α-fetoprotein elevated in >90%

√ nonspecific imaging findings:
√ testicular enlargement without a mass
√ pulmonary metastases (most common site of recurrent disease)

Sex Cord and Stromal Tumors = Interstitial Cell Tumors

Prevalence: 4% of all testicular tumors; 10–30% during childhood

• precocious virilism (children)
• gynecomastia (adults)
• loss of libido (adults)
• impotence (adults)

Rx: orchiectomy; conservative resection under ultrasound guidance
Prognosis: malignant in 10%

Leydig Cell Tumor

Prevalence: 1–3% of all testicular tumors
Origin: interstitial cells forming the fibrovascular stroma
Age: 3–6 years; 20% in patients <10 years; 25% between ages 30 and 50 years; 25% in patients >50 years

• endocrinopathy (in 30%) with secretion of androgens or estrogens by the tumor:
  • precocious virilization
  • gynecomastia (in almost 50%)
  • decreased libido

√ usually small hypoechoic nodule ± cystic areas (from hemorrhage / necrosis)

Prognosis: benign:malignant = 9:1

Sertoli Cell Tumor

Prevalence: <1% of all testicular tumors
Origin: sex cords (derived from Sertoli cells of seminiferous tubules)
Peak age: 1st year of life

• may secrete estrogens (gynecomastia is rare)

√ usually well-circumscribed unilateral round / lobulated hypoechoic nodule
√ multiple bilateral large areas of calcifications in large-cell calcifying Sertoli cell tumors (subtype of pediatric age group)
Associated with: Peutz-Jeghers syndrome, Carney syndrome

Prognosis: benign:malignant = 9:1

Gonadoblastoma

= primitive gonadal stroma tumor (exceedingly rare) containing sex cord-stromal elements + germ cells

• dysgenetic gonads
• abnormal karyotype in 80% (intersex status, phenotypically female)

Nonprimary Testicular Tumors

Metastases to Testis (0.06%)

(a) in adults: prostate > lung > kidney > GI tract, bladder, thyroid, melanoma
◊ More common than germ cell tumors in males >50 years of age!
(b) in children: neuroblastoma, Wilms tumor, rhabdomyosarcoma

√ often multiple and bilateral
√ mostly hypoechoic, occasionally echogenic masses

Lymphoma of Testis

◊ The most common bilateral testicular tumor!

Incidence: 5–6.7% of all testicular tumors; in <1% of patients with lymphoma; most common testicular tumor in men > age 60

Presentation:
(a) primary site of disease
(b) initial manifestation of clinically occult disease
(c) site of recurrent disease

Histo: almost exclusively B-cell lymphoma (most commonly diffuse large cell lymphoma)
Associated with: extranodal involvement of skin, CNS, Waldeyer ring
• painless testicular enlargement
• weight loss, anorexia, fever, weakness (initial complaint in 25%)
Location: bilateral in 38% (metachronous > synchronous)
√ ill-defined diffuse infiltrative process
√ focal hypoechoic mass / masses
√ epididymis + spermatic cord commonly involved
Prognosis: median survival of 13 months; 12–35% 5-year survival

Leukemia of Testis

Incidence:
60–92% on autopsy;
8–16% on clinical examination during therapy;
up to 41% on clinical examination after therapy
◊ Occult testicular tumor often found in patients in bone marrow remission (gonadal barrier = blood-testis barrier to chemotherapy)
√ uni- / bilateral tumors:
√ diffuse / focal
√ hypo- or hyperechoic

Burned-out Tumor of Testis

= AZZOPARDI TUMOR = REGRESSED GERM CELL TUMOR
= widespread metastatic disease + spontaneous regression of testicular malignancy (teratocarcinoma)
Histo: minute amounts of residual tumor / dense deposit of collagen + scattered inflammatory cells
Pathogenesis: tumor with high metabolic rate outgrows its own blood supply
√ small primary tumor:
√ hypoechoic lesion
√ highly echogenic focal lesion (= scarred tumor residue)
√ ± shadowing (= focal calcification)
√ metastases to retroperitoneum, mediastinum, cervical / axillary / supraclavicular lymph nodes, lung, liver

Second Testicular Tumor

Risk for second tumor in cryptorchidism:
15% for inguinal, 30% for abdominal location
Risk for second contralateral tumor:
500–1,000 x ; bilaterality in 1.1–4.4%;
◊ Development interval between 1st + 2nd tumor: 4 months to 25 years
◊ Detected in 47% by 2 years; in 60% by 5 years, in 75% by 10 years
◊ Synchronous contralateral tumor in 1–3%
US: a testicular abnormality is malignant in only 50%!

TRANSITIONAL CELL CARCINOMA

Prevalence: 85% of all urothelial tumors / primary renal pelvic tumors; 7% of all renal neoplasms
Mean age: 68 years; M:F = 2.7:1; Whites > Blacks
Pathogenesis: chemical carcinogens act locally on epithelium (= field of change), action enhanced by length of contact time (eg, stasis / diverticulum)
Risk factors:
(1) tobacco (2–3 x)
(2) aniline dye, benzidine, aromatic amines, azo dyes in textile, rubber, petroleum, printing, plastic manufacturing (lag time of 10 years)
(3) cyclophosphamide therapy (lag time of 6.5 years)
(4) analgesic abuse (8 x increase): phenacetin
(5) Balkan nephritis (= progressive renal failure + development of bilateral and multiple tumors)
(6) recurrent / chronic urinary tract infection
(7) high amounts of coffee consumption
Classification:
(a) papillary lesion (85%) with predominantly exophytic growth = frondlike structure with central fibrovascular core lined by epithelial layer
– broad based
– pedunculated
(b) infiltrating: usually higher grade + less common
(c) carcinoma in situ
Grade: usually correlates with stage
1 = cells slightly anaplastic
2 = intermediate features
3 = marked cellular pleomorphism
Metastases: regional lymph nodes, peritoneum, liver

SYNCHRONOUS TCC
(a) both renal pelves (in 1–2%)
(b) both ureters (in 2–9%)
(c) bladder – in 24% of primary renal pelvic involvement
– in 39% of primary ureteral involvement
– in 2% of primary bladder involvement
• frank / microscopic painless hematuria (72%)
• dull flank pain (22%)
• acute renal colic (due to obstruction)
Location: bladder 30–50 x more common than upper urinary tract

Renal and Ureteral TCC

Staging:

TNM	AJCC	Description
Tis	0	in situ lesion
Ta	...	noninvasive papillary carcinoma
T1	I	invasion of subepithelial connective tissue
T2	II	confined to muscularis layer
T3	III	invasion of renal parenchyma / peripelvic soft tissues
T4	IV	extension beyond renal capsule

@ Kidney
METACHRONOUS TCC IN UPPER TRACT
(a) in 12% of pelvic + ureteral primaries (within 25 months)

(b) in 4% of bladder primaries (2/3 within 2 years, up to 20 years later)

Site: extrarenal part of renal pelvis > infundibulocaliceal region

IVP:
- √ single / multiple sessile / pedunculated mulberry-like filling defects in renal pelvis (35%):
  - √ "stipple sign" = contrast material trapped in interstices (DDx: blood clot, fungus ball)
- √ dilated calyx with filling defect (26%) due to partial / complete obstruction of infundibulum:
  - √ "phantom calyx" = failure to opacify from obstruction
  - √ ± focal delayed increasingly dense nephrogram
  - √ "oncocalyx" = caliceal distension with tumor
- √ caliceal amputation (19%)
- √ absent / decreased excretion with renal atrophy (13%) due to long-standing obstruction of ureteropelvic junction
- √ hydronephrosis with renal enlargement (6%) due to tumor obstruction of ureteropelvic junction
- √ infiltrative invasion of renal parenchyma maintaining a bean-shaped kidney

US:
- √ bulky hypoechoic (similar to renal parenchyma) / hyperechoic mass lesion
- √ infiltrative without disruption of renal contour
- √ splitting / separation of central renal sinus complex
- √ ± caliectasis without pelviectasis

CT (52% accuracy due to overstaging):
- √ sessile filling defect in opacified collecting system
- √ thickening + induration of pelvicaliceal wall
- √ central solid mass in renal pelvis expanding centrifugally
  - √ obliteration / compression of renal sinus fat
- √ invasion of renal parenchyma (infiltrating growth pattern) with preservation of renal contour
- √ coarse punctate calcific deposits (0.7–6.7%) may mimic urinary calculi
- √ variable enhancement of tumor

@ Ureter

Site: lower 1/3 (70%), mid 1/3 (15%), upper 1/3 (15%)

IVP:
- √ nonfunctioning kidney in advanced tumor (46%)
- √ hydronephrosis ± hydroureter (34%)
- √ single / multiple ureteral filling defects (19%)
- √ irregular narrowing of ureteral lumen

Retrograde:
- √ "champagne glass" / "chalice" / "goblet sign" = focal expansion of ureter around + distal to mass (probably secondary to to-and-fro peristalsis of mass)
- √ "Bergman sign" = "catheter-coiling sign" = coiling of catheter on retrograde catheterization below the mass

CT:
- √ intraluminal soft-tissue mass
- √ eccentric / circumferential thickening of ureteral wall

Dx: cytologic analysis of urine (selective lavage, ureteral urine collection, brush biopsy, ureteroscopy

DDx: papilloma (benign lesion, fronds lined by normal epithelium)

Prognosis: 77–80% 5-year survival rate without invasion of muscularis mucosa; 5% 5-year survival rate with invasion of muscularis mucosa

Bladder TCC

Incidence: 50,000 new cases annually; 5% of all new malignant neoplasms; most common tumor of genitourinary tract; 2% of all cancer deaths in United States

Staging

T 1 =	A	= lesions involving mucosa + submucosa
T 2 =	B1	= invasion of superficial muscle layer
T 3a =	B2	= invasion of deep muscular wall
T 3b =	C	= invasion of perivesical fat
T 4a =	D1	= extension to perivesical organs (seminal vesicles, prostate, rectum)
T4b		= invasion of pelvic / abdominal wall
	D2	= distant metastases

Staging accuracy: 50% clinically; 32–80% for CT; 73% for MRI

Overstaging due to: edema following endoscopy / endoscopic resection, fibrosis from radiation therapy

Histo: 80% low-stage superficial papillary neoplasm, (multifocal in 1/3), becoming invasive in 10–20%; 20% invasive (almost always solitary)

Site: lateral wall of bladder, bladder diverticulum (in 0.8–10.8%)

METACHRONOUS TCC OF BLADDER
(a) in 23–40% of primary renal TCC after 15–48 months
(b) in 20–50% of primary ureteral TCC after 10–24 months

IVP (70% accuracy rate):
- √ irregular filling defect with broad base and fronds (DDx: rectal gas marginated by Simpson's white line)
- √ <1% calcified

CT / US:
- √ focal wall thickening
- √ papillary mass protruding into lumen

MR (staging modality of choice):
- √ TCC isointense to bladder muscle on T1WI + hyperintense on T2WI
- √ enhancement differentiates between early enhancing mucosa, submucosa, tumor + nonenhancing muscle

Prognosis: 40–70% recurrence rate

GU

TRAUMA TO KIDNEY

Incidence: 10% of injuries in emergency department

Indications for imaging:

(1) Penetrating injury + hematuria
(2) Blunt trauma + hematuria + hypotension <90 mm Hg
(3) Microscopic hematuria + positive peritoneal lavage
(4) Blunt trauma + known association with renal injury (contusion / hematoma of flank, fracture of lower ribs, fracture of transverse processes, fracture of thoracolumbar spine)

Classification:

I. MINOR RENAL INJURY (75–85%)
√ no / limited perinephric hematoma
DDx: respiratory motion artifact (low-attenuation area surrounding kidney)
√ no extravasation of urine (= no caliceal disruption)

1. Intrarenal hemorrhage / hematoma = **renal contusion**
√ hyperattenuating area of 40–70 HU (= acute clotted blood) on NECT
√ sharply / poorly defined round / ovoid area of decreased enhancement during CECT (DDx: renal infarction with no enhancement)
√ focal area of striation on delayed nephrogram
√ area of persistent contrast material staining on very delayed scan
2. **Subcapsular hematoma**
√ round / lenticular-shaped fluid collection + flattening of subjacent parenchyma
3. **Perinephric hematoma** without extension to collecting system / medulla
√ defects in periphery of renal parenchyma
√ ± limited perinephric hematoma with attenuation values of 45–90 HU
◊ Subcapsular / perinephric hematoma usually proportional to extent of injury
4. **Small subsegmental cortical infarc**t
Cause: stretching + thrombotic occlusion of accessory renal artery / capsular artery / segmental artery
√ sharply demarcated wedge-shaped area of decreased contrast enhancement
Rx: observation

II. MAJOR RENAL LACERATION (10%)
= complete **cortical laceration** / fracture extending to medulla ± collecting system

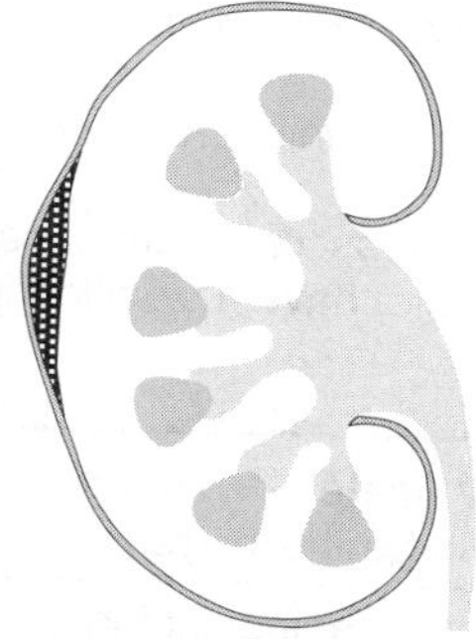

Grade 1
Subcapsular Hematoma

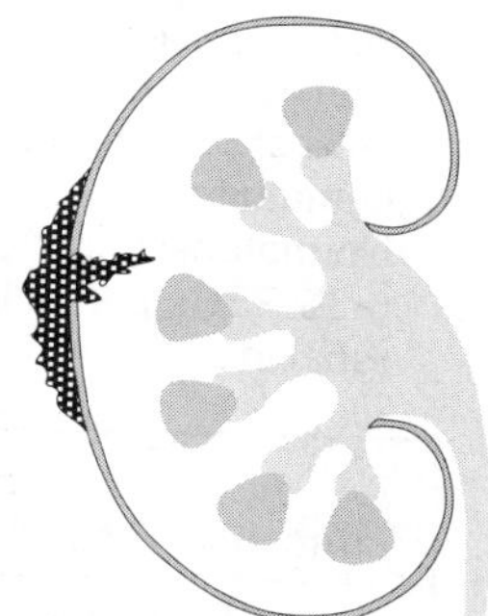

Grade 2
***Superficial* Renal *Laceration* with Perirenal Hematoma**

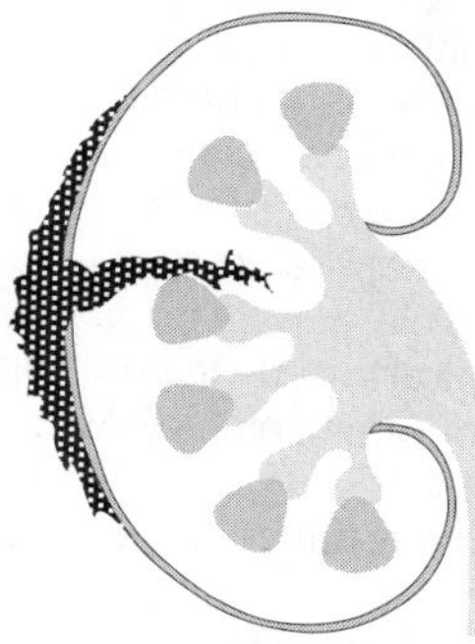

Grade 3
***Deep* Renal *Laceration* without Extension into Collecting System**

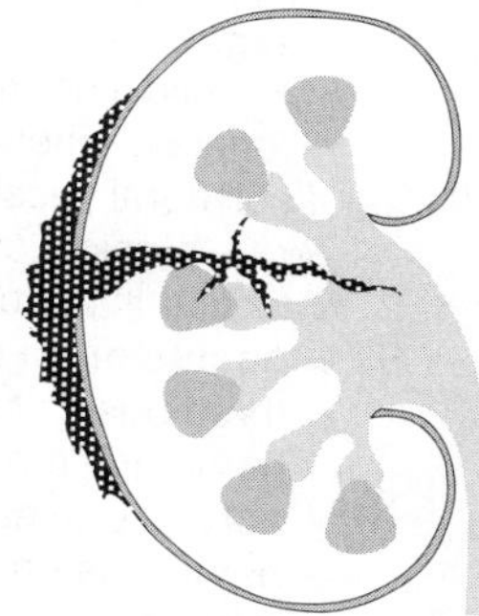

Grade 4
Deep Laceration with Extension *into Collecting System*

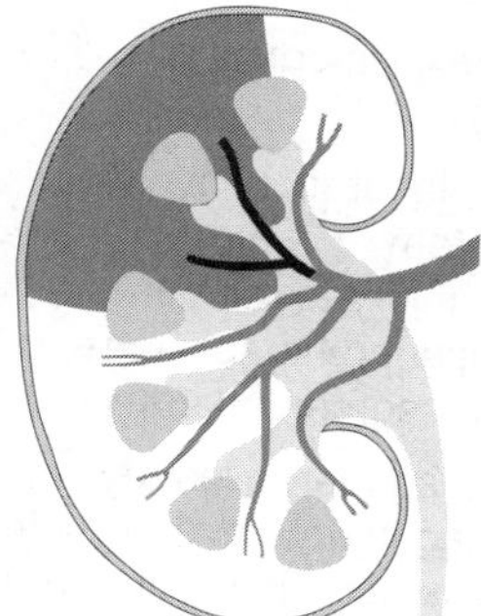

Grade 4
***Thrombosis of Segmental Artery Branch* with Infarction**

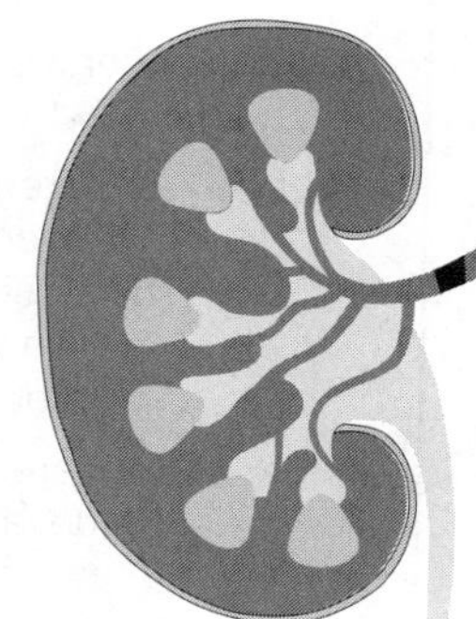

Grade 5
Traumatic *Occlusion of Main Renal Artery* from Intimal Injury

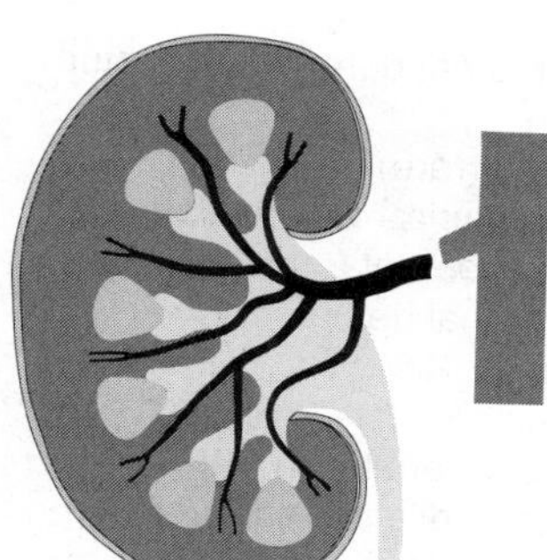

Grade 5
Renal Artery Avulsion

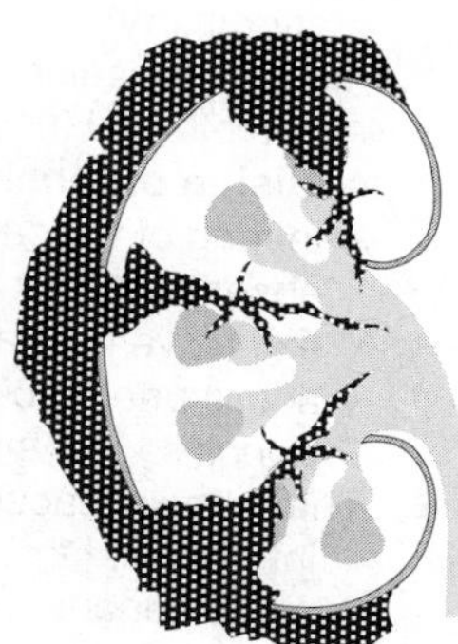

Grade 5
Shattered Kidney

Renal Trauma Grading System (American Association of Surgeons in Trauma)

√ laceration connecting two cortical surfaces = **renal fracture** = separation of renal poles
√ ± devascularization of renal parenchyma
(a) without involvement of collecting system:
  √ nonenhancing deep parenchymal cleft filled with hematoma on CECT
  √ perirenal hematoma from capsular disruption
(b) with involvement of collecting system:
  √ urine extravasation of contrast material on delayed images 3–5 minutes after injection
(c) active hemorrhage / pseudoaneurysm:
  ◊ Hemodynamic decompensation may be imminent in 38%!
  √ intense contrast enhancement within a laceration / hematoma during early phase:
    √ linear / flamelike contrast extravasation of 80–370 HU or within 10–15 HU of aortic density

Rx: variable (clinical judgement required)

III. CATASTROPHIC RENAL INJURY (5%)
√ extravasation of contrast material with patchy areas of 85–370 HU (= active bleeding)
1. Multiple renal lacerations = **shattered kidney**
   √ multiple separate renal fragments
   √ lack of enhancement of part of kidney (due to segmental renal arterial infarctions)
   √ ± cortical rim nephrogram (= enhancement of renal periphery through intact capsular / collateral vessels)
   Rx: surgical exploration / nephrectomy
2. Vascular injury of renal pedicle
   = **occlusion of main renal artery** by intimal flap; thrombosis / laceration of renal vein is RARE
   • hematuria may be absent
   √ abrupt termination of main renal artery just beyond its origin
   √ minimal hematoma around proximal renal a.
   √ absence of perinephric hematoma (HALLMARK)
   √ absent nephrogram on affected side
   √ retrograde opacification of ipsilateral renal vein
   √ cortical rim nephrogram (develops >8 hours after injury)
   Rx: revascularization procedure (in 14% return of renal function)
3. **Avulsion of renal artery** (rare)
   = tearing of tunica muscularis + adventitia
   √ absent contrast enhancement (= global infarct)
   √ extensive medial perirenal hematoma
   √ active arterial bleeding
   Prognosis: life-threatening
4. Thrombosis / laceration of renal vein (rare)
   √ intraluminal thrombus in dilated renal vein
   √ acute venous hypertension:
     √ nephromegaly
     √ diminished nephrogram
     √ delayed nephrographic progression
     √ decreased excretion

IV. INJURY OF THE UPJ (rare)
= laceration (= incomplete tear in 60%) / avulsion (= complete transection) of ureter at UPJ

Mechanism: tension on renal pedicle by sudden deceleration
Age: usually young boys
Associated with: fracture of transverse process (30%)
• gross / microscopic hematuria (53–60%)
N.B.: delayed images to check for urine leak!
√ massive extravasation of contrast material medially in the region of UPJ
√ nonfilling of affected ureter (with avulsion)
√ ± circumferential perinephric urinoma

Cx: posttraumatic renovascular hypertension

Blunt Trauma to Kidney

Incidence: 80–90% of all renal injuries
Cause: motor vehicle accident, contact sports, falls, fights, assaults
Mechanism: direct blow (>80%) often lacerated by lower ribs, acceleration-deceleration (renal artery tear)
Associated with: other organ injury in 75%
• >95% hematuria (>5 RBCs per high-power field):
  N.B.: poor correlation between severity of hematuria + severity of renal injury
  ◊ 25% of patients with gross hematuria have significant injuries!
  ◊ 24% of patients with renal pedicle injury have no hematuria!
  ◊ Normotensive patients with microscopic hematuria (<35 RBCs per high-power field) have a significant renal injury in <0.2%!

Renal Injury Scale (American Association of Surgeons in Trauma)	
Grade 1	hematuria + normal imaging findings; renal contusion; nonexpanding subcapsular hematoma
Grade 2	laceration of cortex (<1 cm deep); nonexpanding perirenal hematoma
Grade 3	laceration of cortex + medulla (>1 cm deep)
Grade 4	(a) parenchyma: laceration involving collecting system (b) vessel injury: injury to renal artery / vein with contained hemorrhage; thrombosis of segmental artery
Grade 5	(a) parenchyma: shattered kidney (b) devascularizing injury: avulsion / in situ thrombosis of main renal artery

Location: simultaneous upper + lower GU tract injury in <5%
Rx: The only absolute indication for surgery is life-threatening active bleeding! Urine leaks will close spontaneously in 87%!

GU

Penetrating Renal Trauma

Incidence: 10–20% of all renal trauma
Cause: gunshot, shrapnel, stab wound
Associated with: multiorgan injuries in 80%
Cx: "bullet colic", "buckshot colic", "birdshot calculus" = ureteral obstruction 2° to migrating missiles

Blunt Trauma to Urinary Bladder

Associated with: pelvic fracture in 70%
Indications for urethrogram:
- blood at urethral meatus
- "floating" prostate
- inability to pass Foley catheter

√ symphysis diastasis

CT cystogram:
√ focal thickening of bladder wall = contusion
√ contrast extravasation

Bladder Contusion *(most common injury)*

= intramural hematoma
√ no extravasation
√ lack of normal distensibility
√ crescent-shaped filling defect in contrast-distended bladder

Interstitial Bladder Injury *(uncommon)*

= bladder tear without serosal involvement

Bladder Rupture

Cystography: diagnostic in >85%; false-negatives if tear sealed by hematoma / mesentery

Extraperitoneal Rupture of Bladder (80%)

Cause: pelvic fracture (sharp bony spicule) or avulsion tear at fixation points of puboprostatic ligaments
Location: usually close to base of bladder anterolaterally
Plain film:
√ "pear-shaped" bladder
√ loss of obturator fat planes
√ paralytic ileus
√ upward displacement of ileal loops
Contrast examination:
√ flame-shaped contrast extravasation into perivesical fat, best seen on postvoid films, may extend into thigh / anterior abdominal wall
US:
√ "bladder within a bladder" = bladder surrounded by fluid collection

Intraperitoneal Rupture of Bladder (20–30%)

Cause:
(a) usually as a result of invasive procedure (cystoscopy), stab wound, surgery
(b) blunt trauma with sudden rise in intravesical pressure (requires distended bladder)
Location: usually at dome of bladder
√ contrast extravasation into paracolic gutters
√ contrast outlining small bowel loops
√ uriniferous ascites

Combined Intra- and Extraperitoneal Rupture (5%)

TUBERCULOSIS

Urogenital tract is the second most common site after lung; almost always affects the kidney first as a hematogenous focus from lung / bone / GI tract
Age: usually before age 50; M > F
Path: organisms lodge in the periglomerular capillaries; breakdown in host immunity results in extensive necrosis + fibrosis (coalescing cortical granulomas); organisms spill down the nephrons and become trapped in the narrow segment of the loop of Henle forming ulcerocavernous papillary lesions, which erode into collecting system
Spread:
(a) contiguous: from renal parenchyma along urothelium to infundibula, renal pelvis, ureter, bladder
(b) hematogenous (rare): epididymis, testis
◊ It is unusual for genitourinary sites to be affected without involvement of kidney first!

- gross / microscopic hematuria
- "sterile" pyuria
- frequency, urgency, dysuria
- history of previous clinical TB (25%) with a lag time of 2–20 years

IVP (abnormal in 85–90%):
@ EXTRARENAL SIGNS ON ABDOMINAL PLAIN FILM
√ osseous / paraspinous changes of TB (diskitis + psoas abscess)
√ calcified granulomas in liver, spleen, lymph nodes, adrenals
@ RENAL TUBERCULOSIS
◊ Renal TB in 5–10% of patients with pulmonary TB!
◊ Radiographic evidence of pulmonary TB in <50% of patients with renal TB (only 5% have active cavitary TB)!
Location: unilateral renal involvement in 75%
√ <u>renal size</u>: enlarged (early) / small (late) / normal (most common):
√ "putty kidney" = tuberculous pyonephrosis from ureteral stricture
√ autonephrectomy = small shrunken scarred nonfunctioning kidney ± dystrophic calcifications
√ cortical scars, often associated with parenchymal calcifications:
√ distortion of collecting system due to adjacent cortical scarring
√ displacement of collecting system secondary to tuberculoma of low attenuation (initial infection)
√ "moth-eaten calyx" = "smudged" papillae = irregular feathery appearance of surface of papilla due to erosion (earliest sign)
√ <u>cavities</u> communicating with collecting system:
√ irregular tract formations from calyx into papilla
√ large irregular cavities with extensive destruction
√ blunted dilated calyces = papillary necrosis

√ strictures of infundibula / renal pelvis:
- √ dilated calices (hydrocalicosis) often with sharply defined circumferential narrowing (infundibular strictures) at one / several sites (most common finding)
- √ caliceal truncation
- √ "phantom calyx" / amputated calyx = incomplete visualization of calyx due to infundibular stenosis
- √ reduced capacity of renal pelvis
- √ Kerr kink = kinking of renal pelvis
- √ mural thickening of collecting system

√ dystrophic amorphous parenchymal calcifications in tuberculomas (in 25%): amorphous / granular / curvilinear / punctate / confluent ("toothpaste") / involving entire kidney ("putty kidney"):
- √ nephrolithiasis (in 10%)

√ globally poor renal function

√ infection may extend into peri- / pararenal space + psoas

@ URETERAL TUBERCULOSIS

Incidence: in 50% of genitourinary TB; always with evidence of renal involvement as it spreads from kidney

Location: either end of ureter (most commonly distal 1/3), usually asymmetric, may be unilateral

√ ureteral filling defects (due to mucosal granulomas)

√ "saw-tooth ureter" = irregular jagged contour secondary to dilatation (from ureterovesical junction obstruction) + multiple small mucosal ulcerations + wall edema (early changes)

√ strictures (late changes):

"beaded ureter" = alternating areas of strictures + dilatations

"corkscrew ureter" = marked tortuosity with strictures + dilatations

"pipestem ureter" = rigid aperistaltic foreshortened thick and straight ureter

√ vesicoureteral reflux through "fixed" patulous orifice

√ ureteral calcifications uncommon (usually in distal portion)

CT:
- √ thickening of ureteral wall with periureteric inflammation

@ BLADDER TUBERCULOSIS

Infection from renal source causing interstitial cystitis

√ thickened bladder wall (= muscle hypertrophy + inflammatory tuberculomas)

√ filling defects (due to multiple granulomas)

√ bladder wall ulcerations

√ "shrunken bladder" = scarred bladder with diminished capacity

√ "thimble bladder" = diminutive irregular bladder

√ bladder wall calcifications (rare)

Cx: fistula / sinus tract / vesicoureteral reflux (due to fibrosis of ureteral orifice)

@ MALE GENITAL TUBERCULOSIS

√ calcifications in 10% (diabetes more common cause)

(1) Tuberculous prostatitis / prostatic abscess:
- √ hypoechoic irregular area in peripheral zone
- √ hypoattenuating prostatic lesion
- √ hypointense diffuse radiating streaky areas on T2WI (= "watermelon sign")
- √ peripheral enhancement

(2) Tuberculous epididymitis
ascending / descending route of infection

(3) Tuberculous orchitis
direct extension from epididymal infection, rarely from hematogenous spread

DDx: brucellosis, fungal infections (identical picture)

@ FEMALE GENITAL TUBERCULOSIS

(1) Salpingitis (94%): mostly bilateral

(2) Tuboovarian abscess: extension into extraperitoneal compartment

UNICALICEAL (UNIPAPILLARY) KIDNEY

Path: OLIGOMEGANEPHRONIA = reduced number of nephrons and enlargement of glomeruli

Associated with: absence of contralateral kidney, other anomalies

- hypertension
- proteinuria
- azotemia

URACHAL ANOMALIES

urachus = median umbilical ligament = thick fibrous cord as the remnant of the allantois (= endodermal outgrowth from yolk sac into stalk), which regresses at 5th month of development

Cx: infection (23%), intestinal obstruction, hemorrhage into cyst, peritonitis from rupture, malignant degeneration

Alternating Sinus

= cystic dilatation of urachus periodically emptying into bladder / umbilicus

Patent Urachus

= fistula between bladder and umbilicus

Incidence: 1:200,000 live births

- urine draining from umbilicus

Urachal Cyst (30%)

= gradually enlarging cyst due to closure of both ends of urachus

Incidence: 1:5,000 (at autopsy)

- asymptomatic in children unless rupture occurs
- symptomatic in adults due to enlargement / infection

√ cystic extraperitoneal mass

Urachal Diverticulum (3%)

= urachus communicates only with bladder dome

Urachal Sinus

= urachus patent only at umbilicus

Associated with: urachal cyst

- umbilical mass / inflammation ± drainage

√ thickened tubular structure with echogenic center

GU

URACHAL CARCINOMA

= rare tumor arising from the urachus (vestigial remnant of cloaca + allantois) within space of Retzius

Incidence: 0.01% of all adult cancers; 0.22–0.34% of all bladder cancers; 20–40% of all primary bladder adenocarcinomas

Cause: epithelial metaplasia in urachal remnant

Histo:

(a) adenocarcinoma (84–90%), in 75% mucin producing
◊ 34% of all bladder adenocarcinomas are urachal in origin

(b) TCC (3%), sarcoma, squamous cell carcinoma
◊ 75% of urachal neoplasms in patients <20 years of age are sarcomas!

Age: 41–70 years; M:F = 3:1

- suprapubic mass, abdominal pain
- hematuria (71%)
- discharge of blood, pus, mucus from umbilicus
- irritative voiding symptoms
- mucous micturition (25%)

Stage:

I cancer limited to urachus
II invasion limited to urachus
III A local invasion of bladder
B invasion of abdominal wall
C invasion of peritoneum
D invasion of other viscera
IV A metastases to local lymph nodes
B distant metastases (liver)

Location: supravesical, midline, anterior (80%), in space of Retzius (bounded by transversalis fascia ventrally + peritoneum dorsally)

√ mass anterosuperior to vesical dome with predominantly muscular / extravesical involvement
√ invasion of bladder dome (88%)
√ low-attenuation mass in 60% (mucin)
√ often peripheral curvilinear / psammomatous PATHOGNOMONIC calcifications (50–70%)
√ markedly increased signal intensity on T2WI

Prognosis: 7–16% 5-year survival rate

URETERAL DUPLICATION

= RENAL DUPLICATION

Complete Duplication of Ureter

Cause: second ureteral bud arising from mesonephric duct leading to complete ureteral duplication

Prevalence: 0.2% of live births; M:F = 1:2; in 15–40% bilateral

Risk of recurrence: 12% in 1st-degree relatives

Embryology: ureters develop from separate ureteric buds originating from a single Wolffian duct

Weigert-Meyer rule

(a) lower moiety ureter
drains lower pole and interpolar portion; is incorporated into developing bladder first, ascends during bladder growth + enters bladder at trigone;

(b) upper moiety ureter
remains with wolffian duct longer, passes through bladder wall + inserts ectopic inferior and medial to lower moiety ureter below the level of the trigone / into any wolffian duct derivative

Cx:
(1) Vesicoureteral reflux (most commonly)
(2) Ectopic ureteral insertion
(3) Ectopic ureterocele
(4) Ureteropelvic junction obstruction of lower pole

UPPER MOIETY URETER

◊ Subject to ureteral obstruction from ectopic ureteral insertion / ectopic ureterocele / aberrant artery crossing!

Associated with: significant renal dysplasia

Site of insertion of ectopic ureter

M: suprasphincteric insertion:
low in bladder, bladder neck, prostatic urethra, vas deferens, seminal vesicle (seminal vesical cyst), ejaculatory duct
- NO ENURESIS in males as insertion is always above external sphincter
- epididymitis / orchitis in preadolescent male
- urge incontinence (insertion into posterior urethra)

F: infrasphincteric insertion:
distal urethra, vaginal vestibule, vagina, cervix, uterus, fallopian tube, rectum
- WETTING in upright females if insertion is below external sphincter (common)
- intermittent / constant dribbling

LOWER MOIETY URETER

◊ Subject to vesicoureteral reflux due to its shortened ureteral tunnel at bladder insertion!

Cx: lower pole of duplex kidney may atrophy (in 50%) secondary to chronic pyelonephritis from reflux nephropathy (= reflux ± infection)
√ clubbed calyces underneath focal scars

√ renal enlargement
√ tortuous dilated lower pole ureter

US:
√ two separate echodense renal sinuses + pelves separated by parenchymal bridge

IVP:
√ poor / nonvisualization of upper pole collecting system (delayed films):
√ "drooping lily sign" = hydronephrosis + decreased function of obstructed upper pole moiety causing downward displacement of lower pole calyces
√ lateral + downward displacement of lower pole collecting system + ureter:
√ "nubbin sign" = scarring, atrophy, and decreased function of lower pole moiety may simulate a renal mass
√ displacement of proximal orifice upward

VCUG:
√ ureterocele
√ reflux into lower moiety (rare)

GU

Incomplete / Partial Duplication of Ureter

= branching of single ureteral bud (common distal ureter + one ureteral orifice) before reaching metanephric blastema

Prevalence: in 0.6% of urograms

Associated with: ureteropelvic junction obstruction of lower renal pole

√ bifid ureter (in early branching)
√ bifid pelvis (in late branching)
√ ureteroureteral reflux = "yo-yo" / "saddle" / "seesaw" peristalsis = urine moves down the cephalad ureter + refluxes up the lower pole ureter and vice versa
√ asymmetric dilatation of one ureteral segment
√ upper pole ureter may end blindly (seen on retrograde injection only)

Cx: urinary tract infections

URETEROCELE

= cystic ectasia of subepithelial segment of intravesical ureter

Prevalence: 1:5,000 to 1:12,000 children

IVP:
√ early filling of bulbous terminal ureter ("cobra head")
√ radiolucent halo (= ureteral wall + adjacent bladder urothelium)

VCUG:
√ round / oval lucent defect near trigone
√ effacement with increased bladder distension
√ ± eversion during voiding

Simple Ureterocele

= ORTHOTOPIC URETEROCELE
= congenital prolapse of dilated distal ureter + orifice into bladder lumen at the usual location of the trigone, typically seen with single ureter

Presentation: incidental finding in adults; M:F = 2:3; bilateral in 33%

Cx:
(1) Pyelocaliceal dilatation
(2) Prolapse into bladder neck / urethra causing obstruction (rare)
(3) Wall thickening secondary to edema from impacted stone / infection

Ectopic Ureterocele

= ureteral bud arising in an abnormal cephalad position from the mesonephric duct and moving caudally resulting in an ureteral orifice distal to trigone within / outside bladder

Incidence: in 10% bilateral

(a) in single nonduplicated system (20%)
M:F = 1:1
• hypoplastic / absent ipsilateral trigone
√ poorly visualized / nonvisualized kidney
√ small / poorly functioning kidney

(b) in upper moiety ureter of duplex kidney (80%)
M:F = 1:4–1:8

Cx:
(1) Bladder outlet obstruction (from ectopic ureterocele prolapsing into bladder neck / urethra)
(2) Contralateral ureteral obstruction (if ectopic ureterocele large)
(3) Multicystic dysplastic kidney (the further the orifice from normal site of insertion, the more dysplastic the kidney!)

Pseudoureterocele

= obstruction of an otherwise normal intramural ureter mimicking ureterocele

Cause:
(a) Tumor
bladder tumor (most common in adults), invasion by cervical cancer, pheochromocytoma of intravesical ureter
(b) Edema
from impacted ureteral calculus (most common in children), radiation cystitis, following ureteral instrumentation, schistosomiasis

√ thick, irregular halo in urinary bladder
√ "cobra head" / "spring onion" appearance of distal ureter
√ NO protrusion of ureter into bladder lumen (oblique views + cystoscopy normal)

URETEROPELVIC JUNCTION OBSTRUCTION

Most common cause of fetal / neonatal hydronephrosis

Cause:
A. Primary UPJ obstruction
(a) intrinsic cause
primarily functional (= adynamic segment) with impaired formation of urine bolus
(1) replacement of UPJ muscle by excessive collagen
(2) abnormal arrangement of junction muscles causing dysmotility (69%)
(3) abnormal intercellular conduction
(4) high ureteral insertion
(5) mucosal folds in upper ureter
(b) extrinsic cause
(1) aberrant vessels to lower pole (in 25–39% of adult patients): anterior to UPJ (90–95%), posterior to UPJ (5–10%)
(2) fixed kinks / angulation
(3) adventitial bands
(4) renal cyst
(5) aortic aneurysm
B. Secondary UPJ obstruction
(1) infection: eosinophilic ureteritis, XGP
(2) stones
(3) ischemia
(4) iatrogenic injury

Associated anomalies (27%):
vesicoureteral reflux, bilateral ureteral duplication, bilateral obstructed megaureter, contralateral nonfunctioning kidney, contralateral renal agenesis, meatal stenosis, hypospadia

M:F = 5:1

• abdominal mass, abdominal pain, hematuria, UTI

Location: left > right side; bilateral (10–40%)

GU

√ large dilated anechoic renal pelvis communicating with calyces, no dilatation of ureter

IVP:
- √ sharply defined narrowing at UPJ
- √ pelvicaliectasis without ureterectasis
- √ anterior rotation of pelvis
- √ broad tangential sharply defined extrinsic compression (in arterial crossing)
- √ longitudinal striae of redundant mucosa (in dehydrated state)
- √ late changes: unilateral renal enlargement, diminished opacification, wasting of kidney substance

NUC: confirm obstruction at UPJ + determine function

OB-US:
- √ enlargement of renal pelvis + branching infundibula + calyces
- √ anteroposterior diameter of renal pelvis ≥10 mm
- √ large unilocular fluid collection (severely dilated collecting system)

DDx: multicystic dysplastic kidney, perinephric urinoma

ADDITIONAL TESTS:
(1) Diuresis excretory urography (Whitfield): accurate in 85%
(2) Diuresis renography (Iodine-131-iodohippurate sodium / Tc-99m-DTPA)
(3) Pressure flow urodynamic study (Whitaker)

Rx: early surgical correction may be needed to preserve renal function

URETHRAL DIVERTICULUM

Age: 26–74 years; 6 x more common in black women
- urinary incontinence (9–32–70%)
- asymptomatic (3–20%)

Congenital Urethral Diverticulum

Cause: ectopic cloacal epithelium; M > F

Acquired Urethral Diverticulum

Prevalence: 0.6–6%; M < F

Cause:
(1) obstruction of paraurethral glands (of Skene) with subsequent infection + rupture into urethra
(2) trauma: catheterization / childbirth

May be associated with: cloacal epithelium, wolffian / müllerian duct remnant

Site: posterolateral aspect of midurethra
- vague urinary tract symptoms mimicking chronic / interstitial cystitis, carcinoma in situ of the bladder, detrusor instability
- dyspareunia
- tender cystic swelling protruding from anterior wall of vagina + expulsion of purulent material
- dribbling after voiding
- frequency / urgency (67%), dysuria (45%)
- recurrent urinary tract infections (40%)

Voiding cystourethrography (65% accurate):
- √ rounded / elongated sac connected to urethra

MR:
- √ multiseptated cystic lesion surrounding urethra
- √ heterogenous hyperintense signal compared with urine on T1WI / fluid-fluid levels on T2WI if inflammation present

Cx:
(1) Infection
(2) Stone formation (in up to 10%)
(3) Malignant degeneration (5% of all urethral carcinomas)

DDx:
(1) Vaginal cyst (Gartner duct cyst, paramesonephric cyst, müllerian duct cyst, epithelial inclusion cyst)
(2) Ectopic ureterocele
(3) Endometrioma
(4) Urethral tumor

URETHRAL TRAUMA

Incidence: in 4–17% of pelvic fractures in males, in <1% of pelvic fractures in females

Associated with: bladder injury in 20%

Types:

I = separation of puboprostatic ligament with craniad displacement of prostate (least common)
- √ elongated narrowed urethra
- √ elevation of bladder (displacement by hematoma)

II = urethral rupture at prostatomembranous junction above urogenital diaphragm
- √ contrast extravasation into true pelvis

III = rupture of proximal bulbous urethra below the urogenital diaphragm (most common injury)
- √ contrast extravasation into perineum ± scrotum

Cx:
(1) Urethral stricture (38–100%)
(2) Impotence (in up to 40%)
(3) Incontinence (30%)

URINOMA

= uriniferous perirenal pseudocyst secondary to tear in collecting system with continuing renal function

Etiology:
(a) nonobstructive: blunt / penetrating trauma, surgery, infection, calculus erosion
(b) obstructive:
  (1) ureteral obstruction (calculus, surgical ligature, neoplasm)
  (2) bladder outlet obstruction (posterior urethral valves)

◊ Augmented by sudden diuretic load of urographic contrast material!

Path: fibroblastic cavity (in 5–12 days), dense connective tissue encapsulation (in 3–6 weeks)
- malaise, nausea, fever
- hematuria (10–50%)
- fluctuant tender mass

Location:
- √ cystic mass in perirenal space = **localized perirenal urinoma** (most common)
- √ cystic mass filling entire perirenal space = **diffuse perirenal urinoma**
- √ sickle-shaped collection = **subcapsular urinoma**

GU

√ encapsulated expanding intrarenal cystic mass separating renal tissue fragments = **intrarenal urinoma**

Plain radiography:
- √ soft-tissue mass obliterating retroperitoneal structures
- √ superior + lateral displacement of kidney

CT:
- √ extravasation of contrast material
- √ smooth thin-walled cavity (−10 to +30 HU)
- √ frequently associated with urine ascites

Cx: retroperitoneal fibrosis, stricture of upper ureter, perinephric abscess
◊ Renal dysplasia of affected kidney in almost 100% when detected in utero!

Dx: aspirated fluid with high urea concentration

DDx: lymphocele, hematoma, abscess, renal cyst, pancreatic pseudocyst, ascites

UROLITHIASIS

= NEPHROLITHIASIS

◊ Most common cause of calcification within the kidney:
- ◊ 12% of population develop a renal stone by age 70
- ◊ 2–3% of population experience an attack of acute renal colic during their lifetime
- ◊ Patients with acute flank pain have ureteral calculi in 67–95%

Annual incidence: 1–2:1,000; M:F = 4:1

Peak age: onset in 3rd decade

Formation theory:

Anderson-Carr-Randall theory of renal stone formation: in the presence of abnormally high calcium excretion exceeding lymphatic capacity, microaggregates of calcium (present in the normal kidney) occur in medulla, increase in size, migrate toward caliceal epithelium, and rupture into calyces to form calculi

(a) nucleation theory
= crystal / foreign body initiates formation in urine supersaturated with crystallizing salt

(b) stone matrix theory
= organic matrix of urinary proteins + serum serves as framework for deposition of crystals

(c) inhibitor theory
= little / no concentration of urinary stone inhibitors (citrate, pyrophosphate, glycosaminoglycan, nephrocalcin, Tamm-Horsfall protein) results in crystal formation

Composition:
- calcium oxalate 75%
- struvite 15%
- calcium phosphate 5%
- uric acid 5%
- cystine 1%

Cause:
◊ 70–80% of patients with first-time stones have a specific metabolic disorder

1. **Hypercalciuria**
   - with hypercalcemia (50%):
     primary hyperparathyroidism, milk-alkali syndrome, hypervitaminosis D, malignant neoplasm, Paget disease, prolonged immobilization, sarcoidosis, adrenal insufficiency, hyper- and hypothyroidism, renal transplantation
   - with normocalcemia (30–60%):
     obstruction, urinary tract infection, vesical diverticulum, horseshoe kidney, medullary sponge kidney, renal tubular acidosis, malignant neoplasm, Paget disease, Cushing syndrome, prolonged immobilization, idiopathic hypercalciuria, acetazolamide therapy, sarcoidosis

Frequency and Radiographic Opacity of Urolithiasis

Mineral Composition	*Frequency (%)*	*Opacity*
A. **Calcium stones**	**70–80**	**+++**
1. Calcium oxalate	20–30	+++
(a) Calcium oxalate monohydrate (= whewellite)		
√ small highly opaque		
(b) Calcium oxalate dihydrate (= wedellite)		
√ may be spiculated / mamillated ("mulberry stone")		
2. Calcium oxalate-phosphate (calcium oxalate plus apatite)	30–40	+++
3. Calcium phosphate (= apatite)	5–10	+++
• rarely pure (= laminated), occasionally forms in infected alkaline urine		
4. Calcium hydrogen phosphate (= brushite)		+++
B. **Struvite stones**	**15–20**	**++**
1. Magnesium ammonium phosphate (= struvite)	1	++
√ laminated, result of urea-splitting organisms (usually Proteus),		
• most common constituent of staghorn calculus		
2. Struvite plus calcium phosphate	15–20	++
• associated with infection		
B. **Cystine**: mildly opaque	**1–3**	**+**
C. **Uric acid**: radiolucent	**5–10**	**-**
D. **Xanthine**: nonopaque	**extremely rare**	**-**
E. **Matrix** (mucoprotein / mucopolysaccharide): nonopaque	**rare**	**-**

GU

(a) absorptive hypercalciuria
= increased intestinal absorption of calcium
Cause: increase in 1,25-dihydroxy-vitamin D levels (50%)
(b) renal hypercalciuria
= abnormal renal calcium leak
Cause: diet high in sodium, urinary tract infection (33%)
(c) resorptive hypercalciuria
= increased bone demineralization secondary to subtle hyperparathyroidism
(d) idiopathic
√ attenuation of calcium stones >1,000 HU similar to bone cortex

2. **Hyperoxaluria**
Physiology:
◊ 85% of urinary oxalate is produced endogenously in liver!
◊ Oxalic acid is present in many foods but poorly absorbed in healthy individuals resulting in increase in urinary oxalate by only 2–3%!
Cause:
(a) congenital = deficiency of an enzyme leading to accumulation of glycolate + oxylate
(b) acquired = increased intake of oxalate / oxalate precursors, excess oxalate absorption from bowel in patients with ileal resection / inflammatory bowel disease
◊ Hyperoxaluria has a stronger correlation to severity of stone disease than hypercalciuria!

3. **Hyperuricosuria**
• uric acid lithiasis (15–20%); stones form in acid urine
• M > F; usually familial
(a) with hyperuricemia:
gout (25–50%) from excessive intake of meat, fish, poultry, myeloproliferative diseases, antimitotic drugs, chemo- / radiation therapy, uricosuric agents, Lesch-Nyhan syndrome
(b) with normouricemia:
idiopathic; occurrence in concentrated acidic urine, which becomes supersaturated with undissociated uric acid (hot climate, ileostomy)
√ bright well-defined of medium-high attenuation (>150 HU [300–500 HU])
Rx: raising urinary pH (potassium citrate / sodium bicarbonate)

4. **Cystinuria** (stones form in acid urine)
= autosomal recessive disorder in renal tubular reabsorption of cystine, ornithine, lysine, arginine
Age of onset: after 10 years
Rx: (1) decreased intake of methionine
(2) alkalinization of urine

5. **Xanthinuria**
= inherited autosomal recessive deficiency of xanthine oxidase (failure of normal oxidation of purines)

6. Urinary tract infection
Cause: urea-splitting organisms (Proteus mirabilis, P. vulgaris, Haemophilus influenzae, S. aureus, Ureaplasma urealyticum) + alkaline environment (pH >7.19)
◊ May lead to magnesium ammonium phosphate = **struvite stones**
Predisposed: women (M:F = 1:2), neurogenic bladder, urinary diversion, indwelling catheter, lower-urinary-tract voiding dysfunction
√ often branching into staghorn calculi
√ most struvite stones are radiopaque, but poorly mineralized matrix stones are not

7. Any condition causing nephrocalcinosis
8. Idiopathic calcium urolithiasis

NONRADIOPAQUE STONES
mnemonic: "SMUX"
Struvite (rarely magnesium ammonium phosphate)
Matrix stone (mucoprotein, mucopolysaccharide)
Uric acid
Xanthine

CALCULI OFTEN ASSOCIATED WITH INFECTION
mnemonic: "S and M"
Struvite (magnesium ammonium phosphate ± calcium phosphate)
Matrix stone (mucoprotein, mucopolysaccharide)

RADIOGRAPHIC SHAPE
√ spiculated stone = child's toy jack
– due to calcium oxalate dihydrate
√ mulberry stone = mamillated contour
– due to calcium oxalate dihydrate
√ seed calculi = small stones all of similar size with lapidary effect (like cut gems):
– forming in small cavity (caliceal diverticulum, cyst, hydronephrosis)
√ milk of calcium (with urine-calcium level)
– due to calcium carbonate:
– forms in any epithelium-lined structure directly communicating with the collecting system (caliceal diverticulum, hydrocalyx, renal cyst)
√ staghorn calculus:
– due to mixture of calcium, magnesium, ammonium, phosphate / cystine stone
– forms with recurrent urinary tract infections

Acute Obstruction by Ureteric Calculi

see also ACUTE HYDRONEPHROSIS
• renal colic = acute colicky flank pain frequently radiating into pelvis / groin / testis
• hematuria
Site: at points of ureteral narrowing
(a) ureterovesical junction (UVJ) in 70%
(b) ureteropelvic junction (UPJ)
(c) iliac vessel crossing

Plain radiography:
◊ 60% of calcifications along expected course of ureter on symptomatic side are ureteric stones!
◊ Stones may be present in 30% of the time when KUB is negative!

GU

IVU (50–70% sensitive):
- √ hydroureteronephrosis
- √ displays degree of obstruction

US:
- √ unilateral pelvicaliectasis (up to 35% false-negative, up to 10% false-positive rate)
- √ resistive index >0.7 in symptomatic kidney
- √ absent ureteral jet on affected side (may be present with partially obstructing calculus)
- √ direct visualization of prevesical calculus by transabdominal, transrectal, transvaginal US

NECT (97% sensitive, 96% specific, 97% accurate):
- ◊ Helical NECT is the most accurate technique for detecting urinary tract calculi!

Advantages:
- (a) visualization of all calculi
- (b) short exam time (3–5 minutes)
- (c) avoidance of IV contrast
- (d) imaging of conditions that mimic renal colic

- √ calcified stone within ureter (PATHOGNOMONIC)
  DDx: phlebolith (no continuity with the ureter):
  - √ all stone compositions readily detectable (except unmineralized stone matrix + stones related to protease inhibitor indinacir [Crixivan®] for HIV treatment)
  - √ stone at ureterovesical junction
    DDx: stone passed into bladder (stone falls anteriorly in prone position)
- √ ureteric rim sign (77%) = thickening of ureteral wall surrounding impacted small ureteric calculus due to edema (92% specific):
  - √ not seen in 33% of stones >5 mm
  - √ in 90% of stones <4 mm
  DDx: gonadal vein phlebolith (in front of upper ureter, lateral to mid ureter); <10% of phleboliths have a soft-tissue rim
- √ secondary signs of urinary tract obstruction:
  - √ asymmetric stranding of perinephric / periureteric fat (76% sensitive, 90% specific) with loss of well-defined fat-kidney interface due to
    - (a) fluid within bridging septa of perinephric fat (due to increased lymphatic pressure)
      - ◊ A higher degree of perinephric edema means a higher degree of obstruction!
    - (b) focal nonlinear fluid collection of extravasated urine as a result of forniceal rupture
  - √ asymmetric dilatation of intrarenal collecting system (80% sensitive, 91% specific) = rounded fluid-filled calices and infundibula partially obliterating the renal sinus fat
    DDx: extrarenal pelvis
  - √ hydroureter above stone (87% sensitive, 90% specific) continuous with renal pelvis
  - √ unilateral renal enlargement (64% sensitive, 89% specific)
  - √ unilateral absence of white pyramid (= loss of the occasional incidental finding of high-attenuation medullary pyramids in normal kidneys)

Cx: xanthogranulomatous pyelonephritis

Rx:
- (1) hydration (within 3 hours after meal, during strenuous physical activity, at bedtime) maintaining urine output of 2–3 L/day
- (2) diet: restrict amounts of protein, sodium, calcium
- (3) drugs: thiazide diuretics (lowers urinary calcium), allopurinol (lowers urate + oxalate excretion)

DDx:
- (1) Recent passage of stone
- (2) Phlebolith ("comet-tail sign" = extension of curvilinear soft-tissue band from stone representing the gonadal vein)

Prognosis:
- (1) Spontaneous passage of ureteral calculi in 93%
  - ◊ Most stones <5 mm will eventually pass!
- (2) Without treatment stone recurrence is 10% at 1 year, 33% at 5 years, 50% at 10 years

VARICOCELE

= dilatation + tortuosity of plexus pampiniformis secondary to retrograde flow into internal spermatic vein

Components of pampiniform plexus:
- (a) internal spermatic vein (ventral location) draining testis
- (b) vein of vas deferens (mediodorsal location) draining epididymis
- (c) cremasteric vein (laterodorsal location) draining scrotal wall

Etiology:
- (1) Incompetent / absent valve at level of left renal vein / IVC on right side
- (2) Compression of left renal vein by tumor, aberrant renal artery, obstructed renal vein
  - ◊ Check left renal vein!

Incidence:
- (a) clinical varicocele: in 8–15% of adult males, in 21–39% of infertile men
- (b) subclinical varicocele: in 40–75% of infertile men

Theoretical causes for infertility:
- (1) Increase in local temperature
- (2) Reflux of toxic substances from adrenal gland (countercurrent exchange of norepinephrine from refluxing renal venous blood into testicular arterial blood at the level of the pampiniform plexus)
- (3) Alteration in Leydig cell function
- (4) Hypoxia of germinative tissue due to venous reflux resulting in venous hypertension + stasis

- • scrotal pain
- • scrotal swelling
- • abnormal spermatogram (impaired motility, immature sperm, oligospermia)

Location: left side (78%), bilateral (16%), right side (6%)

Bidirectional Doppler sonography (erect with quiet breathing):
- (1) SHUNT TYPE (86%): insufficient distal valves allow spontaneous + continuous reflux from internal spermatic vein (retrograde flow) into cremasteric vein + vein of vas deferens (where flow is orthograde) via collaterals

GU

- sperm quality diminished
- clinically plexus type (grade II + III) = medium-sized + large varicoceles

√ continuous reflux during Valsalva maneuver

(2) STOP TYPE / PRESSURE TYPE (14%): intact intrascrotal valves allow only brief period of reflux from spermatic vein into pampiniform plexus under Valsalva maneuver

- sperm quality normal
- clinically central type (grade 0 + I) = subclinical + small varicocele

√ short phase of initial retrograde flow

US:

√ diameter of dominant vein in upright position at inguinal canal

Grading of Varicocele

Grade	Relaxed State	During Valsalva
Normal	2.2 mm	2.7 mm
Small varicocele	2.5–4.0	increase by 1.0 mm
Moderate varicocele	4.0–5.0	increase by 1.2–1.5 mm
Large varicocele	>5.0	increase by >1.5 mm

Dx: documentation of venous reflux

Rx: (1) Ivanissevitch procedure = surgery
(2) Transcatheter spermatic vein occlusion

VESICOURETERIC REFLUX

A. CONGENITAL REFLUX = PRIMARY REFLUX
= incompetence of ureterovesical junction due to abnormal tunneling of distal ureter through bladder wall

Prevalence: in 9–10% of normal Caucasian babies; in 1.4% of school girls; in 30% of children with a first episode of UTI

- short submucosal ureteral tunnel (normally has a length/width ratio of 4:1)
- large laterally located ureteral orifice

Location: uni- / bilateral (frequently involves lower pole ureter in total ureteral duplication)

√ renal scars in 22–50%

Prognosis: disappears in 80%

Cx: reflux atrophy / nephropathy in 22–50%; end-stage renal disease in 5–15% of adults

B. ACQUIRED REFLUX = SECONDARY REFLUX

1. Paraureteric diverticulum = Hutch diverticulum
2. Duplication with ureterocele
3. Cystitis (in 29–50%)
4. Urethral obstruction (urethral valves)
5. Neurogenic bladder
6. Absence of abdominal musculature (prune belly syndrome)

Cx: renal scarring with UTI (30–60%)

GRADES OF REFLUX (VCUG):

Grade I : √ reflux into ureter

Grade II : √ reflux into pelvicaliceal system (without caliceal dilatation / blunting)

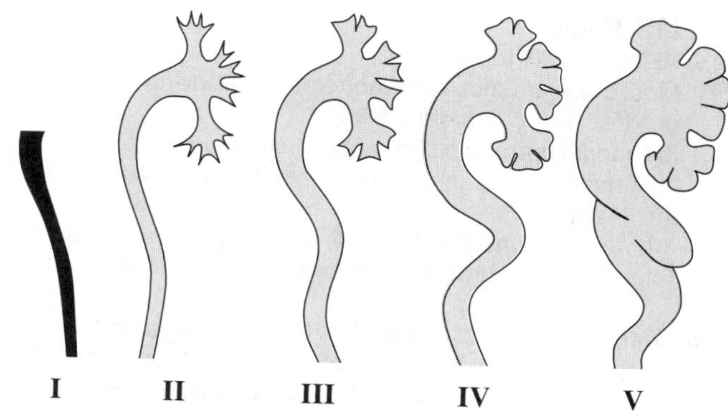

Grading of Vesicoureteral Reflux
(International Reflux System)

Grade III : √ all of the above + mild dilatation of ureter and pelvicaliceal system
√ distinct forniceal angles + papillary impressions

Grade IV : √ reflux into tortuous ureter + moderately dilated pelvicaliceal system
√ blunted forniceal angles
√ distinct papillary impressions

Grade V : √ reflux into markedly dilated and tortuous ureter + markedly dilated pelvicaliceal system
√ obliteration of forniceal angles + papillary impressions

Prognosis:

All grades of reflux can be outgrown:

— 80% of grade I–II and 46% of grade III outgrow reflux within 5 years
— 50% of grade IV continue to have reflux 9 years after initial diagnosis

Renal scarring: >20% chance for grade III–V reflux; 2–3% chance for grade I–II reflux

Rx:

— grade I–III resolve with maturation of the ureterovesical junction
— grade IV–V require surgery to avoid renal scarring + renal impairment + hypertension (except in infants)
— periureteral diverticulum requires surgery (grade of reflux not prognostic)

Radionuclide cystography:

◊ Lower radiation dose to gonads than fluoroscopic cystography (5 mrad)!

US (74% of kidneys with VUR may be normal by US):

√ intermittent hydroureteronephrosis = variable size of collecting system
√ redundant mucosa causing apparent thickening of renal pelvic wall
√ large thin-walled bladder
√ midline-to-orifice distance >7–9 mm has high probability of vesicoureteric reflux

GU

WILMS TUMOR

= NEPHROBLASTOMA

◊ Most common malignant abdominal neoplasm in children 1–8 years old (10%)!

◊ 3rd most common malignancy in childhood (after leukemia + brain tumors; neuroblastoma more common in infancy)!

◊ 3rd most common (87%) of all renal masses in childhood (after hydronephrosis + multicystic dysplastic kidney)!

Incidence: 1:10,000 live births; 450 cases/year in USA; familial in 1–2%; multifocal in 10%; bilateral in 4–13% (with nephrogenic rests in 94–99%)

Age: peak age at 3–4 years (range of 3 months to 11 years); rare during first year; 50% before 3 years, 80% before 5 years; 90% before 8 years; rare in neonates (0.16% of cases) + adults; M:F = 1:1; more common in blacks

Histo: arises from undifferentiated metanephric blastema (= nephrogenic rests) with variable amounts of blastema, stroma, epithelium; occasionally mesodermal derivatives of striated / smooth muscle, fat, bone, cartilage = "teratoid Wilms tumor"

(a) unfavorable histologic character (= presence of anaplasia) in 6.2%: localized / diffuse

(b) favorable histologic character (90%)

◊ Multilocular cystic nephroma, mesoblastic nephroma, nephroblastomatosis are related to the more favorable types of Wilms tumor!

Genetics: multifactorial; abnormal WT1 gene on locus 11p13 with WAGR syndrome (Wilms tumor, aniridia, genitourinary abnormalities, mental retardation) or Drash syndrome; abnormal WT2 gene on locus 11p15 with Beckwith-Wiedemann syndrome or hemihypertrophy; familial Wilms tumor in 1%

In 14% associated with:

(1) Sporadic aniridia (= severe hypoplasia of iris)

◊ 33% of patients with sporadic aniridia develop Wilms tumor!

(2) Beckwith-Wiedemann syndrome = EMG syndrome (exomphalos, macroglossia, gigantism) + hepatomegaly, hyperglycemia from islet cell hyperplasia

◊ 10–20% of patients with Beckwith-Wiedemann syndrome develop Wilms tumor!

(3) Hemihypertrophy: total / segmental / crossed (2.5%);

◊ Ipsilateral or contralateral kidney affected

◊ Increased incidence of all embryonal tumors (adrenal cortical neoplasms, hepatoblastoma)

(4) Genitourinary disorders (4.4%):

(a) Drash syndrome (male pseudohermaphroditism, progressive glomerulonephritis)

(b) Renal anomalies (horseshoe kidney, duplex / solitary / fused kidney)

(c) Genital anomalies: cryptorchidism (2.8%), hypospadia (1.8%), ambiguous genitalia

Screening recommendations (up to age 7 years):
CT at 6 months of age followed by US every 3 months

Stage (National Wilms' Tumor Study Group):

I tumor limited to kidney (renal capsule intact)

II local extension beyond renal capsule into perirenal tissue / renal vessels outside kidney / lymph nodes

III not totally resectable (peritoneal implants, other than paraaortic nodes involved, invasion of vital structures)

IV hematogenous metastases (lung in 85%, liver in 7%, bone in 0.8%, brain [rare]) / lymph node metastases outside abdomen or pelvis

V bilateral renal involvement at diagnosis (4–13%)

- asymptomatic palpable abdominal mass (90%)
- hypertension (in up to 25%) due to renin production by tumor / vascular compression by tumor
- abdominal pain (25%)
- low-grade fever (15%)
- gross hematuria (7–15%) with invasion of renal pelvis
- microscopic hematuria (15–25%)
- hemorrhage after minor trauma
- ascites due to venous obstruction
- varicocele from left-sided tumor

RULE OF 10's:

– 10% unfavorable histology
– 10% bilateral
– 10% vascular invasion
– 10% calcifications
– 10% pulmonary metastases at presentation

√ large tumor (average size 12 cm)

√ expansile growth:

√ sharply marginated with compression of renal tissue = pseudocapsule

√ distorted "clobbered" / dilated calyces

√ displacement of major vessels, rather than encasement

√ curvilinear / phlebolithic calcifications in 5% on plain film, in 15% on CT (DDx: regular stippled calcifications in 85% of neuroblastomas)

√ tumor invasion of renal vein and IVC (4.1–10%); extension into right atrium (in 21% of cases with IVC invasion)

√ tumor may cross midline

√ poor / nonexcretion of IV contrast due to invasion or compression of hilar vessels + collecting system / extensive tumor infiltration of renal parenchyma

US:

√ predominantly solid spherical mass:

√ heterogenous echogenicity (frequent):

√ irregular anechoic areas due to central necrosis + hemorrhage + cyst formation

√ echogenic areas representing fat / calcium

√ fairly evenly echogenic (rare)

CT (preferred modality):
- √ well-circumscribed heterogeneous partially cystic mass due to focal hemorrhage and necrosis (71%), cyst formation, fat, calcification
- √ beak / claw of renal tissue extends partially around mass
- √ tumor less enhancing than renal parenchyma

CECT:
- √ nodal / hepatic metastases
- √ tumor extension into renal vein / IVC
- √ contralateral synchronous tumor/ nephrogenic rests

MR:
- √ hypointense on T1WI
- √ high / variable intensity on T2WI

NUC:
- √ nonfunctioning kidney (10%)
- √ hypo- / iso- / hyperperfusion on radionuclide angiogram
- √ absent tracer accumulation on delayed static images
- √ displacement of kidney + distortion of collecting system

Angio:
- √ hypervascular tumor: enlarged tortuous vessels, coarse neovascularity; small arterial aneurysms, vascular lakes
- √ parasitization of vascular supply

Rx: presurgical chemotherapy + nephrectomy + adjuvant chemotherapy ± radiation therapy

Prognosis: survival rate depending on pathologic pattern, age at time of diagnosis, extent of disease; 4-year relapse-free survival: 91% for stage I; 88% for stage II; 79% for stage III; 78–84% for stage IV

DDx:
(1) Neuroblastoma (encasement / elevation of aorta, regular stippled calcifications)
(2) Cystic partially differentiated nephroblastoma (largely cystic tumor)

WOLMAN DISEASE

= PRIMARY FAMILIAL XANTHOMATOSIS

= rare autosomal recessive lipidosis with accumulation of cholesterol esters and triglycerides in visceral foam cells + various tissues (liver, spleen, lymph nodes, adrenal cortex, small bowel)

Etiology: deficiency of lysosomal acid esterase / acid lipase

- • malabsorption in neonatal period: failure to thrive, diarrhea, steatorrhea, vomiting
- • delayed growth, diminished muscle mass, abdominal distension
- √ hepatosplenomegaly
- √ extensive bilateral punctate calcifications (calcification of fatty-acid soaps) throughout enlarged adrenals (maintaining their normal triangular shape) is DIAGNOSTIC
- √ enlarged fat-containing lymph nodes
- √ small bowel wall thickening (due to infiltration of mucosa of small bowel by lipid-filled histiocytes impairing absorption)
- √ generalized osteoporosis

CT & MR: attenuation + signal intensities consistent with deposition of lipids

Dx: assay of leukocytes / cultured skin fibroblasts

Prognosis: death occurs within first 6 months of life

ZELLWEGER SYNDROME

= CEREBROHEPATORENAL SYNDROME

autosomal recessive

- • muscular hypotonia
- • hepatomegaly + jaundice
- • craniofacial dysmorphism
- • seizures, mental retardation
- √ brain dysgenesis (lissencephaly, macrogyria, polymicrogyria)
- √ renal cortical cysts

Prognosis: death in early infancy

GU

DIFFERENTIAL DIAGNOSIS OF OBSTETRIC AND GYNECOLOGIC DISORDERS

GENERAL OBSTETRICS

Parity Nomenclature (for pregnancies <20 weeks)

example: G_5P_{4004}

Gravida		5 pregnancies
Parity		
mnemonic:	"FPAL"	
Full term		4 full term
Preterm		0 preterm
Abortion		0 abortion
Living		4 living

Level I Obstetric Ultrasound

Indication: MS-AFP ≥2.5 multiples of mean (MoM) between 14 and 18 weeks MA

Limited scope of examination to identify frequent causes of MS-AFP elevation in 20–50% of pregnancies:

1. Gestational age ≥2 weeks more advanced than estimated clinically (18%)
2. Multiple gestations (10%)
3. Unsuspected fetal demise (5%)
4. Obvious fetal NTD / abdominal wall defect

Outcome: no cause identified in 50–80%

Recommendation if level I ultrasound is unrevealing:

(1) amniocentesis for AF-AFP (with normal results in >90%)
(2) level II obstetric ultrasound (skipping amniocentesis)

Level II Obstetric Ultrasound

Indication: AF-AFP ≥2 MoM

Accuracy: identification of abnormal fetuses in 99%

Examination targeted for:

1. Open neural tube defect: anencephaly, encephalocele, open spina bifida, amniotic band syndrome resulting in open neural tube defect
2. Closed neural axis anomaly: hydrocephalus, Dandy-Walker malformation
3. Abdominal wall defect: gastroschisis, omphalocele, gastropleuroschisis from amniotic band syndrome
4. Upper GI obstruction: esophageal atresia ± tracheoesophageal fistula, duodenal obstruction
5. Cystic hygroma
6. Teratoma: sacrococcygeal, lingual, retropharyngeal
7. Renal anomalies: obstructive uropathy, renal agenesis, multicystic dysplastic kidney, congenital Finnish nephrosis

◊ Risk of fetal chromosomal anomaly is only 0.6–1.1% with normal level II sonogram!

MATERNAL SERUM SCREENING

Alpha-fetoprotein

= glycoprotein as major circulatory protein of early fetus

Origin: formed initially by yolk sac + fetal gut (4–8 weeks), later by fetal liver

Detectable in

(a) fetal serum
- concentration peaks at 14–15 weeks followed by progressive decline

(b) amniotic fluid (AF-AFP) is a result of
- – fetal urination
- – fetal gastrointestinal secretions
- – transudation across fetal membranes (amnion, placenta)
- – transudation across immature fetal epithelium
- concentration peaks early in 2nd trimester followed by progressive decline

(c) maternal circulation (MS-AFP) secondary to leakage from amniotic fluid across the placenta
- levels start to rise at 7th week, peak at 32nd week, and decline toward end of pregnancy

◊ Either high / low MS-AFP is associated with 34% of all major congenital defects!

Sample Site	*Approximate Level (ng/mL)*	*Peak*
Maternal serum	30	30th–32nd week
Amniotic fluid	20,000	early 2nd trimester
Fetal plasma	3,000,000	14th–15th week

At the end of the 1st trimester AFP is present:

in fetal plasma in *milligram* quantities
in amniotic fluid in *microgram* quantities
in maternal serum in *nanogram* quantities

Reported in MoM = multiples of mean to standardize interpretation among laboratories

Elevated Alpha-fetoprotein

- screening at 16–18 weeks GA

◊ Values must be corrected for dates, maternal weight, race, presence of diabetes (diabetes has depressing effect on MS-AFP so that lower levels may be associated with NTDs)

(a) Elevation in MATERNAL SERUM (MS-AFP)

= defined as ≥2.5 MoM / equivalent to the 5th percentile; 4.5 MoM for multiple gestations

<u>Power of detection at ≥2.5 MoM cutoff</u>:

98% of gastroschisis
90% of anencephalic fetuses
75–80% of open spinal defects
70% of omphaloceles

Incidence: 2–5% screen-positive rate (in 16% normal MS-AFP on retesting);
6–15% of fetuses have some type of major congenital defect; in 1.3:1,000 tests fetal anomaly detected

◊ The higher the AFP elevation the higher the probability of fetal anomalies

◊ 20–38% of women with unexplained high MS-AFP (ie, in absence of fetal abnormality) suffer adverse pregnancy outcomes (premature birth, preeclampsia, 2–4 x IUGR, 10 x perinatal mortality, 10 x placental abruption)!

(b) Elevation in AMNIOTIC FLUID (AF-AFP)
= defined as ≥2 MoM (<2 MoM has a 97% NPV)
Incidence: <10% of women with elevated MS-AFP and "unrevealing" level I US exam

- amniotic fluid also tested for karyotype + acetylcholinesterase (= neurotransmitter enzyme present when neural tissue is exposed)

◊ 66% of fetuses of women with elevated AF-AFP levels are normal!

◊ A targeted level II ultrasound exam will show fetal anomalies in 33%!

Associated with:

A. LABORATORY ERROR
B. ERRONEOUS DATES (18%): GA ≥2 weeks more advanced sonographically than by clinical estimate (AFP levels rise 15% per week during 16–18-week window)
C. MULTIPLE GESTATIONS (14%)
D. FETAL DEMISE (7%) / fetal distress / threatened abortion
E. FETAL ANOMALIES (61%)
   1. Neural tube defects (51%): [anencephaly (30%), myelomeningocele (18%), encephalocele (3%), forebrain malformation]
      Prevalence: 1.6:1,000 births in USA;
      6:1,000 births in Great Britain
      ◊ In 90% as 1st time event!
      Risk of recurrence: 3% after one affected child; 6% after 2 affected children
   2. Ventral wall defects (21%) (gastroschisis, omphalocele): sensitivity of 50%
   3. Proximal fetal gut obstruction (esophageal / duodenal atresia)
      = diminished AFP degradation in small bowel
   4. Cystic hygroma, teratoma (pharyngeal, sacral)
   5. Amniotic band syndrome (asymmetric cephalocele, gastropleuroschisis)
   6. Renal abnormalities:
      multicystic dysplastic kidney, renal agenesis, pelviectasis, **congenital Finnish nephrosis** (typically ≥10 MoM + negative amniotic fluid acetylcholinesterase)
   7. Oligohydramnios
F. PLACENTAL LESION
   altering the placentomaternal barrier
   1. Chorioangioma
   2. Peri- and intraplacental hematoma resulting in fetomaternal hemorrhage
   3. Placental lakes, infarct, intervillous thrombosis
G. LOW BIRTH WEIGHT
H. Normal pregnancy + MATERNAL DISORDER
   1. Hepatitis
   2. Hepatoma
I. Fetal-maternal blood mixing: collection of MS-AFP samples after amniocentesis

mnemonic: "GEM MINER CO"
Gastroschisis
Esophageal atresia
Multiple gestations
Mole
Incorrect menstrual dates
Neural tube defects
Error (laboratory)
Renal disease in fetus (autosomal recessive polycystic kidney disease, renal dysplasia, obstructive uropathy, congenital Finnish nephrosis)
Chorioangioma
Omphalocele

Low Alpha-fetoprotein

= MS-AFP ≤0.5 / AF-AFP ≤0.72 MoM
Incidence: 3%

1. Autosomal trisomy syndromes (trisomy 21, 18, 13)
   ◊ 20% of trisomy 21 fetuses are found in women with low MS-AFP after adjustment for age!
2. Absence of fetal tissues (eg, hydatidiform mole)
3. Fetal demise
4. Misdated pregnancy
5. Normal pregnancy
6. Patient not pregnant

Use of Karyotyping

Frequency: 11–35% of fetuses with sonographically identified abnormalities have chromosomal abnormalities

A. FETAL ANOMALIES
   1. CNS anomalies: holoprosencephaly (43–59%), Dandy-Walker malformation (29–50%), cerebellar hypoplasia, agenesis of corpus callosum, myelomeningocele (33–50%)
   2. Cystic hygroma (72%): Turner syndrome
   3. Omphalocele (30–40%)
   4. Cardiac malformations
   5. Nonimmune hydrops
   6. Duodenal atresia
   7. Severe early-onset IUGR: trisomy 18, 13, triploidy
   8. Diaphragmatic hernia
   9. Bone-echodense bowel (20%): trisomy 21

B. MATERNAL RISK FACTORS
1. Advanced age
2. Low serum alpha-fetoprotein
3. Abnormal triple screen of maternal serum
4. History of previous chromosomally abnormal pregnancy (1% risk of recurrence)

C. PLANNED INTENSE INTRAUTERINE MANAGEMENT

Fetal anomalies not associated with chromosomal anomalies:
1. Gastroschisis
2. Unilateral renal anomaly
3. Intestinal obstruction distal to duodenal bulb
4. Off-midline unilateral cleft lip
5. Fetal teratoma (sacrococcygeal / anterior cervical)
6. Isolated single umbilical artery

Aneuploid Risk of Major Anomalies

Structural Defect	*Incidence*	*Aneuploidy Risk*	*Aneuploidy Most common*
Cystic hygroma	1:6,000	60–75%	45X,21,18, 13,XXY
Hydrops	1:4,000	30–80%	13,21,18,45X
Holoprosencephaly	1:16,000	40–60%	13,18,18p
Cardiac defects	1:125	5–30%	21,18,13,22
AV canal		40–70%	21
Omphalocele	1:5,800	30–40%	13,18
Duodenal atresia	1:10,000	20–30%	21
Diaphragmatic hernia	1:4,000	20–25%	13,18,21,45X
Bladder outlet obstruction	1:1,000	20–25%	13,18
Limb reduction	1:2,000	8%	18
Club foot	1:830	6%	18,13,4p-, 18q-
Hydrocephalus	1:1,250	3–8%	13,18, triploidy
Facial cleft	1:700	1%	13,18, deletions
Prune belly	1:40,000	low	18,13,45X
Single umb. artery	1:100	minimal	
Bowel obstruction	1:4,000	minimal	
Gastroschisis	1:12,000	minimal	

AMNIOTIC FLUID VOLUME

Production:
(a) 1st trimester: dialysate of maternal + fetal serum across the noncornified fetal skin
(b) 2nd + 3rd trimester: fetal urine (600–800 cm^3/day near term), fetal lungs (600–800 cm^3/day near term), amniotic membrane

Absorption:
fetal swallowing + GI absorption, fetal lung absorption, clearance by placenta

Assessment of amniotic fluid volume by:
(1) Subjective assessment ("Gestalt" method): quick + efficient, accounts for GA-related variations in fluid volume, considered the most accurate if performed by experienced operator, operator + interpreter must be identical, no documentation, variations on serial scans difficult to appreciate
(2) Depth of largest vertical pocket: simple + quick (used in BPP), pockets >2 cm may be found in crevices between fetal parts with moderately severe oligohydramnios, does not account for GA-related variations
(3) Four-quadrant **Amniotic Fluid Index** (AFI): fairly quick, probably correlates better with fluid volume than any single measurement, may not accurately reflect overall fluid volume, may be affected by fetal movement during measurements
(4) Planimetric measurement of total intrauterine volume
(5) Dye / para-amino hippurate dilution technique: 800 cm^3 at 34 weeks, 500 cm^3 >34 weeks

Polyhydramnios

= amniotic fluid volume >1,500–2,000 cm^3 at term
Incidence: 1.1–2–3.5%
√ fetus does not fill the AP diameter of uterus
√ single largest pocket devoid of fetal parts / cord >8 cm in vertical direction
√ AFI ≥20–24 cm
Prognosis: 64% perinatal mortality with severe polyhydramnios

Etiology:
A. IDIOPATHIC (60%)
associated with macrosomia in 19–37%
Suggested cause:
(1) increased renal vascular flow
(2) bulk flow of water across surface of fetus + umbilical cord + placenta + membranes

B. MATERNAL CAUSES (20%)
1. Diabetes (5%)
2. Isoimmunization (Rh incompatibility)
3. Placental tumors: chorioangioma

C. FETAL ANOMALIES (20–63%)
(a) gastrointestinal anomalies (6–16%)
impairment of fetal swallowing (esophageal atresia in 3%); high intestinal atresias / obstruction of duodenum / proximal small bowel (1.2–1.8%), omphalocele, meconium peritonitis
(b) nonimmune hydrops (16%)
(c) neural tube defects (9–16%)
anencephaly, hydranencephaly, holoprosencephaly, myelomeningocele, ventriculomegaly, agenesis of corpus callosum, encephalocele, microcephaly

(d) chest anomalies (12%)
diaphragmatic hernia, cystic adenomatoid malformation, tracheal atresia, mediastinal teratoma, primary pulmonary hypoplasia, extralobar sequestration, congenital chylothorax

(e) skeletal dysplasias (11%)
dwarfism (thanatophoric dysplasia, achondroplasia), kyphoscoliosis, platyspondyly

(f) chromosomal abnormalities (9%)
trisomy 21, 18, 13

(g) cardiac anomalies (5%)
VSD, truncus arteriosus, ectopia cordis, septal rhabdomyoma, arrhythmia

(h) genitourinary malformations
Cause: ? hormonally mediated polyuria
unilateral UPJ obstruction, unilateral multicystic dysplastic kidney, mesoblastic nephroma

(i) miscellaneous (8%)
cystic hygroma, facial tumors, cleft lip / palate, teratoma, amniotic band syndrome, congenital pancreatic cyst

◊ In polyhydramnios efforts to detect fetal anomalies should be directed at SGA fetuses!

mnemonic: "TARDI"
Twins
Anomalies, fetal
Rh incompatibility
Diabetes
Idiopathic

Oligohydramnios

= amniotic fluid volume <500 cm^3 at term

√ single largest pocket devoid of fetal parts / cord ≤1–2 cm in vertical direction

√ AFI ≤5–7 cm

Etiology:
mnemonic: "DRIPP"
Demise of fetus / **D**rugs (Motrin therapy for tocolysis of preterm labor)
Renal anomalies, bilateral (= inadequate urine production): renal agenesis / dysgenesis, infantile polycystic kidney disease, prune belly syndrome, posterior urethral valves, urethral atresia, cloacal anomalies
◊ 20-fold increase in incidence of fetal anomalies with oligohydramnios!
N.B.: bilateral renal obstruction, if combined with intestinal obstruction, may be associated with polyhydramnios
IUGR (reduced renal perfusion)
Premature rupture of membranes (most common)
Postmaturity

Cx: pulmonary hypoplasia, cord compression

Prognosis: 77–100% perinatal mortality with 2nd trimester oligohydramnios

ABNORMAL FIRST TRIMESTER

Time of onset: prior to 8–10 weeks

First Trimester Bleeding

= VAGINAL BLEEDING IN FIRST TRIMESTER

Frequency: 15–25% of all pregnancies, of which 50% terminate in abortion

A. INTRAUTERINE CONCEPTUS IDENTIFIED
1. Threatened abortion
2. Embryonic demise
3. Blighted ovum
4. Gestational trophoblastic disease
5. Implantation bleed (3–4 weeks after last menstrual period)
6. Subchorionic hemorrhage
7. Low-lying placenta previa
8. Twin loss

B. NORMAL ENDOMETRIAL CAVITY
(a) with β-HCG level >1,800 mIU/mL
1. Recent spontaneous abortion
2. Ectopic pregnancy
(b) with β-HCG level <1,800 mIU/mL
1. Very early IUP
2. Ectopic pregnancy

C. SAC VULNERABILITY
1. Leiomyoma
2. Intrauterine contraceptive device

Abnormal Sonographic Findings in 1st Trimester

1. Embryonic demise = abortion (clinical term)
2. Nondevelopment = blighted ovum
3. Maldevelopment = hydatidiform mole

Empty Gestational Sac

1. Normal early IUP between 5 and 7 weeks MA
2. Blighted ovum

DDx: Pseudosac of ectopic pregnancy

Gestational Sac in Low Position

1. Abortion in progress
√ no placental blood flow
2. Cervical ectopic pregnancy
3. Fundal fibroid compressing sac downward

Positive β-HCG without IUP

mnemonic: "HERE"
HCG-producing tumor (rare)
Ectopic pregnancy
Recent / incomplete abortion
Early intrauterine pregnancy

Thickened Central Cavity Complex

1. Intrauterine blood
2. Retained products of conception following an incomplete spontaneous abortion
3. Early intrauterine not yet visible pregnancy
4. Decidual reaction secondary to ectopic pregnancy

Uterus Large for Dates

1. Multiple gestation pregnancy
2. Inaccurate menstrual history
3. Fibroids
4. Polyhydramnios
5. Hydatidiform mole
6. Fetal macrosomia

Intrauterine Membrane in Pregnancy

A. MEMBRANE OF MATERNAL ORIGIN
  1. Uterine septum
     = incomplete resorption of sagittal septum between the fused two müllerian ducts
  2. Amniotic sheet / shelf
     = folding of amniochorionic membrane around uterine synechia
     √ synechia often thins during uterine stretching + disappears as pregnancy progresses

B. MEMBRANE OF FETAL ORIGIN
  1. Intertwin membrane
     = apposing membrane of multiple pregnancy
  2. Amniotic band
     = rent within amnion
  3. Chorioamnionic separation
     = incomplete fusion / hemorrhagic separation of amnion (= inner membrane) and chorion (= outer membrane)
  4. Subchorionic hemorrhage = chorioamnionic elevation
     = separation of chorionic membrane from decidua
     • implantation bleed of early pregnancy

C. FIBRIN STRAND
  Cause: hemorrhage during transplacental amniocentesis

mnemonic: "STABS"
Separation (chorioamnionic)
Twins (intertwin membrane)
Abruption
Bands (amniotic band syndrome)
Synechia

Dilated Cervix

1. Inevitable abortion
2. Premature labor
   = spontaneous onset of palpable, regularly occurring uterine contractions between 20 and 37 weeks MA
3. Incompetent cervix

PLACENTA

Abnormal Placental Size

◊ Placental mass tends to reflect fetal mass!

A. ENLARGEMENT OF PLACENTA = **Placentomegaly**
   = >5 cm thick in sections obtained at right angles to long axis of placenta
  (a) maternal disease
    1. Maternal diabetes (= villous edema)
    2. Chronic intrauterine infections (eg, syphilis)
    3. Maternal anemia (= normal histology)
    4. Alpha-thalassemia
  (b) fetal disease
    1. Hemolytic disease of the newborn (= villous edema + hyperplasia) due to immunologic incompatibility including Rh sensitization
    2. Umbilical vein obstruction
    3. Fetal high-output failure: large chorioangioma, arteriovenous fistula
    4. Fetal malformation: Beckwith-Wiedemann syndrome, sacrococcygeal teratoma, chromosomal abnormality, fetal hydrops
    5. Twin-twin transfusion syndrome
  (c) fetomaternal hemorrhage
  (d) placental abnormailites
    1. Molar pregnancy
    2. Chorioangioma
    3. Inytraplacental hemorrhage

  mnemonic: "HAD IT"
  Hydrops
  Abruption
  Diabetes mellitus
  Infection
  Triploidy

B. DECREASE IN PLACENTAL SIZE
  1. Preeclampsia
     associated with placental infarcts in 33–60%
  2. IUGR
  3. Chromosomal abnormality
  4. Intrauterine infection

Vascular Spaces of the Placenta

1. **"Placental cysts"**
   = large fetal veins located between amnion + chorion anastomosing with umbilical vein
   √ sluggish blood flow (detectable by real-time observation)
2. **Basal veins**
   = decidual + uterine veins
   √ lacy appearing network of veins underneath placenta
   DDx: placental abruption
3. **Intraplacental venous lakes**
   √ intraplacental sonolucent spaces
   √ whirlpool motion pattern of flowing blood

Macroscopic Lesions of the Placenta

1. **Intervillous thrombosis** (36%)
   = intraplacental areas of hemorrhage
   Etiology: breaks in villous capillaries with bleeding from fetal vessels
   √ irregular sonolucent intraplacental lesions (mm to cm range)
   √ blood flow may be observed within lesion
   Significance: fetal-maternal hemorrhage (Rh sensitization, elevated AFP levels)
2. **Perivillous fibrin deposition** (22%)
   = nonlaminated collection of fibrin deposition
   Etiology: thrombosis of intervillous space
   Significance: none

3. **Septal cyst** (19%)
   Etiology: obstruction of septal venous drainage by edematous villi
   √ 5–10-mm cyst within septum
   Significance: none
4. **Placental infarct** (25%)
   = coagulation necrosis of villi
   Etiology: disorder of maternal vessels, retroplacental hemorrhage
   √ not visualized unless hemorrhagic
   √ well-circumscribed mass with hyperechoic / mixed echo pattern
   Significance: dependent on extent + associated maternal condition
5. **Subchorionic fibrin deposition** (20%)
   = laminated collection of fibrin deposition
   Etiology: thrombosis of maternal blood in subchorionic space
   √ subchorionic sonolucent area
   Significance: none
6. **Massive subchorial thrombus**
   = BREUS MOLE = PREPLACENTAL HEMORRHAGE

Placental Tumor

A. TROPHOBLASTIC
   1. Complete hydatidiform mole
   2. Partial hydatidiform mole
   3. Invasive mole
   4. Choriocarcinoma

B. NONTROPHOBLASTIC
   1. Chorioangioma (in up to 1% of placentas)
   2. Teratoma (rare)
   3. Metastatic lesion (rare): melanoma, breast carcinoma, bronchial carcinoma

Unbalanced Intertwin Transfusion

= unbalanced intertwin transfusion through vascular anastomoses between the two circulations of monochorionic twins

A. ACUTE = Twin-embolization syndrome
B. CHRONIC = Twin-twin transfusion syndrome
C. REVERSE = Acardiac twinning

UMBILICAL CORD

Abnormal Cord Attachment

1. Marginal cord attachment (7%)
   = battledore placenta (flat wooden paddle used in an early form of badminton)
   • no clinical significance
2. Velamentous insertion of cord (1%)
3. Vasa previa

Umbilical Cord Lesions

◊ Umbilical cord cysts persisting into 2nd + 3rd trimester are frequently accompanied by fetal anomalies (hernia, intestinal obstruction, urinary tract obstruction, urachal anomalies, omphalocele, cardiac defect, trisomy 18)!

A. DEVELOPMENTAL CORD LESION
1. **Umbilical hernia**
   = protrusion from anterior abdominal wall with normal insertion of umbilical vessels
   Predisposed:
   Blacks, low-birth-weight infants, trisomy 21, congenital hypothyroidism, Beckwith-Wiedemann syndrome, mucopolysaccharidoses
   Prognosis: spontaneous closure in first 3 years of life
2. **Omphalomesenteric duct cyst**
   √ near fetal end of cord + eccentric in cord
3. **Allantoic cyst**
   = remnant of umbilical vesicle / allantois; usually degenerates by 6 weeks
   Histo: lined by single layer of flattened epithelium
   √ near fetal end of cord + in center of cord
4. **Amniotic inclusion cyst**
   = amniotic epithelium trapped within umbilical cord
5. **Mucoid degeneration of umbilical cord**
   = **umbilical cord pseudocyst**
   = liquefaction of Wharton jelly / edema
   √ focal thickening of Wharton jelly, usually near umbilicus
   √ usually resolved by 12 weeks MA
   Associated commonly with omphalocele
6. **Noncoiled "straight" cord**
   counterclockwise:clockwise umbilical cords = 7:1
   right-handed:left-handed persons = 7:1
   Incidence: 3.7–5%
   √ absent vascular coiling for entire length of visible cord
   At risk for: intrauterine death (8%), stillbirth, fetal anomalies (24%), prematurity, intrapartum heart rate decelerations, fetal distress, meconium staining

B. ACQUIRED CORD LESION
1. **False knot**
   (a) exaggerated looping of cord vessels causing focal dilatation of cord
   (b) focal accumulation of Wharton jelly
   (c) varix of umbilical vessel
   √ knoblike protrusion / bulge of cord
2. **True knot**
   Incidence: 1% of pregnancies
   Cause: excessive fetal movements
   Predisposed: long cord, polyhydramnios, small fetus, monoamniotic twins
   √ local distension / thrombosis of umbilical vein near cord knot resembling an umbilical cyst
   √ tortuosity of cord at level of knot
   Cx: vascular occlusion + fetal death in utero
   OB management: expectant
3. **Umbilical cord hematoma**
   = rupture of the wall of the umbilical vein secondary to mechanical trauma (torsion, loops, knots, traction) / congenital weakness of vessel wall

Incidence: 1:5,505 to 1:12,699 deliveries
Location: near fetal insertion of umbilical cord (most common)
√ hyper- / hypoechoic mass 1–2 cm in size, multiple (in 18%)
Cx: rupture into amniotic cavity with exsanguination
Prognosis: 52% overall perinatal fetal mortality

4. Neoplasm
   (a) **Angiomyxoma / hemangioma of cord**
   Incidence: 22 cases in literature
   Histo: multiple vascular channels lined by benign endothelium surrounded by edema + myxomatous degeneration of Wharton jelly
   Associated with: elevated α-fetoprotein level
   Location: more frequently near placental end of umbilical cord
   √ hyperechoic / multicystic mass within cord
   √ may be associated with pseudocyst (= localized collection of edema)
   Cx: premature delivery, stillbirth, hydramnios, nonimmune hydrops, massive hemorrhage due to rupture
   (b) Other tumors: myxosarcoma, dermoid, teratoma
5. **Umbilical vein varix**
   Incidence: <4% of all umbilical cord abnormalities
   Site: intraamniotic, intraabdominal
   √ fusiform dilatation of umbilical vein
   Cx: (1) Thrombosis with subsequent fetal death
   (2) Partial thrombosis with IUGR
   Prognosis: usually no clinical significance
6. Umbilical artery aneurysm

FETAL SKELETAL DYSPLASIA

= DWARFISM
= heterogeneous group of bone growth disorders resulting in abnormal shape + size of the skeleton
◊ More than 200 skeletal dysplasias are known, but only a few are frequent:
- thanatophoric dysplasia
- osteogenesis imperfecta type II
- achondrogenesis
- heterozygous achondroplasia

Birth prevalence:
2.3:10,000–7.6:10,000 births for all skeletal dysplasias;
1.5:10,000 births for lethal skeletal dysplasias
Prognosis: 51% lethal due to hypoplastic lungs:
23% stillbirths, 32% death in 1st week of life

	Birth Prevalence	*Perinatal Deaths*
Thanatophoric dysplasia	0.69:10,000*	1:246
chondroplasia	0.37:10,000	none
ondrogenesis, type I	0.23:10,000*	1:639
ndrogenesis, type II	0.25:10,000*	
Osteogenesis imperf. type II	0.18:10,000*	1:799
Osteogenesis imperf., others	0.18:10,000	none
Asphyxiating thoracic dysplasia	0.14:10,000	1:3,196
Hypophosphatasia	0.10:10,000*	
Chondrodysplasia punctata, rhizo	0.09:10,000*	none
Camptomelic dysplasia	0.05:10,000*	1:3,196
Chondroectodermal dysplasia	0.05:10,000	1:3,196
Cleidocranial dysplasia	0.05:10,000	
Diastrophic dysplasia	0.02:10,000*	

* = lethal dysplasias

Associated with:
√ polyhydramnios
√ small thorax
√ morphologically abnormal bones
√ shortening of long bones (common characteristic)
◊ Femur length >5 mm below 2 standard deviations suggests skeletal dysplasia!
√ femur length/foot length ratio <0.9
√ moderate limb shortening of 40–60% of the mean in thanatophoric dysplasia + OI type II
√ severe limb shortening of >30% of the mean in achondrogenesis
DDx features: mineralization, bowing, fractures, number of digits, fetal movement, thoracic measurement, associated anomalies, age of onset
DDx: constitutionally short limbs, severe IUGR
see also DWARFISM

Fetal Hand Malformation

Polydactyly
trisomy 13, short-rib-polydactyly syndrome, asphyxiating thoracic dystrophy (Jeune syndrome), Smith-Lemli-Opitz syndrome
(a) Postaxial polydactyly
chondroectodermal dysplasia (Ellis-van Creveld syndrome), Meckel-Gruber syndrome, hydrolethalus syndrome
(b) Preaxial polydactyly
orofaciodigital syndrome

Syndactyly
Apert syndrome, triploidy, Roberts syndrome

Clinodactyly
trisomy 21, triploidy

Overlapping Digit
trisomy 18

Hitchhiker's Thumb
diastrophic dysplasia

Flexion Contractures
trisomy 13 + 18, fetal akinesia deformation sequence

Limb Reduction
congenital varicella, hypoglossia-hyperdactyly syndrome

Amputation
amniotic band syndrome

FETAL CNS ANOMALIES
Incidence: 2:1,000 births in USA; 90% as 1st time occurrence
Recurrence: 2–3% after 1st, 6% after 2nd occurrence
√ ventricular atrium + cisterna magna are two sensitive anatomic markers for normal brain development!
A. HYDROCEPHALUS
  1. Aqueductal stenosis
  2. Communicating hydrocephalus
  3. Dandy-Walker malformation
  4. Choroid plexus papilloma
B. NEURAL TUBE DEFECT
  Incidence: 1:500–600 live births
  Risk of recurrence: 3–4%
  1. Spina bifida
  2. Anencephaly
  3. Acrania
  4. Encephalocele (8–15%)
  5. Porencephaly
  6. Hydranencephaly
  7. Holoprosencephaly
  8. Iniencephaly
  9. Microcephaly
  10. Agenesis of corpus callosum
  11. Lissencephaly
  12. Arachnoid cyst
  13. Choroid plexus cyst
  14. Vein of Galen aneurysm
C. INTRACRANIAL NEOPLASM
  1. Teratoma (>50%): benign / malignant
     Location: originate from base of skull
  2. Glioblastoma
  3. Astrocytoma

Fetal Ventriculomegaly
Cause:
A. Morphologic anomaly (70–80%):
  1. Spina bifida (30–65%)
  2. Dandy-Walker malformation
  3. Encephalocele
  4. Holoprosencephaly
  5. Agenesis of corpus callosum
B. Abnormal karyotype (10–20%)
C. Viral infection
◊ 20–40% of concurrent anomalies are missed by ultrasound!
√ "dangling" choroid plexus
√ width of ventricular atrium >10 mm
Prognosis: 21% survival rate; 50% with intellectual impairment; 80% with isolated mild ventriculomegaly (atrial width >10 and ≤15 mm) have normal motor + intellectual function at ≥12 months of age

Prenatal Intracranial Calcifications
1. Toxoplasmosis
2. CMV infection
3. Tuberous sclerosis
4. Sturge-Weber syndrome
5. Venous sinus thrombosis
6. Teratoma

Cystic Intracranial Lesion
mnemonic: "CHAP VAN"
Choroid plexus cyst
Hydrocephalus, **H**oloprosencephaly, **H**ydranencephaly
Agenesis of corpus callosum + cystic dilatation of 3rd ventricle
Porencephaly
Vein of Galen aneurysm
Arachnoid cyst
Neoplasm (cystic teratoma)

Abnormal Cisterna Magna
Normal size between 15 and 25 weeks MA:
>2 to <10 mm (usually 4–9 mm) in 94–97% of fetuses
A. SMALL CISTERNA MAGNA + "banana sign"
  1. Chiari II malformation (with myelomeningocele)
  2. Occipital cephalocele
  3. Severe hydrocephalus
B. LARGE CISTERNA MAGNA
  1. Megacisterna magna
     √ cerebellum + vermis remain intact
  2. Arachnoid cyst
     √ en bloc displacement of cerebellum + vermis
  3. Cerebellar hypoplasia
  4. Dandy-Walker syndrome (with vermian agenesis)

FETAL ORBITAL ANOMALIES
Hypotelorism
1. Holoprosencephaly
2. Chromosomal abnormalities: trisomy 13
3. Microcephaly, trigonocephaly
4. Maternal phenylketonuria
5. Meckel-Gruber syndrome
6. Myotonic dystrophy
7. Williams syndrome
8. Oculodental dysplasia

Hypertelorism
1. Median cleft syndrome: cleft lip/palate
2. Craniosynostosis: Apert /Crouzon syndrome
3. Pena-Shokeir syndrome
4. Frontal / ethmoidal, sphenoidal encephalocele
5. Dilantin / phenytoin effect

Orbital and Periorbital Masses
1. Dacryocystocele
2. Anterior encephalocele
3. Glioma
4. Hemangioma
5. Teratoma

FETAL NECK ANOMALIES

1. Cervical myelomeningocele
2. Occipital cephalocele
3. Cystic hygroma / lymphangioma
4. Teratoma
5. Branchial cleft cyst
6. Enlarged thyroid
7. Sarcoma

Nuchal Skin Thickening

= NUCHAL SONOLUCENCY / FULLNESS / EDEMA
= skin thickening of posterior neck measured between calvarium + dorsal skin margin
(a) ≥3 mm during 9–13 weeks MA
(b) ≥5 mm during 14–21 weeks MA
(c) ≥6 mm during 19–24 weeks MA
◊ The smallest measurement should be used!

Image plane: axial / transverse image (slightly craniad to that of the BPD measurement) that includes cavum septi pellucidi, cerebellar hemisphere and cisterna magna (transcerebellar diameter view)

Incidence: among the most common anomaly in 1st trimester + early 2nd trimester

Causes:

A. NORMAL VARIANT (0.06%)
B. CHROMOSOMAL DISORDERS
   trisomy 21 (in 45–80%), Turner syndrome (45 X0), Noonan syndrome, trisomy 18, XXX syndrome, XYY syndrome, XXXX syndrome, XXXXY syndrome, 18p-syndrome, 13q-syndrome
   ◊ 30–40% of fetuses with Down syndrome have nuchal skin thickening!
C. NONCHROMOSOMAL DISORDERS
   1. Multiple pterygium syndrome = Escobar syndrome
   2. Klippel-Feil syndrome (fusion of cervical vertebrae, CHD, deafness (30%), cleft palate
   3. Zellweger syndrome = cerebrohepatorenal syndrome (large forehead, flat facies, macrogyria, hepatomegaly, cystic kidney disease, contractures of extremities)
   4. Robert syndrome
   5. Cumming syndrome

√ larger lymphangiomas with radiating septations are usually found with trisomy 18
√ nuchal fullness ≥3 mm during 1st trimester is seen in trisomy 21 / 18 / 13 (30–50% PPV)
√ often reverting to normal by 16–18 weeks
√ septations within nuchal translucency carries a 20- to 200-fold risk for chromosomal anomalies compared with normal

Sensitivity: 2–44–75% for detection of trisomy 21
Specificity: 99% for detection of trisomy 21
PPV: 69%
Positive screen: 1.2–3% in general population (exceeding 0.5% risk of amniocentesis)
False positives: 0.5–2–8.5%

OB management: thorough sonographic evaluation at 18–20 weeks MA
DDx: chorioamnionic separation

Protruding Tongue

1. Macroglossia
2. Lymphangioma of the tongue

Macroglossia

1. Beckwith-Wiedemann syndrome
2. Down syndrome
3. Hypothyroidism
4. Mental retardation

FETAL CHEST ANOMALIES

Pulmonary Hypoplasia

Path: absolute decrease in lung volume / weight for gestational age

Cause:

1. Prolonged oligohydramnios (20–25%)
2. Skeletal dysplasia (small thorax)
3. Intrathoracic mass (lung compression)
4. Large hydrothorax (lung compression)
5. Neurologic condition (reduced breathing activity)
6. Chromosomal abnormality
7. CHD with R-sided cardiac obstructing lesion

√ thoracic circumference (TC) <5th percentile for EGA
√ declining TC:AC ratio from >0.80 (75% sensitive, 80–90% specific); not applicable for intrathoracic masses

Intrathoracic Mass

in order of frequency:

1. Diaphragmatic hernia / eventration
2. Cystic adenomatoid malformation
3. Bronchopulmonary sequestration
4. Bronchogenic cyst with bronchial compression
5. Bronchial atresia

Unilateral Chest Mass

1. Congenital diaphragmatic hernia
2. Cystic adenomatoid malformation
3. Bronchopulmonary sequestration
4. Bronchogenic cyst
5. Unilateral bronchial atresia / stenosis

Bilateral Chest Masses

1. Laryngeal / tracheal atresia
2. Bilateral cystic adenomatoid malformation
3. Bilateral congenital diaphragmatic herniae

Mediastinal Mass

1. Goiter
2. Cystic hygroma
3. Pericardial teratoma
4. Neuroblastoma

Cystic Chest Mass
1. Bronchogenic cyst
2. Enteric cyst
3. Neurenteric cyst
4. Cystic adenomatoid malformation (type I)
5. Congenital diaphragmatic hernia
6. Pericardial cyst
7. Mediastinal meningocele

Complex Chest Mass
1. Congenital diaphragmatic hernia
2. Cystic adenomatoid malformation (type I, II, III)
3. Pulmonary sequestration
4. Complex enteric cyst
5. Pericardial teratoma

Solid Chest Mass
1. Congenital diaphragmatic hernia (bowel ± liver)
2. Cystic adenomatoid malformation type III
3. Pulmonary sequestration
4. Obstructed lung from bronchial atresia, laryngeal atresia, bronchogenic cyst
5. Bronchopulmonary foregut malformation
6. Pericardial tumor
7. Heterotopic brain tissue

Regressing Fetal Chest Mass
1. Cystic adenomatoid malformation
2. Bronchopulmonary sequestration

Chest Wall Mass
1. Hemangioma
2. Cystic hygroma
3. Teratoma
4. Hamartoma
5. Thoracic myelomeningocele

Pleural Effusion
1. Primary idiopathic chylothorax (most common)
2. Hydrops fetalis (multiple causes)
3. Chromosome anomaly: trisomy 21, 45 XO (mostly)
4. Pulmonary lymphangiectasia / cystic hygroma
5. Lung mass: cystic adenomatoid malformation, bronchopulmonary sequestration, congenital diaphragmatic hernia, chest wall hamartoma (uncommon)
6. Pulmonary vein atresia
7. Idiopathic

FETAL CARDIAC ANOMALIES
Incidence: 1:125 births = 0.8% of population; most common of all congenital malformations (40%)

◊ 90% occur as isolated multifactorial traits with a recurrence risk of 2–4%
◊ 10% are associated with multiple birth defects
◊ responsible for 50% of childhood deaths from congenital malformations

Antenatal sonographic diagnosis to prompt cardiac evaluation:

A. ABNORMALITIES IN CARDIAC POSITION
B. CNS
   1. Hydrocephalus
   2. Microcephaly
   3. Agenesis of corpus callosum
   4. Encephalocele (Meckel-Gruber syndrome)
C. GASTROINTESTINAL
   1. Esophageal atresia
   2. Duodenal atresia
   3. Situs abnormalities
   4. Diaphragmatic hernia
D. VENTRAL WALL DEFECT
   1. Omphalocele
   2. Ectopia cordis
E. RENAL
   1. Bilateral renal agenesis
   2. Dysplastic kidneys
F. TWINS
   1. Conjoined twins

Prenatal Risk Factors for Congenital Heart Disease
A. FETAL RISK FACTORS
   1. Symmetric IUGR
   2. Arrhythmias
      (a) fixed fetal bradycardia (50%) ≤ 110 bpm
      (b) tachycardia (low risk)
      (c) irregular: PACs, PVCs (low risk)
   3. Abnormal fetal karyotype (CHD in Down syndrome in 40%; in trisomy 18 / 13 in >90%; in Turner syndrome in 35%)
   4. Extracardiac somatic anomalies by US: omphaloceles (20%), duodenal atresia, hydrocephaly, spina bifida, VACTERL
   5. Nonimmune hydrops (30–35%)
   6. Oligo- / polyhydramnios
B. MATERNAL RISK FACTORS
   1. Maternal heart disease (10%)
   2. Insulin-dependent diabetes mellitus (4–5%)
   3. Phenylketonuria (in 15% if maternal phenylalanine >15%)
   4. Collagen vascular disease: SLE
   5. Viral infection: rubella
   6. Drugs
      (a) phenytoin (in 2% PS, AS, coarctation, PDA)
      (b) trimethadione (in 20% transposition, tetralogy, hypoplastic left heart)
      (c) sex hormones (in 3%)
      (d) lithium (7%): Ebstein anomaly, tricuspid atresia
      (e) alcohol (25% of fetal alcohol syndrome): VSD, ASD
      (f) retinoic acid = isotretinoin (?15%)
   7. Paternal CHD (risk uncertain)
C. MENDELIAN SYNDROMES
   1. Tuberous sclerosis
   2. Ellis-van Creveld syndrome
   3. Noonan syndrome

OB&GYN

D. FAMILIAL RISK FACTORS FOR RECURRENCE OF HEART DISEASE
- — overall incidence : 6–8:1,000 live births
- — affected sibling : 1–4% (risk doubled)
- — affected parent : 2.5–4%

◊ In 50% of neonates with CHD there is no identifiable risk factor!

Poor prognostic features:
(1) Intrauterine cardiac failure (hydrops)
(2) Severe trisomy (18, 13)
(3) Hypoplastic left heart + endocardial fibroelastosis
(4) Delivery in center without pediatric cardiology

In Utero Detection of Cardiac Anomalies

A. ABNORMAL HEART POSITION
1. Diaphragmatic hernia
2.. Lung anomaly
3. Pleural effusion
4. Cardiac defect

B. CHAMBER ENLARGEMENT

RA:
1. Tricuspid regurgitation
2. Tricuspid valve dysplasia
3. Ebstein anomaly

RV:
1. Coarctation
2. Normal in 3rd trimester

LA:
1. Mitral stenosis
2. Aortic stenosis

LV:
1. Aortic stenosis
2. Cardiomyopathy

C. ABNORMAL FOUR-CHAMBER VIEW
1. Septal rhabdomyoma
2. Endocardial cushion defect
3. Ventricular septal defect
4. Ebstein anomaly
5. Single ventricle

D. VENTRICULAR DISPROPORTION
1. Hypoplastic right / left ventricle
2. Hypoplastic aortic arch
3. Aortic / subaortic stenosis
4. Coarctation of aorta
5. Ostium primum defect

E. INCREASED AORTIC ROOT DIMENSION
1. Tetralogy of Fallot
2. Truncus arteriosus
3. Hypoplastic left ventricle with transposition

F. DECREASED AORTIC ROOT DIMENSION
1. Coarctation of aorta
2. Hypoplastic left ventricle

◊ 26–80% of serious cardiac anomalies can be detected on four-chamber view!

◊ Increased sensitivity >20 weeks + by including outflow views!

Structural Cardiac Abnormalities & Fetal Hydrops

1. Atrioventricular septal defect + complete heart block
2. Hypoplastic left heart
3. Critical aortic stenosis
4. Cardiac tumor
5. Ectopia cordis
6. Dilated cardiomyopathy
7. Ebstein anomaly
8. Pulmonary atresia

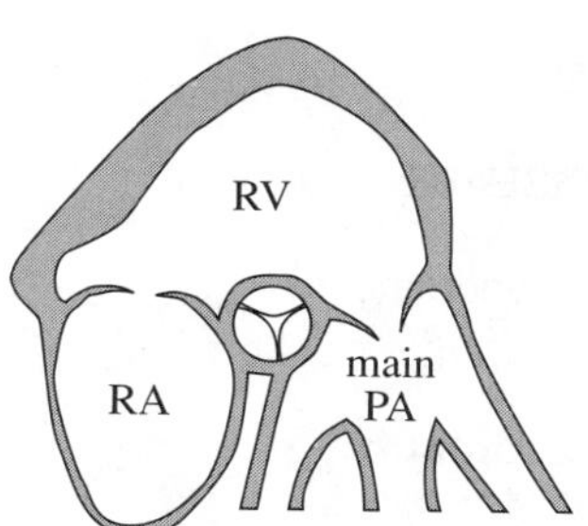

Fetal Short-Axis View

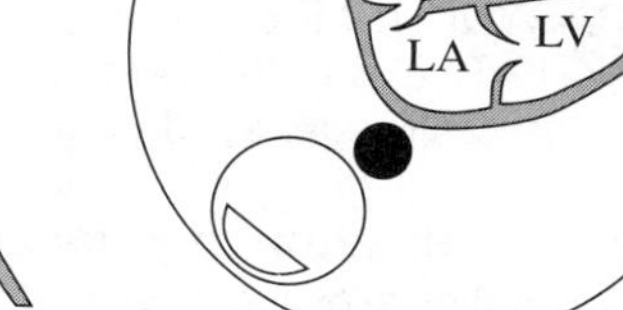

Fetal Four-Chamber View

Fetal Echocardiographic Views

A. FOUR-CHAMBER VIEW
1. Position of heart within thorax
2. Number of cardiac chambers
3. Ventricular proportion
4. Integrity of atrial + ventricular septa
5. Position + size + excursion of AV valves

B. PARASTERNAL LONG-AXIS VIEW
= LEFT VENTRICULAR OUTFLOW TRACT VIEW
1. Continuity between ventricular septum + anterior aortic wall
2. Caliber of aortic outflow tract
3. Excursion of aortic valve leaflets

C. SHORT-AXIS VIEW OF OUTFLOW TRACTS
1. Spatial relationship between aorta + pulmonary artery
2. Caliber of aortic + pulmonary outflow tracts

D. AORTIC ARCH VIEW

<u>Identification of fetal RV</u>
- √ RV lies closest to anterior chest wall
- √ foramen ovale flap seen within LA
- √ prominent moderator band + papillary muscles in RV

FETAL GASTROINTESTINAL ANOMALIES

1. Esophageal atresia ± TE fistula
2. Duodenal atresia
3. Meconium peritonitis
4. Hirschsprung disease
5. Choledochal cyst
6. Mesenteric cyst

Abdominal Wall Defect

Prevalence: 1:2,000 pregnancies
1. Gastroschisis
2. Omphalocele spectrum:
   - — upper abdominal wall defect
     3. Ectopia cordis
     4. Pentalogy of Cantrell
   - — midabdominal wall defect: classic omphalocele
   - — lower abdominal wall defect
     5. Bladder exstrophy
     6. Cloacal exstrophy
7. Amniotic band syndrome
8. Limb-body wall complex

Fetal Hepatomegaly

A. CONGENITAL INFECTIONS
   1. CMV
B. SEVERE HEMOLYTIC DISEASE
C. SYNDROMES
   1. Beckwith-Wiedemann syndrome
   2. Zellweger syndrome

Nonvisualization of Fetal Stomach

◊ Fetal swallowing begins at 11 weeks MA

Normal: stomach is visualized in almost all normal fetuses by 13–14 weeks (definitely by 19 weeks)

Incidence: 2%

Cause:

1. Physiologic gastric emptying / intermittent swallowing
   ◊ Repeat scan after 30 minutes!
2. Oligohydramnios
3. CNS depression / abnormalities impairing swallowing
4. Abnormal position of stomach:
   (a) stomach on contralateral side (situs inversus)
   (b) congenital diaphragmatic hernia
5. Esophageal atresia ± TE fistula
   ◊ Nonvisualization of fetal stomach and polyhydramnios in 33% fetuses with esophageal atresia after 24 weeks MA!
6. Cleft lip / palate (impairing normal swallowing)

Rx: repeat ultrasound scan

Double Bubble Sign

= fluid-filled stomach + proximal duodenum

◊ A persistently fluid-filled duodenum is always abnormal!

1. Duodenal atresia (usually not seen <24 weeks MA)
   Cause: in 30% due to Down syndrome (trisomy 21)
2. Severe duodenal stenosis
3. Duodenal web
4. Annular pancreas
5. Midgut volvulus
6. Preduodenal portal vein
7. Ladd bands
8. Malrotation
9. Duodenal duplication cyst

mnemonic: "LADS"

Ladd bands / malrotation
Annular pancreas
Duodenal atresia
Stenosis (duodenal)

Dilated Bowel in Fetus

1. Meconium ileus
   ◊ All newborns with meconium ileus have cystic fibrosis!
   ◊ 10–15% of newborns with cystic fibrosis present with meconium ileus!
2. "Apple peel" atresia of small bowel
3. Jejunal atresia
4. Megacystis-microcolon-intestinal hypoperistalsis syndrome
5. Colonic aganglionosis = Hirschsprung disease (may be associated with Down syndrome)
6. Anorectal atresia (associated with CNS abnormalities, part of VACTERL complex)

Bowel Obstruction in Fetus

Etiology: intestinal atresia / stenosis secondary to vascular accident, volvulus, meconium ileus, intussusception after organogenesis

Incidence: imperforate anus 1:3,000; small bowel 1:5,000; colon 1:20,000

Pathologic types:

I one / more transverse diaphragms
II blind-ending loops connected by fibrous string
III complete separation of blind-ending loops
IV apple-peel atresia of small bowel (occlusion of SMA branch)

Associated with: GI anomalies in 45% (malrotation, duplication, microcolon, esophageal atresia)

√ multiple distended bowel loops >7 mm in diameter
√ increased peristalsis
√ polyhydramnios (if obstruction above level of mid jejunum; exceptions are esophageal atresia + TE fistula) due to fetal inability to cycle amniotic fluid through gut

Cx: Meconium peritonitis (50%)

DDx: (1) Other cystic masses: duodenal atresia, hydronephrosis, ovarian cyst, mesenteric cyst
(2) Chronic chloride diarrhea

Hyperechoic Fetal Bowel

Definition: bowel echogenicity ≥ bone

Incidence: 0.2–0.6% of 2nd trimester fetuses

Cause: (?) "constipation" in utero due to decreased swallowing, hypoperistalsis, bowel obstruction + increased fluid absorption

1. Normal small bowel variant (especially <20 weeks MA) with resolution on follow-up sonogram toward end of 2nd trimester (55–68%)
2. Meconium ileus
   ◊ Increased abdominal echogenicity is seen in 60–70% of fetuses with cystic fibrosis!
3. Meconium peritonitis
   Cause: (a) intestinal atresia with perforation
   (b) CMV infection
4. Chromosomal abnormality (3–25%)
   (a) Down syndrome (5–14%)
   (b) Trisomy 13, 18
   (c) Turner syndrome
5. Severe IUGR (16%)

Prognosis:

5-fold increase in risk for adverse fetal outcome (due to chromosomal abnormality, other anomalies, placental abruption, perinatal death [8–16%], IUGR [67–23%])

◊ 30–50% of fetuses with echogenic bowel in 2nd trimester will have poor outcome!

Management: parental testing for cystic fibrosis, careful fetal anatomic survey, follow-up for growth assessment

Intraabdominal Calcifications in Fetus

A. PERITONEAL
1. Meconium peritonitis
2. Plastic peritonitis associated with hydrometrocolpos

B. TUMORS
1. Hemangioma / hemangioendothelioma
2. Hepatoblastoma
3. Metastatic neuroblastoma
4. Teratoma
5. Ovarian dermoid

C. CONGENITAL INFECTION
1. Toxoplasmosis
2. Cytomegalovirus

◊ Isolated liver calcifications are relatively frequent and of no clinical significance!

Cystic Mass in Fetal Abdomen

A. POSTERIOR MID ABDOMEN
1. Cysts of renal origin
2. Hydroureteronephrosis
3. Multicystic dysplastic kidney
4. Paranephric collection

B. RIGHT UPPER QUADRANT
1. Liver cyst
2. Choledochal cyst

C. LEFT UPPER QUADRANT
1. Splenic cyst

D. ANTERIOR MID ABDOMEN
1. Gastrointestinal duplication cyst
2. Mesenteric cyst
3. Meconium pseudocyst
4. Dilated bowel
5. Urachal cyst

E. LOWER ABDOMEN
1. Adnexal cyst: follicular cyst (most), corpus luteum cyst, theca lutein cyst, paraovarian cyst, teratoma, cystadenoma
   Cx of large cysts: polyhydramnios, dystocia, torsion, respiratory distress
   Prognosis: 60% resolve within first 6 months of life
2. Hydrometrocolpos
3. Meningocele
4. Sacrococcygeal teratoma

Fetal Ascites

A. ASCITES + FETAL HYDROPS
1. Immune hydrops
2. Nonimmune hydrops

B. ISOLATED ASCITES
1. Urinary ascites
2. Meconium peritonitis
3. Bowel rupture
4. Ruptured ovarian cyst
5. Hydrometrocolpos
6. Glycogen storage disease

FETAL URINARY TRACT ANOMALIES

Incidence: 0.25%–1% liveborn infants (OB-US); 1:100–1:200 neonates (pediatrics)

Types:
1. Bilateral renal agenesis
2. Infantile polycystic kidney disease
3. Adult polycystic kidney disease
4. Multicystic dysplastic kidney
5. Ureteropelvic junction obstruction
6. Megaureter
7. Posterior urethral valves
8. Prune belly syndrome
9. Megacystis-microcolon-intestinal hypoperistalsis syndrome
10. Mesoblastic nephroma
11. Wilms tumor
12. Neuroblastoma

Associated with: chromosome abnormalities in 12% (74% trisomy, 10% deletion, 9% sex chromosome aneuploidy, 6% triploidy)

• fetal urine production: 5 mL/hr at 20 weeks MA; 56 mL/hr at 40 weeks MA

√ bladder volume: 1 mL at 20 weeks MA; 36 mL at 40 weeks MA

√ filling + emptying of fetal urinary bladder occurs every 10–30 (range 7–43) minutes

√ increased renal parenchymal echogenicity indicates renal abnormality in 80%

√ fetal hydronephrosis
= AP diameter of renal pelvis >5 mm at 15–20 weeks, ≥8 mm at 20–30 weeks, ≥10 mm at >30 weeks

GENERAL GYNECOLOGY

Pelvic Features of Estrogen Stimulation

√ increased thickness + volume of uterus
√ fundocervical ratio >2
√ echogenic endometrium
√ appearance of ovaries NOT USEFUL (because of widely varying ovarian volumes + normal visiualization of follicles at all ages)

Precocious Puberty

= complete sexual development with secondary sex characteristics appearing <8 years of age in girls / <9 years of age in boys

• premature thelarche / adrenarche / menarche

Terminology:
(a) <u>isosexual</u> = secondary sex characteristics appropriate for patient's gender
(b) <u>heterosexual</u> = secondary sex characteristics inappropriate for patient's gender
  — virilization in girls
  — feminization in boys
(c) gonadotropin-dependent = <u>true precocious puberty</u>
(d) gonadotropin-independent = <u>pseudoprecocious puberty</u>

Isolated Premature Adrenarche
= pubic hair development due to action of adrenal androgens
- increased levels of adrenal androgens

√ prepubertal uterus + ovaries (0.1–1 cm^3)

Isolated Premature Thelarche
= breast enlargement

◊ May occur without endocrine abnormalities

√ prepubertal uterus + ovaries

Pseudoprecocious Puberty
= PSEUDOSEXUAL PRECOCITY = PERIPHERAL PRECOCIOUS PUBERTY= INCOMPLETE PRECOCIOUS PUBERTY

= pubertal changes occurring independently of the action of pituitary gonadotropins, ie, early development of secondary sex characteristics without ovulation

Cause:
1. Autonomous ovarian follicular cyst (most common cause)
2. Estrogen-secreting ovarian tumor: eg, granulosa theca-cell tumor, gonadoblastoma, thecoma, choriocarcinoma
3. McCune-Albright syndrome
4. Adrenocortical neoplasm
5. Hypothyroidism
6. Neurofibromatosis
7. Hepatoblastoma
8. Estrogen ingestion

- low gonadotropin levels after LHRH stimulation
- high estradiol level
- low levels of FSH and LH
- normal bone age

√ prepubertal uterus + ovaries

√ asymmetric ovarian enlargement (one ovary 2.4–7 cm^3) with macrocysts (>9 mm)

√ ± unilateral follicular ovarian cyst characterized by internal daughter cyst

True Precocious Puberty
= CENTRAL PRECOCIOUS PUBERTY = TRUE ISOSEXUAL PRECOCITY = COMPLETE PRECOCIOUS PUBERTY

= gonadotropin-dependent early development of gonads + secondary sex characteristics with ovulation before 8 years of age

Cause:

(1) Idiopathic activation of hypothalamic-pituitary-gonadal axis (66–80%)

(2) Lesion of pituitary gland / hypothalamus: eg, tuber cinereum hamartoma

(3) Increased intracranial pressure: eg, postmeningitis hydrocephalus

- increased levels of estrogen
- increased gonadotropin levels after LHRH stimulation
- advanced bone age

√ adult-sized ovaries (1.2–12 cm^3)

√ dominance of corpus over cervix length

Rx: long-acting gonadotropin-releasing hormone analogue

Amenorrhea
Primary Amenorrhea
Definition:

(a) no menarche by 16 years of age

(b) no thelarche / adrenarche by 14 years of age

(c) no menarche >3 years after adrenarche + thelarche

Cause:

A. FEMALE ANATOMIC ANOMALIES
= Müllerian (uterovaginal) anomalies (20%)

B. CONGENITAL DISORDERS OF SEXUAL DIFFERENTIATION

(a) pure gonadal dysgenesis = Turner syndrome (33%)
√ bilateral dysfunctional / streak gonads

(b) mixed gonadal dysgenesis
√ testis + streak gonad

Risk: in 25% development of dysgerminoma / gonadoblastoma in dysgenetic gonads with Y chromosome

C. OVARIAN FAILURE / DYSFUNCTION

D. HYPOTHALAMIC / PITUITARY CAUSES (15%)

E. CONSTITUTIONAL DELAY (10%)

F. OTHERS: eg, systemic, psychiatric illness (22%)

√ absent / streak gonads + infantile uterus:
1. Hypogonadotrophic hypogonadism
   - low / normal LH + FSH levels

   (a) hypothalamic dysfunction: hypothalamic tumor, Kallmann disease (= lack of pulsatile GnRH release), systemic illness, constitutional growth delay, extreme physical / psychological / nutritional stress (cystic fibrosis, sickle cell disease, Crohn disease), irradiation

   (b) pituitary dysfunction: disruption of pituitary stalk from child abuse, head trauma
2. Hypergonadotropic hypogonadism
   = ovarian tissue fails to respond to endogenous gonadotropins
   - high LH + FSH levels

   (a) abnormal karyotype: Turner syndrome, XY gonadal dysgenesis

   (b) irradiation, chemotherapy, autoimmune disease (eg, autoimmune oophoritis)

√ absent uterus:
1. Testicular feminization = male intersex = male pseudohermaphroditism (end-organ insensitivity to testosterone)
2. Müllerian dysgenesis (= Mayer-Rokitansky-Küster-Hauser syndrome)
   √ normal fallopian tubes + ovaries
   associated with: unilateral renal abnormality (50%), skeletal abnormality (12%)

√ small infantile uterus:
1. Androgen-producing virilizing tumors of adolescent ovary (usually Sertoli-Leydig cell tumor)
   √ unilateral adnexal mass
2. Turner syndrome
3. In utero exposure to diethylstilbestrol

√ normal uterus + unilateral ovarian tumor:
1. Estrogen-producing ovarian tumor with disruption of menstrual cycle: granulosa cell tumor, thecoma

√ hematometrocolpos:
(a) neonate = congenital uterovaginal obstruction
   1. Urogenital sinus / cloacal malformation
      √ pelviabdominal cystic mass with fluid-debris level in fetal US during 3rd trimester
      √ renal dysplasia / obstruction
(b) teenager
   1. Imperforate hymen
   2. Transverse vaginal septum
      – in upper vagina (45%)
      – in mid vagina (40%)
      – in lower vagina (15%)

√ hematometra
1. Cervical dysgenesis

√ bilateral ovarian enlargement:
1. Polycystic ovary syndrome (= Stein-Leventhal syndrome): most common cause of secondary amenorrhea

Secondary Amenorrhea
1. Pregnancy: most common cause in girls >9 years of age
2. Polycystic ovary syndrome (main pathologic cause)
3. Asherman syndrome
4. All causes of primary amenorrhea

Calcifications of Female Genital Tract
A. UTERUS
   1. Uterine fibroid
   2. Arcuate arteries
B. OVARIES
   1. Dermoid cyst (50%)
   2. Papillary cystadenoma (psammomatous bodies)
   3. Cystadenocarcinoma
   4. Hemangiopericytoma
   5. Gonadoblastoma
   6. Chronic ovarian torsion
   7. Pseudomyxoma peritonei
C. FALLOPIAN TUBES
   1. Tuberculous salpingitis
D. PLACENTA
E. LITHOPEDION

Psammoma Bodies in Tumors
1. Papillary serous cystadenoma / cystadenocarcinoma
2. Mucinous carcinoma of colon
3. Papillary thyroid cancer
4. Meningioma

Free Fluid in Cul-de-sac
1. Follicular rupture
2. Ovulation
3. Ectopic pregnancy
4. S/P culdocentesis
5. Ovarian neoplasm
6. Pelvic inflammatory disease

PELVIC MASS

Frequency of Pelvic Masses

1. Benign adnexal cyst	34%
2. Leiomyoma	14%
3. Cancers	14%
4. Dermoid	13%
5. Endometriosis	10%
6. Pelvic inflammatory disease	8%

Cystic Pelvic Masses
A. CYSTIC ADNEXAL MASS
B. EXTRAADNEXAL CYSTIC MASS
   1. Peritoneal inclusion cyst
   2. Mesenteric cyst
   3. Lymphocele
   4. Bladder diverticulum
   5. Ectopic gestation
   6. Fluid-distended bowel
   7. Loculated pelvic abscess: appendiceal, diverticular, postoperative

Complex Pelvic Mass
mnemonic: "CHEETAH"

Cystadenoma / cystadenocarcinoma
Hemorrhagic cyst
Endometrioma
Ectopic pregnancy
Teratoma (dermoid)
Abscess (from adjacent appendicitis, etc.)
Hematoma in pelvis

Solid Pelvic Masses
1. Pedunculated myoma (most common)
2. Fibroma
3. Adenofibroma
4. Thecoma
5. Brenner tumor

Extrauterine Pelvic Masses
1. Solid adnexal mass
2. Metastatic disease
3. Lymphoma

4. Pelvic kidney
5. Rectosigmoid carcinoma
6. Prostate carcinoma
7. Benign prostatic enlargement
8. Bladder carcinoma
9. Retroperitoneal tumor
10. Intraperitoneal fat
11. Vascular mass / malformation
12. Hematoma
13. Bowel

Pelvic Pain in Pediatric Age Group

1. Ovarian torsion
   (a) of normal ovary
   Cause: excessive mobility of ovary in childhood
   (b) with ovarian mass:
   — functional cyst (60%)
   — neoplasm (40%):
   - benign mature teratoma (66%)
   - malignancy (33%): germ cell tumor (60–75%), epithelial tumor (10–20%), stromal tumor (10%)
2. Hemorrhagic ovarian cyst
3. Pelvic inflammatory disease
4. Ectopic pregnancy

ADNEXA

Adnexal Masses

A. CYSTIC
1. Physiologic ovarian cyst:
   — Graafian follicle: at midcycle <25 mm
   — Corpus luteum: after midcycle <15 mm
2. Functional / retention cyst
3. Endometrioma
4. Tuboovarian abscess
5. Dermoid cyst
6. Ectopic pregnancy
7. Paraovarian cyst / cystadenoma
8. Serous / mucinous ovarian tumor
9. Hyperstimulation cysts
10. Peritoneal inclusion cyst
11. Massive ovarian edema
12. Hydrosalpinx

B. SOLID
1. Ovarian tumor
2. Ovarian torsion
3. Oophoritis
4. Polycystic ovaries
5. Fallopian tube carcinoma

(DDx: pedunculated fibroid)

Hemorrhagic Adnexal Lesion

1. Endometriosis
2. Hemorrhagic ovarian cyst
3. Hemorrhagic foci of adenomyosis
4. Hematosalpinx

OB&GYN

Low-intensity Adnexal Lesion on T1WI

1. Fibroma
2. Fibrothecoma
3. Cystadenofibroma
4. Brenner tumor
5. Wall of chronic pelvic abscess
6. Pedunculated leiomyoma

High-intensity Adnexal Lesion on T1WI

1. Endometrioma
   √ frequently multilocular + bilateral
   √ shading (= signal loss) on T2WI
2. Dermoid
   √ chemical shift artifact
   √ signal drop-out after fat suppression
3. Mucinous cystic neoplasm
   √ signal intensity less than fat / blood
4. Hemorrhagic cyst
   √ unilocular
   √ no shading
   √ resolution with time
5. Ovarian carcinoma
   √ solid components, septations
   √ large size

Adnexal Mass in Pregnancy

Incidence: 0.5–1.2%

A. RESOLVING BY 14–16 WEEKS EGA
1. Corpus luteum cyst
2. Theca lutein cyst

B. PERSISTENT ADNEXAL MASS
1. Benign
   correctly diagnosed by US: 95% of dermoids, 80% of endometriomas, 71% of simple cysts
2. Malignant (0.1–0.8%)

Ovarian Tumors

- pressure symptoms: abdominal discomfort, vomiting, flatulence, dyspnea
- acute pain from torsion, hemorrhage
- chronic pain from slowly enlarging mass, impaction, adhesions
- menstrual irregularity

Radiologic guidelines:

◊ Imaging features of ovarian neoplasms virtually never allow a specific diagnosis. Regardless of further differentiation patients always undergo surgery!

Signs suggestive of benignancy:
√ unilocularity of cyst
√ thin wall <3 mm
√ minimal septations
√ absence of papillary projection

Signs suggestive of malignancy:
√ solid nonfatty nonfibrous tissue (most powerful predictor of malignancy!)
√ many solid-tissue elements in a complex lesion
√ wall thickness >3 mm

√ inner wall irregularities / papillary projections
√ thick septations >3 mm
√ increased echogenicity within a cyst

Age: 13% of neoplasms malignant in premenopause; 45% of neoplasms malignant in postmenopause

Cx: (1) Torsion (in 10–20%)
(2) Rupture (rare)
(3) Infection

Classification:

◊ 75% of ovarian neoplasms are benign
◊ 21% of ovarian neoplasms are malignant
◊ 4% of ovarian neoplasms are borderline malignant

A. TUMORS OF SURFACE EPITHELIUM (60–70%)
= 85–95% of all ovarian cancers
- propensity for early peritoneal + lymphatic spread

√ peritoneal studding
√ omental cake
√ perihepatic diaphragmatic implants

1. Serous ovarian tumor (50%)
2. Endometrioid tumor (15–30%)
3. Mucinous ovarian tumor (15%)
4. Clear cell adenocarcinoma (5%)
5. Undifferentiated carcinoma (<5%)
6. Brenner tumor (2.5%)
7. Cystadenofibroma

B. GERM CELL TUMORS (15–30%)
◊ 40% of germ cell tumors are malignant
(a) benign (10%)
1. Dermoid cyst = mature teratoma (most common)

(b) malignant
account for 75% of ovarian cancers seen in 1st–2nd decade of life; <5% of all ovarian tumors; in order of frequency:
1. Dysgerminoma (1.9%)
2. Immature teratoma (1.3%)
3. Endodermal sinus tumor (1%)
4. Malignant mixed germ cell tumor (0.7%)
5. Embryonal carcinoma (0.1%)
6. Choriocarcinoma (0.1%)

C. SEX CORD-STROMAL TUMORS (5–8%)
usually have more than one cell type + arise from two groups of cells:
— primitive sex cord cells, which form from the coelomic epithelium (= primordial peritoneum) differentiate into granulosa cells + Sertoli cells
— stromal cells (fibroblasts, theca cells, Leydig cells) derive from the genital ridge mesonephros mesenchyma
- broad range of ages
- most present at stage I with good prognosis
- absent tumor markers

◊ Often manifest with tumor-mediated hormonal effects
√ NO papillary projections
√ lack of fat + calcifications
— hyperestrogenic tumors: granulosa cell tumor, thecoma, stromal luteoma
— virilizing tumors: Sertoli-Leydig cell tumor, steroid cell tumor (Sertoli cell tumor, Leydig cell tumor)

(a) Granulosa-stromal cell tumors
1. Juvenile granulosa cell tumor ... multicystic
2. Adult granulosa cell tumor .... solid
3. Thecoma .... solid
4. Fibroma .... solid
5. Fibrosarcoma
6. Sclerosing stromal tumor

(b) Sertoli-stromal cell tumors
1. Sertoli-Leydig tumor .... solid
2. Sertoli cell = arrhenoblastoma .... solid
3. Leydig cell

(c) Steroid cell tumors = lipid cell tumors
1. Stromal luteoma
2. Leydig cell tumor = hilus cell tumor
3. Steroid cell tumor, not otherwise specified

(d) Other
1. Gynandroblastoma
2. Sex cord tumor with annular tubules associated with Peutz-Jeghers syndrome (30% of all tumors with annular tubules)
3. Sclerosing stromal tumor

D. SECONDARY OVARIAN TUMORS (5%)
Metastases from: pelvic organs, upper GI tract, breast, bronchus, reticuloendothelial tumors, leukemia

Subclassification:

	Benign	*Borderline*	*Malignant*
[all types combined	75%	4%	21%]
Serous	60%	15%	25%
Mucinous	80%	10%	10%
Endometrioid	~0%	~0%	~100%
Clear cell	~0%	~0%	~100%
Undifferentiated	0%	0%	100%

Terminology:

prefix "cyst-" : cystic component present
suffix "-fibroma" : >50% fibrous component
"tumor of low malignant potential" : borderline malignant

Solid Ovarian Tumor

1. Fibroma
2. Thecoma
3. Granulosa cell tumor
4. Sertoli-Leydig cell tumor
5. Brenner tumor
6. Sarcoma
7. Dysgerminoma
8. Endodermal sinus tumor
9. Teratoma
10. Metastasis
11. Endometrioma
12. Massive ovarian edema

Proximal Fallopian Tube Obstruction

1. Extensive fibrosis / salpingitis isthmica nodosa (40%)
2. Amorphous debris / minimal adhesions (40%)
3. Tubal spasm (20%)

UTERUS

Prepubertal Vaginal Bleeding

1. Vaginal foreign body
   Incidence: in 18% of children with vaginal bleeding + discharge; in 50% of children with vaginal bleeding + no discharge
2. Vaginal rhabdomyosarcoma
3. Precocious puberty
4. Hemangioma
5. Vascular malformation

Postmenopausal Vaginal Bleeding

1. Endometrial atrophy (in 60–75%)
   • thin atrophic endometrium is prone to superficial ulceration
   √ in 75% endometrial thickness <4–5 mm
   ◊ Patient may forego endometrial biopsy!
   √ in 25% endometrial thickness of 6–15 mm
2. Endometrial hyperplasia
3. Endometrial polyp
4. Submucosal fibroid
   √ hypoechoic mass with an overlying normal echogenic endometrium
   √ ± acoustic attenuation
   √ ± prolapse into endometrial cavity
   Rx: can be removed at hysteroscopy if >50% of mass projects into endometrial cavity
5. Adenomyoma
   √ indistinguishable from submucosal fibroid
6. Endometrial carcinoma (in 7–20%)
7. Estrogen withdrawal

Optimal time of imaging:
immediately after cessation of bleeding when endometrium is presumed to be thinnest

Rx: any focal / generalized thickness >5 mm at transvaginal US requires further investigation (sonohysterography, guided biopsy, hysteroscopy)

Diffusely Thickened Irregular Endometrium

Normal endometrial thickness: *see* Anatomy

Sensitivity for detection of endometrial abnormalities:
80% for transvaginal US; 30% for endometrial biopsy
Time of sonohysterography: day 4, 5, or 6 of menstrual cycle

1. **Endometrial hyperplasia**
   Age: peri- / postmenopausal women
   Cause: prolonged endogenous / exogenous unopposed estrogen stimulation
   √ focal / diffuse endometrial thickening >5–6 mm
   √ formation of polyps of up to 5 cm
   Types:
   (a) glandular-cystic hyperplasia (most common)
   Histo: dilated glands lined by tall columnar / cuboidal epithelium
   √ small cysts within evenly echogenic endometrium
   Prognosis: NO premalignant condition
   (b) adenomatous hyperplasia
   √ endometrium with irregular hypoechoic areas
   Prognosis: precursor of endometrial cancer
2. Secretory endometrium
   ◊ Improve timing of the examination!
3. Endometrial cancer
4. Endometritis
5. Tamoxifen-related endometrial changes
   = nonsteroidal antiestrogen in breast acts as a weak estrogen agonist causing proliferative effects on the endometrium
   Increased prevalence of: endometrial hyperplasia, polyps, carcinoma
   ◊ 50% of women treated with tamoxifen will develop endometrial abnormalities within 6–36 months
   Histo:
   a) endometrial thickness increased to 10.4 mm; 4.2 mm in control subjects
   (b) polyps (36%); 10% in control subjects
   (c) atrophic changes (28%); 87% in control group
   • hemorrhage (requires further evaluation)
   √ endometrial thickening >5–9 mm:
   √ endometrial hyperplasia
   √ endometrial polyp
   √ subendometrial cystic changes (= glandular distension within a polyp / reactivated adenomyosis within inner myometrium)
   MR:
   √ endometrium-myometrium interface (due to endometrial atrophy / proliferative changes):
   √ homogeneously hyperintense on T2WI
   √ signal void + enhancement on T1WI
   √ polyps:
   √ heterogenous intensity on T2WI
   √ laticelike enhancement traversing endometrial canal on T1WI

DDx: normal thickening during secretory phase

Focally Thickened Endometrium

1. **Endometrial polyp**
   = focal hyperplasia of stratum basale; in 20% multiple
   Age: mainly 30–60 years
   Histo: projections of endometrial glands + stroma into uterine cavity
   (a) hyperplastic polyp resembling endometrial hyperplasia
   (b) functional polyp resembling surrounding endometrium (least frequent)
   (c) atrophic polyp
   Frequently associated with: tamoxifen therapy

US:
- √ sessile broad-based / pedunculated well-defined smooth hyperechoic homogeneous intracavitary mass (79%) / variable echogenicity (best seen on sonohysterography):
  - √ cystic spaces (in 59%) due to enlarged dilated glands filled with proteinaceous fluid
  - √ heterogeneous texture suggests infarction, inflammation, hemorrhage
  - √ vessel visualized within stalk on color Doppler

Malignant transformation: in 0.4–3.7%

2. Primary carcinoma of the endometrium
   Risk factors: exposure to unopposed estrogen, obesity, nulliparity, hypertension, diabetes
   Location: predominantly in uterine fundus; 24% in isthmic portion)
   - ◊ 10% cancer rate with endometrial thickness of 6–15 mm
   - ◊ 50% cancer rate with endometrial thickness of >15 mm
   - √ irregular heterogeneous endometrium >5 mm in thickness
   - √ focal / diffuse endometrial thickening (mean thickness of 18.2 mm)
   - √ irregular poorly defined endometrial-myometrial interface
   - √ increased echogenicity in myometrium (= invasive endometrial cancer)
   - √ Doppler waveforms with resistive index <0.7 suggest malignancy
3. Metastatic carcinoma:
   ovary, cervix, fallopian tube, leukemia
4. Hydatidiform mole
   - √ echogenic mass with irregular sonolucent areas
5. Incomplete abortion
6. Submucosal leiomyoma
   - √ mass hypo- / hyperechoic relative to myometrium
   - √ wide attachment to myometrium
   - √ intracavitary margin outlined by echogenic rim of endometrium
   - √ ± acoustic attenuation

   Rx: hysteroscopic removal if >50% of mass projects into endometrial cavity
7. Focal adenomyoma
   - √ hypoechoic mass with an overlying echogenic endometrium

   DDx: indistinguishable from submucosal fibroid
8. Intrauterine synechiae
   - √ echogenic bands extending from one endometrial surface to the other

DDx: adherent blood clots

Fluid Collection within Endometrial Canal

Types: blood, mucus, purulent material

A. PREMENOPAUSAL
1. Infection: endometritis, pyometrium
2. Congenital obstructive lesion: imperforate hymen, vaginal septum, vaginal / cervical atresia
3. Acquired obstructive lesion: cervical stenosis (following instrumentation / cone biopsy / radiation), cervical carcinoma
4. Spontaneous hematometra in bleeding disorders
5. Pregnancy: intrauterine, ectopic, incomplete abortion
6. Endometrial cancer
7. Endometrial polyp, submucosal fibroid
8. Functional: during menstruation

B. POSTMENOPAUSAL
1. Endometrial / cervical cancer
2. Cervical stenosis
3. Normal if amount small

Endometrial Cysts

1. Endometrial cystic atrophy
   Histo: cystically dilated atrophic glands lined by single layer of flattened / low cuboidal epithelium
   - √ very thin endometrium of <4–5 mm
2. Endometrial cystic hyperplasia

Diffuse Uterine Enlargement

1. Diffuse leiomyomatosis
2. Adenomyosis
3. Endometrial carcinoma (15%)

Uterine Masses

A. BENIGN
1. Uterine fibroids (99%)
2. Pyometra
3. Hemato- / hydrocolpos
4. Transient uterine contraction (during pregnancy)
5. Bicornuate uterus
6. Adenomyosis
7. Intrauterine pregnancy
8. Lipoleiomyoma (<50 cases in world literature)

B. MALIGNANT
1. Cervical carcinoma
2. Endometrial carcinoma
3. Leiomyosarcoma
4. Invasive trophoblastic disease

Cervical Mass

1. Fibroid
2. Carcinoma
3. Endometrial polyp
4. Nabothian cyst (= retention cyst related to chronic cervicitis)

Fundic Depression on HSG

1. Bicornuate uterus
2. Septate uterus
3. Arcuate uterus
4. Fundal myoma

Postpartum Hemorrhage

1. Uterine atony
   - • hemorrhage in immediate postpartum period
   - √ normal uterus

2. Retained products of conception
   - hemorrhage several days after delivery
   - √ echogenic intracavitary mass attached to endometrium
   - √ high-velocity flow >21 cm/sec of low resistance (supplying residual trophoblastic tissue)
   - √ calcification of retained products (late finding)

VAGINA

Vaginal Cyst

1. Gartner duct cyst
2. Bartholin gland cyst
   = female homologue of male Cowper glands
   Location: posterolateral portion of lower vagina
3. Paramesonephric / müllerian duct cyst
   = aberrant remnant of paramesonephric duct
   Location: anterior wall of vagina near cervix
4. Epithelial inclusion cyst
   = arise from urogenital sinus
   Histo: lined by transitional epithelium containing thick caseous material

Vaginal Fistula

1. Enterovaginal fistula
   (a) rectovaginal: incomplete healing of perineal laceration from obstetric trauma, radiation therapy
   (b) anovaginal: inflammatory bowel disease (10% of patients with Crohn disease)
   (c) colovaginal: diverticulitis
2. Vesicovaginal fistula: hysterectomy, radiation therapy
3. Ureterovaginal fistula: vaginal hysterectomy

Vaginal & Paravaginal Neoplasm

A. PRIMARY
   1. Cavernous hemangioma of vulva
   2. Pedunculated submucosal leiomyoma prolapsed into vagina
   3. Adenoid cystic carcinoma of Bartholin gland
   4. Vaginal carcinoma
      (a) squamous cell carcinoma (90%)
      (b) adenocarcinoma (3%)
   5. Rhabdomyosarcoma

B. SECONDARY (80% of all vaginal tumors)
   direct extension from bladder, rectum, cervix, uterus

GAS IN GENITAL TRACT

A. UTERUS
   1. Endometritis
   2. Superinfection of leiomyoma: more common in submucosal leiomyoma (insufficient blood supply)
   3. Bacterial metabolism of necrotic neoplastic tissue
   4. Fistula to GI tract: uterine cancer
   5. Pyometra secondary to obstruction by cervical cancer
   6. Gas gangrene: due to clostridial infection from septic abortion

B. OVARY
   1. Superinfected ovarian neoplasm

C. VAGINA
   1. Vaginitis emphysematosa = nonbacterial self-limiting process mostly occurring during pregnancy characterized by numerous gas-filled spaces in submucosa of vagina + exocervix

ANATOMY AND PHYSIOLOGY OF FEMALE REPRODUCTIVE SYSTEM

HUMAN CHORIONIC GONADOTROPIN

= hCG = glycoprotein elaborated by placental trophoblastic cells beginning the 8th day after conception

A. IMMUNOLOGIC PREGNANCY TEST
= indirect agglutination test for hCG in urine; cross-reaction with other hormones / medications possible
Becomes positive at 5 weeks MA
Advantages: readily available, easily + rapidly performed
Disadvantages: frequently false-positive + false-negative results
Sensitivity:
(a) slide: 400–15,000 mIU/mL (2-minute test time)
(b) test tube: 1,000–3,000 mIU/mL (2-hour test time)

B. RADIOIMMUNOASSAY (RIA) PREGNANCY TEST
= measures beta subunit of hCG in serum with a sensitivity as low as 1–2 mIU/mL
◊ Serum β-hCG becomes positive at 3 weeks MA / 7–10 days following conception!
Standards:
(1) Second International Standard (SIS)
(2) International Reference Preparation (IRP)
(3) Third International Standard (TIS)
1 mIU/mL (SIS) = 2 mIU/mL (IRP) = 2 mIU/mL (TIS)
1 ng/mL = 5–6 mIU/mL (SIS)
= 10–12 mIU/mL (IRP or TIS)
◊ Variations of lab values of up to 50% can occur among different laboratories!
◊ 6–15% between-run precision!
Advantages: specific for hCG, sensitive
Disadvantages: requires specialized lab + 3–24 hours for completion
Sensitivity:
(a) qualitative: 25–30 mIU/mL (3 hours test time)
(b) quantitative: 3–4 mIU/mL (24 hours test time)
Rise:
>66% increase of initial β-hCG level over 48 hours in 86% of NORMAL pregnancies
<66% increase of initial β-hCG level over 48 hours in 87% of ECTOPIC pregnancies
◊ β-hCG levels double every 2–3 days during first 60 days of pregnancy!

"1–7–11 Rule":

β–hCG (IRP)	*US Landmarks*	*Gestational Age*
1,000 mIU/mL	gestational sac	32 d (4.5 weeks)
7,200 mIU/mL	yolk sac	36 d (5.0 weeks)
10,800 mIU/mL	embryo + heart motion	40 d (6.0 weeks)

ANATOMY OF GESTATION

Choriodecidua

Chorion
= trophoblast + fetal mesenchyme with villous stems protruding into decidua; provides nutrition for developing embryo
(a) chorion frondosum = part adjacent to decidua basalis, forms primordial placenta
(b) chorion laeve = smooth portion of chorion with atrophied villi
(c) "chorionic plate" = amnionic membrane covering the chorionic plate of the placenta

Decidua
(a) decidua basalis = between chorion frondosum + myometrium
(b) decidua capsularis = portion protruding into uterine cavity
(c) decidua parietalis = decidua vera = portion lining the uterine cavity elsewhere

Gestational Sac

Arises from blastocyst, which implants into secretory endometrium 6–9 days after ovulation (= 20–23 days of MA), surrounded by echogenic trophoblast
◊ GS measures 0.1 mm at time of implantation
√ **intradecidual sign** (earliest sign) = intrauterine fluid collection corresponding to gestational sac completely embedded within decidua (48% sensitive, 66% specific, 45% accurate) at <5 weeks GA
√ **double decidual sac sign** (DDS) [most useful >5 weeks GA] = 2 concentric hyperechoic rings surrounding a portion of the gestational sac:
√ outer echogenic ring (= decidua parietalis)
√ interposed hypoechoic line (apposed endometrial walls)
√ inner echogenic ring (= decidua capsularis)
√ DDS present with a mean sac diameter of 10 mm (= 40 days GA)

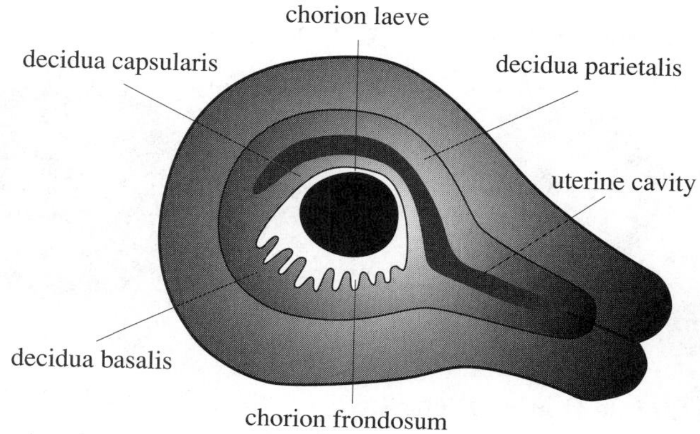

Anatomy of Gestation

◊ A double decidual sac sign correlates with the presence of pregnancy in 98%!

√ GS surrounded by endometrial thickening >12 mm
√ continuous hyperechoic inner rim >2 mm thick
√ spherical / ovoid shape without angulations
√ mean sac diameter grows 1.13 (range 0.71–1.75) mm/day

Gestational Sac Size

linear growth: 10 mm by 5th week MA
60 mm by 12th week MA

fills chorionic cavity by 11–12 weeks MA

Visualization of Gestational Sac

Earliest visualization: mean sac diameter of 2–3 mm

A. GS VISUALIZATION VERSUS β-hCG LEVEL (2nd International Standard):
   (a) on transabdominal scan:
      in 100% with β-hCG levels of >1,800 IU/L
   (b) on transvaginal scan:
      in 20% with β-hCG levels of <500 IU/L
      in 80% with β-hCG levels of 500–1,000 IU/L
      in 100% with β-hCG levels of >1,000 IU/L

B. GS VISUALIZATION VERSUS MENSTRUAL AGE
   (a) on transabdominal scan:
      5.0 ± 1 weeks = 5–10 mm
      5.5 ± 1 weeks = 8.5–13 mm
      6.0 ± 1 weeks = 12–17 mm
   (b) **on transvaginal scan**:
      2.5 weeks = 1 mm
      5.0 ± 1 weeks = 2 mm
      5.5 ± 1 weeks = 6 mm
      6.0 ± 1 weeks = 11 mm

C. GS VISUALIZATION VERSUS VISUALIZATION OF EMBRYO
   (a) on transabdominal scan
      100% visualization if gestational sac ≥27 mm
   (b) on transvaginal scan
      100% visualization if gestational sac ≥12 mm
   ◊ Transvaginal scan not necessary if on transabdominal scan gestational sac >27 mm without evidence of embryo!

Secondary Yolk Sac

= rounded sonolucent structure (outside amniotic cavity) within chorionic sac (= extracoelomic cavity) connected to umbilicus via a narrow stalk; formed by proliferation of endodermal cells; part of yolk sac is incorporated into fetal gut; the rest persists as a sac connected to the fetus by the vitelline duct

Function:
   (a) transfer of nutrients from trophoblast to embryo prior to functioning placental circulation
   (b) early formation of blood vessels + blood precursors on sac wall
   (c) formation of primitive gut
   (d) source of primordial germ cells

Time of formation: at around 28 days MA

Mean size:
   1.0 mm by 4.7 weeks MA; 2.0 mm by 5.6 weeks MA; 3.0 mm by 7.1 weeks MA; 4.0 (2.2–5.3) mm by 10 weeks MA; disappears around 12 weeks MA

◊ First visible structure within gestational sac

Definite visualization on transvaginal scan:
   √ at 5.5 weeks MA
   √ in GS with a mean sac diameter of ≥8 mm

Definite visualization on transabdominal scan:
   √ in GS with a mean diameter of ≥20 mm
   √ at a gestational age of 7 weeks MA

Embryo

Developmental stages:
   Preembryonic period: 2nd–4th week MA
   Trilaminar embryonic disk: during 5th week MA
      3 laminae = ectoderm, endoderm, mesoderm
   Embryonic period: 6th–10th week MA
      physiologic umbilical herniation: 8th–12th week MA
   Fetal period: beginning at 11th week MA

Average growth rate:
   0.7 mm per day / 1.5 mm every 2 days;
   curvilinear growth from 7 mm at 6.3 weeks MA to 50 mm at 12.0 weeks MA

Earliest visualization (on endovaginal scan):
   at 5.4 weeks MA at CRL of 1.2 mm

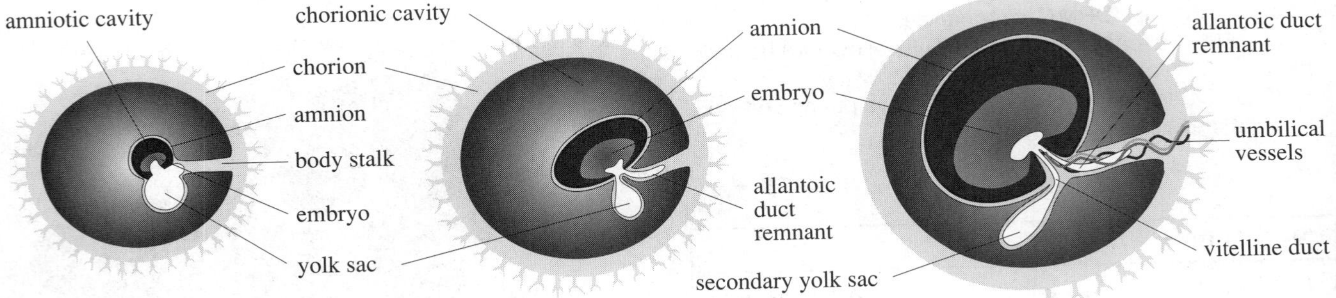

Simple Double Bleb Stage
earliest detection at 5 weeks GA, embryo 2 mm in length

Vitelline Duct
8 weeks GA

Early Coiled Umbilical Cord
9 weeks GA

OB&GYN

Failed pregnancy:
nonvisualization of embryo with mean gestational sac size of ≥18 mm

Cardiac Activity of Embryo

◊ Heart begins to contract at a CRL of 1.5–3 mm = 22 days GA = 36 days MA

Definite visualization on endovaginal scan:
(a) at 46 days GA
(b) mean sac diameter of 16 mm
(c) **CRL ≥ 5 mm CRL = 6.2 weeks**

Definite visualization on transabdominal scan:
(a) at 55 days GA
(b) mean sac diameter of 25 mm

Rate:
- at 5-6 weeks GA .... 101 bpm
- at 8-9 weeks GA .... 143 bpm

Amnionic Membrane

= curvilinear echogenic line within chorionic sac; fills chorionic cavity by 11–12 weeks MA;

Fusion:
— fuses with chorionic membrane at approximately 16 weeks MA to form the chorionic plate
— incomplete fusion with chorion frequent (DDx: subchorionic hemorrhage, twin abortion, coexistent with limb-body wall complex)

Umbilical Cord

Embryology:
- cord forms between 5th and 12th postmenstrual week with contributions from body stalk, omphalomesenteric or vitelline duct, yolk sac, allantois
- junction of the amnion with ventral surface of embryo will form umbilicus
- midgut undergoes physiologic herniation into the base of the umbilical cord 7–12 postmenstrual weeks
- cord grows until end of 2nd trimester: average diameter of 17 mm, length of 50–60 cm

Anatomy:
- 1–2 cm in diameter
- two umbilical arteries = branches of the two internal iliac arteries
- one umbilical vein (remains after regression of right umbilical vein in early embryonic period)
- Wharton jelly = compressible matrix of cord
- covered by amnion
- spiraling of cord with 0–40 twists established by 9 weeks

Placental Grading

according to echo appearance of basal zone, chorionic plate, placental substance

◊ Premature placental calcifications are associated with cigarette smoking, hypertension, IUGR!

◊ Not considered useful because placental grading is imprecise for fetal dating or for fetal lung maturity!

GRADE 0
√ homogeneous placenta + straight line of chorionic plate
Time: <30 weeks MA

GRADE 1
√ undulated chorionic plate + scattered bright placental echoes
Time: seen at any time during pregnancy; in 40% at term
◊ in 68% L/S ratio >2.0

GRADE 2
√ linear bright echoes parallel to basal plate
√ confluent stippled echoes within placenta ± indentations of chorionic plate
Time: rarely seen in gestations <32 weeks MA; seen in 40% at term
◊ in 87% L/S ratio >2.0

GRADE 3
√ calcified intercotyledonary septa, often surrounding sonolucent center
Time: rarely seen in gestations <34 weeks MA; in 15–20% at term
◊ in 100% L/S ratio >2.0 (= strongly correlated with lung maturity)

PREMATURE PLACENTAL SENESCENCE
= grade 3 placenta seen in gestation <34 weeks MA
◊ In 50% suggestive of maternal hypertension / IUGR

Uteroplacental Circulation

By 20 weeks MA trophoblast invades maternal vessels and transforms spiral arteries into distended tortuous vessels = uteroplacental arteries

Histo:
(a) in the decidual portion of spiral arteries: proliferating trophoblast from anchoring villi invades lumen of spiral arteries + partially replaces endothelium
(b) in the myometrial portion of spiral arteries: disintegration of smooth muscle elements (loss of elastic lamina) leads to easily distensible vascular system of low resistance

Uterine Blood Volume Flow

— 50 mL/min shortly after conception
— 500–900 mL/min by term

Intervillous blood flow: 140 ± 53 mL/min (by Xe-133 washout)

Umbilical Artery Doppler

Variables of Doppler measurements:
site of Doppler (close to placenta preferred), fetal heart rate, fetal breathing, drugs (ritodrine hydrochloride decreases S/D ratio)

√ degree of diastolic flow increases as gestation progresses
- S/D ratio between 3.3 and 4.3 at 20 weeks
- S/D ratio between 1.7 and 2.4 at term

√ highly turbulent flow

IUGR Lesions
= narrowing of vascular lumen through
  (a) thrombosis of decidual segments of uteroplacental arteries
  (b) failure of development of myometrial segments of uteroplacental arteries

FETAL MENSURATION
US is more reliable than LMP / physical examination
ULTRASOUND MILESTONES:
- √ gestational sac w/o embryo or yolk sac = 5.0 weeks
- √ gestational sac + yolk sac w/o embryo = 5.5 weeks
- √ heartbeat ± embryo <5 mm = 6.0 weeks

Accuracy: ± 0.5 week

Fetal Age
= GESTATIONAL AGE (GA) = "MENSTRUAL AGE" (MA)
= age of pregnancy based on woman's regular last menstrual period (LMP) projecting the estimated date of confinement (EDC) at 40 weeks
◊ Note the inaccurate clinical usage of "gestational age," which strictly speaking refers to the true age of the pregnancy counting from the day of conception, whereas "menstrual age" refers to the true age of the pregnancy + approximately 2 weeks counting from the first day of the last menstruation!
◊ On subsequent scans GA = GA assigned at 1st ultrasound + number of intervening weeks!

ACCURACY OF CLINICAL ASSESSMENT

menstrual history	±2–3 weeks
1st-trimester exam	±2 weeks
fundal height	±4 weeks

ACCURACY OF BIOMETRY (95% confidence range):

Stage	*Based on*	*Accuracy [weeks]*
1st trimester		
(5–6 weeks)	US milestones	±0.5
(6–13 weeks)	CRL	±0.7
2nd trimester		
(14–20 weeks)	cBPD / HC	±1.2
	BPD / FL	±1.4
(20–26 weeks)	cBPD / HC	±1.9
	BPD / FL	±2.1–2.5
3rd trimester		
(26–32 weeks)	cBPD / HC / FL	±3.1–3.4
	FL	±3.1
(32–42 weeks)	cBPD / HC / FL	±3.5–3.8
	FL	±3.5

Gestational Sac
= average of 3 diameters (craniocaudad, AP, TRV) of anechoic space within sac walls
◊ Used for dating between 6 and 12 weeks MA (identified as early as 5 weeks MA on transabdominal scan)
EGA [in wks] = (GS [in mm] + 25.43) ÷7.02
Accuracy: ± 7 days

Early Embryonic Size
= length of embryo <25 mm on transvaginal scan performed at <11 weeks MA
Gestational age (days) = embryonic size (mm) + 42
Accuracy: ± 3 days

Crown-rump Length (CRL)
= length of fetus; useful up to 12 weeks MA (usually identified by 7 weeks MA on transabdominal scan)
Rule of thumb: MA (in weeks) = CRL (in cm) + 6
Accuracy: ± 5–7 days

Biparietal Diameter (BPD)
= measured from leading edge to leading edge of calvarial table at widest transaxial plane of skull
= level of thalami + cavum septi pellucidi + sylvian fissures with middle cerebral arteries
◊ Excellent means of estimating GA in 2nd trimester >12 weeks MA
Accuracy:
2 mm for "between occasion error"
◊ Most accurate for dating if combined with HC, AC, FL provided body ratios are normal!
◊ Less reliable for dating in 3rd trimester because of increasing biologic variability!

Cephalic Index (CI)
= BPD / OFD; measurements of BPD and occipitofrontal diameter (OFD) are both taken from outer to outer edge of calvarium
◊ Confirms appropriate use of BPD if ratio is between 0.70 and 0.86 (2 SD)

Corrected BPD (cBPD)
= BPD and OFD are used to adjust for variations in head shape

$$cBPD = \sqrt{BPD \times OFD \div 1.26}$$

Head Circumference (HC)
Used if ratio of BPD/OFD outside 0.70–0.86

$$HC = ([BPD + OFD]/2) \times \pi$$
$$= ([BPD + OFD] \times 1.62) \times 3.1417$$

Accuracy: slightly less than for BPD
HC too large: hydrocephalus, hydranencephalus, intracranial hemorrhage, short limb dystrophies, tumor
HC too small: anencephaly, cerebral infarction, synostosis, microcephaly vera

Abdominal Circumference (AC)
= measured at level of vascular junction of umbilical vein with left portal vein ("hockey-stick" appearance) where it is equidistant from the lateral walls in a plane perpendicular to long axis of fetus; measured from outer edge to outer edge of soft tissues
◊ Allows evaluation of head-to-body disproportion
◊ Better predictor of fetal weight than BPD

AC too large: GI tract obstructions, obstructive uropathy, ascites, hepatosplenomegaly, congenital nephrosis, abdominal tumor
AC too small: diaphragmatic hernia, omphalocele, gastroschisis, renal agenesis

Femur Length (FL)
= measurement of ossified femoral diaphysis
Error: "flare" at distal end included in measurement (= reflection from cartilaginous condyle)

Thoracic Circumference (TC)
= measured in axial plane of chest, which includes four-chamber view of heart without inclusion of SQ tissue
◊ Linear growth between 16 and 40 weeks similar to AC
Useful age-independent parameter: TC:AC >0.80

Estimated Fetal Weight (EFW)
based on measurements of head size (BPD / HC), abdominal size (AD / AC), and femur length (FL)
Accuracy:

body part used	95% confidence range
abdomen	±22%
head + abdomen	±17–20%
head + abdomen + femur	±15%

Appearance of Epiphyseal Bone Centers
in 95% of all cases
— distal femoral epiphysis (DFE): >33 weeks GA
— distal femoral epiphysis (DFE) >5 mm: >35 weeks
— proximal tibial epiphysis (PTE): >35 weeks GA
— proximal humeral epiphysis (PHE): >38 weeks GA

CNS Ventricles
width of 3rd ventricle: <3.5 mm (any gestational age)

Diameter of Cisterna Magna
measured from inner margin of occiput to vermis cerebelli: 2–10 mm

DISCORDANT ESTIMATED DATE OF CONFINEMENT (EDC) BY LMP AND BPD:
1. Methodological error in measurement
   (a) wrong axial section
   (b) cranial compression (multiple gestation, breech presentation, oligohydramnios, dolichocephaly)
2. Erroneous LMP
   other measurements (AC, FL) correlate with BPD
3. Abnormal head growth
   (a) BPD less than AC: microcephaly, fetal macrosomia
   (b) BPD more than AC: intracranial abnormality, asymmetric IUGR

ASSESSMENT OF FETAL WELL-BEING

Amniotic Fluid Index
= sum of vertical depths of largest clear amniotic fluid pockets in the 4 uterine quadrants measured in mm

Method: patient supine, uterus viewed as 4 equal quadrants, transducer perpendicular to plane of floor + aligned longitudinally with patient's spine

Variation: 3.1% intraobserver, 6.7% interobserver
Result:
— 95th percentile: 185 mm at 16 weeks GA, rising to 280 mm at 35 weeks, declining to 190 at 42 weeks
— 5th percentile: 80 mm at 16 weeks GA, rising to 100 mm at 23 weeks, declining to 70 mm at 42 weeks

Biophysical Profile (Platt and Manning) = BPP
= in utero Apgar score = assessment of fetal well-being
Gestational age at entry: 25 weeks MA

Observation period: 30 (occasionally 60) minutes; ordinarily <8 minutes needed; in 2% full 30 minutes required

A. ACUTE BIOPHYSICAL VARIABLES
◊ Subject to rhythmic variation coincident with sleep-wake cycle!

1. Fetal breathing movement (FBM):
   √ ≥1 episode of chest + abdominal wall movement for a period lasting 30 seconds (time is arbitrary to avoid confusion with general body movements / maternal respiration)
   stimulated by: glucose, catecholamine, caffeine, prostaglandin synthetase inhibitor
   suppressed by: barbiturates, benzodiazepine, labor, hypoxia, asphyxia, prostaglandin E_2

2. Fetal body movement:
   √ ≥3 discrete movements of limbs / trunk
   influenced by: glucose, gestational age, time of day, maternal drugs, intrinsic rhythm, labor

3. Fetal tone
   upper + lower limbs usually fully flexed with head on chest; least sensitive test parameter
   √ ≥1 episode of opening + closing of hand / extension + flexion of limb

B. CHRONIC FETAL CONDITION
4. Amniotic fluid volume
   √ at least one pocket ≥2 cm in vertical diameter in two perpendicular planes
   ◊ Avoid inclusion of loops of cord!

Score (for each test): 2 points if normal; 0 points if abnormal

Results (including NST for a maximum of 10 points):

Score	*Interpretation*	*Perinatal Mortality*
10	asphyxia rare	0.0%
8 + normal fluid	asphyxia rare	<0.1%
8 + abnormal fluid	chronic compromise	8.9%
6 + normal fluid	equivocal	variable
6 + abnormal fluid	asphyxia probable	8.9%
4	asphyxia highly probable	9.1%
2	asphyxia almost certain	12.5%
0	asphyxia certain	60.0%

False-negative rate: 0.7:1,000

◊ The probability of fetal death within a week of a BPP score of 8/8 is 1:1,000!

Stress Tests

Nonstress Test (*NST*)

◊ Test needed in less than 5% of cases!

√ reactive fetal heart rate tracing (normal) = at least 4 fetal heart accelerations (>15 bpm over baseline lasting >15 seconds) in a 20-minute period subsequent to fetal movement >34 weeks GA

√ nonreactive (abnormal) fetal heart rate tracing = absence of acceleration in a continuous 40-minute observation period

N.B.: no heart accelerations in immaturity, during sleep cycle, with maternal sedative use

Accuracy: false-negative rate of 3.2:1,000 (if done weekly) or 1.6:1,000 (if done biweekly); 50% false-positive rate for neonatal morbidity + 80% for neonatal mortality

Contraction Stress Test (*CST*)

= external monitoring after injection of oxytocin / maternal breast stimulation

√ >3 uterine contractions in 10-minute period

Accuracy: false-negative rate of 0.4/1000; 50% false-positive rate

INVASIVE FETAL ASSESSMENT

Amniocentesis

Indications:

(1) Inadequate sonographic fetal anatomic survey due to fetal position / maternal body habitus
(2) Equivocal sonographic findings (eg, abnormal posterior fossa but spinal defect not seen)
(3) Experienced sonographer not available
(4) Nonlethal anomaly detected on level I sonogram for which karyotype testing is appropriate

A. DIAGNOSTIC AMNIOCENTESIS
1. Genetic studies: karyotype, DNA analysis, biochemical assay
   Timing: early (11–15 weeks), late (15–18 weeks)
2. Neural tube defect: α-fetoprotein, acetylcholinesterase
3. Isoimmunization: Δ-OD 450
4. Fetal lung maturity
5. Intraamniotic infection
6. Confirmation of ruptured membranes

B. THERAPEUTIC AMNIOCENTESIS
1. Polyhydramnios
2. Twin-twin transfusion syndrome

Technique:

√ avoid fetus, placenta, umbilical cord, uterine contraction, fibroid, large uterine vessel

√ use continuous ultrasound guidance

√ inject 2–5 mL of indigo carmine dye in first sac of twin (colorless fluid assures that second sac has been entered)

Risk: fetal loss rate generally quoted as 1:200 (0.5%)

A. FETAL RISK
1. Spontaneous abortion (0.3–1.5%)
2. Amniotic fluid leak
3. Chorioamnionitis
4. Fetal injury: skin dimple, limb gangrene, porencephalic cyst, hemothorax, spleen laceration, orthopedic abnormality, amniotic band syndrome

B. MATERNAL RISK (rare)
1. Bowel perforation
2. Hemorrhage
3. Isoimmunization

Advantage over CVS:
1. Error rate (<1% versus 2%)
2. Culture failure rate (0.6% versus 2.2%)
3. Fetal loss rate (0.6–0.8% less)

Chorionic Villus Sampling (CVS)

= aspiration of cells from chorion frondosum for genetic studies (karyotype, DNA analysis, biochemical assay)

◊ Transabdominal CVS for rapid karyotyping in 2nd + 3rd trimester = **placental biopsy**

Advantage: >2 weeks earlier results compared with amniocentesis

Timing: 9–11 weeks

Approach:

(a) transcervical route = catheter introduced through cervix into chorion frondosum, easier for posterior placenta; contamination by cervical flora possible;
◊ CONTRAINDICATED in cervical infections!

(b) transabdominal route = 20–22-gauge needle inserted from anterior abdominal wall; easier for anterior / fundal placenta; sterile technique

Chromosome analysis:

(a) direct preparation = analysis of cytotrophoblasts (may have different karyotype than fetus)
→ analysis can be performed immediately

(b) villus culture = cells from central mesenchymal core (same karyotype as fetus)
→ cultured for several days before analysis

Errors (2%):
1. Mosaicism = cell line forming cytotrophoblast may develop abnormal karyotype while fetal cell line is normal

OB&GYN

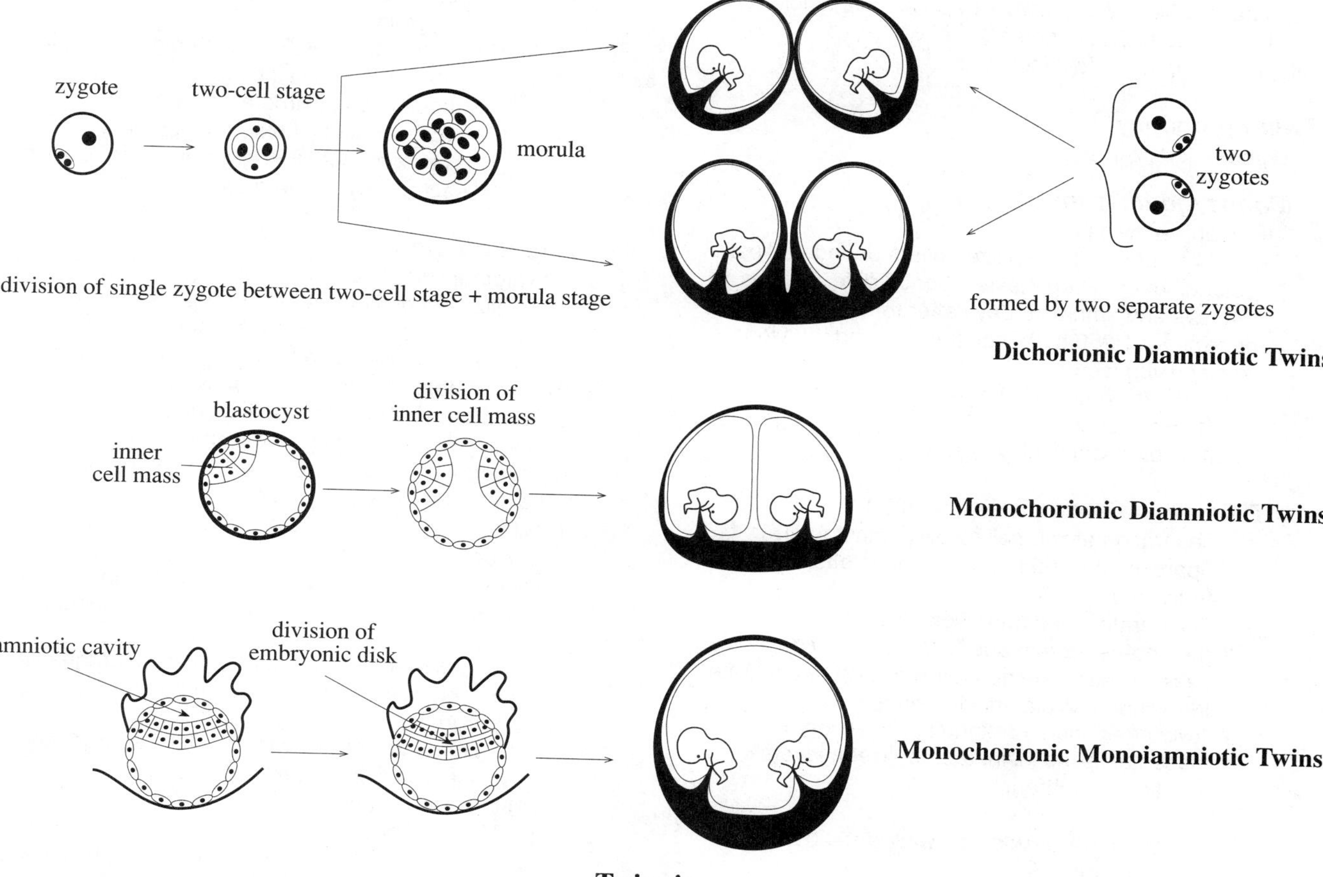

Twinning

2. Maternal contamination = cells from maternal decidua may overgrow mesenchymal core cells

Risks:
1. Spontaneous abortion (1%)
2. Perforation of amniotic sac
3. Infection
4. Teratogenesis: limb reduction defect

Cordocentesis

= PERCUTANEOUS UMBILICAL BLOOD SAMPLING (PUBS)

A. DIAGNOSTIC CORDOCENTESIS
1. Hematocrit
2. Karyotype
3. Immunodeficiency: chronic granulomatous disease, severe combined immunodeficiency
4. Coagulopathy: von Willebrand syndrome, factor deficiency
5. Platelet disorder: alloimmune / idiopathic thrombocytopenic purpura
6. Hemoglobinopathy: sickle cell anemia, thalassemia
7. Infection: toxoplasmosis, rubella, varicella, cytomegalovirus, parvovirus
8. Hypoxia / acidosis

B. THERAPEUTIC CORDOCENTESIS
1. Intravascular fetal transfusion (fresh rh-negative CMV-negative leukodepleted irradiated packed cells compatible with mother infused at 10–15 mL/min)
2. Direct delivery of medication to fetus

Cx:
1. Chorioamnionitis
2. Rupture of membranes
3. Umbilical cord hematoma
4. Umbilical cord thrombosis
5. Bleeding from insertion site
6. Fetal bradycardia

MULTIPLE GESTATIONS

Incidence: 1.2% of all births; in 5–50% clinically undiagnosed at term

Occurrence:

twins	in	1:85	pregnancies (= 85^1)
triplets	in	1:7,600	pregnancies (~ 85^2)
quadruplets	in	1:729,000	pregnancies (~ 85^3)
quintuplets	in	1:65,610,000	pregnancies (~ 85^4)

- uterus large for dates
- may have elevated hCG, HPL (human placental lactogen), AFP levels

Perinatal morbidity & mortality compared with singletons:
twins: up to 5-fold increase
triplets: up to 18-fold increase

Twin Pregnancy

Zygote = fertilized egg

Monozygotic Twins (1/3)

= "identical twins"
= division of a single fertilized ovum during earliest stages of embryogenesis (chorion differentiates 4 days and amnion 8 days after fertilization)

Incidence: 1:250 birth (constant around the world)

Predisposing factors:
(1) Advanced maternal age
(2) In vitro fertilization

√ same sex + identical genotype

Dichorionic Diamniotic Twins (30%)

= separation at two-cell stage (= blastomere) approximately 60 hours / <4 days after fertilization
√ 2 separate fused / unfused placentas
√ membrane >2 mm due to 2 separate chorionic sacs + 2 separate amniotic sacs (92% accurate for dichorionic diamniotic twins)
√ "twin peak" sign = triangular projection of placental tissue insinuated between layers of intertwin membrane

Monochorionic Diamniotic Twins (69–80%)

(most common)
= separation in blastocyst stage between 4th and 7th day after fertilization (chorion already developed and separated from embryo)
√ 2 separate amniotic sacs in single chorionic sac
◊ Common monochorionic placenta has vascular communications in 100%!

Cx: (1) Twin-twin transfusion syndrome
(2) Twin embolization syndrome = DIC in surviving twin from transfer of thromboplastin; 17% morbidity / mortality of survivor after fetal death of twin
(3) Acardiac parabiotic twin

Monochorionic Monoamniotic Twins (1%)

= division of embryonic disk between 8th and 12th day after fertilization (amniotic cavity already developed)
√ common amniotic + chorionic sac, no separating membrane
√ entanglement of cords (the only definitive positive sonographic sign of monoamnionicity)

Cx: double perinatal mortality up to 45%
(1) Entangled umbilical cord (70%)
(2) True knot of cord
(3) Conjoined twins (umbilical cord with >3 vessels, shared fetal organs, continuous fetal skin contour)

Prognosis: 40% survival rate

Cx: (1) perinatal mortality 2.5 times greater than for dizygotic twins
(2) Fetal anomalies 3–7 times higher than in dizygotic twins / singletons (often only affecting one twin): anencephaly, hydrocephalus, holoprosencephaly, cloacal exstrophy, VATER syndrome, sirenomelia, sacrococcygeal teratoma

Dizygotic Twins (2/3)

= "fraternal twins"
(a) fertilization of two ova by two separate spermatozoa during two simultaneous ovulations (occurring either in both ovaries or in one ovary)
(b) superfetation = fertilization of two ova by two separate spermatozoa during two subsequent ovulations (frequency unknown)
(c) superfecundation = two ova fertilized by two different fathers (very rare)

Incidence: 1:80 to 1:90 births

Predisposing factors:
(1) Advanced maternal age (increased up to age 35): reduced gonadal-hypothalamic feedback with increase of FSH levels
(2) Ovulation-inducing agents (multiple pregnancies in 6–17% with clomiphene, in 18– 53% with Pergonal)
(3) Maternal history of twinning (3 times as frequent compared with normal population)
(4) Increased parity
(5) Maternal obesity
(6) Race with inherited predisposition for multiple ovulations (Blacks > Whites > Asians)

√ different phenotypes; same / opposite sex
√ always dichorionic diamniotic

Amnionicity & Chorionicity

Embryologic events in monozygotic twins:

Days after Fertilization	*Embryologic Event*	*Cleavage results in* Chorion	Amnion
1–2	cell divisions → morula	di~	di~
3–4	chorionic differentiation		
6	blastocyst implants in endometrium	mono~	di~
8	amnionic differentiation	mono~	mono~
>13	division of embryonic disk	mono~	mono~ but conjoined

Rules:
◊ Only monozygotic twins can give rise to monochorionic + monoamniotic pregnancies!
◊ All monoamniotic twins must also be monochorionic!
◊ All dizygotic twins must be dichorionic + diamniotic!
◊ 77% of all twin pregnancies are dichorionic (ie, all dizygotics [2/3 of all twins], which equals 67% + 30% of all monozygotics [1/3 of all twins], which equals 10%)

1. GESTATIONAL SACS (<10 weeks MA)
   Accuracy: 100% in 1st trimester, 80–90% in 2nd trimester
   √ 2 gestational sacs, each with a live fetus, indicates dichorionic twinning
   √ single gestational sac with 2 live fetuses indicates monochorionic twins
   √ single extraembryonic coelom indicates monochorionic twins
2. YOLK SAC
   √ number of yolk sacs = number of amnions
3. FETAL GENDER
   √ different genders (in 25% of twin pregnancies) must be dizygotic twins and thus dichorionic! [DDx: testicular feminization demonstrates female external genitalia with a 46,XY karyotype]
4. PLACENTAL SITES
   √ 2 placentas (in 45% of twin pregnancies) indicate dichorionic diamniotic pregnancy
   √ 1 placenta indicates
   (a) monochorionic pregnancy
   (b) dichorionic pregnancy with fused placenta (occurs in 50% of dichorionic twin pregnancies)
5. CHORIONIC PEAK
   √ "twin peak" sign (= triangular projection of placental tissue extending beyond chorionic surface of the placenta + insinuated between layers of intertwin membrane + wider at chorionic surface and tapering to a point some distance inward from surface) indicates dichorionic pregnancy

6. MEMBRANE
   √ separating membrane confirms diamniotic pregnancy, but does not distinguish between mono- or dichorionic pregnancy
   √ dichorionic membrane (two layers of chorion + two layers of amnion) is thicker (>2 mm) than monochorionic membrane (two layers of amnion <1 mm): 88–92% accuracy in 1st trimester, 39–83% accuracy in 2nd + 3rd trimester
   ◊ All membranes appear to be thin in 3rd trimester!
   √ absence of membrane suggests a monoamniotic monochorionic twin pregnancy
   ◊ Nonvisualization of membrane is not sufficient evidence of monoamnionicity due to technical factors!

7. CORD
   √ entanglement of cords is the only definitive positive sonographic sign of monoamnionicity
   √ simultaneous recording of fetal arterial signals at nonsynchronous rates within wide Doppler gate

8. AMNIOGRAPHY
   √ detection of imbibed intestinal contrast in both twins by CT following single sac contrast injection proves monoamniotic monochorionic twin pregnancy

Growth Rates of Twins

Twins should be scanned every 3–4 weeks >26–28 weeks GA

A. Below 30–32 weeks GA
   √ normal individual twins grow at same rate as singletons
   √ BPD growth rates similar to singleton fetuses
B. Beyond 30–32 weeks GA
   √ combined weight gain of both twins equals that of a singleton pregnancy (AC of twins < AC of singleton)
   ◊ Weight of twin fetus falls below that of singleton when combined weight of twins >4,000 g!
   √ BPD + HC growth may / may not be affected (controversial)
   √ FL not affected

Discordant Growth

= weight difference at birth >25%

Cause: (1) Twin-twin transfusion syndrome
(2) IUGR of one fetus

√ BPD difference >5 mm (discordant growth in 20–30%)
√ discordant HC increases probability of IUGR
√ AC is single most sensitive parameter for IUGR
√ EFW is most sensitive set of combined parameters for IUGR
√ >15% S/D ratio difference of umbilical artery Doppler waveforms between twins

Risks in Multiple Gestations

1.	Placental abruption	3-fold
2.	Anemia	2.5-fold
3.	Hypertension	2.5-fold
4.	Congenital anomaly	2–3-fold
5.	Preterm delivery	12-fold
6.	Perinatal mortality	4–6-fold

◊ Risk increases with number of fetuses, monozygosity, monochorionicity

Risk for IUGR

monochorionic-monoamniotic > monochorionic-diamniotic > dichorionic-diamniotic

Risk for Perinatal Mortality

1% for singletons, 9% for diamniotic dichorionic twins, 26% for diamniotic monochorionic twins, 50% for monoamniotic monochorionic twins

Prognosis:
(1) Perinatal mortality 5–10 times that of singleton pregnancy (91–124:1,000 births)
— 9% for dichorionic diamniotic twins
— 26% for monochorionic diamniotic twins
— 50% for monochorionic monoamniotic twins
(a) preterm delivery with birth weight <2,500 g
(b) IUGR (25–32%; 2nd most common cause of perinatal mortality + morbidity)
(c) amniotic fluid infection (60%)
(d) premature rupture of membranes (11%)

(e) twin-twin transfusion syndrome (8%)
(f) large placental infarct (8%)
(g) placenta previa
(h) abruptio placentae
(i) preeclampsia
(j) cord accidents
(k) malpresentations
(l) velamentous cord insertion (7-fold increase compared with singleton pregnancy)

(2) Fetal death in utero (0.5–6.8%; 3 times as often in monochorionic than in dichorionic gestations)
◊ 50% of twin gestations seen at 10 weeks GA will be singletons at birth!

(3) Increased risk of congenital anomalies (23:1,000 births = twice as frequent as in singletons; 3–7 times more frequent in monozygotic twins than in dizygotic twins)

UTERUS

Uterine Size

◊ Overfilling of urinary bladder can modify uterine shape!

A. PREPUBERTAL UTERUS
(a) NEONATAL UTERUS
Length of 2.3–4.6 cm (mean 3.4 cm), fundal width of 0.8–2.1 cm (mean 1.2 cm), cervical width of 0.8–2.2 cm (mean 1.4 cm)
- **spade**-shaped uterus (58%) with cervix often twice as thick as fundus
- **tube**-shaped uterus (32%) with cervical + fundal AP measurements identical
- adult **pear**-shaped uterus (10%) with fundus wider than cervix

√ thin echogenic endometrium
√ endometrial fluid (in 23%) secondary to maternal hormonal stimulation
√ becomes smaller by 4th month of life (2.6–3.0 cm)
◊ Best time to evaluate uterus in child with ambiguous genitalia is first few months of life!

(b) INFANTILE UTERUS
Age: infancy to 7 years of age
Length of 2.5–3.3 cm, fundal width of 0.4–1.0 cm, cervical width of 0.6–1.0 cm
√ cervix occupies 2/3 of uterine length

(c) PREMENARCHAL / PREPUBERTAL UTERUS
Mean length of 4.3 cm
√ usually tubular configuration with fundocervical ratio of 1:1

B. POSTPUBERTAL UTERUS
— nulliparous: 5–8 cm (L); 3 cm (AP); 1.6–3.0 cm (TRV)
— multiparous: 6–11 cm (L); 3–4 cm (AP); 3–5 cm (TRV)
√ fundocervical ratio of 2:1 to 3:1
√ mean uterine volume of 90 cm^3

C. POSTMENOPAUSAL UTERUS
cervix occupies 1/3 of uterine length;
3.5–6.5 cm (L); 2 cm (AP); 1.2–1.8 cm (TRV)

Uterine Zonal Anatomy (on T2WI)

Thickness of zones depends on menstrual cycle + hormonal medication

A. ENDOMETRIUM
√ high signal intensity similar to fat

B. JUNCTIONAL ZONE
= innermost layer of myometrium
Mean thickness: 2–8 mm
Histo: compact smooth muscle fibers with 3-fold increase in number + size of nuclei compared with outer myometrium
√ low signal intensity (lower water content); seen in 40–60%, may not be visible in premenarchal + postmenopausal women

C. MYOMETRIUM
√ intermediate signal intensity, increases during secretory phase

Cervical Zones

(a) Central stripe of high signal intensity on T2WI
Histo: secretions in endocervical canal + cervical mucosa + plicae palmatae
√ arbor vitae / plicae palmatae = irregular branched mucosal pattern of cervical canal

(b) Middle layer of low signal intensity continuous with junctional zone of corpus uteri
Histo: inner zone of fibromuscular stroma with percentage of nuclear area 2.5 times greater than in outer zone

(c) Outer layer of intermediate signal intensity
Histo: outer zone of fibromuscular stroma

Endometrium

Measurements refer to
- AP diameter of both apposed endometrial layers (= bilayer thickness) excluding intrauterine fluid
- the level of the uterine fundus
- midline long-axis image of uterus

◊ Measurements increase by 1–2 mm in patients with large body habitus
◊ If there is a discrepancy between concomitant endometrial + ovarian findings bleeding is usually associated with anovulatory cycles

1. MENSTRUAL PHASE (usually days 1–5)
Thickness: 1–4 mm
√ interrupted thin echogenic line of central interface

2. PROLIFERATIVE PHASE (days 6–14)
Thickness: 5–7 mm

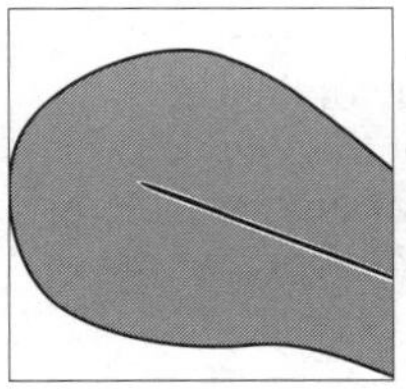
During Menstruation

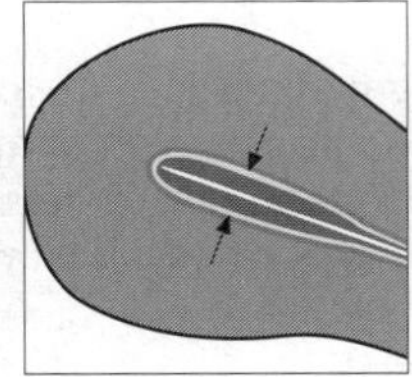
Late Proliferative Phase

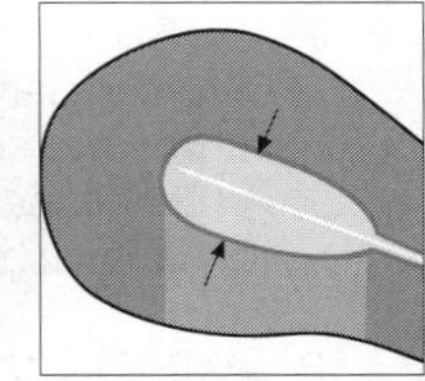
Secretory Phase

Normal Premenopausal Endometrium

√ bright echogenic central line (= apposed borders of endometrial canal)
√ thickened isoechoic to hyperechoic endometrium compared with myometrium (due to development of glands, blood vessels, stroma)

3. PERIOVULATORY PHASE (day 14)
   Thickness: up to 11 mm
   √ "triple ring sign" = multilayered endometrium:
      √ echogenic basal layer
      √ hypoechoic inner functional layer
      √ thin echogenic median layer arising from the central interface
   √ concomitant with mature preovulatory follicle
   √ disappears within 48 hours after ovulation
4. SECRETORY PHASE (days 15–28)
   Thickness: 7–12–16 mm
   √ bright central line
   √ markedly echogenic thick endometrium (due to stromal edema + distended glands filled with mucus and glycogen):
      √ ± posterior acoustic enhancement
      √ maximum thickness during midsecretory phase
      √ concomitant with a corpus luteum
   √ thin hypoechoic halo of inner myometrial zone

Postmenopausal Endometrium

A. NO HORMONAL REPLACEMENT THERAPY
   √ bilayer thickness of <5 mm with a homogeneous echogenic endometrium
   Histo: consistently associated with atrophic inactive endometrium
B. WITH HORMONAL REPLACEMENT THERAPY
   (a) cyclic estrogen + progestin therapy
      √ endometrial thickness may increase to 8 mm:
         √ thickest prior to progestin exposure
         √ thinnest after progestin phase (imaging should be done at the beginning / end of a treatment cycle)
   (b) unopposed estrogen therapy / continuous estrogen + progesterone
      √ endometrial thickness may increase to 15 mm
      Rx: biopsy / D&C recommended if endometrial thickness >8 mm

Normal Postpartum Endometrium

√ endometrial cavity <20 mm in diameter:
   √ small echogenic foci of retained membranes / clot / debris (in up to 24% of healthy patients)
   √ intrauterine air (in up to 21% of healthy patients)
√ cavity wall:
   √ smooth well-defined border
   √ irregular heterogenous lining
   √ endometrial stripe thickness decreases with uterine involution

Pelvic Spaces

1. Rectouterine pouch = cul-de-sac
   Anterior boundary: broad ligaments + uterus
   ◊ Most dependent portion of pelvis in women!
2. Rectovesical recess
   ◊ Most dependent portion of pelvis in men!
3. Vesicouterine recess
4. Inguinal fossa
   located between lateral + medial umbilical folds

Pelvic Ligaments

1. Broad ligament
   Histo: 2 layers of peritoneum
   Origin: uterine peritoneum
   Attachment: pelvic sidewall
   — medial superior free edge: formed by fallopian tube
   — lateral superior free edge: suspensory ligament of ovary
   — lower margin: cardinal ligament
   Contents (= parametrium):
   extraperitoneal connective tissue, smooth muscle, fat, fallopian tube, round ligament, ovarian ligament, uterine + ovarian blood vessels, nerves, lymphatics, mesonephric remnants
2. Round ligament
   = anterior suspensory ligament of uterus
   Histo: band of fibromuscular tissue + lymphatic channels
   Origin: anterolateral uterine fundus, just below + anterior to ovarian ligament
   Attachment: through internal inguinal canal (lateral to deep inferior epigastric vessels) to labia majora
3. Cardinal ligament = transverse cervical ligament
   = Mackenrodt ligament
   Origin: cervix + upper vagina
   Attachment: fascia of obturator internus muscle
   Relationship:
   — uterine artery runs along its superior aspect
   — forms the base of the broad ligament
4. Uterosacral ligament
   Origin: posterolateral cervix + vagina
   Attachment: anterior body of sacrum at S2 or S3
5. Ovarian ligament = round ligament of the ovary
   Origin: medial aspect of ovary
   Attachment: uterus, just inferior + posterior to fallopian tube + round ligament
6. Suspensory ligament of ovary = infundibulopelvic lig.
   Origin: anterolateral aspect of ovary
   Attachment: connective tissue over psoas muscle
   Contents: ovarian artery + vein
7. Lateral umbilical fold / ligament
   = reflection of peritoneum over deep inferior epigastric vessels
8. Medial umbilical fold / ligament
   = reflection of peritoneum over obliterated umbilical arteries
9. Median umbilical ligament
   = reflection of peritoneum over obliterated urachus
   Origin: dome of urinary bladder
   Attachment: umbilicus

OVARIES

Fixation:

fairly mobile with attachments to

anterior pelvic wall	by	broad ligament
uterine body	by	uteroovarian ligament
fallopian tube	by	tuboovarian ligament
lateral pelvic wall	by	infundibulopelvic ligament

Histology:

A. Stromal cells
   - form cortex, medulla, hilus
   - surround all developing follicles
   - cell surface has estrogen-, progesterone-, testosterone-binding sites
   - major source of androgens in postmenopause

B. Cells derived from stroma cells
   1. Fibroblasts
   2. Luteinizing stromal cells containing lipid
   3. Hilus cells
      morphologically similar to Leydig cells in testis; contain intracellular crystalline structures (= crystals of Reinke)
   4. Theca cells
      - surround granulosa cells
      - produce estradiol under control of FSH
      - stimulated by LH after ovulation into theca-lutein cells, which develop lipid-laden cytoplasm involved in steroidogenesis

C. Cells derived from sex cords
   1. Granulosa cells
      - derived from sec cords
      - surround each primordial oocyte
      - form lining of developing follicle
      - granulosa cell layer contains small cystic cavities lined by basal lamina (= Call-Exner bodies)
      - produce estradiol under control of FSH
      - stimulated by LH after ovulation into granulosa-lutein cells, which develop lipid-laden cytoplasm involved in steroidogenesis
   2. Sertoli cells
      not seen in normal ovary

Embryology:

coelomic (surface) epithelium invaginates into mesenchymal substance (= primary sex cords) and incorporates primordial germ cells, which develop into primordial follicles

Ovarian Size

Ovarian volume = length x height x width x 0.523

<3 months:	1.06–3.56 cm^3
4–12 months:	up to 2.71 cm^3
1 year:	1.05 ± 0.7 (S.D.) cm^3
2–6 years:	$\leq 1.0 \pm 0.4$ (S.D.) cm^3
6–10 years:	1.2–2.3 cm^3
11–12 years:	2–4 cm^3
after puberty:	2.5–5 cm (L), 0.6–1.5 cm (H), 1.5–3 cm (W) = 8 (range 2.5–20) cm^3

◊ An ovary >20 cm^3 is enlarged!

◊ An ovary between 15 and 20 cm^3 requires follow-up!

Prepubertal Girls	
Ovarian volume:	4–5 cm^3
Uterine length:	4.5 cm
Uterine thickness:	1 cm

Ovarian Morphology

neonate: √ follicles occasionally fail to involute + undergo growth

<8 years: √ solid ovoid structures with homogeneous / finely heterogeneous texture
√ up to 68–80% of ovaries contain cystic follicles (in 95% <9 mm, in 5% >9 mm)

Visualization of Ovaries

(a) after menopause (average onset at age 50):
   <5 years after menopause: in 78%
   >10 years after menopause: in 64%
   — both ovaries: in 85%
   — one ovary: in 60%

(b) following hysterectomy: in 43%

Ovarian Cycle

1. FOLLICULAR PHASE = days 1–14
   - a number of immature primordial follicles begin to mature in response to FSH

   √ multiple small cysts:
   (a) unstimulated follicles are <2 mm in size
   (b) stimulated follicles grow >2 mm in size

   √ 2–3 follicles in each ovary of day 4 enlarge subsequently to approximately 10 mm
   - 2–3 follicles capture the most FSH and aromatize the most estradiol from their granulosa cells

   √ single "ascendant / **dominant follicle**" of 8–12 mm (= graafian follicle) appears by day 10:
   √ grows by 2 mm/day
   √ subsequently enlarges to 21 (range 17–24) mm by day 14
   - rapidly rising estradiol production triggers the hypothalamic arcuate nucleus to increase GnRH secretion, which prompts the anterior pituitary to disgorge the stored LH over 24 hours
   - LH binds to ovarian receptors + releases cAMP from granulosa cells halting granulosa cell mitosis + increasing peptidase, collagenase, growth factor, angiotensin, prostaglandin as the cause for follicular rupture + conversion to corpus luteum

   √ progressively increasing diastolic flow on the side of maturing follicle
2. OVULATORY PHASE = day 14
   - "Mittelschmerz" = pain just prior to ovulation (pressure of graafian follicle distending ovarian capsule)

   √ sudden decrease in follicular size over minutes / hours (= rupture of mature graafian follicle with extrusion of ovum)

3. LUTEAL PHASE = days 15–28
   ◊ All corpora lutea evolve over days and change size and texture constantly
   ◊ All corpora lutea contain hemorrhage: uncontrolled bleeding into center frequently at time of ovulation + on day 8 when regression begins
   √ round / ovoid bulging protrusion on one side of ovary = **corpus luteum of menstruation**:
      √ mean diameter of 10–25 mm
      √ hyperechoic 1–4-mm thick wall
      √ hyperechoic central blood clot gradually transforming to weblike fibrin net
      √ blood flow in main arteriole supplying the corpus luteum is approximately 100 cm/sec
      √ surrounded by wreath-like color flow
   √ involution + atrophy of corpus luteum on about 24th day of cycle = **corpus luteum atreticum**
   Prognosis: large painful copora lutea will resolve in a week

Graafian Follicle

Size of mature graafian follicle: 17–29 mm
√ growth rate 3 mm/day until the last preovulatory 24 hours followed by a sudden increase in diameter
√ cumulus = 1-mm mural echogenic focus projecting into antrum of follicle + containing oocyte, followed by ovulation within next 36 hours

Signs of Ovulation

√ development of solid echoes within graafian follicle
√ decrease in diameter / sudden collapse of dominant follicle 28–35 hours after LH peak
√ "ring" structure within uterine fundus
√ free fluid appearing in pouch of Douglas

Signs of Ovulatory Failure

√ development of internal echoes prior to 18 mm size
√ continuous cystic enlargement up to 30–40 mm

Ovarian Doppler Signals

A. NONFUNCTIONING OVARY
   √ high-impedance waveform
B. FUNCTIONING OVARY
   — days 1–6:
      √ high-impedance waveform with RI close to 1.0
   — days 7–22 = midfollicular to midluteal phase = developing dominant follicle + ovulation + corpus luteal phase:
      √ continuous diastolic flow with RI close to 0.5
   — days 23–28 = late luteal phase:
      √ high-impedance waveform with RI close to 1.0

Hormonal Status

Thelarche = onset and progress of breast development
Mean age: 8 years

Adrenarche = onset and progress of pubic (pubarche) + axillary hair devlopment
Mean age: 9.8 years

Menarche = first episode of vaginal bleeding originating from the uterus
Mean age: 12.7 years in USA

OB&GYN

OBSTETRIC AND GYNECOLOGIC DISORDERS

ABORTION

= loss of products of conception <20 weeks of MA (definitions may vary)

A. INDUCED ABORTION
 (a) medical / therapeutic abortion
 (b) nonmedical abortion

B. SPONTANEOUS ABORTION

Spontaneous Abortion

= FAILED PREGNANCY = PREGNANCY LOSS
= MISCARRIAGE

Incidence:
— >50% of all fertilized ova (estimate)
— 31–43% of all implantations (estimate)
— 10–25% of clinically diagnosed pregnancies
— 2–4% with normal cardiac activity
— decreases with increasing gestational age

Time of loss: <8–10 weeks MA; the majority occur before 7th week MA

Etiology (usually due to abnormal karyotype):
autosomal trisomy (52%), triploidy (20%), monosomy (15%)

◊ Spontaneous pregnancy loss at <8 weeks gestation occurs in 10–17% of embryos with cardiac activity!

Signs of Abnormal Pregnancy
√ thin decidual reaction of <2 mm
√ abnormally shaped sac
√ gestational sac low in uterus

Impending / Inevitable Abortion

= ABORTION IN PROGRESS
= gestational sac with embryo having become detached from implantation site; leading to spontaneous abortion within next few hours

Clinical triad:
- bleeding >7 days
- persistent painful uterine contractions
- rupture of membranes
- moderate effacement of cervix
- dilated cervix >3 cm

√ sac located low within uterus (DDX: cervical ectopic with closed internal os)
√ progressive migration of sac toward / into cervical canal (on rescanning a short time later)
√ dilated cervix
√ sac surrounded by anechoic zone of blood

Threatened Abortion

= 1st trimester bleeding (after period of implantation bleed at 3–4 weeks MA) with a live embryo

Incidence: 20–25% of all pregnancies

Clinical triad:
- mild bleeding
- cramping
- closed cervix

Nonviability diagnosis with certainty (transvaginal scan):

@ Cardiac activity:
 √ no cardiac activity with a CRL ≥5 mm
 √ no cardiac activity with certain GA ≥6.5 weeks
 √ no cardiac activity with a GS diameter >16 mm

@ Yolk sac:
 √ no yolk sac with a GS diameter ≥20 mm
 √ embryo visualized without demonstrable yolk sac
 √ yolk sac diameter >5.6 mm at <10 weeks MA

@ GS contents:
 √ fibrinous strands / residual embryonic debris (in 25%)

Nonviability diagnosis with high probability (transvaginal scan):

@ Ultrasound milestone not met as expected:
 √ ≥5.0 weeks gestational sac first identifiable
 √ ≥5.5 weeks yolk sac first identifiable
 √ ≥6.0 weeks embryo and FHM first identifiable

@ Yolk sac:
 √ no yolk sac with GS of 6–9 mm
 √ distorted sac configuration

@ Choriodecidua
 √ thinning of choriodecidual reaction with hypoechoic clefts

@ Cardiac activity:
 √ no cardiac activity with GS of ≥9 mm
 √ slow embryonic heart rate (=bradycardia):

≤6.2 Weeks	*≤7.0 Weeks*	*Mortality Rate*
>100 bpm	>120 bpm	11%
90–99 bpm	110–119 bpm	32%
80–89 bpm	100–109 bpm	64%
<80 bpm	<100 bpm	100%

Predictors of poor outcome:

@ Bradycardia
 √ <85 bpm during 5–8 weeks EGA

@ Small sac size = "first-trimester oligohydramnios"
 [misnomer: amnionic cavity is not diminished in size but rather the chorionic cavity]
 = MSD (mean sac diameter) – CRL ≤ 5 mm (with a live embryo at 5.5–9.0 weeks)
 Prognosis: miscarriage in 94%

@ Abnormal yolk sac
 √ failure to visualize YS at 5.5 weeks MA
  = mean diameter of GS ≥8 mm
 √ yolk sac size >5 mm
 √ calcification / debris within yolk sac
 √ double appearance of yolk sac

@ Abnormal amnion
 √ mean diameter of amniotic cavity > CRL

@ Subchorionic hemorrhage
Frequency: in up to 18% of pregnancies during first half
N.B.: significance controversial
Prognosis: 50% develop normally; 15–39% blighted ovum, 4% mole, 4–13% ectopic pregnancy, 0–15% incomplete abortion, 17–57% missed abortion

Complete Abortion

- cervix closed
- abrupt decline of serum β-hCG

√ IUP documented previously
√ thin regular endometrium with apposed surfaces
√ absence of central / eccentric fluid-filled sac
DDx: nongravid state, very early IUP, ectopic pregnancy
Rx: dilatation & curettage may be avoided if IUP was documented previously

Incomplete Abortion

= RETAINED PRODUCTS OF CONCEPTION
= portion of chorionic villi (placental tissue) / trophoblastic tissue (fetal tissue) remaining within uterus

- continued (occasionally massive) genital bleeding (may occur months / years after last abortion / delivery)
- patulous cervix

US (overall accuracy 96%):

Finding		Retained Products
√ gestational sac / collection		100%
√ sac with dead fetus		100%
√ endometrium	>5 mm thick	100%
√ endometrium	2–5 mm thick	43%
√ endometrium	<2 mm thick	14%

√ usually no embryo / fetus seen
√ irregular / angulated small gestational sac containing amorphous echogenic material
√ ragged disrupted choriodecidual reaction
√ subchorionic fluid ± hemorrhage
Cx: endometritis, myometritis, peritonitis, septic shock, diffuse intravascular coagulation (with retention >1 month)
Rx: suction D&C after IV oxytocin
DDx: mole, blighted ovum, embryonic demise, intrauterine fetal death

Placental Polyp

= intrauterine polypoid mass formed by a retained fragment of placental tissue after an abortion / term pregnancy
Predilection in: placenta accreta
MR:
√ hyperintense polypoid mass on T2WI
DDx: arteriovenous malformation, trophoblastic disease, endometrial polyp, submucosal myoma

Missed Abortion

= dead conceptus within uterine cavity ≥8 weeks occurring prior to 28 weeks MA
Time of diagnosis: not before 13 weeks MA

- brownish vaginal discharge
- closed firm cervix

√ no cardiac activity in a well-defined embryo with CRL >9 mm (on abdominal scan) / CRL >5 mm (on transvaginal scan)
√ gestation not in correspondence with menstrual age
√ sac >25 mm in diameter without an embryo (DDx: anembryonic pregnancy)
√ sac >20 mm without yolk sac
√ crenated irregular / distorted angular sac configuration
√ stringlike debris within gestational sac (in 25%)
√ discontinuous / irregular / thin (2 mm) choriodecidual reaction
√ no double decidual sac
√ low sac position
√ subchorionic collection
Cx: coagulopathy secondary to low plasma fibrinogen (after 4 weeks in 2nd trimester pregnancy)
Rx: suction D&C (in 1st trimester); prostaglandin E suppositories (in 2nd trimester)
DDx: blighted ovum

ACARDIA

= ACARDIAC MONSTER = TWIN REVERSED ARTERIAL PERFUSION SEQUENCE (TRAP)
= rare developmental anomaly of monochorionic twinning in which one twin develops without a functioning heart
Incidence: 1:30,000–35,000 births; in 1% of monozygotic twins
Pathophysiology:
normal twin perfuses acardiac twin through *artery-to-artery + vein-to-vein anastomoses* in shared placenta; reversed circulation alters hemodynamic forces, which result in abnormal cardiac morphogenesis
Spectrum:
(1) Holoacardia = no heart at all
(2) Pseudoacardia = rudimentary cardiac tissue
√ proximity of the two cord insertions on placental surface linked by an arterioarterial anastomosis
√ reversed arterial flow in cord toward acardiac twin
√ fused placentas
√ polyhydramnios

A. PUMP TWIN
at increased risk for fetal demise + preterm labor
√ morphologically normal
√ cardiac overload signs: hydrops, IUGR, hypertrophy of right ventricle, increased cardiothoracic ratio, hepatosplenomegaly, ascites

B. PERFUSED TWIN = ACARDIAC TWIN
monochorial placenta (same gender) with vascular anastomosis sustains life of acardiac monster; wide range of associated abnormalities
√ absent / rudimentary heart ("acardius")

√ tiny / absent cranium (acephalus)
√ small upper torso ± absent / deformed upper extremities
√ marked integumentary edema + cystic hygroma

Prognosis: mortality of 100% for perfused twin, 50% for pump twin (increased with increased size of acardiac twin)
Rx: laser ablation of umbilical cord to acardiac twin (up to 20–22 weeks)

ADENOMYOSIS

= ENDOMETRIOSIS INTERNA
= focal / diffuse benign invasion of myometrium by endometrium (heterotopic "endometrial islands"), which incites reactive myometrial hyperplasia

Cause: ? uterine trauma (parturition, myomectomy, curettage), chronic endometritis, hyperestrogenemia
Incidence: 9–31% of hysterectomy specimens
Hormonal dependency:
adenomyosis involves only basal layer of endometrium; largely nonfunctioning due to resistance to hormonal stimulation unlike endometriosis with some degree of proliferative + secretory changes during menstrual cycle
Path: endometrial glands deeper than 1/4 of thickness of junctional zone
Histo: endometrial glands + stroma within myometrium surrounded by smooth muscle hyperplasia
Age: multiparous women >30 years during menstrual life (later reproductive years)
Associated with: endometriosis (in 36–40%)

• asymptomatic in 5–70%
• pelvic pain, menorrhagia, dysmenorrhea (abates after menopause)

A. DIFFUSE ADENOMYOSIS (67%)
  √ smooth uterine enlargement (DDx: diffuse leiomyomatosis)
  √ thickening of junctional zone >10 mm
B. FOCAL ADENOMYOSIS (33%) = "adenomyoma"
  √ mass of 2–7 cm in diameter
  √ oval / elongated shape (DDx: leiomyoma is round)
  √ ill-defined margins (DDx: sharp margin in leiomyoma)
  √ contiguity with junctional zone (DDx: leiomyomas may occur anywhere in myometrium)

MR (86–100% sensitive, 66–100% specific, 85–90% accurate):
  √ myometrial mass with indistinct margins of primarily low signal intensity on all sequences (due to surrounding reactive dense smooth muscle hypertrophy)
  √ diffuse / focal widening of junctional zone (= inner myometrium) ≥12 mm on T2WI, T2-weighted SE images, contrast-enhanced T1WI images
  √ pseudowidening of endometrium (= indistinct foci of endometrial invasion of myometrium)
  √ central high-intensity spots / linear striations on T2WI (due to ectopic endometrial tissue / endometrial cyst / hemorrhagic foci) in 50%
  √ cystic adenomyosis = well-circumscribed cystic myometrial lesions of hemorrhage in different stages of organization (in 40% of diffuse adenomyosis, in 100% of focal adenomyosis)
  √ enhancement always less than adjacent myometrium

US (80–86% sensitive, 50–96% specific, 68–86% accurate):
  √ focal / diffuse heterogenous myometrial echotexture (in 75%)
  √ nodular / linear areas of increased myometrial echogenicity (= heterotopic endometrial tissue)
  √ area of decreased myometrial echogenicity (= smooth muscle hyperplasia)
  √ <5 mm small myometrial cysts (in 50%) due to dilated cystic glands / hemorrhagic foci:
    √ "Swiss cheese" appearance of myometrium in cystic adenomyosis
  √ poor definition of endomyometrial junctional zone (= endometrial tissue extending into myometrium)
  √ pseudowidening of endometrium due to increased myometrial echogenicity
  √ thickening + asymmetry of anterior and posterior myometrial walls
  √ lack of uterine contour abnormality / mass effect

Cx: infertility
DDx:
(1) Leiomyoma (well-defined borders, mass effect, globular shape, large vessels at lesion margin, calcifications, edge shadowing, whorled appearance)
(2) Endometrial carcinoma (error in staging if adenomyosis coexists)
(3) Myometrial contraction (transient nature, distortion of endometrial lining)
(4) Muscular hypertrophy (hypoechoic inner myometrium, diffuse junctional zone thickening)

DDx of cystic adenomyosis:
(1) Leiomyoma with hemorrhagic degeneration
(2) Hematometra

Rx: hysterectomy (the only definitive cure for debilitating adenomyosis)

AMNIOTIC BAND SYNDROME

= EARLY AMNION RUPTURE SYNDROME
= rupture of the amnion exposing the fetus to the injurious environment of fibrous mesodermic bands that emanate from the chorionic side of the amnion

Prevalence: 1:1,200 – 1:2,000 – 1:15,000 live births
√ very thin membrane that flaps with fetal movement or attaches to fetus
√ abnormal sheet / bands of tissue that attach to the fetus (DDx: uterine synechiae, incomplete amniochorionic fusion, amniochorionic separation due to subchorionic hemorrhage, fibrin deposits, venous lakes, residual sac of blighted twin pregnancy, wisps of umbilical cord)

√ restriction of fetal motion secondary to entrapment of fetal parts by bands

Associated with fetal deformities in 77%:

1. Limb defects (multiple + asymmetric)
   √ amputation / constriction rings of limbs / digits
   √ distal syndactyly
   √ clubbed feet (30%)
2. Craniofacial defects
   = asymmetric nonanatomic defects of skull + brain
   √ anencephaly
   √ asymmetric lateral encephalocele
   √ facial clefting of lip / palate
   √ asymmetric microphthalmia
   √ incomplete / absent cranial calcification
   √ ± attachment of head to uterine wall
3. Visceral defects
   √ gastroschisis ± exteriorization of liver
   √ omphalocele
   √ gibbus deformity of spine

DDx: (1) Chorioamnionic separation
(2) Intrauterine synechiae

ANEMBRYONIC PREGNANCY

= BLIGHTED OVUM

= abnormal intrauterine pregnancy with developmental arrest prior to formation of embryo; may occur as a blighted twin

Cause: early arrest of embryonic development related to chromosomal abnormality

- ± vaginal bleeding

√ empty gestational sac (>6.5 weeks MA)
√ yolk sac identified without embryo:
  √ vanishing (passed) yolk sac on serial scans
√ gestational sac small / appropriate / large for dates:
  √ decrease in gestational sac (GS) size
  √ GS fails to grow by >0.6 mm/day on serial scans
√ irregular weakly echogenic decidual reaction of <2 mm
√ distorted sac shape

(a) by transabdominal scan:
GS usually not visualized before 5–5.5 weeks MA; yolk sac forms at 4 weeks MA when GS is 3 mm; embryo usually visualized by 6 weeks MA
  √ GS size ≥10 mm of mean diameter without DDS
  √ GS size ≥20 mm of mean diameter without yolk sac
  √ GS size ≥25 mm of mean diameter without embryo

(b) by transvaginal scan
normal intradecidual GS routinely detected at 4–5 weeks with a mean sac diameter of 5 mm
  √ GS size ≥8 mm of mean diameter without yolk sac
  √ GS size ≥16 mm of mean diameter without cardiac activity

Cx: first trimester bleeding

ARTERIOVENOUS MALFORMATION OF UTERUS

= UTERINE ARTERIOVENOUS FISTULA = UTERINE CIRSOID ANEURYSM

Associated with: dilatation & curettage, endometrial carcinoma, gestational trophoblastic disease

- genital bleeding, often requiring blood transfusions

MR:
√ tortuous tubular signal voids in myometrium / parametrium / protruding into endometrial cavity on T1WI + T2WI
√ vascular lake with sluggish flow hyperintense on T2WI
√ intensely enhancing lesion isointense to vessels on contrast-enhanced dynamic subtraction MR

ASHERMAN SYNDROME

= association of intrauterine synechiae (= adhesions consisting of fibrous tissue or smooth muscle) with menstrual dysfunction + infertility

Cause: sequelae of endometrial trauma (vigorous instrumentation during dilatation & curettage) usually during postpartum or postabortion period / severe endometritis

- hypomenorrhea / amenorrhea
- habitual abortion / sterility

HSG:
√ solitary / multiple filling defects
√ bands of tissue traversing endometrial cavity
√ irregularity of uterine cavity
√ partial / near complete obliteration of uterine cavity (DDx: DES exposure)

Sonhysterography:
√ echogenic bands bridging the uterine cavity
  ◊ Thick fibrotic bands may prevent complete uterine distension

BECKWITH-WIEDEMANN SYNDROME

= EMG SYNDROME (**E**xomphalos = omphalocele, **M**acroglossia, **G**igantism)

= common autosomal dominant overgrowth syndrome with reduced penetrance + variable expressivity related to short arm of chromosome 11; sporadic in 85%

◊ Increased risk of benign + malignant tumors of multiple organs: Wilms tumor > adrenocortical neoplasm > hepatoblastoma

Incidence: 1:13,700 to 1:14,300 live births; M:F = 1:1

- neonatal polycythemia

√ advanced bone age

Constellation:

(1) Hemihypertrophy 13–33%
(2) Hyperplastic visceromegaly: 57%
kidney, liver, spleen, pancreas, clitoris, penis, ovaries, uterus, bladder
(3) Abdominal wall defects
  (a) Omphalocele 76%
  (b) Umbilical hernia 49%
  (c) Diastasis recti 33%
(4) Macroglossia 98%
(5) Facial nevus flammeus 63%
(6) Ear lobe creases and pits 66%
(7) Prominent eyes with intraorbital creases
(8) Infraorbital hypoplasia 81%
(9) Gastrointestinal malrotation 83%
(10) Pancreatic islet hyperplasia
(11) Cardiac anomalies
(12) Natal / postnatal gigantism 77%

@ Adrenal gland
Histo: adrenocortical hyperplasia, hyperplastic adrenal medulla, cystic adrenal cortex, bilateral adrenal cytomegaly (= enlargement of fetal cortical cells)

@ Kidney
Histo: disordered lobar arrangement, medullary dysplasia
√ nephromegaly
√ increased cortical echogenicity (due to glomeruloneogenesis)
√ accentuation of corticomedullary definition
√ medullary sponge kidney
√ pyelocaliceal diverticula

OB-US:
√ LGA fetus with growth along 95th percentile
√ polyhydramnios (51%)
√ thickened placenta
√ long umbilical cord

Cx: (1) Development of malignant tumors (in 10%)
(2) Neonatal hypoglycemia (50–61%)

BRENNER TUMOR

= almost always benign ovarian tumor
Incidence: 1.5–2.5%
Histo: transitional epithelial cells within prominent fibrous connective tissue stroma
Associated with: mucinous cystadenoma / other epithelial tumor in 20–30%
Peak age: 40–70 years
• may have estrogenic activity
√ usually hypoechoic solid homogeneous tumor with well-defined back wall
√ mostly 1–2 cm (up to 30 cm) in diameter
√ ± extensive calcifications
√ bilateral in 5–7%

CERVICAL CANCER

6th most common cause of death from cancer in women; 3rd most common gynecologic malignancy; 13,700 new cases + 4,900 deaths in 1998
Incidence: 12:100,000 women per year
Peak age: 45–55 years
Histo: squamous cell carcinoma (95%), adenocarcinoma (5%), unusual clear cell adenocarcinoma in women exposed to DES in utero
Risk factors: lower socioeconomic class, Black race, early marriage, increased parity, young onset of sexual relations, multiple sexual partners, positive herpes virus type II titers

FIGO stage:

0	Carcinoma in situ (before invasion)
I	Confined to cervix
IA	microinvasion of stroma (<5 mm)
IB	invasion confined to cervix (>5 mm)
IB-1	<4 cm
IB-2	>4 cm
II	Extension beyond cervix but not to pelvic wall / lower one-third of vagina
IIA	vaginal extension excluding lower 1/3
IIB	parametrial invasion excepting pelvic sidewall
III	Extension to pelvic wall / lower third of vagina
IIIA	invasion of lower 1/3 of vagina
IIIB	pelvic wall invasion + hydronephrosis
IV	Located outside true pelvis
IVA	invasion of bladder / rectal mucosa
IVB	spread to distant organs (paraaortic / inguinal nodes, intraperitoneal metastasis)

Significance of tumor size:
>4 cm: nodal metastases (80%), local recurrence (40%), distant metastases (28%)
<4 cm: nodal metastases (16%), local recurrence (5%), distant metastases (0%)

Spread:
(a) direct extension to lower uterine segment + vagina + paracervical space along broad and uterosacral ligaments
(b) lymphatic
(c) hematogenous

Incidence of nodal metastases (77% accuracy for CT, 78% for MR):

0.3%	for stage	0, I A
16%	for stage	I B
33%	for stage	II A
37%	for stage	II B
55%	for stage	IV

• leukorrhea ± vaginal bleeding (<30%)
• postcoital bleeding / metrorrhagia

Location:
centered at level of cervix, originating from
(a) squamocolumnar junction (in young woman)
(b) endocervical canal (older woman)
with protrusion into vagina / invasion of lower myometrium

CT:
@ Primary tumor
√ growth pattern: exophytic, infiltrating, endocervical
√ bulky enlargement of cervix >3.5 cm (DDx: cervical fibroid)
√ iso- (50%) / hypoattenuating (due to necrosis, ulceration, reduced vascularity) after IV contrast
√ gas within tumor (necrosis / prior biopsy)
√ fluid-filled uterus (blood, serous fluid, pus) secondary to obstruction
√ hypoattenuating lesion of myometrium / with vaginal distension

@ Parametrial spread (30–58% accuracy):
√ parametrial soft-tissue mass
√ ureteral encasement
√ thickening of ureterosacral ligaments
√ >4-mm soft-tissue strands of increased attenuation extending from cervix into parametria, cardinal / sacrouterine ligaments
√ obliteration of fat planes
√ ill-defined irregular cervical margins
√ eccentric parametrial enlargement

OB&GYN

DDx: parametrial inflammation due to instrumentation, ulceration, infection, prior pelvic surgery, endometriosis

@ Pelvic side wall disease
- √ tumor <3 mm from side wall
- √ enlarged piriform / obturator internus muscles
- √ encasement of iliac vessels
- √ destruction of pelvic bones

@ Pelvic visceral disease (60% PPV)
- √ loss of perivesical / perirectal fat plane
- √ asymmetric nodular thickening of bladder / rectal wall
- √ intraluminal mass
- √ air in bladder due to fistula

@ Lymphatic spread (65–80% accuracy)
- √ nodes >1 cm in diameter (>7 mm for internal iliac nodes, 9 mm for common iliac nodes, >10 mm for external iliac nodes) with 44% sensitivity
- √ lymph node necrosis (100% PPV)

DDx: adenopathy from secondary tumor infection

MR (76–91% accuracy for staging, 82–94% accuracy for parametrial involvement):
- √ focal bulge / mass:
  - √ mass isointense on T1WI
  - √ hyperintense on T2WI compared with fibrous stroma (DDx: postbiopsy changes, inflammation, nabothian cysts)
  - √ size of tumor accurately depicted (on T2WI rarely overestimated due to inflammation / edema)
  - √ early contrast enhancement on fat-saturated T1WI
- √ blurring + widening of junctional zone secondary to obstruction of cervical os (retained secretions in uterine cavity)
- √ disruption of hypointense vaginal wall by hyperintense thickening on T2WI
- √ disruption of hypointense cervical fibrous stromal ring on T2WI by nodular / irregular tumor signal intensity
- √ linear stranding around cervical mass
- √ tumor extending to involve internal obturator, piriform, levator ani muscles
- √ dilatation of ureter
- √ disruption of hypointense walls of bladder / rectum (DDx: hyperintense thickening of bladder wall on T2WI due to bullous edema)
- √ lymphadenopathy >10 mm, hyperintense compared with muscle / blood vessels on T2WI

Prognosis: depending on tumor stage + volume of primary mass + histologic grade + lymph node metastases; in 30% recurrent / persistent disease (usually within 2 years)

Rx:
(1) Surgery for stages <IIA / tumor <4 cm
(2) Radiation therapy ± chemotherapy for stages >IIB

DDx:
(1) Endometrial polyp / adenocarcinoma (centered in endometrial cavity protruding into endocervical canal)
(2) Prolapsed submucosal fibroid (more hypointense on T2WI)

Recurrent Cervical Carcinoma

= local tumor growth / development of distant metastasis ≥6 months after complete regression

@ Pelvic recurrence

Prevalence: varies with stage, histologic type, adequacy of therapy, host response; 11% in stage IB

Site: cervix, uterus, vagina / vaginal cuff, parametria, ovaries, bladder, ureters, rectum, anterior abdominal wall, pelvic side wall
- • lower extremity swelling (lymphatic obstruction)
- • pain (nerve compression, ureteral obstruction)
- √ hydrometra (obstruction by preserved cervix)
- √ rectovaginal fistula
- √ hydronephrosis (70% by autopsy)
- √ vesicovaginal fistula
- √ pelvic side wall mass

DDx: radiation fibrosis (82% MR accuracy)

@ Nodal recurrence

◊ Prognosis worsens as nodal involvement progresses!

(a) primary: paracervical, parametrial, internal + external iliac, obturator nodes (= medial group of the external iliac nodes)
Frequency: in 75% of adenocarcinoma, in 61% of squamous cell carcinoma (autopsy)

(b) secondary: sacral, common iliac, inguinal, paraaortic nodes
Frequency: in 62% of adenocarcinoma, in 30% of squamous cell carcinoma (autopsy)

@ Solid abdominal organ recurrence

Location: liver (33%) > adrenal gland (15%) > spleen, pancreas, kidney

@ Peritoneal recurrence
1. Peritoneal carcinomatosis (5–27% by autopsy)
2. Tumor deposits in mesentery + omentum

• Sister Joseph nodule = umbilical metastasis developing from anterior peritoneal surface

@ GI tract recurrence

Location: rectosigmoid junction (17%), colon, small bowel
- √ fistula formation
- √ focal bowel wall thickening + tethering
- √ intestinal obstruction (12% by autopsy)

Prognosis: immediate cause of death in 7%

@ Chest recurrence
1. Lung metastases (33–38% by autopsy)
2. Pleural metastases associated with hydrothorax
3. Pericardial metastasis
4. Lymphangitic carcinomatosis (<5%)
5. Mediastinal / hilar adenopathy + pleural lesions / effusion

@ Osseous recurrence

Prevalence: 15–29% by autopsy

Location: vertebra > pelvis > rib > extremity

Mechanism: direct extension from paraaortic nodes (most common) / lymphatic / hematogenous spread

@ Skin + subcutaneous tissue recurrence (in up to 10%)

CHORIOAMNIONIC SEPARATION

(a) normally seen <16 weeks
= incomplete fusion of amniotic membrane with chorionic plate
(b) abnormal >17 weeks MA
= secondary to hemorrhage / amniocentesis (10%)
√ membrane extends over fetal surface + stops at origin of umbilical cord
√ elevated membrane thinner than chorionic membrane
Cx: rupture of amniotic membrane may lead to amniotic band syndrome
DDx: amniotic band syndrome, uterine synechia, fibrin strand after amniocentesis, cystic hygroma (moves with embryo)

CHORIOANGIOMA

= benign vascular malformation of proliferating capillaries (= hamartoma)
Incidence: 1:3,500 to 1:20,000 births
Location: usually near the umbilical cord insertion site
√ well-circumscribed intraplacental mass with complex echo pattern protruding from the fetal surface of the placenta
√ polyhydramnios (in 1/3)
√ arterial signal on Doppler ultrasound in angiomatous chorioangioma
Cx: hemorrhage, fetal hydrops, cardiomegaly, congestive heart failure, IUGR, premature labor, fetal demise (with large lesion)

CHORIOCARCINOMA

Prevalence: 5% of gestational trophoblastic diseases
Age: child-bearing age
Histo: biphasic pattern including syncytiotrophoblastic + cytotrophoblastic proliferation without villous structures; extensive necrosis + hemorrhage; early + extensive vascular invasion
Preceded by: *mnemonic:* "MEAN"

Mole (hydatidiform)	in 50.0%
Ectopic pregnancy	in 2.5%
Abortion, spontaneous	in 25.0%
Normal pregnancy	in 22.5%

• continued vaginal bleeding
• continued elevation of hCG after expulsion of molar / normal pregnancy (25%)
√ mass enlarging the uterus
√ mixed hyperechoic pattern (hemorrhage, necrosis)
Metastases:
(a) hematogenous (usually): lung, kidney (10–50%), brain
√ radiodense pulmonary masses with hazy borders due to hemorrhage + necrosis
√ hyperechoic hepatic foci
(b) lymphatic + direct extension (occasionally): vagina
Prognosis: 85% cure rate (even with metastases); fatal with spread to kidneys + brain
Rx: (1) Chemotherapy: methotrexate, actinomycin D ± cyclophosphamide
(2) Hysterectomy (if at risk for uterine rupture)

DDx mnemonic: "THE CLIP"
True mole
Hydropic degeneration of placenta
Endometrial proliferation
Coexistent mole and fetus
Leiomyoma (degenerated)
Incomplete abortion
Products of conception (retained)

CLEAR CELL NEOPLASM OF OVARY

= MESONEPHROID TUMOR
= almost always invasive carcinoma
Incidence: 2–5–10% of all ovarian cancers
Histo: clear cells (cuboidal cells with clear cytoplasm) + hobnail cells (columnar cells with large nuclei projecting into the lumina of glandular elements); identical to clear cell carcinoma of endometrium, cervix, vagina, kidney; ~100% malignant
Not associated with: in utero DES exposure (like lesions of the vagina + cervix)
• 75% of patients present with stage I disease
√ frequently unilocular cyst + mural nodule(s)
Prognosis: 50% 5-year survival rate (better than for other ovarian cancers)

CONJOINED TWINS

= incomplete division of embryonic cell mass in monozygotic twins occurring at 13–16 days GA but before the 3rd week of gestation
Prevalence: 1:50,000 to 1:200,000 deliveries (1:14,000 to 1:25,000 in Southeast Asia + Africa); 1:600 twin births; M:F = 1:3
Types (classified according to most prominent site of connection):
A. Superior conjunction:
1. Dipygus (<1%) single head, thorax, abdomen + two pelves and four legs
2. Syncephalus (<1%) facial fusion ± thoracic fusion
3. Craniopagus (**2%**) joined between homologous portions of cranial vault
B. Middle conjunction:
1. Thoracopagus (**40%**) between thoracic walls; conjoined hearts (75%)
2. Omphalopagus (**33%**) joined between umbilicus + xiphoid
3. Xiphopagus joined at xiphoid
4. Rachipagus joined at any level of spinal column above sacrum
5. Thoracoomphalopagus
C. Inferior conjunction:
1. Diprosopus (<1%) two faces + one head and body
2. Dicephalus (<1%) two heads + one body
3. Ischiopagus (**6%**) joined by inferior sacrum and coccyx
4. Pygopagus (**19%**) joined by posterolateral sacrum and coccyx

D. Incomplete duplication (10%): duplication of only one part of body

◊ The more fused twins are usually joined laterally, whereas the more separate twins are joined anteriorly, posteriorly, cranially, and caudally!

OB-US (diagnosed as early as 12 weeks GA):
- √ single placenta without separating amniotic membrane (monochorionic, monoamniotic = hallmark of monozygotic twinning)
- √ inseparable fetal bodies + skin contours:
  - √ fetuses commonly face each other
  - √ both fetal heads persistently at same level
  - √ no change in relative position of fetuses
  - √ bibreech (more common) / bicephalic presentation (cephalic-breech presentation is most common presentation for omphalopagus)
  - √ backward flexion of cervical spine (in anterior fusion)
  - √ single cardiac motion (if heart shared)
- √ polyhydramnios (in almost 50%)
- √ single umbilical cord with >3 vessels
- √ fewer limbs than expected

Associated malformations:
- √ omphalocele
- √ congenital heart disease (high frquency in all types of conjoined twinning)

Prognosis: 40–60% stillborn; 35% die within 24 hours of life

Craniopagus
= united at any part of the skull except face / foramen magnum (usually vertical / parietal in >60%)
- √ shared cranium, meninges, dural venous sinuses (brains commonly remain separate ± connecting bridge of neural tissue)

Ischiopagus
= united from umbilicus to large conjoined pelvis, face to face / end to end

Types: tetrapus (4 legs), tripus (3 legs), bipus (2 legs)
- √ usually two sacra ± single symphysis pubis
- √ varying degrees of renal fusion + ectopia
- √ one / two urinary baldders
- √ single external urethral orifice (usually)
- √ shared sex organs (frequently born as females)
- √ lower GI tract usually shared with anal atresia + colovesical fistulas
- √ large pelvic vessel connecting both aortas

Omphalopagus
= joined ventrally in umbilical region, often with inclusion of lower thorax
- √ liver fusion (80%)
- √ shared terminal ileum (join at Meckel diverticulum) + proximal colon (33%)

Parapagus
= side-to-side position with ventrolateral fusion sharing umbilicus, abdomen, pelvis

Types: dithoracic (= separate thoraces), dicephalic (= separate heads)
- √ conjoined pelvis with single symphysis pubis
- √ one / two sacra
- √ multiple other anomalies

Pygopagus
= united dorsally sharing sacrococcygeal + perineal region
- √ fusion of sacral vertebrae (spinal cords usually separate)
- √ single anus ± single rectum
- √ single urinary bladder + urethra (15%)

Thoracopagus
= united from upper thorax to umbilicus
- √ common sternum, diaphragm, upper abdominal wall
- √ common pericardial sac (90%) + some degree of cardiac fusion
- √ fusion of liver (invariably):
  - √ shared biliary system (in 25%)
  - √ ± absent / anomalous hepatic venous drainage
- √ common small intestine (in 50%): joins at duodenum + separates at distal ileum

Prognosis: cardiac fusion precludes successful surgical separation in 75%

CORD PROLAPSE
= prolapse of cord into endocervical canal

Incidence: 0.5% at delivery

Predisposing factors:
nonvertex fetal lie, polyhydramnios, cephalopelvic disproportion, multiple gestation, increased length of umbilical cord

Cx: cord compression with high perinatal mortality
N.B.: MEDICAL EMERGENCY! Alert obstetrician immediately!

OB management:
(1) Patient immediately placed into Trendelenburg / knee-elbow position in radiology department
(2) Cesarean section for term infants
(3) Expectant management for preterm infants

DDx: **Cord presentation** (= umbilical cord between fetus and internal os)

CYSTADENOFIBROMA
= variant of serous cystadenoma, rarely malignant

Prevalence: nearly 50% of all benign ovarian cystic serous tumors; bilateral in 6%

Age: 15–65 (mean 31) years
- • may produce estrogen excess
- √ small multilocular cystic tumor
- √ clusters of short rounded papillary processes

DERMOID
= DERMOID CYST = MATURE CYSTIC TERATOMA
= congenital benign germ cell tumor containing mature tissues from all 3 germ cell layers with predominance of ectodermal component

Incidence: 5 –11–25% of all ovarian neoplasms; 66% of pediatric ovarian tumors; most common ovarian neoplasm
Origin: self-fertilization of a single germ cell after the first meiotic division (= random error in meiosis)
Path: unilocular thin-walled cyst lined by an opaque gray-white wrinkled epidermis from which hair shafts protrude; lumen of cyst filled with sebaceous secretions mixed with hair strands
Histo: mature epithelial elements (skin, hair, teeth, desquamated epithelium); bone; may contain struma ovarii, carcinoid tumor
Age: reproductive life (80%); age peak 20–40 years
• relatively soft pelvic mass (2/3) difficult to palpate
• pelvic pressure / pain due to torsion or hemorrhage
Location: bilateral in 8–15–25%

√ cystic mass with average diameter of 10 cm
√ fat-fluid / hair-fluid level
√ "dermoid plug" = Rokitansky nodule / protuberance
= oval / round mural solid tissue mass (sebaceous material) of 10–65 mm projecting into cyst lumen
Plain film (diagnostic in 40%):
√ tooth / bone
√ fat density (SPECIFIC)
CT:
√ round mass of fat floating in interface between two water-density components (93%)
√ Rokitansky nodule = dermoid plug (81%) of adipose tissue, usually single, may be multiple
√ sebum-rich fat-fluid level in cyst cavity (12%)
√ globular calcifications (tooth) / rim of calcification (56%)
US (77–87% sensitive):
√ complex mass containing echogenic components (66%):
√ "tip of the iceberg" sign = echogenic mass with "dirty" acoustic shadowing (= mixture of sebum + hair strands creates multiple tissue interfaces) in a predominantly cystic mass (25–44%) (DDx: stool-filled rectosigmoid)
√ fat-fluid level
√ predominantly solid mass (10–31%)
√ purely cystic tumor (9–15%)
√ echogenic focus with acoustic shadowing (due to calcification)
MR:
√ hyperintense lipid-laden cyst fluid (within fluid of low signal intensity) on T1WI + of intermediate intensity on T2WI
√ hyperintense mass (fat + serous fluid both with high signal intensity) on T2WI
√ ± chemical shift artifact of bright/ dark bands (along frequency-encoding gradient)
Cx: (1) Malignant degeneration in 1–3% (usually within dermoid plug of tumors >10 cm in diameter in postmenopausal women) into squamous cell carcinoma (most common)
(2) Torsion (4–16%)
(3) Rupture with chemical peritonitis (rare)
(4) Hydronephrosis
Rx: surgery (to avoid torsion / rupture)
DDx: tuboovarian abscess, acute hemorrhagic cyst, atypical endometrioma, bowel gas

Rupture of Ovarian Cystic Teratoma

Cause: torsion, infarction, trauma, infection, malignant change, prolonged pressure during labor, idiopathic
• acute abdomen (due to severe chemical peritonitis)
√ spilled sebaceous material / hair ball on T1WI + fat-suppressed T1WI (DDx to fluid)
√ thickened peritoneum / intraperitoneal adhesions on contrast-enhanced fat-suppressed T1WI
DDx: tubercular peritonitis, carcinomatosis

DIETHYLSTILBESTROL (DES) EXPOSURE

= first reported transplacental carcinogen
@ Vagina: adenosis, septa, ridges, clear-cell adenocarcinoma (in 1:1,000 women exposed in utero to DES, by age 35)
@ Cervix: hypoplasia, stenosis, mucosal displacement, pseudopolyps, hooded / "cockscomb" appearance
@ Uterus: hypoplasia, bands, contour irregularity, "T- shaped" uterus
@ Tubes: deformity, irregularity, obstruction

DYSGERMINOMA

= malignant germ cell tumor of ovary homologous to testicular seminoma
Incidence: 0.5–2% of all malignant ovarian tumors
Peak age: 2nd–3rd decade
• no elevation of AFP / hCG (in 5% syncytiotrophoblastic giant cells present, which can elevate hCG levels)
Location: usually unilateral; bilateral in 15–17%
√ multilobulated solid mass divided by fibrovascular septa
√ speckled pattern of calcifications (rare)
MR:
√ hypo- / isointense septa on T2WI with contrast-enhancement on T1WI
US:
√ hyperechoic solid mass, may have areas of hemorrhage + necrosis
√ prominent arterial color Doppler flow within septa
Rx: highly radiosensitive

ECLAMPSIA

= occurrence of coma ± pre-, intra-, or postpartum convulsions not related to a coincidental neurologic disorder in a preeclamptic patient
Pathophysiology:
A. VASOSPASM THEORY
overregulation of cerebral vasoconstrictive response to acute + severe hypertension progresses to vasospasm; prolonged vasospasm causes local ischemia, increased brain capillary permeability, disruption of blood-brain barrier, arteriolar necrosis, leading to cerebral edema + hemorrhage

OB&GYN

B. FORCED-DILATATION THEORY
with severe arterial hypertension upper limit of cerebral autoregulation is reached + cerebral vasodilatation starts disrupting the blood-brain barrier and resulting in cerebral edema

Time of onset: 2nd half of pregnancy in primigravida; <20th week GA with trophoblastic disease

- severe throbbing frontal headache
- visual disturbance: scotomata, amaurosis, blurred vision
- retinal / cortical blindness
- hyperreflexia, hemi- / quadriparesis, confusion, coma
- seizures: usually tonic-clonic

CT (positive in up to 50%):
- √ bilateral rather symmetric white matter hypodensities without contrast enhancement
- √ ± cerebral edema with compression of lateral ventricles
- √ usually transient + completely reversible cerebral-cortical + basal ganglia hypodensities (= reversible ischemic lesions)
- √ cerebral infarction in prolonged ischemia
- √ intracerebral hemorrhage (major cause of mortality in 10–60%)

MR:
- √ transiently increased T2-signal intensity in cerebral cortex + subcortical white matter frequently in watershed areas of posterior hemispheres

ECTOPIA CORDIS

= fusion defect of anterior thoracic wall / sternum / septum transversum prior to 9th week of gestation

A. THORACIC TYPE (60%)
= heart outside thoracic cavity protruding through defect in sternum

B. ABDOMINAL TYPE (30%)
= heart protruding into abdomen through gap in diaphragm

C. THORACOABDOMINAL TYPE (7%)
= in pentalogy of Cantrell

D. CERVICAL TYPE (3%)
= displacement of heart into cervical region

Associated with:
(1) Facial deformities
(2) Skeletal deformities
(3) Ventral wall defects
(4) CNS malformations: meningocele, encephalocele
(5) Intracardiac anomalies: tetralogy of Fallot, TGA
(6) Amniotic band syndrome

Prognosis: stillbirth / death within first hours / death within first days of life in most case

ECTOPIC PREGNANCY

= implantation outside the endometrial cavity

Incidence: 1.6:1,000 of all pregnancies (increasing); 9.9:10,000 women annually; 73,700 cases in 1986 in United States

Risk of recurrence: 10–15%

Cause: delayed transit of the fertilized zygote (formed on day 14 MA) secondary to
(a) abnormal angulation of oviduct
(b) adhesions or scarring from inflammation
(c) slowed tubal transit from ciliary abnormalities

Risk factors:
(1) Previous tubal surgery (tubal ligation / tuboplasty)
(2) Previous PID (30–50%): esp. Chlamydia
(3) In vitro fertilization / gamete intrafallopian tube transfer
(4) Endometriosis
(5) Previous ectopic pregnancy (prevalence up to 1.1%, 10-fold increase in risk, 25% chance of recurrence)
(6) Current use of IUD
(7) Advanced maternal age
◊ If the pregnancy cannot be documented as intrauterine, the patient should be considered at risk!

Time of manifestation: usually by 7th week of MA

CLASSIC CLINICAL TRIAD (<50%):
- abnormal vaginal bleeding (75–86%)
- pelvic pain (97%)
- palpable adnexal mass (23–41%)

- secondary amenorrhea (61%)
- cervical motion tenderness
- positive urinary pregnancy test (50%)
- progesterone level <25 mg/mL
- β-hCG does not rise >66% within 48 hours (lower levels + slower rise and decline compared with IUP)
  ◊ Most ectopic pregnancies do not exhibit a β-hCG of >6,500 mIU/mL (1st IRP) prior to symptomatology!
  ◊ A β-hCG level above the discriminatory zone with absence of IUP suggests ectopic pregnancy!

Discriminatory zone of β-hCG
(at which a normal IUP should be visualized):
(a) by transabdominal scan:
≥6,500 mIU/mL (IRP) with 100% sensitivity + 96% specificity
(b) by endovaginal scan:
≥2,000–3,000 mIU/mL (IRP)

Caveats: technical quality of exam, multiple gestations, distortion by uterine cavity (leiomyoma), lab error, assay variation

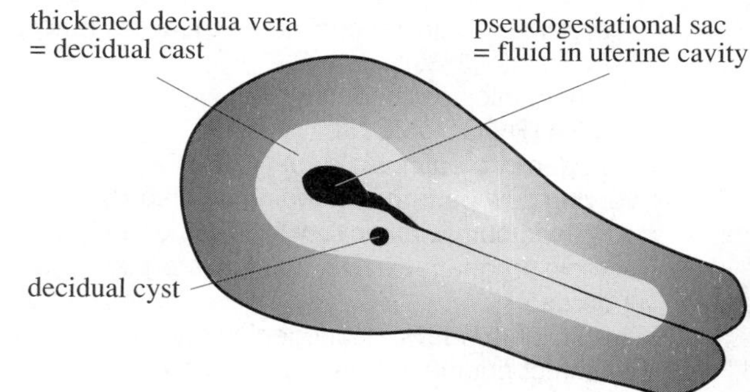

Intrauterine Signs of an Ectopic Pregnancy

Dx: diagnostic laparoscopy (3–4% false negative, 5% false positive)

Location:

(a) tubal (95%): (1) Ampullary ectopic (75–80%)
(2) Isthmic ectopic (10–15%)
(3) Fimbrial ectopic (5%)
(4) Interstitial ectopic (2–4%)

(b) other (5%): (1) Abdominal ectopic
(2) Ovarian ectopic (0.5–1%)
(3) Interligamentary ectopic
(4) Cervical ectopic (0.15%)

Spectrum:

Type 1: unruptured live ectopic + heartbeat
Type 2: early embryonic demise without rupture / embryonic structures / heartbeat
Type 3: ruptured ectopic with blood in pelvis
Type 4: no sonographic signs of ectopic

Transvaginal US (6–20% false-negative rate):
◊ Detected 1 week sooner than by transvesical US!
@ Uterus
√ absence of intrauterine pregnancy (beyond 6 weeks MA / with ß-hCG level >1,000 mIU/mL [2nd IRP])
◊ No IUP by transvesical US = ectopic pregnancy in 43–46%
◊ No IUP by endovaginal US = ectopic pregnancy in 67%
√ thickening of endometrium:
√ hyperechoic endometrial thickening (50%) due to hormonal stimulation from ectopic pregnancy
√ sloughing of endometrium = **decidual cast** (21%)
√ decidual endometrium lacks low-impedance blood flow
√ **decidual cyst** = 1–5-mm cyst at junction of endometrium and myometrium (14%)
√ **pseudogestational sac** (10–20%) = single parietal decidual layer surrounding an anechoic fluid collection in uterine cavity secondary to bleeding
@ Adnexa
√ "tubal ring" = extrauterine hypoechoic saclike structure (40–68%) 1–3 cm in diameter + surrounded by a 2–4-mm concentric ring
√ extrauterine mass of any type (84%):
√ solid / complex adnexal mass = clotted blood free in peritoneal cavity / hematosalpinx (36%)
√ extrauterine gestational sac without live embryo / yolk sac (35%)
√ embryonic heartbeat (6–28%) = PATHOGNOMONIC
√ echogenic "tubal mass" (89–100%)
√ varying flow pattern depending on viability
√ corpus luteum within ovary in >50% on side of ectopic pregnancy (DDx: ectopic pregnancy)
@ Cul-de-sac
√ free fluid (40–83%): echogenic / particulate fluid (= hemoperitoneum) has 93% positive predictive value for ectopic pregnancy
DDx: anechoic fluid in 10–27% of IUP

Doppler-US (low diagnostic impact):
√ high-velocity low-impedance flow around extrauterine gestation in 54% (up to 4 kHz shift with 3 MHz transducer, 0.38 ± 0.2 Pourcelot index, RI = 0.18–0.58)
√ absence of peritrophoblastic flow after 36 days (<0.8 kHz shift with 3 MHz transducer or <1.3 kHz shift with 5 MHz transducer)
DDx of low-impedance flow:
corpus luteum cyst, tuboovarian abscess, fibroid

Probability of ectopic pregnancy in absence of IUP + clinical symptoms of an ectopic pregnancy with:

normal scan / simple cyst in adnexa	5%
complex adnexal mass	92%
tubal ring	95%
live embryo outside uterus	100%

MR:
√ hemosalpinx slightly hyperintense relative to urine on fat-suppressed T1WI
√ bloody ascites
√ heterogenous adnexal mass of mixed signal intensity on fat-suppressed T1WI + T2WI
√ extravasation of contrast material (= bleeding site) on contrast-enhanced dynamic subtraction MR

Prognosis: (1) 3.8:10,000 mortality rate (4% of all maternal deaths)
(2) Infertility (in 40%)

Dx: (1) Laparoscopy (almost 100% accurate)
(2) Culdocentesis (high probability for ectopic with aspiration of nonclotting blood with a hematocrit >15)

Cx: maternal death in 1:1,000; tubal rupture (10–15%)

DDx: (1) Hemorrhagic corpus luteum / hematoma
(2) Adnexal mass: hydrosalpinx, endometrioma, ovarian cyst
(3) Fluid-containing small bowel loop
(4) Eccentrically placed GS in bicornuate / retroflexed / fibroid uterus

Abdominal Ectopic (1:6,000)

◊ >25% may be missed sonographically!
• bloating, abdominal pain (fetal movement / peritoneal irritation due to adhesions)
• bleeding, hypotension, shock
√ extrauterine location of fetus + placenta
√ uterus compressed with visible endometrial cavity line
√ absence of uterine wall between gestation + bladder / abdominal wall
√ anhydramnios
Cx: bowel obstruction / perforation; erosion of pregnancy through abdominal wall

Lithopedion

= "stone child" = very rare obstetric complication consisting of a dehydrated + calcified demised fetus in an extrauterine pregnancy existing for >3 months without infection

Types:
(1) Lithokelyphosis = fetal membranes calcified
(2) Lithokelyphopedion = fetus + membranes calcified
(3) True lithopedion = only fetus calcified

Maternal age at discovery: 23–100 years of age; within 4–20 years of fetal demise

Location: most common in adnexae
√ large densely calcified mass in lower abdomen / upper pelvis
√ CT scan reveals fetal skeleton

DDx: uterine fibroid, calcified ovarian malignancy / cyst, sarcoma

Heterotopic Pregnancy
= ectopic + coexistent intrauterine pregnancy

Incidence: 1:6,800–30,000 pregnancies (higher number of coexisting ectopic with ovulation induction)

◊ An IUP does not preclude a complete pelvic ultrasound evaluation, although depiction of an IUP virtually excludes the diagnosis of an ectopic pregnancy!

Interstitial (Cornual) Ectopic (2–4%)
= ectopic pregnancy with eccentric location in relation to endometrium + close to uterine serosa

◊ Often rupture late because of greater myometrial distensibility compared with other parts of tube!
◊ High likelihood of catastrophic hemorrhage + death due to abundant blood supply by both ovarian + uterine arteries!

Increased risk: previous ipsilateral salpingectomy

- Baart de la Faille sign = broad-based palpable mass extending outward from uterine angle
- Ruge-Simon syndrome = fundus displaced to contralateral side with rotation of uterus + elevation of affected cornu

√ eccentric heterogeneous mass in cornual region (66%)
√ eccentrically placed gestational sac (25%)
√ thinning of myometrial mantle to <5 mm (33%)
√ interstitial line sign = thin echogenic line extending directly up to the center of ectopic pregnancy (= endometrial canal / interstitial portion of fallopian tube) in 92%
√ myometrium between sac and uterine cavity
√ large vascular channels + peritrophoblastic blood flow
√ absence of double decidual sign

Prognosis: massive bleeding from erosion of uterine arteries + veins (pregnancy survives only 12–16 weeks GA); 2-fold mortality compared with other tubal ectopics

DDx: pregnancy within horn of bicornuate uterus; hydatidiform mole; degenerating uterine fibroid

EMBRYONIC DEMISE
Incidence: 20–71% loss rate of one twin <10 weeks

Early Embryonic Demise / Failing Pregnancy
- β-hCG level <2–3 standard deviations below the mean for given MA / GS size / CRL

√ on endovaginal scan:
A. DEFINITE DEMISE
  √ absence of cardiac activity with CRL of ≥5 mm / ≥6.5 weeks GA (repeat scan in 3 days for confirmation)
B. PROBABLY FAILING PREGNANCY
  √ mean sac diameter of ≥16 mm without embryo
  √ mean sac size of ≥8 mm without yolk sac (repeat scan in 3 days for confirmation)
  √ >1,000 mIU/mL (1st IRP) without gestational sac
  √ >7,200 mIU/mL (1st IRP) without yolk sac
  √ >10,800 mIU/mL (1st IRP) without embryo
C. HIGH RISK OF SUBSEQUENT DEMISE
  √ severe bradycardia <80 bpm
  √ small mean gestational sac size (difference between mean sac size and CRL <5 mm is predictive of miscarriage in 94%)
D. MODERATELY HIGH RISK OF DEMISE
  √ bradycardia of 80–90 bpm
  √ large subchorionic hematoma lifting much of placenta
  √ yolk sac >6 mm / abnormal shape

√ mean gestational sac size too small for good clinical dates
√ gestational sac growth ≤ 0.7 mm/day (normal growth rate of 1.13 mm/day determines appropriate time interval for follow-up scan, ie, when sac is expected to be 27 mm)
√ sac position in lower uterine segment / cervix
√ stringlike / granular debris / fluid-fluid level within gestational sac (= intrasac bleeding)

Late Embryonic Demise
√ on endovaginal scan:
  √ wrinkled collapsing amniotic membrane
  √ irregular distorted shape of gestational sac (DDx: compression by bladder, myoma, contraction)
  √ absence of double decidual sac = thin (<2 mm) weakly hyperechoic / irregular choriodecidual reaction

ENDODERMAL SINUS TUMOR OF OVARY
= YOLK SAC TUMOR
= rare but highly malignant tumor

Histo: resembles endodermal sinuses of the rat yolk sac
(a) papillary pattern (most common): contains glomerular structures with central vessel + peripheral mantling of epithelial cells (= Schiller-Duval bodies)

(b) others: reticular, solid, polyvesicular vitelline
— periodic acid-Schiff reaction
— α-fetoprotein–positive hyaline globules

Incidence: <1% of all ovarian carcinomas
Age: usually adolescence
May be associated with: teratoma, dermoid cyst, choriocarcinoma

• frequently abdominal enlargement + pain
• elevated serum AFP (common)
√ predominantly echogenic solid tumor
√ cystic areas (epithelial-lined cysts / cysts of coexisting mature teratoma / hemorrhage / necrosis)
√ bilateral in 1%

Rx: surgery + combination chemotherapy
Prognosis: poor

ENDOMETRIAL CANCER

Most common invasive gynecologic malignancy;
4th most prevalent female cancer in USA women
Incidence: 34,000 new cases per year with 3,000 deaths
Histo: adenocarcinoma (90–95%), sarcoma (1–3%)
Peak age: 55–62 years; 74% > age 50
Risk factors: nulliparity, late menopause, exposure to unopposed estrogen therapy, polycystic ovaries, obesity, hypertension, diabetes mellitus

FIGO stage:

0	In situ
I a	Tumor limited to endometrium
I b	Superficial invasion to <50% of myometrium
I c	Deep invasion to more than half of myometrium
II a	Endocervical glandular involvement only
II b	Cervical stromal invasion
III a	Invasion of serosa / adnexa / peritoneal metastases
III b	Vaginal metastases
III c	Metastases to pelvic / paraaortic lymph nodes
IV a	Invasion of bladder / bowel mucosa
IV b	Distant metastases (lung, brain, bone) including intraabdominal / inguinal lymph nodes

◊ Clinical staging with dilatation & curettage inaccurate in up to 51%!

Histo:
(a) endometrioid carcinoma (75% of all cancers)
(b) serous, mucinous, clear cell carcinoma (less common): similar to ovarian counterpart
(c) squamous (rare): associated with cervical stenosis, pyometra, chronic inflammation
(d) mixed mesodermal tumor: contains elements of epithelial + mesenchymal differentiation

Lymph node metastases: 3% with superficial invasion; 40% with deep invasion

• postmenopausal bleeding without hormonal therapy

Location: predominantly in uterine fundus; 24% in isthmic portion)

US:
√ normal-sized / enlarged uterus
√ focal / diffuse endometrial thickening (mean AP bilayer thickness of 18.2 mm)
◊ any endometrial thickness >5 mm is suspicious (100% negative predictive value, not very specific):
◊ 10% cancer rate with endometrial thickness of 6–15 mm
◊ 50% cancer rate with endometrial thickness of >15 mm
√ irregular heterogeneous echogenic texture with hypoechoic areas:
√ irregular poorly defined endometrial-myometrial interface (= invasive endometrial cancer)
√ increased echogenicity in myometrium (= invasive endometrial cancer)
√ intrauterine fluid collection (DDx: cervical stenosis)

Transvaginal US:
√ apparent distension of endometrial lumen with extrinsic thinning of the myometrium (polypoid tumor)
√ Doppler pulsatility index of <1.5 or resistive index <0.7 suggest malignancy (DDx: endometritis, benign endometrial polyp)
√ areas of venous flow (DDx: endometrial hyperplasia)

MR (82–92% accuracy for staging, 74–87% accuracy for depth of invasion):
√ endometrial cancer has slightly lower signal intensity than endometrium but higher than myometrium on T2WI
√ endometrial thickness abnormal if >3 mm (postmenopausal woman) / >10 mm (under estrogen replacement)
DDx: blood clot, uterine secretions, adenomatous hyperplasia, submucosal leiomyoma
√ disruption / absence of junctional zone (myometrial invasion)
√ hyperintense areas penetrating into myometrium (deep muscle invasion; 74–87% accuracy)

ENDOMETRIOID CARCINOMA OF OVARY

Incidence: 8–15% of all ovarian cancers; 2nd most common malignant ovarian neoplasm (after serous adenocarcinoma)
Associated with: hyperplasia / carcinoma of the uterine endometrium in 20–33%
Path: malignant mixed mesodermal tumor = carcinoma-sarcoma is grouped with endometrioid cancer
Histo: tubular glandular pattern with a pseudostratified epithelium resembling endometrial adenocarcinoma / metastatic colon carcinoma; ~100% malignant

√ solid / complex (= cystic + solid) tumor
√ bilateral in 15% of stage I cases

Prognosis: better than serous / mucinous carcinomas

ENDOMETRIOSIS

= ENDOMETRIOSIS EXTERNA
= encysted functional endometrial epithelium + stroma in an ectopic site outside the uterine cavity / myometrium (internal endometriosis within uterus = adenomyosis)

Prevalence: 5–10% of menstruating women; in 5% of postmenopausal women on estrogen replacement therapy

Etiology:
(1) Metastatic theory:
(a) peritoneal implantation of endometrial cells via retrograde menstruation through fallopian tubes
◊ Up to 90% of women have bloody peritoneal fluid during perimenstrual period
◊ Obstructive müllerian duct anomalies are the most common cause in girls <17 years of age
(b) vascular + lymphatic spread
(c) intraoperative implantation (uterine surgery, amniocentesis, needle biopsy)
(2) Metaplastic theory: transformation of peritoneal epithelium into functioning endometrial tissue
(3) Induction theory: combination of first two

Mean age: 25–29 years

Path:
(a) punctate small foci / stellate patches of <2 cm initiating inflammatory response (as organizing hemorrhage, fibrosis, adhesions)
(b) endometriotic cysts in ovary containing thick dark degenerated blood products = "**chocolate cyst**" (due to repeated cyclic hemorrhage), in up to 50% bilateral

Histo: endometrial glands, stroma, rare smooth muscle fibers; secretory changes during 2nd half of menstrual cycle; stromal decidualization during pregnancy

• infertility:
◊ 20% of infertile women have endometriosis
◊ 30–50% of women with endometriosis are infertile
Cause: involvement of tubes + ovaries (peritubal adhesions causing anatomic distortion, impaired tubal mobility to capture ovum, tubal destruction / occlusion)
• pelvic pain:
◊ 24–33% of women with pelvic pain have endometriosis
• dysmenorrhea, dyspareunia, back pain, rectal discomfort
• chronic pelvic pain (peritoneal adhesions, bleeding)
• localized tenderness along uterosacral ligaments + cul-de-sac + adnexa
• thickened nodular ligaments + rectovaginal masses
• fixed pelvic organs during bimanual exam

Location: ovaries (80%) > uterosacral ligaments > pouch of Douglas > uterine serosal surface > fallopian tube > rectosigmoid

Morphologic types:
1. Diffuse form (70%)
√ often no detectable abnormality (when lesions small + scattered)
√ frequently multiple cysts bilaterally
√ thickened wall + loss of definition of borders of pelvic organs
√ any combination of signal intensities
2. Discrete pelvic mass
Histo: obliterated mostly endometrial gland lining; initially thin wall that becomes fibrotic + thickened with irregular external border
◊ Multiplicity favors the diagnosis of endometrioma

US:
√ unilocular **endometrioma** = cyst of up to 20 cm in diameter (usually 2–5 cm):
√ acoustic enhancement
√ diffuse homogeneous low-level internal echoes (= hemorrhagic debris) in 95% CLASSIC
√ anechoic cyst (rare)
√ may show fluid-fluid / fluid-debris level (due to layering of debris)
√ echogenic wall foci (= cholesterol deposits) in 35% CLASSIC
√ wall nodularity in 20%
√ may contain echogenic material (= blood clot) appearing as a solid tumor floating dependently within cyst cavity
√ multilocular endometrioma = multiple separate cysts:
√ thin / thick septations between loculi
√ hematosalpinx (in 28%)

DDx:
(1) Hemorrhagic ovarian cyst (acute symptoms, more complex cyst with clot retraction, thin fibrin stranding, resolution in 4–6 weeks)
(2) Dermoid cyst (calcification, fat-fluid level, hyperechoic areas)
(3) Cystic neoplasm
(4) Tuboovarian abscess

MR (90–92% sensitive, 91–98% specific with fat suppression):
√ multiple cystic masses <u>typically</u> homogeneously hyperintense on T1WI (similar to fat):
√ additional hyperintensity (like urine) on T2WI (effectively excluding a dermoid cyst):
√ "shading" = faint / complete loss of signal within cyst on T2WI (= high concentrations of iron + protein with cross-linking results in a decrease in T2-relaxation time)
√ hyperintense lesion on all pulse sequences in 47% (DDx: hemorrhagic ovarian cyst)
√ hypointense on all pulse sequences in 27%
√ hypointense thickened wall (DDx: PID)
√ adhesion to surrounding organs

Cx:
1. Adhesions
√ fixed pelvic organs (during bimanual US)
√ obscuration of organ interfaces
√ posterior displacement of uterus (retroverted uterus) and ovaries
√ angulation of bowel loops
√ elevation of posterior vaginal fornix
√ loculated fluid collection
√ hydrosalpinx
2. Malignant transformation (<1%)
endometrioid carcinoma > clear cell carcinoma

Dx: laparoscopy / surgery
Rx: (1) Expectant

(2) Hormonal therapy (for pelvic pain / dyspareunia) to create a state of pseudopregnancy /pseudo-menopause / chronic anovulation: danocrine (Danazol®), GRH agonist (Lupron®), oral contraceptive pills
(3) Surgery (for infertility / intractable pain): implant recurrence in 28% by 18 months + in 40% by 9 years; adhesion recurrence in 40–50%

Atypical Sites of Endometrial Implantation

@ GI tract (12–37%)
- catamenial diarrhea, constipation
- rectal pain / bleeding

Path: initially serosal endometriotic deposits that erode into bowel wall causing hypertrophy + fibrosis of muscularis propria
Location: inferior margin of sigmoid colon + anterior wall of rectosigmoid (72%); rectovaginal septum (14%); distal ileum (7%); cecum (4%); appendix (3%); occasionally multiple lesions
√ single extramucosal mass with crenulated / spiculated mucosal pattern (DDx: drop metastasis)
√ polypoid intraluminal mass / annular constricting lesion (rare appearance)
Cx: adhesion, bowel stricture, GI obstruction

@ GU tract (20%)
- urgency, frequency, hematuria
- urinary obstruction, flank pain

Path: initially serosal endometriotic deposits that may infiltrate into bladder / ureteral wall
√ mass projecting into bladder lumen typically at dome of bladder (DDx: bladder cancer)
√ smooth / tapered / angulated short to medium-length ureteral stricture near inferior aspect of sacroiliac joint

@ Chest
= THORACIC ENDOMETRIOSIS SYNDROME
- pleuritic chest pain, cyclic hemoptysis

Cause: microembolization (via lymphatics or vascular channels), peritoneal-pleural migration (through diaphragmatic defects)
Time of onset: 5 years after pelvic endometriosis
- presenting symptoms:
  - pneumothorax (73%), hemothorax (14%)
  - hemoptysis (7%), lung nodules (6%)

√ almost exclusively right-sided pleural lesions
√ bilateral lung nodules
√ catamenial pneumothorax
√ pleural effusion

@ Cutaneous Tissue
- palpable mass ± catamenial bleeding
- focal pain / tenderness associated with menses

Location: laparotomy scar, cervical biopsy / electrocautery, episiotomy scar, umbilicus
√ well-defined hypoechoic / cystic / solid mass
√ hyperechoic border / tissue stranding (due to inflammatory reaction)
DDx: abscess, hematoma, hernia, sebaceous cyst, lipoma, hemangioma, malignant tumor

@ CNS
- cyclic headaches, seizures

√ subarachnoid hemorrhage

Ruptured Ovarian Endometrioma

= uncommon acute complication
- acute abdomen (due to chemical peritonitis)

√ distorted shape of endometrioma
√ thinned irregular wall component = rupture site
√ markedly hyperintense fluid in free intraperitoneal space on fat-suppressed T1WI
Rx: emergency surgery

FACIAL CLEFTING

Incidence:
0.5:1,000 in Blacks; 1:1,000 live births in white population; 1.5:1,000 in Asians; 3.6:1,000 in American Indians;
13% of all congenital anomalies; second most common congenital malformation; most common craniofacial malformation

Normal embryology:
1st branchial arch develops into maxillary + mandibular prominences; by 5th week the stomadeum is surrounded by 5 prominences: frontal-nasal, paired maxillary, paired mandibular prominences; nasal pits are formed by invagination of nasal placodes on each side of frontal-nasal prominence; the 2 maxillary prominences grow medially to fuse with the 2 medial nasal prominences forming the upper lip; the lateral nasal prominences form the nasal alae

Risk of recurrence: 4% with one affected sibling, 17% with one affected sibling + parent

Median Facial Cleft

= failure of fusion of the 2 medial nasal prominences
Incidence: rare
Cause:
1. median cleft face syndrome = frontonasal dysplasia
   √ brain anomalies rare
2. Holoprosencephaly
3. Majewski syndrome (short rib, polydactyly, median cleft)

Lateral Facial Cleft

Cleft Lip (25%)

Cause: lack of fusion of maxillary prominence with medial nasal prominence (= intermaxillary segment) around 7th week MA
Associated with: anomalies in 20% (most frequently clubfoot); NO chromosomal anomalies
Site: isolated in 8%, bilateral in 20%
√ linear echo-poor region extending from one side of fetal upper lip into nostril
Prognosis: excellent

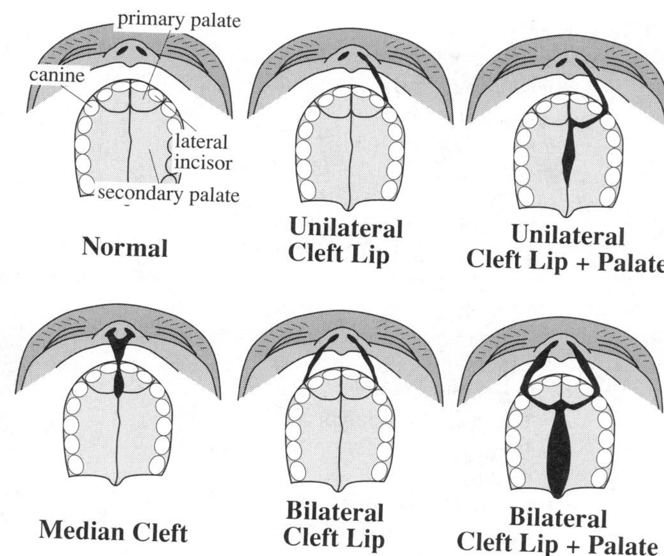

Cleft Lip & Palate (50%)

Cause: incomplete fusion of lip + primary palate with secondary palate

Associated with: 72 abnormalities in 56–80%: most frequently polydactyly; chromosomal anomalies in 20–33%

Location: L > R

Site: unilateral in 23%, bilateral in 30%

√ linear defect extending through alveolar ridge + hard palate reaching the floor of the nasal cavity / orbit (often deeper + longer cleft than in isolated cleft lip)

√ paranasal echogenic mass inferior to nose (= premaxillary protrusion of soft tissue + alveolar process + dental structures) in bilateral cleft lip + palate

Cleft Palate (25%)

= lack of fusion of mesenchymal masses of lateral palatine processes around 8th–9th weeks MA

Associated with: anomalies in 50% (most frequently clubfoot + polydactyly)

√ often missed on prenatal sonograms

√ small fetal stomach + polyhydramnios (due to impaired fetal swallowing)

FETAL CARDIAC DYSRHYTHMIAS

Normal heart rate: 120–160 bpm

Premature Atrial Contractions

= PAC = most common benign rhythm abnormality

√ transient tachycardia

√ transient bradycardia (due to atrial bigeminy if every other beat is nonconducted)

Cx: supraventricular tachycardia (unusual)

Rx discontinue smoking, alcohol, caffeine

Follow-up: biweekly auscultation until arrhythmia resolves

Supraventricular Tachyarrhythmia

Incidence: 1:25,000; most frequent tachyarrhythmia in children

Etiology: viral infection, hypoplasia of sinoatrial tract

Pathogenesis:

(1) Automaticity = irritable ectopic focus discharges at high frequency

(2) Reentry = electric pulse reentering the atria inciting new discharges

Types:

1. Supraventricular tachyarrhythmia (SVT)
   (a) paroxysmal supraventricular tachycardia
   (b) paroxysmal atrial tachycardia
   √ atrial rate of 180–300 bpm + ventricular response of 1:1
2. Atrial flutter
   √ atrial rate of 300–460 bpm + ventricular rate of 60–200 bpm
3. Atrial fibrillation
   √ atrial rate of 400–700 bpm + ventricular rate of 120–200 bpm

Hemodynamics:

fast ventricular rate results in suboptimal filling of heart chambers + decreased cardiac output, overload of RA, CHF

Associated with:

(1) cardiac anomalies (5–10%): ASD, congenital mitral valve disease, cardiac tumors, WPW syndrome, cardiomyopathy

(2) thyrotoxicosis

OB-US:

√ M-mode echocardiography with simultaneous visualization of atrial + ventricular contractions allows inference of atrioventricular activation sequence

Cx: congestive heart failure + nonimmune hydrops

Rx: Intrauterine pharmacologic cardioversion (digoxin, verapamil, propranolol, procainamide, quinidine)

Atrioventricular Block

Incidence: 1:20,000 live births; in 4–9% of all infants with CHD

Etiology: (1) Immaturity of conduction system
(2) Absent connection to AV node
(3) Abnormal anatomic position of AV node

Associated with:

(1) Cardiac structural anomalies (45–50%): corrected transposition, univentricular heart, cardiac tumor, cardiomyopathy

(2) Maternal connective tissue disease: lupus erythematosus

Types:

1. First-degree heart block = simple conduction delay
   √ normal heart rate + rhythm (not reportedly diagnosed in utero)
2. Second-degree heart block
   (a) Mobitz type I
   = progressive prolongation of PR interval finally leading to the block of one atrial impulse (Luciani-Wenckebach phenomenon)

√ a few atrial contractions are not followed by a ventricular contraction

(b) Mobitz type II
= intermittent conduction with a ventricular rate as a submultiple of the atrial rate (eg, 2:1 / 3:1 block)
√ atrial contraction not followed by ventricular contraction in a constant relationship

3. Third-degree heart block = complete heart block
= complete dissociation of atria + ventricles
√ slow atrial + ventricular contractions independent from each other

Cx: decreased cardiac output + CHF

FETAL DEATH IN UTERO

= INTRAUTERINE DEMISE
= fetal death during 2nd + 3rd trimesters

Specific signs:
√ absent cardiac / somatic motion

Nonspecific signs seen not before 48 hours after death:
√ same / decreased BPD measurement compared with prior exam
√ development of dolichocephaly
√ "Spalding sign" = overlapping fetal skull bones
√ distorted fetus without recognizable structures
√ skin edema (epidermolysis) = fetal maceration
√ increased amount of echoes in amniotic fluid (= fetal tissue fragments)
√ gas in fetal vascular system

"Vanishing Twin"

= disappearance of one twin in utero due to complete resorption / anembryonic pregnancy

Incidence: 13–78% (mean 21%) before 14 weeks GA

Time: <13 weeks MA

√ NO sonographic evidence of twin pregnancy later in pregnancy

"Fetus Papyraceus"

= compression + mummification of fetus

Time: in 2nd trimester

Path: resorption of fluid resulting in paperlike fetal body + compression into adjacent membranes

√ compressed mummified fetus plastered against uterine wall

Risk to surviving twin:

A. Dichorionic gestation (minimal risk)
(1) Premature labor
(2) Obstruction of labor by macerated fetus

B. Monochorionic gestation
(1) DIC in response to release of thromboplastin from degenerating fetus
(a) into maternal circulation
(b) into twin fetus through shared circulation (= twin embolization syndrome)

FETAL HYDROPS

Nonimmune Hydrops

= excess of total body water evident as extracellular accumulation of fluid in tissues + serous cavities without antibodies against RBC

Incidence: 1:1,500 to 1:4,000 deliveries

Causes:

1. Cardiac anomalies (40%):
(a) structural heart disease (25%): AV septal defect, hypoplastic left heart, rhabdomyoma
(b) tachyarrhythmia (15%)
2. Hematologic causes: thalassemia, hemolysis, fetal blood loss
3. Idiopathic (25–44%)
4. Twin-twin transfusion (20%)
5. Chromosomal abnormalities (6%): Turner syndrome
6. Skeletal dysplasias: achondroplasia, achondrogenesis, osteogenesis imperfecta, thanatophoric dwarfism, asphyxiating thoracic dysplasia
7. Renal disease (4%): congenital nephrotic syndrome
8. Infections: toxoplasmosis, CMV, syphilis, Coxsackie virus, parvovirus
9. Cervical tumors: teratoma
10. Chest masses: cystic adenomatoid malformation, extralobar sequestration, mediastinal tumor, rhabdomyoma of heart, diaphragmatic hernia
11. Abdominal masses: neuroblastoma, hemangioendothelioma of liver
12. Placental tumors: chorioangioma

Prognosis: 46% death in utero; 17% neonatal death

Immune Hydrops

= ERYTHROBLASTOSIS FETALIS
= lysis of fetal RBCs by maternal IgG antibodies

Prevalence: 35:10,000 live births at risk

Pathophysiology:
rh-negative women (= no D antigen) may become isoimmunized (= alloimmunization) if exposed to paternally derived fetal Rh-positive blood inherited from the father (= D allotype present); maternal IgM antibodies develop initially, later IgG antibodies with ability to cross placenta (= transplacental passage)

Cause of isoimmunization:
fetomaternal hemorrhage during pregnancy / delivery / spontaneous or elective abortion if fetus is D-positive; fetus has a 50% chance of being rh-negative as 56% of RhD-positive fathers are heterozygous for D antigen

At risk:
Caucasians (15%), Blacks (6%), Orientals (1%); absence of D antigen originates in Basques

Determination of extent of disease by:
(1) Optical density shift at 450 nm (= delta OD 450) reflects amount of bilirubin in amniotic fluid; reasonably reliable only >25 weeks MA; unreliable in alloimmunization due to Kell antibodies

OB&GYN

(2) Percutaneous umbilical cord sampling (PUBS) with direct determination of Hct and Hb
• hemolysis + anemia
√ anasarca (= skin edema)
√ fetal ascites in 2nd trimester (indicates severe anemia with Hct <15%, Hb <4 g/dL; present in only 66%)
√ pleural effusion
√ increased diameter of umbilical vein
√ subcutaneous edema (skin thickness >5 mm)
√ polyhydramnios (75%)
√ placentomegaly >6 cm
√ pericardial effusion
√ hepatosplenomegaly
√ increased blood flow in middle cerebral artery (due to increased cardiac output + decline in blood viscosity)

Prophylaxis:
Rh immune globulin (RhoGAM® = antibody against D antigen) blocks antigen sites on Rh-positive cells in maternal circulation to prevent initiation of maternal antibody production; Rh immune globulin given at 28 weeks to all rh-negative women

OB management:
regular monitoring from 18 weeks on when maternal anti-D concentration exceeds 4 IU/mL (severe anemia unlikely if maternal antibodies <15 IU/mL)

Prognosis: (if untreated) 45–50% mild anemia, 25–30% moderate anemia (with neonatal problems only), 20–25% develop hydrops (death in utero / neonatally)

Rx: umbilical vein transfusion during PUBS (necessary in only 10% before 34 weeks GA)

FETAL TRAUMA

Incidence: 7% of pregnant patients sustain accidental injury (greatest frequency during 3rd trimester); 0.3–0.4% are admitted to a hospital

Cause: motor vehicle accident (66%), physical abuse (10%)

Type of injury to pregnancy:
1. Uterine rupture (0.6%)
2. Complete (6–66%) / incomplete (30–80%) placental separation

US: evaluate fetal motion, breathing, heart rate, placenta

◊ The major cause of fetal death is maternal death!

GARTNER DUCT CYST

Frequency: 1–2%

Origin: remnant of vaginal portion of mesonephric / wolffian duct with incomplete involution + persistent glandular secretion

Histo: lined by flat cuboidal / columnar epithelium

May be associated with: complex renal + urogenital malformations
(1) Herlyn-Werner-Wunderlich syndrome = ipsilateral renal agenesis + ipsilateral blind vagina
(2) Ectopic ureter inserting into Gartner duct cyst

• usually asymptomatic

Location: anterolateral aspect of proximal third of vaginal wall extending into ischiorectal fossa

√ well-defined round lesion with fluid contents
√ large cysts may displace ureter upward / protrude through introitus

Cx: dyspareunia; interference with vaginal delivery

GASTROSCHISIS

= paramedian full-thickness abdominal fusion defect usually on right side of umbilical cord; may involve thorax; bowel is nonrotated and lacks secondary fixation to dorsal abdominal wall

Incidence: 1–2:10,000 live births (same as omphalocele), sporadic

Cause:
(a) abnormal involution of right umbilical vein resulting in rupture of anterior abdominal wall at area of weakness
(b) premature interruption of right omphalo-mesenteric artery (normally persists proximally as superior mesenteric artery) resulting in ischemic damage to abdominal wall

Age of occurrence: 37 days (5 weeks) of embryonic life

Age of detection: difficult <20 weeks GA due to small size of defect (1–3 cm) + lack of bowel dilatation

Associated anomalies (5%):
intestinal atresia / stenosis (25%; small size of opening leads to compression or torsion of vessels); ectopia cordis (rare)

• MS-AFP ≥2.5 MoM in 77–100%

√ exteriorized bowel = thick-walled edematous freely floating loops outside fetal abdomen (due to lack of peritoneal covering)
√ dilated intra- / extraperitoneal bowel
√ <2–5 cm paraumbilical defect, usually on right side of cord insertion
√ normal insertion of umbilical cord
√ no fetal ascites
√ polyhydramnios may be present
√ liver / spleen may herniate infrequently
√ malrotation / nonrotation of bowel

Cx before birth:
(1) Bowel obstruction
(2) Peritonitis (exposure of bowel to fetal urine / meconium)
(3) Perforation (from peritonitis)
(4) Fetal growth restriction (38–77%) secondary to nutritional loss from exposed bowel

Cx after birth: malrotation, jejunal / ileal atresia (18%), bowel necrosis, necrotizing enterocolitis, hyperalimentation hepatitis, prolonged intestinal motility dysfunction, chronic short-gut syndrome

Mortality rate: 17%

Survival rate: 87–100% after surgical treatment (during 1st day of life, not influenced by mode of delivery); death from premature delivery / sepsis / bowel ischemia

GERM CELL TUMOR OF OVARY

= malignant (except for mature teratoma) ovarian tumors of varying histology

Age: 14 years on average

- pelvic / abdominal pain + mass
- elevated alpha-fetoprotein (60% in immature teratoma; 100% in endodermal sinus tumor)
- elevated β-hCG (30% of endodermal sinus tumors)

√ average diameter of 15 cm
√ unilateral, rarely bilateral
√ calcifications (40%)
√ homogeneously solid (3%), predominantly solid (85%), predominantly cystic (12%)

GESTATIONAL TROPHOBLASTIC DISEASE

= group of disorders as a result of an aberrant fertilization event arising from trophoblastic elements of the developing blastocyst with invasive tendency

Components of trophoblast:

1. Cytotrophoblast = stem cell with high mitotic activity
2. Syncytiotrophoblast = synthesis of β-hCG
3. Intermediate trophoblast = responsible for endometrial invasion + implantation

- increased levels of β-hCG

Incidence: <1% of all gynecologic malignancies

Associated with: molar pregnancy (most), post abortion, ectopic pregnancy, term pregnancy

Spectrum:
1. Benign hydatidiform mole (80–90%)
2. Invasive mole (5–8–10%)
3. Choriocarcinoma (1–2–5%)
4. Placental site trophoblastic tumor (rare)

Cytogenesis:
= fertilization of one egg by two sperm = chromosomes completely / predominantly of paternal origin

1. Diploid karyotype
   - 46,XX = from fertilization of ovum by two 23,X sperm after loss of maternal haploid chromosomes
   - 46,XY = from fertilization of a chromosomally empty ovum by two different sperm:
   - in complete hydatidiform mole (almost 100%), invasive mole (almost 100%), choriocarcinoma (50%)
2. Triploid karyotype (69,XXX; 69 XXY; 69,XYY)
   = fertilization of a normal ovum (23,X) by 2 different sperm thus containing 2/3 paternal chromosomes
   - occurs in partial hydatidiform mole

At risk: maternal age >35 years and <20 years, previous molar gestation, previous spontaneous abortions

GRANULOSA CELL TUMOR

= most common hormone-active estrogenic tumor of ovary

Incidence: 1–2–3% of all ovarian neoplasms

Origin: from cells surrounding developing follicles

Age: puberty (5%), reproductive age (45%), postmenopausal (50%)

Path:
(a) large encapsulated smooth / lobulated multicystic mass with thick irregular septa + solid components; multiple blood-filled cysts (due to hemorrhage / cystic degeneration when tumor gets larger)
(b) unilocular cyst (rare) apt to manifest with virilization

- abdominal pain (acute hemorrhage into tumor / rupture into peritoneal cavity)
- palpable adnexal mass

Location: unilateral in 90–95%; bilateral in 5%

√ multilocular mass containing cystic spaces with fluid / blood (most frequently) + solid components:
  √ thick irregular septations but NO intracystic papillary projections
  √ usually large with sizes up to 40 cm in diameter
√ predominantly solid small hypoechoic mass simulating fibroid (less common)
√ calcifications (rare)

MR:
  √ hyperintense on T1WI (hemorrhage within tumor cysts)
  √ "spongelike" appearance of mostly solid intermediate signal intensity with innumerable cystic spaces

Estrogenic effects:
  √ uterine enlargement
  √ endometrial thickening / hemorrhage
  √ endometrial hyperplasia / polyps / carcinoma

Pattern of dissemination:
  √ local extension
  √ peritoneum-based metastases similar to epithelial neoplasm (rare)
  √ cystic liver metastases

Rx: uni- / bilateral salpingo-oophorectomy ± postoperative chemotherapy

DDx: serous / mucinous ovarian tumor (intracystic papillary projections)

Adult Granulosa Cell Tumor

◊ Most common estrogenic ovarian tumor! (occasionally produces androgen)

Incidence: 95% of all GCT; 5–10% of solid ovarian tumors

Age: in peri- and postmenopausal women; peak prevalence at 50–55 years

Histo: macrofollicular (multiple cysts resembling follicles), microfollicular (with Call-Exner bodies), insular, trabecular, cylindromatous, watered silk, diffuse type; frequently accompanied by theca cells + fibroblasts

- irregular menstruation cycles, menorrhagia
- postmenopausal bleeding
- amenorrhea
- 90% present at stage I (confined to ovary)

Cx:
(1) Malignant transformation (5–25%)
(2) Low-grade endometrial carcinoma (3–25%)
(3) Recurrence (raised serum aromatase + estradiol levels)

Recurrence: common even decades after resection with slow growth

Juvenile Granulosa Cell Tumor

Incidence: 5% of all GCT; more common than adult GCT in patients <30 years old
Mean age: 13 years; 3% in women >30 years of age
Histo: larger cells with hyperchromatic nuclei + lack of characteristic nuclear groves (compared with adult GCT)
Associated with: Ollier disease, Mafucci syndrome
• sexual pseudoprecocity (estrogen effect without ovulation)
◊ GCT accounts for 10% of cases of precocious puberty
Cx: malignant degeneration (rare)
Prognosis: 80–93% cure rate after surgery
Recurrence: unusual after simple resection for stage Ia / Ib tumors

HELLP SYNDROME

= **H**emolysis, **E**levated **L**iver enzymes, **L**ow **P**latelets
Prevalence: 4–12% of patients with severe preeclampsia / eclampsia; higher in White women (24%), with delayed diagnosis of preeclampsia / delayed delivery (57%), in multiparous patients (14%)
Time of onset: before / immediately after birth
Histo: portal areas surrounded by deposited fibrin + hemorrhage + hepatocellular necrosis
• epigastric / RUQ pain (90%)
• nausea + vomiting (45%), occasionally jaundice
• headache (50%)
• demonstrable edema (55%)
• tender hepatomegaly
√ fatty infiltration of liver (peak at 35th week)
√ intraparenchymal hemorrhage of liver leading to subcapsular hematoma / rupture into peritoneal cavity
√ hepatic necrosis
√ subcapsular hematoma of kidney
√ ascites + pleural effusions
√ vitreous hemorrhage
Cx: (1) Perinatal mortality (8–60%)
(2) Maternal death (3–24%) from hepatic necrosis, hemorrhagic liver infarction, liver rupture, DIC, abruptio placentae, acute renal failure, sepsis

HYDATIDIFORM MOLE

= MOLAR PREGNANCY

Complete / Classic Mole

= fertilization of ovum by two 23,X sperm after loss of maternal haploid chromosomes (46,XX) or occasionally fertilization of an "empty egg" (= ovum with no active chromosomal material) by 2 different sperm (46,XY)
Frequency: 1:1,200 to 1:2,000 pregnancies; <5% of abortions
Histo: generalized hydropic swelling of all chorionic villi with prominent acellular space centrally; pronounced trophoblastic proliferation of syncytio- and cytotrophoblast
• severe eclampsia prior to 24 weeks
• uterus too large for dates (in 50%)
• 1st trimester bleeding
• marked elevation of β-hCG with hyperemesis
• passing of grapelike vesicles per vagina
• hyperthyroidism (due to thyroid-stimulating properties of β-hCG)
• anemia (secondary to plasma volume expansion + vaginal bleeding)
• diploid karyotype, almost always paternal XX chromosomes
√ hyperechoic to moderately echogenic central uterine mass interspersed with punctate hypoechoic areas
√ numerous discrete cystic spaces (= hydropic villi) within a central area of heterogeneous echotexture
√ in 25% atypical appearance:
 √ large hyperechoic areas (blood clot) + areas of cystic degeneration resembling incomplete abortion
 √ single large central fluid collection with hyperechoic rim mimicking an anembryonic gestation / abortion
√ no fetal parts / no chorionic membrane
√ bilateral theca lutein cysts (18–37–50%), which may take 4 months to regress after evacuation of a molar pregnancy
Prognosis: in 80–85% benign, in 15–20% invasive mole / choriocarcinoma
Rx: dilatation + suction curettage (curative in 85%)
DDx: (1) Hydropic degeneration of the placenta (associated with incomplete / missed abortions)
(2) Degenerated uterine leiomyoma
(3) Incomplete abortion = retained products with hemorrhage
(4) Choriocarcinoma
(5) Hydropic changes of the placenta

Complete Mole with Coexistent Fetus (1–2%)

= molar degeneration of one conceptus of a dizygotic twin pregnancy with same risk of malignant degeneration as in classic mole
• vaginal bleeding in 2nd trimester
• uterus large for dates
• abnormally elevated serum β-hCG
• amniocentesis with normal diploid karyotype excludes diagnosis of partial mole
√ normal gestation with placenta + separate typical echogenic material of a hydatidiform mole
√ ovarian theca lutein cysts
Prognosis: fetal survival unlikely due to maternal complications from coexistent mole

Invasive Mole

= CHORIOADENOMA DESTRUENS
Histo: excessive trophoblastic proliferation with presence of villous structure + invasion of myometrium
Preexisting condition: complete / partial hydatidiform mole
• history of previous molar gestation / missed abortion (75%)

- continued uterine bleeding
- persistently elevated β-hCG levels (with failure of β-hCG to return to undetectable levels after treatment of a complete hydatidiform mole)

√ hyperechoic tissue with punctate lucencies
√ irregular focal hyperechoic region within myometrium
√ bilateral theca lutein cysts, 4–8 cm in size
√ myometrial invasion occasionally demonstrable

Rx: chemotherapy, hysterectomy (if at risk for uterine perforation)

Partial Mole

= areas of molar change alternating with normal villi + fetus with significant congenital anomalies

Histo: focal proliferations of syncytiotrophoblast; normal villi interspersed with hydropic villi

- triploid karyotype (66% XXY; 33% XXX) due to fertilization of single ovum with 2 sperm
- early onset of preeclampsia

√ nearly always coexistent fetus with severe abnormalities
√ placenta with numerous cystic spaces

Prognosis:
(1) frequently spontaneous abortion (unrecognized as mole for lack of karyotyping of the abortus)
(2) no survival of triploid fetus
(3) 3% risk of persistent gestational trophoblastic neoplasia

HYDRO- / HEMATOMETROCOLPOS

= accumulation of sterile fluid (hydro~) / blood (hemato~) / pus (pyo~) within uterus (~metria) + vagina (~colpos);
(a) premenarcheally = secretions + mucus
(b) postmenarcheally = blood

Incidence: 1:16,000 female births

Etiology:

A. CONGENITAL OBSTRUCTION
(a) persistent urogenital sinus = single exit chamber for bladder + vagina; separate orifice for anus; caused by virilization of female fetus / intersex anomaly / arrest of normal vaginal development
Frequently associated with: ambiguous genitalia
Age: newborn period
(b) cloacal malformation = single perineal orifice for bladder + vagina + rectum; caused by early embryologic arrest
Frequently associated with: duplex genital tract
Age: newborn period
(c) imperforate hymen, transverse vaginal septum, segmental vaginal atresia, imperforate cervix, blind horn of bicornuate uterus, Mayer-Rokitansky-Küster-Hauser syndrome (= agenesis of uterus + vagina with active uterine anlage)
◊ Hematometrocolpos / hematocolpos are due to imperforate hymen / transverse vaginal septum
◊ Hematometra is due to cervical dysgenesis + vaginal agenesis / Mayer-Rokitansky-Küster-Hauser syndrome / obstructed uterine horn

- primary amenorrhea = "delayed menarche"
- cyclical abdominal pain
- interlabial mass

Age: puberty
May be associated with:
imperforate anus, hydronephrosis, renal agenesis / dysplasia, polycystic kidneys, duplication of vagina + uterus, sacral hypoplasia, esophageal atresia

B. ACQUIRED OBSTRUCTION
neoplastic obstruction of endocervical canal / vagina, postpartum infection, attempted abortion, cervical stenosis after radiotherapy, postsurgical scarring (eg, dilatation & curettage, traumatic delivery), senile contraction

- vague pelvic discomfort
- pain during defecation / urination
- asymptomatic

√ smooth symmetric enlargement resulting in pear-shaped uterus ± distended vagina
√ varying amounts of low-level internal echoes centrally within uterus continuous with vaginal canal
√ hematosalpinx ± endometriosis

OB-US:
√ cystic / midlevel echogenic retrovesical mass (mucous secretions secondary to stimulation by maternal estrogens during fetal life)
√ cystic mass ± fluid-debris level (distended vagina)
√ bladder often not identified (compression by distended vagina)

DDx: ovarian cyst, duplication cyst, meconium cyst, mesenteric cyst, rectovesical fistula, anterior meningocele, cystic tumor, trophoblastic disease, degenerating leiomyoma / leiomyosarcoma

Cx: endometritis, myometritis, parametritis (= pelvic lymphangitis), pelvic abscess, septic pelvic thrombophlebitis, urinary tract infection

IMMATURE TERATOMA OF OVARY

= EMBRYONAL TERATOMA = MALIGNANT TERATOMA
= SOLID TERATOMA

Histo: immature tissue resembling those of the embryo; grade 0–3 reflect amount of immature neuroectodermal tissue

May be associated with: gliomatosis peritonei = multiple peritoneal implants of mature glial tissue

- elevated AFP levels (50%)
- no elevation of serum hCG levels

√ predominantly solid tumor with numerous cysts of varying size
√ scattered calcifications (due to invariable association with mature teratoma)

INCOMPETENT CERVIX

= gaping cervix usually develops during 2nd trimester / early 3rd trimester

Predisposed: cervical trauma (D & C, cauterization), DES exposure in utero with cervical hypoplasia, estrogen medication

- physical examination tends to underestimate the true length of the cervix

◊ Appearance of cervix may change during course of sonographic examination!

Cause: uterine contraction / manual pressure on fundus / patient erect (stress test of cervix) / degree of bladder distention

√ dilatation of cervical canal beginning at internal os + extending toward external os:
  √ beaking / funneling of cervical canal
  √ bulging of membranes through external os (= amniotic fluid within dilated endocervical canal)
  √ visualization of fetal parts within dilated endocervical canal

√ shortening of cervix to <25 mm

Normal Cervical Length			
		Transabdominal	*Transvaginal*
1st trimester	(<14 wks)	53 ± 17	40 ± 8 mm
2nd trimester	(14–28 wks)	44 ± 14	42 ± 10 mm
3rd trimester	(≥ 28 wks)	40 ± 10	32 ± 12 mm

◊ Distended bladder improves visualization but increases cervical length on transabdominal US!

◊ Difference between nulli- and multiparous women 10%!

Prognosis: 14th–18th week best time for Rx prior to significant cervical dilatation

INFERTILITY

= failure to conceive after 1 year of unprotected intercourse

Incidence: affects 10–15% of couples

Etiology:

(a) female factors (55%):
  - Tubal disease (10–20–40%): congenital anomalies, DES exposure, pelvic inflammatory disease, salpingitis isthmica nodosa, endometriosis, postoperative factors, polyp, neoplasm, ectopic pregnancy
  - Uterine factors (2–5%): bicornuate uterus, septate uterus, DES exposure, intrauterine adhesions, endometrial inflammation / infection, uterine neoplasm, complications after pregnancy, leiomyoma
  - Ovulatory disorder (10–20%)
  - Pelvic factors (20–25%)
  - Cervical factors (5–10%)

(b) male factors (40%)

(c) combination of factors (15–25%)

(d) unknown cause (5–10%)

Tests:
- history + physical examination
- laboratory tests (mainly hormonal)
- basal body temperature measurement
- postcoital test
- cervical culture
- endometrial biopsy
- sonographic monitoring of ovaries
- sperm agglutination studies
- in vitro mucus penetration test
- laparoscopy + hysteroscopy
- hysterosalpingography

INTRAUTERINE CONTRACEPTIVE DEVICE

√ double echogenic line with plastic IUD

√ reverberation echoes with metal IUD

Types of IUD:

1. Lippes loop
   √ 4–5 echogenic dots on SAG view
   √ horizontal line / dot on TRV view
2. Saf-T-coil
   √ echogenic solid line on SAG view
   √ series of echoes / dot on TRV view
3. Copper 7 / Copper T / Progestasert
   √ dot in fundus + solid line in corpus on SAG view
   √ solid line in fundus + dot in corpus on TRV view
4. Dalkon shield (no longer produced)

Cx: pelvic inflammatory disease (2–3-fold risk compared with that of non-IUD users) in 35%; actinomycosis with IUD in place for >6 years

"Lost IUD"

= locator device not palpated

Cause:
1. expulsion of IUD
2. migration of thread
3. detachment of thread
4. uterine perforation of IUD

◊ Abdominal plain film is indicated if IUD not identified by US!

IUD & Pregnancy

√ IUD may not be visualized after 1st trimester (as uterus grows IUD is drawn into cavity)

Prognosis: high risk of septic abortion

Rx: early removal of IUD if string remained in vagina

INTRAUTERINE GROWTH RESTRICTION

= FETAL GROWTH RETARDATION

= perinate with a weight at/below the 10th percentile for gestational age occurring as a result of a pathologic process inhibiting expression of normal intrinsic growth potential

<u>for twin pregnancy</u>: discordant weight >25%

◊ Fetal weight at/below 10th percentile for age will classify 7% of normal fetuses as growth retarded!

◊ IUGR is primarily an ultrasound diagnosis!

Prevalence: 3–7% of all deliveries; in 12–47% of all twin pregnancies; in 25% of fetuses following birth of a growth-retarded sibling / stillborn

Etiology:

A. UTEROPLACENTAL INSUFFICIENCY (80%)
   = injury during period of cell hypertrophy resulting in decreased cell size with features of intrauterine starvation + protective cardiac output redistribution reflex

- absence of body fat
- diminished liver and muscle glycogen

1. Maternal causes:
   √ asymmetric IUGR / symmetric IUGR (in severe cases)
   (a) deficient supply of nutrients:
   cyanotic heart disease, severe anemia (in 10–25% of sickle cell anemia), maternal starvation, life in high altitudes, drugs (anticonvulsants, methotrexate, warfarin), alcohol abuse (dose related), illicit drugs (up to 50% with heroine addiction, 30% with cocaine abuse), uterine anomaly, multiple gestation (in 15–20%)
   (b) maternal vascular disease resulting in inadequate placental perfusion:
   nicotine-induced release of catecholamines, preconceptual diabetes, preeclampsia, chronic renal disease collagen vascular disease (SLE)
   (c) maternal demographics:
   maternal age (adolescence / advanced), nulliparous mother, small short habitus, racial influence (Asians)
2. Primary placental causes:
   Extensive placental infarctions, chronic partial separation (abruption), partial mole, Breus mole, chorioangioma, placenta previa, low implantation, placental metastases (breast, melanoma), placentitis (luetic, malaria)
   Histo: reduction in placental villous surface area + in number of capillary vessels
   √ asymmetric growth failure

B. PRIMARY FETAL CAUSES (20%)
   = injury during the period of cell hyperplasia (= embryogenesis) producing profound reduction in cell number across all cell lines
   √ symmetric IUGR (globally decreased intrinsic growth)
   √ normal / increased amniotic fluid volume

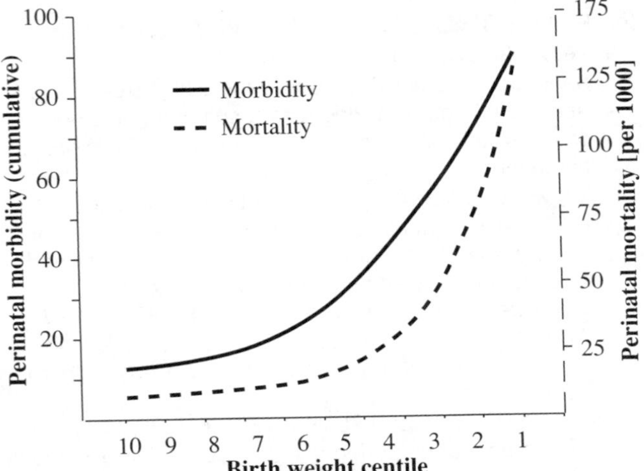

Effect of Birth Weight on Perinatal Morbidity and Mortality

1. Chromosomal abnormalities (in 2–6%):
   triploidy, tetraploidy, trisomy 13 + 18 + 21, aneuploidy (Turner syndrome), partial deletion (4-p, 5-p [cri du chat], 13-q), partial trisomy (4-p, 18-p, 10-q, 18-q), unbalanced translocation (chromosomes 4 + 15), balanced translocation (chromosomes 5 + 11)
2. Structural anomalies: congenital heart disease, genitourinary anomalies, CNS anomalies, dwarfism
3. Viral infection: rubella (in 40–60%), CMV, varicella (in 40%)

◊ All fetuses with IUGR need to have a detailed and often repeated search for structural anomalies!

- fundal height as screening test (37–60% true positive, 40–55% false negative; 26–60% false positive)

Sequence of events in fetal hypoxia:
nonreactive CST > absence of fetal breathing > nonreactive NST > diminished fetal movements > absence of fetal movements > absence of fetal tone

PHENOTYPES

1. **Pure symmetric IUGR** = decreased–cell-number IUGR = early-insult IUGR = low-profile IUGR
   = proportionate reduction of all fetal measurements due to
   (a) intrinsic alteration in growth potential (usually due to chromosomal abnormalities)
   (b) severe nutritional deprivation overwhelming protective brain-sparing mechanism occurring prior to 26 weeks MA + persisting until delivery
   √ proportionate decrease in HC and AC maintaining normal HC:AC ratios
   √ estimated fetal weight <10th percentile for age by middle of 2nd trimester
2. **Mixed IUGR**
   = onset of IUGR during period of mixed hyperplasia / hypertrophy with near normal inherent fetal growth potential but decreased size + impaired function of placenta
   √ impaired fetal growth ± asymmetry
   √ abnormal Doppler umbilical artery flow velocity (due to increased placental vascular resistance)
   √ progressive oligohydramnios
3. **Asymmetric IUGR** = decreased–cell-size IUGR
   = late-onset IUGR = late-flattening IUGR (75%)
   = disproportionate reduction of fetal measurements due to uteroplacental insufficiency with preferential shunting of blood to fetal brain occurring after 26 weeks GA

◊ IUGR usually not detectable before 32–34 weeks GA (time of maximal fetal growth)!

Effective time for screening: 34 weeks MA
Routine surveillance: every 4 weeks beginning at 26 weeks MA

√ AC >2 SD below the mean for age = highly suspicious; AC >3 SD below mean for age = diagnostic (AC single most effective fetal parameter for detection of asymmetric IUGR)

√ high HC/AC and FL/AC ratios (head size + femur length less affected)
√ fetal weight percentile useful for follow-up
√ accelerated placental maturity
√ decreased amniotic fluid volume
√ elevated umbilical artery S/D ratio
◊ FL/AC ratio + umbilical artery S/D ratio are the only effective techniques to screen for IUGR on a single exam with late prenatal care in 3rd trimester!

DIAGNOSTIC ULTRASOUND METHODS

◊ An accurate fix on fetal age dictates accuracy of diagnosis of IUGR (early US exam, clinical dates, early physical exam, pregnancy test)!
◊ Every effort needs to be made to determine the underlying cause for growth failure as it effects management + perinatal morbidity and mortality!

1. Fetal morphometric indices
   The three key parameters for diagnosing IUGR are
   (1) low estimated fetal weight (EFW),
   (2) low amniotic fluid volume (AFV),
   (3) maternal hypertension (HBP)!

Sonographic criteria for IUGR	*PPV [%]*	*NPV [%]*
Advanced placental grade	16	94
Elevated FL/AC	18–20	92–93
Abnormal UA waveform	17–37	
Low total intrauterine volume	21–24	92–97
Small BPD	21–44	92–98
Slow BPD growth rate	35	97
Low EFW	45	99
Oligohydramnios	55	92
Elevated HC/AC	62	98

   (a) intrafetal proportions
      √ elevated HC:AC ratio for dysmature IUGR (overall 36% sensitive, 90% specific, 67% PPV, 72% NPV; 93% sensitive in fetus >28 weeks MA with severe dysmature IUGR)
      ◊ Early-onset dysmature IUGR not detectable!
      ◊ May not be used in anomalous fetuses!
   (b) rate of growth = growth velocity
      √ HC, AC, FL measurements allow DDx between erroneous dates + normal small fetus + fetus with intrinsic abnormality
      √ plot growth curves
      ◊ Minimum time interval of 2 weeks necessary!
2. Amniotic fluid volume
   ◊ Screening for decreased amniotic fluid is of value in the fetus with dysmature IUGR (60–84% sensitive, 79–100% accurate)!
   √ normal amniotic fluid does not exclude IUGR
   √ oligohydramnios means dysmature IUGR in a fetus with normal GU tract until proven otherwise (DDx: trisomy 13 + 18)
3. Fetal morphologic assessment + fat distribution
   √ diminished thigh circumference
   √ absent paraspinal fat pad (posterior neck)
   √ reduced / absent malar fat pads
   √ disproportionately small liver size
   √ increased small bowel echogenicity (= absent omental fat)
4. Placental assessment
   √ increased placental calcium deposition
5. Doppler blood flow velocities
   a. Nonstress test (NST)
   b. Contraction stress test (CST)
   c. Umbilical artery waveform
      ◊ Not useful with unknown dates / for screening!
      Pathophysiology: fewer terminal villi due to developmental defect / villous infarction
      √ elevated systolic:diastolic ratio (S/D ratio >3.0 beyond 30–34 weeks GA) indicates an increase in vascular resistance within placental circulation
      √ absent diastolic flow = 50–90% mortality rate
      √ reverse diastolic flow = impending fetal collapse (due to severe fetal hypoxia)
      Note: S/D ratio increases with sampling site closer to fetus + increasing fetal heart rate; S/D ratio decreases with advancing gestational age; S/D ratio may decrease in lateral recumbent position
   d. Uterine artery waveform (measured at its point of overlap with external iliac artery)
      √ S/D ratio >2.6 after 26 weeks GA
      √ persistence of early diastolic notch
      Pathophysiology: lack of trophoblastic invasion of spiral arteries
      Rules:
      – Trophoblastic invasion may not occur until 20–22 weeks GA in some patients
      – An abnormal waveform at 24 weeks GA will never become normal
      – A normal waveform will never revert to a high resistive waveform
      – Both / one uterine artery may be abnormal
   e. Fetal aortic flow volume (no proven usefulness)
      √ decrease in blood flow to <185–246 mL/kg/min
   f. Fetal middle cerebral artery
      Pathophysiology: preferential shunting of blood to brain ("brain sparing")
      √ S/D ratio 2.5 to 3.0 (normally about 6.0)
6. Biophysical profile
   Accuracy: false-negative fetal death rate of 0.645/1000 fetuses within 1 week of the last normal BPP; 33% sensitivity, 17% positive predictive value
7. Invasive fetal testing: fetal blood analysis for karyotyping, hypoxemia, hypercapnia, acidemia, hypoglycemia, hypertriglyceridemia

Cx: increased risk for perinatal asphyxia, meconium aspiration, electrolyte imbalance from metabolic acidosis, polycythemia

Neonatal Cx: pulmonary hemorrhage + vasoconstriction, persistent fetal circulation, intracranial hemorrhage, bowel ischemia, necrotizing enterocolitis, acute renal failure

Prognosis: 6–8-fold increase in risk for intrapartum death + neonatal death
◊ 20% of all stillborn fetuses are growth retarded!

DDx of fetus small for gestational age (SGA):

Definition: generic clinical term describing a group of perinates at/below the 10th percentile for gestational age without reference to etiology

(1) Small normal fetus = constitutionally small fetus (80–85%)
◊ No indication for surveillance / intervention!

(2) Small abnormal fetus = primary growth failure associated with karyotype anomaly / fetal infection (5–10%)
◊ Active intervention is of no benefit!

(3) Dysmature fetus = growth failure as a result of compromised placental function (10–15%)
◊ Intensive management is likely of benefit!

KRUKENBERG TUMOR

= ovarian tumors from GI tract cancer (colon:stomach = 2:1) now including pancreatic + biliary primaries; 2% of females with gastric cancer develop Krukenberg tumor

◊ Krukenberg tumors antedate the discovery of the primary lesion in up to 20%!

Age: any age, most common in 5th–6th decade

√ in 80% bilateral hypo- / hyperechoic mass ± cystic degeneration

LIMB-BODY WALL COMPLEX

Prevalence: 1:10,000 live births

Cause: ? severe form of amniotic band syndrome; ? early vascular disruption; ? embryonic dysplasia due to malformation of ectodermal placodes

A. EXTERNAL DEFECTS
1. Ventral wall anomaly
√ large eccentric defect
Location: L:R = 3:1 (DDx: gastroschisis)
2 Craniofacial defects: anencephaly, cephalocele, facial cleft
3. Limb reductions
4. Spinal defects: dysraphism, scoliosis

B. INTERNAL DEFECTS (in 95%)
1. Cardiac defects
2. Diaphragmatic absence
3. Bowel atresia
4. Renal abnormalities: agenesis, hydronephrosis, dysplasia

√ persistence of extraembryonic coelom (= separation of amnion + chorion)

Prognosis: invariably fatal shortly after birth

MACROSOMIA

= FETAL GROWTH ACCELERATION
= fetus large for gestational age (LGA) with EFW >90th percentile for age / >4,000 g at term

√ AC >3 SD above the mean for age (most reliable + largest measurement)
√ estimated fetal weight (EFW) including fetal head, abdomen, femur length >90th percentile (± 15% accuracy)
√ low FL:AC ratio
√ low HC:AC ratio
√ enlarged thigh circumference
√ low FL:thigh circumference ratio
√ greater than expected interval growth
√ polyhydramnios

Risk: shoulder dystocia, prolonged labor, meconium aspiration

MASSIVE OVARIAN EDEMA

= tumorlike condition with marked enlargement of one / (occasionally) both ovaries due to accumulation of edema fluid in stroma

Age: 6–33 (average 21) years

Cause:
(1) partial / intermittent torsion (obstruction to ovarian lymphatic + venous drainage)
(2) ovarian stromal proliferation with enlargement of ovary susceptible to torsion

Histo: edematous ovarian stroma + extensive fibromatosis surrounding primordial follicles, luteinized cells

• acute / intermittent lower abdominal pain for month
• masculinization (in chronic phase)

√ solid / multicystic adnexal mass
√ ovarian diameter of 5–40 (mean 11.5) cm

Rx: oophorectomy / salpingo-oophorectomy / wedge resection with ovarian suspension

MUCINOUS OVARIAN TUMOR

Incidence: 20% of all ovarian tumors; 2nd most common benign epithelial neoplasm of ovary (after serous ovarian neoplasm)

Histo: single layer of nonciliated tall columnar epithelium with clear cytoplasm of high mucin content (similar to endocervix + intestinal epithelium)

Age: middle adult life, rare before puberty + after menopause

Cx: rupture may lead to pseudomyxoma peritonei

DDx: serous ovarian tumor (smaller, unilocular)

Mucinous Cystadenoma (80%)

Prevalence: 20% of all benign ovarian neoplasms

Age: 3rd–5th decade of life

√ multilocular cyst with numerous thin septa
√ cysts frequently have high protein content:
√ low-level echoes in cysts
√ high attenuation on CT
√ hyperintense on T1WI
√ usually unilateral, bilateral in 5%

Borderline Malignant Mucinous Cystadenoma
(10%)

Mucinous Cystadenocarcinoma (10%)
Histo: mucoid material in cysts, sometimes accompanied by hemorrhagic / cellular debris; difficult to differentiate from benign variety + metastasis from intestinal primary
√ multilocular with numerous smooth thin-walled cysts
√ solid tissue areas: thick septa + other soft-tissue elements within septated cyst
√ usually unilateral; bilateral in 5–10% of stage I cases
√ capsular infiltration with loss of definition + fixation
CT:
√ multiseptated tumor of low attenuation
√ high-attenuation proteinaceous material (20–30 HU) in some loculi
MR:
√ variable signal intensity in different loculi (proteinaceous / mucinous content, hemorrhage)

NUCHAL CORD
= umbilical cord encircling fetal neck: single loop > two loops (2–3%) > 3 or more loops (<1%)
Incidence: 25% of pregnancies; frequently transient
Associated with: increased cord length, small fetus, vertex presentation, polyhydramnios
• generally not of clinical significance: no difference in 5-minute Apgar score, no increase in infant mortality

√ two adjacent cross sections of cord on longitudinal view of neck (diagnosis facilitated by color Doppler flow)
√ indentation of skin by nuchal cord suggests tight loop
Risk: signs of fetal distress (fetal bradycardia, variable decelerations, depressed 1-minute Apgar score)
OB management:
1. Assess fetal well-being (biophysical profile biweekly, NST, fetal growth)
2. Vaginal delivery permissible if without evidence of fetal compromise
3. Intervention only for signs of fetal distress

OMPHALOCELE
= midline defect of anterior abdominal wall due to failure to form the umbilical ring during 3rd to 4th week of gestation with herniation of intraabdominal contents into base of umbilical cord
Prevalence: 1:4,000 to 1:5,500 pregnancies
Cause:
(a) migration failure of lateral mesodermal body folds:
√ omphalocele contains liver
(b) persistence of primitive body stalk beyond 12th week MA:
√ omphalocele contains primarily bowel
Age: earliest detection at 12 weeks menstrual age

High incidence of ASSOCIATED ANOMALIES (45–88%):
1. Chromosomal (10–30–58%): trisomy 13, 18, 21, Turner syndrome (13% with liver in omphalocele, 77% with bowel in omphalocele), triploidy
2. Genitourinary (40%): bladder exstrophy
◊ OEIS complex = **O**mphalocele + bladder **E**xstrophy + **I**mperforate anus + **S**pinal anomalies
3. Cardiac (16–30–47%): VSD, ASD, tetralogy of Fallot, ectopia cordis in pentalogy of Cantrell, DORV
4. Neural tube defects (4–39%): holoprosencephaly, encephalocele, cerebellar hypoplasia
5. IUGR (20%)
6. Beckwith-Wiedemann syndrome (5–10%)
7. GI tract:
intestinal atresia (vascular compromise); malrotation; abnormal fixation of liver, esophageal atresia, facial cleft, diaphragmatic hernia
8. Limb-body wall deficiency; cystic hygroma

• MS-AFP ≥2.5 in 40–70%

√ midline central defect at base of umbilical cord insertion:
√ defect over entire ventral abdominal wall (mean size 2.5–5 cm)
√ widened cord where it joins the skin of the abdomen
√ cord inserting at apex of defect
√ herniation of abdominal viscera at base of umbilical cord: liver (27%) ± stomach ± bowel
√ covering amnioperitoneal membrane (inner layer = peritoneum; outer layer = amnion); may rupture in up 15% of cases
√ hypoechoic loose mesenchymal tissue (= Wharton jelly) between layers of membrane
√ ascites within herniated sac (common)
√ polyhydramnios (occasionally oligohydramnios)

mnemonic: "OMPHALOCele"
Other anomalies (common)
Membrane surrounding viscera
Perfectly midline
Heart anomalies
Ascites
Liver commonly herniated
O for "zero" bowel complications
Chromosomal abnormalities (common)

Cx: (1) Infection, inanition
(2) Immaturity (23%)
(3) Rupture of hernia sac
(4) Intestinal obstruction

Mortality rate: 10% mortality if isolated abnormality; 80% with one / more concurrent malformations; nearly 100% with chromosomal + cardiovascular abnormalities

DDx: (1) Gastroschisis (usually right-sided defect)
(2) Limb-body wall complex (usually left-sided defect)

Pseudo-omphalocele

(1) Deformation of fetal abdomen by transducer pressure coupled with an oblique scan orientation may give the appearance of an omphalocele
  √ obtuse angle between pseudomass and fetal abdominal wall
(2) Physiologic herniation of midgut into umbilical cord between 8th and 12th week of gestation
  √ herniated sac never contains liver
  √ herniated sac usually <7 mm
  √ disappears by 12th week GA

OMPHALOMESENTERIC DUCT CYST

Etiology: persistence + dilatation of a segment of the omphalomesenteric / vitelline duct joining the embryonic midgut and the primary yolk sac, which is formed during the 3rd week and closed by the 16th week of gestation

Histo: cyst lined by columnar mucin-secreting gastrointestinal epithelium

M:F = 3:5

Location: usually in close proximity to fetus

√ umbilical cord cyst up to 6 cm in diameter
√ beneath amniotic surface of cord (= eccentric)

Cx: (1) Compression of umbilical vessels by expanding cyst
(2) Erosion of umbilical vein from acid-producing gastric mucosal lining

DDx: allantoic cyst, umbilical cord hematoma

OVARIAN CANCER

8th leading cause of cancer in women (4% of all cancers among women); 2nd most common gynecologic malignancy; 5th leading cause of cancer deaths in women after lung, breast, colon, pancreas (leading cause of cancer deaths of all female cancers); accounts for 50% of cancer deaths of female genital tract

◊ 1:70 women will develop ovarian cancer (lifetime risk)
◊ 1:100 women will die of ovarian cancer

Etiology: ovarian surface epithelium proliferates temporarily to repair defect after rupture of ovum, which may result in an "inclusion body" / "cystoma"; an error in DNA replication within inclusion body may occur resulting in inactivation / loss of a tumor-suppressor gene

Incidence: affects 1:2,000 women; 50 cases per year per 100,000 women (33 cases per year per 100,000 women > age 50); 26,700 new cases + 14,500 deaths in 1996

Age: increasing with age; peaking at 55–59 years (80% of cases in women >50 years)

Histo:
The proportion of malignant tumors increases with age:
<20 years of age 4%
>50 years of age 40%

A. MALIGNANT EPITHELIAL TUMORS (85%)
= arising from surface epithelium / mesothelium
Age peak: 6th–7th decade; rare before puberty
(a) serous tumor resembling ciliated columnar cells of the fallopian tubes (60–80%)
(b) mucinous tumor similar to endocervical canal epithelium (15%)
(c) endometrioid tumor similar to endometrial adenocarcinoma (8–15%)
(d) clear cell carcinoma = mesonephroid tumor (5%)
(e) undifferentiated tumor (4%) = cellular dedifferentiation does not allow categorization
(f) Brenner tumor (2.5%)

	Benign	*Borderline*	*Malignant*
[all types combined	75%	4%	21%]
Serous	60%	15%	25%
Mucinous	80%	10%	10%
Endometrioid	~0%	~0%	~100%
Clear cell	~0%	~0%	~100%
Undifferentiated	0%	0%	100%

B. MALIGNANT GERM CELL TUMORS (7%)
Frequency: 2/3 of ovarian malignancies in females <20 years of age
Age: 4–27 years
(a) mature teratoma (10%) = the only benign variety
(b) dysgerminoma (1.9%)
(c) immature teratoma (1.3%)
(d) endodermal sinus tumor (1%)
(e) malignant mixed germ cell tumor (0.7%)
(f) choriocarcinoma (0.1%)
(g) embryonal carcinoma (0.1%)

C. METASTASES (5–10%)

D. SEX CORD STROMAL TUMORS (7%)

Size versus risk of malignancy: <5 cm in 3%
5–10 cm in 10%
>10 cm in 65%

Epidemiology:
(1) sporadic: "ovulation hypothesis" = risk of ovarian cancer is a direct function of the number of ovulatory cycles during a woman's life span
(2) hereditary (1–5%) = defined as ovarian cancer occurring in at least two 1st-degree relatives
  ◊ 50% lifetime probability to develop ovarian cancer
  (a) breast cancer-ovarian cancer syndrome
  (b) ovarian cancer only syndrome
  (c) Lynch type II cancer family syndrome
  = inheritance of nonpolyposis colorectal cancer, endometrial cancer and (rarer) ovarian cancer

Increased risk:
nulliparity, early menarche, late menopause, Caucasian race, higher socioeconomic group, positive family history for ovarian cancer (risk factor of 3 with one close relative, risk factor of 30 with two close relatives affected with ovarian cancer), history of breast cancer (risk factor of 2) / early colorectal cancer (risk factor of 3.5)

Decreased risk = protective effect:
multiparity, use of oral contraceptives, breast-feeding

OB&GYN

Stage (FIGO system) based on staging laparotomy

- I Limited to ovary
  - I a limited to one ovary
  - I b limited to both ovaries
  - I c + positive peritoneal lavage / ascites
- II Limited to pelvis
  - II a involvement of uterus / fallopian tubes
  - II b extension to other pelvic tissues
  - II c + positive peritoneal lavage / ascites
- III Limited to abdomen = intraabdominal extension outside pelvis / retroperitoneal or inguinal nodes / extension to small bowel / omentum
  - III a microscopic abdominal peritoneal seeding
  - III b ≤2 cm implants of abdominal peritoneum
  - III c >2 cm implants of abdominal peritoneum
- IV Hematogenous disease (liver parenchyma) / spread beyond abdomen

◊ 50–70–75% of patients have stage III / IV disease at time of diagnosis!

Staging laparotomy = abdominal hysterectomy + bilateral salpingo-oophorectomy + omentectomy + random peritoneal biopsy + lymph node biopsy

Spread:

(1) direct extension through subperitoneal space (sigmoid mesocolon on left, cecum + distal ileum on right), uterus, fallopian tubes, broad ligament

(2) intraperitoneal implantation = exfoliation of tumor cells from ovarian capsule into peritoneal space (often microscopic)

with frequent seeding to:
- posterior cul-de-sac in pouch of Douglas
- infundibulopelvic ligaments
- omentum
- superior aspect of sigmoid
- right paracolic gutter
- termination of small bowel mesentery
- undersurface of right hemidiaphragm

with less frequent seeding to:
- Morison pouch
- liver surface
- porta hepatis
- intrahepatic fissure

(3) lymphatic spread
- craniad parallel to gonadal veins in infundibulo-pelvic ligament terminating at level of renal vessels
- laterally through broad ligament terminating at pelvic side wall: external iliac, obturator, hypogastric chains

√ lymph node short-axis diameter of >1 cm (in 88% positive for ovarian cancer)
√ hydronephrosis (2nd most common form of tumor-related morbidity after bowel obstruction)
√ thoracic adenopathy (paracardiac lymph nodes >5 mm in 28% of stage II/III disease + in 29% mediastinal lymphadenopathy at autopsy)

(4) hematogenous dissemination (% at autopsy): liver (45–48%), lung (34–39%), adrenal gland (15–21%), pancreas (11–21%), spleen (15–20%), bone (11%), kidney (7–10%), skin (5%), brain (3–6%)

√ malignant pleural effusion (pleural metastases in 28–60%, lung parenchymal metastases in 7%, pericardial metastases in 5%)

- often "silent" without obvious signs / symptoms
- occasional pelvic-abdominal pain
- constipation, urinary frequency
- early satiety
- ascites
- paraneoplastic hypercalcemia
- elevated CA-125 levels (= cancer-associated marker = high-molecular-weight glycoprotein with normal level of <35 units/mL):
  - >35 U/mL in 29–50% of stage I disease
  - >65 U/mL in 21% of stage I disease

  ◊ CA-125 levels elevated in 80% of ovarian cancers (60% of mucinous + 20% of nonmucinous tumors) and in 40% of patients with advanced intraabdominal nonovarian malignancy!

  ◊ CA-125 levels elevated in 30% of benign processes (in 1% of healthy individuals, fibroid, first-trimester pregnancy, menstruation, endometriosis, PID, benign ovarian tumors, liver cirrhosis, pancreatitis)!

Limitations of imaging:

◊ Microscopic peritoneal disease not detectable!

Benefit of imaging:

◊ Second-look surgery can be avoided if there is evidence for residual / recurrent tumor!

US:

◊ Screening finds adnexal cysts in 1–15% of postmenopausal women; only 3% of ovarian cysts <5 cm are malignant!

@ Morphologic tumor criteria (85–97% sensitive, 56–95% specific, 99% NPV):
√ thick irregular walls and thick septations (DDx: endometrioma, abscess, peritoneal cyst, cystadenofibroma, mucinous cystadenoma)
√ papillary projections ≥3 mm (in 67%, 38%, 9% of borderline, malignant, benign neoplasm)
√ solid / moderately echogenic loculi
√ postmenopausal ovarian volume >9 cm^3

@ Doppler tumor criteria (50–100% sensitive, 46–100% specific, 49% PPV; more sensitive + specific in postmenopausal women):
√ presence of color flow (in 93% of malignant + 35% of benign tumors) usually within thick wall, septa, papillary projections, solid inhomogeneous areas
√ low-resistance Doppler waveform (due to lack of muscular layer of arterial wall + presence of arteriovenous shunts in neoplasms):
RI <0.40, PI <1.0 (37–47% PPV)
false positive: physiologic alteration of ovarian blood flow during menstrual cycle, benign tumor, acute inflammatory disease, endometriosis

@ Metastatic disease
√ omental / peritoneal masses ("omental cake")
√ pseudomyxoma peritonei (with tumor rupture)
√ liver metastases
√ ascites

CT (70–90% preoperative staging accuracy):
- @ Primary tumor:
  - √ lesion diameter >4 cm
  - √ enhancing papillary projections
  - √ septa and walls >3 mm thick
  - √ partially solid, partially cystic mass
  - √ lobulated solid mass
  - √ tumor vessels on contrast-enhanced images
- @ Local extension:
  - √ localized distortion of uterine contour
  - √ irregular interface between tumor and myometrium
  - √ loss of tissue plane between tumor and wall of sigmoid colon / bladder
  - √ encasement of sigmoid colon
  - √ tumor distance from pelvic side wall <3 mm
  - √ iliac vessels surrounded / displaced by tumor
- @ Secondary findings:
  - √ <u>ascites:</u>
    - √ often lesser sac ascites with displacement of fundus and posterior wall of stomach anteriorly (DDx to benign ascites) + gastrosplenic ligament laterally
    - √ loculated ascites due to adhesions
  - √ >10-mm nodular / plaquelike <u>peritoneal implants:</u>
    - √ indentation of hepatic / splenic surface
    - √ ± calcifications
  - √ <u>lymphadenopathy</u>, may be calcified
  - √ <u>omental implants:</u>
    - √ small nodules / strands of hyperdense soft tissue increasing the attenuation of omental fat / marked omental thickening ("omental cake")
    - √ fat plane obscured between anterior abdominal wall + intestinal wall
  - √ <u>mesenteric deposits:</u>
    - √ round / irregular ill-defined masses / stellate lesions of small bowel mesentery
    - √ tethering of small bowel loops
  - √ <u>invasion of bowel:</u>
    - √ bowel obstruction (most common form of ovarian-cancer associated morbidity)
    - √ nodular / plaquelike lesions along / projecting from peritoneal surfaces
    - √ bowel wall thickening
  - √ <u>pseudomyxoma peritonei</u>

MR (combines best features of US and CT)

BE:
- √ serosal spiculation / tethering
- √ annular constriction / complete obstruction

Rx:
- stage I: total abdominal hysterectomy (TAH) + bilateral salpingo-oophorectomy (BSO) ± melphalan / intraperitoneal P-32
- stage >I: TAH/BSO + surgical cytoreduction (debulking) + 6 cycles of chemotherapy (cyclophosphamide + cisplatin)

Prognosis (without change in past 60 years):
46% overall 5-year survival rate, 5–8% for stage IV, 14–30% for stage III, 50% for stage II, 80–90% for stage I

DDx: tuboovarian abscess, dermoid cyst, endometrioma

OVARIAN CYST

Functional / Retention Cyst

Cause:
- (a) failure of involution of follicle / corpus luteum with changes in the menstrual cycle
- (b) excessive hormonal stimulation of follicles preventing normal follicular regression (eg, theca-lutein cysts)

Prognosis: spontaneous regression is common but unpredictable; typically resolve within 2 menstrual cycles (less likely if cyst >5 cm)

Cx: torsion

Rx:
- (1) Hormonal manipulation
- (2) Surgery (absolutely indicated if cyst enlarges)
- (3) Percutaneous aspiration (if chance of malignancy is nil as in infants)

DDx: cystic teratoma, simple benign epithelial neoplasm, endometrioma in resolution, paraovarian cyst, quiescent hydrosalpinx

Follicular Cyst (from preovulatory follicle)

Cause:
- (a) unruptured Graafian follicle from failure to ovulate
- (b) Graafian follicle with failure to regress / involute
- (c) ruptured Graafian follicle that sealed immediately (after continued stimulation)

- • may elaborate estrogen, extremely common
- • sign of anovulatory cycle

Predisposed: patients during puberty + menopause; S/P salpingectomy

- √ thin-walled, unilocular cyst
- √ size usually >2.5 cm / occasionally up to 10 cm
- √ usually multiple / may be single
- √ low-level internal echoes / fluid-debris level / septations / predominantly hyperechoic = hemorrhagic cyst (DDx: teratoma, abscess, torsion, malignancy, ectopic pregnancy)

Prognosis: usually disappears after 1–2 menstrual cycles

Corpus Luteum Cyst (from postovulatory follicle)

= hemorrhage into mature corpus luteum

Types:

1. **Corpus luteum of menstruation**
   = formed after rupture of follicle + increasing in size until 22nd day of menstrual cycle
   - √ usually >12–17 mm in size
   - • elaborates progesterone causing delayed menstruation / persistent bleeding

   Prognosis: resolves within 1–2 menstrual cycles
2. **Corpus luteum of pregnancy**
   = caused by hCG stimulation during pregnancy
   - • may be temporarily painful
   - √ usual size 30–40 mm, may grow up to 15 cm in diameter
     - ◊ Excessively large cysts with thin wall suggest poor function (= low progesterone levels)
   - √ reaches maximum size after 8–10 weeks
   - √ occurs on same side as ectopics in 85%

Prognosis: resolves by 12–16 weeks, occasionally persists past 1st trimester

√ high diastolic flow component
√ thin-walled usually unilateral cyst
√ echogenic (organized clot) / sonolucent (resorbed blood)
√ low-level internal echoes frequent (= hemorrhage)

Cx:
(1) Enlarging hemorrhagic corpus luteum with
- severe pelvic adhesions preventing ovulation of luteinized follicles
- NSAIDs which may cause luteinized unruptured follicle syndrome
- excessive anticoagulation
- endometriosis

(2) Rupture with intraperitoneal life-threatening hemorrhage at ovulation

DDx: endometrioma, ovarian tumor, organized clot in any enclosed space

Corpus Albicans Cyst

= from corpus luteum following regression of luteal tissue; no hormone production

Theca Lutein Cyst

= multiple bilateral corpus luteum cysts
- in hyperstimulated ovary from ovary-stimulating drugs, twins, trophoblastic disease
- elaborates estrogen

Surface Epithelial Inclusion Cyst

common in postmenopausal women

Age: any; in newborns (influence of maternal estrogen)

Incidence: 3–5–17% in postmenopausal women
- usually asymptomatic
- acute unilateral pelvic pain (from hemorrhage / pressure)

√ up to 8–10 cm in diameter

Imaging Classification of Ovarian Cyst

A. SIMPLE CYST
√ unilocular smooth-walled cyst + thin sharply defined wall of <3 mm
√ contents anechoic = NO internal septations / mural nodules
√ posterior acoustic enhancement
√ Doppler flow in cyst wall (detected in 19–61%) with pulsatility index >1.0 / RI >0.4 (unreliable!)
√ isointense to urine on T1WI + T2WI

DDx: serous cystadenoma

B. HEMORRHAGIC CYST
= functional cysts that developed internal hemorrhage

US:
√ echogenic mass (= solid clot)
√ whirled pattern of mixed echogenicity
√ "ground-glass" pattern = diffuse low-level echoes
√ "fishnet weave" pattern = fine interdigitating septations / lacelike reticular echoes
√ NO color Doppler signals inside cyst

MR:
√ intermediate / high intensity on T1WI
√ intermediate / high intensity with distinct central area of hypointensity on T2WI

Cx: rupture into intraperitoneal space

C. COMPLEX CYST
= does not satisfy criteria for hemorrhagic cysts / endometrioma
√ internal septations / mural nodules / internal echoes
√ mixed signal intensity, hyperintense on T2WI

Management of Ovarian Cyst

A. NEONATAL
√ change in position between exams suggests pedunculation with potential for torsion
√ fluid debris level / low-level echoes / retracting clot suggest torsion

B. PREMENOPAUSAL
1. Unilocular cyst ≤2.5 cm ± hemorrhage
   Rx: no follow-up unless on birth control pills
2. Unilocular thin-walled cyst 2.5–6 cm without hemorrhage
   Rx: clinical / sonographic follow-up in 1–2 months ± addition of hormones
3. Unilocular cyst 2.5–6 cm with hemorrhage
   Rx: sonographic follow-up in 1 month ± addition of hormones
4. Unilocular cyst >6 cm
   Rx: surgery

N.B.: All follow-up scans should take place in the immediate postmenstrual period, when follicular cysts should not be present!

C. POSTMENOPAUSAL
◊ Screening of 1,300 symptomatic women:
— in 2.5% abnormalities on US
— in 1.9% benign ovarian tumors
— in 0.15% ovarian cancers

1. Unilocular nonseptated thin-walled cyst <3 cm
   Incidence: 15–17%
   √ high resistive index (RI) of >0.7 (resistive index <0.40 is suspect for malignancy!)
   Prognosis: 56% decrease in size / disappear; 28% remain unchanged for up to 2 years
   DDx: serous ovarian cyst, peritubal cyst, hydrosalpinx
   Rx: serial follow-up
2. Septated cyst / cyst >3 cm / cyst with low RI
   ◊ 18% of complex cysts are malignant!
   Rx: CA-125 determination + surgical exploration

OVARIAN FIBROMA

Incidence: 3–4% of all ovarian tumors; bilateral in <10%
◊ Most common of the sex cord-stromal tumors!

Age: primarily >40 years
Path: solid firm white mass
Histo: pure mesenchymal tumor consisting of intersecting whorled bundles of spindle-shaped fibroblasts + collagen; varying degrees of edema often separate cells
Association: fibromas occur in 17% of patients with the basal cell nevus syndrome (Gorlin) syndrome (commonly bilateral calcified tumors + mean age of 30 years)

- usually asymptomatic (pure fibromas are not estrogenic, admixture of theca cells causes estrogenic effect)
- Meigs syndrome (in only 1%):
  - √ ascites (in 10–40% of tumors >10 cm)
  - √ pleural effusion (rare)
  - √ ascites + pleural effusion resolve after removal of tumor

Location: bilateral in 4–8%
√ ± cystic degeneration and edema in larger lesions
US:
- √ solid hypoechoic mass with marked sound attenuation
- √ occasionally hyperechoic / with increased through-transmission

MR:
- √ well-circumscribed low-signal-intensity mass on T1WI + T2WI less than or equal to myometrium due to abundant collagen content (FAIRLY DIAGNOSTIC)
- √ scattered high-signal-intensity areas (edema / cystic degeneration)

CT:
- √ well-defined solid homogeneous / slightly heterogeneous slightly hypoattenuating mass
- √ poor delayed contrast enhancement

DDx: pedunculated uterine leiomyoma, Brenner tumor, adenofibroma, malignant ovarian neoplasm

OVARIAN HYPERSTIMULATION SYNDROME

Incidence: severe OHSS in 1.5–6% under Perganol therapy
Etiology:
(1) Induced by hCG therapy with human menopausal gonadotropin (Perganol), occasionally with clomiphene (Clomid)
(2) Hydatidiform mole
(3) Chorioepithelioma
(4) Multiple pregnancies

Path: enlarged ovaries with multiple follicular + theca lutein cysts, edematous stroma (fluid shift secondary to increased capillary permeability)

- abdominal pain (100%) + distension (100%)
- nausea (100%), vomiting (36%)
- acute abdomen (17%)
- dyspnea (16%)
- thrombophlebitis (11%)
- marked hemoconcentration
- fainting (11%)
- blurred vision (5%)
- anasarca (5%)
- hydrothorax
- enhanced fertility

√ ovary >5 cm in longest dimension containing large geometrically packed follicles
√ ovarian cyst >10 cm (100%): usually disappear after 20–40 days; may persist for 12–16 weeks during pregnancy
√ ascites (33%)
√ pleural effusion (5%)
√ hydroureter (11%)
Cx: (related to volume depletion)
(1) Hypovolemia + hemoconcentration
(2) Oliguria, electrolyte imbalance, azotemia
(3) Death from intraabdominal hemorrhage / thromboembolic event

OVARIAN VEIN THROMBOSIS

Etiology:
(1) Bacterial seeding from puerperal endometritis with secondary thrombosis (pregnancy + puerperium are hypercoagulable states)
= **puerperal ovarian vein thrombophlebitis**
(2) Pelvic inflammatory disease
(3) Gynecologic surgery
(4) Malignant tumors
(5) Chemotherapy

Incidence: 1:600–1:2,000 deliveries

- presents on 2nd / 3rd postpartum day
- lower abdominal / flank pain (>90%)
- palpable ropelike tender abdominal mass (50%)
- fever if diagnosis delayed

Location: right ovarian vein (80%), bilateral (14%), left ovarian vein (6%)
CT:
- √ tubular structure in location of ovarian vein with low-density center + peripheral enhancement

Cx: IVC thrombosis; pulmonary embolism (25%); septicemia; metastatic abscess formation
Mortality: 5%
Rx: IV antibiotics + heparin; ligation of involved vessel at most proximal point of thrombosis after failure to improve after 3–5 days
DDx: appendicitis, broad-ligament phlegmon / hematoma, torsion of ovarian cyst, urolithiasis, pyelonephritis, degenerated pedunculated leiomyoma, pelvic cellulitis, pelvic / abdominal abscess

PARAOVARIAN CYST

= vestigial remnant of wolffian duct in mesosalpinx
Frequency: 10% of all pelvic masses
Embryology:
wolffian body (= mesonephros) consists of
(a) mesonephric duct (= wolffian duct)
in female degenerates into vestigial structures of epithelial-lined cysts (= canals / duct of Gartner)
Location: at lateral edge of uterus and vagina extending from broad ligament to vestibule of vagina

(b) mesonephric tubules
in female degenerates into vestigial structures of
1. EPOÖPHORON (at lateral part of fallopian tube)
2. PAROÖPHORON: (at medial part of fallopian tube)

Location: between the tube and hilum of the ovary within the two peritoneal layers of broad ligament

1. **Gartner duct cyst**: inclusion cyst lateral to vagina + uterine wall
2. **Paroöphoron**: medial location between tube + hilum of ovary
3. **Epoöphoron**: lateral location between tube + hilum of ovary
4. **Hydatids of Morgagni** (= appendices vesiculosae): most lateral + outer end of Gartner duct
   √ ≥1 vesicle(s) attached to fringes of tube + filled with clear serous fluid

√ thin-walled unilocular cyst, up to 18 cm in diameter
√ may arise out of pelvis (if pedunculated + mobile)
√ ± low-level internal echoes (from hemorrhage)

DDx: functional cyst, cystic teratoma, benign epithelial neoplasm

PARAOVARIAN CYSTADENOMA

May be associated with: von Hippel-Lindau disease
Location: typically unilateral
√ simple cyst
√ one / more small nodules along a smooth inner wall (86%)
√ ± septations

Cx: malignant degeneration in 2–3%

DDx:
(1) Hydrosalpinx (tubular shape, folds / short echogenic lines protruding into lumen)
(2) Peritoneal inclusion cyst (surrounding much of the ovary, history of surgery / PID)
(3) Cystic neoplasm of fallopian tube (more solid components)
(4) Paraovarian cyst with blood clot (resolution of clot on follow-up sonogram)
(5) Exophytic complex ovarian mass

PELVIC INFLAMMATORY DISEASE

= PID
= acute clinical syndrome associated with ascending spread of microorganisms ("canalicular spread") from vagina / cervix to uterus, fallopian tubes, and adjacent pelvic structures, not related to surgery / pregnancy

Incidence: 10% of women in reproductive age (17% in Blacks); 1 million American women/year

Risk factors: early age at sexual debut, multiple sexual partners, history of sexual transmitted disease, douching

Predisposed: formerly married > married > never married; intrauterine contraceptive device (1.5–4-fold increase in risk)

Etiology:
(a) bilateral: venereal disease, IUD, S/P abortion
(b) unilateral = nongynecologic: rupture of appendix, diverticulum, S/P pelvic surgery

Organisms:
(1) Chlamydia trachomatis + Neisseria gonorrhoeae (>50% with high prevalence of coinfection) damage protective barrier of endocervical canal with spread to tubes (30–50%) producing fibrosis + adhesions
(2) Aerobes: Streptococcus, Escherichia coli, Haemophilus influenzae
(3) Anaerobes: Bacteroides, Peptostreptococcus, Peptococcus
(4) Mycobacterium tuberculosis (hematogenous)
(5) Actinomycosis in IUD users
    = chronic suppurative infection characterized by multiple abscesses, abundant granulation tissue, fibrosis
(6) Herpesvirus hominis type 2, Mycoplasma

May be associated with: **Fitz-Hugh-Curtis syndrome** (= gonorrheal perihepatitis)

Sexually Transmitted Diseases (STD)

Disease	%	Disease	%
Chlamydia	33%	Human papillomavirus (warts)	6%
Trichomoniasis	25%	Genital herpes simplex	4%
Nonspecific urethritis	10%	Hepatitis B virus	1.2%
Gonorrhea	9%	Syphilis	1%
Mucopurulent cervicitis	8%	HIV	0.3%

- usually bilateral lower abdominal pain (due to peritoneal irritation)
- abnormal vaginal discharge / uterine bleeding
- dysuria, dyspareunia, nausea, vomiting
- lower abdominal + adnexal + cervical motion tenderness
- fever, leukocytosis, elevated ESR
- elevated blood level of C-reactive protein

MR:
√ ill-defined hyperintense area on fat-suppressed T2WI + intense enhancement on contrast-enhanced fat-suppressed MR (= extent of inflammation)

Dx: clinically, laparoscopically
◊ Imaging employed only to differentiate between medical + surgical condition!

Cx:
(1) Infertility due to tubal occlusion (25%): 8% after single episode, 20% after 2 episodes, 40% after ≥3 episodes of PID
(2) Ectopic pregnancy (6 x as frequent)
(3) Chronic pelvic pain (from pelvic adhesions)

Prognosis: infertility, ectopic pregnancy, chronic pelvic pain

DDx: acute appendicitis, endometriosis, hematoma of corpus luteum, ectopic pregnancy, paraovarian cyst

Endometritis

√ endometrial prominence
√ small amount of fluid within uterine lumen
√ gas reflection within uterine cavity (most specific)
√ pain over uterus

Postpartum Endometritis

Incidence: 2–3% of vaginal deliveries; up to 85% of cesarean sections

Associated with: prolonged labor, premature rupture of membranes, retained clots, retained products of conception

• fever (most common cause of postpartum fever)

√ normal ultrasound

√ thickened heterogenous endometrium

√ intracavitary fluid

√ intrauterine air

Salpingitis

◊ NOT depicted by imaging techniques

• often beginning during / immediately after menstruation (due to less effective barrier of mucus at cervix)

MR:

√ thickened wall of dilated fallopian tube + tubal contents of low signal intensity on T2WI

√ debris / hemorrhage in fluid component most conspicuously hypointense to urine on heavily T2WI

Salpingitis Isthmica Nodosa

Etiology: unknown; commonly associated with pelvic inflammatory disease, infertility, ectopic pregnancy

• nodular thickening of isthmic portion of tube

√ tubal irregularity + multiple diverticula / tubal obstruction on HSG

Hydro- / hemato- / pyosalpinx

= continued secretion of tubal epithelium into lumen of a fallopian tube obstructed at two sites

Cause: infection, endometriosis, adhesions, microtubal surgery, ectopic pregnancy

Location: ampullary / infundibular portion of tube

√ undulating / folded tubular structure in extraovarian location filled with sterile fluid / debris / pus

√ short linear echoes protruding into lumen (= tall ramified mucosal plicae)

√ longitudinal folds in ampullary portion

US (sensitivity of 34%):

√ thickened fluid-filled tubes

HSG:

√ absence of peritoneal spill

MR:

√ high-signal intensity of fluid on T1WI due to hematosalpinx

√ well-enhancing wall, thicker than in hydrosalpinx

Cx: tubal torsion

DDx: dilated uterine / ovarian vein, TOA, neoplasm, endometrioma, developing follicle

Tuboovarian abscess (TOA)

Cause: sexually transmitted disease, IUD (20%), diverticulitis, appendicitis, pelvic surgery, gynecologic malignancy

Organism: anaerobic bacteria become dominant

Location: usually in posterior cul-de-sac extending bilaterally

√ multilocular complex mass often with debris, septations, irregular thick wall

√ may contain fluid-fluid levels or gas

√ intense contrast enhancement of abscess wall

DDx: endometrioma, ovarian tumor, infected cyst, abscess from other sources (eg, Crohn disease, appendicitis)

PENA-SHOKEIR PHENOTYPE

= autosomal recessive syndrome (45% sporadic, 55% familial) characterized by fetal akinesia

Cause: decreased / absent fetal motion secondary to abnormalities of fetal muscle / nerves / connective tissue ("fetal akinesia deformation sequence")

Time of first detection: 16–18 weeks MA

@ Spine: scoliosis, kyphosis, lordosis

@ Thorax: pulmonary hypoplasia, cardiac anomalies

@ Kidney: renal dysplasia

@ Limbs: limited movement, knee + hip ankylosis (arthrogryposis), abnormal shape + position, demineralization, camptodactyly, clubfeet

√ craniofacial anomalies

√ polyhydramnios

√ IUGR

√ short umbilical cord

Prognosis: still birth

DDx: multiple pterygium syndrome, Neu-Laxova syndrome, restrictive dermopathy, Larsen syndrome, trisomies 13 + 18

PENTALOGY OF CANTRELL

= sporadic very rare abnormality

Cause: failure of lateral body folds to fuse in the thoracic region with variable extension inferiorly

1. Omphalocele + defect of lower sternum
2. Ectopia cordis
3. Deficiency of anterior diaphragm (herniation of intraabdominal organs into thoracic cavity is rare)
4. Deficiency of diaphragmatic pericardium
5. Cardiovascular malformation: atrioventricular septal defect (50%), VSD (18%), tetralogy of Fallot (11%)

Associated with: trisomies

√ exteriorization of heart

Prognosis: death within a few days after birth

PERITONEAL INCLUSION CYST

= PERITONEAL PSEUDOCYST = ENTRAPPED OVARIAN CYST

Cause: from previous abdominal surgery (time delay of 6 months to 20 years) / trauma / pelvic inflammatory disease / endometriosis

Pathogenesis: extensive pelvic adhesions result in impaired peritoneal clearing of fluid normally produced by an active ovary

Path: cyst adherent to surface of ovary

Histo: cyst lined by hyperplastic mesothelial cells + fibroglandular tissue with chronic inflammation

√ single / multiloculated cyst contiguous with ovary
Cx: infertility
Rx: surgery (30–50% risk of recurrence)
DDx: paraovarian cyst (ovoid cyst outside ovary), hydrosalpinx (visible folds, located outside ovary), ovarian neoplasm, lymphangioma

PLACENTAL ABRUPTION

= PLACENTAL HEMORRHAGE
= premature separation of placenta from the myometrium secondary to maternal hemorrhage into decidua basalis between 20th week and birth

Incidence: 0.5–1.3% of gestations
Risk factors: *mnemonic:* "VASCULAR"
Vascular disease + hypertension
Abruption (previous history)
Smoking
Cocaine
Unknown (idiopathic)
Leiomyoma
Anomaly (fetal malformation)
Reckless driving (trauma)

Associated with: intraplacental infarction / hematoma

- vaginal bleeding (80%): bright red (acute), brownish red (chronic)
- abdominal pain (50%)
- consumptive coagulopathy = DIC (30%)
- uterine rigidity (15%)

Echogenicity of hemorrhage:
√ hyperechoic / isoechoic hematoma (initially difficult to distinguish from placenta):
√ abnormally thick + heterogenous placenta (if blood isoechoic)
√ hypoechoic / complex collection between uterine wall + placenta in 50% within 1 week (hematoma / placental infarction)
√ anechoic collection within 2 weeks

◊ A normal ultrasound does not rule out abruption if
(a) separation occurs WITHOUT hematoma
(b) hematoma isoechoic to placenta

Prognosis:
(1) Only large hematomas (occupying >30–40% of the maternal surface) result in fetal hypoxia
(2) Abruptions with contained hematoma have worse prognosis
(3) Responsible for up to 15–25% of all perinatal deaths
(4) Normal term deliveries in 27% of hematomas detected >20 weeks GA
(5) Normal delivery in 80% of intrauterine hematomas detected <20 weeks GA

Cx: (1) Perinatal mortality (20–60%), up to 15–25% of all perinatal deaths
(2) Fetal distress / demise (15–27%)
(3) Premature labor + premature delivery (23–52%) (3-fold increase)
(4) Threatened abortion during first 20 weeks
(5) Infant small-for-gestational age (6–7%)

DDx: (1) Normal draining basal veins
(2) Normal uterine tissue
(3) Retroplacental myoma
(4) Focal contraction
(5) Chorioangioma
(6) Coexistent mole

Retroplacental Hemorrhage (16%)

= ABRUPTIO PLACENTAE
= accumulation of blood beneath placenta

Pathophysiology:
high-pressure bleed due to rupture of spiral arteries; hemorrhage may dissect into placenta / myometrium; associated with hypertension + vascular disease

Incidence: 4.5%; 16% of all placental abruptions

- external bleeding

√ thickened heterogeneous appearing placenta (hematoma of similar echogenicity as placenta)
√ rounded placental margins + intraplacental sonolucencies

Cx: (1) Precipitous delivery
(2) Coagulopathy
(3) Fetal demise (accounts for 15–25% of all perinatal deaths); risk for fetal demise with hematomas >60 mL: 6% before 20 weeks GA; 29% after 20 weeks GA

Subchorionic Hemorrhage (79%)

= MARGINAL PLACENTAL HEMORRHAGE
= SUBMEMBRANOUS PLACENTAL HEMORRHAGE
= separation of chorionic membrane from decidua with accumulation of blood in subchorionic space (placental membranes are more easily stripped from myometrium than from placenta)

Pathophysiology: low-pressure bleed due to tears of marginal veins; associated with cigarette smoking
Incidence: 79% of all placental abruptions; in 91% before 20 weeks MA

- may lead to vaginal hemorrhage after dissection through decidua (18% of all causes of 1st-trimester bleeding)

√ placental margin detached from adjacent myometrium (60%):
√ separation / rounding of placental margin
√ elevation of chorioamnionic membrane (DDx: incomplete chorioamnionic fusion during 2nd trimester, blighted twin)
√ hematoma contiguous with placental margin (100%)
√ predominant hemorrhage often separate from placenta, even on opposite side of placenta

Prognosis: worsens with (1) increased maternal age, (2) earlier gestational age, (3) size of hematoma; 9% overall miscarriage rate; risk of fetal demise doubles once hematoma reaches 2/3 of circumference of chorion

Preplacental Hemorrhage

= BREUS MOLE = SUBCHORIAL HEMORRHAGE
= variant of placental abruption with progressive slow intracotyledonary bleeding

Incidence: in 4% of all placental abruptions

Etiology: massive pooling + stasis due to extensive venous obstruction
Time of onset: 18 weeks MA
√ total loss of normal placental architecture
√ gelatinous character of placenta elicited by fetal movement / abdominal jostling
√ severe symmetric IUGR
Risk for fetal demise: 67% overall; 100% for hematomas >60 mL

PLACENTA ACCRETA

= underdeveloped decidualization with chorionic villi growing into myometrium
Incidence: 1:2,500–7,000 deliveries; in 5% of placenta previa patients
Risk of placenta accreta vs. cesarean section:
in 10% of placenta previa; in 24% of placenta previa + 1 cesarean section; in 48% of placenta previa + 2 cesarean sections; in 67% of placenta previa + 4 cesarean sections
Predisposed: areas of uterine scarring with deficient decidua: previous dilatation + curettage, endometritis, submucous leiomyoma, Asherman syndrome, manual removal of placenta, adenomyosis, increasing parity
Associated with: placenta previa (20%)
Types:
1. PLACENTA ACCRETA (76%) = chorionic villi in direct contact with myometrium
2. PLACENTA INCRETA (18%) = villi invade myometrium
3. PLACENTA PERCRETA (6%) = villi penetrate through uterine serosa

US (78–86% sensitive, 92–94% specific):
√ thinning to <1 mm / absence of hypoechoic myometrial zone between placenta + echodense uterine serosa / posterior bladder wall (retroplacental hypoechoic zone of decidua + myometrium + dilated periuterine venous channels measures 9.5 mm thick >18 weeks GA)
√ thinning / irregularity / focal disruption of linear hyperechoic boundary echo (= uterine serosa-bladder wall interface)
√ focal masslike elevations / extensions of echogenic placental tissue beyond uterine serosa
√ >6 irregular intraplacental lacunae (= vascular spaces)

MR:
√ heterogeneous hyperintense placenta on T2WI
√ interruption of junctional zone
√ focal thinning of myometrium

Cx: (1) Retention of placental tissue
(2) Life-threatening hemorrhage in 3rd stage of labor necessitating emergent hysterectomy
(3) Persistent postpartum bleeding
(4) Maternal death

Rx: (1) Hysterectomy
(2) Conservative measures: curettage, oversewing of placental bed, ligation of uterine arteries

PLACENTA EXTRACHORIALIS

= chorionic plate smaller than basal plate; ie, the transition of membranous to villous chorion occurs at a distance from the placental edge that is smaller than the basal plate radius

A. CIRCUMMARGINATE PLACENTA
Incidence: up to 20% of placentas
• No clinical significance
√ placental margin not deformed

B. CIRCUMVALLATE PLACENTA
= attachment of fetal membranes form a folded thickened ring with underlying fibrin + often hemorrhage
Incidence: 1–2% of pregnancies
Cx: premature labor, threatened abortion, increased perinatal mortality, marginal hemorrhage

PLACENTA MEMBRANACEA

= presence of well-vascularized placental villi in the peripheral membranes
Cause: ? endometritis, endometrial hyperplasia, extensive vascularization of decidua capsularis, previous endometrial damage by curettage
• repeated vaginal bleeding extending into 2nd trimester + abortion at 20–30 weeks
• postpartum hemorrhage
√ thickened outline over whole gestational sac (0.2–3.0 cm)
√ may show additional distinct disk of placenta

PLACENTA PREVIA

= abnormally low implantation of ovum with the placenta covering all / part of internal cervical os
Incidence: 0.5% of all deliveries; in 7–11% of women with 2nd + 3rd trimester vaginal bleeding; in 0.26% with unscarred uterus
Risk for placenta previa vs. cesarean section:
0.65% after 1 section, 1.8% after 2 sections, 3% after 3 sections, 10% after 4 sections
Cause: defective decidual vascularization in areas of endometrial scarring causing compensatory placental thinning; placenta occupies a greater surface of the uterus with increased probability for encroachment upon internal os
Predisposed:
(1) Previous uterine incision (cesarean section, myomectomy)
(2) Older women
(3) Multiparous women
Types on clinical examination:
1. Central / total previa (1/3) = complete covering of internal os
2. Partial previa = internal os partially covered by placenta
3. Low-lying placenta = low placental edge without extension over internal os; palpable by examining finger

• painless vaginal bleeding in 93% (usually 3rd trimester / as early as 20 weeks)

◊ 3–5% of all pregnancies are complicated by 3rd trimester bleeding; of these 7–11% are due to placenta previa!

US - FALSE POSITIVES (5–7%):

1. Placental "migration" / rotation
   = differential growth rates between lower uterine segment + placenta
   ◊ 63–93% will have normal implantation at term!
   — conversion to normal position: anterior wall > posterior wall of uterus
   — NO conversion if placenta attaches to both posterior + anterior walls
2. Overfilled urinary bladder
   bladder-induced compression leads to apposition of the lower anterior + posterior uterine walls (cervical length >3.5–4 cm) simulating a placenta previa
3. Focal myometrial contraction (myometrial thickness >1.5 cm) in the region of the lower uterine segment

mnemonic: "ABCD and F"
Abruption (may mimic placenta previa)
Bladder (must be empty)
Contraction (may have to wait 15–20 minutes)
Dates (be wary in 1st half of pregnancy)
Fibroid

US - FALSE NEGATIVES (2%):

1. Obscuring fetal head
   remedied by Trendelenburg position / gentle upward traction on fetal head
2. Lateral position of placenta previa; remedied by obtaining oblique scans
3. Blood in region of internal os mistaken for amniotic fluid

Cx: (secondary to premature detachment of placenta from lower uterine segment)
(1) Maternal hemorrhage (blood from intervillous space)
(2) Premature delivery
(3) IUGR
(4) Perinatal death (5%)

Rx: precludes vaginal delivery + pelvic examination

PLACENTAL SITE TROPHOBLASTIC DISEASE

= very rare neoplasm (? type of choriocarcinoma)
Path: microscopic tumor / diffuse nodular replacement of myometrium
Histo: proliferation of predominantly intermediate trophoblasts but no syncytio- or cytotrophoblasts

• abnormal bleeding / amenorrhea
• low β-hCG levels (due to lack of syncytiotrophoblastic proliferation)
√ cystic / solid lesions ± central component
√ myometrium usually invaded

Prognosis: benign / highly malignant course
Rx: hysterectomy

POSTMATURITY SYNDROME

= inability of aging placenta to support demands of fetus
Incidence: in 15% of all postterm gravidas

• meconium-stained amniotic fluid
√ grade 3 placenta (in 85%), grade 2 (in 15%), grade 1 (in 0%)
√ decreased subcutaneous fat + wrinkling of skin
√ long fingernails
√ decreased vernix

Cx: meconium aspiration, perinatal asphyxia, thermal instability

Postterm Fetus

= fetus undelivered by 42nd week MA
Incidence: 7–12% of all pregnancies
Risk of perinatal mortality:
2-fold at 43 weeks MA, 4–6-fold at 44 weeks MA

PREECLAMPSIA

= TOXEMIA OF PREGNANCY
Incidence: 5% of pregnancies, typically during 3rd trimester
Clinical triad:
• pregnancy-induced / -aggravated hypertension
• proteinuria
• peripheral edema + weight gain

Histo: blunted invasion of vasa media of spiral arterioles + focal vasculitis + atheromatous degeneration + fibrin deposits in intima of maternal placental arterioles

√ heavy calcium deposition (in areas of placental degeneration)
√ IUGR (6% with late-onset preeclampsia, 18% with early-onset preeclampsia)

Cx:
@ CNS
@ Liver: hematoma, infarction
@ Kidney

ECLAMPSIA
• convulsions + coma

PREMATURE RUPTURE OF MEMBRANES

= spontaneous rupture of chorioamnionic membranes before the onset of labor
Types:
(a) Preterm premature rupture of membranes (PPROM) <37 weeks GA
(b) Term premature rupture of membranes (TPROM) >37 weeks GA

Incidence: overall 2.1–17.1%; PPROM 0.9–4.4%; in 29% of all preterm deliveries; in 18% of all term deliveries
Risk of recurrence: 21% of women with PPROM
Cause: ? infection of membranes
Cx:
(a) TPROM:
   — >24 hours may result in intrapartum fever
   — >72 hours may result in chorioamnionitis + still-birth
(b) PPROM: respiratory distress syndrome (9–43%), neonatal sepsis (2–19%)

PRIMARY OVARIAN CHORIOCARCINOMA

= NONGESTATIONAL CHORIOCARCINOMA

Incidence: extremely rare; 50 cases in world literature

Age: <20 years

• elevated serum hCG

√ predominantly solid tumor with areas of hemorrhage + necrosis

DDx: metastasis to ovary from gestational choriocarcinoma (reproductive age)

SECKEL SYNDROME

= BIRD-HEADED DWARFISM

= rare autosomal recessive disorder (44 cases)

• proportionate postnatal short stature

• characteristic stance: slight flexion of hips and knees

• mental retardation

• simian crease

• cryptorchidism

@ Skull

√ severe microcephaly

√ receding forehead, large beaked nose, micrognathia

@ Skeleton

√ dislocation of radial head + hypoplasia of proximal end of radius

√ absence of phalangeal epiphysis

√ clinodactyly of 5th digit

√ gap between 1st and 2nd toe

√ hip dislocation

√ hypoplasia of proximal fibula

√ absence of patella

√ 11 pairs of ribs

OB-US:

√ severe IUGR

√ oligohydramnios

√ decreased bone length (femur, tibia, fibula)

√ decreased AC, HC

SEROUS OVARIAN TUMOR

◊ Most common neoplasm in benign + malignant category

Incidence: 30% of all ovarian tumors; 60–80% of all malignant ovarian neoplasms

Path: areas of solid tissue components + hemorrhage and necrosis (more common in malignant tumors)

Histo: lined by tall columnar epithelial cells (like fallopian tubes), filled with serous fluid, psammoma bodies (= microscopic calcifications in up to 30% of malignant tumors);

Age: 20–50 years (malignant variety later)

Serous Cystadenoma (60%)

second most common benign tumor of the ovary (after dermoid cyst); 20% of all benign ovarian neoplasms

√ usually unilocular (occasionally multilocular) thin-walled cyst up to 20 cm in diameter

√ only small amount of solid tissue: occasional septum / mural nodule (papillary projections in 9%)

√ bilateral in 7–20–30%

Borderline Malignant Serous Cystadenoma (15%)

√ papillary projections within cyst (in 67%)

Serous Cystadenocarcinoma (25%)

= 60–80% of all ovarian carcinomas

√ multilocular cyst with large amount of solid tissue: papillomatous excrescences within cyst (= papillary serous carcinoma) in 38%

√ may have calcifications

√ bilateral in 50–70%

√ loss of capsular definition + tumor fixation

√ ascites secondary to peritoneal surface implantation

√ lymph node enlargement (periaortic, mediastinal, supraclavicular)

CT:

√ psammomatous calcifications (12%)

SERTOLI–STROMAL CELL TUMOR OF OVARY

= ANDROBLASTOMA = ARRHENOBLASTOMA

Origin: from hilar cells of ovary

Incidence: <0.5%

Age: any age; most common in 2nd–3rd decade

Histo: components of Sertoli cells, Leydig cells, fibroblasts

• androgenic

√ hypoechoic mass simulating fibroid

√ may have cystic / hemorrhagic degeneration

Sertoli-Leydig Cell Tumor

◊ Most common virilizing tumor of ovary!

Incidence: 0.5% of all ovarian neoplasms

Age peak: 25–45 years (range 15–66 years); 75% occur in patients <30 years of age

Path: solid ± cystic areas; hemorrhage is rare

Histo: 6 subtypes; tissues are so varied that it is frequently confused with other tumors

• virilization (30%): amenorrhea, male secondary sexual characteristics

• estrogenic (20%); no hormonal manifestations (50%)

√ small mass often difficult to visualize by US / CT

√ solid mass with cystic components (hemorrhage ± necrosis)

√ well-defined hypoechoic mass ± intratumoral cysts

√ calcifications are unusual

√ contrast enhancement

√ unilateral (95%), up to 27 cm in diameter

Cx: malignant transformation in 10–18%

Prognosis: good when detected as stage I (in 92%); tend to recur soon after initial diagnosis

DDx: granulosa cell tumor (spongelike multicystic with areas of hemorrhage)

SINGLE UMBILICAL ARTERY

Etiology:

(1) Primary agenesis of one umbilical artery (usually first appears in 5th menstrual week)

(2) Secondary atrophy / atresia of one umbilical artery

(3) Persistence of original single allantoic artery of the body stalk

Incidence: 0.2–1% of singleton births; 5% in dizygotic twins; 2.5% in abortuses; increased incidence in trisomy D / E, diabetic mothers, White patients, spontaneous abortions

Associated with:
(a) Congenital anomalies (21%):
1. CHD (most frequent): VSD, conotruncal anomalies
2. Abdomen: ventral wall defect, diaphragmatic hernia
3. CNS: hydrocephalus, holoprosencephaly, spina bifida
4. GU: hydronephrosis, dysplastic kidney
5. Esophageal atresia, cystic hygroma, cleft lip
6. Polydactyly, syndactyly
(b) IUGR
(c) Premature delivery
(d) Perinatal mortality (20%): stillbirth (66%)
(e) Marginal (18%) / velamentous (9%) insertion of umbilical cord
(f) Chromosomal anomalies (67%): trisomy 18 > trisomy 13 > Turner syndrome > triploidy

Site: left artery slightly more often absent than right
√ axial view of cord shows 2 vessels
√ single umbilical artery nearly as large as umbilical vein (umbilical vein-to-umbilical artery ratio < 2)
√ incurvation of distal aorta toward common iliac artery on the side of patent umbilical artery
√ ipsilateral hypoplastic common iliac artery
√ absence of abdominal portion of umbilical artery on ipsilateral side of missing umbilical artery
√ color flow imaging permits earlier (15–16 weeks) + more confident diagnosis

Prognosis:
(1) 4-fold increase in perinatal mortality (14%) with concurrent major abnormality
(2) Isolated single umbilical artery does not affect clinical outcome

DDx:
(1) Normal variant = two arteries at fetal end may fuse near placental end into single umbilical artery (umbilical arteries normally unite with allantoic artery near placental insertion)
(2) Arterial convergence of 2 into 1 umbilical a.

STEIN-LEVENTHAL SYNDROME

= POLYCYSTIC OVARY SYNDROME

Incidence: 2.5% of all women

Etiology: deficient aromatase activity (catalyst for conversion of androgen into estrogen) results in androgen excess; exaggerated pulsatile release of LH stimulates continued ovarian androgen secretion at the expense of estradiol; reduction of local estrogen impairs FSH activity; this results in accumulation of small- + medium-sized atretic follicles without final maturation into graafian follicles

Path: pearly white ovaries with multiple cysts below the capsule, which are lined by a hyperplastic theca interna layer showing pronounced luteinization; granulosa cells are absent / degenerating; corpora lutea are absent

Age: late 2nd decade

Associated with: Cushing syndrome, basophilic pituitary adenoma, postpill amenorrhea, virilizing ovarian / adrenal tumor

- reduced infertility / sterility
- mild facial / severe generalized hirsutism
- obesity
- secondary amenorrhea (most common cause)
- menstrual irregularities / oligomenorrhea
- cystic acne
- cephalic hair loss
- periodic abdominal discomfort
- elevated LH levels without LH surge + normal / decreased FSH = increased LH/FSH ratio
- elevated androstenedione / testosterone levels
- elevated estrone / estradiol

√ bilaterally enlarged ovaries >15 cm^3 (70%)
√ normal ovarian size (in 30%), polycystic ovaries have a volume of 6–30 cm^3
√ excessive number of developing follicles:
  √ multiple (more than 5) small cysts of 5–8 mm in subcapsular location (40%)
  √ hypoechoic ovaries (25%)
  √ isoechoic ovaries (5%)

Cx: endometrial cancer <40 years of age (due to unopposed chronic estrogen stimulation)

DDx: ovaries in congenital adrenal hyperplasia, normal ovaries

Rx: (1) Ovulation induction with clomiphene (Clomid) / menotropins (Perganol)
(2) Wedge resection (transient effect only)

STEROID CELL TUMORS

= LIPID / LIPOID CELL TUMORS
= characterized by cells resembling typical steroid-secreting cells (lutein cells, Leydig cells, adrenocortical cells)

Incidence: 0.1–0.2% of all ovarian tumors

Age: wide range of ages; usually 5th–6th decade

Types: stromal luteoma, Leydig / hilus cell tumor, steroid tumor not otherwise specified

Path: usually <3 cm yellow nodule with rich vascularity; rarely cystic

Histo: abundant clear cytoplasm + varying amounts of lipid resembling adrenocortical cells

- virilizing (majority): amenorrhea, hirsutism
- Cushing syndrome (rare)

√ unilateral solid tumor
√ cystic change / necrosis (rare)

MR:
  √ high-signal intensity on T1WI (lipid content)
  √ intense contrast enhancement (high tumor vascularity)

Prognosis: clinically malignant (33%)

STUCK TWIN

= one twin with IUGR residing within an oligo- / anhydramniotic sac of a diamniotic twin pregnancy
√ amnion invisible secondary to close contact with fetal parts

√ fetus fixed relative to the uterine wall without change during shift in maternal position
√ diminished / absent active fetal motion
√ absence of intermingling of fetal parts between twins
Prognosis: fetal death in utero

SUCCENTURIATE LOBE OF PLACENTA

= ACCESSORY LOBE
= separate mass of chorionic villi connected to main placenta by vessels within membrane
Cause: placental villi atrophy in area of inadequate blood supply + proliferate in two opposite directions (trophotropism) with fetal vessels remaining at the site of villous atrophy
Incidence: 0.14–3%
Cx: (1) Retained in utero with postpartum hemorrhage
(2) Placenta previa with intrapartum hemorrhage
(3) Vasa previa = succenturiate vessels traversing internal os, which may rupture resulting in fetal blood loss

TERATOMA OF NECK

= germ cell tumor of neck (oropharynx, tongue)
√ polyhydramnios in 30% (from esophageal obstruction)
√ complex mass in cervical region
Cx: airway obstruction
DDx: cystic hygroma, goiter, branchial cleft cyst, cervical meningocele, neuroblastoma of neck, hemangioma of neck

TERATOMA OF OVARY

= immature derivatives of all 3 germ cell layers
Incidence: rare
Age: childhood / adolescence
√ cystic / complex mass (most frequently)
√ usually large solid mass with internal echoes

THECA CELL TUMOR OF OVARY

= THECOMA = FIBROSED THECOMA = FIBROTHECOMA
= spectrum of tumors with varying amounts of theca cells (lipid-rich with estrogenic activity) + fibroblasts
Histo: theca cells contain intracellular lipids
Incidence: 4–6% of all ovarian neoplasms; 50% of all gonadal-stromal tumors
Age: mean age of 59 years;
>30 years (30%), postmenopausal (70%)
May be associated with: endometrial hyperplasia / ca.
• estrogenic with uterine bleeding
√ hypoechoic mass with sound attenuation
√ unilateral
MR:
√ low signal intensity on T2WI for fibrotic component
√ high signal intensity on T2WI for components with little / no fibrosis

Luteinized Thecoma

= rare subtype of fibrothecomas associated with virilization rather than estrogenic activity

THECA LUTEIN CYST

= multiple bilateral corpus luteum cysts as a form of ovarian hyperstimulation
• associated with abnormally high levels of β-hCG secondary to
(a) multiple gestations
(b) gestational trophoblastic disease (in 40%)
(c) fetal hydrops
(d) pharmacologic stimulation with β-hCG
(e) normal pregnancy (uncommon)
√ multiloculated cysts, often bilateral
√ ovaries several cm in size
√ involution within a few months after source of gonadotropin removed

TORSION OF OVARY

= result of rotation of ovary ± tube on its axis producing arterial, venous, and lymphatic stasis
Cause:
(1) Enlarged ovary (large cyst / tumor, paraovarian cyst)
◊ Benign cystic teratoma is most common neoplasm
(2) Hypermobility of adnexa (more frequent in younger children + during pregnancy), excessively long mesosalpinx, tubal spasm
Associated with: ipsilateral ovarian lesion (in 50–81%)
Age: usually affects prepubertal girls, may occur prenatally, increased risk during pregnancy
Path: hemorrhagic necrosis
Pathophysiology: cicrculatory stasis is initially venous; becomes arterial as torsion + edema progress; complete obstruction of arterial blood supply leads to gangrenous + hemorrhagic necrosis
• gradual / sudden onset of severe lower abdominal pain
• nausea, vomiting, fever
• palpable mass in 50%
Location: R:L = 3:2 (? protective effect of sigmoid mesentery)
√ deviation of uterus toward side of torsion (36%)
√ engorgement of blood vessels on side of torsion
√ small amount of clear (64%) / hemorrhagic (8%) ascites
US:
√ markedly enlarged hypo- / hyperechoic midline mass
√ multiple peripheral cysts (= transudation of fluid into follicles) measuring 8–12 mm in diameter (64–74%)
√ good sound transmission (vascular engorgement + stromal edema)
√ free fluid in cul-de-sac (32%)
√ absence of arterial Doppler waveforms (not always reliable due to dual blood supply by ovarian + uterine artery
√ "whirlpool sign" = twisted ovarian pedicle
√ ± complex mass (if secondary to cyst / tumor)
CT:
√ amorphous / tubular masslike structure (84%) between adnexal mass + uterus due to tube thickening >10 mm
N.B.: the diameter of the normal tube measures up to 4 mm at isthmic, 8 mm at ampullary, 10 mm at infundibular portion

√ whorled structure abutting ovarian mass (= twisted vascular pedicle)
√ cystic ovarian mass with smooth wall thickening (76%):
  √ >10 mm thickness suggests hemorrhagic infarction
√ obliteration of fat planes around torsed ovary
√ attenuation >50 HU means hemorrhagic infarction on NECT
√ lack of enhancement of solid component

MR:
√ thickened cyst wall / mural nodule
√ high signal intensity on fat-suppressed T1WI (= hemorrhage / vascular congestion)
√ no enhancement of solid component on contrast-enhanced dynamic subtraction MR
√ tube thickening (SAG image improves detection)

Prognosis:
(1) Spontaneous detorsion is common (history of prior similar episodes = intermittent torsion)
(2) Infection of torsed ovary with local peritonitis ± bowel obstruction

Rx: immediate surgery (most ovaries not salvageable)

TRIPLOIDY

= 69 chromosomes

Incidence: 1% of conceptions; 0.04% of 20-week fetuses

NO obvious pattern!

√ early severe asymmetric IUGR (MOST PROMINENT FEATURE); cephalocorporal disproportion
√ oligohydramnios
√ large hydropic placenta with scattered vesicular spaces (partial hydatidiform mole)
√ congenital heart disease: ASD, VSD
√ brain anomalies: hydrocephalus, holoprosencephaly, neural tube defect
√ cleft lip / palate
√ syndactyly of fingers
√ omphalocele
√ renal abnormalities

Prognosis: most ending in spontaneous abortion

TRISOMY 13

= PATAU SYNDROME

Incidence: 1:5,000 births

@ OB: severe IUGR, hydramnios
@ CNS: alobar holoprosencephaly, posterior encephalocele, neural tube defect
@ Face: midline labial cleft, proboscis, hypotelorism, cyclopia, anophthalmia
@ Skeleton: postaxial polydactyly, rocker-bottom foot
@ Heart: (CHD in 90%) VSD, echogenic chordae tendineae, hypoplastic ventricle, tetralogy of Fallot, transposition
@ Kidney: polycystic kidney, horseshoe kidney
@ GI: omphalocele (occasionally)

Prognosis: few infants live more than a few days / hours

DDx: Meckel-Gruber syndrome

TRISOMY 18

= EDWARD SYNDROME

Incidence: 3:10,000 births

• triple-marker screening test:
  • decreased maternal alpha-fetoprotein
  • decreased hCG (DDx: increased in Down syndrome)
  • decreased estriol

@ OB: severe symmetric IUGR (28% <24 weeks MA), single umbilical artery (30%), polyhydramnios (occasionally)
@ Face: micrognathia, hypotelorism, facial cleft (10–40%)
@ Head: strawberry-shaped head (50%), cystic hygroma
@ CNS: holoprosencephaly, choroid plexus cyst (30–75%), small cerebellum with prominent cisterna magna, myelomeningocele
@ Hand: clenched hand with overlapping of index finger (>60%, HIGHLY CHARACTERISTIC)
@ Arm: shortened radial ray, clubbed forearm
@ Foot: clubbed foot, rocker-bottom foot
@ Heart: (CHD in 90%) VSD, complete AV canal, DORV
@ GI: diaphragmatic hernia, omphalocele (30–40%), TE fistula
@ Kidney: polycystic kidney, horseshoe kidney, UPJ obstruction

Prognosis: usually delivered by emergency cesarean section due to IUGR + fetal distress, if not detected prenatally

TWIN EMBOLIZATION SYNDROME

= rare complication of monochorionic pregnancy following the death of one twin whose blood pressure falls to zero

Pathophysiology:
1. Acute reversal of transfusion to co-twin at time of intrauterine demise of one twin with ischemic changes in survivor
2. Embolization of thromboplastin-enriched blood / detritus from the dead to the living twin through vascular anastomoses in placenta

Embolized organs: CNS (72%), GI tract (19%), kidneys (15%), lungs

√ ventriculomegaly, cortical atrophy, porencephalic cyst, cystic encephalomalacia within 2 weeks of death of co-twin

TWIN-TWIN TRANSFUSION SYNDROME

= FETO-FETAL TRANSFUSION SYNDROME
= MONOVULAR TWIN TRANSFUSION = INTRAUTERINE PARABIOTIC SYNDROME

= complication of monozygotic twinning with one placenta or one fused placenta of mono- / dizygotic twins

Incidence: 5–18% of twin pregnancies; 5–15% of monozygotic multiple pregnancies; 15–30% of monochorionic twin gestations

Cause: unbalanced intrauterine shunting of blood through shared placental vessels

Time of onset: 2nd trimester with discordant amniotic fluid volumes

Path: large communication between arterial circulation of one twin and venous circulation of the other twin through *arteriovenous* shunt (= common villous district) deep within placenta

√ discrepant amniotic fluid volume (75%)

√ discordant BPD by >5 mm (57%)
√ discordant estimated fetal weight >25% (67–100%)

A. DONOR TWIN
   = twin that transfuses the recipient twin + remains itself underperfused
   • anemia + hypovolemia
   • high output cardiac failure + hydrops (rare)
   √ oligohydramnios (75–80%) / "stuck twin" = severe oligohydramnios (60%) from oliguria
   √ intrauterine growth restriction (common) diagnosed by discordant EFW of >25%
   √ morphologically normal

B. RECIPIENT TWIN
   • polycythemia (higher hemoglobin)
   • plethora = hypervolemia (volume overload)
   √ polyhydramnios (70–75%) from increased fetal urination
   √ fetal hydrops (10–25%): pericardial + pleural effusions, ascites, skin thickening
   √ organomegaly
   √ fetus papyraceus = macerated dead fetus
   √ velamentous cord insertion (64%)

Prognosis: 80–100% perinatal mortality if presenting <28 weeks MA and left untreated
Cx: amniorrhexis, preterm labor
Rx: elective termination, volume-reduction amniocentesis of polyhydramniotic sac (decreasing mortality rates to 34%), selective feticide, laser ablation of vascular anastomoses
DDx: IUGR of one dizygotic twin (two separate placentas, two different sexes)

UTERINE ANOMALIES

= anomalies of fusion of paramesonephric duct (= müllerian duct) completed by 18th week of fetal life

Incidence: 0.1–3%

◊ Uterine anomalies are found in 9% of women with infertility / repeated spontaneous abortions!
◊ 25% of women with uterine abnormalities have fertility problems!

Associated with: urinary tract anomalies in 20–50%; possibly increased familial occurrence of limb reduction

Embryology:
(a) müllerian ducts develop at 5–6 weeks GA from coelomic epithelium and form uterovaginal canal by **lateral fusion** at 7–9 weeks GA
(b) by 8 weeks the uterovaginal canal reaches the urogenital sinus at the müllerian tubercle while a vaginal plate develops distally resulting in **vertical fusion** (upper 2/3 to 4/5 of vagina are of müllerian duct origin, lower 1/3 or 1/5 of vagina originate from urogenital sinus)

Classification:
[classes in parenthesis refer to the classification of the American Fertility Society]

A. ARRESTED MÜLLERIAN DUCT DEVELOPMENT
   1. bilateral: **Uterine agenesis / hypoplasia** (class I)
      Incidence: 1:5,000
      Often associated with: vaginal agenesis / hypoplasia
      Age of detection: menarche
      √ small uterus with small endometrial canal
      √ poor zonal differentiation + abnormal T2-hypointense myometrium
   2. unilateral: **Unicornuate uterus** = Uterus unicornis unicollis (class II)
      (a) with contralateral rudimentary horn
      (b) without rudimentary horn
      Incidence: 3–6–13% of uterine anomalies
      May be associated with: ipsilateral renal agenesis
      • infertility in 5–20%
      • ? pregnancy wastage
      √ reduced uterine volume
      √ asymmetric ellipsoidal uterine configuration
      √ rudimentary horn may contain endometrium + may communicate with main uterine cavity
      √ solitary fusiform "banana-shaped" uterine cavity with lateral deviation within pelvis terminating in a single fallopian tube on HSG
      Cx: cryptomenorrhea within endometrium-containing rudimentary horn that does not communicate with endometrium cavity

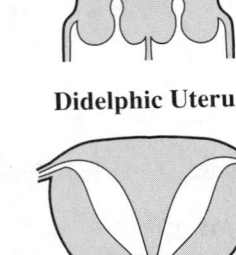

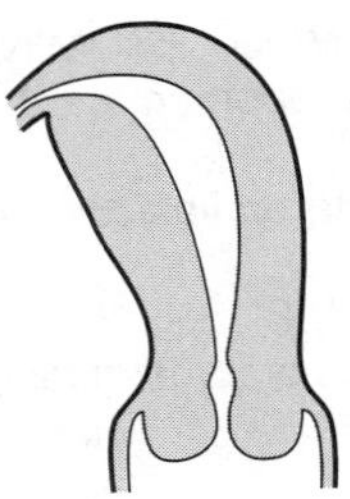
Unicornuate Uterus

Didelphic Uterus

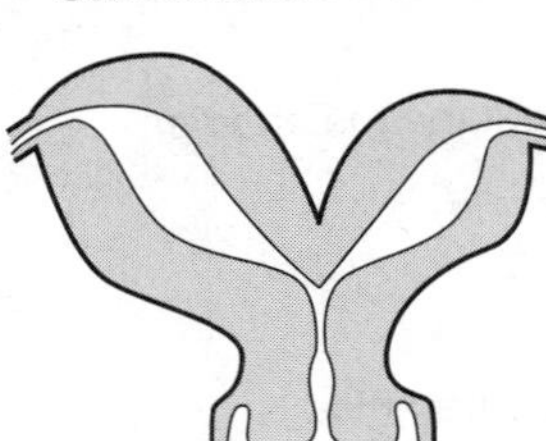
Bicornuate Uterus

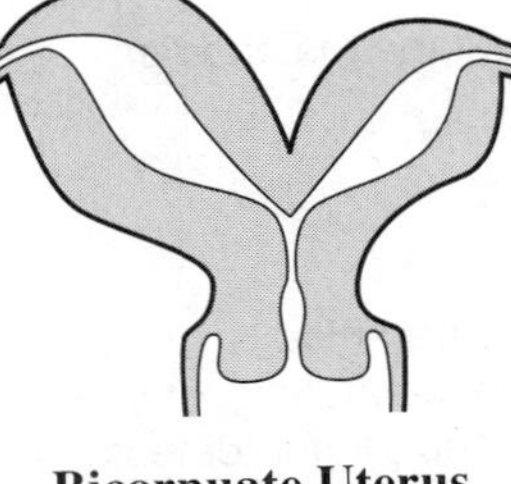
Septate Uterus (complete)

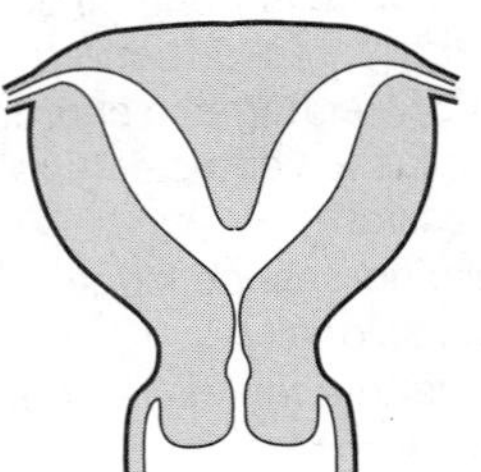
Septate Uterus (partial)

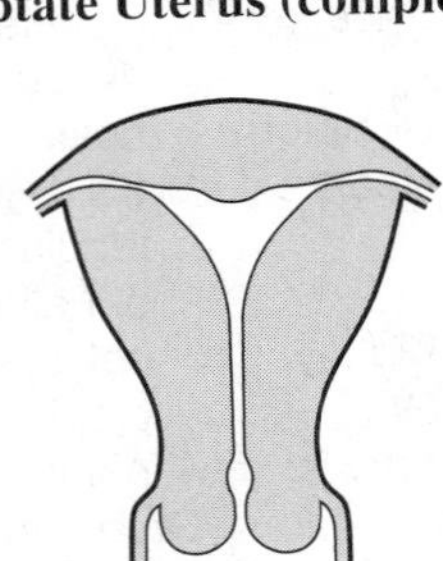
Arcuate Uterus

Uterine Anomalies

3. **Mayer-Rokitanski-Küster-Hauser syndrome**
   (1) vaginal agenesis / hypoplasia of proximal + middle segments
   (2) intact normal ovaries + fallopian tubes
   (3) variable anomalies of uterus (agenesis / hypoplasia, uni- or bicornuate), urinary tract (renal agenesis, pelvic kidney in 40–50%), skeletal system (12%)

   Frequency: 1:4,000–1:5,000
   Cause: lack of müllerian development
   • normal external genitalia
   • shallow distal vaginal pouch (derived from urogenital sinus)
   • amenorrhea
   • cyclic pelvic pain (secondary to functioning endometrium within rudimentary uterine tissue) in 6–10%
   ◊ 2nd most common cause of primary infertility
   Rx: neovaginoplasty

B. TOTAL / PARTIAL FAILURE OF MÜLLERIAN DUCT FUSION = duplication defects = disorders of lateral fusion (75% of uterine anomalies)

1. **Uterus didelphys** (class III)
   = complete duplication with 2 vaginas + 2 cervices + 2 uterine horns
   May be associated with: renal agenesis
   • usually asymptomatic
   √ two widely spaced uterine corpora, each with a single fallopian tube
   √ separate divergent uterine horns
   √ large fundal cleft
   √ cervical duplication
   √ horizontal septum of upper vagina (ipsilateral to renal agenesis)
   √ opacification of single deviated horn on HSG
   Cx: unilateral hydro- / hematocolpos (if transverse vaginal septum present) with reflux endometriosis
   Rx: surgery is rarely performed
2. **Bicornuate uterus** = uterus bicornis (class IV)
   = lack of fusion of corpus
   (a) bicornis bicollis = complete with division down to internal os
   (b) bicornis unicollis = partial
   √ concave / heart-shaped external fundal contour due to a large fundal cleft >1–2 cm deep
   √ separation of uterine horns
   √ intercornual angle of >75–105° (demonstrated on luteal-phase US in conjunction with HSG)
   √ intercornual distance (= distance between maximum lateral extent of hyperintense endometrium on transaxial image) >4 cm
   √ divider between cornua comprised of myometrium / fibrous tissue / both
   √ fusiform shape of each uterine horn with lateral convex margins
   √ discrepancy in size of the 2 uterine horns
   √ elongation + widening of cervical canal + isthmus

   Laparoscopy: typical external fundal indentation
   Cx: repeated spontaneous abortions (frequently in 2nd–3rd trimester), premature rupture of membranes, premature labor, SGA infant, persistent malpresentations (transverse lie)
   Rx: transabdominal surgery to fuse uterine horns (abdominal metroplasty)

C. NONRESORPTION OF SAGITTAL UTERINE SEPTUM

1. **Septate uterus** (class V)
   Most common anomaly (almost 50%) associated with reproductive failure in 67%
   Path: septum may be composed of fibrous tissue (low-signal intensity), myometrium (intermediate-signal intensity), or both
   √ convex / flat / minimally indented (≤1 cm) external fundal contour
   √ distal portion of septum hypoechoic to myometrium (= fibrous tissue)
   √ acute angle of <75° between uterine cavities
   √ duplication of uterine horns on HSG (DDx to bicornuate uterus unreliable)
   √ endometrial canals completely separated by tissue isoechoic to myometrium extending into endocervical canal
   Types:
   (a) Uterus septus
   = complete septum extending to internal os
   (b) Uterus subseptus
   = partial septum involving endometrial canal
   Cx: 90% abortion rate (poor septal vascularity)
   Rx: hysteroscopic metroplasty (= excision of septum)
2. **Uterus arcuatus** (class VI)
   Most common anomaly unassociated with reproductive failure
   √ NO division of uterine horns
   √ normal fundal contour
   √ smooth indentation of fundal endometrial canal
   √ increased transverse diameter of uterine cavity
   √ single uterine canal with saddle-shaped fundus on HSG

D. INADEQUATE HORMONAL STIMULATION DURING FETAL DEVELOPMENT
= DES (= diethylstilbestrol)-related abnormalities (class VII)
• synthetic hormone used in 1950s + 1960s to prevent miscarriage
• may cause abnormal uterine morphology (with decreased fertility)
• increased risk of vaginal malignancy

1. **Uterine hypoplasia**
   associated with DES exposure in utero
   √ mean uterine volume = 50 cm^3

2. **T-shaped uterus**
   encountered in 15% of women exposed to DES in utero
   √ low uterine volume
   √ uterine fundus thinner than cervix
   √ greater width than depth of corpus + fundus over cervix
   √ T-shaped lumen on hysterosalpingogram

UTERINE LEIOMYOMA

= FIBROID = MYOMA
= benign overgrowth of smooth muscle + connective tissue
◊ Most common gynecologic neoplasm! Commonest cause for uterine enlargement after pregnancy!

Incidence: in 20–25% of White women; in 50% of Black women; Black:White women = 3:1–9:1; 0.3–2.6% during pregnancy; account for 30% of all hysterectomies in USA

Path: whorl-like trabeculated tumor surrounded by pseudocapsule; may outgrow its blood supply resulting in:
(a) hyaline degeneration (>60%) = homogeneous eosinophilic bands / plaques of proteinaceous material in extracellular space
(b) myxoid degeneration = gelatinous intratumoral foci of hyaluronic acid-rich mucopolysaccharides
(c) cystic degeneration (4%) = extreme sequelae of edema
(d) red / hemorrhagic / carneous degeneration = massive hemorrhagic infarction due to venous thrombosis / rupture of intratumoral arteries; often during pregnancy / during use of oral contraceptives
(e) calcification (4%) = dense amorphous calcifications within hyalinized tissue

Specific types:
(1) **Lipoleiomyoma** (0.8%) = substantial amount of fat due to fatty metamorphosis
(2) **Myxoid leiomyoma** = rare soft translucent mass due to abundant myxoid material between smooth muscle cells, may be clinically malignant
(3) **Intravenous leiomyomatosis** = wormlike masses growing within pelvic veins
(4) Benign metastasizing leiomyoma
(5) **Diffuse leiomyomatosis** = development of innumerable small leiomyomas
   √ symmetric enlargement of uterus
(6) **Peritoneal disseminated leiomyomatosis**
   • frequently associated with pregnancy
   √ multiple nodules on peritoneal surface

Histo: monoclonal proliferation of smooth muscle cells (NOT myometrial hyperplasia) separated by variable amounts of fibrous connective tissue

Hormonal dependency:
◊ Uterine smooth muscle cells have an abundance of estrogen receptors!
(1) Growth during pregnancy in 15–32% by a mean volume of 12 ± 6% within the 1st trimester (NOT during remainder of pregnancy)
   ◊ The larger the myoma, the greater the likelihood of growth!
(2) Shrinkage in puerperium + after menopause

Age: usually >30 years
• asymptomatic in 70–75%
• palpable abdominopelvic mass
• pelvic pressure:
  • urinary frequency (due to compression of bladder)
  • constipation (due to impingement on rectosigmoid)
• pain (30%) due to acute hemorrhagic infarction + necrosis, torsion of pedunculated subserosal fibroid, prolapse of pedunculated submucosal fibroid
• dysmenorrhea (= colicky pelvic pain with menstruation)
• abnormal uterine bleeding:
  • menorrhagia (= heavy + prolonged menstrual flow)
  • metrorrhagia (= uterine bleeding outside time of menstruation)
• infertility (infrequent)

Location: mostly in fundus + corpus; 3–8% in cervix

Classification by location:
1. **Intramural fibroid** (within confines of uterine outline) in 95%
   • asymptomatic (mostly)
   • occasionally menorrhagia (due to interference with normal uterine contractility)
   • occasionally infertility (due to compression of interstitial portion of fallopian tube / distortion of endometrial cavity)
2. **Subserosal / exophytic fibroid**
   • usually asymptomatic
   • pain from infarction due to torsion
   (a) **intraligamentous fibroid** (lateral growth between folds of broad ligament)
      • simulates ovarian mass
      • occasionally infertility (due to compression of isthmic / ampullary portion of fallopian tube)
      Cx: hydroureteronephrosis (due to compression of ureter)
   (b) **parasitic fibroid** = subserosal fibroid, which has become detached secondary to circulatory occlusion of vessels in pedicle; revitalized through omental / mesenteric blood supply
3. **Submucosal fibroid** (5%) = projecting into endometrial canal
   • dysmenorrhea, menorrhagia, infertility
   • increased prevalence of early abortion
     ◊ Most frequently symptomatic type of fibroid!
   (a) fibroid polyp (2.5%) = partial / complete extrusion of pedunculated submucosal fibroid into cervical canal / vagina

√ uterine enlargement
√ lobulated / nodular distortion of uterine outline (subserosal leiomyoma) + indentation of urinary bladder
√ distortion / obliteration of the contour of the uterine cavity (submucosal leiomyoma)

√ intramural soft-tissue mass (most frequent), usually multiple, solitary in 2%
√ speckled / ringlike / popcorn calcification

US (60% sensitivity, 99% specificity, 87% accuracy):
√ hypoechoic solid concentric mass (<33%) (= muscle component prevails)
√ echogenic attenuating mass (= dense fibrosis prevails)
√ sharp discrete refractory shadows (from borders between fibrous tissue and smooth muscle, margins of leiomyoma with normal myometrium, edges of whorls, bundles of smooth muscle)
√ anechoic features (secondary to internal degeneration: atrophic, hyaline, cystic, myxomatous, lipomatous, calcareous, carneous, necrobiotic, hemorrhagic, proteolytic degeneration)
√ acoustic shadowing (= calcifications)
◊ Presence of a prominent artery by color Doppler suggests potential for growth during pregnancy

CT:
√ hypo- / iso- / hyperdense mass containing mixed hyperechoic areas

MR (86–92% sensitive, 100% specific, 97% accurate; most accurate + desirable for planning myomectomy):
N.B.: subserosal, intramural and submucosal classification enabled by uterine zonal anatomy
@ Nondegenerated leiomyoma
√ well-circumscribed mass of homogeneously low signal intensity on T2WI compared with myometrium (for leiomyoma with variable amounts of collagen)
√ slightly higher signal intensity + contrast enhancement on T2WI (for cellular leiomyoma with little / no collagen)
@ Degenerated leiomyoma
√ low signal intensity on T2WI (for hyaline / calcific degeneration)
√ high signal intensity on T2WI (for cystic degeneration) without enhancement of cystic areas
√ very high signal intensity on T2WI (for myxoid degeneration) with minimal enhancement
√ variable signal intensity on T1WI + low signal intensity on T2WI (for hyaline / coagulative necrosis)
√ peripheral / diffuse high signal intensity on T1WI (due to proteinaceous content of blood) + variable signal intensity on T2WI (for red degeneration)
√ hyperintense rim on T2WI in 33% (= pseudocapsule of dilated lymphatics / veins / edema)
√ enhancement pattern (usually later than myometrium): 65% hypointense, 23% isointense, 12% hyperintense to myometrium

Hysterosalpingography (9% sensitive, 97% specific, 76% accurate)

Cx:
(1) Infertility in 35%
(a) narrowing of isthmic portion of tube
(b) impingement on endometrium interfering with implantation; infertility rates highest for submucosal leiomyomas
(2) Complications in pregnancy
◊ Significantly increased for myomas >6 cm in size / multiple in number / myomas >200 cm³ and when fibroid is retroplacental
(a) increased frequency of spontaneous abortions
(b) increased frequency of ectopic pregnancies
(c) increased frequency of IUGR
(d) preterm labor in 7% + premature rupture of membranes
(e) placental abruption
(f) uterine dyskinesia, uterine inertia during labor
(g) dystocia, obstruction of birth canal during vaginal delivery (if near internal os)
(h) abnormal presentation
(i) postpartum hemorrhage
(j) retained products of conception
(3) Hydroureteronephrosis
(4) Malignant transformation (in 0.2%)

Rx: (1) Hysterectomy for pain, menorrhagia, visceral compression (after childbearing completed)
(2) Myomectomy for 2nd trimester fetal loss / anemia due to hypermenorrhea / pelvic pain
◊ Submucosal leiomyomas may be treated with hysteroscopic myomectomy
(3) Uterine artery embolization for symptomatic fibroids

DDx of necrotic leiomyoma:
(1) Ovarian mass (ovarian cyst, hemorrhagic cyst, endometrioma, cystic dermoid, cystadenoma, malignancy)
(2) Ectopic interstitial pregnancy
(3) Intrauterine gestational sac
(4) Intrauterine fluid collection
(5) Hydatidiform mole
(6) Myometrial contraction (lasts for 15–30 minutes)
(7) Cervical tumor
(8) Hematoma of broad ligament

DDx of pedunculated subserosal leiomyoma:
(1) Ovary: use transvaginal US / MR to identify follicles!

DDx of leiomyoma by MR:
(1) Adenomyosis
(2) Solid adnexal mass (Brenner tumor, fibroma)
(3) Focal myometrial contraction (transient)
(4) Uterine leiomyosarcoma

Benign Metastasizing Leiomyoma

= smooth muscle tumors in lung, lymph nodes, abdomen

Incidence: <60 cases

Classification:
(1) Benign metastasizing leiomyoma
Origin: uterus in mature women; progression with estrogen + regression with progesterone
• benign uterine leiomyoma removed many years earlier
Rx: hysterectomy, bilateral oophorectomy, long-term hormone therapy; good prognosis

(2) Metastatic leiomyoma
Origin: extrauterine primary in men + children (? slow-growing sarcoma)
Rx: surgical resection with mixed success
(3) Multiple fibroleiomyomatous hamartoma
Origin: lung; totally benign behavior

Spread: lymph nodes outside the pelvis, peritoneal surface, venous channels, lung, heart

- asymptomatic in most cases
- fever, mild nonproductive cough

Histo: well-differentiated benign-appearing smooth muscle cells

√ multiple pulmonary nodules
√ miliary pattern
√ pedunculated pulmonary leiomyoma with cyst formation
√ giant cyst

UTERINE LEIOMYOSARCOMA

Cause: (a) de novo growth independent of leiomyoma!
(b) sarcomatous transformation of preexisting leiomyoma (rare)

Histo: infiltrative margins, nuclear atypia, increased mitotic figures

- rapidly enlarging uterus (<3%)

√ mass with irregular margin

Dx: often first established by pathologist

UTERINE RUPTURE IN PREGNANCY

= disruption of all layers surrounding the fetus (membranes, decidua, myometrium, serosa)

Prevalence: 3–5% for classic cesarean sections; 1–2% for lower segment operations

Classification:
1. Spontaneous rupture during labor
2. Traumatic rupture during delivery
3. Rupture due to myometrial scars / disease

Predisposed:
previous uterine surgery, previously excessively long / difficult labor

Location: (a) corpus with rupture before onset of labor
(b) lower uterine segment during labor, L > R

Cx: hypofibrinogenemia (triggered by excessive blood loss, trauma, amniotic fluid embolism)

Mortality: 2–20% maternal mortality; 10–25% fetal mortality

DDx: Uterine dehiscence = rupture of only myometrium

UTERINE TRAUMA DURING PREGNANCY

Incidence: 6–7%

Cause: motor vehicle accident (70%), physical abuse (10%)

1. Placental abruption: complete (6–66%) / incomplete (30–80%)
2. Uterine rupture (0.6%)
3. Fetal injury (eg, cerebral injury)
4. Fetal death

◊ The major cause for fetal death is maternal death

US: evaluate fetal motion, breathing, heart rate, placenta

VAGINAL AGENESIS

2nd most common cause of primary amenorrhea

Incidence: 1:4,000–5,000 women

- cyclic abdominal pain

May be associated with:
(1) Uterine + partial tubal agenesis (90%)
(2) Unilateral renal agenesis / ectopia (34%)
(3) Skeletal malformations (12%)
(4) McKusick-Kaufman syndrome (hydrometrocolpos + polydactyly + heart defects)
(5) Ellis-van Creveld syndrome

VASA PREVIA

= rare type of velamentous cord insertion in which umbilical vessels cross the internal os
(a) vessels connecting separate succenturiate lobe to main portion of placenta
(b) cord vessels of velamentous (membranous) cord insertion from low-lying placenta
(c) aberrant chorionic vessels in association with marginal cord insertion from low lying placenta

Cx: (1) Bleeding from torn fetal vessels
(2) Cord compression by presenting part during labor
(3) Cord prolapse

Risk: 50–100% fetal mortality

VELAMENTOUS CORD INSERTION

= umbilical cord insertion into membranes before entering placenta = attachment of cord to chorion laeve

Incidence: 0.09–1.8%

Associated with:
(a) multiple gestation, uterine anomaly, IUD
(b) congenital anomalies (in 5.9–8.5%): asymmetric head shape, spina bifida, esophageal atresia, obstructive uropathy, VSD, cleft palate

Cx: (1) IUGR
(2) Preterm labor

Risk: (1) Cord compression
(2) Rupture of cord with traction during delivery

NUCLEAR MEDICINE

TABLE OF DOSE, ENERGY, HALF-LIFE, RADIATION DOSE

Organ	Pharmaceutical	Dose	keV	$T_{1/2}$ phys	$T_{1/2}$ bio
Brain	Tc-99m pertechnetate	10–30 mCi	140	6 h	
	Tc-99m DTPA	10 mCi	140	6 h	
	Tc-99m glucoheptonate	10 mCi	140	6 h	
	Tc-99m Ceretec	20 mCi	140	6 h	
	I-123 Spectamine	3–6 mCi	159	13.6 h	
CSF	In-111 DTPA	500 μCi	173, 247	2.8 d	
	Tc-99m DTPA	1 mCi	140	6 h	
Cardiac	Tl-201	1–2 mCi	**72**, 135, 167	73 h	
	Tc-99m pyrophosphate	15 mCi	140	6 h	
	Tc-99m pertechnetate	15–25 mCi	140	6 h	
	Tc-99m–labeled RBCs	10–20 mCi	140	6 h	
	Tc-99m sestamibi	25 mCi	140	6 h	
	Tc-99m teboroxime	30 mCi	140	6 h	
Liver	Tc-99m sulfur colloid	3–5 mCi	140	6 h	
	Tc-99m DISIDA	4–5 mCi	140	6 h	
Lung	Xe-127	5–10 mCi	172, 203, 375	36.4 d	13 s
	Xe-133	10–20 mCi	81, 161	5.3 d	20 s
	Kr-81m	20 mCi	176, 188, 190	13 s	
	Tc-99m MAA aerosol	3 mCi	140	6 h	8 h
Kidney	Tc-99m DTPA	15–20 mCi	140	6 h	
	Tc-99m DMSA	2–5 mCi	140	6 h	
	Tc-99m glucoheptonate	15–20 mCi	140	6 h	
	Tc-99m mercaptoacetyltriglycine	10 mCi	140	6 h	
	I-131 Hippuran	250 μCi	365*	8 d	18 min
	I-123 Hippuran	1 mCi	159	13.2 h	
Thyroid	Tc-99m pertechnetate	5–10 mCi	140	6 h	
	I-123	50–200 μCi	159	13.2 h	
	I-125	30–100 μCi	27, 35	60 d	
	I-131	30–100 μCi	365*	8 d	
Testes	Tc-99m pertechnetate	10 mCi	140	6 h	
Gastric mucosa	Tc-99m pertechnetate	50 μCi / kg	140	6 h	
Gallium	Ga-67 citrate	3–5 mCi	93, 184, 296, 388	3.3 d	
WBC	In-111 oxine	550 μCi	173, 247	2.8 d	
	Tc-99m Ceretec	10–20 mCi	140	6 h	

mnemonic: * = as many days as in a year

RADIATION DOSE

	Critical Organ	*rad/mCi*
I-131	Thyroid	1,000
I-125	Thyroid	900
In-111 oxine WBC	Spleen	26
I-123	Thyroid	15
In-111 DTPA	Spinal cord	12
Tl-201	Kidney	1.5
Ga-67 citrate	Colon	1.0
Tc-99m MAA	Lung	0.4
Tc-99m albumin microspheres	Lung	0.4
Tc-99m DISIDA	Large bowel	0.39
Tc-99m sulfur colloid	Liver	0.33
Tc-99m pertechnetate	Intestine	0.3
	Thyroid	0.15
Tc-99m glucoheptonate	Kidney	0.2
Tc-99m pertechnetate (+ perchlorate)	Colon	0.2
Tc-99m pyrophosphate	Bladder	0.13
Tc-99m phosphate	Bladder	0.13
Tc-99m DTPA	Bladder	0.12
Tc-99m–tagged RBCs	Spleen	0.11
Tc-99m albumin	Blood	0.015
Xe-133	Trachea	

PEDIATRIC DOSE

Actual doses for pediatric patients may vary in different institutions based on empirical data. As rough guidelines use:

1. Clark's rule (body weight): $Dose_{Ped}$ = Body weight [in lbs] / 150 x $Dose_{Adult}$
2. Young's rule (child up to age 12): $Dose_{Ped}$ = Age of child / (Age of child + 12) x $Dose_{Adult}$
3. Surface area: $Dose_{Ped}$ = (weight [in kg]$^{0.7}$ / 11) / 1.73 x $Dose_{Adult}$

Lactating Patients

1. Nursing mothers must be counseled about the need to interrupt / discontinue breast feeding
2. Pumped milk may be refrigerated and used after the radioactivity has decayed

<u>Complete cessation of breast feeding</u>:

Ga-67 citrate
I-131 sodium iodide therapy

<u>Interruption of breast feeding for 12 hours</u>:

Tc-99m macroaggregated albumin
Tc-99m–labeled RBCs (in vivo labeling)
In-111–labeled WBCs

<u>Interruption of breast feeding for 24 hours</u>:

Tc-99m pertechnetate
I-123 metaiodobenzylguanidine
Tc-99m–labeled WBCs

<u>Interruption of breast feeding for 168 hours</u>:

Tl-210 chloride

QUALITY CONTROL

◊ Quality control logs should be kept for 3 years!

RADIOPHARMACEUTICALS

Production of Radionuclides

Reactor-produced Radionuclides

◊ Not carrier free = contamination with other forms
» Thermal neutrons captured by stable nuclides
» Used to produce standard generators

(1) Mo-99/Tc-99m generator

(parent)		(daughter)				
^{99}Mo	→	^{99m}Tc	→	^{99}Tc	→	^{99}Ru
67 hours		6 hours		2.1×10^5 years		stable

glass column filled with aluminum (Al_2O_3); parent and daughter isotopes are firmly absorbed onto aluminum at top of column; daughter isotope can be separated / eluted by passing isotonic oxidant-free NaCl through the column

(2) Kr-81m generator

(parent)		(daughter)		
^{81}Rb	→	^{81m}Kr	→	^{81}Kr
4.7 hours		13 seconds		stable

Accelerator / Cyclotron-produced Radionuclides

◊ Generally carrier-free product
- collision of charged particles (protons, deuterons, helium, alpha particles) with target nuclide
- used to produce Ga-67, I-123, Tl-201

Fission-produced Radionuclides

◊ Carrier-free product
- splitting of a heavy nucleus into smaller nuclei
- used to produce I-131, Mo-99

Radionuclide Impurity

= amount (µCi) of radiocontaminant per amount (µCi/mCi) of desired radionuclide

Mo-99 Breakthrough Test:

Test frequency: with every elution

(a) NRC allowable contamination of 1:1,000 = 1 µCi Mo-99 per 1 mCi of Tc-99m
(b) USP limit of 0.15 µCi Mo-99 per 1 mCi Tc-99m
(c) <5 µCi Mo-99 per administered dose (NRC dropped this requirement, but nonagreement states may still require this)
(d) chemical evaluation: Mo-99 contaminated eluate forms colored complexes with phenylhydrazine (for reactor product generators)

- measured in dose calibrator with lead shielding of vial (filters 140 keV but permits 740 and 780 keV of Mo-99 to pass through

Effect of impurity:
increased radiation dose, poor image quality

Radiochemical Impurity

Test frequency: with every elution

Precise registration of different compounds of Tc-99m, eg,

— hydrolyzed reduced technetium (HR Tc) a radiocolloid $[TcO(OH)_2 \cdot H_2O]$
Limit: <2% (presently no legal limit)
— free pertechnetate $[TcO^4]^{-1}$

- can be monitored by paper chromatography

Effect of impurity with hydrolyzed reduced Tc:
RES uptake, poor image quality, increased radiation dose

Chemical Impurity

Chemicals from elution process are restricted in their amount (NRC limit):

Tc-99m: <10 µg Al^{3+} per 1 mL eluate if radionuclide from fission generator;
<20 µg Al^{3+} per 1 mL eluate if radionuclide from thermal activation generator

Aluminum Ion Breakthrough Test:

Test frequency: with every elution

- one drop of generator eluate placed on one end of special test paper containing aluminum reagent
- equal-sized drop of a standard solution of Al^{3+} (10 ppm) is placed on other end of strip
- if color at center of drop eluate is lighter than that of standard solution, the eluate has passed the colorimetric test

Effect of impurity: degradation of image quality

Radiopharmaceutical Sterility and Pyrogenicity

USP XX Test

Monitor rectal temperature of 3 suitable rabbits after injection of material through ear vein

Acceptable results: no rabbit shows a rise of >0.6°C; total rise for all three rabbits <1.4°C

Limulus Amoebocyte Lysate Test (LAL)

Highly specific for Gram-negative bacterial endotoxins, sensitivity 10 x greater than USP XX test

Quality Control for Dose Calibrators

Test	*When*	*Limit*	*Test Isotopes*
Constancy	daily,*	<±5%	Cs-137
Channel check	daily,*	<±5%	Cs-137
Linearity	quarterly,*	<±5%	Tc-99m
Accuracy	annually,*	<±5%	Cs-137, Co-57, Ba-133
Geometry	*	<±1.6%	Tc-99m

* = after install / repair

Amoebocyte = primitive blood cell of horseshoe crab (Limulus polyphebus); lysate formed by hydrolysis of amoebocyte

Positive result: in the presence of minute amounts of endotoxin LAL forms an opaque gel; response to other pyrogens (particulate contaminations, chemicals) doubtful

CALIBRATORS

Dose Calibrator

= gas ionization chamber that transforms photon flux into current with digital readout

Disadvantages:

(1) open top geometry
(2) nonlinearity between photon energy and measured current (corrected with a calibration factor)

Constancy = Precision

= reproducibility over time

Test frequency: daily

Method: measurement of a long-lived source, usually a Cs-137 standard

Evaluation: measurement must fall within ± 5% of the calculated activity

Linearity

= accurate measurement over large range of activity levels

Test frequency: 4 x per year

Method: 1 mCi source activity is measured every 4 hours for 10 / more measurements (down to 10–100 μCi)

Evaluation: measurements must fall within ± 5% of the calculated physical decay curve

Accuracy

Test frequency: annually

Method: measurements of three different activity standards whose amount is certified by the National Bureau of Standards (NBS); standard values are decayed mathematically to calibrator date

Tc-99m: 140 keV, half-life of 6.01 hours
Co-57: 123 keV, half-life of 270 days
Ba-133: 356 keV, half-life of 10.5 years
Cs-137: 662 keV, half-life of 30.1 years

Evaluation: measurements must fall within expected range

Geometry

= to ensure that measurement is not dependent upon location of tracer within ionization chamber, usually done by manufacturer

Test frequency: at installation / after factory repair / recalibration

Method: 0.5 mL of Tc-99m (activity 25 mCi) is measured in a 3-mL syringe; syringe contents are then diluted with water to 1.0 mL, 1.5 mL, and 2.0 mL and each level remeasured; test is repeated with a 10-mL glass vial

SCINTILLATION CAMERA

Peaking

= ensures that window of pulse height selector is correctly set to desired photopeak

(a) for Tc-99m source: between 137 and 143 keV
(b) for Co-57 source: between 117 and 123 keV

Frequency of quality control: daily

Field Uniformity

= ability of camera to reproduce a uniform radioactive distribution = variability of observed count density with a homogeneous flux

(a) Integral uniformity = maximum deviation
(b) Differential uniformity = maximum rate of change over a specified distance (5 pixels)

Causes for nonuniformity:

(1) High kilovoltage drift of photomultiplier (PM) tubes
(2) Physical damage to collimator
(3) Improper photopeak setting
(4) Contamination

Frequency of quality control: daily

A. INTRINSIC FIELD UNIFORMITY TEST (without collimator)

1. Remove collimator + replace with lead ring (to eliminate edge packing)
2. Place a point source at a distance of at least 5 crystal diameters from detector (4–5 feet for small, 7–9 feet for large crystals)
3. Point source contains 200–400 μCi of Tc-99m for minimal personnel exposure (avoid contamination of crystal)
4. Set count rate below limit of instrument (<30,000 counts)
5. Adjust the pulse height selector to normal window settings by centering at 140 keV with a window of 15% (for Tc-99m studies only)

Quality Control for Gamma Cameras

Test	*When*	*Test Result*
Peaking	daily	Tc-99m and Co-57
Energy resolution	daily	<14% at FWHM
Extrinsic field uniformity	daily	<5% RMS variation
Bar phantom	weekly	visual assessment
Field uniformity	monthly	visual assessment
Center of rotation	monthly	visual assessment
Jaczak phantom	quarterly	visual assessment

6. Use the same photographic device
7. Acquire 1.25 million counts for a 10" field of view, 2.5 million counts for a 15" field of view
8. Register counts, time, CRT intensity, analyzer settings, initials of controller

B. EXTRINSIC FIELD UNIFORMITY TEST (with collimator on)
1. Collimator is kept in place
   ◊ Only 1 of 2,000 gamma rays that reach the collimator are transmitted to the sodium iodide crystal!
2. Sheet source / flood of 2–10 mCi activity is placed on collimator
   (a) fillable floods: mix thoroughly, avoid air bubbles, check for flat surface
   (b) nonfillable: commercially available Co-57 source
3. Other steps as described above

Evaluation:
(1) Compare uncorrected with corrected images. Note acquisition time!
(2) Store correction flood
(3) Rerecord image with corrected flood + check for uniformity
(4) Variation in image should be <5% RMS

Spatial Resolution / Linearity

A. SPATIAL RESOLUTION
= parameter of scintillation camera that characterizes its ability to accurately determine the original location of a gamma ray on an X,Y plane; measured in both X and Y directions; expressed as full width at half maximum (FWHM) of the line spread function in mm
(a) intrinsic spatial resolution
(b) system spatial resolution

B. INTRINSIC SPATIAL LINEARITY
= parameter of a scintillation camera that characterizes the amount of positional distortion caused by the camera with respect to incident gamma events entering the detector
(a) differential linearity = standard deviation of line spread function peak separation (in mm)
(b) absolute linearity = maximum amount of spatial displacement (in mm)

Frequency of quality control: every week
1. Mask detector to collimated field of view (lead ring)
2. Lead phantom is attached to front of crystal
   (a) Four-quadrant bar pattern (3 pictures each after 90° rotation to test entire crystal)
   (b) Parallel-line equal-spacing (PLES) bar pattern [2 pictures]
      ◊ Change bar direction angles weekly
   (c) Smith orthogonal hole test pattern (OHP) [one picture only]
   (d) Hine-Duley phantom [2 pictures]
3. Set symmetric analyzer window to width normally used
4. Place a point source (1–3 mCi) at a fixed distance of at least 5 crystal diameters from detector on central axis (remove all sources from immediate area so that background count rate is low)
5. Acquire 1.25 million counts for a small field, 2.5 million counts for a large field on the same media used for clinical studies
6. Record counts, time, CRT intensity, analyzer setting, initials of controller

(All new cameras are equipped with a spatial distortion correction circuit)

Evaluation:
Visual assessment of
(1) Spatial resolution over entire field
(2) Linearity

Intrinsic Energy Resolution

= ability to distinguish between primary gamma events and scattered events; performed without collimator; expressed as ratio of photopeak FWHM to photopeak energy (in %)

Limit: 11% for SPECT, 14% for some planar cameras

Frequency of quality control: daily (may be weekly for some cameras)

CRT-output / Photographic Device

(1) Check for dirt, scratches, burnt spots on CRT face plates
(2) Adjust gray scale + contrast settings to suit film

SPECT QUALITY CONTROL

= SINGLE PHOTON EMISSION COMPUTED TOMOGRAPHY
= gamma cameras rotating about a pallet supporting the patient obtain 60–120 views over 180° / 360° rotation with typically a field of view of 40–50 cm across the patient and 30–40 cm in axial direction

Spatial resolution: ~8 mm for high-count study

SPECT Uniformity

1. 64 x 64 word matrix = 30 million count flood with collimator, orientation and magnification same as patient study
2. Co-57 sheet source with <1% uniformity variance is necessary
3. 128 x 128 word matrix = 120 million count flood with collimator, orientation, and magnification same as patient study

Frequency of quality control: weekly

Center of Rotation (COR)

1. Tc-99m–filled line source (5–8 mCi) positioned 3–5 cm off the center of rotation while keeping scanning palette out of field of view
2. Direction of rotation to be the same as patient study
3. Number of steps (32, 64, or 128) to be the same as in patient study

4. Time per step such that at least 100K counts are acquired
5. COR must be done with same collimator, orientation, and magnification as patient study

Frequency of quality control: weekly

Jaczak Phantom SPECT Study
tests multiple camera systems with a final image
- phantom contains multiple objects of various sizes (hot and cold rods and cold balls)
- final reconstructed image is visually assessed

SPECT Sources of Artifacts
1. Scanning palette in field of view
2. Collimator shifting + rotation on camera face
3. Noncircular orbit of camera head
4. PM tube failure
5. PM tube uncoupling
6. Cracked crystal
7. Improper peaking of camera

SOURCES OF ARTIFACTS
A. ATTENUATOR BETWEEN SOURCE AND DETECTOR
   Materials: cable, lead marker, solder dropped into collimator during repair, belt buckle / watch / key on patient, defective collimator
   (a) at time of correction flood procedure:
      √ hot spot
   (b) after correction flood procedure:
      √ cold spot

B. CRACKED CRYSTAL
   √ white band with hot edges

C. PMT FAILURE + LOSS OF OPTICAL COUPLING BETWEEN PMT AND CRYSTAL
   √ cold defect

D. PROBLEMS DURING FILM EXPOSURE + PROCESSING
   1. Double exposed film
   2. Light leak in multiformat camera
   3. Water lines from film processing
   4. Frozen shutter:
      √ part of film cut off
   5. Variations in film processing

E. IMPROPER WINDOW SETTING
   1. Photopeak window set too high:
      √ hot tubes
   2. Photopeak window set too low:
      √ cold tubes

F. ADMINISTRATION OF WRONG ISOTOPE
   √ atypically imaged organs

G. EXCESSIVE AMOUNTS OF FREE TC-99M PERTECHNETATE
   √ too much uptake in choroid plexus, salivary glands, thyroid, stomach

H. FAULTY INJECTION TECHNIQUE
   eg, inadvertently labeled blood clot in syringe leading to iatrogenic pulmonary emboli

I. CONTAMINATION WITH RADIOTRACER
   on patient's skin, stretcher, collimator, crystal

J. CRT PROBLEMS
   1. Burnt spot on CRT phosphor
   2. Dirty / scratched CRT face plates

POSITRON EMISSION TOMOGRAPHY

= PET = technique that permits noninvasive in vivo examination of metabolism, blood flow, electrical activity, neurochemistry

Concept:
measurement of distribution of a biocompound as a function of time after radiolabeling and injection into patient

Labeling:
PET compounds are radiolabeled with positron-emitting radionuclides

Physics:
positron matter-antimatter annihilation reaction with an electron results in formation of annihilation photons, which are emitted in exactly opposite directions (511 keV each); detected by coincidence circuitry through simultaneous arrival at detectors (bismuth germanate-68) on opposite sides of the patient (= electronic collimation through coincidence circuit); lead collimators not necessary (= advantages in resolution + sensitivity over SPECT); spatial reconstruction similar to transmission CT

Radionuclide production:
in nuclide generator / particle accelerator (positive / negative ion cyclotron; linear accelerator)
Expected amount of radionuclide: 500–2,000 mCi
Generator characteristics:
beam energy (radionuclide production rate increases monotonically with beam energy), beam current (production rate directly proportional to beam current), accelerated particle, shielding requirement, size, cost

Radiopharmaceutical production:
(1) Initialize accelerator, setup
(2) Irradiation
(3) Synthesis
(4) Sterility test, compounding

Sensitivity:
= fraction of radioactive decays within the patient that are detected by the scanner as true events (measured in counts per second per microcurie per milliliter)
◊ 30–100 times more sensitive than SPECT (due to electronic collimation as opposed to lead collimation)!

Resolution:
= resolving power = smallest side-by-side objects that can be distinguished as separate objects in images with an infinite number of counts (measured in mm);
determined by
- distance a positron travels before annihilation occurs (usually 0.5–2 mm depending on energy)
- angle variation from 180° (±5° = 0.5 mm)
- physical size of detector (1–3 mm)

◊ Typical spatial resolution: 4–7 mm

Measurement of radioactivity distribution:
Pixel values proportional to radioactivity per volume
Unit: mg of glucose per minute per 100 g tissue
Imaging time: 1–10 minutes

Organ-specific concentration:
(a) heart, brain: contain little glucose-6-phosphatase resulting in high concentrations of F-18 fluorodeoxyglucose
- metabolic rate of glucose is proportional to phosphorylation rate of FDG

(b) liver: abundance of glucose-6-phosphatase + low levels of hexokinase resulting in rapid clearing of FDG
(c) neoplasm: enhanced glycolysis with increased activity of hexokinase + other enzymes

FDG PET Imaging in Oncology

FDG = glucose analogue tracer 2-[fluorine-18] fluoro-2-deoxy-D-glucose
Physical half-life: 110 minutes

Isotope		Use	Half-life (min)	Average Positron Energy (keV)	Typical Reaction	Yield at 10 MeV (mCi/μA EOSB)
Rubidium	Rb-82		1.23	1,409	Sr/Rb generator	—
Fluorine	F-18	glucose metabolism	109	242	O-18(p,n)F-18	120
Oxygen	O-15	O_2, H_2O, CO_2, CO	2.1	735	N-15(p,n)O-15	70
Nitrogen	N-13	perfusion of NH_3	10	491	C-13(p,n)N-13	110
Carbon	C-11	carbon metabolism	20.3	385	N-14(p,α)C-11	85

p = proton injected; n = neutron ejected; α = alpha particle; EOSB = end of saturated bombardment (infinitely long irradiation at which time the numbers of radionuclides produced equals the number of radionuclides that are decaying) per microampere of beam current (= number of particles per second emerging from accelerator and impinging on target material)

Pathophysiology:
serum glucose competes with FDG for entry into tumor cells; trapped intracellularly as FDG-6-phosphate; malignant cells have a high rate of glycolysis

Preparation: fasting for 4–18 hours (FDG tumor uptake is diminished by an elevated serum glucose level)

Dose: 10 mCi (370 MBq)

Imaging time: 50–70 minutes after administration (trade-off between decreasing background activity and declining counting statistics)

Distortion correction in whole-body imaging:
attenuation correction can be achieved with a transmission scan before / after emission image acquisition at each corresponding bed position

Standardized uptake value (SUV):
= normalized target-to-background measure to allow comparison within and between different patients and diseases

$$SUV = FDG_{region} / (FDG_{dose}/WT)$$

FDG_{region} = decay-corrected regional radiotracer concentration
FDG_{dose} = injected radiotracer dose
WT = body weight in kilograms (corrected for body fat as it elevates SUV spuriously)

Typical values:

soft tissue	0.8
blood pool (at 1 hour)	1.5–2.0
liver	2.5
renal cortex	3.5
malignant neoplasm	2–20
non-small cell lung cancer	8.2
breast cancer	3.2

Distribution:
Intense accumulation in: brain, myocardium, intrarenal collecting system + ureter + bladder
Moderate accumulation in: liver, spleen, bone marrow, renal cortex, mediastinal blood pool

Sites of variable physiologic uptake:
@ Digestive tract
stomach: SUV usually <3.8, may be as high as 5.6
small bowel: isolated foci with SVU <4
colon: right colon may have an SVU as high as 10
@ Thyroid gland
moderate / intense uptake in 1/3 of euthyroid patients
@ Skeletal muscle
extraocular muscles, paravertebral muscles in neck + thorax (patient anxiety), laryngeal muscle (speech)
@ Myocardium
related to glycolytic metabolism (extended fasting switches to dominantly fatty acid metabolism)
@ Genitourinary tract
pooling in upper pole calyx, dilated redundant ureter, bladder diverticulum, endometrial uptake, testes (young patients)

Sites of benign pathologic uptake:
@ Healing bone
@ Lymph nodes
active granulomatous disease (TB, sarcoidosis), infection, recent instrumentation
@ Joints
degenerative / inflammatory joint disease (often in sternoclavicular + acromioclavicular + shoulder joints)
@ Infection / inflammation
leukocytic infiltration in abscess, pneumonia, sinusitis, acute pancreatitis, healing by secondary intention, wound repair, resorption of necrotic debris, hematoma

Indications:
1. Lung cancer
   √ tumor uptake > mediastinal uptake of FDG (94–97% sensitive, 87–89% specific, 92% accurate)
   √ FDG can differentiate adrenal "incidentaloma" from metastasis
2. Breast cancer
3. Colon cancer recurrence
4. Lymph node metastases from head and neck cancer (91% sensitive, 88% specific)
5. Brain tumor:
   (a) necrosis versus residual / recurrent tumor
       √ decreased FDG uptake in necrosis
   (b) response to chemo- / radiation therapy
   (c) prediction of patient's average survival in pediatric primary brain tumors:
       ≤6 months if FDG uptake ≥ gray matter
       1–2 years if FDG uptake > white matter
       2.5 years if FDG uptake = white matter
       3 years if FDG uptake < gray matter
6. Pancreatic cancer (96% sensitive + specific)
7. Lymphoma staging with whole-body scan

IMMUNOSCINTIGRAPHY

= imaging with monoclonal antibodies [= homogeneous antibody population directed against a single antigen (eg, cancer cell)], which are labeled with a radiotracer

Hybridoma technique:
antibody-producing B lymphocytes are extracted from the spleen of mice that were immunized with a specific type of cancer cell; B lymphocytes are fused with immortal myeloma cells (= hybridoma)

Agents:
Indium-111 satumomab pendetide = indium-111 CYT-103 (OncoScint® CR/OV) = murine monoclonal antibody product derived by site-specific radiolabeling of the antibody B27.3-GYK-DTPA conjugate with indium-111

Use: detection + staging of colorectal + ovarian cancers

Dose: 1 mg of antibody radiolabeled with 5 mCi of indium-111 injected IV

Biodistribution: liver, spleen, bone marrow, salivary glands, male genitalia, blood pool, kidneys, bladder

Imaging: 2 sets of images 2–5 days post injection + 48 hours apart

LYMPHANGIOSCINTIGRAPHY

Technique:
Tc-99m albumin solution injected intradermally to raise a wheal in 1st interdigital web space of both feet / hands
Dose: 500 µCi (18.5 MBq); 92–98% of albumin are tightly bound to Tc-99m
Volume: 0.05 mL; >98% of albumin macromolecules (molecular weight of 60 kDa) enter lymphatic vessels
Imaging: at 1 minutes, 10–40 minutes and 3–5 hours with parallel-hole collimator passing over patient
Transport Index Score (TIS)
= semiquantitive measurement of objective + subjective criteria of peripheral lymphatic radiotracer transport

$$\text{TIS} = K + D + 0.04T + N + V$$

K = transport kinetics = degree of transport delay
D = radionuclide distribution pattern = degree of dermal backflow
T = timing of radionuclide appearance in regional lymph nodes (in minutes normalized for 200 minutes as maximal delay)
N = demonstration + intensity of lymph nodes
V = demonstration + intensity of lymphatic collectors

LYMPH FLOW DISORDERS

Primary Lymphatic Dysplasia

• uni- / bilateral swelling of lower / upper extremities resembling other angiodysplastic syndromes
1. Klippel-Trenaunay-Servelle syndrome
   = venous + lymphatic abnormalities
2. Klippel-Trenaunay-Weber syndrome
   = venous + lymphatic + arterial disturbances
3. Milroy disease
   = inherited autosomal disorder with high penetrance characterized by lymphedema of one / both lower /upper extremities, face, other body parts

Secondary Lymphatic Dysplasia

= obstruction of lymph flow from an acquired cause
Cause:
1. Treatment of cancer: obliteration of lymph nodes by excision or irradiation
   ◊ Lymphedema may appear months to years after treatment due to gradual deterioration in intrinsic contractile force of lymphatic wall / valve incompetence
2. Filariasis
   = nematode (Wuchereria bancrofti, Brugia malayi) resides within peripheral lymphatic vessels + nodes + obstructs lymph flow
   • elephantine / pachydermatous extremities / genitalia
   • chyluria, hydrocele, chylous reflux (chylometrorrhagia, chylous vesicles), genital edema, massive breast engorgement
3. Long-standing venous disease / following venous stripping
4. Lymphatic obstruction by cancer, Kaposi sarcoma
5. Lymphatic inflammation: topical use of cantharone (for eradication of plantar warts); injection treatment of varicosities
6. Minor trauma to soft tissue / bone
7. Sedentary condition: eg, confinement to wheelchair
8. Morbid obesity
9. Lymphedema tarda
   = congenital lymphedema with delayed manifestation secondary to superimposed secondary cause

Primary Lymphedema

• no history of cancer chemotherapy, nodal extirpation / irradiation, severe trauma
Age: birth to >25 years
Cause: primary / acquired lymphatic disorder
√ complete absence / delay of radiotracer transport
√ absence / paucity of lymphatic collectors (truncal flow)
√ intense dermal dispersion / backflow
√ lymphatic dysplasia may involve viscera
  • chylous skin vesicles
  • external leakage of milky lymph
Pitfall: subcutaneous injection leads to factitious failure of radiotracer movement

Congenital Lymphedema

Age: birth to 5 years

Lymphedema Precox

Age: puberty to 25 years
(a) congenital
  √ lack of lymph collectors, dermal diffusion, delayed transport
(b) acquired
  √ intact collectors, rapid regional transport, delayed dermal diffusion

Secondary Lymphedema

√ prominent lymphatic trunks:
  √ long-standing lymphatic obstruction leads to "die-back" (obliteration) of lymphatics due to intraluminal coagulum-gel deposition / reactive inflammation
√ dermal diffusion (backflow) of variable intensity
√ delayed radiotracer transport
√ faintly visualized regional lymph nodes

NON-ORGAN–SPECIFIC WHOLE BODY SCINTIGRAPHY

Indications for Non-organ–specific Whole Body Imaging:

1. Tumor
   Agents: Ga-67 citrate, I-131 MIBG,
   In-111 pentetreotide (Octreoscan®),
   In-111 antiprostate antibody (ProstaScint®),
   In-111 Oncoscint,
   Tc-99m anti-CEA antibody (CEA-Scan®),
   F-18 deoxyglucose
2. Inflammation / infection
   Agents: Ga-67 citrate, In-111 oxime labeled WBC,
   Tc-99m HMPAO labeled WBC

GALLIUM-67 CITRATE

Ga-67 acts as an analogue of ferric ion; used as gallium citrate (water-soluble form)

Production: bombardment of zinc targets (Zn-67, Zn-68) with protons (cyclotron); virtually carrier-free after separation process

Decay: by electron capture to ground state of Zn-67

Energy levels:
- (a) used: 93 keV (38%), 184 keV (24%), 296 keV (16%), 388 keV (8%)
- (b) unused: 91 keV (2%), 206 keV (2%)

Physical half-life: 3.3 days (= 78 hours)

Biologic half-life: 2–3 weeks

Adult dose: 3–6 mCi or 50 μCi/kg

Radiation dose:
0.3 rads/mCi for whole body; 0.9 rads/mCi for distal colon (= critical organ); 0.58 rads/mCi for red marrow; 0.56 rads/mCi for proximal colon; 0.46 rads/mCi for liver; 0.41 rads/mCi for kidney; 0.24 rads/mCi for gonads

Physiology:
Ga-67 is bound to iron-binding sites of various proteins (strongest bond with transferrin in plasma, lactoferrin in tissue); multiexponential + slow plasma disappearance; competitive iron administration (Fe-citrate) enhances target-to-background ratio by increasing Ga-67 excretion

Binding Sites

(a) fluid spaces
1. Transferrin, haptoglobin, albumin, globulins in blood serum (90%)
2. Interstitial fluid space (increased capillary permeability and hyperemia in inflammation + tumor)
3. Lactoferrin in tissue

(b) cellular binding
1. Viable PMNs incorporate 10% of Ga-67 (bound to lactoferrin in intracytoplasmic granules)
2. Nonviable PMNs + their protein exudate (iron-binding proteins are deposited at sites of inflammation; these remove iron from the extracellular space; iron is no longer available for bacterial growth)
3. Lymphocytes have lactoferrin-binding surface receptors
4. Phagocytic macrophages engulf protein-iron complexes
5. Bacteria + fungi (siderophores = lysosomes = low-molecular–weight chelates produced by bacteria) have iron-transporting protein mechanism
6. Tumor cell-associated transferrin receptor + transportation into cells (lymphocytes bind Ga-67 less avidly than PMNs; RBCs do not bind Ga-67)

mnemonic: "LFT'S"
Lactoferrin (WBCs)
Ferritin
Transferrin
Siderophores (bacteria)

Uptake

at 24 hours: most intense in RES, liver, spleen (4%), bone marrow (lumbar spine, sacroiliac joints), bowel wall (chiefly colonic activity on delayed images), renal cortex, nasal mucosa, lacrimal + salivary glands, blood pool (20%), lung (<3% = equivalent to background activity), breasts

at 72 hours: 75% of dose remains in body its activity equally distributed among soft tissue (orbit, nasal mucosa, large bowel), liver, bone or bone marrow (occiput); kidney activity no longer detectable; lacrimal + salivary glands may still be prominent

Excretion

(a) via urinary tract (10–25% within 24 hours)
no activity in kidneys + urinary bladder after 24 hours

(b) via GI tract (10–20%)
hepatobiliary pathway + colonic mucosal excretion
- ◊ Enemas + laxatives promote clearing of bowel activity!
- ◊ Bowel cleansing not optimal as gallium lies also within colonic wall

(c) via various body fluids
eg, human milk (mandates to stop nursing for 2 weeks)

Imaging

usually [6, 24], 48–72 hours (up to 7 days)
- ◊ Best target-to-background ratio generally at 72 hours
- ◊ Optimal target-to-background ratio at 6–24 hours for abscess
- ◊ Optimal target-to-background ratio at 24–48 hours for tumor
- 500,000 count spot views / whole body
- SPECT useful

Degrading Factors of Imaging

√ lesions <2 cm are not detectable
√ photon scatter within overlying tissues
√ physiologic high activity of liver, spleen, bones, kidney, GI tract may obscure lesion

Normal Variants of Ga-67 Uptake

1. Breasts: increased uptake under stimulus of menarche, estrogens, pregnancy, lactation, phenothiazine medication, renal failure, hypothalamic lesion
2. Liver: suppressed uptake by chemotherapeutic agents / high levels of circulating iron / irradiation / severe acute liver disease
3. Lung: prominent uptake after lymphangiography
4. Spleen: increased uptake in splenomegaly
5. Thymus: uptake in children
6. Salivary glands: uptake within first 6 months after radiation therapy to neck (may persist for years)
7. Epiphyseal plates in children
8. Previous steroid therapy, chemotherapy, and radiation therapy may decrease Ga uptake
9. Healing surgical incision

No Ga-67 Uptake

most benign neoplasms; hemangioma; cirrhosis; cystic disease of the breast, liver, thyroid; reactive lymphadenopathy; inactive granulomatous disease

Indications

A. INFECTION
   Gallium has been largely replaced with WBC imaging but can be used in chronic infection
   1. Inflamed / infarcted bowel (eg, Crohn disease)
      DDx: normal bowel excretions (must be cleared by enema; bowel pathology shows persistent activity)
   2. Diffuse lung uptake
      sarcoidosis, diffuse infections (TB, CMV, PCP), lymphangitic metastases, pneumoconioses (asbestosis, silicosis), diffuse interstitial fibrosis (UIP), drug-induced pneumonitis (bleomycin, cyclophosphamide, busulfan), acute radiation pneumonitis, recent lymphangiographic contrast
   3. Lymph node involvement
      sarcoidosis, TB, MAI, Hodgkin disease
      DDx: NOT seen in Kaposi sarcoma, a useful distinction in AIDS patients with hilar nodes

B. TUMOR
   Neoplastic uptake is variable; prominent uptake is usually seen in:
   1. Non-Hodgkin lymphoma (especially Burkitt)
   2. Hodgkin disease
   3. Hepatoma
   4. Melanoma

   Useful in:
   — detection of tumor recurrence
   — DDx of focal cold liver lesions on Tc-99m sulfur colloid scan

Gallium in Bone Imaging

Increased activity in:

1. Active osteomyelitis (90% sensitivity is higher than for Tc-99m MDP)
2. Sarcoma
3. Cellulitis (bone scan followed by gallium scan)
4. Septic arthritis, rheumatoid arthritis
5. Paget disease
6. Metastases (65% sensitivity, less than for bone agents)

Gallium in Tumor Imaging

Particularly useful in evaluating extent of known tumor disease + in detection of tumor recurrence

A. USEFUL CATEGORY
   1. Lymphoma
      (a) Hodgkin disease: 74–88% sensitivity
      (b) NHL: sensitivity varies
         — histiocytic form: 85–90% sensitivity
         — lymphocytic well-diff.: 55–70% sensitivity
         95% sensitivity for mediastinal disease, 80% sensitivity for cervical + superficial lesions; poor sensitivity below diaphragm
   2. Burkitt lymphoma: almost 100% sensitivity
   3. Rhabdomyosarcoma: >95% sensitivity
   4. Hepatoma: 85–95% sensitivity
   5. Melanoma: 69–79% sensitivity

B. POSSIBLY USEFUL
   1. NHL: good for large + mediastinal lesions
   2. Nodal metastases from seminoma + embryonal cell carcinoma: 87% sensitivity
   3. Non-small cell lung cancer: 85% sensitivity for primary of any histologic type, 90% probability for uptake in mediastinal nodes, 67% probability for uptake in normal mediastinal nodes, 90% probability for uptake in extrathoracic metastases

C. NOT USEFUL
   head & neck tumors, GI tumors (especially adenocarcinomas; 35–40% sensitivity), breast tumor (52–65% sensitivity), gynecologic tumors (<26% sensitivity), pediatric tumors

Gallium in Lung Imaging

◊ Scans obtained at 48 hours, because 50% of normals show activity at 24 hours

A. FOCAL UPTAKE
   1. Primary pulmonary malignancy (>90% sensitivity)
   2. Benign disorders: granuloma, abscess, pneumonia, silicosis

B. MULTIFOCAL / DIFFUSE UPTAKE
   (a) Infection
      1. Tuberculosis
         √ intense uptake in active lesions (97%) = parameter of activity
         √ diffuse uptake in miliary TB + rapidly progressive TB pneumonia
      2. Pneumocystis carinii
         √ increased uptake at time when physical signs, symptoms, and roentgenographic changes are unimpressive

3. Cytomegalovirus
(b) Inflammation
1. Sarcoidosis
70% sensitivity for active parenchymal disease, 94% sensitivity for hilar adenopathy
= indicator of therapeutic response to steroids
2. Interstitial lung disease
pneumoconiosis, idiopathic pulmonary fibrosis, lymphangitic carcinomatosis
3. Exudative stage of radiation pneumonitis
(c) Drugs
1. Bleomycin toxicity
2. Amiodarone
(d) Contrast lymphangiography (in 50%)

C. GALLIUM UPTAKE + NORMAL CHEST FILM
1. Pulmonary drug toxicity
2. Tumor infiltration
3. Sarcoidosis
4. Pneumocystis carinii

Gallium in Renal Imaging

Abnormal uptake on delayed images at 48–72 hours

A. RENAL TUMOR
1. Primary renal tumor (variable uptake)
2. Lymphoma / leukemia
3. Metastases (eg, melanoma)

B. RENAL INFLAMMATION
1. Acute pyelonephritis (88% sensitivity):
√ diffuse / focal uptake
2. Lobar nephronia
3. Renal abscess

C. OTHERS
1. Collagen-vascular disease, vasculitis, Wegener granulomatosis
2. Amyloidosis, hemochromatosis
3. Hepatic failure
4. Administration of antineoplastic drugs

D. TRANSPLANT
1. Acute / chronic rejection
2. Acute tubular necrosis

E. URINARY BLADDER
1. Cystitis
2. Tumor

mnemonic: "CHANT An OLD PSALM"
Chemotherapy
Hemochromatosis, **H**epatorenal failure
Acute tubular necrosis, **A**cute lobar nephronia
Neoplasm
Transfusion, **T**uberous sclerosis
Abscess
Obstruction
Lymphoma
Drugs (Fe, drugs causing ATN)
Pyelonephritis, **P**olyarteritis nodosa
Sarcoidosis
Amyloidosis, **A**llograft
Leukemia
Metastasis, **M**yeloma

Gallium Imaging in Lymphoma

= chief use of gallium in tumor imaging before + after chemo- / radiation therapy:
√ persisting Ga-67 uptake indicates residual tumor
√ reversion to normal of a previously Ga-67 avid mass indicates fibrosis
√ new Ga-67 uptake during therapy indicates tumor progression

A. HODGKIN DISEASE
50–70% average sensitivity dependent on size, location, technique

B. NON-HODGKIN LYMPHOMA
30% sensitivity for lymphocytic subtype,
70% sensitivity for histiocytic subtype
Sensitivity:
90% for mediastinal nodes
80% for neck nodes
48% for periaortic nodes
47% for iliac nodes
36% for axillary nodes

Gallium Imaging in Malignant Melanoma

Types:
1. Lentigo maligna: low invasiveness, low metastatic potential
2. Superficial spreading melanoma: intermediate prognosis
3. Nodular melanoma: most lethal

Prognosis (level of invasion versus 5-year survival):

Level	I	(in situ)	100%
Level	II	(within papillary dermis)	100%
Level	III	(extending to reticular dermis)	88%
Level	IV	(invading reticular dermis)	66%
Level	V	(subcutaneous infiltration)	15%

Ga-67:
>50% sensitivity for primary + metastatic sites; detectability versus tumor size:
73% sensitivity >2 cm; 17% sensitivity <2 cm

Bone, brain, liver scintigraphy:
show very low yield in detecting metastases at time of preoperative assessment and are not indicated

AGENTS FOR INFLAMMATION

Ga-67 citrate

overall 58–100% sensitivity; 75–100% specificity (lower for abdominal inflammation because of problematic abdominal activity)

Indication: Ga-67 mostly limited to
(a) chest: interstitial pneumonia, opportunistic infection, sarcoidosis, drug toxicity
(b) bone: osteomyelitis

Pathophysiology:
leakage of protein-bound Ga-67 into extracellular space secondary to hyperemia + increased capillary permeability; Ga-67 is preferentially bound to nonviable PMNs + macrophages
1. Leukocyte incorporation (rich in lactoferrin)

2. Bacterial uptake (iron-chelating siderophores)
3. Inflammatory tissue stimulates lactoferrin production

GALLIUM IN CHRONIC ABDOMINAL INFLAMMATION

67% sensitivity, 64% specificity, 13% false-negative rate, 5% false-positive rate

Dose: 5 mCi

Imaging: routine at 48–72 hours (after clearance of high background activity); optional at 6–24 hours (prior to renal + gastrointestinal excretion); delayed images as needed

√ diffuse uptake in peritonitis

√ localized uptake in acute pyogenic abscess, phlegmon, acute cholecystitis, acute pancreatitis, acute gastritis, diverticulitis, inflammatory bowel disease, surgical wound, pyelonephritis, perinephric abscess

Labeled Leukocyte Imaging

= primary imaging method for inflammation / infection

Indication:

(1) Fever of unknown origin / bacteremia
(2) Abdominal infection / abscess
(3) Osteomyelitis
(4) Inflammatory bowel disease
(5) Vascular graft infection

Preparation (3-hour time):

- 30–40 mL of whole blood drawn into syringe containing an anticoagulant
- syringe stands in upright position for 1–2 hours with addition of hydroxyethyl starch (for sedimentation of RBCs)
- under centrifugation leukocytes form a pellet at bottom of tube (allows separation of leukocytes from platelets)

Requirements:

1. WBC count >2,000/mm^3
2. Neutrophil-mediated inflammatory process

Physiologic uptake:

@ Granulation wounds = healing by secondary intention (eg, ostomies, skin graft)
◊ Leukocytes do not accumulate in normally healing wounds

@ Lung
√ physiologic diffuse lung uptake up to 4 hours
◊ Lung uptake >24 hours due to pneumonia / ARDS
√ physiologic diffuse lung uptake in severely septic patient (due to cytokine release at site of infection + subsequent activation of pulmonary vascular endothelium)

In-111–labeled WBC

= In-111-oxime–labeled autologous leukocytes with 80% sensitivity; 97% specificity, 91% accuracy (superior to Ga-67 citrate); no activity in intestinal contents / urine

Indications:

occult sepsis (postoperative fever), acute pyogenic infection, abdominal + renal abscess, inflammatory bowel disease, nonpulmonary infection with HIV positivity, prosthetic graft infection (bone / cardiovascular graft), acute + chronic + complicated bone / joint infection

Technique:

chelating agents (oxime = 8-hydroxyquinoline / tropolone) used for labeling of leukocytes; lipophilic oxime-indium complex penetrates cell membrane of white cells; intracellular proteins scavenge the indium from oxime; oxime diffuses out from cell; requires 2 hours of preparation time

Recovery rate: 30% at 1–4 hours after injection

Limitations: 19 gauge IV access, leukopenia, impaired chemotaxis, abnormal WBCs, children

Dose: 0.5 mCi

Half-life: 67 hours

Useful photopeaks: 173 keV (89%), 247 keV (94%)

Radiation dose:

13–18 rad/mCi for spleen; 3.8 rad/mCi for liver; 0.65 rad/mCi for red marrow; 0.45 rad/mCi for whole body; 0.29 rad/mCi for testes; 0.14 rad/mCi for ovaries (compared with Ga-67 higher dose to spleen, but lower dose to all other organs)

Biodistribution: spleen, liver, bone marrow; blood clearance halftime of 6–7 hours; NO bowel activity

Imaging:

best at 18–24 hours following injection of cell preparation; optional at 2–6 hours (eg, in inflammatory bowel disease); delayed images as needed; bone marrow uptake provides useful landmarks

- SPECT imaging >> standard planar imaging

√ focal activity greater than in spleen is typical for abscess (comparison based on liver, spleen, bone marrow activity)

√ activity equal to liver (significant inflammatory focus)

√ abdominal activity is always abnormal (eg, pseudomembranous / ischemic colitis, inflammatory bowel disease, GI bleeding)

False positives:

@ Chest: CHF, RDS, embolized cells, cystic fibrosis, vascular access lines, dialysis catheter

@ Abdomen: accessory spleen, colonic accumulation, renal transplant rejection, active GI hemorrhage, vasculitis, ischemic bowel disease, following CPR, uremia, postradiation therapy, Wegener granulomatosis, ALL, lumbar puncture

@ Miscellaneous: IM injection, histiocytic lymphoma, cerebral infarction, arthritis, skeletal metastases, thrombophlebitis, hematoma, hip prosthesis, cecal carcinoma, postsurgical pseudoaneurysm, necrotic tumors that harvest WBCs

False negatives:
chronic infection, aortofemoral graft, LUQ abscess, infected pelvic hematoma, splenic abscess, hepatic abscess (occasionally)

Disadvantages:
2-day procedure, low-quality images especially of extremities

Advantages:
no activity in normal GI / GU tract (preferred in postoperative patient + vascular grafts); simultaneous WBC + sulfur colloid bone marrow scan possible

Tc-99m–HMPAO Labeled WBC

Optimal use: osteomyelitis in extremities

Biodistribution: bone marrow, little soft tissue, spleen > liver, renal + bladder activity

Excretion: in bile + urine

Advantages over In-111 WBC imaging:
(a) improved photon flux with lower dose
(b) earlier imaging (same day)

Disadvantages:
(1) Biliary excretion leads to bowel activity, which may obscure abdominal / graft abscess if not imaged early
(2) Heart and blood pool activity
(3) Nonspecific accumulation in lung may obscure lung disease

Technique:
chelating agents (exametazine oxime) used for labeling of leukocytes; Tc-99m Ceretec binds with autologous WBCs and is reinjected

Dose: up to 10 mCi

Imaging:
30 minutes (optimum for use in abdomen), 60 minutes, 3–4 hours, 4–8 hours (optimum outside abdomen); 24 hours (optional)

False positives:
may be due to unusual marrow distribution, correlation with bone marrow (sulfur colloid) scan may be necessary

BONE SCINTIGRAPHY

BONE AGENTS

A. POLYPHOSPHATES = LINEAR PHOSPHATES = CONDENSED PHOSPHATES
First agents described; contain up to 46 phosphate residues; simplest form contains 2 phosphates = pyrophosphate (PYP)

B. DIPHOSPHONATES
Organic analogs of pyrophosphate characterized by P-C-P bond; chemically more stable; not susceptible to hydrolysis in vivo; most widely used agents:
1. ethylene hydroxydiphosphonate (EHDP) = ethane-1-hydroxy-1,1-diphosphonate
2. methylene diphosphonate (MDP)

C. IMIDODIPHOSPHONATES (IDP)
Characterized by P-N-P bond

Indications:
1. Imaging of bone, myocardial / cerebral infarct, ectopic calcifications, some tumors (neuroblastoma)
2. Rx for Paget disease, myositis ossificans progressiva, calcinosis universalis (inhibits formation + dissolution of hydroxyapatite crystals)

Usual dose: 20 mCi (740 MBq)
Radiation dose: 0.13 rad/mCi for bladder (critical organ), 0.04 rad/mCi for bone, 0.01 rad/mCi for whole body

Imaging:
@ Bone: 2–3 hours post injection
◊ Fractures may not show positive uptake until 3–10 days depending on age of patient
@ Myocardium: 90–120 minutes post injection
◊ Ideal imaging time is 1–3 days post infarction

Labeling: Tc (VII) is eluted as a pertechnetate ion; chemical reduction with Sn (II) chloride; chelated into a complex of Tc-99m (IV)-tin-phosphate

Quality Control:
(1) <10% Tc-99m tin colloid / free Tc-99m pertechnetate (a good preparation is 95% bound)
(2) Agent should not be used prior to 30 minutes after preparation
(3) Avoid injection of air in preparation of multidose vials (oxidation results in poor Tc bond)
(4) Kit life is 4–5 hours after preparation

Uptake:
(a) rapid distribution into ECF (78% of injected dose with biologic half-life of 2.4 minutes) directly related to blood flow + vascularity; blood clearance rate determines ECF (= background) activity (at 4 hours 1% for diphosphonates, 5% for pyrophosphate / polyphosphate secondary to greater degree of protein binding)
(b) chemisorbs on hydroxyapatite crystals in bone + in calcium crystals in mitochondria; MDP concentration at 3 hours is directly proportional to calcium contents of tissues (14–24% calcium in bone, 0.005% calcium in muscle); 50–60% (58% for MDP, 48% for EHDP, 47% for PYP) are localized in bone by approx. 3 hours depending on blood flow + osteoblastic activity; 2–10% of the dose are present within soft tissues; myocardial uptake depends on at least some revascularization of infarcted muscle

Excretion:
via urinary tract by 6 hours in 68% of MDP/EHDP, in 50% of PYP, in 46% of polyphosphates
◊ Forcing fluids + frequent voiding reduces radiation dose to bladder!

THREE-PHASE BONE SCANNING
over area of interest
1. Rapid sequence flow study (2–5 seconds/frame) = early arterial flow = 1st phase
2. Immediate postflow images (1 million counts for central body + 0.5 million counts for extremities) = blood pool = 2nd phase
3. Delayed images (0.5–1.0 million counts) between 3–4 hours following injection = 3rd phase

BONE MARROW AGENTS

for assessment of hematopoiesis / phagocytosis by RES

1. Tc-99m sulfur colloid (10% uptake in bone marrow)
2. In-111 chloride
3. Tc-99m MMAA
= mini-microaggregated albumin colloid for liver, spleen, hematopoietic marrow
Particle size: 30–100 µm
Dose: 10 mCi
Marrow dose: 0.55 rad
Marrow accumulation at 1 hour:
6 x higher than for sulfur colloid
3 x higher than for antimony-sulfur colloid

Indications:
(a) expansion of hematopoietically active bone marrow
1. Hematologic disorders to reveal presence of peripheral expansion of functional marrow
(b) focal defect due to displacement by infiltrating disease
1. Marrow replacement disorders: eg, Gaucher disease
2. Bone infarction: eg, sickle cell anemia (DDx from osteomyelitis)
3. Avascular necrosis in children

Pediatric Indications for Bone Scan

A. BACK PAIN
   1. Diskitis
   2. Pars interarticularis defect: SPECT imaging adds sensitivity
   3. Osteoid osteoma: can be used intraoperatively to ensure removal of nidus
   4. Sacroiliac infection

B. NONACCIDENTAL TRAUMA

Superscan

A. METABOLIC
   1. Renal osteodystrophy
   2. Osteomalacia
      √ randomly distributed focal sites of intense activity = Looser zones = pseudofractures = Milkman fractures (most characteristic)
   3. Hyperparathyroidism
      √ focal intense uptake corresponds to site of brown tumors
   4. Hyperthyroidism
      rate of bone resorption more increased than rate of formation (= decrease in bone mass)
      - hypercalcemia (occasionally)
      - elevated alkaline phosphatase
      √ NOT visible on radiographs
      √ susceptible to fracture

B. WIDESPREAD BONE LESIONS
   1. Diffuse skeletal metastases (most frequent) from prostate, breast, multiple myeloma, lymphoma, lung, bladder, colon, stomach
   2. Myelofibrosis / myelosclerosis
   3. Aplastic anemia, leukemia
   4. Waldenström macroglobulinemia
   5. Systemic mastocytosis
   6. Widespread Paget disease

√ diffusely increased activity in bones: particularly prominent in axial skeleton, calvarium, mandible, costochondral junctions (= "rosary beading"), sternum (= "tie sternum"), long bones
√ increased metaphyseal + periarticular activity
√ increased bone-to-soft-tissue ratio
√ "absent kidney sign" = little / no activity in kidneys but good visualization of urinary bladder
√ femoral cortices become visible
CAVE: scan may be interpreted as normal, particularly in patients with poor renal function!

Hot Bone Lesions

mnemonic: "NATI MAN"

Neoplasm
Arthropathy
Trauma
Infection
Metastasis
Aseptic **N**ecrosis

Long Segmental Diaphyseal Uptake

A. BILATERALLY SYMMETRIC
   1. Hypertrophic pulmonary osteoarthropathy
   2. Thigh / shin splints = mechanical enthesopathy
   3. Ribbing disease
   4. Engelmann disease = progressive diaphyseal dysplasia

B. UNILATERAL
   1. Inadvertent arterial injection
   2. Melorheostosis
   3. Chronic venous stasis
   4. Osteogenesis imperfecta
   5. Vitamin A toxicity
   6. Osteomyelitis
   7. Paget disease
   8. Fibrous dysplasia

Photon-deficient Bone Lesion

= decreased radiotracer uptake

A. INTERRUPTION IN LOCAL BONE BLOOD FLOW
   = vessel trauma or vascular obstruction by thrombus / tumor
   1. Early osteomyelitis
   2. Radiation therapy
   3. Posttraumatic aseptic necrosis
   4. Sickle cell crisis

B. REPLACEMENT OF BONE BY DESTRUCTIVE PROCESS
   1. Metastases (most common cause): central axis skeleton > extremity, most commonly in carcinoma of kidney + lung + breast + multiple myeloma
   2. Primary bone tumor (exceptional)

mnemonic: "HM RANT"

Histiocytosis X
Multiple myeloma
Renal cell carcinoma
Anaplastic tumors (reticulum cell sarcoma)
Neuroblastoma
Thyroid carcinoma

Benign Bone Lesions

A. NO TRACER UPTAKE
   1. Bone island
   2. Osteopoikilosis
   3. Osteopathia striata
   4. Fibrous cortical defect
   5. Nonossifying fibroma

B. INCREASED TRACER UPTAKE
   1. Fibrous dysplasia
   2. Paget disease
   3. Eosinophilic granuloma
   4. Melorheostosis
   5. Osteoid osteoma
   6. Enchondroma
   7. Exostosis

Soft-tissue Uptake

A. PHYSIOLOGIC
1. Breast
2. Kidney: accentuated uptake with dehydration, antineoplastic drugs, gentamicin
3. Bowel: surgical diversion of urinary tract

B. FAULTY PREPARATION WITH RADIOCHEMICAL IMPURITY
(a) free pertechnetate (TcO^{4-})
Cause: introduction of air into the reaction vial
√ activity in mouth (saliva), salivary glands, thyroid, stomach (mucus-producing cells), GI tract (direct secretion + intestinal transport from gastric juices), choroid plexus
(b) Tc-99m MDP colloid
Cause: excess aluminum ions in generator eluate / patient ingestion of antacids; hydrolysis of stannous chloride to stannous hydroxide, excess hydrolyzed technetium
√ diffuse activity in liver + spleen

C. NEOPLASTIC CONDITIONS
(a) Benign tumor
1. Tumoral calcinosis
2. Myositis ossificans
(b) Primary malignant neoplasm
1. Extraskeletal osteosarcoma / soft-tissue sarcoma: bone forming
2. Neuroblastoma (35–74%): calcifying tumor
3. Breast carcinoma
4. Meningioma
5. Bronchogenic carcinoma (rare)
6. Pericardial tumor
(c) Metastases with extraosseous activity
1. to liver: mucinous carcinoma of colon, breast carcinoma, lung cancer, osteosarcoma
mnemonic: "LE COMBO"
Lung cancer
Esophageal carcinoma
Colon carcinoma
Oat cell carcinoma
Melanoma
Breast carcinoma
Osteogenic sarcoma
2. to lung: 20–40% of osteosarcomas metastatic to lung demonstrate Tc-99m MDP uptake
3. Malignant pleural effusion, ascites, pericardial effusion

D. INFLAMMATION
1. Inflammatory process (abscess, pyogenic / fungal infection):
(a) adsorption onto calcium deposits
(b) binding to denatured proteins, iron deposits, immature collagen
(c) hyperemia
2. Crystalline arthropathy (eg, gout)
3. Dermatomyositis, scleroderma
4. Radiation: eg, radiation pneumonitis
5. Necrotizing enterocolitis
6. Diffuse pericarditis
7. Bursitis
8. Pneumonia

E. TRAUMA
1. Healing soft-tissue wounds
2. Rhabdomyolysis: crush injury, surgical trauma, electrical burns, frostbite, severe exercise, alcohol abuse
3. Intramuscular injection sites: especially Imferon (= iron dextran) injections with resultant chemisorption; meperidine
4. Ischemic bowel infarction (late uptake)
5. Hematoma: soft tissue, subdural
6. Heterotopic ossification
7. Myocardial contusion, defibrillation, unstable angina pectoris
8. Lymphedema

F. METABOLIC
1. Hypercalcemia (eg, hyperparathyroidism):
(a) uptake enhanced by alkaline environment in stomach (gastric mucosa), lung (alveolar walls), kidneys (renal tubules)
(b) uptake with severe disease in myocardium, spleen, diaphragm, thyroid, skeletal muscle
2. Diffuse interstitial pulmonary calcifications: hyperparathyroidism, mitral stenosis
3. Amyloid deposits

G. ISCHEMIA WITH DYSTROPHIC SOFT-TISSUE CALCIFICATIONS
= necrosis with dystrophic calcification
@ Spleen: infarct (sickle cell anemia in 50%), microcalcification secondary to lymphoma, thalassemia major, hemosiderosis, glucose-6-phosphate-dehydrogenase deficiency
@ Liver: massive hepatic necrosis
@ Heart: transmural myocardial infarction, valvular calcification, amyloid deposition
@ Muscle: traumatic / ischemic skeletal muscle injury
@ Brain: cerebral infarction (damage of blood-brain barrier)
@ Kidney: nephrocalcinosis
@ Vessels: calcified wall, calcified thrombus

Abnormal Uptake within Kidneys

1. Effect of chemotherapeutic drugs: bleomycin, cyclophosphamide, doxorubicin, mitomycin C, 6-mercaptopurine
2. S/P radiation therapy
3. Metastatic calcification
4. Pyelonephritis
5. Acute tubular necrosis
6. Iron overload
7. Multiple myeloma
8. Renal vein thrombosis
9. Ureteral obstruction

Abnormal Uptake within Breast

1. Breast carcinoma
2. Prosthesis
3. Drug-induced

Abnormal Uptake in Ascitic, Pleural, Pericardial Effusion

1. Uremic renal disease
2. Infection
3. Malignant effusion

Incidental Urinary Tract Abnormalities

>50% of injected dose of Tc-99m MDP is excreted by 3 hours

A. BILATERAL DIFFUSE INCREASED UPTAKE
   = uptake greater than that of lumbar spine
   (a) excess tissue calcium
      1. Hyperparathyroidism
      2. Hypercalcemia
      3. Osteosarcoma metastatic to kidney
   (b) tissue damage
      1. Drug-induced nephrotoxicity
         (a) Chemotherapy (eg, cyclophosphamide, vincristine, doxorubicin, bleomycin, mitomycin-C, S-6-mercaptopurine, mitoxantrone)
         (b) aminoglycosides
         (c) amphotericin B
      2. Radiation therapy
      3. Necrotic renal cell carcinoma (rare)
      4. Renal metastasis (rare)
      5. Acute pyelonephritis
      6. Acute tubular necrosis
      7. Multiple myeloma
   (c) iron overload
      1. Sickle cell anemia
      2. Thalassemia major

   mnemonic: "RICH CON"
   Radiation therapy to kidney
   Iron overload
   Chemotherapy (cytoxan, vincristine, doxorubicin)
   Hyperparathyroidism
   Calcification (metastatic), **C**arcinoma
   Obstruction (urinary)
   Nephritis, **N**ormal variant

B. BILATERAL DECREASED RENAL UPTAKE
   (a) loss of renal function
      1. End-stage renal disease
   (b) increased osteoblastic activity (= superscan)

C. FOCALLY DECREASED RENAL UPTAKE
   (a) space-occupying lesion replacing normal renal parenchyma
      1. Abscess
      2. Cyst
      3. Primary / metastatic renal neoplasm
   (b) scar
      1. Infarct
      2. Chronic pyelonephritis
      3. Partial nephrectomy

D. UNI- / BILATERAL FOCALLY INCREASED GU UPTAKE
   (a) urine accumulation
      1. normal upper pole calices (supine position)
      2. Urinary tract diversion / ileal conduit
      3. Urinoma

E. CHANGE IN LOCATION OF KIDNEY
   1. Congenital anomaly (eg, pelvic kidney)

BRAIN SCINTIGRAPHY

RADIONUCLIDE ANGIOGRAPHY

Increased perfusion in:

1. Primary / metastatic brain tumor
2. AVM, large aneurysm, tumor shunting
3. Luxury perfusion after infarction
4. Infections (eg, herpes simplex encephalitis)
5. Extracranial lesions: bone metastasis, fibrous dysplasia, Paget disease, eosinophilic granuloma, fractures, burr holes, craniotomy defects

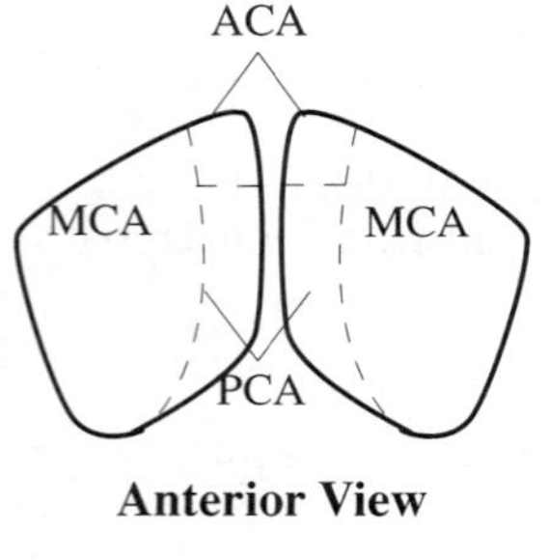

Anterior View

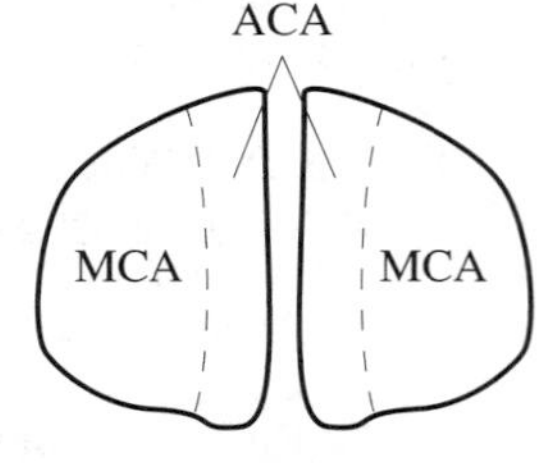

Posterior View

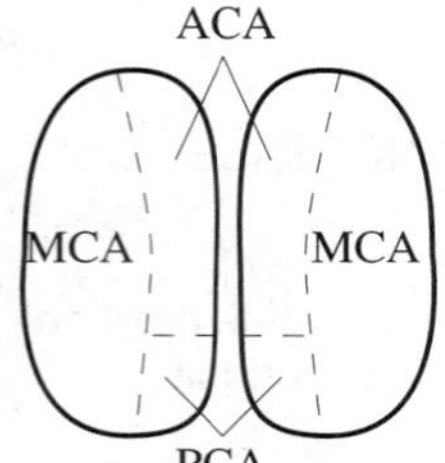

High Axial View

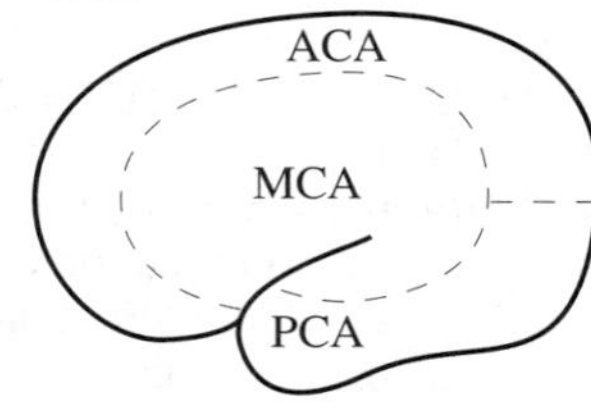

Left Lateral View

Blood-Brain Barrier Agents

= old-style agents requiring a disruption of blood-brain barrier to diffuse into brain

A. Tc-99m glucoheptonate
15–20 mCi bolus injection in <2 mL saline; 30 flow images of 2 seconds' duration; static image of 1 million counts after 4 hours; delayed image after 24 hours (higher target-to-background ratio than DTPA)

B. Tc-99m DTPA

C. Thallium-201: best predictor for tumor burden

Brain Perfusion Agents

= lipophilic agents rapidly crossing blood-brain barrier with accumulation in brain

Applications:
any disease in- / decreasing regional perfusion

1. Brain death (most common)
2. Refractory seizure disorder
3. Dementia

potential: stroke, receptor imaging, activation studies, tumor recurrence

Tc-99m HMPAO

= hexamethylpropylene amine oxime = exametazime
Product: Ceretec®
Dose: 10–30 mCi
Imaging: as early as 15 minutes post injection
Pharmacokinetics:
lipophilic radiopharmaceutical distributing across a functioning blood-brain barrier proportional to cerebral blood flow; no redistribution
Indication:
acute cerebral infarct imaging before evidence of CT / MRI pathology; positive findings within 1 hour of event

Tc-99m ECD

= ethyl cysteinate dimer = bicisate
Product: Neurolite®
Dose: 10–30 mCi
Imaging: 30–60 minutes post injection

I-123 Iofetamine

= N-isopropyl-p[123I]iodoamphetamine iodine = I-123-IMP
Product: Spectamine®
Pharmacokinetics:
initially distributes proportional to regional cerebral blood flow with increased flow to basal ganglia and cerebellum; homogeneous uptake in gray matter; decreased activity in white matter; redistribution over time
√ activity in an area of initial deficit on reimaging (after 4 hours) implies improved prognosis

Indications for Radionuclide Angiography

Seizures

Abnormal cerebral radionuclide angiography within 1 week of seizure activity even without underlying organic lesion
Etiology:
(1) 35% cerebral tumors (meningioma in 34%, metastases in 17%)
(2) Cerebrovascular disease (more common in age >50 years)
(3) Trauma, inflammation, CNS effects of systemic disease
√ transient hyperperfusion of involved hemisphere

SEIZURE FOCUS IMAGING
for localizing intractable seizures
√ focal hypoperfusion during interictal injection of tracer (less sensitive)
√ focal hyperperfusion during ictal injection of tracer (better detection)

Alzheimer Disease

√ bilateral temporoparietal hypoperfusion

Brain Tumor

Etiology:

√ good correlation between hyperperfusion and enlarged supplying vessels:
(1) Meningioma (increased activity in 60–80%);
(2) Metastases (increased activity in 11–23%);
(3) Vascular metastases: thyroid, renal cell, melanoma, anaplastic tumors from lung / breast

√ asymmetric decreased perfusion in mass lesions:
(1) Tumor
(2) Hemorrhage
(3) Subdural hematoma

Cerebral Death

Pathophysiology:
increased intracranial pressure results in markedly decreased cerebral perfusion, thrombosis, total cerebral infarction

Path: severe brain edema, diffuse liquefactive necrosis

√ carotid arteries visualized (= confirmation of good bolus)
√ activity stops abruptly at the skull base
√ sagittal sinus not visualized
√ activity in arteries of face + scalp with "hot nose" sign

DDx by EEG:
severe barbiturate intoxication may produce a flat EEG response in the absence of brain death

Arterial Stenosis

◊ Radionuclide angiography of limited value!

√ asymmetric decreased perfusion in acute / chronic cerebrovascular disease:
(1) Complete occlusion / >80% stenosis of ICA: 53–80% sensitivity
(2) 50–80% stenosis of ICA: 50% sensitivity
(3) <50% stenosis of ICA: 10% sensitivity

Problematic lesions:
(1) Bilaterally similar degree of stenosis
(2) Occlusion of MCA + unilateral ACA
(3) Vertebrobasilar occlusive disease (20% sensitivity)

Stroke

√ "flip-flop" phenomenon (= decreased perfusion in arterial phase, equalization of activity in capillary phase, increased activity in venous phase) secondary to late arrival of blood via collaterals + slow washout

POSITRON EMISSION TOMOGRAPHY

A. REGIONAL CEREBRAL BLOOD FLOW
(a) breathing of carbon monoxide (C-11 and O-15), which concentrates in RBCs
(b) Xe-133 inhalation / injection into ICA / IV injection after dissolution in saline: volume distribution is in the water space of the brain; no correction for recirculation necessary because all Xe is exhaled during lung passage, but correction for scalp + calvarial activity is required (for inhalation method)

√ washout rate of gray matter:white matter = 4–5:1

B. GLUCOSE METABOLISM
for measurements of metabolic rate + mapping of functional activity
(a) C-11 glucose: rapid uptake, metabolization, and excretion by brain
(b) F-18 fluorodeoxyglucose (FDG): diffuses across blood-brain barrier + competes with glucose for phosphorylation by hexokinase, which traps FDG-6-phosphate within mitochondria; FDG-6-phosphate cannot enter most metabolic pathways (eg, glycolysis, storage as glycogen) and accumulates proportional to intracellular glycolytic activity; FDG-6-phosphate is dephosphorylated slowly by glucose-6-phosphatase and then escapes cell

Indications:

1. Focal epilepsy prior to seizure surgery
   √ interictal decreased uptake of FDG of >20% at seizure focus (70% sensitivity, 90% for temporal lobe hypometabolism)
   √ hypermetabolism within 30 minutes of seizure
   √ measurement of opiate receptor density with C-11-labeled carfentanil (= high-affinity opium agonist) uptake by μ receptors (found in thalamus, striatum, periaqueductal gray matter, amygdala), which mediate analgesia and respiratory depression
2. Alzheimer disease
   • clinical diagnosis false positive in 35%
   √ bilateral temporoparietal hypoperfusion + hypometabolism resulting in decreased FDG uptake (92–100% sensitive)
   √ sparing of sensory and motor cortex + basal ganglia + thalamus
   DDx: frontal lobe dementia, primary progressive aphasia without dementia, normal-pressure hydrocephalus, multi-infarct dementia
3. Parkinson disease
   = deficient presynaptic terminals with normal postsynaptic dopaminergic receptors
   • clinical diagnosis in 50–70% accurate
   DDx: drug-induced chorea, Huntington disease, tardive dyskinesia, progressive supranuclear palsy, Shy-Drager syndrome, striatonigral degeneration, alcohol-related cerebellar dysfunction, olivopontocerebellar atrophy
4. Huntington disease, senile chorea
   √ hypometabolism of basal ganglia
5. Schizophrenia
   √ abnormally reduced glucose activity in frontal lobes
   √ dopamine receptors in caudate / putamen elevated to 3 x that of normal levels
6. Stroke, cerebral vasospasm
   √ disassociated oxygen metabolism + brain blood flow

RADIONUCLIDE CISTERNOGRAPHY

Indications:
1. Suspected normal pressure hydrocephalus
2. Occult CSF rhinorrhea / otorrhea
3. Ventricular shunt
4. Porencephalic cyst, leptomeningeal cyst, posterior fossa cyst

Technique:
1. Measurement of spinal subarachnoid pressure
2. Sample of CSF for analysis
3. Subarachnoid injection of radiotracer

Normal study (completed within 48 hours):
symmetric activity sequentially from basal cisterns, up the sylvian fissures + anterior commissure, eventual ascent over cortices with parasagittal concentration
- √ image lumbar region immediately after injection to ensure subarachnoid injection
- √ activity in basal cistern by 2–4 hours
- √ activity at vertex by 24–48 hours
- √ no / minimal lateral ventricular activity (may be transient in older patients)

Agents:
1. **Indium-111 DTPA**
   Physical half-life: 2.8 days
   Gamma photons: 173 keV (90%), 247 keV (94%) detected with dual pulse height analyzer
   Dose: 250–500 μCi
   Radiation dose: 9 rads/500 μCi for brain + spinal cord (in normal patients)
   Imaging: at 10-minute intervals / 500,000 counts up to 4–6 hours; repeat scans at 24, 48, 72 hours
2. **Technetium-99m DTPA**
   Not entirely suitable for imaging up to 48–72 hours; DTPA tends to have faster flow rate than CSF; used for shunt evaluation + CSF leak study since leak increases CSF flow
   Dose: 4–10 mCi
   Radiation dose: 4 rads for brain + spinal cord
3. **Iodine-131 serum albumin** (RISA)
   prototype agent; beta emitter
   Physical half-life: 8 days; high radiation dose of 7.1 rads/100 μCi; no longer used secondary to pyrogenic reactions
4. **Ytterbium-169 DTPA**
   Physical half-life: 32 days
   Gamma decay: 63 keV; 177 keV (17%); 198 keV (25%); 308 keV; dual pulse height analyzer set for 177 + 198 keV
   Dose: 500 μCi
   Radiation dose: 9 rads/500 mCi for brain + spinal cord (in normal patients)

CSF Leak Study

Purpose: localization of origin of CSF leak in patient with CSF rhinorrhea / otorrhea

Causes of dural fistula:
- (a) traumatic: in 30% of basilar skull fractures
- (b) nontraumatic: brain, pituitary and skull tumors; skull infections; congenital defects

Location of dural fistula:
cribriform plate > ethmoid cells > frontal sinus

Method:
1. Weigh cotton pledgets
2. Pledgets placed by ENT surgeon in the anterior and posterior turbinates bilaterally
3. Radiopharmaceutical injected intrathecally via lumbar puncture; immediate postinjection view of lumbar region to ensure intrathecal placement
4. Pledgets removed and weighed 4–6 hours after lumbar injection
5. Pledget activity counted + indexed to weight
6. Results compared with 0.5-mL serum specimens drawn at the time of pledget removal
7. Pledget to serum count ratio of >1.5 is evidence of CSF leak
8. With active leak patient should be placed in various positions with various maneuvers to accentuate leak

Hydrocephalus

A. NORMAL-PRESSURE HYDROCEPHALUS
- √ reversal of normal CSF flow dynamic = tracer moves from basal cisterns into 4th, 3rd, and lateral ventricles
- √ loss of w sign

B. OBSTRUCTIVE HYDROCEPHALUS
- √ delay (up to 48 hours) for tracer to surround convexities + reach arachnoid villi
- √ positive w sign

THYROID AND PARATHYROID SCINTIGRAPHY

THYROID SCINTIGRAPHY

Indications:

(1) Evaluation of solitary / dominant nodule
(2) Evaluation of upper mediastinal mass
(3) Classification of hyperthyroidism
(4) Detection and staging of postoperative thyroid cancer
(5) Evaluation of neonatal hypothyroidism
(6) Evaluation of developmental anomalies

A. SUPPRESSION SCAN
= to define autonomy of a nodule
√ suppression of a hot nodule following T_3 / T_4 administration is proof that autonomy does not exist

B. STIMULATION SCAN
= to demonstrate thyroid tissue suppressed by hyperfunctioning nodule
√ administration of TSH documents functioning thyroid tissue (rarely done)

C. PERCHLORATE WASHOUT TEST
= to demonstrate organification defect
√ repeat measurement of radioiodine uptake following oral potassium perchlorate shows lower values if organification defect present

Tc-99m Pertechnetate

Physical decay: 10 mCi Tc-99m decays to 2.7×10^{-7} mCi Tc-99
Physical half-life: 2×10^5 years
Biologic half-life: 6 hours
Decay: by photon emission of 140 keV
Quality control:
(1) <0.1% Mo-99 (= 1 μCi/mCi), maximum of Mo-99 at 5 μCi
(2) <0.5 mg aluminum/10 mCi Tc-99m
(3) <0.01% radionuclide impurities
Administration: oral / IV
Dose: 3–5 mCi administered IV 20 minutes prior to imaging (100–300 mrad/mCi)
Pharmacokinetics:
Uptake: in thyroid, salivary glands, gastric mucosa, choroid plexus
Excretion: mostly in feces, some in urine

Thyroid Agents

	I-131	*I-123*	*Tc-99m*
Physical half-life	8 days	13 hours	6 hours
Main photopeak	364 keV	159 keV	140 keV
Usual dose	50–100 μCi	100–300 μCi	2–10 mCi
Absorbed dose	50–100 rad	2–5 rad	0.2–1.8 rad
Administration	PO	PO	IV
Interval to image	24 hours	6 hours	20 minutes

Uptake in thyroid:
0.5–3.7% at 20 minutes (time of maximum uptake) assessment of trapping function only; NO organification; may be almost completely discharged by perchlorate
Imaging:
(a) Collimator: usually with pinhole collimator for image magnification (5-mm hole)
(b) Distance: selected so that organ makes up 2/3 of field of view; significant distortion of organ periphery occurs if detector too close
(c) Counts: 200,000–300,000 counts are usually acquired within 5 minutes after a dose of 5–10 mCi of Tc-99m pertechnetate
(d) Image must include markers for scale + anatomic landmarks + palpatory findings
Advantages:
(1) Low cost
(2) Reduced radiation exposure
(3) Greater photon flux than iodine = detectability of small thyroid lesions (>8 mm) is improved
(4) Excellent physical characteristics
Disadvantages:
(1) High neck background (target-to-background ratio less favorable than with iodine)
(2) Lesions with pertechnetate-iodine discordance (= hot on Tc-99m pertechnetate + cold on radioiodine) are very rare + due to Tc-99m–avid cancer
(3) Poor for substernal evaluation

Iodine-123

◊ Agent of choice for thyroid imaging!
Production:
in accelerator; contamination with I-124 dependent on source (Te-122 in ~ 5%, Xe-123 in ~ 0.5%); contamination with I-125 increases with time elapsed after production
Physical half-life: 13.3 hours
Decay: by electron capture with photon emission at 159 keV (83% abundance) + x-ray of 28 keV (87% abundance)
Dose: 200–400 μCi orally 24 hours prior to imaging (radiation dose of 7.5 mrad/μCi)
Uptake: iodine readily absorbed from GI tract (10–30% by 24 hours), distributed primarily in extracellular fluid spaces; trapped + organified by thyroid gland; trapped by stomach + salivary glands
Excretion: via kidneys in 35–75% during first 24 hours + GI tract

Advantages:
(1) Low-radiation exposure
(2) Excellent physical characteristics
(3) Uptake + scan with one agent (organified)

Disadvantages compared with Tc-99m pertechnetate:
(1) More expensive
(2) Less available with short shelf-life
(3) More time-consuming
(4) Radionuclide impurities
(5) Higher dose to thyroid (but less to whole body)

Iodine-131

Indication: thyroid uptake study, thyroid imaging, treatment of hyperthyroidism, treatment of functioning thyroid cancer, imaging of functioning metastases
Production: by fission decay
Physical half-life: 8.05 days (allows storing for long periods)
Decay: principal gamma energy of 364 keV (82% abundance) + significant beta decay fraction of a mean energy of 192 keV (92% abundance)

Dose: 30–50 μCi (1.2 rad/μCi = 50 rad for thyroid)
Radiation dose:
(90% from beta decay, 10% from gamma radiation)
0.6 mrad/mCi for whole body; 1.2 mrad/μCi for thyroid (critical organ)
Pharmacokinetics: identical to I-123
Advantages:
(1) Low cost
(2) Ectopic tissue search
(3) Uptake and scan at same time
Disadvantages:
(1) Too energetic for gamma camera, well suited for rectilinear scanner with limited resolution
(2) High radiation exposure (due to beta decay) prohibits use for diagnostic purposes
(3) Ectopic thyroid tissue just as well detectable with I-123 or Tc-99m pertechnetate

Iodine Fluorescence Imaging

Technique:
collimated beam of 60 keV gamma photons from an Am-241 source is directed at thyroid, which results in production of K-characteristic x-rays of 28.5 keV; x-rays are detected by semiconductor detector
Advantages:
(1) No interference with flooded iodine pool / thyroid medication
(2) Measures total iodine content
(3) Low radiation exposure (15 mrad) acceptable for children + pregnant women
Disadvantage: dedicated equipment necessary

Thyroid Uptake Measurements

Agents: I-123 / I-131 (easier to use), Tc-99m pertechnetate (requires calibration)
Method:
» orally administered isotope of iodine is absorbed from upper GI tract
» tracer mixes with intravascular iodine pool
» iodine is cleared by thyroid in competition with kidneys
» uptake parallels thyroidal clearance of plasma inorganic iodide
» all measurements are taken for 3 minutes at 4 and 24 hours (measurements at both 4 and 24 hours prevent missing the occasional rapid-turnover hyperthyroid patient returning to normal by 24 hours)

Radioactive Iodine Uptake (RAIU):
RAIU = Thyroid Counts* / Capsule Counts˘
* = background corrected (thigh) + decay corrected
˘ = decay corrected

Interpretation:
(a) normal: <25% at 4 hours, <35% at 24 hours
(b) increased: in Graves disease
(c) decreased: in subacute thyroiditis
N.B.: Uptake values do not diagnose hyperthyroidism, which is done with laboratory values (T_4, T_3, TSH) and clinical history

PARATHYROID SCINTIGRAPHY

for the evaluation of primary hyperparathyroidism after other causes for hypercalcemia have been excluded

Technetium-thallium Subtraction Imaging

= DUAL ISOTOPE SCINTIGRAPHY
Sensitivity: 72–92% (depending on size, smallest adenoma was 60 mg)
Specificity: 43% (benign thyroid adenomas, focal goitreous changes, Hashimoto thyroiditis, parathyroid carcinoma, cancer metastatic to neck, lymphoma, sarcoidosis, lymph nodes also concentrate thallium)
Method:
(1) IV injection of 1–3.5 mCi Tl-201 chloride; images recorded for 15 minutes with 2-mm pinhole collimator
√ concentrates in normal thyroid + enlarged parathyroid glands (extraction proportional to regional blood flow + tissue cellularity)
(2) IV injection of 1–10 mCi Tc-99m pertechnetate; images recorded at 1-minute intervals for 20 minutes
√ pertechnetate concentrates only in thyroid
(3) Computerized subtraction
√ focal / multifocal excess Tl-201
Limitations:
(1) unfavorable dosimetry + poor-quality images of Tl-201 (up to 3.5 mCi, 80 keV photons)
(2) prolonged patient immobilization (motion artifact)
(3) processing artifacts (eg, over- / undersubtraction)

(4) poor Tc-99m thyroid uptake from interfering medications / recent iodinated contrast media
(5) parathyroid pathology may be mimicked by coexisting thyroid disease (eg, nonfunctioning adenoma, multinodular goiter)

Indications:
Localization of one / more parathyroid adenoma (hyperplasia not visualized), may be more sensitive than CT / MRI in detection of ectopic mediastinal parathyroid tissue and in postoperative context

Technetium-99m Sestamibi

= Tc-99m MIBI

Sensitivity: 88–100% (smallest adenoma weighed 150 mg); 91% for early SPECT imaging
◊ For unknown reasons even large tumors (2 g) may not accumulate sufficient MIBI for detection!

Pharmacokinetics:
MIBI localizes in myocardium + mitochondria-rich tumors proportional to regional blood flow + cellular metabolic activity; MIBI washes out of thyroid quickly, but is retained in abnormal parathyroids (= need for dual-phase study)

Method:
1. IV injection of 20–25 mCi Tc-99m MIBI
2. 10–30 minutes after injection anterior cervicothoracic images (5 minutes/view) with large-field-of-view camera equipped with low-energy high-resolution parallel-hole collimator
3. Repeat set of images at 2–4 hours post injection (10 minutes/view)
4. Adjunctive dual phase imaging with thyroid-selective agent for computer-aided subtractions is optional (I-123, Tc-99m)

Advantages (over thallium):
A. Physical properties:
— optimal gamma emission (140 keV)
— abundant photons (high dose of 20 mCi)
— favorable dosimetry
— high parathyroid-to-thyroid ratio
— unaffected by medications / iodinated contrast

B. Technical features:
— Single readily available radiopharmaceutical
— Simple protocol of early + delayed images
— No prolonged patient immobilization
— No subtraction study / computer processing
— SPECT / multiple projections possible

C. Scan interpretation
— sharp images
— clear visualization of abnormal parathyroid glands
— ectopic sites surveyed

LUNG SCINTIGRAPHY

PERFUSION AGENTS

Tc-99m Macroaggregated Albumin (MAA)

Preparation:
human serum albumin (HSA) is heat-denatured + pH adjusted; added stannous chloride precipitates albumin into tin-containing macroaggregates; lyophilization prolongs stability; added Tc-99m pertechnetate is reduced by $SnCl_2$ and tagged onto the MAA particles

Quality control (USP guidelines):
(1) 90% of particles should have a diameter between 10 and 90 µm
(2) No particle should exceed 150 µ
(3) Should be at least 90% pure (by ascending chromatography)
(4) A batch of Tc-99m MAA should not be used >8 hours after preparation
(5) Preparation should not be backflushed with blood into syringe, causes "hot spots" on lungs

Physical half-life: 6 hours
Biologic half-life: 6 hours
Dose: approximately 2–4–6 mCi + 0.14 µg/kg albumin, which corresponds to >60,000 particles (recommended number of particles is 200,000–700,000 particles for even spatial distribution + good image quality)

- IV injection <u>in supine position</u> to give an even distribution between base + apex of lung (ventral to posterior gradient persists)
- imaging in upright position to allow maximum expansion of lung, especially at lung bases

N.B.: reduce number of particles to 50,000–80,000 in
(a) critically ill patients with severe COPD, on mechanical ventilator support, documented pulmonary arterial hypertension, significant left-to-right cardiac shunts need reduction in number of particles but not tagged activity!
(b) children up to age 5 need reduction in number of particles + tagged activity!

Radiation dose (rads/mCi):
0.013 for whole body, 0.25 for lung (critical organ), 0.01 for gonads

Physiology:
90% of MAA particles act as microemboli and will be trapped in lung capillaries on first pass; there are an estimated 600 million pulmonary arterioles small enough to trap the particles; the effect is insignificant physiologically as only 500,000 particles are injected per study; 0.22% of capillaries become occluded (= 2 of 1,000); protein is lysed within 6–8 hours and taken up by RES; particles <1 µm are phagocytized by RES in liver + spleen

IMAGING
Large-field-of-view scintillation camera + parallel-hole low-energy collimator with identical recording times for corresponding views
Views:
– anterior, posterior
– posterior oblique (LPO, RPO): additional information in 50% due to segmental delineation of basal segments and separation of both lungs
– anterior oblique (LAO, RAO): additional information in 15%
– lateral: "shine through" from contralateral lung
◊ Oblique views reduce equivocal findings from 30% to 15%

Counts: 750,000–1,000,000 counts for each image

Tc-99m Human Albumin Microspheres

Particle size: 20–30 µm
Biologic half-life: 8 hours

VENTILATION AGENTS

Xe-133, Xe-127, Xe-125, Kr-81m, N-13, O_2-15, CO_2-11, CO-11, radioactive aerosol (Tc-99m–DTPA, Tc-99m-PYP, Tc-99m–labeled ultrafine dry dispersion of carbon "soot")

Xenon-133

Fission product of U-235
Decay: to stable Cs-133 under emission of beta particle (374 keV), <u>gamma ray</u> (81 keV), x-ray (31 keV); beta-component responsible for high radiation dose of 1 rad to lung)
Physical half-life: 5.24 days
Biologic half-life: 2–3 minutes
Physical properties: highly soluble in oil + grease, absorbed by plastic syringe
Administration: injection into mouth piece of a disposable breathing unit at the beginning of a maximal inspiration
Dose: 15–20 mCi

TECHNIQUE
Ventilation study preferably done <u>before</u> perfusion scan to avoid interference with higher-energy Tc-99m (Compton scatter from Tc-99m into lower Xe-133 photopeak); [may be feasible after perfusion scan if dose of Tc-99m MAA is kept below 2 mCi + concentration of Xe-133 is above 10 mCi/L of air and if Xe-133 acquisition times for washing, equilibrium, washout images are kept to about 30 seconds]
◊ Posterior imaging routine, ideally in upright position

<u>Phase 1 = single-breath image</u>:
= inhalation of 10–20 mCi Xe-133 to vital capacity with breath-holding over 10–30 seconds (65% sensitivity for abnormalities)
√ cold spot is abnormal

Phase 2 = equilibrium phase:
= tidal breathing = closed-loop rebreathing of Xe-133 + oxygen for 3–5 minutes for tracer to enter poorly ventilated areas; also functions as internal control for air leaks; posterior oblique images + posterior images are obtained to improve correlation with perfusion scan.
√ activity distribution corresponds to aerated lung

Phase 3 = washout phase:
= clearance phase after readjusting intake valves of spirometer permitting patient to inhale ambient air and to exhale Xe-133 into shielded charcoal trap; washout phase should last >5 minutes
• images taken at 30–60-sec intervals for >5 minutes
√ rapid clearance within 90 seconds with slight retention in upper zones is normal
√ tracer retention (hot spot) at 3 minutes reveals areas of air-trapping

√ poor image quality secondary to significant scatter
√ abnormal scan:
(a) COPD / acute obstructive disease:
√ delayed wash-in (during initial 30 seconds of tidal breathing)
√ tracer accumulation on equilibrium views (partial obstruction with collateral air drift + diffusion into affected area via bloodstream)
√ delayed washout = retention >3 minutes due to air trapping
√ tracer retention in regions not seen on initial single-breath view (from collateral airdrift into abnormal lung zones)
(b) consolidated lung disease
√ no tracer uptake throughout imaging sequence

Xenon-127

cyclotron-produced with high cost
Physical half-life: 36.4 days
Photon energies: 172 keV (22%), 203 keV (65%)
Advantages:
(1) High photon energy allows ventilation study following perfusion study
(2) Decreased radiation dose (0.3 rad)
(3) Storage capability because of long physical half-life

Krypton-81m

insoluble inert gas; eluted from Rb-81 generator (half-life of 4.7 hours); decays to Kr-81 by isomeric transition
Physical half-life: 13 seconds
Biologic half-life: <1 minute
Principal photon energy: 190 keV (65% abundance)
Advantages:
(1) Higher photon energy than Tc-99m so that ventilation scan can be performed following perfusion study
(2) Each ventilation scan can be matched to perfusion scan without moving patient
(3) Can be used in patients on respirator (no contamination due to short half-life)
(4) Low radiation dose (during continuous inhalation for 6–8 views 100 mrad are delivered)

Disadvantages:
(1) High cost
(2) Limited availability (generator good only for one day, so weekend availability may not be possible
(3) No washout images possible due to short half-life
(4) Decreased resolution due to septal penetration with low-energy collimators

√ lack of activity = abnormal area (tracer activity is proportional to regional distribution of tidal volume because of short biologic half-life, washout phase not available)

Tc-99m DTPA Aerosol

= Tc-99m diethylenetriaminepentaacetic radioaerosol
= UltraVent®
Biological half-life: 55 minutes
Administration: delivery through a nebulizer during inspiration
Dose: 30–50 mCi in 2–3 mL of saline added to nebulizer unit and connected to wall oxygen at a flow rate of 8–10 L/min

PHYSIOLOGY
radioaerosols are small particles that become impacted in central airways, sediment in more distal airways, experience random contact with alveolar walls during diffusion in alveoli; cross respiratory epithelium with rapid removal by bloodstream
◊ Less physiologic indicator of ventilation + subject to nebulization technique
◊ Erect position preferable for basilar perfusion defects (dependent lung region receives more ventilation + radiotracer)

TECHNIQUE
◊ Aerosol applied ideally before perfusion; postperfusion aerosol imaging possible to assess for “fill-in” of aerosol in region of perfusion defect
• breathe from nebulizer for 3–5 minutes
• images recorded in multiple projections, each for 100,000 counts

√ abnormal scan:
(a) COPD
√ decreased activity in peripheral lung (slow and turbulent airflow prevents a normal amount of aerosol to reach the involved lung)
√ central airway deposition (aerosol sticks to trachea + bronchial walls)
(b) consolidated lung disease
√ absent tracer

Carbon Dioxide Tracer

O-15–labeled carbon dioxide
Physical half-life: 2 minutes (requires on-site cyclotron)

PHYSIOLOGY:
inhalation of carbon dioxide; rapid diffusion across alveolar-capillary membrane; clearance from lung within seconds

√ cold spot due to failure of tracer entry into airway
= airway disease
√ hot spot due to delayed / absent tracer clearance
= perfusion defect (87% sensitivity, 92% specificity)

Indications:
1. Emboli can be detected in preexisting cardiopulmonary disease
2. Equivocal / indeterminate V/Q studies

TUMOR IMAGING

Positron Emission Tomography

Dose: 10 mCi FDG

Technique:
- patient fasts for 4 hours
  ◊ Elevated serum glucose may cause a decrease in FDG uptake!
- imaging 30–60 minutes after IV injection in 30–45 image planes (15 cm axial field of view; resolution of 5 mm)
- calculation of standardized uptake ratio (SUR) in region of interest (ROI) = mean activity in ROI [mCi/mL] divided by injected dose [mCi]

◊ SUR >2.5 indicates malignant disease

Indications:
(1) Focal pulmonary abnormality
accurate differentiation of benign and malignant lesions as small as 1 cm
√ low FDG uptake = benign
√ increased FDG uptake = cancer, active TB, histoplasmosis, rheumatoid nodule
(2) Staging lung cancer
◊ Occult metastases detected in up to 40% of cases!
(a) intrathoracic lymph nodes
√ lymph node with short-axis diameter > 1 cm by CT + not FDG avid = 100% NPV
√ small lymph node by CT + intense FDG uptake = 100% PPV
(b) adrenal metastasis: 100% sensitive, 80% specific
(3) Recurrent disease
√ increased FDG uptake at sites of residual radiographic abnormality >8 weeks after completion of therapy

QUANTITATIVE LUNG PERFUSION IMAGING

Indication:
determination of postresection pulmonary function when combined with pulmonary function testing (FEV_1)

Technique:
1. Acquire posterior and anterior perfusion (MAA) image and calculate geometric mean
2. Separate into right + left and into 2 equal lung zones from top to bottom, which yields 4 segments (upper left, bottom right, etc)

Result:
activity in each segment is compared with total activity, which yields % perfusion to each lung field

Unilateral Lung Perfusion

Incidence: 2%

A. PULMONARY EMBOLISM (23%)
B. AIRWAY DISEASE
(a) Unilateral pleural / parenchymal disease (23%)
(b) Bronchial obstruction
1. Bronchogenic carcinoma (23%)
2. Bronchial adenoma
3. Aspirated endobronchial foreign body
C. CONGENITAL HEART DISEASE (15%)
D. ARTERIAL DISEASE
1. Swyer-James syndrome (8%)
2. Congenital pulmonary artery hypoplasia / stenosis
3. Shunt procedure to pulmonary artery (eg, Blalock-Taussig)
E. ABSENT LUNG
1. Pneumonectomy (8%)
2. Unilateral pulmonary agenesis

mnemonic: "SAFE POEM"
Swyer-James syndrome
Agenesis (pulmonary)
Fibrosis (mediastinal)
Effusion (pleural)
Pneumonectomy, **P**neumothorax
Obstruction by tumor
Embolus (pulmonary)
Mucous plug

Perfusion Defects

A. VASCULAR DISEASE
(a) Acute / previous pulmonary embolus
1. Pulmonary thromboembolic disease
2. Fat embolism
√ nonsegmental perfusion defect
3. Air embolism
√ characteristic decortication appearance in uppermost portion on perfusion scintigraphy
4. Embolus of tumor / cotton wool / balloon for occlusion of AVM / obstruction by Swan-Ganz catheter, other foreign body
5. Dirofilaria immitis (dog heartworm): clumps of heartworms break off cardiac wall + embolize pulmonary arterial tree
6. Sickle cell disease
(b) Vasculitis
1. Collagen vascular disease: sarcoidosis
2. IV drug abuse
3. Previous radiation therapy:
√ defect localized to radiation port
4. Tuberculosis
(c) Vascular compression
1. Bronchogenic carcinoma:
√ perfusion defect depending on tumor size + location
2. Lymphoma / lymph node enlargement
3. Pulmonary artery sarcoma
4. Fibrosing mediastinitis due to histoplasmosis

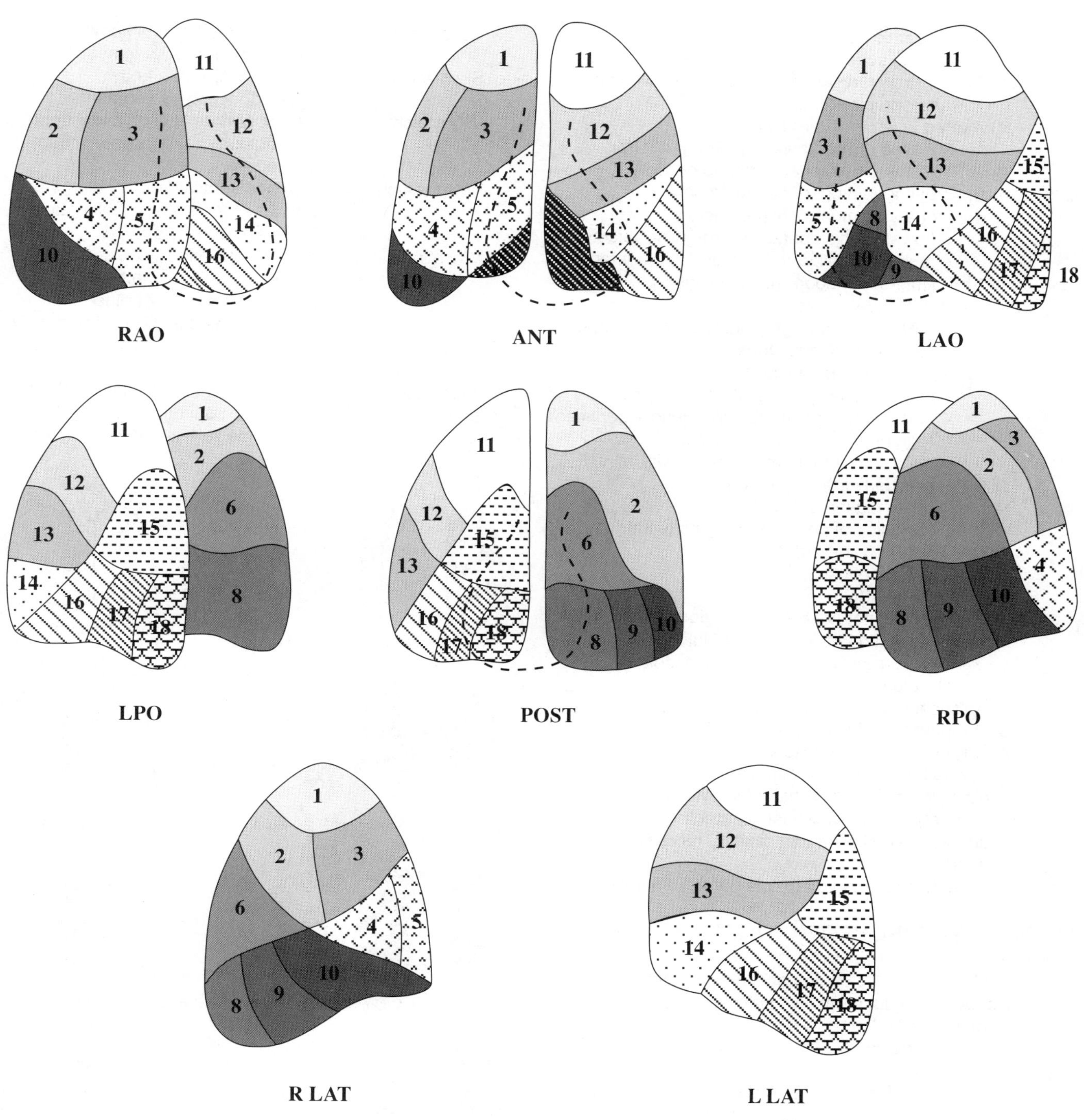

Lung Segments

RUL

1 apical
2 posterior
3 anterior

RML

4 lateral
5 medial

RLL

6 superior
7 mediobasal
8 posterobasal
9 laterobasal
10 anterobasal

LUL

11 apicoposterior
12 anterior
13 superior lingual
14 inferior lingual

LLL

15 superior
16 anteromedial basal
17 laterobasal
18 posterobasal

5. Idiopathic pulmonary fibrosis:
   √ small subsegmental defects in both lungs
6. Aortic aneurysm (large saccular / dissecting)
7. Intrathoracic stomach

(d) Altered pulmonary circulation
1. Absence / hypoplasia of pulmonary artery
2. Peripheral pulmonary artery stenosis
3. Bronchopulmonary sequestration
4. Primary pulmonary hypertension
   √ upward redistribution + large hilar defects
   √ multiple small peripheral perfusion defects
5. Pulmonary venoocclusive disease
6. Mitral valve disease
   √ predilection for right middle lobe + superior segments of lower lobes
7. Congestive heart failure
   √ diffuse nonsegmental VQ mismatch
   √ enlargement of cardiac silhouette + perihilar regions
   √ reversed distribution: more activity anteriorly than posteriorly
   √ accentuation of fissures
   √ flattening of posterior margins of lung (lateral view)
   √ pleural effusion

B. AIRWAY DISEASE
◊ Nearly all pulmonary disease produces decreased pulmonary blood flow to affected lung zones!
1. Asthma, chronic bronchitis, bronchospasm, mucus plugging
2. Bronchiectasis (bronchiolar destruction)
3. Emphysema (bulla / cyst)
4. Pneumonia / lung abscess
5. Lymphangitic carcinomatosis

√ perfusion defects in area of hypoxia (autoregulatory reflex vasoconstriction)
√ abnormal ventilation to a similar / more severe degree
√ mostly nonanatomic multiple defects (in 20%)

PULMONARY THROMBOEMBOLISM

Rationale for ventilation-perfusion scan:

◊ A pulmonary embolus presents as segmentally hypoperfused but normally ventilated lung (V/Q mismatch).
◊ A normal perfusion scan excludes an embolus for practical purposes.
◊ A perfusion defect requires further evaluation with a ventilation scan and CXR to determine the most likely etiology.
◊ If ventilation scan and CXR are normal an embolus must be suspected.
◊ A ventilation scan detects obstructive lung disease because a CXR is insensitive for this entity.

Terminology:

Nonsegmental = does not conform to a lung segment (eg, enlarged hilar structures / aorta, small pleural effusion, elevated hemidiaphragm, cardiomegaly);

Subsegmental = involves 25–75% of a known bronchopulmonary segment;

Segmental = involves >75% of a known bronchopulmonary segment;

V/Q match = area of abnormal ventilation identical to perfusion defect in size, shape, and location;

Triple match = matched ventilation-perfusion defect with an associated matching area of increased opacity on CXR;

V/Q mismatch = normal ventilation / normal CXR in region of perfusion defect or perfusion defect larger than ventilation defect / CXR abnormality;

Probabilities:

high = >85%

intermediate = perfusion abnormality falling short of diagnostic confidence for PE (eg, single segmental mismatch);

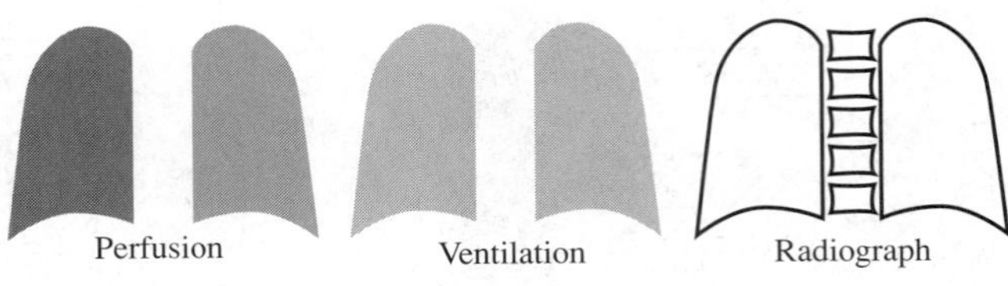

Normal

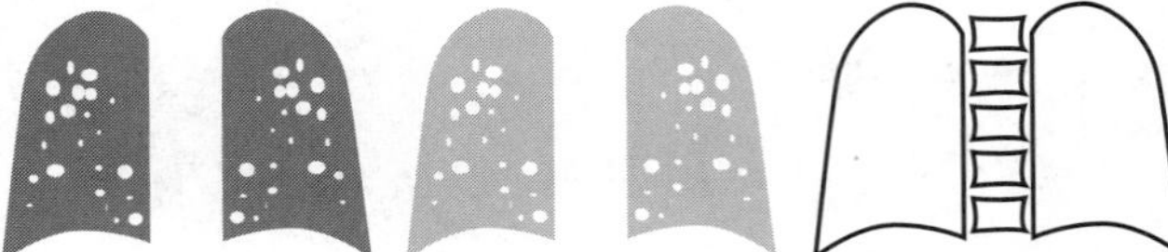
Matching nonsegmental V/Q defects & normal CXR = **low probability**

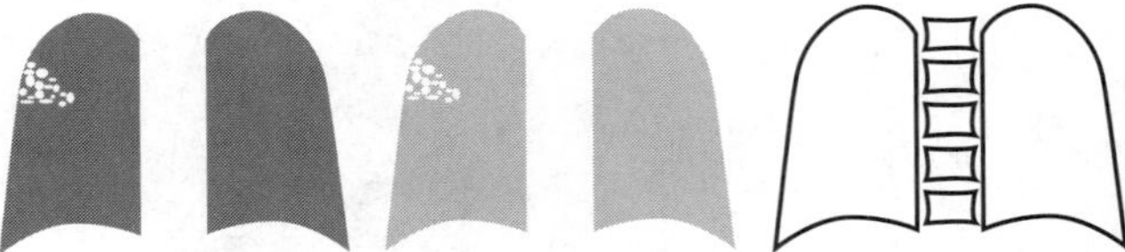
No definite V/Q mismatch & normal CXR = **moderate probability**

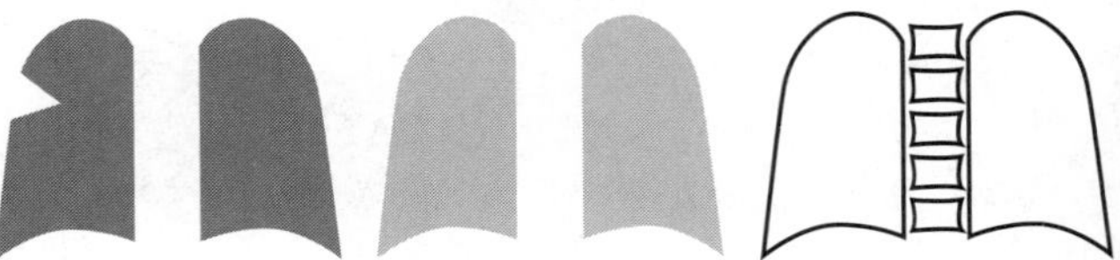
Segmental perfusion defect & normal ventilation = **high probability**

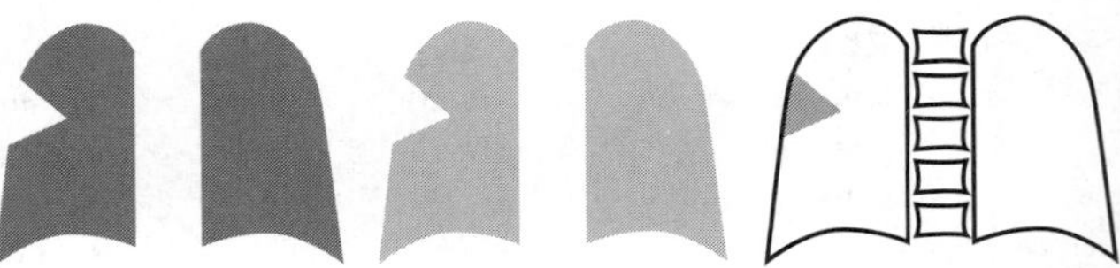
Matching segmental V/Q defect & CXR opacity = **indeterminate**

Interpretation Criteria for V/Q Lung Scans		
Probability of PE	*Modified Biello Criteria*	*Modified PIOPED Criteria*
Normal	√ normal perfusion	√ normal perfusion
Low (0–19%)	√ small (<25% segment) V/Q mismatches √ focal V/Q matches without corresponding CXR consolidation √ perfusion defects substantially smaller than CXR abnormality	√ small perfusion defects regardless of number / ventilation scan finding / CXR finding √ perfusion defect substantially smaller than CXR abnormality; ventilation findings irrelevant √ V/Q match in ≤50% of one lung / ≤75% of upper / mid / lower lung zone; CXR normal / nearly normal √ single moderate perfusion defect with normal CXR; ventilation findings irrelevant √ nonsegmental perfusion defects
Indeterminate Intermediate (25 – 50%)	√ severe COPD with perfusion defects √ perfusion defect with corresponding CXR consolidation of √ single moderate / large V/Q mismatch without corresponding CXR abnormality	√ 1 large(segmental) ± 1 moderate (subsegmental) V/Q mismatch √ 1–3 moderate (subsegmental) V/Q mismatches √ 1 matched V/Q with normal CXR
High (>85%)	√ perfusion defects substantially larger than CXR abnormalities √ ≥2 moderate (25–90% segment) / ≥2 large (>90% segment) V/Q mismatches; no corresponding CXR abnormality	√ ≥2 large (segmental) perfusion defects without match √ >2 large (segmental) perfusion defects substantially larger than matching ventilation / CXR abnormality √ ≥2 moderate (subsegmental) + 1 large (segmental) perfusion defect without match √ ≥4 moderate (subsegmental) perfusion defects; ventilation + CXR findings normal

indeterminate = lungs cannot be adequately evaluated because of underlying consolidation / obstructive disease
low = <15%

Perfusion images will detect:
(a) 90% of emboli that completely occlude a vessel >1 mm in diameter
(b) 90% of surface perfusion defects that are larger than 2 x 2 cm
(c) 26% of emboli that partially occlude a vessel
- A history of prior PE decreases probability of acute embolism because small V/Q mismatches never resolve!

Therapeutic implications:
(a) high probability scan : treat for PE
(b) indeterminate scan : pulmonary angiogram
(c) low probability scan : consider other diagnosis, unless clinical suspicion very high

Interpretative algorithm:
- no perfusion defect
  Diagnosis: normal
  Interpretation: no PE
- perfusion defect without lung disease (= normal ventilation + normal CXR = V/Q mismatch)
  Diagnosis: PE
  Interpretation: high probability for PE, >1 perfusion defect needed to increase certainty
- perfusion defect with lung disease
  (a) ventilation abnormality + clear CXR:
  Diagnosis: COPD
  Interpretation: low probability for PE
  (b) absent ventilation + consolidation on CXR:
  Diagnosis: lung infarction / pneumonia / atelectasis
  Interpretation: indeterminate

Probability of PE:
PIOPED (Prospective Investigation of Pulmonary Embolism Diagnosis) study results:

Probability of PE	*in*	*Angiogram Positive in*
High	13%	88%
Intermediate	39%	33%
Low	34%	16%
Normal	14%	9%

Effect of a priori suspicion for pulmonary embolus
— increased in patients with risk factors (immobilization, recent surgery, known hypercoagulable state, malignancy, previous pulmonary embolus, DVT, estrogen therapy)
— incidence of PE for a low probability scan increases from 15% to 40% in patients with a high clinical risk!

Overall accuracy:
68% for perfusion scan only,
84% for ventilation-perfusion scan
◊ 100% sensitivity in detection of PE is due to the occurrence of multiple emboli (usually >6–8), at least one of which causes a perfusion defect!
◊ A normal perfusion scan virtually excludes PE!
◊ In an individual <45 years of age a subsegmental perfusion defect + pleuritic chest pain in the same region is indicative of pulmonary embolism in 77%! (DDx: idiopathic / viral pleurisy)
◊ 73–82% of patients have equivocal perfusion scans (ie, low and intermediate probability)!
◊ Interobserver variability for intermediate- and low-probability scans is 30%!

False-positive scans: nonthrombotic emboli, IV drug abuse, vasculitis, redistribution of flow, acute asthma (due to mucus plugging)
False-negative scans: saddle embolus

√ "stripe sign" = rim of preserved peripheral activity to a perfusion defect usually indicates
(a) nonembolic cause
(b) old / resolving pulmonary embolism

Indications for pulmonary angiography:
1. Embolectomy is a therapeutic option
2. Indeterminate V/Q scan with high clinical suspicion + risky anticoagulation therapy
3. Specific diagnosis necessary for proper management (vasculitis, drug induced, lung cancer with predominant vascular involvement)

TEMPORAL RESOLUTION
(1) abnormality resolves within weeks / months (in most)
(2) abnormality may last permanently
◊ Baseline study necessary to detect new emboli!

CORRELATION WITH CXR:
(CXR should be taken within 6–12 hours of scan)

CXR Category	*Nondiagnostic V/Q Scan*
No acute abnormality	12%
Linear atelectasis	12%
Pulmonary edema	12%
Pleural effusion	36%
Parenchymal consolidation	82%

Criteria for Very Low Probability Interpretation of V/Q Lung Scans (<10% PPV for thromboembolism)

Criterion	*PPV [%]*
Nonsegmental perfusion abnormality	8
Perfusion defect smaller than corresponding radiographic defect	8
Stripe sign	7
Triple matched defect in upper / middle lung zone	4
Matched ventilation-perfusion defects in 2 / 3 zones of a single lung + normal CXR	3
1 to 3 small segmental perfusion defects	1

Indeterminate V/Q Lung Scans

Criterion	*PPV [%]*
Q defect << CXR consolidation	14
Q defect equal to CXR	26
Q defect >> CXR consolidation	89

√ focal lung opacity + not ventilated + not perfused = "indeterminate scan"
Cause: pneumonia, pulmonary embolism with infarction, segmental atelectasis
√ perfusion defect larger than CXR opacity = high probability for PE
√ perfusion defect substantially smaller than CXR opacity = low probability for PE
√ perfusion defect of comparable size = intermediate probability
√ focal lung opacity (not changed >1 week) + not ventilated + not perfused = low probability for PE
◊ When there is lung opacity, evaluate well-aerated areas for perfusion defects!
◊ COPD does not diminish usefulness of V/Q scan, but does increase likelihood of an indeterminate result!
◊ 75% of patients with pulmonary edema + without pulmonary embolism have a normal perfusion scan!

INFLUENCE OF CLINICAL ESTIMATE:

V/Q scan	*Clinical Probability*	*PE Present*
High-probability	>80%	96%
Low-probability	<20%	4%
Indeterminate	DVT present	93%

INFLUENCE OF CARDIOPULMONARY DISEASE (CPD):

V/Q Probability	*Normal CXR*	*No prior CPD*	*Any prior CPD*	*COPD*
High	67%	93%	83%	100%
Intermediate	24%	39%	26%	22%
Low	17%	15%	14%	6%
Near normal	3%	4%	4%	0%

HEART SCINTIGRAPHY

CARDIAC IMAGING CHOICES

1. PLANAR imaging
   - √ tracer defect may be visible on only one image projection
   - √ 15–20% regional tracer intensity variation is normal

2. SPECT imaging
   improves object contrast by removing overlying tissues; cinematic display of wall motion; EF calculation
   - √ tracer defect should be visible on more than one image set
   - √ up to 30% regional tracer intensity reduction compared with peak activity is normal

   (a) Standard
   180° acquisition extending from 45° RAO to 45° LPO for single-head camera

   (b) Gated SPECT
   tomographic data acquired gated to ECG (8 frames per cardiac cycle)
   - √ viable although hypoperfused myocardium may demonstrate systolic contraction + wall thickening
   - √ geometric EF calculation based on ROIs drawn on end-systolic + end-diastolic frames (different from blood pool scans)

3. QUANTITATIVE analysis
   = circumferential profiles
   = plotting of average counts along equally spaced radii emanating from center of LV makes interpretation more objective + reproducible

LEFT VENTRICULAR ANATOMY AND PROJECTIONS

A. AP
   - √ displays anterolateral wall, apex, inferior wall
   - √ decreased activity at apex of LV due to thinning in 50%

B. LEFT LATERAL
   - √ displays inferior + anterior wall

C. LAO 40° / LAO 70°
   - ◊ Most often used projection; for all exercise studies
   - √ displays interventricular septum, posterior wall, inferior wall
   - √ best projection to separate right + left ventricles
   - √ best projection to evaluate septal + posterior LV wall motion

D. RAO 45°
   - √ displays anterior + inferior ventricular wall
   - √ useful during 1st-pass studies with temporal separation of ventricles

E. LPO 45° (rarely used)
   10° caudal tilt minimizes LA contamination of LV region
   - √ displays anterior + inferior ventricular wall
   - √ preferred over RAO 45° because LV is closer to camera

F. Angled LAO (slant-hole collimator / caudal tilt)
   - √ separates ventricular from atrial activity
   - √ highlights apical dyskinesis

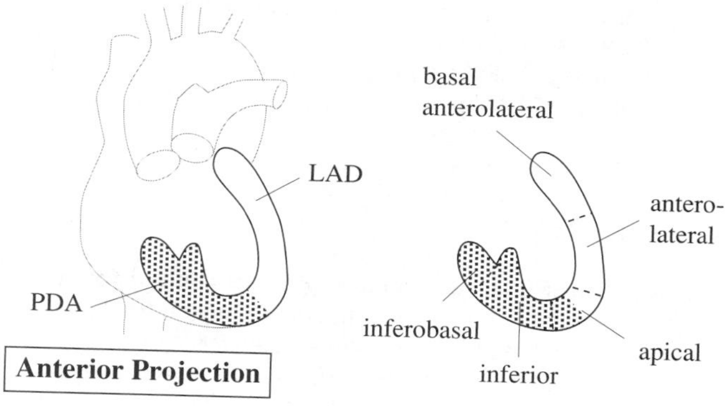

Anterior Projection

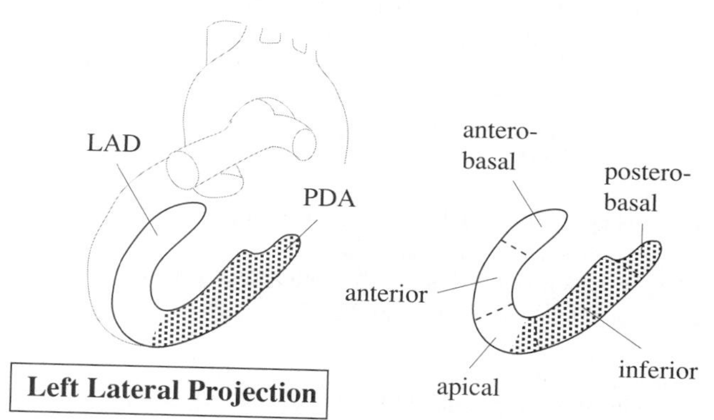

Left Lateral Projection

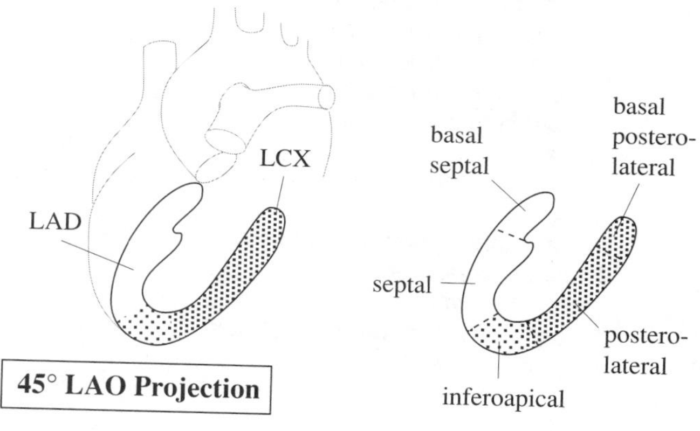

45° LAO Projection

Planar Reconstruction Planes

LAD supplies:	upper 2/3 of interventricular septum, anterior wall + part of lateral wall, apex of left ventricle (in most patients)
LCX supplies:	posterior portion of left ventricle (in 10%) lateral portion of left ventricle
RCA supplies:	lower 1/3 of interventricular septum, inferior wall of LV + entire RV
PDA supplies:	(through RCA) posterior wall (in 90%)

NucMed

MYOCARDIAL ISCHEMIA & VIABILITY

Imaging of Coronary Artery Disease

(1) DIRECTLY with **myocardial perfusion imaging** providing a pictorial representation of the relative perfusion of viable myocardial tissue using exercise + rest physiology images
 (a) Tl-201 chloride SPECT imaging (92% sensitive, 68% specific)
 (b) Tc-99m sestamibi / tetrofosmin SPECT imaging (89% sensitive, 90% specific)
 (c) PET

(2) INDIRECTLY with **imaging of ventricular function**, i.e., evaluation of wall motion + ejection fraction
 (a) multigated acquisition studies (MUGA)
  – Tc-99m–labeled RBCs
  – Tc-99m human serum albumin
 (b) first-pass radionuclide angiography
  – sodium pertechnetate
  – diethylenetriamine pentaacetic acid (DTPA)
  – sulfur colloid
  – gold-195 m
  – iridium-191m

(3) SIMULTANEOUS assessment of myocardial perfusion + ventricular function
 = first-pass radionuclide angiography + gated SPECT perfusion imaging

Interpretation:
Normal myocardium:
 √ homogeneous perfusion
 √ similar appearance at rest + with exercise
Ischemic viable myocardium:
 √ normal perfusion at rest
 √ relative hypoperfusion with exercise (= reversible defect)
 DDx:
  (1) Reversible septal defect in left bundle branch block
  (2) Differing soft-tissue attenuation artifact
Myocardial infarction:
 √ reduced muscle mass
 √ absent / reduced uptake at rest + with exercise (= fixed defect)
 DDx:
  (1) "Hibernating myocardium" = chronic myocardial hypoperfusion producing abnormal regional ventricular function
  (2) Soft-tissue attenuation artifacts
   √ marked variability in LV tracer uptake of inferior wall (diaphragmatic attenuation) + anterior wall (breast attenuation)
  (3) Infiltrative disorders

DDx of a mild fixed defect:
 (1) Scar
 (2) Hibernating myocardium
 (3) Attenuation artifact

Location of Perfusion Defects on Planar Images

(1) Right coronary artery (RCA)
 best seen on left LAT / AP projections
 √ inferior + posteroseptal segments
(2) Circumflex branch of left coronary artery (LCX)
 best seen on LAO projection
 √ posterolateral segment
(3) Anterior descending branch of left coronary artery (LAD)
 √ anteroseptal, anterior, anterolateral segments

N.B.: decreased activity in apical + posterior segments is not reliably correlated with disease of any vessel!

Myocardial Viability Assessment

1. Perfusion
 Tl-201 rest injection with redistribution images preferable to sestamibi
 √ uptake >50% of maximum
2. Metabolic activity
 FDG may provide best assessment (normal myocardium uses fatty acids as chief metabolic substrate, but can switch to glucose metabolism)
 √ enhanced glucose uptake by ischemic but viable myocardium

EJECTION FRACTION

Ejection fraction (EF) = stroke volume (SV) divided by end-diastolic volume (EDV)

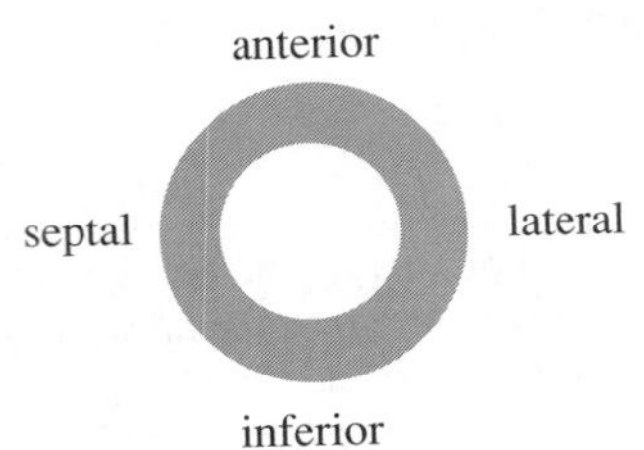

Short Axis

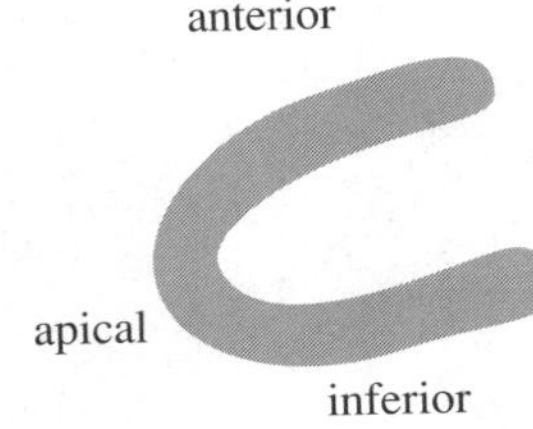

Vertical Long Axis

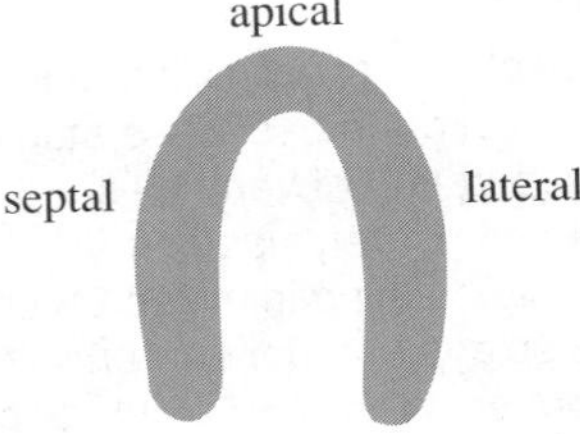

Horizontal Long Axis

SPECT Reconstruction Planes

stroke volume = end-diastolic volume (EDV) minus end-systolic volume (ESV)

$$EF = [EDV - ESV] / [EDV]$$

$$= [ED_{counts} - ES_{counts}] / [ED_{counts} - BKG_{counts}]$$

sensitive indicator of left ventricular function

@ Left ventricle
- calculated on shallow LAO view

Normal value	50–65% (5% variation)
Definitely abnormal	<50%
Hypertrophic myocardium	>65%

◊ Peak exercise LVEF is an independent predictor of coronary artery disease

@ Right ventricle
mean normal value >45%
(RV ejection fraction is smaller than for LV because RV has greater EDV than LV but the same stroke volume)

Accuracy in detection of coronary artery disease:
(a) Exercise EF: 87% sensitivity; 92% specificity
(b) Exercise ECG: 60% sensitivity; 81% specificity

Interpretation:
◊ Ventricular function at rest is insensitive to CAD!
(1) at rest
√ EF may be decreased in CAD
DDx: cardiomyopathy, valvular disease
√ correlates well with clinical severity + regional distribution of myocardial infarction
(2) during exercise
√ reduced (hypokinetic) / absent (akinetic) / paradoxical (dyskinetic) wall motion indicate varying degrees of CAD / myocardial infarction
√ focal akinetic / dyskinetic area = aneurysm
√ paradoxical septal motion (= septal movement to right in systole) may reflect septal infarction, left bundle branch block, after bypass surgery

Shortcoming:
poor study in patients with atrial fibrillation because of inability to achieve adequate cardiac gating (exercise MUGA can yield more sensitive assessment of coronary artery disease)
False-positive with (a) inadequate exercise
(b) recent ingestion of meal

BLOOD POOL AGENTS

Tc-99m DTPA / Tc-99m Sulfur Colloid

preferred for cardiac first-pass studies as they allow multiple studies with little residual from any preceding study

Tc-99m–labeled Autologous RBCs

= agent of choice because of good heart-to-lung ratio

Technique:
(1) IN VIVO LABELING
- IV injection of reducing agent stannous pyrophosphate (1 vial PYP diluted with 2 mL sterile saline = 15 mg sodium pyrophosphate containing 3.4 mg anhydrous stannous chloride)
- 15–20–30 minutes later injection of Tc-99m pertechnetate (+7), which binds to "pretinned" RBCs (reduction to Tc-99m [+4])

◊ Least time-consuming + easiest method!
◊ Worst labeling efficiency (30% not tagged to RBCs + excreted in urine)!

(2) IN VIVTRO LABELING
= MODIFIED IN VIVO METHOD
◊ Preferred over in vivo because of high labeling efficiency within syringe, which reduces exposure to plasma constituents + creates little free pertechnetate!
- IV injection of 1 mg stannous pyrophosphate
- 10 minutes later 2–5–10 mL of blood are drawn into a heparinized syringe
- 10–20-minute incubation period with Tc-99m pertechnetate
- reinjection of preparation in 3-way stopcock technique

N.B.: poor tagging in
(a) heparinized patient
(b) injection through IV line (adherence to wall)
(c) syringe flushed with dextrose instead of saline

(3) IN VITRO LABELING
◊ Most reliable labeling method!
- 50 mL drawn blood incubated with Tc-99m reduced by stannous ion; RBCs washed and reinjected

N.B.: Labeling kit (with chelating + oxidizing substances) allows excellent in vitro labeling with only 3 mL of blood and 15-minute incubation period!

Dose: 15–20–30 mCi (larger dose required for stress MUGA + obese patients);
for children: 200 μCi/kg (minimum dose of 2–3 mCi)
Radiation dose: 1.5 rad for heart, 1.0 rad for blood, 0.4 rad for whole body

Tc-99m HSA

HSA = human serum albumin
Indication: drug interference with RBC labeling (eg, heparinized patient)
Physiology: (a) albumin slowly equilibrates throughout extracellular space
(b) poorer heart-to-lung ratio than with labeled RBCs

VENTRICULAR FUNCTION

First-pass Ventriculography

= FIRST-PASS RADIONUCLIDE ANGIOGRAPHY = FIRST TRANSIT

= recording of initial transit time of an intravenously administered tight Tc-99m bolus through heart + lungs; limited number of cardiac cycles available for interpretation; additional projections / serial studies require additional bolus injection

Accuracy: good correlation with contrast ventriculography

Agents: pertechnetate, pyrophosphate, albumin, DTPA, sulfur colloid (almost any Tc-99m–labeled compound except lung scanning particles), Tc-99m–labeled autologous RBCs

Indications:

(1) Only 15 seconds of patient cooperation required
(2) Calculation of cardiac output + ejection fraction (RBCs)
(3) Subsequent first-pass studies within 15–20 minutes of initial study possible (DTPA)
(4) Separate assessment of individual cardiac chambers in RAO projection (temporal separation without overlying atria, pulmonary artery, aortic outflow tract), eg, for right ventricular EF and intracardiac shunts

Minimal dose: 10 mCi

Technique:

- cannulation of antecubital / external jugular vein with ≥20 ga needle attached to 3-way stopcock and two syringes:
  - syringe 1 contains ≤1 mL of radiotracer
  - syringe 2 contains a saline flush (10–20 mL)
- injection of radiotracer is followed by a strong flush of saline

Gating:

Improved images obtained by selection of time interval corresponding only to RV passage of bolus averaged over several (3–5) individual beats; gating may be done intrinsically or with ECG guidance

Imaging:

Region of interest (ROI) over RV silhouette in RAO projection; background activity taken over horseshoe-shaped ventricular wall; counts in ROI displayed as function of time; 25 frames/second for 20–30 seconds

Normal passage of bolus: SVC, RA, RV, lungs, LA, LV, aorta

R-to-L shunt: tracer appears in left side of heart before passage through lungs

Evaluation of:

1. Obstruction in SVC region
2. Reflux from RA into IVC / jugular vein
3. Stenosis in pulmonary outflow tract
4. R-L shunt
5. Contractility of RV
6. Sequential beating of RA and RV
7. Ejection fraction of RV and LV

Equilibrium Images

= "blood pool" radionuclide angiography

Agents: Tc-99m–labeled autologous RBCs (most commonly) / human serum albumin

Imaging: after thorough mixing of radiotracer throughout vascular space

- acquisition of images during selected portions of cardiac cycle triggered by R-wave; each image is composed of >200,000 counts (2–10 minutes) obtained over 500–1,000 beats after equilibrium has been reached; high-quality images can be obtained in different projections
- gated acquisition from 16–32 equal subdivisions of the R-R cycle (electronic bins) allows display of synchronized cinematic images (assembled to composite single-image sequence) of an "average" cardiac cycle
  √ may be displayed as time activity curves reflecting changes in ventricular counts throughout R-R interval
  — measured functional indices: preejection period (PEP), left ventricular ejection time (LVET), left ventricular fast filling time ($LVFT_1$), left ventricular slow filling time ($LVFT_2$), PEP/LVET ratio, rate of ejection + filling of LV
- at rest: count density 200–250 counts/pixel requires generally 7–10 minutes acquisition time for 200,000–250,000 counts/frame
- during exercise: 100,000–150,000 counts/frame requires an acquisition time of 2 minutes

Evaluation of:

1. LV ejection fraction
2. Regional wall motion
3. Valvular regurgitation

Interpretation:

1. Heart failure: decreased EF, prolongation of PEP, shortening of LVET, decreased rate of ejection
2. Hypertensive heart: normal systolic indices, normal EF, prolonged LVT_1
3. Hypothyroidism: prolonged PEP, normal EF
4. Aortic stenosis: mild reduction of EF, prolonged LV emptying time, decreased rate of ejection, normal rate of filling

√ area of decreased periventricular uptake secondary to
(a) pleural effusion >100 mL
(b) ventricular hypertrophy

Gated Blood Pool Imaging

= MULTIPLE GATED ACQUISITION (MUGA)
= gated equilibrium images depict average cardiac contraction by summation over several minutes

Recording of:

(1) Ejection fraction (EF) of left ventricle before + after exercise (>6 million counts, 32 frames)
(2) Regional wall motion of ventricular chambers (>4.5 million counts, 24 frames)
  (a) at rest : myocardial infarction, aneurysm, contusion
  (b) during exercise : ischemic dyskinesia (detectable in 63%)

(3) Regurgitant index

Projection:

(a) best septal view (usually LAO 45°) for EF; often requires some cephalad tilting of detector head

(b) two additional views for evaluation of wall motion (usually anterior + left lateral views)

Imaging:

Physiologic trigger provided by R-R interval of ECG ("bad beat" rejection program desirable); R-R interval divided into typically about 20 frames; several hundred cardiac contractions are summed (depending on count density) for each planar projection

(a) gated images obtained for 5 minutes

(b) 2-minute image acquisition time for each stage of exercise

PROs: (1) Higher information density than 1st-pass method

(2) Assessment of pharmacologic effect possible

(3) "Bad beat" rejection possible

CONs: (1) Significant background activity

(2) Inability to monitor individual chambers in other than LAO 45° projection

(3) Plane of AV valve difficult to identify

Radiation dose: 1.5 rad for heart; 1.0 rad for blood; 0.4 rad for whole body

Qualitative evaluation:

(1) chamber size

(2) wall thickness

(3) regional wall motion

MYOCARDIAL PERFUSION IMAGING AGENTS

Potassium-43

Not suitable for clinical use because of its high energy

Thallium-201 Chloride

= cation produced in cyclotron from stable Tl-203

= image agent of choice to assess myocardial viability

Cyclotron: by (p,3n) reaction to radioactive Pb-201 (half-life of 9.4 hours), which decays by electron capture to Tl-201

Decay: by electron capture to Hg-201

Energy spectrum: 69–83 keV of Hg-K x-rays (98% abundance); 135 keV (2%) + 167 keV (8% abundance) gamma photons

Physical half-life: 74 hours

Biologic half-life: 10 ± 2.5 days

Dose: low dose of 3–4 mCi (the larger dose for SPECT) because of long half-life and slow body clearance

Radiation dose:

3 rad for kidneys (critical organ) (1.2 rad/mCi); 1.2 rad for gonads (0.6 rad/mCi); 0.7 rad for heart + marrow (0.34 rad/mCi); 0.5 rad for whole body (0.24 rad/mCi)

Quality control: should contain <0.25% Pb-203, <0.5% Tl-202 (439 keV)

Indications:

1. Acute myocardial infarction
2. Coronary artery disease

particularly useful over ECG in:

(a) conduction disturbances (eg, bundle branch block, preexitation syndrome)

(b) previous infarction

(c) under drug influence (eg, digitalis)

(d) left ventricular hypertrophy

(e) hyperventilation

(f) ST depression without symptoms

(g) if stress ECG impossible to obtain

Thallium uptake & distribution

– intracellular uptake via Na/K-ATPase (analogue to ionic potassium), but less readily released from cells than potassium

– distribution is proportional to regional blood flow

– uptake depends on

(1) quality of regional perfusion

(2) viable cells with integrity of Na/K pump

@ Blood pool

<5% remain in blood pool 15 minutes post injection

@ Myocardium

uptake depends on

(a) myocardial perfusion

(b) myocardial mass

(c) myocardial cellular integrity

◊ First-pass extraction efficiency is 88%! REMEMBER: 90% in 90 seconds!

– 4% of total dose localizes in myocardium at rest (myocardial blood flow = 4% of cardiac output)

– peak myocardial activity occurs at 5–15 minutes after injection

– uptake can be increased to 8–10% with dipyridamole stress

– clearance from myocardium is proportional to regional perfusion + begins within a few minutes after injection ("wash out"); zones of initially higher uptake wash out more rapidly than areas of low uptake (= "redistribution")

@ Skeletal muscle + splanchnicus:

first-pass extraction efficiency is 65%

– accumulate 40% of injected dose

– 4–6 hours fast + exercise decreases flow to splanchnicus and increases cardiac uptake

@ Lung:

10% of total dose localizes in lung

– augmented pulmonary extraction with left ventricular dysfunction, bronchogenic carcinoma, lymphoma of lung

√ <5% activity over lung is normal

√ heart-to-lung ratio decreased with triple-vessel disease

@ Kidney:

accumulates 4% of injected dose

– excretion of 4–8% within 24 hours

@ Thyroid:

√ increased uptake >1% in Graves disease + thyroid carcinoma

@ Brain:

√ uptake only if blood-brain barrier disrupted

Technique:
A. Single dose method
- 3 mCi injected at peak exercise for exercise image immediately + rest image 3 hours later

B. Split dose method
- 2 mCi injected for exercise image
- 1 mCi reinjected at rest after 3 hours with rest image taken 30 minutes later

C. Booster reinjection technique
- reinjection of thallium followed by imaging after 18–24–72 hours augments blood concentration of isotope

= late reversibility provides evidence of regional myocardial ischemia + viability not appreciated even on very delayed (24–72 hours) redistribution images; predicts scintigraphic improvement post intervention
Reasoning: 50% of irreversible persistent defects improve significantly after booster reinjection

Imaging:
1. EXERCISE IMAGE = DISTRIBUTION IMAGE
   = stress thallium image
   = map of regional perfusion obtained within minutes after injection at peak exercise; initial distribution proportional to myocardial blood flow, arterial concentration of radioisotope, and muscle mass; 300,000–400,000 counts / view (approximately 5–8 minutes sampling time), should be completed by 30 minutes

2. REDISTRIBUTION IMAGE
   = equilibrium between tracer uptake and efflux dependent on blood flow + mass of viable tissue + concentration gradients
   = map of hypoperfused ischemic but viable myocardium obtained at rest after 2–3–4–6 hours; washout half-life from normal myocardium is 54 minutes

3. DELAYED IMAGE (optional)
   = viability study at 24 hours

Interpretation of Stress Thallium Images

Immediate Image	*Delayed Image*	*Diagnosis*
Normal	normal	normal
Defect	fill-in	exertional ischemia
Defect	persistent	myocardial scar
Defect	partial fill-in	scar + ischemia / persistent ischemia

Interpretation:
√ "apical thinning" = less myocardial mass of cardiac apex as a normal finding
√ normally diminished tracer uptake at basal portions of ventricle (near plane of mitral valve) due to more fibrous tissue + less muscle mass
√ variation in tracer intensity by 15–20% between regions on planar images may be normal (due to soft-tissue attenuation artifacts from subdiaphragmatic abdominal contents or breast tissue)

1. Initial phase = first-pass extraction
   √ temporary defect accentuated by exercise
   √ defect >15% of ventricular surface suggests >50% stenosis of coronary artery
   √ right heart well seen during stress test, tachycardia, volume / pressure overload
   √ dilated heart cavity on stress images (but not on rest images) due to exercise-induced LV dysfunction
2. Redistribution phase (on 2–4-hour images)
   √ washout in normal areas
   √ slow continued accumulation of tracer for areas of greatly reduced perfusion
   √ increased uptake in viable ischemic zones ("redistribution")
   √ permanent defect = nonviable myocardium as in myocardial infarction / fibrosis
   √ increased lung activity (ie, >50% of myocardial count) indicative of
   (a) left ventricular failure due to severe LCA disease / myocardial infarction
   (b) pulmonary venous hypertension due to cardiomyopathy / mitral valve disease
   √ right heart faintly visualized during rest (15% of perfusion to right side); increased activity in RV due to
   (a) increase in ventricular systolic pressure
   (b) increase in mean pulmonary artery pressure
   (c) increase in total pulmonary vascular resistance

Sensitivity: overall 82–84% for stress Tl-201 (60–62% for exercise ECG)
(a) increased with:
   (1) severity of stenosis (86% + 67% sensitive with stenosis >75% + <75%)
   (2) greater number of involved arteries
   (3) stenosis of left main > LAD > RCA > LXC
   (4) prior infarction
   (5) high work load during exercise testing in patients with single-vessel disease
(b) decreased with:
   (1) presence of collateral
   (2) beta blockers
   (3) time delay for poststress images

Specificity: overall 91–94% for stress Tl-201 (81–83% for exercise ECG)

False-positive thallium test (37–58%):
A. INFILTRATING MYOCARDIAL DISEASE
   1. Sarcoidosis
   2. Amyloidosis
B. CARDIAC DYSFUNCTION
   1. Cardiomyopathy
   2. IHSS

3. Valvular aortic stenosis
4. Mitral valve prolapse (rare)

C. DECREASED CARDIAC PERFUSION OTHER THAN MYOCARDIAL INFARCTION
1. Cardiac contusion
2. Myocardial fibrosis
3. Coronary artery spasm
(severe unstable angina may cause defect after stress + on redistribution images, but will be normal at rest!)

D. NORMAL VARIANT
1. Apical myocardial thinning
2. Attenuation due to diaphragm, breast, implant, pacemaker

mnemonic: "I'M SIC"
Idiopathic hypertrophic subaortic stenosis
Myocardial infarct without coronary artery disease
Scarring, **S**pasm, **S**arcoidosis
Infiltrative / metastatic lesion
Cardiomyopathy

False-negative thallium test:
1. Under influence of beta-blocker (eg, propranolol)
2. "Balanced ischemia" = symmetric 3-vessel disease
3. Insignificant obstruction
4. Inadequate stress
5. Failure to perform delayed imaging
6. Poor technique

mnemonic: "3NMRS COR"
3-vessel disease (rare)
Noncritical stenosis
Medications interfering
Right coronary lesion (isolated)
Submaximal exercise
Collateral (coronary) blood vessels
Overestimation of stenosis on angiography
Redistribution (early / delayed)

Advantages compared with Tc-99m compounds:
(1) Higher total accumulation in myocardium
(2) Provides redistribution information

Disadvantages:
(1) Low energy x-rays result in poor resolution (improved with SPECT)
(2) Dose is limited by its long half-life
(3) Half-value thickness of 3 cm results in less avid appearing myocardium: inferior wall (deeper part of myocardium) / anterolateral wall (overlain by breast)
(4) Imaging must be completed by 45 minutes post injection or redistribution occurs

Tc-99m MIBI (Sestamibi)

= cationic lipophilic isonitrile complex, which associates with myocyte mitochondria

Pharmacokinetics:
- relatively rapid clearance from circulation (40% first-pass extraction) due to passive diffusion across cell membranes
- high myocardial accumulation (4%) with nonlinear uptake proportional to regional perfusion (fall-off in extraction at higher rates of flow)
- slow washout with long retention time in myocardium and little recirculation
- significant hepatic + gallbladder activity

Excretion: through biliary tree (give milk after injection and before imaging to decrease GB activity)
Dose: 25–30 mCi (Cardiolite®)
Imaging: optimum images 1 hour after injection (may be imaged up until 3 hours)

Technique: separate injections for stress and rest studies because of slow washout

A. 1-DAY PROTOCOL (rest-stress protocol)
Improved detection of reversibility compared with stress-rest protocol
- inject of 5–8 mCi Tc-99m sestamibi
- rest images 60–90 minutes after injection
- wait 0–4 hours
- stress patient followed by injection of 15–25 mCi Tc-99m sestamibi at peak stress (increased myocardial blood flow means increased myocardial uptake)
- image 30–60 minutes later (optimum imaging time of stress-induced defects)

B. 2-DAY PROTOCOL (impractical stress-rest protocol):
- stress images on 1st day: Tc-99m sestamibi given at peak stress; imaging after 30–60 minutes' delay to allow some clearing of liver activity
- repeat on 2nd day if stress views abnormal

C. DUAL TRACER STRATEGY
- Tl-201 for initial injection
- Tc-99m sestamibi as 2nd injection immediately afterwards (as its higher energy photons are unaffected by residual Tl-201

Advantages over thallium:
(1) Low radiation dose related to shorter half-life allowing larger doses with less patient radiation
(2) Excellent imaging characteristics due to
(a) improved photon flux, which means faster imaging + ability for cardiac gating
(b) higher photon energy means less attenuation artifact from breast tissue / diaphragm + less scatter
(3) NO redistribution
(4) Temporal separation of injection and imaging allows injection during acute myocardial infarct when patient may not be stable for imaging; after stabilization + intervention (angioplasty / urokinase) imaging can demonstrate the pre-intervention defect
(5) Low cost
(6) Easy availability
(7) Flexible scheduling
(8) Increased patient throughput

Disadvantage: less well suited to assess viability

Tc-99m Teboroxime

= neutral boronic acid oxime complex

Pharmacokinetics:

- very rapid clearance time from circulation (rapid uptake by myocardium with high extraction efficiency)
- distribution proportional to cardiac blood flow EVEN at high blood flow levels (sestamibi + thallium plateau at high levels of flow)
- biexponential washout from myocardium
- high background from lung + liver

Dose: 25–30 mCi (Cardiotec®)

Imaging: must begin immediately post injection due to rapid washout; rest image can immediately follow stress image

Tc-99m Tetrofosmin

= diphosphine complex (Myoview®)

Related compounds: Q12 (furifosmin), Q3

Pharmacokinetics:

- lower first-pass extraction and accumulation than thallium
- slow myocardial washout
- rapid background clearance
- quicker liver excretion than sestamibi

Positron Emission Tomography

Perfusion agents: N-13 ammonia, O-15 water, Rb-82 (available from a strontium generator)

Metabolic agents: Fluorine-18-deoxyglucose = FDG (glycolysis), carbon-11-palmitate (beta-oxidation), carbon-11-acetate (tricarboxylic acid cycle)

Pathophysiology:

in myocardial ischemia glycolysis (utilization of glucose) increases while mitochondrial β-oxidation of fatty acids decreases!

Sensitivity: >95%

Technique:

- give oral glucose load
- inject 10 mCi FDG
- image after 30 minutes

Variation: simultaneously injection of perfusion tracer

Interpretation:

√ mismatched defect (= decreased perfusion but enhanced metabolism indicated by FDG uptake) indicates viable myocardium (= dysfunctional myocardium salvageable by revascularization procedure)

√ matched defect (= flow + FDG accumulation both decreased) indicate nonviable myocardium

◊ 80–90% of matching defects do not improve after bypass

√ 11-C-acetate superior to FDG (accurately reflects overall oxidation metabolism, not influenced by myocardial substrate utilization)

Comparison with thallium:

accuracy for fixed lesions similar; higher for reversible ischemia

STRESS TEST

Rationale:

◊ Rest-injected images can separate viable from nonviable myocardium + detect very severe ischemia (with stenosis of >90–95%), but cannot detect most coronary artery disease (CAD)!

Exercise increases myocardial work and oxygen requirement; at peak exercise blood flow may rise 5-fold from baseline through coronary artery dilatation + increase in heart rate; exercise will unveil CAD-related regional hypoperfusion relative to normal regions, if coronary artery stenosis >50%.

Physical Stress Test

◊ Exercise in erect position (peak heart rate lower if supine) on treadmill or bicycle; isometric handgrip exercise raises blood pressure less (but adequate for evaluation)

◊ Starting point of workload selected according to preliminary exercise results (at an average of 200 kilowatt pounds)

Bruce treadmill protocol:

- grade of exercise incrementally increased by inclination + belt speed (200 kilowatt pounds)
- graded exercise in 3-minute stages of increasing workload
- endpoints for discontinuing exercise:
  (1) attainment of 85% of predicted maximal heart rate = 220 – age in years
  (2) Inability to continue due to fatigue, dyspnea, leg cramps, dizziness, chest pain
  (3) Severe angina / hypotension
  (4) Severe ECG ischemic changes / arrhythmia
  (5) Fall in BP >10 mm Hg below previous stage
  (6) Ventricular tachycardia
  (7) Run of 3 successive premature ventricular beats
  ◊ Cardiologist with crash cart should be available!

Problems with exercise imaging:

(1) Sensitivity to detect ischemic lesions decreases with suboptimal exercise (in particular for older population)
(2) Higher false-positive tests in women (artifacts from overlying breast tissue)
(3) Propranolol (beta blocker) interferes with stress test, should be discontinued 24–48 hours prior to testing

Pharmacologic Stress Test

Advantages:

(1) Reproducibility
(2) Independent from patient motivation
(3) Freedom from patient infirmities, eg, severe peripheral vascular disease, arthritis, pain

NucMed

Drugs:

A. VASODILATORS

Action: binding to A2 receptors affects the intracellular cyclic AMP, GMP, and calcium levels resulting in coronary hyperemia

N.B.: Discontinue use of caffeine, tea, chocolate, cola drinks for 24 hours prior to test

◊ Cannot be used in patients on theophylline!

(1) IV infusion of 140 μg/kg/min dipyridamole (= Persantine®) causes 3–5-fold increase in coronary artery blood flow

Total dose: 0.84 mg/kg

Drug action: 30 minutes

Side effects: flushing, nausea, bronchospasm (reversible with aminophylline)

- dipyridamole injection over 4 minutes
- wait 10 minutes for maximum effect
- inject radiotracer

◊ Prolonged supervision after test necessary

(2) IV infusion of 140 μg/kg/min adenosine (= Adenocard®, Adenoscan®)

Drug action: 2–3 minutes (half life of 15 seconds)

Side effects: flushing, nausea, transient AV block, bronchospasm

Drug reversal: theophylline

- continuous IV infusion for 3 minutes
- radiotracer injection
- continue infusion for additional 3 minutes

◊ Supervision after test not needed

Contraindication: significant pulmonary disease requiring use of inhalers

B. INOTROPES

Action: beta-1 agonist increasing myocardial contractility + work thus oxygen demand

Candidates: patients with COPD, asthma, allergy to vasodilators, patients on theophylline preparations

(1) IV infusion of 5 μg/kg/min dobutamine for 5 minutes, increased in steps of 5 μg/kg every 5 minutes to a maximum infusion rate of 30–40 μg/kg/min titrated to patient's response

- radiotracer injected at onset of significant symptoms / ECG changes / achievement of maximal rate of infusion or heart rate
- infusion maintained for an additional 2 minutes with dose adjusted to patient's condition

(2) IV infusion of arbutamine with its own computerized delivery system titrating dose rate automatically

Contraindication: severe hypertension, atrial flutter / fibrillation

Applied to:

1. THALLIUM IMAGING (redistribution images after stress test):
   - injection of 1.5–2 mCi of Tl-201 during peak exercise, continuation of exercise for additional 60 seconds before imaging commences

   Clues for stress images:

   √ RV myocardium well visualized

   √ little pulmonary background activity

   √ little activity in liver, stomach, spleen

   √ distribution more uniform after stress than during rest

   ◊ Degree of liver uptake useful as direct measure of level of exercise!

   Sources of technical errors:

   mnemonic: "ABCDE PS"

   Attenuation from overlying breast / diaphragm

   Background oversubtraction

   Camera field nonuniformity

   Drugs, **D**elayed (excessively) imaging, **D**ose infiltration

   Eating / **E**xercising between stress + delayed images

   Positioning variation between stress + delayed images

   Submaximal exercise
2. GATED BLOOD POOL IMAGING (response of EF)

   √ increase in ejection fraction from 63–93% in normals

   √ increase in ventricular wall motion (anterolateral > posterolateral > septal)

INFARCT-AVID IMAGING

= hot spot imaging

Agent: Tc-99m pyrophosphate (standard), Hg-203 chlormerodrin, Tc-99m tetracycline, Tc-99m glucoheptonate, F-18 sodium fluoride, Indium-111 antimyosin (murine monoclonal antibodies to myosin), Tc-99m antimyosin Fab fragment

Tc-99m Pyrophosphate

Pathophysiology in MYOCARDIAL INFARCTION:

Pyrophosphate is taken up by myocardial necrosis through complexation with calcium deposits >10–12 hours post infarction

- requires presence of residual collateral blood flow
- 30–40% maximum accumulation in hypoxic cells with a 60–70% reduction in blood flow (greater levels of occlusion reduce uptake)

Uptake post infarction:

- earliest uptake by 6–12–24 hours;
- peak uptake by 48–72 hours;
- persistent uptake seen up to 5–7 days with return to normal by 10–14 days

Sensitivity: 90% for transmural infarction, 40–50% for subendocardial (nontransmural) infarction

Specificity: as low as 64%

Dose: 15–20 mCi IV (minimal count requirement of 500,000/view)

Imaging: at 3–6 hours (60% absorbed by skeleton within 3 hours)

Indications:
1. Lost enzyme pattern = patient admitted 24–48 hours after infarction
2. Equivocal ECG + atypical angina:
   (a) left ventricular bundle branch block
   (b) left ventricular hypertrophy
   (c) impossibility to perform stress test
   (d) patient on digitalis
3. ST depression without symptoms
4. Equivocal enzyme pattern + equivocal symptoms
5. S/P cardiac surgery (perioperative infarction in 10%, enzymes routinely elevated, ECG always abnormal), requires preoperative baseline study as 40% are preoperatively abnormal
6. For detection of right ventricular infarction

NOT HELPFUL:
1. In differentiating multiple- from single-vessel disease
2. Typical angina
3. Normal ECG stress test + NO symptoms

Scan interpretation:
[Grade 2+ and above are positive]

Grade 0	no activity
Grade 1+	faint uptake
Grade 2+	slightly less than sternum, equal to ribs
Grade 3+	equal to sternum
Grade 4+	greater than sternum

√ "doughnut" pattern = central cold defect (necrosis in large infarct) usually in cases of large anterior + anterolateral wall infarctions
√ uptake in inferior wall extending behind sternum (anterior projection) suggests RV infarction
  ◊ SPECT imaging improves sensitivity (eliminates rib overlap)
√ diffuse uptake can be seen in angina, cardiomyopathy, subendocardial infarct, pericarditis and normal blood pool (normal blood pool can be eliminated with delayed imaging)

FALSE POSITIVES (10%)
A. Cardiac causes
   1. Recent injury: myocardial contusion, resuscitation, cardioversion, radiation injury, Adriamycin cardiotoxicity, myocarditis, acute pericarditis
   2. Previous injury: left ventricular aneurysm, mural thrombus, unstable angina, previous infarct with persistent uptake
   3. Calcified heart valves / calcified coronary arteries (rare) / chronic pericarditis
   4. Cardiomyopathy: eg, amyloidosis
B. Extracardiac causes:
   1. Soft-tissue uptake: breast tumor / inflammation, chest wall injury, paddle burns from cardioversion, surgical drain, lung tumor
   2. Osseous: calcified costal cartilage (most common), lesions in rib / sternum
   3. Increased blood pool activity secondary to renal dysfunction / poor labeling technique (improvement on delayed images)

mnemonic: "SCUBA"
Subendocardial infarction (extensive)
Cardiomyopathy / myocarditis
Unstable angina
Blood pool activity
Amyloidosis

FALSE NEGATIVES (5%)
Myocardial metastasis

PERSISTENTLY POSITIVE SCAN (>2 weeks)
= ongoing myocardial necrosis indicating poor prognosis, may continue on to cardiac aneurysm, repeat infarction, cardiac death
— in 77% of persistent / unstable angina pectoris
— in 41% of compensated congestive heart failure
— in 51% of ECG evidence of ventricular dyssynergy

Prognosis: the larger the area, the worse the mortality + morbidity

Tc-99m Antimyosin Fab Fragments
= specific marker for myocyte damage
= Fab fragments of an antibody raised against water-insoluble heavy chains of cardiac myosin that are exposed due to necrosis

Sensitivity: 95%
√ uptake ONLY in acute infarct with decreasing intensity as the infarct heals

NONAVID INFARCT IMAGING
= Cold spot imaging
= myocardial perfusion study for acute myocardial infarct

Agent: Tl-201 (at rest)

Sensitivity after onset of symptoms:
96% within 6–12 hours, 79% after 48 hours, 59% in remote infarction; sensitivity for SPECT (seven pinhole tomography) 94% > planar scintigraphy 75%
√ fixed permanent defect in acute infarction
√ fixed permanent defect at rest + on stress thallium + redistribution images in old infarction
√ "cold defect" at rest may represent transient ischemia in unstable angina

N.B.: Tl-201 cannot distinguish between recent + remote infarction!

INTRACARDIAC SHUNTS
Blood-pool agents administered by peripheral IV injection:
Tc-99m pertechnetate, DTPA, sulfur colloid, macroaggregated albumin, labeled RBCs

Method:
C2/C1-method measures hemodynamic significance of a shunt; raw data obtained from pulmonary activity curve (gamma variate method, Q_p:Q_s ratio = two-area ratio method, count method); accuracy depends on the shape of the input bolus (single peak of <2 seconds' duration); measuring C1, C2, T1, T2

A. NORMAL
C2/C1 is <32%
B. L-R SHUNT
Indication: ASD, VSD, AV canal, aortopulmonic window, rupture of sinus of Valsalva aneurysm
√ C2/C1 >35% (area A = primary pulmonary circulation; area B = L-R shunt; area (A - B) = systemic circulation; Q_P / Q_S = area A / area (A - B) >1.2)
C. R-L SHUNT
Indication: Tetralogy of Fallot, transposition, truncus, Ebstein anomaly
√ early arrival of tracer in left side of heart + aorta (first-pass method) prior to arrival of activity from lungs to LV
√ quantification possible only by registration of sum of activity of trapped macroaggregate / microspheres in brain + kidneys

Causes of abnormal nonshunt-related activity:
(1) Radiopharmaceutical breakdown
√ free pertechnetate activity in salivary glands, gastric mucosa, thyroid, kidney
(2) Hepatic cirrhosis
abnormal pulmonary vascular channels bypassing the lung (in 10–70%)
(3) Pulmonary AVM

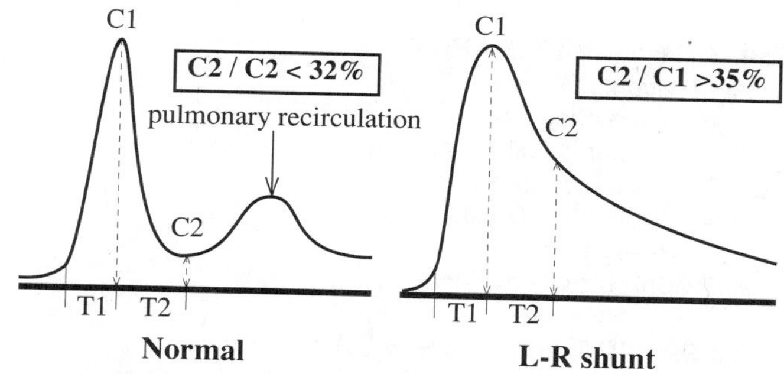

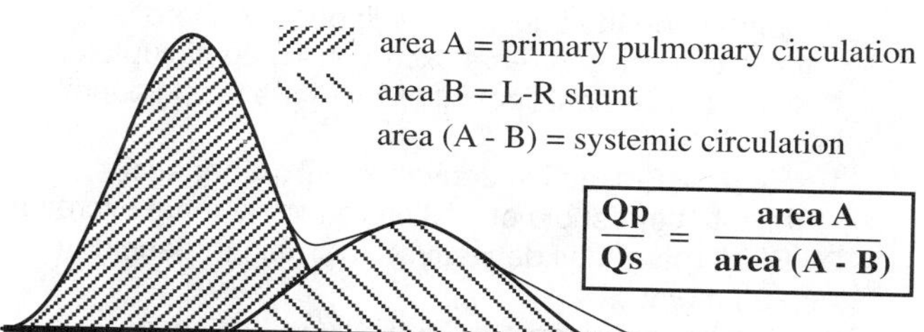

Two-Area Ratio Method
Pulmonary Activity Curves

LIVER AND GASTROINTESTINAL TRACT SCINTIGRAPHY

BILIARY SCINTIGRAPHY

Application:

1. Acute cholecystitis
2. Congenital biliary atresia
3. Evaluation of bile leak
4. Choledochal cyst
5. Biliary-enteric fistula
6. Chronic GB dysfunction

Tc-99m IDA analogs = HIDA agents

= Tc-99m acetanilide iminodiacetic acid analogs (IDA)

Dependent on the substance's lipophility, there is a trade-off between renal excretion + hepatic uptake (BIDA is the most lipophilic, HIDA the least lipophilic)

1. HIDA (2,6-dimethyl derivative): [H = hepatic] bilirubin threshold of <18 mg/dL; 15% renal excretion
2. BIDA (parabutyl derivative): bilirubin threshold of <20 mg/dL
3. PIPIDA (paraisopropyl derivative): 2% renal excretion
4. DIDA (diethyl derivative)
5. DISIDA (diisopropyl derivative) = Disida®, Disofenin®, Hepatolite®: bilirubin threshold of <30 mg/dL
6. TMB-IDA (m-bromotrimethyl IDA) = Mebrofenin®, Choletec®: $T_{1/2}$ uptake is 6 minutes, $T_{1/2}$ excretion is 14 minutes in normals; bilirubin levels may be as high as 30 mg/dL

Quality control: the final compound should contain

— 90–100% Tc-99m IDA
— <10% Tc-99m tin colloid
— <10% Tc-99m sodium pertechnetate

Pharmacokinetics:

@ Bloodstream
tracer binds predominantly to albumin, which decreases renal excretion (renal excretion seen in most normals); dissociation of albumin + Tc-99m-IDA takes place at space of Disse

@ Liver
peak liver activity 5–15 minutes post injection = hepatic phase; 85% extracted by hepatocytes; tracer enters anion pathway of bilirubin
◊ Delayed liver uptake implies hepatocyte dysfunction / CHF (less likely)
◊ Look for liver lesions on early images

@ Bile
secretion by hepatocytes without conjugation; CBD + cystic duct visualized within 10–30 minutes (not always visualized in normals); GB visualized by 20–60 minutes
◊ Activity in right paracolic gutter / intraperitoneal space implies postoperative bile leak

@ Bowel
excretion into duodenum by 30 minutes; bowel visualized within 1 hour; no enterohepatic recirculation

Dose: 2–8 mCi for adults

Radiation dose: 2 rad for upper large bowel; 0.55 rad for gallbladder; 3 rad/mCi for small bowel; 0.01 rad/mCi for whole body

Patient preparation:

1. Narcotics (opiates) + sedatives increase tone of sphincter of Oddi and are stopped 6–12 hours before exam
2. Fasting for at least (2–)4 hours but <24 hours to avoid a contracting or overdistended GB
3. Injection of 0.02 μg/kg Kinevac® over >3 minutes to empty gallbladder about 30 minutes before tracer injection in patients on prolonged fasting

Equipment:

Large field-of-view scintillation camera fitted with LEAP collimator; spectrometer set at 140 keV with 20% window

Computer software for deconvolutional analysis allows determination of percent of hepatic arterial and percent of portal venous blood flow to liver (helpful in assessment of liver transplants)

Imaging:

at 5–10-minute intervals for 60 minutes; if gallbladder not visualized for at least up to 4 hours; RLAT, RAO, LAO projections to confirm gallbladder position
◊ Look for enterogastric reflux as a cause of biliary gastritis!

IV morphine sulfate (0.04 mg/kg or up to 3 mg):
contracts sphincter of Oddi + raises intrabiliary pressure with retrograde filling of gallbladder; maximal effect 5 minutes post injection; shortens study time in cases of nonvisualization of gallbladder; increases accuracy from 88% to 98% and specificity from 83% to 100%
√ inject at 45–60 minutes if tracer in bowel
√ image for 45 minutes after injection

Normals:

√ gallbladder appearance within 60 minutes (90% within 30 minutes)
◊ excludes diagnosis of acute cholecystitis
√ gallbladder visualization within 30 minutes after administration of morphine
√ small bowel activity within 90 minutes (80% within 60 minutes)

False-positive DISIDA Scan

mnemonic: "F2C PAL"

Food (recent meal)
Fasting (prolonged)
Cystic duct cholangiocarcinoma
Pancreatitis
Alcoholism
Liver dysfunction

False-negative DISIDA Scan

mnemonic: "ADA"

Acalculous cholecystitis
Duodenal diverticulum simulating GB
Accessory cystic duct

Gallbladder Ejection Fraction (GBEF)

$$GBEF = [GB_{initial} - GB_{post}] \div GB_{initial}$$

Indications:
(1) to increase sensitivity of study for acute (acalculous) cholecystitis
(2) in patients with atypical GB pain and no cholelithiasis

Technique:
1. Select ROI about GB
2. Administer Sincalide 1 hour post HIDA in a dose of 0.02 µg/kg body weight IV over 30 minutes (with infusion pump)
3. Image acquisition for 30 more minutes

Normal result: >30% GBEF

LIVER SCINTIGRAPHY

Technetium-99m Sulfur Colloid

= LIVER-SPLEEN SCAN

Indications: liver, spleen, bone marrow, acute rejection in renal transplant, lower GI bleeding, gastric emptying

Physiology: small colloid particles are phagocytosed by reticuloendothelial system (RES); 90% of RES function lies within liver + spleen, 10% primarily within bone marrow

Preparation:
Tc-99m pertechnetate and sodium trisulfate are heated in a water bath (95 ± 5°C) for 10 ± 2 minutes; sulfur atoms aggregate to form a "colloid" (average particle size 0.1–1 µm with a range of 0.001–1 µm; true colloid has a particle size of 0.001–0.5 µm); gelatin is added to prevent further growth of particles

Quality control:
(a) >92% remain at origin of ascending chromatography
(b) upper limit for particle size is 1 µm
— Usual cause for poor preparation is excessive / prolonged heating or a pH >7
— Preparation should not be used >6 hours (agglomeration of particles with aging)

Dose: usually 3–6 mCi (8 mCi for SPECT)

Radiation dose: 0.3 rad/mCi for liver (critical organ); 0.02 rad/mCi for whole body; 0.025 rad/mCi for bone marrow

Imaging: 15–30 minutes post IV injection

Pharmacokinetics:
accumulation in liver (85%), spleen (10%), bone marrow (5%); lung localization is rare (presumably secondary to circulating endotoxins + macrophage infiltration)

A. RETICULOENDOTHELIAL LOCALIZATION
√ colloid shift away from liver in diffuse hepatic dysfunction / decreased hepatic perfusion
√ increased bone marrow activity in hemolytic anemia
√ increased splenic activity in hypersplenism of splenomegaly / cancer / systemic illness

B. BONE MARROW LOCALIZATION
Hematopoietic system extends into long bones in children; recedes to axial skeleton, femora, and humeri with age
◊ Bone marrow distribution cannot be used to determine sites of erythropoiesis!

C. ABSCESS LOCALIZATION
Sulfur colloid phagocytized by PMNs + monocytes
Labeling:
(a) in vivo: small labeling yield
(b) in vitro: 40% labeling efficiency, but difficult + time-consuming preparation

Colloid Shift

= increased uptake of injected colloid by bone marrow

A. HEPATIC DYSFUNCTION
1. Cirrhosis
2. Hepatitis
3. Chronic passive congestion

B. AUGMENTED PERFUSION OF SPLEEN + BONE MARROW
1. Hematopoietic disorders
2. Long-term corticosteroid therapy

Focal Hot Liver Lesion

1. IVC / SVC obstruction
   √ increased perfusion of quadrate lobe located at posterior aspect of medial segment left hepatic lobe (collateral pathway via umbilical vein)
2. Budd-Chiari syndrome
   √ "increased" perfusion of caudate lobe (actually decrease of activity elsewhere in liver)
3. FNH (varying amount of Kupffer cells)
   √ hot (DIAGNOSTIC) / cold / isoactive with surrounding parenchyma
4. Regenerating nodules of cirrhosis

Defects in Porta Hepatis

1. Normal variant (thinning of hepatic tissue overlying portal veins + gallbladder)
2. Biliary causes: dilatation of bile ducts, gallbladder hydrops
3. Enlarged portal lymph nodes
4. Metastases
5. Hepatic cyst
6. Hepatic parenchymal disease (pseudotumor)
7. Hepatic compression by adjacent extrinsic mass
8. Postsurgical changes following cholecystectomy

Focal Liver Defects

A. NEOPLASTIC
   (a) primary liver tumor: hepatoma, hemangioma, hepatic adenoma, FNH
   (b) metastases: 85% sensitivity, 75–80% specificity (for lesion >1–2 cm)
B. INFECTIOUS DISEASE / ABSCESS
C. BENIGN CYST
D. TRAUMA
E. PSEUDOTUMOR = normal variant

mnemonic: "L'CHAIM
Lymphoma
Cyst
Hematoma
Abscess
Infarct
Metastasis

Mottled Hepatic Uptake

1. Cirrhosis
2. Acute hepatitis
3. Lymphoma
4. Amyloidosis
5. Granulomatous disease (sarcoid, fungal, viral, parasitic)
6. Chemo- / radiation therapy

SPLENIC SCINTIGRAPHY

1. Tc-99m sulfur colloid: 3–5 mCi
2. Tc-99m heat-denatured erythrocytes

Indication:
(1) Splenic trauma
(2) Accessory + ectopic spleen

Technique:
20–30 minutes after injection of pyrophosphate IV
15–20 mL of blood are drawn + incubated with 2 mCi of pertechnetate; blood is heated to 49.5°C for 35 minutes and reinjected
◊ Fragmentation of RBCs from overheating increases hepatic uptake!

Imaging: 20 minutes post injection

Hyposplenism

= no uptake of Tc-99m sulfur colloid

A. ANATOMIC ABSENCE OF SPLEEN
   1. Congenital asplenia = Ivemark syndrome
   2. Splenectomy
B. FUNCTIONAL ASPLENIA
   = marked decrease in splenic phagocytic function despite presence of splenic tissue within the body
   1. Circulatory disturbances:
      occlusion of splenic artery / vein, hemoglobinopathies (sickle cell disease, hemoglobin-SC disease, thalassemia), polycythemia vera, idiopathic thrombocytopenic purpura
   2. Altered RES activity:
      thorotrast, irradiation, combined splenic irradiation + chemotherapy, replacement of RES by tumor / infiltrate, splenic anoxia (cyanotic congenital heart disease), sprue
   3. Autoimmune disease
      Cx: children at risk for pneumococcal pneumonia (liver partially takes over immune response later in life)
C. FUNCTIONAL ASPLENIA + SPLENIC ATROPHY
   Ulcerative colitis, Crohn disease, celiac disease, tropical sprue, dermatitis herpetiformis, thyrotoxicosis, idiopathic thrombocytopenic purpura, thorotrast
D. FUNCTIONAL ASPLENIA + NORMAL / LARGE SPLEEN
   Sarcoidosis, amyloidosis, sickle cell anemia (if not infarcted), after bone marrow transplantation

• RBC (acanthocytes, siderocytes)
• lymphocytosis, monocytosis
• Howell-Jolly bodies (intraerythrocytic inclusions)
• thrombocytosis

√ spleen not visualized on Tc-99m sulfur colloid
√ Tc-99m heat-damaged RBCs / In-111 labeled platelets may demonstrate splenic tissue if Tc-99m sulfur colloid does not

Cx: increased risk of infection (pneumococcus, meningococcus, influenza)

GASTROINESTINAL SCINTIGRAPHY

Radionuclide Esophagogram

Preparation: 4–12 hours fasting; imaging in supine / erect position
Dose: 250–500 μCi Tc-99m sulfur colloid in 10 mL of water taken through straw
Imaging: when swallowing begins

√ normal transit time: 15 seconds with 3 distinct sequential peaks progressing aborally
√ prolonged transit time: achalasia, progressive systemic sclerosis, diffuse esophageal spasm, nonspecific motor disorders, "nutcracker" esophagus, Zenker diverticulum, esophageal stricture + obstruction

Difficult interpretation in: hiatal hernia, GE reflux, Nissen fundoplication

Gastroesophageal Reflux

89% correlation with acid reflux test

Cause:
(1) Decreased pressure of lower esophageal sphincter
   (a) transient-complete relaxation of LES
   (b) low resting pressure of LES
(2) Transient increase in intraabdominal pressure
(3) Short intraabdominal esophageal segment

Age of population: usually 6–9 months, up to 2 years

• poor weight gain
• vomiting, aspiration, choking
• asthmatic episodes, stridor, apnea

Detection: upper GI examination with barium, distal esophageal sphincter pressure measurements, 24-hour pH probe measurement in distal esophagus (gold standard), radionuclide examination

Preparation: 4 hours / overnight fasting; abdominal sphygmomanometer (for adults)
Dose: 0.5–1.0 mCi Tc-99m sulfur colloid in 300 mL of acidified orange juice (150 mL juice + 150 mL 0.1 N hydrochloric acid) followed by "cold" acidified orange juice
Imaging: at 30–60-second intervals for 30–60 minutes, images taken in supine position from anterior; sphygmomanometer inflated at 20, 40, 60, 80, 100 mm Hg
Interpretation:
Reflux (in %) = ([esophageal counts – background] / gastric counts) x 100
√ up to 3% magnitude reflux is normal
√ evidence of pulmonary aspiration (valuable in pediatric age group)

Cx: reflux esophagitis secondary to
(a) delayed clearance time of esophageal acid load: tertiary / repetitive esophageal contractions, supine position of refluxor, aspiration of saliva, stimulation of salivary flow, stretched phrenoesophageal membrane in hiatal hernia
(b) delayed gastric emptying: increased intragastric pressure (gastric outlet obstruction), viral gastropathy, diabetes

Prognosis:
(1) Self-limiting process with spontaneous resolution by end of infancy (in majority of patients)
(2) Persistent symptoms until age 4 (1/3 of patients)
(3) Death from inanition / recurrent pneumonia (5%)
(4) Cause of recurrent respiratory infections, asthma, failure to thrive, esophagitis, esophageal stricture, chronic blood loss, sudden infant death syndrome (SIDS)

Rx:
(1) Conservative therapy:
avoidance of food + drugs that decrease pressure in LES, elevation of head during sleep, acid neutralization, cimetidine / ranitidine (reduction of acid production), metoclopramide / domperidone (increase sphincter pressure + promote gastric emptying)
(2) Antireflux surgery

Gastric Emptying

◊ Rates of gastric emptying vary widely between subjects and even in the same subject at different times

Dose: 0.5–1 mCi
(a) Tc-99m sulfur colloid cooked with egg white / liver pâté as solid food
(b) In-111 DTPA in milk, water, formula, juice for simultaneous measurement of liquid phase

Imaging: 1-minute anterior abdominal images obtained at 0, 10, 30, 60, 90 minutes in erect position if dual-head camera available; anterior and posterior imaging performed with geometric mean activity calculated

Pharmacokinetics:
79% tracer activity in stomach for solid phase at 10 minutes; 65% at 30 minutes; 33% at 60 minutes; 10% at 90 minutes

Normal result: 50% of activity in stomach at time zero; should empty by 60 ± 30 minutes
√ acutely delayed emptying in stress (pain, cold), drugs (morphine, anticholinergics, levo-dopa, nicotine, β-adrenergic antagonists), postoperative ileus, acute viral gastroenteritis, hyperglycemia, hypokalemia
√ chronically delayed gastric emptying in gastric outlet obstruction, postvagotomy, gastric ulcer, chronic idiopathic intestinal pseudoobstruction, GE reflux, progressive systemic sclerosis, dermatomyositis, spinal cord injury, myotonia dystrophica, familial dysautonomia, anorexia nervosa, hypothyroidism, diabetes mellitus, amyloidosis, uremia
√ abnormally rapid gastric emptying in gastric surgery, ZE syndrome, duodenal ulcer disease, malabsorption (pancreatic exocrine insufficiency / celiac sprue)

Gastrointestinal Bleeding

Detection depends on:
(1) Rate of hemorrhage
◊ If bleeding not detectable by RBC scintigraphy, it will not be detectable by angiography!
• RBC scan detects bleeding of 0.1 mL/min
• Angiography detects bleeding of 0.5 mL/min:
63% sensitive for upper GI bleed
39% sensitive for lower GI bleed
(2) Continuous versus intermittent bleeding (most GI hemorrhages are intermittent)
(3) Site of hemorrhage
(4) Characteristics of radionuclide agent

Tc-99m–labeled RBCs (In Vivtro Labeling Preferred)

◊ Generally preferred and accepted most sensitive imaging method for lower GI bleeding
◊ Serves to triage patients for angiography as a negative exam predicts a negative arteriogram

Indications: acute / intermittent bleeding (0.35 mL/min); NOT useful in occult bleeding
— Remains in vascular system for prolonged period
— Liver + spleen activity are low allowing detection of upper GI tract hemorrhage
— Low target-to-background ratio (high activity in great vessels, liver, spleen, kidneys, stomach, colon; probably related to free pertechnetate fraction)

Dose: 10–20 mCi
Imaging:
(a) every 2 seconds for 64 seconds
(b) static images for 500,000–1,000,000 counts at 2, 5, and every consecutive 5 minutes up to 30 minutes + every 10 minutes until 90 minutes
(c) delayed images at 2, 4, 6, 12 hours up to 24/36 hours

Localization of bleeding site:
may be difficult secondary to rapid transit time (bowel motility reduced with 1 mg glucagon IV) or too widely spaced time intervals; overall 83% positive correlation with angiography
√ progressive tracer accumulation over time in abnormal location
√ bleeding site conforms to bowel anatomy (localizing information may be misleading due to forward / backward peristalsis)
√ change in appearance over time consistent with bowel peristalsis

Sensitivity:
in 83–93% correctly identified bleeding site (50–85% within 1st hour, may become positive in 33% only after 12–24 hours); collection as small as 5 mL may be detected; superior to sulfur colloid
— 50% sensitivity for blood loss <500 mL/24 hours
— >90% sensitivity for blood loss >500 mL/24 hours

False positives (5%):
(a) free pertechnetate fraction: physiologic uptake in stomach + intestine, renal pelvis + bladder uptake
(b) hepatic hemangioma, varices, inflammation, isolated vascular process (AVM, venous / arterial graft)

False negatives:
9% for bleeding of <500 mL/24 hours

Tc-99m Sulfur Colloid

Indication: bleeding must be active at time of tracer administration; length of active imaging can be increased by fractionating dose
— Disappearance half-life of 2.5–3.5 minutes (rapidly cleared from blood by RES + low background activity)
— Active bleeding sites detected with rates as low as 0.05–0.1 mL/min
— Not useful for upper GI bleeding (interference from high activity in liver + spleen) or bleeding near hepatic / splenic flexure

Dose: 10 mCi (370 MBq)

Imaging:
every image should be for 500,000–1,000,000 counts with oblique + lateral images as necessary
(a) every 5 seconds for 1 minute ("flow study" = radionuclide angiogram)
(b) 60-second images at 2, 5, 10, 15, 20, 30, 40, 60 minutes; study terminated if no abnormality up to 30 minutes
(c) delayed images at 2, 4, 6, 12 hours

√ extravasation of tracer seen in active bleeding

Specificity: almost 100% (rare false-positives due to ectopic RES tissue)

False positives: transplanted kidney, ectopic splenic tissue, modified marrow uptake, male genitalia, arterial graft, aortic aneurysm

Tc-99m Pertechnetate

Indication: bleeding from functioning gastric mucosa in Meckel diverticulum / intestinal duplication; consider in adults up to age 25; independent of bleeding rate

Pathophysiology: tracer accumulation in mucus-secreting cells

◊ Avoid barium GI studies + endoscopy + irritating bowel preparation prior to study!

Dose: 5–10 mCi (185–370 MBq)

Imaging:
(a) radionuclide angiogram 2–3 seconds/frame for 1st minute
(b) sequential 5-minute images up to 20 minutes with 500,000–1,000,000 counts per image

Sensitivity: >80%
enhanced by
— fasting for 3–6 hours to reduce gastric secretions passing through bowel
— nasogastric tube suction to remove gastric secretions
— premedication with pentagastrin (6 µg/kg SC 15 minutes before study) to stimulate gastric secretion of pertechnetate
— premedication with cimetidine (300 mg qid x 48 hours) to reduce release of pertechnetate from mucosa
— voiding just prior to injection

False positives:
Barrett esophagus, duodenal ulcer, ulcerative colitis, Crohn disease, enteric duplication, small bowel, hemangioma, AV malformation, aneurysm, volvulus, intussusception, urinary obstruction, uterine blush

False negatives:
ulcerated epithelium

Levine / Denver Shunt Patency

Technique:
sterile injection of 0.5–1 mCi Tc-99m MAA / sulfur colloid via paracentesis

Imaging:
over abdomen (or chest) to detect uptake in liver (or lung), which confirms patency

RENAL AND ADRENAL SCINTIGRAPHY

RENAL AGENTS

1. Agents for renal function: Tc-99m DTPA, I-131 Hippuran
2. Renal cortical agent: Tc-99m DMSA
3. Renal combination agent: Tc-99m glucoheptonate

Tc-99m DTPA

= Tc-99m diethylenetriamine pentaacetic acid
= agent of choice for assessment of
(1) Perfusion
(2) Glomerular filtration = relative GFR
(3) Obstructive uropathy
(4) Vesicoureteral reflux

Pharmacokinetics:
chelating agent; 5–10% bound to plasma protein; extracted with 20% efficiency on each pass through kidney (= filtration fraction); excreted exclusively by glomerular filtration (similar to inulin) without reabsorption / tubular excretion / metabolism
Time-activity behavior:
— abdominal aorta (15–20 seconds)
— kidneys + spleen (17–24 seconds); liver appears later because of portal venous supply
— renal cortical activity (2–4 minutes): mean transit time of 3.0 ± 0.5 minutes; static images of cortex taken at 3–5 minutes
— renal pelvic activity (3–5 minutes): peak at 10 minutes; asymmetric clearance of renal pelvis in 50%; accelerated by furosemide

Biologic half-life: 20 minutes
Dose: 10–20 mCi
Radiation dose: 0.85 rad/mCi for renal cortex; 0.6 rad/mCi for kidney; 0.5 rad/mCi for bladder; 0.15 rad/mCi for gonads; 0.15 rad/mCi for whole body

Adjunct:
Lasix administration (20–40 mg IV) 20 minutes into exam allows assessment of renal pelvic clearance with accuracy equal to Whitaker test (DDx of obstructed from dilated but nonobstructed pelvicaliceal system)

[Tc-99m Glucoheptonate]

largely replaced by Tc-99m MAG3
Pharmacokinetics:
rapid plasma clearance + urinary excretion with excellent definition of pelvicaliceal system during 1st hour; extracted by (a) glomerular filtration and (b) tubular excretion (30–45% within 1st hour); 5–15% of dose accumulates in tubular cells by 1 hour, 15–25% by 3 hours; cortical accumulation remains for 24 hours
Imaging:
(a) collecting system within first 30 minutes
(b) renal parenchyma after **1**–2 hours (interfering activity in collecting system)

Biologic half-life: 2 hours
Dose: 15 (range 10–20) mCi
Radiation dose: 0.17 rad/mCi for kidney; 0.008 rad/mCi for whole body; 0.015 rad/mCi for gonads

Tc-99m DMSA

= Tc-99m dimercaptosuccinic acid
= suitable for imaging of functioning cortical mass: pseudotumor versus lesion

Renal Scintigraphic Agents

MORPHOLOGIC AGENTS			
Tc-99m GHA	5 mCi	proximal tubular uptake + glomerular filtration	collecting system visualized on delayed images
Tc-99m DMSA	2–5 mCi	proximal + distal tubular uptake	limited availability, relatively high radiation dose, collecting system not visualized on delayed images
FUNCTIONAL AGENTS			
I-131 OIH	200–400 μCi	80% secreted, 20% filtered	routinely used for ERPF measurement, analog of PAH, highest renal extraction fraction, poor image detail, high radiation dose, requires high-energy collimator
Tc-99m DTPA	10–15 mCi	nearly 100% filtered	GFR calculation, delayed time-to-peak with slow clearance
Tc-99m MAG_3	2–10 mCi	99% secreted	ERPF estimate, good cortical detail, high target-to background ratio

Pharmacokinetics:
high protein-binding + slow plasma clearance; 4% extracted per renal passage; 4–8% glomerular filtration within 1 hour and 30% by 14 hours; 50% of dose accumulates in proximal + distal renal tubular cells by 3 hours (= cortical agent)

Imaging: after 1– **3**–24 hours (optimal at 34 hours); improved sensitivity to structural defects with SPECT
Biologic half-life: >30 hours
Dose: 5–10 mCi
Radiation dose: 0.014 rad/mCi for gonads; 0.015 rad/mCi for whole body

[I-131 OIH]

largely replaced by Tc-99m MAG3
= I-131 orthoiodohippurate (Hippuran®)
= good for evaluation of renal tubular function / effective renal plasma flow; agent with highest extraction ratio without binding to renal parenchyma; visualizes kidney even in severe renal failure

Pharmacokinetics:
80% secreted by proximal tubules; 20% filtered by glomeruli; maximal renal concentration within 5 minutes; normal transit time of 2–3 minutes; approximately 2% free iodine
◊ Lugol's solution is administered to protect thyroid

Imaging:
in 15–60-second intervals for 20 minutes; renal uptake determined from images obtained by 1–2 minutes (patient in supine position for equidistance of kidneys to camera)
Biologic half-life: 10 minutes (with normal renal function)
Dose: 200 (range 150–300) μCi
Radiation dose: 0.06 rad/200 μCi for bladder; 0.02 rad/200 μCi for kidney; 0.02 rad/200 μCi for whole body; 0.02 rad/200 μCi for gonads

Tc-99m Mercaptoacetyltriglycine (MAG_3)

= renal plasma flow agent similar to OIH but with imaging benefits of Tc-99m label (improved dosimetry)

Pharmacokinetics:
correlates with renal plasma flow; clearance is less than Hippuran
Dose: 10 mCi
Evaluation:
true renal plasma flow = MAG_3 flow (obtained off renogram curve) multiplied by a constant (varies between 1.4 and 1.8)

ACE Inhibitor Scintigraphy

= screening for renovascular hypertension with angiotensin-converting enzyme inhibitor (ACEI) challenge

Pharmacology:
the affected kidney responds to decreased arteriolar flow by releasing angiotensin II (= extremely potent vasoconstrictor acting on the efferent renal arteriole to increase filtration pressure); ACE inhibitors (eg, captopril, enalapril) block the angiotensin-converting enzyme which reduces GFR (51–96% sensitive, 80–93% specific)

Enalaprilat (Vasotec®)-enhanced Renography

Technique:
- Blood pressure check (to prevent testing excessively hypertensive patients) -4d
- Discontinue captopril / lisinopril -2 d
- Discontinue enalaprilat -1 d
- Stop any other antihypertensive medications overnight (except for β-blockers) -9 hrs
- Fasting (liquids acceptable) -4 hrs
- Bladder catheterization to monitor urinary output -40 min
- 1/2 normal saline IV drip at 75 mL/hr at a dose of 10 mL fluid/kg body weight (to ensure adequate hydration) -30 min
- Furosemide (= Lasix®) IV -5 min
  20 mg if serum creatinine <1.5 mg/dL,
  40 mg if serum creatinine >1.5 mg/dL,
  60 mg if serum creatinine >3.0 mg/dL
  (not to exceed 1.0 mg/kg)
- 2.5–5 mCi Tc-99m MAG_3 IV for baseline study 0 min
  (a) flow phase with 1 sec/frame for 60 frames
  (b) tracer kinetic (dynamic) phase with 15 sec/frame for 120 frames
- Rehydration with 1/2 normal saline keeping a 250–300 mL negative fluid balance +30 min
- Postvoid image (or Foley catheter with PVR)
- 0.04 mg/kg enalaprilat IV (up to a maximum of 2.5 mg) infused over 5 minutes + blood pressure and heart rate checks q 5 minutes +105 min
- Repeat furosemide (= Lasix®) IV +115 min
- 5–7.5 mCi Tc-99m MAG_3 IV [or 10 mCi Tc-99m MAG_3 IV single post-enalaprilat study for patients already on ACEI therapy] +120 min
- Image acquisition at 1–2-minute intervals for 22 minutes

Captopril (Capoten®)-enhanced Renography

Dose: 1 mg/kg PO for pediatric patient, 25 or 50 mg PO for adult patient
Technique: radiopharmaceutical injected 60 minutes after ingestion of captopril

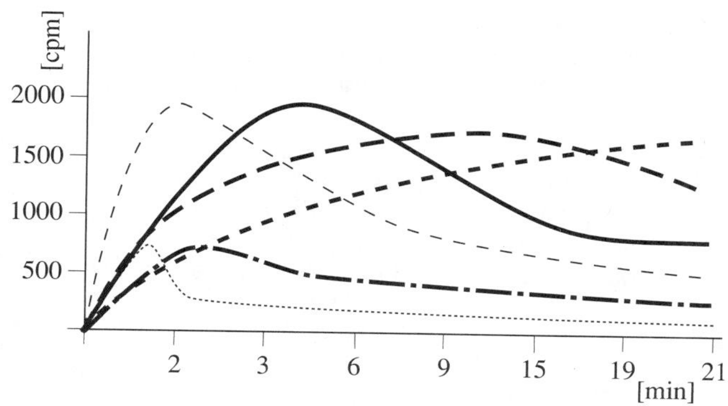

Tc-99m MAG$_3$ Scintigram after ACE Inhibition

- (solid line) minor abnormalities with T_{max} >5 minutes and 20-minute/peak uptake ratio >0.3
- (long dashes) marked delayed excretion with preserved washout phase
- (short dashes) accumulation curve = delayed excretion without washout phase
- (dash-dot) renal failure pattern with measurable renal uptake
- (dotted) renal failure pattern without measurable renal uptake = bloodpool background
- (thin dashes) normal postvasotec renogram

√ change from baseline grade 0 / 1 by >1 grade
  = high probability for renal artery stenosis
√ abnormal baseline curve without change
  = indeterminate for renovascular hypertension
√ functional improvement following ACEI challenge
  = low probability for renovascular hypertension

<u>Semiquantitative interpretation of time-activity renograms</u>:
- √ normal ACE inhibitor scintigram (<10% probability for renovascular hypertension)

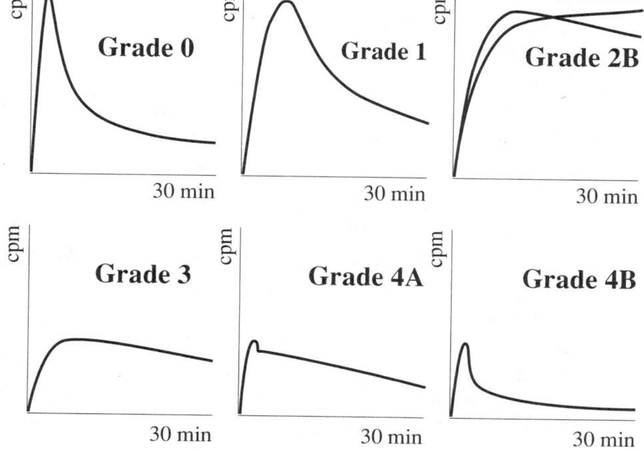

Grading of Differential Renal Function

- √ criteria for high probability (>90%):
  - √ worsening of scintigraphic curve
  - √ reduction in relative uptake with >10% change after ACE inhibition
  - √ prolongation of parenchymal transit time with >2 minutes delay of excretion into renal pelvis
  - √ increase in 20-min/peak uptake ratio >0.15 (reduced GFR results in reduced urinary output and increased radiotracer retention)
  - √ prolongation of T_{max} of >2 minutes
- √ asymmetry of renal uptake <40% of total renal uptake

Decreased accuracy with:
(1) bilateral renal artery stenosis
(2) impaired renal function
(3) urinary obstruction
(4) chronic ACE inhibitor therapy

Cold Defect on Renal Scan

mnemonic: "CHAT SIN"

Cyst
Hematoma
Abscess
Tumor
Scar
Infarct
Neoplasm

DIFFERENTIAL RENAL FUNCTION

Agents:
(1) <u>Tc-99m DTPA</u>:
measurements prior to excretion within first 1–3 minutes; images taken at 1.5-second intervals for 30 seconds followed by serial images for next 30 minutes
(2) <u>I-131 Hippuran</u>:
measurements prior to excretion within first 1–2 minutes

Evaluation: generation of time-activity curves
- √ upslope (= accretion phase)
- √ peak activity (maximal uptake phase)
- √ downslope (excretion phase)

√ increased hepatic + soft-tissue uptake with impaired renal function
√ measurements usually not significantly affected with differences in renal depth
√ measurements are accurate in renal obstruction if obtained within 1–3 minutes
√ prediction about functional recovery not possible following surgical relief of obstruction

RADIONUCLIDE CYSTOGRAM

Use: evaluation of bladder volume at reflux, volume of refluxed urine, residual urine volume, ureteral reflux drainage time

Technique:
(a) indirect: IV injection of Tc-99m DTPA
(b) direct: instillation of 0.5–1 mCi Tc-99m pertechnetate-saline mixture into bladder (more sensitive for reflux during filling phase, which occurs in 20%)

Imaging:
posterior upright views throughout filling and voiding phases; review on cinematic loop helpful; residual bladder volume can be calculated

Advantage:
lower radiation dose to gonads than fluoroscopic contrast cystography (5 mrad)!

ADRENAL SCINTIGRAPHY

A. ADRENOCORTICAL IMAGING AGENTS
1. NP-59
2. Selenium-75 6-β-selenomethylnorcholesterol (Scintadrin®)

B. SYMPATHOADRENAL IMAGING AGENTS
1. I-131 / I-123 metaiodobenzylguanidine (MIBG)

I-131 Metaiodobenzylguanidine (MIBG)

Indications:
APUDomas = tumors of neural crest origin (C cells of thyroid, melanocytes of skin, chromaffin cells of adrenal medulla, pancreatic cells, Kulchitsky cells), which share the presence of neurosecretory granules capable of accumulating I-131 MIBG
(1) Pheochromocytoma (80–90% sensitivity, >90% specificity); tumors as small as 0.2 g have been detected
(2) Neuroblastoma, carcinoid, medullary thyroid carcinoma, nonfunctioning retroperitoneal neuroendocrine tumor, middle mediastinal paraganglioma, adrenal metastasis of choriocarcinoma, Merkel (skin) tumor

Pharmacokinetics:
Chemically similar to norepinephrine, which is synthesized by adrenergic neurons + cells of the adrenal medulla; localizes in storage granules of adrenergic tissue by means of energy- and sodium-dependent uptake mechanism; not metabolized to any appreciable extent;
Normal activity is seen in liver, spleen, bladder, salivary glands, myocardium, lungs; 85% of injected dose is excreted unchanged by kidneys

Method:
Lugol solution administered orally (50 mg of iodine per day) for 4–5 days starting the day before injection (to block thyroid uptake of free iodine)

Dose: 0.4–0.5 mCi/1.73 square meters of body surface MIBG, up to 500 μCi

Radiation dose: 35 rad/mCi for adrenal medulla, 1.0 rad/mCi for ovaries, 0.4 rad/mCi for liver, 0.22 rad/mCi for whole body

Imaging: 24–48–(72) hours after injection with 100,000 counts / 20 minutes per image

False-negative scan:
uptake blocked by reserpine, imipramine, other tricyclic depressants, amphetamine-like drugs

I-123 Metaiodobenzylguanidine

agent of choice, also allows SPECT imaging

Dose: 10 mCi

Radiation dose: 2.76 rad/mCi for adrenals,
0.07 rad/mCi for ovaries,
0.05 rad/mCi for liver,
0.02 rad/mCi for whole body

Imaging: at 6 and 24 hours

Indium-111 Pentetreotide

= Octreotide® = somatostatin analogue

Indication: pituitary tumor, gastrinoma, paraganglioma, carcinoid, neuroblastoma, small cell lung cancer, pheochromocytoma

Dose: 3–6 mCi

Imaging: 4–24–(48) hours

Distribution: kidneys, spleen, liver, bladder, intestines, thyroid, pituitary gland

Advantage: superior to MIBG

Iodocholesterol

Agent: I-131 6-β-iodomethyl-19-norcholesterol (NP-59); NO FDA approval (available as investigational new drug)

Indications: adrenocortical imaging
(1) ACTH-independent Cushing syndrome (adenoma, cortical nodular hyperplasia)
(2) Adrenocortical carcinoma
√ spectrum from nonfunctioning to functioning
(3) Primary aldosteronism (adenoma, bilateral adrenal hyperplasia) improved scintigraphic discrimination requires dexamethasone suppression before + during imaging
(4) Hyperandrogenism (adrenal adenoma, zona reticularis hyperplasia, polycystic ovary disease, ovarian stromal hyperplasia, androgen-secreting ovarian neoplasm)
(5) Incidentaloma (= adrenal mass)
√ localization to side of CT-depicted adrenal mass (= concordant uptake) suggests hyperfunctioning adenoma
√ markedly diminished / absent uptake (= discordant uptake) or symmetric uptake (= nonlateralization) suggests space-occupying mass (eg, cyst) / malignant adrenal mass

Pharmacokinetics:
NP-59 is incorporated into low-density lipoproteins (LDL), circulates to adrenal cortex, absorbed from LDL complex by low-density lipoprotein receptors, esterified in adrenal cortex; adrenocortical uptake affected by adrenocortical secretagogues (corticotropin, angiotensin II);

Enterohepatic excretion may obscure adrenals (prior laxative administration beneficial)

Dose: 1 mCi (37 MBq) with slow IV injection

Radiation dose: 26 rad/mCi for adrenals, 8.0 rad/mCi for ovaries, 2.4 rad/mCi for liver, 2.3 rad/mCi for testes, 1.2 rad/mCi for whole body

Method: Lugol solution administered orally (50 mg of iodine per day) for 4–5 days starting the day before injection (to block thyroid uptake of free iodine); mild laxative administered to decrease bowel activity

Imaging:

(a) 5–7-day interval between injection + imaging;

(b) 3–5-day interval between injection + imaging in case of dexamethasone suppression (1 mg four times daily for 7 days prior to and throughout 4–5 days of postinjection imaging interval)

STATISTICS

Incidence = number of diseased people per 100,000 population per year

Prevalence = number of existing cases per 100,000 population at a target date

Mortality = number of deaths per 100,000 population per year

Fatality = number of deaths per number of diseased

Decision Matrix:

TEST	GOLD STANDARD normal	abnormal	subtotal	
normal	TN	FN	T-	NPV
abnormal	FP	TP	T+	PPV
subtotal	D-	D+		total
	spec	sens		acc

TP = test positive in diseased subject
FP = test positive in nondiseased subject
FN = test negative in diseased subject
TN = test negative in nondiseased subject
T+ = abnormal test result
T- = normal test result
D+ = diseased subjects
D- = nondiseased subjects

Sensitivity

= ability to detect disease
= probability of having an abnormal test given disease
= number of correct positive tests / number with disease
= true positive ratio = TP / (TP + FN) = TP / D+
• D+ column in decision matrix
◊ Independent of prevalence

Specificity

= ability to identify absence of disease
= probability of having a negative test given no disease
= number of correct negative tests / number without disease
= true negative ratio = TN / (TN + FP) = TN / D-
• D- column in decision matrix
◊ Independent of prevalence

Accuracy

= number of correct results in all tests
= number of correct tests / total number of tests
= (TP + TN) / (TP + TN + FP + FN) = (TP + TN) / total
◊ Depends much on the proportion of diseased + nondiseased subjects in studied population
◊ Not valuable for comparison of tests

Example: same test accuracy of 90% for two tests A and B

Test A

TEST	GOLD STANDARD *normal*	*abnormal*	*subtotal*
normal	**90**	10	100
abnormal	10	**90**	100
subtotal	100	100	**200**

Test B

TEST	GOLD STANDARD *normal*	*abnormal*	*subtotal*
normal	**170**	20	190
abnormal	0	**10**	10
subtotal	170	30	**200**

Positive Predictive Value

= positive test accuracy
= likelihood that a positive test result actually identifies presence of disease
= number of correct positive tests / number of positive tests
= TP / (TP + FP) = TP / T+
• T+ row in decision matrix
◊ Dependent on prevalence
◊ PPV increases with increasing prevalence for given sensitivity + specificity
◊ PPV increases with increasing specificity for given prevalence

Negative Predictive Value

= negative test accuracy
= likelihood that a negative test result actually identifies absence of disease
= number of correct negative tests / number of negative tests
= TN / (TN + FN) = TN / T-
• T- row in decision matrix
◊ Dependent on prevalence
◊ NPV increases with decreasing prevalence for given sensitivity + specificity
◊ NPV increases with increasing sensitivity for given prevalence

False-positive Ratio

= proportion of nondiseased patients with an abnormal test result
• D- column in decision matrix
= FP / (FP + TN) = FP / D-
= 1 – specificity = (TN + FP - TN) / (TN + FP)

False-negative Ratio

= proportion of diseased patients with a normal test result
• D+ column in decision matrix
= FN / (TP + FN) = FN / D+
= 1 – sensitivity = (TP + FN - TP) / (TP + FN)

Disease Prevalence

= proportion of diseased subjects to total population
= (TP + FN) / (TP + TN + FP + FN) = D+ / total
◊ Sensitivity + specificity are independent of prevalence
◊ Affects predictive values + accuracy of a test result

Example:

Test A: **90%** sensitivity + ***90%*** specificity

		GOLD STANDARD		
T		*normal*	*abnormal*	*subtotal*
E	*normal*	***90***	**10**	100
S	*abnormal*	***10***	**90**	100
T				
	subtotal	100	100	200

NPV = 90%
PPV = 90%

Test B: prevalence of **10%**, 90% sensitivity + specificity

		GOLD STANDARD		
T		*normal*	*abnormal*	*subtotal*
E	*normal*	162	2	164
S	*abnormal*	18	18	36
T				
	subtotal	180	**20**	**200**

NPV = 99%
PPV = 50%

Test C: prevalence of **90%**, 90% sensitivity + specificity

		GOLD STANDARD		
T		*normal*	*abnormal*	*subtotal*
E	*normal*	18	18	36
S	*abnormal*	2	162	164
T				
	subtotal	20	**180**	**200**

NPV = 50%
PPV = 99%

BAYES'S THEOREM

= the predictive accuracy of any test outcome that is less than a perfect diagnostic test is influenced by
(a) pretest likelihood of disease
(b) criteria used to define a test result

RECEIVER OPERATING CHARACTERISTICS (ROC)

= degree of discrimination between diseased + nondiseased patients using varying diagnostic criteria instead of a single value for the TP + TN fraction
= curvilinear graph generated by plotting TP ratio as a function of FP ratio for a number of different diagnostic criteria (ranging from definitely normal to definitely abnormal)

Y-axis: true-positive ratio = sensitivity
X-axis: false-positive ratio = 1 – specificity; reversing the values on the X-axis results in an identical "sensitivity-specificity curve"

Use: variations in diagnostic criteria are reported as a continuum of responses ranging from definitely abnormal to equivocal to definitely normal due to subjectivity + bias of individual radiologist
◊ A minimum of 4–5 data points of diagnostic criteria are needed!

Difficulty: subjective evaluation of image features; subjective diagnostic interpretation; data must be ordinal (= discrete rating scale from definitely negative to definitely positive)

Interpretation:
◊ Increase in sensitivity leads to decrease in specificity!
◊ Increase in specificity leads to decrease in sensitivity!
◊ The most sensitive point is the point with the highest TP ratio
— equivalent to "overreading" by using less stringent diagnostic criteria (all findings read as abnormal)

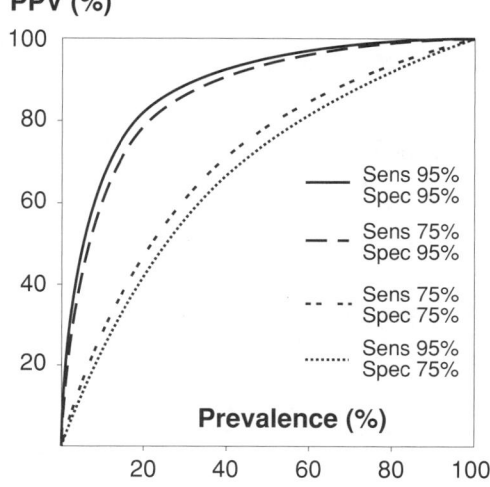

PPV (%)
100
80
60
40
20
Sens 95% Spec 95%
Sens 75% Spec 95%
Sens 75% Spec 75%
Sens 95% Spec 75%
Prevalence (%)
20 40 60 80 100

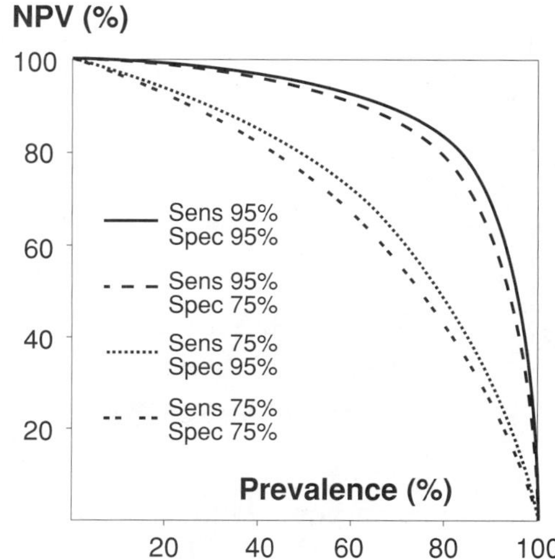

◊ The most specific point is the point with the lowest FP ratio
  — equivalent to "underreading" by using more strict diagnostic criteria (all findings read as normal)
◊ The ROC curve closest to the Y-axis represents the best diagnostic test
◊ Does not consider disease prevalence in the population

KAPPA (κ)

measures concordance between test results and gold standard
◊ Analogous to Pearson correlation coefficient (r) for continuous data!

GOLD STANDARD

T	A_1	$M_2M'_2$	$M_3M'_3$	$M_4M'_4$	M_1
E	$M_2M'_1$	A_2	$M_2M'_3$	$M_2M'_4$	M_2
S	$M_3M'_1$	$M_3M'_2$	A_3	$M_3M'_4$	M_3
T	$M_4M'_1$	$M_4M'_2$	$M_4M'_3$	A_4	M_4
	M'_1	M'_2	M'_3	M'_4	N

$$P_o = \frac{\Sigma_1^4 A}{N} \qquad P_c = \frac{\Sigma_1^4 MM'}{N^2}$$

$$\kappa = \frac{P_o - P_c}{1 - P_c}$$

Example: κ = 0.743

GOLD STANDARD

T	18	3	0	0	21
E	2	20	5	2	29
S	1	4	20	3	28
T	0	0	5	17	22
	21	27	30	22	100

Predictive value of κ:

0.00 — 0.20	little or none
0.20 — 0.40	slight
0.40 — 0.60	group
0.60 — 0.80	some individual
0.80 — 1.0	individual

CONFIDENCE LIMIT

= degree of certainty that the proportion calculated from a sample of a particular size lies within a specific range (binomial theorem)
◊ Analogous to the mean ± 2 SD

CLINICAL EPIDEMIOLOGY

= application of epidemiologic principles + methods to problems encountered in clinical medicine with the purpose of developing + applying methods of clinical observation that will lead to valid clinical conclusions

Epidemiology = branch of medical science dealing with incidence, distribution, determinants in control of disease within a defined population

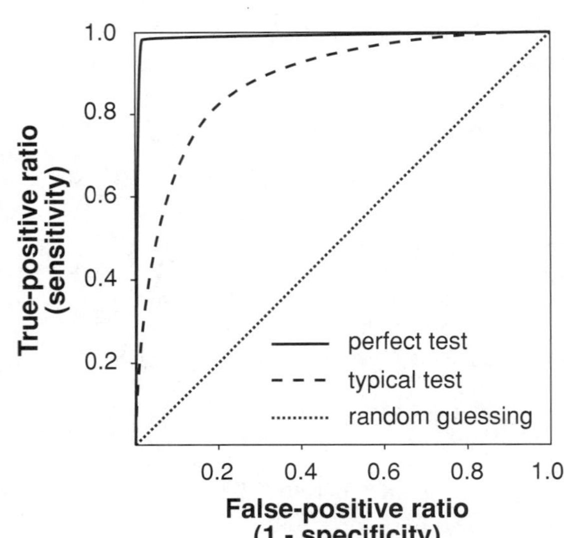

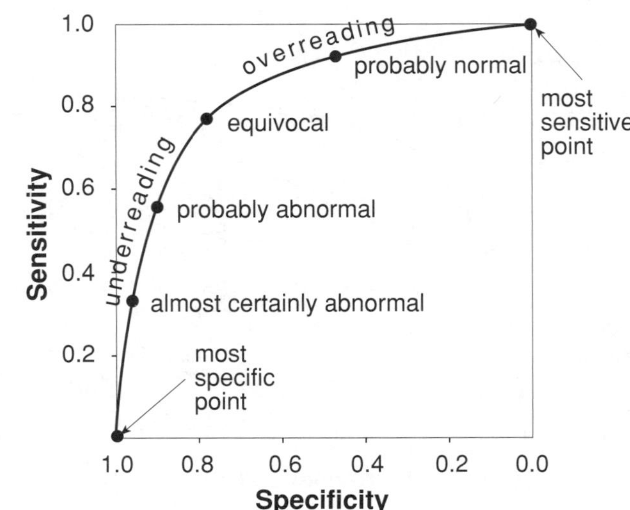

Screening Techniques

Principle question: can early detection influence the natural history of the disease in a positive manner?

Outcome measure: early detection + effective therapy should reduce morbidity + mortality, ie, increase survival rates (observational study)!

Biases:

Lead time = interval between disease detection at screening + the usual time of clinical manifestation; early diagnosis always appears to improve survival by at least this interval, even when treatment is ineffective

Length time = differences in growth rates of tumors:
- (a) slow-growing tumors exist for a long time before manifestation thus enhancing the opportunity for detection
- (b) fast-growing tumors exist for a short time before manifestation thus providing less opportunity for detection at screening "interval cancers" = clinically detected between scheduled screening exams are likely fast-growing tumors; patients with tumors detected by means of screening tests will have a better prognosis than those with interval cancers

Self-selection = decision to participate in screening program; usually made by patients better educated + more knowledgeable + more health-conscious; mortality rates from noncancerous causes can be expected to be lower than in general population

Overdiagnosis = detection of lesions of questionable malignancy, eg, in situ cancers, which might never have been diagnosed without screening + have an excellent prognosis

Randomized Trials

Design: two arms consisting of (a) study group and (b) control group with patients assigned to each arm on randomized basis

Endpoint: difference in mortality rates of both groups

Power: study must be of sufficient size + duration to detect a difference, if one exists; analogous to sensitivity of a diagnostic test

Impact on effective size of groups:

Compliance = proportion of women allocated to screening arm of trial who undergo screening

Contamination = proportion of women allocated to control group of trial who do undergo screening

Case-control Studies

Retrospective inquiry, which is less expensive, takes less time, is easier to perform:
- (a) determine the number of women who died from breast cancer
- (b) chose same number of women of comparable age who have not died from breast cancer
- (c) ascertain the number of women who were screened + who were not screened in both arms

Calculation of odds ratio = ad / bc :

	cases of deaths from breast cancer	controls not died from breast cancer
screened	a	b
not screened	c	d

WATER-SOLUBLE CONTRAST MEDIA

Ionic = dissociation in water
Nonionic = soluble in water (hydrophilic); no dissociation in solution

Iodine-to-particle ratio:
= quotient of iodine atoms (attenuation of x rays) and number of particles (osmotoxic effect)

- ratio 1.5 agents = high-osmolar contrast media (HOCM)
- ratio 3.0 agents = low-osmolar contrast media (LOCM)
- ratio 6.0 agents = isotonic contrast media (IOCM)

IONIC MONOMERS

= monoacidic salts composed of benzoic acid derivatives, with 3 hydrogen atoms replaced by iodine atoms + 3 hydrogen atoms replaced by simple amide chains

in solution: strong organic acid completely dissociated (ionized) into negatively charged ions / anions

Conjugated cations:
(1) sodium
(2) methylglucamine (meglumine)
(3) combination of above

Iodine concentration: up to 400 mg/mL
Iodine-to-particle ratio: 3:2 or 1.5:1
Osmolality: 1,400–2,100 mOsm/kg = HOCM

Acetrizoate
The parent triiodinated contrast medium in first clinical use; the benzene ring is attached to a carboxyl (COO-) group at the 1-carbon position and conjugated with sodium / meglumine

Diatrizoate
The unsubstituted hydrogen of acetrizoate has been exchanged for another acetamido unit leading to higher biologic tolerance through higher degree of protein binding

IONIC DIMERS

Construction:
2 iodinated benzene rings containing 6 iodine atoms, one of which contains an ionizing carboxyl group; benzene rings are connected by a common amide side chain

Conjugation with: sodium + meglumine
Compound: ioxaglate (the only available)

Ioxaglate (Hexabrix®)
Sodium + meglumine are conjugated with the carboxyl group.

Iodine concentration: 320 mg/mL
Iodine-to-particle ratio: 6:2 or 3:1
Osmolality: 600 mOsm/kg = LOCM

NONIONIC MONOMERS

Construction:
benzoic acid carboxyl group replaced by amide; side chains have been modified by adding 4–6 hydroxyl (OH) groups, which allows solubility in water

Iodine concentration: up to 350 mg/mL
Iodine-to-particle ratio: 3:1
Compounds: iohexol, iopamidol, ioversol, iopental, iopromide (Ultravist®), iobitridol (Xenetix®), ioxilan (Oxilan®)
Osmolality: 616–796 mOsm/kg

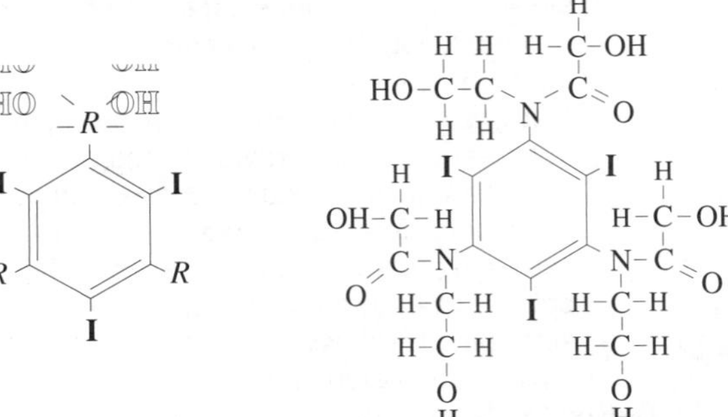

Metrizamide
The first compound with 4 hydroxyl groups positioned at one end of the molecule on the glucosamide moiety.

Iohexol (Omnipaque®)
contains 6 hydroxyl (OH) groups more evenly distributed around the molecule improving subarachnoid toxicity.

Iopamidol (Isovue®)
This nonionic monomer contains 5 hydroxyl (OH) groups.

Ioversol (Optiray®)
This nonionic monomer contains 6 hydroxyl (OH) groups.

NONIONIC DIMERS

Construction:

contain up to 12 hydroxyl groups to eliminate ionicity, increase hydrophilicity, lower osmotoxicity, and increase iodine atoms per molecule

Iotrolan (Iotrol®)

This nonionic dimer contains 12 hydroxyl (OH) groups.

Compounds: iodecol, iotrolan (Isovist®), iodixanol (Visipaque®)

Iodine-to-particle ratio: 6:1

Osmolality: hypo- / isoosmolar

Excretory Urography

Clearance: >99% of contrast material eliminated through kidney (<1% through liver, bile, small and large intestines, sweat, tears, saliva); vicarious excretion with renal insult / failure (may be unilateral as in obstructive uropathy)

Halftime: 1–2 hours (doubled in dialysis patients)

Concentration: 60% by weight

(a) Sodium-containing HOCM

√ less distension of collecting system

(b) Meglumine-only HOCM

√ improved distension of collecting system (due to decreased tubular resorption of water)

Physicochemical Properties of Commonly Used Radiographic Contrast Media

Contrast Media	*Compound*	*mOsm/kg H_2O*	*Viscosity (cps) at 37°C*	*Iodine mg/mL*
Ionic monomers				
URORADIOLOGICAL				
Cysto-Conray® II (Mallinckrodt)	Meglumine-iothalamate	1,300	4	202
GASTROINTESTINAL				
Hypaque® Sodium Oral Solution (Nycomed Amersham)	Na diatrizoate	1,300	4	249
Gastrografin® (Bracco)	Na-meglumine diatrizoate	1,940	8.4	370
INTRAVASCULAR				
Renovue®-DIP (Bracco)	Meglumine iodamide	433	1.8	111
Conray-60®(Mallinckrodt)	Meglumine iothalamate	1,400	4	282
Renografin®-60 (Bracco)	Na-meglumine diatrizoate	1,450	4	292
Ionic dimers				
Hexabrix® (Mallinckrodt)	Na-meglumine ioxaglate	600	7.5	320
Nonionic monomers				
Oxilan® 300 (Cook)	ioxilan	585	5.1	300
Ultravist® 300 (Berlex)	iopromide	607	4.9	300
Isovue® 300 (Bracco)	iopamidol	616	4.7	300
Optiray® 300 (Mallinckrodt)	ioversol	651	5.5	300
Omnipaque® 300 (Nycomed Amersham)	iohexol	672	6.3	300
Omnipaque® 140 (Nycomed Amersham)	iohexol	322	1.5	140
Omnipaque® 240 (Nycomed Amersham)	iohexol	520	3.4	240
Omnipaque® 350 (Nycomed Amersham)	iohexol	844	10.4	350
Nonionic dimers				
Iotrol®300 (Schering AG)	iotrolan	~310	9.1	300
Visipaque®-320 (Nycomed Amersham)	iodixanol	290	11.8	320

Δ Osmolality of human serum is 290 mOsm/kg!

Δ The higher the number of hydroxyl groups, the larger the size + the higher the viscosity + the higher the hydrophilicity! This decreases protein- and tissue-binding properties making the compound biologically more inert!

(c) LOCM
√ denser nephrogram + slightly denser pyelogram than HOCM (due to higher tubular concentration)

Angiography

Burning sensation:
(a) intense with concentration of 60–76% HOCM
(b) reduced with concentration of ≤30% HOCM / LOCM
◊ Overall incidence of adverse allergic-type reactions is (for unknown reasons) much less with intra-arterial than with intravenous use of contrast media!

Venography

(1) Foot / calf discomfort or pressure or burning
(a) ~24% with 60% HOCM
(b) ~5% with 40% HOCM / 300 mg iodine/mL LOCM
◊ The addition of 10–40 mg lidocaine/50 mL of contrast media decreases patient discomfort!

(2) Postphlebography deep vein thrombosis
(a) 26–48% with 60% HOCM
(b) 0–9% with dilute HOCM / LOCM
◊ Infusion of 150–200 mL of 5% dextrose in water / 5% dextrose in 0.45% saline / heparinized saline through injection site immediately after examination reduces likelihood of DVT!

CONTRAST MATERIAL IN PEDIATRICS

Conventional dose: 1 mL / pound up to 150 mL
Maximum dose: 280–300 mgI/mL

ADVERSE CONTRAST REACTIONS

Prevalence:

	Ionic High-osmolar	Nonionic Low-osmolar
Non–life-threatening reaction	1–2%	0.2–0.4%
Life-threatening reaction	0.2%	0.04%
Mortality	1:100,000	1:100,000
Late reaction		6%

A. Nonidiosyncratic (= dose-related) reactions
Cause: direct chemotoxic / hyperosmolar effect
- nausea, vomiting
- cardiac arrhythmia
- renal failure
- pulmonary edema
- cardiovascular collapse

B. Idiosyncratic (= anaphylactoid) reactions
= reactions occurring unpredictably + independently of dose / concentration = not a true antigen-IgE antibody-mediated reaction nor a reaction to iodine / iodide
Cause: unknown
- hives, itching
- facial / laryngeal edema
- bronchospasm, respiratory collapse
- circulatory collapse

C. Delayed reactions
- erythematous rashes, pruritus
- fever, chills, flulike symptoms
- joint pain
- loss of appetite, taste disturbance
- headache, fatigue, depression
- abdominal pain, constipation, diarrhea

Risk Factors and Incidence of Adverse Reactions for High- and Low-Osmolality Contrast Media

Type of Reaction	*HOCM [%]*	*LOCM [%]*
Overall incidence		
Australia (Palmer et al.)	3.80	1.20
United States (Wolf et al.)	4.20	0.70
Japan (Katayama et al.)	12.70	3.10
Severe adverse reactions	0.22	0.04
Severe allergies to drugs, foods, etc.	23.40	6.90
Asthma	19.70	7.80
Repeat reaction to contrast media	16–44	4.1–11.2

Significant underlying medical conditions
(a) renal disease
(b) cardiac disease
(c) blood dyscrasias
(d) pheochromocytoma
(e) increased symptoms with COPD plus pulmonary hypertension
(f) increased sickling in patients with sickle-cell disease
◊ Approximately 20–40% of population are at increased risk for adverse reaction to contrast media!
◊ In patients with adverse reactions to HOCM repeated reactions will be lowered to 5% by using LOCM
◊ No direct correlation / association to povidone-iodine skin cleansing solution (Betadine®)

NEPHROTOXICITY

Nonoliguric Transient Renal Dysfunction

= transient decline of renal function
- serum creatinine level peaks on days 3–5
- serum creatinine returns to baseline values within 14–21 days
- fractional excretion of sodium <0.01 (DISTINCTIVE CHARACTERISTIC compared with other causes)

Acute Renal Failure

= sudden + rapid deterioration of renal function
= increase in serum creatinine of >25% or to >2 mg/dL within 2 days of receiving contrast material
Frequency: 1–30%; 3rd most common cause of in-hospital renal failure after hypotension and surgery
Risk factors:
1. Preexisting renal insufficiency (serum creatinine >1.5 mg/dL)

2. Diabetes mellitus with renal insufficiency (possibly related to dehydration / hyperuricemia)
   ◊ Ratio 3 nonionic LOCM appear to be 50% less nephrotoxic than ratio 1.5 ionic HOCM
   ◊ Diabetics with normal renal function are not at increased risk!
3. Dehydration
4. Cardiovascular disease
5. Use of diuretics
6. Advanced age >70 years
7. Multiple myeloma (in dehydrated patients)
8. Hypertension
9. Hyperuricemia / uricosuria
10. High dose of contrast material

CAVE:
- ◊ Small decreases in renal function may greatly exacerbate the mortality caused by the underlying condition!
- ◊ Metformin (Glucophage®) should be discontinued for 48 hours after contrast medium administration (accumulation of metformin may result in lactic acidosis, which is fatal in 50%)!
  - ◊ It is not necessary to stop metformin after gadolinium administration because gadolinium is not nephrotoxic!
- ◊ Avoid concomitant use of nephrotoxic drugs (eg, gentamycin, NSAIDs)

Proposed mechanisms:
- contrast agents are concentrated in nephrons + collecting tubules

1. Vasoconstriction
   (a) increase in intrarenal pressure induced by hypertonicity
   (b) intrarenal smooth muscle contraction in response to hypertonic substances
2. RBC aggregation in medullary circulation
3. Direct tubular cell injury

Potential antidotes:
Hydration (0.9% saline at 100 mL/h) 12 hours before + 12 hours after angiography
- ◊ Extracellular volume expansion is the most effective + widely recommended measure!

√ immediate dense nephrogram persisting for up to 24 hours (in 75%)
√ gradually increasing dense nephrogram resembling bilateral acute ureteral obstruction (in 25%):
- √ bilaterally enlarged smooth kidneys
- √ poor opacification of urine-conducting structures
- √ effacement of collecting system (interstitial edema)

Cx: 34% mortality (0.4% of all patients)
Rx: 0.1% require renal replacement therapy

Assessment of Patients before Contrast Injection

A. General status
   Assess hemodynamic, neurologic, general nutritional, anxiety status
B. History of significant allergies
   1. Prior anaphylactic response to any allergen
   2. Asthma
C. Renal disease
   1. Renal dysfunction: obtain baseline BUN + creatinine
   2. Diabetes mellitus
   3. Multiple myeloma
   ◊ Hydrate patients and limit contrast dose!
D. Cardiac disease
   1. Angina
   2. CHF with minimal exertion
   3. Severe aortic stenosis
   4. Primary pulmonary hypertension
   5. Severe cardiomyopathy
   ◊ Limit contrast dose!

TREATMENT OF CONTRAST REACTIONS

◊ 94–100% of severe + fatal anaphylactoid reactions occur within 20 minutes of contrast medium injection
- ⇒ use a plastic cannula for IV access
- ⇒ maintain IV access for 30 minutes
- ⇒ have emergency drugs close to the room where contrast injections are done
- ⇒ post a listing of available medications + their common doses in the room

Oral Steroid Premedication Protocol

- ⇒ 32 mg methylprednisolone (Medrol®) PO 12 and 2 hours prior to contrast injection
- ⇒ 50 mg prednisone PO 13 + 7 + 1 hour prior to contrast injection, *plus*
  50 mg diphenhydramine (Benadryl®) IV/IM/PO 1 hour prior to contrast injection
- ⇒ nonionic low-osmolality contrast agent

Indication: previous respiratory adverse contrast reaction, history of significant allergies / severe asthma

Caution in patients with: active tuberculosis, diabetes mellitus, peptic ulcer disease

◊ Antihistamines alone have not proved to be effective!

Treatment of Premedicated Patients

A. Patient on β-blocker
   if response to epinephrine inadequate
   ⇒ 1–5 mg glucagon IV + subsequent slow drip of 5 mg glucagon over 60 min
B. Patient on calcium channel blocker (eg, nifedipine, nicardipine)
   ⇒ calcium IV
C. Excessive vasoconstriction on epinephrine IV
   ⇒ infusion of 0.5–10 μg/kg/min of reconstituted sodium nitroprusside (Nipride®) (50 mg in 500–1000 mL of 5% dextrose wrapped in metal foil during use to protect solution from light)
D. Metformin (Glucophage®)
   ⇒ Stop metformin medication at time of contrast injection + for subsequent 48 hours
   ⇒ Reinstate metformin medication if renal function remains normal
   ◊ Contrast material is contraindicated if patient is in renal failure because of risk of lactic acidosis!

Useful Medications

1. Alpha- and β-adrenergic agents:
   Action: vasoconstriction, increased cardiac output
   - **Epinephrine**
     - 1 mL glass vials of epinephrine 1:1,000
       Adult dose: 0.1–0.2 mL epinephrine (1:1,000) (= 0.1–0.2 mg) SQ
       Pediatric dose: 0.01 mL/kg up to 0.3 mL/dose
       Repeat in 15–30 minutes if needed
       Indications: bronchospasm, facial edema, severe urticaria, laryngospasm
     - prepackaged 10-mL syringes of epinephrine 1:10,000
       Adult dose: 1–3 mL epinephrine (1:10,000) (= 0.1 mg) slowly IV
       Pediatric dose: 0.1 mL/kg slowly IV
       Repeat every 5–15 minutes if needed
       Indications: bronchospasm / laryngospasm with peripheral vascular collapse
       Maximum dose: 1.0 mg
   - **Dopamine** (Inotropin®)
     Adult dose: 2–5 pg/kg/min IV; rarely need to exceed 20 pg/kg/min
     Indications: hypotension
   Cx: arrhythmia, myocardial ischemia, nausea, vomiting, tremulousness, headache

2. **Atropine sulfate**
   Adult dose: 0.6–1.0 mg slowly IV
   Pediatric dose: 0.02 mg/kg slowly IV (0.2 mg/kg of the 0.1 mg/mL solution); min dose of 0.1 mg (children) + 1.0 mg (adolescents)
   Repeat after 5 min
   Maximum dose: 0.04 mg/kg (2–3 mg) in adults
   Indications: bradycardia, hypotension
   Cx: angina, myocardial infarction

3. Metered-dose inhalers of β-adrenergic bronchodilators
   - **Metaproteranol** (Alupent®)
   - **Terbutaline** (Brethaire®)
   - **Albuterol** (Proventil®, Ventolin®)
   Dose: 2 puffs every 20–30 minutes, as needed

4. H_1 antagonists = antihistamines
   - **Diphenhydramine** (Benadryl®)
     Adult dose: 25–50 mg PO/IM/IV
     Pediatric dose: 1–2 mg/kg IV, up to 50 mg
   - **Hydroxyzine** (Vistaril®)
     Dose: 25–50 mg PO/IM/IV
   Indications: hives, rash, itching
   Cx: hypotension, sedation

5. H_2 receptor blockers
   - **Cimetidine** (Tagamet®)
     Dose: 300 mg PO / slowly IV (diluted in 10 mL D5W solution)
   - **Ranitidine** (Zantac®)
     Dose: 50 mg PO / slowly IV (diluted in 10 mL D5W solution)
   Indications: hypotension; bronchospasm

6. **Aminophylline**
   - 250 mg in 250 mL of 5% dextrose
   Dose: 6 mg/kg IV in D5W over 15–20 minutes (loading dose); then 0.4–1.0 mg/kg/hour
   Indications: bronchospasm, pulmonary edema
   Cx: hypotension, cardiac arrhythmia

7. **Terbutaline**
   - 0.25–0.50 mg IM/SQ

8. Sedatives
   - **Midazolam** (Versed®)
     Dose: 0.5–1.0 mg IV; short acting
     Indications: sedation
   - **Diazepam** (Valium®)
     Dose: 2–10 mg IV
     Indications: seizures
   - **Pentobarbital** (Nembutal®)
     Dose: <50 mg/min IV; 150–200 mg IM
     Indications: toxic convulsions
   Cx: respiratory depression, apnea, laryngospasm, hypotension

9. Pain
   - **Fentanyl**
     Dose: 25–50 mg IV; short acting
   - **Morphine**
     Dose: 1–3 mg IV
     Indications: pain; pulmonary edema
   - **Demerol**
     Cx: respiratory depression

10. Volume expander
    - **Crystalloid solution** as 0.9% saline
    - **Hydroxylethyl starch** (high-molecular-weight colloid)

11. **Furosemide** (Lasix®)
    Adult dose: 20–40 mg IV slow push / PO
    Pediatric dose: 1 mg/kg/dose IV up to 40 mg
    Effect: 5–15 minutes after IV; 60 minutes after PO
    Indications: acute pulmonary edema, CHF, hypertensive emergency

12. Corticosteroids
    - **Methylprednisolone** (Solu-Medrol®)
      Dose: (a) 32 mg PO; 12 & 2 hours prior
      (b) 100–1,000 mg (anaphylaxis with shock)
      Indications: allergy prophylaxis; severe anaphylaxis with shock

INDEX

A

B

C

D

E

F

G

I

M

Q

R

S

U

V

X

Y

Z